DIAGNOSIS and TREATMENT of UVEITIS

C. STEPHEN FOSTER, M.D.

Professor of Ophthalmology
Harvard Medical School
Director, Immunology and Uveitis Service
Massachusetts Eye and Ear Infirmary
Boston, Massachusetts

ALBERT T. VITALE, M.D.

Chief, Uveitis Division
Member, Vitreoretinal Division
King Khaled Eye Hospital
Riyadh, Saudi Arabia

W.B. SAUNDERS COMPANY

A Harcourt Health Sciences Company

Philadelphia   London   New York   St. Louis   Sydney   Toronto

W.B. SAUNDERS COMPANY
A Harcourt Health Sciences Company

The Curtis Center
Independence Square West
Philadelphia, Pennsylvania 19106

Library of Congress Cataloging-in-Publication Data

Diagnosis and treatment of uveitis / C. Stephen Foster, Albert T. Vitale.

p. cm.

ISBN 0–7216–6338–9

1. Uveitis.   I. Vitale, Albert T.   II. Title.   [DNLM: 1. Uveitis—diagnosis.
  2. Uveitis—therapy.   WW 240 F754d 2001]

RE351.F67   2001   617.7'2—dc21

DNLM/DLC   00-058356

Acquisitions Editor: Richard Lampert
Manuscript Editor: Carol DiBerardino
Senior Production Manager: Natalie Ware
Illustration Specialist: Lisa Lambert

DIAGNOSIS AND TREATMENT OF UVEITIS   ISBN 0–7216–6338–9

Printed in the United States of America.

Last digit is the print number: 9   8   7   6   5   4   3   2   1

To my wife, Frances Barrett Foster, without whom nothing would get done; she is my everything.

C. STEPHEN FOSTER, M.D.

To my teachers: patients, colleagues, wife, children, and parents. Most especially, I offer a lifetime of gratitude to my Dad, dedicated and compassionate physician, loving father and husband, my first mentor and best friend.

ALBERT T. VITALE, M.D.

NOTICE

Medicine is an ever-changing field. Standard safety precautions must be followed, but as new research and clinical experience broaden our knowledge, changes in treatment and drug therapy may become necessary or appropriate. Readers are advised to check the most current product information provided by the manufacturer of each drug to be administered to verify the recommended dose, the method and duration of administration, and contraindications. It is the responsibility of the treating physician, relying on experience and knowledge of the patient, to determine dosages and the best treatment for each individual patient. Neither the publisher nor the editor assumes any liability for any injury and/or damage to persons or property arising from this publication.

THE PUBLISHER

CONTRIBUTORS

MEHRAN A. AFSHARI, M.D., M.P.H.
Assistant Professor of Ophthalmology, Retina Service, Yale University School of Medicine, New Haven, Connecticut
Schistosomiasis (Bilharziasis)

NASRIN AFSHARI, M.D.
Assistant Professor of Ophthalmology, Cornea Service, Duke University School of Medicine, Durham, North Carolina
Schistosomiasis (Bilharziasis)

WILLIAM AYLIFFE, F.R.C.S., Ph.D.
University of London; Croydon Eye Unit, Mayday University Hospital, London, England
Retinal Vasculitis

JOHN C. BAER, M.D.
Omni Eye Specialists, Baltimore, Maryland
Borrelliosis

STEFANOS BALTATZIS, M.D.
Associate Professor of Ophthalmology, Department of Ophthalmology, Athens University Medical School; General Hospital of Athens, University Eye Clinic, Athens, Greece
Ophthalmia Nodosa

NEAL P. BARNEY, M.D.
Associate Professor, Department of Ophthalmology and Visual Sciences, University of Wisconsin Medical School, Madison, Wisconsin
Diffuse Unilateral Subacute Neuroretinitis

RICHARD BAZIN, M.D., F.R.C.S.
Clinical Professor of Ophthalmology, Faculté de Médecine de l'Université Laval; Member of the Cornea and External Diseases Service, Laval University Hospital Center, Quebec City, Quebec, Canada
Rickettsial Diseases

MARGARITA CALONGE, M.D.
Full Professor of Ophthalmology, University of Valladolid, Valladolid, Spain
Medication-Induced Uveitis

BARBARA L. CARTER, M.D.
Professor of Radiology, Tufts University School of Medicine; Chief of ENT Radiology, New England Medical Center, Boston, Massachusetts
Diagnostic Imaging Studies for Inflammatory Systemic Diseases with Eye Manifestations

PIK SHA CHAN, M.D.
Active Consultant, Retina Service, St. Luke's Medical Center, Institute of Ophthalmology, Quezon City; Asian Eye Institute, Makati City, Philippines
Systemic Lupus Erythematosus; Multiple Evanescent White Dot Syndrome

ROXANNE CHAN, M.D.
Clinical Fellow in Radiology, Tufts University School of Medicine, Boston, Massachusetts
Diagnostic Imaging Studies for Inflammatory Diseases with Eye Manifestations; Ocular Whipple's Disease

LOUIS J. CHORICH III, M.D.
Assistant Professor of Ophthalmology, Ohio State University, Columbus, Ohio
Diagnosis of Uveitis; Bartonellosis

ISABELLE COCHEREAU, M.D.
Professor, University of Angers; Chief of Infectious Disease Department, Angers Hospital, Angers, France
Pneumocystosis; Human Immunodeficiency Virus–Associated Uveitis

M. REZA DANA, M.D., M.P.H.
Assistant Professor, Harvard Medical School; Director, Cornea/External Disease and Ocular Immunology, Brigham and Women's Hospital; Associate Scientist, Laboratory of Immunology, Schepens Eye Research Institute, Boston, Massachusetts
Leptospirosis

ANTHONY S. EKONG
Ophthalmology Department, Health Partners, Minneapolis, Minnesota
Scleroderma

TAMER EL-HELW
Formerly, Department of Radiology, New England Medical Center, Boston, Massachusetts
Diagnostic Imaging Studies for Inflammatory Systemic Diseases with Eye Manifestations

YOSUF EL-SHABRAWĪ, M.D.
Department of Ophthalmology, Karl-Franzens University, Graz, Austria
Loiasis

MELANIE FIEDLER, M.D.
Assistant Professor, Department of Urology, University of Essen, Essen, Germany
Herpesviruses

MARTIN FILIPEC, M.D., Ph.D.
Assistant Professor, Charles University; Chairman and
Director, Cornea and Immunology Service and Department
of Ophthalmology, Prague, Czech Republic
Onchocerciasis

C. STEPHEN FOSTER, M.D., F.A.C.S.
Professor of Ophthalmology, Harvard Medical School;
Director, Immunology and Uveitis Service, Massachusetts
Eye and Ear Infirmary, Boston, Massachusetts
**Introduction; The Uvea: Anatomy, Histology, and
Embryology; Definition, Classification, Etiology, and
Epidemiology; General Principles and Philosophy; Basic
Immunology; Diagnosis of Uveitis; Diagnostic Imaging
Studies for Inflammatory Systemic Diseases with Eye
Manifestations; Treatment of Uveitis—Overview;
Corticosteroids, Mydriatic and Cycloplegic Agents;
Nonsteroidal Anti-inflammatory Drugs;
Immunosuppressive Chemotherapy; Diagnostic Surgery;
Therapeutic Surgery: Cornea, Iris, Cataract, Glaucoma,
Vitreous, Retinal; Syphilis; Tuberculosis; Ocular
Whipple's Disease; Measles; Rubella; Sporotrichosis;
Ocular Toxocariasis; Masquerade Syndromes:
Malignancies; Masquerade Syndromes: Endophthalmitis;
Nonmalignant, Noninfectious Masquerade Syndromes;
Scleroderma; Giant Cell Arteritis; Adamantiades-
Behçet Disease; Antiphospholipid Syndrome;
Sarcoidosis; Tubulointerstitial Nephritis and Uveitis
Syndrome; Lens-Induced Uveitis**

NICOLETTE GION
Ev. Krankenhaus Muelheim a. d. Ruhr, Augenklinik,
Muelheim a. d. Ruhr, Germany
**The Uvea: Anatomy, Histology, and Embryology;
Tubulointerstitial Nephritis and Uveitis Syndrome**

STEPHANIE L. HARPER
Assistant Professor of Ophthalmology, Director of Residency
Program, Howard University, Washington, D.C.
Diagnosis of Uveitis

KATERINA HAVRLIKOVA-DUTT, M.D.
SCRA, Parexel, Prague, Czech Republic
Cryptococcosis

ARND HEILIGENHAUS, Priv. Doz., M.D.
Department of Ophthalmology, University of Essen School
of Medicine, Essen; Head, Department of Ophthalmology,
Inflammatory Eye Diseases, St. Franziskus Hospital,
Muenster, Germany
Herpesviruses

HORST HELBIG, Priv. Doz., M.D.
Head, Retina Service, Kantonsspital St. Gallen, St. Gallen,
Switzerland
Herpesviruses

RAMZI K. HEMADY, M.D.
Associate Professor, Program Director and Co-director
Cornea, Uveitis, and Refractive Surgery Services,
Department of Ophthalmology, University of Maryland
School of Medicine; Chief of Ophthalmology, Veterans
Administration Hospital, Baltimore, Maryland
Rift Valley Fever

THANH HOANG-XUAN, M.D.
Professor, University of Paris; Chief of Ophthalmology,
Bichar Hospital and Fondation Rothschild, Paris, France
**Pneumocystosis, Human Immunodeficiency
Virus–Associated Uveitis**

FREDERICK A. JAKOBIEC, M.D., D.Sc.(Med.)
Henry Willard Williams Professor of Ophthalmology,
Professor of Pathology, and Chairman of Ophthalmology,
Harvard Medical School; Chief of Ophthalmology,
Massachusetts Eye and Ear Infirmary, Boston, Massachusetts
Foreword

JAMES KALPAXIS, M.D.
Private Practice, Austin, Texas
Multifocal Choroiditis and Panuveitis

ADAM H. KAUFMAN, M.D., F.A.C.S.
Director, Uveitis Service; Director, Corneal and Refractive
Surgery Service; Associate Professor of Clinical
Ophthalmology, University of Cincinnati College of
Medicine; Cornea and Uveitis Specialist, Cincinnati Eye
Institute, Cincinnati, Ohio
Cysticercosis

ERIK LETKO, M.D.
Harvard Medical School; Fellow, Ocular Immunology and
Uveitis Service, Massachusetts Eye and Ear Infirmary,
Boston, Massachusetts
Measles; Rubella

CHARALAMPOS LIVIR-RALLATOS, M.D.
Clinical Vitreoretinal Fellow, Tulane University, New
Orleans, Louisiana
Fuchs' Heterochromic Iridocyclitis

NIKOS N. MARKOMICHELAKIS, M.D.
Attending Ophthalmologist, Athens Medical School; Head
of Ocular Immunology and Inflammation, Department of
Ophthalmology, General Hospital of Athens, Athens,
Greece
Multiple Sclerosis

JESUS MERAYO-LLOVES, M.D., Ph.D., M.B.A.
Principal Investigator, Chief of Refractive Surgery Unit,
Instituto de Oftalmobiologia Aplicada (IOBA), Universidad
de Valladolid, Valladolid; CEO and Consultant, Ocular
Immunology and Refractive Surgery, Centro de
Especialidades Oftalmologicas, Madrid
Free-Living Amebas and Amebiasis

ELISABETH M. MESSMER, M.D.
Attending, Department of Ophthalmology, Ludwig-
Maximilians University Hospital, Munich, Germany
Ocular Leprosy; Candidiasis

**SHAWKAT SHAFIK MICHEL, F.R.C.S.(Ed.), D.O.,
M.B.Ch.B**
Private Practice, Alberta, Canada
**Definition, Classification, Etiology, and Epidemiology;
Lens-Induced Uveitis**

ELISABETTA MISEROCCHI, M.D.
University of Milan—Italy, Ospedale San Raffaele, Milano,
Italy
Antiphospholipid Syndrome

RON NEUMANN
Formerly Fellow, Massachusetts Eye and Ear Infirmary,
Boston, Massachusetts
Giardia Lamblia

QUAN DONG NGUYEN, M.D., M.Sc.
Assistant Professor of Ophthalmology, Vitreoretina Service,
Wilmer Ophthalmological Institute, Johns Hopkins
University School of Medicine, Baltimore, Maryland
Traumatic Uveitis

E. MITCHEL OPREMCAK, M.D.
Clinical Associate Professor, Department of Ophthalmology,
Ohio State University; Physician and Surgeon, The Retina
Group, Columbus, Ohio
**Diagnostic Surgery; Therapeutic Surgery: Cornea, Iris,
Cataract, Glaucoma, Vitreous, Retinal;
Ophthalmomyiasis**

FERNANDO ORÉFICE, M.D., Ph.D.
Professor of Ophthalmology, Universidade Federal de
Minas Gerais, Belo Horizonte, Minas Gerais, Brazil
Toxoplasmosis

TOMAS PADILLA, Jr, M.D.
Clinical Associate Professor, Department of Ophthalmology,
University of the Philippines–Manila, Manila; Associate
Active Staff Member, Institute of Ophthalmology, St. Luke's
Medical Center, Quezon City; Visiting Staff, Department of
Ophthalmology, Makati Medical Center, Makati City,
Philippines
Trypanosomiasis

CARL H. PARK, M.D.
Resident in Ophthalmology, Tufts University School of
Medicine; Resident in Ophthalmology, New England Eye
Center, New England Medical Center, Boston,
Massachusetts
Punctate Inner Choroidopathy

BENALEXANDER A. PEDRO
Formerly Fellow, Massachusetts Eye and Ear Infirmary,
Boston, Massachusetts
Acute Retinal Pigment Epitheliitis

MIGUEL PEDROZA-SERES, M.D., Ph.D.
Professor, Universidad Nacional Autonoma De Mexico;
Staff, Department of Ocular Immunology and Uveitis
Service, Instituto de Oftalmologia, Conde de Valenciana,
Mexico City, Mexico
**Acute Posterior Multifocal Placoid Pigment
Epitheliopathy**

ANDRÉA PEREIRA DA MATA, M.D.
Doctoral Candidate, Universidade Federal de Minas Gerais,
Belo Horizonte, Minas Gerais, Brazil; Clinical Research
Ophthalmologist, Cincinnati Eye Institute, Cincinnati, Ohio
Toxoplasmosis

VAKUR PINAR
Formerly Fellow, Massachusetts Eye and Ear Infirmary,
Boston, Massachusetts
Tubulointerstitial Nephritis and Uveitis Syndrome

**WILLIAM J. POWER, F.R.C.S., F.R.C.Ophth.,
M.C.H.**
Consultant Ophthalmologist, Royal Victoria Eye and Ear
Hospital, Dublin, Ireland
Sympathetic Ophthalmia

MICHAEL B. RAIZMAN, M.D.
Associate Professor of Ophthalmology, Tufts University
School of Medicine; Ophthalmologist, Ophthalmic
Consultants of Boston; New England Medical Center,
Boston, Massachusetts
Punctate Inner Choroidopathy

TATIANA ROMERO RANGEL, M.D.
Formerly Fellow Massachusetts Eye and Ear Infirmary
Boston, Massachusetts
Ocular Toxocariasis

LAWRENCE A. RAYMOND, M.D.
Associate Professor of Clinical Ophthalmology, University of
Cincinnati College of Medicine; Director, Retina-Vitreous
Service, University of Cincinnati Medical Center; Retinal-
Vitreous Surgeon, Cincinnati Eye Institute, Cincinnati,
Ohio
Cysticercosis

ALEJANDRO RODRIGUEZ-GARCIA, M.D.
Associate Professor, Director, Immunology and Uveitis
Service, Department of Ophthalmology, Hospital San
Jose—TEC de Monterrey (ITESM), Monterrey, Nuevo
Leon, Mexico
Serpiginous Choroiditis

BLANCA ROJAS, M.D., Ph.D.
Associate Professor of Ophthalmology, Facultad de
Medicina, Universidad Complutense; Ophthalmologist,
Instituto de Investigaciones Oftalmologicas Ramon
Castroviejo, Madrid, Spain
Subretinal Fibrosis and Uveitis Syndrome

MANOLETTE RANGEL ROQUE, M.D.
Formerly, Department of Ophthalmology, Massachusetts
Eye and Ear Infirmary, Boston, Massachusetts
Sporotrichosis

MAITE SAINZ DE LA MAZA, M.D., Ph.D.
Professor, Central University of Barcelona School of
Medicine; Clinical Associate Professor of Ophthalmology,
Hospital Clinico, Barcelona, Spain
Seronegative Spondyloarthropathies

C. MICHAEL SAMSON, M.D.
Assistant Clinical Instructor, New York Medical College,
Valhalla, New York; Assistant Clinical Instructor, The New
York Eye and Ear Infirmary, New York, New York
**Syphilis; Tuberculosis; Masquerade Syndromes:
Endophthalmitis**

VIRENDER S. SANGWAN, M.S.(Ophthalmol.)
Director, Uveitis and Ocular Immunology Service, L.V.
Prasad Eye Institute, L.V. Prasad Marg, Banjara Hills,
Hyderabad, India
Ascariasis

GURINDER SINGH, M.D., M.H.A.
Associate Clinical Professor, Department of Ophthalmology,
University of Kansas Medical Center; Chief of
Ophthalmology, Providence Medical Center, Kansas City,
Kansas
Presumed Ocular Histoplasmosis Syndrome

AARON L. SOBOL, M.D.
Cornea Fellow, Tulane University School of Medicine, New
Orleans, Louisiana
Rift Valley Fever

MASOUD SOHEILIAN, M.D.
Clinical Associate Professor of Ophthalmology and
Vitreoretinal Surgery, Shaheed Beheshti University of
Medical Sciences School of Medicine; Director, The
Immunology and Uveitis Clinic, and Associate Clinical
Director of Vitreoretinal Service, Ophthalmology
Department and Eye Research Center, Labbafinejad
Medical Center, Tehran, Iran
Polyarteritis Nodosa

SARKIS H. SOUKIASIAN, M.D.
Associate Clinical Professor, Tufts University School of
Medicine, Boston; Director: Cornea/External Diseases
Service, Ocular Inflammation and Uveitis Service, Lahey
Clinic Medical Center, Eye Institute, Burlington,
Massachusetts
Wegener's Granulomatosis

PANAGIOTA STAVROU, F.R.C.S.
Consultant Ophthalmic Surgeon, Birmingham and Midland
Eye Centre, City Hospital NHS Trust, Birmingham, United
Kingdom
Sarcoidosis

J. WAYNE STREILEIN, M.D.
Charles L Schepens Professor of Ophthalmology, Harvard
Medical School; President, Schepens Eye Research Institute,
Boston, Massachusetts
Basic Immunology

RICHARD R. TAMESIS, M.D.
Assistant Professor, Department of Ophthalmology,
University of Nebraska Medical Center, Omaha, Nebraska
Coccidioidomycosis

KHALED A. TAWANSY
Assistant Professor of Ophthalmology, Retina/Vitreous
Service, Vanderbilt University School of Medicine,
Nashville, Tennessee
**Diagnostic Studies for Inflammatory Systemic Diseases
with Eye Manifestations**

NATTAPORN TESAVIBUL, M.D.
Instructor in Ophthalmology, Pramongkutklao Medical
School; Chief of Ocular Immunology Service, Department
of Ophthalmology, Pramongkutklao Hospital, Bangkok,
Thailand
Vogt-Koyanagi-Harada Syndrome

HARVEY SIY UY, M.D.
Clinical Associate Professor, University of the Philippines
College of Medicine, Manila; Active Consultant, Retina and
Uveitis Services, St. Luke's Medical Center Institute of
Ophthalmology, Quezon City, and Asian Eye Institute,
Makati City, Philippines

**Systemic Lupus Erythematosus; Multiple Evanescent
White Dot Syndrome**

ALBERT T. VITALE, M.D.
Chief, Uveitis Division, Member, Vitreoretinal Division, King
Khaled Eye Specialist Hospital, Riyadh, Saudi Arabia
**Treatment of Uveitis—Overview; Corticosteroids;
Mydriatic and Cycloplegic Agents; Nonsteroidal Anti-
Inflammatory Drugs; Immunosuppressive
Chemotherapy; Brucellosis; Free-Living Amebas and
Amebiasis; Birdshot Retinochoroidopathy; Multifocal
Choroiditis and Panuveitis; Intermediate Uveitis**

CINDY M. VREDEVELD
Clinical Research Coordinator, Ocular Immunology and
Uveitis Service, Massachusetts Eye and Ear Infirmary,
Harvard Medical School, Boston, Massachusetts
Free-Living Amebas and Amebiasis

NADIA KHALIDA WAHEED, M.D.
Resident in Ophthalmology, Massachusetts Eye and Ear
Infirmary, Harvard Medical School, Boston, Massachusetts
Masquerade Syndromes: Malignancies

RICHARD PAUL WETZIG, M.D.
Associate Clinical Attending, Department of
Ophthalmology, University of Colorado, Denver, Colorado
**Eye Disease and Systemic Correlates in Relapsing
Polychondritis**

HELEN WU, M.D.
Assistant Professor of Ophthalmology, Tufts University
School of Medicine; Director, Refractive Surgery Service;
Ophthalmologist, Cornea and Anterior Segment Service,
New England Eye Center, Boston, Massachusetts
Acute Zonal Occult Outer Retinopathy

LIJING YAO, M.D.
Clinical Fellow, Department of Ophthalmology, Children's
National Medical Center, Washington, D.C.
Nonmalignant, Noninfectious Masquerade Syndromes

JEAN YANG, M.D.
State University of New York—Health Science Center at
Brooklyn, Brooklyn, New York
Giant Cell Arteritis

PANAYOTIS ZAFIRAKIS, M.D.
General Hospital of Athens, Athens, Greece
Adamantiades-Behçet Disease

MANFRED ZIERHUT, M.D.
Professor of Ophthalmology, University Eye Clinic,
Department of Ophthalmology, University of Tübingen,
Tübingen, Germany
Intermediate Uveitis

FOREWORD

The uvea is the highly pigmented, vascularized middle tissue or tunic of the eye, sandwiched on the inside by the neuroretina and on the outside by the collagenous sclera. If the sclera is topographically an extension of the dura of the optic nerve, then the uvea is an extension of the pia-arachnoid, whereas the axons of the optic nerve are extensions from the innermost gangion cells of the retina. The uvea comprises, posteriorly, the choroid; more anteriorly, the smooth muscle of the ciliary body; and up front, the stroma of the iris. The choroid can leak on inflammatory or immunologic provocation to create an effusion; inflammations situated primarily in the sclera and less often the retina may also cause secondary choroidal inflammations and effusions. It is interesting to note that large cell lymphoma of the retina and brain elicits an intense non-neoplastic chronic nongranulomatous inflammation of the choroid and other parts of the uvea. On the other hand, in systemic nodal lymphoma, the neoplastic lymphocytes settle in the choroid and hardly ever in the retina, and do not typically incite a secondary reactive inflammatory response.

In addition to its abundant blood vessels, the choroid possesses scattered melanocytes and fibroblasts, the latter basically unable to proliferate as scar tissue in the wake of inflammation or infection. (The sclera also has limited powers of healing.) Most true scar production featuring collagen within the eye is the result of fibrous metaplasia of the retinal pigment epithelium (itself, curiously, a neuroectodermal derivative), which is on the retinal side of Bruch's membrane. The lobular arrangement of the fenestrated choriocapillaris, which nourishes the outer retina and is situated right next to Bruch's membrane on the choroidal side, can be the focus of inflammations and infections, sometimes leading to proliferations of the pigment epithelium such as Dalen-Fuchs nodules in sympathetic ophthalmia. There are no lymphatics in the choroid, and none in either the retina or the sclera; thus, immunologic events in the eye may deviate from those elsewhere in the body ("immune privilege"). The uveal tissues of the choroid, ciliary body and iris are all derivatives of the neural crest, owing to the fact that there are no paired paraxial mesodermal somites in the head and neck region.

It is against the foregoing unusual anatomic and reparative features of the choroid and other parts of the uvea that one must analyze the idiopathic inflammations and infectious diseases that cause uveitis. This textbook, edited by Drs. C. Stephen Foster and Albert Vitale, is the most comprehensive, scholarly and up-to-date effort at encompassing the diagnosis, etiopathogenesis, and therapy for this often arcane spectrum of diseases. There is no doubt that this textbook, containing 79 chapters encompassing 867 pages, will become the dominant reference and touchstone for those with a sophisticated and deeply committed interest in uveitis. (Dr. Foster's earlier textbook on the *Sclera* [Springer-Verlag, 1994] has already become a classic.) Having read through many chapters of this textbook in galleys, I can testify to the richness, accuracy, and pure pleasure attendant on reading a treatise that brings the greatest degree of scientific precision to dissipate the miasma that too often envelops the subspecialty of uveitis.

This textbook would have been unthinkable and undoable without its impresario Dr. C. Stephen Foster harnessing the energy and knowledge of many of his past and present trainees, including his coeditor Dr. Vitale. I have long been an admirer of Dr. Foster's intellect and accomplishments, and my other colleagues locally, regionally, nationally, and internationally often regard his as the court of last appeal for totally enigmatic and "hopeless" cases. I can think of no one else who combines his intellectual capacity, knowledge, experience, surgical skills, and powers of communication in dealing with all facets of uveitis; he is probably in the company of no more than six individuals internationally who can manage these difficult problems. Through his training in ophthalmology, internal medicine, and immunology, and his highly systematic approach to the patient, he has mastered the cabalistic field of uveitis. Consequently, he has been able to restore vision to innumerable patients who otherwise would have lost their sight. Dr. Foster's inquisitive mind propels him to produce continually new laboratory and clinical research at the highest levels, with enormous patient relevancy and applicability. This textbook is a treasure, and will further enlighten the ophthalmic community about many recondite infectious and autoimmune diseases. Moreover, it also demonstrates the unsurpassed skills of one of the world's foremost ophthalmologists, Dr. C. Stephen Foster.

FREDERICK A. JAKOBIEC, M.D., D.Sc.(Med.)
Henry Willard Williams Professor of Ophthalmology,
Professor of Pathology, and Chairman of Ophthalmology,
Harvard Medical School; Chief of Ophthalmology,
Massachusetts Eye and Ear Infirmary

PREFACE

When the invitation came from W.B. Saunders Company, nearly a decade ago, to write this textbook, it contained three primary charges: (1) that the textbook should be comprehensive, even "encyclopedic"; (2) that it should emphasize more modern, aggressive approaches to treating uveitis that have evolved over the past 20 years; (3) that it should be a single-authored text. And although this invitation was incredibly tempting, I was unprepared and unwilling to take on the task single-handedly. Eventually, agreement was reached that one of my former fellows, Dr. Albert Vitale, would coedit a multiauthored textbook with me, and that the opportunity would be exploited to reconnect with former fellows and colleagues who share our therapeutic philosophy: an attempt at total control of all inflammation and freedom from all relapses, while at the same time eliminating the need for chronic use of corticosteroids.

The challenge posed by the charge from the publisher has been enormous. Other books on the subject of uveitis have met this challenge by increasing their focus on particular matters, avoiding the problems posed by being encyclopedic. In particular, textbooks by Opremcak,[1] by Smith and Nozik,[2] by Kraus-MacKiw and O'Connor,[3] by Nussenblatt, Palestine, and Whitcup,[4] and by BenEzra[5] are all excellent textbooks addressing the issue of diagnosis and therapy of uveitis. We have met the challenge posed by the publisher through the participation of 74 contributors, all of whom have had a relationship with the Massachusetts Eye and Ear Infirmary Ocular Immunology and Uveitis Service, and all of whom share in our basic philosophy of a complete intolerance to chronic, even low-grade intraocular inflammation, and at the same time a philosophy of steroid-sparing anti-inflammatory therapy.

The overriding philosophical principles that underpin the writings within this textbook are as follows: (1) Diagnosis matters; we advocate a comprehensive approach to diagnosing the underlying cause of a patient's uveitis. (2) Intolerance to chronic, even great low-grade inflammation; history abundantly teaches that, eventually, such chronic inflammation produces permanent damage to structures within the eye that are critical to good vision. (3) Intolerance to the chronic use of corticosteroids in an effort to control inflammation; history shows and all physicians agree that such chronic use of corticosteroids inevitably produces damage itself. (4) A stepladder algorithmic approach to achieve the goal: *no* inflammation on *no* steroids. (5) Collaboration with a rheumatologist or other individual who is, by virtue of training and experience, truly expert in the use of immunomodulatory medications, so that *no* significant drug-induced side effects occur in the exploitation of the stepladder algorithmic approach to achieving the goal of no inflammation on no steroids.

The experience of writing this textbook has been indescribable. The knowledge gained has been worth the effort itself. The reconnection with former fellows and colleagues has doubled the pleasure. Working with Dr. Albert Vitale has made it all infinitely easier, and indeed has made it possible. The effort has also refocused and sharpened my attention to many aspects in the care of our patients.

The Immunology and Uveitis Service of the Massachusetts Eye and Ear Infirmary was established in 1977. The first Research Fellow was accepted into the Laboratory in 1980. The first Clinical Fellow arrived in 1984. During this same year, a generous donation from Ms. Susan Hilles, a patient of the Service, provided for the construction of a new, state-of-the-art immunology laboratory: the Hilles Immunology Laboratory. A second gift from Mr. Richard Rhodes, another of the Service's patients, enabled us to equip an additional laboratory, the Rhodes Molecular Immunology Laboratory, in 1990. These laboratories are described as applied research laboratories—that is, we have attempted to bring to the clinic as soon as practicable the discoveries and lessons learned from the laboratory.

Our hope in producing this textbook is that a new generation of ophthalmologists will not only learn the lessons of the past with respect to diagnosis and treatment of uveitis in the usual way, with corticosteroids, but will also learn that the prevalence of blindness from uveitis, unchanged since the improvements occurring after the introduction of cortiocsteroids, can be further reduced by the adoption of the therapeutic principles espoused herein.

C. STEPHEN FOSTER, M.D.

References

1. Opremcak EM: Uveitis: A Clinical Manual for Ocular Inflammation. New York, Springer-Verlag, 1995.

2. Smith RE, Nozik RM: Uveitis: A Clinical Approach to Diagnosis and Management. Baltimore, Williams & Wilkins, 1989.
3. Kraus-MacKiw E, O'Connor GR: Uveitis: Pathophysiology and Therapy. New York, Thieme Verlag, 1986.
4. Nussenblatt RB, Whitcup SM, Palestine AG: Uveitis: Fundamentals and Clinical Practice. St. Louis, Mosby–Year Book, 1996.
5. BenEzra D: Ocular Inflammation: Basic and Clinical Concepts. London, Blackwell Science, 1999.

It has been an honor and a privilege to participate in the creation of this text. This work represents much more than the concerted efforts and efficient teamwork of a group of individuals dedicated to a multi-authored book; it is the product of an extended family bound by similar philosophical values in their care for patients with ocular inflammatory disease. Indeed, the essence of this philosophy, the pleasure of reconnecting and collaborating with the current and former fellows of the Ocular Immunology and Uveitis Service of the Massachusetts Eye and Ear Infirmary, and the refocusing and crystallization of the state of the art with respect to many aspects of patient care as a result of this effort have all been articulated in Dr. Foster's preface. What is not mentioned is the personal and professional respect and gratitude that I, myself, and the members of this extended family share for our association with Dr. Foster. The ultimate and most important beneficiaries, of course, are our patients who suffer from uveitis.

ALBERT T. VITALE, M.D.

ACKNOWLEDGMENTS

We wish to thank here the thousands of patients with uveitis who have entrusted their care to us. It is through them that the inspiration for this textbook arises, and it is for them primarily to whom this textbook is dedicated. We also acknowledge and thank the support staff at the Massachusetts Eye and Ear Infirmary, its clinics and its operating rooms, for their loyalty and support in our care of patients. In particular, Ms. Cindy Vredeveld and Ms. Audrey Melanson are acknowledged and thanked for their assistance, Cindy for her unstinting dedication to editorial assistance and organizational efforts in this multi-authored text, and Audrey for her help in assembling many of the photographs employed in the text. We acknowledge the help of and are grateful to the many fellows who participate on the Ocular Immunology and Uveitis Service; without their help the day's work could not be done. We also acknowledge the help of Dr. Tongzhen Zhao, Chief Technician in the Hilles Immunology Laboratory, whose help in processing tissue and fluid specimens for analysis is invaluable. Finally, we would like to extend our thanks and acknowledgment to all the referring physicians, not only in New England but across the United States and throughout Europe, who have consistently referred patients to this Service.

C. Stephen Foster, M.D.

I would like to thank the medical staff secretaries of the King Khaled Eye Specialist Hospital, especially Mrs. Yvonne Brinc, for their tireless dedication and support in preparing the manuscript for this work.

Albert T. Vitale, M.D.

CONTENTS

Part IV

THE UVEITIS SYNDROMES—
Masquerade Syndromes

Part V

THE UVEITIS SYNDROMES—
Traumatic

Part VI

THE UVEITIS SYNDROMES—
Autoimmune

Part VII

THE UVEITIS SYNDROMES—
Medication Induced

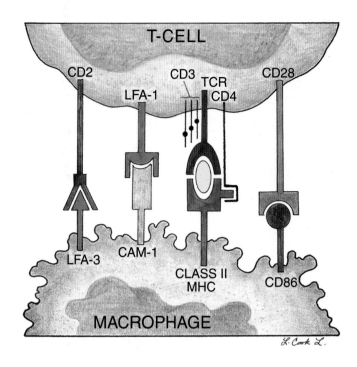

COLOR FIGURE 5–4. Antigen presentation, macrophage to CD4+ T cell. Note the oval-shaped (yellow) peptide fragment from the macrophage-phagocytosed integrated antigen in the groove of the Class II MHC molecule on the surface of the macrophage, being presented to the T cell receptor in the context of the helper- or inducer-specific CD4 molecule. Note also the attachment complex interactions between CD2 and LFA-3, and between LFA-1 and CAM-1, ensuring appropriate cell-to-cell contact and stability during antigen presentation. Note also the costimulatory molecule interactions between CD28 and CD86, ensuring a "correct" presentation of the antigen to the T cell such that an active, proinflammatory immune response will ensue. (Original drawing courtesy of Laurel Cook Lhowe).

COLOR FIGURE 5–5. Signal transduction: intracellular and intranuclear. With antigen-presenting cell presentation of antigen to the T cell (green peptide fragment in the MHC Class II groove of the macrophage), an extraordinary cascade of events occurs, through the cell membrane, into the cytoplasm, and subsequently into the nucleus, to the level of specific genes on the chromosomes of the nucleus. Specifically, tyrosine-rich phosphorylases result in phosphorylation of a series of intracellular proteins, with resultant liberation of calcium stores, and production of the calcineurin-calmodulin complex, which then facilitates the production of nuclear factor–AT_C, capable of being transported through one of the nuclear pores into the nucleus, where interaction then with specific foci on the gene results in induction of gene transcription (in this instance, transcription of production of messenger RNA for ultimate synthesis of the protein interleukin 2). (Original drawing courtesy of Laurel Cook Lhowe.)

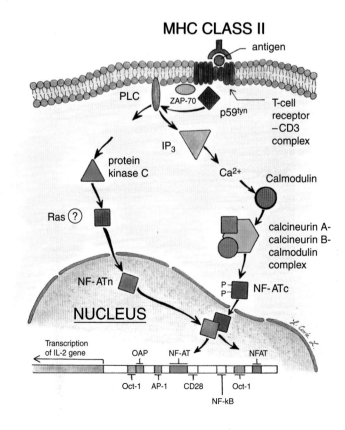

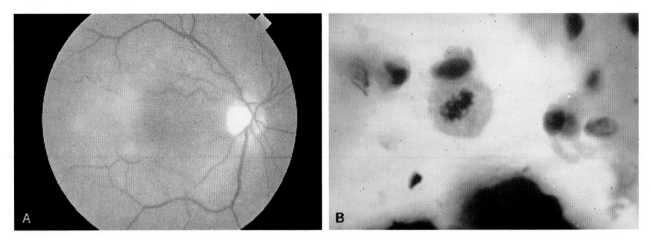

COLOR FIGURE 13–2. *A,* Fundus photograph of a 65-year-old patient with chronic, medically unresponsive vitritis and multifocal, subretinal infiltrates. *B,* Photomicrograph of a vitreous biopsy showing neoplastic cells with mitotic figures establishing a diagnosis of intraocular, non-Hodgkin's lymphoma.

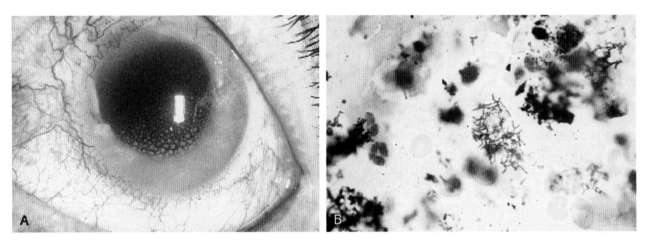

COLOR FIGURE 13–3. *A,* Anterior segment photograph from a patient with low-grade uveitis, 4 weeks following cataract surgery, showing "dirty" keratic precipitates. *B,* Photomicrograph of a Gram's stain of a vitreous aspirate from the same patient showing gram-positive, pleomorphic bacilli. Anaerobic cultures grew *Propionibacterium granulosum* after an 8-day incubation.

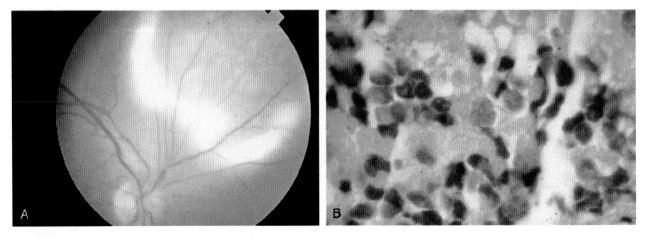

COLOR FIGURE 13–4. *A,* Fundus photograph from an immunosuppressed patient with a progressive, brushfire-like retinitis of unknown etiology that was unresponsive to antiviral therapy. *B,* Photomicrograph of a retinal biopsy showing toxoplasmosis of organisms and tissue cysts. The vitreous specimen did not show toxoplasmosis organisms.

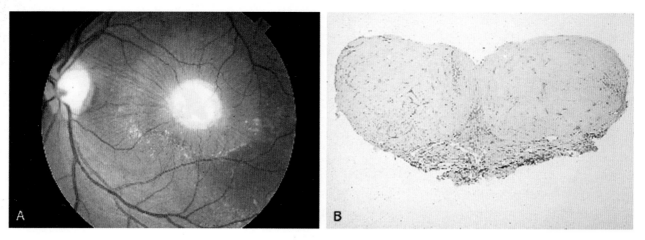

COLOR FIGURE 13–5. *A,* Fundus photograph of a submacular lesion in a 24-year-old patient with vitritis and a subretinal lesion who was referred for ocular cysticercosis. *B,* Photomicrograph of the submacular lesion showing a fibrovascular scar. *Cysticercus* sp. was not found in serial sections and the etiology of the inflammatory scar was unknown.

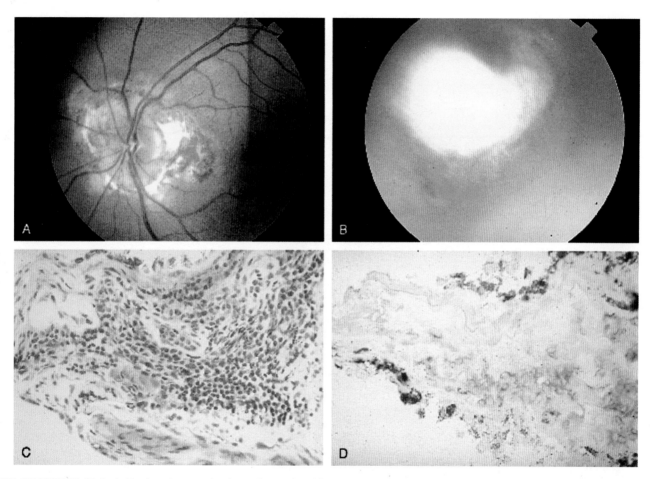

COLOR FIGURE 13–6. *A,* Fundus photograph of a patient with a 15-year history of multifocal choroiditis and panuveitis (MCP) of unknown etiology. The patient was intolerant of corticosteroid agents. The right eye was NLP and the left eye had active MCP and a progressive, macula threatening lesion. *B,* Fundus photograph of the superior chorioretinal biopsy site showing the underlying sclera. The retina remained attached following surgery. *C,* Photomicrograph of a chorioretinal biopsy specimen showing choroidal infiltration with epithelioid cells, plasma cells, eosinophils, and a Dalen-Fuchs nodule, which support a diagnosis of sympathetic ophthalmia. Infectious organisms were not identified. Following the operation, the patient recalled traumatic, strabismus surgery as a child that may have been the original trauma inducing the uveitis. *D,* Immunohistochemical staining of the same biopsy specimen showing activated CD4 +, helper T cells (red-stained mononuclear cells) supporting an active, cellular immune response.

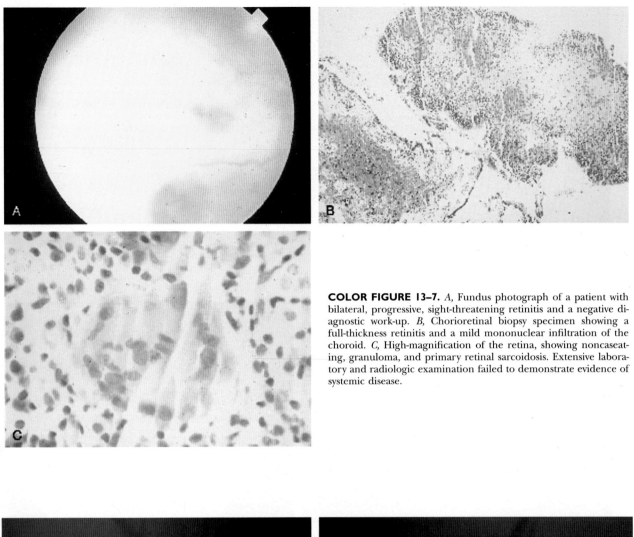

COLOR FIGURE 13–7. *A*, Fundus photograph of a patient with bilateral, progressive, sight-threatening retinitis and a negative diagnostic work-up. *B*, Chorioretinal biopsy specimen showing a full-thickness retinitis and a mild mononuclear infiltration of the choroid. *C*, High-magnification of the retina, showing noncaseating, granuloma, and primary retinal sarcoidosis. Extensive laboratory and radiologic examination failed to demonstrate evidence of systemic disease.

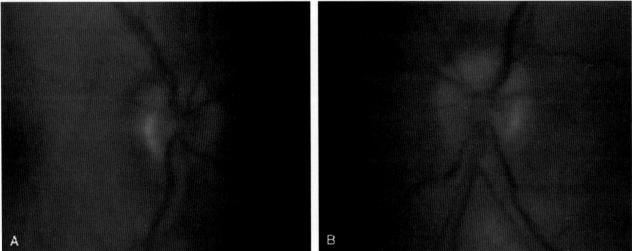

COLOR FIGURE 16–2. *A*, A young woman complaining of bilateral floaters was noted to have bilateral vitritis and papillitis. Visual acuity was 20/20 OU. Lyme serology was positive. *B*, The vitritis and papillitis cleared promptly after antibiotic treatment. Convalescent titer confirmed the diagnosis.

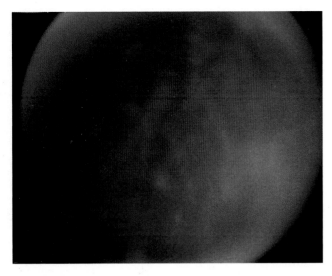

COLOR FIGURE 16–3. Vitreous "snowballs" are present in the inferior vitreous cavity of a patient with Lyme borreliosis. (Courtesy of William W. Culbertson, M.D.)

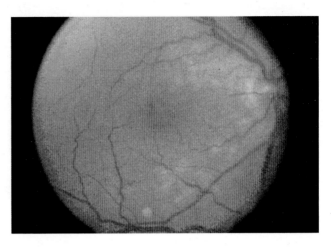

COLOR FIGURE 21–1. Case #1: Multiple faint, white choroidal lesions.

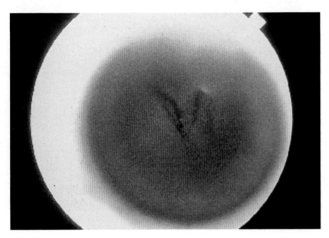

COLOR FIGURE 21–3. Case #3: Vitreous strands.

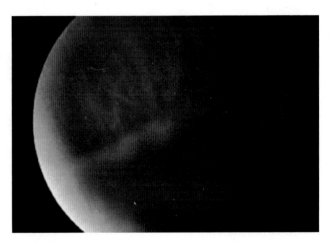

COLOR FIGURE 21–4. Case #3: Diffuse, fluffy, white infiltrate.

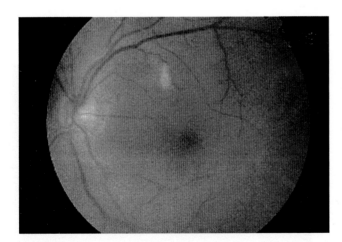

COLOR FIGURE 21–5. Case #3: Cotton-wool spot in superior macula.

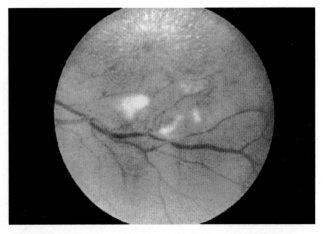

COLOR FIGURE 22–1. Retinal involvement in rickettsiosis. Note the periarteritis, the macular star exudate, and the retinal infiltrates. (Courtesy of C. Stephen Foster, M.D.)

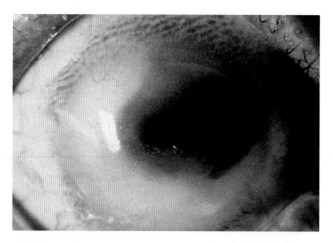

COLOR FIGURE 23–1. Lepromatous uveitis with corneal edema, retrocorneal fibrovascular membrane formation, mutton-fat keratic precipitates, 3+ anterior chamber inflammation, and secluded pupil.

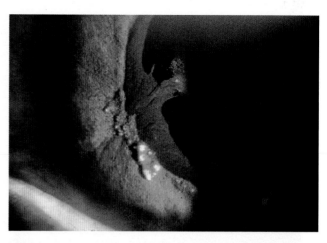

COLOR FIGURE 23–2. Iris granuloma formation (so-called iris pearls) in lepromatous uveitis. (From Messmer EM, Raizman MB, Foster CS: Lepromatous uveitis diagnosed by iris biopsy. Graefes Arch Clin Exp Ophthalmol 1998;236:717–719.)

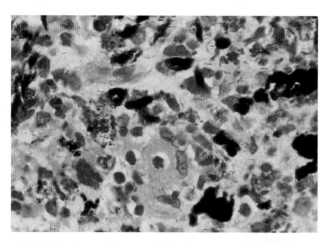

COLOR FIGURE 23–3. Iris biopsy in patient with lepromatous uveitis disclosed abundant Wade-Fite–positive intracellular and extracellular organisms consistent with *Mycobacterium leprae* (Wade-Fite stain, ×330). (From Messmer EM, Raizman MB, Foster CS: Lepromatous uveitis diagnosed by iris biopsy. Graefes Arch Clin Exp Ophthalmol 1998;236:717–719.)

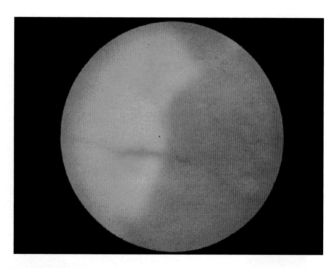

COLOR FIGURE 24–3. Clinical appearance of acute retinal necrosis with vitritis, yellowish white retinal infiltrates, and vasculitis.

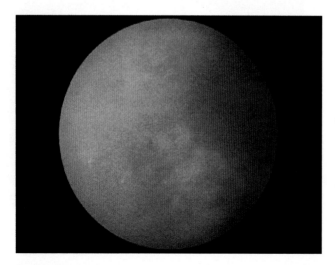

COLOR FIGURE 24–4. Regression of acute retinal necrosis with "Swiss cheese pattern" and retinal atrophy.

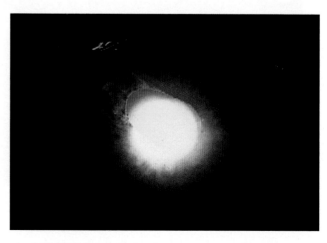

COLOR FIGURE 24–5. Iris atrophy in a patient with HSV.

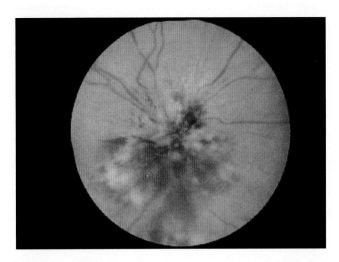

COLOR FIGURE 24–6. Clinical appearance of CMV retinitis: fluffy, dense, white confluent retinal infiltrations, multiple retinal hemorrhages, and perivasculitis.

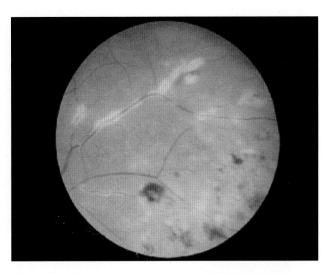

COLOR FIGURE 24–7. Clinical appearance of CMV retinitis: frosted branch angiitis.

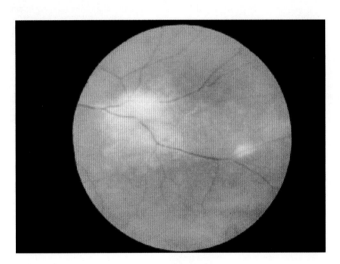

COLOR FIGURE 24–8. Clinical appearance of CMV retinitis: granular, less-opaque lesions.

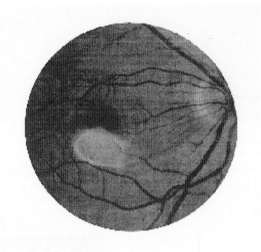

COLOR FIGURE 26–1. Ophthalmoscopic photograph, right macula. Note the well circumscribed, deep retinal opacification inferior to the fovea, with faint nerve fiber layer swelling extending from the lesion to the optic disk. (From Park DW, Boldt HC, Massicotte SJ, et al: Subacute sclerosing panencephalitis manifesting as viral retinitis: Clinical and histopathologic findings. Am J Ophthalmol 1997;123:533–543. With permission from Elsevier Science.)

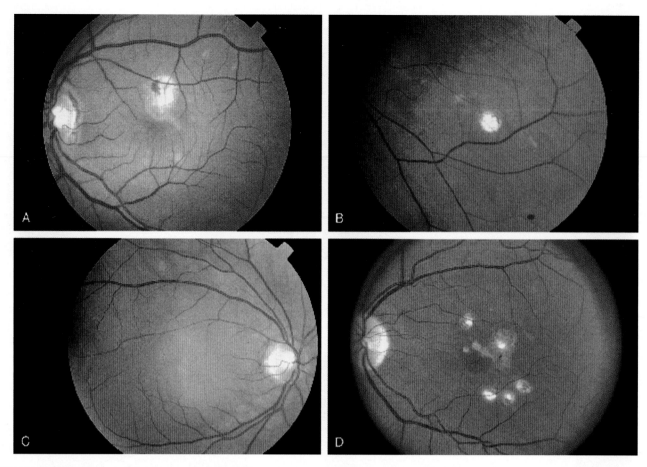

COLOR FIGURE 28–1. *A,* Color fundus photograph illustrating juxtafoveal punched-out typical "histo spot." *B,* Peripheral "histo spot" in the same eye. *C,* Ground-glass–like macular "atypical histo spot" with ill-defined edges. *D,* Multiple macular "histo spots" in another patient.

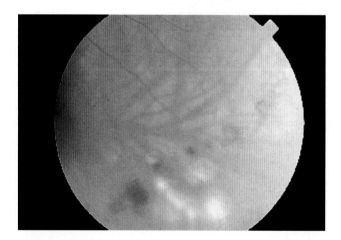

COLOR FIGURE 28–2. Color fundus photograph illustrating a clump of histo spots arranged in linear fashion in peripheral retina to constitute linear streaks.

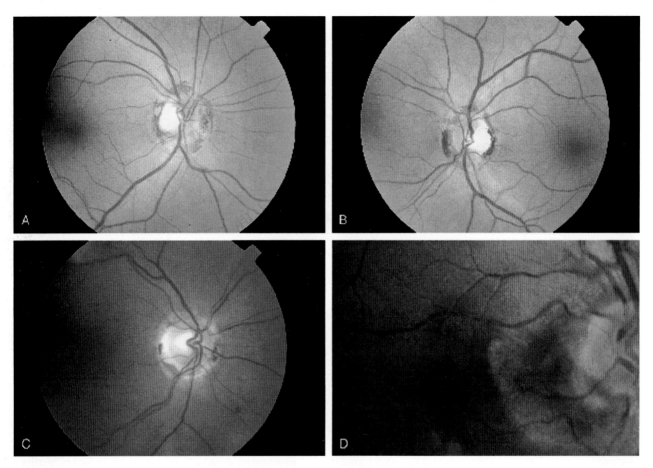

COLOR FIGURE 28–3. *A*, and *B*, Color fundus photographs illustrating bilateral peripapillary chorioretinal degeneration in POHS. *C*, Peripapillary chorioretinal degeneration in another patient. *D*, Peripapillary CNV causing subretinal hemorrhage extending into the macular area.

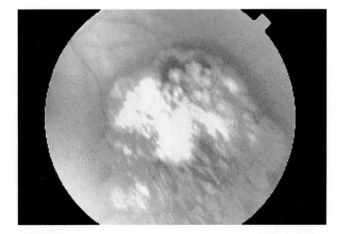

COLOR FIGURE 28–4. Color fundus photograph illustrating disciform macular scar in POHS.

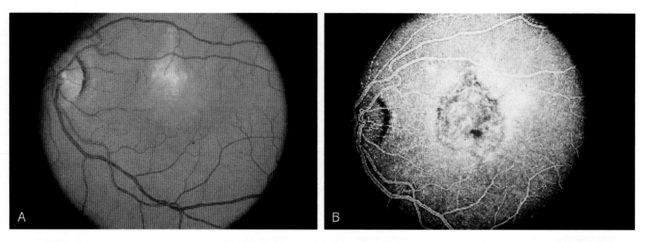

COLOR FIGURE 28–5. *A,* Color photograph illustrating macular chorioretinal neovascularization (CNV) in POHS. *B,* Flourescein angiogram of the same eye to show CNV.

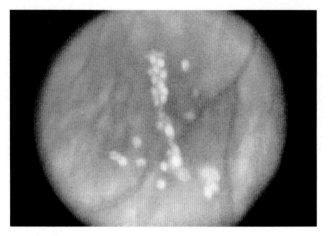

COLOR FIGURE 29–1. "String of pearls" appearance to the vitreal exudates in a patient with endogenous *Candida* endophthalmitis.

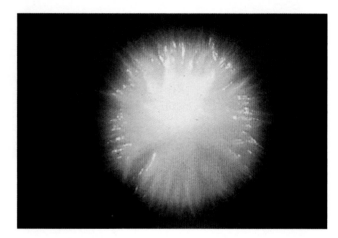

COLOR FIGURE 32–1. Young colonies of *Sporothrix schenckii* remain white for some time at 25°C or when incubated at 37°C to induce its yeast phase. (Reprinted from *http://fungusweb.utmb.edu/mycology/sporothrix.html,* with permission from Medical Mycology Research Center, Department of Pathology, University of Texas Medical Branch.)

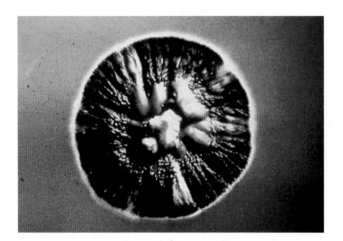

COLOR FIGURE 32–2. Older colonies of *Sporothrix schenckii* turn black due to the production of dark conidia that arise directly from the hyphae. (Reprinted from *http://fungusweb.utmb.edu/mycology/sporothrix.html,* with permission from Medical Mycology Research Center, Department of Pathology, University of Texas Medical Branch.)

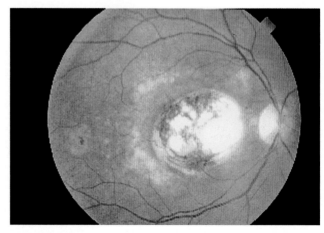

COLOR FIGURE 33–5. Classic macular retinochoroidal lesion of congenital toxoplasmosis.

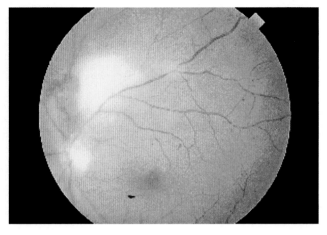

COLOR FIGURE 33–7. Active toxoplasma retinitis adjacent to a pigmented juxtapapillary scar. Note also the small, active lesion along the superior branch of the temporal arcade.

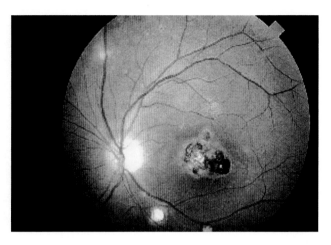

COLOR FIGURE 33–8. Recurrent active retinitis distant from the primary pigmented lesion. Note the primary lesion in the macula with evidence of prior recurrences along the inferotemporal arcade, as well as a small, active lesion along the supranasal arcade.

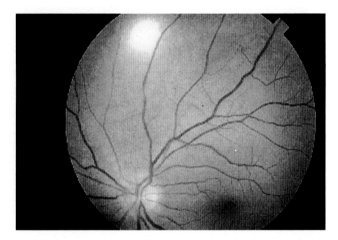

COLOR FIGURE 33–9. Unilateral, solitary, active lesion without evidence of chorioretinal scarring typical of acquired toxoplasmosis.

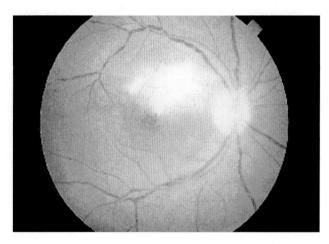

COLOR FIGURE 33–10. Active toxoplasma retinitis. Note the yellowish white appearance of the lesion with ill-defined borders due to surrounding retinal edema. There is associated phlebitis of the supratemporal arcade.

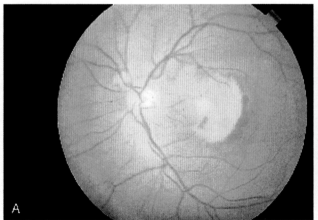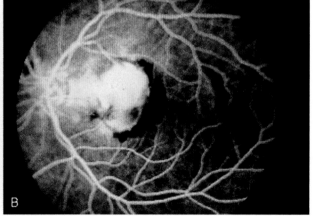

COLOR FIGURE 33–11. *A*, Macular toxoplasma scar complicated by a choroidal neovascular membrane. Note the hemorrhage around the neovascular membrane. *B*, Late fluorescein angiogram hyperfluorescence of a choroidal neovascular membrane and blockage by the surrounding hemorrhage.

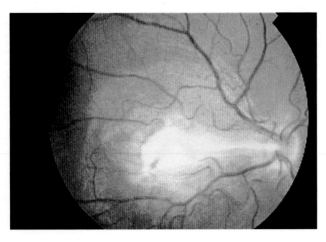

COLOR FIGURE 33–12. Franceschetti's syndrome, a traction band from the toxoplasma macular lesion to the optic nerve.

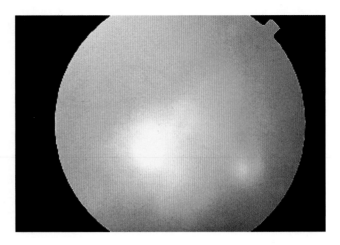

COLOR FIGURE 33–13. Active toxoplasma retinitis with marked vitritis producing the classic appearance of a headlight in the fog. (Courtesy of Maria Elenir F. Péret, M.D., COMG, Brazil.)

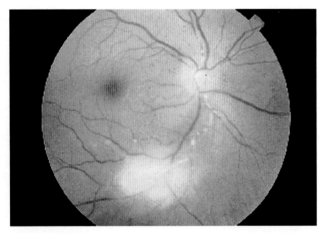

COLOR FIGURE 33–14. Segmental arteritis associated with an active toxoplasma lesion in the vicinity of the vessel. The localized perivascular inflammatory accumulations may line up around the vessels and resemble a rosary.

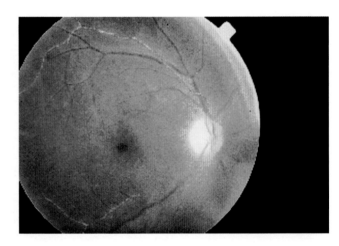

COLOR FIGURE 33–15. Toxoplasma periarterial plaques known as kyrieleis arteriolitis.

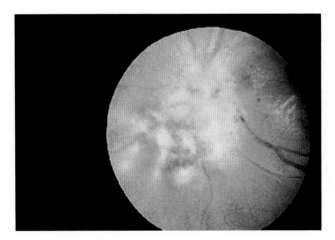

COLOR FIGURE 33–18. Juxtapapillary active toxoplasma lesion with severe involvement of the optic nerve. Note the severe papillitis and retinitis with hemorrhages.

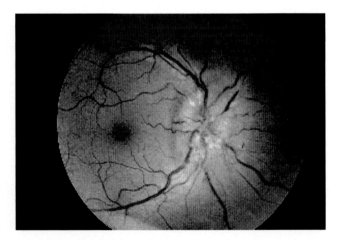

COLOR FIGURE 33–19. Initial presentation of toxoplasma neuroretinitis. Note papillitis with disc hemorrhages and venous engorgement prior to the development of retinochoroiditis.

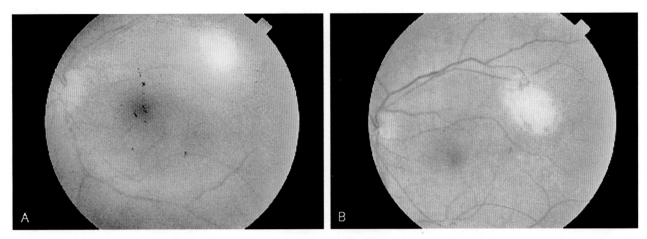

COLOR FIGURE 33–24. *A,* Active toxoplasma lesion resistant to prolonged medical therapy. Note that the visual acuity measured 20/70. *B,* The same eye after laser photocoagulation. Note the well-defined, slightly pigmented borders of the lesion. The visual acuity improved to 20/30. (Courtesy of Professor Suel Abujamra, USP, Brazil.)

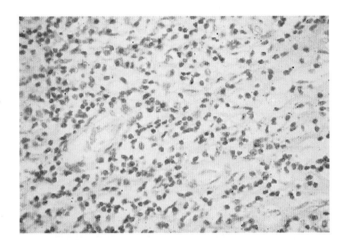

COLOR FIGURE 38–1. Histopathology of chorioretinal granuloma in a patient whose eye was enucleated secondary to chronic endophthalmitis and irreparable retinal detachment, ultimately shown to be secondary to toxocariasis. Note the complete loss of choroidal or retinal architecture with the granulomatous inflammatory infiltrate.

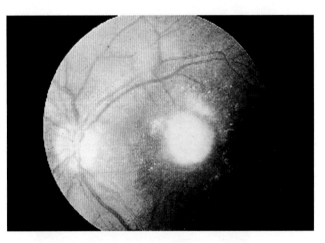

COLOR FIGURE 38–2. Posterior granuloma, macular, in a patient with toxocara chorioretinitis. Exuberant vitritis has been controlled with systemic prednisone.

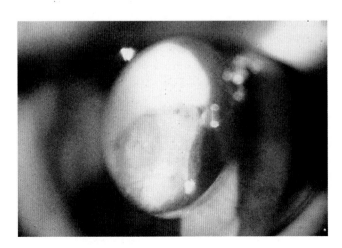

COLOR FIGURE 38–3. Peripheral retinitis and retinal detachment in a patient with a peripheral toxocara granuloma. This eye was eventually enucleated and was the source of the histopathology shown in Figure 38–1.

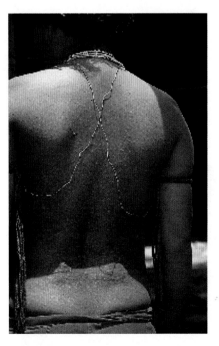

COLOR FIGURE 40–4. Acute papular onchodermatitis in an 18-year-old Yanomami girl, Venezuela.

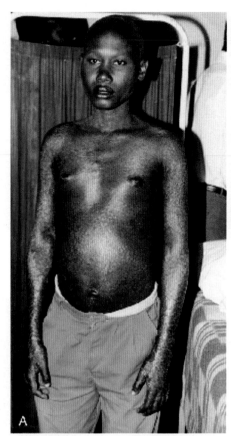

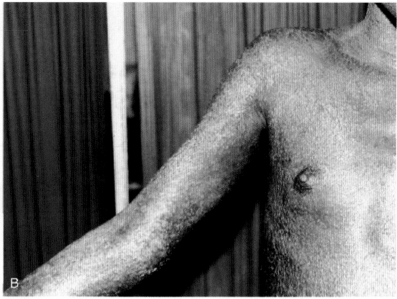

COLOR FIGURE 40–5. Chronic papular onchodermatitis (CPOD). (Photo courtesy of E.M. Pedersen.)

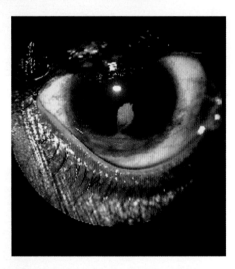

COLOR FIGURE 40–10. Sclerosing keratitis: opacification of the inferior cornea with pupillary aperture drawn inferiorly and cataract. (Photo courtesy of A. Rothova.)

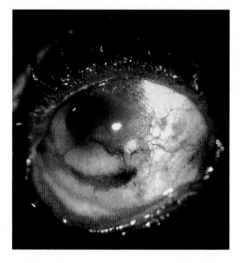

COLOR FIGURE 40–11. Advanced sclerosing keratitis with extended opacification of the cornea. (Photo courtesy A. Rothova.)

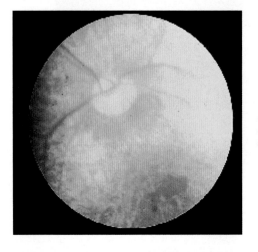

COLOR FIGURE 40–12. Fundus changes in onchocerciasis: optic nerve atrophy, diffuse chorioretinal atrophy, and secondary pigmentary changes, pigment clumping in the macular area. (Photo courtesy A. Rothova.)

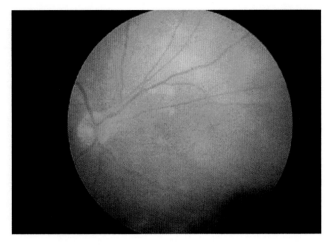

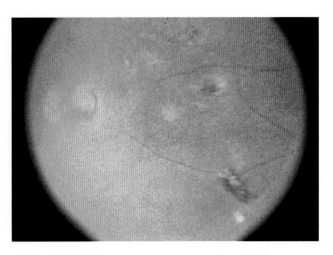

COLOR FIGURE 43–1. Early-stage diffuse unilateral subacute neuro-retinitis: vitritis, disc margin swelling, and multiple yellow-white lesions at the level of the retinal pigment epithelium and outer retina. (Courtesy of Donald Gass, M.D.)

COLOR FIGURE 43–2. Late-stage diffuse unilateral subacute neuro-retinitis: vessel attenuation and chorioretinal scars. (Courtesy of Donald Gass, M.D.)

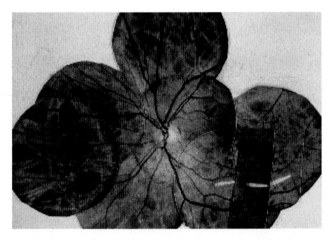

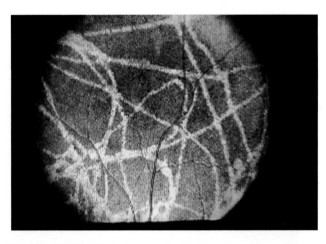

COLOR FIGURE 45–1. Composite "collage" fundus photograph demonstrating the etiologic agent of ophthalmomyiasis, the botfly maggot. (From Stereoscopic Atlas of Macular Disease, 3rd ed. St. Louis, CV Mosby, 1987. Courtesy of Constance Fitzgerald, MD, with permission from J. Donald Gass, MD, and Mosby Publishers.)

COLOR FIGURE 45–2. Fundus photograph of a patient with long-standing ophthalmomyiasis, demonstrating the extensive RPE loss in "track" fashion, evidence of the very extensive amount of migration and travel of the maggot. (From Stereoscopic Atlas of Macular Disease, 3rd ed. St. Louis, CV Mosby, 1987. Courtesy of J. Donald Gass, MD, with permission from Mosby Publishers.)

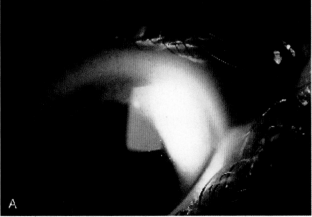

COLOR FIGURE 46–2. *A,* Slit-lamp photograph of a patient with ophthalmia nodosa, with keratitis secondary to a tarantula hair. *B,* Ophthalmia nodosa with both keratitis and uveitis. (Courtesy of Dr. E. Mitchel Opremcak.)

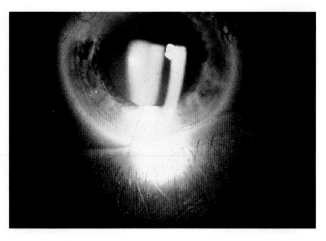

COLOR FIGURE 46–3. Ophthalmia nodosa with hypopyon uveitis. (Courtesy of Dr. E. Mitchel Opremcak.)

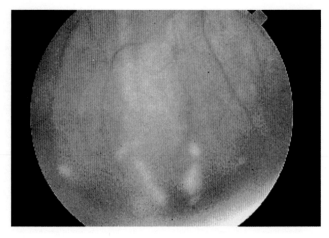

COLOR FIGURE 46–4. Ophthalmia nodosa, with intraocular penetration of tarantula hair, with production of posterior uveitis and the formation of vitreal infiltrates, both in the form of snowballs and in the form of a snowman (central figure). (Courtesy of Dr. E. Mitchel Opremcak.)

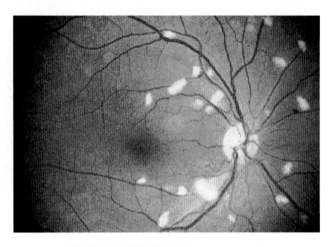

COLOR FIGURE 47–2. HIV microangiopathy.

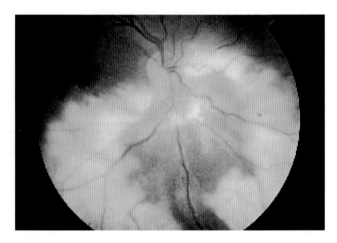

COLOR FIGURE 47–3. Fulminant CMV retinitis.

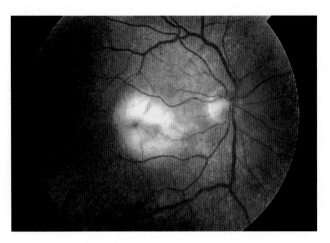

COLOR FIGURE 47–6. VZV retinitis: cherry-red spot macula.

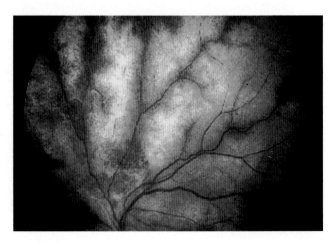

COLOR FIGURE 47–7. VZV retinitis: cracked mud appearance.

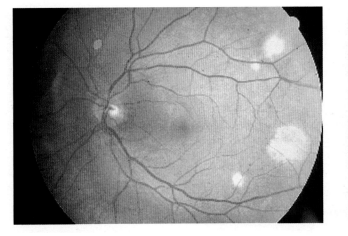

COLOR FIGURE 47–8. Pneumocystosis.

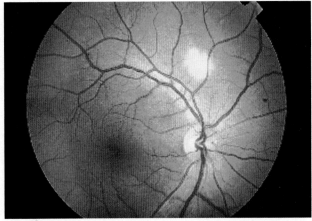

COLOR FIGURE 47–9. Ocular tuberculosis.

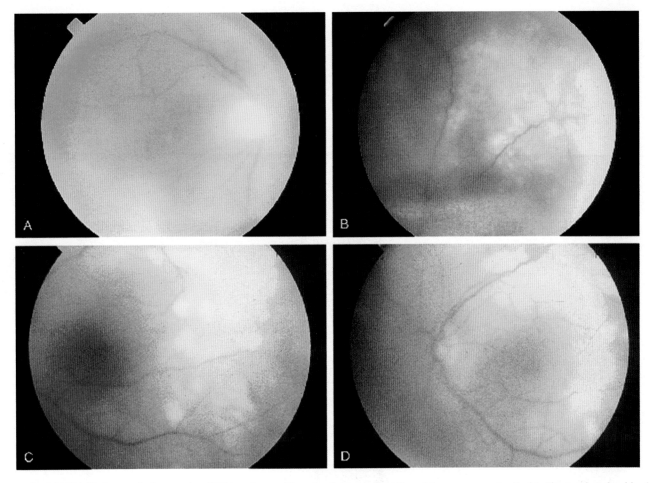

COLOR FIGURE 48–1. *A* to *D*, Intraocular–CNS lymphoma. Note the dense vitritis *(A)*, and the presence of retinal infiltrates that should raise the suspicion of intraocular–CNS lymphoma.

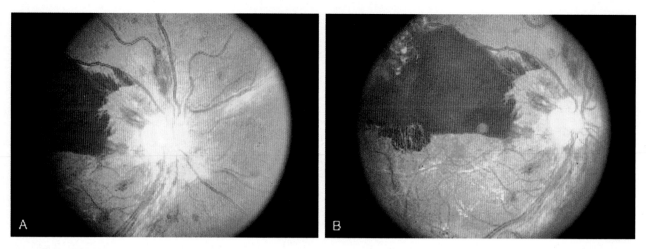

COLOR FIGURE 48-2. *A* and *B,* Fundus photographs in a patient with leukemia. Flame-shaped nerve fiber layer hemorrhages and large subhyaloid hemorrhages can be seen.

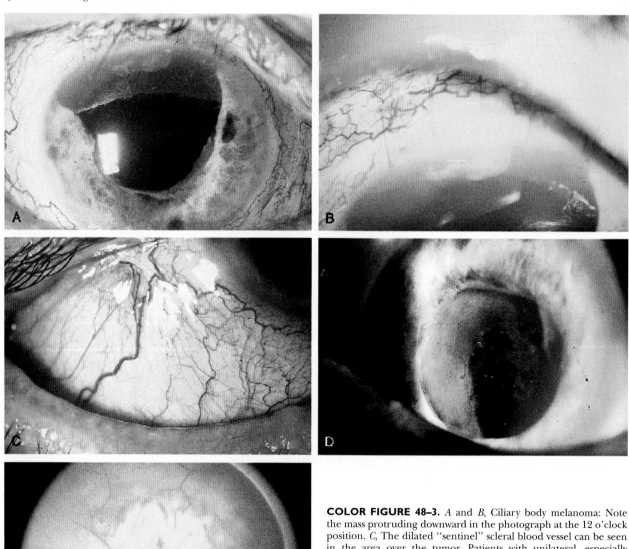

COLOR FIGURE 48-3. *A* and *B,* Ciliary body melanoma: Note the mass protruding downward in the photograph at the 12 o'clock position. *C,* The dilated "sentinel" scleral blood vessel can be seen in the area over the tumor. Patients with unilateral, especially sectorial, conjunctivitis should always have a dilated examination to rule out an intraocular tumor. *D,* Cataract in a patient with ciliary body melanoma. *E,* Malignant melanoma. The large, elevated dome shape of the tumor seen in this picture is characteristic. Tumors may also show breaks in the Bruch's membrane, giving a collar-button appearance. Although most tumors are pigmented, nearly 25% can be nonpigmented.

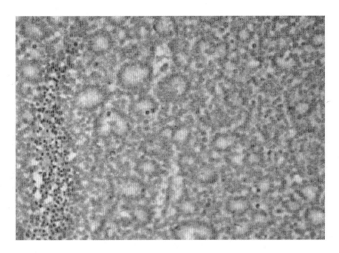

COLOR FIGURE 48–4. Flexner-Wintersteiner rosettes, which are characteristic of retinoblastoma. (Courtesy of Thadeus P. Dryja, MD)

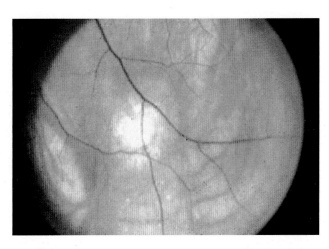

COLOR FIGURE 48–5. Metastases to the choroid. Note the multiple lesions and irregular outline. Choroidal metastases are typically multiple, have an irregular outline, are yellow-gray to pink-white in color with edematous and detached overlying retina, are generally several disc diameters in size, and may have overlying clumps of pigment.

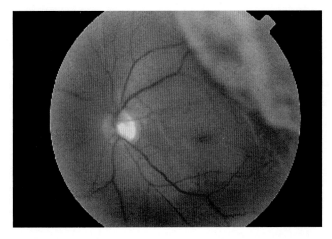

COLOR FIGURE 50–1. Peripheral retinal detachment. The detachment has progressed to the point at which it is now quite obvious. However, it has existed for approximately 6 weeks and has slowly progressed to this point. Once the detachment was repaired and the peripheral retinal break was successfully closed, the "chronic uveitis" vanished without further (medical) treatment.

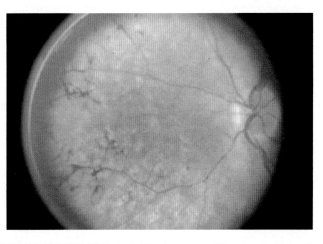

COLOR FIGURE 50–2. Retinitis pigmentosa. Note in particular the bone-spicule mid and far peripheral retinal pigmentary changes, and retinal arteriolar narrowing. This patient had had chronic vitritis for 2 years before the appearance of the characteristic, diagnostic retinal pigmentary changes.

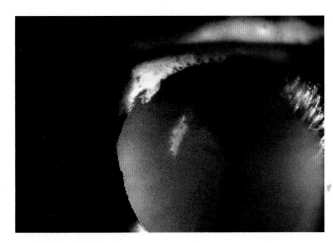

COLOR FIGURE 50–3. Foreign body imbedded in the crystalline lens. Note also the small tear of the iris sphincter. This intraocular foreign body had caused chronic intraocular inflammation.

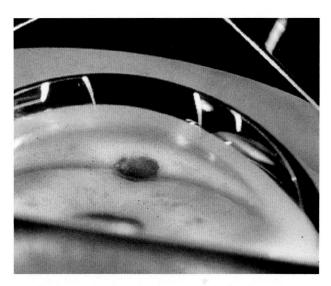

COLOR FIGURE 50–4. A tiny pebble of sand resting in the inferior angle. Its presence was not inert but rather created continuing iris trauma with stimulation of chronic anterior chamber cells.

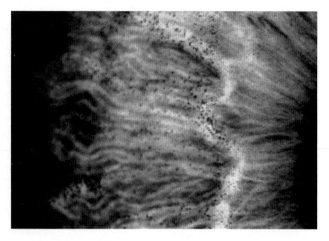

COLOR FIGURE 50–6. A patient with pigmentary dispersion syndrome. Note the pigmentary granules deposited on the iris surface. This patient had been treated for multiple episodes of recurrent uveitis. In fact, the cells in the anterior chamber were pigment granules.

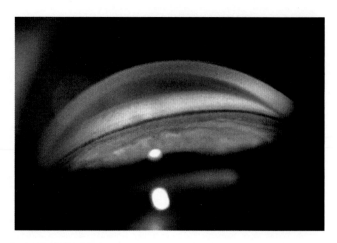

COLOR FIGURE 50–7. Another patient with pigmentary dispersion syndrome. Note the diagnostic presence of extreme amounts of pigment deposited in the angle.

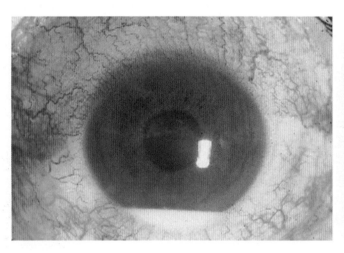

COLOR FIGURE 52–2. Hypopyon, in a patient with HLA-B27–associated uveitis in the context of ankylosing spondylitis.

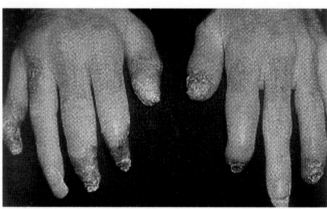

COLOR FIGURE 52–3. Dactylitis, with so-called sausage digit formation in a patients with Reiter's syndrome.

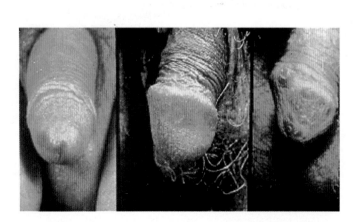

COLOR FIGURE 52–5. Circinate balanitis in three patients with Reiter's syndrome.

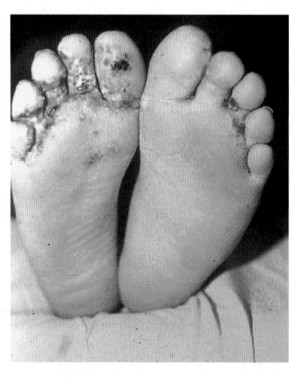

COLOR FIGURE 52–6. Keratosis blennorrhagica in a patient with Reiter's syndrome.

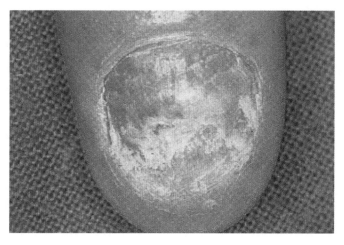

COLOR FIGURE 52–7. Onycholysis in a patient with Reiter's syndrome.

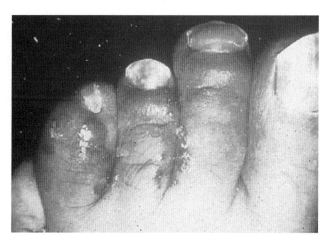

COLOR FIGURE 52–8. Psoriatic arthritic nail changes with so-called sausage digits and onycholysis.

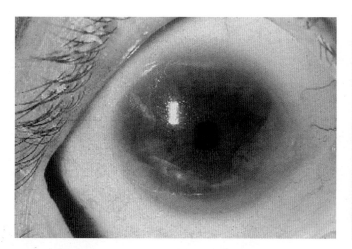

COLOR FIGURE 52–9. The typical quiet eye of a patient with active juvenile rheumatoid arthritis–associated iridocyclitis with an undilatable pupil secondary to dense posterior synechial formation.

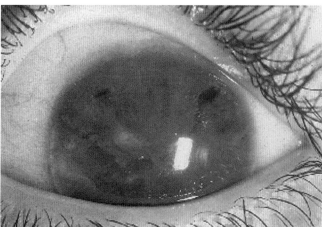

COLOR FIGURE 52–12. Left eye of a young woman with juvenile rheumatoid arthritis–associated iridocyclitis, status post cataract extraction with implantation of a posterior chamber lens implant. Note not only the pupillary seclusion but also the obvious inflammatory membrane cocoon around the lens implant. Contraction of this membrane is displacing the lens implant anteriorly and is detaching the ciliary body, producing progressive hypotony.

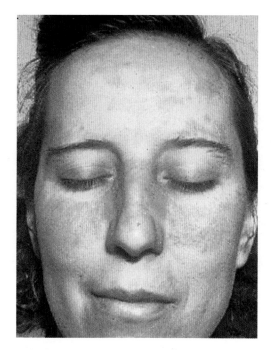

COLOR FIGURE 53–1. Lupus mask or butterfly rash. Note the erythematous dermatitis over the malar eminences of the cheeks and the bridge of the nose.

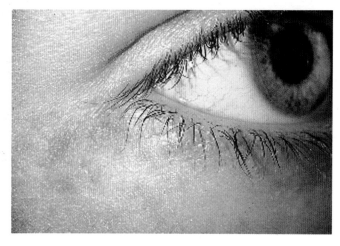

COLOR FIGURE 53–2. Discoid lupus in a patient with chronic blepharitis. Note the subtle erythematous lesions of the skin of the lower eyelid.

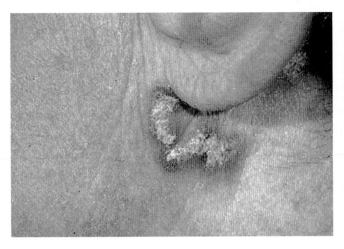

COLOR FIGURE 53–3. Hypertrophic discoid lupus. Note the hypertrophic lesion under the patient's left ear, with silvery keratinization on the surface.

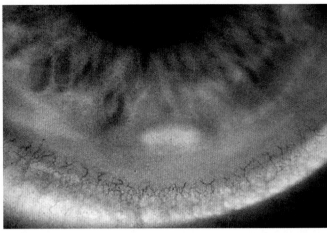

COLOR FIGURE 53–4. Peripheral keratitis in a patient with systemic lupus erythematosus. Note the perilimbal, circumferential mid to deep stromal infiltrate in the corneal stroma.

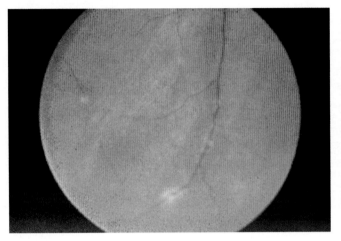

COLOR FIGURE 53–5. Retinal arteritis in a patient with systemic lupus erythematosus. Note the periarteriolar inflammatory cell infiltrate.

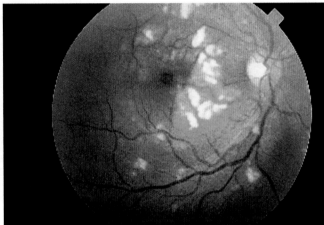

COLOR FIGURE 53–7. Extensive lupus retinopathy, with arteriolitis, arteriolar occlusion, and retinal infarcts, with extensive cotton-wool lesions in the nerve fiber layer of the retina.

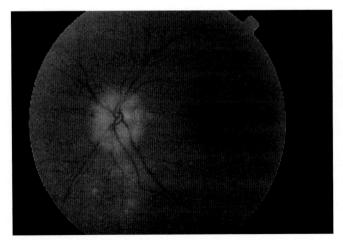

COLOR FIGURE 55–2. Giant cell arteritis, in a patient who demonstrates the chalky white form of disc edema. (Courtesy of Joseph F. Rizzo III, MD.)

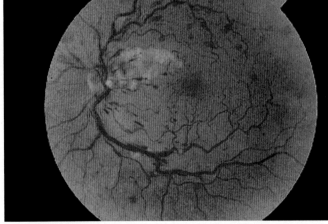

COLOR FIGURE 55–3. Giant cell arteritis with occlusion of a cilioretinal artery, and associated intraretinal hemorrhages. (Courtesy of John I. Loewenstein, MD.)

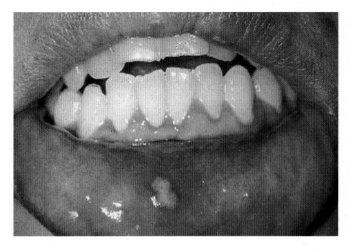

COLOR FIGURE 56–1. Aphthous oral ulcer on the inner surface of the inferior lip.

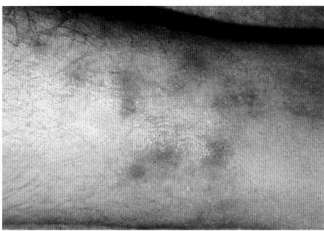

COLOR FIGURE 56–2. Erythema nodosum–like lesions on anterior tibial surface.

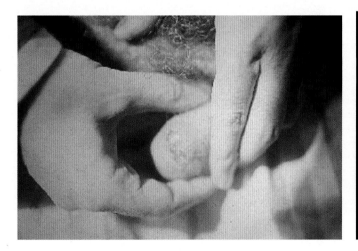

COLOR FIGURE 56–4. ABD lesion on the penis.

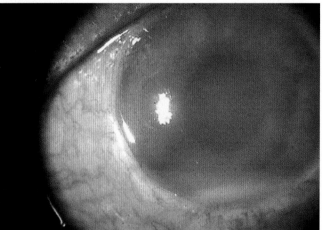

COLOR FIGURE 56–5. Hypopyon in a patient with ABD.

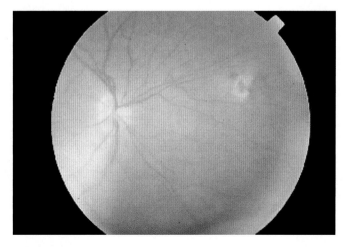

COLOR FIGURE 56–6. Fundus photograph of a retinal lesion with accompanying intraretinal hemorrhages and vasculitis.

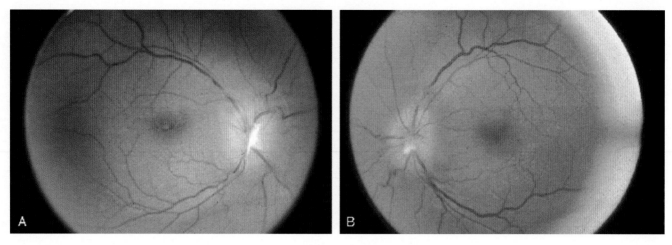

COLOR FIGURE 56–8. *A* and *B*, Bilateral optic disc edema in a patient with ABD.

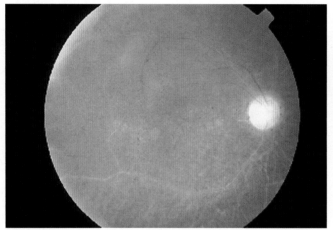

COLOR FIGURE 56–9. End stage of repeated ABD attacks of posterior pole. Note the retinal atrophy associated with vessel attenuation and an optic disc atrophy.

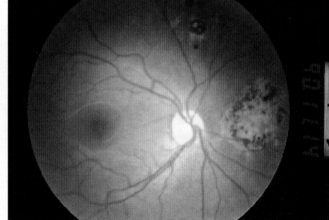

COLOR FIGURE 56–10. Fundus photograph from a patient with repeated attacks of ABD showing a scar in the nasal area of the posterior pole.

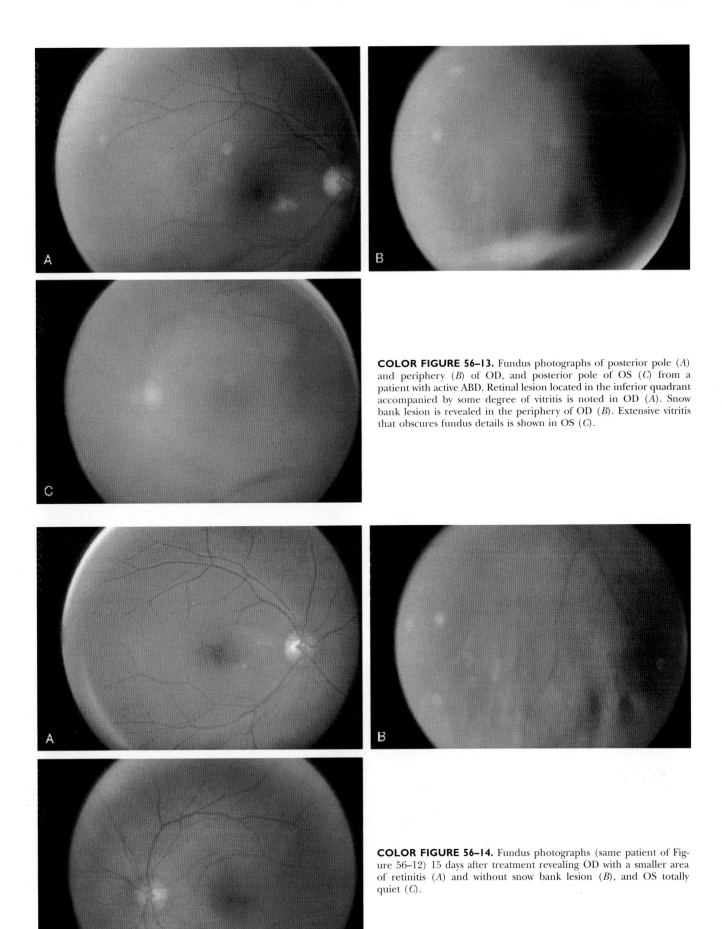

COLOR FIGURE 56–13. Fundus photographs of posterior pole (*A*) and periphery (*B*) of OD, and posterior pole of OS (*C*) from a patient with active ABD. Retinal lesion located in the inferior quadrant accompanied by some degree of vitritis is noted in OD (*A*). Snow bank lesion is revealed in the periphery of OD (*B*). Extensive vitritis that obscures fundus details is shown in OS (*C*).

COLOR FIGURE 56–14. Fundus photographs (same patient of Figure 56–12) 15 days after treatment revealing OD with a smaller area of retinitis (*A*) and without snow bank lesion (*B*), and OS totally quiet (*C*).

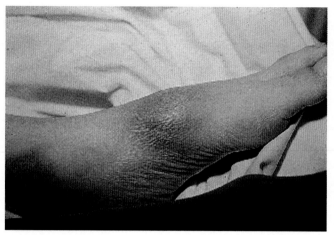

COLOR FIGURE 57–1. Subcutaneous nodule, dorsal aspect of the foot of a patient who subsequently was biopsied (see Figure 57–7), with histopathologically proven polyarteritis nodosa. (Courtesy of C. Stephen Foster, M.D.)

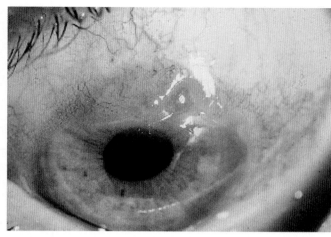

COLOR FIGURE 57–3. Left eye of patient described in Figure 57–2, with resolving scleritis but now with the onset of peripheral ulcerative keratitis prior to the institution of adequate doses of cyclophosphamide therapy. (Courtesy of C. Stephen Foster, M.D.)

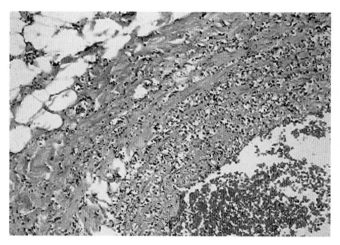

COLOR FIGURE 57–7. Histopathology, H&E section, 800 ×, from the biopsy of the subcutaneous nodule of the patient shown in Figure 57–1. Note the neutrophil invasion of the media of this artery, with fibrinoid necrosis of the vessel wall. (Courtesy of C. Stephen Foster, M.D.)

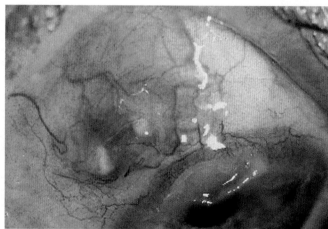

COLOR FIGURE 58–4. Necrotizing scleritis with associated peripheral keratitis in a patient with Wegener's granulomatosis.

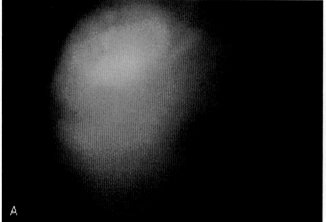

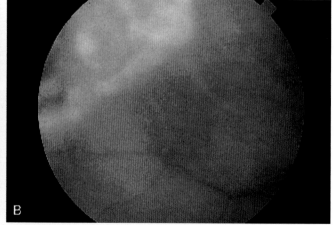

COLOR FIGURE 58–5. *A,* Posterior uveitis, with retinal vasculitis and frank retinal infarct in a patient with Wegener's granulomatosis. Note in particular the hazy view as a consequence of cells in the vitreous. *B,* Same patient as in Figure 58–5*A,* with partial resolution after institution of cyclophosphamide therapy. Note the clearing of the vitreous and a clearer view of the area of retina, which has now been destroyed through infarction.

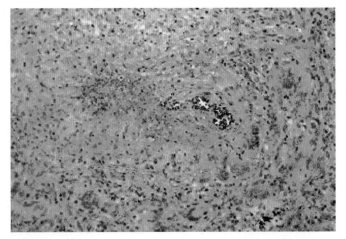

COLOR FIGURE 58–6. Lung biopsy demonstrating granulomatous inflammation in a patient with Wegener's granulomatosis.

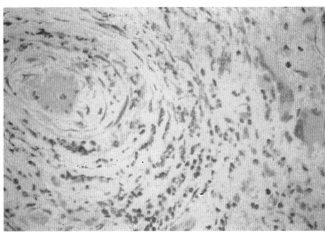

COLOR FIGURE 58–7. Photomicrograph of scleral tissue from a patient with limited Wegener's granulomatosis demonstrating granulomatous foci with collagen necrosis.

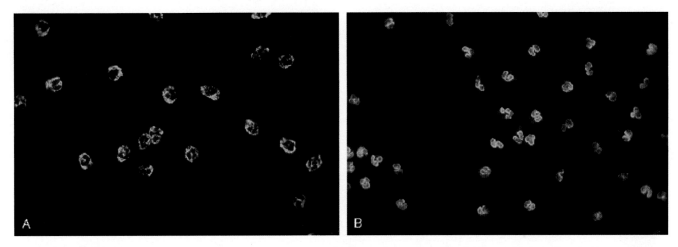

COLOR FIGURE 58–8. *A,* Photomicrograph showing a positive cANCA pattern of staining on ethanol-fixed neutrophils by indirect immunofluorescence. This centrally accentuated cytoplasmic pattern of staining is characteristic for patients with Wegener's granulomatosis and is almost always due to antibodies directed against proteinase 3 (PR3). *B,* This photomicrograph demonstrates a pANCA (paranuclear) pattern of staining by indirect immunofluorescence. A variety of target antigens can produce this pattern of staining including those that are nonspecific. Myeloperoxidase (MPO) is the target antigen (as demonstrated by ELISA) with the most utility, because it is frequently associated with Wegener's granulomatosis, microscopic polyangiitis, and pauci-immune glomerulonephritis.

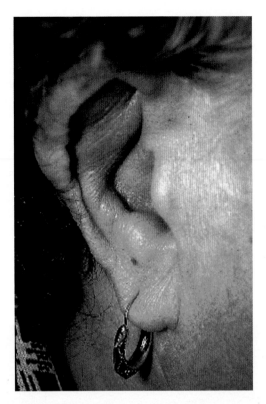

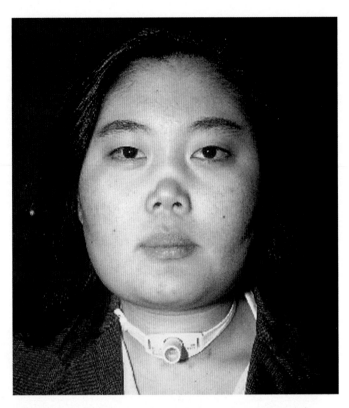

COLOR FIGURE 59–1. Active chondritis of the external ear, with "floppiness" of that same ear as a consequence of prior episodes of chondritis with loss of cartilage. (Courtesy of C. Stephen Foster, MD.)

COLOR FIGURE 59–2. Relapsing polychondritis with obvious destruction of nasal cartilage, with collapse and saddle nose deformity. Note also that the patient has developed tracheal involvement as a consequence of undertreatment, with resultant need for permanent tracheostomy. (Courtesy of C. Stephen Foster, MD.)

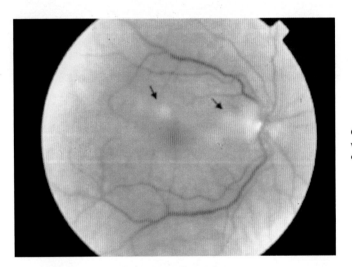

COLOR FIGURE 60–2. Posterior segment involvement in a patient with antiphospholipid syndrome. The arrows show presence of retinal cotton-wool spots.

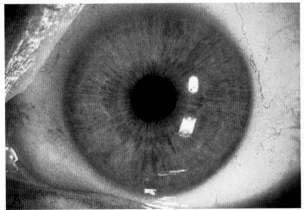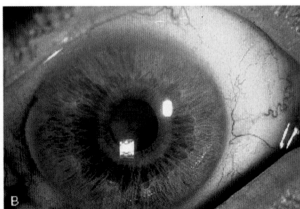

COLOR FIGURE 61–1. Right and left eye of a patient with Fuchs' heterochromic iridocyclitis (right eye, *A*; left eye, *B*). Note the difference in apparent color of the irides. The left eye is the eye with the iridocyclitis. (Courtesy of C. Stephen Foster, MD.)

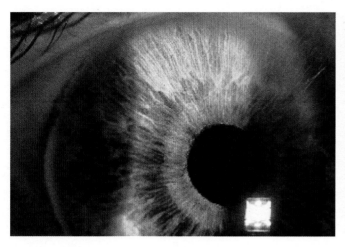

COLOR FIGURE 61–2. Higher magnification of the left eye shown in Figure 61–1*B.* Note the loss of iris substance in the anterior layers of the iris, allowing the pigment epithelium to be more apparent. (Courtesy of C. Stephen Foster, MD.)

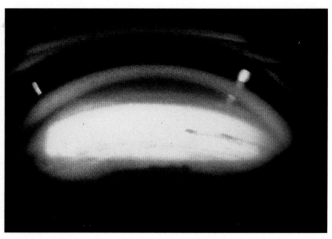

COLOR FIGURE 61–3. Gonioscopic photograph of a patient with Fuchs' heterochromic iridocyclitis. Note the very subtle vascular anomalies in the angle. (Courtesy of C. Stephen Foster, MD.)

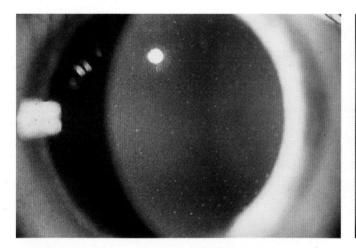

COLOR FIGURE 61–4. Typical keratic precipitate (KP) distribution and configuration in a patient with Fuchs' heterochromic iridocyclitis. Note that the KPs are distributed throughout the entire extent of the corneal endothelium and that many have a fibrillar or stellate character to them. (Courtesy of C. Stephen Foster, MD.)

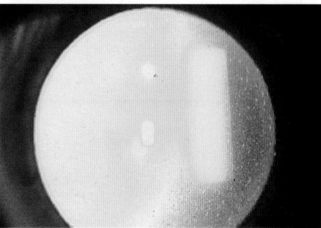

COLOR FIGURE 61–5. Same eye as shown in Figure 61–4; retroillumination photo, which allows one to see slightly more clearly the small fibrils that connect adjacent KPs. (Courtesy of C. Stephen Foster, MD.)

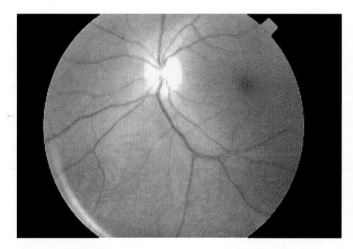

COLOR FIGURE 62–1. Optic nerve pallor following optic neuritis.

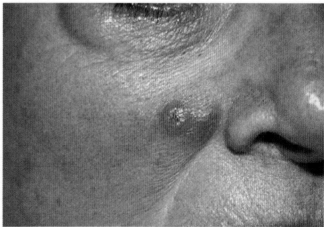

COLOR FIGURE 63–2. Umbilicated sarcoid skin lesion in a patient who presented with uveitis.

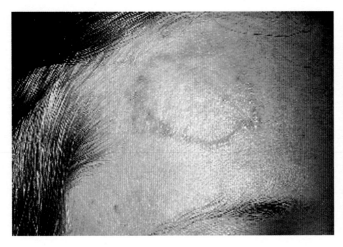

COLOR FIGURE 63–3. Sarcoid plaque-like skin lesion in a patient with sarcoidosis.

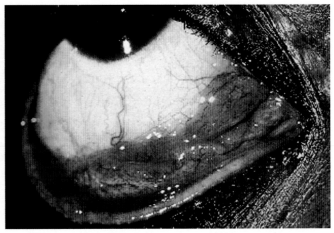

COLOR FIGURE 63–4. Conjunctival nodules in sarcoidosis.

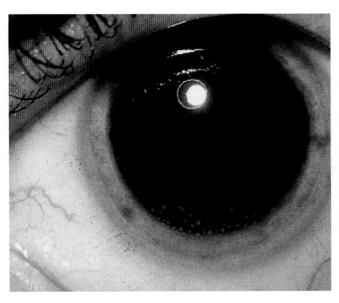

COLOR FIGURE 63–5. Mutton fat keratic precipitates.

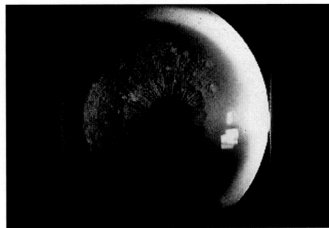

COLOR FIGURE 63–6. Busacca iris nodules.

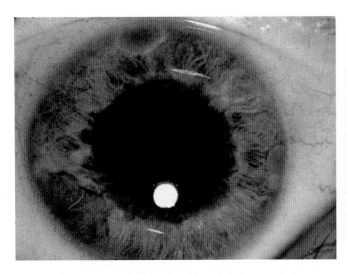

COLOR FIGURE 63–7. True iris nodule in sarcoidosis.

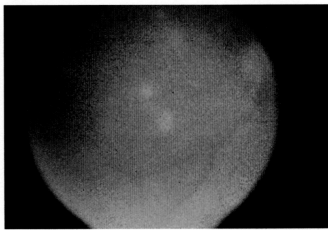

COLOR FIGURE 63–8. Vitritis, snow balls, and perivenular exudates in a patient with sarcoidosis.

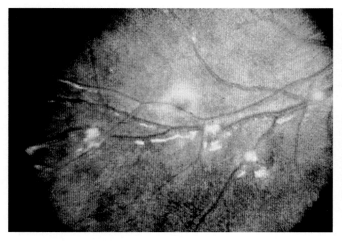

COLOR FIGURE 63–9. Perivenular exudates in sarcoidosis.

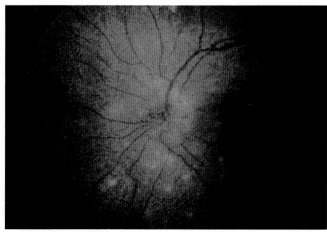

COLOR FIGURE 63–10. Vitritis, disc edema, disc neovascularization, nerve fiber layer hemorrhages, and multiple atrophic chorioretinal lesions in sarcoidosis.

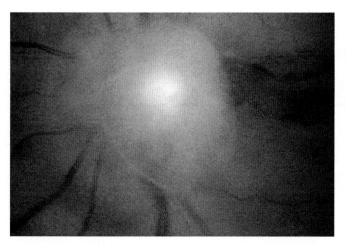

COLOR FIGURE 63–11. Optic nerve granuloma in a patient with sarcoidosis.

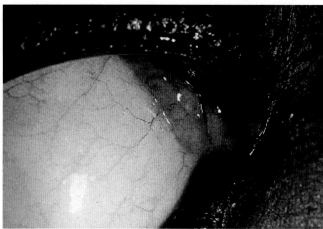

COLOR FIGURE 63–12. Lacrimal gland enlargement in a patient with sarcoidosis.

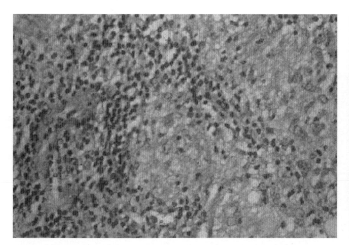

COLOR FIGURE 63–13. Non-necrotizing granuloma in sarcoidosis. Histiocytes, epithelioid cells, and multinucleated giant cells are surrounded by lymphocytes, plasma cells, and fibroblasts.

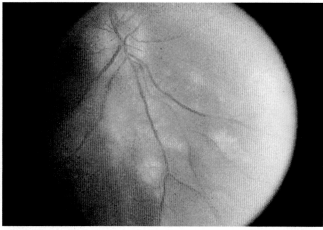

COLOR FIGURE 65–1. Typical appearance of birdshot lesions in the posterior pole consisting of scattered cream-colored spots varying in size from 50 to 1500 μm.

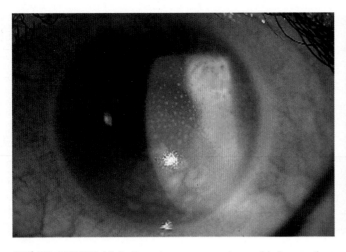

COLOR FIGURE 66–1. Granulomatous anterior uveitis in a patient with acute sympathetic ophthalmia.

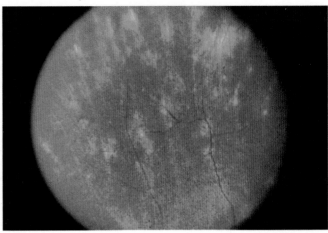

COLOR FIGURE 66–2. Multiple cream-colored lesions scattered throughout the midequatorial region of the fundus in a patient with sympathetic ophthalmia.

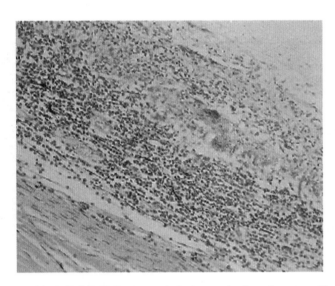

COLOR FIGURE 66–5. Histopathologic examination of an eye with sympathetic ophthalmia shows an intense mononuclear cell infiltrate in the choroid with relative sparing of the choriocapillaris. (H&E original magnification × 80.)

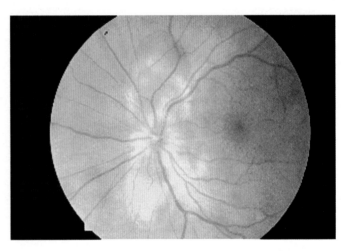

COLOR FIGURE 67–1. Optic disc edema and exudative retinal detachment in early VKH syndrome.

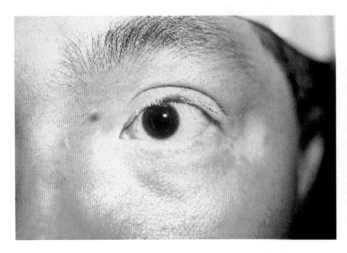

COLOR FIGURE 67–3. Periocular vitiligo in an Asian patient with VKH syndrome. Note also the poliosis of cilia nasally, upper lid.

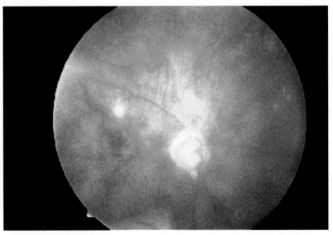

COLOR FIGURE 67–4. "Blond" appearance of fundus in Asian patient after the active inflammatory stage of VKH syndrome.

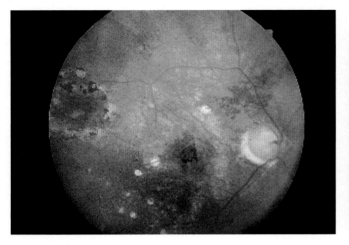

COLOR FIGURE 67–5. Fundus photo from the same patient demonstrating advanced glaucomatous optic disc cupping, severe chorioretinal scar with severe RPE alteration, and old Dalen-Fuchs nodules.

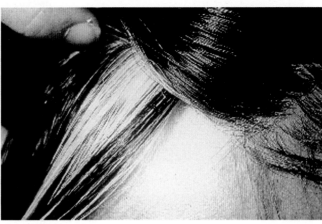

COLOR FIGURE 67–6. Vitiligo of hair (white forelock) in a patient with VKH. (Courtesy of C. Stephen Foster, M.D.)

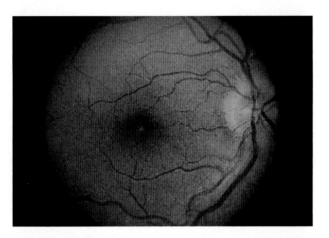

COLOR FIGURE 69–1. Fundus photograph of a patient with MEWDS. Note the deep, slightly indistinct, yellow-white lesions in the posterior pole.

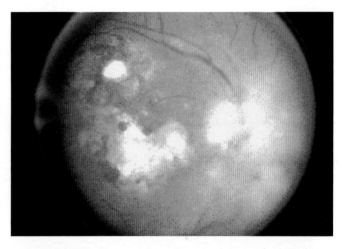

COLOR FIGURE 72–1. Serpiginous choroiditis, with both active and inactive lesions. Note the peripapillary involvement, with active foci nasal to the disc and the inactive areas of chorioretinal scarring in the macula. (Courtesy of C. Stephen Foster, MD.)

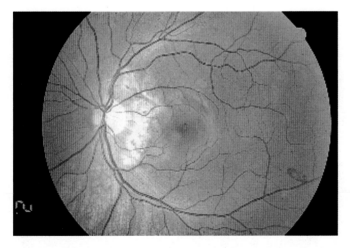

COLOR FIGURE 72–2. Residuum of the earliest lesions of serpiginous choroiditis around the disc. Note, however, that the disease is now inactive and that the vitreous is crystal clear. (Courtesy of C. Stephen Foster, MD.)

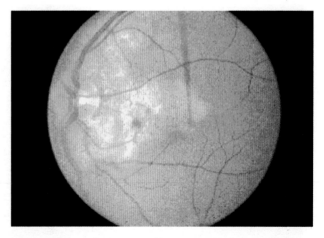

COLOR FIGURE 72–3. Progressive, active serpiginous choroiditis, which first began in the peripapillary region but now has spread in a serpiginous way superiorly and temporally in this left eye, now involving the macula. (Courtesy of C. Stephen Foster, MD.)

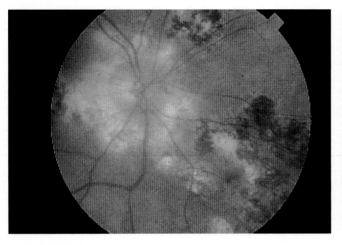

COLOR FIGURE 73–1. Soft yellow-white subretinal lesions, at the level of the choroid, of various ages and stages. (Courtesy of C. Stephen Foster, MD.)

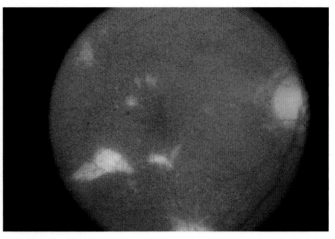

COLOR FIGURE 73–2. Fibrotic scar formation in the area of former soft choroidal lesions. (Courtesy of C. Stephen Foster, MD.)

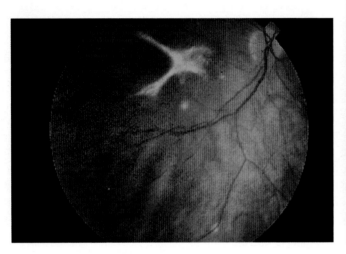

COLOR FIGURE 73–3. Expanding fibrotic bands, now beginning to contract in a patient with SFU. (Courtesy of C. Stephen Foster, MD.)

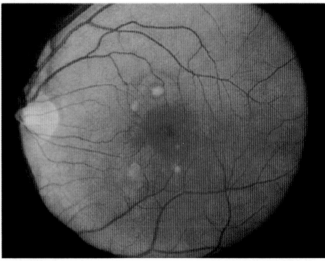

COLOR FIGURE 74–1. Case 1. Thirty-two-year-old white, myopic woman presented with a 2-week history of metamorphopsia OS. Fundus examination revealed several punctate chorioretinal lesions with overlying neurosensory retinal detachments.

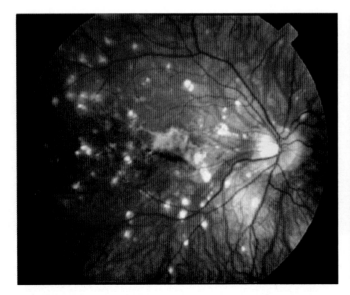

COLOR FIGURE 74–2. Case 2. Twenty-three-year-old white, myopic woman was referred with a 3-month history of central vision loss OD. Fundus examination showed numerous punctate, white chorioretinal atrophic lesions in the posterior pole. A fibrovascular CNVM was evident in the macular. (Courtesy of Jay S. Duker, M.D.)

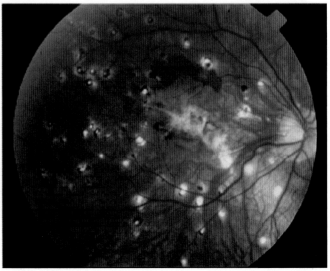

COLOR FIGURE 74–3. Case 2. One year later, the patient returned for a follow-up examination. Note that many of the chorioretinal lesions have become pigmented. A new CNVM with an associated subretinal hemorrhage is evident superior to the old macular scar.

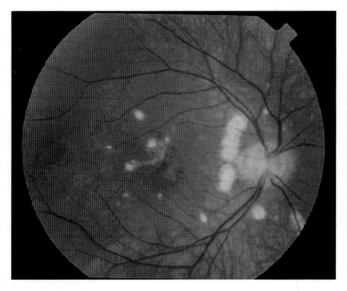

COLOR FIGURE 74–4. Case 3. Twenty-four-year-old white, myopic woman was referred with an 8-month history of a central scotoma. Fundus examination revealed multiple, punctate perifoveal lesions with a fibrovascular CNVM in the fovea. (Courtesy of Jay S. Duker, M.D.)

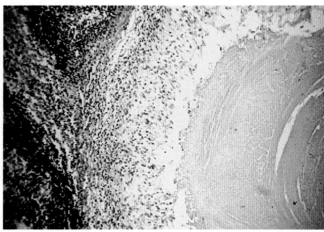

COLOR FIGURE 76–1. Pathology of phacogenic uveitis: epithelioid and multinucleated giant cells engulfing lens material.

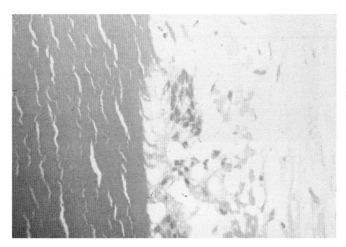

COLOR FIGURE 76–2. Pathology of phacogenic uveitis: zonal inflammation around the lens, especially at the site of capsular rupture. Mononuclear cells are seen together with epithelioid cells and giant cells.

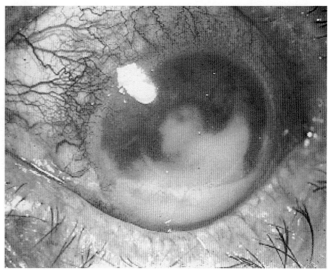

COLOR FIGURE 76–3. A case of phacogenic uveitis showing lens material in the anterior chamber. The uveitis in this patient did not respond to topical steroids but dramatically improved after complete surgical removal of lens material.

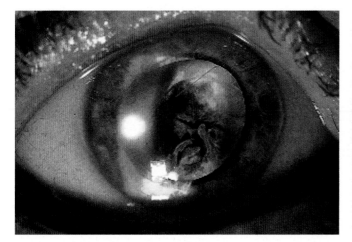

COLOR FIGURE 76–4. Significant amount of residual lens matter following extracapsular cataract extraction with lens implantation. This patient is at higher risk of developing phacogenic uveitis.

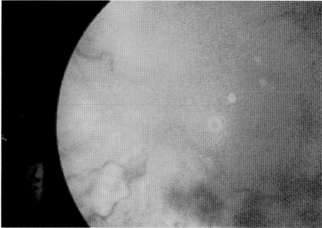

COLOR FIGURE 77–5. Recurrent vitreous hemorrhage in a patient with periphlebitis of Eales' disease.

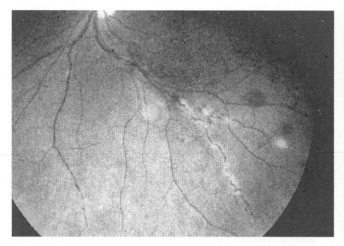

COLOR FIGURE 77–6. The fundus of a patient with sarcoidosis and retinal vasculitis showing creamy white sheathing of the retinal veins.

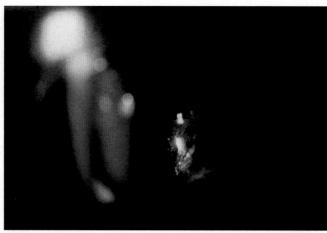

COLOR FIGURE 78–1. Vitreous inflammation, with dense vitreal cellular infiltrate seen on slit-lamp biomicroscopy.

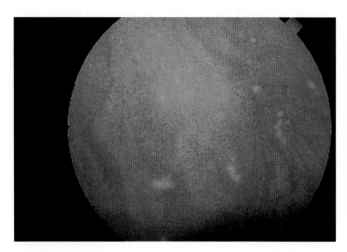

COLOR FIGURE 78–2. Vitreal cellular aggregates anterior to the retina ("snowballs").

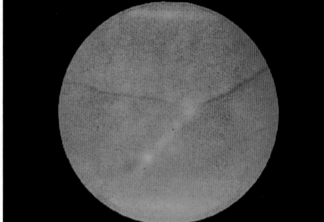

COLOR FIGURE 78–3. Vasculitis of peripheral retinal vein in a patient with intermediate uveitis.

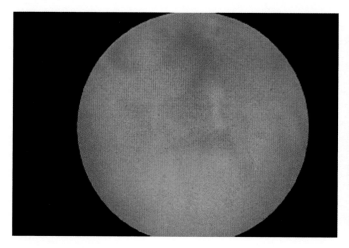

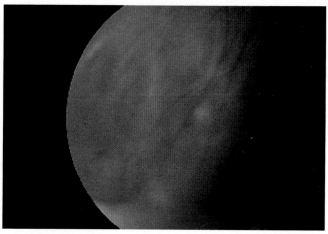

COLOR FIGURE 78–4. Neovascularization after occlusive vasculitis in intermediate uveitis.

COLOR FIGURE 78–5. White collagen band at pars plana.

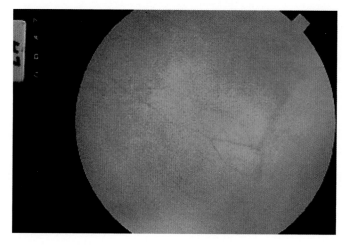

COLOR FIGURE 78–7. Exudative retinal detachment in intermediate uveitis, demonstrated by fluorescein angiography.

Part I

BASIC PRINCIPLES

1 INTRODUCTION

C. Stephen Foster

The problem of inflammation of the eye, including uveitis, was known to the ancient Egyptians. The Edwin Smith surgical papyrus, now in the library of the New York Academy of Medicine, is the oldest known existing ophthalmic document.[1] It dates from 1700 BC, but it makes clear that it is based on, among other things, writings from the time of Imhotep, the physician and architect of the first step pyramid at Saqqara (2640 BC). And while it appears to be primarily a manual on wound treatment (perhaps for an army doctor), it also contains references to inflammatory conditions of the eye. It is known that physicians with special interest in the eye were identifiable as early as the 6th Egyptian Dynasty (2400 BC), and indeed the most ancient identifiable ophthalmologist was the Royal Oculist, Pepi-Ankh-Or-Iri, whose stele (an upright stone slab bearing identifying markings) has been discovered in a tomb near the Great Pyramid of Cheops. He was physician to the Pharaoh and chief of the court medical corps, bearing the titles "palace eye physician" and "guardian of the anus." And while we in modern ophthalmology have by-and-large given up the role of "guardian of the anus," we must remember that physician preoccupation with purgative therapy, the concept of whdw (ukedhu)—"the rotten stuff par excellence," and cleansing the body of noxious elements did not leave ophthalmic practice in general and treatment of uveitis in particular until the first half of the 20th century.

But Egyptian ophthalmology contributed considerably more than expurgation to therapy of uveitis. Indeed, Egyptian medicine in general was recognized throughout the ancient world as the most advanced healing art; Cambyses the Elder (Great), King of another very advanced ancient civilization (Persia), wrote to Amasis in 560 BC requesting an ophthalmologist who "should be the best in all of Egypt."

The Ebers papyrus (1500 BC) is essentially a pharmacopia and treatment manual for a variety of ocular problems including uveitis.[2, 3] It was translated by Georg Moritz Ebers (1837–1898), a German Egyptologist and novelist, in 1874. It is now in the University of Leipzig (Germany) library. And although many of the remedies of the time detailed in this papyrus clearly, in light of current knowledge, are ineffective, some are now known to have a solid basis for efficacy. For example, dried leaves of myrtle (which we now know are rich in salicylates) were applied to the back and abdomen of women "to extract pain from the womb." One hundred of the 237 medication recipes in the Ebers papyrus are for eye disease, with zinc, antimony, and copper predominant but with aloe, yellow ochre, red ochre, myrrh, malachite, ink powder, galena, and djaret especially represented in recipes employed for treating eye inflammation. For constriction of the pupil or occlusion of the pupil (possibly, uveitis synechiae) the recommended treatment was compresses with a lotion made of saltpeter and ebony wood shavings.

Hippocrates, Galen, and Aëtius were also faced with the need to care for patients with uveitis, but despite their building upon their knowledge of the Egyptian approaches, it was not until the 18th century that more "modern" therapy for intraocular inflammation become well entrenched in the medical community. Scarpa, in his 1806 text,[1] describes "a strong country-woman, 35 years old" who "was brought into this hospital towards the end of April 1796, on account of a violent, acute ophthalmia in both her eyes, with which she had been afflicted three days, with great tumefaction of the eyelids, redness of the conjunctiva, acute pain, fever, and watchfulness." Scarpa then described the presence of hypopyon and his treatment of same:

I took away blood abundantly from the arm and foot, and also locally by means of leeches applied near both the angles of the eyes, and I also purged her. These remedies were attended with some advantage, inasmuch as they contributed to abate the inflammatory stage of the violent ophthalmia. Nevertheless an extravacation of yellowish glutinous lymph appeared in the anterior chamber of the aqueous humor, which filled out one-third of that cavity.[1]

Adjunctive therapy, common to the times, was then used: "The uninterrupted application of small bags of gauze filled with emollient herbs boiled in milk . . . and repeated mild purges with a grain of the antimonium tartarizatum dissolved in a pint of the decoction of the root of the triticum repens." The symptoms of the inflammation were entirely relieved, and "on the eleventh day the patient was able to bear a moderate degree of light." Additional therapies mentioned in Scarpa's text[1] include drops of vitriolic collyrium, with mucilage of quince-seed, bags of tepid mallows, a few grains of camphire, and blister production of the neck. Scarpa's text makes clear that these therapies were accepted as best medical practice for the time.

By 1830, as outlined in MacKenzie's text on diseases of the eye,[5] dilation of the pupil with tincture of belladonna had been added to bloodletting, purging, and blistering therapy. Also added was the use of antimony and other nauseants, opiates for relief of pain, and mercury as an adjunctive antiphlogistic agent. Fever therapy, induced by intramuscular injection of milk or intravenous injection of triple typhoid H antigen, became fashionable in the first half of the 20th century. This "stimulatory" treatment, effective only if the patient's temperature was raised to about 40°C three or four times in succession, persisted into the early 1950s. Its effectiveness was undisputed, although its mechanism is unknown. Possible mechanisms include stimulation of endogenous cortisol production and effects on regulatory cytokines. The treatment, however, was sometimes fatal.

The next major advance in the care of patients with inflammatory disease was not made until 1950 with the discovery of the effectiveness of corticosteroid therapy for uveitis.[6]

Despite the advances made in the past 50 years with the discovery and development of nonsteroidal anti-inflammatory agents, and both cytotoxic and noncytotoxic immunomodulatory agents, a significant proportion of patients with uveitis are still treated suboptimally by ophthalmologists unfamiliar with the effective and safe use of such drugs. It is regrettable that, still today, fully 10% of all blindness occurring in the United States alone results from inadequately treated uveitis.

It is our fervent hope that the following chapters will contribute to a "sea change" in the attitudes of ophthalmologists regarding tolerance or not of low-grade chronic inflammation that continues, eventually, to rob children and adults of precious vision. We believe strongly in a paradigm of zero tolerance for chronic intraocular inflammation and further believe that a stepwise algorithm to achieve that goal is highly effective in reducing ocular morbidity secondary to uveitis.

References

1. Breasted J: The Edwin Smith Surgical Papyrus. Chicago, University of Chicago Press, 1930.
2. Ebbell B: Die altägyptische Chirurgie. Die chirurgischen Abschnitte des Papyrus E. Smith und Papyrus Ebers. Oslo, Dybwad, 1939.
3. Hirschberg J: The History of Ophthalmology, Vol. 1. Antiquity. Bonn, Wayenborgh Verlag, 1982.
4. Scarpa A: Practical Observations on the Principal Diseases of the Eyes. London: Strand, 1806, pp 292–321.
5. MacKenzie W: A Practical Treatise on the Diseases of the Eye. London, Longman, Rees, Orme, Brown & Green, 1830, pp 422–457.

2 | THE UVEA: ANATOMY, HISTOLOGY, AND EMBRYOLOGY

C. Stephen Foster and Nicolette Gion

UVEAL TRACT

Uvea is the Latin word for grape. The term *uveal tract* has been given to the vascular middle layer of the eye because its structure is brown and spherical, and it resembles a grape, with the optic nerve forming the stalk.[1]

The uveal tract is located between the corneosclera and the neuroepithelium; it consists of the iris anteriorly, the ciliary body in the middle, and the choroid posteriorly (Fig. 2–1). Embryologically, it is derived from the neuroectoderm, neural crest cells, and vascular channels.[1, 2]

Ciliary arteries, which originate from the ophthalmic artery, supply blood to the whole vascular tunic; the iris and ciliary body are supplied by the anterior and long posterior ciliary arteries via the major arterial circle of the iris, located posterior to the anterior chamber angle recess, within the ciliary body. The circulation of the anterior choroid arises from recurrent and perforating branches of these arteries and from branches of the ciliary intramuscular artery.[2, 3] Most blood to the choroid is supplied by the short posterior ciliary arteries.

Venous drainage of the uvea is provided by the vortex veins (venae vorticosae) primarily, and by the scleral and episcleral venous system.

The long and short ciliary nerves innervate the iris and choroid.[1] The long ciliary nerves originate from the nasociliary nerve, a branch of the ophthalmic division of the trigeminal nerve. They contain sensory fibers that ascend to the trigeminal nerve and postganglionic sympathetic fibers from the superior cervical sympathetic ganglion. The short ciliary nerves arise from the ciliary ganglion and carry postganglionic parasympathetic and some sympathetic nerve fibers. The ciliary muscle is innervated by the postganglionic parasympathetic fibers derived from the oculomotor nerve, which reach the muscle via the short ciliary nerves.

Because of its extreme vascularity, the uveal tract is often involved in general systemic diseases and may be a site for circulatory metastases. Furthermore, the structures of the uveal tract share a common blood supply and together are often involved in inflammatory processes. Inflammation of the ciliary body and iris is associated with boring eye pain and with ciliary injection (dilation of the anterior ciliary arteries).

Iris

Development

The development of the iris in about the sixth week of gestation is associated with the formation of the anterior part of the tunica vasculosa lentis.[4] The vascular channels of this structure grow from the annular vessels that encircle the rim of the optic cup and extend to the mesenchymal anterior surface of the lens, which is incorporated into the iris stroma.[5]

The vessels at the periphery of the tunica vasculosa lentis are joined by branches coming from the long posterior ciliary arteries in the nasal and temporal regions of the ciliary body. These vessels, later accompanied by branches from the plexus of the anterior ciliary arteries, form the major arterial circle. The anterior region of the tunica vasculosa lentis is replaced by the pupillary membrane, which obtains its blood supply from the major arterial circle and the long posterior ciliary arteries. At the end of the third month, after the ciliary folds have formed, both walls of the neuroectodermal optic cup grow forward and separate the peripheral part of the tunica vasculosa lentis from the vessels of the pupillary membrane.[5, 6] By the end of the fourth month, two vascular iris layers are formed: the vessel layer of the tunica vasculosa lentis posteriorly, and the vessel layer of the iridopupillary membrane anteriorly.[3] During the fifth month, branches of the long ciliary arteries reach the mesenchyme in the mid-region of the iris, which includes the superficial pupillary membrane, the iris stroma, and the sphincter muscle. Development of the collarette in the iris stroma is secondary to the arteriovenous loops of the pupillary membrane, which are arranged over the sphincter muscle.

Mesenchymal cells at the anterior iris surface form the anterior border layer. Later in gestation, pigmented cells accumulate beneath the anterior border layer. Some mesenchymal cells in the developing stroma differentiate into

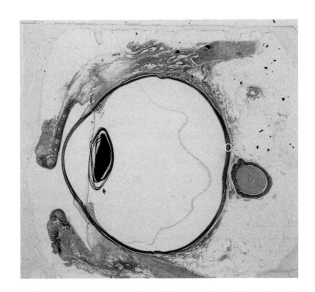

FIGURE 2–1. Photomicrograph of horizontal meridional section of entire human globe. The uveal tract consists of the iris (i), the ciliary body (cb), and the choroid (c). (Nuclei, red blood cells, collagenous tissue, muscle, and epithelium and nerve tissue, are shown.) (Stain: Masson's trichrome, magnification: 2×.) (From The Russell L. Carpenter Collection for the Study of Ophthalmic Histology, Department of Pathology, Massachusetts Eye and Ear Infirmary, Boston.)

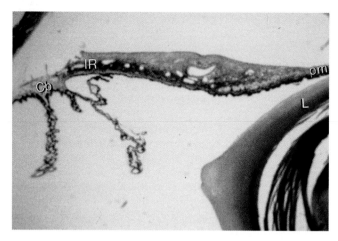

FIGURE 2–2. Photomicrograph of horizontal meridional section of human iris. The iris root (IR) is attached to the ciliary body (Cb), and the pupillary margin (pm) rests on the anterior surface of the lens (L). See also Figure 2–3. sm: sphincter muscle. (Stain: Masson's trichrome, magnification: 20×.) (From The Russell L. Carpenter Collection for the Study of Ophthalmic Histology, Department of Pathology, Massachusetts Eye and Ear Infirmary, Boston.)

fibroblast-like cells that secrete collagen fibrils and other components of the extracellular matrix.[6]

Sphincter and dilator muscles are formed by further growth and differentiation of the two neuroectodermal layers of the optic cup. In contrast to the dilator muscle, the sphincter pupilla is invaded by connective tissue and blood vessels during the sixth month of gestation and comes to lie free in the posterior iris stroma during the eighth month.[5, 6]

The posterior pigmented iris epithelium develops as a continuation of both the nonpigmented ciliary body layer and the neuroectoderm that forms the neural retina. The epithelial cells gradually become pigmented (seventh month).

At birth, the iris is not yet fully developed; the stroma is very thin, the extracellular framework is not completed, and the collarette is very close to the pupil.

Gross Appearance

The iris, the most anterior part of the uvea, lies between anterior and posterior chamber and is suspended in aqueous humor. The periphery of the iris, called the *root*, is attached to the anterior surface of the ciliary body. The iris, which measures about 12 mm in diameter and has a circumference of 38 mm, is thickest (0.6 mm) at the pupillary margin (the so-called *collarette*), and is thinnest (0.5 mm) at the ciliary margin (Fig. 2–2).[3] The pupil, which circumscribes the optical axis, is the central aperture of the iris diaphragm. The pupillary margin rests lightly on the anterior surface of the lens.

Iris color varies from light blue to dark brown, depending on the amount of pigment produced in the melanocytes. The blue color results from the absorption of light with long wavelengths and the reflection of shorter blue waves, which can be seen by the observer. The iris color is inherited; brown is a dominant trait, and blue is recessive. In whites, the iris is usually blue at birth owing to a paucity of stromal melanocytes. By the age of 3 to 5 months, it becomes darker as more melanin

accumulates in the superficial melanocytes. In black races, the stroma is denser and pigmented melanocytes are more numerous. The albino iris is characterized by an absence of pigmented melanocytes, which causes the blood vessels of the iris and retina to transmit as a reddish glow. In some individuals, the iris color is different between the two eyes (heterochromia).

Macroscopic Appearance

ANTERIOR SURFACE

The collarette, a circular ridge lying about 1.6 mm from the pupillary margin, divides the anterior surface of the iris into the outer ciliary zone and the inner pupillary zone. The collarette overlies the incomplete minor vascular circle of the iris, which is formed both by anastomoses of blood vessel branches from the major arterial circle (emanating from the ciliary region), and by the vessels of this circle (emanating from the ciliary body). The iris surface has a trabecular structure, most pronounced in the collarette region, that encloses large, pitlike depressions, called *Fuchs' crypts*. These crypts communicate with the tissue spaces of the iris.

The posterior pigmented layer of the iris extends anteriorly around the edge of the pupil as the *pupillary ruff*. The radial folds of the posterior iris surface give the ruff its crenated appearance. In blue irides, the iris sphincter is visible as a muscle that encircles the pupil. The central zone of the outer iris is smooth, but peripherally, several contraction furrows occur concentrically with the pupil; these deepen as the pupil dilates.[3]

POSTERIOR SURFACE

The posterior surface of the iris is dark brown and shows a number of radial contraction folds, which are most prominent in the pupillary zone (Schwalbe's contraction folds). Circular folds are also present in the periphery (Fig. 2–3).

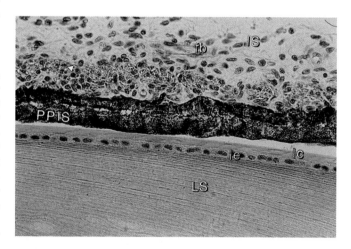

FIGURE 2–3. Photomicrograph of horizontal meridional section through human fetal (7 months) iris and lens. The epithelial cells of the posterior pigmented iris epithelium gradually become pigmented during the seventh month of gestation. (fb, fibroblasts; ppie, posterior pigmented iris epithelium; IS, iris stroma; lc, lens capsule; le, lens epithelium; LS, lens substance; *arrow*, clump cells) (Stain: Masson's trichrome, magnification: 850×.) (From The Russell L. Carpenter Collection for the Study of Opthalmic Histology, Department of Pathology, Massachusetts Eye and Ear Infirmary, Boston.)

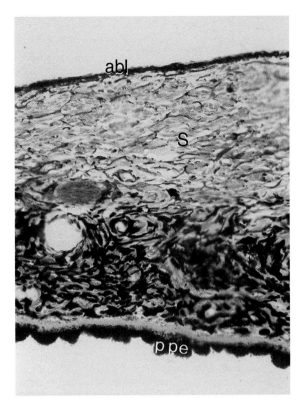

FIGURE 2–4. Photomicrograph of horizontal meridional section of human iris. The four layers of the iris. (ABL, anterior border layer; S, stroma; ppe, posterior pigmented epithelium. See also Figures 2–5 and 2–6). (Stain: Masson's trichrome, magnification: 500×.) (From The Russell L. Carpenter Collection for the Study of Ophthalmic Histology, Department of Pathology, Massachusetts Eye and Ear Infirmary, Boston).

Histology

Microscopically, the iris consists of four layers: (1) the anterior border layer, (2) the stroma with the sphincter muscle, derived from mesenchyme, (3) the anterior epithelium with the dilator muscle, and (4) the posterior pigment epithelium, derived from neural ectoderm (Fig. 2–4).

ANTERIOR BORDER LAYER

The anterior border layer consists of loose connective tissue and pigment cells. Peripherally, the anterior border layer ends abruptly at the iris root, except where it extends into the drainage angle as fine iris processes, which continue toward Schwalbe's line. Fibroblasts form a fairly continuous sheet of cells and interlacing processes, stretching from the iris root to the pupil.[3] Pigmented uveal melanocytes lie deep to the fibroblasts. Three types of intercellular junctions are reported between cells of like type in the anterior border layer, including gap junctions, intermediate junctions, and discontinuous tight junctions.[7, 8] Capillaries and venules as well as numerous nerve endings are found in this layer, which is responsible for the iris color; it is thick and densely pigmented in the brown eye, and thin and rarely pigmented in the blue eye.

STROMA AND SPHINCTER MUSCLE

The stroma consists of pigmented and nonpigmented cells and a loose collagenous network lying in a matrix

of mucopolysaccharides.[9] The collagen is generally arranged in cylindric groupings or bundles around cells, nerves, or blood vessels. The bundles are interlaced and form clockwise and counterclockwise curved arcades, which are attached to the iridial muscles, the anterior border layer, and the ciliary body. There are wide spaces in the stroma, which permit a free diffusion of aqueous and large molecules (up to 200 μm) into the stroma.[3]

The cellular elements of the stroma include fibroblasts, melanocytes, clump cells, and mast cells (Fig. 2–5). Fibroblasts, the most common stromal cells, are found around blood vessels, nerves, and muscle tissue and throughout the iris substance. Melanocytes form plexuses with each other that are arranged around the adventitia of vessels. In the pupillary portion of the iris, clump cells are found; these are believed to represent macrophages filled with melanin granules and partly displaced neuroectodermal cells containing melanocyte granules.[10] Mast cells, also found in the stroma, are round cells with villous processes and contain characteristic amorphous inclusions.

Lying in the pupillary zone of the iris stroma is a ring of smooth muscle, 1 mm wide, known as the *sphincter pupillae*. It is separated from the anterior layer by a sheet of connective tissue to which it is firmly bound. The muscle fibers contain melanin granules of neuroepithelial type. The arrangement of the muscle cells in a concentric way allows the pupil to constrict when the muscle contracts. Parasympathetic nerve fibers, originating in the Edinger-Westphal nucleus, innervate the iris sphincter, but sympathetic innervation has also been shown.[5]

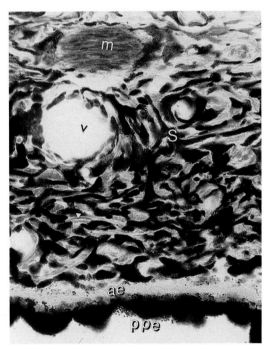

FIGURE 2–5. Photomicrograph of horizontal meridional section of human iris. Note the great amount of pigment cells of the posterior pigmented epithelium. (S, stroma; ae, anterior epithelium; ppe, posterior pigmented epithelium; m, muscle; v, vessel; *arrow*, collagenous fibers.) (Stain: Masson's trichrome, magnification: 850×.) (From The Russell L. Carpenter Collection for the Study of Ophthalmic Histology, Department of Pathology, Massachusetts Eye and Ear Infirmary, Boston.)

ANTERIOR EPITHELIUM AND DILATOR MUSCLE

The anterior epithelium is about 12.5 mm thick and adjoins apically the posterior epithelium.[3] Its cuboidal pigmented cell bodies remain at the basal portion in continuity with the fibers of the dilator muscle, which derives from these cells. The dilator muscle demarcates the posterior boundary of the iris stroma, peripheral to the sphincter muscle. When the muscle elements, which are arranged in an overlapping manner, contract, their radial direction causes pupillary dilation. The dilator muscle is innervated by the sympathetic nerve via the long ciliary nerves.

POSTERIOR PIGMENT EPITHELIUM

The double layer of pigment epithelium that covers the posterior iris surface is derived from the internal layer of the optic cup.

The anterior border layer is separated from the pupil by a ridge of more heavily pigmented cells, the pigment ruff, which is the clinically visible portion of the iris pigment epithelium.[9] The ruff folds up like an accordion on pupillary constriction and stretches to form an almost smooth ridge that lines the pupillary margin on wide dilation. The cytologic bases of the pigmented cuboidal cells of the anterior layer expand and specialize into the overlapping smooth muscle cells that make up the dilator muscle, except in the region behind the sphincter muscle where dilator muscle is lacking. In this region, a thin basement membrane is present. The anterior layer continues in the layer of pigmented epithelium of the ciliary body and in the retinal pigment epithelium.

The posterior layer of pigment epithelium is continuous with the nonpigmented epithelium of the ciliary body and ultimately with the neural retina (Fig. 2–6). Its columnar cells are arranged apex-to-apex with the cells of the anterior layer. This arrangement provides a multilaminar basement membrane on the posterior surface and clusters of apical villi on the anterior surface that project into small spaces between the two layers of epithelium.[11] A tight adhesion between the anterior and posterior epithelial layer is provided by well-developed desmosomes between the lateral and apical surfaces of the two layers. Adjacent posterior pigmented epithelial cells of the iris are joined by an apicolateral junctional complex, consisting of zonula occludens, zonula adherens, and gap junction.[12] The abundant melanin granules of the pigment epithelium are spherical, membrane bound, and much larger than those of the melanocytes.[13]

Vascular Supply and Innervation

The arteries of the iris arise mainly from the major arterial circle; some come from the anterior ciliary arteries.[3, 14] Entering the iris stroma at the attachments of the ciliary processes, they form a series of vascular arcades converging radially from ciliary to pupillary margin. At the collarette, some anastomoses occur, which, with corresponding venous anastomoses, form the incomplete circulus arteriosus iridis minor. Most vessels reach the pupillary margin where they bend around into the veins, after breaking up into capillaries (Fig. 2–7).

The iridial vessels consist of two tubular structures, one within the other. The outer tube is the adventitia

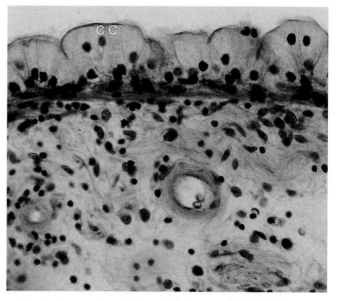

FIGURE 2–6. Photomicrograph of depigmented vertical meridional section of human iris. The melanin and fuchsin pigments are removed in this section to make evident structure that is otherwise masked by these brown pigments. Note the single layer of tall columnar (cc) cells (with the spherical nucleus lying in the basal part of the cell) of the posterior pigmented layer from which the pigment has been bleached. Remarkable also is the architecture of the anterior pigmented layer. The cells that make up the pigment epithelium of the ciliary body continue into the iris as a single layer and assume a long spindle shape, the oval nucleus remaining in the central thicker belly of the cell, whereas in the anterior portion of the cells, they develop contractile myofibrils that extend in either direction in spindle processes. The spindle processes collectively comprise the dilatator pupillae muscle. Their pigmented cell bodies constitute the anterior pigment layer. (Nuclei collagenous tissue and muscle and epithelium are shown.) (Stain: Masson's trichrome, magnification: 850×.) (From The Russell L. Carpenter Collection for the Study of Ophthalmic Histology, Department of Pathology, Massachusetts Eye and Ear Infirmary, Boston.)

proper, which is made up of fine connective tissue fibers; the inner one is the essential blood channel, consisting of endothelial lining and, in the case of arteries, muscle cells and elastic fibers. Between these two zones lies the tunica media, made up of loose collagen. The arteries and veins can be distinguished by the structure of the inner tube, which is much thicker in arteries. In these, the media consists of circular, nonstriated muscle cells that can be followed to the capillaries and elastic fibers in the intima.

Experimental studies show that smooth muscle cells are absent in human iris vessels, in contrast to capillaries.[15] The vascular endothelium of the iris is not fenestrated, and there are two types of intercellular junctions between the endothelial cells: zonular tight junctions and gap junctions.[15–17] The pericytes of the iris vessels are similar to those found elsewhere.[18]

The veins of the iris accompany the arteries, anastomose with each other, and enter the ciliary body to join the veins of the ciliary processes leading to the venae vorticosae. The two superior vorticose veins open into the superior ophthalmic vein either directly or via its muscular or lacrimal tributaries. The two inferior veins open into the inferior ophthalmic vein or into its anastomotic connection with the superior ophthalmic vein.

The anterior surface of the iris and its stroma are freely accessible to the diffusion of fluid and solute from the aqueous humor in the anterior chamber; the posterior iris epithelium is impermeable and secludes the posterior chamber.[23] In the normal eye, the continuous, nonfenestrated vascular endothelium of the iris capillaries prevents the entry of proteins and tracer materials (e.g., horseradish peroxidase) from the vessel lumen into the iris stroma (in contrast to the permeable ciliary capillaries).[24, 25] This barrier breaks down in a condition of inflammation (iritis) and allows proteins to pass into the aqueous, where it becomes visible by slit-lamp microscopy as aqueous flare. Freddo and Sacks-Wilner observed simplification and disruption of endothelial tight junctions in endotoxin-induced uveitis in rabbits, leading to a leakage of tracer material through the vessels.[26]

Ciliary Body

Development

The ciliary epithelium differentiates behind the advancing margin of the optic cup from its two layers of neuroectoderm.[4] Longitudinally oriented indentations juxtaposed to small blood vessels in the choroid are observed in the outer pigmented layer late in the third month. At this stage, the nonpigmented epithelium is smooth, but between the third and fourth months, it starts to fold so that it follows the contour of the pigmented layer. Some of these radial folds develop further and form later on the ciliary processes. During the fourth month, the mesenchymal core of the developing processes is invaded by capillaries, which are found in the growing tips of endothelial cells. The intracytoplasmic vesicles of the endothelial cells are supposed to fuse with the intercellular spaces to form lumina. The endothelial cells secrete a basal lamina on their abluminal surfaces and develop fenestrations in their cytoplasm.[6] In the fifth month, the juxtaposed apical surfaces of the double-layered ciliary epithelium become connected by gap junctions, desmosomes, and fasciae adherens complexes. Golgi complexes found in the cytoplasm during the fifth month of gestation indicate the synthesis of aqueous humor.

The ciliary muscle starts to grow during the 10th week as an accumulation of mesenchymal cells between the anterior scleral condensation and the primitive ciliary epithelium in the region of the optic cup margin. Dense bodies, arranged as plaques along the plasmalemma and surrounded by myofilaments, can be found during the 12th week of gestation in the cytoplasm of the differentiating cells.[27] Individual cells are surrounded by a discontinuous basal lamina. As gestation continues, the outer part of the ciliary muscle increases in size; the cells become elongated and arranged parallel to the anterior sclera. By the fourth month of gestation, fibroblasts are present in addition to smooth muscle cells. At the end of the fifth month, these cells become organized and ensheath the ciliary muscle bundles.[27] The meridional muscle cells organize into a characteristic triangular shape, and the ends of the muscle fibers continue with the developing scleral spur. The fibers of the inner part of the ciliary muscle cells next become established as the circular portion of the ciliary muscle. However, the devel-

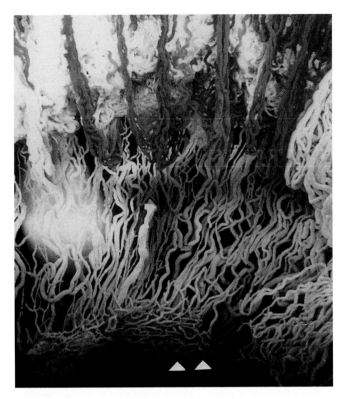

FIGURE 2–7. Ultrastructure of ciliary processes (cp) and iris from posterior view. Arrowheads, iris margins, vascular cast. (SEM ×29.) (From Fryczkowski AW, Hodes BL, Walker J: Diabetic choroidal and iris vasculature scanning electron microscopy findings. Int Ophthalmol 1989;13:560–568.)

The iris nerves derive from the long and short ciliary nerves, which accompany the corresponding arteries, pierce the sclera, and run forward between the sclera and choroid to the ciliary plexus.[3, 4, 19, 20] Here, they branch and form plexuses in the anterior border layer, around blood vessels, and anterior to the dilator pupillae. Their fibers supply nerve filaments to all layers except the posterior pigmented epithelium. The dilator nerve receives sympathetic innervation, and the sphincter muscle, parasympathetic innervation, but both adrenergic and cholinergic innervation have been shown in both muscles.[21]

Function

The pupil regulates the entry of light into the eye: It is very small in bright sunlight and widely dilated in the dark. The range of pupil diameter lies between 1.5 and 8 mm (with mydriatic drops, it is over 9 mm).[22] The sphincter pupillae are innervated by parasympathetic nerve endings and constrict the pupil (miosis). The dilator muscle is sympathetically innervated, and its contraction dilates the pupil (mydriasis). These muscles show a reciprocal innervation.

Pupil constriction occurs during accommodation for near focus and improves the depth of field while reducing spherical aberration. It can be observed also after injury or during inflammation, in response to fifth nerve stimulation and the release of mediator substances such as prostaglandin.

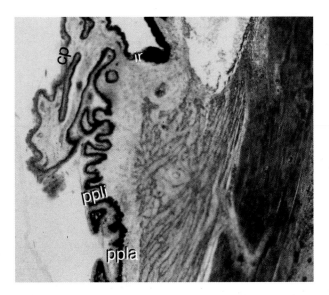

FIGURE 2–8. Photomicrograph of vertical meridional section of human ciliary body. (cp, ciliary processes; ppli, pars plicata; ppla, pars plana; ir, iris root). (Stain: Masson's trichrome, magnification: 100×.) (With permission from The Russell L. Carpenter Collection for the Study of Ophthalmic Histology, Department of Pathology, Massachusetts Eye and Ear Infirmary, Boston.)

opment of the circular muscle continues for at least 1 year after birth. Soon after the beginning of the differentiation of the circular component, the radial portion of the ciliary muscle, lying between the circular and meridional fibers, develops. Endothelial cells that line the vessels of the ciliary muscle form a continuous layer and are joined by tight junctions.

Gross Appearance and Macroscopic Appearance

The triangular, black-colored ciliary body has its base at the iris root anteriorly, and its apex at the ora serrata, the dentate limit of the retina, posteriorly (about 6 mm in anteroposterior width) (Fig. 2–8). Considered as a whole, the ciliary body is a complete ring that runs around the inside of the anterior sclera. On the outside of the eyeball, the ciliary body extends from a point about 1.5 mm posterior to the corneal limbus to a point 7.5 mm posterior to this point on the temporal side and 6.5 mm posterior on the nasal side.[1] The anterior part of the ciliary body becomes a part of the anterior chamber angle, and the uvea continues anteriorly as the uveal trabecular meshwork and the iris root. At the ora serrata, posteriorly, the ciliary body joins the posterior continuation of the uvea, the choroid. The ora serrata exhibits forward extensions, which are well defined on the nasal side and less so temporally. These dentate processes are usually directed toward a minor ciliary process.

The neuroretina and retinal pigment epithelium, derived from the two layers of the optic cup, become the internal layers of the ciliary body, the pigmented and nonpigmented epithelium, respectively; the vasculature of the choroid is replaced by that of the ciliary body.[3, 4, 19, 20] Externally, it is formed from the intermediate portion of the mesodermal uveal tract.

The ciliary body is divisible into two parts: the smooth

pars plana (orbiculus ciliaris) posteriorly and the pars plicata (corona ciliaris) anteriorly. The width of the pars plicata is about 2 mm, and that of the pars plana, about 4 mm. The pars plana is a relatively avascular zone, which is important surgically in the pars plana approach to the vitreous space.

PARS PLANA

The internal surface of the pars plana shows dark ridges, the ciliary striae of Schultze, which converge from the dentate processes of the ora serrata to the valleys between the ciliary processes. The pars plana is usually not uniformly pigmented, but there is often a dark band in front of and following the contours of the ora serrata (Fig. 2–9). Posterior zonular fibers take their origin from a band of the pars plana, lying 1.5 mm anterior to the ora, and pass along the lateral edges of the striae to the ciliary valleys. The vitreous base gains attachment to the epithelium of the pars plana over a band extending forward from the ora.

PARS PLICATA

The name of the pars plicata derives from a ring of ciliary processes (around 70 major crests) that are meridionally arranged and project from the anterior portion of the ciliary body.[19] In the valleys between the crests lie smaller, accessory processes, which vary in size and become longer with age.[28] In the intervals between the ciliary processes, the suspensory ligaments of the lens pass to attach to the surface of the pars plicata. The equator of the lens lies about 0.5 mm from the ciliary processes.

The internal surface of the corona ciliaris is formed

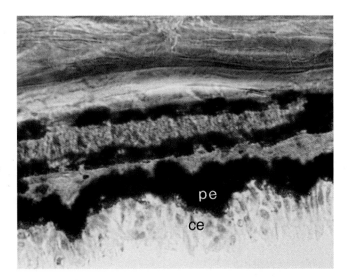

FIGURE 2–9. Photomicrograph of equatorial section through human pars plana. The ciliary epithelium (ce) rests on the pigment epithelium (pe). The clear cells of the ciliary epithelium are high columnar in shape over the pars plana but gradually decrease in height to become cuboidal over the crests of the ciliary processes. See also Figure 2–13. The pigment epithelium is a single layer of cells, in which the melanin granules are darker, round, and more densely packed than in the same retinal layer. (Stain: Masson's trichrome, magnification: 850×.) (With permission from The Russell L. Carpenter Collection for the Study of Ophthalmic Histology, Department of Pathology, Massachusetts Eye and Ear Infirmary, Boston.)

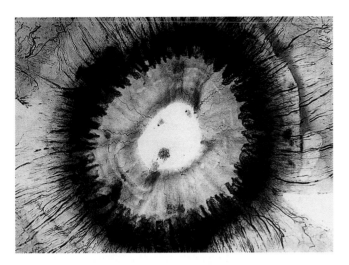

FIGURE 2–10. Microangiogram from human ciliary body, pars plana and processes ciliares, view from behind. Two types of the ciliary processes can be recognized. (Magnification: 8×.) (Courtesy of Andrzej W. Fryczkowski, MD, PhD, DSc.)

from the ciliary epithelium, which is the secretory source of the aqueous humor.

The ciliary processes contain no muscle and are the most vascular region of the whole eye. The vascular core is a continuation of the pars plana and consists of veins and capillaries. The capillary endothelium is fenestrated and permeable to plasma proteins and tracer material (Fig. 2–10).

Histology

From inside to outside, the ciliary body consists of the ciliary epithelium, the ciliary stroma, the ciliary muscle, and the supraciliary layer.

CILIARY EPITHELIUM

The ciliary epithelium is made up of two layers of cuboidal cells that cover the inner surface of the ciliary body. There is an outer pigmented layer and an inner nonpigmented layer.

Specialized connections exist within and between the cell layers, which are important for their ability to secrete aqueous humor.

The pigmented epithelium secretes the anterior basement membrane, which continues posteriorly with the basement membrane of the retinal pigment epithelium and anteriorly with the basement membrane of the dilator muscle of the iris. Over the pars plicata, the anterior basement membrane is separated by a little space from the capillaries; over the pars plana, it is related to stromal collagen and veins.

The cells of the pigmented epithelium are 8 to 10 μm wide and contain dark, pigmented granules that are three to four times larger than those of the choroid and retina.[19] Ultrastructural studies show the cells to be rich in organelles and to contain tonofilaments.[29] The basal membranes of the cells are related to the anterior basal membrane, the lateral membranes interdigitate with each other, and the apical membranes are apposed to those of the nonpigmented epithelium.

The nonpigmented epithelium continues anteriorly

with the posterior epithelium of the iris at the iris root. Its cells are cuboidal over the pars plicata (12 to 15 μm wide) and columnar over the pars plana (6 to 9 μm wide). Electron microscopic studies show abundant organelles, like mitochondria (increasing with age), and a well-developed, rough endoplasmic reticulum.[17, 30, 31] Apically, the surfaces of the cells are connected to those of the pigmented epithelium and, laterally, intercellular glycosaminoglycan-like material containing spaces is found. The basal surfaces are deeply infolded at the perimeter of each cell in the pars plicata region. These basal infoldings and lateral interdigitations of the plasma membrane increase the surface area of the cells, and thus the aqueous humor secretion capacity.[32]

The cellular junctions found between the pigmented and nonpigmented epithelia are zonulae occludentae, gap junctions, desmosomes, and puncta adherentia.[33] These connecting structures are important for the secretory role of the ciliary processes: the zonulae occludentae form a tight barrier, which is impermeable to the diffusion of macromolecular tracers across the epithelium, but anastomosing strands at the interfaces of the cells allow water and small ions to penetrate.[34] However, different concentrations of certain ions and molecules (e.g., ascorbate, bicarbonate in a higher concentration, calcium, and urea in a lower concentration) in the aqueous humor, in comparison to their concentration in a plasma filtrate, indicate a selective transport.[35, 36] It is presumed that the ciliary epithelial cells act as a functional syncytium through their gap junctions, ensuring the coordination of the secretory activity.

The internal limiting membrane is formed by the basal lamina of the nonpigmented epithelium on its basal (vitreal) surface; it is posteriorly in continuation with the inner retinal basement membrane and anteriorly, with the inner basement membrane of the iris. It gives origin to parts of the suspensory lens ligament.

CILIARY STROMA

The ciliary stroma consists of bundles of loose connective tissue, rich in blood vessels and melanocytes, containing the embedded ciliary muscle.[1] The connective tissue extends into the ciliary processes, forming a connective tissue core. Ciliary arteries, veins, and capillary networks make up the stromal blood vessels, which can be found mainly in the inner stromal layer. At the iris periphery, just in front of the circular portion of the ciliary muscle, lies the major arterial circle, which is formed by branches of the long posterior ciliary arteries.

CILIARY MUSCLE

The ciliary muscle consists of three layers (longitudinal, radial, and circular) of nonstriated muscle fibers. Anteriorly, the muscle is attached by collagenous tendons into the scleral striata and to the iris wall; posteriorly, it gains attachment by an elastic tendon into the pars plana (Fig. 2–11). It is the contraction of the ciliary muscle, especially of the longitudinal and circular fibers, that pulls the ciliary muscle forward during accommodation. This forward movement is responsible for relieving the tension in the suspensory lens ligament, making the elastic lens

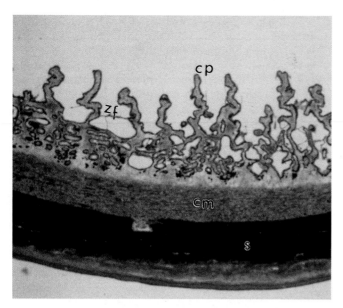

FIGURE 2–11. Photomicrograph of equatorial section through human pars plicata. Notice the ring of ciliary processes (cp) and the attachments of the zonular fibers (zf) to the processes. (cm: ciliary muscle; s: sclera.) (Stain: Masson's trichrome, magnification: 75×.) (From The Russell L. Carpenter Collection for the Study of Ophthalmic Histology, Department of Pathology, Massachusetts Eye and Ear Infirmary, Boston.)

more convex and thereby increasing the refractive power of the lens.

Postganglionic parasympathetic fibers, derived from the oculomotor nerve, reach the muscle via the short ciliary nerves and innervate it.

SUPRACILIARY LAYER

This layer, resembling the suprachoroidea of the choroid, consists of melanocyte- and fibroblast-rich tissue and collagen strands derived from the longitudinal layer of the ciliary muscle. The collagen enters and mingles with the collagen fibers of the overlying sclera. The supraciliary layer forms a potential space, allowing the aqueous humor to exit via the "unconventional" pathway.[37] Furthermore, this space may be expanded pathologically by transudate or exudate associated with ciliary body detachment.[38]

Vascular Supply and Innervation

The circulus iridis major, formed predominantly by the long posterior ciliary arteries, is located in the ciliary body (Fig. 2–12). The intramuscular vascular circle of the ciliary muscle is formed by penetrating branches of the anterior ciliary arteries and supplies the outer and superficial part of the muscle. The inner and anterior part is fed by arterioles derived from the major arterial circle. Venules join the parallel veins from the ciliary processes and drain into the ciliary valleys, or they join the anterior ciliary veins.

The arteries of the ciliary processes spring from the major arterial circle. Each process usually receives a separate artery. These arteries pierce the ciliary muscle to enter the ciliary processes anteriorly, where they form a dense capillary plexus (Fig. 2–13). Their veins drain into the vortex veins, which lie in the ciliary muscle. The ciliary blood flow is autoregulated, and it is probable that blood-shunting between major processes exists.

The ciliary body is innervated by posterior ciliary nerves, which lie in the choroid and branch near the ora serrata to form a plexus of myelinated and unmyelinated nerves. Parasympathetic fibers, coming from the Edinger-Westphal nucleus with the oculomotor nerve, are mixed with nerve fibres from the ciliary ganglion and form a plexus in the ciliary muscle.

Sympathetic fibers come from the cervical sympathetic trunk, synapse in the superior cervical ganglion, and run to the ciliary muscle via the long ciliary nerve.[39] The sensory fibers, coming from the nasociliary branch of the trigeminal nerve, also run in the long ciliary nerve to the ciliary body and terminate in the ciliary muscle.

Function

Aqueous humor is secreted into the posterior chamber, mainly by active transport across the ciliary epithelium, creating an osmotic gradient and leading to waterflow. The nonpigmented cells of the epithelium are supposed to selectively absorb sodium ions from the ciliary stroma and transport them into the intercellular clefts.[40] This process, regulated by intramembranous ATPase, leads to hyperosmolarity in the clefts, creating an osmotic flow of water from the stroma into the clefts and a continuous flow of fluid into the posterior chamber.

Accommodation is a complex constellation of sensory, neuromuscular, and biophysical phenomena by which the refracting power of the eye changes rapidly to focus clearly on the retina objects at different viewing distances.[41] The lenticular rounding and flattening (accommodation and disaccommodation) are accomplished

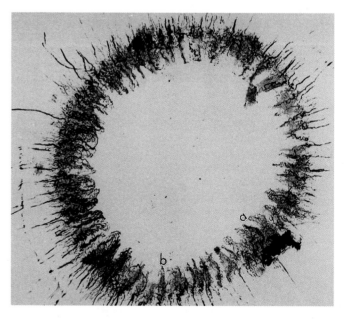

FIGURE 2–12. The human ciliary bodies and processes ciliares, view from behind. Two main types of processes: (1) wide, angulated and broad, developed, (2) thin with sharp angle. Specimen injected by microthrast, superimposed photograph, microangiogram. (Magnification: 8×.) (Courtesy of Andrzej W. Fryczkowski, MD, PhD, DSc.)

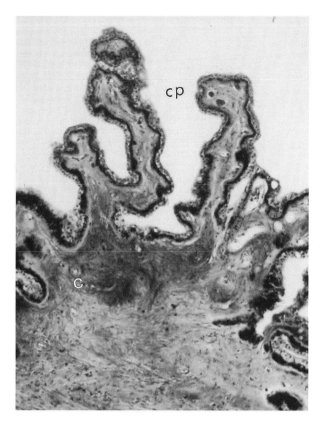

FIGURE 2–13. Photomicrograph of equatorial section through human pars plicata. Remarkable are the wide capillaries (c) and the reduction of pigment in the crests of the ciliary processes (cp). (Stain: Masson's trichrome, magnification: 250×.) (With permission from The Russell L. Carpenter Collection for the Study of Ophthalmic Histology, Department of Pathology, Massachusetts Eye and Ear Infirmary, Boston.)

through the action of the ciliary muscle. When the outer longitudinal muscle fibers contract under parasympathetic innervation, the main mass of the muscle slides forward along the curved inner wall of the sclera toward the scleral spur. By sliding away from the equator along the curved surface of the spherical globe, diametrically opposite points on the muscle move toward one another.

This narrowing may be further augmented by contraction of the circular muscle fibers. These changes lead to a more spherical lens and serve to increase the refracting power of the accommodating system.

Regarding shifts from near to distant objects, the sequence of changes is reversed: parasympathetic input into the ciliary muscle decreases, and the muscle relaxes.

Choroid

Development

Neural crest cells condense and differentiate into the cells of the ensheathing choroidal stroma. This mesenchymal tissue is invaded early by endothelium-lined blood spaces, which form the embryonic annular vessel.[6] During the fourth week of gestation, the choriocapillaris differentiates. At the beginning of the sixth week, the human eye is already completely invested with a primitive layer of capillaries.[42] The endothelial cells contain numerous vesicles, which are presumed to have a secretory function.

The characteristic fenestrations of the choriocapillaris are first seen after the seventh week of gestation.[4] Their development parallels an enlargement of the vessel lumen, thinning of the endothelium, and an increase in the number of intracellular vesicles.[5] Concomitantly, the basal lamina become well defined, continuous, and thicker. Branches of the future short posterior ciliary arteries and rudimentary vortex veins can be distinguished by the end of the second month[4] (Fig 2–14). During the third month, the outer, large vessel layer (von Haller) and the inner, mainly venous capillary layer (choriocapillaris), which connects the vortex veins, develop. A third middle layer, the stromal arteriolar layer (Sattler's), develops between the choriocapillaris and the outer capillary layer during the fifth month. The choroidal stroma contains collagen fibers, fibroblasts, elastic tissue, and melanocytes, which determine the pigmentation of the choroid.

Another layer of the choroid, Bruch's membrane (lamina vitrea), derives from the choriocapillaris and the retinal pigment epithelium.[4] Four of the five layers of Bruch's membrane are distinguishable by the end of the ninth

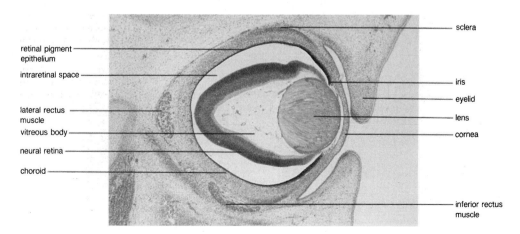

FIGURE 2–14. Photomicrograph of a sagittal section of the eye of an embryo (50×) at Carnegie stage 23, about 56 days. Observe the developing neural retina and the retinal pigment epithelium. The intraretinal space normally disappears as these two layers of the retina fuse. (From Moore KL, Pesaud TVN, Shiota K: Color Atlas of Clinical Embryology. Philadelphia, WB Saunders, 1994.)

week (inner basal lamina, two layers of collagen, and a layer of elastin). The outermost component, the basal lamina of the endothelial cells of the choriocapillaris, is the last to be organized.[42]

Gross Appearance and Macroscopic Appearance

The choroid is a soft, thin, brown, extremely vascular layer, lining the inner surface of the sclera. It extends posteriorly from the optic nerve to the ora serrata anteriorly. The smooth inner surface is firmly attached to the pigmented epithelium of the retina; the rough outer surface is attached to the sclera in both the region of the optic nerve and the region where the vortex veins exit the eyeball. These attachment points are the characteristic, smooth configuration seen ophthalmoscopically during "choroidal" detachment. At the optic nerve, the choroid becomes continuous with the pia and arachnoid.

The choroid can be divided into three superimposed major strata: the outer stromal layer of large and medium vessels, the layer of capillaries (choriocapillaris), and, between the choriocapillaris and the retinal pigment epithelium, the noncellular inner surface of the choroid, Bruch's membrane, extending from the optic disc to the ora serrata. It presents a smooth, brown, glistening, transparent aspect.

The suprachoroid lamina (lamina fusca) is a pigmented sheet overlying the perichoroidal space, which lies between the sclera and choroid and contains the long and short posterior ciliary arteries and nerves.

The thickness of the choroid has been estimated at about 100 to 220 μm, with the greatest thickness noted over the macula (500 to 1000 μm) (Fig. 2–15).[20, 43]

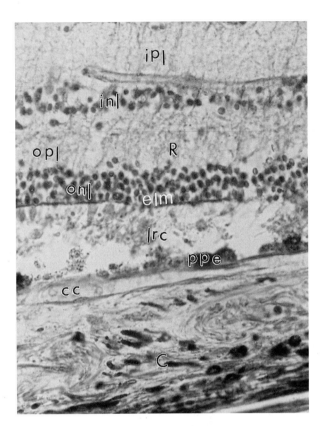

FIGURE 2–16. Photomicrograph of horizontal meridional section of human choroid and retina. Note the layers of the retina and the choroid (cc, choriocapillaris.) (ppe, posterior pigmented epithelium; lrc: layer of rods and cones; elm: external limiting membrane; onl: outer nuclear layer; opl: outer plexiform layer; inl: inner nuclear layer; ipl: inner plexiform layer.) (Stain: Masson's trichrome, magnification: 850×.) (From The Russell L. Carpenter Collection for the Study of Ophthalmic Histology, Department of Pathology, Massachusetts Eye and Ear Infirmary, Boston.)

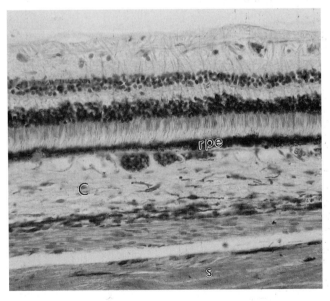

FIGURE 2–15. Photomicrograph of vertical meridional section of human choroid and retina. Note the attachment of the choroid (C) to the retinal pigmented epithelium (rpe) and to the sclera (s). (Stain: Masson's trichrome, magnification: 500×.) (With permission from The Russell L. Carpenter Collection for the Study of Ophthalmic Histology, Department of Pathology, Massachusetts Eye and Ear Infirmary, Boston.)

Histology

LAMINA FUSCA

The lamina fusca is 10 to 34 μm thick and consists of pigmented (melanocytes) and nonpigmented uveal cells (fibrocytes), a musculoelastic system, and a mesh of collagen fibers forming pigmented bands, which run from the sclera anteriorly to the choroid.[9]

CHOROIDAL STROMA

This layer contains vessels, nerves, cells (melanocytes, fibrocytes, macrophages, mast cells, and plasma cells), and connective tissue (Fig. 2–16).[20]

The brown color of the stromal layer is characterized by dendritic melanocytes. They form an almost continuous interconnecting lamellar arrangement in the outer choroid, outlining the vessels. On surface view, the choroid is least pigmented where the larger vessels are located and most pigmented in the spaces between the vessels. Melanocyte nuclei are round; they show an even chromatin dispersal and no nucleolus.

Associated with these cells are varying amounts of collagen fibrils and watery mucinous intercellular materials (Fig. 2–17).

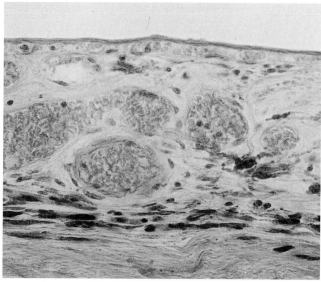

FIGURE 2–17. Photomicrograph of horizontal meridional section of human choroid. The suprachoroid layer consists of a network of branching, flat strands of elastic fibers that course mostly lengthwise in long spirals parallel to the choroidal surface. (Elastic fibers, nuclei, and collagenous tissue are shown.) (Stain: Masson's trichrome, magnification: 850×.) (From The Russell L. Carpenter Collection for the Study of Ophthalmic Histology, Department of Pathology, Massachusetts Eye and Ear Infirmary, Boston.)

The vessels and nerves of this layer will be described in the section "Vascular Supply and Innervation."

CHORIOCAPILLARIS

The choriocapillaris shows a lobular organization of wide-lumen capillaries, supplying an independent segment of choriocapillaries and lying in a single plane.[44–46] The lobular network is well developed at the posterior pole and is less regular more anteriorly towards the ora serrata. The submacular choroid is fed by 8 to 16 precapillary arterioles, which show frequent interarteriolar anastomoses.

Fryczkowski showed that the lobular anatomy is "veno-centric," with the feeding arteriole located peripherally, and one or more draining venules located centrally (Fig. 2–18).[47, 48] The lobules are arranged in a mosaic, with little anastomosis between them, creating vascular water-

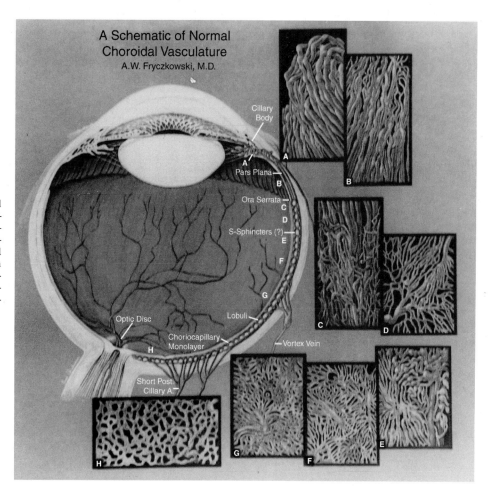

FIGURE 2–18. Schematic of the normal choroidal vasculature showing differences with the appearance of the choriocapillaris in different areas from the optic nerve head to the periphery. Based on vascular cast and SEM images. (From Fryczkowski AW, Sato SE: Scanning electron microscopy of the ocular vasculature in diabetic retinopathy. Contemporary Ophthalmic Forum 1986;4:39–50.)

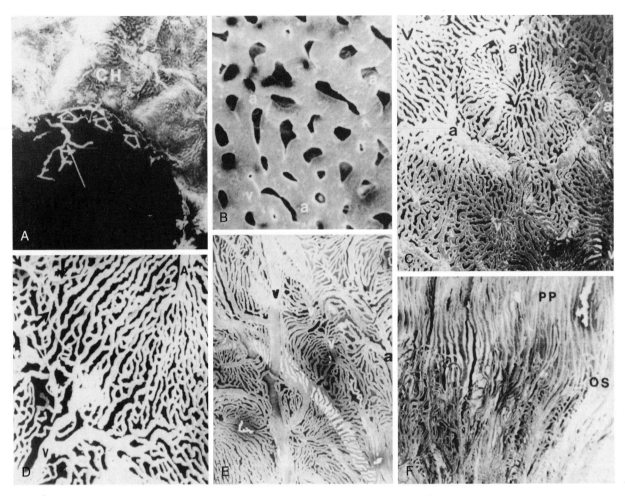

FIGURE 2–19. Human choriocapillaris, posterior pole, retinal view, vascular cast. Montage of the SEM images from periphery to peripheral areas. *A,* Peripapillary area; *B,* submacular area; *C,* lobular area; *D, E, F,* equatorial areas. Arterioles (a) and venules (v), choriocapillaris (CH), ora serrata (OS), pars plana (PP), and lobuli (boxed). (SEM ×39.) (From Fryczkowski AW: Anatomical and functional lobuli. Int Ophthalmol 1994;18:131–141.)

sheds that may lead to occlusive events in the choroid and at the optic nerve (Fig. 2–19).[20] The ischemia produced by such occlusions gives rise to pale lesions seen ophthalmoscopically as *Elschnig spots.*

The endothelial cells of the choriocapillaris are fenestrated and surrounded by a basal membrane. They show junctions of the zonula adherens type, but a zonula occludens appears to be poorly formed.[23] This structural characteristic may lead to "leakiness" of the choriocapillaris in fluorescein angiography.

Bruch's Membrane

This thin (2 to 4 μm), noncellular lamina consists of five layers[20]:

1. The inner basal lamina is in continuity with the basal lamina of the ciliary epithelium. It is separated from the retinal pigment epithelium by a 100-mm-wide zone.
2. The inner collagenous zone is composed of interweaving collagen fibers and is 1 μm in thickness.
3. The elastic zone shows a dense cortex and a homogenous core of interwoven bands of elastic fibers.
4. The outer collagenous zone shows a similar structure to the inner zone.

5. The outer basal lamina forms a noncontinuous sheet across Bruch's membrane.

Vascular Supply and Innervation

The choroid receives its blood primarily from the short posterior ciliary arteries and to a small extent from recurrent branches of the anterior ciliary arteries.[1] All these arteries are branches of the ophthalmic artery.

The short ciliary arteries pierce the sclera and run in the suprachoroid space to the choroid, where they bifurcate and eventually divide into the choriocapillaris. Branches from the short posterior ciliary arteries, lying in Haller's layer, give rise to the choroidal arterioles of Sattler's layer.[20]

The short posterior ciliary arteries supply the posterior choroid up to the equator, and the temporal long posterior ciliary arteries supply a small temporal sector of the choroid. The anterior part of the choroid is supplied by recurrent ciliary arteries arising from the circulus iridis major and from the long posterior and anterior ciliary arteries. These vessels run back into the pars plana, where they divide to supply the anterior choriocapillaris.

The choroidal veins form the venae vorticosae. They show four tributaries: two superior (posterior) and two inferior (anterior) veins. Their posterior tributaries arise from the posterior choroid, the optic nerve head, and the peripapillary retina; the anterior tributaries from the iris, the ciliary processes, the ciliary muscle, and the anterior choroid. Some branches of the posterior tributaries do not follow the courses of the corresponding arteries, but run from around the optic disc directly to the venae vorticosae. The veins draining the anterior choroid run parallel with each other in the pars plana but turn at the ora obliquely toward the corresponding vortex veins.

The stems of the vortex veins undergo ampulliform dilatation just before they enter the sclera. Here, they are joined by radial and curved tributaries, which give the whole a whorl-like appearance. It is this appearance that gives the venae vorticosae their names.

The choroid is innervated by the long and short ciliary nerves. The long ciliary nerves carry sensory nerve fibers and sympathetic fibers (vasoconstrictor function). The short ciliary nerves carry parasympathetic and sympathetic fibers.

The nerves pierce the sclera around the optic nerve and run forward in the perichoroidal space.[1] Branches are given off to the choroid to form perivascular and ganglionic neural plexuses.

Function

The principal function of the choroid lies in the blood nourishment of the outer layers of the retina.[1] It is thought that changes in blood flow in the choroidal vessels may serve to produce heat exchange from the retina. Another suggestion is that the blood flow in the choroidal arteries helps in regulating intraocular pressure. Further, the large number of choroidal pigment cells prevents reflection by absorbing excess light penetrating the retina.

References

1. Snell RS, Lemp MA: The eyeball. In: Snell RS, Lemp MA, eds: Clinical Anatomy of the Eye, 2nd ed. Malden, MA, Blackwell Science, 1998, pp 140–156.
2. Rao NA, Forster DJ: Basic principles. In: Podos SM, Yanoff M, eds: The Uvea, Uveitis and Intraocular Neoplasms, vol. 2. New York, Gower Medical Publications, 1992, pp 1–17.
3. Bron AJ, Tripathi RC, Tripathi BJ: The iris. In: Bron AJ, Tripathi RC, Tripathi BJ, eds: Wolff's Anatomy of the Eye and Orbit, 8th ed. London, Chapman & Hall Medical, 1997, pp 308–334.
4. Bron AJ, Tripathi RC, Tripathi BJ: The posterior chamber and the ciliary body. In: Bron AJ, Tripathi RC, Tripathi BJ, eds: Wolff's Anatomy of the Eye and Orbit, 8th ed. London, Chapman & Hall Medical, 1997, pp 335–370.
5. Tripathi BJ, Tripathi RC, Wisdom J: Embryology of the anterior segment of the human eye. In: Ritch R, Shields MB, Krupin T, eds: The Glaucomas, 2nd ed. St Louis, Mosby, 1995.
6. Ozanics V, Jakobiec FA: General topographic anatomy of the eye. Arch Ophthalmol 1982;1:1.
7. Freddo TF, Townes-Anderson E, Raviola G: Rod-shaped bodies and crystalloid inclusions in ocular vascular endothelia of adult and developing Macaca mulatta. Anat Embryol 1980;158:121.
8. Raviola G, Sagaties MJ, Miller C: Intercellular junctions between fibroblasts in connective tissues of the eye in Macuaque monkeys. Invest Ophthalmol Vis Sci 1987;28:834.
9. Fine BS, Yanoff M: Ocular histology. In: Fine BS, Yanoff BS, eds: Ocular Histology, 2nd ed. Hagerstone, MD: Medical Department, Harper & Row Publishers, 1972, pp 197–246.
10. Wobman PR, Fine BS: The clump cells of Koganei. A light and electron microscopic study. Am J Ophthalmol 1972;73:90.
11. Lim WC, Webber WA: A light and transmission electron-microscopic study of the rat iris in pupillary dilation and constriction. Exp Eye Res 1975;21:433.
12. Freddo TF: Intercellular junctions of the iris epithelia in Macaca mulatta. Invest Ophthalmol Vis Sci 1984;25:1094.
13. Feeney L, Grieshaber JA, Hogan MJ: Studies on human ocular pigment. In: Rohen JW, ed: The Structure of the Eye. Stuttgart, Schattauer, 1965, p 535.
14. Woodlief NF: Initial observations on the ocular microcirculation in man. Arch Ophthalmol 1980;98:1268.
15. Ikui H, Minutsu T, Maeda J, et al: Fine structure of the blood vessels of the iris; light and electron microscopic studies. Kyushu J Med Sci 1960;11:113.
16. Vegge T, Ringvold A: Ultrastructure of the wall of the human iris vessels. Z Zellforsch Mikrosk Anat 1969;94:19.
17. Hogan MJ, Weddell JE, Alvarado JA: Histology of the Human Eye. Philadelphia, WB Saunders, 1971.
18. de Oliviera F: Pericytes in diabetic retinopathy. Br J Ophthalmol 1966;50;134.
19. Bron AJ, Tripathi RC, Tripathi BJ: The choroid and uveal vessels. In: Bron AJ, Tripathi RC, Tripathi BJ, eds: Wolff's Anatomy of the Eye and Orbit, 8th ed. London, Chapman & Hall Medical, 1997, pp 371–410.
20. Bron AJ, Tripathi RC, Tripathi BJ: Development of the human eye. In: Bron AJ, Tripathi RC, Tripathi BJ, eds: Wolff's Anatomy of the Eye and Orbit, 8th ed. London, Chapman & Hall Medical, 1997, pp 620–664.
21. Lowenstein O, Loewenfeld IE: The pupil. In: Davson H, ed: The Eye, 2nd ed. New York, Academic Press, 1969, p 231.
22. Yanoff M, Fine BS: Ocular Pathology: A Text and Atlas, 3rd ed. Philadelphia, Lippincott, 1989.
23. Raviola G: The structural basis of the blood ocular barriers. Exp Eye Res Suppl 1977;27:27.
24. Vegge T: An electron microscopic study of the permeability of iris capillaries to horseradish peroxidase in the velvet monkey. Zellforsch Mikrosk Anat 1971;121:74.
25. Raviola G: Effects of paracentesis on the blood-aqueous barrier. Invest Ophthalmol 1974;13:828.
26. Freddo TF, Sacks-Wilner R: Interendothelial junctions of the rabbit iris vasculature in anterior uveitis. Invest Ophthalmol Vis Sci 1989;30:1104.
27. Sellheyer K, Spitznas M: Differentiation of the ciliary muscle in the human embryo and fetus. Graefe's Arch Clin Exp Ophthalmol 1988;226:281.
28. Reese AB: Ciliary processes; their relationship to intra-ocular surgery. Am J Ophthalmol 1934;17:422.
29. Misotten L: L'Ultrastructure des tissues oculaires. Bull Soc Belge Ophthalmol 1964;136:199.
30. Holmberg A: Differences in the ultrastructure of normal human and rabbit ciliary epithelium. Arch Ophthalmol 1959;62:952.
31. Fine BS, Zimmermann LE: Light and electron microscopic observations on the ciliary epithelium in man and rhesus monkey. Invest Ophthalmol 1963;2:105.
32. Ohnishi Y, Kuwabara T: Breakdown site of blood-aqueous barrier in the ciliary epithelium. RVO Suppl: Invest Ophthalmol Vis Sci 1979;18:241.
33. Raviola G: The fine structure of the ciliary zonule and ciliary epithelium with special regard to the organization and insertion of the zonular fibrils. Invest Ophthalmol 1971;10:851.
34. Noske W, Stamm CC, Hirsch M: Tight junctions of the human ciliary epithelium: Regional morphology and implications on trans-epithelial resistance. Exp Eye Res 1994;59:141.
35. Cole DF: Secretion of the aqueous humor. Exp Eye Res Suppl 1977;1:161.
36. Cole DF: Ocular fluids. In: Davson H, ed: The eye, 3rd ed. New York, Academic Press, 1984, p 269.
37. Laties AM: Central retinal artery innervation. Absence of adrenergic innervation to the intraocular braches. Arch Ophthalmol 1967;77:405.
38. Bill A: Basic physiology of the drainage of aqueous humor. Exp Eye Res 1977;25:291.
39. Ruskell GL: Sympathetic innervation of the ciliary muscle in monkey. Exp Eye Res 1973;16:183.

40. Cole DF, Tripathi RC: Theoretical consideration on the mechanism of the aqueous outflow. Exp Eye Res 1971;12:25.

41. Salzmann M: The Anatomy and Histology of the Human Eyeball in the Normal State. Its Development and Senescence. Chicago, University of Chicago Press, 1912.

42. Sellheyer K: Development of the choroid and related structures. Eye 1990;4:255.

43. Coleman DJ, Lizzi FL: In vivo choroidal thickness measurement. Am J Ophthalmol 1979;88:369.

44. Torczynski E, Tso MOM: The architecture of the choriocapillaris at the posterior pole. Am J Ophthalmol 1976;81:428.

45. Yoneya S, Tso MOM: Patterns of the choriocapillaris. Invest Ophthalmol 1984;6:95.

46. Yoneya S, Tso MOM: Angioarchitecture of the human choroid. Arch Ophthalmol 1987;105:681.

47. Fryczkowski AW: Blood vessels of the eye and their changes in diabetes. In: Motta PM, Murakami T, Fujita H, eds: Scanning Electron Microscopy of Vascular Casts: Methods and Applications. Boston: Kluwer Academic Publishers, 1992, p 293.

48. Fryczkowski AW: Choroidal microvascular anatomy. In: Yanuzzi LA, Flower RW, Slakter JS, eds: ICG Indocyanine Green Angiography. New York: Thieme, 1993, p 29.

DEFINITION, CLASSIFICATION, ETIOLOGY, AND EPIDEMIOLOGY

Shawkat Shafik Michel and C. Stephen Foster

DEFINITION

The uvea (from the Latin, uva or grape) is composed of iris, ciliary body, and choroid. Each of these components of the uvea has a unique histology, anatomy, and function. The uvea is the intermediate of the three coats of the eyeball, sandwiched between the sclera and the retina in its posterior (choroid) portion. Anteriorly, the iris controls the amount of light that reaches the retina, whereas the ciliary body is primarily responsible for aqueous humor production. The ciliary muscle is the only effector muscle of accommodation, changing the curvature of the lens through the fibers of the zonular ligament of the lens. In addition, contraction of the ciliary muscle opens the spaces of the trabecular meshwork, facilitating aqueous outflow. The choroid, with its rich vascular plexuses and high flow rates, is the sole blood supply to the avascular outer part of the retina (branches of the central retinal vessels run in the nerve fiber layer).

Uveitis, or inflammation of the uvea, may occur as a consequence of diverse stimuli. Inflammation[1] is a protective response. The ultimate goal of inflammation is to rid the individual of both the initial cause of cell injury (e.g., microbes and toxins) and the consequences of such injury, the necrotic cells and tissue. Inflammation and repair are closely intertwined. However, both inflammation and repair may be potentially harmful, as is commonly seen in allergic and autoimmune diseases. Components of both innate (essentially neutrophils, other granulocytes, macrophages, and the complement system) and specific immunity (B and T lymphocytes through their antibodies and cytokines) may not only damage inflamed target tissues but also may participate in the "innocent bystander injury" of surrounding normal tissues.

Inflammation may be acute, subacute or chronic. Acute inflammation is the immediate and early response to an injurious agent developing within minutes to a few days at most. The cardinal signs of acute inflammation include pain, redness, swelling, warmth, and impaired function. Acute inflammation has three components: (1) vasodilation and increased blood flow, (2) structural changes in the microvasculature that permit extravasation of plasma proteins and leukocytes (e.g., induction or increased expression of leukocyte adhesion molecules on the vascular endothelium), and (3) emigration of the leukocytes, mainly neutrophils or eosinophils, in cases of allergy, from the microcirculation and their accumulation in the focus of injury. Edema fluid in acute inflammation may be characterized as either an exudate or a transudate. An exudate has a high protein concentration, copious cellular debris, and a specific gravity above 1.020. This finding implies a significant alteration in the normal permeability of small blood vessels. A transudate has a low protein content (most of which is albumin) and a specific gravity of less than 1.012. Essentially, it is an ultrafiltrate of blood plasma. The process of leukocyte emigration and attraction to the site of injury, whether it be an infectious or immune response, is called chemotaxis and is mediated by special cytokines known as chemokines. Chemokines are mainly secreted by activated macrophage phagocytes and activated T lymphocytes. During the process of chemotaxis and phagocytosis, or during antigen-antibody reactions, leukocytes, mast cells, and macrophages release their granules in the interstitial tissue. The chemical mediators of acute inflammation originate from cells, the blood plasma, or both. These mediators include vasoactive amines, plasma proteases (kinins, components of the complement and coagulation systems), arachidonic acid metabolites (prostaglandins and leukotrienes) derived from cell membrane phospholipids, platelet-activating factor, cytokines (lymphokines and monokines), nitric oxide, lysosomal constituents, oxygen-derived free radicals and other mediators (e.g., substance P and growth factors) (Table 3–1). Histopathologically, acute inflammation is dominated by neutrophils and other granulocytes, in addition to eosinophils in allergic reactions.

Chronic inflammation by definition has a prolonged duration. It develops within weeks or months and may persist for years. In this category of inflammation, active

TABLE 3–1. CHEMICAL MEDIATORS OF INFLAMMATION

CHEMICAL MEDIATOR	SOURCE	MAJOR CELLULAR SOURCES
Histamine	Cells, preformed	Mast cells, platelets
Serotonin	Cells, preformed	Platelets, mast cells
Lysosomal enzymes	Cells, preformed	Neutrophils, macrophages
Prostaglandins	Cells, newly synthesized	All leukocytes, platelets, endothelium
Leukotrienes	Cells, newly synthesized	All leukocytes
Platelet-activating factor	Cells, newly synthesized	All leukocytes
Cytokines	Cells, newly synthesized	Macrophages, endothelium
Nitric oxide	Cells, newly synthesized	Macrophages, endothelium
C3a	Plasma, complement activation	
C5a	Plasma, complement activation	
C5b-9	Plasma, complement activation	
Kinin system (bradykinin)	Plasma, Hageman factor activation	
Coagulation/ fibrinolysis system	Plasma, Hageman factor activation	

inflammation, tissue destruction, and attempts at healing proceed simultaneously. Chronic inflammation is characterized by (1) infiltration with mononuclear cells, including macrophages, lymphocytes, and plasma cells (a reflection of a persistent reaction to injury); (2) tissue destruction, largely induced by these inflammatory cells; and (3) attempted tissue repair through angiogenesis and fibrosis. Chronic inflammation may follow acute inflammation or may begin insidiously as a low-grade, smoldering, and often asymptomatic response. Granulomatous inflammation is a distinctive type of chronic inflammatory reaction in which the predominant cell type is an activated macrophage with a modified epithelial-like appearance (epithelioid). A granuloma is a focal area of granulomatous inflammation consisting of an aggregation of macrophages (some of which may be epithelioid cells or may fuse into syncytium-like multinucleated giant epithelioid cells), which may or may not be surrounded by a collar of mononuclear leukocytes, principally lymphocytes and occasionally plasma cells. The histopathology of chronic inflammation is dominated by lymphocytes, plasma cells and mononuclear phagocytes, epithelioid cells, and sometimes, epithelioid giant cells.

Two features that are unique to the eye must also be defined; the blood-retina barrier and the immune privilege of the eye. The blood-retina barrier[2] is important for optimum function of the retina. Disturbances in the integrity of this barrier are common causes of retinal pathology and dysfunction, for example, cystoid macular edema, which may be seen after cataract extraction and in many inflammatory conditions. The blood-retina barrier is composed of two components. The tight junction complex of the retinal pigment epithelium forms the outer part of the blood-retina barrier; the retinal vascular endothelium forms the inner part of this barrier. The blood-retina barrier is similar to the blood-brain barrier (both the retinal pigment epithelium and the sensory neuroretina develop as an outpouching of the forebrain neuroectoderm). During fluorescein angiography, the normal fenestrated choriocapillaries are permeable to fluorescein, whereas the overlying retinal pigment epithelium (RPE) prevents the extravasation of dye into the subneurosensory retinal space. Normal retinal capillaries are not permeable to fluorescein, features that are at once a reflection of the blood-retina barrier concept and a marker for disease resulting in a breakdown of blood-retina barrier.

The eye has specific, unique immunologic features. Ocular immune privilege[3, 4, 5] is defined as follows: foreign tissues placed in the anterior chamber, the vitreous cavity (in the vitreous, only soluble but not particulate), the subretinal space or the corneal stroma experience extended or indefinite survival compared with similar tissues placed subcutaneously (a conventional immunizing, sensitizing site). Immune privilege is an active, antigen-specific process that produces immunologic tolerance. This systemic, antigen-specific, active immunologic tolerance is mediated by specific class I major histocompatibility complex (MHC)–restricted regulatory T lymphocytes. A wide variety of antigens have been injected into the anterior chamber (AC), and the immune response has generally been stereotypical. For example, this antigen-specific active immunologic tolerance enables rats pretreated with allogeneic lymphoid cells in the AC to accept for extended periods orthotopic skin grafts syngeneic with the AC-injected cells. The term AC-associated immune deviation (ACAID), was coined to describe this phenomenon and is characterized by the following features:

1. Suppressed helper T cell-mediated delayed-type hypersensitivity
2. Suppressed secretion by specific B lymphocytes of complement-fixing antibodies
3. Unimpaired development of primed cytotoxic T-cell responses mediated by CD8+ T lymphocytes
4. Unimpaired development of immunoglobulin G (IgG) non-complement–fixing serum antibodies

The regulatory mechanisms of ACAID can also suppress preformed memory and effector T cells that mediate delayed hypersensitivity. A systemic response identical to ACAID is also evoked when a soluble antigen is injected into the vitreous cavity or in the subretinal space. ACAID develops because intraocular antigen-presenting cells (APCs), under the influence of local immunomodulatory factors, capture intraocular antigenic material and migrate with it to the spleen via the blood stream (the eye is virtually devoid of lymphatics). In the spleen, these "deviant" APCs process and present antigen in a unique fashion, which enables them to present and activate distinct regulatory class I MHC-restricted T lymphocytes. These APCs do not activate delayed hypersensitivity class II MHC-restricted T cells. It has been experimentally shown that class I MHC molecules are indispensable for the genesis of ACAID.

The immunomodulatory properties of the AC are due to passive and active features. The passive features include the blood-ocular barrier, virtual absence of lymphatics and aqueous humor drainage to the blood stream; and reduced expression of class I and II MHC molecules. The active features that promote ACAID include the constitutive expression of inhibitory cell surface molecules on all cells surrounding the AC and immunomodulatory constituents of the aqueous humor. The constitutively expressed inhibitory cell surface molecules are Fas ligand, promoting apoptosis of activated T lymphocytes or any leukocytes exhibiting the Fas molecule; decay-accelerating factor (DAF); and CD59 and CD46.[6] DAF is a membrane protein that accelerates degradation of C3- and C5-convertase enzymes of both the classic and alternative complement pathways, and thus prevents further activation of the complement system. CD46, or membrane cofactor protein (MCP), is another membrane protein that acts as a cofactor for factor I–mediated proteolysis of C3b and C4b, and thus helps to down-regulate the activity of the complement system. CD59 (also called membrane inhibitor of reactive lysis) is a membrane protein and is the major membrane inhibitor of the membrane attack complex (MAC) of the complement system.

Soluble immunomodulatory constituents of the aqueous humor include transforming growth factor-β (TGF-β), alpha melanocyte stimulating hormone (α-MSH), vasoactive intestinal peptides (VIP), calcitonin gene–related peptide (CGRP), macrophage migration inhibition factor

TABLE 3–2. FEATURES OF IMMUNE PRIVILEGES IN THE EYE

PASSIVE FEATURES	ACTIVE FEATURES
Blood-ocular barrier	Constitutive expression of inhibitory cell surface molecules: Fas ligand, DAF, CD59, CD46
Deficient efferent lymphatics	Immunosuppressive microenvironment: TGF-β, α-MSH, VIP, CGRP, MIF, free cortisol
Aqueous drainage into the blood Reduced expression of major histocompatibility class I and II molecules	

DAF, decay-accelerating factor; TGF, transforming growth factor; VIP, vasoactive intestinal peptide; MIF, migration inhibition factor; CD46 is also called membrane cofactor protein; CD59 is also called membrane inhibitor of reactive lysis; CD, cluster of differentiation; MSH, melanocyte stimulating hormone; CGRP, calcitonin gene related peptide.

(MIF), and a high concentration of free cortisol (due to the impermeability of the blood-ocular barrier to cortisone-binding globulin) (Table 3–2).

ACAID is probably an evolutionary adaptation meant to provide the eye with those immune mechanisms that interfere with vision as little as possible by attenuating the potentially destructive "innocent bystander" effect of the immune inflammatory response to foreign antigen. It also helps avoid autoimmune diseases to unique ocular antigens, such as retinal S antigen. The extraordinary success of corneal allografts and intraocular retinal cells and transplants are partly explained by ACAID. On the other hand, ACAID has been implicated in the unfortunate progressive growth of intraocular tumors, the pathogenesis of stromal keratitis, and acute retinal necrosis due to the herpes virus.

CLASSIFICATION

Classification of uveitis is important for the following reasons:

1. The uvea consists of three continuous but distinct parts. One or more parts of the uvea may be inflamed, but others may not. In some cases, all three parts of the uvea are affected.
2. Uveitis may be caused by a vast number of highly variable conditions. Treatment and prognosis of one entity may be completely different from that of another (e.g., infectious uveitis and autoimmune uveitis).
3. Uveitis may be one of the features of a serious or life-threatening systemic disease (e.g., systemic vasculitis). In some cases, uveitis is the presenting feature of such a disease. Proper diagnosis and treatment of the uveitis and of the systemic condition can enormously enhance quality of life and reduce mortality.
4. Uveitis is an entity for which no causative agent may be found, despite the most thorough diagnostic investigations, in a number of cases. Accurately describing, characterizing, and classifying such cases may eventually help researchers and clinicians in elucidating the nature of such diseases.
5. Proper classification is essential if one is to avoid con-

fusion and misinterpretation. The anatomic classification should not be confused or overlap with the etiologic classification. Both classifications are required and important, but they are distinct and different.

Anatomic Classification

Uveitis may be classified anatomically into anterior, intermediate, posterior, and panuveitis. Different researchers and clinician groups have chosen, admittedly arbitrarily, to separate some of the various uveitic entities into these anatomic classification groups differently. For example, the International Uveitis Study Group (IUSG)[7] "partitions" the ciliary body into anterior and posterior layers, places iridocyclitis and anterior cyclitis into the "anterior" uveitis category, and reserves the "intermediate" uveitis category for patients with posterior cyclitis, pars planitis, and peripheral uveitis (Table 3–3). Retinal vasculitis is provided no anatomic home in the uveitis kingdom by the IUSG, although it is clear that patients with retinal vasculitis (for example, secondary to systemic lupus erythematosus or sarcoidosis) suffer from intraocular inflammation and are typically cared for by uveitis experts. Tessler[8] specifically recognized this in his classification system (see Table 3–3). In our Immunology and Uveitis Service of the Massachusetts Eye and Ear Infirmary (MEEI), we use the classification shown in Table 3–4. This is not to say that the world needs yet another anatomic classification scheme, nor that ours is better than theirs. However, we were urged to publish this text by others, with emphasis on how we do it at Harvard and MEEI; and because we find this system useful in organizing our thoughts in designing diagnostic and therapeutic strategies, we share it here with the readers. For us, anterior uveitis includes cases of iritis. Intermediate uveitis includes iridocyclitis, cyclitis, phacogenic (lens-induced) uveitis, pars planitis, Fuchs' heterochromic uveitis, and peripheral uveitis. Posterior uveitis includes focal, multifocal, or diffuse choroiditis; chorioretinitis; retinochoroiditis; retinal vasculitis; and neuroretinitis.

TABLE 3–3. ANATOMIC CLASSIFICATION OF UVEITIS

INTERNATIONAL UVEITIS STUDY GROUP (IUSG)	TESSLER
—	Sclerouveitis
—	Keratouveitis
Anterior uveitis: Iritis Anterior cyclitis Iridocyclitis	Anterior uveitis: Iritis Iridocyclitis
Intermediate uveitis (formerly known as pars planitis): Posterior cyclitis Hyalitis Basal retinochoroiditis	Intermediate uveitis: Cyclitis Vitritis Pars planitis
Posterior uveitis: Focal, multifocal, or diffuse choroiditis Chorioretinitis Retinochoroiditis Neurouveitis Panuveitis	Posterior uveitis: Retinitis Choroiditis

In his classification of uveitis into granulomatous and nongranulomatous forms, Tessler mentioned vascular sheathing as a possible fundus finding in both granulomatous and chronic nongranulomatous uveitis.

TABLE 3–4. ANATOMIC CLASSIFICATION OF UVEITIS IMMUNOLOGY AND UVEITIS SERVICE, MASSACHUSETTS EYE AND EAR INFIRMARY HARVARD MEDICAL SCHOOL

Anterior uveitis	Iritis
Intermediate uveitis	Iridocyclitis
	Cyclitis
	Fuchs' heterochromic iridocyclitis
	Phacogenic uveitis
	Pars planitis
	Peripheral uveitis
Posterior uveitis	Focal, multifocal, or diffuse choroiditis
	Chorioretinitis
	Retinochoroiditis
	Retinal vasculitis
	Neuroretinitis
Panuveitis	Inflammation of all three regions of the uvea
Sclerouveitis	Uveitis and scleritis
Keratouveitis	Uveitis and keratitis

Panuveitis is the term used to denote inflammation affecting all three of these anatomic regions of the eye.

In some diseases, uveitis may be accompanied by keratitis or scleritis (keratouveitis or sclerouveitis), giving another clue to the etiologic diagnosis, and hence, it is useful to clinicians to pay very careful attention to whether or not these areas of the outer ocular coat are specifically inflamed.

Pathologic Classification

Uveitis may also be classified as granulomatous or nongranulomatous on the basis of the predominant pathologic characteristics, with distinct etiologies, features, sequelae, and treatment for each category. Mutton fat keratic precipitates (KPs) composed predominantly of macrophages, Koeppe (pupillary border granulomas) and Busacca (iris stroma granulomas) nodules, large vitreous "snowballs" (clumps of macrophages and lymphocytes in the vitreous), retinal vascular "candle wax drippings" (clumps of inflammatory exudates along vessels), and granulomas in the choroid are characteristics of granulomatous inflammation typical of classic granulomatous diseases such as leprosy, tuberculosis, syphilis, sarcoidosis, sympathetic ophthalmia, and other disorders known to cause granulomatous inflammation. Other examples of such disorders include toxoplasmosis, toxocariasis, multiple sclerosis, Lyme disease, cat-scratch disease, Vogt-Koyanagi-Harada disease, leptospirosis, brucellosis, trypanosomiasis, histoplasmosis, actinomycosis, blastomycosis, coccidiodimycosis, aspergillosis, mucormycosis, onchocerciasis, hookworm disease, cysticercosis, and *Taenia solium* or *saginata* infection. And although this is a long list of possible etiologies for granulomatous uveitis, most clinicians would agree that characterizing a patient's uveitis as granulomatous is helpful in narrowing the diagnostic search to within the collection of known causes of granulomatous inflammation. The patient's history generally enables the ophthalmologist to eliminate further many unusual causes, such as fungi, parasites, and leprosy.

Onset and Course

Uveitis may also be categorized usefully according to its time course of onset and duration. The IUSG[7] has recommended the descriptors acute, subacute, chronic, and recurrent, with each episode evaluated separately, onset described as insidious or sudden, and duration considered acute (less than 3 months) or chronic (more than 3 months).

Unilateral vs. Bilateral

Some uveitic entities commonly occur bilaterally (e.g., acute posterior multifocal placoid pigment epitheliopathy [APMPPE]), whereas others commonly occur unilaterally (e.g., acute retinal pigment epitheliitis [ARPE]). This observation can obviously be helpful when one is considering two entities that share some similar characteristics, one of which has historically always been reported to be unilateral, whereas the other has always been bilateral. Careful examination of both eyes cannot be overstressed (Table 3–5).

Age, Race, and Sex

The patient's age, race, and sex may also help the clinician narrow the diagnostic possibilities, or at least help him or her take into consideration the probability of one disorder versus another. For example, juvenile rheumatoid arthritis–associated uveitis and *Toxocara* uveitis are common in young patients, whereas birdshot retinochoroidopathy and serpiginous choroiditis are not, but are more common in middle-aged individuals. Although intraocular lymphoma is usually a disease of older individuals (mean age 59 in one of the studies), the wise clinician remembers that odds are just odds and not, certainty. Patients in their teens and twenties who have been treated for extended periods for uveitis actually turned out to have the infamous uveitis masquerade, intraocular large cell lymphoma.

The patient's racial characteristics may also help focus the clinician's attention. Vogt-Koyanagi-Harada disease, for example, is much more common in darkly pigmented individuals (especially those with Asian background genetics), whereas presumed ocular histoplasmosis is very uncommon in such individuals.

Similarly, the patient's sex may be of some help in one's diagnostic confidence and in vigilance for evolution

TABLE 3–5. WHITE-DOT SYNDROMES

USUALLY BILATERAL	USUALLY UNILATERAL
Acute posterior multifocal placoid pigment epitheliopathy (APMPPE)	Acute retinal pigment epitheliitis (ARPE). *75% Unilateral*
Punctate inner choroiditis (PIC)	Multiple evanescent white-dot syndrome (MEWDS). *80% Unilateral*
Multifocal choroiditis and panuveitis (MCP). *82% Bilateral*	Diffuse unilateral subacute neuroretinitis (DUSN)
Subretinal fibrosis and uveitis syndrome (SFU). *Only women.*	Ophthalmomyasis
Presumed ocular histoplasmosis syndrome (POHS). *62% Bilateral*	
White dot fovea. *90% Bilateral*	
Birdshot retinochoroidopathy. *85% Bilateral*	
Serpiginous choroidopathy	

The following white-dot syndromes may be unilateral or bilateral:
AMN, acute macular neuroretinopathy; AIBSE/AIBESES, acute idiiopathic blind spot enlargement syndrome; AZOOR, acute zonal occult outer retinopthy.

of extraocular problems. For example, the male patient with unilateral recurrent non-granulomatous anterior uveitis, who is fluorescent treponemal antigen absorption (FTA-abs)-negative but human leukocyte antigen (HLA)–B27 positive and whose review of systems is negative should be advised to report any onset of joint or spine symptoms, because such individuals are at higher risk than the general population for spondyloarthropathies.

Etiologic Classification

Uveitis may also be classified and organized etiologically and pathophysiologically according to the following mechanisms:

- Traumatic
- Immunologic
- Infectious
- Masquerade

Much of this text is devoted to the specific syndromes and causes of uveitis, grouped into these four major categories for organizational and study purposes.

EPIDEMIOLOGY

Uveitis may affect individuals of any age from infancy on.[9, 10, 11] It also affects people from all parts of the world, and it is a highly significant cause of blindness.[12, 13, 14] The differential diagnosis of uveitis is extensive, changes with time, and is highly variable.[11, 15] It is influenced by numerous factors including genetic, ethnic, geographic, and environmental factors. Availability and quality of diagnostic investigations, diagnostic criteria, referral patterns (patient selection), and clinician's interests are other factors that contribute to the great diversity of etiology and reported epidemiologic profiles from various centers.[11, 15, 16]

The incidence[17] of uveitis in the United States is approximately 15 cases per 100,000 population per year or a total of some 38,000 new cases per year. The prevalence[10] in the United States and Western countries is 38 per 100,000. The incidence in other developed countries is very close to that of the United States: 14 in 100,000 per year in Denmark[18] and 17 per 100,00 per year in Savoy, France. There are no accurate estimates of the incidence and prevalence of uveitis in developing countries.

An examination of reported studies from different parts of the world[9, 11, 15, 20–26] shows that the mean age at presentation is approximately 40 years (Table 3–6). It also demonstrates that uveitis can affect people at virtually any age. Many patients in the pediatric age group, younger than 16 years, suffer devastating complications of uveitis (see later discussion). The peak age at onset of uveitis, in the third and fourth decades, magnifies the socioeconomic impact of uveitis on the individual and on the community.

Comparison of the percentage contribution of the different types of uveitis, from tertiary referral centers in different parts of the world (Table 3–7), shows that anterior uveitis is the most common form, followed by posterior or panuveitis; intermediate uveitis is the least common form but still comprises a significant number of cases (4% to 17% of all cases of uveitis).

Data from tertiary referral centers also reveals that

- Chronic uveitis is more common than acute and recurrent uveitis. Chronic uveitis is especially common in patients with intermediate uveitis.
- Nongranulomatous uveitis occurs more frequently than does granulomatous uveitis, especially in patients with anterior uveitis.
- Noninfectious uveitis is more common than is infectious uveitis, particularly among patients with panuveitis and anterior uveitis.
- Bilateral uveitis is more common than is unilateral uve-

TABLE 3–6. MEAN AGE, PEAK AGE AT PRESENTATION AND MALE:FEMALE RATIO

AUTHORS PLACE OF STUDY, AND TIMING OF THE STUDY	MEAN AGE AT PRESENTATION (RANGE)	PEAK AGE AT PRESENTATION	MALE:FEMALE RATIO	TOTAL NUMBER OF PATIENTS
Guyton and Woods, Baltimore (1925–39)	Younger than 1 year to 90 years	Third, fourth and fifth decades	312:250	562
Perkins and Folk, London and Iowa, (London 1956 to 1960, Iowa ? 1980)	Not available	Not available	3:2 (acute anterior uveitis)	1718 +172
James et al, London (1963 to 1974)	4 y to older than 60 y	Third and fourth decade	1:1	368 all are inpatients
Weiner and BenEzra, Israel (1982 to 1988)	6 to 75 years	Not available	1.4:1	400
Rothova et al, The Netherlands (1984 to 1989)	42 years (3 to 91 years)	Third and fourth decade	1:1	865
Rosenthal et al, Leicester, UK (1985 to 1995)	39.2 (1.7 to 95 years)	Not available	52.1:47.9	712
Foster et al, New England, USA (1982 to 1992)	37.2 years (1 to 79 years)	Not available	1:1.4	1237
Baarsma and Vries, Rotterdam (? 1990 to 1992)	(5 y–85 y) children mostly excluded	Third and fourth decade	48:52	750
Merrill and Jaffe, southeast USA (1989 to 1994)	(6 to 86 years)	Not available	38:62	385
Biswas and Ganesh, India (Jan 1992 to Dec 1994)	Younger than 10 years to older than 60 years	Fourth decade	62:38	1273

TABLE 3–7. SUMMARIZES THE PERCENTAGE CONTRIBUTION OF THE DIFFERENT ANATOMIC TYPES OF UVEITIS IN DIFFERENT PARTS OF THE WORLD

AUTHORS (YEAR OF PUBLICATION)	ANTERIOR UVEITIS (%)	INTERMEDIATE UVEITIS (%)	POSTERIOR UVEITIS (%)	PANUVEITIS (%)	TOTAL NUMBER
Guyton and Woods; Maryland, USA. 1941	37.3	Not available	27.4	35.2	562
Perkins; Iowa, USA, 1984	59.0	5.0	21	16	172
Henderly et al; California, USA, 1987	28.0	15.0	38.0	18.0	600
Palmers et al; Portugal, 1990	60.0	4.0	24.0	12.0	450
Karaman K, et al; Yugoslavia, 1990	61.8	5.3	18.4	14.5	152
Weiner and BenAzra; Israel, 1991	45.8	15.2	14.2	24.5	400
Opermack; Ohio, USA, 1992	36.0	17.0	28.0	19.0	854
Rothova et al; Holland, 1992	54.5	8.8	16.4	20.3	865
Vassileva; Bulgaria, 1992	51.0	3.0	25.0	21.0	315
Soylu et al; Turkey, 1993	39.9	7.7	16.8	35.5	363
Li and Yang; China, 1994	45.7	11.0	9.3	34.0	Not available
Trant et al; Switzerland, 1994	61.0	10.0	21.0	7.0	558
Pivetti-Pezzi et al; Italy, 1996	49.1	12.4	22.1	16.4	1,417
Foster et al; New England, USA, 1996	51.6	13.0	19.4	16	1,237
Merrill et al; southeast USA, 1997	25.0	12.0	24.0	38.0	385
Juberias and Calonge; Spain, 1997	50.2	10.1	29.6	10.1	297

itis in patients with panuveitis and intermediate uveitis. Anterior and posterior uveitis cases have approximately equal distribution of unilateral and bilateral cases.

- The mean age at onset is clearly younger in patients with intermediate uveitis, 30.7 year (± 15.1).
- Despite the huge advance in diagnostic techniques and the determination of ophthalmologists worldwide to reach an etiologic diagnosis, many cases remain in the idiopathic category (35% to 50%). The term idiopathic uveitis denotes that the intraocular inflammation could not be attributed to a specific ocular cause or to an underlying systemic disease, and it was not characteristic of a recognized uveitic entity.
- The most common causes of anterior uveitis are idiopathic, 37.8%; seronegative HLA-B27–associated ar-

thropathies, 21.6% (mainly nonspecific arthropathy, ankylosing spondylitis, Reiter's disease and inflammatory bowel disease [ulcerative colitis, Crohn's disease, and Whipple's disease]; psoriatic arthropathy also contributed a small proportion to this group); juvenile rheumatoid arthritis, 10.8%; herpetic uveitis, 9.7% (herpes simplex and herpes zoster); sarcoidosis, 5.85%; Fuchs' heterochromic iridocyclitis, 5.0%; systemic lupus erythematosus, 3.3%; intraocular lens–induced persistent uveitis, 1.2%; Posner-Schlossman syndrome, 0.9%; rheumatoid arthritis, 0.9%. Syphilis, tuberculosis, phacogenic uveitis, Lyme disease, and collagen vascular disease (Wegener's granulomatosis, polyarteritis nodosa, and relapsing polychondritis) caused some cases of anterior uveitis (Fig. 3–1).

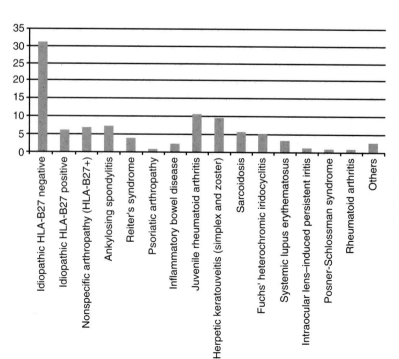

FIGURE 3–1. Relative frequency of the most common causes of anterior uveitis. (Data from Rodriguez A, Calonge M, Foster CS, et al: Referral patterns of uveitis in a tertiary eye care center. Arch Ophthalmol 1996;114:593–596.)

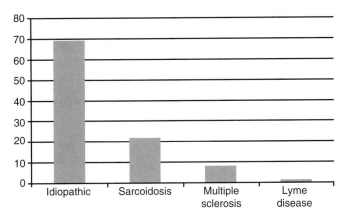

FIGURE 3–2. Relative frequency (%) of the most common causes of intermediate uveitis. (Data from Rodriguez A, Calonge M, Foster CS, et al: Referral patterns of uveitis in a tertiary eye care center. Arch Ophthalmol 1996;114:593–596.)

- The most common causes of intermediate uveitis are idiopathic, 69.1%; sarcoidosis, 22.2%; multiple sclerosis, 8.0%; and Lyme disease, 0.6% (Fig 3–2).
- The most common causes of posterior uveitis are toxoplasmosis, 24.6%; idiopathic, 12.3%; cytomegalovirus retinitis, 11.6%; systemic lupus erythematosus, 7.9%; birdshot retinochoroidopathy, 7.9%; sarcoidosis, 7.5%; acute retinal necrosis syndrome, 5.5%; Epstein-Barr virus retinochoroiditis, 2.9%; toxocariasis, 2.5%; Adamantiades-Behçet's disease (ABD), 2.0%; syphilis, 2.0%; acute posterior multifocal placoid pigment epitheliopathy (APMPPE), 2.0%; and serpiginous choroidopathy, 1.65%. Other causes of posterior uveitis include punctate inner choroidopathy (PIC), multiple evanescent white-dot syndrome (MEWDS), multiple sclerosis, temporal arteritis, presumed ocular histoplasmosis, fungal retinitis, and leukemia (Fig. 3–3).

- The most common causes of panuveitis are idiopathic, 22.2%; sarcoidosis, 14.1%; multifocal choroiditis and panuveitis, 12.1%; ABD, 11.6%; systemic lupus erythematosus, 9.1%; syphilis, 5.5%; Vogt-Koyanagi-Harada syndrome, 5.5%; HLA-B27 associated, 4.5%; sympathetic ophthalmia, 4.0%; tuberculosis, 2.0%; fungal retinitis, 2.0%. Other causes of panuveitis include bacterial panophthalmitis, intraocular lymphoma, relapsing polychondritis, polyartertitis nodosa, leprosy, dermatomyositis and progressive systemic sclerosis (Fig. 3–4).

The above-mentioned percentages and figures were obtained from a study of 1237 uveitis patients referred to the Uveitis and Immunology Service of the MEEI,[11] Harvard Medical School, from 1982 to 1992. The study was published in 1996. These figures were found to be similar to the results of other studies of tertiary referral centers from different parts of the world,[9, 11, 19, 25] especially those of developed countries.

Most uveitis cases are first seen and treated by the general (comprehensive) ophthalmologists, who may or may not refer the patients to a uveitis specialist. In a study[26] comparing the epidemiologic differences between community-based patients (seen by comprehensive ophthalmologists) and university referral patients (seen by a uveitis sub-specialist) in the University of California at Los Angeles (UCLA) community (Table 3–8), the results showed that anterior uveitis was much more common in the community-based population, whereas the other anatomic types of uveitis were more common in the university referral patients, highlighting the referral bias of the more difficult, vision-threatening cases to the specialist (Fig. 3–5). There were no significant differences in the mean age at presentation or sex and race distribution.[26]

The influence of genetic factors on the etiopathogenesis of uveitis is clearly shown by the close relationship of some specific uveitic entities and the MHC. Some

FIGURE 3–3. Relative frequency (%) of the most common causes of posterior uveitis. (Data from Rodriguez A, Calonge M, Foster CS, et al: Referral patterns of uveitis in a tertiary eye care center. Arch Ophthalmol 1996;114: 593–596.)

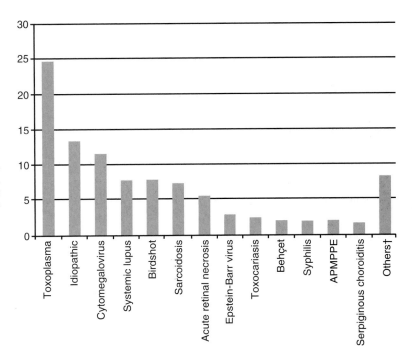

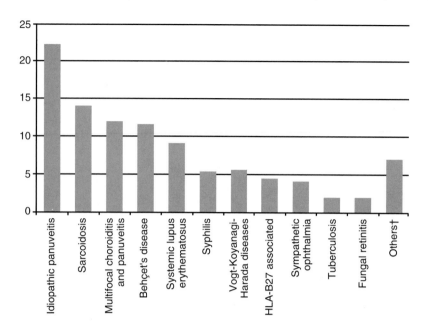

FIGURE 3–4. Relative frequency (%) of the most common causes of panuveitis (Data from Rodriguez A, Calonge M, Foster CS, et al: Referral patterns of uveitis in a tertiary eye care center. Arch Ophthalmol 1996;114:593–596.)

histocompatibility genes[6, 18] appear to act as a "first-hit" immune response gene (*IR* gene) conspiring with a "second-hit," mostly yet unidentified, environmental factor for the development of a specific uveitis entity. HLA-A29 + individuals[19] have at least a 50 times higher chance of developing birdshot retinochoroidopathy than do individuals who did not inherit this HLA gene. HLA-A29 is a class I MHC molecule with a frequency of 7% to 8% in the population of Europe and the United States. Similarly, HLA-B27 genotype is clearly associated with an increased risk of developing inflammation in the eye, the spine, the bowel, or any combination thereof. ABD[18] and HLA-B51, a subtype of HLA-B5, is another example for the influence of genetics on the risk for development of a uveitic entity (ABD). Adamantiades-Behçet's disease is especially common in areas in which the HLA-B51 gene is prevalent in the gene pool (e.g., Asia and the Middle East).

The relative diagnostic frequencies of uveitis continue to change with time, possibly because of a better understanding of the different uveitic entities associated with systemic diseases, evolution of better diagnostic techniques, and real changes in disease frequency. The classic infectious causes of uveitis, tuberculosis and syphilis, which had been dramatically suppressed with the dawn of the antibiotic era, are now re-emerging as increasingly important causes of uveitis. New atypical mycobacteria resistant to most antibiotics are becoming more common. The acquired immunodeficiency syndrome (AIDS) epidemic is responsible for many opportunistic viral, bacterial, fungal, and parasitic infections, and in general, it appears as if infectious causes of uveitis may be emerging as increasingly important, epidemiologically, in the uveitis population.

The epidemiologic importance of uveitis in children deserves special mention. Patients with uveitis starting before the age of 16 years[15] represent 5% to 10% of the total uveitis population. Uveitis is a serious, potentially

TABLE 3–8. FREQUENCY OF GENERAL UVEITIS CASES (EXCLUDING CYTOMEGALOVIRUS RETINOPATHY) BASED ON ANATOMIC LOCATION

	COMMUNITY-BASED PATIENTS (N = 213) (%)	UNIVERSITY REFERRAL PATIENTS (N = 213) (%)	P VALUE
Anterior uveitis:			
Total	193 (90.6)	129 (60.6)	<.0001
Cases with specific diagnosis	83 (43.0)	66 (51.2)	.15
Intermediate uveitis:			
Total	3 (1.4)	26 (12.2)	<.0001
Cases with specific diagnosis	3 (100)	18 (69.2)	.54
Posterior uveitis:			
Total	10 (4.7)	31 (14.6)	<.0006
Cases with specific diagnosis	9 (90)	25 (80.6)	.66
Panuveitis:			
Total	3 (1.4)	20 (9.4)	<.0003
Cases with specific diagnosis	3 (100)	13 (65.0)	.53
Other types			
Total	4 (1.9)	7 (3.3)	.36
Cases with specific diagnosis	3 (75)	1 (14.3)	.09

Other types includes endophthalmitis, isolated vitreous reaction and inflammation involving more than one anatomic location.

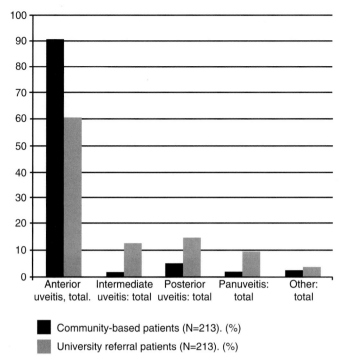

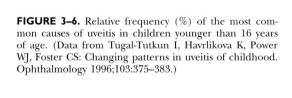

Community-based patients (N=213). (%)

University referral patients (N=213). (%)

FIGURE 3–5. Comparison of the frequency of the different types of uveitis in tertiary referral centers and general ophthalmology clinic (community based patients). (Data from McCannel CA, Holland GN, Helm CJ et al: Causes of uveitis in the general practice of ophthalmology. UCLA Community-Based Uveitis Study Group. Am J Ophthalmol 1996;121:35–46.)

vision-robbing problem for anyone. But it is an especially cruel[15, 28] disease in children and is associated with unique problems. The manner of initial presentation and treatment options differ significantly from those of adults. Children with uveitis may be asymptomatic due to the preverbal age of the child, or they may actually be asymptomatic because of the insidious nature of the disease.

Consequently, the child may already have serious complications of chronic uveitis at initial presentation to the ophthalmologist. Furthermore, the adverse effects of prolonged topical steroid use and the risks of systemic treatment must be considered carefully in young patients who have developing skeletal and reproductive systems. In our study[28] of 130 patients 16 years of age and younger, referred to the Uveitis and Immunology Service of the MEEI, Harvard Medical School, between 1982 to 1992, the causes of uveitis were as follows:

• Juvenile rheumatoid arthritis (JRA)–associated uveitis was the largest group (41.5%), followed by idiopathic uveitis (21.5%) and pars planitis (15.3%). Toxoplasmosis accounted for 7.7%; toxocariasis, 3.1%; sarcoidosis, 2.3%; Vogt-Koyanagi-Harada syndrome, 2.0%; acute retinal necrosis syndrome, 2.0%; HLA-B27+–associated uveitis, 1.0%; Reiter's syndrome, 1.0%, and also 1.0% each for systemic lupus erythematosus, Adamantiades-Behçet's disease, Fuchs' heterochromic iridocyclitis, tubulointerstitial nephritis and uveitis syndrome (TINU); and chickenpox (Fig. 3–6).

Uveitis in developing countries[13, 19, 29, 30] has distinct epidemiologic features. Uveitis as a cause of significant visual loss and blindness is often underestimated in these countries.[13, 29] Common complications of uveitis, such as cataract and glaucoma, were cited as the main causes of visual loss and blindness in many statistical studies from regions where proper ophthalmic care is often deficient. The fact that uveitis is the primary offender is often overlooked.

Onchocerciasis, a parasitic infection, is an important cause of uveitis in central Africa, extending into Yemen. About 17.5 million persons are infected in this area; 270,000 are blind from the disease. It is caused by infection with *Onchocerca volvulus* through the bite of an infected black fly, *Simulium damnosum*, which breeds in fast-flowing rivers. An adult worm can live up to 17 years in

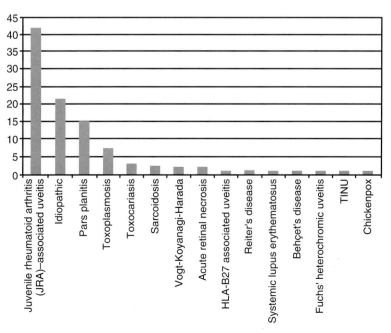

FIGURE 3–6. Relative frequency (%) of the most common causes of uveitis in children younger than 16 years of age. (Data from Tugal-Tutkun I, Havrlikova K, Power WJ, Foster CS: Changing patterns in uveitis of childhood. Ophthalmology 1996;103:375–383.)

nodules in the skin or other organs of an infected person, producing millions of microfilariae in its lifetime. These microfilariae can migrate through the body and tend to concentrate in the skin or the eye, where they cause inflammation. Onchocerciasis causes anterior uveitis, posterior uveitis, or panuveitis. It also may cause snowflake opacities in the cornea, sclerosing keratitis, glaucoma, retinal vasculitis, and optic atrophy. Uveitis is the second leading cause of blindness in developing countries.

Uveitis is also a significant cause of blindness[12, 14] and visual impairment in developed countries. It accounts for 10% to 15%[12] of all cases of blindness in the United States. In a study by Rothova and associates[14] published in 1996 on 582 uveitis patients in the Netherlands, 35% suffered from significant visual loss in a mean follow-up period of 4.3 years. Bilateral legal blindness developed in 4.0%; 4.5% had one blind eye, with visual impairment of the other; and 1.5% had bilateral visual impairment. Unilateral visual loss occurred in 25.0%, unilateral blindness in 14%, and unilateral visual impairment in 11.0%. Legal blindness was defined as a best-corrected visual acuity of 0.1 for the better eye; visual impairment was defined as best-corrected visual acuity equal to or less than 0.3 for the eye with better vision. The final visual acuity (not the worst visual acuity at any visit) was used for evaluation. The most important causes of visual loss were irreversible cystoid macular edema, macular inflammatory lesions, retinal vascular abnormalities, and retinal detachment. The systemic diseases associated with the worst visual prognoses were juvenile chronic arthritis and sarcoidosis.

SUMMARY

Uveitis affects patients of all ages. It is prevalent all over the globe, and it is one of the leading causes of visual loss worldwide. The peak age at onset (third and fourth decades) during highly productive years, and the potential for severe visual loss (10% to 15% of all cases of blindness in the United States is due to uveitis) underscores the gravity and devastating impact of uveitis on patients and communities. Awareness of the characteristic clinical and epidemiologic features of the different uveitic entities is essential in making an accurate diagnosis and instituting early appropriate treatment in an effort to minimize the damage caused by the disease (uveitis is caused by a vast number of completely different conditions, and the treatment of each entity may be accordingly different). Uveitis patients from infancy to the age of 16 years compose 5% to 10% of the total uveitis population; the disease is particularly cruel to this group. Pediatricians should be aware of this important fact, especially because the disease is usually silent and asymptomatic. Pediatricians and teachers, from preschool through secondary school, should routinely perform vision screening.

References

1. Cotran RS, Kumar V, Robbins SL, eds: Pathologic Basis of Disease, 5th ed. Philadelphia, W.B. Saunders, 1994, p 51.
2. Albert DM, Jakobiec FA, eds: Principles and Practice of Ophthalmology. Philadelphia, WB Saunders, 1994.
3. Streilein JW: Anterior chamber associated immune deviation: The privilege of immunity in the Eye. Surv Ophthalmol 1990;35:67–73.
4. Streilein JW, Foster CS: Immunology; An overview. In: Albert DM, Jakobiec FA, eds: Principles and Practice of Ophthalmology, 2nd ed. Philadelphia, WB Saunders, 1999, pp 47–49.
5. Streilein JW, Foster CS: Regulation of immune responses. In: Albert DM, Jakobiec FA, eds: Principles and Practice of Ophthalmology, 2nd ed. 1999, Section II, Ch 10, pp 83–84.
6. Abbas AK, Lichtman AH, Pober JS: Cellular and Molecular Immunology, 3rd ed. Philadelphia, WB Saunders, 1997.
7. Bloch-Michel E, Nussenblatt RB: International Uveitis Study Group recommendations for the evaluation of intraocular inflammatory disease. Am J Ophthalmol 1987;103:234–235.
8. Tessler HH: Classification and symptoms and signs of uveitis. In: Duane TD, Jeager EA, eds: Clinical Ophthalmology, Revised ed, Vol 4. Philadelphia, Lippincott Williams & Wilkins, 1998, pp 1–9.
9. Guyton JS, Woods AC: Etiology of uveitis; a clinical study of 562 cases. Arch Ophthalmol 1941;26:983–1018.
10. Thean LH, Thompson J, Rosenthal AR: A uveitis register at the Leicester Royal Infirmary. Ophthalmic Epidemiology 1996–1997;3–4:151–158.
11. Rodriguez A, Calonge M, Pedroza-Seres M, et al: Referral pattern of uveitis in a tertiary eye care center. Arch Ophthalmol 1996;114:593–599.
12. Suttorp MSA, Rothova A: The possible impact of uveitis in blindness: a literature survey. Br J Ophthalmol 1996;80:844–848.
13. Ronday MJH, Stilma JS, Rothova A: Blindness from uveitis in a hospital population in Sierra Leone. Br J Ophthalmol 1994;9:690–693
14. Rothova A, Suttorp-van Schulten MSA, Treffers WF, et al: Causes and frequency of blindness in patients with intraocular inflammatory disease. Br J Ophthalmol 1996;4:332–336.
15. Foster CS, Tugal-Tutkun I, Havrlikova K, Power WJ: Changing patterns in uveitis of childhood. Ophthalmology 1996;103:375–383.
16. Rothova A, Buitenhuis HJ, Meenken C, et al: Uveitis and systemic diseases. Br J Ophthalmol 1992;70:137–141.
17. Silverstein A: Changing trends in the etiological diagnosis of uveitis. Documenta Ophthalmologica 1997;94:25–37.
18. Baarsma GS. The epidemiology and genetics of endogenous uveitis; a review. Curr Eye Res 1992;11(Suppl):1–9.
19. Biswas J, Narain S, Das D, et al: Pattern of uveitis in a referral uveitis clinic in India. Int Ophthalmol 1996;20:223–228.
20. Merrill PT, Kim J, Cox TA, et al: Uveitis in the southeastern United States. Curr Eye Res 1997;9:865–874.
21. Perkins ES, Folk J: Uveitis in London and Iowa. Ophthalmologica 1984;189:36–40
22. Smit RLMJ, Baarsman GS, DeVries J: Classification of 750 consecutive uveitis patients in the Rotterdam Eye Hospital. Int Ophthalmol 1993;17:71–75
23. James DG, Friedmann AI, Graham E: Uveitis; A series of 368 patients. Trans Ophthalmol Soc UK 1976;6:108–112
24. Henderly DE, Genstler AJ, Smith RE, Rao NA: Changing patterns of uveitis. Am J Ophthalmol 1987;103:131–136
25. Weiner A, BenEzra D: Clinical patterns and associated conditions in chronic uveitis. Am J Ophthalmol 1991;112:151–158.
26. McCannel CA, Holland GN, Helm CJ, et al: Causes of uveitis in the general practice of ophthalmology. Am J Ophthalmol 1996;121:35–46.
27. Nussenblatt RB, Palestine AG, eds: Uveitis: Fundamentals and Clinical Practice, Mosby, St. Louis, 1989.
28. Dana MR, Merayo-Lloves J, Schaumberg DA, Foster CS: Visual outcomes prognosticators in juvenile rheumatoid arthritis–associated uveitis. Ophthalmology 1997;104:236–244.
29. Darrell RW, Wagener HP, Kurland LT: Epidemiology of uveitis. Arch Ophthalmol 1962;68:502–515.
30. Ronday M: Uveitis in Africa, with Emphasis on Toxoplasmosis. Amsterdam, Netherlands Ophthalmic Research Institute of the Royal Netherlands Academy of Arts and Sciences, Dept. of Ophthalmology, 1996.

4 GENERAL PRINCIPLES AND PHILOSOPHY

C. Stephen Foster

Uveitis is such a small word, and yet in common usage in most medical circles it encompasses the entire spectrum of intraocular inflammation: iritis, iridocyclitis, pars planitis, posterior uveitis, choroiditis, retinitis, retinal vasculitis. It is such a small word, and yet, like cancer, the condition itself can devastate not only the life of the patient with it but the lives of the patient's family as well. And it does so not only through its capacity to rob people of eyesight but also through its protracted evolution, with the financial and emotional toll that comes with a slowly progressive yet ocularly pernicious problem. It is estimated that the United States federal budget costs for the uveitic blind (no medical costs, but simply the federal and state benefits to which legally blind individuals are entitled) annually amounts to approximately 242.6 million dollars, a figure nearly identical to that for diabetic patients.[1] Suttorp-Schulten and Rothova, in their brilliant analysis of the role which uveitis plays in world blindness, have emphasized that among the 2.3 million individuals in the United States alone with uveitis each year, many have an underlying systemic disease, which, if left undiagnosed, may be potentially lethal.[2] These authors also point out that, although uveitis accounts for 10% of the blindness in the United States, it accounts for even greater numbers of patients who, although not legally blind, have substantial visual impairment. They have estimated that perhaps as many as 35% of patients with uveitis have visual impairment of one type or another.[3] One might have thought that we would have done better than this over the past 50 years, since the introduction of corticosteroids for medical care.

THE PROBLEM

The problem of uveitis is a problem of truly epic proportions. It is worldwide, it is prevalent, it is an important cause of permanent structural damage that produces irrevocable blindness, it can occur as a consequence of many causes (indeed, this textbook contains at least 65 chapters devoted to specific individual causes of uveitis), and it does not lend itself to the quick diagnosis, elucidation, and eradication of the underlying cause to which ophthalmologists have grown accustomed in modern ophthalmic practice. Instead, care of the patient with uveitis is much more akin to the practice of internal medicine than it is to ophthalmology. And ophthalmologists, in general, are not terribly enthusiastic about the vagaries, uncertainties, and protracted diagnostic hunt and chronic therapy inherent to an internist's life.

Ocular immunologists are committed to this type of life and to the care of patients with ocular inflammatory disease. Happily, a great many more training programs for the training of ocular immunologists exist today than existed just two decades ago. Although the number of ophthalmologists interested in the care of patients with uveitis was quite small in the 1960s (the American Uveitis Society began in the 1970s with just 40 members), the number today is considerably larger; the current membership in the American Uveitis Society is 159. We believe this expanding resource for the comprehensive ophthalmologist is likely to make a significant difference in the prevalence of blindness secondary to uveitis in the future. But this will be true only if general mindsets of comprehensive ophthalmologists in developed countries change, philosophically, with respect to therapeutic vigor and diagnostic efforts. As long as large numbers of ophthalmologists continue to harbor the beliefs that "you rarely find the underlying cause, and so making a big effort to find the cause is useless," and "it's too dangerous to consider systemic chemotherapy for a patient who just has uveitis," too few referrals to ocular immunologists will be made, and uveitis will continue to be a major cause of preventable blindness 50 years from now.

PHILOSOPHY

Two major philosophical principles have guided our service and have distinguished it from many others over the past 25 years: diagnostic vigor and therapeutic aggressiveness. We believe that the diagnosis of a patient's underlying uveitis matters a great deal, and therefore, we make a serious effort to diagnose the underlying cause of the patient's uveitis. We do so primarily through an extensive review of systems health questionnaire and through the ocular examination. We expand beyond this minimum work-up if the patient has more than three episodes of uveitis, if the patient's uveitis is granulomatous, if we find positive diagnostic leads from the review of systems questionnaire, if the patient has posterior uveitis or retinal vasculitis, or if the patient does not improve (and certainly if the patient worsens) on steroid therapy. Our approach to these matters is addressed in great detail in Chapter 6, Diagnosis of Uveitis.

Our guiding therapeutic principles are to treat specifically for treatable diseases (e.g., administering penicillin for syphilis, and radiation and chemotherapy for lymphoma), and to use steroids as the first step on a therapeutic stepladder algorithm except in the instance of a patient with infectious disease and in patients with potentially lethal disease who need to go to the final step on the ladder immediately (e.g., cyclophosphamide for a patient whose retinal vasculitis is secondary to Wegener's granulomatosis or to polyarteritis nodosa). We use steroids through all routes required for abolition of active inflammation. We use them aggressively, subsequently tapering to total discontinuation (Tables 4–1 to 4–3). The long-term chronic use of steroid therapy is to be abhorred; the consequences of such long-term therapy are far too well known now for reasonable ophthalmologists to accept this form of therapy indefinitely.

TABLE 4–1. OPHTHALMIC TOPICAL CORTICOSTEROID PREPARATIONS

DRUG/PREPARATION	COMMON TRADE NAME	FORMULATION
Dexamethasone		
Alcohol	Maxidex (Alcon)	0.1% suspension
Sodium phosphate	Decadron Phosphate (MSD)	0.1% solution, 0.05% ointment
Prednisolone		
Acetate	Pred Forte (Allergan), Econopred Plus (Alcon), AK-Tate (Akorn)	1.0% suspension
	Pred Mild (Allergan), Econopred (Alcon)	0.12% suspension
Sodium phosphate	Inflamase Forte (CIBA Vision, Duluth, GA); AK-Pred (Akorn),	1% solution
Metreton	(Schering); Hydeltrasol (MSD)	0.5% solution
	Inflamase Mild (CIBA Vision), AK-Pred (Akorn) Hydeltrasol	0.125% solution
	(MSD)	0.25% ointment
Fluoromethalone		
Alcohol	FML (Allergan)	0.1% suspension, 0.1% ointment
Medroxyprogesterone		
Acetate	Provera	1% suspension
Medrysone		
Alcohol	HMS (Allergan)	1.0% suspension
Rimexolone	Vexol (Alcon)	
Loteprednol	Lotemax (Bausch & Lomb)	0.5% suspension

If a patient with recurrent noninfectious uveitis continues to experience recurrences each time steroids are discontinued, we typically offer that patient advancement to the second rung on our therapeutic ladder, provided no contraindications exist to such therapy: chronic use of an oral nonsteroidal anti-inflammatory drug (NSAID).

Our experience has been that many patients (e.g., approximately 70% of patients with recurrent idiopathic uveitis or with recurrent HLA-B27–associated uveitis) can be maintained in long-term remission with such chronic NSAID use. The usual caveats pertain but particularly now with the availability of the Cox-2–specific NSAIDs,

TABLE 4–2. SYSTEMIC CORTICOSTEROID PREPARATIONS

DRUG	COMMON TRADE NAME	ORAL FORMULATION	FORMULATION
Hydrocortisone	Cortef (Upjohn, Kalamazoo, MI)	5- to 20-mg tablet 10-mg/5-ml suspension	25- and 50-mg suspension IM
Sodium phosphate	Hydrocortone Phosphate (MSD, West Point, PA)		50-mg/ml solution IM/IV
Sodium succinate	Solu-Cortef (Upjohn)		100- to 1000-mg powder IM/IV
Prednisone	Deltasone (Upjohn)	1.0- to 50-mg tablet	
	Meticorten (Shering, Kenilworth, NJ)		
	Drasone (Solvay, Marietta, GA)		
	Liquid Pred (Muro, Tewksbury, MA)	5-mg/ml solution	
Prednisolone	Delta-Cortef (Upjohn)	1- to 5-mg tablet	
	Prelone (Muro)	15-mg/5-ml syrup	
Acetate	Predalone (Forest, St. Louis, MO)		25- to 100-mg/ml suspension IM
Sodium phosphate	Hydeltrasol (MSD)		20-mg/ml solution IM/IV
Methylprednisolone	Medrol (Upjohn)	2- to 32-mg tablet	
Acetate	Depo-Medrol (Upjohn)		20- to 80-mg/ml suspension IM
Sodium succinate	Solu-Medrol (Upjohn)		40- to 1000-mg powder IM/IV
Triamcinolone			
Diacetate	Kenacort (Apothecon, Princeton, NJ)	4-mg/5-ml syrup	
Dracetate	Aristocort (Fujisawa, Deerfield, IL)	1- to 8-mg tablet	40-mg/ml suspension IM
Acetonide	Kenalog (Westwood-Squibb, Princeton, NJ)		10- and 40-mg/ml suspension IM
Dexamethasone sodium	Decadron (MSD)	0.25- to 6.0-mg tablet 0.5-mg/5-ml elixir 0.5-mg/5-ml solution	
Dexamethasone			
Sodium phosphate	Decadron Phosphate (MSD)		24-mg/ml solution IV
Acetate	Decadron-LA (MSD)		8-mg/ml suspension
Betamethasone	Celestone (Schering)	0.6-mg tablet 0.6-mg/5-ml syrup	
Sodium phosphate	Celestone Phosphate (Schering)		3-mg/ml solution IV
Acetate and sodium phosphate	Celestone Soluspan (Schering)		3 × 3 mg/ml suspension

IM, intramuscular; IV, intravenous.

TABLE 4–3. REGIONAL CORTICOSTEROID PREPARATIONS

DRUG	COMMON TRADE NAMES	FORMULATION	ROUTE AND TYPICAL DOSE
Hydrocortisone	Hydrocortisone Sodium Succinate (MSD, West Point, PA)	100–1000-mg powder	Subconjunctival/Tenon 50–125 mg
Methylprednisolone			
Sodium succinate	Solu-Medrol (Upjohn, Kalamazoo, MI)	40-mg/ml, 125-mg/ml, 2-g/30-ml solution	Subconjunctival/Tenon 40–125 mg
Acetate	Depo-Medrol (Upjohn)	20- to 80-mg/ml (depot) suspension	Transseptal, retrobulbar 40–80 mg/0.5 ml
Triamcinolone			
Diacetate	Aristocort (Fujisawa, Deerfield, IL)	25- and 40-mg/ml suspension	Subconjunctival/Tenon 40 mg
Acetonide	Kenalog (Westwood-Squibb, Princeton, NJ)	10- and 40-mg/ml suspension	Transseptal 40 mg
Dexamethasone			
Acetate	Decadron-LA (MSD)	8- to 16-mg/ml suspension	Subconjunctival/Tenon 4–8 mg, Transseptal 4–8 mg
Sodium phosphate	Decadron Phosphate (MSD)	4-, 10-, 24-mg/ml solution	Retrobulbar, intravitreal 0.4 mg
Betamethasone acetate and sodium phosphate	Celestone Soluspan (Schering, Kenilworth, TX)	3-mg/ml suspension	Subconjunctival/Tenon, transseptal, 1 mg

Subconjunctival/Tenon, subconjunctival or sub-Tenon injection.

the risk-benefit therapeutic ratio has shifted even further toward the benefit side of chronic use of such medication (Table 4–4).

Immunomodulatory therapy is offered next to the patient who continues to experience recurrences of uveitis despite the chronic use of an oral NASID, and within this category of immunomodulators, a "ladder" exists with respect to the risk-benefit ratio (Table 4–5). All of these matters are addressed in detail in Chapters 8 to 12. Clearly, the comprehensive ophthalmologist will not want or need the aggravation associated with taking primary responsibility for monitoring of potential toxicity in a patient on systemic medication, immunomodulators, and perhaps, even the NSAIDs. He or she may want to refer the patient to an ocular immunologist for monitoring. Alternatively, the ophthalmologist may be able to establish a productive collaboration with a hematologist, oncologist, or rheumatologist who would be willing to take on the responsibility of chemotherapeutic monitoring, who, in turn, would take guidance from the ophthalmologist regarding the patient's ocular status and the need for more vigorous therapy because of incomplete resolution

TABLE 4–4. SYSTEMIC NONSTEROIDAL ANTI-INFLAMMATORY AGENTS

DRUG CLASS	DRUG Generic	DRUG Trade Name	SUPPLIED (mg)	TYPICAL ADULT DAILY DOSE (mg)
Salicylates	Aspirin	Multiple	325–925	650 every 4 h
	Diflunisal	Dolobid (MSD, West Point, PA)	250, 500	250–500 bid
Fenamates	Mefenamate	Pronstel (Parke-Davis, Morris Plains, NJ)	250	250 qid
Indoles	Indomethacin	Indocin (MSD)	25, 50, 75(SR)	25–50 tid–qid, 75 bid
	Sulindac	Clinoril (MSD)	150, 200	150–200 bid
	Tolmetrin	Tolectin (McNeil, Raritan, NJ)	200, 400, 600	400 tid
Phenylacetic acids	Diclofenac	Voltaren (Geigy, Summit, NJ)	25, 50, 75, 100	50–75 bid
Phenylalkanoic acids	Fenoprofen	Nalfon (Lilly, Indianapolis, IN)	200, 300, 600	300–600 tid
	Ketoprofen	Oridus (Wyeth, Philadelphia, PA)	25, 50, 75	50 qid–75 tid
	Piroxicam	Feldene (Pfizer, New York, NY)	10, 20	10 bid, 20 qd
	Flurbiprofen	Ansaid (Upjohn, Kalamazoo, MI)	50, 100	100 tid
	Ketorolac	Toradol (Syntex, Nutley, NJ)	10	10 qid
	Naproxen	Naprosyn (Syntex)	250, 375, 500	250–500 bid
		Anaprox (Syntex)	275, 550	275–550 bid
	Ibuprofen	Motrin (Upjohn)	200, 300, 400, 600, 800	400–800 tid
		Rufen (Boots, Whippany, NJ)	400, 600, 800	
		Advil (Whitehall, Madison, NJ)	200	
		Nuprin (Bristol Meyers, Princeton, NJ)	200	
Pyrazolones	Phenylbutazone	Butazolidin (Geigy)	100	100 tid-qid
		Azolid (USV, Westborough, MA)		
	Oxyphenylbutazone	Tendearil (Geigy)	100	100 tid-qid
		Osalid (USV)		
para-Aminophenols	Acetaminophen	Multiple	80, 325, 500, 650	650 every 4 h
Cox-2 inhibitors	Celecoxib	Celebrex (Pharmacia, Peapack, NJ)	100, 200	100 bid, 200 bid
	Rofecoxib	Vioxx (Merck, Whitehouse Station, NJ)	12.5, 25, 50	12.5 qd, 25 qd, 50 qd

TABLE 4–5. IMMUNOSUPPRESSIVE DRUGS: CLASS, DOSAGE, AND ROUTE OF ADMINISTRATION

CLASS/DRUG	DOSE AND ROUTE
Alkylating agents	
Cyclophosphamide	1–3.0 mg/kg/day, PO, IV
Chlorambucil	0.1 mg/kg/day, PO
Antimetabolites	
Azathioprine	1–3.0 mg/kg/day, PO
Methotrexate	0.15 mg/kg once weekly, PO, SC/IM
Antibiotics	
Cyclosporine	2.5–5.0 mg/kg/day, PO
FK 506	0.1–0.15 mg/kg/day, PO
Rapamycin	
Dapsone	25–50 mg, 2–3 times daily, PO
Adjuvants	
Bromocriptine	2.5 mg, 3–4 times daily, PO
Ketoconazole	200 mg, 1–2 times daily, PO
Colchicine	0.5–0.6 mg, 2–3 times daily, PO

of the ocular inflammation, and being responsible for drug dose reduction or choosing an alternative medication in the event that the chosen immunomodulator is not tolerated at doses sufficient to induce remission of the uveitis.

The history of immunomodulatory therapy for ocular inflammatory disease began in Spain, with the 1951 publication by Roda-Perez describing the treatment of a patient with progressive, steroid-resistant uveitis with nitrogen mustard.[4] A treatise on this new approach to treating such cases appeared, again in the Spanish literature, the following year by the same author,[5] but the matter gained little attention and laid dormant for more than a decade. Wong and associates, from the National Institute of Neurological Diseases (one of the Institutes of Health, from which arose the current National Eye Institute) next reported on the use of methotrexate in the care of a series of patients with uveitis.[6] This report was then followed by a series of papers in the American ophthalmologic literature reporting on small series of patients with ocular inflammatory disease treated with immunomodulation. Newell and Krill[7] described their experience with azathioprine. Moore[8] reported on treatment of sympathetic ophthalmia with azathioprine. Buckley and Gills[9] described the use of cyclophosphamide in the care of patients with pars planitis. Mamo,[10] and later Godfrey and associates,[11] described the effectiveness of chlorambucil in the care of larger numbers of patients with uveitis secondary to Adamantiades-Behçet disease and other steroid-resistant causes. Andrasch and associates described their experience with a large series of patients with treatment-resistant uveitis who were treated with azathioprine.[12] Meanwhile, Martenet was reporting similar successes in the European ophthalmologic literature in her care of patients with progressive ocular damage secondary to uveitis that could not be sufficiently controlled with corticosteroids.[13–18]

Why is it, then, that despite this series of publications from Europe and America extending over a 15-year period, so few ophthalmologists followed the lead of these pioneers in ocular inflammatory disease treatment? In the succeeding 20 years, from 1980 to the present, 10 or fewer centers in America have devoted resources and

personnel, as a matter of specific policy, to dedicated services for the care of patients with ocular inflammatory diseases, and specifically to the "tertiary" care of such patients, including care through immunomodulatory therapy. And fewer such centers have been developed in Europe and in Asia. Why would it be that in spite of the abundant published evidence from all developed countries, the prevalence of blindness secondary to uveitis has not been reduced during the past 40 years?

I believe that two factors account for this lack of progress: (1) A legacy of ignorance. Ophthalmologists, in general, are not knowledgeable about the safety and efficacy record of immunosuppressive immunomodulatory therapy for patients with nonmalignant autoimmune diseases, yet they remember the side effects and risks of the medications used for cancer chemotherapy. Therefore, not only do they not know the real risk-benefit data for the treatment approach advocated herein but often actually mislead patients and parents of patients on the subject, dissuading them from pursuing consultation with another physician whose treatment approach to uveitis includes the use of such medications. (2) A failure to lead. Regrettably, too few leaders in ophthalmology have had the vision to recruit modern trained ocular immunologists onto their faculties, with the resultant training of generation after generation of ophthalmology residents in the old tradition of steroid therapy alone for the care of patients with uveitis. And this failure to lead persists to the present, despite the fact that the American Academy of Ophthalmology has, in its home study teaching guides, prominently highlighted the immunomodulatory alternative therapy approach and has even reproduced tables from the recommendations of the International Uveitis Study Group,[19] which admonish ophthalmologists to refer patients for immunosuppressive chemotherapy as first-line therapy for certain ocular inflammatory diseases, rather than as a therapy of last resort.

Happily, increasing numbers of ophthalmologists throughout the world are beginning to realize what rheumatologists and dermatologists have known for 30 years or more: Immunomodulatory immunosuppressive chemotherapy can be sight saving in patients with various types of ocular inflammatory disease. Also, the side effects of such therapy are typically trivial, especially compared with those of chronic steroid use, provided, of course, that the therapy is managed by an individual who is, by virtue of training and experience, truly expert in the proper and safe use of such drugs, the monitoring of the patient for emergence of subclinical side effects which, when detected early and treated, are reversible, and who is expert in the treatment of any such detected side effects. Clearly, most ophthalmologists are not trained to do this, but they certainly are trained to assess the eye and its inflammation and can therefore guide the chemotherapist with whom they collaborate in the care of the patient and in determining the need for more vigorous immunomodulation.

A pivotal publication on this subject has now appeared in the American Journal of Ophthalmology,[20] in which a panel of experts, comprised of 12 ocular immunologists, rheumatologists, and pediatricians, assessed the world's literature and met multiple times over the course of a year to discuss the strength of the evidence supporting the view that immunosuppressive chemotherapy has been shown to be both safe and effective in the care of patients with ocular inflammatory diseases. The conclusions of this group of experts confirmed and extended the assessment of the International Uveitis Study Group 15 years earlier. And we vigorously support this philosophical position throughout this textbook, believing that the prevalence of blindness secondary to uveitis will be reduced from its current level only if increasing numbers of ophthalmologists embrace this therapeutic philosophy of a limit to the total amount of steroid used and a stepladder escalation of systemic therapeutic vigor in the effort to achieve the goal: The patient should have no inflammation and should be off all steroids. A summary of this therapeutic philosophy is presented in Figure 4–1.

Detailed discussions of each of the chemotherapeutic agents and the use of these drugs for specific diseases is found elsewhere in this text. But two additional matters warrant attention here, because misconceptions on these two points are widespread among ophthalmologists: sterility and malignancy associated with the use of the medications recommended for the care of patients with ocular inflammatory diseases. None of the nonalkylating drugs

we use is associated with impairment of fertility. The alkylating drugs (chlorambucil and cyclophosphamide) do impair spermatogenesis and induce early menopause, especially if they are used for more than 6 to 12 months. We have employed a technique, borrowed from the cancer chemotherapy specialists, which usually is successful in preserving ovarian function through the artificial induction of menopause, with ovarian stimulation after the cessation of the alkylating therapy.[20] Cryopreservation of sperm for later use is the only technique for later procreation available to men who need prolonged alkylating therapy. Most of the chemotherapeutic drugs are potentially teratogenic (or at least insufficient data exist to exclude that possibility), and so effective contraception should be used during therapy with such medications.

The alkylating drugs also increase the likelihood that an individual will develop a malignancy later in life if the drugs are used in sufficient doses and for a prolonged duration. The level of increased risk probably increases with increasing doses and with increasing duration of use, although the data on this matter are imperfect. Most of the studies on this subject come from the cancer and from the autoimmune disease literature. Also, of course, it should be well known by all that individuals with cancer,

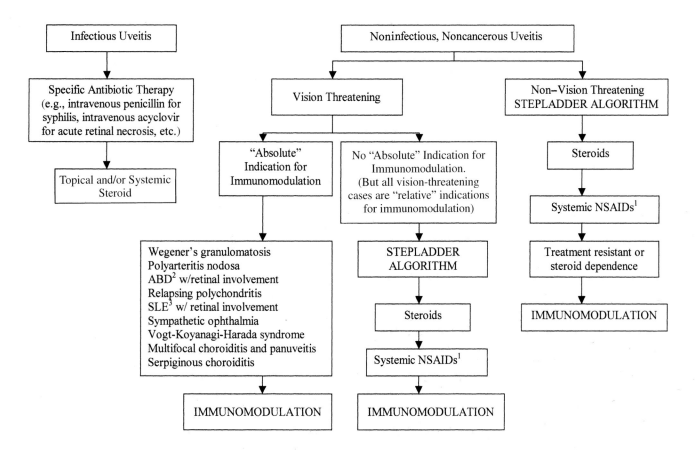

1. Nonsteroidal anti-inflammatory drugs
2. Adamantiades-Behçet disease
3. Systemic lupus erythematosus

FIGURE 4–1. Treatment of uveitis.

and individuals with many of the autoimmune diseases are, even without exposure to immunomodulatory drugs, more likely to develop a malignancy later in life than are those individuals without these diseases. Therefore, even when one evaluates the question of the development of malignancy in patients with rheumatoid arthritis who are treated with an immunosuppressant, interpretation of the data may not be straightforward. However, if one analyzes such patients, excluding those who are infected with Epstein-Barr virus and taking into consideration the fact that patients with rheumatoid arthritis who are not treated with an immunosuppressant have a higher prevalence of malignancy than do individuals in the general population, any additional risk conferred by exposure to a nonalkylating immunosuppressant appears to be small. Additionally, the author has shown, in an analysis of 543 patients with ocular inflammatory disease and treated with a variety of immunomodulatory agents, including alkylating agents, and followed for a total of 1261 patient-years, that there was not a significant increase in the prevalence of malignancy in the study sample, compared with both the expected malignancy rate in the general population and the rate of occurrence of malignancy in a comparison group of patients treated with steroids.[21]

Therefore, we believe the available evidence indicates that, used properly, the immunosuppressive chemotherapeutic agents presented and advocated here for the care of patients with chronic or recurrent uveitis are both effective and safe, with the usual caveats as outlined herein.

Of course, we want to do no harm. Of course, we are eager for the arrival of newer and better and safer drugs. We wait with great hope for selective immunomodulation and for protein, oligonucleotide, and gene therapy and for successful retolerization techniques. We wait for the discovery of prions and slow viruses and mollecutes and other moieties that can be expunged to effect outright cure. And although it is true that 50 years from now, scientists will undoubtedly look with amazement at the crude treatments employed by our generation, the fact remains that comparison outcomes studies now show unequivocally that immunosuppressive chemotherapy should have a much more prominent role in the care of patients with uveitis than it does at present. Our hope is that this text will stimulate increasing numbers of ophthalmologists and directors of ophthalmology training programs to more seriously consider this therapeutic alternative in the 21st century.

OTHER MATTERS

Finally, I would like to mention matters that are probably important but for which little scientific proof exists. For example, it is the widespread impression among uveitis specialists and their patients that stress can provoke a recurrent attack of uveitis in an individual who has had uveitis. We have attempted, thus far without success, to design an appropriate study to address this issue, and we are continuing to search for an appropriate proxy serologic marker for stress that could be longitudinally monitored easily in patients with a history of recurrent uveitis, so that an appropriately designed study could be performed in an effort to study the relationship of stress to

the provocation of uveitis recurrence. In the meantime, it is probably prudent to counsel patients with uveitis on the possible relationship of stress to flare-ups, and to emphasize to them the general health-promoting benefits of stress-reduction efforts, exercise, smoking cessation, and alcoholic drink and diet moderation.

Knox has promulgated the idea that smoking and alcohol consumption are potential provocateurs of uveitis recurrence, and that caffeine, refined sugar (''junk food''), and milk protein also provoke recurrences in some patients.[22] I am not convinced that there is reasonable evidence for this conclusion, but I do not discount its possibility. It would be enlightening if Knox or others would conduct a scientifically sound study of this matter. The same may be said of the idea of Hamel and colleagues that allergy (to food or to environmental material) can cause or aggravate uveitis in some patients.[23] We, too, are impressed that some of our patients with uveitis present with flare-ups year after year at the same time of the year at each occurrence and so do not discount the possibility that such patients are stimulated to have a recurrence through contact with an environmental material at some specific time of the year. This is an area of great vagueness, and designing the appropriately sound study is very challenging.

And finally there is the matter of hormonal influence on recurrent inflammation, another gray area of great scientific difficulty. Some women with recurrent uveitis remark that, although they do not have an attack of uveitis every month, each attack that they do have is always at precisely the same point in their menstrual cycle. In one instance, one of my patients was able to substantiate this impression through basal body temperature charting and recording of recurrences of uveitis. Longitudinal plasma hormonal studies by a gynecologic endocrinologist confirmed an ''imbalance'' in relative levels of estrogen and progesterone at exactly the time of uveitis recurrence, and therapy with an oral contraceptive was associated with a cessation of the attacks of uveitis.

Caring for patients with uveitis is a complex business. It lacks the glamour and quick gratification of keratorefractive or even cataract surgery. But what it lacks in glamour it makes up for in challenge and (usually) delayed gratification. The rewards are enormous. We hope that the reader will enjoy them as much as we do.

References

1. Chang Y, Bassi LJ, Javitt JC: Federal budgetary costs of blindness. The Millbank Q 1992;70:319–340.
2. Suttorp-Schulten MSA, Rothova A: The possible impact of uveitis in blindness: A literature survey. Br J Ophthalmol 1996;80:844–848
3. Rothova A, Suttorp-Schulten MSA, Treffers WF, Kijlstra A: Cause and frequency of blindness in patients with intraocular inflammatory disease. Br J Ophthalmol 1996;80:332–326.
4. Roda-Perez E: Sobre un caso de uveitis de etiologia ignota tratado con mostaza nitrogenada. Rev Clin Esp 1951;40:265–267.
5. Roda-Perez E: El tratamiento de las uveitis de etiologia ignota con mostaza nitrogenada. Arch Soc Oftal Hisp-Amer 1952;12:131–151.
6. Wong VG, Hersh EM: Methotrexate therapy of patients with pars planitis. Trans Am Acad Ophthalmol Otolaryngol 1965;69:279.
7. Newell FW, Krill AE: Treatment of uveitis with azathioprine. Trans Ophthalmol Soc UK 1967;87:499–511.
8. Moore CE: Sympathetic ophthalmitis treated with azathioprine. Br J Ophthalmol 1968;52:688–690.
9. Buckley CE, Gills JP: Cyclophosphamide therapy of peripheral uveitis. Arch Intern Med 1969;124:29–35.

10. Mamo JG, Azzam SA: Treatment of Behçet's disease with chlorambucil. Arch Ophthalmol 1970;48:446–450.
11. Godfrey WA, Epstein WV, O'Connor GR, et al: The use of chlorambucil in intractible idiopathic uveitis. Am J Ophthalmol 1974;78:415.
12. Andrasch RH, Pirofsky B, Burns RP: Immunosuppressive therapy for severe chronic uveitis. Arch Ophthalmol 1978;96:247–251.
13. Martenet AC: Indications de l'immunosuppression par cytostatique en ophtalmologie. Ophthalmologica 1976;172:106–115.
14. Martenet AC: Echecs des cytostatiques en ophtalmologie. Klin Monatsbl Augenheilkd 1980;176:648–651.
15. Martenet AC: Les immunosuppresseurs en ophtalmologie. Journal of Head and Neck Pathology 1988;266–272.
16. Martenet AC: Immunodépresseurs classiques. Bull Soc Belge Ophtalmol 1989;230:135–141.
17. Martenet AC, Paccolat F: Traitement immunodépresseur du syndrome Behçet. Résultats à long terme. Ophtalmologie 1989;3:40–42.
18. Martenet AC: Immunosuppressive therapy of uveitis: Mid- and long-term follow-up after classical cytostatic treatment. Ocular Immunology Today 1990:443–446.
19. Bloch-Michel E, Nussenblatt RB: International Uveitis Study Group recommendations for the evaluation of intraocular inflammatory disease. Am J Ophthalmol 1987;103:234–235.
20. Jabs DA, Rosenbaum JT, Foster CS, et al: Guidelines for the use of immunosuppressive drugs in patients with ocular inflammatory disorders: Recommendations of an expert panel. Am J Ophthalmol 2000;140:492–513.
21. Lane L, Tamesis R, Rodriguez A, et al: Systemic immunosuppressive therapy and the occurrence of malignancy in patients with ocular inflammatory disease. Ophthalmology 1995;102:1530–1535.
22. Knox DL: Glaucomatocyclitic crises and systemic disease: Peptic ulcer and other gastrointestinal disorders, allergy and stress. Trans Am Ophthalmol Soc 1988;86:473–495.
23. Hamel CP, DeLuca H, Billotte C, et al: Nonspecific immunoglobulin E in aqueous humor: Evaluation in uveitis. Graefe's Arch Clin Exp Ophthalmol 1989;227:489–493.

BASIC IMMUNOLOGY

C. Stephen Foster and J. Wayne Streilein

CELLS OF THE IMMUNE SYSTEM

The cellular components of the immune system include lymphocytes, macrophages, Langerhans' cells, neutrophils, eosinophils, basophils, and mast cells. Many of these cell types can be further subdivided into subtypes and subsets. For example, lymphocytes include T lymphocytes, B lymphocytes, and non-T, non-B (null) lymphocytes. Each subtype can be further subcategorized, both by functional differences and by differences in cell surface glycoprotein specialization and uniqueness. The latter differentiating aspect of cell types and cell-type subsets has been made possible through the development of hybridoma-monoclonal antibody technology[1, 2] (Table 5–1).

Lymphocytes

Lymphocytes are mononuclear cells that are round, 7 to 8 μm in diameter, and found in lymphoid tissue (lymph node, spleen, thymus, gut-associated lymphoid tissue, mammary-associated lymphoid tissue, and conjunctiva-associated lymphoid tissue) and in blood. They ordinarily constitute approximately 30% of the total peripheral white blood cell count. The lymphocyte is the premier character in the immune drama; it is the primary recognition unit for foreign material, the principal specific effector cell type in immune reactions, and the cell exclusively responsible for immune memory.

T lymphocytes, or thymus-derived cells, compose 65% to 80% of the peripheral blood lymphocyte population, 30% to 50% of the splenocyte population, and 70% to 85% of the lymph node cell population. B lymphocytes compose 5% to 15% of peripheral blood lymphocytes, 20% to 30% of splenocytes, and 10% to 20% of lymph node cells.

T cells possess cell surface receptors for sheep erythrocytes and for the plant-derived mitogens concanavalin A and phytohemagglutinin. They do not possess surface immunoglobulin or surface membrane receptors for the Fc portion of antibody—two notable cell surface differences from B lymphocytes, which do possess these two entities. B cells also exhibit cell surface receptors for the third component of complement, for the Epstein-Barr virus, and for the plant mitogen known as pokeweed mitogen, as well as for the purified protein derivative of *Mycobacterium tuberculosis* and for lipopolysaccharide.

Null cells are lymphocytes that possess none of the aforementioned cell surface antigens characteristic of T cells or B cells. This cell population is heterogeneous, and some authorities include natural killer (NK) cells among the null cell population, even though the origin of NK cells may be in monocyte/macrophage precursor lines rather than the lymphocyte lineage. Nonetheless, the morphologic characteristics and behaviors of NK cells, along with the ambiguity of their origin, enables their inclusion under the null cell rubric. NK cells are nonadherent (unlike macrophages, they do not stick to the surface of plastic tissue culture dishes) mononuclear cells present in peripheral blood, spleen, and lymph node. The most notable function of these cells is the killing of transformed (malignant) cells and virus-infected cells. Because they do this without prior sensitization, they are an important component of the early natural response in the immune system. The cytotoxicity of NK cells is not major histocompatibility complex (MHC)–restricted, a dramatic contrast with cytotoxic T cells. (More about the MHC and the products of those gene loci will be provided later.) But they do have recognition structures that detect class I MHC molecules; when these receptors engage class I MHC molecules on target cells, the NK *fails* to trigger cytolysis of that target cell. The large granules present in NK cells (the cells are sometimes called *large granular lymphocytes*) contain perforin and perhaps other cell membrane–lysing enzymes; it is the enzymes in these granules that are responsible for the lethal-hit cytolysis for which NK cells are famous.

Killer cells are the other notable null cell subpopulation. These cells do have receptors for the Fc portion of immunoglobulin G (IgG) and thus can attach themselves to the Fc portion of IgG molecules. Through this receptor, they are a primary cell responsible for cytolysis in the so-called antibody-dependent, cell-mediated cytotoxicity reaction. These cells probably participate in type II Gell and Coombs hypersensitivity reactions and are involved in immune removal of cellular antigens when the target cell is too large to be phagocytosed.

It is clear that both B cells and T cells can be further divided into specialized subsets. B cells, for example, are subdivided into the B cells that synthesize the five separate classes of immunoglobulin (IgG, IgA, IgM, IgD, and IgE). All B cells initially produce IgM specific for an antigenic determinant (epitope) to which it has responded, but some subsequently switch from synthesis of IgM to synthesis of other immunoglobulin classes. The details of the control of antibody synthesis and class switching are discussed later in this chapter. Less known is the fact that functionally distinct subsets of B cells exist, in addition to the different B cells involved in antibody class synthesis. The field of B-cell diversity analysis is embryonic, but it is clear that the exploitation of monoclonal antibody technology will distinguish, with increasingly fine specificity, differences in B-cell subpopulations. It is clear, for example, that a subpopulation of B lymphocytes possess the CD5 glycoprotein on the cell surface plasma membrane (a CD glycoprotein not ordinarily present on B lymphocytes but rather on the cell surfaces of T cells).[3] These cells appear to be associated with autoantibody production.[4]

It is also clear now that B cells are functionally important as antigen-presenting cells (APCs) for previously primed or memory (not naive) T cells, a fact that startles most physicians who studied immunology before 1991. T-cell receptors (TCRs) cannot react with native antigen;

TABLE 5–1. CLUSTERS OF DIFFERENTIATION (CD) DESIGNATIONS

CLUSTERS	CELL SPECIFICITY	FUNCTION
CD1	Thymocytes, Langerhans' cells	
CD2	T cells, NK subset	CD58 receptor/sheep erythrocyte receptor; adhesions molecule—binds to LFA-3
CD3	T cells	T-cell antigen-complex receptor
CD4	Helper-inducer T cells	MHC class II immune recognition; HIV receptor
CD5	T cells, B-cell subset	
CD6	T-cell subset	?
CD7	T cells, NK cells, platelets	?Fc receptor IgM
CD8	Cytotoxic suppressor T cells	MHC class I immune recognition
CD9	Pre–B cells	?
CD10	Pre–B cells, neutrophils	Neutrophil endopeptidase
CD11a	Leukocytes	Adhesion molecule (LFA-1) binds to ICAM-1
CD11b	Monocytes, granulocytes, NK cells	α-Chain of complement receptor CR3
CD11c	Monocytes, granulocytes, NK cells	Adhesion
CD13	Monocytes, granulocytes	Aminopeptidase N
CD14	Macrophages	Lipopolysaccharide receptor
CD15	Neutrophils, activated T cells	
CD16	Granulocytes, macrophages, NK cells	Fc receptor IgG (Fc-γ RIII); activation of NK cells
CD19	B cells	B-cell activation
CD20	B cells	B-cell activation
CD21	B cells	Complement receptor CR2—Epstein-Barr virus receptor
CD22	B cells	Adhesion; B-cell activation
CD23	Activated B cells, macrophages	Low-affinity Fc-ε receptor, induced by IL-4
CD25	Activated T cells, B cells	IL-2 receptor
CD28	T cells	Receptor for co-stimulator molecules B7-1 and B7-2
CD30	Activated B and T cells	?
CD31	Platelets, molecules, and B cells	Role in leukocyte-endothelial adhesion
CD32	B lymphocytes, granulocytes, macrophages, eosinophils	Fc receptor IgG (Fc-γ RIII) ADCC
CD35	B cells, erythrocytes, neutrophils, mononuclear cells	Complement receptor CR1
CD37	B cells	
CD38	Activated T and plasma cells	?
CD40	B cells	B-cell activation by T-cell contact
CD41	Megakaryocytes, platelets	Gp11b/11a platelet aggregation; Fc receptor
CD42	Megakaryocytes, platelets	Gp1b—platelet adhesion
CD43	Leukocytes	T-cell activation
CD44	Leukocytes	Pgp1 (Hermes) receptor; homing receptor for matrix components (e.g., hyaluronate)
CD45	All leukocytes	Leukocyte common antigen—signal transduction (tyrosine phosphatase)
CD45RA	Naive cells	
CD45RO	Activated/memory T cells	
CD45RB	B cells	
CD49 (VLA)	T cells, monocytes	Adhesion to collagen, laminin, Fc, VCAM
CD54 (ICAM-1)	Activated cells	Adhesion to LFA-1 and MAC
CD56	NK	NCAM-adhesion
CD58 (LFA-3)	B cells, antigen-presenting cells	Binds to CD2
CD62E E-selectin, ELAM-1	Endothelial cells	Adhesion
CD62L L-selectin, LAM-1	T cells	Adhesion
CD62P P-selectin, PADGEM	Platelets, endothelial cells	Adhesion
CD64	Monocytes, macrophages	Adhesion, Fc-γ receptor; ADCC
CD69	Activated lymphocytes	
CD71	Proliferating cells	Transferrin receptor
CD72	B cells	Ligand for CD5; B cell–T cell interactions
CD80 (B7-1)	B cells; dendritic cells, macrophages	Ligand for CD28; co-stimulator for T-cell activation
CD89 (Fc-α receptor)	Neutrophils, monocytes	IgA-dependent cytotoxicity
CD95 (Fas)	Multiple cell types	Role in programmed cell death
CD102 (ICAM-2)	Endothelial cells, monotypes	Ligand for LFA-1 integrin
CD103 (HML-1)	T cells	Role in T cell homing to mucosae
CD106 (VCAM-1)	Endothelial cells, macrophages	Receptor for VLA-4 integrin; adhesion

ADCC, antibody-dependent cell-mediated cytotoxicity; B, bursal equivalent influenced; ELAM, endothelial leukocyte adhesion molecule; HIV, human immunodeficiency virus; HML, human mucosal lymphocyte; ICAM, intercellular adhesion molecule; LAM, leukocyte adhesion molecule; LFA, leukocyte function–associated antigen; MAC, Mac-1; MHC, major histocompatibility complex; NCAM, neural cell adhesion molecule; NK, natural killer; PADGEM, platelet activation–dependent granule—external membrane; T, thymus influenced; VCAM, vascular cell adhesion molecule; VLA, very late antigen.

rather, they respond to processed antigenic determinants of that antigen. APCs phagocytose the antigen, process it, and display denatured, limited peptide sequences of the native antigen on the cell surface of the APC in association with cell surface class II MHC glycoproteins. B cells, as well as classic APCs, such as macrophages and Langerhans' cells, can perform this function. The antigen is endocytosed by the B cell and processed in the B-cell endosome (possibly through involvement of cathepsin D) to generate short, denatured peptide fragments, which are then transported to the B-cell surface bound to class II glycoprotein peptides; here, the antigenic peptides are "presented" to CD4 helper T lymphocytes.

Finally, regarding B-cell heterogeneity, it is becoming apparent that some B lymphocytes also have suppressor or regulatory activity. The emerging data on B-cell functional and cell surface heterogeneity will be exciting to follow in the coming years.

Much more widely recognized, of course, is that subsets of T lymphocytes exist. Helper (CD4) T cells "help" in the induction of an immune response, in the generation of an antibody response, and in the generation of other, more specialized components of the immune response. Cytotoxic (CD8) T cells, as the name implies, are involved in cell killing or cytotoxic reactions. Delayed-type hypersensitivity (CD4) T cells are the classic participants in the chronic inflammatory responses characteristic of certain antigens such as mycobacteria. Regulatory T cells (CD8) are responsible for modulating immune responses, thereby preventing uncontrolled, host-damaging inflammatory responses. It is even likely that there are sub-subsets of these T cells. Excellent evidence exists, for example, that there are at least three subsets of regulatory T cells and at least two subsets of helper T cells.

Mosmann and Coffman[5] described two types of helper (CD4) T cells with differential cytokine production profiles. T_H1 cells secrete interleukin-2 (IL-2) and interferon-γ (IFN-γ) but do not secrete IL-4 or IL-5, whereas T_H2 cells secrete IL-4, IL-5, IL-10, and IL-13, but not IL-2 or IFN-γ. Furthermore, T_H1 cells can be cytolytic and can assist B cells with IgG, IgM, and IgA synthesis but not IgE synthesis. T_H2 cells are not cytolytic but can help B cells with IgE synthesis, as well as with IgG, IgM, and IgA production.[6] It is becoming clear that CD4 T_H1 or CD4 T_H2 cells are selected in infection and in autoimmune diseases. Thus, T_H1 cells accumulate in the thyroid of patients with autoimmune thyroiditis,[7] whereas T_H2 cells accumulate in the conjunctiva of patients with vernal conjunctivitis.[8] The T cells that respond to *M. tuberculosis* protein are primarily T_H1 cells, whereas those that respond to *Toxocara canis* antigens are T_H2 cells. Romagnani has proposed that T_H1 cells are preferentially "selected" as participants in inflammatory reactions associated with delayed-type hypersensitivity reactions and low antibody production (as in contact dermatitis or tuberculosis), and T_H2 cells are preferentially selected in inflammatory reactions associated with persistent antibody production, including allergic responses in which IgE production is prominent.[9] Further, it is now clear that these two major CD4 T-lymphocyte subsets regulate each other through their cytokines. Thus, T_H2 CD4 lymphocyte cytokines (notably IL-10) inhibit T_H1 CD4 lymphocyte proliferation and cytokine secretion, and T_H1 CD4 lymphocyte cytokines (notably IFN-γ) inhibit T_H2 CD4 lymphocyte proliferation and cytokine production.

Macrophages

The macrophage ("large eater") and dendritic cells are the preeminent professional APCs. Macrophages are 12 to 15 μm in diameter, the largest of the lymphoid cells. They possess a high density of class II MHC glycoproteins on their cell surfaces, along with receptors for complement components, the Fc portion of Ig molecules, receptors for fibronectin, interferons -α, -β, and -γ, IL-1, tumor necrosis factor, and macrophage colony–stimulating factor. These cells are widely distributed throughout various tissues (when found in tissue, they are called histiocytes); the microenvironment of the tissue profoundly influences the extent of expression of the various cell surface glycoproteins as well as the intracellular metabolic characteristics. It is clear that further compartmentalization of macrophage subtypes occurs in the spleen. Macrophages that express a high density of class II MHC glycoproteins are present in red pulp, and macrophages with significantly less surface class II MHC glycoprotein expression are in the marginal zone, where intimate contact with B cells exists. It is likely that, just as in the murine system,[10] so too in humans, one subclass of macrophage preferentially presents antigen to one particular subset of helper T cells responsible for induction of regulatory T-cell activation, whereas a different subset of macrophage preferentially presents antigen to a different helper T-cell subset responsible for cytotoxic or delayed-type hypersensitivity effector functions.

Macrophages also participate more generally in inflammatory reactions. They are members of the natural (early defense) immune system and are incredibly potent in their capacity to synthesize and secrete a variety of powerful biologic molecules, including proteases, collagenase, angiotensin-converting enzyme, lysozyme, IFN-α, IFN-β, IL-6, tumor necrosis factor-α, fibronectin, transforming growth factor-β, platelet-derived growth factor, macrophage colony-stimulating factor, granulocyte-stimulating factor, granulocyte-macrophage colony-stimulating factor, platelet-activating factor, arachidonic acid derivatives (prostaglandins and leukotrienes), and oxygen metabolites (oxygen free radicals, peroxide anion, and hydrogen peroxide). These cells are extremely important, even pivotal, participants in inflammatory reactions and are especially important in chronic inflammation. The epithelioid cell typical of so-called granulomatous inflammatory reactions evolves from the tissue histiocyte, and multinucleated giant cells form through fusion of many epithelioid cells.

Specialized macrophages exist in certain tissues and organs, including the Kupffer cells of the liver, dendritic histiocytes in lymphoid organs, interdigitating reticular cells in lymphoid organs, and Langerhans' cells in skin, lymph nodes, conjunctiva, and cornea.

Langerhans' Cells

Langerhans' cells are particularly important to the ophthalmologist. They probably are the premier APC for the external eye. Derived from bone marrow macrophage precursors, like macrophages, their function is basically identical to that of the macrophage in antigen presentation. They are rich in cell surface class II MHC glycoproteins and have cell surface receptors for the third component of complement and for the Fc portion of IgG. Langerhans' cells are abundant in the mucosal epithelium of the mouth, esophagus, vagina, and conjunctiva. They are also abundant at the corneoscleral limbus, less so in the peripheral cornea; they are normally absent from the central third of the cornea.[11] If the center of the cornea is provoked through trauma or infection, the peripheral cornea Langerhans' cells quickly "stream" into the center of the cornea.[12] These CD1-positive dendritic cells possess a characteristic racket-shaped cytoplasmic granule on ultrastructural analysis, the Birbeck granule, whose function is unknown.

Polymorphonuclear Leukocytes

Polymorphonuclear leukocytes (PMNs) are part of the natural immune system. They are central to host defense through phagocytosis, but if they accumulate in excessive numbers, persist, and are activated in an uncontrolled manner, the result may be deleterious to host tissues. As the name suggests, they contain a multilobed nucleus and many granules. PMNs are subcategorized as neutrophils, basophils, or eosinophils, depending on the differential staining of their granules.

Neutrophils

Neutrophils account for more than 90% of circulating granulocytes. They possess surface receptors for the Fc portion of IgG (CD16) and for complement components, including C5a (important in chemotaxis), CR1 (CD35), and CR3 (CD11b) (important in adhesion and phagocytosis). When appropriately stimulated by chemotactic agents (complement components, fibrinolytic and kinin

system components, and products from other leukocytes, platelets, and certain bacteria), neutrophils move from blood to tissues through margination (adhesion to receptors or adhesion molecules on vascular endothelial cells) and diapedesis (movement through the capillary wall). Neutrophils release the contents of their primary (azurophilic) granules (lysosomes) and secondary (specific) granules (Table 5–2) into an endocytic vacuole, resulting in: (1) phagocytosis of a microorganism or tissue injury, (2) type II antibody-dependent, cell-mediated cytotoxicity, or (3) type III hypersensitivity reactions (immune complex–mediated disease). Secondary granules release collagenase, which mediates collagen degradation. Aside from the products secreted by the granules, neutrophils produce arachidonic acid metabolites (prostaglandins and leukotrienes), as well as oxygen free radical derivatives.

Eosinophils

Eosinophils constitute 3% to 5% of the circulating PMNs. They possess surface receptors for the Fc portion of IgE (low affinity) and IgG (CD16) and for complement components, including C5a, CR1 (CD35), and CR3 (CD11b). Eosinophils play a special role in allergic conditions and parasitoses. They also participate in type III hypersensitivity reactions or immune complex–mediated disease, following attraction to the inflammatory area by products from mast cells (eosinophil chemotactic factor of anaphylaxis), complement, and other cytokines from other inflammatory cells. Eosinophils release the contents of their granules to the outside of the cell after fusion of the intracellular granules with the plasma membrane (degranulation). Table 5–3 shows the known secretory products of eosinophils; the role these products of inflammation play, even in nonallergic diseases (such as Wegener's granulomatosis), is underappreciated.

TABLE 5–2. NEUTROPHIL GRANULES AND THEIR CONTENTS

AZUROPHIL GRANULES	SPECIFIC GRANULES	OTHER GRANULES
Myeloperoxidase	Alkaline phosphatase	Acid phosphatase
Acid phosphatase	Histaminase	Heparinase
5′-Nucleotidase	Collagenase	β-Glucosaminidase
Lysozyme	Lysozyme	α-Mannosidase
Elastase	Vitamin B$_{12}$-binding proteins	Acid proteinase
Cathepsins B, D, G	Plasminogen activator	Elastase, gelatinase
	Lactoferrin	
Proteinase 3		Glycosaminoglycans
β-Glycerophosphatase		
β-Glucuronidase		
N-acetyl-β-glucosaminidase	Cytochrome	
α-Mannosidase		
Arylsulfatase		
α-Fucosidase		
Esterase		
Histonase		
Cationic proteins		
Defensins		
Bactericidal permeability-increasing protein (BPI)		
Glycosaminoglycans		

HIV, human immunodeficiency virus; ICAM, intercellular adhesion molecules; IL, interleukin; NCAM, neural cell adhesion molecule; NK, natural killer; MHC, major histocompatibility complex; LFA, leukocyte function–associated antigen; VCAM, vascular cellular adhesion molecules; VLA, very late antigen.

TABLE 5–3. GRANULAR CONTENT OF EOSINOPHILS

Lysosomal hydrolases	Cathepsin
Arylsulfatase	Histaminase
β-Glucuronidase	Peroxisomes
Acid phosphatase	Major basic proteins
β-Glycerophosphatase	Eosinophil cationic protein
Ribonuclease	Eosinophil peroxidases
Proteinases	Phospholipases
Collagenase	Lysophospholipases

Basophils

Basophils account for less than 0.2% of circulating granulocytes. They possess surface receptors for the Fc portion of IgE (high affinity) and IgG (CD16) and for complement components, including C5a, CR1 (CD35), and CR3 (CD11b). Their role, other than perhaps as tissue mast cells, is unclear.

Mast Cells

The mast cell is indistinguishable from the basophil in many respects, particularly its contents. There are at least two classes of mast cells, based on their neutral protease composition, T-lymphocyte dependence, ultrastructural characteristics, and predominant arachidonic acid metabolites (Table 5–4). Mucosa-associated mast cells (MMC or MC-T) contain primarily tryptase as the major protease (hence, some authors designate these MC-T, or mast cells–tryptase) and prostaglandin D_2 as the primary product of arachidonic acid metabolism. MMCs are T cell–dependent for growth and development (specifically IL-3–dependent), and they are located predominantly in mucosal stroma (e.g., gut). MMCs are small and short-lived (<40 days). They contain chondroitin sulfate but not heparin, and their histamine content is modest (Table 5–5). MMCs degranulate in response to antigen-IgE triggering but not to exposure to compound 48/80, and they are not stabilized by disodium cromoglycate. They are formalin-sensitive, so formalin fixation of tissue eliminates or greatly reduces our ability to find these cells using staining technique. With special fixation techniques, MMC granules stain with Alcian blue but not with safranin.

Connective tissue mast cells (CTMCs) contain both

TABLE 5–4. MAST CELL TYPES AND CHARACTERISTICS

CHARACTERISTICS	MUCOSAL MAST CELL (MC-T, MMC)	CONNECTIVE TISSUE, MAST CELL (MC-TC, CTMC)
MORPHOLOGY		
Size	Small, pleomorphic	Large, uniform
Nucleus	Unilobed or bilobed	Unilobed
Granules	Few	Many
LOCATION	Gut	Peritoneum
HISTOCHEMISTRY		
Protease	Tryptase	Tryptase and chymase
Proteoglycans	Chondroitin sulfate	Heparin
Histamine	<1 pg/cell	≥5 pg/cell
IgE	Surface and cytoplasmic	Heparin
Formalin-sensitive	Yes	No
IN VITRO EFFECT OF:		
Compound 48/80	Proliferation	Degranulation
Polymyxin	Proliferation	Degranulation
SECRETAGOGUES		
Antigen	Yes	Yes
Anti-IgE	Yes	Yes
Compound 48/80	No	Yes
Bee venom	No	Yes
Con A	Yes	Yes
STAINING		
Alcian blue	Yes	Yes
Safranin	No	Yes
Berberine sulfate	No	Yes
ANTIALLERGIC COMPOUNDS		
Cromoglycate	No	Yes
Theophylline	No	Yes
Doxantrile	Yes	Yes
ENHANCEMENT OF SECRETION		
Phosphatidyl serine	No	Yes
Adenosine	Yes	Yes
PREDOMINANT ARACHIDONIC ACID METABOLITE	Prostaglandin D_2	Leukotrienes B_4, C_4, D_4
ULTRASTRUCTURAL FEATURES OF GRANULES	Lattice	Scroll

TABLE 5–5. MAST CELL CONTENTS

Histamine
Serotonin
Rat mast cell protease I and II
Heparin
Chondroitin sulfate
β-Hexosaminidase
β-Glucuronidase
β-D-Galactosidase
Arylsulfatase
Eosinophil chemotactic factor for anaphylaxis (ECF-A)
Slow reactive substance of anaphylaxis (SRS-A)
High-molecular-weight neutrophil chemotactic factor
Arachidonic acid derivatives
Platelet-activating factor

tryptase and chymase (so some authors designate them MC-TC), as well as leukotrienes B$_4$, C$_4$, and D$_4$, as the primary products of arachidonic acid metabolism. CTMCs are T cell–independent. They are larger than MMCs and are located principally in skin and at mucosal interfaces with the environment. They contain heparin and large amounts of histamine, and they degranulate in response to compound 48/80 in addition to antigen-IgE interactions. CTMCs are stabilized by disodium cromoglycate. They stain with alkaline Giemsa, with toluidine blue, Alcian blue, safranin, and berberine sulfate.

The ultrastructural characteristics of MMCs and CTMCs are also different. Electron microscopy shows that the granules of MMCs contain lattice-like structures; the granules of CTMCs contain scroll-like structures. Mast cells play a special role in allergic reactions—they are the preeminent cell in the allergy drama. However, they also can participate in type II, III, and IV hypersensitivity reactions. Their role in these reactions, aside from notable vascular effects, is not well understood. Non–IgE-mediated mechanisms (e.g., C5a) can trigger mast cells to release histamine, platelet-activating factor, and other biologic molecules when antigen binds to two adjacent IgE molecules on the mast cell surface. Histamine and other vasoactive amines cause increased vascular permeability, allowing immune complexes to become trapped in the vessel wall.

Platelets

Blood platelets, cells well adapted for blood clotting, also are involved in the immune response to injury, which is a reflection of their evolutionary heritage as myeloid (inflammatory) cells. They possess surface receptors for the Fc portion of IgG (CD16) and IgE (low affinity), for class I histocompatibility glycoproteins (human leukocyte antigen-A, -B, or -C), and for factor VIII. They also carry molecules such as Gp11b/111a (CDw41), which binds fibrinogen, and Gp1b (CDw42), which binds von Willebrand factor.

After endothelial injury, platelets adhere to and aggregate at the endothelial surface, releasing permeability-increasing molecules from their granules (Table 5–6). Endothelial injury may be caused by type III hypersensitivity. Platelet-activating factor released by mast cells after antigen-IgE antibody complex formation induces platelets to aggregate and release their vasoactive amines.

These amines separate endothelial cell tight junctions and allow immune complexes to enter the vessel wall. Once the immune complexes are deposited, they initiate an inflammatory reaction through activation of complement components and neutrophil lysosomal enzyme release.

Ontogeny of the Immune System

Cells of the hematologic system are derived from primordial stem cell precursors of the bone marrow. Embryonically, they originate in the blood islands of the yolk sac.[13] These cells populate embryonic liver and bone marrow.[14] All blood elements are derived from the primordial stem cells: erythrocytes, platelets, PMNs, monocytes, and lymphocytes. These primordial stem cells are pluripotential; the exact details of the influences that are responsible for a particular pluripotential primordial stem cell evolving along one differentiation pathway (e.g., into a monocyte) as opposed to some other differentiation pathway (e.g., into a lymphocyte) are incompletely understood. It appears, however, that special characteristics of the microenvironment within the bone marrow, particularly with respect to a stem cell's association with other resident cells in the bone marrow, contribute to or are responsible for the different pathways of maturation and differentiation. For example, specific cells in the bone marrow in the endosteal region promote the differentiation of hematopoietic stem cells into B lymphocytes.[15] In birds, primordial pluripotential stem cells that migrate to a gland near the cloaca of the chicken known as the bursa of Fabricius (for reasons of probable stimuli in the bone marrow as yet not understood) are influenced by the epithelial cells in that gland to terminally differentiate into B lymphocytes.[16, 17] Interestingly, various candidates for the so-called bursal equivalent that is responsible for B-cell differentiation in humans were proposed for many years before the role of the bone marrow itself for this function became evident. Extra–bone marrow tissues that had been proposed as bursal equivalent candidates included the appendix, tonsils, liver, and Peyer's patch.

TABLE 5–6. PLATELET GRANULES AND THEIR CONTENTS

α-Granules
  Fibronectin
  Fibrinogen
  Plasminogen
  Thrombospondin
  von Willebrand factor
  α$_2$-Plasmin inhibitor
  Platelet-derived growth factor (PDGF)
  Platelet factor 4 (PF4)
  Transforming growth factor (TGF)-α and -β
  Thrombospondin
  β-Lysin
  Permeability factor
  Factors D and H
  Decay-accelerating factor
Dense granules
  Serotonin
  Adenosine diphosphate (ADP)
Others
  Arachidonic acid derivatives

T-cell development results from pluripotential hematopoietic stem cell migration (stimulus unknown) from the bone marrow to the thymus. Thymic hormones (at least 20 have been preliminarily described) produced by the thymic epithelium initiate the complex series of events that result not only in differentiation of the hematopoietic stem cells into T lymphocytes but in subdifferentiation of T lymphocytes into their various functional subsets; helper function, killer function, and suppressor function are acquired while the T cells are still in the thymus. Table 5–7 lists the four thymic hormones most rigorously studied to date. Note that all are involved in T-cell differentiation and in the development of helper T-cell function, and that three of the four can be involved or are involved in the acquisition of suppressor T-cell activity. Clearly, the story is considerably more complex than the part we currently understand, and additional factors are undoubtedly responsible for the final differentiation of T lymphocytes into their functionally distinct subsets. These various hormones are also undoubtedly responsible for the induction of cell surface glycoprotein expression on the surfaces of T cells. The cell surface expression of the various glycoproteins changes during T-cell maturation in the thymus. For example, the CD2 glycoprotein is the first that can be identified on the differentiating T cell, but this is eventually joined by CD5; these are both eventually replaced (CD2 completely and CD5 partially) by CD1 glycoprotein, which in turn is lost and replaced by the mature CD3 marker. CD4 and CD8 glycoproteins are acquired prior to emigration from the thymus of helper and cytotoxic-regulatory T cells, respectively.

Monocytes, NK cells, and killer cells evolve from pluripotential hematopoietic stem cells through influences that are incompletely understood. All three types of cells do arise from a common monocyte precursor and later subdifferentiate under unknown influences.

Primary (Central) Lymphoid Organs

The primary or central lymphoid organs are the bone marrow, thymus, and liver. The peripheral lymphoid organs include lymph nodes, spleen, gut-associated lymphoid tissue, bronchus-associated lymphoid tissue, and conjunctiva-associated lymphoid tissue. The anatomic characteristics of the thymus, lymph node, and spleen are described briefly.

The thymus consists of a medulla that contains thymic epithelial tissue and lymphocytes, and a surrounding cortex densely packed with small, proliferating T lymphocytes (Fig. 5–1). The cells in the cortex emigrate from the thymus: the cell population turns over completely every 3 days. Only about 1% of the cells produced in the thymus, however, actually emigrate from it; 99% are destroyed locally, probably in a process designed to prevent autoreactive T lymphocytes from gaining access to the extrathymic regions of the organism. Thymic nurse cells, epithelial cells in the cortical region, may be responsible in part for some of the later events in T-lymphocyte differentiation (e.g., into helper and regulatory T cells).

Lymph nodes (Fig. 5–2) are also composed of medulla and cortex. The medulla, rich in the arterial and venous components of the lymph node, contains reticular cells that drain into the efferent lymphatic vessels. The cortex contains the primary lymphoid follicles, which comprise mature, resting B cells, secondary lymphoid follicles with their germinal centers (full of antigen-stimulated B cells and dendritic cells) and mantle, and lymphocytes. The paracortical region close to the medulla is rich in T cells, particularly CD4 + T cells.

The arrangement of the spleen is similar to that of the thymus and lymph node, although lymph node–type follicles are not so clearly distinguished (Fig. 5–3). The lymphoid follicles and surrounding lymphocytes are called the *white pulp* of the spleen. The red pulp of the spleen is composed of the sinusoidal channels that typically contain a relatively large number of red blood cells. Papiernik has described the white pulp as being organized as a lumpy cylindric sheath surrounding central arterioles. The arterioles curve back on the white pulp to develop it as the marginal sinus, which separates the white pulp from the red.[18] B cells predominate in the marginal zone, but CD4 + T cells are present as well. T cells are clustered tightly around the central arteriole, where about 70% of the T cells are CD4 +. B cells also predominate in the lumpy eccentric follicle of white pulp. Table 5–8 summarizes the categorization of the primary and the secondary lymphoid organs. The spleen is the primary site of immune responses to intravenous and anterior chamber–introduced antigens.

Lymphoid Traffic

Lymphatic vessels and blood vessels connect these lymphatic organs to one another and to the other organs of the body. Lymphatic vessels drain every organ except the nonconjunctival parts of the eye, internal ear, bone marrow, spleen, and cartilage, and some parts of the central nervous system. The interstitial fluid and cells entering the lymphatic system are propelled (predominantly by skeletal muscle contraction) to regional lymph nodes. Efferent lymphatics draining these regional nodes converge to form large lymph vessels that culminate in the thoracic duct and in the right lymphatic duct. The thoracic duct empties into the left subclavian vein, carrying approximately three quarters of the lymph, whereas the right lymphatic duct empties into the right subclavian vein.

The subject of lymphocyte traffic, like so many areas of immunology, has undergone intensive reexamination since the 1980s; since then, discoveries relating to homing receptors, addressins, and other adhesion molecules have revolutionized our understanding of how lymphoid cells migrate into and out of specific areas. For example, it is clear that one or more homing receptors is present on the surfaces of all lymphoid cells. These receptors can be regulated, induced, and suppressed. Furthermore, induc-

TABLE 5–7. THYMIC HORMONES

HORMONE	NUMBER OF AMINO ACIDS
Thymosin	28
Thymopoietin	49
Thymic humoral factor	31
Facteur thymique serique	9

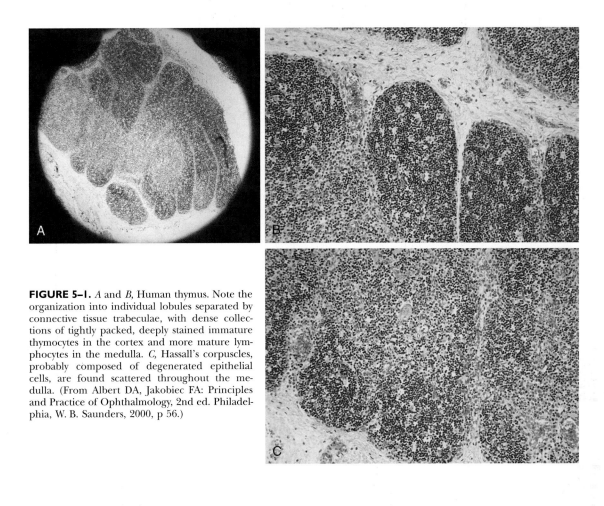

FIGURE 5–1. *A* and *B,* Human thymus. Note the organization into individual lobules separated by connective tissue trabeculae, with dense collections of tightly packed, deeply stained immature thymocytes in the cortex and more mature lymphocytes in the medulla. *C,* Hassall's corpuscles, probably composed of degenerated epithelial cells, are found scattered throughout the medulla. (From Albert DA, Jakobiec FA: Principles and Practice of Ophthalmology, 2nd ed. Philadelphia, W. B. Saunders, 2000, p 56.)

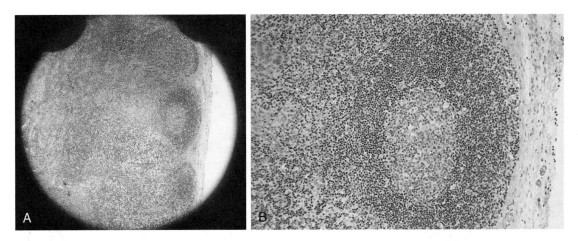

FIGURE 5–2. *A,* Human lymph node. Note the organization, in some respects similar to that of the thymus, into two predominant areas—the cortex and the medulla. The cortex is rich in B cells; the medulla contains cords of lymphoid tissue that contain both B and T cells; and an intermediate zone called the paracortex is rich in T cells. The paracortex, in addition to being rich in T cells, contains antigen-presenting cells. *B,* the medulla contains macrophages and plasma cells as well as B and T cells. The cortex contains the primary and secondary follicles, the distinction between the two being the germinal center (site of activity proliferating B cells) in the secondary follicles. (From Albert DA, Jakobiec FA: Principles and Practice of Ophthalmology, 2nd ed. Philadelphia, W. B. Saunders, 2000, p 57.)

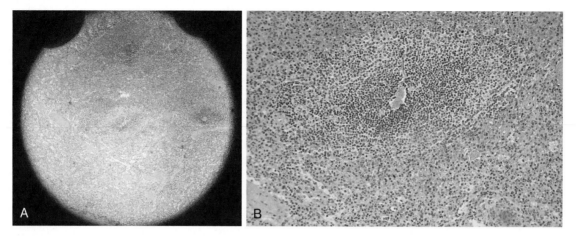

FIGURE 5–3. *A,* Human spleen. Note the red pulp, primarily involved in destruction of old red blood cells containing immune complexes, and white pulp, organized primarily around central arterioles and hence forming a "follicle" or a periarticular lymphoid sheath (PALS). *B,* T cells are particularly rich around the central arteriole of the PALS. B cells are particularly rich in the periphery of the PALS. The far periphery of the PALS, adjoining the red pulp, contains macrophages as well as B cells. (From Albert DA, Jakobiec FA: Principles and Practice of Ophthalmology, 2nd ed. Philadelphia, W. B. Saunders, 2000, p 57.)

tion and suppression of other cell surface moieties that may regulate lymphoid cell exit from one location or another occurs. For example, cortical thymocytes rich in peanut agglutinin on their surface have a paucity of homing receptors, a fact that might ordinarily allow them to migrate out of the thymus to some other location. Butcher and Weissman have hypothesized that "terminal sialidation could release formerly peanut agglutinin–positive thymocytes from hypothetical peanut agglutinin–like lectins in the thymus, providing 'exit visas' for their release from the thymus."[19] In any event, one thing is clear: mature T cells emerging from the thymus cortex toward the medulla are rich either in cell surface or plasma membrane–homing receptors, or adhesion molecules or "adhesomes," which are ligands for various addressins or adhesion molecules at other, remote loci. In the mouse, homing receptors on the surfaces of mature T cells have been identified for the lymph node (MEL-14 or L-selectin [LFA-1]) and for Peyer's patch (LPAM-1 $\alpha_4\beta_7$ integrin, CD44). Equivalent homing receptors undoubtedly exist in humans, but work in this area is currently embryonic. A 90-kDa glycoprotein designated Hermes-3, however, has been identified as a specific heterotypic recognition unit on lymphocytes.[20] The Hermes glycoprotein has been shown to be identical to the CD44 molecule.[21] Antibodies to this glycoprotein prevent binding of lymphocytes to mucosal lymph node high endothelial venules.[22]

Table 5–9 summarizes many of the currently recognized adhesion molecules and their homing receptor ligands.

Immune Response

Professional APCs phagocytose foreign material (antigens), process it through protease endosomal-lysosomal

degradation, "package" it with MHC molecules, and transport the peptide-MHC complex to the cell surface. B cells and dendritic cells (including Langerhans' cells) perform this function too, but differences in protease types and class II MHC molecules among these APCs may influence the type of T cell activated by an antigen. It is this unit of antigenic peptide determinant and self-MHC glycoproteins, along with the aid of adhesion molecules (ICAM-1 [CD54] and LFA-3 [CD58]) and co-stimulatory molecules (B7 [CD80]), that forms the recognition unit for T-cell antigen receptors (TCRs) specific for the antigenic epitope of the foreign material. The TCR is composed of recognition units for the epitope and for the autologous MHC glycoprotein. Endogenous antigens, such as endogenously manufactured viral protein, typically collect in cytoplasm, associate with class I MHC

TABLE 5–9. ADHESION MOLECULES

LFA-1α	(CD11a)
MAC	(CD11b)
GP150,95	(CD11c)
LFA-1β	(CD18)
Integrin α4	(CD49c)
TCRαβ	
TCRγ/δ	
LFA-2	(CD2)
CD22	
NCAM	(CD56)
ICAM-1	(CD54)
LFA-3	(CD58)
LECAM-1	
CD5	
HCAM	(CD44)
HPCA-2	(CD34)
CD28	
88-1	
PECAM	(CD31)
GMP140	(CD62)
HNK-1	(CD57)

GMP, granule membrane protein; HCAM, homing–associated cell adhesion molecule; HNK, human natural killer; HPCA, human progenitor cell antigen; ICAM, intercellular adhesion molecule; LECAM, lectin adhesion molecule; LFA, leukocyte function–associated antigen; MAC, Mac-1 (macrophage differentiation antigen); NCAM, neural cell adhesion molecule; PECAM, platelet-endothelial cell adhesion molecule; TCR, T-cell receptor.

TABLE 5–8. LYMPHOID ORGANS

PRIMARY	SECONDARY
Thymus	Lymph nodes
Bone marrow	Spleen
	Mucosa-associated lymphoid tissue

molecules, and are transported to the surface of the APC, where the class I MHC-peptide complex preferentially associates with the TCR of CD8+ cells. As described earlier, exogenous antigens that are phagocytosed typically associate, in the endosomal, endocytic, and exocytic pathways, with class II MHC molecules; this complex preferentially associates with CD4+ TCRs.

The αβ heterodimer of the TCR is associated with CD3 and ζη proteins and (for CD4 cells) the CD4 molecule, thus forming the TCR complex. Antigen presentation can then occur as the TCR complex interacts with the antigenic determinant/MHC complex on the macrophage, with simultaneous CD28-CD80 interaction. Macrophage secretion of IL-1 during this cognitive "presentation" phase of the acquired immune response to CD4 T cells completes the requirements for successful antigen presentation to the helper T cell (Fig. 5–4; see also color insert).

The CD3 and ζη proteins are the signal-transducing components of the TCR complex; transmembrane signaling via this pathway results in activation of several phosphotyrosine kinases, including those of the tyk/jak family, and other signal transduction and activation of transcription molecules and phosphorylation of tyrosine residues in the cytoplasmic tails of the CD3 and ζη proteins, leading to the creation of multiple sites that bind proteins

(enzymes), like phosphatidylinositol phospholipase C-γ1 (PI-PLC-γ1) with SH2-binding domain. PI-PLC-γ1 in turn is phosphorylated (and thereby activated), and it catalyzes hydrolysis of plasma membrane phosphatidylinositol 4,5 bisphosphate into inositol 1,4,5-triphosphate (IP_3), and diacylglycerol. IP_3 then provokes the release of calcium from its endoplasmic reticulum storage sites. The increased intracellular calcium concentration that results from the release from storage in turn results in increased binding of calcium to calmodulin; this then activates the phosphatase, calcineurin. Calcineurin catalyzes the conversion of phosphorylated nuclear factor of activated T cells, cytoplasmic component (NFATc) to free NFATc. This protein (and probably others) then enters the cell nucleus, where gene transcription of cellular proto-oncogene/transcription factor genes, cytokine receptor genes, and cytokine genes is then activated and regulated by it (them). For example, NFATc translocates to the nucleus, where it combines with AP-1 proteins; this complex then binds to the NFAT-binding site of the IL-2 promoter. This, coupled with NFκB binding by proteins *possibly* induced by the events stimulated by CD28-CD80 signal transduction, results in IL-2 gene transcription typical of T-cell activation (see Fig. 5–5; see also color insert). Thus, this activation phase of the acquired immune response is characterized by lymphocyte proliferation and cytokine production.

Expression of Immunity

The emigration of hematopoietic cells from the vascular system typically occurs at the region of postcapillary high endothelial venule cells. These cells are rich in the constitutive expression of so-called addressins, which are tissue- or organ-specific endothelial cell molecules involved in lymphocyte homing. These adhesion molecules are lymphocyte-binding molecules for the homing receptors on lymphocytes. Thus, the mucosal addressin[21] specifically binds to the Hermes 90-kDa glycoprotein. In the murine system, a 90-kDa glycoprotein (designated MECA-79) is a peripheral lymph node addressin specifically expressed by high endothelial venules in peripheral lymph nodes.[23] MECA-367 and MECA-89 are additional addressin glycoproteins in the murine system that are specific for mucosal vascular high endothelial venules. Along with the constitutive expression of addressins or adhesion molecules, expression of additional adhesion molecules is induced by a panoply of proinflammatory cytokines. It is this directed trafficking of inflammatory cells via adhesion molecules that gives the expression of an immune response its focus, its specifically directed, targeted expression.

Lymphocytes, monocytes, and neutrophils preferentially migrate or "home" to sites of inflammation because of this upregulation of cytokines and the induction of adhesion molecules promoted by them. Thus, L-selectin (CD62L) on the neutrophil cell surface membrane does not adhere to normal vascular endothelium, but ICAM and ELAM (CD62E) expression on the vascular endothelial cell surface induced by IFN-α, IFN-γ, IL-1, IL-17, or a combination thereof results in low-affinity binding of CD62L, with resultant slowing of neutrophil transit through the vessel, neutrophil "rolling" on the endothe-

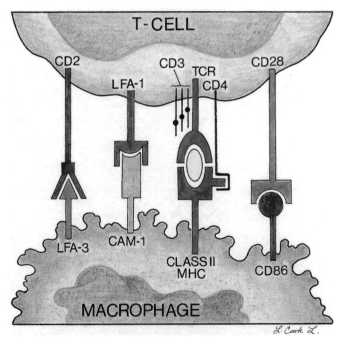

FIGURE 5–4. Antigen presentation, macrophage to CD4+ T cell. Note the oval-shaped (yellow) peptide fragment from the macrophage-phagocytosed integrated antigen in the groove of the Class II MHC molecule on the surface of the macrophage, being presented to the T-cell receptor in the context of the helper- or inducer-specific CD4 molecule. Note also the attachment complex interactions between CD2 and LFA-3, and between LFA-1 and CAM-1, ensuring appropriate cell-to-cell contact and stability during antigen presentation. Note also the costimulatory molecule interactions betwen CD28 and CD86, ensuring a "correct" presentation of the antigen to the T-cell such that an active, proinflammatory immune response will ensue. (Original drawing by Laurel Cook Lhowe). (See color insert.)

MHC CLASS II

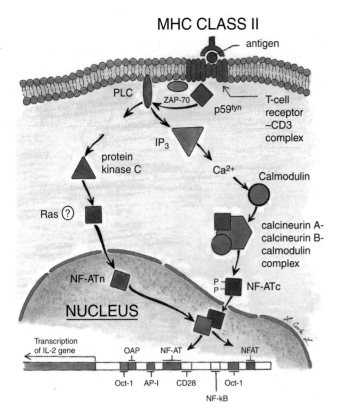

FIGURE 5–5. Signal transduction: intracellular and intranuclear. With antigen-presenting cell presentation of antigen to the T-cell (green peptide fragment in the MHC Class II groove of the macrophage), an extraordinary cascade of events occurs, through the cell membrane, into the cytoplasm, and subsequently into the nucleus, to the level of specific genes on the chromosomes of the nucleus. Specifically, tyrosine-rich phosphorylases result in phosphorylation of a series of intracellular proteins, with resultant liberation of calcium stores, and production of the calcineurin-calmodulin complex, which then facilitates the production of nuclear factor-AT_C, capable of being transported through one of the nuclear pores into the nucleus, where interaction then with specific foci on the gene result in induction of gene transcription (in this instance, transcription of production of messenger RNA for ultimate synthesis of the protein interleukin 2). (Original drawing by Laurel Cook Lhowe.) (See color insert.)

lial surface, and (with complement split product and IL-8–driven chemotaxis of increasing numbers of neutrophils) neutrophil margination in the vessels of inflamed tissue. Neutrophil LFA-1 (CD11a, CD18)–activated expression (stimulated by IL-6 and IL-8) then results in stronger adhesion of the neutrophil to endothelial cell ICAM molecules, with resultant neutrophil spreading and diapedesis into the subendothelial spaces and into the surrounding tissue.

Immunologic Memory

The anamnestic capacity of the acquired immune response system is one of its most extraordinary properties. Indeed, it is this remarkable property that was the first to be recognized by the Chinese ancients and (later) by Jenner. We take it axiomatic that our immunization in childhood with killed or attenuated smallpox and poliovirus provoked not only a primary immune response but also the development of long-lived "memory" cells that immediately produce a rapid, vigorous secondary im-

mune response whenever we might encounter smallpox or poliovirus, thereby resulting in specific antibody- and lymphocyte-mediated killing of the microbe and defending us from the harm the virus would otherwise have done. But just what do we know about the cells responsible for this phenomenon? What special characteristics enable memory cells to live for prolonged periods in the absence of continued or repeated antigen exposure?

Niels Jerne first hypothesized a clonal selection theory to explain at once the specificity and the diversity of the acquired immune response, and Frank Macfarlane Burnet expanded on Jerne's original hypothesis, clearly predicting the necessary features that would prove the theory; many subsequent studies have done so. Clones are derived from the development of antigen-specific clones of lymphocytes arising from single precursors prior to and independent from exposure to antigen. Approximately 10^9 such clones have been estimated to exist within an individual, allowing him or her to respond to all currently known or future antigens. Antigen contact results in preferential activation of the preexisting clone with the cell surface receptors specific for it, with resultant proliferation of the clone and differentiation into effector and memory cells. The secondary or anamnestic immune response is greater and more rapid in onset than is the primary immune response because of the large number of lymphocytes derived from the original clone of cells stimulated by primary contact with antigen, and because of the long-lived nature of many of the cells (memory cells). The memory cells can survive for very long periods, even decades. They express certain cell surface proteins not expressed by nonmemory cells (CD45RO). In memory cells, the level of cell surface expression of peripheral lymph node homing receptors is low compared with the population of such receptors on the surfaces of nonmemory cells; in contrast, the population of other adhesion molecules on the surfaces of memory cells is much greater than that on the surfaces of nonmemory cells. These adhesion molecules include CD11a, CD18 (LFA-1), CD44, and VLA molecules. Because of the constitutive expression of the cell surface adhesion molecules, memory T cells rapidly home to sites of inflammation, "looking" for antigen to which they might respond.

Summary

The evolutionary advantage of the immune system is obvious. The complexity of the system that has evolved to protect us, however, is extraordinary, and our understanding of the immune system is far from complete. The major cell types of the system are well known, but subtypes and sub-subtypes are still being identified. The primary products of one of the major cell types, the B lymphocytes, have been well characterized (antibody), but additional cellular products or cytokines from these cells, which in the 1980s were believed to secrete only immunoglobulins in their mature (plasma cell) state, are being discovered. Thus, the 18 interleukins and other cytokines listed in Table 5–10 will be an incomplete list of the known cytokines of the immune system by the time this edition is published. The seemingly never-ending story of immunologic discovery is at once as fascinating

TABLE 5–10. CYTOKINES AND TARGET CELLS

CYTOKINE	SOURCE	TARGET CELLS
IL-1	Mφ, T$_H$, FB, NK, B, Nφ, EC	Pluripotent stem cells, T$_C$T$_H$, B, Mφ, FB, Nφ
IL-2	T$_H$1	T$_C$T$_H$, B, NK
IL-3	BM, T$_H$, MC	T$_C$T$_H$, B, MC, stem cells
IL-4	T$_H$2, MC	T$_H$1, B, Mφ, MC, T$_H$2, NK, FC
IL-5	T$_H$2, MC, Eφ	T$_C$T$_H$, B, Eφ
IL-6	BM, Mφ, MC, EC, B, T$_H$2, FB	Pluripotent stem cells, T$_C$T$_H$, B, FB, Nφ
IL-7	FB, BM	Subcapsular thymocytes, T$_C$T$_H$, FB
IL-8	BM, FB, EC, Mφ, Nφ, Eφ	T$_C$T$_H$, Mφ, Nφ
IL-9	T$_H$2	Pluripotent stem cells, T$_C$T$_H$, MC
IL-10	T$_H$2, B, Mφ	T$_{CD2}$, T$_C$, T$_H$1, MC
IL-11	BM	Pluripotent stem cells, T$_C$T$_H$, B
IL-12	Mφ, Nφ	NK, T$_H$-T$_H$1
IL-13	T$_H$2	T$_H$1, Mφ, B
IL-14	T	B
IL-15	Mφ, FB, BM	T, NK, B
IL-16	T, Eφ	T
IL-17	T$_H$	FB, T
IL-18	Mφ	T, NK
TNF-α	Mφ	T$_C$T$_H$, B, Mφ, FB
TNF-β	T$_C$, T$_H$1	EC, Nφ
GM-CSF	T$_H$, Mφ, MC, null cells, FB	T$_C$T$_H$, Eφ, Nφ
G-CSF	BM, Mφ, FB	T$_C$T$_H$, FB, Nφ
M-CSF	BM, Mφ, FB	
LIF	BM	Myeloid progenitor
SCF	BM	Myeloid progenitor, cortical thymocytes
IFN-γ	NK, T$_H$1	NK, T$_C$, T$_H$2, B, FB, MC
IFN-α	Mφ	T$_C$T$_H$, B
IFN-β	FB	T$_C$T$_H$
TGF-β	Mφ	T$_C$T$_H$, B, Mφ, FB

B, B cell; BM, bone marrow; CSF, colony-stimulating factor; Eφ, eosinophil; EC, endothelial cell; FB, fibroblast; GM, granulocyte, macrophage; IFN, interferon; IL, interleukin; LIF, leukocyte inhibitory factor; Mφ, macrophage; MC, mast cell; Nφ, neutrophil; NK, natural killer cell; SCF, stem cell factor; T, T cell; T$_C$, cytotoxic T cell; TGF, transforming growth factor; T$_H$, helper T cell; TNF, tumor necrosis factor.

as any Shakespearean play and as frustrating as attempting to understand the universe and the meaning of life. Each year, a chapter brings new knowledge and new questions, and the wise physician realizes that schooling never ends in immunology, as in so many other biologic sciences. Stay tuned.

B-LYMPHOCYTE RESPONSES

B-lymphocyte development from pluripotential bone marrow stem cells influenced by endosteal region bone marrow interstitial cells is introduced earlier in this chapter. This cell, thus committed, has been designated a *pre–B lymphocyte.* It contains cytoplasmic, but not membrane, immunoglobulin M (IgM) heavy chains that associate with "surrogate light chains" devoid of variable regions. These primitive immunoglobulin molecules in pre–B cells, composed of complete, mature heavy chains and surrogate light chains, are critical to the further development of the B cell into the immature B lymphocyte containing complete κ or λ light chains with suitable variable regions. IgM is then expressed on the immature B-cell surface. Interleukin-7 is important in the process of B-cell development, as is src family tyrosine kinase in bone marrow stromal cells and stem cells. When an antigen encounters cell surface IgM that has binding specificities for the antigen (e.g., self-antigens), tolerance to the antigen is the typical result if such an encounter precedes emigration of the B cell from the bone marrow.

Once the immature B cell has acquired its "exit visa" (complete surface IgM), it leaves the bone marrow, resid-ing primarily in the peripheral lymphoid organs (and blood), where it further matures to express both IgM and IgD on its cell surface. It is now a mature B cell, responsive to antigen with proliferation and antibody synthesis.

The hallmark of the vertebrate immune system is its ability to mount a highly specific response against virtually any foreign antigen, even those never before encountered. The ability to generate a diverse immune response depends on the assembly of discontinuous genes that encode the antigen-binding sites of immunoglobulin and T-cell receptors during lymphocyte development. Diversity is generated through the recombination of various germline gene segments, the imprecise joining of segments with insertion of additional nucleotides at the junctions, and somatic mutations occurring within the recombining gene segments. Other factors, such as the chromosomal position of the recombining gene segments and the number of homologous gene segments, may play a role in determining the specificities of the antigen-recognizing proteins produced by a maturing lymphocyte.

Antibody Diversity

The paradox of an individual possessing a limited number of genes but the capability to generate an almost infinite number of different antibodies remained an enigma to immunologists for a considerable time. The discovery of distinct variable (V) and constant (C) regions in the light and heavy chains of immunoglobulin molecules (Fig. 5–6) raised the possibility that immunoglobu-

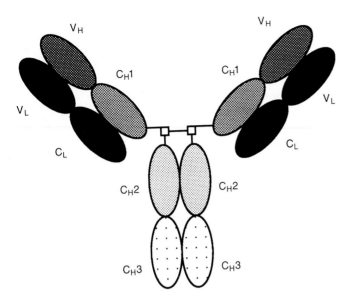

FIGURE 5–6. Structure of IgG showing the regions of similar sequence (domains). (From Albert DA, Jakobiec FA: Principles and Practice of Ophthalmology, 2nd ed. Philadelphia, W. B. Saunders, 2000, p 66.)

lin genes possess an unusual architecture. In 1965, Dreyer and Bennett proposed that the V and C regions of an immunoglobulin chain are encoded by two separate genes in embryonic (germline) cells (germline gene diversity).[24] According to this model, one of several V genes becomes joined to the C gene during lymphocyte development. In 1976, Hozumi and Tonegawa discovered that variable and constant regions are encoded by separate, multiple genes far apart in germline DNA that become joined to form a complete immunoglobulin gene active in B lymphocytes.[25] Immunoglobulin genes are thus translocated during the differentiation of antibody-producing cells (somatic recombination) (Fig. 5–7).

Structure and Organization of Immunoglobulin Genes

The V regions of immunoglobulins contain three hypervariable segments that determine antibody specificity

(Fig. 5–8).[26] Hypervariable segments of both the light (L) and heavy (H) chains form the "antigen-binding" site. Hypervariable regions are also called "complementarity-determining regions" (CDRs). The V regions of L and H chains have several hundred gene segments in germline DNA; the exact number of segments is still being debated but is estimated to range between 250 and 1000 segments.

LIGHT-CHAIN GENES

A complete gene for the V region of a light chain is formed by the splicing of an incomplete V-segment gene with one of several J (joining)-segment genes, which encodes part of the last hypervariable segment (Fig. 5–9).[27–29] Additional diversity is generated by allowing V and J genes to become spliced in different joining frames (junctional diversity) (Fig. 5–10).[28] There are at least three frames for the joining of V and J. Two forms of light chain exist: kappa (κ) and lambda (λ). For κλ chains, assume that there are approximately 250 V-segment genes and four J-segment genes. Therefore, a total of $250 \times 4 \times 3$ (for junctional diversity), or 3000, kinds of complete VJ genes can be formed by combinations of V and J.

HEAVY-CHAIN GENES

Heavy-chain V-region genes are formed by the somatic recombination of V, an additional segment called D (diversity), and J-segment genes (Fig. 5–11). The third CDR of the heavy chain is encoded mainly by a D segment. Approximately 15 D segments lie between hundreds of V_H and at least four J_H gene segments. A D segment joins a J_H segment; a V_H segment then becomes joined to the DJ_H to form the complete V_H gene. To further diversify the third CDR of the heavy chain, extra nucleotides are inserted between V and D, and between D and J (N-region addition) by the action of terminal deoxyribonucleotidyl transferase.[30] Introns, which are noncoding intervening sequences, are removed from the primary RNA transcript.

The site-specific recombination of V, D, and J genes is mediated by enzymes (immunoglobulin recombinase) that recognize conserved nonamer and palindromic heptamer sequences flanking these gene segments.[31, 32] The nonamer and heptamer sequences are separated by either 12–base pair (bp) or 23-bp spacers (Fig. 5–12). Re-

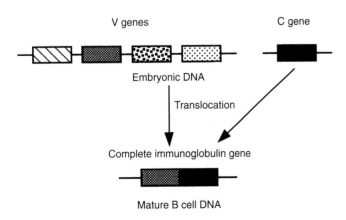

FIGURE 5–7. Translocation of a V-segment gene to a C gene in the differentiation of an antibody-producing B cell. (From Albert DA, Jakobiec FA: Principles and Practice of Ophthalmology, 2nd ed. Philadelphia, W. B. Saunders, 2000, p 67.)

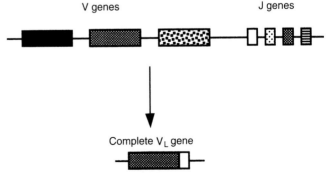

FIGURE 5–8. Hypervariable or complementarity-determining regions (CDRs) on the antigen-binding site of the variable regions of IgG. (From Albert DA, Jakobiec FA: Principles and Practice of Ophthalmology, 2nd ed. Philadelphia, W. B. Saunders, 2000, p 67.)

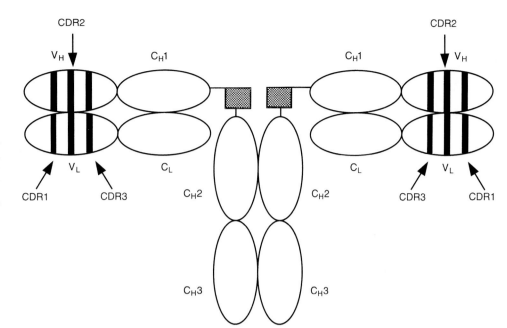

FIGURE 5–9. A V gene is translocated near a J gene in forming a light-chain V region gene. (From Albert DA, Jakobiec FA: Principles and Practice of Ophthalmology, 2nd ed. Philadelphia, W. B. Saunders, 2000, p 67.)

combination can occur only between the 12- and 23-bp spacers but not between two 12-bp types or two 23-bp types (called the 12/23 rule of V-gene-segment recombination). For example, V_H segments and J_H segments are flanked by 23-bp types on both their 5′ and 3′ ends. Consequently, they cannot recombine with each other or among themselves. Instead, they recombine with D segments, which are flanked on both 5′ and 3′ ends by recognition sequences of the 12-bp type.

Sources of Immunoglobulin Gene Diversity

For 250 V_H, 15 D_H, and 4 J_H gene segments that can be joined in three frames, at least 45,000 complete V_H genes

can be formed. Therefore, more than 10^8 different specificities can be generated by combining different V, D, and J gene segments and by combining more than 3000 L chains and 45,000 H chains. If the effects of N-region addition are included, more than 10^{11} different combinations can be formed. This is large enough to account for the immense range of antibodies that can be synthesized by an individual.

Far fewer V genes than Vκ genes encode light chains. However, many more V amino-acid sequences are known.[33–35] It is therefore likely that mutations introduced somatically give rise to much of the diversity of λ light chains (somatic hypermutation).[28] Likewise, somatic hy-

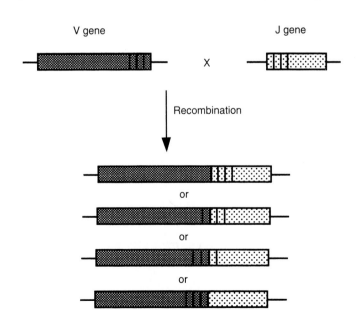

FIGURE 5–10. Imprecision in the site of splicing of a V gene to a J gene (junctional diversity). (From Albert DA, Jakobiec FA: Principles and Practice of Ophthalmology, 2nd ed. Philadelphia, W. B. Saunders, 2000, p 68.)

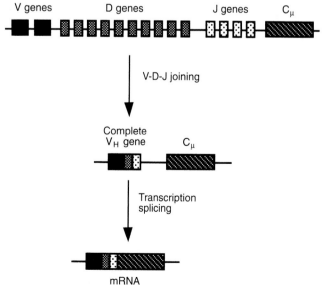

FIGURE 5–11. The variable region of the heavy chain is encoded by V-, D-, and J-segment genes. (From Albert DA, Jakobiec FA: Principles and Practice of Ophthalmology, 2nd ed. Philadelphia, W. B. Saunders, 2000, p 68.)

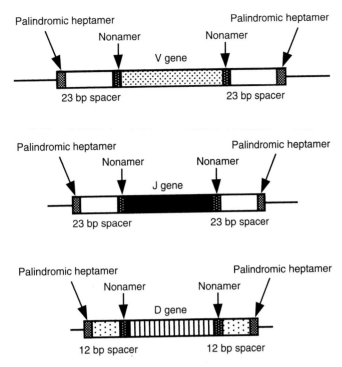

FIGURE 5–12. Recognition sites for the recombination of V-, D-, and J-segment genes. V and J genes are flanked by sites containing 23-bp spacers, whereas D-segment genes possess 12-bp spacers. Recombination can occur only between sites with different classes of spacers. (From Albert DA, Jakobiec FA: Principles and Practice of Ophthalmology, 2nd ed. Philadelphia, W. B. Saunders, 2000, p 68.)

permutation further amplifies the diversity of heavy chains. To summarize, four sources of diversity are used to form the almost limitless array of antibodies that protect a host from foreign invasion: germline gene diversity, somatic recombination, junctional diversity, and somatic hypermutation.

Regulation of Immunoglobulin Gene Expression

An incomplete V gene becomes paired to a J gene on only one of a pair of homologous chromosomes. Successful rearrangement of one heavy-chain V region prevents the process from occurring on the other heavy-chain allele. Only the properly recombined immunoglobulin gene is expressed. Therefore, all of the V regions of immunoglobulins produced by a single lymphocyte are the same. This is called *allelic exclusion*.[36, 37]

There are five classes of immunoglobulins. An antibody-producing cell first synthesizes IgM and then IgG, IgA, IgE, or IgD of the same specificity. Different classes of antibodies are formed by the translocation of a complete V_H (V_{HDH}) gene from the C_H gene of one class to that of another.[38] Only the constant region of the heavy chain changes; the variable region of the heavy chain remains the same (Fig. 5–13). The light chain remains the same in this switch. This step in the differentiation of an antibody-producing cell is called class switching and is mediated by another DNA rearrangement called single-stranded *(SS) recombination* (Fig. 5–14).[39] This process is regulated by cytokines produced by helper T cells.[28] For

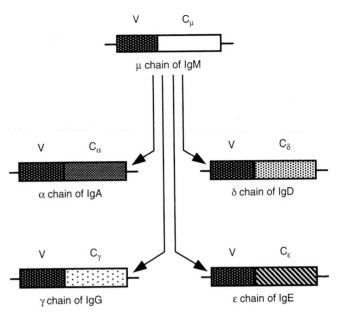

FIGURE 5–13. The V_H region is first associated with C_μ and then with another C region to form an H chain of a different class in the synthesis of different classes of immunoglobulins. (From Albert DA, Jakobiec FA: Principles and Practice of Ophthalmology, 2nd ed. Philadelphia, W. B. Saunders, 2000, p 69.)

example, switching to IgE class immunoglobulin production is provoked by the CD4 T_H2 cytokine, IL-4.

Determination of B-Cell Repertoire

V-segment genes can be grouped into families based on their DNA sequence homologies. In general, variable

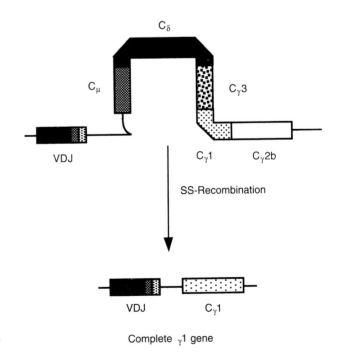

FIGURE 5–14. The V_HDJ_H gene moves from its position near C_μ to one near $C_\gamma1$ by SS recombination. (From Albert DA, Jakobiec FA: Principles and Practice of Ophthalmology, 2nd ed. Philadelphia, W. B. Saunders, 2000, p 69.)

genes sharing greater than 80% nucleotide similarity are defined as a family.[40] Currently, there are 11 known V_H gene families in the mouse[40–43] and 6 in humans.[44–47] At least 29 families are known for the V of murine light-chain genes.[48, 49] In fetal pre–B cells, chromosomal position is a major determinant of V_H rearrangement frequency, resulting in a nonrandom repertoire that is biased toward use of V_H families closest to the J_H segments.[50–53] In contrast, random use of V_H families based on the number of members in each family occurs in mature B cells without bias toward J_H proximal families.[54–56] The preferential V_H gene rearrangement frequency seen in pre–B cells presumably becomes normalized when contact of the organism with a foreign antigen selects for the expression of the entire V_H gene repertoire. One can speculate that members of V_H families preferentially used in the pre–B cell encode antibody specificities that are needed in the early development of the immune system.[57]

Immunoglobulins are serum proteins that migrate with the globulin fractions by electrophoresis.[25] Although they are glycoproteins, primary functions of the molecules are determined by their polypeptide sequence.[26] At one end of the immunoglobulin is the amino terminus, a region that binds a site (epitope) on an antigen with great specificity. At the other end is the carboxyl terminus, a non–antigen-binding region responsible for various functions, including complement fixation and cellular stimulation via binding to cell surface Ig receptors. The generalized structure of immunoglobulin is best understood initially by examining its most common class, IgG (see Fig. 5–6).

IgG is composed of four polypeptide chains: two identical heavy chains and two identical light chains. Heavy chains weigh about twice as much as light chains. The identical heavy chains are covalently linked by two disulfide bonds. One light chain is associated with each of the heavy chains by a disulfide bond and noncovalent forces. The two light chains are not linked. Asparagine residues on the heavy chains contain carbohydrate groups. The amino terminals of one light chain and its linked heavy chain compose the region for specific epitope binding. The carboxyl termini of the two heavy chains constitute the non–antigen-binding region.

Each polypeptide chain, whether light or heavy, is composed of regions that are called constant (C) or variable (V). A variable region on a light chain is called V_L, the constant region of a heavy chain is called C_H, and so forth. If the amino-acid sequence of multiple light or heavy chains is compared, the constant regions vary little, whereas the variable regions differ greatly. The light chains are divided approximately equally into a constant (C_L) and a variable (V_L) region at the carboxyl and amino terminals, respectively. The heavy chains also contain a similar length of variable region (V_H) at the amino terminals, but the constant region (C_H) is three times the length of the variable region (V_H). The variable regions are responsible for antigen binding, and it is this variability that accounts for the ability to bind to millions of potential and real epitopes.[27] Because each antibody molecule has two antigen-binding sites with variable regions, cross linking of two identical antigens may be performed

by one antibody. The constant regions carry out effector functions common to all antibodies of a given class (e.g., IgG) without the requirement of unique binding sites.

The functions of various regions of the immunoglobulin molecule were determined in part by the use of proteolytic enzymes that digest these molecules at specific locations. These enzymes have also been exploited for the development of laboratory reagents. The enzyme papain splits the molecule on the amino terminal side of the disulfide bonds that link the heavy chains, resulting in three fragments: two identical Fab fragments (each composed of the one entire heavy chain and a portion of the associated heavy chain) and one Fc fragment composed of the linked carboxyl terminal ends of the two heavy chains. In contrast, treatment with the enzyme pepsin results in one molecule composed of two linked Fab fragments known as F(ab').[25] The Fc fragment is degraded by pepsin treatment.

Within some classes of immunoglobulins, whole molecules may combine with other molecules of the same class to form polymers with additional functional capabilities. J chains facilitate the association of two or more immunoglobulins (Fig. 5–15), most notably IgA and IgM. Secretory component is a polypeptide synthesized by nonmotile epithelium found near mucosal surfaces. This polypeptide may bind noncovalently to IgA molecules,

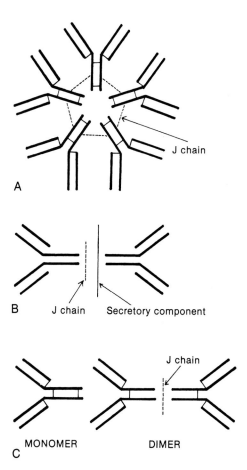

FIGURE 5–15. Schematic diagram of polymeric human immunoglobulins. (From Albert DA, Jakobiec FA: Principles and Practice of Ophthalmology, 2nd ed. Philadelphia, W. B. Saunders, 2000, p 70.)

allowing their transport across mucosal surfaces to be elaborated in secretions.

Five immunoglobulin classes are recognized in humans: IgG, IgM, IgA, IgE, and IgD (see Table 5–4). Some classes are composed of subclasses as well. The class or subclass is determined by the structure of the heavy-chain constant region (C_H).[28] The heavy chains γ, μ, α, ε, and δ are found in IgG, IgM, IgA, IgE, and IgD, respectively. Four subclasses of IgG and two subclasses of both IgA and IgM exist (see Table 5–5). The two light chains on any immunoglobulin are identical and, depending on the structure of their constant regions, may be designated kappa (κ) or lambda (λ). Kappa chains tend to predominate in human immunoglobulins regardless of the heavy chain–determined class. Whether an immunoglobulin is composed of two κ or two λ chains does not determine its functional capabilities. Heavy chain–determined class does dictate important capacities.[29]

Immunoglobulin G (IgG)

The most abundant of the human classes in serum, IgG constitutes about three quarters of the total serum immunoglobulins. Respectively, IgG_1 and IgG_2 make up about 60% and 20% of the total IgG. IgG_3 and IgG_4 are relatively minor components. IgG is the primary immunoglobulin providing immune protection in the extravascular compartments of the body. IgG is able to fix complement in the serum, an important function in inducing inflammation and controlling infection. IgG_3 and IgG_1 are most adept at complement fixation. IgG is the only immunoglobulin class to cross the placenta, an important aspect in fetal defense. Via their Fc portions, IgG molecules bind Fc receptors found on a host of inflammatory cells. Such binding activates cells such as macrophages and natural killer cells, enhancing cytotoxic activities important in the immune response.

Immunoglobulin M (IgM)

Less abundant in the serum than IgG, IgM typically exists as a pentameric form, stabilized by J chains, theoretically allowing the binding of 10 epitopes. (In vivo, this is usually limited by steric considerations.) IgM appears early in the immune response to antigen and is especially efficient at initiating agglutination, complement fixation, and cytolysis. IgM probably preceded IgG in the evolution of the immune response and is the most important antibody class in defending the circulation.

Immunoglobulin A (IgA)

IgA is found in secretions of mucosal surfaces as well as in the serum. In secretions, it exists as a dimer coupled by J chain and stabilized by secretory component. IgA protects mucosal surfaces from infection but may also be responsible for immunologic surveillance at the site of first contact with antigen. IgA in secretion is hardy, able to withstand the ravages of proteolytic degradation.

Immunoglobulin D (IgD)

IgD is present in minute amounts in the serum and is the least stable of the immunoglobulins. Its function is not known, but it probably serves as a differentiation marker. IgD is found on the surfaces of B lymphocytes (along with IgM) and may have a role in class switching and tolerance.

Immunoglobulin E (IgE)

IgE is notable for its ability to bind to mast cells; when cross-linked by antigen, it causes a variety of changes in the mast cell, including release of granular contents and membrane-derived mediators. Although IgE is recognized as a component of the allergic response, its role in protective immunity is speculative.

Immunoglobulin Intraclass Differences

Differences among the immunoglobulin classes are known as isotypes because all normal individuals in a species possess all of the classes. Allotype refers to antigenic structures on immunoglobulins that may differ from one individual to another within a species. Idiotype refers to differences among individual antibodies and is determined by the variable domain. Just as the variable domain allows for antibodies to recognize many antigens (epitopes), these differences also allow individual antibodies to be recognized on the basis of idiotype. In fact, antibodies directed against antibodies exist and are called anti-idiotypic antibodies. These anti-idiotypic antibodies are crucial to the regulation of the antibody response and constitute the basis for Jerne's idiotype network.

Complement

The complement system functions in the immune response by allowing animals to recognize foreign substances and defend themselves against infection.[46] The pathways of complement activation are complex (Fig. 5–16).[47] Activation begins with the formation of antigen-antibody complexes and the ensuing generation of peptides that lead to a cascade of proteolytic events. The particle that activates the system accumulates a protein complex on its surface that often leads to cellular destruction via disruption of membranes.

Two independent pathways of complement activation are known. The classic pathway is initiated by IgG- and IgM-containing immune complexes. The alternative pathway is activated by aggravated IgA or complex polysaccharides from microbial cell walls.[49] One component, C3, is crucial to both pathways and in its proactive form can be found circulating in plasma in large concentrations. Deficiency or absence of C3 results in increased susceptibility to infection.[50] Cleavage of C3 may result in at least seven products (lettered *a* through *g*), each with biologic properties related to cellular activation and immune and nonimmune responses.[51] C3a, for instance, causes the release of histamine from mast cells, neutrophil enzyme release, smooth muscle contraction, suppressor T-cell induction, and secretion of macrophage IL-1, prostaglandin, and leukotriene.[52] C3e enhances vascular permeability. C3b binds to target cell surfaces and allows opsonization of biologic particles.

The alternative pathway probably is a first line of defense because, unlike the classic pathway, it may neutralize foreign material in the absence of antibody. The initiating enzyme of this pathway, factor D, circulates in an active form and may protect bystander cells from

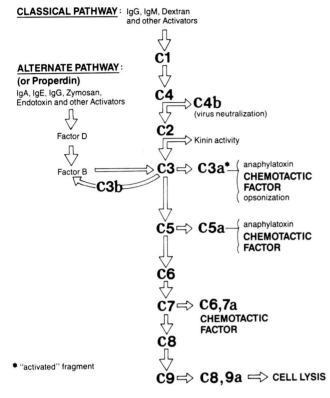

COMPLEMENT CASCADE

CLASSICAL PATHWAY: IgG, IgM, Dextran and other Activators

ALTERNATE PATHWAY: (or Properdin)
IgA, IgE, IgG, Zymosan, Endotoxin and other Activators

Factor D

Factor B

C1

C4 → C4b
(virus neutralization)

C2 → Kinin activity

C3 → C3a* anaplylatoxin **CHEMOTACTIC FACTOR** opsonization

C3b

C5 → C5a anaphylatoxin **CHEMOTACTIC FACTOR**

C6

C7 → C6,7a **CHEMOTACTIC FACTOR**

C8

* "activated" fragment

C9 → C8,9a ⇒ CELL LYSIS

FIGURE 5–16. Simplified schematic of steps in classic and alternate complement cascades. (From Albert DA, Jakobiec FA: Principles and Practice of Ophthalmology, 2nd ed. Philadelphia, W. B. Saunders, 2000, p 72.)

inadvertent destruction following activation of the pathway.

The final step of both pathways is membrane damage leading to cytolysis. Both pathways require the assembly of five precursor proteins to effect this damage: C5, C6, C7, C8, and C9. The mechanism of complement-mediated cell lysis is similar to that of cell-mediated cytotoxicity (as with natural killer cells). Membrane lesions result from insertion of tubular complexes into the membranes, leading to uptake of water with ion-exchange disruption and eventual osmotic lysis.

The complement system interfaces with a variety of immune responses, as outlined earlier, and with the intrinsic coagulation pathways.[53] Complement activity is usually measured by assessing the ability of serum to lyse sensitized sheep red blood cells.[54] Values are expressed as 50% hemolytic complement units per millimeter. The function of an individual component may be studied by supplying excess quantities of all other components in a sheep red blood cell lysis assay.[55] Components are quantitated by radial diffusion or immunoassay. Complement may be demonstrated in tissue sections by immunofluorescence or enzymatic techniques.

Complement plays a role in a number of human diseases. Complement-mediated cell lysis is the final common pathologic event in type III hypersensitivity reactions. Deficiencies of complement exist in the following human disorders: systemic lupus erythematosus, glomeru-

lonephritis, Raynaud's phenomenon, recurrent gonococcal and meningococcal infections, hereditary angioedema, rheumatoid disease, and others.[50]

B-Cell Response to Antigen

Primary Response

Naive B cells respond to protein antigen in much the same way that T cells do, through the help of antigen-presenting cells and "helper" T cells. An antigen-presenting cell (usually a macrophage or dendritic cell) processes the antigen and presents it to an antigen-specific helper (CD4) T cell, generally in the T cell–rich zones of the required lymph node. The T cell is thus activated, expresses the membrane protein gp39, secretes cytokines (e.g., IL-2 and IL-6), and binds to similarly activated antigen-specific B cells (activated by the binding cross linking of antigen to surface IgM- and IgD-binding sites). The T-cell/B-cell proliferation and a cascade of intracellular protein phosphorylation events, together with T-cell cytokine signals, result in production of transcription factors that induce transcription of various B-cell genes, including those responsible for production of IgM light and heavy chains with paratopes specific to the antigen epitopes that initiated this primary B-cell response. The proliferating B cells form germinal centers in the lymph node follicles, and somatic hypermutation of the IgM genes in some of these cells results in the evolution of a collection of B cells in the germinal center with surface IgM of even higher antigen-binding affinity. This phenomenon is called affinity maturation of the primary antibody response. Those cells with the greatest antigen-binding affinity survive as this primary B-cell response subsides, persisting as long-lived memory cells responsible for the classic distinguishing characteristics of the secondary humoral immune response.

Secondary Response

The development of the secondary humoral immune response is markedly accelerated compared with the primary response, and it is greatly amplified in terms of magnitude of antibody production (Fig. 5–17). The secondary response differs from the primary one in the isotype or isotypes of antibody produced, as well as in the avidity of the paratopes for the epitopes on the elicited antigen. IgG, IgA, and IgE isotypes may now be seen in the effector phase of this secondary humoral immune response, and the binding affinities of these antibodies are usually greater than that of the IgM elicited in the primary response.

The cellular and molecular events of the secondary B-cell response are considerably different from those of the primary response. Memory B cells themselves become the preeminent antigen-binding, processing, and presenting cells, presenting peptide fragments (antigenic determinants) to CD4 helper T cells in typical major histocompatibility complex–restricted fashion, with "processed" peptide/human leukocyte antigen/DR motifs interacting with the appropriate elements of the T-cell receptor for antigen at the same time that B-cell CD40 and T-cell gp39 signaling occurs.[58] Additionally, various T-cell cytokines induce the memory B cells to divide, proliferate, produce

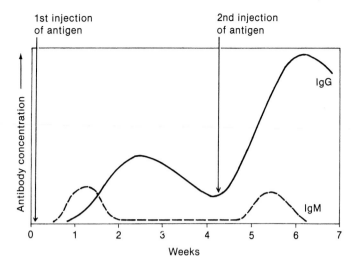

FIGURE 5–17. Relative synthesis of IgG and IgM following initial and subsequent antigen injection. (From Albert DA, Jakobiec FA: Principles and Practice of Ophthalmology, 2nd ed. Philadelphia, W. B. Saunders, 2000, p 72.)

antibody, and switch the class of antibody being produced, depending on the sum total message being received by the B cell, that is, the nature of the antigenic stimulus, the amount and the site of stimulation, and the sites of cells involved in the cognitive and activation phases of the secondary response. Memory cells of each immunoglobulin isotype involved in the secondary response, of course, persist after devolution of the response.

T-LYMPHOCYTE RESPONSES

T lymphocytes stand at the center of the adaptive immune response.[59] In the presence of T cells, the entire array of immune effector responses and tolerance are possible, but in the absence of T cells, only primitive antibody responses and no cell-mediated immune responses can be made. T cells are leukocytes that originate from lymphocyte precursors in the bone marrow. The majority of T cells undergo differentiation in the thymus gland and, upon reaching maturity, disseminate via the blood to populate secondary lymphoid organs and to circulate among virtually all tissues of the body. A second population of T cells undergoes differentiation extrathymically; these cells have a somewhat different (and not yet completely defined) set of functional properties. T cells are exquisitely antigen-specific, a property conferred on them by unique surface receptors that recognize antigenic material. Once activated, T cells initiate or participate in the various forms of cell-mediated immunity, humoral immunity, and tolerance.

T-Lymphocyte Development

From the pluripotent hematopoietic stem cell, a lineage of cells emerges that becomes the oligopotent lymphocyte progenitor.[59] During fetal life, this lineage of cells is observed first in the liver, but as the fetus matures, the lymphocyte progenitors shift to the bone marrow. According to developmental signals not completely understood, lymphocyte progenitors in the bone marrow differentiate into (at least) three distinct lineages of committed precursor cells: pre-thymocytes, pre–B lymphocytes, and pre–natural killer lymphocytes. Pre-thymocytes, which give rise eventually to T lymphocytes, escape from the bone marrow (or fetal liver) and migrate via the blood

primarily to the thymus where cell adhesion molecules on microvascular endothelial cells direct them into the cortex. The differentiation process that thymocytes experience within the thymus accomplishes several critical goals in T-cell biology: (1) each cell acquires a unique surface receptor for antigen, (2) cells with receptors that recognize antigen molecules in the context of "self" class I or class II molecules (encoded b genes within the histocompatibility complex [MHCT]) are positively selected,[60] (3) cells with receptors that recognize self-antigenic molecules in the context of self-MHC molecules are negatively selected (deleted or inactivated),[61] and (4) each mature cell acquires unique effector functions—the capacity to respond to antigen by secreting immunomodulatory cytokines or by delivering to a target cell a "lethal hit."[58]

Differentiation in the Thymic Cortex

Within the thymic cortex, pre-thymocytes receive differentiation signals from resident thymic epithelial cells and thus initiate the process of maturation.[59] A unique set of genes is activated, including: (1) genes that commit the cells to proliferation, (2) genes that encode the T-cell receptors for antigen, and (3) genes that code accessory molecules that developing and mature T cells use for antigen recognition and signal transduction. The genes that make it possible for T cells to create surface receptors for antigen are the structural genes that encode the four distinct polypeptide chains (α, β, γ, δ) from which the T-cell receptor (TCR) for antigen is composed, as well as the genes that create genetic rearrangements that confer an extremely high degree of diversity on TCR molecules. Each TCR is a heterodimer of transmembrane polypeptides ($\alpha\beta$ or $\gamma\delta$). The portion of the TCR that is involved in antigen recognition resides at the ends of the peptide chains distal to the cell surface and is called the "combining site." The accessory genes encode, on the one hand, the CD3 molecular complex (γ, δ, ϵ, ζ), which enables a TCR that has engaged antigen to signal the T cell across the plasma membrane and, on the other hand, the CD4 and CD8 molecules that promote the affinity of the TCR for antigenic peptides in association with class I and II molecules, respectively, of the MHC. Thus, within the thymic cortex, individual pre-thymocytes proliferate, come to express a unique TCR, and simultaneously express CD3, CD4, and CD8 on the cell surface. Each day, a very large number of thymocytes is generated; therefore, an enormous diversity of TCR is also generated. Conservative estimates place the number of novel TCRs produced each day in excess of 10^9!

Nature of Antigen Recognition by T Cells

Understanding the nature of the antigenic determinants detected by individual T-cell receptors for antigen is central to understanding the differentiation process that occurs among thymocytes in the thymus gland. Thymocytes acquire one of two types of T-cell receptors: αβ-TCRs are heterodimers composed of polypeptides encoded by the TCR-α and TCR-β chain genes; γδ-TCRs are heterodimers composed of polypeptides encoded by the TCR-γ and TCR-δ chain genes.[62] Because much is known about αβ-TCR, whereas much remains to be learned about γδ-TCR, this discussion is limited to the former. The αβ–T-cell receptor for antigen does not recognize a protein antigen in its native configuration. Rather, the TCR recognizes peptides (ranging in size from 7 to 22 amino acids in length) derived from limited proteolysis of the antigen, and it recognizes these peptides when they are bound noncovalently to highly specialized regions of antigen-presenting molecules.[63] Two types of antigen-presenting molecules exist, and both are encoded within the MHC.[64] Class I molecules are transmembrane proteins expressed on antigen-presenting cells (APCs). These molecules possess on their most distal domains a platform of two parallel α-helices separated by a groove. This groove accommodates peptides (generated by regulated proteolysis of antigenic proteins) ranging from seven to nine amino acids in length. Class II molecules are also transmembrane proteins expressed on APC; the platforms on their distal domains contain similar grooves, which accept peptides of 15 to 22 amino acids in length. The "combining site" of an individual TCR possesses three contact points: a central point that interacts directly with an antigenic peptide in the groove, and two side points that interact directly with the platform (α-helices) of class I or class II molecules. Thus, the conditions that must be met for successful recognition of antigen by TCR are: (1) a class I or class II molecule must be available on an APC, and (2) a peptide must occupy the groove of the presenting molecule's platform.

Other molecules promote the affinity of TCR binding with antigenic peptides associated with class I and class II MHC molecules.[65] CD4 molecules that are expressed on certain T cells and thymocytes have the ability to bind class II molecules at a site distinct from the antigen presentation platform. As a consequence, CD4-bearing T cells whose TCR has engaged a peptide-containing class II molecule are much more likely to be stimulated than T cells with similar receptors that don't express CD4. Similarly, CD8-bearing T cells whose TCR has engaged a peptide-containing molecule are much more likely to be stimulated than T cells without CD8.

Within the thymic cortex, epithelial cells express class I and class II molecules encoded by the individual's own MHC genes.[59, 60] When TCR-bearing thymocytes are generated in the cortex, cells with TCR that recognize peptide-containing self–class I or –class II molecules are induced to undergo successive rounds of proliferation, leading to clonal expansion. By contrast, TCR-bearing thymocytes that fail to recognize peptide-containing class I or class II molecules are not activated within the cortex. In the absence of this cognate signal, all such cells enter a default pathway, which ends inevitably in cell death (apoptosis). This process is called *positive selection* because thymocytes with TCR that have an affinity for self-MHC molecules (plus peptide) are being selected for further clonal expansion. Unselected cells simply die by apoptosis. At the completion of their sojourn in the thymic cortex, large numbers of positively selected TCR+, CD3+, CD4+, and CD8+ thymocytes migrate into the thymic medulla.

Differentiation in the Thymic Medulla

In addition to epithelial cells, the thymic medulla contains a unique population of bone marrow–derived cells called *dendritic cells*.[61, 66] These nonphagocytic cells express large numbers of class I and class II molecules and actively endocytose proteins within their environment. Peptides derived from these proteins by proteolysis are loaded into the grooves of MHC-encoded antigen presentation platforms. Within the thymic medulla, the vast majority of such endocytosed proteins are "self" proteins. As thymocytes enter the medulla from the cortex, a subpopulation expresses TCR that recognize peptides of "self" proteins expressed on "self" class I or class II molecules. By contrast, another subpopulation fails to recognize "self" class I or class II molecules because the TCR is specific for a peptide not included among peptides from "self" proteins. The former population, comprising cells that recognize "self" exclusively, engage self-derived peptides plus MHC molecules on medullary dendritic cells. This engagement delivers a "death" signal to the T cell, and all such cells undergo apoptosis. This process is called *negative selection* because thymocytes with TCR that have an affinity for self-peptides in self-MHC molecules are being eliminated. In part, this process plays a major role in eliminating autoreactive T cells that would be capable of causing autoimmunity if they should escape from the thymus. Many other thymocytes that enter the medulla express TCRs that are unable to engage self–class I or –class II molecules on dendritic cells because the relevant peptide does not occupy the antigen-presenting groove. T cells of this type proceed to downregulate expression of either CD4 or CD8 and acquire the properties of mature T cells. The T cells that are ready at this point to leave the thymus are TCR+, CD3+, and either CD4+ or CD8+ (but not both). Moreover, they are in G_0, of the cell cycle, that is, resting. The number of such cells exported from the thymus per day is very large; in humans, it is estimated that more than 108 new mature T cells are produced daily. These cells are fully immunocompetent and are prepared to recognize and respond to a large diversity of foreign antigens that are degraded into peptides and presented on self–class I or –class II molecules on tissues outside the thymus. It is estimated that the number of different antigenic specificities that can be recognized by mature T cells (i.e., the T-cell repertoire for antigens) exceeds 10^9.

Properties and Functions of Mature T Lymphocytes

Mature, resting T cells with αβ-TCR migrate from the thymus to any and all tissues of the body, but there are vascular specializations (postcapillary venules) in secondary lymphoid organs (lymph nodes, Peyer's patches, tonsils) that promote the selective entry of T cells into these tissues.[67] More than 99% of T cells in blood that traverse a lymph node are extracted into the parafollicular region of the cortex. This region of the nodal cortex is designed to encourage the interaction of T cells with APC. Because the encounter of any single, antigen-specific T cell with its antigen of interest on an APC is a rather rare event, most T cells that enter a secondary lymphoid organ fail to find their antigen of interest. In this case, the T cells disengage from resident APC and migrate into the effluent of the node, passing through lymph ducts back into the general blood circulation. An individual T cell may make journeys such as this numerous times during a single day, and countless journeys are accomplished during its lifetime (which may be measured in tens of years). Remarkably, this monotonous behavior changes dramatically if and when a mature T cell encounters its specific antigen via recognition of the relevant peptide in association with a class I or class II molecule on an APC in a secondary lymphoid organ. It is this critical encounter that initiates T cell–dependent, antigen-specific immune responses.

T-Cell Activation by Antigen

There is a general rule regarding the minimal requirements for activation of lymphocytes, including T cells, which are normal in a resting state: two different surface signals received simultaneously are required to arouse the cell out of G_0.[65] One signal (referred to as "signal 1") is delivered through CD3 and is triggered by successful engagement of the TCR with its peptide in association with an MHC molecule. The other signal (referred to as "signal 2") is delivered through numerous cell surface molecules other than the TCR. Signals of this type are also referred to as co-stimulation, and co-stimulation is usually the result of receptor/ligand interactions in which the receptor is on the T cell and the ligand is expressed on the APC. For example, B7-1 (CD80) and B7-2 (CD81) are surface molecules expressed on APC; these molecules engage the receptor CD28 on T cells, thus delivering an activation signal to the recipient cells. Similarly, CD40 ligand on T cells and CD40 on APC function in a costimulatory manner. Another example of co-stimulation occurs when a cytokine produced by an APC, such as interleukin-1 (IL-1) or IL-2, is presented to T cells expressing the IL-1 or IL-2 receptor, respectively. When both conditions are met—signal 1 (TCR binds to peptide plus MHC molecule) and signal 2 (e.g., CD80 binds to CD28)—the T cell receives coordinated signals across the plasma membrane, and these signals initiate a cascade of intracytoplasmic events that lead to dramatic changes in the genetic and functional programs of the T cells.

Antigen-Activated T-Cell Responses

When a T cell encounters its antigen of interest along with a satisfactory signal 2, it escapes from G_0. Under

these circumstances, the genetic program of the cell shifts in a direction that makes it possible for the cell to proliferate and to undergo further differentiation. *Proliferation* results in emergence of a "clone" of cells, all of the identical phenotype, including the TCR. This process is called clonal expansion, results from the elaboration of growth factor (e.g., IL-2), is one hallmark of the process of immunization or sensitization, and accounts for why the number of T cells able to recognize a particular antigen increases dramatically after sensitization has taken place. The signal that triggers proliferation arises first from the APC, but sustained T-cell proliferation takes place because the responding T cell activates its own IL-2 and IL-2R receptor genes.[68, 69] IL-2 is a potent growth factor for T cells, and T cells expressing the IL-2R respond to IL-2 by undergoing repetitive rounds of replication. IL-2 is not the only growth factor for T cells; another important growth factor is IL-4, which is also made by T cells. Thus, once activated, T cells have the capacity to autocrine stimulate their own proliferation—so long as their TCRs remain engaged with the antigen (plus MHC) of interest.

In addition to proliferation, antigen-activated T cells proceed down pathways of further *differentiation*. The functional expressions of this differentiation include: (1) secretion of lymphokines that promote inflammation or modify the functional properties of other lymphoreticular cells in their immediate environment, and (2) acquisition of the cytoplasmic machinery required for displaying cytotoxicity, that is, the ability to lyse target cells.[70] The list of lymphokines that an activated mature T cell can make is long: IL-2, IL-3, IL-4, granulocyte-macrophage colony-stimulating factor (GM-CSF), IL-5, IL-6, IL-10, interferon-γ (IFN-γ), tumor necrosis factor-α (TNF-α), and transforming growth factor-β (TGF-β). The range of biologic activities attributable to these cytokines is extremely broad, and no single T cell produces all of these factors simultaneously. The pattern of cytokines produced by a T cell accounts in large measure for the functional phenotype of the cell (see later discussion).

The ability of antigen-activated T cells to lyse antigen-bearing target cells is embodied in specializations of the cell cytoplasm and cell surface. Cytotoxic T cells possess granules in their cytoplasm that contain a molecule, perforin, that can polymerize and insert into the plasma membrane of a target cell, creating large pores. The granules also contain a series of lytic enzymes (granzymes) that enter the target cell, perhaps through the perforin-created pores, and trigger programmed cell death. There is a second mechanism by which T cells can cause death of neighboring cells. Activated T cells express Fas or CD95, a cell surface glycoprotein. The co-receptor for Fas is called (appropriately) Fas ligand or CD95 ligand. It is a member of the TNF receptor superfamily, and its cytoplasmic tail contains a "death domain." After sustained activation, T cells also express Fas ligand; when Fas interacts with Fas ligand, the cell bearing Fas undergoes programmed cell death. Thus, Fas+ ligand T cells can trigger apoptotic death in adjacent cells that are Fas+, including other T cells. In fact, the ability of antigen-activated T cells to elicit apoptosis among neighboring similarly activated T cells may serve to downregulate the immune response to that particular antigen, that is, by eliminating responding T cells.

Imperfect Antigen-Activated T-Cell Responses

On occasion, T cells may encounter their antigen of interest (in association with an MHC molecule) under circumstances wherein an appropriate "signal 2" does not exist.[71] This can be arranged in vitro, for example, by using paraformaldehyde-fixed APC. Not surprisingly, delivery of "signal 1" alone fails to activate the T cells in question. However, if these same T cells are reexposed subsequently to the same antigen/MHC signal 1 on viable APC capable of delivering a functional "signal 2," activation of the T cells *still fails*. The inability of T cells first activated by signal 1 in the absence of signal 2 to respond subsequently to functional signal 1 and signal 2 is referred to as *anergy*. Although the phenomenon just described was described in vitro, there is evidence that anergy occurs in vivo and that this process is important in regulating the immune response and some forms of tolerance.

T-Lymphocyte Heterogeneity

The adaptive immune response is separable into a cell-mediated immune arm and an antibody or humoral immune arm.[58] T cells themselves initiate and mediate cell-mediated immunity, and they play a dominant role in promoting antibody-mediated responses. There is heterogeneity among T cells that function in cell-mediated immunity, and there is heterogeneity among T cells that promote humoral immunity.

Cell-mediated immunity arises when effector T cells are generated within secondary lymphoid organs in response to antigen-induced activation. Two types of effector cells are recognized: (1) T cells that elicit delayed hypersensitivity (DH), and (2) T cells that are cytotoxic for antigen-bearing target cells. T cells that elicit delayed hypersensitivity recognize their antigen of interest on cells in peripheral tissues and, upon activation, they secrete proinflammatory cytokines such as IFN-γ and TNF-α. These cytokines act on microvascular endothelium, promoting edema formation and recruitment of monocytes, neutrophils, and other leukocytes to the site. In addition, monocytes and tissue macrophages exposed to these cytokines are activated to acquire phagocytic and cytotoxic functions. Because it takes hours for these inflammatory reactions to emerge, they are called "delayed." It is generally believed that the T cells that elicit delayed hypersensitivity reactions are CD4+ and recognize antigens of interest in association with class II MHC molecules. However, ample evidence exists to implicate CD8+ T cells in this process (especially in reactions within the central nervous system). Although the elicitation of delayed hypersensitivity reactions is antigen-specific, the inflammation that attends the response is itself nonspecific. This feature accounts for the high level of tissue injury and cell destruction that is found in DH responses. By contrast, effector responses elicited by cytotoxic T cells possess much less nonspecific inflammation. Cytotoxic T cells interact directly with antigen-bearing target cells and deliver a "lethal hit" that is clean and highly specific;

there is virtually no innocent bystander injury in this response.

Humoral immunity arises when B cells produce antibodies in response to antigenic challenge.[58] Although antigen alone may be sufficient to activate B cells to produce IgM antibodies, this response is amplified in the presence of helper T cells. Moreover, the ability of B cells to produce more differentiated antibody isotypes, such as IgG or IgE, is dependent on helper signals from T cells. Within the past 10 years, immunologists have appreciated that helper T cells provide "help" in the form of lymphokines and that the pattern of lymphokines produced by a helper T cell plays a key role in determining the nature of the B-cell antibody response. For example, one polar form of helper T cell—called Th1—responds to antigen stimulation by producing IL-2, IFN-γ, and TNF-α.[72] In turn, these cytokines influence B-cell differentiation in the direction of producing complement-fixing antibodies. By contrast, Th2 cells (the other polar form of helper T cell) respond to antigen stimulation by producing IL-4, IL-5, IL-6, and IL-10. In turn, these cytokines influence B-cell differentiation in the direction of producing non–complement-fixing IgG antibodies or IgA and IgE antibodies. The discovery of two polar forms of helper T cells (as well as numerous intermediate forms) has already had a profound impact on our understanding of the immune response and its regulation. Although the Th1/Th2 dichotomy was first described for CD4+ T cells, recent evidence strongly suggests that a similar difference in cytokine profiles exists for subpopulations of CD8+ T cells. Moreover, there is good experimental evidence to suggest that Th1-type cells mediate delayed hypersensitivity reactions and thus can function as effector cells, as well as helper cells. Th2-type cells do not mediate typical delayed hypersensitivity reactions, but these cells are not without immunopathogenic potential because they have been implicated in inflammatory reactions of both immediate and intermediate types. Much still remains to be learned about helper–T cell subsets, but it is already clear that Th1-dependent immune responses are particularly deleterious in the eye.

T Cell–Dependent Inflammation

Primarily by virtue of the lymphokines they produce, T cells can produce immunogenic inflammation if they encounter their antigens of interest in a peripheral tissue. This is equally true for CD4+ and CD8+ cells, although much more is known about the former. The requirement for signal 1 (peptide plus MHC class I or II molecules) must be fulfilled in order for effector T cells to be activated by antigen in the periphery. If the responding T cell is CD4+, then an MHC class II–bearing professional APC (bone marrow derived dendritic cell or macrophage) is usually responsible for providing signal 1. If the responding T cell is of the Th1 type, it produces IFN-γ along with other proinflammatory molecules. IFN-γ is a potent activator of microvascular endothelial cells and macrophages. Activated endothelial cells become "leaky," permitting edema fluid and plasma proteins to accumulate at the site. Activated endothelial cells also promote the immigration of blood-borne leukocytes, including monocytes, into the site; it is the activated macrophages that provide much of the "toxicity" at the inflammatory site. These cells respond to IFN-γ by upregulating the genes responsible for nitric oxide (NO) synthesis. NO, together with newly generated reactive oxygen intermediates, creates much of the local necrosis associated with immunogenic inflammation. Because Th2 cells do not make IFN-γ in response to antigenic stimulation, one might expect that Th2 cells would not promote inflammatory injury, but this does not appear to be the case. Th2 cells have been directly implicated in immune inflammation, including that found in the eye. The offending lymphokine may be IL-10, although other cytokines may also participate.

T Cells in Disease: Infectious, Immunopathogenic, Autoimmune

T cells were presumably created via evolution to aid in the process by which invading pathogens are prevented from causing disease. It is generally believed that T cells were designed to detect intracellular pathogens, a belief based on the ability of T cells to detect peptides derived from degradation of intracellular or phagocytosed pathogens. This property is most obviously revealed in viral infections in which CD8+ T cells detect peptides on virus-infected cells derived from viral proteins in association with class I molecules. Once recognition has occurred, a "lethal hit" is delivered to the target cell, and lysis aborts the viral infection. T-cell immunity is also conferred when CD4+ T cells detect peptides derived from other bacteria (or other pathogens) that have been phagocytosed by macrophages. Recognition in this case does not result in delivery of a "lethal hit"; instead, proinflammatory cytokines released by the activated T cells cause the macrophages to acquire phagocytic and cytotoxic functions that lead to the death of the offending pathogen.

To a limited extent with CD8+ cells, but to a greater extent with CD4+ cells, the inflammation associated with the immune attack on the invading pathogen can lead to injury of surrounding tissues.[73] If the extent of this injury is of sufficient magnitude, disease may result from the inflammation itself, quite apart from the "toxicity" of the pathogen. This is the basis of the concept of T cell–dependent immunopathogenic disease. As previously mentioned, certain organs and tissues, especially the eye, are particularly vulnerable to immunopathogenic injury. In tissues of this type, the immune response may prove to be more problematic than the triggering infection.

In some pathologic circumstances, T cells mistake "self" molecules as "foreign," thus mediating an autoimmune response that can eventuate into disease. Although this idea is conceptually sound, it is often (usually) difficult to identify the offending "self" antigen. Because of this difficulty, it is frequently impossible to determine whether a particular inflammatory condition, initiated by T cells, is immunopathogenic in origin (and therefore, triggered by an unidentified pathogen) or autoimmune in origin. This is a particularly common problem in the eye.

IMMUNE-MEDIATED TISSUE INJURY

The immune response of an organism to an antigen may be either helpful or harmful. If the response is excessive or inappropriate, the host may incur tissue damage. The term *hypersensitivity reactions* has been applied to such excessive or inappropriate immune responses. Four major types of hypersensitivity reaction are described, and all can occur in the eye (Table 5–11). The necessary constituents for these reactions are already present in, or can be readily recruited into, ocular tissues. Immunoglobulins, complement components, inflammatory cells, and inflammatory mediators can, under certain circumstances, be found in ocular fluids (i.e., tears, aqueous humor, and vitreous) and in the ocular tissues, adnexa, and orbit. Unfortunately, these tissues (especially the ocular tissues) can be rapidly damaged by inflammatory reactions that produce irreversible alterations in structure and function. Some authors have described a fifth type of hypersensitivity reaction, but this adds little to our real understanding of disease mechanisms and is unimportant to us as oph-

TABLE 5–11. GELL, COOMBS, AND LACKMANN HYPERSENSITIVITY REACTIONS

TYPE	PARTICIPATING ELEMENTS	SYSTEMIC EXAMPLES	OCULAR EXAMPLES
Type I	Allergen, IgE, mast cells	Allergic rhinitis, allergic asthma, anaphylaxis	Seasonal allergic conjunctivitis, vernal keratoconjunctivitis, atopic keratoconjunctivitis, giant papillary conjunctivitis
Type II	Antigen, IgG, IgG3, or IgM, complement, neutrophils (enzymes), macrophages (enzymes)	Goodpasture's syndrome, myasthenia gravis	Ocular cicatricial pemphigoid, pemphigus vulgaris, dermatitis herpetiformis
Type III	Antigen, IgG, IgG3, or IgM, complement-immune complex, neutrophils (enzymes), macrophages (enzymes)	Stevens-Johnson syndrome, rheumatoid arthritis, systemic lupus erythematosus, polyarteritis nodosa, Behçet's disease, relapsing polychondritis	Ocular manifestations of diseases listed in systemic examples
Type IV	Antigen, T cells, neutrophils, macrophages	Transplant rejection, tuberculosis, sarcoidosis, Wegener's granulomatosis	Contact hypersensitivity (drug allergy), herpes disciform keratitis, phlyctenulosis, corneal transplant rejection, tuberculosis, sarcoidosis, Wegener's granulomatosis, uveitis, herpes simplex virus stromal keratitis, river blindness

thalmologists in the study and care of patients with destructive ocular inflammatory diseases. For this reason, this discussion is confined to the classic four types of hypersensitivity reactions that were originally proposed by Gell, Coombs, and Lackmann.

Injury Mediated by Antibody

Type I Hypersensitivity Reactions

The antigens typically responsible for type I (immediate) hypersensitivity reactions are ubiquitous environmental allergens such as dust, pollens, danders, microbes, and drugs. Under ordinary circumstances, exposure of an individual to such materials is associated with no harmful inflammatory response. The occurrence of such a response is considered, therefore, out of place (Greek, *a topos*) or inappropriate; it is for this reason that Cocoa and Cooke coined the word "atopy" in 1923 to describe the predisposition of individuals who develop such inappropriate inflammatory or immune responses to ubiquitous environmental agents.[74] The antibodies responsible for type I hypersensitivity reactions are homocytotropic antibodies, principally immunoglobulin E (IgE) but sometimes IgG4 as well. The mediators of the clinical manifestations of type I reactions include histamine, serotonin, leukotrienes (including slow-reacting substance of anaphylaxis [SRS-A]), kinins, and other vasoactive amines. Examples of type I hypersensitivity reactions include anaphylactic reactions to insect bites or to penicillin injections, allergic asthma, hay fever, and seasonal allergic conjunctivitis. It should be emphasized that in real life, the four types of hypersensitivity reactions are rarely observed in pure form, in isolation from each other; it is typical for hypersensitivity reactions to have more than one of the classic Gell and Coombs responses as participants in the inflammatory problem. For example, eczema, atopic blepharokeratoconjunctivitis, and vernal keratoconjunctivitis have hypersensitivity reaction mechanisms of both type I and type IV. The atopic individuals who develop such abnormal reactions to environmental materials are genetically predisposed to such responses. The details of the events responsible for allergy (a term coined in 1906 by von Pirquet, in Vienna, meaning "changed reactivity") are clearer now than they were even a decade ago.[75]

Genetically predisposed allergic individuals have defects in the population of suppressor T lymphocytes responsible for modulating IgE responses to antigens. After the initial contact of an allergen with the mucosa of such an individual, abnormal amounts of allergen-specific IgE antibody are produced at the mucosal surface and at the regional lymph nodes. This IgE has high avidity, through its Fc portion, to Fc receptors on the surfaces of mast cells in the mucosa. The antigen-specific IgE antibodies, therefore, stick to the receptors on the surfaces of the tissue mast cells and remain there for unusually long periods. Excess locally produced IgE enters the circulation and binds to mast cells at other tissue locations as well as to circulating basophils. A subsequent encounter of the allergic individual with the antigen to which he or she has become sensitized results in antigen binding by the antigen-specific IgE molecules affixed to the surfaces

of the tissue mast cells. The simultaneous binding of the antigen to adjacent IgE molecules on the mast cell surface results in a change in the mast cell membrane and particularly in membrane-bound adenyl cyclase (Fig. 5–18). The feature common to all known mechanisms that trigger mast cell degranulation (including degranulation stimulated by pharmacologic agents or anaphylatoxins like C3a and C5a and antigen-specific IgE-mediated degranulation) is calcium influx with subsequent aggregation of tubulin into microtubules, which then participate in the degranulation of vasoactive amines (see Fig. 5–16). In addition to the degranulation of the preformed media-

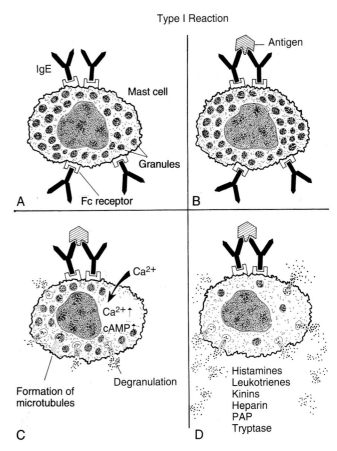

Type I Reaction

FIGURE 5–18. Type I hypersensitivity reaction mechanism. *A,* Mast cell Fcε receptors have antigen-specific IgE affixed to them by virtue of the patient's being exposed to the antigen and mounting an inappropriate (atopic) immune response to that antigen, with resultant production of large amounts of antigen-specific IgE antibodies. The antibodies have found their way to the mucosal mast cell and have bound to the mast cells but have not provoked allergic symptoms because the patient is no longer exposed to the antigen. *B,* Second (or subsequent) exposure to the sensitizing antigen or allergen results in a "bridging" binding reaction of antigen to two adjacent IgE antibodies affixed to the mast cell plasma membrane. *C,* The antigen-antibody bridging reaction shown in B results in profound changes in the mast cell membrane, with alterations in membrane-bound adenyl cyclase, calcium influx, tubulin aggregation into microtubules, and the beginning of the degranulation of the preformed mast cell mediators from their storage granules. *D,* The degranulation reaction proceeds, and newly synthesized mediators, particularly those generated by the catabolism of membrane-associated arachidonic acid, begin. The array of liberated and synthesized proinflammatory mediators is impressive. (From Albert DA, Jakobiec FA: Principles and Practice of Ophthalmology, 2nd ed. Philadelphia, W. B. Saunders, 2000, p 75.)

tors such as histamine, induction of synthesis of newly formed mediators from arachidonic acid also occurs with triggering of mast cell degranulation (Table 5–12). The preformed and newly synthesized mediators then produce the classic clinical signs of a type I hypersensitivity reaction: wheal (edema), flare (erythema), itch, and in many cases, the subsequent delayed appearance of the so-called late-phase reaction characterized by subacute signs of inflammation.

CONTROL OF IgE SYNTHESIS

The Th2 subset of helper T cells bearing Fc receptors produce, in addition to interleukin-4 (IL-4), IgE-binding factors after stimulation by interleukins produced by antigen-specific helper T cells activated by antigen-presenting cells and antigen. The two known types of IgE-binding factor that can be produced are IgE-potentiating factor and IgE-suppressor factor; both are encoded by the same codon, and the functional differences are created by post-translational glycosylation. The glycosylation is either enhanced or suppressed by cytokines derived from other T cells. For example, glycosylation-inhibiting factor (identical to migration inhibitory factor) is produced by antigen-specific suppressor T cells. Glycosylation-enhancing factor is produced by an Fc receptor helper T cell (Fig. 5–19). The relative levels of these factors control the production of IgE-potentiating factor and IgE-suppressor factor by the central helper T cell and, thus, ultimately control the amount of IgE produced (see Fig. 5–19). They probably do so through regulation of IgE B-lymphocyte proliferation and synthesis of IgE by these cells.

MAST CELL SUBPOPULATIONS

It has become increasingly clear that at least two subpopulations of mast cells exist. Connective tissue mast cells (CTMCs) contain heparin as the major proteoglycan, produce large amounts of prostaglandin D_2 in response to stimulation, and are independent of T cell–derived interleukins for their maturation, development, and function. These cells stain brilliantly with toluidine blue in formalin-fixed tissue sections.

Mucosal mast cells (MMCs) do not stain well with toluidine blue. They are found primarily in the subepithelial mucosa in gut and lung; they contain chondroitin sulfate as the major proteoglycan; they manufacture leukotriene C4 as the predominant arachidonic acid metabo-

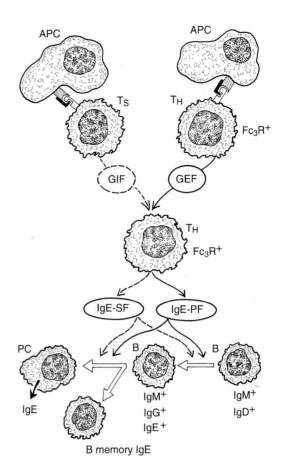

FIGURE 5–19. IgE synthesis. Glycosylation-enhancing factor, glycosylation-inhibiting factor, IgE-promoting factor, IgE suppressor factor, and the helper and suppressor T lymphocytes specific for regulation of IgE synthesis are shown. (From Albert DA, Jakobiec FA: Principles and Practice of Ophthalmology, 2nd ed. Philadelphia, W. B. Saunders, 2000, p 76.)

lite after stimulation; and they are dependent on IL-3 (and IL-4) for their maturation and proliferation. Interestingly, MMCs placed in culture with fibroblasts rather than T cells transform to cells with the characteristics of CTMCs. Disodium cromoglycate inhibits histamine release from CTMCs but not from MMCs. Steroids suppress the proliferation of MMCs, probably through inhibition of IL-3 production.

ATOPY GENETICS AND THE ROLE OF THE ENVIRONMENT

Both genetic and environmental components are clearly involved in the allergic response. Offspring of marriages in which one parent is allergic have approximately 30% risk of being allergic, and if both parents are allergic, the risk to each child is greater than 50%. At least three genetically linked mechanisms govern the development of atopy: (1) general hyperresponsiveness, (2) regulation of serum IgE levels, and (3) sensitivity to specific antigens. General hyperresponsiveness, defined as positive skin reactions to a broad range of environmental allergens, is associated with HLA-B8/HLA-DW3 phenotypy, and this general hyperresponsiveness appears not to be IgE class–specific. Total serum IgE levels are also controlled geneti-

TABLE 5–12. MAST CELL MEDIATORS

PREFORMED IN GRANULES	NEWLY SYNTHESIZED
Histamine	LTB4
Heparin	LTC4
Tryptase	LTD4
Chymase	Prostaglandins
Kinins	Thromboxanes
Eosinophil chemotactic factor	Platelet-activating factor
Neutrophil chemotactic factor	
Serotonin	
Chondroitin sulfate	
Arylsulfatase	

LTB4, leukotriene B4; LTC4, leukotriene C4; LTD4, leukotriene D4.

cally, and family studies indicate that total IgE production is under genetic control. Finally, experimental studies using low-molecular-weight allergenic determinants disclose a strong association between IgE responsiveness to such allergens and HLA-DR/DW2 type, whereas for at least some high-molecular-weight allergens, responsiveness is linked to HLA-DR/DW3. In mice at least, gene regulation of IgE production occurs at several levels, including: (1) regulation of antigen-specific, IgE-specific suppressor T cells, (2) manufacture of glycosylation-inhibiting factor or of glycosylation-enhancing factor by helper T cells, (3) at the level of IL-4, regulation of class switching to IgE synthesis, and (4) at the level of IgE binding, factors such as IgE-potentiating factor and IgE-suppressor factor.

The environment plays a major role in whether or not a genetically predisposed individual expresses major clinical manifestations of atopy. The "dose" of allergens to which the individual is exposed is a critical determinant of whether or not clinical expression of an allergic response develops. Less well recognized, however, is the fact that the general overall quality of the air in an individual's environment plays a major role in whether clinical expression of allergic responses to allergens to which the individual is sensitive does or does not develop. It has become unmistakably clear that, as the general quality of the air in urban environments has deteriorated and as the air has become more polluted, the prevalence in the population of overt atopic clinical manifestations has increased dramatically. On a global level, the immediate environment in which an individual finds himself much of the time, the home, plays an important part in the expression of allergic disease. Allergically predisposed persons whose household includes at least one member who smokes cigarettes, have enhanced sensitivity to allergens such as house dust, mites, and molds, among others. It is probably also true that the overall health and nutritional status of an individual influence the likelihood of that person developing a clinically obvious allergy.

DIAGNOSIS OF TYPE I REACTIONS

The definite diagnosis of type I hypersensitivity reactions requires the passive transfer of the reaction via a method known as the Prausnitz-Küstner reaction. Intradermal injection of the serum of a patient suspected of having a type I hypersensitivity–mediated problem into the skin of a volunteer is followed by injection of varying dilutions of the presumed offending antigen at the same intradermal sites as the patient's serum injection. A positive Prausnitz-Küstner reaction occurs when local flare-and-wheal formation follows injection of the antigen. This method for proving type I reactions is not used clinically; therefore, diagnosis of type I mechanisms contributing to a patient's inflammatory disorder is always based on a collection of circumstantial evidence that strongly supports the hypothesis of a type I reaction. A typical history (e.g., a family history of allergy or a personal history of eczema, hay fever, asthma, or urticaria) elicitation of allergic symptoms following exposure to suspected allergens involves itching as a prominent symptom, elevated IgE levels in serum or other body fluids, and blood or tissue eosinophilia.

THERAPY FOR TYPE I REACTIONS

Therapy for type I reactions must include scrupulous avoidance of the offending antigen. This is not easy, and it is a component of proper treatment that is often neglected by the patient and the physician alike. It is crucial, however, for a patient with an incurable disease such as atopy to recognize that, throughout a lifetime, he or she will slowly sustain cumulative permanent damage to structures affected by atopic responses (e.g., lung, eye) if he or she is subjected to repetitive triggering of the allergic response. Pharmacologic approaches to this disorder can never truly succeed for careless patients who neglect their responsibility to avoid allergens. A careful environmental history is, therefore, a critical ingredient in history taking, and convincing education of the patient and family alike is an essential and central ingredient in the care plan.

A careful environmental history and meticulous attention to environmental details can make the difference between relative stability and progressive inflammatory attacks that ultimately produce blindness. Elimination of pets, carpeting, feather pillows, quilts, and wool blankets and installation of air-conditioning and air-filtering systems are therapeutic strategies that should not be overlooked.[76]

One of the most important advances in the care of patients with type I disease during the past two decades has been the development of mast cell–stabilizing agents. Disodium cromoglycate, sodium nedocromil, lodoxamide, and olopatidine are four such agents. Topical administration is both safe and effective in the care of patients with allergic eye disease.[77, 78] This therapeutic approach is to be strongly recommended and is very much favored over the use of competitive H_1 antihistamines. Clearly, if the mast cells can be prevented from degranulating, the therapeutic effect of such degranulation-inhibiting agents would be expected to be vastly superior to that of antihistamines, simply by virtue of preventing liberation of an entire panoply of mediators from the mast cell rather than competitive inhibition of one such mediator, histamine.

Histamine action inhibition by H_1 antihistamines can be effective in patients with ocular allergy, especially when administered systemically. The efficacy of such agents when given topically is marginal in some atopic individuals, and long-term use can result in the development of sensitivity to ingredients in the preparations. The consistent use of systemic antihistamines, particularly the newer noncompetitive antihistamines such as astemizole, however, can contribute significantly to long-term stability. Additionally, slow escalation of the amount of hydroxyzine used in the care of atopic patients can help to interrupt the itch-scratch-itch psychoneurotic component that often accompanies eczema and atopic blepharokeratoconjunctivitis.

Generalized suppression of inflammation, through use of topical corticosteroids, is commonly used for treatment of type I ocular hypersensitivity reactions, and this is appropriate for acute breakthrough attacks of inflammation. It is, however, completely inappropriate for long-term care. Corticosteroids have a direct effect on all inflammatory cells, including eosinophils, mast cells, and basophils. They are extremely effective, but the risks of long-term topical steroid use are considerable and unavoidable, thus such use is discouraged.

Although desensitization immunotherapy can be an important additional component to the therapeutic plan for a patient with type I hypersensitivity, it is difficult to perform properly. The first task, of course, is to document to which allergens the patient is sensitive. The second task is to construct a "serum" containing ideal proportions of the allergens that induce the production of IgG-blocking antibody and stimulate the generation of antigen-specific suppressor T cells. For reasons that are not clear, the initial concentration of allergens in such a preparation for use in a patient with ocular manifestations of atopy must often be considerably lower than the initial concentrations usually used when caring for a person with extraocular allergic problems. If the typical starting concentrations for nonocular allergies are employed frequently, a dramatic exacerbation of ocular inflammation immediately follows the first injection of the desensitizing preparation.

Plasmapheresis is an adjunctive therapeutic maneuver that can make a substantial difference in the care of patients with atopy, high levels of serum IgE, and documented *Staphylococcus*-binding antibodies.[76] This therapeutic technique is expensive, is not curative, and must be performed at highly specialized centers, approximately three times each week, indefinitely. It is also clear, from our experience, that the aggressiveness of the plasmapheresis must be greater than that typically employed by many pheresis centers. Three to four plasma exchanges per pheresis session typically are required to achieve therapeutic effect for an atopic person.

Intravenous or intramuscular gamma globulin injections may also benefit selected atopic patients. It has been recognized that, through mechanisms that are not yet clear, gamma globulin therapy involves much more than simple passive "immunization" through adoptive transfer of antibody molecules. In fact, immunoglobulin therapy has a pronounced immunomodulatory effect, and it is because of this action that such therapy is now recognized and approved as effective therapy for idiopathic thrombocytopenic purpura.[79] The use of gamma globulin therapy is also being explored for other autoimmune diseases, including systemic lupus erythematosus and atopic disease.

Cyclosporine is being tested in patients with certain atopic diseases. Preliminary evidence suggests that topical cyclosporine can have some beneficial effect on patients with atopic keratoconjunctivitis and vernal keratoconjunctivitis.[80] Furthermore, in selected desperate cases of blinding atopic keratoconjunctivitis, we have demonstrated that systemic cyclosporine can be a pivotal component of the multimodality approach to the care of these complex problems.[76]

Finally, appropriate psychiatric care may be (and usually is) indicated in patients with severe atopy (and family members). It is not hyperbole to state that, in most cases, patients with severe atopic disease and the family members with whom they live demonstrate substantial psychopathology and destructive patterns of interpersonal behavior. The degree to which these families exhibit self-destructive, passive-aggressive, and sabotaging behaviors is often astonishing. Productive engagement in psychiatric care is often difficult to achieve, but it can be extremely rewarding when accomplished successfully. Table 5–13 summarizes the components of a multifactorial approach to the care of atopic patients.

Type II Hypersensitivity Reactions

Type II reactions require the participation of complement-fixing antibodies (IgG1, IgG3, or IgM) and complement. The antibodies are directed against antigens on the surfaces of specific cells (i.e., endogenous antigens). The damage caused by type II hypersensitivity reactions, therefore, is localized to the particular target cell or tissue. The mediators of the tissue damage in type II reactions include complement as well as recruited macrophages and other leukocytes that liberate their enzymes. The mechanism of tissue damage involves antibody binding to the cell membrane with resultant cell membrane lysis or facilitation of phagocytosis, macrophage and neutrophil cell-mediated damage (Fig. 5–20), and killer cell damage to target tissue through antibody-dependent cell-mediated cytotoxicity (ADCC) reaction (see Fig. 5–20). It is important to remember (particularly in the case of type II hypersensitivity reactions that do not result in specific target cell lysis through the complement cascade with eventual osmotic lysis) that neutrophils are prominent effectors of target cell damage. Neutrophil adherence, oxygen metabolism, lysosomal enzyme release, and phagocytosis are tremendously "upregulated" by IgG-C3 complexes and by the activated split product of C5a. As mentioned in the description of type I hypersensitivity reactions, mast cells also participate in nonallergic inflammatory reactions, and type II hypersensitivity reactions provide an excellent example of this. The complement split products C3a and C5a both produce mast cell activation and degranulation, with resultant liberation of preformed vasoactive amines and upregulation of membrane synthesis of leukotriene B4 (and other cytokines [e.g., TNF-α] with known chemoattractant activity for neutrophils even more potent than IL-8/rantes), eosinophil chemotactic factor, and other arachidonic acid metabolites. Neutrophils and macrophages attracted to this site of complement-fixing IgG or IgM in a type II hypersensitivity reaction cannot phagocytose entire cells and target tissues; they thus liberate their proteolytic and collagenolytic enzymes and cytokines in "frustrated phagocytosis." It is through this liberation of tissue digestive enzymes that the target tissue is damaged. Direct target cell damage (as opposed to "innocent bystander"

TABLE 5–13. THERAPY FOR THE ATOPIC PATIENT

Environmental control
Mast cell stabilizers
Systemic antihistamines
Topical steroids (for acute intervention only)
Desensitization immunotherapy
Plasmapheresis
Intravenous gamma globulin
Cyclosporine (systemic and topical)
Psychiatric intervention for the patient and family

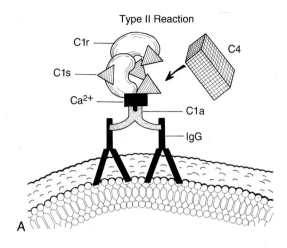

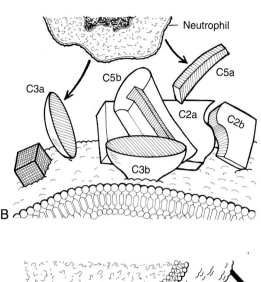

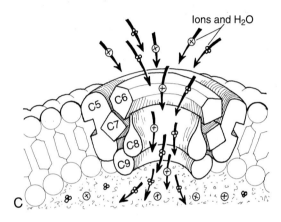

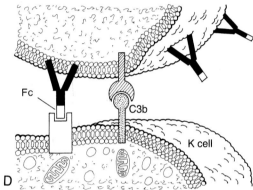

FIGURE 5–20. Type II hypersensitivity. *A,* A "synthesized" cell with two antibodies specific for antigenic determinants on the cell surface has attached to the target cell. C1q, C1r, and C1s complement components have begun the sequence that will result in the classic cascade of complement factor binding. *B,* The complement cascade has progressed to the point of C5 binding. Note that two anaphylatoxin and chemotactic split products, C3a and C5a, have been generated, and a neutrophil is being attracted to the site by virtue of the generation of these two chemotactic moieties. *C,* The complement cascade is complete, with the result that a pore has been opened in the target cell membrane, and osmotic lysis is the nearly instantaneous result. *D,* A variant type II hypersensitivity reaction is the antibody-dependent cellular cytotoxicity (ADCC) reaction. Target-specific antibody has attached to the target cell membrane, and the Fc receptor on a neutrophil, a macrophage, or a killer (K) cell is attaching to that membrane-affixed antibody. The result is lysis of the target cell. (From Albert DA, Jakobiec FA: Principles and Practice of Ophthalmology, 2nd ed. Philadelphia, W. B. Saunders, 2000, p 78.)

damage caused by liberation of neutrophil and macrophage enzymes) in type II hypersensitivity reactions may be mediated by killer (K) cells through the antibody-dependent cytotoxicity reaction. In fact, definitive diagnosis of type II reactions requires the demonstration of fixed antitissue antibodies at the disease site, as well as demonstration of in vitro killer cell activity against the tissue. No ocular disease has been definitively proved to represent a type II reaction, but several candidates, including ocular cicatricial pemphigoid, exist.

The classic human autoimmune type II hypersensitivity disease is Goodpasture's syndrome. Many believe ocular cicatricial pemphigoid is analogous (in mechanism at least) to Goodpasture's syndrome, in which complement-fixing antibody directed against a glycoprotein of the glomerular basement membrane fixes to the glomerular basement membrane. This action causes subsequent damage to the membrane by proteolytic and collagenolytic enzymes liberated by phagocytic cells, including macrophages and neutrophils.

THERAPY FOR TYPE II REACTIONS

Therapy for type II reactions is extremely difficult, and immunosuppressive chemotherapy has, in general, been the mainstay of treatment. Experience with ocular cicatricial pemphigoid has been especially gratifying in this regard.[81–83] Progressive cicatricial pemphigoid affecting the conjunctiva was, eventually, almost universally blinding before the advent of systemic immunosuppressive chemotherapy for this condition. With such therapy available now, however, 90% of cases of the disease are arrested and vision is preserved.[84]

Type III Hypersensitivity Reactions

Type III reactions, or immune complex diseases, require, like type II hypersensitivity reactions, participation of complement-fixing antibodies (IgG1, IgG3, or IgM). The antigens participating in such reactions may be soluble and diffusible antigens, microbes, drugs, or autologous antigens. Microbes that cause such diseases are usually those that cause persistent infections in which both the infected organ and the kidneys are affected by the immune complex–stimulated inflammation. Autoimmune-immune complex diseases are the best known of these hypersensitivity reactions—the classic collagen vascular diseases and Stevens-Johnson syndrome. Kidney, skin, joints, arteries, and eyes are frequently affected in these disorders. Mediators of tissue damage include antigen-antibody-complement complexes and the proteolytic and collagenolytic enzymes from phagocytes such as macrophages and neutrophils. As with type II reactions, the C3a and C5a split products of complement exert potent chemotactic activity for the phagocytes and also activate mast cells, which through degranulation of their vasoactive amines and TNF-α increase vascular permeability and enhance emigration of such phagocytic cells. It is again through frustrated phagocytosis that the neutrophils and macrophages liberate their tissue-damaging enzymes (Fig. 5–21).

Arthus' reaction, a special form of type III hypersensitivity, is mentioned for completeness. Antigen injected into the skin of an animal or individual previously sensitized with the same antigen, and with circulating antibodies against that antibody, results in an edematous, hemorrhagic, and eventually necrotic lesion of the skin. A passive Arthus reaction can also be created if intravenous injection of antibody into a normal host recipient is followed by intradermal injection of the antigen. An accumulation of neutrophils develops in the capillaries and venule walls after deposition of antigen, antibody, and complement in the vessel walls.

Immune complexes form in all of us as a normal consequence of our "immunologic housekeeping." Usually, however, these immune complexes are continually removed from the circulation. In humans, the preemi-

nent immune complex–scavenging system is the red blood cells, which have a receptor (CR1) for the C3b and C4b components of complement. This receptor binds immune complexes that contain complement, and the membrane-bound complexes are removed by fixed tissue macrophages and Kupffer cells as the red blood cells pass through the liver. Other components of the reticuloendothelial system, including the spleen and the lung, also remove circulating immune complexes. Small immune complexes may escape binding and removal; not surprisingly, smaller immune complexes are principally responsible for immune complex–mediated hypersensitivity reactions. It is also true that IgA complexes (as opposed to IgG or IgM complexes) do not bind well to red blood cells. They are found in the lung, brain, and kidney rather than in the reticuloendothelial system.

The factors that govern whether or not immune complexes are deposited into tissue (and if so, where) are complex and rather incompletely understood. It is clear that the size of the immune complex plays a role in tissue deposition. It is also clear that increased vascular permeability at a site of immune system activity or inflammation is a major governor of whether or not immune complexes are deposited in that tissue. Additionally, it is clear that immune complex deposition is more likely to occur at sites of vascular trauma; this includes trauma associated with the normal hemodynamics of a particular site, such as the relatively high pressure inside capillaries and kidneys, the turbulence associated with bifurcations of vessels, and obviously, sites of artificial trauma as well. Excellent examples of the latter include the areas of trauma in the fingers, toes, and elbows of patients with rheumatoid arthritis, in which subsequent vasculitic lesions and rheumatoid nodules form, and the surgically traumatized eyes of patients with rheumatoid arthritis or Wegener's granulomatosis, wherein immune complexes are deposited subsequently and necrotizing scleritis develops.[85] It is likely that addressins or other attachment factors in local tissue play a role in the "homing" of a particular immune complex. Antibody class and immune complex size are also important determinants of immune complex localization at a particular site, as is the type of basement membrane itself.

THERAPY FOR TYPE III REACTIONS

Therapy for type III reactions consists predominantly of large doses of corticosteroids, of immunosuppressive chemotherapeutic agents, or both. Cytotoxic immunosuppressive chemotherapy may or may not be necessary to save both the sight and the life of a patient with Behçet's disease, but it is categorically required to save the life of a patient with either polyarteritis nodosa[86] or Wegener's granulomatosis.[87] In the case of rheumatoid arthritis–associated vasculitis affecting the eye, it is likely that systemic immunosuppression will also be required if death from a lethal extra–articular, extraocular, vasculitic event is to be prevented.[88]

Injury Mediated by Cells

Type IV Hypersensitivity Reactions: Immune-Mediated Injury Due To Effector T Cells

The original classification of immunopathogenic mechanisms arose in an era when considerably more was known

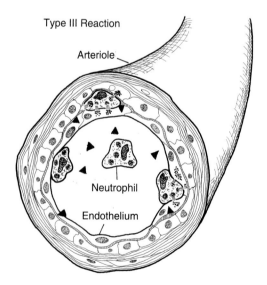

FIGURE 5–21. Type III hypersensitivity reaction. Circulating immune complexes (shown here as triangle-shaped moieties in the vascular lumen) percolate between vascular endothelial cells but become trapped at the vascular endothelial basement membrane. Neutrophils and other phagocytic cells are attracted to this site of immune complex deposition. These phagocytic cells liberate their proteolytic and collagenolytic enzymes and damage not only the vessel but also the surrounding tissue. (From Albert DA, Jakobiec FA: Principles and Practice of Ophthalmology, 2nd ed. Philadelphia, W. B. Saunders, 2000, p 79.)

Type III Reaction

Arteriole

Neutrophil

Endothelium

about antibody molecules and serology than about T cells and cellular immunity. Out of this lack of knowledge, T cell–mediated mechanisms were relegated to the "type IV" category, and all types of responses were unwittingly grouped together[89] (Fig. 5–22). We now know that T cells capable of causing immune-based injury exist in at least three functionally distinct phenotypes: cytotoxic T cells (typically CD8+) and two populations of helper T cells (typically CD4+). Because cytotoxic T lymphocytes (CTLs) were discovered well after the original Gell and Coombs classification, they were never anticipated in that classification system. As mentioned previously, CD4+ T cells can adopt one of two polar positions with regard to their lymphokine secretions.[72] Th1 cells secrete IL-2, IFN-γ, and lymphotoxin, whereas Th2 cells were identified in the 1940s and 1950s as the initiators of delayed hypersensitivity reaction. The latter cells, in addition to providing helper factors that promote IgE production, mediate tissue inflammation, albeit of a somewhat different type than that with Th1 cells.

IMMUNOPATHOGENIC T CELLS

CTLs exhibit exquisite antigen specificity in their recognition of target cells; the extent of injury that CTLs effect is usually limited to target cells that bear the relevant instigating antigens. Therefore, if a CTL causes tissue injury, it is because host cells express an antigen encoded by an invading pathogen, an antigen for which the TCR on the CTL is highly specific. Delivery of a cytolytic signal eliminates hapless host cells, and in so doing aborts the intracellular infection. Assuming that the infected host

cell is one of many and can thus be spared (e.g., epidermal keratinocytes), there may be little or no physiologic consequence of this CTL-mediated loss of host cells. However, if the infected cell is strategic, is limited in number, or cannot be replaced by regeneration (e.g., neurons, corneal endothelial cells), then the immunopathogenic consequences may be severe.

CD4+ effector cells also exhibit exquisite specificity in recognition of target antigens. However, the extent of injury that these cells can effect is diffuse and is not limited to cells that bear the target antigen. CD4+ effector cells secrete cytokines that possess no antigen specificity in their own right. Instead, these molecules indiscriminately recruit and activate macrophages, natural killer cells, eosinophils, and other mobile cells that form the nonspecific host defense network. It is this defense mechanism that leads to eradication and elimination of the offending pathogen. In other words, CD4+ effector cells protect by identifying the pathogen antigenically, but they cause elimination of the pathogen by enlisting the aid of other cells. The ability of CD4+ effector cells to orchestrate this multicellular response rests with the capacity of these cells to secrete proinflammatory cytokines to arm inflammatory cells with the ability to "kill." Once armed, these "mindless assassins" mediate inflammation in a nonspecific manner that leads often, if not inevitably, to "innocent bystander" injury to surrounding tissues. For an organ that can scarcely tolerate inflammation of even the lowest amount, such as the eye, "innocent bystander" injury is a formidable threat to vision.

AUTOIMMUNE T CELLS

The foregoing discussion addresses immunopathogenic injury due to T cells that develops among host tissues invaded by pathogenic organisms. However, there is another dimension to immunopathology. T cells can sometimes make a mistake and mount an immune attack on host tissues simply because those tissue cells express self molecules (i.e., autoantigens). Although an enormous amount of experimental and clinical literature is devoted to autoimmunity and autoimmune diseases, very little is known in a "factual" sense that enables us to understand this curious phenomenon. What seems clear is that T cells with receptors that recognize "self" antigens, as well as B cells bearing surface antibody receptors that recognize "self" antigens, exist under normal conditions.[89] Moreover, there are examples of T and B cells with "self"-recognizing receptors that become activated in putatively normal individuals. Thus, immunologists have learned to distinguish an autoimmune response (not necessarily pathologic) from an autoimmune disease. Whereas all autoimmune diseases arise in a setting in which an autoimmune response has been initiated, we understand little about what causes the latter to evolve into the former. Whatever the pathogenesis, autoimmune disease results when effector T cells (or antibodies) recognize autoantigens in a fashion that triggers a destructive immune response.[90, 91]

The eye comprises unique cells bearing unique molecules. Moreover, the internal compartments of the eye exist behind a blood-tissue barrier. The very uniqueness

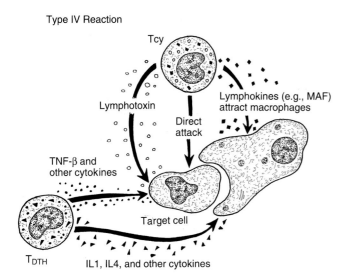

Type IV Reaction

Tcy

Lymphotoxin

Direct attack

Lymphokines (e.g., MAF) attract macrophages

TNF-β and other cytokines

Target cell

T_DTH   IL1, IL4, and other cytokines

FIGURE 5–22. Type IV hypersensitivity reaction. DTH (CD4) T lymphocytes and cytotoxic (CD8 and CD4) T lymphocytes directly attack the target cell or the organism that is the target of the type IV hypersensitivity reaction. Surrogate effector cells are also recruited through the liberation of cytokines. The most notable surrogate or additional effector cell is the macrophage, or tissue histiocyte. If the reaction becomes chronic, certain cytokines or signals from mononuclear cells result in the typical transformation of some histiocytes into epithelioid cells, and the fusion of multiple epithelioid cells produces the classic multinucleated giant cell. (From Albert DA, Jakobiec FA: Principles and Practice of Ophthalmology, 2nd ed. Philadelphia, W. B. Saunders, 2000, p 80.)

of ocular molecules and their presumed sequestration from the systemic immune system have provoked immunologists to speculate that ocular autoimmunity arises when, via trauma or infection, eye-specific antigens are "revealed" to the immune system. Sympathetic ophthalmia is a disease that almost fits this scenario perfectly. Trauma to one eye, with attendant disruption of the blood-ocular barrier and spillage of ocular tissues and molecules, leads to a systemic immune response that is specific to the eye. This response is directed not only at the traumatized eye but also at its putatively normal fellow eye. However, even in sympathetic ophthalmia, not every case of ocular trauma leads to this outcome; in fact, only in a few cases does this type of injury produce inflammation in the undamaged eye. Suspicion is high that polymorphic genetic factors may be responsible for determining who will, and who will not, develop sympathetic ophthalmia following ocular injury. However, environmental factors may also participate.

Range of Hypersensitivity Reactions Mediated by T Cells

Because a wealth of new information about T cell–mediated immunopathology has accrued within the past decade, our ideas about the range of hypersensitivity reactions that can be mediated by T cells have expanded. But, as yet, any attempt to classify these reactions must necessarily be incomplete. In the past, four types of delayed hypersensitivity reactions were described: (1) tuberculin, (2) contact hypersensitivity, (3) granulomatous, and (4) Jones-Mote (Table 5–14). Delayed hypersensitivity reactions of these types were believed to be caused by IFN-γ–producing CD4+ T cells and to participate in numerous ocular inflammatory disorders, ranging from allergic keratoconjunctivitis, through Wegener's granulomatosis, to drug contact hypersensitivity. Based on recent knowledge concerning other types of effector T cells, this list must be expanded to include cytotoxic T cells and proinflammatory, but not IFN-γ–secreting, Th2-type cells, such as the cells that are believed to cause corneal clouding in river blindness.[92]

Herpes Simplex Keratitis as an Example of T Cell–Mandated Ocular Inflammatory Disease

Infections of the eye with herpes simplex virus (HSV) are significant causes of morbidity and vision loss in developed countries. Although direct viral toxicity is damaging to the eye, the majority of intractable herpes infections appear to be immunopathogenic in origin. That is, the immune response to antigens expressed during a herpes infection leads to tissue injury and decompensation, even though the virus itself is directly responsible for little pathology. Herpes stromal keratitis (HSK) is representative of this type of disorder.[93]

Numerous experimental model systems have been developed in an effort to understand the pathogenesis of HSK. Perhaps the most informative studies have been conducted in laboratory mice. Evidence from these model systems indicates that T cells are central to the corneal pathology observed in HSK.[84] At least four different pathogenic mechanisms have been discovered, each of which alone can generate stromal keratitis. Genetic factors of the host seem to play a crucial role in dictating which mechanism will predominate. First, HSV-specific cytotoxic T cells can cause HSK and do so in several strains of mice. Second, HSV-specific T cells of the Th1 type, which secrete IFN-γ and mediate delayed hypersensitivity, also cause HSK, but in genetically different strains of mice. Third, HSV-specific T cells of the Th2 type, which secrete IL-4 and IL-10, correlate with HSK in yet a different strain of mice. Fourth, in association with HSK, T cells have been found that recognize an antigen uniquely expressed in the cornea. The evidence suggests that this corneal antigen is unmasked during a corneal infection with HSV, and an autoimmune response is evoked in which the cornea becomes the target of the attack.

Only time will tell whether similar immunopathogenic mechanisms will prove to be responsible for HSK in humans, but the likelihood is very great that this will be the case. Furthermore, it is instructive to emphasize that quite different pathologic T cells can be involved in ocular pathology, which implies that it will be necessary to devise different therapies in order to meet the challenge of preventing immunopathogenic injury from proceeding to blindness.

Summary

Faced with a patient who is experiencing extraocular or intraocular inflammation, the thoughtful ophthalmologist will try, to the best of his or her ability, to diagnose the specific cause of the inflammation, or at the very least to investigate the problem so that the mechanisms responsible for the inflammation are understood as completely as possible. Armed with this knowledge, the ophthalmologist is then prepared to formulate an appropriate therapeutic plan rather than to indiscriminately prescribe corticosteroids. It is clear as we move into the 21st century that the past four decades of relative neglect of ocular immunology by mainstream ophthalmic practitioners are coming to an end. Most ophthalmologists are no longer satisfied to cultivate practices devoted exclusively to the "tissue carpentry" of cataract surgery, or even to a broad-based ophthalmic practice that includes "medical ophthalmology" but is restricted to problems related exclusively to the eye (e.g., glaucoma) yet divorced from the eye as an organ in which systemic disease is often manifested. More ophthalmologists than ever before are demanding the continuing education they need to satisfy intellectual curiosity and to prepare for

TABLE 5–14. TYPES OF DELAYED HYPERSENSITIVITY REACTIONS

REACTION TYPE	EXAMPLE	PEAK REACTION
Tuberculin contact	Tuberculin skin test	48–72 hr
Contact	Drug contact hypersensitivity	48–72 hr
Granulomatous	Leprosy	14 days
Jones-Mote	Cutaneous basophil hypersensitivity	24 hr

modern care of the total patient when a patient presents with an ocular manifestation of a systemic disease. It is to these doctors that this chapter is directed. The eye can be affected by any of the immune hypersensitivity reactions; acquiring an understanding of the mechanism of a particular patient's inflammatory problem lays the ground work for correct treatment. In the course of the average ophthalmologist's working life, the diagnostic pursuit of mechanistic understanding will also result in a substantial number of instances when the ophthalmologist has been responsible for diagnosing a disease that, if left undiagnosed, would have been fatal.

REGULATION OF IMMUNE RESPONSES

Immunization with an antigen leads, under normal circumstances, to a robust immune response in which effector T cells and antibodies are produced with specificity for the initiating antigen. Viewed teleologically, the purpose of these effectors is to recognize and combine with antigen (e.g., on an invading pathogen) in such a manner that the antigen and pathogen are eliminated. Once the antigen has been eliminated, there is little need for the persistence of high levels of effector cells and antibodies; what is regularly observed is that levels of these effectors in blood and peripheral tissues fall dramatically. Only the T cells and B cells that embody antigen-specific memory (anamnesis) are retained.

The ability of the immune system to respond to an antigenic challenge in a sufficient and yet measured manner such as this is a dramatic expression of the ability of the system to regulate itself. An understanding of the mechanisms of immune regulation is extremely important. Examples abound of unregulated immune responses that led to tissue injury and disease; therefore, an understanding of the basis of immune regulation is an important goal.

Regulation by Antigen

Antigen itself is a critical factor in the regulation of an immune response.[94] When nonreplicating antigens have been studied, it has been found that the high concentration of antigen required for initial sensitization begins to fall through time. In part, this occurs because antibodies produced by immunization interact with the antigen and cause its elimination. As the antigen concentration falls, the efficiency with which specific T and B cells are stimulated to proliferate and differentiate also falls; eventually, when antigen concentration slips below a critical threshold, further activation of specific lymphocytes stops. Thus, antigen proves to be a central player in determining the vigor and duration of the immune response. As a corollary, immune effectors (specific T cells and antibodies) also play a key role in terminating the immune response, in part by removing antigen from the system. The use of anti-Rh antibodies (RhoGAM) to prevent sensitization of Rh-negative women bearing Rh-positive fetuses is a clear, clinical example of the ability of antibodies to terminate (and in this particular case, even prevent) a specific (unwanted) immune response.

Regulation by Th1 and Th2 Cells

There are other, more subtle and more powerful, regulatory mechanisms that operate to control immune responses. More than 20 years ago, experimentalists discovered that certain antigen-specific T lymphocytes are capable of suppressing immune responses,[95] and the mechanism of suppression was found to be unrelated to the simple act of clearing antigen from the system. Although immunologists first suspected that a functionally distinct population of T lymphocytes (analogous to helper and killer cells) was responsible for immune suppression, it is now clear that there is a broad range of T cells that, depending on the circumstances, can function as suppressor cells. Moreover, the mechanisms by which these different T cells suppress are also diverse.

The concept has previously been introduced that helper T cells exist, cells that are responsible for enabling other T and B cells to differentiate into effector cells and antibody-producing cells, respectively. And it is now evident that the effectors of immunity include functionally diverse T cells (delayed hypersensitivity, cytotoxic) and antibodies (immunoglobulin [Ig]M, IgG1, IgG2, IgG3, IgG4, IgA, IgE). Any particular immunizing event does not necessarily lead to the production of the entire array of effector modalities; one of the reasons for this is that helper T cells tend to polarize into one or the other of two distinct phenotypes.[72] Th1 cells provide a type of help that leads to the generation of T-cell effectors that mediate T cell–dependent inflammatory responses (e.g., delayed hypersensitivity), as well as B cells that secrete complement-fixing antibodies. The ability of Th1 cells to promote these types of immune response rests with their capacity to secrete a certain set of cytokines—IFN-γ, TNF-β, large amounts of TNF-α, and IL-2. It is these cytokines, acting on other T cells, B cells, and macrophages, that shape proinflammatory responses. By contrast, Th2 cells provide a type of help that leads to the generation of B cells that secrete non–complement-fixing IgG antibodies, as well as IgA and IgE. Once again, the ability of Th2 cells to promote these types of antibody response rests with their capacity to secrete a different set of cytokines—IL-4, IL-5, IL-6, and IL-10. These cytokines act on other antigen-specific B and T cells to promote the observed responses.

As it turns out, Th1 and Th2 cells can cross-regulate each other. Thus, Th1 cells with specificity for a particular antigen secrete IFN-γ, and in the presence of this cytokine, Th2 cells with specificity for the same antigen fail to become activated. Moreover, they are unable to provide the type of help for which they are uniquely suited. Similarly, if Th2 cells respond to a particular antigen by secreting their unique set of cytokines (especially IL-4 and IL-10), Th1 cells in the same microenvironment are prevented from responding to the same antigen. Thus, precocious activation of Th1 cells to an antigen, such as ragweed pollen, may prevent the activation of ragweed-specific Th2 cells and thereby prevent the production of ragweed-specific IgE antibodies. Alternatively, precocious activation of Th2 cells to an antigen (e.g., urushiol—the agent responsible for poison ivy dermatitis) may prevent the activation of urushiol-specific Th1 cells and thus eliminate the threat of dermatitis when the skin is exposed to the leaf of the poison ivy plant.

The discovery of Th1 and Th2 cell diversity has led to a profound rethinking of immune regulation. It is still too early to know, on the one hand, whether the extent to which sensitization leads to polarization in the direction of Th1- or Th2-type responses is responsible for human inflammatory diseases and, on the other hand, whether the extent to which the ability to influence an immune response toward the Th1 or Th2 phenotype will have therapeutic value in humans.

Regulation by Suppressor T Cells

Suppressor T cells are defined operationally as cells that suppress an antigen-specific immune response. Cells of this functional property were described before the discovery of Th1 and Th2 cells. It is now apparent that at least some of the phenomena previously attributed to suppressor T cells initially are explained by the cross-regulating abilities of Th1 and Th2 cells. However, it is also abundantly clear that there remain forms and examples of suppression of immune responses that depend on T cells that are neither Th1 nor Th2 cells.

Various experimental maneuvers have been described that lead to the generation of suppressor T cells. The list includes (but is not limited to): (1) injection of soluble heterologous protein antigen intravenously, (2) application of a hapten to skin previously exposed to ultraviolet B radiation, (3) ingestion of antigen by mouth, (4) injection of allogeneic hematopoietic cells into neonatal mice, (5) injection of antigen-pulsed antigen-presenting cells (APCs) that have been treated in vitro with transforming growth factor (TGF)-β (or aqueous humor, cerebrospinal fluid, or amniotic fluid), and (6) engraftment of a solid tissue (e.g., heart, kidney) under cover of immunosuppressive agents.[96, 97] In each of these examples, T cells harvested from spleen or lymph nodes of experimentally manipulated animals induce antigen-specific unresponsiveness when injected into immunologically naive recipient animals. Cell transfers such as this have helped to define different types of suppressor cell activity. Because the immune response is functionally divided into its afferent phase (induction) and efferent phase (expression), it is no surprise that certain suppressor T cells suppress the afferent process by which antigen is first detected by specific lymphocytes, and other suppressor T cells inhibit the expression of immunity. Moreover, different suppressor T cells act on different target cells. Some suppressor cells inhibit the activation of CD4+ helper or CD8+ cytotoxic T cells, whereas other suppressor cells interfere with B-cell function. There are even suppressor cells that inhibit the activation and effector functions of macrophages and other APCs.

The mechanisms by which suppressor T cells function remain ill-defined. Certain suppressor T cells secrete immunosuppressive cytokines, such as TGF-β, whereas other suppressor cells inhibit only when they make direct cell surface contact with target cells. The notion that suppressor cells act by secreting suppressive factors (other than known cytokines) has been challenged and is a controversial topic in immunology. There is convincing evidence that suppressor T cells play a key role in regulating the normal immune response. The decay in immune response that is typically observed after antigen has been successfully neutralized by specific immune effectors correlates with the emergence of antigen-specific suppressor T cells, and these cells have been found to be capable of secreting TGF-β.

Tolerance as an Expression of Immune Regulation

Immunologic tolerance is defined as the state in which immunization with a specific antigen fails to lead to a detectable immune response. In a sense, tolerance represents the ultimate expression of the effectiveness of immune regulation because active mechanisms are responsible for producing the tolerant state. In another sense, tolerance is the obverse of immunity; the fact that an antigen can induce either immunity or tolerance, depending on the conditions at the time of antigen exposure, indicates the vulnerability of the immune system to manipulation.

Originally described experimentally in the 1950s,[98, 99] but accurately predicted by Ehrlich and other immunologists at the end of the 19th century, immunologic tolerance has been the subject of considerable experimental study during the past 50 years. It has been learned that several distinct mechanisms contribute singly, or in unison, to creation of the state of tolerance. These mechanisms include clonal deletion, clonal anergy, suppression, and immune deviation.

Mechanisms Involved in Tolerance

The term *clonal* refers to a group of lymphocytes that all have identical receptors for a particular antigen. During regular immunization, a clone of antigen-specific lymphocytes responds by proliferating and undergoing differentiation. *Clonal deletion* refers to an aberration of this process, in which a clone of antigen-specific lymphocytes responds to antigen exposure by undergoing apoptosis (programmed cell death).[100] Deletion of a clone of cells in this manner eliminates the ability of the immune system to respond to the antigen in question (i.e., the immune system is tolerant of that antigen). Subsequent exposures to the same antigen fail to produce the expected immune response (sensitized T cells and antibodies) because the relevant antigen-specific T and B cells are missing.

Clonal anergy resembles clonal deletion in that a particular clone of antigen-specific lymphocytes fails to respond to antigen exposure by proliferating and undergoing differentiation.[101] However, in clonal anergy, the lymphocytes within the clone are not triggered to undergo apoptosis by exposure to antigen. What has been learned experimentally is that lymphocytes exposed to their specific antigen under specialized experimental conditions enter an altered state in which their ability to respond is suspended, but the cells are protected from programmed cell death. Even though these cells survive this encounter with antigen, subsequent encounters still fail to cause their expected activation; that is, the immune system is tolerant of that antigen, and the tolerant cell is said to be anergic.

Antigen-specific *immune suppression,* as described earlier, is another mechanism that has been shown to cause immunologic tolerance. As in clonal deletion and anergy, immune suppression creates a situation in which subsequent encounters with the antigen in question fail to lead to signs of sensitization. However, in suppression, the failure to respond is actively maintained. Thus, suppressor cells actively inhibit antigen-specific lymphocytes from responding, even though the antigen-specific cells are present at the time antigen is introduced into the system.

Immune deviation is a special form of immune suppression.[102] Originally described in the 1960s, immune deviation refers to the situation wherein administration of a particular antigen in a particular manner fails to elicit the expected response. In the first such experiments, soluble heterologous protein antigens injected intravenously into naive experimental animals failed to induce delayed hypersensitivity responses. Moreover, subsequent immunization with the same antigens plus adjuvant injected subcutaneously also failed to induce delayed hypersensitivity. With respect to delayed hypersensitivity, one could say that the animals were tolerant. However, the sera of these animals contained unexpectedly large amounts of antibody to the same antigen, indicating that the so-called tolerance was not global. Thus, in immune deviation, a preemptive exposure to antigen in a nonimmunizing mode prejudices the quality of subsequent immune responses to the same antigen. In other words, the immune response is deviated from the expected pattern, hence the term *immune deviation*.

Factors That Promote Tolerance Rather Than Immunity

Experimentalists have defined various factors that influence or promote the development of immunologic tolerance. The earliest description of tolerance occurred when antigenic material was injected into newborn (and therefore developmentally immature) mice. This indicates that exposure of the developing immune system to antigens before the system has reached maturity leads to antigen-specific unresponsiveness. In large part, maturation of the thymus gland during ontogeny correlates positively with development of resistance to tolerance induction. Much evidence reveals that the mechanism responsible for tolerance in this situation is clonal deletion of immature, antigen-specific thymocytes. In large measure, because cells within the thymus gland are normally expressing self-antigens, the thymocytes that are deleted represent those cells with T-cell receptors of high affinity for self-antigens. This mechanism undoubtedly contributes to the success with which the normal immune system is able to respond to all biologically relevant molecules, except those expressed on self-tissues—and therefore avoids autoimmunity.

However, tolerance can also be induced when the immune system is developmentally mature. The factors that are known to promote tolerance under these conditions include: (1) the physical form of the antigen, (2) the dose of antigen, and (3) the route of antigen administration. More specifically, soluble antigens are more readily able to induce tolerance than particulate or insoluble antigens. Very large doses of antigens, as well as extremely small quantities of antigens, are also likely to induce

tolerance. This indicates that the immune system is disposed normally to respond to antigens within a relatively broad, but nonetheless defined, range of concentrations or amounts. Antigen administered in quantities above or below this range can induce tolerance. Injection of antigen intravenously also favors tolerance induction, whereas injection of antigen intracutaneously favors conventional sensitization. In a similar, but not identical, manner, oral ingestion of antigen produces a kind of immune deviation in which, on the one hand, delayed hypersensitivity to the antigen is impaired (i.e., tolerance), but on the other hand, IgA antibody production to the antigen is exaggerated. (See the following discussion of ocular surface immunity.[103]) In addition, antigens injected with adjuvants induce conventional immune responses, whereas antigens administered in the absence of adjuvants may either promote tolerance or elicit no response whatever.

Additional factors influencing whether tolerance is induced concern the status of the immune system itself. For example, antigen X may readily induce tolerance when injected intravenously into a normal, immunologically naive individual. However, if the same antigen is injected into an individual previously immunized to antigen X, then tolerance will not occur. Thus, a prior state of sensitization mitigates against tolerance induction. Alternatively, if a mature immune system has been assaulted by immunosuppressive drugs, by debilitating systemic diseases, or by particular types of pathogens (the human immunodeficiency virus is a good example), it may display increased susceptibility to tolerance. Thus, when an antigen is introduced into an individual with a compromised immune response, tolerance may develop and be maintained, even if the immune system recovers.

Regional Immunity and the Eye

All tissues of the body require immune protection from invading or endogenous pathogens. Because pathogens with different virulence strategies threaten different types of tissues, the immune system consists of a diversity of immune effectors. The diversity includes at least two different populations of effector T cells (that mediate delayed hypersensitivity and kill target cells) and seven different types of antibody molecules (IgM, IgG1, IgG2, IgG3, IgG4, IgA, and IgE). Thus, evolution has had to meet the challenge of designing an immune system that is capable of responding to a particular pathogen or antigen in a particular tissue with a response that is effective in eliminating the threat, while at the same time not damaging the tissue itself. Different tissues and organs display markedly different susceptibilities to immune-mediated tissue injury.[104, 105] The eye is an excellent example. Because integrity of the microanatomy of the visual axis is absolutely required for accurate vision, the eye can tolerate inflammation to only a very limited degree. Vigorous immunogenic inflammation, such as that found in a typical delayed hypersensitivity reaction in the skin, wreaks havoc with vision, and it has been argued that the threat of blindness has dictated an evolutionary adaptation in the eye that limits the expression of inflammation.

The conventional type of immunity that is generated

when antigens or pathogens enter through the skin is almost never seen in the normal eye. Therefore, almost by definition, any immune responses that take place in or on the eye are regulated. On the ocular surface, immunity resembles that observed on other mucosal surfaces, such as the gastrointestinal tract, the upper respiratory tract, and the urinary tract. Within the eye, an unusual form of immunity is observed; a description of this follows under "Intraocular Immunology: Ocular Immune Privilege."

Ocular Surface Immunity—Conjunctiva, Lacrimal Gland, Tear Film, Cornea, and Sclera

The normal human conjunctiva is an active participant in immune defense of the ocular surface against invasion by exogenous substances. The presence of blood vessels and lymphatic channels fosters transit of immune cells that can participate in the afferent and efferent arms of the immune response. The marginal and peripheral palpebral arteries and anterior ciliary arteries are the main blood suppliers of the conjunctiva. The superficial and deep lymphatic plexuses of the bulbar conjunctiva drain toward the palpebral commissures, where they join the lymphatics of the lids. Lymphatics of the palpebral conjunctiva on the lateral side drain into the preauricular and parotid lymph nodes. Lymphatics draining the palpebral conjunctiva on the medial side drain into the submandibular lymph nodes. Major immune cells found in normal human conjunctiva are dendritic cells, T and B lymphocytes, mast cells, and neutrophils. Dendritic cells, Langerhans' and non-Langerhans', have been detected in different regions of the conjunctiva.[106] Dendritic cells act as APCs to T lymphocytes and may stimulate antigen-specific class II region–mediated T-lymphocyte proliferation.[107] T lymphocytes, the predominant lymphocyte subpopulation in conjunctiva, are represented in the epithelium and in the substantia propria. T lymphocytes are the main effector cells in immune reactions such as delayed hypersensitivity or cytotoxic responses. B lymphocytes are absent except for rare scattered cells in the substantia propria of the fornices. Plasma cells are detected only in the conjunctival accessory lacrimal glands of Krause or in minor lacrimal glands.[108] T and B lymphocytes and plasma cells are also present between the acini of the major lacrimal gland. Plasma cells from major and minor lacrimal glands synthesize Igs, mainly IgA.[109, 110] IgA is a dimer that is transported across the mucosal epithelium bound to a receptor complex. IgA dimers are released to the luminal surface of the ducts associated with a secretory component after cleavage of the receptor and are excreted with the tear film. Secretory IgA is a protectant of mucosal surfaces. Although secretory IgA does not seem to be bacteriostatic or bactericidal, it may blanket cell surface receptors that might otherwise be available for viral and bacterial fixation,[111] and it may modulate the normal flora of the ocular surface.[112] Foreign substances can be processed locally by the mucosal immune defense system. Somehow, after exposure to antigen, specific IgA helper T lymphocytes stimulate IgA B lymphocytes to differentiate into IgA-secreting plasma cells. Dis-

persed T and B lymphocytes and IgA-secreting plasma cells of the conjunctiva and lacrimal gland are referred to as the conjunctival and lacrimal gland–associated lymphoid tissue (CALT).[113] CALT is considered part of a widespread mucosa-associated lymphoid tissue (MALT) system, including the oral mucosa and salivary gland–associated lymphoid tissue, the gut-associated lymphoid tissue (GALT),[114] and the bronchus-associated lymphoid tissue (BALT).[115] CALT drains to the regional lymph nodes in an afferent arc; effector cells may return to the eye via an efferent arc.

The adaptive and the innate immune responses form part of an integrated system. Immunoglobulins and lymphokines produced by the lymphoid tissue of the conjunctiva help neutrophils and macrophages to destroy antigens. Macrophages in turn help the lymphocytes by transporting the antigens from the eye to the lymph nodes. Some immunoglobulins (e.g., IgE) bind to mast cells; others (IgG, IgM) bind complement. Mast cells and complement facilitate the arrival of neutrophils and macrophages.

Mast cells are located mainly perilimbally, although they can also be found in bulbar conjunctiva. Their degranulation in response to an allergen or an injury results in the release of vasoactive substances such as histamine, heparin, platelet-activating factor, and leukotrienes, which can cause blood vessel dilation and increased vascular permeability.[116]

The tears contain several substances known to have antimicrobial properties. Lysozyme, immunoglobulins, and lactoferrin may be synthesized by the lacrimal gland. Lysozyme is an enzyme capable of lysing bacteria cell walls of certain gram-positive organisms.[117] Lysozyme may also facilitate secretory IgA bacteriolysis in the presence of complement.[118] The tear IgG has been shown to neutralize virus, lyse bacteria, and form immune complexes that bind complement and enhance bacterial opsonization and chemotaxis of phagocytes.[119] The tear components of the complement system enhance the effects of lysozyme and immunoglobulins.[120] Lactoferrin, an iron-binding protein, has both bacteriostatic and bactericidal properties.[121, 122] Lactoferrin may also regulate the production of granulocyte- and macrophage-derived colony-stimulating factor,[123] may inhibit the formation of the complement system component C3 convertase,[124] and may interact with specific antibody to produce an antibacterial effect more powerful than that of either lactoferrin or antibody alone.[125]

Autoimmune disorders that involve the conjunctiva include cicatricial pemphigoid, pemphigus vulgaris, erythema multiforme, and collagen vascular diseases. Autoimmune disorders that involve the lacrimal gland include Sjögren's syndrome. The mechanisms by which immunopathologic damage occurs in these diseases vary, depending on whether they are or are not organ-specific. When the antigen is localized in a particular organ, type II hypersensitivity reactions appear to be the main mechanisms (cicatricial pemphigoid and pemphigus vulgaris). In non–organ-specific diseases, type III and type IV hypersensitivity reactions are more important (erythema multiforme, collagen vascular diseases).

The unique anatomic and physiologic characteristics

of the human cornea explain, on the one hand, its predilection for involvement in various immune disorders and, on the other hand, its ability to express immune privilege. The peripheral cornea differs from the central cornea in several ways. The former is closer to the conjunctiva in which blood vessels and lymphatic channels provide a mechanism for the afferent arc of corneal immune reactions. Blood vessels derived from the anterior conjunctival and deep episcleral arteries extend 0.5 mm into the clear cornea.[126] Adjacent to these vessels, the subconjunctival lymphatics drain into regional lymph nodes. The presence of this vasculature allows diffusion of some molecules, such as immunoglobulins and complement components, into the cornea. IgG and IgA are found in similar concentrations in the peripheral and central cornea; however, more IgM is found in the periphery, probably because its high molecular weight restricts diffusion into the central area.[127] Both classical and alternative pathway components of complement and their inhibitors have been demonstrated in normal human corneas. However, although most of the complement components have a peripheral-to-central cornea ratio of 1.2:1.0, C1 is denser in the periphery by a factor of 5. The high molecular weight of C1, the recognition unit of the classical pathway, may also restrict its diffusion into the central area.[128, 129] Normal human corneal epithelium contains small numbers of Langerhans' cells, which are distributed almost exclusively at the limbus; very few cells are detected in the central cornea.[130] The peripheral cornea also contains a reservoir of inflammatory cells, including neutrophils, eosinophils, lymphocytes, plasma cells, and mast cells.[126] The presence of antibodies, complement components, Langerhans' cells, and inflammatory cells makes the peripheral cornea more susceptible than the central cornea to involvement in a wide variety of autoimmune and hypersensitivity disorders, such as Mooren's ulcer and collagen vascular diseases. A discussion of corneal antigens and immune privilege follows.[131]

The sclera consists almost entirely of collagen and proteoglycans. It is traversed by the anterior and posterior ciliary vessels but retains a scanty vascular supply for its own use. Its nutrition is derived from the overlying episclera and underlying choroid[132]; similarly, both classical and alternative pathway components of complement are derived from these sources.[133] Normal human sclera has few if any lymphocytes, macrophages, Langerhans' cells, or neutrophils.[134] In response to an inflammatory stimulus in the sclera, the cells pass readily from blood vessels of the episclera and choroid. Because of the collagenous nature of the sclera, many systemic autoimmune disorders, such as the collagen vascular diseases, may affect it.[134]

Intraocular Immunology: Ocular Immune Privilege

For more than 100 years, it has been known that foreign tissue grafts placed within the anterior chamber of an animal's eye can be accepted indefinitely.[135] The designation of this phenomenon as immune privilege had to await the seminal work of Medawar and colleagues, who discovered the principles of transplantation immunology in the 1940s and 1950s. These investigators studied immune privileged sites—the anterior chamber of the eye, the brain—as a method of exploring the possible ways to thwart immune rejection of solid tissue allografts.[136–139] It had been learned that transplantation antigens on grafts were carried to the immune system via regional lymphatic vessels and that immunization leading to graft rejection took place within draining lymph nodes. Because the eye and brain were regarded at the time as having no lymphatic drainage, and because both tissues resided behind a blood-tissue barrier, Medawar and associates postulated that immune privilege resulted from immunologic ignorance—although this was not a term that was used at the time. What these investigators meant was that foreign tissues placed in immune privileged sites were isolated by physical vascular barriers from the immune system and that they never alerted the immune system to their existence. During the past 25 years, immunologists who have studied immune privilege at various sites in the body have learned that this original postulate is basically untrue.[140–147] First, some privileged sites possess robust lymphatic drainage pathways—the testis is a good example. Second, antigens placed in privileged sites are known to escape and to be detected at distant sites, including lymphoid organs such as lymph nodes and the spleen. Third, antigens in privileged sites evoke antigen-specific, systemic immune responses, albeit of a unique nature. Thus, the modern view of immune privilege states that privilege is an actively acquired, dynamic state in which the immune system conspires with the privileged tissue or site in generating a response that is protective, rather than destructive. In a sense, immune privilege represents the most extreme form of the concept of regional immunity.

Immune Privileged Tissues and Sites

Immune privilege has two different manifestations: privileged sites and privileged tissues (Table 5–15). Immune privileged sites are regions of the body in which grafts of foreign tissue survive for an extended, even indefinite, time, compared with nonprivileged, or conventional sites. Immune privileged tissues, compared with nonprivileged tissues, are able to avoid, or at least resist, immune rejection when grafted into conventional body sites. The eye contains examples of both privileged tissues and privileged sites, of which the best studied site is the anterior chamber, and the best studied tissue is the cornea.

Much has been learned about the phenomenon of immune privilege during the past two decades. The forces

TABLE 5–15. IMMUNE PRIVILEGE

SITES	TISSUES
Eye	
Cornea, anterior chamber	Cornea
Vitreous cavity, subretinal space	Lens
Brain	Cartilage
Pregnant uterus	Placenta/fetus
Testis	Testis
Ovary	Ovary
Adrenal cortex	Liver
Hair follicles	
Tumors	Tumors

that confer immune privilege have been shown to act during both induction and expression of the immune response on antigens placed within, or expressed on, privileged sites and tissues. The forces that shape immune privileged sites and tissues include an ever-expanding list of microanatomic, biochemical, and immunoregulatory features. A short list of privilege-promoting features is displayed in Table 5–16. The eye expresses virtually every one of these features. Although passive features such as blood-ocular barrier, lack of lymphatics, and low expression of major histocompatibility complex (MHC) class I and II molecules are important, experimental attention has focused on immunomodulatory molecules expressed on ocular tissues and present in ocular fluids.

Regulation of Immune Expression in the Eye

As mentioned previously, activated T cells that express Fas on their surfaces are vulnerable to programmed cell death if they encounter other cells that express Fas ligand.[148] Constitutive expression of Fas ligand on cells that surround the anterior chamber has been shown to induce apoptosis among T cells and other leukocytes exposed to this ocular surface.[149] More important, Fas ligand expressed by cells of the cornea plays a key role in rendering the cornea resistant to immune attack and rejection.[150, 151] Similarly, constitutive expression on corneal endothelial cells, as well as iris and ciliary body epithelium, of several membrane-bound inhibitors of complement activation is strategically located to prevent complement-dependent intraocular inflammation and injury.[152]

The realization that the intraocular microenvironment is immunosuppressive arises chiefly from studies of aqueous humor and secretions of cultured iris and ciliary body. Transforming growth factor-β_2, a normal constituent of aqueous humor,[153–155] is a powerful immunosuppressant that inhibits various aspects of T-cell and macrophage activation. However, it is by no means the only (or perhaps even the most) important inhibitor present. Although the list is still incomplete, other relevant factors in aqueous humor include α-melanocyte–stimulating hormone,[156] vasoactive intestinal peptide,[157] calcitonin gene–related peptide,[158] and macrophage migration inhibitory factor.[159] These factors account in part for the immunosuppressive properties of aqueous humor: inhibition of T-cell activation (proliferation) and differentiation (secre-

tion of lymphokines such as IFN-γ) after ligation of the T-cell receptor for antigen; suppression of macrophage activation (phagocytosis, generation of nitrous oxide)[160]; and inhibition of natural killer (NK) cell lysis of target cells.[161] It is important to point out that aqueous humor does not inhibit all immune reactivity. For example, antibody neutralization of virus infection of target cells is not prevented in the presence of aqueous humor.[160] Moreover, cytotoxic T cells that are fully differentiated are fully able to lyse antigen-bearing target cells cultured in aqueous humor. The ability of the immune system to express itself within the eye is highly regulated by the factors just described; suppression of immune expression that leads to inflammation and damage is one important dimension of ocular immune privilege.

Regulation of Induction of Immunity to Eye-Derived Antigens

Another dimension to immune privilege is the ability of the eye to regulate the nature of the systemic immune response to antigens placed within it. It has been known for more than 20 years that injection of alloantigenic cells into the anterior chamber of rodent eyes evokes a distinctive type of immune deviation—now called anterior chamber–associated immune deviation (ACAID).[162–164] In ACAID, eye-derived antigens elicit an immune response that is selectively deficient in T cells that mediate delayed hypersensitivity and B cells that secrete complement-fixing antibodies. There is not, however, a global lack of response because animals with ACAID display a high level of antigen-specific serum antibodies of the non–complement-fixing varieties,[165, 166] as well as primed cytotoxic T cells.[167, 168] In ACAID, regulatory T cells are also generated that, in an antigen-specific manner, suppress both induction and expression of delayed hypersensitivity to the antigen in question.[169–172] ACAID can be elicited by diverse types of antigens, ranging from soluble protein to histocompatibility to virus-encoded antigens. A deviant systemic response similar to ACAID can even be evoked by antigen injected into the anterior chamber of the eye of an individual previously immunized to the same antigen.

Induction of ACAID by intraocular injection of antigen begins within the eye itself.[172–177] After injection of antigen into the eye, local APCs capture the antigen, migrate across the trabecular meshwork into the canal of Schlemm, and then traffic via the blood to the spleen. In the splenic white pulp, the antigen is presented in a unique manner to T and B lymphocytes, resulting in the spectrum of functionally distinct antigen-specific T cells and antibodies found in ACAID. The ocular microenvironment sets the stage for this sequence of events by virtue of the immunoregulatory properties of aqueous humor. This ocular fluid or, more precisely, TGF-β_2, confers upon conventional APCs the capacity to induce ACAID. Thus, the ocular microenvironment not only regulates the expression of immunity within the eye, but it also regulates the functions of eye-derived APCs and thus promotes a systemic immune response that is deficient in those immune effector modalities most capable of inducing immunogenic inflammation—delayed hypersensitivity T cells and complement-fixing antibodies.

TABLE 5–16. FEATURES OF IMMUNE PRIVILEGED SITES

PASSIVE

Blood-tissue barriers
Deficient efferent lymphatics
Tissue fluid that drains into blood vasculature
Reduced expression of major histocompatibility complex class I and
  II molecules

ACTIVE

Constitutive expression of inhibitory cell surface molecules:
  Fas ligand, DAF, CD59, CD46
Immunosuppressive microenvironment: TGF-β, α-MSH, VIP, CGRP,
  MIF, free cortisol

CGRP, calcitonin gene–related peptide; DAF, decay accelerating factor; MIF, migration inhibitory factor; MSH, melanocyte stimulating hormone; TGF, transforming growth factor; VIP, vasointestinal peptide.

Relationship Between Immune Privilege and Intraocular Inflammatory Diseases

The rationale of immune privilege is that all tissues, including the eye, require immune protection. Immune privilege represents the consequence of interactions between the immune system and the eye in which local protection is provided by immune effectors that do not disrupt the eye's primary and vital function—vision. Because maintenance of a precise microanatomy is essential for vision, privilege allows for immune protection that is virtually devoid of immunogenic inflammation.

At the experimental level, ocular immune privilege has been implicated in: (1) the extraordinary success of corneal allografts,[178-181] (2) progressive growth of intraocular tumors,[182] (3) resistance to herpes stromal keratitis,[183] and (4) suppression of autoimmune uveoretinitis.[184-186] When immune privilege prevails within the eye, corneal allografts succeed, trauma to the eye heals without incident, and ocular infections are cleared without inflammation. However, in this case, ocular tumors may then grow relentlessly, and uveal tract infections may persist and recur.

The consequences of failed immune privilege have been explored experimentally and considered clinically. When privilege fails in the eye, blindness is a likely outcome. As examples, ocular trauma may result in sympathetic ophthalmia, ocular infections may produce sight-threatening inflammation, and corneal allografts may fail.

Corneal Transplantation Immunology

The cornea is an immune privileged tissue and, in part, this attribute accounts for the extraordinary success of orthotopic corneal allografts in experimental animals and also in humans. It is pertinent that the corneal graft forms the anterior surface of a site that is also typically immune privileged (the anterior chamber). Despite the advances that have been made in corneal tissue preservation and surgical techniques, a significant proportion of grafts eventually fail.[187-190] The main cause of transplant failure now is immune-mediated graft rejection, which occurs in 16% to 30% of recipients in a large series after several years of follow-up. Certain recipients seem to be at increased risk of graft rejection.[191-193] Corneal vascularization, either preoperative from recipient herpetic, interstitial, or traumatic keratitis, or stimulated by silk or loose sutures, contact lenses, infections, persistent epithelial defects, and other disorders associated with inflammation, has been widely recognized as a clear risk factor for decreased graft survival. It is estimated that the failure rate is 25% to 50% in vascularized corneas and 5% to 10% in avascular ones. Other factors that increase the risk of allograft rejection include: (1) a history of previous graft loss,[194-196] (2) eccentric and large grafts, and (3) glaucoma. The reasons why corneal bed neovascularization is a dominant risk factor for cornea graft rejection remain to be elucidated. Evidence indicates that neovascularized corneas also contain neolymphatic vessels.[197] Moreover, the graft bed is heavily infiltrated with APCs, especially Langerhans' cells. These factors are probably important for increasing the immunogenic potential of the allogeneic corneal graft.

Transplantation Antigen Expression on Corneal Tissue

In outbred species, such as humans, transplants of solid tissue grafts usually fail unless the recipient is immunosuppressed; the reason for failure is the development of an immune response directed at so-called transplantation antigens displayed on cells of the graft. Immunologists have separated transplantation antigens into two categories, major and minor, primarily because major antigens induce more vigorous alloimmunity than do minor antigens.[198] The genes that encode the major transplantation antigens in humans are located within the MHC, called *human leukocyte antigen (HLA)*. Minor histocompatibility antigens are encoded at numerous loci spread throughout the genome. The HLA complex, which is a large genetic region, is situated on the short arm of the sixth human chromosome. HLA genes that encode class I and class II antigens are extremely polymorphic. Similarly, minor histocompatibility loci contain highly polymorphic genes. In the aggregate, polymorphisms at the major and minor histocompatibility loci account for the observation that solid tissue grafts exchanged between any two individuals selected at random within a species are acutely rejected.

The expression of HLA antigens on corneal cells is somewhat atypical.[199-203] Class I MHC antigens are expressed strongly on the epithelial cells of the cornea, comparable in intensity to the expression of epidermal cells of skin. Keratinocytes express less class I than conventional fibroblasts, and corneal endothelial cells express small amounts of class I antigen under normal circumstances. Except at the periphery near the limbus, the cornea contains no adventitial cells (i.e., cells of bone marrow origin).[204, 205] In most solid tissues, class II HLA antigens are expressed primarily on these types of cells.[206] Therefore, under normal conditions, the burden of class II MHC antigens on corneal grafts is minimal. Corneal epithelial and endothelial cells resemble other cells of the body in responding to IFN-γ by upregulation of class I antigen expression. Among IFN-γ–treated epithelial cells, class II antigens are also expressed. However, corneal endothelial cells resist expression of class II antigens. Because class II antigens, especially those expressed on bone marrow–derived cells, are extremely important in providing solid tissue grafts with their ability to evoke transplantation immunity, the deficit of these antigens on corneal cells offers a significant barrier to sensitization.

A major accomplishment of modern immunology is the ability of contemporary clinical pathology laboratories to tissue-type for HLA class I and class II antigens. With most solid tissue allografts, tissue typing that identifies HLA matching between a graft donor and a recipient correlates with improved graft survival.[207] Thus, HLA-matched kidney grafts survive with fewer rejection episodes and with a reduced need for immunosuppressive therapy, compared to HLA-mismatched grafts. The evidence that HLA tissue typing similarly improves the fate of matched corneal allografts is conflicting.[208-215] There seems to be no controversy regarding the influence of tissue typing on grafts placed in eyes of patients with low risk. In this situation, virtually no studies suggest a positive typing effect. The rate of graft success is so high in low-risk situations with unmatched grafts that there is little opportunity for a matching effect to be seen. However, in high-risk situations, the literature contains reports that claim: (1) HLA matching, especially for class I antigens, has a powerful positive effect on graft outcome; (2) HLA matching has no effect on graft outcome; or (3) HLA matching may have a deleterious effect on graft outcome.

The reasons for confusion about the effects of HLA matching on corneal allograft success may relate to studies on orthotopic corneal allografts conducted in mice. It has been reported that minor transplantation antigens offer a significant barrier to graft success in rodents.[216–218] In fact, corneal allografts that display minor, but not major, transplantation antigens are rejected more vigorously and with a higher frequency than grafts that display MHC, but not minor, transplantation antigens. Two factors seem to be important in this outcome. First, the reduced expression of MHC antigens on corneal grafts renders these grafts less immunogenic than other solid tissue grafts. Second, corneal antigens are detected by the recipient immune system only when the recipient's own APCs infiltrate the graft and capture donor antigens. Graft cells are the source of donor antigens and, apparently in the cornea, minor transplantation antigens are quantitatively more numerous than MHC antigens. Therefore, the recipient mounts an immune response directed primarily at minor transplantation antigens. Because tissue typing is unable at present to match organs and donors for minor histocompatibility antigens, it is no surprise that current tissue typing has proved to be ineffectual at improving corneal allograft success.

Corneal Allograft Acceptance— When Immune Privilege Succeeds

The normal cornea is an immune privileged tissue, and several features are known to contribute to this privileged status. First, as mentioned earlier, expression of MHC class I and class II molecules is reduced and impaired, especially on the corneal endothelium. The net antigenic load of corneal tissue is thus reduced compared with other tissues, which has a mitigating effect on both induction and expression of alloimmunity. Second, the cornea lacks blood and lymph vessels. The absence of these vascular structures isolates the corneal graft in a manner that prevents antigenic information from escaping from the tissue while at the same time prevents immune effectors from gaining access to the tissue. Third, the cornea is deficient in bone marrow–derived cells, especially Langerhans' cells. Mobile cells of this type are one way in which antigenic information from a solid tissue graft alerts the immune system in regional lymph nodes to its presence. The absence of APCs from the cornea dramatically lengthens the time it takes for the recipient immune system to become aware of the graft's existence. Fourth, cells of the cornea constitutively secrete molecules with immunosuppressive properties.[219–223] Cells of all three corneal layers secrete TGF-β, as well as yet-to-be-defined inhibitory molecules. In addition, corneal epithelial cells and keratinocytes constitutively produce an excess of IL-1 receptor antagonist, compared with the endogenous production of IL-1γ.[221] These immunosuppressive molecules have powerful modulatory effects on APC, T cells,

B cells, NK cells, and macrophages and can act during induction and expression of alloimmunity to prevent or inhibit graft rejection. Fifth, cells of the cornea constitutively express surface molecules that inhibit immune effectors. Corneal endothelial cells display on their surfaces DAF, CD59, and CD46—molecules that inhibit complement effector functions.[222] These inhibitors protect corneal endothelial cells from injury by complement molecules generated during an alloimmune response. Corneal cells have been found to express CD95L (Fas ligand), and expression of this molecule on mouse cornea grafts has been formally implicated in protecting the grafts from attack by Fas+ T cells and other leukocytes.[150, 151, 223] Finally, the corneal graft forms the anterior surface of the anterior chamber; antigens released from the graft endothelium escape into aqueous humor. Experimental evidence indicates that allogeneic corneal grafts induce donor-specific ACAID in recipients,[216, 224] and the inability of these recipients to acquire donor-specific delayed hypersensitivity plays a key role in maintaining the integrity of accepted grafts.

When placed in low-risk (normal) eyes of mice, a high proportion of corneal allografts with the features listed earlier experience prolonged, even indefinite, survival in the complete absence of any immunosuppressive therapy. This dramatic expression of immune privilege is mirrored by the success of keratoplasties performed in low-risk situations in humans. However, neither in mice nor in humans are all such grafts successful. This observation indicates that immune privilege is by no means absolute and irrevocable.

Pathogenesis of Corneal Allograft Rejection—When Immune Privilege Fails

The high rate of failure of corneal allografts in high-risk situations in humans resembles the high rate of failure of orthotopic corneal allografts placed in high-risk mouse eyes.[225] Studies of the rejection process in experimental animals have begun to unravel the pathogenic mechanisms responsible. Sensitization develops in recipient animals with surprising rapidity when grafts are placed in high-risk eyes. Within 7 days of engraftment, immune donor-specific T cells can be detected in lymphoid tissues. Similar grafts placed in low-risk mouse eyes do not achieve T-cell sensitization until at least 3 weeks after engraftment. The reason for rapid sensitization when grafts are placed in high-risk eyes appears to be the speed with which recipient APCs (chiefly Langerhans' cells) migrate into the graft from the periphery. Whereas migration of Langerhans' cells into allografts placed in low-risk eyes is detectable between 1 and 2 weeks after grafting, Langerhans' cells can be detected in grafts in high-risk eyes within a few days of engraftment. It is very likely that the vulnerability to rejection of grafts placed in high-risk eyes is dictated by the efficiency with which recipient APCs enter the graft, capture antigens, and migrate to the regional lymph nodes where recipient T cells are initially activated. Support for this view is provided by the observation that Langerhans' cell migration into the graft can be inhibited by topical application of IL-1 receptor antagonist.[226] Experiments indicate that grafts that have been treated with IL-1Ra take longer to induce donor-specific sensitization, and the majority of such grafts avoid immune rejection.

When normal corneal grafts are placed in high-risk eyes, they are typically rejected. In this case, the inherent immune privileged status of the graft is clearly insufficient to overcome the fact that the graft site (a neovascularized eye) can no longer act as an immune privileged site. It is also possible to show that grafts that have lost their immune privileged status are vulnerable to rejection, even when placed in normal, low-risk eyes (which display immune privilege). Langerhans' cells can be induced to migrate into the central corneal epithelium by several different experimental maneuvers. When grafts containing Langerhans' cells are placed in low-risk eyes, rapid recipient sensitization occurs, and the grafts are rejected. The tempo and vigor of rejection of these grafts strongly resemble the fate of normal grafts placed in high-risk eyes. These results indicate that both the privileged tissue (the corneal graft) and the privileged site (the low-risk eye) make important contributions to the success of orthotopic corneal allografts.

Summary and Conclusion

The eye is defended against pathogens, just as is every other part of the body. Components of both the natural and the acquired immune systems respond to pathogens in the eye, but the responses are different from those following antigen encounter in most other places in the body, perhaps as a result of evolutionary pressures that have led to the survival of those species and members of species in which a blinding, exuberant inflammatory response was prevented by "regulation" of the response. In any event, we are left for the moment with an organ (the eye) in which special immunologic responsiveness allows us to enjoy a degree of "privileged" tolerance to transplanted tissue not experienced by other organs. It is clear now that this tolerance is an active process, not simply a passive one derived from the "invisibility" of the transplant to the recipient's immune system.

References

1. Kohler J, Milstein C: Continuous cultures of fused cells secreting antibody of predefined specificity. Nature 1975; 256:495.
2. Reinherz EL, Schlossman SF: The differentiation and function of human T lymphocytes. Cell 1980; 19:821.
3. Hardy RR, Hayakawa K, Parks DR, Herzenberg LA: Murine B cell differentiation lineages. J Exp Med 1984; 1959:1169.
4. Hardy RR, Hayakawa K, Schimizu M, et al: Rheumatoid factor secretion from human Leu-1 B cells. Science 1987; 236:81.
5. Mosmann TR, Coffman R: Two types of mouse helper T cell clones: Implications from immune regulation. Immunol Today 1987; 8:233.
6. Coffman R, O'Hara J, Bond MW, et al: B cell stimulatory factor-1 enhances the IgE response of lipopolysaccharide-activated B cell. J Immunol 1986; 136:4538.
7. Mariotti S, del Prete GF, Mastromauro C, et al: The autoimmune infiltrates of Basedow's disease: Analysis of clonal level and comparison with Hashimoto's thyroiditis. Exp Clin Endocrinol 1991; 97:139.
8. Maggi E, Biswas P, del Prete GF, et al: Accumulation of TH2-like helper T cells in the conjunctiva of patients with vernal conjunctivitis. J Immunol 1991; 146:1169.
9. Romagnani S: Human TH1 and TH2 subsets: Doubt no more. Immunol Today 1991; 12:256.
10. Murphy DB, Mamauchi K, Habu S, et al: T cells in a suppressor circuit and non-T:non-B cells bear different I-J determinants. Immunogenetics 1981; 13:205.
11. Gillette TE, Chandler JW, Greiner JV: Langerhans cells of the ocular surface. Ophthalmology 1982; 89:700.
12. Tagawa Y, Takeuchi T, Saga T, et al: Langerhans cells: Role in ocular surface immunopathology. In: O'Connor GR, Chandler JW, eds: Advances in Immunology and Immunopathology of the Eye. New York, Masson, 1985, pp 203–207.
13. Le Douarin NM: Ontogeny of hematopoietic organ studies in avian embryo interspecific chimeras. In: Clarkson D, Marks PA, Till JE, eds: Cold Spring Harbor Meeting on Differentiation of Normal and Neoplastic Hematopoietic Cells. Cold Spring Harbor, NY, Cold Spring Harbor Laboratory, 1978, pp 5–32.
14. Metcalf D, Moore MAS: Hematopoietic cells. In: Neuberger A, Tatum EL, eds: Frontiers of Biology, vol. 24. Amsterdam, Elsevier North-Holland, 1971.
15. Hermans MJA, Hartsuiker H, Opstaelten D: An insight to study of B lymphocytopoiesis in rat bone marrow: Topographical arrangement of terminal yatsi nucleotidal transferase positive cells and pre-B cells. J Immunol 1989; 44:67.
16. Szengerg A, Warner ML: Association of immunologic responsiveness in fowls with a hormonally arrested development of lymphoid material. Nature 1962; 194:146.
17. Cooper MD, Peterson RD, South MA, Good RA: The functions of the thymus system and the bursa system in the chicken. J Exp Med 1966; 123:75.
18. Papiernik M: Lymphoid organs. In: Bach JF, ed: Immunology, 2nd ed. New York, John Wiley & Sons, 1982, pp 15–37.
19. Butcher EC, Weissman IL: Lymphoid tissues and organs. In: Paul W, ed: Fundamental Immunology, 2nd ed. New York, Raven Press, 1989, pp 117–137.
20. Berg EL, Goldstein LA, Jutila MA, et al: Homing receptors and vascular addressins: Cell adhesion molecules that direct lymphocyte traffic. Immunol Rev 1989; 108:5.
21. Picker LJ, de los Toyos J, Tellen MJ, et al: Monoclonal antibodies against the CD 44 and Pgp-1 antigens in man recognize the Hermes class of lymphocyte homing receptors. J Immunol 1989; 142:2046.
22. Holzmann B, McIntyre BW, Weissman IC: Identification of a murine Peyer's patch–specific lymphocyte homing receptor as an integrin molecule with an alpha chain homologous to human VLA-4 alpha. Cell 1989; 56:37.
23. Streeter PR, Rause ET, Butcher EC: Immunohistologic and functional characterization of a vascular addressin involved in lymphocyte homing into peripheral lymph nodes. J Cell Biol 1988; 107:1853.
24. Dreyer WJ, Bennett JC: The molecular basis of antibody formation: A paradox. Proc Natl Acad Sci U S A 1965; 54:864.
25. Hozumi N, Tonegawa S: Evidence for somatic rearrangement of immunoglobulin genes coding for variable and constant regions. Proc Natl Acad Sci U S A 1976; 73:3628.
26. Wu TT, Kabat EA: An analysis of the sequences of the variable regions of Bence Jones proteins and myeloma light chains and their implications for antibody complementarity. J Exp Med 1970; 132:211.
27. Leder P: The genetics of antibody diversity. Sci Am 1982; 246:102.
28. Tonegawa S: Somatic generation of antibody diversity. Nature 1983; 302:575.
29. Honjo T, Habu S: Origin of immune diversity: Genetic variation and selection. Annu Rev Biochem 1985; 54:803.
30. Alt FW, Baltimore D: Joining of immunoglobulin heavy chain gene segments: Implications from a chromosome with evidence of three D-JH fusions. Proc Natl Acad Sci U S A 1982; 79:4118.
31. Early P, Huang H, Davis M, et al: An immunoglobulin heavy chain variable region gene is generated from three segments of DNA: VH, D and JH. Cell 1980; 12:981.
32. Sakano H, Huppi K, Heinrich G, Tonegawa S: Sequences at the somatic recombination sites of immunoglobulin light-chain genes. Nature 1979; 280:288.
33. Weigert MG, Cesari IM, Yondovich SJ, Cohn M: Variability in the lambda light chain sequences of mouse antibody. Nature 1970; 228:1045.
34. Brack C, Hirama M, Lenhard-Schuller R, Tonegawa S: A complete immunoglobulin gene is created by somatic recombination. Cell 1978; 15:1.
35. Bernard O, Hozumi N, Tonegawa S: Sequences of mouse immunoglobulin light chain genes before and after somatic changes. Cell 1978; 15:1133.

36. Pernis BG, Chiappino G, Kelus AS, Gell PGH: Cellular localization of immunoglobulins with different allotypic specificities in rabbit lymphoid tissues. J Exp Med 1965; 122:853.

37. Cebra J, Colberg JE, Dray S: Rabbit lymphoid cells differentiated with respect to alpha-, gamma-, and mu-heavy polypeptide chains and to allotypic markers for Aa1 and Aa2. J Exp Med 1966; 123:547.

38. Kataoka T, Kawakami T, Takahasi N, Honjo T: Rearrangement of immunoglobulin g1-chain gene and mechanism for heavy-chain class switch. Proc Natl Acad Sci U S A 1980; 77:919.

39. Gritzmacher CA: Molecular aspects of heavy-chain class switching. Crit Rev Immunol 1989; 9:173.

40. Brodeur PH, Riblet R: The immunoglobulin heavy chain variable region (Igh-V) locus in the mouse I. One hundred Igh-V genes comprise seven families of homologous genes. Eur J Immunol 1984; 14:922.

41. Winter EA, Radbruch A, Krawinkel U: Members of novel VH gene families are found in VDJ regions of polyclonally activated B lymphocytes. EMBO J 1985; 4:2861.

42. Kofler R: A new murine Ig VH family. J Immunol 1988; 140:4031.

43. Reininger L, Kaushik A, Jaton JC: A member of a new VH gene family encodes anti-bromelinised mouse red blood cell autoantibodies. Eur J Immunol 1988; 18:1521.

44. Rechavi G, Bienz B, Ram D, et al: Organization and evolution of immunoglobulin VH gene subgroups. Proc Natl Acad Sci U S A 1982; 79:4405.

45. Rechavi G, Ram D, Glazer R, et al: Evolutionary aspects of immunoglobulin heavy chain variable region (VH) gene subgroups. Proc Natl Acad Sci U S A 1983; 80:855.

46. Matthyssens G, Rabbitts TH: Structure and multiplicity of genes for the human immunoglobulin heavy chain variable region. Proc Natl Acad Sci U S A 1980; 77:6561.

47. Berman JE, Mellis SJ, Pollock R, et al: Content and organization of the human Ig VH locus: Definition of three new VH families and linkage to the Ig CH locus. EMBO J 1988; 7:727.

48. Potter M, Newell JB, Rudikoff S, Haber E: Classification of mouse VK groups based on the partial amino acid sequence to the first invariant tryptophan: Impact of 14 new sequences from IgG myeloma proteins. Mol Immunol 1982; 12:1619.

49. D'Joostelaere LA, Huppi K, Mock B, et al: The immunoglobulin kappa light chain allelic groups among the Igk haplotypes and Igk crossover populations suggest a gene order. J Immunol 1988; 141:652.

50. Yancopoulos GD, Desiderio SV, Pasking M, et al: Preferential utilization of the most JH-proximal VH gene segments in pre-B cell lines. Nature 1984; 311:727.

51. Perlmutter RM, Kearney JF, Chang SP, Hood LE: Developmentally controlled expression of immunoglobulin VH genes. Science 1985; 227:1597.

52. Reth M, Jackson N, Alt FW: VHDJH formation and DJH replacement during pre-B differentiation: Non-random usage of gene segments. EMBO J 1986; 5:2131.

53. Lawler AM, Lin PS, Gearhart PJ: Adult B-cell repertoire is biased toward two heavy-chain variable region genes that rearrange frequently in fetal pre-B cells. Proc Natl Acad Sci U S A 1987; 84:2454.

54. Yancopoulos GD, Malynn B, Alt FW: Developmentally regulated and strain-specific expression of murine VH gene families. J Exp Med 1988; 168:417.

55. Dildrop R, Krawinkel U, Winter E, Rajewsky K: VH-gene expression in murine lipopolysaccharide blasts distributes over the nine known VH-gene groups and may be random. Eur J Immunol 1985; 15:1154.

56. Schulze DH, Kelsoe G: Genotypic analysis of B cell colonies by in situ hybridization. Stoichiometric expression of the three VH families in adult C57BL/6 and BALB/c mice. J Exp Med 1987; 166:163.

57. Krawinkel U, Cristoph T, Blankenstein T: Organization of the Ig *VH* locus in mice and humans. Immunol Today 1989; 10:339.

58. Janeway CA Jr, Travers P, eds: Immunobiology: The Immune System in Health and Disease, 3rd ed. New York, Current Biology/Garland Publishing, 1997.

59. Von Boehmer H: The developmental biology of T lymphocytes. Annu Rev Immunol 1993; 6:309.

60. Moller C, ed: Positive T cell selection in the thymus. Immunol Rev 1993; 135:5.

61. Nossal CJV: Negative selection of lymphocytes. Cell 1994; 76:229.

62. Havran WL, Boismenu R: Activation and function of $\gamma\delta$ T cells. Curr Opin Immunol 1994; 6:442.

63. Germain RN: MHC-dependent antigen processing and peptide presentation: Providing ligands for T lymphocyte activation. Cell 1994; 76:287.

64. Fremont DH, Rees WA, Kozono H: Biophysical studies of T cell receptors and their ligands. Curr Opin Immunol 1996; 8:93.

65. Janeway CA, Bottomly K: Signals and signs for lymphocyte responses. Cell 1994; 76:275.

66. Sprent J, Webb SR: Intrathymic and extrathymic clonal deletion of T cells. Curr Opin Immunol 1995; 7:196.

67. Picker LJ, Butcher EC: Physiological and molecular mechanisms of lymphocyte homing. Annu Rev Immunol 1993; 10:561.

68. Jain J, Loh C, Rao A: Transcription regulation of the IL-2 gene. Curr Opin Immunol 1995; 7:333.

69. Minami Y, Kono T, Miyazaki T, Taniguchi T: The IL-2 receptor complex: Its structure, function, and target genes. Annu Rev Immunol 1993; 11:245.

70. Griffiths GM: The cell biology of CTL killing. Curr Opin Immunol 1995; 7:343.

71. Mueller DL, Jenkins MK: Molecular mechanisms underlying functional T cell unresponsiveness. Curr Opin Immunol 1995; 7:325.

72. Mosmann TR, Coffman RL: Th1 and Th2 cells: Different patterns of lymphokine secretion lead to different functional properties. Ann Rev Immunol 1989; 7:145.

73. Maggi E, Romagnani S: Role of T cells and T cell-derived cytokines in the pathogenesis of allergic diseases. Ann N Y Acad Sci 1994; 725:2.

74. Cocoa AF, Cooke RA: On the classification of the phenomena of hypersensitiveness. J Immunol 1923; 8:163.

75. von Pirquet C: Allergie. Munch Med Wochenschr 1906; 53:1457.

76. Foster CS, Calonge M: Atopic keratoconjunctivitis. Ophthalmology 1990; 97:992.

77. Foster CS, Duncan J: Randomized clinical trial of disodium cromoglycate therapy in vernal keratoconjunctivitis. Am J Ophthalmol 1980; 90:175.

78. Foster CS: Evaluation of topical cromolyn sodium in the treatment of vernal keratoconjunctivitis. Ophthalmology 1988; 95:194.

79. Bussel JB, Kimberly RP, Inamen RD, et al: Intravenous gamma globulin treatment of chronic idiopathic cytopenic purpura. Blood 1983; 62:480.

80. Bleik JH, Tabbara KS: Topical cyclosporine in vernal keratoconjunctivitis. Ophthalmology 1991; 98:1679.

81. Foster CS: Cicatricial pemphigoid. Thesis of the American Ophthalmological Society. Trans Am Ophthalmol Soc 1986; 84:527.

82. Foster CS, Wilson LA, Ekins MB: Immunosuppressive therapy for progressive ocular cicatricial pemphigoid. Ophthalmology 1982; 89:340.

83. Tauber J, Sainz de la Maza M, Foster CS: Systemic chemotherapy for ocular cicatricial pemphigoid. Cornea 1991; 10:185.

84. Neumann R, Tauber J, Foster CS: Remission and recurrence after withdrawal of therapy for ocular cicatricial pemphigoid. Ophthalmology 1991; 98:868.

85. Sainz de la Maza M, Foster CS: Necrotizing scleritis after ocular surgery: A clinical pathologic study. Ophthalmology 1991; 98:1720.

86. Leib ES, Restivo C, Paulus AT: Immunosuppressive and corticosteroid therapy of polyarteritis nodosa. Am J Med 1979; 67:941.

87. Wolf SM, Fauci AS, Horn RG, Dale DC: Wegener's granulomatosis. Ann Intern Med 1974; 81:513.

88. Foster CS, Forstot SL, Wilson LA: Mortality rate in rheumatoid arthritis patients developing necrotizing scleritis or peripheral ulcerative keratitis. Ophthalmology 1984; 91:1253.

89. Janeway CA Jr, Travers P, eds: Immunobiology: The Immune System in Health and Disease, 3rd ed. New York, Current Biology/Garland Publishing, 1997.

90. Steinman L: Escape from "horror autotoxicus": pathogenesis and treatment of autoimmune disease. Cell 1995; 80:7.

91. Tan EM: Autoantibodies in pathology and cell biology. Cell 1991; 67:841.

92. Pearlman E, Lass HJ, Bardenstein DS, et al: Interleukin 4 and T helper type 2 cells are required for development of experimental onchocercal keratitis (River Blindness). J Exp Med 1995; 182:931.

93. Streilein JW, Dana MR, Ksander BR: Immunity causing blindness: Five different paths to herpes stromal keratitis. Immunol Today 1997; 18:443.

94. Janeway CA Jr, Travers P: Immunobiology. Current Biology, 3rd ed. New York, Limited/Garland Publishing, 1997.

95. Qin S, Cobbold SP, Pope H, et al: Infectious transplantation tolerance. Science 1993; 259:974.

96. Asherson GL, Collizi V, Zembala M: An overview of T-suppressor cell circuits. Ann Rev Immunol 1986; 4:37.

97. Groux H, O'Garra A, Bigler M, et al: A CD4+ T-cell subset inhibits antigen-specific T-cell responses and prevents colitis. Nature 1997; 389:737.

98. Billingham RE, Brent L, Medawar PB: Actively acquired tolerance of foreign cells. Nature 1953; 172:603.

99. Burnet FM: The Clonal Selection Theory of Acquired Immunity. Cambridge, Cambridge University Press, 1959.

100. Kappler JW, Roehm N, Marrack P: T cell tolerance by clonal elimination in the thymus. Cell 1987; 49:273.

101. Jenkins MK, Pardoll DM, Mizuchi J, et al: RH: Molecular events in the induction of a non-responsive state in interleukin-2 producing helper lymphocyte clones. Proc Natl Acad Sci U S A 1987; 84:5409.

102. Asherson GL, Stone SH: Selective and specific inhibition of 24-hour skin reactions in the guinea-pig. I: Immune deviation: Description of the phenomenon and the effect of splenectomy. Immunology 1965; 9:205.

103. Khoury SJ, Hancock WW, Weiner HL: Oral tolerance to myelin basic protein and natural recovery from experimental autoimmune encephalomyelitis are associated with downregulation of inflammatory cytokines and differential upregulation of transforming growth factor β, interleukin 4, and prostaglandin E expression in the brain. J Exp Med 1992; 176:1355.

104. Streilein JW: Regional immunology of the eye. In: Pepose JW, Holland GN, Wilhemus KR, eds: Ocular Infection and Immunity. Philadelphia, Mosby–Year Book, 1996, pp 19–33.

105. Streilein JW: Regional immunology. In: Dulbecco R, ed: Encyclopedia of Human Biology, 2nd ed, vol. 4. San Diego, Academic Press, 1997, pp 767–776.

106. Sacks E, Rutgers J, Jakobiec FA, et al: A comparison of conjunctival and nonocular dendritic cells utilizing new monoclonal antibodies. Ophthalmology 1986; 93:1089.

107. Murphy GF: Cell membrane glycoproteins and Langerhans cells. Hum Pathol 1985; 16:103.

108. Sacks E, Wieczorek R, Jakobiec FA, et al: Lymphocytic sub-populations in the normal human conjunctiva. Ophthalmology 1986; 93:1276.

109. Franklin RM, Remus LE: Conjunctival-associated lymphoid tissue: Evidence for a role in the secretory immune system. Invest Ophthalmol Vis Sci 1984; 25:181.

110. Wieczorek R, Jakobiec FA, Sacks E, et al: The immunoarchitecture of the normal human lacrimal gland. Ophthalmology 1988; 95:100.

111. Tomasi TB: The Immune System of Secretion. Englewood Cliffs, Prentice-Hall, 1976.

112. Gibbons RJ: Bacterial adherence to the mucosal surfaces and its inhibition by secretory antibodies. Adv Exp Med Biol 1974; 45:315.

113. Jackson DE, Lally ET, Nakamura MC, et al: Migration of IgA-bearing lymphocytes into salivary glands. Cell Immunol 1981; 63:203.

114. Parrott DM: The gut as a lymphoid organ. Clin Gastroenterol 1976; 5:211.

115. Bienenstock J, Johnston N, Percy DYE: Bronchial lymphoid tissue. I: Morphologic characteristics. Lab Invest 1973; 28:686.

116. Allansmith MR: The Eye and Immunology. St. Louis, CV Mosby, 1982.

117. Allansmith MR: Defense of the ocular surface. Int Ophthalmol Clin 1979; 12:93.

118. Fleming A: On a remarkable bacteriolytic element found in tissues and secretions. Proc R Soc Lond (Biol) 1922; 93:306.

119. Strober W, Hague HE, Lum LG, et al: IgA-Fc receptors on mouse lymphoid cells. J Immunol 1978; 121:2140.

120. Bluestone R: Lacrimal immunoglobulins and complement quantified by counterimmunoelectrophoresis. Br J Ophthalmol 1975; 59:279.

121. Masson PL, Heremans JF, Prignot JJ, et al: Immunohistochemical localization and bacteriostatic properties of an iron-binding protein from bronchial mucus. Thorax 1966; 21:358.

122. Arnold RR, Cole MF, McGhee JR: A bactericidal effect for human lactoferrin. Science 1977; 197(297):263.

123. Badgy GC: Interaction of lactoferrin monocytes and lymphocyte subsets in the regulation of steady-state granulopoiesis in vitro. J Clin Invest 1981; 68:56.

124. Kijlstra A, Jeurissen SHM: Modulation of classical C_3 convertase of complement by tear lactoferrin. Immunology 1982; 47:263.

125. Bullen JJ, Rogers HJ, Leigh L: Iron-binding proteins in milk and resistance of Escherichia coli infection in infants. BMJ 1972; 1:69.

126. Hogan MJ, Alvarado JA, Weddell JE: The limbus. In: Histology of the Human Eye: An Atlas and Textbook. Philadelphia, WB Saunders, 1971, pp 112–182.

127. Allansmith MR, McClellan BH: Immunoglobulins in the human cornea. Am J Ophthalmol 1975; 80:123.

128. Mondino BJ, Ratajczak HV, Goldberg DB, et al: Alternate and classical pathway components of complement in the normal cornea. Arch Ophthalmol 1980; 98:346.

129. Mondino BJ, Brady KJ: Distribution of hemolytic complement in the normal cornea. Arch Ophthalmol 1981; 99:1430.

130. Klaresjkog L, Forsum U, Tjernlund VM, et al: Expression of Ia antigen-like molecules on cells in the corneal epithelium. Invest Ophthalmol Vis Sci 1979; 18:310.

131. Mondino BJ: Inflammatory diseases of the peripheral cornea. Ophthalmology 1988; 95:463.

132. Watson PG, Hazleman BL: The Sclera and Systemic Disorders. Philadelphia, WB Saunders, 1976.

133. Brawman-Mintzer O, Mondino BJ, Mayer FJ: Distribution of complement in the sclera. Invest Ophthalmol Vis Sci 1989; 30:2240.

134. Fong LP, Sainz de la Maza M, Rice BA, et al: Immunopathology of scleritis. Ophthalmology 1991; 98:472.

135. van Dooremall JC: Die entwickelung der in fremden grund versetzten lebenden gewebe. Graefes Arch Clin Exp Ophthalmol 1873; 19:358.

136. Medawar P: Immunity to homologous grafted skin. III: The fate of skin homografts transplanted to the brain, to subcutaneous tissue and to the anterior chamber of the eye. Br J Exp Pathol 1948; 29:58.

137. Barker CF, Billingham RE: Immunologically privileged sites. Adv Immunol 1977; 25:1.

138. Streilein JW: Immune privilege as the result of local tissue barriers and immunosuppressive microenvironments. Curr Opin Immunol 1993; 5:428.

139. Streilein JW: Perspective: Unraveling immune privilege. Science 1995; 270:1158.

140. Streilein JW: Immune regulation and the eye: A dangerous compromise. FASEB J 1987; 1:199.

141. Niederkorn JY: Immune privilege and immune regulation in the eye. Adv Immunol 1990; 48:191.

142. Tompsett E, Abi-Hanna D, Wakefield D: Immunological privilege in the eye: A review. Curr Eye Res 1990; 9:114.

143. Ksander BR, Streilein JW: Regulation of the immune response within privileged sites. In: Granstein R, ed: Mechanisms of Regulation of Immunity Chemical Immunology. Basel, Switzerland, Karger, 1993, pp 117–145.

144. Streilein JW: Ocular regulation of systemic immunity. Reg Immunol 1994; 6:143.

145. Streilein JW: Ocular immune privilege and the Faustian dilemma. Invest Ophthalmol Vis Sci 1996; 37:1940.

146. Streilein JW, Ksander BR, Taylor AW: Commentary: Immune privilege, deviation and regulation in the eye. J Immunol 1997; 158:3557.

147. Streilein JW, Takeuchi M, Taylor AW: Immune privilege, T cell tolerance, and tissue-restricted autoimmunity. In: Burlingham W, ed: Proceedings of Ray Owens Symposium on Tolerance. Hum Immunol 1997; 52:138.

148. Nagata S, Golstein P: The Fas death factor. Science 1995; 267:1449.

149. Griffith TS, Brunner T, Fletcher SM, et al: Fas ligand-induced apoptosis as a mechanism of immune privilege. Science 1995; 270:1189.

150. Stuart PM, Griffith TS, Usui N, et al: CD95 ligand (FasL)-induced apoptosis is necessary for corneal allograft survival. J Clin Invest 1997; 99:396.

151. Yamagami S, Kawashima H, Tsuru T, et al: Role of Fas/Fas ligand interactions in the immunorejection of allogeneic mouse corneal transplantation. Transplantation 1997; 64:1107.

152. Bora NS, Gobleman CL, Atkinson JP, et al: Differential expression of the complement regulatory proteins in the human eye. Invest Ophthalmol Vis Sci 1993; 34:3579.

153. Granstein R, Stszewski R, Knisely T, et al: Aqueous humor contains transforming growth factor-β and a small (<3500 daltons) inhibitor of thymocyte proliferation. J Immunol 1990; 144:302.

154. Cousins SW, McCabe, MM, Danielpour D, et al: Identification of transforming growth factor-beta as an immunosuppressive factor in aqueous humor. Invest Ophthalmol Vis Sci 1991; 32:2201.

155. Jampel HD, Roche N, Stark WJ, Roberts AB: Transforming growth factor-β in human aqueous humor. Curr Eye Res 1990; 9:963.

156. Taylor AW, Streilein JW, Cousins SW: Identification of alpha-melanocyte stimulating hormone as a potential immuno-suppressive factor in aqueous humor. Curr Eye Res 1992; 11:1199.

157. Taylor AW, Streilein JW, Cousins SW: Vasoactive intestinal peptide (VIP) contributes to the immunosuppressive activity of normal aqueous humor. J Immunol 1994; 153:1080.

158. Wahlestedt C, Beding N, Ekman R: Calcitonin gene-related peptide in the eye: Release by sensory nerve stimulation and effects associated with neurogenic inflammation. Regul Pept 1986; 16:107.

159. Apte RS, Niederkorn JY: MIF: A novel inhibitor of NK cell activity in the anterior chamber (AC) of the eye. J Allergy Clin Immunol 1997; 99:S467.

160. Kaiser CJ, Ksander BR, Streilein JW: Inhibition of lymphocyte proliferation by aqueous humor. Reg Immunol 1989; 2:42.

161. Apte RS, Niederkorn JY: Isolation and characterization of a unique natural killer cell inhibitory factor present in the anterior chamber of the eye. J Immunol 1996; 156:2667.

162. Kaplan HJ, Streilein JW: Immune response to immunization via the anterior chamber of the eye. I: F$_1$ lymphocyte-induced immune deviation. J Immunol 1977; 118:809.

163. Kaplan HJ, Streilein JW: Immune response to immunization via the anterior chamber of the eye. II: An analysis of F$_1$ lymphocyte induced immune deviation. J Immunol 1978; 120:689.

164. Streilein JW, Niederkorn JY, Shadduck JA: Systemic immune unresponsiveness induced in adult mice by anterior chamber presentation of minor histocompatibility antigens. J Exp Med 1980; 152:1121.

165. Niederkorn JY, Streilein JW: Analysis of antibody production induced by allogeneic tumor cells inoculated into the anterior chamber of the eye. Transplantation 1982; 33:573.

166. Wilbanks GA, Streilein JW: Distinctive humoral responses following anterior chamber and intravenous administration of soluble antigen: Evidence for active suppression of IgG2a-secreting B-cells. Immunology 1990; 71:566.

167. Niederkorn JY, Streilein JW: Alloantigens placed into the anterior chamber of the eye induce specific suppression of delayed type hypersensitivity but normal cytotoxic T lymphocyte responses. J Immunol 1983; 131:2670.

168. Ksander BR, Streilein JW: Analysis of cytotoxic T cell responses to intracameral allogeneic tumors. I: Quantitative and qualitative analysis of cytotoxic precursor and effector cells. Invest Ophthalmol Vis Sci 1989; 30:323.

169. Waldrep JC, Kaplan HJ: Anterior chamber-associated immune deviation induced by TNP-splenocytes (TNP-ACAID). II: Suppressor T cell networks. Invest Ophthalmol Vis Sci 1983; 24:1339.

170. Streilein JW, Niederkorn JY: Characterization of the suppressor cell(s) responsible for anterior chamber associated immune deviation (ACAID) induced in BALB/c mice by P815 cells. J Immunol 1985; 134:1381.

171. Ferguson TA, Kaplan HJ: The immune response and the eye. II: The nature of T suppressor cell induction of anterior chamber-associated immune deviation (ACAID). J Immunol 1987; 139:346.

172. Wilbanks GA, Streilein JW: Characterization of suppressor cells in anterior chamber-associated immune deviation (ACAID) induced by soluble antigen: Evidence of two functionally and phenotypically distinct T-suppressor cell populations. Immunology 1990; 71:383.

173. Kosiewicz MM, Okamoto S, Miki S, et al: Imposing deviant immunity on the presensitized state. J Immunol 1994; 153:2962.

174. Wilbanks GA, Streilein JW: Studies on the induction of anterior chamber associated immune deviation (ACAID). I: Evidence that an antigen-specific, ACAID-inducing, cell-associated signal exists in the peripheral blood. J Immunol 1991; 146:2610.

175. Wilbanks GA, Mammolenti MM, Streilein JW: Studies on the induction of anterior chamber associated immune deviation (ACAID). II: Eye-derived cells participate in generating blood borne signals that induce ACAID. J Immunol 1991; 146:3018.

176. Wilbanks GA, Mammolenti MM, Streilein JW: Studies on the induction of anterior chamber-associated immune deviation (ACAID). III: Induction of ACAID depends upon intraocular transforming growth factor-β. Eur J Immunol 1992; 22:165.

177. Hara Y, Okamoto S, Rouse B, et al: Evidence that peritoneal exudate cells cultured with eye-derived fluids are the proximate antigen presenting cells in immune deviation of the ocular type. J Immunol 1993; 151:5162.

178. Maumanee AE: The influence of donor-recipient sensitization on corneal grafts. Am J Ophthalmol 1951; 34:142.

179. Sonoda Y, Streilein JW: Orthotopic corneal transplantation in mice: Evidence that the immunogenetic rules of rejection do not apply. Transplantation 1992; 54:694.

180. Streilein JW: Anterior chamber privilege in relation to keratoplasty. In: Zierhut M, ed: Immunology of Corneal Transplantation. Buren, Aeolus Press, 1994, pp 117–134.

181. Streilein JW: Immune privilege and the cornea. In: Pleyer U, Hartmann C, Sterry W, eds: Proceedings of Symposium: Bullous Oculo-Muco-Cutaneous Disorders. Buren, Aeolus Press, 1997, pp 43–52.

182. Niederkorn J, Streilein JW, Shadduck JA: Deviant immune responses to allogeneic tumors injected intracamerally and subcutaneously in mice. Invest Ophthalmol Vis Sci 1980; 20:355.

183. McLeish W, Rubsamen P, Atherton SS, et al: Immunobiology of Langerhans cells on the ocular surface. II: Role of central corneal Langerhans cells in stromal keratitis following experimental HSV-1 infection in mice. Reg Immunol 1989; 2:236.

184. Mizuno K, Clark AF, Streilein JW: Induction of anterior chamber associated immune deviation in rats receiving intracameral injections of retinal S antigen. Curr Eye Res 1988; 7:627.

185. Hara Y, Caspi RR, Wiggert B, et al: Suppression of experimental autoimmune uveitis in mice by induction of anterior chamber associated immune deviation with interphotoreceptor retinoid binding protein. J Immunol 1992; 148:1685.

186. Gery I, Streilein JW: Autoimmunity in the eye and its regulation. Curr Opin Immunol 1994; 6:938.

187. Khodadoust AA: The allograft rejection reaction: The leading cause of late failure of clinical corneal grafts. In: Porter R, Knight J, eds: Corneal Graft Failure. Ciba Foundation Symposium 15. Amsterdam, Associated Science Publishers, 1973.

188. Stark WJ: Transplantation immunology of penetrating keratoplasty. Trans Am Ophthalmol Soc 1978; 78:1079.

189. Epstein RJ, Seedor JA, Dreizen NG, et al: Penetrating keratoplasty for herpes simplex keratitis and keratoconus: Allograft rejection and survival. Ophthalmology 1987; 94:935.

190. Wilson SE, Kaufman HE: Graft failure after penetrating keratoplasty. Surv Ophthalmol 1990; 34:325.

191. Paque J, Poirier RH: Corneal allograft reaction and its relationship to suture site neovascularization. Ophthalmic Surg 1977; 8:71.

192. Vlker-Dieben HJM, D'Amaro J, Kok-van Alphen CC: Hierarchy of prognostic factors for corneal allograft survival. Aust N Z J Ophthalmol 1987; 15:11.

193. Boisjoly HM, Bernard P-M, Dube I, et al: Effect of factors unrelated to tissue etching on corneal transplant endothelial rejection. Am J Ophthalmol 1989; 107:647.

194. Donshik PC, Cavanagh HD, Boruchoff SA, et al: Effect of bilateral and unilateral grafts on the incidence of rejections after keratoconus. Am J Ophthalmol 1979; 87:823.

195. Khodadoust AA, Karnema Y: Corneal grafts in the second eye. Cornea 1984; 3:17.

196. Meyer RF: Corneal allograft rejection in bilateral penetrating keratoplasty: Clinical and laboratory studies. Trans Am Ophthalmol Soc 1986; 84:664.

197. Dana M-R, Streilein JW: Loss and restoration of immune privilege in eyes with corneal neovascularization. Invest Ophthalmol Vis Sci 1996; 37:2485.

198. Klein J: Natural History of the Major Histocompatibility Complex. New York, Wiley, 1986.

199. Fujikawa LS, Colvin RB, Bhan AK, et al: Expression of HLA-A/B/C and -DR locus antigens on epithelial, stromal and endothelial cells of the human cornea. Cornea 1982; 1:213.

200. Mayer DL, Daar AS, Casey TA, et al: Localization of HLA-A, B, C and HLA-DR antigens in the human cornea: Practical significance for grafting technique and HLA typing. Transplant Proc 1983; 15:126.

201. Whitsett CF, Stulting RD: The distribution of HLA antigens on human corneal tissue. Invest Ophthalmol Vis Sci 1984; 25:519.
202. Treseler PA, Foulks GN, Sanfilippo F: The expression of HLA antigens by cells in the human cornea. Am J Ophthalmol 1984; 98:763.
203. Abi-Hanna D, Wakefield D, Watkins S: HLA antigens in ocular tissues. I: In vivo expression in human eyes. Transplantation 1988; 45:610.
204. Streilein JW, Toews GB, Bergstresser PR: Corneal allografts fail to express Ia antigens. Nature 1979; 282:326.
205. William KA, Ash JK, Coster DJ: Histocompatibility antigen and passenger cell content of normal and diseased human cornea. Transplantation 1985; 39:265.
206. Austyn JM, Larsen CP: Migration patterns of dendritic leukocytes: Implications for transplantation. Transplantation 1990; 48:1.
207. Martin S, Dyer PA: The case for matching MHC genes in human organ transplantation. Nat Genet 1993; 5:210.
208. Batchelor JR, Casey TA, Gibbs DC, et al: HLA matching and corneal grafting. Lancet 1976; 1:551.
209. Kissmeyer-Nielsen F, Ehlers N: Corneal transplantation and matching for HLA-A and B. Scand J Urol Nephrol 1977; 42(suppl):44.
210. Foulks GN, Sanfilippo FP, Locascio JA, et al: Histocompatibility testing for keratoplasty in high-risk patients. Ophthalmology 1983; 90:239.
211. Stark WJ, Taylor HR, Datiles M, et al: Transplantation antigens and keratoplasty. Aust J Ophthalmol 1983; 11:333.
212. Sanfilippo F, MacQueen JM, Vaughn WK, et al: Reduced graft rejection with good HLA-A and -B matching in high-risk corneal transplantation. N Engl J Med 1986; 315:29.
213. Boisjoly HM, Bernard P-M, et al: Association between corneal allograft reactions and HLA compatibility. Ophthalmology 1990; 97:1689.
214. Stark W, Stulting D, Maguire M, et al: The Collaborative Corneal Transplantation Studies (CCTS): Effectiveness of histocompatibility matching of donors and recipients in high risk corneal transplantation. Arch Ophthalmol 1992; 110:1392.
215. Gore SM, Vail A, Bradley BA, et al: HLA-DR matching in corneal transplantation. Transplantation 1995; 60:1033.
216. Sonoda Y, Streilein JW: Impaired cell mediated immunity in mice bearing healthy orthotopic corneal allografts. J Immunol 1993; 150:1727.
217. Sonoda Y, Sano Y, Ksander B, et al: Characterization of cell mediated immune responses elicited by orthotopic corneal allografts in mice. Invest Ophthalmol Vis Sci 1995; 36:427.
218. Sano Y, Ksander BR, Streilein JW: Murine orthotopic corneal transplantation in "high-risk" eyes: Rejection is dictated primarily by weak rather than strong alloantigens. Invest Ophthalmol Vis Sci 1991; 38:1130.
219. Wilson SE, Lloyd SA: Epidermal growth factor and its receptor, basic fibroblast growth factor, transforming growth factor beta-1, and interleukin 1 alpha messenger RNA production in human corneal endothelial cells. Invest Ophthalmol Vis Sci 1991; 32:2747.
220. Kawashima H, Prasad SA, Gregerson DS: Corneal endothelial cells inhibit T cell proliferation by blocking IL-2 production. J Immunol 1994; 153:1982.
221. Kennedy MC, Rosenbaum JT, Brown J: Novel production of interleukin-1 receptor antagonist peptides in normal human cornea. J Clin Invest 1995; 95:82.
222. Bora NS, Gobleman CL, Atkinson JP: Differential expression of the complement regulatory proteins in the human eye. Invest Ophthalmol Vis Sci 1993; 34:3579.
223. Mohan RR, Liang Q, Kim W-J, et al: Apoptosis in the cornea: Further characterization of Fas/Fas ligand system. Exp Eye Res 1997; 65:575.
224. Yamada J, Streilein JW: Induction of anterior chamber–associated immune deviation by corneal allografts placed in the anterior chamber. Invest Ophthalmol Vis Sci 1997; 38:2833.
225. Sano Y, Ksander BR, Streilein JW: Fate of orthotopic corneal allografts in eyes that cannot support ACAID induction. Invest Ophthalmol Vis Sci 1995; 36:2176.
226. Dana M-R, Yamada J, Streilein JW: Topical IL-1 receptor antagonist promotes corneal transplant survival. Transplantation 1997; 63:1501.

Part II

PRINCIPLES OF DIAGNOSIS AND THERAPY

6 — DIAGNOSIS OF UVEITIS

Stephanie L. Harper, Louis J. Chorich III, and C. Stephen Foster

THE PROBLEM

Uveitis is defined as inflammation of the uveal tract, the vascular coat of the eye composed of the iris, ciliary body, and choroid. Inflammation of these structures is frequently accompanied by involvement of the surrounding ocular tissues, including the cornea, sclera, vitreous, retina, and optic nerve. Therefore, in common practice, uveitis refers to inflammation involving any intraocular structure. Because these structures are vital for visual function or globe integrity, or both, tissue biopsy is rarely a primary method used to establish the etiology of uveitis in a patient presenting with intraocular inflammation. Instead, the diagnosis is made based on an extensive review of a patient's family and personal history, a detailed review of medical systems, systemic and ocular examinations, and a targeted laboratory investigation based on suggestive historical and clinical findings. Indeed, the character of a uveitis specialty practice is much more that of an internal medicine practice rather than a surgical one.

The diagnosis of uveitis has been influenced by the availability of diagnostic tools, understanding of the relationship between uveitis and systemic disease, and recognition of new diseases that are characterized by uveitis. In the 19th and early 20th centuries, intraocular inflammation was thought to be largely infectious in etiology; the tuberculous bacillus and *Treponema pallidum* were the commonly implicated pathogens. As diagnostic capabilities were expanded and with widespread implementation of the Wasserman reaction, the number of literature reports attributing uveitis to *T. pallidum* decreased.[1] Development of the tuberculin skin test and the finding of positivity in patients without active disease helped to curb early enthusiasm with respect to *Mycobacterium tuberculosis* and its relationship to uveitis. The organism responsible for brucellosis, a known cause of abortions in cattle, was thought to be a major cause of uveitis, and a summary of ocular manifestations was published in 1939,[2] soon after human infection was recognized. Repeated failure to isolate the causative organism using the diagnostic modalities available at that time virtually eliminated this organism as a serious diagnostic contender.

The relationship between intraocular inflammation and systemic disease was suggested by the concept of focal infection, which described the ability of infection at extraocular sites to provoke ocular inflammation. The theory regarded the spread of infection or toxins from an extraocular source as the origin of intraocular inflammation.[3, 4]

. . . for it is obvious that some possible causes of uveitis will be missed entirely if adequate investigation is not carried out, and it is equally obvious that some possible source of focal infection will be found in the majority of patients if an adequate search is made for it.[3]

Common sources of focal infection reported to be associated with uveitis were the teeth and tonsils.[1, 5] The cause of uveitis was believed to be determined after a site of systemic infection was identified, and treatment was directed at elimination of the extraocular infection.

Eventually, noninfectious conditions with systemic manifestations, like sarcoidosis and the rheumatic diseases, were associated with uveitis. Early work demonstrating a relationship between sarcoidosis and uveitis was conducted by Walsh in 1939; he described several cases of systemic sarcoidosis in association with ocular inflammation in one patient population between 1925 and 1939, with an increase from 0.5% then to 7.5% between 1939 and 1943.[6, 7] Reiter's disease helped focus attention on the relationship between uveitis and rheumatologic disease, and as disease markers have been identified, the association with uveitis has become more established.[8, 9]

The description of new disease entities, such as acute posterior multifocal placoid pigment epitheliopathy (APMPPE), birdshot retinochoroidopathy (BSRC), and multifocal choroiditis and panuveitis (MCP) has helped expand the spectrum of diagnostic possibilities. The clinical and angiographic findings in APMPPE were initially described in 1968 from three cases reporting the disease features and course of resolution.[10] BSRC was first described in 1980 as a chorioretinitis with multifocal cream-colored lesions distributed throughout the fundus, vitritis, and macular edema.[11] Since its initial description, a genetic predisposition to BSRC development has been discovered, facilitating diagnosis.[12] Multifocal choroiditis with panuveitis (MCP) was appreciated as an entity similar to the presumed ocular histoplasmosis syndrome but with distinguishing features in 1984, establishing MCP as a new diagnostic entity.[13] The ever-evolving list of conditions associated with uveitis, coupled with the re-emergence of old conditions, such as syphilis and tuberculosis, can make the diagnosis of the specific cause of uveitis extremely challenging (Table 6–1).

TABLE 6–1. DIFFERENTIAL DIAGNOSIS BY ANATOMIC LOCATION

ANTERIOR UVEITIS	INTERMEDIATE UVEITIS	POSTERIOR UVEITIS
Seronegative spondyloarthropathies	Sarcoidosis	Toxoplasmosis
Juvenile rheumatoid arthritis	Lyme disease	Histoplasmosis
Herpes simplex uveitis	Cat-scratch disease	Lyme disease
Varicella zoster uveitis	Multiple sclerosis	Cat scratch disease
Sarcoidosis	Toxocariasis	Herpetic retinitis—herpes simplex, varicella zoster
Fuchs' heterochromic iridocyclitis	Pars planitis	Cytomegalovirus
Posner-Schlossman syndrome	Masquerades—intraocular foreign body, ophthalmia nodosa, amyloid, lymphoma	Acute retinal necrosis
Kawasaki's disease		Adamantiades-Behçet disease
Syphilis		Systemic lupus erythematosus
Traumatic		Birdshot retinochoroidopathy
Inflammatory bowel disease		Diffuse unilateral subacute neuroretinitis
Lens-associated uveitis		Vogt-Koyanagi-Harada syndrome
Ocular ischemia		Sympathetic ophthalmia
Sjögren's syndrome		Serpiginous
Lyme disease		White dot syndromes—multiple evanescent white-dot syndrome, acute posterior multifocal placoid pigment epitheliopathy, punctate inner choroidopathy, multifocal choroiditis and panuveitis, subretinal fibrosis and uveitis syndrome, acute retinal pigment epitheliitis
Leptospirosis		Toxocariasis
Amoebiasis		Whipple's disease
Giardiasis		Infectious endophthalmitis
Adamantiades-Behçet disease		Rubella/measles
Polyarteritis nodosa		Trypanosomiasis
Relapsing polychondritis		Acanthamoeba
Tuberculosis		Giardiasis
Toxoplasmosis		Relapsing polychondritis
Leprosy		Crohn's disease
Brucella		Wegener's granulomatosis
Helminthic		Polyarteritis nodosa
Gonococcal		Scleroderma
Onchocerciasis		Dermatomyositis
Schistosomiasis		Cryoglobulinemia
Drug-induced uveitis		Sjögren's syndrome
Masquerades—intraocular lymphoma, leukemia, juvenile xanthogranuloma, pigment dispersion		Eales' disease
		Multiple sclerosis
		Radiation vasculitis
		Coccidioidomycosis
		Helminthic
		Ascariasis
		Onchocerciasis
		Cysticercosis
		Schistosomiasis
		Microfilial
		Masquerades—intraocular lymphoma, leukemia, endophthalmitis, familial exudative vitreoretinopathy, retinitis pigmentosa, amyloid, tumors

We reviewed the records of 1237 patients who received care on the Ocular Immunology and Uveitis Service of the Massachusetts Eye and Ear Infirmary (MEEI) between 1982 and 1992.[14] A definitive diagnosis in these patients was made in only 17% on initial evaluation. Following a thorough review of past medical history, a complete review of systems, and a targeted serologic, aqueous or vitreous evaluation when indicated, the identification of a local ocular disease or the diagnosis of a specific condition was made, and appropriate treatment and longitudinal care was initiated. A diagnosis was eventually established in 65% of the patients (see later).

CASE I

A 31-year-old woman with unilateral granulomatous uveitis associated with elevated intraocular pressure was referred to the MEEI for further management of her uncontrolled uveitis and glaucoma. Additional examinations and findings revealed decreased corneal sensation. Clinical history and examination suggested herpetic uveitis and this was subsequently confirmed at the time of urgent trabeculectomy with aqueous humor analysis. Systemic and topical therapy was instituted, and the patient has remained inflammation free on prophylactic antiviral therapy.

However challenging the task of arriving at a diagnosis, it is incumbent on the treating physician to embark on the journey toward a definitive diagnosis, because different uveitic conditions require different therapy, and uveitis is frequently associated with occult systemic disease or is a harbinger of the development of systemic illness. Case I describes the course of a patient who had a suggestive history and confirmatory initial laboratory evaluation resulting in immediate determination of the cause of her uveitis. More often, however, in the majority of patients, diagnostic gratification is delayed and comes only after a relentless pursuit, using re-evaluation (sometimes multiple evaluations) ultimately to disclose the local ocular or systemic disease responsible for the patient's uveitis.

THE CONFUSION
Uveitis can be the first manifestation of a systemic disease, or it may be the diagnosis-clinching disease feature. If this is so (and it is), why is it that referral to an internist and extensive laboratory testing is so often unrevealing of any systemic disease that is causing the uveitis? In our previously mentioned review of 1237 patients with uveitis, only 17% of patients had a definitive diagnosis made on initial presentation, yet the diagnosis was ultimately confirmed (57%) or strongly suspected (8%) in a total of 805 patients (65%). In 85% of those with a confirmed diagnosis, the definitive diagnosis was made during the longitudinal care of the patients based on repeated clinical and laboratory evaluations. This is to be expected, as conditions associated with uveitis are frequently characterized by an evolving course. The diagnosis of systemic lupus erythematosus (SLE), for example, is based on a constellation of findings. All of the criteria required to make the diagnosis, although strongly suspected, may not manifest until later in the course of disease as the condition evolves. In other cases, a specific positive finding, like a positive tissue biopsy in the case of sarcoidosis, may be required to make a definitive diagnosis; consequently, the diagnosis is "presumed" unless tissue is obtained. Thus, when the initial evaluation is unrevealing, continued follow-up is warranted because the clinical picture may evolve to include disease-defining characteristics and involvement of other structures that may lend themselves to further diagnostic investigations.

THE FRUSTRATION
Negative work-ups do occur in the evaluation of patients with uveitis. The label "idiopathic uveitis" was given to approximately 35% of patients in our report. The actual number of idiopathic cases, however, may be lower because a significant percentage (41%) of these patients had only one visit with us and longitudinal follow-up may have revealed an associated condition. Nevertheless, there are patients with uveitis who reveal no clues to the diagnosis despite careful and repeat review of their medical history, review of medical symptoms, ocular and systemic examinations, and serologic screening. These patients can be a source of frustration for the diligent ophthalmologist. All too often, repeat negative work-ups have led some physicians to abandon searching for associated disease in the patient with intraocular inflammation. This is tragic, because neglect of targeted diagnostic strategies can do great harm.

CASE II
An 81-year-old woman presented to the MEEI with a history of chronic uveitis and resulting corneal decompensation with band keratopathy, secluded pupils, and dense cataracts contributing to visual acuities of light perception and 20/200 of right and left eyes, respectively. She had uveitis for 30 years before she presented to us. A serologic screen revealed a positive fluorescent treponemal antibody absorption test (FTA-ABS). She received intravenous penicillin, and the uveitis vanished and has remained quiescent. This patient had had untreated latent syphilis for 30 years.

These preamble remarks are made in an effort to emphasize the difficulty and the incredible challenge an ophthalmologist faces in pursuit of a diagnosis in a patient with uveitis, and to forewarn the reader against any illusion that this text contains secrets that are revealed that enable the clinician to diagnose and treat uveitis easily. It does not. Truthfully, the business of uveitis is a hard business, filled with the kind of daily activity that characterizes an internist's life: uncertainty, frustration, and delayed gratification. One must love such a life to endure it. For those who do, the gratifications are enormous.

A SYSTEMATIC APPROACH TO ESTABLISHING A DIAGNOSIS
Classifications of Uveitis
In order to develop a targeted strategy for definitively diagnosing the causes of uveitis, we use descriptive categories to aid in our development of a differential diagnosis. The descriptive categories that we find most helpful are the location of uveitis, course and onset of intraocular inflammation, clinicopathologic features, patient age, social and geographic characteristics, and the source of ocular inflammation. The patient's symptoms are not included in the diagnostic categories because all sources of intraocular inflammation cause similar symptoms—anterior uveitis is usually characterized by redness, pain, and photophobia, whereas posterior uveitis results in blurred vision and floaters with or without pain and with or without redness. Although these complaints may assist in making the diagnosis of anterior or posterior uveitis, they do little to distinguish between causative entities. The location, course, clinicopathologic characteristics, patient age, social and geographic characteristics and source of inflammation also individually afford little assistance in establishing a definitive diagnosis. However, when used simultaneously, in the setting of relevant medical and laboratory information, these factors can provide the clinician with a wealth of data on which to make a definitive diagnosis.

Location of Uveitis
The International Uveitis Study Group proposed a classification system based on anatomic location (Table 6–2 definitions appended) in an attempt to unify the description of intraocular inflammatory diseases.[15] Tessler used a classification system that included anatomic localization with consideration of adjacent nonuveal (cornea and sclera) tissue involvement.[16] Because uveal inflammation frequently involves inflammation of adjacent structures, which often provides additional insight into the diagnosis,

TABLE 6–2. CLASSIFICATION OF UVEITIS BY LOCATION

TYPE	DESCRIPTION
Anterior uveitis	Inflammatory cells in the anterior chamber with minimal spillover into the retrolental space
Intermediate uveitis	Inflammatory cells in the anterior vitreous
Posterior uveitis	Inflammation of the retina or choroid primarily, but involvement of both structures can occur as a retinochoroiditis or a chorioretinitis
Panuveitis	All above-mentioned locations involved

TABLE 6–3. EXPANDED CLASSIFICATION OF UVEITIS

TYPE	CLINICAL DESCRIPTION
Anterior uveitis	Iritis
Intermediate uveitis	Iridocyclitis
	Cyclitis
	Phacogenic uveitis
	Pars planitis
	Vitritis
	Fuchs' heterochromic iridocyclitis
	Peripheral uveitis
Posterior uveitis	Choroiditis
	Retinochoroiditis
	Retinal vasculitis
	Neuroretinitis
Panuveitis	Inflammation involving all anatomic segments of the uvea
Keratouveitis	Uveal inflammation with associated corneal involvement
Sclerouveitis	Uveal inflammation with an associated scleritis

we consider nonuveal involvement (sclera, cornea, retinal vasculature) in our classification system (Table 6–3). The anatomic classification of uveitis can provide the framework on which to build the most likely and reasonable diagnostic considerations.

Most reports suggest that uveitis most commonly involves the anterior segment of the eye.[17–21] This has indeed been our experience; 51% of our patients reviewed had anterior uveitis. Anterior uveitis is also the most common form seen in community-based ophthalmology practices.[22] Some referral centers report that panuveitis or posterior uveitis occurs more frequently in their patient populations.[22, 23]

Anterior uveitis (Figs. 6–1, 6–2) is typically noninfectious (80% in our experience). The experience of other practitioners is similar.[17, 18] The most common noninfectious inflammatory diseases associated with anterior uveitis are the seronegative spondyloarthropathies (21.6%) and juvenile rheumatoid arthritis (10.8%). Viral uveitis (herpetic in 9.7% of our patients) is the most common infectious cause of anterior uveitis.[18, 22–24] Thus, simply identifying uveitis as solely involving the anterior segment of the eye suggests that the cause is likely noninfectious. Furthermore, a significant percentage of these patients have uveitis and associated systemic findings, the most common of which is an arthropathy (present in 32% of our patient population). We find that anterior uveitis

is the most common form of uveitis in both children and adults.

Posterior uveitis (Figs. 6–3 to 6–11) is the next most common form of uveitis, seen in 19% of our patients. There is widespread agreement that posterior uveitis more commonly has an infectious etiology in contrast to inflammation of the other anatomic locations, which has a noninfectious etiology. *Toxoplasma gondii* is the most common culprit. Twenty-five percent of our patients with posterior uveitis had toxoplasma retinochoroiditis. Other centers have estimated toxoplasma to be the etiology in approximately 40% of posterior uveitis patients.[20–24] One group, in comparing uveitis in two different regions of the world, found the incidence of toxoplasmosis in acute posterior uveitis to be 70% in London and 65% in Iowa.[19] Thus, when only the posterior segment of the eye is involved, an infectious etiology for the inflammation is increasingly likely. A special consideration is the category of retinal vasculitis, which in our experience, when present as the predominant feature of posterior uveitis, is more frequently associated with systemic inflammatory

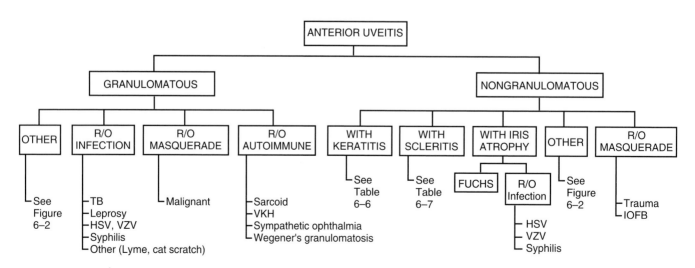

FIGURE 6–1. HSV, Herpes simplex virus; IOFB, intraocular foreign body; TB, tuberculosis; VKH, Vogt-Koyanagi-Harada syndrome; VZV, varicella-zoster virus.

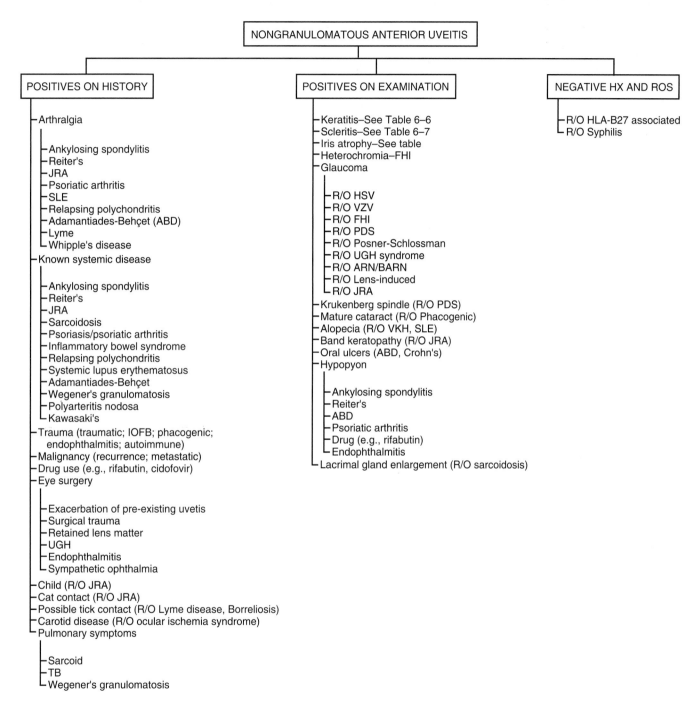

FIGURE 6–2. ARN, Acute retinal necrosis; BARN, bilateral acute retinal necrosis; FHI, Fuchs' heterochromic iridocyclitis; HSV, herpes simplex virus; IOFB, intraocular foreign body; JRA, juvenile rheumatoid arthritis; PDS, pigment dispersion syndrome; SLE, systemic lupus erythematosus; TB, tuberculosis; UGH, uveitis glaucoma hyphema syndrome; VZV, varicella zoster virus.

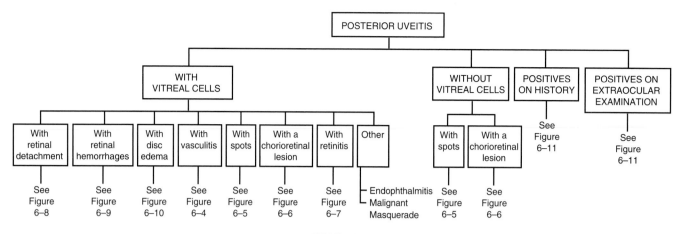

FIGURE 6–3

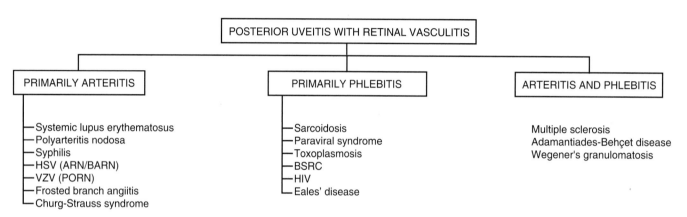

FIGURE 6–4. ARN, Acute retinal necrosis; BARN, bilateral acute retinal necrosis; BSRC, birdshot retinochoroidopathy; HIV, human immunodeficiency virus; HSV, herpes simplex virus; PORN, progressive outer retinal necrosis; VZV, varicella-zoster virus.

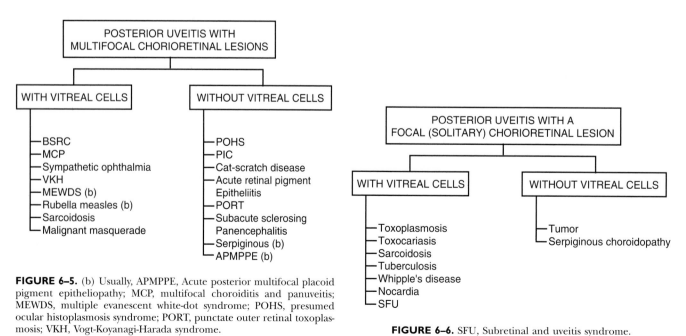

FIGURE 6–5. (b) Usually, APMPPE, Acute posterior multifocal placoid pigment epitheliopathy; MCP, multifocal choroiditis and panuveitis; MEWDS, multiple evanescent white-dot syndrome; POHS, presumed ocular histoplasmosis syndrome; PORT, punctate outer retinal toxoplasmosis; VKH, Vogt-Koyanagi-Harada syndrome.

FIGURE 6–6. SFU, Subretinal and uveitis syndrome.

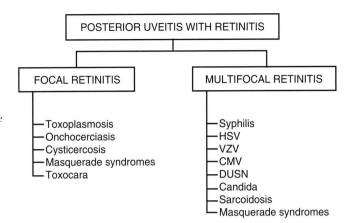

FIGURE 6–7. CMV, Cytomegalovirus; DUSN, diffuse unilateral subacute neuroretinitis; HSV, herpes simplex virus; VZV, varicella-zoster virus.

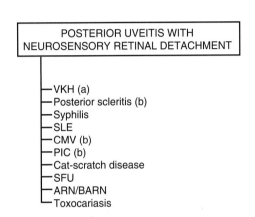

FIGURE 6–8. (a) Typically bilateral. (b) Typically without significant vitritis. ARN, Acute retinal necrosis; BARN, bilateral acute retinal necrosis; CMV, cytomegalovirus; PIC, punctate inner choroidopathy; SFU, subretinal fibrosis and uveitis syndrome; SLE, systemic lupus erythematosus; VKH, Vogt-Koyanagi-Harada syndrome.

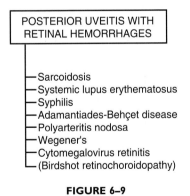

FIGURE 6–9

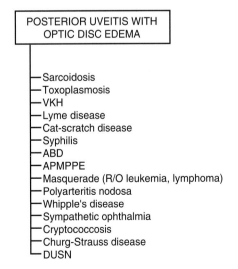

FIGURE 6–10. ABD, Admantiades-Behçet disease; APMPPE, acute posterior multifocal placoid pigment epitheliopathy; DUSN, diffuse unilateral subacute neuroretinitis; VKH, Vogt-Koyanagi-Harada syndrome.

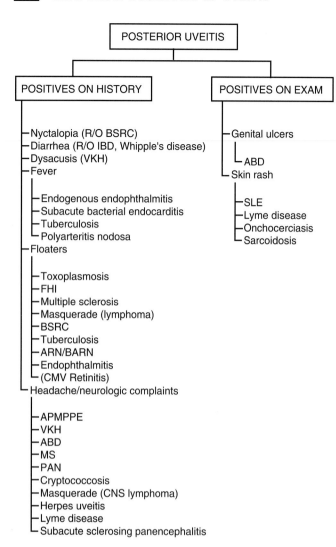

FIGURE 6–11. ABD, Adamantiades-Behçet disease; APMPPE, acute posterior multifocal placoid pigment epitheliopathy; ARN, acute retinal necrosis; BARN, bilateral acute retinal necrosis; BSRC, birdshot retinochoroidopathy; CMV, cytomegalovirus; FHI, Fuchs' heterochromic iridocyclitis; IBD, inflammatory bowel disease; VKH, Vogt-Koyanagi-Harada syndrome.

conditions (e.g., sarcoidosis, SLE, Adamantiades-Behçet disease, polyarteritis nodosa, and multiple sclerosis [MS]) and can represent more than 50% of all idiopathic posterior segment inflammations.

Intermediate uveitis (Fig. 6–12) occurs in at least 13% of uveitis patients and is most commonly noninfectious in etiology. It is usually idiopathic in origin (69%), but it can be associated with conditions such as sarcoidosis (22%), MS (8%), Lyme disease, cat-scratch disease, and toxocariasis (see Table 6–1). Thus, identifying intraocular

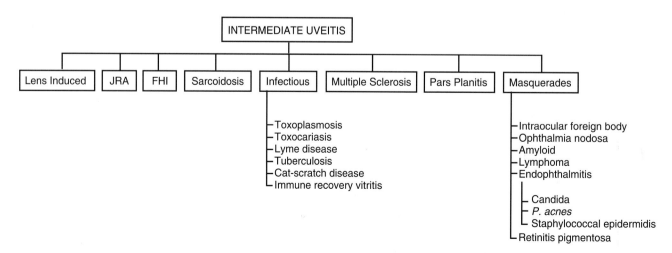

FIGURE 6–12. FHI, Fuchs' heterochromic iridocyclitis; JRA, juvenile rheumatoid arthritis.

inflammation as intermediate uveitis narrows the diagnostic possibilities substantially. Simply realizing that the intermediate segment of the eye is the primary focus of inflammation instantly reduces the list of potential diagnoses from more than 75 items (see Table 6–1) down to less than 10.

Panuveitis (Fig. 6–13) occurred in 16% of our patients with uveitis, consistent with other published series that note panuveitis in 15% to 25% of patients.[17, 18, 20, 21, 23] Our experience suggests that panuveitis may be idiopathic (22%) or may result from Adamantiades-Behçet disease (12%) and other infectious and sterile inflammatory processes with local ocular or systemic manifestations. A report from a tertiary care institution with a high percentage of black patients (31%) noted that the most common form of uveitis in this population was idiopathic panuveitis, occurring in 28% of their black patients with uveitis.[24] In pediatric patients from Turkey, panuveitis has been reported to be the most frequent form of uveitis, representing 34% of pediatric cases followed in an ocular immunology clinic.[25]

Course and Onset of Inflammation

The course of inflammation can provide clues to the diagnosis (Table 6–4). Acute inflammation resolves within 6 weeks; inflammation occurring for a period greater than 6 weeks is considered chronic. Acute uveitis with an explosive onset (even with hypopyon) is more typical of the seronegative spondyloarthropathies, endophthalmitis, and Adamantiades-Behçet disease rather than, for example, sarcoidosis and juvenile rheumatoid arthritis. Posterior synechiae are frequently a manifestation of chronic inflammation; however, patients with Fuchs' hetero-

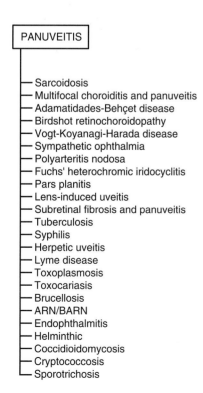

FIGURE 6–13. ARN, Acute retinal necrosis; BARN, bilateral acute retinal necrosis.

TABLE 6–4. COURSE OF INFLAMMATION

ACUTE

Explosive Onset
Seronegative spondyloarthropathies
Posner-Schlossman syndrome
Toxoplasmosis
Endophthalmitis
Adamantiades-Behçet Disease

CHRONIC
Juvenile rheumatoid arthritis
Fuchs' heterochromic iridocyclitis
Sarcodosis
Syphilis
Masquerades

RECURRENT
Herpetic uveitis
Seronegative spondyloarthropathies

WHITE EYE
Juvenile rheumatoid arthritis
Fuchs' heterochromic iridocyclitis
Posner-Schlossman syndrome
Kawasaki's syndrome
Intermediate uveitis
Posterior uveitis

chromic iridocyclitis, which is characterized by chronic inflammation, usually do not develop posterior synechiae. Chronic uveitis in a white eye would be more typical of Posner-Schlossman syndrome, juvenile rheumatoid arthritis, Kawasaki's disease, Fuchs' heterochromic iridocyclitis, and intermediate uveitis rather than uveitis associated with the seronegative spondyloarthropathies, herpetic eye disease, and sarcoidosis. The seronegative spondyloarthropathies and herpetic uveitis are also characterized by multiple recurrences, the former involving both eyes (unilateral alternating symptoms and signs) and the latter occurring primarily unilaterally.

Clinicopathologic Characteristics of the Inflammation

Pathologic classification divides inflammation into an acute form, characterized by a predominant neutrophil response, and a chronic form, characterized by a mononuclear response.[26] Further division separates acute inflammation into a suppurative-type with necrotic and degenerated neutrophils, including a sanguinopurulent form characterized by hemorrhage and pus. Acute nonsuppurative inflammation includes a serous response, a fibrinous response, and a hemorrhagic response. Chronic inflammation is classified as granulomatous or nongranulomatous. Granulomas take the form of zonal accumulations of inflammatory cells around a stimulus and diffuse or discrete cellular collections. These histologic findings are useful features in the diagnosis from tissue specimens. For instance, zonal granulomas are quite characteristic of lens-induced uveitis specimens with inflammatory cell infiltration around lens fragments. They are also seen as inflammatory cells surrounding collagen fragments in the sclerouveitis of rheumatoid arthritis. Discrete granulomas characterize sarcoidosis, and diffuse granulomatous infiltration of the choroid is seen in sympathetic ophthalmia and in Vogt-Koyanagi-Harada (VKH) syndrome.

Two histopathologic features can be seen on clinical examination and thus can be used to classify uveitis further through the slit lamp. Granulomatous inflammation, typified by large, fatty-appearing keratic precipitates (KPs) or nodules, or granulomas of the iris, classically characterize the disease entities in Table 6–5. Therefore, the diagnostic possibilities in a patient with granulomatous uveitis can be reduced from the list of all 75 causes of uveitis to these 10 entities.

Hypopyon uveitis is characterized by an outpouring of inflammatory cells and fibrin sufficient to cause accumulation in the inferior portion of the anterior chamber angle. Conditions associated with hypopyon formation include Adamantiades-Behçet disease, the seronegative spondyloarthropathies, leukemia, necrosis of intraocular tumors, metastatic lesions, infectious endophthalmitis, phacogenic uveitis, and corneal ulcers with sterile hypopyon formation (for example, *Acanthamoeba, Candida albicans, Pseudomonas aeruginosa*). Certain drugs can cause hypopyon uveitis; these drugs include rifabutin, an antimycobacterial agent used to prevent disseminated *Mycobacterium avium* complex disease in patients with acquired immunodeficiency syndrome (AIDS).

Sanguinopurulent inflammation may occur in seronegative spondyloarthropathy-associated uveitis, and a hemorrhagic response with hyphema formation can occur in herpetic uveitis, Fuchs' heterochromic iridocyclitis, gonorrheal iridocyclitis, vascularized tumors of the iris, and trauma. Anterior segment neovascularization from any cause can masquerade as uveitis and result in hyphema. Juvenile xanthogranuloma, a skin condition with ocular involvement, is characterized by the accumulation of histiocytes in tissues with resultant granuloma formation. Iris nodules can form in association with delicate vasculature that may rupture, producing spontaneous hyphema.

Age of the Patient

Uveitis occurs in patients of all ages, but several conditions have a predilection for certain age groups. It has been our experience at the MEEI that the most common form of uveitis in patients younger than 16 years of age is that associated with juvenile rheumatoid arthritis (41.5%), followed by idiopathic uveitis (21.5%), pars planitis (15.3%), and toxoplasmosis (7.7%).[27] Kanski and associates[28] analyzed 340 cases of systemic uveitis syndromes, and Giles[29] reviewed cases from four tertiary referral centers. Both groups found that juvenile arthropathies were the most common entities in patients younger than 16 years of age. Sarcoidosis-associated uveitis was the next most frequent condition in pediatric uveitis patients in our series and the reports of the previously mentioned authors. Masquerade syndromes in this age group include retinoblastoma, juvenile xanthogranuloma, intraocular foreign bodies, intraocular leukemia, and retinal detachment.

The most common causes of uveitis in young adults are HLA-B27–associated uveitis, Fuchs' heterochromic iridocyclitis, sarcoidosis, the white-dot syndromes, pars planitis, and histoplasmosis. Common masquerade syndromes in this age group include occult intraocular foreign body, pigmentary glaucoma, ghost cell glaucoma, and retinal detachment.

Older adults with uveitis are more likely than younger patients to have a systemic illness such as SLE, polyarteritis nodosa, and late latent syphilis. Other causes of uveitis in this group include ocular ischemia, VKH syndrome, serpiginous choroiditis, and BSRC. Masquerade syndromes in older patients with uveitis can be the result of metastatic disease, primary central nervous system (CNS) lymphoma, uveal melanoma, retinitis pigmentosa, and other retinal degenerations.

Social and Geographic Characteristics

Many social factors can influence intraocular inflammatory diseases. Demographic characteristics, such as race and ancestry, can be predispositions to the development of specific conditions. For example, the incidence of sarcoidosis is higher in blacks compared to whites in the United States. Evaluation of posterior uveitis in a Native American patient requires a search for alopecia, poliosis, vitiligo, and detailed testing for auditory nerve dysfunction and meningeal signs, because VKH syndrome is a more common cause of posterior uveitis in Native Americans. Posterior uveitis in an immunocompromised person or in an intravenous drug abuser generates concern for infectious causes including fungal and opportunistic pathogens. However, in an Asian or an individual of Middle-Eastern or Mediterranean basin genetic heritage (e.g., Greece, Turkey, Lebanon, or Iran) with posterior uveitis or panuveitis and associated retinal vasculitis, Adamantiades-Behçet disease (ABD) would be a prime suspect as a cause for the inflammation, and so one would pay careful attention to the patient's medical review of systems regarding extraocular foci with potential for involvement in ABD (e.g., mucosal ulceration).

Patients who own dogs or cats, or are handlers of these animals (groomers) may be exposed to the intestinal parasites *Toxoplasma gondii* and *Toxocara canis* after ingestion of contaminated food sources or contact with soil. The colonized patient may develop intermediate, posterior, or panuveitis. Plumbers and sewer workers are at an increased risk of leptospirosis, which is transmitted by a spirochete in sewer water and rat urine.

Geographic considerations include places of residence and recent or distant travel. Epidemiologic and histopathologic data suggest that residents of areas where *Histoplasma capsulatum* is endemic—Mississippi and Ohio River valleys, the San Joaquin Valley and parts of Maryland—are at increased risk for the development of the presumed ocular histoplasmosis syndrome (POHS). Although other features of this disease are frequently as helpful in making this diagnosis (punched out chorioretinal scars, the absence of vitreal inflammation), the characteristic lesions in a resident from these geographic areas strongly support the diagnosis. An example is the

TABLE 6–5. GRANULOMATOUS INFLAMMATION

Sarcoidosis	Syphilis
Herpetic uveitis	Lepromatous uveitis
Tuberculosis	Fungal
Sympathetic ophthalmia	Helminthic
Vogt-Koyanagi-Harada syndrome	Masquerade syndromes

outdoorsman who recently returned from a camping trip in the woods of New England and who now complains of photophobia and blurred vision. The evaluation of this patient clearly raises suspicion of Lyme disease and so requires detailed inquiry into a history of a tick bite, rash, and arthralgias. Uveitis in a patient who has visited Central or South America raises the concern of cysti-cercosis, whereas a visit to West Africa (below the Sahara) increases concern for onchocerciasis. Thus, attention to the social and geographic factors can influence diagnostic possibilities and shape subsequent laboratory evaluation.

Source of Inflammation

Uveitis can result from exogenous or endogenous stimuli with invasion of intraocular tissues by inflammatory cells. Exogenous stimuli generally (although not always) cause intraocular inflammation usually due to a break in the eyewall as a result of nonsurgical or surgical trauma or contiguous involvement from an adjacent source of infection or inflammation (for example, the sinuses). Traumatic uveitis can represent sterile inflammation occurring solely as a response to tissue injury, or it can occur after the introduction of foreign substances into the eye. Endogenous stimuli can be hematogenously spread to the eye from an active source of infection elsewhere in the body (15% of all cases of infectious endophthalmitis), or they may be ocular antigens to which the patient has become sensitized. Endogenous infectious endophthalmitis accounts for 2% to 15% of all cases of infectious endophthalmitis. Host factors that predispose to the development of infectious endogenous endophthalmitis include diabetes, renal failure, immunosuppression and systemic infection. Endogenous host intraocular antigens can serve as a stimulus for uveitis in autoimmune diseases, such as in sympathetic ophthalmia, VKH syndrome, BSRC, phacoantigenic endophthalmitis, and probably many other uveitides.

Associated Involvement of the Cornea and Sclera

Uveitis can occur in association with inflammation of the cornea or the sclera. Guyton and associates[6] reported that the cornea was secondarily involved in anterior uveitis (27.7%) and panuveitis (19.2%) more than in posterior uveitis (2%) in their 1941 case series. Interstitial keratitis was the most common finding they observed. Sclero-uveitis occurred most commonly in their patients with panuveitis (7.1%) as compared with anterior uveitis (2%) and posterior uveitis (0.7%).

Keratouveitis may involve the corneal epithelium, stroma, or endothelium. We believe that uveitis associated with involvement of any corneal layer is a manifestation of herpetic disease until proven otherwise. Herpetic keratouveitis usually takes the form of anterior uveitis and an associated stromal keratitis. The stroma can be involved in a diffuse fashion, with inflammatory cell infiltration, or as a sector keratitis with keratopathy limited to a sector of the cornea. Interstitial keratitis can also be seen in the keratouveitis associated with congenital and acquired syphilis, Cogan's syndrome, tuberculosis, and leprosy. Herpetic epithelial disease most commonly manifests as a dendrite that is small with terminal bulbs in herpes

TABLE 6–6. KERATOUVEITIS

Herpes simplex virus	Systematic lupus erythematosus
Varicella zoster virus	Leprosy
Lyme disease	Systematic vasculitis
Sarcoidosis	Collagen vascular disease
Tuberculosis	Inflammatory bowel disease
Syphilis	Mumps
Cogan's syndrome	

simplex virus infection, and large without terminal bulbs in herpes zoster. Repeat clinical and subclinical keratopathy results in corneal hypoesthesia, a clue to the diagnosis of herpetic ocular disease. Another corneal clue is the presence of unexplained corneal scars, which are more common with herpes simplex as opposed to herpes zoster. A superficial punctate epithelial keratitis can be seen in other viral keratouveitides and in association with SLE. Linear endotheliitis is associated with herpes simplex virus, presenting as a line of keratic precipitates on the endothelium accompanied by corneal edema. Other causes of keratouveitis can be found in Table 6–6.

Scleral involvement can occur as diffuse or sectorial scleritis (Table 6–7). Sclerouveitis is seen in vasculitic conditions, such as SLE, polyarteritis nodosa, syphilis, Adamantiades-Behçet disease, sarcoidosis, Wegener's granulomatosis, and Reiter's syndrome. Therefore, the identification of keratitis or scleritis in addition to the uveitis narrows the list of potential diagnostic contenders considerably.

DIAGNOSTIC APPROACH TO THE UVEITIS PATIENT

Taking the History

A comprehensive ocular and systemic history, including an extensive review of medical systems, is probably the most important component of the uveitis work-up. In no other discipline in ophthalmology is a patient more likely to have ocular disease in association with a systemic condition. In fact, 83% of our patients with a confirmed diagnosis of uveitis have been shown to have an associated systemic disease. Perhaps more importantly, we frequently find that the ocular manifestation brings attention to occult systemic disease.

CASE III

A 42-year-old woman presented to the MEEI with acute granulomatous uveitis. A review of the patient's systems revealed a history of intermittent shortness of breath.

TABLE 6–7. SCLEROUVEITIS

Systemic lupus erythematosus	Leprosy
Wegener's granulomatosis	Crohn's disease
Polyarteritis nodosa	Adamantiades-Behçet disease
Reiter's syndrome	Psoriatic arthritis
Herpes simplex virus	Relapsing polychondritis
Varicella zoster virus	Polyarteritis nodosa
Syphilis	Cogan's syndrome
Tuberculosis	Mumps
Toxoplasmosis	Lyme
Sarcoidosis	Vasculitis

Testing for elevated angiotensin-converting enzyme levels was positive. The chest x-ray study showed hilar enlargement and radiopaque densities consistent with granulomas. Biopsy of hilar nodes confirmed the presence of noncaseating granulomas, and systemic therapy was instituted.

Because the information revealed by way of the ocular and systemic histories is critical to the care of the patient with uveitis, it is imperative that standard questions are asked of all patients so that no information is neglected. We have found that the most accurate and efficient way to collect this large amount of data is by using a diagnostic survey. Our diagnostic survey is a questionnaire completed by a patient and reviewed in detail during the patient-doctor encounter (see Appendix A). It solicits detailed information regarding the patient's family and personal medical history, including demographic information, geographic history, past medical history, habits, and occupational exposures. This questionnaire is followed by an extensive review of medical systems. The diagnostic survey is completed by all patients on initial presentation to our service. We use the gathered data to identify diagnostic clues that require further exploration.

Clinical Examination

The Ocular Examination and Findings

VISUAL ACUITY, PUPILS, AND EXTRAOCULAR MOTILITY

A comprehensive eye examination is a requirement for all patients with uveitis, beginning with an assessment of the patient's best-corrected visual acuity. The most common method used to assess visual acuity is the Snellen acuity chart. Although this method works well in most adults, picture (for example, Allen figures) or letter optotypes (for example, HOTV or illiterate E) may be necessary for children and adults who cannot identify letters. Preverbal children may require assessment of acuity based on their response to light (blinks to light); their ability to fix, follow, and maintain central and steady fixation; or their performance on specialized tests of grading acuity, such as vernier acuity cards or the preferential looking test. Other methods of acuity assessment include tests that use interference fringe instruments to project two beams of light through two small areas of the pupil, forming an image on the retina. Tests that use this method are useful in the assessment of visual potential in patients with media opacities.

Pupil assessment includes the evaluation of both direct and consensual responses. Neurosyphilis is a major consideration when an Argyll Robertson (AR) pupil is identified. The AR pupil is miotic and irregular and demonstrates light-near dissociation. Other causes of light-near dissociation include MS and sarcoidosis. Miotic and irregular pupils can also be seen in patients with posterior synechiae, but the response of the pupil to light and near is symmetric. A relative afferent pupillary defect (RAPD), seen in diseases with asymmetric optic nerve involvement, occurs with disc edema due to uveitis, papillophlebitis, hypotony, orbital disease, hereditary and compressive optic neuropathies, and severe retinal vascular dysfunction

(for example, ischemic central retinal vein occlusion). Herpetic uveitis can produce sectorial iris paralysis, resulting in irregular constriction of the pupil in response to light.

Important findings on ocular motility examination can lend evidence to support the diagnosis of a specific uveitis entity. Accommodative insufficiency can be seen in sympathetic ophthalmia. Pain on eye movements, with or without limitation of ductions and versions, may occur in patients with uveitis associated with posterior scleritis or an associated orbital inflammatory process, such as orbital inflammation due to varicella zoster virus, Wegener's granulomatosis, and idiopathic orbital inflammatory disease. Pain with eye movements may also be a feature of optic neuritis associated with MS. Intranuclear ophthalmoplegia, caused by lesions involving the medial longitudinal fasciculus (MLF), should also raise the suspicion of MS, especially if the condition is bilateral.

CONJUNCTIVA, EPISCLERA, AND SCLERA

Examination of the anterior surface of the eye should first be performed in ambient illumination because subtle color differences are best discerned in daylight. Inflammation on the conjunctiva and episclera appear bright red in daylight. Scleritis, however, gives a bluish gray tinge to the eye, a violaceous hue, especially prominent perilimbally. White, avascular areas are seen in necrotizing scleritis.

Slit-lamp examination frequently reveals conjunctival injection that involves the perilimbal area more than the palpebral and fornical conjunctiva when the iris or ciliary body is inflamed. This is in contrast to the more benign inflammation of the conjunctiva, which is characterized by diffuse injection of conjunctival vessels. Conjunctival granulomas (sarcoidosis) and vascular abnormalities (anterior segment ischemia) may give clues to the cause of the patient's uveitis. Scleritis may be overlooked unless the observer is specifically attuned to the cues and clues that speak to its presence in addition to the conjunctival vascular dilatation secondary to the uveitis: deep episcleral vascular plexus dilation and tenderness to palpation.

CORNEA

Uveitis KPs are usually located on the inferior corneal endothelium as a result of aqueous convection currents in an area referred to as Arnt's triangle. These precipitates generally exhibit the typical features of either nongranulomatous KPs (small, round, and white) or granulomatous KPs (large, yellow-white color). Corneal endothelial deposits other than these types should alert the clinician to some specific syndrome. For example, fine pigmented KP in the Krukenberg spindle pattern may suggest that the patient with alleged episodes of uveitis has, in fact, a history of pigment granule and cell showers during pigmentary dispersion syndrome provocations. Diffuse KPs can be seen in Fuchs' heterochromic iridocyclitis, herpes simplex uveitis, and cytomegalovirus (CMV) retinitis. Star-shaped KPs, or KPs with fine fibrils extending from them and distributed over the entire endothelium, are pathognomonic of Fuchs' heterochromic iridocyclitis.

Dendritic epithelial keratitis and superficial punctate keratitis may accompany viral uveitis. Ocular findings in SLE also include a keratouveitis characterized by a superficial punctate keratitis. Uveitides with accompanying interstitial keratitis (necrotizing and non-necrotizing) include viral uveitis (herpes, mumps), syphilis, leprosy, onchocerciasis, acanthamoebiasis, psoriasis, and inflammatory bowel disease. Bilateral keratitis is seen in congenital syphilis, Cogan's syndrome, mumps, sarcoidosis, collagen vascular diseases, systemic vasculitis, onchocerciasis, psoriasis, and inflammatory bowel disease. Band keratopathy, characterized by the deposition of calcium complexes at the level of Bowman's membrane, occurs in juvenile rheumatoid arthritis and sarcoidosis. Endothelial damage and guttata formation may follow chronic uveitis.

ANTERIOR CHAMBER

The common pathologic event in all forms of uveitis is breakdown of the blood-ocular barrier. In anterior uveitis, increased permeability of the nonpigmented layer of the ciliary epithelium, posterior iridial epithelium, and the iris vessel endothelial cells results in accumulation of inflammatory cells and protein in the anterior chamber. Thus, the presence of cells and protein (visible to the examiner as flare) in the anterior chamber is a marker for iris and ciliary body inflammation. The severity of blood-aqueous barrier disruption can be estimated by using a standard grading system to indicate the extent of anterior chamber cell and protein accumulation as a result of iris and ciliary body inflammation. We grade anterior chamber cells using a 0.2mm × 0.2mm light beam directed obliquely into the anterior chamber with the light tower tilted forward. We then document the number of cells and flare as shown in Tables 6–8 and 6–9.

Using this system, we are able to follow the course of the patient's uveitis and adjust our therapeutic strategies as required to achieve the goal of finding no cells. In chronic forms of uveitis, permanent breakdown of the blood-aqueous barrier occurs, resulting in a chronic flare that is unresponsive to corticosteroid therapy. Severe blood-aqueous barrier breakdown can cause substantial leakage of inflammatory constituents including fibrin (fibrinoid aqueous response) and white blood cells (hypopyon). Other features of anterior chamber inflammation that may provide diagnostic value are the presence of sanguinopurulent inflammation or hyphema.

IRIS

Important findings on iris examination include the presence of posterior synechiae, iris atrophy, iris nodules, abnormal iris vessels, and heterochromia. Posterior synechiae, characterized by iris apposition to the anterior lens capsule, occur in chronic anterior uveitis. Posterior synechiae can be extensive and produce seclusio pupillae, which increases the patient's risk of iris bombé and angle-closure glaucoma. Iris atrophy is a diagnostic feature of herpetic uveitis. Varicella zoster virus generally produces sector iris atrophy due to a vaso-occlusive vasculitis, whereas herpes simplex virus usually produces patchy iris atrophy. Both conditions, however, can produce either manifestation. Other causes of atrophy include anterior segment ischemia, syphilis, and previous attacks of angle-closure glaucoma. Iris atrophy associated with syphilis is a diffuse atrophy of all iris layers, making the iris tissue very thin and friable. This is most obvious at the time of surgery in the patient with late latent syphilis and seclusio pupillae because attempts at synechiae lysis can result in tissue disintegration. Pathologically, granulomatous uveitis is characterized by the accumulation of mononuclear phagocytes, epithelioid cells, and multinucleated giant cells. Infiltration of plasma cells and lymphocytes also occurs and surrounds the accumulated mononuclear cells, usually aggregating into granulomas. Tissue necrosis and fibrosis ensue. Granulomas may be prominent in the iris stroma or the choroid. Iris nodules are most common at the pupillary margin, described as Koeppe's nodules, or on the iris surface, where they are referred to as Busacca's nodules. Iris nodules differ from granulomas in that they are accumulated deposits of epithelioid cells and lymphocytes that have been deposited onto the iris without tissue destruction.[31] In Fuchs' heterochromic iridocyclitis, iris nodules can occasionally be seen on the anterior iris surface or on the pupillary margin. Normal radial iris vessels can be dilated, producing iris hyperemia. Angiogenic factors can produce new, abnormal iris vessels in the process of neovascularization. Heterochromia can be hypochromia (abnormal eye is lighter than fellow eye), as in Fuchs' heterochromic iridocyclitis or hyperchromic (abnormal eye is darker than fellow eye), as in rubeosis irides.

ANTERIOR CHAMBER ANGLE

Gonioscopic evaluation of the anterior chamber angle may reveal peripheral anterior synechiae sufficient to account for elevated intraocular pressure (IOP). Additionally, one may find angle KPs, a small hypopyon, and inflammatory debris, suggesting an additional mechanism of IOP elevation from occlusion of filtering trabecular meshwork. Abnormal iris vessels, including thick trunklike vessels (neovascularization) or fine branching vessels (Fuchs' heterochromic iridocyclitis) are easily identified by gonioscopy, and their presence can direct

TABLE 6–9. GRADING AQUEOUS FLARE

GRADE	AMOUNT OF AQUEOUS FLARE
0	No flare
1+	Faint
2+	Moderate (iris and lens clear)
3+	Marked (iris and lens hazy)
4+	Intense (fibrin, plastic aqueous)

TABLE 6–8. GRADING AQUEOUS CELLS

GRADE	AMOUNT OF AQUEOUS CELLS
0	No cells
½+	1–5
1+	6–15
2+	16–25
3+	26–60
4+	Greater than 60

subsequent therapy. In cases in which traumatic uveitis is suspected, angle recession may provide confirmation.

LENS

Important lenticular findings include cataract; lenticular deposits composed of inflammatory debris or pigment, or both; and infarcted lens epithelial cells with degenerated cortex (glaukomflecken). The presence of cataract or the rapid progression of lenticular opacification can be a manifestation of chronic intraocular inflammation or the result of corticosteroid therapy and glaucoma medications (cholinergic agents) used in the management of uveitis and uveitic glaucoma. In a patient with recently diagnosed uveitis, the presence of cataract can provide insight into the chronic duration of the disease. The most common type of cataract in uveitis patients is the posterior subcapsular opacity. Anterior lens changes may also occur, often in association with lens capsule thickening at a site of iris adhesion. The presence of pigment on the anterior lens capsule suggests past iris-capsule adhesion. Chronic subclinical active inflammation can manifest as the steady accumulation of lenticular inflammatory debris on the surface of an intraocular lens in the absence of other signs of uveitis. Anterior lens opacities following extreme elevations in intraocular pressure (glaukomenflecken) provide insight into a history of acute uveitic glaucoma.

INTRAOCULAR PRESSURE

The IOP in patients with uveitis is most commonly decreased owing to impaired production of aqueous by the nonpigmented ciliary body epithelium. This, however, is not always true because final IOP is also based on the facility of outflow and episcleral venous pressure. It is the balance of these factors that determines the ultimate IOP. Factors that can affect IOP include the accumulation of inflammatory material and debris in the trabecular meshwork with obstruction of aqueous outflow, inflammation of the trabecular meshwork (trabeculitis), obstruction of venous return, and steroid therapy. For unknown reasons, elevated IOP is frequently associated with infectious uveitis, for example, herpetic uveitis. In the patient with uveitis, intraocular pressure should be assessed before the instillation of fluorescein to prevent obscuration of anterior chamber details due to the production of a greenish hue after fluorescein penetration into the anterior chamber. Repeat measurements should be taken at each visit because the effects of uveitis on IOP can vary over the course of the inflammatory episode.

VITREOUS

Inflammatory cell accumulation in the vitreous is the result of inflammatory processes in other intraocular structures, such as the ciliary body, retina, and choroid. Rarely is vitritis a manifestation of a primary vitreous process. Various methods of vitreous evaluation have been suggested. Nussenblatt and associates proposed a grading system based on vitreous haze because they believe that it combines the optical effects of protein leakage and cellular infiltration. They developed standardized color photographs and recommend viewing the vitreous by indirect ophthalmoscopy using a 20-diopter lens to assess

TABLE 6–10. GRADING VITREOUS CELLS

GRADE	NUMBER OF VITREOUS CELLS
0	No Cells
½+	1–10
1+	11–20
2+	20–30
3+	30–100
4+	Greater than 100

the disc and posterior retina, and then comparing the view of the patient's vitreous with the standard photo to arrive ultimately at a grading for the vitritis.[12] Other groups use a grading system that assigns value to the amount of vitreous cells and flare present at the time of the examination.

Our system also grades vitreous cells and flare with modifications based on the knowledge that cells in the vitreous can be living and dead, and both can become immutably affixed to vitreous fibers (Table 6–10). Therefore, in addition to the amount of vitreous pathology as judged by fundus observation, we try to pay attention to the free-floating, active cells in the vitreous and grade these cells as well. In active vitritis, cells appear white and are evenly distributed between the liquid and formed vitreous. Old cells are small and pigmented, whereas debris tends to be pigmented but larger in size. Active cells can be found in locations that can be helpful diagnostically. A localized pocket of vitritis may suggest underlying focal retinal or retinochoroidal disease. Focal accumulation of inflammatory cells around vessels is seen in active retinal vasculitis. Inflammatory cells that accumulate in clumps (snowballs) may precipitate onto the peripheral retina, usually inferiorly, for example, in intermediate uveitis, associated with sarcoidosis. Cells may accumulate in the retrovitreal space following contraction of vitreous fibrils and posterior vitreous detachment.

It is important to recognize that the amount of cells in the vitreous will affect the grade of vitreous haze to the extent that they contribute to visual obscuration of the fundus. If a more detailed assessment of vitreous haze is desired, the examiner may indicate whether first, second, or third order retinal vessels are visible. Using a 1×3 mm light beam, we apply the grading system found in Tables 6–11 and 6–12.

RETINA AND CHOROID

The blood-retinal barrier is composed of tight junctions between the retinal pigment epithelial cells and the endothelium of the retinal vessels. Increased permeability at

TABLE 6–11. GRADING VITREOUS FLARE

GRADE	AMOUNT OF VITREOUS FLARE/HAZE
0	No flare
1+	Clear optic disc and vessels Hazy nerve fiber layer
2+	Hazy optic disc and vessels
3+	Only optic disc visible
4+	Optic disc not visible

TABLE 6–12. TARGETED APPROACH TO THE DIAGNOSIS

CLINICAL SETTING	DIAGNOSTIC CONCERN	TARGETED INVESTIGATION
Recurrent uveitis with a history of low back stiffness upon awakening each morning	Ankylosing spondylitis	HLA-B27 Lumbosacral spine films
Child with recurrent or chronic iridocyclitis	Juvenile rheumatoid arthritis	ANA (on both Hep-2 and rat substrates) HLA-B8
Retinochoroiditis adjacent to a pigmented scar	Toxoplasmosis	Antitoxoplasma IgG and IgM
Recurrent uveitis with a history of episodic diarrhea, possibly sometimes with mucous or blood in the stool	Inflammatory bowel disease	Gastroenterology consult with endoscopy and biopsy
Retinal vasculitis with a history of subacute sinusitis	Wegener's granulomatosis	Chest x-ray study, sinus films, urine analysis, serum ANCA
Elderly woman with new onset "vitritis," partially steroid responsive	Intraocular lymphoma	Vitreal biopsy for culture, cytology, and cytokines
Female with intermediate uveitis and on review of systems, a history of paresthesias	Multiple sclerosis	MRI scanning of the brain, spinal tap
Retinal vasculitis and a history, on review of systems, of recurrent aphthous ulcers and pretibial skin lesions	Adamantiades-Behçet disease	HLA-B51

ANCA, Antineutrophil cytoplasmic antibody; MRI, magnetic resonance imaging.

the level of the blood-retinal barrier results in inflammatory cell accumulation and tissue destruction in the retina with or without involvement of the choroid. Retinitis presents with a yellow-white appearance and poorly defined edges, often associated with hemorrhage and exudation. Involvement may be focal or multifocal. Retinal vasculitis can involve the arteries (Wegener's granulomatosis, toxoplasmosis, SLE) or veins (sarcoidosis) as inflammatory cells accumulate around the involved vessels. Primary retinal vasculitis refers to vasculitis due to direct involvement of the vasculature, for example, in diseases characterized by immune complex deposition to the vessel wall. An occlusive vasculitis may result, producing retinal opacification, edema, and infarction. Secondary retinal vasculitis is due to egress of inflammatory cells through vessel walls with a resulting periphlebitis. Neovascularization of the retina can be a manifestation of ischemic uveitis. Accumulation of fluid in the outer plexiform and inner nuclear layers can result in cystoid macular edema with a petaloid pattern on fluorescein angiography.

Choroidal inflammation can also be focal or multifocal. It frequently is not associated with vitritis due to intact retinal pigment epithelial cells that prevent inflammatory cell migration. There may be an overlying associated retinitis. The inflamed choroid can appear thickened, and prominent infiltrates and granulomas may be present. Choroidal neovascularization can occur with chronic inflammation and breaks in Bruch's membrane. Retinal pigment epithelial (RPE) disturbance can produce hyperpigmentation associated with choroidal and retinal disease, and decompensation of the RPE can alter the permeability of the blood-ocular barrier, resulting in a neurosensory retinal detachment.

Pars Plana

Examination of the peripheral retina and pars plana usually requires scleral depression or use of a three-mirror Goldmann contact lens. Exudate, fibroglial band formation (snowbanking), and neovascularization are pathologic processes that occur at the pars plana. The findings

are usually more prevalent inferiorly. Causes of inflammation in the intermediate segment of the eye include sarcoidosis, tuberculosis, Lyme disease, cat-scratch disease, and MS.

Optic Disc

Optic disc inflammation can occur with or without other signs of uveitis. Optic disc involvement takes the form of papillitis or disc edema, neovascularization, infiltration, and cupping. Papillitis is characterized by vascular congestion and hyperemia, absence of the cup, and blurring of the margins. Neovascularization occurs in ischemic states and is characterized by fragile vessels that are easily ruptured. Sarcoidosis and leukemia can infiltrate the disc tissue, producing an appearance similar to papillitis. Cupping of the optic nerve head can occur in association with uveitic glaucoma.

Extraocular Examination

Extraocular examination of the uveitis patient begins with a mental status assessment. Systemic vasculitis processes (for example, lupus cerebritis, syphilis, Lyme disease) and aseptic meningitis (for example, sarcoidosis, VKH syndrome, Adamantiades-Behçet disease) can occur with alteration in a patient's mentation—for example, cognition, thought formulation, emotional stability. One may need to speak with the patient's accompanying family member about changes in the mental abilities or thought processes for verification and a more detailed evaluation of possible central nervous system involvement.

The physical signs of extraocular disease can add evidence to support the diagnostic considerations entertained as a result of the history and ocular examination findings. Frequently, the findings may have escaped recognition by the patient or may have been recognized but deemed insignificant. Thus, it is important for the ophthalmologist caring for the uveitis patient to routinely evaluate patients for evidence of extraocular disease.

Epidermal changes (skin and appendages) occur in conditions associated with uveitis. Whitening of hair in-

TABLE 6–13. INITIAL WORK-UP WITH NEGATIVE MEDICAL HISTORY

HISTORY	WORK-UP
First episode of nongranulomatous uveitis Unrevealing history and review of medical systems and examination	No work-up
Second episode of nongranulomatous anterior uveitis Unrevealing history and review of medical systems and examination	Complete blood count with differential Erythrocyte sedimentation rate Fluorescent treponemal antibody absorption Human lymphocyte antigen-B27 Soluble interleukin-2 receptor
Granulomatous uveitis	Complete blood count with differential Erythrocyte sedimentation rate Angiotensin-converting enzyme Lysozyme Fluorescent treponemal antibody absorption Purified protein derivative with anergy panel Chest x-ray study
Intermediate uveitis	Lyme titers and western blot Angiotensin-converting enzyme Fluorescent treponemal antibody absorption Toxocara titers Cat-scratch titers Magnetic resonance imaging
Posterior uveitis or involvement of posterior segment (panuveitis)	Complete blood count with differential Erythrocyte sedimentation rate Soluble interleukin-2 receptor Toxoplasma titers
Retinal vasculitis	Complete blood count with differential Erythrocyte sedimentation rate Soluble interleukin-2 receptor Raji Cell Assay C1Q binding immune complex assay
Positive history or review of systems	As guided by responses on questionnaire or history

cluding eyebrows and lashes, is characteristic of VKH syndrome. Loss of hair can occur in SLE, VKH syndrome, and syphilis. Hypopigmentation of the skin is seen in leprosy, sympathetic ophthalmia, and VKH syndrome. A rash can be a manifestation of a vasculitic disease, and is seen in SLE, ABD, herpes zoster, syphilis, and Lyme disease. Vesicular lesions appearing in a dermatomal distribution or as a vesicular blepharoconjunctivitis suggest herpetic disease. An outbreak of tender, violaceous subcutaneous nodules primarily on the lower extremities characterizes erythema nodosum and can be associated with Epstein-Barr virus, inflammatory bowel disease, sarcoidosis, tuberculosis, and ABD. Scaling of the skin can be a manifestation of SLE, psoriatic arthritis, syphilis, and Reiter's syndrome. Discoid lesions are seen with SLE, sarcoidosis, and tuberculosis. Nail abnormalities are seen in psoriatic arthritis, Reiter's syndrome, and vasculitic diseases.

Mucosal surface ulceration can involve the oral or urogenital surfaces. Adamantiades-Behçet disease and Reiter's syndrome are associated with both oral and genital lesions. Oral ulcers alone are seen in SLE and inflammatory bowel disease, whereas syphilis is associated with genital lesions. Other nasopharyngeal manifestations include sinusitis, which may occur in Wegener's granulomatosis, sarcoidosis, Whipple's disease, and mucormycosis. The mucosal surface of the bladder can be involved as a cystitis in Whipple's disease and Reiter's disease. Other urogenital manifestations can include urethral discharge, seen in Reiter's syndrome, syphilis, herpes simplex, and gonococcal urethritis. Epididymitis oc-

curs in Adamantiades-Behçet disease, and prostatitis is seen in Whipple's disease, Reiter's syndrome, ankylosing spondylitis, and gonococcal disease. Nephritis can be a manifestation of vasculitis (Wegener's granulomatosis, SLE, ABD), sarcoidosis, tuberculosis, and tubulointerstitial nephritis-uveitis (TINU) syndrome.

Arthropathy and cartilage loss may occur in various uveitic conditions. Articular abnormalities, arthralgias, and arthritis are components of the seronegative spondyloarthropathies, juvenile rheumatoid arthritis, ABD, sarcoidosis, SLE, relapsing polychondritis, syphilis, Lyme disease, and gonococcal disease. Specific involvement of the sacroiliac joint characterizes the seronegative spondyloarthropathies—ankylosing spondylitis, Reiter's syndrome, and inflammatory bowel disease. Cartilage loss from the nose can result in saddle-nose deformity, which is seen in relapsing polychondritis, Wegener's granulomatosis, and syphilis. In patients with relapsing polychondritis, cartilage is also lost from the ear resulting in floppy ears.

Other important signs include the enlargement of lymph nodes and organs, neuropathy, and impaired hearing. Enlargement of lymph nodes and organs may be seen in sarcoidosis, Epstein-Barr virus infection, and lymphoma, all of which can involve salivary and lacrimal tissue. Sarcoidosis, tuberculosis, and lymphoma can also be associated with lymphoid organ enlargement. Neuropathy can affect the cranial nerves and the peripheral nerves. Cranial nerves are more likely to be affected in syphilis, Lyme disease, and sarcoidosis. Peripheral nerves

TABLE 6–14. COMMON TESTS USED IN UVEITIS

TEST	DESCRIPTION
Erythrocyte sedimentation rate	A nonspecific marker of tissue injury, inflammation, and infection
Angiotensin-1-converting enzyme (ACE)	Synthesized by epithelioid cells and endothelial cells primarily, but under certain conditions, ACE can be synthesized by macrophages
Anti-neutrophil cytoplasmic antibodies (ANCA)	An indirect immunofluorescent test for antinuclear cytoplasmic antibodies. Positive staining occurs in a perinuclear (P-ANCA) or cytoplasmic (C-ANCA) pattern. ELISA testing is performed when a positive result occurs to confirm the presence of antibodies to myeloperoxidase or proteinase-3.
Antinuclear antibodies	Tested on two substrates (rat and Hep-2 cells). Found in multiple autoimmune diseases. Followed up with other nuclear antibodies as appropriate.
Antiphospholipid antibodies Complement proteins (C3, C4, total complement)	Low values confirm complement fixation in vivo. Hypocomplementemia is seen in SLE, cryoglobulinemia, glomerulonephritis, and septicemia.
Properdin factor B	Tests for elevated concentration of C3b:Bb:Properdin complex. After binding C3, this complex becomes the alternative pathway C5 convertase. Elevated levels occur in autoimmune disease and gram-negative sepsis. Hyperconsumption indicates activation of the alternative complement pathway.
Soluble interleukin-2 receptor	Determines the presence of the interleukin-2 receptor alpha subunit soluble domain. The extracellular soluble domain is shed by activated cells during an immune response.
Raji cell assay	Assays for IgG-containing circulating immune complexes
C1q binding assay	Assays for IgM-containing circulating immune complexes
C-reactive protein	An acute-phase protein used to monitor acute-phase responses to inflammatory disorders
α_1-Acid glycoprotein	An acute-phase protein used to monitor acute-phase responses to inflammatory disorders
Human lymphocyte antigen typing	Detects the gene products of the human major histocompatibility complex and can provide support for a disease diagnosis based on the known associations between genetic makeup and autoimmune diseases
Rheumatoid factor	Autoantibodies reactive with the Fc fragment of IgG; IgM, IgA, and IgG isotypes can be involved.
Fluorescent treponemal antibody absorption test (FTA-ABS)	A treponemal test for the detection of antibodies reactive with *T. pallidum*
Microhemagglutination assay antibodies to *Treponema pallidum* (MHA-TP)	A treponemal test for the detection of antibodies reactive with *T. pallidum*
Interleukin levels	Helpful in distinguishing inflammatory processes and lymphoma. IL-10 can be elevated in intraocular lymphoma while IL-6, IL-8, and IL-12 may be increased in inflammation.
Toxoplasma titers	Acutely, IgM is elevated. IgG is elevated chronically.
Lyme titers	Confirm positive titers with western blot
Hepatitis serology	Forty percent of polyarteritis nodosa cases follow hepatitis B infections.
Polymerase chain reaction (PCR)	PCR on aqueous and vitreous samples can detect viral, bacterial, and protozoan DNA (e.g., HSV, VZV, CMV, EBV, TB, syphilis, toxoplasma, lyme disease).
Purified protein derivative (PPD)	Skin test for tuberculosis
Fluorescein angiography	Helpful in the diagnosis of retinal and choroidal disease including retinal vasculitis and cystoid macular edema
Indocyanine green angiography (ICG)	Particularly helpful in the identification of choroidal pathology
Gallium scan	Nuclear medicine test to identify foci of inflammation. Often helpful in subtle sarcoidosis.
Ultrasonography	
Electroretinography (ERG)	Helpful in diagnosis and monitoring of retinal autoimmune disorders such as birdshot retinochoroidopathy
Chest x-ray study	Tuberculosis, sarcoidosis, Wegener's granulomatosis
Lumbosacral spine films	Seronegative spondyloarthropathies, particularly Reiter's syndrome and ankylosing spondylitis
Magnetic resonance imaging (MRI)	Multiple sclerosis, lymphoma
CT scan	Foreign body, lymphoma
Biopsy and cytology	Helpful in distinguishing inflammatory processes from neoplasms

CMV, Cytomegalovirus; CT, computed tomography; EBV, Epstein-Barr virus; ELISA, enzyme-linked immunosorbent assay; HSV, herpes simplex virus; PCR, polymerase chain reaction; SLE, systemic lupus erythematosus; TB, tuberculosis; VZV, varicella-zoster virus.

are involved in Lyme, leprosy, herpes zoster, sarcoidosis, and MS. Hearing loss occurs in VKH syndrome and sarcoidosis.

Laboratory Evaluation

Once a thorough history is obtained, including a review of medical systems, and a comprehensive examination is performed, the data are synthesized into a list of most likely and possible diagnoses (i.e., the differential diagnosis). It is at this point that selected laboratory studies may be indicated. Testing is generally parsimonious, limited to those studies most likely to be of some reasonable diagnostic value for a given patient, rather than the performance of some general battery of tests. Indiscriminant testing can result in false-positive results, with more confusion than enlightenment. For example, using Bayes' theorem to predict the probability of a given diagnosis based on disease prevalence and the sensitivity and specificity of a diagnostic test, Rosenbaum and associates found that screening all patients with uveitis for antinuclear antibodies would result in approximately 100 false-positive results for every one positive test in an individual with SLE.[30] Therefore, to increase the pretest likelihood of diagnosing a condition (for example, SLE), disease-specific testing should be performed only in those in whom the clinical suspicion is high.

Extensive and indiscriminate laboratory testing or referral to a primary medical doctor with instructions to "search for any underlying systemic disease" is not recommended. This approach is time consuming and inconvenient for the patient. It is also not cost effective, and with the limitations in resources experienced by all health systems, it is a wasteful practice.

After the appropriate history has been taken and the examination performed, most patients with uveitis will require only a targeted laboratory evaluation in the form of a complete blood count with a differential and an FTA-ABS (or microhemagglutination assay–*Treponema pallidum* [MHA-TP]). A more extensive work-up is required for the patient with recurrent uveitis (three or more attacks), granulomatous uveitis, posterior uveitis, or positive items on the review of systems. Examples of how to use the history and review of medical systems to arrive at a targeted investigation strategy can be found in Table 6–6.

When there are no diagnostic leads provided by the history, review of medical symptoms, or examination, no work-up is required for a patient with his or her first episode of nongranulomatous uveitis. These patients should be followed regularly with repeated queries about the development of new symptoms or signs that may provide a hint at the diagnosis. We typically have the patient complete additional diagnostic questionnaires during the course of follow-up. A third episode of intraocular inflammation warrants investigation. In the absence of clues from the history and examination, a combination of FTA-ABS, HLA-B27, complete blood count (CBC), erythrocyte sedimentation rate (ESR), and soluble interleukin 2 receptor (SIL2R) and PPD skin test should be performed (see Table 6–14). Subsequent investigation is based on the results of the initial screen or the introduction of additional information. The patient with suggestive information provided on the initial encounter

requires a detailed, but targeted, evaluation. A list of potential investigational tools can be found in Table 6–7.

Differential Diagnosis

Putting it all together thus far, we are able to form a provisional list of diagnostic contenders, and based on this list, a targeted approach to laboratory testing can be pursued. We have prepared differential diagnosis reference tables for the major diagnostic considerations. The tables are not meant as shortcuts to distract from the process of complete evaluation of the patient with uveitis. Instead, they are provided to supplement the generation of diagnostic possibilities. The items listed under each heading ideally should be simultaneously considered as one evaluates the patient.

The evaluation and, thus, the development of the differential diagnosis, starts when the patient enters the examination room, and it is developed during the clinical encounter. After the preliminary information is obtained and reviewed with the help of the diagnostic survey, the diagnostic possibilities being considered guide further questioning and direct the examination. As more information is revealed, the differential diagnosis is contracted or supplemented. For example, a 30-year-old man who reports that he is healthy is referred by his optometrist because of decreased vision and the discovery of anterior uveitis with a unilateral cataract. The review of the diagnostic survey is consistent with the patient's report of good health, and the involved eye appears "white and quiet." The patient denies previous ocular pain, photophobia or redness. The examination confirms suboptimal vision OD. There are stellate KPs on the corneal endothelium, nongranulomatous anterior uveitis, and subtle asymmetry in the iris color, with the right iris lighter than the left. The intraocular pressure is elevated in the right eye. Gonioscopy reveals fine, branching angle vessels. A summary of these significant findings enables one to generate a differential diagnosis, with the most likely diagnosis of Fuchs' heterochromic iridocyclitis. If the patient were a young girl reported to be healthy by the accompanying adult, and one noted a "white and quiet" eye, the primary diagnostic considerations and approach to this patient would be different. But the same method of data acquisition with attention to specific historical information (fever, rash, arthritis) and detailed examination (synechiae, cataract, band keratopathy) followed by a targeted laboratory evaluation (antinuclear antibody [ANA], Rheumatoid factor) enables one to generate a list of diagnostic contenders and then the most likely specific etiology.

References

1. Silverstein AM: Changing trends in the etiologic diagnosis of uveitis. Doc Ophthalmol 1997;94:25.
2. Green J: Ocular manifestations of brucellosis (undulant fever). Arch Ophthalmol 1939;21:51.
3. Billings F: Focal Infections. New York, London, D. Appleton and Company, 1916.
4. Stanworth A, McIntyre H: Aetiology of uveitis. Br J Ophthalmol 1957;41:25.
5. Walsh F: Ocular importance of sarcoidosis. Arch Ophthalmol 1939;21:421.
6. Guyton JS, Woods AC: Etiology of uveitis. Arch Ophthalmol 1941;26:983.

7. Woods AC, Guyton JS: Role of sarcoidosis and of brucellosis in uveitis. Arch Ophthalmol 1944;31:469.
8. Stanworth A: Rheumatism and uveitis. Trans Ophthalmol Soc UK 1956;76:287.
9. Brewerton DA, Webley M, Ward AM: Acute anterior uveitis and the HLA-B27. Lancet 1973;2:994.
10. Gass JDM: Acute posterior multifocal placoid pigment epitheliopathy. Arch Ophthalmol 1968;80:177.
11. Ryan SJ, Maumenee AE: Birdshot retinochoroidopathy. Am J Ophthalmol 1980;89:31.
12. Nussenblatt RB, Mittal KK, Ryan S, Green, et al: Birdshot retinochoroidopathy associated with HLA-A29 antigen and immune responsiveness to retinal S-antigen. Am J Ophthalmol 1982;94:147.
13. Dreyer RF, Gass JDM: Multifocal choroiditis and panuveitis. Arch Ophthalmol 1984;102:1776.
14. Rodriguez A, Calonge M, Pedrosa-Seres M, et al: Referral patterns of uveitis in a tertiary eye care center. Arch Ophthalmol 1996;114:593.
15. Bloch-Michel E, Nussenblatt RB: International uveitis study group recommendations for the evaluation of intraocular inflammatory disease. Am J Ophthalmol 1987;102:234.
16. Tessler HH: Classification of symptoms and clinical signs of uveitis. In: Clinical Ophthalmology, Vol 4. Philadelphia, J.B. Lippincott, 1987, p 1.
17. Weiner A, BenEzra D: Clinical patterns and associated conditions in chronic uveitis. Am J Ophthalmol 1991;112:151.
18. Rothova A, Buitenhuis HJ, Meencken C, et al: Uveitis and systemic disease Br J Ophthalmol 1992;72:137.
19. Perkins ES, Folk J. Uveitis in London and Iowa. Ophthalmologica 1984;189:36.
20. Paola P, Massimo A, LaCava M, et al. Endogenous uveitis: An analysis of 1,417 cases. Ophthalmologica 1996;210:234.
21. Baarsma GS: The epidemiology and genetics of endogenous uveitis: A review. Curr Eye Res 1991;11(Suppl):1.
22. McCannel CA, Holland GN, Helm CJ, et al: Causes of uveitis in the general practice of ophthalmology. Am J Ophthalmol 1996;121:35.
23. Henderly DE, Genstler AJ, Smith RE, et al: Changing patterns in uveitis. Am J Ophthalmol 1987;103:131.
24. Merrill PT, Kim J, Cox TA, et al: Uveitis in the southeastern United States. Curr Eye Res 1997;16:865.
25. Soylu M, Ozdemir G, Anli A: Pediatric uveitis in Southern Turkey. Ocul Immunol Inflamm 1997;5:197.
26. Coté MA, Rao NA: The role of histopathology in the diagnosis and management of uveitis. Intern Ophthalmol 1990;14:309.
27. Tugal-Tutkun I, Havrlikova K, Power WJ, et al: Changing patterns in uveitis of childhood. Ophthalmology 1995;103:375.
28. Kanski JJ, Shun-Shin GA: Systemic uveitis syndromes in childhood: An analysis of 340 cases. Ophthalmology 1984;91:1247.
29. Giles CL: Uveitis in childhood—part I anterior. Ann Ophthalmol 1989;21:13.
30. Rosenbaum JT, Wernick R: The utility of routine screening for systemic lupus erythematosus or tuberculosis. Arch Ophthalmol 1990;108:1291.
31. Duke-Elder S, Perkins EJ: System of Ophthalmology. Diseases of the Uveal Tract. London, Henry Kimpton, 1966.

APPENDIX A.

This a **confidential** survey. Please respond to all questions by circling the proper answer.

Patient Name: _____

Address: _____

_____

Telephone Number: (   ) _____

Referring Physician: _____

Physician's Address: _____

_____

Physician's Telephone Number: (   ) _____

FAMILY HISTORY

These questions refer to your grandparents, parents, aunts, uncles, brothers and sisters, children, or grandchildren

Has anyone in your family ever had any of the following?

Cancer	Yes	No
Diabetes	Yes	No
Allergies	Yes	No
Arthritis or Rheumatism	Yes	No
Syphilis	Yes	No
Tuberculosis	Yes	No
Sickle cell disease or trait	Yes	No
Lyme Disease	Yes	No
Gout	Yes	No

Has anyone in your family had any of the medical problems listed below?

Eyes	Yes	No
Skin	Yes	No
Kidneys	Yes	No
Lungs	Yes	No
Stomach or bowel	Yes	No
Nervous system or brain	Yes	No

DATE: _____ **MD SIGNATURE:** _____

SOCIAL HISTORY:

Age (Years): _____ Current Job: _____		
Have you ever lived outside of the USA?	Yes	No
If yes, where? _____		
Have you ever owned a dog?	Yes	No
Have you ever owned a cat?	Yes	No
Have you ever eaten raw meat or uncooked sausage?	Yes	No
Have you ever had unpasteurized milk or cheese?	Yes	No
Have you ever been exposed to sick animals?	Yes	No
Do you drink untreated stream, well, or lake water?	Yes	No
Do you smoke cigarettes?	Yes	No
Have you ever used intravenous drugs?		
Have you ever had bisexual or homosexual relationships?		
Have you ever taken birth control pills?		

PERSONAL MEDICAL HISTORY:

Are you allergic to any medications?	Yes	No

If yes, which medications? _____

Please list the medications that you are currently taking, including non-prescription drugs such as aspirin, Advil, antihistamines, etc.

_____

_____

_____

_____

PERSONAL MEDICAL HISTORY:

Please list all the eye operations you have had (including laser surgery) and the dates of the surgeries:

_____

_____

_____

_____

_____

_____

Please list all operations you have had and the dates of the surgeries:

_____

_____

_____

_____

_____

Have you ever been told that you have the following conditions?

Anemia (Low Blood Count)	Yes	No
Cancer	Yes	No
Diabetes	Yes	No
Hepatitis	Yes	No
High Blood Pressure	Yes	No
Pleurisy	Yes	No
Pneumonia	Yes	No
Ulcers	Yes	No

Herpes (cold sores)	Yes	No
Chickenpox	Yes	No
Shingles (Zoster)	Yes	No
German Measles (Rubella)	Yes	No
Measles (Rubeola)	Yes	No
Mumps	Yes	No
Chlamydia or Trachoma	Yes	No
Syphilis	Yes	No
Gonorrhea	Yes	No
Any other sexually transmitted disease	Yes	No
Tuberculosis (TB)	Yes	No
Leprosy	Yes	No
Leptospirosis	Yes	No
Lyme Disease	Yes	No
Histoplasmosis	Yes	No
Candida or Moniliasis	Yes	No
Coccidioidomycosis	Yes	No
Sporotrichosis	Yes	No
Toxoplasmosis	Yes	No
Toxocariasis	Yes	No
Cysticercosis	Yes	No
Trichinosis	Yes	No
Whipple's Disease	Yes	No
AIDS	Yes	No
Hay Fever	Yes	No
Allergies	Yes	No
Vasculitis	Yes	No
Arthritis	Yes	No
Rheumatoid Arthritis	Yes	No
Lupus (Systemic Lupus Erythematosus)	Yes	No
Scleroderma	Yes	No

Have you ever had any of the following illnesses?

Reiter's Syndrome	Yes	No
Colitis	Yes	No
Crohn's Disease	Yes	No
Ulcerative Colitis	Yes	No
Adamatiades-Behçet Disease	Yes	No
Sarcoidosis	Yes	No
Ankylosing Spondylitis	Yes	No
Erythema Nodosa	Yes	No
Temporal Arteritis	Yes	No
Multiple Sclerosis	Yes	No
Serpiginous Choroiditis	Yes	No
Fuchs' Heterochromic Iridocyclitis	Yes	No
Vogt-Koyanagi-Harada Syndrome	Yes	No

Have you ever had any of the following illnesses?

GENERAL HEALTH:

Chills	Yes	No
Fevers (persistent or recurrent)	Yes	No

Night Sweats	Yes	No
Fatigue (tire easily)	Yes	No
Poor Appetite	Yes	No
Unexplained Weight Loss	Yes	No
Do you feel sick?	Yes	No

HEAD:

Frequent or Severe Headaches	Yes	No
Fainting	Yes	No
Numbness or Tingling in Your Body	Yes	No
Paralysis in Parts of Your Body	Yes	No
Seizures or Convulsions	Yes	No

EARS:

Hard of Hearing or Deafness	Yes	No
Ringing or Noises in Your Ears	Yes	No
Frequent or Severe Ear Infections	Yes	No
Painful or Swollen Ear Lobes	Yes	No

NOSE AND THROAT:

Sore in Your Nose or Mouth	Yes	No
Severe or Recurrent Nosebleeds	Yes	No
Frequent Sneezing	Yes	No
Sinus Trouble	Yes	No
Persistent Hoarseness	Yes	No
Tooth or Gum Infections	Yes	No

SKIN:

Rashes	Yes	No
Skin Sores	Yes	No
Sunburn Easily (Photosensitivity)	Yes	No
White Patches of Skin or Hair	Yes	No
Loss of Hair	Yes	No
Tick or Insect Bites	Yes	No
Painfully Cold Fingers	Yes	No
Severe Itching	Yes	No

RESPIRATORY:

Severe or Frequent Colds	Yes	No
Constant Coughing	Yes	No
Coughing Up Blood	Yes	No
Recent Flu or Viral Infection	Yes	No
Wheezing or Asthma Attacks	Yes	No
Difficulty Breathing	Yes	No

Have you ever had any of the following symptoms?

CARDIOVASCULAR:

Chest Pain	Yes	No
Shortness of Breath	Yes	No
Swelling of Your Legs	Yes	No

BLOOD:

Frequent or Easy Bruising	Yes	No
Frequent or Easy Bleeding	Yes	No
Have You Received Blood Transfusions	Yes	No

GASTROINTESTINAL:

Trouble Swallowing	Yes	No
Diarrhea	Yes	No
Bloody Stools	Yes	No
Stomach Ulcers	Yes	No
Jaundice or Yellow Skin	Yes	No

BONES AND JOINTS:

Stiff Joints	Yes	No
Painful or Swollen Joints	Yes	No
Stiff Lower Back	Yes	No
Back Pain While Sleeping or Awakening	Yes	No
Muscle Aches	Yes	No

GENITOURINARY:

Kidney Problems	Yes	No
Bladder Trouble	Yes	No
Blood in Your Urine	Yes	No
Urinary Discharge	Yes	No
Genital Sores or Ulcers	Yes	No
Prostatitis	Yes	No
Testicular Pain	Yes	No

Are You Pregnant?	Yes	No
Do You Plan to Be Pregnant in the Future?	Yes	No

APPENDIX B. DIFFERENTIAL DIAGNOSIS TABLES

CLINICAL FEATURE	DIAGNOSTIC CONSIDERATIONS	CLINICAL FEATURE	DIAGNOSTIC CONSIDERATIONS
Iris atrophy	Herpes simplex virus Varicella zoster virus Anterior segment ischemia Other: Syphilis, leprosy, tuberculosis, onchocerciasis	Synechiae	Juvenile rheumatoid arthritis Sarcoidosis Syphilis Seronegative spondyloarthropathies Varicella zoster virus
Band keratopathy	Juvenile rheumatoid arthritis Sarcoidosis Other: Multiple myeloma, chronic uveitis in children, chronic retinal detachment	Cotton-wool spots	Systemic lupus erythematosus Vasculitis HIV retinopathy
		Vitreous hemorrhage	Pars planitis Ocular histoplasmosis Vogt-Koyanagi-Harada syndrome
Heterochromia	Fuchs' heterochromic iridocyclitis Rubeosis irides Siderosis	Choroidal granuloma	Tuberculosis Toxocariasis Sarcoidosis Toxoplasmosis
Glaucoma	Herpes simplex virus Varicella zoster virus Fuchs' heterochromic iridocyclitis Posner-Schlossman syndrome Juvenile rheumatoid arthritis Sarcoidosis Rubeosis irides		Syphilis *Pneumocystis carinii*
		Focal retinitis	Toxoplasmosis
		Multifocal retinitis	Syphilis Herpes simplex virus Cytomegalovirus Sarcoidosis Birdshot retinochoroidopathy Fungal
Hyphema	Fuchs' heterochromic iridocyclitis Herpes simplex uveitis Varicella zoster uveitis Trauma Rubeosis irides Juvenile xanthogranuloma	Focal choroiditis	Toxocariasis Tuberculosis Lymphoma
Hypopyon	Seronegative spondyloarthropathies Adamantiades-Behçet disease Endophthalmitis IOL-related uveitis	Multifocal choroiditis	Histoplasmosis Sympathetic ophthalmia Sarcoidosis Serpiginous choroidopathy *Pneumocystitis carinii* Lymphoma Punctate inner choroidopathy Miliary tuberculosis
Iris nodules	Sarcoidosis Tuberculosis Syphilis Leprosy		
Keratitis	Herpes simplex virus Varicella zoster virus Lyme disease Sarcoidosis Tuberculosis Syphilis Cogan's syndrome Systemic lupus erythematosus Leprosy Systemic vasculitis Collagen vascular disease Inflammatory bowel disease Mumps	Postoperative uveitis	Acute endophthalmitis Surgical traumatic iritis Retained crystalline lens material Sympathetic ophthalmia Exacerbation of pre-existing uveitis
		Retinal "wipeout"	Adamantiades-Behçet disease DUSN Acute retinal necrosis
Scleritis	Systemic lupus erythematosus Wegener's granulomatosis Polyarteritis nodosa Reiter's syndrome Herpes simplex virus Varicella zoster virus Syphilis Tuberculosis Toxoplasmosis Sarcoidosis Leprosy Crohn's disease Adamantiades-Behçet disease Psoriatic arthritis Relapsing polychondritis Cogan's syndrome Mumps Lyme disease Vasculitis		

DUSN, Diffuse unilateral subacute neuroretinitis; HIV, human immunodeficiency virus.

7 — DIAGNOSTIC IMAGING STUDIES FOR INFLAMMATORY SYSTEMIC DISEASES WITH EYE MANIFESTATIONS

Roxanne Chan, Khaled A. Tawansy,
Tamer El-Helw, C. Stephen Foster,
and Barbara L. Carter

Imaging studies, when correlated with the appropriate laboratory test results, clinical findings, and pathology, help confirm the suspected diagnosis or limit the differential diagnosis of a patient with inflammatory eye disease. The evolution of radiology with new imaging modalities has resulted in a high degree of sophistication, allowing significantly more wide-ranging opportunities for establishing the diagnosis.

Types of imaging studies include plain film, ultrasound, computed tomography (CT), magnetic resonance imaging (MRI), and radioactive tracer studies. Each of these modalities has specific advantages, but there is also significant overlap of the information provided. Because the evaluation of a patient with inflammatory eye disease can be wide ranging and costly given the extensive differential diagnosis of ocular inflammatory disease, directed parsimonious laboratory testing, as described previously, and selective imaging, as discussed herein, maximizes cost effectiveness as well as providing the most prudent diagnostic approach. The alternative is indiscriminate testing or gate-keeping negligence.

This chapter is divided into three parts: (1) imaging modalities; (2) case presentations of several common systemic diseases that can cause ocular inflammation, which illustrate the utility of imaging studies in the management of each; and (3) fluorescein and indocyanine green angiography. Appropriate selection of an imaging modality to maximize the relevant information requires an understanding of the regional anatomy, clinical history, ophthalmologic examination, and advantages and disadvantages of each test.

Imaging Modalities

Computed Tomography

Thin-section, multiplanar high-resolution CT permits exquisite delineation of disease entities affecting soft tissue and osseous structures. The eyes, optic nerves, orbital walls, extraocular muscles, paranasal sinuses, vasculature, and lacrimal glands can be studied. CT also permits evaluation of patients with space-occupying lesions and differentiation of localized hemorrhage from solid intraorbital masses.[1]

The utility of CT is ever expanding. Advanced generations of CT scanners, including helical imaging, permits faster image acquisition and decreased motion artifact. Measurements to quantify shapes and sizes from CT scans can be extracted from the digital image data stored in the computer. Computerized thin-section CT images can also be reconstructed in three dimensions to illustrate spatial relationships and contours better; however, these reconstructed coronal and sagittal images have less optimal image quality and resolution than the nonreconstructed (direct) axial and coronal images. Contrast material injected through a peripheral vein enhances visualization of scleral thickening, alteration of vascular structures, inflammatory disease, and tumors; therefore, contrast should be requested when these abnormalities are present, but if the clinician is unsure, scans with and without contrast may be obtained. Increased enhancement and soft tissue disease involvement generally correlates with increased tissue vascularity. Digital subtraction, in which the background is subtracted from contrast-filled vasculature, is also used to optimize contrast.

The advantages of CT include sensitivity for calcium detection, high-resolution bone detail, optimal reformatting capabilities, and the ability to obtain intracranial as well as orbital data.[2] Technical advantages include short acquisition time and improved processing after examination.[2] CT is also often fast enough to be performed without anesthesia in young children, although sedation is often helpful.[2]

Limitations include relative nonspecificity with respect to tissue characterization and potential misdiagnosis of conditions such as subretinal or posterior hyaloid hemorrhage (i.e., vitreous hemorrhage).[3] Disadvantages of CT include suboptimal soft tissue imaging; radiation exposure; artifacts due to high atomic number materials of adjacent structures such as dental amalgam, and due to potential allergic reaction to iodinated contrast material (which can also cause damage to the kidneys in patients with borderline renal failure); and claustrophobia. The radiation dose to the lens depends on the total number of "slices," particularly on the number of transorbital sections, the KVp energy, collimation, detector sensitivity, and overlapping slices. The acute dose is 2 to 4 Gy, above that of a plain film series and less than that that induces cataract.[2, 4] This dose was measured to be less than 4% of the acute dose associated with cataract formation.[4] The potential biologic hazard of ionizing radiation exposure during the CT examination must also be taken into consideration.

Magnetic Resonance Imaging

MRI signal intensity depends on the magnetic properties and concentration of atomic nuclei with an odd number of protons or neutrons. Hydrogen molecules, which have a single proton in their nucleus and are the most abundant in the body, interact with pulsed radio frequency (RF) energy in the presence of a steady magnetic field

TABLE 7–1. NORMAL MR SIGNAL CHARACTERISTICS

TISSUE	T1	T2
Cortical bone	Dark	Dark
Muscle	Intermediate	Intermediate
Ligaments and tendons	Dark	Dark
Fibrocartilage (menisci)	Dark	Dark
Hyaline cartilage (articular)	Dark	Bright
Fat (subcutaneous tissue, marrow)	Bright	Intermediate
Fluid (effusion)	Dark/intermediate	Bright
Vitreous	Dark	Bright
Melanin	Bright	Dark

TABLE 7–3. HEMORRHAGE EVOLUTION AND IRON METABOLISM

		T1	T2
Fe^{+2}	Oxyhemoglobin (oxygenation)	Dark	Bright
	Deoxyhemoglobin (deoxygenation)	Dark	Bright
Fe^{+3}	Methemoglobin, hemichromes (extracellular—red blood cell lysis)	Bright	Bright
	Transferrin, lactoferrin (extracellular)	Bright	Bright
	Ferritin, hemosiderin (intracellular—phagocytes)	Intermediate	Dark

based on the physical principles of proton excitation and relaxation times.[5] Absorbed RF energy is re-emitted, resulting in relaxation times, which are characteristic for each type of tissue (Table 7–1). Differences between the relaxation times of different tissues are what give rise to the exceptional contrast in MRI images. T1-relaxation characterizes the environment of excited nuclei and magnetic field strength, whereas T2-relaxation times express the spin-spin interactions between excited and adjacent nuclei. T1 has a strong dependence on the magnetic field strength, whereas T2 has a negligible dependency.[5, 6] High T1 signal can be seen in many entities (Table 7–2). Pulse sequences can emphasize either T1 or T2 relaxation properties and are called T1- and T2-weighted images, respectively. Spin density images are a third type of weighting, which depends on the concentration of hydrogen nuclei. Fat is bright on T1-weighted images. Hemorrhage age can be estimated due to the magnetic properties of iron and its effect on surrounding water molecules (Table 7–3). Other pulse sequences besides T1 and T2 are also routinely used.

Multiplanar imaging is acquired directly with the patient in a supine position. The data can also be modified later by manipulation, as is done with CT. Image characteristics depend on the various pulse sequences used, signal-to-noise ratio, motion artifacts, field of view, spatial resolution, and the interdependence of these factors. Higher field strength magnets (1 to 2 Tesla) generally have a higher signal-to-noise ratio.[5, 6] Optimization of these variables allows the use of MRI to diagnose disease and to facilitate surgical planning with high resolution.

MRI has clear advantages over CT for superior soft tissue detail in the study of ocular and orbital anatomy as fine as muscles, connective tissue structures, and nerves, which all have different image signal intensity based on

TABLE 7–2. ENTITIES BRIGHT ON T1

Fat
Proteins
Hemorrhage
Melanin
Gadolinium/other new contrast agents
Iron deposition in metabolic disorders
Free radicals
Increased proton density
Flow phenomena
Artifacts

the number of mobile hydrogen atoms.[7–9] Advantages also include the use of nonionizing radiation and excellent tissue specificities based on individual tissue response to various pulse sequences, some of which are specific for structures such as iron, intracellular and extracellular hemoglobin, and melanin. For example, vitreous appears dark on T1-weighted images and bright on T2-weighted images, whereas melanin appears bright on T1-weighted images and dark on T2-weighted images (see Table 7–1). In addition, multiplanar images can be reconstructed, without significant loss of resolution, with the use of MR volume imaging.[10] There is excellent tissue contrast when pulse sequences are selected carefully, which exploits anatomy having high orbital fat content.[11, 12]

Gadolinium dimeglumine or gadolinium diethylenetriamine pentaacetic acid (Gd-DTPA) is a paramagnetic contrast material that shortens T1, leading to increased signal intensity on T1 sequences.[13] Therefore, this contrast agent is occasionally used to provide additional soft tissue detail or tumor enhancement.[11, 13] One should request gadolinium when looking for tumor, infection, granulomatous disease, or causes of increased vascularity.

The sharpest and best anatomic detail is obtained with specially designed orbit surface coils, (which bring the MRI coil closer to the area of interest [increases the signal and decreases the noise], than if a head coil were used), and T1-weighted spin echo sequences. The resultant contrast between the orbital lesions, such as melanoma or pseudotumor, and adjacent normal structures is better with MRI than with high-resolution CT.[14] These orbit coils are optimal for imaging inflammatory lesions, such as optic neuritis, especially when combined with contrast-enhanced fat suppression sequences, and are superior to conventional T1-weighted contrast enhanced images alone.[15] MRI with surface coils allows differentiation of Coats' disease from retinoblastoma and tumors from subretinal fluid.

The differentiation of Coats' disease from retinoblastoma, for example, is very important and is facilitated by MRI findings. Subretinal lipoprotein and blood accumulation from leaky telangiectatic vessels appear bright on T1- and T2-weighted images that enhance on post–Gd-DPTA images. Retinoblastoma, on the other hand, usually exhibits moderate brightness on T1-weighted images and is dark on T2-weighted images. Although Coats' disease may also have dark T2 signal, its diagnosis is favored by enhancement of the sensory retina and absence of an intraocular mass with contrast.

Fat-suppression sequences significantly improve intraocular MRIs by eliminating high fat signal to increase visualization of adjacent structures, decreases volume averaging artifact, and eliminates chemical shift misregistration artifact. These fat-suppression sequences include short T1-inversion recovery (STIR), frequency selection postsuppression (ChemSat), Dixon and Chopper methods, and the hybrid method.[11] Fat-suppression T2-sequences improves lesion detection and lymph node evaluation.[11] However, fat suppression still cannot distinguish inflammatory optic neuritis and ischemic neuritis from other causes of optic nerve demyelination, such as multiple sclerosis (MS).[12, 16] Precontrast- and postcontrast-enhanced T1-weighted images with fat-suppression technique are most helpful in detecting and differentiating small intraocular tumors and other small benign masses with a thickness of more than 1.8 mm; entities measuring less than 1.8 mm may be missed.[17] Now, volume imaging with 0.5mm slice thickness is possible.

Images of the intraorbital and extraorbital parts of the optic nerve and chiasm, and of the entire visual pathway permits the detection of demyelination, ischemia, microinfarct, tumor extension, and hemorrhage.[10] Localized inflammatory pseudotumor versus nodular or diffuse posterior scleritis in proptosis, or choroidal tumors versus subretinal mass may be differentiated.[18] Hemorrhage age, which depends on the state of hemoglobin; vitreous opacity, which is believed to be related to protein exudation into the vitreous; retinal and posterior hyaloid detachment; deformity; cicatrization; and focal deformities can be evaluated.[19–21] Tumors causing choroidal folds and retinal striae, which are also signs of posterior scleritis, can be successfully detected by MRI. The diagnostic accuracy of thin-section MRI in intraocular tumor detection as compared with that of ultrasound is uncertain.[22]

Biochemical activity and composition mapping is now possible with MR spectroscopy. Magnetic resonance angiography (MRA) provides noninvasive vascular evaluation of larger vessels; however, Doppler ultrasound instead of MRA is used for smaller blood vessels. Acute inflammatory muscle changes are differentiated best from chronic fibrosis with high-resolution MRI with T2-weighted sequences. Although it is not routinely used directly, MRI can also be used to evaluate the lacrimal drainage system with enhanced soft tissue detail, as compared with dacryoscintigraphy and dacryocystography, and less ionizing radiation, as compared with CT or radiography.[15, 23]

Limitations of MRI include patient claustrophobia (less of a problem with an open magnet); motion artifact due to longer time for acquiring the images (several minutes depending on the pulse sequence, and T1 imaging requires less time than T2 imaging), sensitivity to paramagnetic material such as eye make-up, high cost, less specificity for imaging bony structures, and problems with dental braces, which may seriously degrade the images. Contraindications to MR have been studied, and the list is constantly updated. These contraindications include metallic structures adjacent to the globe or optic nerve, which can cause blindness; aneurysmal clips, which may result in death due to tearing of the carotid

artery by torsion; pacemakers; and defibrillators.[24] Sedation (i.e., chloral hydrate or pentobarbital [Nembutal]) may be necessary for CT and MRI of pediatric patients who have clinical questions that remain unanswered by ultrasound or plain films.

Plain Films

Radiography has been the most frequently used imaging technique, especially before the advent of CT, and it is still routinely performed for the evaluation of bones and to screen for certain diseases owing to its low cost and superior spatial resolution. Chest, sinus, sacroiliac joint, extremity, temporomandibular joint, and skull films are a few examples. X-ray studies can visualize entities such as bone erosions, soft tissue calcifications or swelling, subluxation or misalignment, periosteal bone absorption, and changes in interosseous articular spaces. However, plain films are poor in the evaluation of noncalcified soft tissues and may give unacceptable false-positive or false-negative results compared with CT in patients with chronic sinusitis.[4] Although plain films are now less often used because CT and MRI eclipse the relatively sparse information provided, plain films play an important role in patient management and should not be overlooked either as a diagnostic modality in or as a baseline study for future monitoring.

Because many inflammatory eye diseases are a manifestation of systemic disease, imaging of extraocular structures with plain films should be considered. Chest X-ray studies are of diagnostic importance in diseases such as tuberculosis, sarcoidosis, Wegener's granulomatosis, and allergic granulomatous angiitis (Churg-Strauss syndrome). Sinus films may reveal mucosal thickening or destruction, or both, as that seen in Wegener's granulomatosis. The arthritides are another group of diseases of importance to ocular inflammation; sacroiliac and extremity films are useful in assessing involvement caused by ankylosing spondylitis, Reiter's syndrome, psoriatic arthritis, and arthritis associated with inflammatory bowel disease. Extremity films are used to evaluate rheumatoid arthritis (RA) and juvenile rheumatoid arthritis (JRA). Arthrography, with single or double contrast, helps provide information about the integrity of intraarticular structures and the presence of joint bodies or synovial cysts.

Nuclear Medicine

Radionuclide scintigraphy is the most sensitive test for very early physiologic changes, including synovial inflammation, as well as hilar, parotid, and submandibular involvement in sarcoidosis. In fact, this modality plays an important adjunctive role in the work-up and diagnosis of patients with ocular inflammatory diseases suspected of having sarcoidosis. The entire body can be scanned at a moderate cost.

Improved gamma camera technology, with higher sensitivity and resolution, has allowed better imaging of dynamic blood flow, enlargement of the vascular pool, and early tissue hyperemia from capillary leak. The rate of bone formation can be evaluated with diphosphonate complexes, such as technetium 99m (Tc^{99m})–methylene diphosphonate (Tc^{99m}–MDP) and Tc^{99m}–hydroxymethylene diphosphonate (Tc^{99m}-HDP), which can then be used to differentiate soft tissue from osseous pathology.[25] Single photon emission computed tomography (SPECT) is used to evaluate smaller body parts, such as facet and temporomandibular joints, owing to its increased anatomic detail and improved contrast enhancement that allows differentiation of radioactivity in inflamed tissue from overlying normal tissue. Gallium citrate or indium 111–labeled white blood cells (WBCs) increase specificity for inflammation, such as infectious lesions. An evolving and experimental area of nuclear medicine is immune complex scintigraphy with monoclonal and polyclonal antibodies. SPECT three-step radioimmunoscintigraphy with Tc^{99m}-labeled antimelanoma monoclonal antibodies, for example, can be used to detect uveal melanoma.[26]

However, nuclear medicine still has poor spatial resolution and anatomic detail, which may be improved by increasing imaging time, magnification scintigraphy with pinhole, electronic "zoom," or converging collimators.[25] A pitfall of the high sensitivity of nuclear medicine studies is the possibility of false-positive results.

Salivary Gland Radiology

Sialography involves the use of fluoroscopy and spot radiographs, suitable contrast materials, and instruments to delineate salivary gland ducts and disease. The glands studied are primarily parotid and submandibular. Contraindications include acute infection, contrast allergy, and anticipated thyroid function tests after sialography.[27] Patients with Sjögren's syndrome may have abnormal sialogram results, indicating salivary gland involvement, particularly of the parotid. There may be persistent punctate pooling of contrast in salivary gland acini after drainage from the tubules and ducts has occurred.

Upper Gastrointestinal Series/Barium Enema

Single or double contrast upper gastrointestinal (UGI) series with or without small bowel follow-through (SBFT) or barium enema (BE) permit better evaluation of mucosal surfaces and luminal contours than other modalities, such as CT. Patients with gastrointestinal diseases, such as Crohn's disease and ulcerative colitis, may need evaluation of the gastrointestinal tract mucosa.

Ultrasound

Ophthalmic ultrasound uses higher frequencies than abdominal ultrasound. Tissues have various echogenicities (Table 7–4). A- and B-scan ultrasound is most suitable for evaluating more superficial tissues that contain fluid. An A-scan is unidimensional, whereas a B-scan creates a two-dimensional image of the scanned cross section. Advantages include low cost, rapidity, real-time imaging, multiple scan planes, and lack of biologic hazards. Limitations include operator dependency, contact with the globe or eyelid (which may not be tolerated by a patient with eye pain), depth of focus, interference from overlying bone, calcification or air-containing structures, findings limited to the number of images, diffuse vitreous hemorrhage, and inferior spatial resolution when compared with CT or MRI.

Overall, common indications include detection of joint

TABLE 7–4. TISSUE ECHOGENICITY ON ULTRASOUND

TISSUE	CHARACTERISTICS
Tendons	Very echogenic (very bright) and linear
Bone	Very echogenic
Muscle	Hypoechoic (moderately dark), multiple fine linear echogenic bands
Fibrocartilage	Echogenic
Hyaline cartilage	Hypoechoic
Simple fluid	Anechoic (homogenous and dark)
Complex fluid	Dark with internal echoes or septations

From Schumacher HR Jr, ed: Primer on Rheumatic Diseases, 10th ed. Atlanta Arthritis Foundation, 1993, pp 74.

effusions, tendinous and ligamentous lesions, and minimal surface irregularities of cartilage; ophthalmic indications include posterior scleritis, which manifests as flattening of the posterior aspect of the globe and thickening of the posterior layers of the eye (choroid and sclera). Retinal and choroidal detachment may also be detected. The combined use of A- and B-scan techniques produces the most useful results in distinguishing posterior scleritis from orbital, choroidal, and retinal diseases, which may clinically mimic scleritis. Retrobulbar edema surrounding the optic nerve, causing squaring off of the normally rounded nerve with extension of edema along the adjacent sclera, is called the "T" sign.[18]

Extrascleral extension of tumors, such as choroidal melanoma, can be evaluated, for example.[28] B-scan plays an extremely important role in the diagnosis of choroidal melanoma, and the modality demonstrates specific findings that differentiate it from other simulating lesions, such as choroidal hemangioma. Ultrasound characteristics of choroidal melanoma include acoustic hollowing, choroidal excavation, low-to-moderate internal reflectivity. Choroidal hemangioma, on the other hand, shows high internal reflectivity without choroidal excavation.

Doppler ultrasound allows selective and noninvasive imaging of the vascular perfusion of organs and vessels.[29] *Color Doppler imaging* permits combined anatomic and velocity data to increase sensitivity and specificity, as compared with gray-scale Doppler imaging.[30] Color Doppler imaging adds useful information to many ultrasound examinations, including those performed for the evaluation of inflammation, trauma, vascular disease, and tumors of the globe and orbit. More specifically, imaging of retinal vascular diseases, pseudotumor, and retrobulbar vasculature (central retinal artery and vein, posterior ciliary arteries, ophthalmic artery) is possible.[30, 31] Doppler spectral analysis allows blood flow velocity assessment.[30] However, there are still remaining inherent limitations imposed by the laws of physics, such as spatial, temporal, and frequency resolution, aliasing, depth ambiguity, angle of insonation, and transducer geometry.[32]

Recent advances include *three-dimensional ultrasound imaging* and image reconstruction, which can be used for improved visualization of ocular pathologies and their physical characteristics.[33] Advantages include imaging of the entire region of interest in oblique and coronal planes. For example, three-dimensional ultrasound can be used to measure extrascleral extension from choroidal

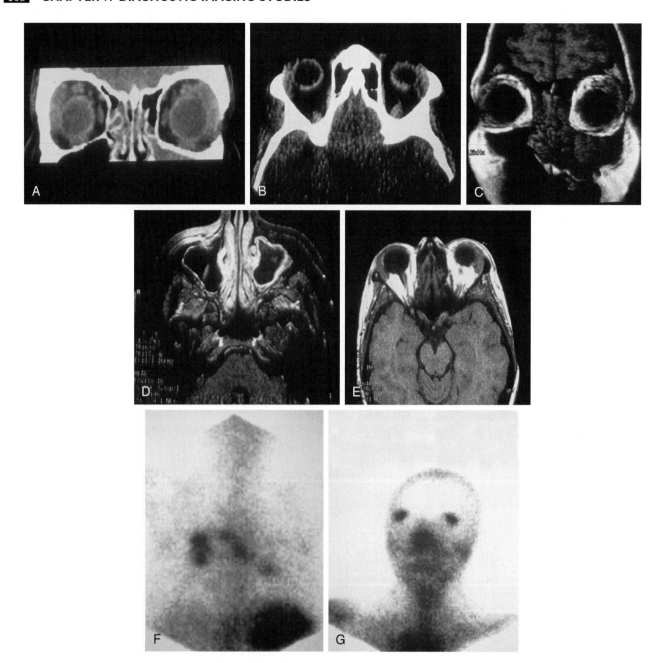

FIGURE 7–I. *A* and *B,* Sarcoid suspect. Coronal and axial CT of orbits. *C* to *E,* Coronal and axial MRI of orbits and sinuses. CT and MRI show bilateral lacrimal gland enlargement, and left maxillary and bilateral ethmoid disease without bone destruction. *F* and *G,* Gallium-67 citrate is intensely localized in the lacrimal glands and hilar-mediastinal lymph nodes. A diagnosis of sarcoidosis was made by conjunctival biopsy. (Courtesy of Elizabeth Oates, M.D.)

melanoma.[28] Other representative advances are tissue characterization, measurement of membrane thickness, parameter imaging, and high-frequency imaging. Detailed discussion of all of these capabilities are beyond the scope of this chapter.

Ultrasound biomicroscopy (UBM) is the newest development in ultrasound that involves the use of 40 to 100 MHz frequencies.[34] The most common current ophthalmic transducers operate at about 10 MHz, in which resolution in the beam direction (axial) is 0.2 to 0.5 mm transverse to the beam (lateral).[34] This increased frequency of UBM allows better resolution, which is analogous to the observation of living tissue at near-microscopic resolution and also visualization of regions not easily accessible by conventional clinical examination.

However, this resolution is at the expense of imaging depth. The maximal depth for a 10 MHz transducer is about 50 mm, and the maximal depth for one of 60 MHz is about 5 mm, the approximate depth of the anterior segment.[34] Other impediments besides decreased depth that limit the effectiveness of ocular sonography include hemorrhage, vitritis, and dense calcification.[3]

This imaging technique can be used to study various aspects of glaucoma, pupillary block, plateau iris syndrome, anterior synechiae, filtering surgery, anterior segment tumors, iris nevi, iris melanoma, ciliary body tumors, and cysts.[34, 35] UBM may eventually be a useful imaging modality for the evaluation of intermediate uveitis in a region where clinical examination is difficult and hampered by media opacities or when the diagnosis is not yet apparent. The diseases that cause intermediate uveitis include systemic diseases, such as multiple sclerosis (MS) and sarcoidosis; however, correlation of the UBM imaging characteristics with pathology is still uncertain.[36]

Other Modalities

There are other important imaging techniques, including fluorescein angiography and indocyanine green angiography, which are described later in this chapter.

IMMUNOLOGIC DISEASES

CASE 1: SARCOID SUSPECT

A 41-year-old woman presents with bilateral granulomatous uveitis. The chest x-ray study (CXR) revealed a bilateral interstitial process and hilar adenopathy compatible with, but not diagnostic of, sarcoidosis. Angiotensin-converting enzyme (ACE) was 77 U/L (normal range 8 to 52). Chest CT showed extensive mediastinal lymphadenopathy and bilateral hilar adenopathy with multiple ill-defined nodules, predominantly along the upper lobes with some right upper lobe airspace disease. CT (Fig. 7–1A and B) and MRI (see Fig. 7–1C to E) of the orbits and sinuses were also obtained. Pathology from conjunctival biopsy was compatible with sarcoidosis.

Discussion

Sarcoidosis is a diagnosis of exclusion, which must be correlated with biopsies of easily accessible sites, such as the conjunctiva, skin, and lacrimal and salivary glands. The pathologic hallmark is noncaseating granulomas with central epithelioid cells and macrophages, and surrounding lymphocytes, plasma cells, and mast cells. The most common extrathoracic manifestation is ophthal-

mic, which is present in 25% of patients.[37, 38] Sarcoid uveitis presenting for the first time in the elderly is not uncommon.[39]

Increased ACE levels and immunoglobulins are associated with active sarcoidosis. ACE may be negative outside the 20- to 40-year age group for sarcoidosis, and if ACE and CXR are negative, then conjunctival biopsy and whole-body gallium scanning may be indicated in patients with an elevated ACE, but with presumed birdshot retinochoroidopathy (BSRC) or multifocal choroiditis and panuveitis (MCP).[40] A positive whole-body gallium-67 scan indicates active disease, which in combination with a positive serum ACE level, increases the diagnostic specificity for sarcoidosis without affecting sensitivity in patients with clinically suspicious ocular sarcoidosis who have normal or equivocal chest radiographs.[41]

Patients with granulomatous uveitis, mildly elevated ACE, and a normal or nonspecific CXR present a diagnostic challenge. These studies may be correlated with CT or gallium-67 scanning, or both, which may help differentiate the etiologies (Fig. 7–2). However, no one clinical finding, or laboratory or radiographic test is sensitive and specific enough to provide a definitive diagnosis of sarcoidosis; these tests may also occasionally be negative even though the patient has the disease.[37, 42]

Because the lung and mediastinum are almost always involved, CXR of patients with clinical eye manifestations only may also have abnormalities. Approximately 80% to 90% of patients with sarcoidosis have an abnormal CXR during the course of their disease.[38, 42] A patient with classic CXR findings does not require a tissue diagnosis because they are unlikely to have any other disorder. Hilar adenopathy is present in about 90% of patients with sarcoidosis and is usually accompanied by paratracheal adenopathy, with or without lung parenchymal abnormalities, such as infiltrates and end-stage pulmonary fibrosis.[37] CXR is less sensitive during

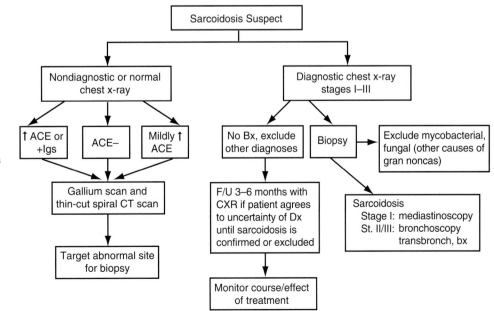

FIGURE 7–2. Diagnostic algorithm for suspected sarcoidosis.

the early stages of sarcoidosis. Other diagnoses, such as inflammation, tuberculosis, primary lung cancer, and lymphoma, must be excluded. The possibility of these other diseases may decrease the specificity of CXR. Equivocal (Case 1) or normal cases warrant additional testing with CT, MRI, or gallium scanning, which better visualize parenchymal lung and mediastinal changes.[43]

Gallium-67 citrate scanning is the most sensitive imaging modality for detecting abnormalities in patients with sarcoidosis. This radioactive tracer depends on the character and extent of active inflammation in which macrophages and their evolutionary progeny, the epithelioid cells, participate. These cells are abundant in normal liver, bone, lung, and spleen. Abnormal lung uptake is also present in silicosis, leprosy, and tuberculosis. Some authors believe that there is relatively little added diagnostic value of gallium-67 scanning owing to lack of specificity.[37, 42] However, a highly specific pattern for sarcoidosis is gallium uptake in intrathoracic lymph nodes (right paratracheal and hilar) in a pattern resembling the λ.[44] Bilateral hilar uptake is seen in sarcoidosis and is less likely in lymphoma, which tends to have peripheral lymph node involvement (see Fig. 7–1F).[45] Abnormal uptake can be targeted for biopsy. Gallium scans should include the head, because one study revealed 53/61 (87%) of patients with sarcoidosis have gallium-67 lacrimal gland uptake, which seems to be independent of the presence of ocular disease (see Fig. 7–1G).[42, 46] The classic finding of lacrimal gland uptake accompanied by parotid and submandibular uptake is called the panda sign.[46, 47] Lacrimal gland uptake in sarcoidosis should be differentiated from patients with orbital pseudotumor, Sjögren's syndrome, systemic lupus erythematosus (SLE), tuberculosis, and lymphoma.

High-resolution CT (HRCT) may guide therapy in patients with lung disease. There may be ground glass, nodular and irregular linear opacities, and interlobular septal thickening (potentially reversible) or cystic spaces and architectural distortion (irreversible).[48] HRCT shows patchy densities and central crowding of bronchi and vessels, and better differentiates nodules from septal thickening than CXR.[49] CT may be used to confirm pulmonary disease and examine eye disease (Case 1). In this case, Gallium-67 scanning was not used because an overall screening site for inflammatory activity to biopsy was not needed and CT was used to delineate better the anatomy of disease in a specific known site.

The study of choice for the evaluation of optic nerve or neurosarcoid is MRI. The most informative is the gadolinium-enhanced T1-weighted sequence with fat suppression.[50] Images may show scleritis, nodules, or optic nerve sheath enhancement on MRI; sarcoidosis may have MRI characteristics that are very similar to pseudotumor, with enlargement of the extraocular muscles that may also resemble Graves' disease (Case 3).[38] The differential diagnosis of sarcoidosis should be included in patients with optic nerve enhancement on CT or MRI.

CASE 2: SCLERITIS

A 56-year-old man presents with a complaint of unilateral eye redness, pain, decreased vision, and double vision for 3 weeks. Similar episodes have occurred over the past 7 years and in both eyes. CT of the orbits was obtained (Fig. 7–3A and B). Findings were consistent with diffuse scleritis.

Discussion

The differential diagnosis of scleritis includes infectious and noninfectious causes. Noninfectious scleritis may be found in association with many systemic vasculitic diseases and the connective tissue diseases (polyarteritis nodosa [PAN], allergic granulomatous angiitis [Churg-Strauss syndrome], Wegener's granulomatosis, RA, SLE, Adamantiades-Behçet disease, giant cell arteritis, Cogan's syndrome, relapsing polychondritis) and seronegative spondyloarthropathies (ankylosing spondylitis, Reiter's syndrome, psoriatic arthritis, and inflammatory bowel disease). Scleritis in systemic vasculitic diseases may be a sign of poor general prognosis because it heralds potentially lethal systemic complications. The prognosis also depends on the specific systemic vasculitic disease.[51] RA is, by far, the most common systemic condition associated with scleritis.

Although autoimmune diseases are the main possibilities, other etiologies, such as infection are possible rare causes of scleritis. The most common infectious etiology is herpes zoster. Others include herpes simplex, tuberculosis, syphilis, toxocariasis, aspergillosis, and local infections. However, regardless of whether the scleral inflammation is associated with vasculitis or autoimmune diseases, follows surgical or accidental trauma, or is idiopathic, the pathologic morphology contains the same

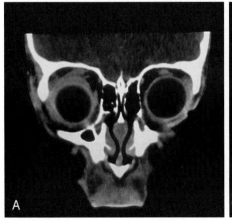
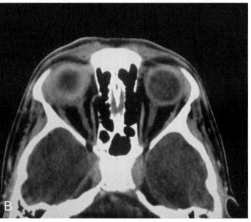

FIGURE 7–3. *A* and *B*, Diffuse scleritis of the right globe. Coronal and axial contrast-enhanced CT (CECT) scan shows thickening of the sclera with enhancement of the uveoscleral coat.

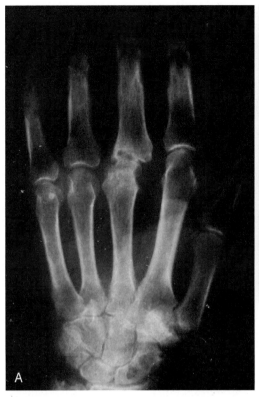
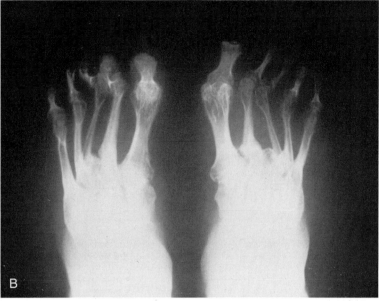

FIGURE 7–4. *A,* Rheumatoid arthritis. Radiograph of the hand demonstrates a symmetric process involving the radiocarpal, intercarpal and carpometacarpal joints. These changes, along with marginal erosions, are consistent with rheumatoid arthritis. The third metacarpal-phalangeal joint shows subchondral cyst formation and narrowed joint spaces. *B,* Juvenile rheumatoid arthritis. Radiograph of the feet demonstrates a bilateral symmetric process with intertarsal and tarsometatarsal joint destruction.

characteristics. Necrotizing scleritis shows chronic granulomatous inflammation.[18, 51]

On identification of scleritis by CT, ultrasound, or another imaging modality, further diagnostic testing, as described later, can be used to exclude, diagnose, or monitor the particular suspected disease. Evaluation of the retina, choroid, posterior scleral or extraocular muscle thickening, lacrimal gland enlargement, and sinus tissue involvement is important to distinguish posterior scleritis from orbital inflammatory diseases, trauma, and neoplasms.[18]

Juvenile Rheumatoid Arthritis and Rheumatoid Arthritis

JRA and RA are idiopathic disorders with chronic erosive synovitis in a symmetric distribution. Chronic uveitis is a hallmark manifestation in 14% to 17% of children with JRA.[52] Iridocyclitis seen in 10% to 50% of these patients with JRA is often insidious and may or may not be associated with the onset of joint pain, which may begin 5 to 10 years later.[53]

RA is thought to be an autoimmune disease with antibodies against the Fc receptor of immunoglobulin G (IgG). Extra-articular manifestations of disease include episcleritis, which is often benign and self-limited; scleritis, which is associated with a high rate of morbidity; and scleral inflammation that resembles rheumatoid nodules, potentially leading to scleromalacia perforans. The onset of necrotizing scleritis, the most severe type of scleritis, and peripheral ulcerative keratitis may indicate the presence of systemic, potentially lethal vasculitis.

Systemic disease severity and progression in JRA and RA can be documented by imaging.[25, 54] Baseline plain films are used to follow bone growth or damage and are not diagnostic nor specific, except to reveal late characteristic changes of articular damage with bone destruction, decreased joint space, and deformity (Fig. 7–4A and B). Cervical spine films may reveal the atlantoaxial subluxation associated with RA. MRI can be used to evaluate structural sequelae (erosion, cartilage damage, and tendon/ligament disruption) and inflammation (fibrovascular pannus and effusion).[55] Gallium lung scans are a controversial indicator of inflammation in rheumatic lung disease. Tc^{99m}-labeled human serum albumin (Tc^{99m}-HSA) is useful for imaging JRA. Bone densitometry dual-energy x-ray absorptiometry (DXA) permits evaluation of regional and whole-body bone mineral content and density, which is especially useful to follow patients treated chronically with corticosteroids.[25] UGI or BE may show gastritis and peptic ulcer disease, a major complication of nonsteroidal anti-inflammatory agents, and of corticosteroid administration, both of which may lead to significant morbidity and mortality if left undetected and untreated.

Vasculitides

Wegener's granulomatosis is thought to be a multisystemic immune-complex–mediated vasculitic disease characterized by necrotizing granulomas of the upper and lower respiratory tract, focal segmental glomerulonephritis, and systemic arteritis. Increased serum antineutrophil cytoplasmic antibodies are 90% specific for Wegener's

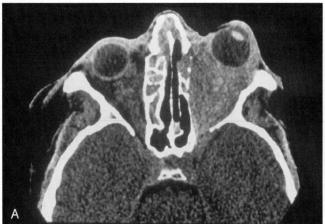 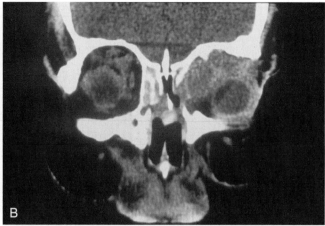

FIGURE 7–5. *A* and *B,* Wegener's granulomatosis of both orbits. A 3-mm axial and coronal CT of the left orbit after decompressive surgery of the medial and lateral orbital wall, with demonstrable mass effect in the orbit, left more than right. The left globe is proptotic secondary to a heterogenous mass, which extends posteriorly through the superior orbital fissure and into the middle cranial fossa. The optic nerve and extraocular muscles are all encased within the mass and are not identifiable as separate entities. A mass is present within the right orbit but the optic nerve, medial, and lateral rectus muscles can still be discerned. Slight irregularity of the globe could be related to scleritis.

granulomatosis, microscopic PAN, and crescentic glomerulonephritis.[56] The essential feature is the presence of bone destruction in the nose and paranasal sinuses without a large soft tissue mass (to differentiate Wegener's granulomatosis from malignancy). Eye involvement includes episcleritis, uveitis, and proptosis secondary to orbital granulomas in 40% to 50% of patients (Fig. 7–5A and B).[57, 58] The majority of patients have nonspecific or no plain film abnormalities. For those that do have CXR findings, nodules and infiltrates that cavitate may be seen. CT is optimal for visualization of bone destruction in the nose and paranasal sinuses and soft tissue orbital involvement. Granulations on MRI have a bright T2-weighted signal (enhance on T1 and T2 post gadolinium), whereas dense fibrous tissue have low T1- and T2-weighted signals on inversion recovery sequences. Common sites of biopsy are the nasal and sinus mucosa and orbit.[58] An inflammatory process (e.g., fungus or mycobacteria), angiocentric T-cell lymphoma, midline lethal granuloma syndrome or a poorly differentiated carcinoma, cocaine abuse, and Churg-Strauss syndrome should be a part of the differential diagnosis.

Other vasculitic diseases besides Wegener's granulomatosis include *Takayasu's arteritis,* which is a chronic vasculitis that involves the aorta and its branches. Arteriography generally confirms the diagnosis and shows smooth, tapered narrowing or occlusions or aneurysms of the aorta and its proximal branches. Digital subtraction angiography resolution is less distinct, with the vessel wall outlining a more restricted survey of the arterial tree; this study may occasionally be adequate. CT and MRI show luminal narrowing and mural thickening in vessels, which is useful support for the angiographic findings and for patient follow-up. A widened thoracic aorta may be detected on radiography.[56] PAN affects the small and medium-sized muscular arteries of any organ, even though peripheral involvement is most common. Mesenteric arteriography may be useful if there is abdominal pain, increased hepatic enzymes, and no readily identifiable and accessible biopsy site. There

are multiple arterial aneurysms, with segmental tapered narrowings and irregularities of the vessel walls and branch points. Ocular disease most commonly affects the choroidal vessels and can be the earliest presenting manifestation.[59, 60] These findings may be similar to those in Churg-Strauss syndrome, Wegener's granulomatosis, and SLE vasculitis and noninflammatory connective tissue disorders such as fibromuscular dysplasia. Giant cell (temporal) arteritis must also be included in the differential diagnosis of Wegener's granulomatosis, PAN, and amyloidosis.

Churg-Strauss syndrome is differentiated from PAN by the presence of lung involvement, which must then be separated from Löffler's syndrome, hypersensitivity vasculitis, and Wegener's granulomatosis. The CXR findings show patchy or nodular infiltrates of diffuse interstitial disease.[56] Abdominal angiography findings are similar to PAN. The diagnosis of *Adamantiades-Behçet disease* involves the presence of two mouth ulcers and two of the following: recurrent genital ulcers, eye lesions (anterior or posterior uveitis, retinal vasculitis), skin lesions (erythema nodosum, pseudofolliculitis, papulopustular lesions, acneiform nodules), or a positive pathergy test (pustule formation 24 to 48 hours after a skin test).[61]

Connective Tissue Diseases

Autoimmune production of antibodies to the cell nucleus components is characteristic of *SLE,* a disease with marked variability in clinical presentation affecting primarily young females. Eye manifestations involve the conjunctiva, sclera, or cornea, and cotton-wool spots and retinal hemorrhages from microangiopathy.[59] SLE patients with the chronic noninflammatory Jaccoud's arthritis usually do not have visible erosions or decreased articular space on plain films, even when subluxations are present (Fig. 7–6). Radionuclide imaging has not been uniformly helpful; however, positron emission tomography (PET) shows areas of low attenuation that may be due to disturbed cerebral circulation and metab-

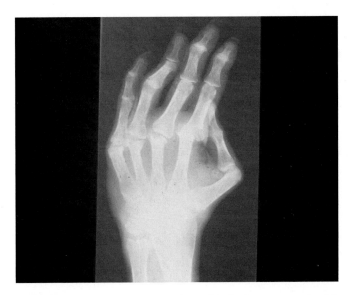

FIGURE 7–6. Lupus arthritis. Radiographic findings are compatible with the typically nonerosive lupus arthritis, Jaccoud's arthritis, with marked demineralization, marked narrowing of joint spaces, sclerosis, subluxation (ulnar deviation), and joint deformity (swan neck).

olism. Some patients may have CT findings of cerebral infarction, hemorrhage, and cortical atrophy and MRI findings of diffuse brain manifestations, including small focal areas of increased signal in the gray and white matter potentially due to inflammatory edema.[56] These findings may be followed after corticosteroid treatment.

Sjögren's syndrome is a chronic slowly progressive autoimmune exocrinopathy that results in lacrimal and salivary gland inflammation. Primary (sicca complex) disease manifests as keratoconjunctivitis sicca and xerostomia. Secondary Sjögren's syndrome is associated with connective tissue disease, including RA, SLE, scleroderma, polymyositis, and PAN. Lacrimal gland enlargement secondary to lymphoid cell infiltration is evident with imaging. Bilateral, symmetric lacrimal gland enlargement is seen in Sjögren's syndrome, sarcoidosis, lymphoproliferative disease, leukemia, nonspecific orbital inflammation, syphilis, and tuberculosis. Parotid sialography is abnormal in patients with Sjögren's syndrome who have xerostomia. Scintigraphy with Tc[99m] may show decreased activity relative to the thyroid, indicating delayed clearance of activity from the glands.[44] Biopsy of minor salivary glands of the lips establishes the diagnosis of Sjögren's syndrome.

Relapsing polychondritis is a recurring inflammatory disorder of unknown etiology, characterized by an inflammatory reaction in cartilaginous structures, including the nose, ears, trachea, and joints. Intraocular disease includes iridocyclitis and retinal vasculitis. Extraocular disease may involve periorbital edema, extraocular muscle palsy, conjunctivitis, keratitis, scleritis, episcleritis, and rarely, proptosis. CT is helpful in delineating tracheal and bronchial inflammatory changes in relapsing polychondritis; the presence of localized or diffuse strictures can also be evaluated. Tracheal involvement is serious, owing to the risk of collapse of the tracheal rings.[62, 63]

Crystal Disease

Gout is caused by the deposition of monosodium urate crystal in tissues, leading to nonspecific changes, such as soft tissue swelling, osteopenia, and joint effusion. Associated problems may include gouty arthritis, tophi, neuropathy, renal calculi, and eye findings. Tophi may occasionally manifest in the eyelids, cornea, and sclerae. The scleritis of gout must be differentiated from that caused by bacterial, fungal, or viral etiologies, and from diseases such as RA, PAN, SLE, and relapsing polychondritis. The eye may be acutely inflamed or show chronic crystal deposition in the cornea.[64]

Soft tissue nodules may be seen on plain film studies of the extremities but are usually not of any positive diagnostic value during the initial gouty attack.[65, 66] Plain films may be useful to exclude septic arthritis in more advanced cases, and chondrocalcinosis or calcific periarthritis, which may clinically resemble acute gouty arthritis.[59] The chronic tophaceous stage is manifest as disease with polyarticular tophi. Articular tophi of chronic later gout tends to produce irregular asymmetric soft tissue nodules that may calcify. Joint spaces are preserved until late stages. Advanced stages of gout have a similar appearance to osteoarthritis and RA with osseous round or oval, and well-circumscribed intra- or periarticular oval bony erosions with sclerotic margins (Fig. 7–7). Thin overhanging edges may be seen in about 40% of those with erosive changes.[67] Joint spaces and bone density is preserved until articular changes are advanced.

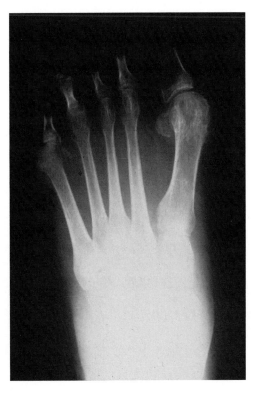

FIGURE 7–7. Gout. The left foot demonstrates radiographic findings of gout, with multiple subchondral cysts involving the first metacarpophalangeal joint as well as erosions involving the medial aspect of the distal first metatarsal heads with significant overlying soft tissue swelling.

TABLE 7–5. PLAIN FILM FINDINGS OF SERONEGATIVE SPONDYLOARTHROPATHIES

	ANKYLOSING SPONDYLITIS	PSORIATIC ARTHRITIS	REITER'S SYNDROME	INFLAMMATORY BOWEL DISEASE
Enthesopathy	Yes	Yes	Yes	Yes
Sacroiliitis	Yes	Yes	Yes	Yes
Spondylitis	Yes	Yes	Yes	Yes
Osteopenia	Yes	No	No	
Location	Axial	Asymmetric, appendicular	Asymmetric, appendicular	Axial, less often appendicular
Extraskeletal manifestations	Aortic Insufficiency, cauda equina syndrome			
Keywords	Osteitis pubis, pseudoarthrosis, Romanus' lesions or shiny corners, vertebral body squaring, bamboo spine, sausage digits, Anderson's lesion, stress fracture, whiskering	Ivory phalanx, pencil in cup, fluffy bone formation, "mouse ears," sausage digits, distal interphalangeal joint erosive disease	Sausage digits, asymmetric comma-shaped ossification (also in psoriasis), fluffy and linear periostitis	Sausage digits

CASE 3: SUSPECTED SERONEGATIVE SPONDYLOARTHROPATHIES

A 32-year-old HLA-B27–positive man presented with uveitis and low back pain. Sacroiliac films were negative. A bone scan revealed increased uptake in both sacroiliac joints, compatible with sacroiliitis.

Discussion

The seronegative spondyloarthropathies include ankylosing spondylitis, Reiter's syndrome, psoriatic arthritis, and arthritis associated with inflammatory bowel disease (IBD). These diseases have in common HLA-B27 association. Anterior uveitis is seen in 20% to 30% of patients with psoriasis, 2% to 11.8% of those with idiopathic IBD, and in 25% to 30% of patients with ankylosing spondylitis.[52, 64, 68–70]

Enthesitis, inflammation at insertion sites of tendons or ligaments, results in bony and fibrocartilage proliferation, and finally, ankylosis or ossification of adjacent bones. There is a spinal predilection that manifests as spondylitis and sacroiliitis, the pathologic hallmark, and the earliest and most consistent finding. These bony changes of sacroiliitis, spondylitis and enthesopathy are eventually seen on plain films, which can be used to help differentiate the seronegative spondyloarthropathies (Table 7–5), for example, from psoriasis (Fig. 7–8). Patients with other diseases, including relapsing polychondritis, Adamantiades-Behçet disease, and Whipple's disease, also may have sacroiliitis and spondylitis.

CT is more sensitive than MRI or plain films for the detection of bony disease; and technetium bone scan-

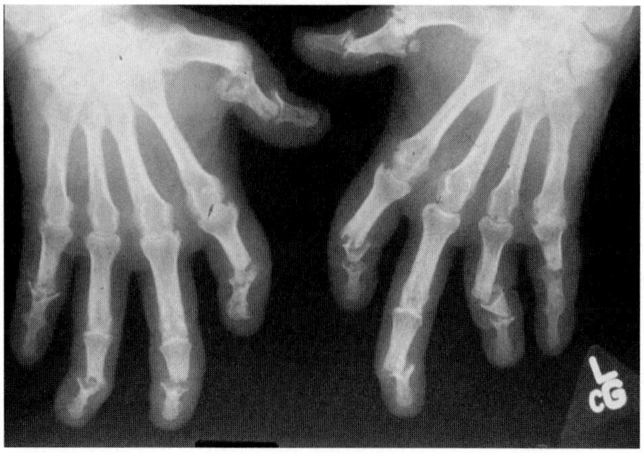

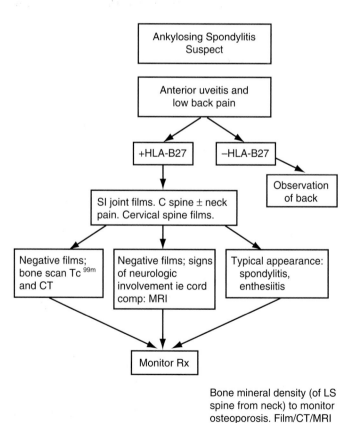

FIGURE 7–8. Psoriasis. Radiograph of both hands shows distal interphalangeal erosive disease with terminal whittling of the fourth and fifth proximal phalanges and "pencil-in-cup" appearance. There is marked soft tissue swelling.

FIGURE 7–9. Diagnostic algorithm for suspected ankylosing spondylitis.

Ankylosing Spondylitis Suspect
↓
Anterior uveitis and low back pain
↓
+HLA-B27 / –HLA-B27
–HLA-B27 → Observation of back
+HLA-B27 →
SI joint films. C spine ± neck pain. Cervical spine films.
↓
Negative films; bone scan Tc 99m and CT
Negative films; signs of neurologic involvement ie cord comp: MRI
Typical appearance: spondylitis, enthesiitis
↓
Monitor Rx

Bone mineral density (of LS spine from neck) to monitor osteoporosis. Film/CT/MRI to dx, follow complications.

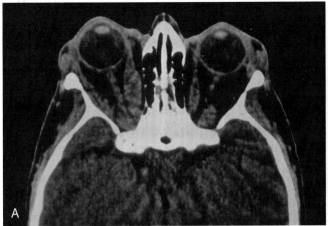

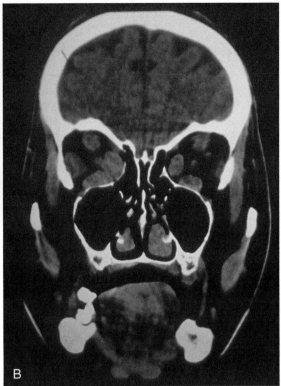

FIGURE 7–10. *A* and *B*, Graves' ophthalmopathy. Axial and coronal sections through the orbits demonstrate enlargement of the extraocular muscles (not superior oblique and not left lateral rectus) primarily involving the central belly portions and not their tendinous insertions. Significant proptosis and right optic nerve compression near the apex of the orbit is present. These findings are compatible with Graves' ophthalmopathy.

ning can detect early sacroiliitis before plain film or CT scan changes occur (Case 3) (Fig. 7–9). MRI is preferable to evaluate stress fractures that may cause spinal cord compression and cauda equina syndrome, and to show the findings of enthesitis. UGI or BE is used to evaluate mucosal lesions caused by the inflammatory bowel disorders.

Case 4: Pseudotumor versus Graves' Disease

In this case, two examples of patients with Graves' disease are provided (Fig. 7–10A and B). Also, Graves' disease after orbital decompression is examined in another patient (Fig. 7–11A and B), and a third patient with pseudotumor (Fig. 7–12).

Discussion
Graves' Disease

Graves' disease is an autoimmune disease affecting the thyroid gland, extraocular muscles of the eyes, and the skin. Eye disease results from swollen enlarged extraocular muscles, up to but not including the tendinous attachments, resulting in eyelid retraction, corneal exposure, proptosis, diplopia, and optic neuropathy.[71] MRI is more reliable than CT for imaging the optic nerve at the orbital apex in Graves' optic neuropathy. Compression of the optic nerve by enlargement of the extraocular muscles or fat causes ischemia and inflammation, which is relieved by orbital decompression (see Fig. 7–11A and B).[72] The Werner classification describes patients with Graves' disease who are more likely to

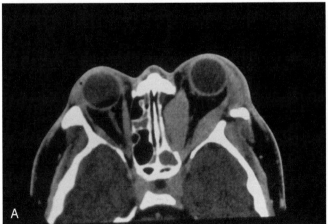

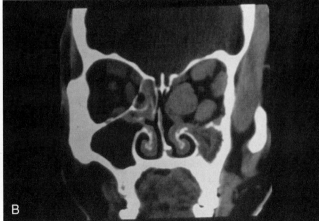

FIGURE 7–11. *A* and *B*, Graves' disease after orbital decompression. Axial and coronal CT images reveal enlargement of almost all extraocular muscle bellies and sparing of the tendinous insertions. Surgical defects are seen in the medial, inferior, and lateral orbital walls of the left orbit statuspost orbital decompression.

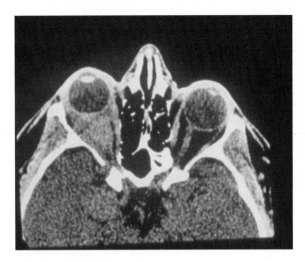

FIGURE 7–12. Pseudotumor. Axial orbit CT showing intracranial mass effect up to the right orbital apex.

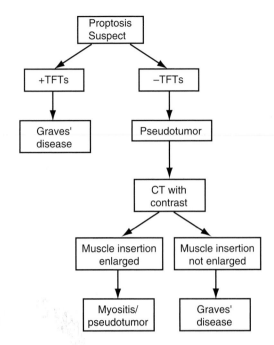

FIGURE 7–13. Diagnostic algorithm for suspected proptosis.

have fat effacement (measure of optic nerve compression) and minimal optic neuritis index (measure of optic nerve thickness).[73] Other than optic nerve imaging, CT and MR are about the same in terms of excellence for imaging Graves' disease. CT shows muscle enlargement even in the early stages of disease. In Graves' orbitopathy, as opposed to orbital myositis, tendinous insertions are not enlarged.[74] B-scan and MRI can also show muscle enlargement but provide no advantage over CT (see Fig 7–11).[71]

Orbital Pseudotumor

A diagnosis of exclusion, orbital pseudotumor represents nongranulomatous inflammation in the orbital soft tissues or eye.[58] The differential diagnosis includes sarcoidosis, Wegener's granulomatosis, Grave's ophthalmopathy, infection, masquerade syndromes, connective tissue diseases, Erdheim-Chester disease, and vasculitis. Unilateral orbital structure enlargement is seen as an infiltrating or, less often, masslike inflammation on CT or MRI. Enlargement of the extraocular muscles simulates Graves' disease except that the enlargement may include some of the tendinous insertions (Fig. 7–13). Pseudotumor may also extend beyond the orbit as an infiltrating mass. It may go beyond the superior orbital fissure to the cavernous sinus or through the inferior orbital fissure to the pterygopalatine fossa (see Fig. 7–12). Pseudotumor may also cause enlargement of the lacrimal glands. The MRI characteristics of pseudotumor are like sarcoidosis.

CASE 5: MASQUERADE SYNDROMES

A 66-year-old man presents with uveitis. A large cell lymphoma masquerade syndrome is suspected (Fig. 7–14).

Discussion

Both CT and MRI may uncover tumor in a patient presenting with uveitis. The masquerade syndromes are a group of diseases that may infiltrate the eye and present as ocular inflammation. This group includes the lymphoproliferative disorders, metastases (Fig. 7–15A

and B), MS, intraocular foreign bodies, retinal detachment, childhood carcinomas (retinoblastoma, leukemia, medulloepithelioma, juvenile xanthogranuloma) (Fig. 7–16), and uveal melanoma.[75–77] CT and MRI should be performed with contrast to enhance visualization of infiltration, hyperplasia, or mass; the principle use of imaging is to identify and monitor tumor extension (Fig. 7–17).[5, 6] Bone windows on CT may reveal any bony destruction and intralesional calcium that favors retinoblastoma. MR has been added to the CT and ultrasound armamentarium to diagnose intraocular lesions. MRI, which should include T1 pre- and postgadolinium enhancement with fat suppression, T2-weighted sequences

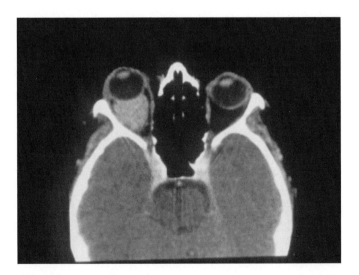

FIGURE 7–14. Large cell lymphoma masquerade. Axial contrast-enhanced CT of the midglobe demonstrates an enhancing soft tissue mass encasing the optic nerve.

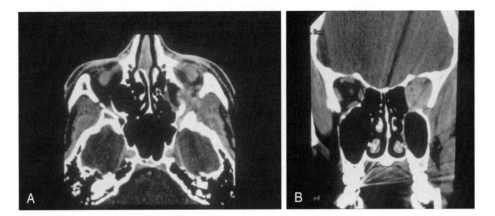

FIGURE 7–15. *A* and *B*, Metastases. Axial and coronal CT with tumor extending to the left pterygopalatine fossa.

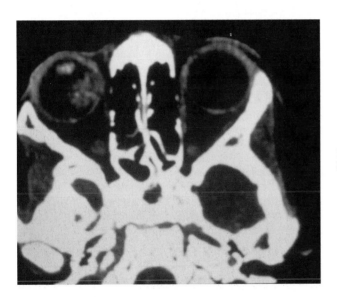

FIGURE 7–16. Retinoblastoma. Axial CT image of a large calcified intraocular mass in the vitreous chamber deforming and expanding the right globe.

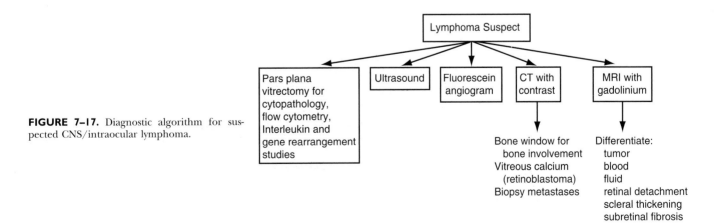

FIGURE 7–17. Diagnostic algorithm for suspected CNS/intraocular lymphoma.

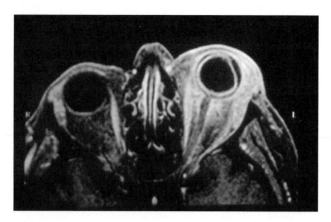

FIGURE 7–18. Choroidal detachment. Axial T1-weighted images with fat saturation after IV administration of contrast reveals marked left eye proptosis, diffuse soft tissue enhancement, and choroidal detachment.

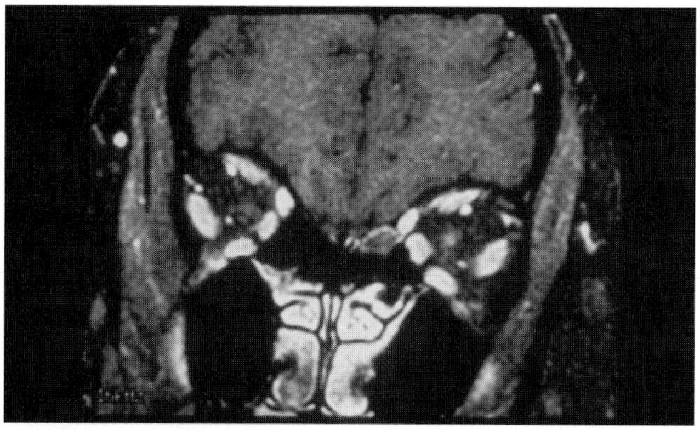

FIGURE 7–19. Multiple sclerosis. Coronal T1-weighted MRI post-gadolinium showing left-greater-than-right optic neuritis with optic nerve enhancement.

in axial, coronal, and perhaps, sagittal images, to permit differentiation of tumor from hemorrhage (variable depending on iron metabolism [see Table 7–3]) and fluid collections (dark/intermediate on T1; bright on T2).

Even though both MRI and CT are sensitive for detecting orbital lesions, MRI is somewhat more specific. MRI shows retinal detachment and scleral thickening, subretinal fluid, Tenon's capsule, orbital, and intracranial and optic disk tumor invasion to better advantage. Therefore, MRI is valuable in differentiating uveal melanoma from associated subretinal effusion, choroidal hemangioma, choroidal metastases, hemorrhagic, and serous detachments (Fig. 7–18).[5, 6, 78, 79] Uveal melanomas, which may masquerade as uveitis, have characteristic signal secondary to the paramagnetic properties of melanin causing reduction of both T1- and T2-weighted relaxation times.[7, 10, 16, 22, 79–81] This then results in bright T1 and dark T2 images compared with the vitreous body, except for the amelanotic melanomas.[1, 80] Amelanotic lesions lack melanin granules that aid in delineation of this tumor.

Fluorescein angiography and ultrasonography are also useful adjuncts to these other imaging modalities for intraocular disease. These tests are useful, for example, to differentiate a masquerade syndrome from Coats' disease, which is an idiopathic disorder characterized by retinal telangiectasias that eventually progress to massive subretinal exudation and detachment, associated with rubeosis iridis, subretinal mass, uveitis, cataract, phthisis bulbi, and neovascular glaucoma, and must be differentiated from retinoblastoma by MRI, CT, or ultrasound.[21, 77]

Imaging findings are also important for the differentiation of these diseases from orbital pseudotumor. MRI is helpful in differentiating orbital pseudotumor and metastases, which are slightly bright on T1-weighted images and slightly dark on T2-weighted images relative to the vitreous and are moderately enhanced with gadolinium.[82] Metastatic orbital CT diagnosis is based primarily on CT findings and biopsy.[82] Goldberg and associates have organized typical findings of metastatic disease into four groups: (1) a mass lesion often contiguous with other structures (e.g., bone and muscle); (2) diffuse enhancement of orbital tissue, loss of normal architec-

ture, and enophthalmos (breast cancer); (3) primarily bone involvement (e.g., prostate and thyroid carcinoma); and (4) primarily muscle involvement with enlargement and often a nodular appearance (e.g., melanoma and breast cancer).[83]

MS is a relapsing and remitting demyelinating central nervous system (CNS) disorder of unknown etiology. Ocular abnormalities are common, including optic neuritis (Fig. 7–19), retrobulbar neuritis, chiasmal and retrochiasmal demyelination, oculomotor abnormalities (internuclear ophthalmoplegia, skew deviation, dysmetria, nystagmus, and cranial nerve palsies).[84] MRI is one of the best ways to aid diagnosis of MS because it is more sensitive in detecting demyelinating lesions, especially T2-weighted FLAIR or STIR sequences, than CT (Fig. 7–20). MRI is also useful for detecting active disease in patients with relapsing-remitting disease.[85] Systematic studies have shown that MRI is positive in 70% to 95%

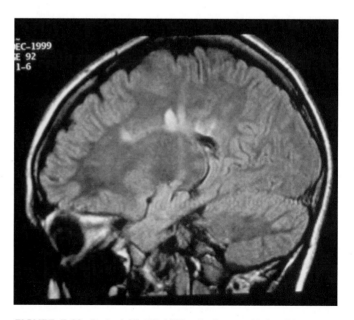

FIGURE 7–20. Sagittal FLAIR MRI revealing multiple white matter increased signal, some of which are oriented perpendicular to the ventricular system (so-called Dawson's fingers). Extensive involvement of the corpus callosum is present.

TABLE 7–6. APPROPRIATE IMAGING STUDIES FOR VARIOUS SUSPECTED INFLAMMMATORY DISEASES

| SUSPECTED DISEASE | MRI | | CT SCAN | | GALLIUM SCAN | TECHNETIUM SCAN |
	With Gadolinium	Without Gadolinium	With Contrast	Without Contrast		
Sarcoidosis		√		√	√	
CNS lymphoma	√	√	√	√		
Wegener's granulomatosis				√		
Ankylosing spondylitis			√			√
Multiple sclerosis	√	√				

of patients with clinically definite MS.[86–88] Dissemination in time can be demonstrated in follow-up scans.[89] Failure to find white matter lesions in patients with clinical symptoms does not rule out MS.[84] MRI is not specific for MS.[89]

Table 7–6 summarizes the most appropriate imaging strategies for a few of the masquerade and inflammatory disorders one might encounter in the case of patients with uveitis.

FLUORESCEIN AND INDOCYANINE GREEN ANGIOGRAPHY

Angiography of the retinal and choroidal circulation is second in importance only to stereoscopic biomicroscopy in the evaluation of posterior segment disorders. Its value cannot be overstated in the management of ocular inflammatory diseases. In this section, we contrast the differences between fluorescein and indocyanine green angiography (ICGA), and show examples of their usefulness. Readers unfamiliar with the basics of interpretation are referred to an outstanding monograph published by the American Academy of Ophthalmology.[90]

The technique of fluorescein angiography (FA) was introduced 40 years ago by MacLean and Maumenee.[90, 91] In the past two decades, the technique has helped define inflammatory disorders such as acute multifocal placoid pigment epitheliopathy, multiple evanescent white dot syndrome (MEWDS), Harada's disease, and serpiginous choroidopathy. The technique of ICGA was introduced

by Flower and Hochheimer in the early 1970s and was adapted to digital imaging by Yannuzzi and others in the late 1980s and early 1990s. Although our ability to interpret ICGA is still limited, it has advanced our understanding of such conditions as birdshot retinochoroidopathy (BSRC) and the subtypes of choroidal neovascularization.[92–94]

Both fluorescein and indocyanine green respect the blood-retinal barriers found at the retinal pigment epithelium (RPE) and retinal vessels. The functional differences between the two dyes depend on their affinity for serum proteins and the wavelengths of emitted light.

Fluorescein absorbs light with a wavelength of 465 to 490 nm and emits light with a wavelength of 520 to 530 nm.[90, 95] If appropriate filters are used, only the emitted light will be detected. Approximately 80% of fluorescein binds to serum proteins, meaning that 20% freely traverses the fenestrated choriocapillaris and Bruch's membrane. The resulting diffuse fluorescence from the sub-pigment epithelial space prohibits evaluation of the large choroidal vessels.

Visible pigment found in blood and pigment epithelium absorbs much of the light emitted from the choriocapillaris. Hence, the retinal vasculature can normally be visualized in exquisite detail on a background of relative choroidal hypofluorescence. The slightest inflammation of the retinal vessels will alter their endothelial tight junctions and allow fluorescein to impregnate the vessel wall and surrounding tissues, well before the inflammation can be seen clinically (Fig. 7–21).[95, 96] Fine defects of

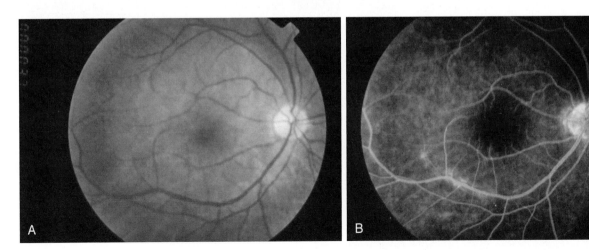

FIGURE 7–21. Idiopathic uveitis and retinal vasculitis. *A*, Fundus photo shows minimal dilation of the inferotemporal macular vein that may be overlooked. *B*, The FA demonstrates segmental staining, confirming a focus of vasculitis.

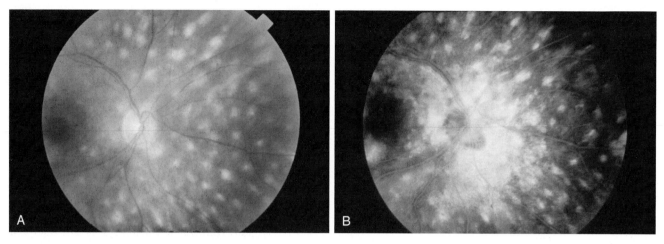

FIGURE 7–22. Chronic inactive birdshot retinochoroidopathy *A,* Note the numerous atrophic, white, oval chorioretinal lesions, most prominently nasal to the disc. *B,* On FA, the lesions manifest as sharply defined window defects.

the RPE barrier that are not otherwise visible may be recorded. For example, atrophic spots that are often a sequela of inflammatory nodules appear as sharply defined hyperfluorescent transmission defects during early dye transit (Fig. 7–22). Choroidal new vessels that have broken through Bruch's membrane into the sub-RPE or subretinal space fill with dye early; they have a characteristic pattern of hyperfluorescence with fuzzy margins that expands through the transit into reperfusion (Fig. 7–23).

The accumulation of blood, fibrin, or pigment will

necessarily prevent study of any underlying structures by FA. This limitation is avoided by indocyanine green, which operates in the infrared range.[90, 93] ICG absorbs light maximally around 790 nm and emits around 830 nm. Pigmented tissues have little, if any, impact on its transmission. Furthermore, a full 98% of the dye is rapidly bound to plasma proteins, and it remains in the circulation until it is excreted unchanged by the liver. (Fluorescein is mostly eliminated after its first passage through the kidneys and is not detected by angiography

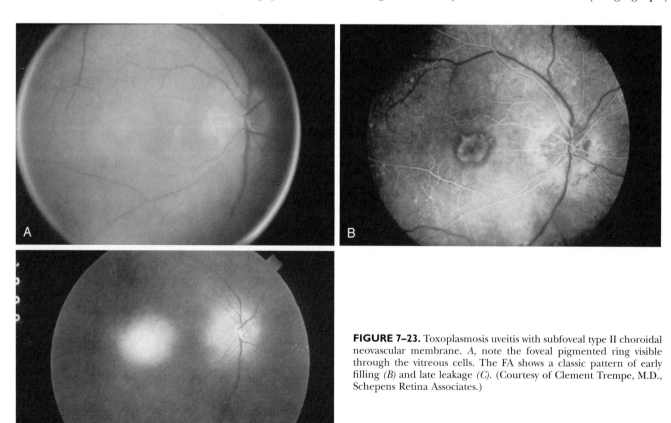

FIGURE 7–23. Toxoplasmosis uveitis with subfoveal type II choroidal neovascular membrane. *A,* note the foveal pigmented ring visible through the vitreous cells. The FA shows a classic pattern of early filling *(B)* and late leakage *(C).* (Courtesy of Clement Trempe, M.D., Schepens Retina Associates.)

after the second pass.) This high protein binding prevents it from easily passing through the walls of the choriocapillaris. A slow study of the choroidal circulation unfolds, allowing visualization of filling patterns of the large vessels and points of protein leakage in the choriocapillaris.[90, 96, 97] ICGA has great potential in the evaluation of inflammation or ischemia of the large and small choroidal vasculature, and space-occupying lesions of the choroidal stroma. Indeed, there is a growing literature describing ICG angiographic features of inflammatory choroidopathies. Because small disturbances of the retinal vessels or RPE do not alter the transmission properties of ICG, it is a poor marker for inflammation in these areas.

In the contemporary management of ocular inflammatory diseases, retinal and choroidal angiography has three roles: (1) the diagnosis of conditions with stereotypic findings on FA or ICGA; (2) the identification of macular complications of anterior or posterior uveitis, such as cystoid macular edema, retinal or choroidal ischemia, choroidal neovascularization, or epiretinal membranes; and (3) the detection of subtle retinal vasculopathy or choroidopathy that may be more apparent on angiography than on clinical examination. Following are categories of diseases in which FA and ICGA have characteristic findings that can be helpful in diagnosis.

Acute Posterior Multifocal Placoid Pigment Epitheliopathy

In 1968, Gass described acute posterior multifocal placoid pigment epitheliopathy (APMPPE), a syndrome of young, otherwise healthy patients who develop rapid loss of vision in one or both eyes from multiple flat, circumscribed, gray-white subretinal lesions in the posterior pole.[95] Some patients have associated viral syndromes or systemic autoimmune phenomena, including thyroiditis, cerebral vasculitis, episcleritis, and Wegener's granulomatosis.[95, 98, 99]

In the acute phase of APMPPE, the FA shows a characteristic pattern of blocked fluorescence in a sharply defined area corresponding to the active white lesions.[95, 100] Mid- and late-phase angiograms demonstrate diffuse, even staining of the acute lesions (Fig. 7–24). Typically, these lesions resolve spontaneously over weeks, with a delayed but reliable improvement in visual acuity to a subnormal level.[95] In its wake, there are variable degrees of RPE atrophy that manifest as geographic hyperfluorescent window defects. These defects may be accompanied by corresponding field defects.

The ICG angiogram in acute APMPPE shows marked choroidal hypofluorescence in the distribution of the lesion, especially in the late phases.[100, 101] The underlying large choroidal vessels are well visualized, suggesting that the choriocapillaris is responsible for the hypofluorescence. In healed APMPPE, a smaller and more clearly delineated area of hypofluorescence persists. These findings have revived a debate. Does inflammatory debris and cloudiness of the cytoplasm of the RPE cause blockage of fluorescence, or is there transient occlusion of the choroidal arterioles that creates a filling defect? The idea of transient occlusion is not consistent with the good visual recovery usually seen, whereas the idea of the blockage

of fluoescence does not explain the persistence of hypofluorescence in the healed phase of the ICGA. Park, Schatz, and coauthors have suggested a theory of partial or relative choroidal vascular obstruction, which is compatible with the angiographic findings and clinical behavior.[100, 102]

Serpiginous Choroiditis

An inflammatory condition of the inner choroid and RPE closely resembling APMPPE is serpiginous choroiditis, also known as geographic choroiditis or helicoid peripapillary choroidopathy. By angiographic criteria, the two conditions cannot be distinguished in the acute phase.[95] Both show hypofluorescence in the early transit and late staining, although the staining is more likely to begin at the edge of the lesion in serpiginous. Also serpiginous is more likely to begin in the peripapillary area and to spread centrifugally over months to years in a series of recurrent episodes.[95] FA should show heavier leakage at the active margins. The convalescent stage is associated with deeper atrophy of the RPE that often includes the choriocapillaris and is associated with permanent field defects (Fig. 7–25). The extent of destruction determines the characteristics on FA. Deep lesions that eliminate the choriocapillaris become hypofluorescent early, whereas RPE defects transmit early. In both cases, there is late scleral staining.

On ICG angiography, active serpiginous lesions display marked hypofluorescence throughout the study.[103] The borders of the lesion are poorly defined early, becoming sharp late. Some lesions are surrounded by a faint rim of hyperfluorescence. The deeper and larger choroidal vessels are not seen in the lesion, possibly owing to a filling defect. Some arteries seem to vanish at the edge of the lesions. In the healed phase, there may be delayed choroidal filling, but the patches of hypofluorescence resolve, at least partially and the deep choroidal vessels are better visualized.[103]

If the macula is spared as the disease spreads in its serpentine path, it is unlikely to be involved later. Nonetheless, the patient may not infrequently be robbed of central vision by late expansion of pigment epithelial atrophy or by growth of a type II choroidal neovascular membrane at the edge of the scar. FA is most useful in distinguishing this situation from a new focus of active chorioretinitis, which is critical in the management paradigm (see Fig. 7–25). In some patients, the choroidal lesions may follow the distribution of the major retinal veins, and a rare patient may develop an obliterative retinal vasculitis with neovascularization.[95, 103] The notion of a herpetic etiology for this condition is still debated, but numerous authors have treated successfully with immunosuppression alone.

Multiple Evanescent White-Dot Syndrome

MEWDS was described in 1984 independently by Jampol and associates[104] in the United States and by Takeda and colleagues[105] in Japan. The typical patient is a young woman who presents with acute monocular blurring of central vision, bothersome photopsias, paracentral scotomas or enlargement of the blind spot, and headaches.

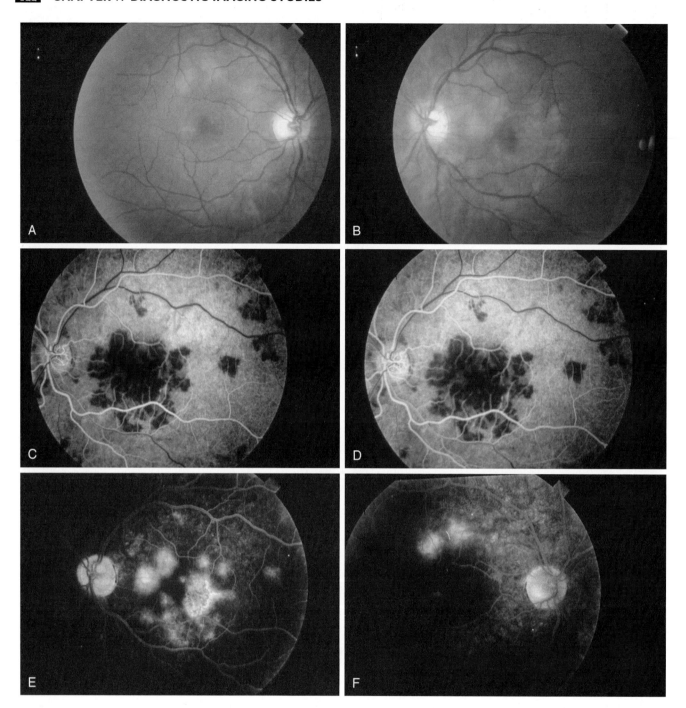

FIGURE 7–24. Acute posterior multifocal placoid pigment epitheliopathy. *A* and *B*, note the plaquelike lesions at the level of the RPE in both eyes. *C* and *D*, FA transit of the left eye shows absence of choroidal fluorescence at the lesions due to blockage by edematous RPE cells or nonfilling of the choriocapillaris. *E* and *F*, There is late staining of the active lesions in both eyes.

Symptoms resolve spontaneously over 2 months. The ophthalmoscopic findings can be easily overlooked. These findings may include mild anterior chamber and vitreous cells, mild disc edema, and multiple transient small white patches in the temporal macula and posterior pole at the level of the RPE. The fovea is spared of these patches but displays granularity of its RPE and often a cluster of tiny white or orange dots.[95, 104] FA of the white patches shows early wreathlike punctate hyperfluorescent lesions, which are more numerous than seen on fundus examination.

Late in the FA, the lesions and the optic disc show increased staining (Fig. 7–26).

ICGA in the acute phase of MEWDS is characteristic, with numerous hypofluorescent spots throughout the posterior pole and periphery at about 10 minutes.[106] These spots are larger than those seen on FA. In some patients, there is a ring of hypofluorescence around the optic nerve that seems to correlate with the presence of blind-spot enlargement.[106] Patients with MEWDS may be at risk for the subsequent development of multifocal cho-

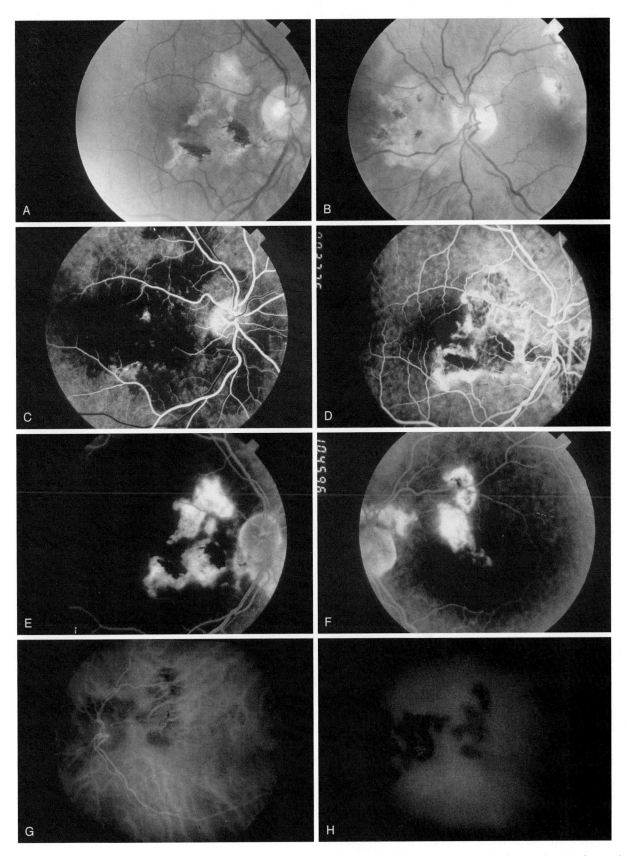

FIGURE 7–25. Bilateral chronic serpiginous choroiditis. *A* and *B,* Note the peripapillary chorioretinal scars, some having pigment clumps. A gray fibrotic neovascular membrane is present inferior to the fovea in the right eye *(A).* Early FA of the right eye shows hypofluorescence in the distribution of the lesion *(C).* Later in the transit, the staining begins at the edge of the lesion *(D).* Staining is most intense at the neovascular membrane, which could be confused for a site of reactivation. *E* and *F,* In the reperfusion stage, the hyperfluorescence persists in both eyes and has expanded from the edges to fill the lesions. *G* and *H,* Note the corresponding jigsaw pattern of hypoflorescent patches in all phases of the ICGA.

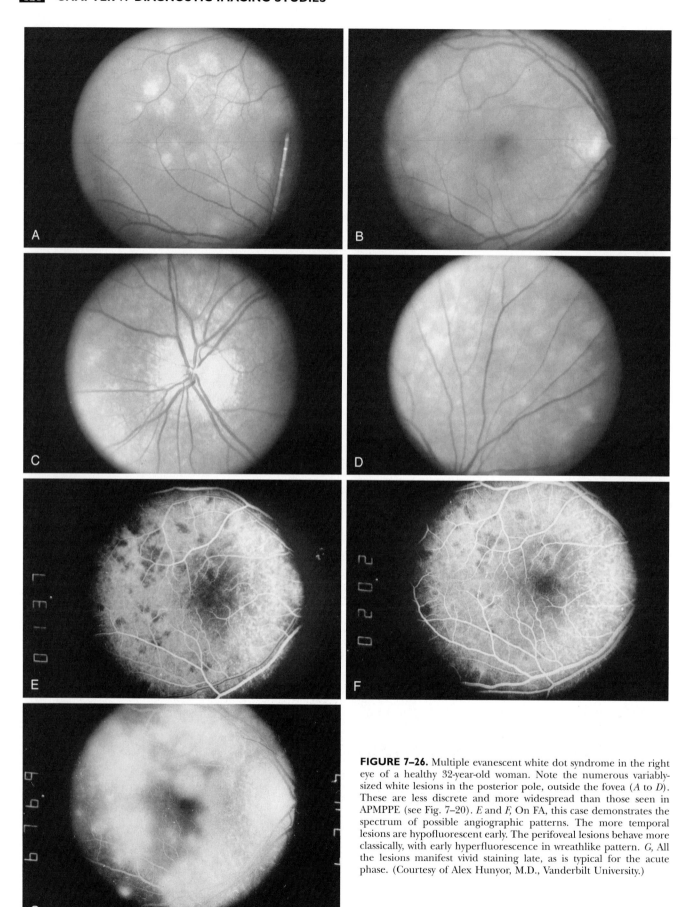

FIGURE 7–26. Multiple evanescent white dot syndrome in the right eye of a healthy 32-year-old woman. Note the numerous variably-sized white lesions in the posterior pole, outside the fovea (*A* to *D*). These are less discrete and more widespread than those seen in APMPPE (see Fig. 7–20). *E* and *F,* On FA, this case demonstrates the spectrum of possible angiographic patterns. The more temporal lesions are hypofluorescent early. The perifoveal lesions behave more classically, with early hyperfluorescence in wreathlike pattern. *G,* All the lesions manifest vivid staining late, as is typical for the acute phase. (Courtesy of Alex Hunyor, M.D., Vanderbilt University.)

roiditis and panuveitis, punctate inner choroidopathy, or acute zonal occult outer retinopathy.

Harada's Disease and Sympathetic Uveitis

Harada's disease and sympathetic uveitis are both T–cell mediated, diffuse or multifocal granulomatous inflammations of the choroid. A preponderance of lymphocytes, plasma cells, and giant cells is seen on histology of both conditions.[95] There may be more involvement of the choriocapillaris in Harada's disease. Both types of patients present with vitritis or iridocyclitis and commonly lose vision from serous retinal detachments. In the early stages, especially in lightly pigmented individuals, both groups may display scattered, gray-white nodules at the level of the RPE (Dalen-Fuchs nodules, Fig. 7–27). These can resemble lesions of APMPPE, although the lesions of APMPPE tend to be larger and less sharply defined.[95, 107] After resolution of the exudative detachment, both Harada's and sympathetic uveitis leave RPE defects that may be patchy or linear (see Figs. 7–27 and 7–28). These defects manifest as hyperfluorescent window defects on FA and set the stage for late choroidal neovascularization.

The history is paramount in distinguishing these processes. Patients with Harada's disease are usually heavily pigmented, often Asian, Latino, or Native American, and may develop neurologic or cutaneous manifestations such as headaches, nausea, paresthesias, dysacousis, poliosis, vitiligo, alopecia, or localizing neurologic defects (Vogt-Koyanagi-Harada Disease). Patients with sympathetic uveitis have, by definition, a previous history of ocular injury, either traumatic or surgical.

Fluorescein angiography in both conditions demonstrates a delay in choroidal perfusion, with possible blockage created by the choroidal infiltrate. On this background, there are multiple pinpoint areas of fluorescein leakage from the RPE, giving a picture sometimes described as a "starry night." The points of hyperfluorescence expand, pooling into the subretinal space in areas of serous detachment. The fluorescence increases during the recirculation phase and progressively outlines the extent of the detachment (Figs. 7–28 and 7–29). In those without detachment, it is easier to see patchy staining of infiltrates at the inner choroid and RPE in a cobblestone pattern. Leakage at the optic disc and perivenous staining are also common. Similar angiographic findings may occur in posterior scleritis or lymphoma.

In these conditions, ICGA typically shows hypofluorescent spots in the early and midphases, correlating in location with the subretinal nodules.[107–109] These spots are most numerous posteriorly, in excess of those seen clinically and on FA.[107, 108] They may obscure filling of the large choroidal vessels. Whether these areas represent filling defects or blockage caused by infiltrates is subject to debate. The late ICGA findings vary with the stage

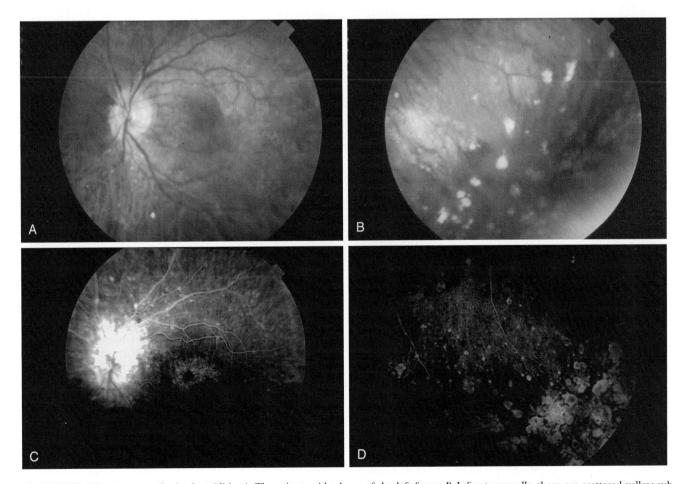

FIGURE 7–27. Chronic sympathetic choroiditis. *A,* There is cystoid edema of the left fovea. *B,* Inferotemporally, there are scattered yellow sub-RPE Dalen-Fuchs nodules. *C* and *D,* FA shows a petaloid pattern of foveal leakage diagnostic of CME and late staining of the nodules.

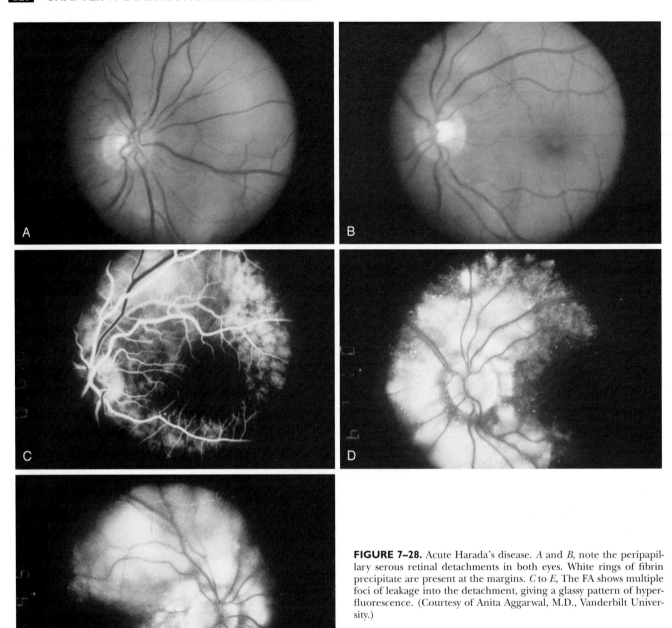

FIGURE 7–28. Acute Harada's disease. *A* and *B,* note the peripapillary serous retinal detachments in both eyes. White rings of fibrin precipitate are present at the margins. *C* to *E,* The FA shows multiple foci of leakage into the detachment, giving a glassy pattern of hyperfluorescence. (Courtesy of Anita Aggarwal, M.D., Vanderbilt University.)

of disease. In those with acute and active disease, the hypofluorescent spots may fade and be replaced with ill-defined areas of hyperfluorescence that do not necessarily correlate with the areas of detachment or choroidal nodules.[107, 108] Resolution of disease is met with disappearance of the areas of late hyperfluorescence. In a minority of cases with a serous retinal detachment, there is an impressive area of late hypofluorescence whose margins outline the detachment.[109–111]

Posterior Scleritis

Often related to RA, posterior scleritis may occur in focal or diffuse forms. Approximately 15% of cases are limited to the posterior potions of the globe and present with

pain, choroidal thickening, and an exudative retinal detachment. There may be one or several foci of white subretinal exudates that resemble Dalen-Fuchs nodules of sympathetic uveitis or Harada's disease. If it is exuberant, the inflammatory response may lead to a subretinal hypopyon or an expanding subretinal mass.[95] Choroidal effusions may occur in chronic cases. Ultrasonography is most useful in demonstrating thickening of the sclera and choroid. FA shows small foci of leakage at the RPE, again similar to Harada's disease but localized to the area of inflammation.[112] Choroidal melanoma may give similar findings on FA but is differentiated by the absence of scleral thickening or Tenon's edema on ultrasound.

Auer and colleagues performed ICGA on eight pa-

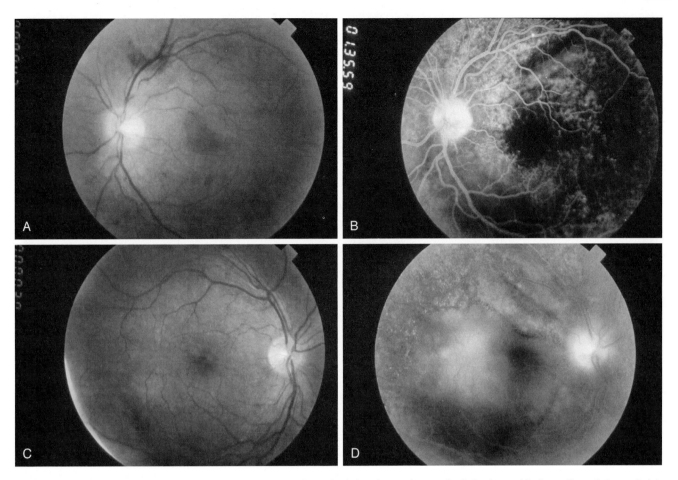

FIGURE 7–29. Resolving Harada's disease. *A,* In the left eye, the retinal detachment has resolved, leaving residual mottling of the underlying RPE. *B,* This is manifest as window defects on FA. *C* and *D,* In the right eye, a small amount of fluid remains in the macula, seen as late leakage on the FA.

tients with posterior scleritis.[113] All showed zonal hyperfluorescence in the mid and late phases, which regressed at least partially after treatment. Five of eight had early hypofluorescent dark dots, smaller and more irregular in distribution than those seen in patients with Harada's disease. They disappeared by the late frames. A delay in choroidal filling was also noted in five patients. The authors found ICGA to be useful in the diagnosis and monitoring of these patients.

Adamantiades-Behçet Retinal Vasculitis

Adamantiades-Behçet disease is a multiorgan inflammation of small vessels and a major cause of blindness in Japan and the Mediterranean basin.[114] Systemic features include aphthous ulcers of the mouth and genitalia, erythema nodosum, cerebral vasculitis, and uveitis. Approximately 50% of patients manifest some form of retinal vasculitis.[114] This condition can be associated with focal areas of necrotizing retinitis, arterial and venous occlusion, papillitis, and retinal neovascularization. FA is ideal for outlining areas of capillary nonperfusion, retinal edema, and vascular staining representative of active inflammation (Figs. 7–30 and 7–31).[95, 114] Leakage of retinal capillaries around the fovea and optic nerve is common and may be related to the deposition of immune complexes. With chronic disease, there may be hyalinized thickening of the vessel wall and perivascular fibrosis. In

the context of adjusting treatment with immunomodulating and cytotoxic agents, FA may give a measure of the level of vascular inflammation that is not appreciated clinically (see Figs. 7–21 and 7–30). This is especially true in the presence of media opacities.

A minority of patients have choroidal inflammation or ischemia. One study of ICGA on 53 eyes showed hyperfluorescent zones in the late phase of 57%, suggesting choroidal vascular hyperpermeability, but the true significance of this finding is yet uncertain.[115]

Presumed Ocular Histoplasmosis and Pseudo–Presumed Ocular Histoplasmosis

The (presumed) ocular histoplasmosis syndrome (POHS) has as its primary features a triad of peripheral punched-out chorioretinal scars, peripapillary atrophy, and submacular choroidal neovascularization. The choroidal neovascularization is responsible for the acute onset of blurred vision, central scotoma, and metamorphopsia that plagues these patients, often at a young age. Clinically, one may observe a localized serous or hemorrhagic detachment of the sensory macula as a sign of a type II neovascular membrane.[95] Additional clues are the presence of a pigment ring of proliferating RPE cells that surround the membrane and its location on the edge of an old scar. In some cases, the neovascular membrane may be too small to be perceived.

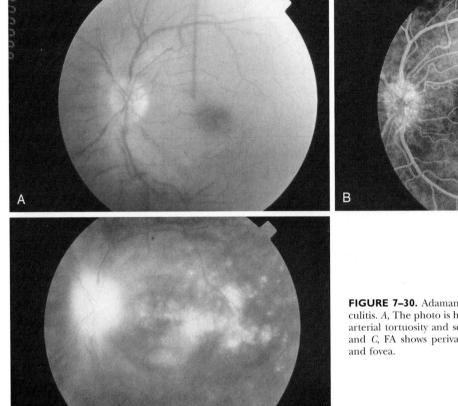

FIGURE 7–30. Adamantiades-Behçet disease with active retinal vasculitis. *A,* The photo is hazy due to the presence of vitritis, but retinal arterial tortuosity and segmental venous dilatation is appreciable. *B* and *C,* FA shows perivascular staining and late leakage at the disc and fovea.

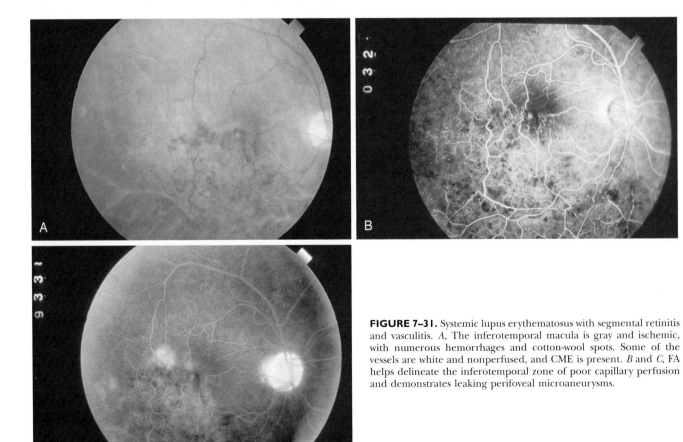

FIGURE 7–31. Systemic lupus erythematosus with segmental retinitis and vasculitis. *A,* The inferotemporal macula is gray and ischemic, with numerous hemorrhages and cotton-wool spots. Some of the vessels are white and nonperfused, and CME is present. *B* and *C,* FA helps delineate the inferotemporal zone of poor capillary perfusion and demonstrates leaking perifoveal microaneurysms.

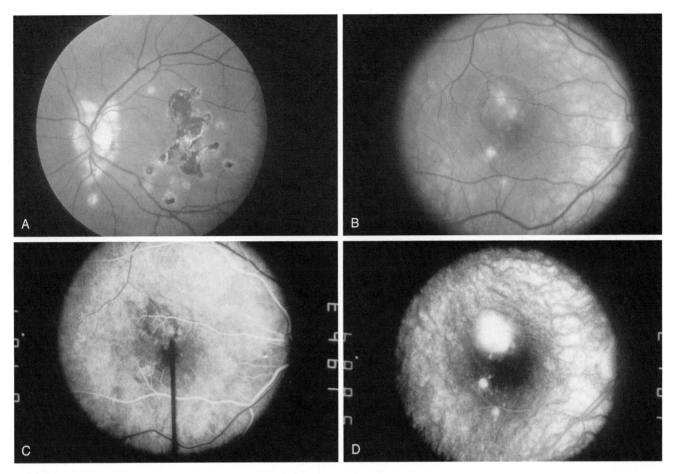

FIGURE 7–32. Punctate inner choroidopathy (PIC) in a healthy myopic woman. *A,* note the numerous old peripapillary and macular scars of the left eye. *B,* The right eye has several acute yellow infiltrative choroidal lesions. The superior fovea has a localized serous detachment, suggestive of a fresh type II neovascular membrane. *C* and *D,* The FA confirms this membrane by demonstrating a classic pattern of early filling and late leakage.

Fluorescein angiography can be critical in differentiating an acute membrane from an inactive scar. The classic lesion displays a cartwheel-shaped pattern of early hyperfluorescence that progressively leaks and stains the surrounding subretinal exudates (Fig. 7–32). An inactive scar with loss of choriocapillaris will manifest as a filling defect with sharp borders that becomes hyperfluorescent late as dye stains the fibrotic lesion and underlying sclera. Accurate angiographic localization of these lesions is key to their proper categorization relative to the center of the fovea and treatment. If a lesion is very fresh, only intense staining may be visible without a definable vessel.[90, 95, 116] Membranes distant from the fovea can be observed for spontaneous fibrosis, but threatening lesions should be promptly photocoagulated.

Multifocal choroiditis and panuveitis (MCP), one of the pseudo-POHS syndromes of unknown etiology, clinically mimics ocular histoplasmosis with some notable exceptions. The vitreous, anterior chamber, and choroid are infiltrated with cells. The peripheral chorioretinal scars are smaller and often clustered, although in both conditions, they can be arranged in a curvilinear pattern (Fig. 7–33).[117, 118] Most patients with MCP are from areas nonendemic for histoplasmosis and have negative skin tests to histoplasmin. The ERG is frequently subnormal,

and there can be large field defects that are not explained by the fundus findings. Both conditions are associated with punched-out posterior pole scars that predispose the patient to subretinal neovascularization (Figs. 7–32 and 7–34).

Recent ICGA reports on acutely symptomatic patients with both MCP and ocular histoplasmosis syndrome reveal the presence of hypofluorescent spots late in the study that resolve in tandem with the patients' symptoms.[117, 119] These spots do not correlate with visible fundus abnormalities but may correlate with visual disturbances or field changes and suggest more widespread choroidal involvement than previously recognized.

Birdshot Retinochoroidopathy

BSRC, also known as vitiliginous chorioretinitis, is an affliction of otherwise healthy middle-aged and older persons who present with bilateral vitritis and patches of chorioretinitis in an eye that appears externally quiet.[95, 120] There is a predilection for female involvement and a strong association with HLA A29.2, occurring in up to 96% of reported patients. The characteristic depigmented patches in the fundus may be subtle early in the disease. The patches are creamy and yellow-white with indistinct borders, and they contain no pigment and no

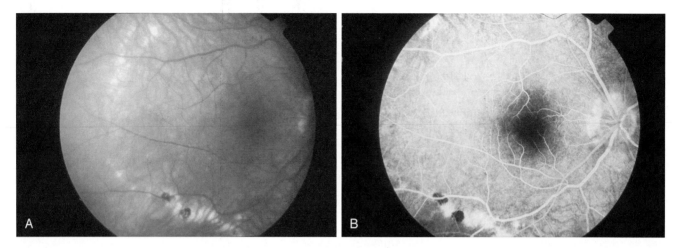

FIGURE 7–33. Presumed ocular histoplasmosis syndrome. *A,* The fundus has peripapillary RPE atrophy and a curvilinear zone of atrophic chorioretinal scars temporal to the macula. *B,* Both of these classic features manifest as RPE window defects without leakage on FA.

atrophy of the underlying choriocapillaris or overlying retina. Although a shotgun "birdshot" distribution is the hallmark, the nasal retina between the equator and the posterior pole is typically involved first, whereas the macula is often spared or involved late. Often, the lesions radiate outward from the disc in lines that seem to follow the choroidal vessels. There can be varying degrees of

papilledema and cystoid macular edema, the primary cause of visual loss.[95]

FA shows delayed retinal vascular filling and variable, unexplained late vascular staining and leakage.[95, 121] The angiographic characteristics of the spots depends on their stage in the disease. Early, when there is choroidal infiltration with minimal RPE atrophy, the spots are hypoflu-

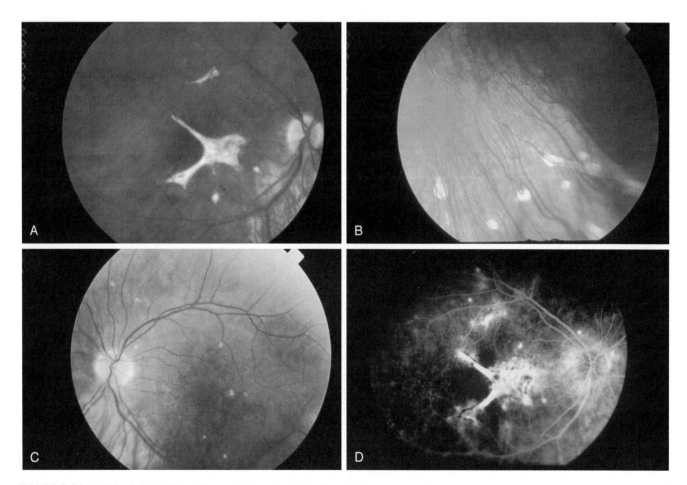

FIGURE 7–34. Multifocal choroiditis with panuveitis. *A* to *C,* Note the macular and peripheral atrophic lesions in both eyes, and chronic vitritis. *D,* The subretinal neovascular membrane of the right eye has involuted to a fibrotic scar that displays minimal fluorescein leakage.

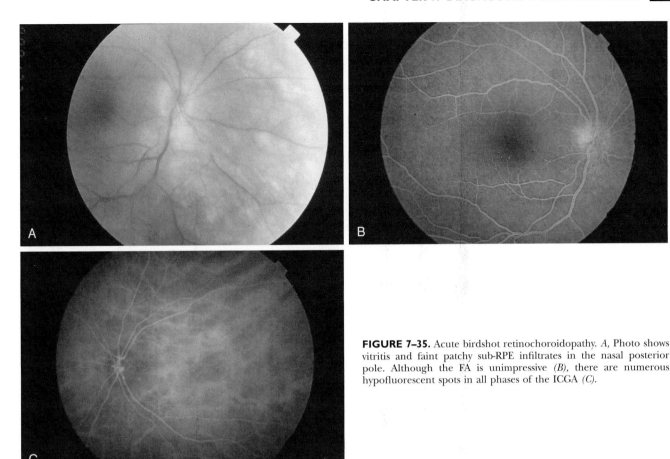

FIGURE 7–35. Acute birdshot retinochoroidopathy. *A,* Photo shows vitritis and faint patchy sub-RPE infiltrates in the nasal posterior pole. Although the FA is unimpressive *(B),* there are numerous hypofluorescent spots in all phases of the ICGA *(C).*

orescent on the transit and stain in the late phases, much like a granulomatous lesion. As RPE atrophy ensues, the spots may show no early alteration of fluorescence or a hyperfluorescent window defect, followed by late staining.[120] More spots are seen clinically than on FA (Figs. 7–35 and 7–36). In the late stages, there can be optic atrophy and narrowing of the retinal vessels.[95] At this stage, the patient complains of nyctalopia and color deficits, and the electroretinogram is permanently impaired.

Rarely, choroidal neovascularization can occur (Fig. 7–37).

Of all the inflammatory choroidopathies, BSRC has benefited the most from study with ICGA. There is a characteristic early pattern of scattered hypofluorescent, well-delineated, round-to-oval spots. In contrast to the hyperfluorescent spots of FA, the hypofluorescent spots of ICGA are more numerous than those seen clinically (see Fig. 7–35).[120, 121] They persist throughout the study.

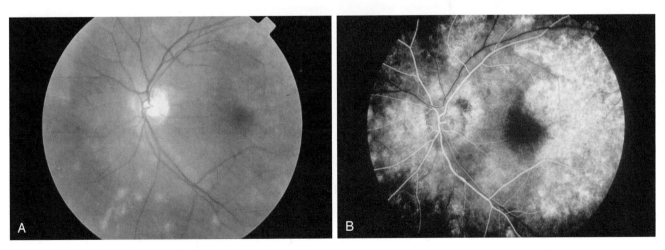

FIGURE 7–36. Chronic birdshot retinochoroidopathy. *A,* Note the secondary RPE changes. A large temporal zone of atrophy splits the macula, and there are considerable peripapillary changes. *B,* These areas manifest as geographic hyperfluorescent window defects on FA. The yellow spots inferior to the disc show minimal angiographic changes.

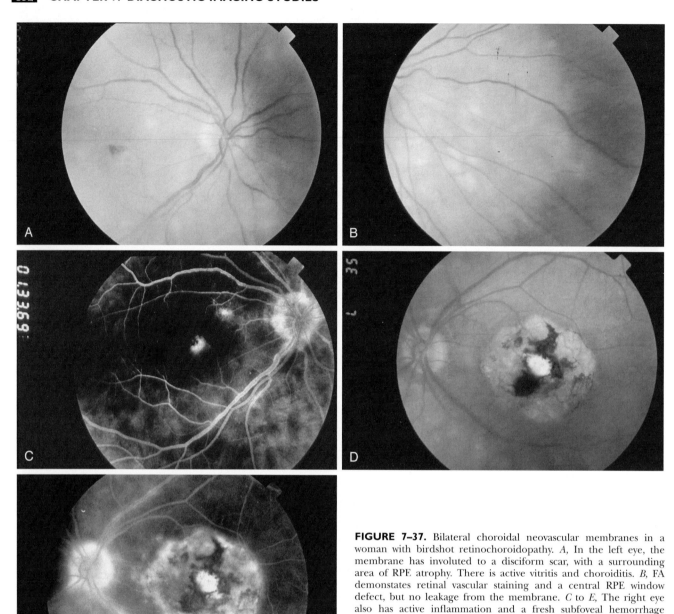

FIGURE 7–37. Bilateral choroidal neovascular membranes in a woman with birdshot retinochoroidopathy. *A,* In the left eye, the membrane has involuted to a disciform scar, with a surrounding area of RPE atrophy. There is active vitritis and choroiditis. *B,* FA demonstates retinal vascular staining and a central RPE window defect, but no leakage from the membrane. *C* to *E,* The right eye also has active inflammation and a fresh subfoveal hemorrhage heralding a new choroidal neovascular membrane. (Courtesy of Joan Miller, M.D., Massachusetts Eye and Ear Infirmary.)

Furthermore, they are present early in the course of the disease and remain throughout convalescence, making for a useful diagnostic clue. Chang and coauthors studied patients from 6 months to 7 years after onset and found hypofluorescent spots in all.[120]

Sarcoid Chorioretinopathy

Sarcoidosis is a systemic granulomatous inflammatory disease with a predilection for ocular involvement. Approximately one third of those with uveitis will have posterior segment disease. The classic fundus findings are the perivenous exudates or "candle wax drippings."[112] FA delineates the altered vascular permeability. Additional findings highlighted by angiography may include branch vein

occlusions with associated regions of nonperfusion, retinal or optic disc neovascularization, or papillitis.[95, 112] There may be vitreous opacities arranged in a string-of-pearls pattern or vitreous hemorrhage. Some sarcoid patients may present with focal choroidal granulomas, typically in the posterior pole, sometimes at the optic nerve. These are creamy yellow nodules or masses with an overlying exudative detachment that may simulate metastasis, melanoma, or tuberculoma. It is unclear whether the predilection for the macula relates to its higher blood flow, or whether more peripheral lesions are asymptomatic and less likely to present. The typical FA shows a mass that is hypofluorescent on the transit, then stains and leaks late in the study. Some of these lesions may contain neovascular membrane with a typical cartwheel or "lacy" pattern of fluorescence. The lacy pattern may resolve spontaneously or with immunosuppression, or it may progress to subretinal fibrosis and severe vision loss.[95]

Viral Retinitis

Acute retinal necrosis is characterized by the spontaneous onset of vitritis and occlusive retinal arteritis that rapidly progresses to necrosis in a typically healthy patient. Herpes zoster and simplex are likely etiologies.[95, 114] The patches of retinal whitening often begin peripherally and become confluent. There is vascular occlusion, hemorrhage, and perivascular infiltration. Fluorescein angiography will demonstrate perfusion defects, capillary leakage, venous staining, and focal choroidal infiltration.[112] In addition, it can demonstrate occlusions of the central retinal and choroidal vessels that result in precipitous loss of vision, which are especially common in immunocompromised patients.

Toxoplasmosis Retinochoroiditis

Toxoplasmosis is the most frequent cause of focal necrotizing retinitis in immunocompetent persons throughout the world.[95, 114] Histopathologic data suggest that the encysted organism lies dormant in the sensory retina, adjacent to or remote from a chorioretinal scar. The organisms may become unencysted to ignite a full-thickness infiltrative lesion, with an overlying vitritis and an under-lying granulomatous choroiditis and scleritis. Those lesions concentrated in the outer retina are frequently accompanied with serous detachment.[122] The active focus of retinitis usually expands for about 2 weeks before resolving, leaving a deep, atrophic, and pigmented chorioretinal scar. One or more of these excavated scars can be seen in the posterior pole of otherwise healthy children as a consequence of congenital infection (Fig. 7–38).

Typical fluorescein angiographic findings include intense staining in the focus of retinitis, which has fuzzy, poorly defined borders, and leakage from the adjacent retinal veins and optic disc. Sometimes edema blocks fluorescence early. Fluorescein pools late into areas of serous detachment. Choroidal neovascularization, a known complication, may be difficult to exclude (Figs. 7–38 and 7–39). Retinal vessels near the lesion may become secondarily inflamed, leading to leakage and arterial and venous obstructions. An interesting finding described by Kyrieleis that simulates arterial emboli may occur either near to or remote from the retinitis; these are focal periarterial exudates and atheromatous plaques that show no alteration of flow on FA (Fig. 7–40).[112, 123] These plaques fade after the retinitis resolves.

The healed scar is often a deep crater devoid of choriocapillaris (see Fig. 7–38). On FA, the large choroidal vessels may be seen on a bed of hypofluorescence. Surrounding pigment clumps show darker hypofluorescence, sometimes with a hyperfluorescent rim at their margins.

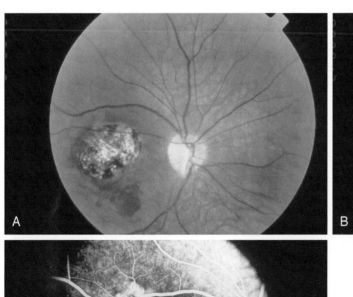

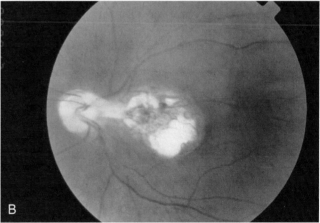

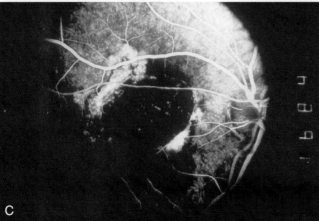

FIGURE 7–38. Congenital bilateral toxoplasmosis chorioretinitis. *A* and *B*, Typical bilateral deeply excavated chorioretinal scars with hyperpigmented margins. *C*, FA of the right eye shows absence of filling of the choriocapillaris in the crater and leakage from active neovascular membranes at the superotemporal and inferonasal edges. Fresh blood is present inferiorly. (Courtesy of Chris Blodi, M.D.)

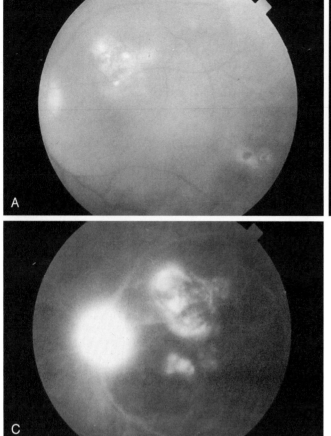

FIGURE 7–39. Active toxoplasmosis chorioretinitis with vitritis. *A* and *B*, An old scar is present superior to the fovea, which does not fill on the FA. The margins are active and stain by midtransit. The inferior border is suspicious for a neovascular membrane, but there is no significant expansion of fluorescence in the late frame *(C)*. The disc and peripapillary vessels stain late.

Late in reperfusion, the sclera stains, giving hyperfluorescence to the entire lesion.

An ICGA study of 25 cases of acute toxoplasmosis showed early choroidal hypofluorescence under the focus of reactivation in all, that usually extended beyond the limits of the lesion seen clinically.[122] In 89% of cases, this hypofluorescence persisted late. More interesting was the

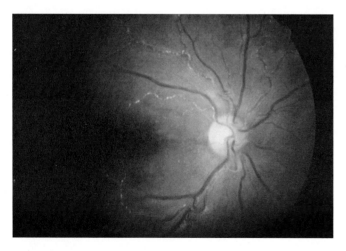

FIGURE 7–40. Resolved toxoplasmosis chorioretinitis. Vitritis has resolved, but there are residual periarterial exudates (Kyrieleis vasculitis). These typically are not associated with filling defects on FA and fade with observation. (Courtesy of J. D. M. Gass, M.D., Vanderbilt University.)

presence of hypofluorescent "satellite dark dots" in 75% of patients. Both lesions tended to resolve with therapy and suggest a greater degree of choroidal involvement than previously appreciated.

In the following situations, FA may help diagnose macular complications of ocular inflammation.

Cystoid Macular Edema

A major cause of visual morbidity from ocular inflammation of any cause is cystoid macular edema (CME). Presumably, there is a localized breakdown of capillary tight junctions in the fovea and at the disc. Early detection and aggressive treatment with periocular and systemic steroids, nonsteroidal anti-inflammatory agents, methotrexate, or cyclosporin A offers maximal chance of resolution. Some unfortunate cases resist treatment. There is a polycystic pattern of expansion of the extracellular space created by serous exudate.

Fluorescein angiography detects CME before biomicroscopy.[90, 95] FA is helpful when no explanation for vision loss is evident.[95, 124] There is perifoveal leakage of dye from the retinal capillaries that accumulates in the cystoid spaces and classically resembles petals of a flower (Fig. 7–41). In the late frames, the dye will continue to diffuse at the fovea and also stain the disc.

Macular Ischemia

A minority of patients with posterior uveitis lose central vision despite adequate suppression of their inflamma-

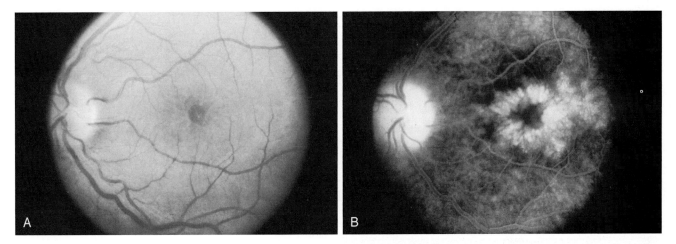

FIGURE 7–41. Idiopathic uveitis with cystoid macular edema. *A,* The fovea has an abnormal reflex. Cystic changes surround an orange spot. *B,* Note the petaloid pattern of fluorescein accumulation and late disc staining that has reduced visual acuity to 20/60.

tion. In this situation, it is prudent to look for choroidal neovascular membranes and macular ischemia. In a retrospective review of 135 patients with active nonocclusive retinal vasculitis, Bentley and associates identified 12 patients who lost macular function owing to capillary nonperfusion.[125] These patients had one of three diagnoses: Adamantiades-Behçet disease, sarcoidosis, or idiopathic vasculitis. Over an average of 3 years' follow-up, visual acuity either deteriorated or failed to improve in all. The FA was predictive. Closure of perifoveal vessels manifests as an enlarged or irregular ("moth-eaten") foveal avascular zone, best seen in the early venous phase (Fig. 7–42). The combination of ischemia and edema resembled that seen in retinal vein occlusion, but these patients had no definable vascular events.

Epiretinal Membrane

Any inflammatory disease creating vitreous cellular infiltrates can lead to the formation of epiretinal membranes, with radiating retinal folds or pucker, capillary leakage, and hemorrhage, and retinal edema or serous exudate.

When the fovea is involved primarily or is secondarily distorted by tractional forces, the patient may complain of metamorphopsia or reduced acuity. Soon after onset of the pucker, FA usually demonstrates leakage from the retinal vessels. Owing to retinal distortion, the dye accumulates in irregular patterns, not typical of classic cystoid macular edema (Fig. 7–43). Leakage is most common soon after the membrane contracts and in eyes more likely to progress; within weeks to months, the leakage slows down as the retinal folds dry up.[95] The chronic cases are less likely to gain acuity with membrane peeling, so FA can help in the timing of surgical intervention.

Choroidal Neovascularization

Patients with chorioretinal scars from any cause are prone to the ingrowth of neovascular membranes from the choroid to the subretinal space at the edge of the scar (see Figs. 7–23, 7–25, 7–32, 7–34, 7–37, 7–39, and 7–43). Gass has elucidated the histology of these type II membranes, which are typically walled off by a proliferation of RPE cells (Fig. 7–44).[126] Their loose connections to the overly-

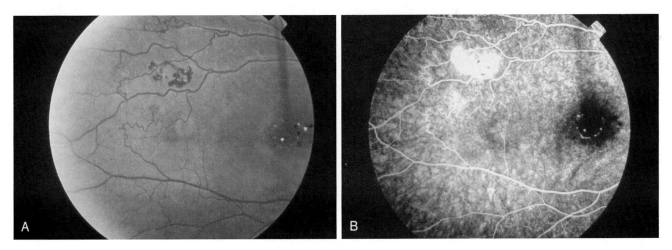

FIGURE 7–42. Resolved dermatomyositis-related retinal vasculitis with macular ischemia. *A,* Note the absence of macular vessels and the foveal pigment accumulation. There is remodeling of the vasculature temporally with venous collaterals and a patch of neovascularization, which went on to hemorrhage. *B,* The FA demonstrates irregularity of the foveal capillary-free zone and early leakage from the incompetent new vessels. Sectoral retinal photocoagulation resulted in regression of these vessels.

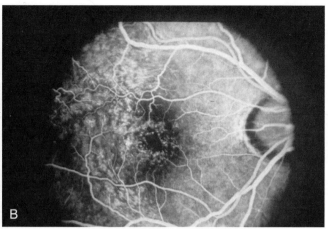

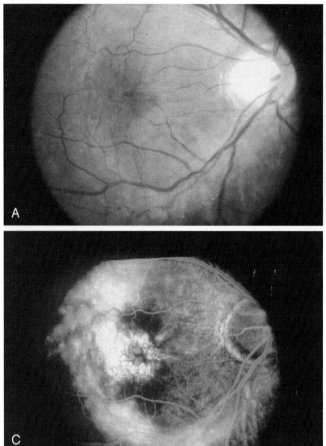

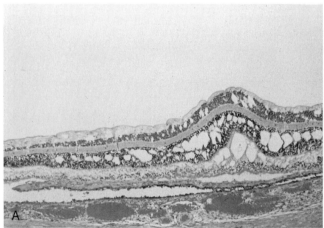

FIGURE 7–43. Vitreomacular traction syndrome. *A,* This patient has a taut posterior hyaloidal membrane secondary to smoldering intermediate uveitis. Macular edema reduced visual acuity to 20/400. *B* and *C,* FA shows significant retinal capillary leakage along the major arcades and at the temporal fovea. (Courtesy of Tatsuo Hirose, M.D., Schepens Retina Associates.)

ing neurosensory retina and underlying native RPE makes them suitable for surgical excision. This is more successful when the site of ingrowth is extrafoveal, as demonstrated by Melberg and colleagues.[127] Patients with inflammatory choroidopathies are particularly prone to this complication, possibly because prostaglandins and interleukins are stimuli for angiogenesis. Inflammatory membranes differ from those associated with macular degeneration in that they are typically pigmented and not associated with drusen, pigment epithelial detachment, or a large degree of hemorrhage (Fig. 7–45). Ocular histoplasmosis syndrome, discussed earlier, is the prototypical example. When the FA is inconclusive or shows an atypical pattern of leakage, in some cases, ICGA may

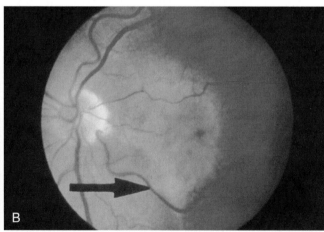

FIGURE 7–44. Type II choroidal neovascular membrane in a patient with POHS. *A,* Histopathology demonstrates that a reactive layer of RPE has covered the posterior surface of the membrane, separating it from the native RPE and choroid. The membrane has yet to extend over the anterior surface. The detached neurosensory retina is only loosely adherent to the membrane. *B,* As is typical with inflammatory disorders, the membrane enters the subretinal space at the edge of a chorioretinal scar *(arrow).* (From Gass JDM: Biomicroscopic and histopathologic considerations regarding the feasibility of surgical excision of subfoveal neovascular membranes. Am J Ophthal 1994;118:285–298.)

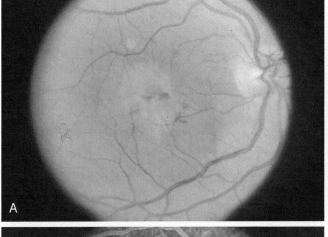

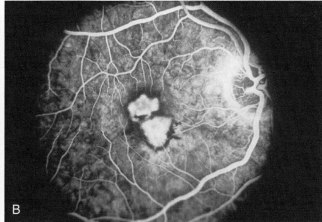

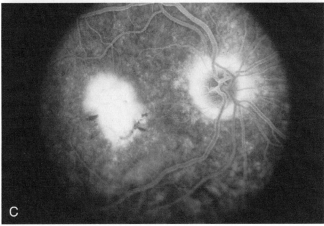

FIGURE 7–45. Lyme disease retinitis with a dumbbell-shaped neovascular membrane. *A,* Notice the pigment ring demarcating the membrane and the surrounding turbid subretinal fluid with minimal hemorrhage. *B* and *C,* The FA shows a classic pattern of well-defined early hyperfluorescence that expands late with fuzzy margins.

demonstrate a "hot spot" representing the focus of leakage.

Retinal Angiography To Monitor Systemic Disease

Patients with a systemic inflammatory disorder may have ocular complaints that cannot be easily explained by the ophthalmoscopic findings. Fluorescein angiography should be used prudently in this situation and may occasionally be revealing. Matsuo and Yamaoka studied five consecutive patients with inflammatory bowel disease referred for ocular examination.[128] One patient had cystoid macular edema in one eye, but the remainder had normal funduscopic examinations and acuities of 1.2 or better. All five patients demonstrated fluorescein leakage from peripheral retinal capillaries and from the optic discs of both eyes, and one showed segmental phlebitis in both peripheral fundi.

We commonly survey patients with Adamantiades-Behçet disease with wide-field FA at the first complaint of visual changes despite a stable appearing fundus on ophthalmoscopy. Late staining of the retinal or choroidal vessels is a reliable warning of early local or systemic reactivation of Adamantiades-Behçet disease activity. The same is true in patients with SLE (see Fig. 7–30).

References

1. Rubin PA, Remulla HD: Orbital venous anomalies demonstrated by spiral computed tomography. Ophthalmology 1997;104:1463–1470.
2. O'Brien JM, Char DH, Tucker N, et al: Efficacy of unanesthetized spiral computed tomography in initial evaluation of childhood leukocoria. Ophthalmology 1995;102:1345–1350.
3. Tonami H, Tamamura H, Kimizu K, et al: Intraocular lesions in patients with systemic disease: findings on MR imaging. AJR Am J Roentgenol 1990;154:385–389.
4. Sillers MJ, Kuhn FA, Vickery CL: Radiation exposure in paranasal sinus imaging. Otolaryngol Head Neck Surg 1995;112:248–251.
5. Kolodny NH, Gragoudas ES, D'Amico DJ, et al: Proton and sodium 23 magnetic resonance imaging of human ocular tissues: A model study. Arch Ophthalmol 1987;105:1532–1536.
6. Kolodny NH, Gragoudas ES, D'Amico DJ, Albert DM: Magnetic resonance imaging and spectroscopy of intraocular tumors. Surv Ophthalmol 1989;33:512–514.
7. Ettl A, Salomonowitz E, Koornneef L, Zonneveld FW: High-resolution MR imaging anatomy of the orbit. Radiol Clin North Am 1998;36:1021–1045.
8. Langer BG, Mafee MF, Pollack S, et al: MRI of the normal orbit and optic pathway. Radiol Clin North Am 1987;25:429–446.
9. Pykett IL, Newhouse JH, Buonanno FS, et al: Principles of nuclear magnetic resonance imaging. Radiology 1982;143:157–168.
10. Mafee MF, Peyman GA, Peace JH, et al: Magnetic resonance imaging in the evaluation and differentiation of uveal melanoma. Ophthalmology 1987;93:341–348.
11. Tien RD: Fat-suppression MR imaging in neuroradiology: techniques and clinical application. AJR Am J Roentgenol 1992; 158:369–379.
12. Lee DH, Simon JH, Szumowski J, et al: Optic neuritis and orbital lesions: Lipid-suppressed chemical shift MR imaging. Radiology 1991;179:543–46.
13. Bond JB, Haik BG, Mihara F, Gupta KL: Magnetic resonance imaging of choroidal melanoma with and without gadolinium contrast enhancement. Ophthalmology 1991;98:459–466.
14. Bilaniuk LT, Schenck JF, Zimmerman RA, et al: Ocular and orbital lesions: Surface coil MR imaging. Radiology 1985;156:669–674.

15. Rubin PA, Bilyk JR, Shore, et al: MRI of the lacrimal drainage system. Ophthalmology 1994;101:235–243.
16. Guy J, Mao J, Bigwood WD Jr, et al: Enhancement and demyelination of the intraorbital optic nerve: Fat suppression magnetic resonance imaging. Ophthalmology 1992;99:713–719.
17. De Potter P, Flanders AE, Shields JA, et al: The role of fat-suppression technique and gadopentetate dimeglumine in magnetic resonance imaging evaluation of intraocular tumors and simulating lesions. Arch Ophthalmol 1994;112:340–348.
18. Foster CS, Sainz de la Maza M: The Sclera, 1st ed. New York, Springer-Verlag, 1994, pp 81–88.
19. Gomori JH, Gorssman RI, Goldberg HI, et al: Intracranial hematomas: Imaging by high-field MR. Radiology 1985;157:87–93.
20. Gonzalez RG, Cheng HM, Barnett P: Nuclear magnetic resonance imaging of the vitreous body. Science 1984;223:399–400.
21. Haik BG, Saint Louis L, Smith ME, et al: Magnetic resonance imaging in the evaluation of leukocoria. Ophthalmology 1985;92:1143–1152.
22. Raymond WR IV, Char DH, Norman D, Protzko EE: Magnetic resonance imaging evaluation of uveal tumors. Am J Ophthalmol 1991;111:633–641.
23. Goldberg RA, Heinz GW, Chiu L: Gadolinium magnetic resonance imaging dacryocystography. Am J Ophthalmol 1993;115:738–741.
24. Shellock FG: Pocket Guide to MR Procedures and Metallic Objects: Update 1997. Philadelphia, Lippincott-Raven Publishers, 1997.
25. Harcke HT, Mandell GA, Cassell ILS: Imaging techniques in childhood arthritis. Rheum Dis Clin North Am 1997;23:523–544.
26. Magnani P, Paganelli G, Modorati G, et al: Quantitative comparison of direct antibody labeling and tumor pretargeting in uveal melanoma. J Nucl Med 1996;37:967–971.
27. Rabinov K, Weber AL: Radiology of the Salivary Glands, 1st ed. Boston, GK Hall Medical Publishers, 1985, pp 1–42.
28. Romero JM, Finger PT, Iezzi R, et al: Three-dimensional ultrasonography of choroidal melanoma: Extrascleral extension. Am J Ophthalmol 1998;126:842–844.
29. Taylor KJ and Holland S: Doppler US. Part I. Basic principles, instrumentation and pitfalls. Radiology 1990;174:297–307.
30. Lieb WE: Color doppler imaging of the eye and orbit. Radiol Clin North Am 1998;36:1059–1071.
31. Williamson TH, Harris A: Color doppler ultrasound imaging of the eye and orbit. Surv Ophthalmol 1996;40:255–67.
32. Mitchell DG: Color doppler imaging: Principles, limitations and artifacts. Radiology 1990;177:1–10.
33. Coleman DJ, Silverman RH, Daly SM, Rondeau MJ: Advances in ophthalmic ultrasound. Radiol Clin North Am 1998;36:1073–1082.
34. Pavlin CJ, Foster FS: Ultrasound biomicroscopy: High-frequency ultrasound imaging of the eye at microscopic resolution. Radiol Clin North Am 1998;36:1047–1058.
35. Marchini G, Pagliarusco A, Toscano A, et al: Ultrasound biomicroscopic and conventional ultrasonographic study of ocular dimensions in primary angle-closure glaucoma. Ophthalmology 1998;105:2091–2098.
36. Haring G, Nolle B, Wiechens B: Ultrasound biomicroscopic imaging in intermediate uveitis. Br J Ophthalmol 1998;82:625–629.
37. Newman LS, Rose CS, Maier LA: Sarcoidosis. N Engl J Med 1997;336:1224–1234.
38. Carmody RF, Mafee MF, Goodwin JA, et al: Orbit and optic pathway sarcoidosis: MR findings. AJNR Am J Neuroradiol 1994;15:775–783.
39. Chatzistefanou K, Markomichelakis NN, Christen W, et al: Characteristics of uveitis presenting for the first time in the elderly. Ophthalmology 1998;105:347–352.
40. Vrabec TR, Augsburger JJ, Fischer DH, et al: Taches de bougie. Ophthalmology 1995;102:1712–1721.
41. Power WJ, Neves RA, Rodriguez A, et al: The value of combined serum angiotensin-converting enzyme and gallium scan in diagnosing ocular sarcoidosis. Ophthalmology 1995;102:2007–11.
42. Krystolik M, Power WJ, Foster CS: Diagnostic and therapeutic challenges of sarcoidosis. Int Ophthalmol Clin 1998;38:61–76.
43. Kosmorsky GS, Meisler DM, Rice TW, et al: Chest computed tomography and mediastinoscopy in the diagnosis of sarcoidosis-associated uveitis. Am J Ophthalmol 1998;126:132–134.
44. Mettler FA, Guiberteau MJ: Essentials of Nuclear Medicine Imaging, 4th ed. Philadelphia, WB Saunders, 1998.
45. Selavik SB, Spencer RP, Weed DA, et al: Recognition of distinctive patterns of gallium-67 distribution in sarcoidosis. J Nucl Med 1990;31:909–914.
46. Weinreb RN, Yavitz EQ, O'Connor GR: Lacrimal gland uptake of gallium citrate Ga 67. Am J Ophthalmol 1981;92:16–20.
47. Karma A, Poukkula AA, Ruokonen AO: Assessment of activity of ocular sarcoidosis by gallium scanning. Br J Ophthalmol 1987;71:361–367.
48. Murdoch J, Muller NL: Pulmonary sarcoidosis: Changes on follow-up CT examination. AJR Am J Roentgenol 1992;159:473–477.
49. Lynch DA, Webb WR, Gamsu G, et al: Computed tomography in pulmonary sarcoidosis. J Comput Assist Tomogr 1989;13:405–410.
50. Mafee MF, Dorodi S, Pai E: Sarcoidosis of the eye, orbit and central nervous system. Radiol Clin North Am 1999;37:73–87.
51. Sainz de la Maza M, Foster CS, Jabbur NS: Scleritis associated with systemic vasculitis diseases. Ophthalmology 1995;102:687–92.
52. Harper SL, Foster CS: The ocular manifestations of rheumatoid disease. Int Ophthalmol Clin 1998;38:1–19.
53. Hemady RK, Baer JC, Foster CS: Immunosuppressive drugs in the management of progressive, corticosteroid-resistant uveitis associated with juvenile rheumatoid arthritis. Int Ophthalmol Clin 1992;32:241–52.
54. Weissman BNW: Imaging techniques in rheumatoid arthritis. J Rheumatol 1994;21(Suppl 42):14–19.
55. Graham TB, Blebea JS, Gylys-Morin V, Passo MH: Magnetic resonance imaging in juvenile rheumatoid arthritis. Semin Arthritis Rheum 1997;27:161–168.
56. Schumacher HR Jr, ed: Primer on Rheumatic Diseases, 10th ed. Atlanta, Arthritis Foundation, 1993.
57. Straatsma BR: Ocular manifestations of Wegener's granulomatosis. Am J Ophthalmol 1957;44:789–799.
58. Weber AL, Romo LV, Sabates NR: Pseudotumor of the orbit: Clinical, pathologic, and radiologic evaluation. Radiol Clin North Am 1999;37:151–168.
59. Kim RY, Loewenstein JI: Systemic disease manifesting as exudative retinal detachment. Int Ophthalmol Clin 1998;38:177–195.
60. Akova YA, Jabbur NS, Foster CS: Ocular presentation of polyarteritis nodosa. Clinical course and management with steroid and cytotoxic therapy. Ophthalmology 1993;100:1775–1781.
61. Tunaci A, Berkman YM, Gokmen E: Thoracic involvement in Behçet's disease: Pathologic, clinical, and imaging features. AJR Am J Roentgenol 1995;164:51–56.
62. Booth A, Dleppe PA, Goddard PL, et al: The radiological manifestations of relapsing polychondritis. Clin Radiol 1989;40:147–149.
63. Mendelson DS, Som PM, Crane R, et al: Relapsing polychondritis studied by computed tomography. Radiology 1985;157:489–490.
64. You TT, Young LH: Retinal manifestations of gastrointestinal conditions. Int Ophthalmol Clin 1998;38:197–220.
65. Watt I, Middlemiss H: The radiology of gout. Clin Radiol 1975;26:27–36.
66. Rubenstein J, Pritzker KPH: Crystal-associated arthropathies. AJR Am J Roentgenol 1989;152:685–695.
67. Martel W: The overhanging margin of bone: A roentgenologic manifestation of gout. Radiology 1968;91:755–756.
68. Lambert JR, Wright V: Eye inflammation in psoriatic arthritis. Ann Rheum Dis 1976;35:354–356.
69. Rosenbaum T: Characterization of uveitis associated with spondyloarthritis. J Rheumatol 1989;16:792–796.
70. Rosenbaum JT: Acute anterior uveitis and spondyloarthropathies. Rheum Dis Clin North Am 1992;18:143–152.
71. Coday MP, Dallow RL: Managing Graves' orbitopathy. Int Ophthalmol Clin 1998;38:103–115.
72. Nianiaris N, Hurwitz JJ, Chen JC, Wortzman G: Correlation between computed tomography and magnetic resonance imaging in Graves' orbitopathy. Can J Ophthalmol 1994;29:9–12.
73. Werner SC: Modification of the classification of eye changes in Graves' disease. Am J Ophthalmol 1977;83:725–727.
74. Enzmann DR, Donaldson SS, Kriss JP: Appearance of Graves' disease on orbital computed tomography. J Comput Assist Tomography 1979;3:815.
75. Kaufman LM, Mafee MF, Song CD: Retinoblastoma and simulating lesions. Radiol Clin North Am 1998;36:1101–1117.
76. Hidayat AA, Mafee MF, Lauer NV, Noujaim S: Langerhans' cell histiocytosis and juvenile xanthogranuloma of the orbit: Clinico-pathologic CT and MR imaging features. Radiol Clin North Am 1998;36:1229–1240.

77. Mafee MF: Uveal melanoma, choroidal melanoma, and simulating lesions. Radiol Clin North Am 1998;36:1083–1099.

78. Edward DP, Mafee MF, Garcia-Valenzuela E, Weiss RA: Coats' disease and primary hyperplastic primary vitreous: Role of MR imaging and CT. Radiol Clin North Am 1998;36:1119–1131.

79. Mafee MF, Goldberg MF: Persistent hyperplastic primary vitreous (PHPV): Role of computed tomography and magnetic resonance imaging. Radiol Clin North Am 1987;25:667–692.

80. Peyster RG, Augsburger JJ, Shields JA, et al: Intraocular tumors: Evaluation with MR imaging. Radiology 1988;168:773–779.

81. Peyman GA, Mafee MF: Uveal melanoma and simulating lesions: The role of magnetic resonance imaging and computed tomography. Radiol Clin North Am 1987;25:471–476.

82. Watkins LM, Rubin PAD: Metastatic tumors of the eye and orbit. Int Ophthamol Clin 1998;38:107–128.

83. Goldberg RA, Rootman J, Cline RA: Tumors metastatic to the orbit: A changing picture. Surv Ophthalmol 1990;35:1.

84. Davis EA, Rizzo JF: Ocular manifestations of multiple sclerosis. Int Ophthalmol Clin 1998;38:129–139.

85. Harris JO, Frank JA, Patronas N, et al: Serial gadolinium-enhanced magnetic resonance imaging scans in patients with early, relapsing-remitting multiple sclerosis: Implications for clinical trials and natural history. Ann Neurol 1991;29:548–555.

86. Lukes SA, Crooks LE, Aminoff MJ, et al. Nuclear magnetic resonance imaging in multiple sclerosis. Ann Neurol 1983;13:592–601.

87. Gebarski SS, Gabrielson TO, Gilman S, et al: The initial diagnosis of multiple sclerosis: Clinical impact of magnetic resonance imaging. Ann Neurol 1985;17–74.

88. Robertson WD, Li D, Mayo J, et al: Magnetic resonance imaging in the diagnosis of multiple sclerosis. J Neurol 1985;232 (Suppl 1):58.

89. Paty DW, Oger JJF, Kastrukoff CF, et al: Magnetic resonance imaging in the diagnosis of multiple sclerosis: A prospective study with comparison of clinical evaluation, evoked potential, oligoclonal banding, and computed tomography. Neurology 1988;38:180–185.

90. Berkow JW, Flower RW, Orth DH, Kelley JS: Fluorescein and indocyanine green angiography: Technique and interpretation. American Academy of Ophthalmology, 1997.

91. MacLean AL, Maumenee AE: Hemangioma of the choroid. Am J Ophthal 1960;50:3–11

92. Flower RW, Hochheimer BF: A clinical technique and apparatus for simultaneous angiography of the separate retinal and choroidal circulations. Invest Ophthal 1973;12:248–261.

93. Yannuzzi LA, Slakter JS, Sorenson JA, et al: Digital indocyanine green videoangiography and choroidal neovascularization. Retina 1992;12:191–223.

94. Destro M, Puliafito CA: Indocyanine green videoangiography of choroidal neovascularization. Ophthalmology 1989;96:846–853.

95. Gass JDM: Stereoscopic Atlas of Macular Diseases: Diagnosis and Treatment. St. Louis, Mosby, 1997.

96. Herbort CP: Posterior uveitis: New insights provided by indocyanine green angiography. Eye 1998;12:757–759.

97. Howe L, Stanford M, Graham E, et al: Indocyanine green angiography in inflammatory eye disease. Eye 1998;12:761–767.

98. Chiquet C, Lumbroso L, Denis P, et al: Acute posterior multifocal pigment epitheliopathy associated with Wegener's granulomatosis. Retina 1999;19:309–313.

99. Borruat FX, Piquet B, Herbort CP: Acute posterior multifocal placoid pigment epitheliopathy following mumps. Ocul Immunol Inflamm 1998;6:189–193.

100. Schatz H, Park D, McDonald HR, Johnson RN: Acute multifocal posterior placoid pigment epitheliopathy. In: Yannuzzi LA, Flower RW, Slakter JS: Indocyanine Green Angiography. St. Louis, Mosby, 1997, pp 239–246.

101. Bohlender T, Weindler J, Ratzkova A, Ruprecht KW: Indocyanine green angiography in acute posterior multifocal placoid pigment epitheliopathy. Klin Monatsbl Augenheilkd 1998;212:170–174.

102. Park D, Schatz H, McDonald HR, Johnson RN: Acute multifocal posterior placoid pigment epitheliopathy: A theory of pathogenesis. Retina 1995;15:351–352.

103. Mones JM, Slakter JS: Serpiginous choroidopathy. In: Yannuzzi LA, Flower RW, Slakter JS: Indocyanine Green Angiography. St. Louis, Mosby, 1997, pp 247–252.

104. Jampol LM, Seiving PA, Pugh D: Multiple evanescent white dot syndrome. Clinical Findings. Am J Ophthalmol 1984;102:671–674.

105. Takeda M, Kimura S, Tamiya M: Acute disseminated retinal pigment epitheliopathy. Folia Ophthalmol Jpn 1984;35:2613–2620.

106. Darmakusuma IE, Yannuzzi LA, Slakter JA: Multiple evanescent white dot syndrome. In: Yannuzzi LA, Flower RW, Slakter JS: Indocyanine Green Angiography. St. Louis, Mosby, 1997, pp 253–258.

107. Freund KB, Yannuzzi LA: Vogt-Koyanagi-Harada syndrome. In: Yannuzzi LA, Flower RW, Slakter JS: Indocyanine Green Angiography. St. Louis, Mosby, 1997, pp 259–269.

108. Bernasconi O, Auer C, Zografos HC: Indocyanine green angiographic findings in sympathetic ophthalmia. Graefes Arch Clin Exp Ophthalmol 1998;236:635–638.

109. Kohno T, Miki T, Shiraki K, et al: Substraction ICG angiography in Harada's disease. Br J Ophthalmol 1999;83:822–833.

110. Pece A, Bolognesi G, Introini V, Brancato R: Indocyanine green angiography in Vogt-Koyanagi-Harada-type disease. Arch Ophthalmol 1997;115:804–806.

111. Harada T, Kabara Y, Takeuchi T, et al: Exploration of Vogt-Koyanagi-harada syndrome by infrared choroidal angiography with indocyanine green. Eur J Ophthalmol 1997;7:163–170.

112. De Laey JJ: Fluorescein angiography in posterior uveitis. Int Ophthalmol Clin 1995;35:33–58.

113. Auer C, Ottavio B, Herbort CP: Indocyanine green angiography features in toxoplasmic retinochoroiditis. Retina 1999;19:22–29.

114. Tabbara KF, Nussenblatt RB: Posterior Uveitis: Diagnosis and Management. Boston, Butterworth-Heinemann, 1994.

115. Atmaca L S, Batioglu F: Indocyanine green videoangiography and color doppler imaging in Behçet's disease. Acta Ophthalmol Scand 1999;77:444–447.

116. Jalkh AE, Celorio JM: Atlas of Fluorescein Angiography. Philadelphia, W.B. Saunders, 1993.

117. Slakter JS, Giovannini A: Multifocal choroiditis and the presumed ocular histoplasmosis syndrome. In: Yannuzzi LA, Flower RW, Slakter JS: Indocyanine Green Angiography. St. Louis, Mosby, 1997, pp 271–278.

118. Slakter JS, Giovannini A, Yannuzzi LA, et al: Indocyanine green angiography of multifocal choroiditis. Ophthalmology 1997;104:1813–1819.

119. Weinberger AWA, Kube T, Wolf S: Dark spots in late-phase indocyanine green angiographic studies in a patient with presumed ocular histoplasmosis syndrome. Graefes Arch Clin Exp Ophthalmol 1999;237:524–526.

120. Chang B, Lumbroso L, Rabb MF, Yannuzzi LA: Birdshot chorioretinopathy. In: Yannuzzi LA, Flower RW, Slakter JS: Indocyanine Green Angiography. St. Louis, Mosby, 1997, pp 231–238.

121. Guex-Crosier Y, Herbort CP: Prolonged retinal arterio-venous circulation time by fluorescein but not by indocyanine green angiography in birdshot chorioretinopathy. Ocul Immunol Inflamm 1997;5:203–206.

122. Auer C, Herbort CP: Indocyanine green angiographic features in posterior scleritis. Am J Ophthalmol 1998;126:471–475.

123. Kyrieleis W: Über atypischenGefasstuberkulose der Netxhaut. Arch Augenheilkd 1993;107:182–190.

124. Cunha-Vaz JG, Travassos AM: Breakdown of the blood-retinal barriers and cystoid macular edema. Surv Ophthal 1984;28:485–492.

125. Bentley CR, Stanford MR, Shilling JS, et al: Macular ischemia in posterior uveitis. Eye 1993;7:411–414.

126. Gass JDM: Biomicroscopic and histopathologic considerations regarding the feasibility of surgical excision of subfoveal neovascular membranes. Am J Ophthal 1994;118:285–298.

127. Melberg NS, Thomas MA, Burgess DB: The surgical removal of subfoveal choroidal neovascularization. Ingrowth site as a predictor of visual outcome. Retina 1996;16:190–195.

128. Matsuo T, Yamaoka A: Retinal vasculitis revealed by fluorescein angiography in patients with inflammatory bowel disease. Jpn J Ophthalmol 1998;42:398–400.

Albert T. Vitale and C. Stephen Foster

The problem of inflammation of the eye, including uveitis, was known to the ancients (Hippocrates, Galen, Aetius), but not until the 18th century did truly "modern" therapy for intraocular inflammation become well entrenched in the medical community. Scarpa, in his 1806 text,[1] describes "a strong country-woman, 35 years old" who "was brought into this hospital towards the end of April 1796, on account of a violent, acute ophthalmia in both her eyes, with which she had been afflicted three days, with great tumefaction of the eyelids, redness of the conjunctiva, acute pain, fever, and watchfulness." Scarpa then described the presence of hypopyon and his treatment of same:

I took away blood abundantly from the arm and foot, and also locally by means of leeches applied near both the angles of the eyes, and I also purged her. These remedies were attended with some advantage, inasmuch as they contributed to abate the inflammatory stage of the violent ophthalmia. Nevertheless an extravasation of yellowish glutinous lymph appeared in the anterior chamber of the aqueous humor, which filled out one-third of that cavity.[1]

Adjunctive therapy, common to the times, was then used: "The uninterrupted application of small bags of gauze filled with emollient herbs boiled in milk . . . and repeated mild purges with a grain of the antimonium tartarizatum dissolved in a pint of the decoction of the root of the triticum repens." The symptoms of the inflammation were entirely relieved, and "on the eleventh day the patient was able to bear a moderate degree of light." Additional therapies mentioned in Scarpa's text[1] include drops of vitriolic collyrium, with mucilage of quince-seed, bags of tepid mallows, a few grains of camphire, and blister production of the neck. Scarpa's text makes clear that these therapies were accepted as best medical practice for the time.

By 1830, as outlined in MacKenzie's text on diseases of the eye,[2] dilation of the pupil with tincture of belladonna had been added to bloodletting, purging, and blistering therapy. Also added was the use of antimony and other nauseants, opiates for relief of pain, and mercury as an adjunctive antiphlogistic agent. Fever therapy, induced by intramuscular injection of milk or intravenous injection of triple typhoid H antigen, became fashionable in the first half of the 20th century. This "stimulatory" treatment, effective only if the patient's temperature was raised to about 40°C three or four times in succession, persisted into the early 1950s. Its effectiveness was undisputed, although its mechanism is unknown.

The next major advance in the care of patients with inflammatory disease was not made until 1952 with the discovery of the effectiveness of corticosteroid therapy. It is with this class of drugs that we begin our discussion of the pharmacology of treating intraocular inflammation. We then address the issue of cycloplegic therapy; then, we introduce the reader to the more modern advances in the care of patients with inflammatory disease: the use of nonsteroidal anti-inflammatory drugs and of immunosuppressive agents.

Clearly, despite the advances made in the past 30 years with the discovery and development of these two additional classes of anti-inflammatory agents, a significant proportion of patients with uveitis are still treated suboptimally by ophthalmologists unfamiliar with the effective and safe use of such drugs. It is regrettable that, still today, fully 10% of all blindness occurring in the United States alone results from inadequately treated uveitis.

It is our fervent hope that the following will contribute to a "sea change" in the attitudes of ophthalmologists regarding the tolerance of low-grade chronic inflammation that continues, eventually, to rob children and adults of precious vision. We believe strongly in a paradigm of zero tolerance for chronic intraocular inflammation and further believe that a stepwise algorithm to achieve that goal is highly effective in reducing ocular morbidity secondary to uveitis.

References

1. Scarpa A: In: Cadell T, Davies W, eds: Practical Observations on the Principle Diseases of the Eyes. London, Strand, 1806, pp 292–321.
2. MacKenzie WA: Practical Treatise on the Diseases of the Eye. London, Longman, Rees, Orme, Brown & Green, 1830, pp 422–457.

9 | CORTICOSTEROIDS

Albert T. Vitale and C. Stephen Foster

INTRODUCTION AND HISTORY

The isolation of cortisone (compound E) in 1935 by Edward C. Kendall and the subsequent clinical demonstration of the dramatic beneficial effects of this compound and of adrenocorticotropic hormone (ACTH) in the treatment of acute rheumatoid arthritis by Hench and colleagues[1] in 1950 marked a revolution in modern medical therapeutics. Today, the synthetic congeners of the naturally occurring corticosteroids produced by the adrenal cortex are as indispensable to medical practice as antibiotics are.

In 1950, Gordon and McLean[2] extended the use of corticosteroids and ACTH to ophthalmic practice. Cortisone and hydroxycortisone were subsequently introduced for systemic and topical use by 1952.[3] Their attendant success in the treatment of ocular inflammation catalyzed a search for better synthetic analogues of these steroids with more potent anti-inflammatory effects, better ocular penetration, and enhanced bioavailability. A variety of formulations for topical, regional (subconjunctival and retrobulbar), and systemic use were developed over the next decade. By 1956, it had become evident that topical prednisolone minimized systemic adverse effects and was more efficacious in the treatment of anterior segment inflammation, whereas systemic prednisone was preferable for posterior disease.[4, 5] As experience with these medications grew, an understanding of their potent anti-inflammatory and immunosuppressive properties emerged, together with an appreciation of their capability for producing many potentially serious ocular and systemic complications. At present, corticosteroids remain the mainstay of management of ocular inflammatory and immune-mediated disease. A wide variety of synthetic preparations are currently available, the efficacy and toxicities of which depend on the formulation; the dose, frequency, and route of administration; and the therapeutic strategy used.

OFFICIAL DRUG NAME AND CHEMISTRY

Corticosteroids (glucocorticoids and mineralocorticoids) may occur naturally in response to ACTH-induced conversion of cholesterol to pregnenolone in the adrenal cortex or as synthetic congeners of cortisol (hydroxycortisone). All corticosteroids comprise 21 carbon molecules consisting of a cyclopentoperhydrophenathrene nucleus, as well as three hexane rings and one pentane ring, designated A, B, C, and D. Modifications in this basic structure at various sites result in compounds with different biologic properties (i.e., duration of action, relative anti-inflammatory activity, sodium-retaining activity [Table 9–1], and transcorneal penetration). These alterations, in turn, determine the overall effectiveness of the compounds in a particular clinical condition or route of administration and influence the occurrence of systemic

or ocular side effects. Modifications in the structure-activity relationship include the following[6]:

1. Most glucocorticoids are 17-α-hydroxy compounds, distinguishing them from androgenic steroids, which are 19-carbon, 17-α-keto molecules. Medrysone is an exception.
2. All naturally occurring steroids and most synthetic congeners have a hydroxyl group attached to carbon 21 (C-21), ring D.
3. All biologically active corticosteroids have a double bond at the C-4,5 position and a ketone group at C-3, ring A. Cortisone, which is an inactive form, contains, in addition to the basic nucleus, a ketone group at C-11, ring C. It is converted to its active 11-hydroxyl form, cortisol (hydroxycortisone), through hepatic 11-B hydroxylation.
4. The addition of a 1,2 double bond in ring A to the basic nucleus results in prednisolone and prednisone (with an 11I-keto group). This modification results in a decreased rate of degradation (prolonged half-life [t½]) and enhanced carbohydrate-regulating capacity.
5. Methylprednisolone is formed by the addition of a 6-methyl carbon group in ring B with slightly more anti-inflammatory activity than prednisolone.
6. Although fluorination at the 9-α position in ring B leads to enhanced anti-inflammatory potency, it produces excessive mineralocorticoid activity. Most fluorinated topical steroids have this basic structure, and the mineralocorticoid effect is diminished by masking the 16- or 17-hydroxy group with various esters.[7]
7. 9-α-Fluorohydrocortisone, together with the 1,2 double bond in ring A, can be further modified by the addition of a 16-α-hydroxy, a 16-α-methyl, or a 16-β-methyl group to produce triamcinolone, dexamethasone, or betamethasone, respectively. Systemically, these glucocorticoids have enhanced anti-inflammatory but minimal mineralocorticoid activity.

PHARMACOLOGY

The mechanism by which corticosteroids are believed to act ultimately entails control of the rate of protein synthesis at both a cellular and a molecular level.[6, 8] After passively entering a target cell, the glucocorticoid molecule rapidly binds to a specific cytoplasmic steroid receptor protein. The cytoplasmic steroid receptor complex then becomes activated, undergoing a conformational change that allows it to cross the nuclear membrane and bind to DNA directly at sites known as glucocorticoid response elements (GREs). GRE binding controls the transcription of specific genes, which in turn either promote or inhibit the production of specific mRNAs. As a consequence, the rates of translation and production of specific protein products encoded by their mRNAs are changed, thereby mediating the response of a particular cell to corticoster-

TABLE 9–1. BIOLOGIC HALF-LIFE, RELATIVE ANTI-INFLAMMATORY ACTIVITY, SYSTEMIC EQUIVALENT, AND SODIUM-RETAINING ACTIVITY OF SYSTEMIC STEROIDS

DRUG	COMMON TRADE NAME	BIOLOGIC HALF-LIFE (hr)	RELATIVE ANTI-INFLAMMATORY ACTIVITY	SYSTEMIC EQUIVALENT (mg)	RELATIVE NA⁺ RETENTION
SHORT-ACTING					
Hydrocortisone	Cortef (Upjohn, Kalamazoo, MI) Hydrocortone Phosphate (MSD, West Point, PA)	8–12	1.0	20	1.0
Cortisone	Cortone Acetate (MSD)	8–12	0.8	25	0.8
INTERMEDIATE-ACTING					
Prednisone	Deltasone (Upjohn) Meticorten (Schering, Kenilworth, NJ) Orasone (Solvay, Marietta, GA)	18–36	4.0	5	0.8
Prednisolone	Delta-Cortef (Upjohn)	18–36	4.0	5	0.8
Methylprednisolone	Medrol (Upjohn)	18–36	5.0	4	0.0
Triamcinolone	Aristocort (Fujisawa, Deerfield, IL)	18–36	5.0	4	0.0
Fludrocortisone	Florinef (Apothecon, Princeton, NJ)	18–36	10	1.5	125
LONG-ACTING					
Paramethasone	Haldrone (Lilly, Indianapolis, IN)	36–54	10	2	0.0
Dexamethasone	Decadron (MSD)	36–54	25	0.75	0.0
Betamethasone	Celestone (Schering)	36–54	25	0.75	0.0

oids. Corticosteroid receptors have been identified in the iris, ciliary body, and adjacent corneoscleral tissue.[9]

Clinical Pharmacology

Corticosteroids produce a multiplicity of important biochemical and physiologic effects on many tissues throughout the body. These effects not only mediate the anti-inflammatory and immunosuppressive actions of corticosteroids, but also account for the potentially undesirable adverse effects that occur during the course of systemic or topical therapy.

Hypothalamic-Pituitary-Adrenal Axis

With the exogenous administration of corticosteroids, the release of both corticotropin-releasing factor (CRF) from the hypothalamus and ACTH from the anterior pituitary is suppressed, resulting in decreased cortisol production by the adrenal cortex. This feedback inhibition is very sensitive and occurs within minutes after administration of a systemic corticosteroid. It is progressive, in both a dose- and time-dependent manner, affects basal and stress-stimulated release, and is reversible.[10] Administration of a large dose of corticosteroids may suppress the hypothalamic-pituitary-adrenal (HPA) axis for a few hours, whereas more prolonged exposure is associated with profound suppression and an extended recovery time for normal HPA axis functioning.

Carbohydrate, Protein, and Lipid Metabolism

The principal biochemical actions of corticosteroids include stimulation and induction of protein synthesis and gluconeogenesis in the liver and inhibition of peripheral tissue protein synthesis.[11] In addition, corticosteroids produce peripheral insulin resistance, inhibiting glucose uptake in most target tissues (except brain, heart, and liver)

and in erythrocytes. Hepatic glycogen storage is enhanced, and lipid stores are stimulated to undergo lipolysis. The net effect is a corticosteroid-induced catabolic state with hyperglycemia, ketosis, and hyperlipidemia, which, in normal subjects, is blunted by a compensatory increase in insulin release.[10] These physiologic effects of corticosteroids on intermediary metabolism may explain some of the more conspicuous manifestations of excessive and prolonged steroid therapy: fat redistribution characteristic of Cushing's syndrome, thinning of the skin, development of striae, osteoporosis, poor wound healing, and corticosteroid-induced myopathy.

Calcium Metabolism

Corticosteroids affect calcium metabolism in a complex manner, resulting in a net reduction in total body calcium stores and osteopenia. Corticosteroids inhibit intestinal absorption, promote renal excretion of calcium, and inhibit osteoblast function. In addition, osteoblasts are stimulated by the compensatory increase in parathyroid hormone levels.[10, 12]

Central Nervous System

Transient mood disturbances ranging from euphoria to depression, as well as anxiety and frank psychosis, are well-known complications of systemic glucocorticoid administration that vary considerably between patients. Although the mechanism or mechanisms underlying these changes are poorly understood, corticosteroids have been suggested to cross the blood-brain barrier (BBB) and either act directly on the brain or mediate these effects indirectly through changes in cerebral blood flow or through perturbations in local electrolyte concentrations.[6]

Electrolyte and Fluid Balance

Synthetic corticosteroids with mineralocorticoid activity (see Table 9–1) may significantly alter the patient's fluid and electrolyte balance. Aldosterone, the prototypical, naturally occurring mineralocorticoid hormone, stimulates active reabsorption of sodium in exchange for potassium at the proximal convoluted tubule in the kidney. Water follows sodium passively while potassium is excreted, which may result in hypokalemia when there is an excessive mineralocorticoid effect. The renin-angiotensin system (RAS) and plasma potassium levels are chiefly responsible for primary mineralocorticoid control.[12]

Cardiovascular System

Hypertension and increased cardiac output may occur after systemic administration of corticosteroids. Indeed, high-dose corticosteroids may restore circulatory function in various states of shock. Although these actions may be due in part to mineralocorticoid effects, myocardial tissue contains high-affinity glucocorticoid receptors and exhibits a positive ionotropic response to corticosteroids.[10, 11]

Gastrointestinal System

Corticosteroids inhibit DNA synthesis in the gastrointestinal (GI) tract and enhance gastric secretions. This increases the risk of formation of duodenal ulcers and contributes to the development of gastritis, particularly when higher doses are used.[10]

Anti-Inflammatory and Immunosuppressive Effects

Corticosteroids have both anti-inflammatory and immunosuppressive effects that are nonspecific, that is, they act to ameliorate the cardinal signs of inflammation (rubor, calor, dolor, and edema), irrespective of the inciting inflammatory stimulus or disease process. Corticosteroids mediate their anti-inflammatory and immunosuppressive effects by many different mechanisms.[6, 11, 13–16] A description of these follows:

1. Induction of lymphocytopenia. In humans, corticosteroids are not cytotoxic to lymphocytes. Instead, the distribution of these cells, particularly the T-helper subset, is altered so that they are sequestered from the intravascular circulation and become concentrated in the bone marrow. Consequently, fewer immunoreactive cells are recruited to the site of inflammation. After administration of a single large dose of corticosteroid, blood lymphocytes are maximally reduced within 1 to 6 hours. Small to moderate doses preferentially affect T lymphocytes, whereas long-term high dosing may affect B lymphocytes and thus antibody production.
2. Neutrophilic leukocytosis. Corticosteroids simultaneously induce production of large numbers of neutrophils by the bone marrow while preventing the adherence of these cells to the vascular endothelium, thereby impeding their migration from the intravascular space to the site of inflammation.
3. Reduction of circulating eosinophils and monocytes.
4. Inhibition of macrophage recruitment with consequent alterations in cell-mediated immune responses (i.e., reduced skin-test reactivity).
5. Inhibition of macrophage migration and reduction of antigen-processing capability. Corticosteroids suppress the action of certain lymphokines (e.g., macrophage migration inhibitory factor) and prevent vascular endothelial adhesion. In this way, the macrophage is denied access to sites at which antigens are initially deposited.
6. Attenuation of bactericidal activity of macrophages and monocytes.
7. Stabilization of intracellular lysozomal membranes. With inhibition of neutrophil degranulation, the surrounding tissues are spared the potentially damaging effects of the liberated lysozomal enzymes.
8. Stabilization of mast cell and basophilic membranes. Degranulation of these cells is inhibited, thereby preventing release of various inflammatory mediators such as histamine, bradykinin, platelet-activating factor (PAF), slow-reacting substance of anaphylaxis (SRS-A), and eosinophilic chemotactic factor (ECF).
9. Inhibition of prostaglandin synthesis. Corticosteroids, through a protein called *macrocortin,* inhibit the enzyme phospholipase A_2 and thus the conversion of phospholipid to arachidonic acid (AA). (See Figure 11–2 in Chapter 11, Nonsteroidal Anti-Inflammatory Drugs.) Consequently, the synthesis of both prostaglandins (through the cyclooxygenase pathway) and leukotrienes (through the lipoxygenase pathway) is prevented.
10. Reduction of capillary permeability and suppression of vasodilation in the setting of acute inflammation. As a consequence, transudation of fluid, protein, and inflammatory cells into the target site is reduced.
11. Suppression of fibroplasia.

PHARMACEUTICS

Topical Corticosteroid Preparations

A variety of corticosteroid preparations are available for topical use in the treatment of inflammatory ocular disease. These are listed in order of ascending anti-inflammatory potency in Table 9–2 and are discussed briefly herein.

Dexamethasone

Dexamethasone is formulated as a 0.1% alcohol suspension/0.1% sodium phosphate solution and as a 0.05% ointment. It is the most potent commercially available topical steroid, and thus poses a concomitant increased risk of untoward ocular adverse effects.

Prednisolone

Prednisolone is available as a 0.12% or 1% acetate suspension, as a 0.12%, 0.5%, or 1% sodium phosphate solution, and as a 0.25% phosphate ointment. Although acetate preparations, with their biphasic solubility, achieve better penetration into and through an intact cornea than do water-soluble phosphate vehicles, this difference is not clinically significant when intraocular inflammation exists; degree of penetration depends more on concentration and dosage frequency[17] (described in the section, "Pharmacokinetics, Concentration-Effect Relationship, and Metabolism"). Moreover, suspensions require thorough mixing to ensure maximal steroid concentrations with each delivery, introducing a potential compliance

TABLE 9–2. OPHTHALMIC TOPICAL CORTICOSTEROID PREPARATIONS

DRUG/ PREPARATION	COMMON TRADE NAME	FORMULATION
Dexamethasone		
Alcohol	Maxidex (Alcon)	0.1% suspension, 0.05% ointment
Sodium phosphate	Decadron Phosphate (MSD)	0.1% solution, 0.05% ointment
Prednisolone		
Acetate	Pred Forte (Allergan), Econopred Plus (Alcon), AK-Tate (Akorn)	1.0% suspension
	Pred Mild (Allergan), Econopred (Alcon)	0.12% suspension
Sodium phosphate	Inflamase Forte (CIBA Vision, Duluth, GA) AK-Pred (Akorn)	1% solution
	Metreton (Schering)	0.5% solution
	Inflamase Mild (CIBA Vision)	0.12% solution
	AK-Pred (Akorn)	
Phosphate	Hydeltrasol (MSD)	0.5% 0.25% ointment
Fluorometholone		
Alcohol	FML (Allergan)	0.1% suspension, 0.1% ointment
Medroxyprogesterone		
Acetate	Provera	1% suspension
Medrysone		
Alcohol	HMS (Allergan)	1.0% suspension
Rimexolone	Vexol (Alcon)	1% suspension
Lodeprednol etabonate	Lotemax (Pharmos)	0.5% suspension
	Alrex (Bausch & Lomb)	0.2% suspension

problem, which may make solutions preferable in clinical practice. The bioavailability and potency of prednisolone not only make it an efficacious anti-inflammatory agent, but also increase the likelihood of dose-dependent ocular toxicity.

Fluorometholone and Medrysone

Fluorometholone (FML) (0.1% or 0.25%) and medrysone (HMS) (1.0%) are supplied as ophthalmic suspensions. Fluorometholone is also available as a 0.1% ointment. These are weak anti-inflammatory agents and are the least likely to produce steroid-related ocular damage (cataract and glaucoma).

Medroxyprogesterone

Medroxyprogesterone is not available commercially for ophthalmic use, but may be prepared by the hospital pharmacy from a 1% solution used parenterally. This agent is particularly useful in certain peripheral ulcerative, inflammatory, external ocular diseases because it not only reduces inflammation but also decreases the production of collagenase, and it interferes less with collagen synthesis than do other steroids.[18] Its relative potency is slightly less than that of 0.12% prednisolone.

Systemic and Regional Corticosteroid Preparations

Corticosteroids used in systemic and regional (subconjunctival, sub-Tenon, transseptal, and retrobulbar) ther-

apy of ocular inflammatory disease are presented in order of increasing anti-inflammatory potency in Tables 9–3 and 9–4, respectively, and are discussed herein.

Hydrocortisone

Hydrocortisone is formulated in 5-, 10-, and 20-mg tablets, and as a 10-mg/5-ml suspension for oral (PO) use. In addition, intramuscular (IM), intravenous (IV), and regional injectable preparations are available in concentrations including 25, 50, 100, 250, and 1000 mg/ml. Subconjunctival doses range from 50 to 125 mg, whereas systemic therapy may be initiated at 20 to 240 mg, depending on the severity of inflammation.

Prednisone

Prednisone is supplied in tablet form in doses of 1, 2.5, 5, 10, 20, 25, and 50 mg and as a 5-mg/ml oral solution. It is commonly used in therapy of severe ocular inflammatory disease, with a typical initial dose of 1.0 to 1.5 mg/kg and subsequent tapering, depending on the clinical response (described in section "Therapeutic Use").

Prednisolone

Prednisolone is available in 5-mg tablets and as a 15-mg/ml syrup for oral use; however, it is used far more often as a topical agent. It has four times the inflammatory potency of hydrocortisone (see Table 9–1), with common systemic dosages ranging from 5 mg every other morning to 50 mg daily in divided doses.[19]

Methylprednisolone

Methylprednisolone is available in 2- to 32-mg tablets for oral use, as an acetate suspension (20 to 80 mg/ml), and as a sodium succinate (40- to 100-mg powder) solution for IM or IV administration. Its relative inflammatory potency is four times that of hydrocortisone (see Table 9–1). The sodium succinate formulation is used regionally, with typical doses ranging from 40 to 125 mg per injection. A methylprednisolone acetate depot is available for subconjunctival, sub-Tenon, or retrobulbar administration in doses ranging from 40 to 80 mg/0.5 ml; this provides prolonged local release of steroid. Finally, methylprednisolone sodium succinate is occasionally used in IV pulse therapy (1 g/day for 3 days) in cases of severe bilateral, sight-threatening uveitis (described in the section, "Therapeutic Use").

Triamcinolone

Triamcinolone tablets are available in strengths of 1, 2, 4, and 8 mg; a 4-mg/5-ml syrup is also available for oral use. Triamcinolone has essentially no mineralocorticoid activity, yet has five times more anti-inflammatory activity than hydrocortisone (see Table 9–1). Triamcinolone acetonide and diacetate suspensions (10 to 40 mg/ml) are also available for IM injection and are frequently administered through the sub-Tenon, subconjunctival, and transseptal routes in the regional management of uveitis (see Table 9–4).

Dexamethasone

Dexamethasone sodium tablets are formulated in strengths of 0.25, 0.5, 0.75, 1.5, 4, and 6 mg; it is also

TABLE 9–3. SYSTEMIC CORTICOSTEROID PREPARATIONS

DRUG	COMMON TRADE NAME	ORAL	FORMULATION
Hydrocortisone	Cortef (Upjohn, Kalamazoo, MI)	5- to 20-mg tablet 10-mg/5-ml suspension	25- and 50-mg suspension IM
	Hydrocortone Phosphate (MSD, West Point, PA) Solu-Cortef (Upjohn)		50-mg/ml solution IM/IV 100- to 1000-mg powder IM/IV
Prednisone	Deltasone (Upjohn) Meticorten (Shering, Kenilworth, NJ) Drasone (Solvay, Marietta, GA) Liquid-Pred (Muro, Tewksbury, MA)	1.0- to 50-mg tablet 5-mg/ml solution	
Prednisolone	Delta-Cortef (Upjohn) Prelone (Muro)	1- to 5-mg tablet 15-mg/ml syrup	
Acetate	Predalone (Forest, St. Louis, MO)		25- to 100-mg/ml suspension IM
Sodium phosphate	Hydeltrasol (MSD)		20-mg/ml solution IM/IV
Methylprednisolone	Medrol (Upjohn)	2- to 32-mg tablet	
Acetate	Depo-Medrol (Upjohn)		20- to 80-mg/ml suspension IM
Sodium succinate	Solu-Medrol (Upjohn)		40- to 1000-mg powder IM/IV
Triamcinolone			
Diacetate	Kenacort (Apothecon, Princeton, NJ) Aristocort (Fujisawa, Deerfield, IL)	4-mg/5-mg syrup 1- to 8-mg tablet	40-mg/ml suspension IM
Acetonide	Kenalog (Westwood-Squibb, Princeton, NJ)		10- and 40-mg/ml suspension IM
Dexamethasone sodium	Decadron (MSD)	0.25- to 6.0-mg tablet 0.5-mg/5-ml elixir 0.5-mg/5-ml solution	
Dexamethasone sodium phosphate	Decadron Phosphate (MSD)		4- to 24-mg/ml solution IV
Acetate	Decadron-LA (MSD)		8-mg/ml suspension IM
Betamethasone	Celestone (Schering)	0.6-mg tablet 0.6-mg/5-ml syrup	
Sodium phosphate	Celestone Phosphate (Schering)		3-mg/ml solution IV
Acetate and sodium phosphate	Celestone (Schering) Soluspan		3- and 6-mg/ml suspension IM

IM, intramuscular; IV, intravenous.

available as a 0.5-mg/ml elixir and as a 0.5-mg/5-ml solution for oral use. Initial doses range from 0.75 mg to 9 mg PO daily, depending on the severity of inflammation.[19] Dexamethasone acetate suspension (9 mg/ml) and sodium phosphate solution (4, 10, and 24 mg/ml) are available for IM and IV administration, respectively. The latter may also be injected regionally or intravitreally at initial doses of 40 mg and 0.4 mg, respectively (see Table 9–4). Dexamethasone is 25 times more potent than hydrocortisone and has little sodium-retaining or potassium-wasting activity (see Table 9–1).

Betamethasone

Betamethasone is the most potent synthetic steroid, with an anti-inflammatory and mineralocorticoid profile similar to that of dexamethasone. It is formulated as 0.6-mg

TABLE 9–4. REGIONAL CORTICOSTEROID PREPARATIONS

DRUG	COMMON TRADE NAMES	FORMULATION	ROUTE AND TYPICAL DOSE
Hydrocortisone	Hydrocortisone Sodium Succinate (MSD, West Point, PA)	100- to 1000-mg powder	Subconjunctival/Tenon 50–125 mg
Methylprednisolone			
Sodium succinate	Solu-Medrol (Upjohn, Kalamazoo, MI)	40-mg/ml, 125-mg/ml, 2-g/30-ml solution	Subconjunctival/Tenon 40–125 mg
Acetate	Depo-Medrol (Upjohn)	20- to 80-mg/ml (depot) suspension	Transseptal, retrobulbar 40–80 mg/0.5 ml
Triamcinolone			
Diacetate	Aristocort (Fujisawa, Deerfield, IL)	25- and 40-mg/ml suspension	Subconjunctival/Tenon 40 mg
Acetonide	Kenalog (Westwood-Squibb, Princeton, NJ)	10- and 40-mg/ml	Transseptal 40 mg
Dexamethasone			
Acetate	Decadron-LA (MSD)	8- to 16-mg/ml suspension	Subconjunctival/Tenon 4–8 mg, Transseptal 4–8 mg
Sodium phosphate	Decadron Phosphate (MSD)	4, 10-, 24-mg/ml solution	Retrobulbar, intravitreal 0.4 mg
Betamethasone acetate and sodium phosphate	Celestone Soluspan (Schering, Kenilworth, TX)	3-mg/ml suspension	Subconjunctival/Tenon, transseptal, 1 mg

Subconjunctival/Tenon, subconjunctival or sub-Tenon injection.

tablets and as a 0.6-mg/5-ml syrup for oral use. The sodium phosphate solution (3 mg/ml) and the acetate–sodium phosphate suspension (3 and 6 mg/ml) are available for IV and IM administration, respectively. The latter may be given by the subconjunctival, sub-Tenon, or transseptal route at a dose of 1 mg per injection (see Table 9–4). Initial systemic doses range from 0.5 to 9 mg/day, depending on disease severity. As with all systemically administered steroids (orally or intravenously), gastrointestinal (GI) prophylaxis should be instituted concomitantly (described in the sections, "Therapeutic Use" and "Adverse Effects and Toxicity").

PHARMACOKINETICS, CONCENTRATION-EFFECT RELATIONSHIP, AND METABOLISM

Systemic Corticosteroids

Orally administered corticosteroids (prednisone) are readily absorbed in the upper jejunum, have a bioavailability ≤90%, and reach peak plasma concentrations 30 minutes to 2 hours after ingestion. Parenteral (IM) administration of corticosteroids in suspension has prolonged effects.[8] Concomitant food ingestion delays absorption, but does not reduce the amount of drug absorbed. Corticosteroids are widely distributed throughout most body tissues. In the plasma, 80% to 90% of corticosteroids are protein bound; the remaining free fraction represents the biologically active form. Two steroid-binding proteins exist: a high-affinity, low-capacity, cortisol-binding globulin (CBG) and a low-affinity, high-capacity protein, albumin. CBG levels are decreased by hypothyroidism, liver and kidney disease, and obesity, thereby increasing the free fraction. Conversely, the relative amount of free steroid is reduced by entities that increase CBG levels (e.g., pregnancy, estrogen therapy, and hyperthyroidism).[6] Corticosteroids compete with each other for binding sites on the CBG. Synthetic congeners or cortisol binds less avidly than the endogenous molecule, thereby increasing the available free fraction of steroid. Prednisolone reportedly binds with greater affinity than do other synthetic compounds, resulting in the replacement of endogenous cortisol from the protein-binding sites.[12] Prolonged and/or high-dose corticosteroid therapy consequently produces a greater proportion of free steroid in the body.

All biologically active corticosteroids have a double bond in the C-4,5 position and a ketone group at the C-3 position. Cortisone and prednisone have no inherent glucocorticoid activity, and they depend on the reversible action of 11-β-hydroxydehydrogenase in the liver to convert them to the active analogues hydroxycortisone and prednisolone. Patients with hepatic disease may have impaired glucocorticoid interconversions and clearance. In such circumstances, administration of prednisolone rather than prednisone is more appropriate.[6] Hepatic reduction of the C-4,5 double bond and the C-3 ketone group results in an inactive metabolite, which is then conjugated with glucuronide to form a soluble product that is excreted by the kidney.[6]

There is a poor correlation between the duration of biologic activity and the plasma t½ of the various synthetic corticosteroids.[8] Their biologic t½ varies: short-acting hydrocortisone, 8 to 12 hours; intermediate-acting triamcinolone, 18 to 36 hours; and long-acting dexamethasone, 36 to 54 hours (see Table 9–1). In contrast, the plasma t½ ranges only from 1 hour (cortisone and prednisone) to 5 hours (triamcinolone).

The intraocular penetration of systemically administered corticosteroids is limited by the blood-ocular barrier. IM administration of cortisone has been shown to penetrate the vitreous in appreciable quantities, although it does not quite reach the aqueous concentrations after topical therapy.[5] In contrast, topical applications yield the lowest vitreous concentrations. Peak concentrations of dexamethasone, triamcinolone, and methylprednisolone have been determined in the aqueous humor of rabbits 1 hour after IV administration of 25 mg of steroid; slightly higher levels of drug are attained when it is applied topically.[20]

Topical and Regional Corticosteroids

Several interdependent factors influence the overall efficacy of a particular topical steroid preparation in the treatment of ocular inflammatory disease, including (1) its ability to penetrate into and through the cornea, sclera, or blood-ocular barrier; (2) its relative anti-inflammatory potency and duration of action in the cornea, aqueous humor, or vitreous cavity; (3) the dose and frequency of administration; and (4) the adverse effect profile.[16, 21]

Early ocular penetration studies demonstrated the presence of 0.97% prednisolone acetate in the aqueous humor of rabbits within 5 minutes of a single topical dose, a peak concentration by 30 minutes, and a nadir by 240 minutes.[22] Similarly, radiolabeled 0.1% dexamethasone phosphate was shown to penetrate the intact cornea and aqueous of rabbits within 10 minutes and to remain in the eye for as long as 24 hours.[23] In the same study, a surprising degree of systemic absorption was observed after topical application, as manifested by the presence of radioactivity in the urine, plasma, kidneys, and liver of the animals. With regard to ocular tissues, the highest concentrations of steroid 30 minutes after topical application have been detected in the cornea and conjunctiva, followed by the sclera, choroid, and aqueous, with very little drug detectable in the lens or vitreous.[24, 25]

Ocular tissues themselves may play an important role in local steroid metabolism and thus determine to some degree the efficacy of a particular topical preparation. Systemically administered cortisone is rendered biologically active (converted to hydroxycortisone) by hydroxylation at C-11 in the liver. The clinical anti-inflammatory efficacy results of topically applied cortisone and prednisone suggest inherent 11-hydroxylase activity in the cornea and, possibly, other ocular tissues.[26] Phosphate derivatives may be converted into more active alcohol forms by corneal phosphatase activity.[27] Steroid reaching the eye may depend in part on degradative enzyme systems such as "A" ring reductase in the iris, cornea, and ciliary body.[28] Long-acting synthetic congeners such as dexamethasone are more resistant to such inactivation.

Variability in ocular penetration among topical steroids is due not only to differences in their formulation, but also to variable intrinsic properties of the cornea. Phosphate preparations, marketed as solutions, are highly water-soluble and would be expected to penetrate lipophilic barriers (the corneal epithelium and endothelium) relatively poorly. In contradistinction, alcohol-based and, in particular, acetate suspensions exhibit biphasic solubility and thus theoretically are better able to penetrate all corneal layers to reach the anterior chamber. Similarly, the presence or absence of the corneal epithelium is expected to affect the intracorneal and intraocular bioavailability of various steroid preparations. The experimental data, however, are not as clear-cut as the theoretical expectations.

In one study, in which a rabbit model of clove oil–induced keratitis was used, the corneal drug concentration after topical administration, when epithelium was intact, was greatest for prednisolone acetate, followed by prednisolone sodium phosphate and dexamethasone alcohol; however, in corneas denuded of epithelium, the concentration of prednisolone phosphate was greatest, followed by prednisolone acetate and dexamethasone alcohol. For each condition, these trends were mirrored in the levels of specific drug detected in the aqueous.[29–33] Results of another study supported the superior penetration of prednisolone sodium phosphate in rabbit corneas denuded of epithelium; however, equal corneal penetration by prednisolone acetate, sodium phosphate, and fluorometholone was demonstrated when epithelium was intact.[34] More recent work, in which the potentially confounding effect of stromal clove oil was eliminated, has demonstrated better penetration of topically applied prednisolone phosphate through an intact rabbit corneal epithelium than might be expected, given its limited lipid solubility.[35] Both in vivo and in vitro studies comparing the permeability of prednisolone phosphate and prednisolone acetate across intact corneal epithelium in rabbits have shown steady-state conditions for penetration and similar fluxes for both drugs with respect to prednisolone, and similar bioavailability in the aqueous humor as measured directly by high-performance liquid chromatography (HPLC).[36, 37] With similar concentrations of drug in the anterior chamber, the differential penetration of phosphate solutions versus acetate suspensions themselves may not be the crucial determinant of therapeutic efficacy in the treatment of intraocular inflammation. Other factors, such as inherent anti-inflammatory activity, glucocorticoid receptor–binding efficacy, metabolic interconversion, and intraocular clearance of a particular steroid preparation, as well as dosing frequency, may be more important in the therapy of uveitis.

The anti-inflammatory activity of various corticosteroids varies considerably (see Table 9–1). Potency is influenced by many factors, including glucocorticoid receptor–binding affinity, formulation, route of administration, and the experimental model used to evaluate the drug. These data on anti-inflammatory potency were obtained from monocular experimental models in which drug was systemically administered; thus they cannot be directly extended to topical ocular human use.[17] Therefore, Leibowitz and Kupferman[17] quantitatively evaluated the anti-inflammatory effects of different topical steroid preparations in a rabbit model of clove oil–induced keratitis by

TABLE 9–5. DECREASE IN CORNEAL INFLAMMATORY ACTIVITY AFTER TOPICAL THERAPY WITH VARIOUS CORTICOSTEROID DERIVATIVES IN RABBITS

	CORNEAL EPITHELIUM	
PREPARATION	**Intact (%)**	**Absent (%)**
Prednisolone acetate 1.0%	51	53
Dexamethasone alcohol 0.1%	40	42
Prednisolone phosphate 1.0%	28	47
Dexamethasone phosphate 0.1%	19	22
Dexamethasone phosphate 0.05% (ointment)		
Fluorometholone alcohol 0.1%	31	37

Adapted from Leibowitz HM, Kupferman A: Int Ophthalmol Clin 1980;20: 117–134.

measuring the decrease in radioactively labeled neutrophils in the cornea. Their work demonstrated that prednisolone acetate 1% was the most potent anti-inflammatory agent for the suppression of inflammation in corneas with or without an intact epithelium (Table 9–5). The two commercially available forms of this drug were identical both in their bioavailability in the cornea and in their anti-inflammatory efficacy.

Although it may be tempting to assume that increased bioavailability of a particular steroid preparation at the site of anterior segment inflammation will provide proportionately enhanced anti-inflammatory activity, Leibowitz and associates showed that this is not the case with respect to intracorneal inflammation.[38] For example, although the corneal concentrations of dexamethasone acetate and alcohol were significantly lower than those of the phosphate preparation, the former demonstrated superior anti-inflammatory activity irrespective of epithelial integrity (Table 9–6). These data suggest that different derivatives of the same corticosteroid base are not equivalent in their anti-inflammatory properties in the therapy of keratitis. Indeed, when assayed for its ability to compete for glucocorticoid receptors, dexamethasone alcohol was shown to be 15 times more potent than dexamethasone phosphate,[39] which may explain in part the apparently diminished topical anti-inflammatory effect associated with phosphate preparations in a keratitis model.[26] Extension of these findings to intraocular inflammation has yet to be confirmed experimentally. Ocular tissue phosphatases might convert the phosphate de-

TABLE 9–6. CORNEAL BIOAVAILABILITY AND ANTI-INFLAMMATORY EFFECTIVENESS OF DIFFERENT DEXAMETHASONE PREPARATIONS

	ANTI-INFLAMMATORY EFFECT (%)		CORNEAL BIOAVAILABILITY (mg/min/g)	
CORTICOSTEROID	**Epithelium Intact**	**Absent**	**Epithelium Intact**	**Absent**
Dexamethasone acetate 0.1%	55	60	111	118
Dexamethasone alcohol 0.1%	40	42	543	1316
Dexamethasone phosphate 0.1%	19	22	1068	4642

Adapted from Leibowitz HM, Kupferman A: Int Ophthalmol Clin 1980;22:117–134.

rivative to the more active alcohol form once the steroid has reached the anterior chamber, thus enhancing the anti-inflammatory effect observed clinically.

More practical considerations may dictate the choice between derivatives of the same steroid base in clinical practice. Acetate suspensions must be adequately shaken to distribute insoluble drug particles so that the maximal concentration of steroid is delivered with each dose. Poor patient compliance has been demonstrated in persons who were instructed to shake their suspension eyedrops before topical instillation.[40] Therefore, a good rationale exists for the selection of phosphate solutions that provide more consistent drug dosage.

Increasing the concentration and dosage frequency of a particular steroid enhances both its bioavailability in the cornea and anterior chamber and its anti-inflammatory efficacy. However, raising the concentration of a drug such as prednisolone acetate beyond 1% does not offer additional anti-inflammatory benefit in the cornea but increases the potential for toxicity.[41] Likewise, hourly administration of prednisolone acetate is five times more effective than instillation every 4 hours in suppressing corneal inflammation (Table 9–7).[42] Although it is clinically impractical, maximal inflammatory suppression was achieved with an every-5-minute regimen.[42]

Rimexolone 1% suspension was introduced for ophthalmic use, including the treatment of mild to moderate uveitis, in 1996. It was shown, in two separate, double-masked, randomized, multicenter trials, to be equivalent in efficacy to 1% prednisolone acetate in reducing anterior chamber flare and cell number in patients with uveitis of initial severity of 2+ anterior chamber cells or fewer. Rimexolone was additionally shown to be considerably less likely to provoke significant rises in intraocular pressure,[43] making this drug a good choice for patients who are steroid responders and who have mild to modest uveitis requiring steroid therapy for several weeks.

Loteprednol etabonate (0.5% suspension) was introduced for ophthalmic use in 1998, and it too is touted for its reduced propensity to provoke rises in intraocular pressure by virtue of its rapid metabolism to an inactive metabolite. Although a clinically meaningful reduction in signs and symptoms of uveitis was noted in both treatment groups in the randomized, masked, multicenter studies comparing loteprednol etabonate 0.5% with prednisolone acetate 1%, loteprednol etabonate was less effective than prednisolone acetate.[44]

Two other less potent topical corticosteroids are commercially available for ocular use: FML and HMS. Although the corneal penetration of 0.1% FML is poor in comparison with that of 1% prednisolone acetate, no significant difference in anti-inflammatory efficacy was observed between the two steroids in the treatment of corneal inflammation.[45] The therapeutic efficacy of FML in the cornea, despite a reduced concentration, may be explained by its mildly hydrophobic properties, which allow achievement of saturation levels in the corneal epithelium before the drug is diffused through the more hydrophilic stroma.[16] In addition, FML has a high affinity for the glucocorticoid receptor; this, combined with its poor corneal penetration, may enhance its "local" corneal anti-inflammatory effect while reducing its propen-

TABLE 9–7. OPHTHALMIC INDICATIONS FOR USE OF CORTICOSTEROIDS

Eyelids
  Contact dermatitis
  Blepharitis
  Discoid lupus
  Chalazion
  Chemical burns
Conjunctiva
  Allergic disease (atopic, seasonal, vernal, GPC)
  Viral (herpetic, EKC)
  Mucocutaneous (graft versus host, erythema multiforme, toxic epidermal necrolysis, ocular cicatricial pemphigoid)
  Chemical burns
Cornea
  Keratitis
    Herpes zoster
    Disciform herpes simplex
    Immune infiltrates
    Interstitial
    Superficial punctate
    Peripheral ulcerative (Wegener's polyarteritis nodosa, Mooren's ulcer)
    Reiter's syndrome, Lyme disease, sarcoid
    Acne rosacea
    Graft rejection
    Chemical burns
Sclera
  Scleritis
Orbit
  Pseudotumor
  Graves' orbitopathy
Uvea
  Anterior uveitis
  Intermediate uveitis (pars planitis)
  Posterior uveitis
  Sympathetic ophthalmia
  Vogt-Koyanagi-Harada syndrome
  Endophthalmitis
Retina
  Cystoid macular edema
  Vasculitis
  Choroiditis
  Retinitis
  Acute retinal necrosis
Optic nerve
  Optic neuritis
  Temporal arteritis
Postoperative care
  Trauma
Extraocular muscles
  Ocular myasthenia gravis

GPC, giant papillary conjunctivitis; EKC, epidemic keratoconjunctivitis.

sity for steroid-induced ocular complications.[26] For the same reasons, the poor corneal penetration of FML makes it less effective than other more potent steroids in the treatment of intraocular inflammation.

HMS has weak anti-inflammatory effects and poor corneal penetration and is the least likely of all topical ophthalmic steroid preparations to produce a steroid-induced increase in intraocular pressure (IOP). It has no place in the treatment of intraocular inflammation.

The emergence of newly formulated "soft steroids" may provide enhanced anti-inflammatory efficacy while minimizing the potential for untoward steroid-induced adverse effects. These agents are inert until activated locally in the eye and are rapidly degraded in the anterior chamber or bloodstream; thus, intraocular or systemic toxicity is limited.[46] One such drug, loteprednol etabonate, a congener of prednisolone, has been shown to be useful in the treatment of giant papillary conjunctivitis in humans.[47]

The drug vehicle has impact on the therapeutic efficacy of topically applied corticosteroids. Although ointments might be presumed to be superior to collyria because of the prolonged contact time between the drug and the ocular surface, dexamethasone phosphate ointment produces lower drug levels in the cornea and anterior chamber than does the solution. The petrolatum vehicle of the ointment is believed to retain drug and thus retard its release.[48] Nevertheless, steroid ointments are a practical alternative to frequent dosing when use of the latter is impossible (during sleep).

Finally, high-viscosity gels[49] and depot preparations in the form of cotton pledgets[50] and collagen shields[51] have been used in an attempt to enhance the ocular bioavailability and anti-inflammatory effects of topically applied corticosteroids. Depot preparations have the advantage of providing slow, steady release of drug over the ocular surface.[16]

Regional therapy of ocular inflammatory disease may be instituted with periocular injection (subconjunctival, sub-Tenon, transseptal, or retrobulbar) of steroid, providing rapid delivery of high concentrations of drug to the target tissues. With the exception of hydrocortisone, the preparations shown in Table 9–3 are of moderate to high potency. Their formulation is likely to affect the rate of release and duration of action of drug administered as subconjunctival or sub-Tenon depots.[26] Water-soluble preparations (methylprednisolone sodium succinate), which diffuse from the depot more rapidly, are short-acting, even when steroids with a prolonged biological t½ (e.g., dexamethasone sodium phosphate) are used.[52] Although less soluble formulations (e.g., methylprednisolone acetate and triamcinolone acetonide) have a longer duration of action, they pose an increased risk of development of steroid-induced ocular toxicity. The site of injection (subconjunctival versus retrobulbar) and the distribution of drug into the surrounding tissues also affect the duration of action and ocular bioavailability; for example, in experiments in which radiolabeled methylprednisolone acetate (Depo-Medrol) was injected by the retrobulbar route, high levels of drug were produced in the sclera, choroid, retina, and vitreous for 1 week or longer.[53] Wine and coworkers[54] showed that higher intraocular concentrations and more rapid ocular penetration of hydrocortisone were achieved after subconjunctival administration than after injection into the anterior orbital fat.

Although the site of injection varies with the location of the inflammatory process (anterior versus posterior segment) and the clinician's individual preference, the clear-cut superiority of a single method of regional injection has not been established. Even though hydroxycortisone may be detected in the anterior chamber almost immediately after subconjunctival injection, controlled experiments have demonstrated that topical instillation of steroids produces a significantly greater reduction in the number of neutrophils infiltrating the cornea than does subconjunctival injection.[55] Concurrent administration of topical and subconjunctival steroids has an additive effect and thus would be expected to demonstrate enhanced therapeutic efficacy in cases of severe anterior segment inflammation. Sub-Tenon, transseptal, and retrobulbar injections were shown to deliver significant sustained levels of drug to the posterior uvea, retina, optic nerve, and vitreous, although these routes were not directly compared.[56–59]

The mechanism of steroid delivery into intraocular tissues is unclear. McCartney and colleagues[60] propose that in rabbits, transscleral diffusion is the major route of penetration after subconjunctival or sub-Tenon injection and emphasize the importance of placing the corticosteroid immediately adjacent to the site of intraocular inflammation. More recent work comparing subconjunctival and retrobulbar injection of dexamethasone in the rabbit eye showed that hematogenous absorption was primarily responsible for drug delivery to the choroid, aqueous, and vitreous with both routes, whereas a combination of hematogenous and transscleral mechanisms was operative in drug delivery to the retina. Retrobulbar injections provided sustained long-term steroid levels, whereas hematogenous delivery of dexamethasone following subconjunctival injection peaked earlier in the choroid and presumably in other ocular tissues.[61]

THERAPEUTIC USE

Steroids are the most widely used anti-inflammatory and immunosuppressant drugs in ophthalmology in general, and are the mainstay of therapy for patients with uveitis. Ophthalmic indications for the use of corticosteroids are shown in Table 9–7: these indications may be grouped into three broad therapeutic categories: (1) postoperative inflammatory control, (2) abnormalities of immune regulation, and (3) entities with a combined immune and inflammatory mechanism.[16] Our philosophy concerning the longitudinal care of patients with uveitis has been one of complete intolerance of recurrent or persistent inflammation, coupled with implementation of a stepladder algorithm for control of inflammation in an effort to limit permanent structural damage to the ocular structures that are critical to good vision. Although this goal may be difficult to achieve in selected cases, it is almost always attainable through use of this stepladder approach to selecting the appropriate aggressiveness of therapy. This algorithm consists of (1) steroids (topical, regional, and systemic), (2) nonsteroidal anti-inflammatory drugs (NSAIDs), (3) peripheral retinal cryopexy in selected patients with pars planitis, (4) systemic immunosuppressive chemotherapy, and (5) pars plana vitrectomy with intraocular steroid injection.

The diagnosis of active inflammation should be based solely on the presence of inflammatory cells in the anterior chamber or vitreous. Aqueous flare should never guide therapy because it represents vascular incompetence from the iris and ciliary body and is usually chronic. Although anterior chamber inflammatory cells are relatively easy to detect, their presence in the vitreous may be extremely difficult to discern. Eyes with chronic or recurrent iridocyclitis or posterior uveitis usually have vitreous pathology that includes the presence of cells, fibrin, and cellular aggregates trapped in vitreous fibrils and fibers. These cannot be eliminated even with the most aggressive anti-inflammatory therapy. The clear spaces, or *lacunae*, in the vitreous are typically devoid of cells in patients with inactive uveitis. Therefore, the diagnosis of active anterior vitreal inflammation is made by careful biomicroscopic examination of the lacunae for the presence of inflammatory cells and by evaluation of the vitreous exudates, or "snowballs." (Sharp borders and no changes over time are characteristic of old, inactive fixed clumps of material, whereas hazy edges of the exudates are more characteristic of acute inflammatory material.)

Topical steroids alone are usually effective in the management of anterior segment inflammation and have little activity against intermediate or posterior uveitis in the phakic eye. The anterior uveitides comprise a heterogenous group of diseases, which include idiopathic anterior uveitis, traumatic and postoperative iritis, HLA-B27–associated diseases, lens-induced uveitis, juvenile rheumatoid arthritis, sclerouveitis, keratouveitis, Adamantiades-Behçet disease, and anterior chamber inflammatory "spillover" from primarily posterior segment disease. Although topical steroids are the first rung in the anti-inflammatory stepladder for most of these entities, important exceptions include ocular inflammation associated with Adamantiades-Behçet disease, Wegener's granulomatosis, polyarteritis nodosa, relapsing polychondritis with renal involvement, sympathetic ophthalmia, Vogt-Koyanagi-Harada (VKH) syndrome, and rheumatoid arthritis, for which systemic immunosuppression, alone or in combination with systemic steroids, is mandatory first-line treatment.[52, 62]

A sensible approach to the use of topical steroids in anterior uveitis is to treat the patient aggressively with a potent agent during the initial stage of inflammation, re-evaluate the patient at frequent intervals, and then taper the drug slowly, as dictated by the clinical response. In very severe cases of anterior uveitis, prednisolone acetate 1% or dexamethasone alcohol 0.1% may be required hourly around the clock, together with periocular and/or oral corticosteroids as adjunctive therapy. Although corticosteroid ointments may be used at night in lieu of 24-hour dosing, these preparations are less potent than steroid drops. In addition, if steroid suspensions (e.g., prednisolone acetate) are used, the patient must be instructed to shake the bottle sufficiently with each administration to ensure delivery of maximal concentration of steroid. We prefer to avert this potential compliance problem (particularly when frequent dosing is required) by using steroid solutions (e.g., prednisolone phosphate).

We and other investigators[15] believe that most treatment failures with topical steroids are due to poor patient compliance, inadequate dosing, or abrupt or rapid tapering schedules. The latter two factors may result in part from the reluctance of some clinicians to expose their patients unduly to potential steroid-induced ocular complications such as cataract formation and glaucoma. Ironically, the effort to do no harm, with less frequent dosing or a switch to a "softer" agent, allows low-grade inflammation to continue, the long-term consequence of which is permanent ocular structural damage (e.g., cystic macula). Again, the goal of therapy is control of intraocular inflammation. Aggressive anti-inflammatory therapy, together with use of antiglaucomatous agents in the short term and with cycloplegic agents to keep the pupil dilated, may limit irreversible damage that even the most elegant surgical procedure cannot repair. One must be prudent in applying topical corticosteroids in cases of anterior uveitis in which the etiology is suspected to be infectious because these agents may potentiate the underlying disease. Active herpetic dendritic keratitis and uveitis associated with suspected fungal keratitis are contraindications to the use of topical corticosteroids. The reactivation of herpes keratitis is potentiated by the use of topical agents, a problem of particular importance in patients undergoing penetrating keratoplasty. Topical steroids should be used judiciously in patients with anterior uveitis associated with disciform keratitis or bacterial corneal ulcers, and always in conjunction with appropriate antibiotic or antiviral "cover."

Topical corticosteroids are not particularly effective in the treatment of Fuchs' heterochromic iridocyclitis and should be used sparingly, if at all, in cases of episcleritis and scleritis (NSAIDs are first-line treatment for most cases of simple, diffuse, or nodular scleritis; immunosuppressive chemotherapy is used for scleritis that is necrotizing or associated with collagen vascular disease). Chronic flare associated with juvenile rheumatoid arthritis–associated iridocyclitis, as in any case of anterior uveitis regardless of etiology, should never be an indication for treatment. Reflexive administration of topical steroids in the aforementioned instances merely increases the risk of steroid-induced ocular morbidity.

Because topical steroids penetrate the posterior segment poorly, they are ineffective in the treatment of intermediate and posterior uveitis. Periocular corticosteroid injection (subconjunctival, anterior or posterior sub-Tenon, transseptal, and retrobulbar) is effective in such instances, particularly in unilateral cases; it provides rapid delivery of high concentrations of drug to the site of inflammation. In cases of severe anterior uveitis, subconjunctival or anterior sub-Tenon injection of corticosteroid serves as a useful adjunct to topical therapy, maximizing the concentration of drug in the anterior segment. The purported superiority of posterior sub-Tenon versus transseptal versus retrobulbar administration for posterior segment inflammation has yet to be established; the choice of delivery method is largely one of individual preference, with each route having its own particular advantage.

Retrobulbar injection, although it provides high concentrations of drug to the posterior segment, poses the risk of inadvertent penetration of the globe, optic nerve, or both. Posterior sub-Tenon injection by the temporal approach, as initially described by Schlaegel[63] and as detailed by Smith and Nozik,[64] decreases the potential for ocular penetration and places the medication in contact with the sclera in the region of the macula. Indeed, proximity of repository steroid to the macular area has been shown to correlate with an improvement in macular function.[65] We prefer the transseptal approach because it reduces the risk of ocular penetration (we believe), is better tolerated, and delivers high concentration of drug to the desired location. Steroid is thoroughly mixed with local anesthetic in a 3-ml syringe with a 30-gauge, 5/8-

inch needle. The patient is instructed to look superonasally, the globe is elevated above the inferior orbital rim with the nondominant index finger, and the needle is introduced between the globe and the lateral third of the orbital margin, then advanced to the hub through the lower lid and orbital septum. A quick wiggle of the syringe assures one, in the absence of any globe movement, of nonpenetrance of the globe. Steroid is then injected quickly to avoid precipitation, and mild pressure is held over the closed lid for approximately 2 minutes. To monitor any adverse reactions, the patient is observed for at least 1 hour if the injection is given in an outpatient setting, and a mild analgesic is administered as needed. As opposed to the posterior sub-Tenon method, in which a side-to-side circumferential motion of the needle is required to verify the proper location of the needle tip between Tenon's capsule and the sclera, no such movement is necessary with the transseptal approach, as the clinician is aware, tactilely, of the location of the needle tip beneath the globe. Although premedication with topical anesthesia such as proparacaine or tetracaine is sufficient for adults, periocular injection in children and infants usually requires general anesthesia.

Corticosteroids available for periocular injection are shown in Table 9–4; they range from short-acting preparations (methylprednisolone sodium succinate) to long-acting depots (methylprednisolone acetate [Depo-Medrol]). Postinjection glaucoma syndrome is a potential hazard after sub-Tenon repository steroid injections; in certain cases, surgical excision of the depot may be required. In clinical practice, however, the occurrence of this complication after posterior sub-Tenon injection (rather than subconjunctival or anterior sub-Tenon injection) is distinctly uncommon, even in steroid responders.[64] Nevertheless, we do not generally use depot preparations unless prior treatment with steroid drops and transseptal injections has not been associated with increased IOP and shorter-acting regional steroids have been only transiently effective. We prefer the aqueous suspension of diacetate (Aristocort) in a concentration of 40 mg/ml. This formulation has little tendency to cause scar formation, extraocular muscle fibrosis, or hypersensitivity to the vehicle.[64]

After periocular injection with triamcinolone, a treatment effect is usually apparent within 2 to 3 days. Injections may be repeated every 2 to 4 weeks, as dictated by the clinical response. We administer a maximum of four injections over an 8- to 10-week period before declaring a treatment failure. Periocular injections are contraindicated in patients with uveitis associated with toxoplasmosis and in patients with necrotizing scleritis.

Systemic corticosteroids are used when, in the clinician's judgment, the inflammatory response is of such severe degree that it warrants this therapeutic approach, usually in cases of bilateral sight-threatening uveitis or in patients with severe unilateral disease who have failed or are intolerant of periocular injections. Although steroids in general remain the first-line agents for treatment of intraocular inflammatory disease, important exceptions exist that require immunosuppressive chemotherapy, alone or in combination with systemic steroids.

Our tolerance for the use of systemic steroids is extremely limited because of our experience[66] and that of other investigators[67] in which highly undesirable effects were associated with their prolonged use. Except in patients with steroid-dependent sarcoidosis, it is extremely unusual for us to continue administering systemic steroids for longer than 6 months. As we do when we initiate topical or periocular therapy, we inform the patient regarding the prognosis, duration, and potential adverse effects of systemic steroid administration for a given diagnosis. The initial dosage and duration of treatment with systemic steroids depend on the nature and severity of the inflammatory disease and the clinical response. Gordon's[68] very early dictum, "use enough, soon enough, to accomplish the goal of complete suppression of inflammation, then taper and discontinue," is as sound today as it was in the early 1960s. Indeed, using too little, too late, and then gradually increasing the dose of steroids generally produces little benefit and potentiates adverse effects.

Accordingly, we initiate therapy with 1.0 to 2.0 mg/kg of prednisone daily as a single morning dose, a regimen that is easily tolerated and produces less suppression of the HPA axis than do divided dose schedules. Other researchers advocate splitting the initial dose to enhance its therapeutic efficacy or dividing it into four parts (dosing every 6 hours) to facilitate a rapid taper if treatment is given for less than 2 weeks.[64] Prednisone and triamcinolone are the preferred preparations because they offer the maximal flexibility required for uveitis therapy by virtue of their anti-inflammatory potency, their intermediate duration of action, and the lack of sodium-retaining activity in the latter.

This relatively high dose is maintained, barring untoward complications, for a short time (7 to 14 days) until a clinical response is noted. A slow and steady taper is then begun at a rate dictated by the clinical condition so that a recurrence of inflammation is not precipitated, until a dose of 20 mg/day prednisone is reached. Some patients require only a periodic short course of systemic steroids, but others require more protracted therapy. In the latter, if inflammatory quiescence has been achieved at the 20-mg/kg level, we frequently use an alternate-day dosage schedule, as described by Fauci.[69] The daily maintenance dose of 20 mg/kg is doubled to 40 mg/kg every other day, which is continued for at least 2 weeks, after which time it is further tapered to 30 mg every other day for 2 additional weeks. If there is no further recurrence of inflammation, the dose is reduced to 20 mg every other day for 2 weeks, with continued tapering on an every-other-week basis to 15 mg every other day, 10 mg every other day, 7.5 mg every other day, and 5 mg every other day, after which time the drug is discontinued. Alternate-day therapy produces less severe and fewer steroid-induced adverse effects and does not disturb the HPA axis.[19] Adrenal suppression is possible, however, and as with any long-term steroid regimen, the medication should never be abruptly discontinued owing to the risk of precipitating an addisonian crisis.

When long-term therapy with systemic corticosteroids is anticipated, another useful approach entails addition of a second, steroid-sparing agent. This strategy reduces the total amount of steroid required to maintain quiescence or to prevent inflammatory recurrence. We frequently use azathioprine or oral NSAIDs to this end; the latter have been shown to reduce ocular inflammation after cataract extraction and may help reduce cystoid macular edema.[70] Systemic steroids combined with cyclosporine have also been shown to be effective in the treatment of noninfectious endogenous uveitis of various etiologies.[71, 72]

Finally, intravenous pulse steroid therapy is an alternative to daily therapy in patients with severe, bilateral, sight-threatening posterior uveitis. Patients receiving such treatment must undergo a thorough medical evaluation before pulse therapy is initiated because serious adverse effects such as perforation of a peptic ulcer, systemic hypertension, aseptic necrosis of the hip, and even sudden death have been reported.[73] Pulse therapy may induce a rapid and prolonged therapeutic effect while avoiding some of the chronic adverse effects associated with daily therapy. A commonly used regimen consists of intravenous methylprednisolone 1 g/day for 3 days, repeated as frequently as once a month.[74]

Patients treated with systemic steroids, particularly those receiving long-term therapy, in contrast to those receiving concomitant NSAIDs, are at risk of gastritis, GI mucosal ulceration, and bleeding. To prevent such adverse effects, patients should be instructed to take oral steroids with milk, food, antacids, or gastric mucosal coating material such as sucralfate (Carafate), and to take calcium supplements to reduce the drug's calcium-leeching effects. In treating patients with a past or current history of such symptoms, we add an H2 receptor blocker such as ranitidine hydrochloride (Zantac); we add misoprostol (Cytotec) to the regimen of any patient with a documented history of peptic ulcer disease or any patient receiving concurrent NSAID therapy.

Systemic corticosteroids are absolutely contraindicated in patients with known or suspected systemic fungal infection and a known hypersensitivity to the components of the steroid formulation.[75] As with topical or periocular therapy, systemic steroids should be avoided in patients in whom an infectious etiology for intraocular inflammation has not been adequately excluded or appropriately covered with antimicrobial therapy. Examples are ocular syphilis, toxoplasmosis, herpes, candidiasis, and tuberculosis, in which disease activity is reactivated or exacerbated by systemic steroids alone. In addition, use of systemic steroids before diagnostic vitrectomy in patients in whom intraocular lymphoma is suspected may confound cytologic interpretation and delay the diagnosis because steroids are cytotoxic to lymphoma cells.[76] Other relative contraindications to systemic steroid therapy are severe cardiovascular (hypertension, congestive heart failure), psychiatric (depression, previous psychosis), GI (active peptic ulcer disease), metabolic (poorly controlled diabetes mellitus), and musculoskeletal (osteoporosis) disease, as well as pregnancy.[75]

ADVERSE EFFECTS AND TOXICITY

Corticosteroid therapy produces both ocular and systemic adverse effects, irrespective of the route of administration. Although topical or periocular administration may result in significant systemic absorption, untoward sys-

TABLE 9–8. NONOCULAR COMPLICATIONS OF CORTICOSTEROID THERAPY

Endocrine
  Adrenal insufficiency
  Cushing's syndrome
  Growth failure
  Menstrual disorders
Neuropsychiatric
  Pseudotumor cerebri
  Insomnia
  Mood swings
  Psychosis
Gastrointestinal
  Peptic ulcer
  Gastric hemorrhage
  Intestinal perforation
  Pancreatitis
Musculoskeletal
  Osteoporosis
  Vertebral compression fractures
  Aseptic hip necrosis
Cardiovascular
  Hypertension
  Sodium and fluid retention
Metabolic
  Secondary diabetes mellitus
  Hyperosmotic, hyperglycemic, or nonketonic coma
  Centripetal obesity
  Hyperlipidemia
Dermatologic
  Acne
  Striae
  Hirsutism
  Subcutaneous tissue atrophy
Immunologic
  Impaired inflammatory response
  Delayed tissue healing

temic complications are far more likely after oral or parenteral therapy, and their frequency is both dose and duration dependent. These are shown in Table 9–8 and are discussed in the section, "Clinical Pharmacology."

In our experience in the care of 402 patients with ocular inflammatory disease treated with systemic corticosteroids alone or in combination with immunosuppressive agents, neuropsychiatric and endocrine adverse effects were the most common complications attributed to prednisone. It is noteworthy that 17 of these patients developed pathologic fractures involving the hip and spine.[66]

The most clinically significant ocular complication of corticosteroid therapy is development of cataract and secondary glaucoma. Other important adverse effects produced by all routes of corticosteroid administration include mydriasis, ptosis, susceptibility to infection, and impaired wound healing (Table 9–9).

Secondary open-angle glaucoma is most likely to occur after prolonged topical therapy with potent steroids. In one study, approximately 30% of normal volunteers treated for 6 weeks with topical betamethasone had an IOP of 20 mm Hg or more, and 4% had an IOP greater than 31 mm Hg.[77] IOP usually returns to baseline values within 2 weeks after drug discontinuation. A more pronounced steroid-induced IOP increase is noted in patients with open-angle glaucoma, in diabetic patients, and in those with high myopia.[78] The increase in IOP may occur as early as 1 week into treatment, or it may be

TABLE 9–9. OCULAR COMPLICATIONS OF TOPICAL, PERIOCULAR, AND SYSTEMIC CORTICOSTEROID THERAPY

Topical
  Blurred vision
  Allergy to vehicle
  Punctate keratopathy
  Paralysis of accommodation
  Potentiation of collagenase
  Altered corneal thickness
  Anterior uveitis
Periocular
  Globe penetration
  Proptosis
  Atrophy and fibrosis of extraocular muscles and periorbita
  Central retinal artery occlusion
  Hemorrhage
  Optic nerve injury
  Limbal dellen
Systemic
  Myopia
  Pseudotumor
  Exophthalmia
  Central serous chorioretinopathy
Common to all routes
  Glaucoma
  Cataract
  Susceptibility to infection
  Impaired wound healing
  Mydriasis
  Ptosis

delayed for years after the initiation of therapy; therefore, all patients treated with corticosteroid medications should be monitored periodically. The exact mechanism for this phenomenon is unclear; however, evidence shows that corticosteroids enhance the deposition of mucopolysaccharide in the trabecular meshwork.[79] Although some topical preparations such as FML and HMS are less apt to produce an increase in IOP, their poor corneal penetration makes them less suitable for treatment of intraocular inflammation than are more potent steroids (described in the section, "Pharmacokinetics, Concentration-Effect Relationship, and Metabolism"). Intractable glaucoma may result after repository steroid injections, requiring surgical excision of the depot (described in the section, "Therapeutic Use").

Posterior subcapsular cataracts (PSCs) arise in a dose- and duration-dependent manner after long-term corticosteroid therapy, although individual susceptibility appears to vary. Children and patients with diabetes are more prone to develop this complication.[80] In one study of patients treated with systemic prednisone for rheumatoid arthritis for 1 to 4 years, 11% treated with 10 to 15 mg/day developed cataracts, as did 78% of those receiving more than 16 mg/day.[81] In another study, 50% of patients treated with topical steroids after undergoing keratoplasty for keratoconus developed PSC after receiving 765 drops of 0.1% dexamethasone in 10.5 months.[82] Once established, the opacity is generally not reversible. However, regression of PSC has been reported in children after therapy is discontinued.[80] The mechanism of corticosteroid-induced cataract formation is believed to involve the binding of glucocorticoids to lens fibers, leading to bio-

chemical alterations with protein aggregation in the cells and a change in the refractive index.[83]

Susceptibility to microbial infections is enhanced by corticosteroids because these agents suppress the inflammatory response. Herpetic, bacterial (particularly pseudomonal), and fungal keratitis may be potentiated by corticosteroid therapy unless the appropriate antiviral or antibiotic is administered concomitantly. Likewise, posterior segment inflammatory conditions such as ocular syphilis, tuberculosis, and toxoplasmosis should always be treated with appropriate anti-infective agents before corticosteroid treatment is instituted.

Corneal epithelial and stromal healing is inhibited by all corticosteroids, with the possible exception of medroxyprogesterone. Manifestations may be as trivial as superficial punctate staining of the cornea or as serious as relentless corneal-scleral melting and perforation. Corticosteroids retard collagen synthesis by fibroblasts[84] and enhance collagenase activity.[85] Cognizance of the effects of steroids on wound healing is particularly important in the presence of corneal-scleral ulceration or thinning or minor trauma, and during the postoperative period. Mild mydriasis and ptosis are often common complications of topical steroid therapy.[86] An increase of 1 mm in the papillary diameter may be observed as early as 1 week after initiation of therapy, with return to normal diameter when steroid treatment is discontinued. Agents in the vehicle mixture rather than the steroids themselves have been suggested to mediate these effects.[87]

After topical therapy, paradoxical anterior uveitis may be induced by the corticosteroid itself rather than by the vehicle.[88] The incidence is apparently greater in blacks than in whites[89]; patients present with signs and symptoms typical of acute iritis, which abate once the steroid is discontinued. The development of corticosteroid-induced uveitis has been suggested to be related to an activation of latent spirochetes in the eye, although no direct proof substantiates this.[18]

Other adverse effects of topical steroid therapy such as blurred vision and punctate keratopathy may relate to ocular irritation arising from mechanical effects of the steroid particles in suspension, allergy to the vehicle, or the underlying inflammatory condition. In addition, refractive changes, paralysis of accommodation, and altered corneal thickness have been reported.[90] Central serous retinopathy has been reported in association with systemic steroid therapy,[91] whereas pseudotumor cerebri, especially in children, may occur after abrupt discontinuation or reduction of therapy.[92]

Periocular injection of steroids is associated with adverse effects and complications unique to the mode of delivery, in addition to those previously described for the drugs themselves. These are shown separately in Table 9–9 and include the following: (1) inadvertent penetration of the globe, (2) proptosis, (3) subdermal fat atrophy and fibrosis of the extraocular muscles and surrounding periorbital tissues, (4) central retinal artery obstruction from drug embolization, (5) subconjunctival or retrobulbar hemorrhage after anterior and posterior injections, respectively, (6) optic nerve injury from retrobulbar injection, (7) limbal dellen after anterior injections, and (8) unsightly white steroid repository after anterior injections in the palpebral fissure.[64]

High-Risk Groups

Corticosteroids are contraindicated in patients with systemic fungal infection or known hypersensitivity to the drug formulation and should be used with great caution in patients with a history of excessive alcohol consumption, oral steroid use, peptic ulcer disease, various infectious diseases, diabetes mellitus, severe hypertension or congestive heart failure, psychiatric problems, and osteoporosis. Postmenopausal women and the elderly receiving prolonged therapy with corticosteroids are at particularly high risk of developing osteoporosis and attendant serious complications such as compression fractures of the vertebral column. Alternate-day regimens in normal adults and dosage reduction to as little as 10 mg/day in the elderly are still associated with insidious osteopenia.[93, 94] Routine screening of such patients with baseline bone mineral density measurements and consideration of bone mineral preservation strategies for anyone who is likely to be on systemic steroids for longer than 6 weeks is appropriate.[8, 93] We prescribe 1.5 g of calcium per day, 800 IU of vitamin D per day, and 10 mg of alendronate sodium (Fosamax) per day, and encourage and engage patients in conversations about daily weight-bearing exercise programs (e.g., walking). Postmenopausal females are referred for consideration of estrogen replacement therapy. Other bone preservation strategies may be preferred by the reader's consultants, but the point is that a program to prevent steroid-induced osteoporosis should be instituted.

Use of corticosteroids in children suppresses normal growth, retarding both epiphyseal maturation and long bone growth (which is particularly problematic during puberty, when epiphyseal closure is accelerated under the influence of sex hormones) and possibly resulting in permanent loss in height.[8] Inhibition or arrest of growth cannot be overcome with exogenous growth hormone.

Newborns of mothers who have received systemic corticosteroids during pregnancy, although not at increased teratogenic risk, should be monitored for adrenal insufficiency during the neonatal period. Furthermore, systemic corticosteroids are excreted in breast milk, placing infants who are breast fed at risk for growth retardation and suppression of endogenous steroid production.[75]

DRUG INTERACTIONS

Concurrent administration of medications that increase microsomal enzymes, such as phenobarbital, phenytoin, carbamazepine, ephedrine, and rifampin, decreases the pharmacologic effects of corticosteroids by enhancing their metabolism.[8] Cholestyramine and antacids decrease the GI absorption of corticosteroids.[75] On the other hand, erythromycin may impair elimination of methylprednisolone, whereas cyclosporine reduces the clearance of prednisone in renal transplant patients. Likewise, the dose of corticosteroids should be reduced when isoniazid and ketoconazole, both of which reduce steroid metabolism, or oral contraceptives, which increase protein binding and impair elimination, are administered concurrently.[75] Corticosteroids enhance the clearance of salicylates and reduce the activity of anticholinesterases and antiviral eye preparations.[95] Finally, corticosteroids diminish the effectiveness of anticoagulant therapy by either increasing or decreasing clotting.[6]

MAJOR CLINICAL TRIALS

Although the efficacy of corticosteroid therapy in the control of intraocular inflammation is tacitly accepted by most clinicians, few well-controlled, randomized clinical trials have clearly demonstrated a treatment effect, much less an optimal dosing regimen. Postoperative inflammation is probably the most common indication for topical steroid use today; however, early randomized, controlled trials failed to demonstrate a significant reduction in intraocular inflammation after uncomplicated intracapsular cataract extraction in eyes treated with topical steroids once to three times daily versus placebo.[96, 97] Suggesting that a treatment benefit might be demonstrable with more frequent dosing, Corboy[92] conducted a randomized, double-blind, multicenter clinical trial, in which topical betamethasone phosphate 0.1% was used five times daily for 2 weeks after uncomplicated intracapsular cataract extraction. This regimen was more effective than placebo in the reduction of postoperative inflammation, with none of the ocular complications associated with corticosteroid treatment.

The efficacy of topical corticosteroids in the treatment of acute unilateral nongranulomatous anterior uveitis was evaluated by Dunne and Travers,[98] who conducted a controlled, double-blind trial comparing betamethasone phosphate 0.1%, clobetasone butyrate 0.1%, and placebo. Both steroids were equivalent in improving clinical symptoms during the initial stage of treatment; however, only betamethasone phosphate was significantly better than placebo in reducing signs of inflammation.

Godfrey and associates[99] retrospectively evaluated the effectiveness of corticosteroids in the treatment of 173 patients with pars planitis who received either no therapy, topical steroids only, systemic steroids, or periocular steroids. Although their findings were inconclusive, periocular administration of steroids appeared to be efficacious in the treatment of cystoid macular edema associated with pars planitis, with a 70% improvement in vision.

The first controlled, double-masked clinical trial in the United States that provided therapeutic success data for systemic corticosteroids was conducted by Nussenblatt and coworkers.[72] Fifty-six patients were randomized to treatment with either cyclosporin A or prednisolone for severe, noninfectious uveitis. Therapeutic efficacy was remarkably similar for both treatment groups; however, improvement in visual acuity in either group was less than 50%. A subgroup of patients who had failed monotherapy with either drug were subsequently treated with a combination of steroid and cyclosporine; some exhibited improvement in visual acuity.[72]

Most recently, a 28-day double-masked, randomized, active-controlled, parallel-group, multicenter study was conducted to evaluate the efficacy of a new soft steroid, rimexolone 1% ophthalmic suspension, as compared with 1% prednisolone acetate in 160 patients with uveitis for whom topical steroid was indicated.[100] Rimexolone 1% suspension was equivalent to 1% prednisolone acetate in controlling anterior chamber inflammation; increased IOP (increased by 10 mm Hg or more as compared with baseline) was reported approximately 50% less frequently in the rimexolone-treated patients. This promising agent is currently undergoing phase III clinical trials.

References

1. Hench PS, Kendall EC, Slocomb CH, et al: Effects of cortisone acetate and pituitary ACTH on rheumatoid arthritis, rheumatic fever, and certain other conditions: Study in clinical physiology. Arch Intern Med 1950;85:545–666.
2. Gordon DM, McLean JM: Effects of pituitary adrenocorticotropin hormone (ACTH) therapy in ophthalmologic conditions. JAMA 1950;142:1271–1276.
3. Thygeson P: Historical observations on herpetic keratitis. Surv Ophthalmol 1976;21:82–90.
4. Gordon DM: Prednisone and prednisolone in ocular disease. Am J Ophthalmol 1956;41:593–600.
5. Leopold IH, Maylath R: Intraocular penetration of cortisone and its effectiveness against experimental corneal burns. Am J Ophthalmol 1952;42:1125–1134.
6. Haynes RC: Adrenocorticotropic hormone; adrenocorticotropic steroids and their synthetic analogs; inhibitors of the synthesis and actions of adrenocortical hormones. In: Gilman AG, Rall TW, Nies AS, Taylor P, eds: Goodman and Gilman's The Pharmacological Basis of Therapeutics. New York, Pergamon Press, 1990, pp 1431–1462.
7. Gallant C, Kenny P: Oral glucocorticoids and their complications: A review. J Am Acad Dermatol 1986;14:161–177.
8. Feldman SR: The biology and clinical application of systemic glucocorticoids. In: Callen JP, ed: Current Problems in Dermatology. St. Louis, Mosby–Year Book, 1992, pp 211–234.
9. Southren LA, Dominguez MO, Gordon GO, et al: Nuclear translocation of cytoplasmic glucocorticoid receptor in the iris-ciliary body and adjacent corneoscleral tissue of the rabbit following topical administration of various glucocorticoids. Invest Ophthalmol Vis Sci 1983;24:147–152.
10. Tyrell JE, Baxter JD: Disorders of the adrenal cortex. In: Wyngaarden JB, Smith LH, Bennett JC, eds: Cecil Textbook of Medicine. Philadelphia, WB Saunders, 1992, pp 1271–1279.
11. Melby JC: Clinical pharmacology of systemic corticosteroids. Ann Rev Pharmacol Toxicol 1977;17:511–527.
12. Wolverton SE: Glucocorticosteroids. In: Wolverton SE, Wilkin JK, eds: Systemic Drugs for Skin Diseases. Philadelphia, WB Saunders, 1991, pp 86–124.
13. Friedlander MH: Corticosteroid therapy of ocular inflammation. Int Ophthalmol Clin 1983;23:175–182.
14. Mondino BJ, Alfuss DH, Farley MK: Steroids. In: Lamberts DW, Potter DE, eds: Clinical Ophthalmic Pharmacology. Boston, Little, Brown, 1987, pp 157–162.
15. Nussenblatt RB, Palestine AF: Uveitis. Fundamental and Clinical Practice. Chicago, Year Book Medical Publishers, 1989, pp 107–117.
16. Abelson MB, Butrus S: Corticosteroids in ophthalmic practice. In: Albert DM, Jakobiec FA, eds: Principles and Practice of Ophthalmology: Basic Sciences. Philadelphia, WB Saunders, 1994, pp 1013–1022.
17. Leibowitz HM, Kupferman A: Anti-inflammatory medications. Int Ophthalmol Clin 1980;20:117–134.
18. Friend J: Physiology of the cornea: metabolism and biochemistry. In: Smolon G, Thoft RA, eds: The Cornea. Scientific Foundations and Clinical Practice. Boston, Little, Brown, 1987, pp 116–138.
19. Pavan-Langston D, Dunkel EL: Handbook of Ocular Drug Therapy and Ocular Side Effects of Systemic Drugs. Boston, Little, Brown, 1991, pp 182–217.
20. Kroman HS, Leopold IL: Studies upon methyl- and fluorosubstituted prednisolones in the aqueous humor of rabbit. Am J Ophthalmol 1961;52:77–81.
21. Leopold IH, Gaster BN: Ocular inflammation and anti-inflammatory drugs. In: Kaufman HE, Barron BA, McDonald MB, Waltman SR, eds: The Cornea. New York, Churchill Livingstone, 1988, pp 67–79.
22. Murdick PW, Keates RH, Donovan EF, et al: Ocular penetration studies. II. Topical administration of prednisolone. Arch Ophthalmol 1966;76:602–603.
23. Rosenblum C, Denglor RE, Geoffory RF: Ocular absorption of dexamethasone sodium phosphate disodium by the rabbit. Arch Ophthalmol 1967;77:234–237.
24. Hamashige S, Potts A: The penetration of cortisone and hydrocortisone into the ocular structures. Am J Ophthalmol 1955;40:211–216.
25. James RG, Stiles JF: The penetration of cortisol into normal and pathologic rabbit eyes. Am J Ophthalmol 1963;56:84–90.
26. Polansky JR, Weinres RN: Anti-inflammatory agents, steroids as anti-inflammatory agents. In: Sears ML, ed: Pharmacology of the Eye. Berlin, Springer-Verlag, 1984, pp 460–538.
27. Sugar J, Burde RM, Sugar A, et al: Tetrahydrotriamcinolone and triamcinolone. I. Ocular penetration. Invest Ophthalmol Vis Sci 1972;11:890–893.
28. Soutaren AL, Altman K, Vittek J, et al: Steroid metabolism in ocular tissues of the rabbit. Invest Ophthalmol Vis Sci 1976;15:222–228.
29. Cox WV, Kupferman A, Leibowitz HM: Topically applied steroids in corneal disease. I. The role of inflammation in stromal absorption of dexamethasone. Arch Ophthalmol 1972;88:308–313.
30. Kupferman A, Pratt MV, Suckewer K, Leibowitz HM: Topically applied steroids in corneal disease. III. The role of drug derivative in stromal absorption of dexamethasone. Arch Ophthalmol 1974;91:373–376.
31. Kupferman A, Leibowitz HM: Topically applied steroids in corneal disease. IV. The role of drug concentration in stromal absorption of prednisolone acetate. Arch Ophthalmol 1974;91:377–380.
32. Kupferman A, Leibowitz HM: Topically applied steroids in corneal disease. V. Dexamethasone alcohol. Arch Ophthalmol 1974;92:329–330.
33. Kupferman A, Leibowitz HM: Topically applied steroids in corneal disease. VI. Kinetics of prednisolone phosphate. Arch Ophthalmol 1974;92:331–334.
34. Hull DS, Hine JE, Edelhauser HF, Hyndiuk RA: Permeability of isolated rabbit cornea to corticosteroids. Invest Ophthalmol Vis Sci 1974;13:457–459.
35. Olejnick O, Weisbecker CA: Ocular bioavailability of topical prednisolone preparations. Clin Ther 1990;12:2–11.
36. Musson DG, Bidgood AM, Olejnick O: Assay methodology for prednisolone, prednisone acetate, and prednisolone sodium phosphate in rabbit aqueous humor and ocular physiologic solutions. J Chromatogr A 1991;565:89–102.
37. Musson DG, Bidwood AM, Olejnick O: An in vitro comparison of the permeability of prednisolone, prednisolone sodium phosphate, and prednisolone acetate across the NZW rabbit cornea. J Ocul Pharmacol Ther 1992;8:139–150.
38. Leibowitz HM, Stewart RH, Kupferman A: Evaluation of dexamethasone acetate as a topical ophthalmic formulation. Am J Ophthalmol 1978;86:418–423.
39. Ballard PL: Delivery and transport of glucocorticoids to target cells. In: Baxter JD, Rousseau GG, eds: Glucocorticoid Hormone Action. Berlin, Springer-Verlag, 1979, p 25.
40. Apt L, Henrick A, Silverman LM: Patient compliance with the use of topical ophthalmic corticosteroid suspensions. Am J Ophthalmol 1979;87:210–214.
41. Leibowitz HM, Kupferman A: Kinetics of topically applied prednisolone acetate optimal concentration for treatment of inflammatory keratitis. Arch Ophthalmol 1976;94:1387–1389.
42. Leibowitz HM: Management of inflammation in the cornea and conjunctiva. Ophthalmology 1980;87:753–758.
43. Foster CS: Rimexolone is the first new corticosteroid for ophthalmic use in 20 years—Its use controls inflammation without significantly raising intraocular pressure. Ocul Surg News 1996;14:124–125.
44. The Loteprednol Etabonate US Uveitis Study Group: Controlled evaluation of loteprednol etabonate and prednisolone acetate in the treatment of acute anterior uveitis. Am J Ophthalmol 1999;127:537–544.
45. Kupferman A, Leibowitz HM: Therapeutic effectiveness of fluorometholone in inflammatory keratitis. Arch Ophthalmol 1975;93:1011–1014.
46. Liebowitz HM, Kupferman A, Ryan WJ, et al: Corneal anti-inflammatory steroidal "soft drug." Invest Ophthalmol Vis Sci 1991;32(suppl):735.
47. Laibowitz RA, Ghormley NR, Insler MS, et al: Treatment of giant

papillary conjunctivitis with loteprednol etabonate, a novel corticosteroid. Invest Ophthalmol Vis Sci 1991;32(suppl):734.

48. Cox WV, Kupferman A, Leibowitz HM: Topically applied steroids in corneal disease. II. The role of the drug vehicle in stromal absorption of dexamethasone. Arch Ophthalmol 1972;88:549–552.

49. Schoenwald RD, Boltralik JS: A bioavailability comparison in rabbits of two steroid formulations as high viscosity gels and reference aqueous preparations. Invest Ophthalmol Vis Sci 1979;18:61–66.

50. Katz IM, Blackman WM: A soluble sustained-release artificial ophthalmic delivery unit. Am J Ophthalmol 1977;83:728–734.

51. Hwang DG, Stern WH, Hwang PH, et al: Collagen shield enhancement of topical dexamethasone penetration. Arch Ophthalmol 1989;107:1375–1380.

52. Hemady R, Tauber J, Foster CS: Immunosuppressive drugs in immune and inflammatory disease. Surv Ophthalmol 1991;35:369–385.

53. Cloes RS, Krohn DL, Breslin H, Braunstein R: Depo-Medrol in the treatment of inflammatory diseases. Am J Ophthalmol 1962;54:407–411.

54. Wine NA, Gornall AG, Bass RP: The ocular uptake of subconjunctivally injected C14 hydrocortisone. Part I. Time and major route of penetration in a normal eye. Am J Ophthalmol 1964;58:362–366.

55. Leibowitz HM, Kupferman A: Periocular injection of corticosteroids. Arch Ophthalmol 1977;95:311–314.

56. Hyndiuk RA, Reagan MG: Radioactive depot corticosteroid penetration into monkey ocular tissue. I. Retrobulbar and systemic administration. Arch Ophthalmol 1968;80:499–503.

57. Hyndiuk RA: Radioactive depot corticosteroid penetration into ocular tissue. II. Subconjunctival administration. Arch Ophthalmol 1969;82:259–263.

58. Levine ND, Aronson SB: Orbital infusion of steroids in the rabbit. Arch Ophthalmol 1970;83:599–607.

59. Jennings T, Rusin MM, Tessier HH, Cunha-Vaz JG: Posterior sub-Tenon's injections of corticosteroids in uveitis patients with cystoid macular edema. Jpn J Ophthalmol 1988;32:385–391.

60. McCartney HJ, Drysdale JO, Gomal AG, Basu PK: An autoradiographic study of the penetration of subconjunctivally injected hydrocortisone into the normal and inflamed rabbit eye. Invest Ophthalmol Vis Sci 1965;4:247–302.

61. Bodker FS, Ticho BA, Feist RM, Lam TT: Intraocular dexamethasone penetration via subconjunctival or retrobulbar injections in rabbits. Ophthalmic Surg 1993;24:453–457.

62. Biswas J, Rao NA: Management of intraocular inflammation. In: Ryan SJ, ed: Retina, vol 2. St. Louis, CV Mosby, 1989, pp 139–146.

63. Schlaegel TF Jr: Essentials of Uveitis. Boston, Little, Brown, 1969, pp 41–42.

64. Smith RE, Nozik RA: Uveitis: A Clinical Approach to Diagnosis and Management. Baltimore, Williams & Wilkins, 1989, pp 51–76.

65. Freeman WR, Green RL, Smith RE: Echographic localization of corticosteroids after periocular injection. Am J Ophthalmol 1987;103:281–288.

66. Tamesis RR, Rodriguez A, Akova YA, et al: Systemic drug toxicity trends in immunosuppressive therapy of immune and inflammatory ocular disease. Ophthalmology 1996;103:769–775.

67. Dave VK, Vickers CHF: Azathioprine in the treatment of mucocutaneous pemphigoid. Br J Ophthalmol 1974;90:183–186.

68. Gordon DM: Diseases of the uveal tract. In: Gordon DM, ed: Medical Management of Ocular Disease. New York, Harper and Row, 1964, pp 245–271.

69. Fauci AS: Alternate-day corticosteroid therapy. Am J Med 1978;64:729–731.

70. Flach AJ: Cyclooxygenase inhibitors in ophthalmology. Surv Ophthalmol 1992;36:259–284.

71. Towler HMA, Whiting PH, Forrester JV: Combination low dose cyclosporin A and steroid therapy in chronic intraocular inflammation. Eye 1990;4:514–520.

72. Nussenblatt RB, Palestine AG, Chan LC, et al: Randomized double masked study of cyclosporine compared to prednisolone in the treatment of endogenous uveitis. Am J Ophthalmol 1991;112:138–146.

73. Bocanegra TS, Castaneda MD, Espinoza LR, et al: Sudden death after methylprednisolone pulse therapy. Ann Intern Med 1981;95:122.

74. Rosenbaum JT: Immunosuppressive therapy of uveitis. Ophthalmol Clin North Am 1993;6:167–175.

75. AMA Drug Evaluations. Chicago, American Medical Association, 1994, pp 1871–1913.

76. Whitcup SM, de Smet MD, Rubin BI, et al: Intraocular lymphoma, clinical and histopathologic diagnoses. Ophthalmology 1993;100:1399–1406.

77. Becker B: Intraocular pressure response to topical corticosteroids. Invest Ophthalmol Vis Sci 1965;4:198–205.

78. Hoskins HD Jr, Kass M: Becker-Schaffe's Diagnosis and Therapy of the Glaucomas. St. Louis, CV Mosby, 1989, pp 115–116.

79. Francois J: The importance of the mucopolysaccharides in intraocular pressure regulation. Invest Ophthalmol Vis Sci 1975;14:173–176.

80. Urban RC Jr, Cotlier E: Corticosteroid-induced cataracts. Surv Ophthalmol 1986;31:102–110.

81. Black RL, Oglesby RB, von Sailmann L, et al: Posterior subcapsular cataracts induced by corticosteroids in patients with rheumatoid arthritis. JAMA 1960;174:166–171.

82. Donshik PL, Cavanaugh HD, Boruchoff DA, et al: Posterior subcapsular cataracts induced by topical steroids following keratoplasty for keratoconus. Ann Ophthalmol 1981;13:29–32.

83. Rubin B, Palestine AG: Complications of corticosteroids and immunosuppressive drugs. Int Ophthalmol Clin 1989;29:159–171.

84. Ashton N, Cook C: Effect of cortisone on healing of corneal wounds. Br J Ophthalmol 1951;35:708–717.

85. Leopold IH: The steroid shield in ophthalmology. Trans Am Acad Ophthalmol Otolaryngol 1967;71:273–289.

86. Armaly MF: Effects of corticosteroids on intraocular pressure and fluid dynamics. I. The effect of dexamethasone in the normal eye. Arch Ophthalmol 1963;70:482–491.

87. Newsome DA, Wong UG, Cameron TP, Anderson RL: "Steroid-induced" mydriasis and ptosis. Invest Ophthalmol Vis Sci 1971;10:424–429.

88. Krupin T, LeBlanc RP, Becker B, et al: Uveitis in association with topically administered corticosteroid. Am J Ophthalmol 1970;70:883–885.

89. Martins JC, Wilensky JT, Asseth CF, et al: Corticosteroid induced uveitis. Am J Ophthalmol 1974;77:433–437.

90. Jaanus SD: Anti-inflammatory drugs. In: Bartlett JD, Jaanus SD, eds: Clinical Ocular Pharmacology. Boston, Butterworths, 1989, pp 163–197.

91. Wakakura M, Ishikawa S: Central serous chorioretinopathy complicating corticosteroid treatment. Br J Ophthalmol 1984;68:329–331.

92. Corboy JM: Corticosteroid therapy for the reduction of postoperative inflammation after cataract extraction. Am J Ophthalmol 1976;82:923–927.

93. Thomas TPL: The complications of systemic corticosteroid therapy in the elderly. Gerontology 1984;30:60–65.

94. Gluck OS, Murphy WA, Hahn TJ, Hahn B: Bone loss in adults receiving alternate-day glucocorticoid therapy: A comparison with daily therapy. Arthritis Rheum 1981;24:892–898.

95. Fraunfelder FT: Drug-Induced Ocular Side Effects and Drug Interactions, 3rd ed. Philadelphia, Lea & Febiger, 1989, pp 321–328.

96. Burde RM, Waltman SR: Topical corticosteroids after cataract surgery. Ann Ophthalmol 1972;4:290–293.

97. Mustakallio A, Kaufman HE, Johnston G, et al: Corticosteroid efficacy in postoperative uveitis. Ann Ophthalmol 1973;6:719–730.

98. Dunne JA, Travers JP: Double-blind clinical trial of topical steroids in anterior uveitis. Br J Ophthalmol 1979;63:762–767.

99. Godfrey WA, Smith RE, Kimura SJ: Chronic cyclitis: corticosteroid therapy. Trans Am Ophthalmol Soc 1976;74:178–187.

100. Foster CS, Drake M, Turner FD, et al: Efficacy and safety of 1% rimexolone ophthalmic suspension vs. 1% prednisolone acetate (Pred Forte) for treatment of uveitis. Am J Ophthalmol 1996;122:171–182.

HISTORY AND SOURCE

Topical cycloplegics and mydriatics have a broad spectrum of clinical utility in diagnostic ophthalmology and serve as important adjunctive medications in the management of anterior chamber inflammation. Specifically, these agents, when used in concert with appropriate anti-inflammatory therapy, are effective in the prevention and treatment of debilitating ocular inflammatory sequelae (e.g., pain arising from ciliary spasm, anterior and posterior synechiae, iris bombé, pupillary block, and secondary angle closure).

The most commonly used drugs fall into two broad categories: those with antimuscarinic activity (cholinergic antagonists such as atropine, scopolamine, homatropine, cyclopentolate, and tropicamide) and the α_1-adrenergic agonists (e.g., phenylephrine). Because the mechanism of action is different for each of the two categories, in clinical practice, these medications are frequently used in combination to achieve maximal therapeutic efficacy; however, for the sake of discussion, each group is considered separately herein.

The naturally occurring belladonna alkaloids, atropine (DL-hyoscyamine) and scopolamine (hyoscine), are derived from the Solanaceae plants: *Atropa belladonna* and *Hyoscyamus niger* respectively.[1] The pharmacologic, medicinal, and toxic properties of these drugs have been well known since antiquity to maidens, physicians, and villains alike. The name belladonna reflects the alleged use of atropine by Italian women to dilate their pupils, thereby imparting to them a flattering, "wide-eyed" appearance, whereas in the Middle Ages these drugs were the agents of choice of professional poisoners.[2] Since the isolation of pure atropine by Mein in 1831,[1] the inhibitory effects of the belladonna alkaloids on the actions of acetylcholine (ACh) in the brain, heart, smooth muscle, and glands have been well characterized. In ophthalmology, these agents have been used since the middle of the 19th century to facilitate examination of the posterior segment and to paralyze accommodation so that a true estimate of the eye's total refractive power could be made.[3] Since then, many semisynthetic congeners (homatropine) of the belladonna alkaloids and synthetic antimuscarinic compounds (cyclopentolate and tropicamide) have been prepared, primarily with the objective of providing adequate mydriasis or cycloplegia, or both, together with a faster onset, a relatively shorter duration of action, and a reduced side effect profile as compared with their naturally occurring counterparts. Cyclopentolate was introduced into clinical practice in 1951,[4] and tropicamide became available for ocular use in 1959.[5] Phenylephrine, a synthetic sympathomimetic amine, was introduced in 1936 principally as a vasoconstrictor and mydriatic.[6, 7]

OFFICIAL DRUG NAME AND CHEMISTRY

The full chemical, nonproprietary names of the most frequently used topical mydriatic-cycloplegic agents, along with the common trade names, manufacturers, and available formulations, are shown in Table 10–1. The corresponding structural formulas of these drugs are shown in Figure 10–1.

The naturally occurring belladonna alkaloids atropine and scopolamine are organic esters formed by the combination of a tropic acid, an aromatic acid, and complex organic bases, either scopine or tropine.[1] The intact ester of tropine and tropic acid and a free hydroxyl (OH) group in the acid portion of the ester are important for antimuscarinic activity. These tertiary ammonium compounds penetrate the blood-brain barrier (BBB) well, with scopolamine providing more significant central nervous system (CNS) effects than atropine.[6] Homatropine is a semisynthetic antimuscarinic agent produced by the combination of mandelic acid with the base tropine.[1] The addition of a second methyl group to nitrogen results in the corresponding quaternary ammonium derivatives, methylatropine nitrate, methscopolamine bromide, and homatropine methylbromide, which, while exhibiting reduced CNS permeability, produce significant nicotinic blocking activity and are of little value in ophthalmology.[1, 6] In contrast, the synthetic congeners cyclopentolate and tropicamide are structurally very different from the natural alkaloids (see Fig. 10–1) and are indispensable in ophthalmic practice owing to their rapid onset and relatively short duration of action.

Phenylephrine is a synthetic analogue of epinephrine. It differs from epinephrine only in lacking an OH group in the number 4 position on the benzene ring.[1] Its potency as an α-adrenoceptor agonist is less than that of epinephrine.

PHARMACOLOGY

Anticholinergic drugs block the actions of ACh and other cholinergic agonists by competing for a common binding site on the muscarinic receptor. This antagonism may be overcome by sufficiently increasing the concentration of ACh at the receptor site of the target tissue. Although three subtypes of muscarinic receptor have been identified pharmacologically (M_1 in sympathetic ganglia and cerebral cortex, M_2 in cardiac muscle, and M_3 in smooth muscle and various glands) and five structural variants have been established by molecular cloning techniques, the anticholinergic agents used in ophthalmology are nonselective.[1] Antimuscarinic drugs have little action at the neuromuscular junction except at very high concentrations; however, they may exert significant effects in sympathetic ganglia, which contain the M_1 muscarinic receptor subtype.[6]

Adrenergic mydriatics such as phenylephrine act directly on α_1-adrenoceptors but have little or no effect on β-adrenoceptors. A minor component of its pharmacologic action, as opposed to that of hydroxyamphetamine, may be due to the release of norepinephrine (NE) from presynaptic adrenergic nerve terminals.[1]

TABLE 10–1. MYDRIATIC-CYCLOPLEGIC AGENTS

GENERIC NAME/TRADE NAME (MANUFACTURER)		CONCENTRATION (%)
Atropine SO$_4$		
Atropine Sulfate Ophthalmic	(Various)	Ointment (1)
Atropine Sulfate S.O.P.	(Allergan, Irvine, CA)	Ointment (0.5, 1)
Atropair	(Texas)	Solution (1)
Atropine Care	(Akorn, Abita Springs, CA)	Solution (1)
Atropisol	(Iolab, Claremont, CA)	Solution (0.5, 1, 2)
Isopto Atropine	(Alcon, Fort Worth, TX)	Solution (0.5, 1, 3)
Ocuo Tropine	(Ocumed, Roseland, NJ)	Solution (1)
Scopolamine HBr		
Isopto Hyoscine	(Alcon)	Solution (0.25)
Homatropine HBr		
Homatropine Ophthalmic	(Various)	Solution (5)
AK-Homatropine	(Akorn)	Solution (5)
Isopto Homatropine	(Alcon)	Solution (2.5)
Cyclopentolate HCl		
Cyclogyl	(Akorn)	Solution (0.5, 1, 2)
AK-Pentolate	(Akorn)	Solution (0.5, 1)
Ocu-Pentolate	(Ocumed)	Solution (1)
Pentolair	(Texas)	Solution (1)
Cyclopentolate HCl and		Solution (1)
Phenylephrine HCl		
Cyclomydril	(Akorn)	Solution (0.2)
Tropicamide		
Mydriacil	(Alcon)	Solution (0.5, 1)
Mydriafair	(Texas)	Solution (0.5, 1)
Ocu-Tropic	(Ocumed)	Solution (0.5)
Tropicacyl	(Akorn)	Solution (0.5)
Phenylephrine HCl		
AK-Dilate	(Akorn)	Solution (2.5, 10)
Dilatir	(Texan)	Solution (2.5)
Mydrifin	(Alcon)	Solution (2.5)
Neo-Synephrine	(Sanofi Winthrop, New York, NY)	Solution (2.5, 10)
Ocu-Phrin	(Ocumed)	Solution (2.5, 10)
Phenylephrine HCl	(Iolab)	Solution (2.5, 10)

CLINICAL PHARMACOLOGY

General systemic effects of antimuscarinic drugs relate to the site of parasympathetic neuroeffector inhibition at various organs and include vasoconstriction; decreased sweating; bronchial, salivary, and gastric secretions; inhibition of cardiac vagal tone with tachycardia; CNS depression; and decreased gastric and urinary bladder tonus.[1] Ocular effects are mediated by the blockage of postganglionic parasympathetic innervation to the longitudinal muscle of the ciliary body and the iris sphincter, with consequent cycloplegia and mydriasis, respectively. In addition, topically applied anticholinergic agents produce conjunctival and uveal arteriole dilation and reduced permeability of the blood-aqueous barrier.[8]

The major systemic consequence of direct activation of α_1-adrenoceptors in vascular smooth muscle (VSM) is increased peripheral vascular resistance and increased blood pressure (BP).[1] In the eye, phenylephrine acts on α-adrenoceptors on the sympathetically innervated iris dilator muscle, arterioles, and Müller's muscle to produce pupillary dilation without cycloplegia, vasoconstriction, and lid elevation.[8]

The relative potencies of the commonly used topical antimuscarinic and adrenergic agents, as reflected by the onset of and recovery from mydriasis and cycloplegia, are listed in descending order in Table 10–2. In general, mydriasis occurs more rapidly, persists longer, and can be achieved at lower concentrations with the anticholinergic agents.[6]

The ocular effects of topical atropine, the most potent

TABLE 10–2. POTENCY OF MYDRIATIC-CYCLOPLEGIC AGENTS

DRUG	STRENGTH (%)	MYDRIASIS		CYCLOPLEGIA	
		Maximal (min)	Recovery (days)	Maximal (hr)	Recovery (days)
Atropine	1.0	30–40	7–10	1–3	7–12
Scopolamine	0.5	20–30	3–7	½–1	5–7
Homatropine	1.0	40–60	1–3	½–1	1–3
Cyclopentolate	0.5–1.0	30–60	1	½–1	1
Tropicamide	0.5–1.0	20–40	¼–1	½	<¼
Phenylephrine	0.5–1.0	20–60	3–6	None	None

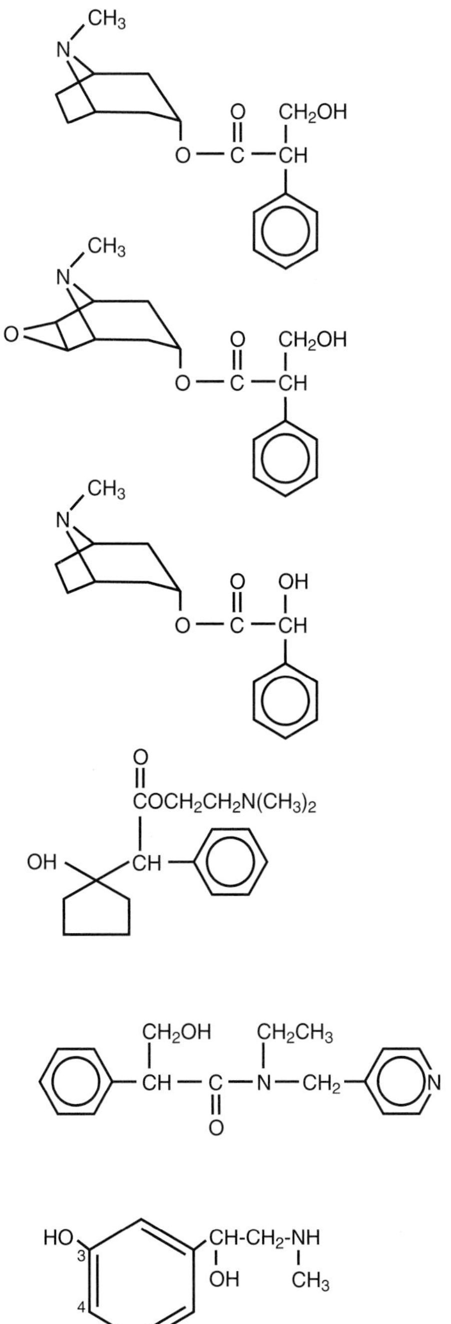

FIGURE 10–1. Structural formulas of atropine, scopolamine, homatropine, cyclopentolate, tropicamide, and phenylephrine.

cycloplegic and mydriatic agent, were first systematically studied by Federsen in 1844.[9] The onset of mydriasis was observed within 12 minutes of topical application of one drop of a 1% solution, reaching a maximum in 26 minutes, with recovery of preinstillation pupillary size by day 10. Cycloplegia began in 12 to 18 minutes and peaked at 160 minutes; full accommodative recovery was achieved by day 8. Although a single drop of atropine may have a prolonged mydriatic or cycloplegic effect in an otherwise healthy patient, eyes with active intraocular inflammation are much more resistant to atropinization and may re-

quire more frequent instillation (two to three times daily), together with supplemental 10% phenylephrine to achieve adequate mydriasis.[2]

Individual variations in response to topical atropine administration is also related to iris pigmentation; mydriasis and cycloplegia have slower onset and longer duration in patients with dark irides than in those with light irides.[2, 10] Pigment binding is believed to reduce the bioavailability of initially administered atropine while providing a prolonged release effect of accumulated drug over time to the muscarinic receptors of the iris and ciliary body.

Scopolamine differs from atropine in that it exerts a more potent antimuscarinic action on the iris, ciliary body, secretory glands, and CNS on a weight basis and has a shorter duration of mydriasis and cycloplegia than atropine at dosage levels used clinically.[11] After instillation of 0.5% solution of scopolamine, maximal pupillary dilation occurred by 20 minutes and was sustained for 90 minutes and with pupils recovered to preinstillation size by day 8. Maximal cycloplegia was achieved by 40 minutes, with accommodative recovery by day 3.[12]

Homatropine is approximately one tenth as potent as atropine, with maximal mydriasis occurring within 40 minutes, after topical instillation of a 1% solution and recovery in 1 to 3 days.[13] Its cycloplegic activity is significantly less pronounced than that of atropine or scopolamine (see Table 10–2).

The onset of maximal mydriasis and cycloplegia after topical administration of either two drops of a 0.5% solution or one drop of 1% solution of cyclopentolate in white patients has been shown to occur in 20 to 30 and 30 to 60 minutes, respectively, with full recovery of each by 24 hours.[4] In contrast, instillation of similar concentrations of drug in black patients or white patients with dark irides produced less effective mydriasis and cycloplegia.[13, 14] In addition, cyclogel did not alter intraocular pressure (IOP) in normal eyes.[14] Its usefulness as an adjunctive agent in management of intraocular inflammatory disease may be limited, however, because it has been shown to be a chemoattractant to inflammatory cells.[15] Various other mydriatic agents, including atropine, homatropine, scopolamine, and tropicamide, failed to produce a similar dose-dependent increase in the migration of neutrophils when tested in vitro.[16]

Tropicamide is the shortest-acting cycloplegic, with a greater mydriatic than cycloplegic effect (see Table 10–2). It has been shown to provide adequate mydriasis for routine ophthalmoscopy at concentrations as low as 0.25%,[17] and pupillary dilation appears to be independent of iris pigmentation.[18] Maximum mydriasis has been shown to occur within 25 to 30 minutes of instillation of either a 0.5% or 1% solution, with recovery of preinstillation pupillary size by 6 hours.[5] Cycloplegia was also achieved in 30 minutes; however, the effect appeared to be dose related, with significant differences between the 0.25% and 1% solutions but not among the 0.5%, 0.75%, or 1% concentrations.[19]

The mydriatic and cycloplegic efficacy of tropicamide has been compared with that of cyclopentolate, homatropine, and phenylephrine.[5] The degree of mydriasis at 30 minutes after instillation of 0.5% or 1% tropicamide was greater than that produced by either 1% cyclopentolate,

5% homatropine, or 10% phenylephrine. Although the maximal cycloplegic action of 1% tropicamide at 30 minutes was more pronounced than that observed with 1% cyclopentolate or 5% homatropine, the effect was not sustained at later timepoints.

Phenylephrine produces maximal mydriasis, with virtually no cycloplegia, in 45 to 60 minutes, depending on the concentration used, with recovery from mydriasis in approximately 6 hours.[20, 21] Dose-response curves demonstrate an increased mydriatic effect with concentrations of phenylephrine to 5% but little additional benefit at concentrations approaching 10%.[22] Clinical studies comparing pupillary dilation with 1.5% and 10% preparations in patients selected at random and not controlled for age or iris color failed to demonstrate significantly greater mydriasis at the higher concentration of phenylephrine.[23, 24] Mydriasis varies with iris color and anterior chamber depth; blue eyes with shallow chambers are more responsive than deep chambers and dark irides.[25] Finally, topical administration of phenylephrine has been shown to decrease IOP in both normal eyes and those with open-angle glaucoma, although the effect is less pronounced than that produced by epinephrine.[26]

PHARMACEUTICS

The various dosage forms and manufacturers of the most commonly used mydriatic-cycloplegic agents are shown in Table 10-1. Prolonged exposure of phenylephrine solutions to air, light, or heat may cause oxidation and a consequent brown discoloration. To prolong the shelf life of phenylephrine, an antioxidant, sodium bisulfite, is frequently added to the vehicle, and refrigeration of the solution is recommended.[11]

PHARMACOKINETICS AND METABOLISM

Topically applied mydriatic agents reach their targets in the eye by diffusing through the cornea, whereas they are absorbed systemically primarily through the conjunctival vessels and nasal mucosa. At a physiologic pH, the pKa values of atropine, homatropine, cyclopentolate, and tropicamide are 9.8. 9.9, 8.4, and 5.37, respectively. A predominance of nonionized molecules exists at lower pKa values, promoting greater diffusibility through the lipid layer of the corneal epithelium and thus greater bioavailability,[11] which may explain the more rapid onset and shorter duration of action of tropicamide as compared with those of other antimuscarinic drugs.

Prior instillation of a topical anesthetic enhances the mydriatic and cycloplegic effect of anticholinergic agents.[27, 28] Likewise, the mydriatic response of phenylephrine is facilitated by use of topical anesthetic agents.[29] Moreover, these pharmacologic effects are amplified by trauma or procedures such as tonometry or gonioscopy, which can disturb corneal epithelial integrity.[30] Gentle lid closure for 5 minutes after instillation of mydriatic drops not only prolongs corneal contact time but also reduces the action of the nasolacrimal pump, thereby enhancing intraocular absorption while minimizing systemic access through the nasolacrimal duct.[31]

The intraocular distribution of atropine has been studied after subconjunctival injection of radiolabeled drug in rabbits.[32] Significant radioactivity was present in the cornea, aqueous, and vitreous; concentrations were lower in the iris, ciliary body, and retina 90 minutes after injection; and 75% of the radioactivity had dissipated from the eye in 5 hours.

Anticholinergic drugs are readily absorbed by the gastrointestinal (GI) tract and distributed throughout the body. Atropine has a half life (t1/2) of approximately 4 hours, with 50% of a single dose being hydrolyzed in the liver and the remainder excreted unchanged in the urine.[1] Phenylephrine, in comparison, is rapidly conjugated and oxidized in the GI mucosa and liver, with only a small fraction being excreted in the urine of normal persons.[33]

THERAPEUTIC USE

The clinical applications of mydriatic-cycloplegic agents in ophthalmology are numerous (Table 10-3), with drug selection depending on the indication and the degree of effect desired; for example, tropicamide 1% alone may provide adequate dilation with minimal cycloplegia and thus obviate residual blurring of vision during routine funduscopic screening.[34] However, reflex contraction of the iris sphincter due to exposure to light during prolonged ophthalmoscopy may require the addition of an adrenergic agent to achieve wide mydriasis. The combination of phenylephrine 2.5% and tropicamide 0.5% or 1% or cyclopentolate 0.5% in a single solution or separately is effective in achieving this end. It also provides adequate mydriasis in patients with dark irides and diabetes (who may respond poorly to topical anticholinergics alone).[35] In contrast, cycloplegia for refraction in children older than 5 years is often achieved by premedication with atropine 0.5% ointment or solution three times daily for 3 days preceding examination and once on the day of refraction. In adults, one drop of 1% cyclopentolate (2% in patients with dark irides) every 15 minutes for one to two doses is frequently sufficient to provide adequate cycloplegia.[36]

In the management of uveitis, the choice of mydriatic-cycloplegic agent used in concert with appropriate anti-inflammatory therapy depends on the nature, severity, location, and duration of inflammation. These agents are most often used in the presence of a clinically significant anterior chamber inflammatory response irrespective of

TABLE 10–3. CLINICAL APPLICATIONS OF MYDRIATIC-CYCLOPLEGIC AGENTS

Dilated funduscopy
Cycloplegic refraction
Pre- and postoperative dilation
Anterior uveitis
Lysis of posterior synechiae
Secondary glaucomas
    Associated with inflammation
    Ciliary block glaucoma
    Lens subluxation
Suppression of amblyopia
Accommodative esotropia
Diagnostic testing
    Horner's syndrome
    Provocative test for angle-closure glaucoma

the location of the primary disease focus (anterior versus posterior uveitis). The principal goals of therapy include complete control of inflammation while limiting permanent ocular structural damage, specifically, prevention of anterior and posterior synechiae formation, iris and ciliary body blood vessel incompetence, secondary cataract, cystic macula, and phthisis bulbi.

Mydriatic-cycloplegic drugs are particularly valuable in both prevention of posterior synechiae, by keeping the pupil in motion until ocular inflammation has been controlled, and in disruption of synechiae that have already formed.[37] The choice of agent, drug combination, frequency, and route of administration depends largely on the severity of uveitis and degree of intraocular pathology. Because the duration of action of mydriatic-cycloplegic agents varies between eyes and with the degree of inflammation, these choices must be made in the context of the individual patient. For example, in patients who present with very mild iridocyclitis and ocular discomfort, 1% tropicamide twice daily in combination with topical corticosteroids may suffice to relieve ciliary spasm without prolonged paralysis of accommodation. In contrast, frequent instillation of atropine 2% may be required in patients with severe ocular pain and a plasmoid anterior chamber. There is little evidence to support the efficacy of mydriatic-cycloplegic agents in reducing either inflammation itself or photophobia in patients with uveitis; rather, aggressive therapy with topical steroids is essential to their mitigation.

We prefer not to use long-acting agents such as atropine and scopolamine routinely, because these drugs cause prolonged paralysis of accommodation, do not keep the pupil moving, and may be associated with unpleasant CNS side effects (scopolamine). However, long-term dilation with these agents may be of value, even during periods of remission, in patients with chronic disease such as juvenile rheumatoid arthritis–associated iridocyclitis and sarcoidosis, in which inflammatory exacerbations are often frequent and severe, and may occur without warning.[37]

Use of cyclopentolate may be contraindicated in patients with uveitis, because it has been shown to be a chemoattractant to inflammatory cells in vitro (described in the Clinical Pharmacology section).[16] In moderate iridocyclitis, phenylephrine or tropicamide alone provide inadequate protection, because the attenuated mydriatic effect of these drugs is further reduced in the presence of inflammation.

Most cases of active iridocyclitis may be adequately treated supplementally with homatropine 5% at a frequency titrated to the anterior chamber inflammatory response (as much as one drop every 2 hours).[37] Alternatively, a combination of phenylephrine 2.5% and tropicamide 1% may be used in a similar fashion to move the pupil during anterior uveitis, or instilled, one drop every 20 minutes for three to four doses, to break recently formed or weak posterior synechiae.[8] Phenylephrine 10% applied to the cornea, usually preceded by a topical anesthetic, has also been used to break recently formed posterior synechiae; however, this agent must be used with caution because of its potential to produce adverse cardiovascular effects.[38] For more tenacious iridolenticular adhesions, frequent applications (one drop every 5 minutes) of a potent mydriatic-cycloplegic (atropine) may be tried.

Should synechialysis fail with the regimens already described, a cotton pledget soaked in a "dynamite cocktail" mixture of various dilating agents may be applied to the topically anesthetized eye in proximity to the area where the synechiae are most extensive and left in place for 10 to 15 minutes. We have successfully used a mixture of equal parts of cocaine 4%, epinephrine 1:1,000, and atropine 1%; other investigators have advocated a filtered mixture of 0.4% homatropine, 0.5% phenylephrine, and 1.0% proparacaine in 100 ml sterile water.[37] With use of these mixtures, complete synechialysis may not be apparent until the following day. Finally, a small volume (0.25 ml) of the homatropine, phenylephrine, and atropine mixture may be injected subconjunctivally at the junction of the adhesion and the freely mobile pupil if synechiae still remain.[37] Again, attention must be paid to potential untoward cardiovascular effects, particularly in elderly patients, because the mixture contains phenylephrine.

SIDE EFFECTS AND TOXICITY

The adverse side effects resulting from topical administration of anticholinergic medications may be local, directly affecting the eye and ocular adnexa, or systemic, due to absorption through the conjunctival lacrimal duct.

Atropine

Systemic toxic effects of atropine are dose dependent with considerable variation between patients.[1] A single drop of a 1% solution provides 0.5 mg of drug[39]; a lethal dose is contained in 200 drops for adults and in 20 drops for children.[1] Signs and symptoms of atropine toxicity include fever, tachycardia, dermal flushing, dryness of the skin and mouth, irritability (the foregoing are particularly common in children), confusional psychosis (especially in the elderly), drowsiness, ataxia, urinary retention, convulsions, even death.[36] Systemic absorption of atropine or of any topically applied solution can be minimized by nasolacrimal occlusion or gentle lid closure for 5 minutes after instillation (which is described in the Pharmacokinetics section).[31]

The ocular and local side effects of topical atropine administration are numerous and clinically significant. Acute, chronic follicular or papillary conjunctivitis and contact dermatitis may arise from direct irritation or hypersensitivity to the drug preparation itself.[2, 11] Atropine, as well as other topical anticholinergic drugs, increases IOP pressure to some degree in 25% to 30% of eyes with open-angle glaucoma.[40] This effect is transient, does not occur in normal eyes, and is believed to arise from a decreased facility of outflow associated with a loss of ciliary muscle tonus.[2] In addition, these agents increase the risk of precipitating acute angle-closure glaucoma in eyes with anatomically narrow angles or a plateau iris configuration.[25] Finally, atropine causes photophobia and blurred vision owing to its prolonged mydriatic effect and paralysis of accommodation. Systemic administration of atropine in conventional doses (0.6 mg) has little ocular effect, but scopolamine in equivalent amounts can cause mydriasis and loss of accommodation.[1]

Scopolamine

The ocular side effects of scopolamine are, with the exception of a shorter duration of action, almost the same as those of atropine. Although systemic effects after topical application are fewer, CNS toxicity appears to be more common, particularly in the elderly, with scopolamine use as compared with atropine use.[41] Black children are apparently more sensitive to the systemic effect of scopolamine.[39]

Homatropine

The side effect profile of homatropine is indistinguishable from that of atropine.[42] However, because it is a less potent drug with a shorter duration of action, it has one fiftieth of the toxicity of atropine and is tolerated in much larger doses than atropine.[39] IOP increase in patients with open-angle glaucoma occurs more often with homatropine than with atropine or scopolamine.[8]

Cyclopentolate

Transient stinging on instillation is the most common ocular side effect of cyclopentolate, occurring more frequently at higher concentrations.[43] Other ocular reactions are similar to those described for atropine.

Likewise, the evolution of systemic toxicity after topical use of cyclopentolate is dose related and parallels that of atropine, except that cyclopentolate is associated with a high incidence of CNS side effects.[39] These side effects may occur at any age but occur more often in the very young and in the elderly. In children, CNS effects are particularly common with use of the 2% solution or after multiple instillations of 1% cyclopentolate and include ataxia, restlessness, memory loss, visual hallucinations, psychosis, disorientation, and irrelevant speech.[44] Although these reactions are typically transient, possible serious neurologic sequelae may develop, including generalized seizures.[45] In addition, GI dysfunction has been reported in premature infants after topical administration of either 1% or 0.5% cyclopentolate.[46]

Tropicamide

Because of short duration of action, adverse ocular side effects are rare with topical application tropicamide but may include hypersensitivity reactions, blurred vision, angle-closure glaucoma in the anatomically predisposed, and a slight increase in IOP.[8] For similar reasons, systemic toxicity is distinctly uncommon, although psychotic reactions, cardiorespiratory collapse, and a transient episode of unconsciousness and muscular rigidity in a child have been reported.[47]

Anticholinergic Overdosage

Treatment of anticholinergic overdosage is both supportive and specific. Adequate hydration and measures to prevent hyperpyrexia may be combined with the specific antidote for CNS toxicity-physostigmine—if these symptoms are severe. A dose of 1 to 4 mg physostigmine salicylate in adults and 0.5 mg in children is administered parenterally and repeated every 15 minutes as necessary.[1] Diazepam is a suitable alternative, providing both sedation and control of convulsions, if specific therapy is not available.[39]

Phenylephrine

Local adverse reactions to topical phenylephrine include transient pain, lacrimation, keratitis, and allergic dermatoconjunctivitis.[48, 49] Angle-closure glaucoma in an anatomically predisposed eye, as well as a transient increase in IOP due to the release of pigment granules from the posterior surface of the iris epithelium with obstruction of the trabecular meshwork, may occur after therapy with topical phenylephrine.[50] This phenomenon is more common in older patients with dark irides and in those with pigment dispersion and pseudoexfoliation syndromes. Lid retraction may be observed because of the adrenergic effect of the drug on Müller's muscle. Rebound miosis has been reported 24 hours after instillation of phenylephrine in patients older than 50 years of age, with attenuation of the mydriatic response on subsequent dosing.[22] Corneal stromal edema and endothelial toxicity may occur, particularly when phenylephrine is administered concomitantly with a topical anesthetic in corneas denuded of epithelium.[51]

Systemic side effects occur more commonly when stronger concentrations, such as phenylephrine 10%, are instilled repeatedly.[25] These reactions include the following: tachycardia, hypertension, reflex bradycardia, angina, ventricular arrhythmia, myocardial infarction, cardiac failure, cardiac arrest, and subarachnoid hemorrhage. Although the overall incidence of severe transient systemic hypertension observed in association with 10% phenylephrine may be low, infants and the elderly appear to be those most susceptible to its administration.[52] Adverse cardiovascular effects can be avoided by using a 2.5% solution.[48] The risk of systemic toxicity in neonates and infants can be reduced by decreasing the drop volume[53] or by using a solution containing cyclopentolate 0.2% and phenylephrine (Cyclomydril), which has been shown to achieve safe and effective mydriasis in premature infants.[54]

HIGH-RISK GROUPS

Both anticholinergic and adrenergic mydriatics present a risk of angle-closure glaucoma in patients with anatomically narrow angles and in eyes with plateau iris configuration[25]; therefore, long-acting agents such as atropine and scopolamine are contraindicated in such eyes and shorter-acting agents, including phenylephrine, should be used cautiously if at all. Hypersensitivity to other anticholinergic or adrenergic agents is an absolute contraindication to the use of atropine, scopolamine, or phenylephrine.

Patients with Down syndrome, keratoconus, spastic paralysis, brain damage, and light irides are particularly sensitive to the mydriatic and systemic side effects of anticholinergic drugs; atropine and scopolamine should be used judiciously in such patients.[55]

Systemic reactions are more frequent after topical administration of both anticholinergic and adrenergic mydriatics in infants, children, and the elderly. These agents should be used at the minimal effective concentration and not more often than is absolutely necessary in such patients. Of the topical anticholinergic drugs, atropine, scopolamine, and cyclopentolate 2% (especially in children) are the most frequent offenders, with scopolamine and cyclopentolate associated with a preponderance of CNS toxicity in all age groups[36] (which is described in the Side Effects and Toxicity section).

Phenylephrine 10% should be used cautiously, if at all, in patients previously treated with atropine, those with coronary artery disease, systemic hypertension (especially those receiving reserpine, methyldopa, or guanethidine), orthostatic hypertension, insulin-dependent diabetes, or aneurysms and should be avoided in neonates and in the elderly.[56–58] It has been suggested that patients at risk of an undue increase in systemic BP or other adverse cardiovascular effects be monitored for 20 to 30 minutes after instillation of even reduced concentrations (2.5%) of phenylephrine drops.[59] Other patients at risk of an increased BP response to topical phenylephrine include those treated with monoamine oxidase inhibitors and tricyclic antidepressants.[36] β-Adrenergic blocking agents failed to demonstrate such an effect in a controlled study of patients with hypertension.[60]

In general, mydriatic agents should be used during pregnancy only when absolutely necessary. Use of atropine and homatropine during the first trimester of pregnancy may cause minor, non–life-threatening malformations, as is the case with phenylephrine, which has been associated with clubfoot and inguinal hernia in particular.[61] Parenteral administration of phenylephrine late in pregnancy may induce fetal hypoxia, as manifested by tachycardia,[62] and scopolamine administered systemically at term may have adverse fetal effects, as reflected by decreased heart rate variability and deceleration.[63]

Whether systemically administered sympathomimetics or anticholinergics are distributed in breast milk is not known with certainty. Because infants are exquisitely sensitive to anticholinergic agents, breast feeding should probably be suspended if these agents must be applied topically to nursing mothers, and use of phenylephrine, which can precipitate severe hypertension, may be contraindicated.[64]

DRUG INTERACTIONS

Analgesics, antihistamines, monoamine oxidase inhibitors, phenothiazines, and tricyclic antidepressants all promote the activity of anticholinergic agents. Anticholinergic drugs themselves enhance the activity of phenothiazines and diminish that of anticholinesterases, and have a variable effect on analgesics.[25]

Concomitant use of phenylephrine 2.5% with echothiophate has been suggested during treatment of accommodative esotropia or open-angle glaucoma because this combination prevents the formation of miotic cysts.[65] The mechanism by which phenylephrine mediates this effect is unknown. Monoamine oxidase inhibitors and tricyclic antidepressants enhance the systemic BP response of concomitantly administered topical phenylephrine[36] (which is described in High-risk Groups section). In patients treated with such drugs for whom phenylephrine is deemed a medical priority, psychiatric medications should be discontinued for at least 21 days before topical therapy is initiated.[8] Finally, phenylephrine itself diminishes the activity of adrenergic blockers and phenothiazines.

MAJOR CLINICAL TRIALS

No high-quality, randomized controlled clinical trials have established the definitive efficacy of mydriatic-cycloplegic agents in reducing or preventing of the adverse sequelae of intraocular inflammation.

References

1. Brown JH: Atropine, scopolamine, and related drugs. In: Gilman AG, Rail TW, Nies AS, Taylor P, eds: Goodman and Gilman's The Pharmacological Basis of Therapeutics. New York, Pergamon Press, 1990, pp 150–165.
2. Havener WA: Ocular Pharmacology. St. Louis, C.V. Mosby, 1983, pp 475–491.
3. Beitel RJ: Cycloplegic refraction. In: Tasman W, Jaeger EA, eds: Duane's Clinical Ophthalmology, Vol. 1. Philadelphia, J.B. Lippincott, 1992, pp 1–4.
4. Priestly BS, Medine MM: A new mydriatic and cycloplegic drug. Am J Ophthalmol 1951;34:572–575.
5. Merrill OL, Goldberg B, Zavel S: Tropicamide, a new parasympatholytic. Curr Ther Res 1960;2:43–50.
6. Liv JHK, Erickson K: Cholinergic agents. In: Albert DM, Jakobiec FA, eds: Principles and Practice of Ophthalmology: Basic Sciences. Philadelphia, W.B. Saunders, 1994, pp 985–992.
7. Heath P: Neosynephrine hydrochloride. Some uses and effects in ophthalmology. Arch Ophthalmol 1936;16:839–846.
8. Pavan-Langston D, Dunkel EC: Handbook of Ocular Drug Therapy and Ocular Side Effects of Systemic Drugs. Boston, Little, Brown, 1991, pp 226–239.
9. Federsen IM. Beitrag zur Atropinvergiftung. Inaug Dissert Berlin; Franke O. 1884, as cited by Marron J: Cycloplegia and mydriasis by use of atropine, scopolamine, and homatropine-paradrine. Arch Ophthalmol 1940;23:340–350.
10. Wolf AV, Hodge AC: Effects of atropine sulfate, methylatropine nitrate (metropine) and homatropine hydrobromide on adult human eyes. Arch Ophthalmol 1946;32:293–301.
11. Jaanus SD, Pagano VT, Bartlett JO: Drugs affecting the autonomic nervous system, In: Bartlett JD, Jaanus SD, eds: Clinical Ocularpharmacology. Boston, Butterworths, 1989, pp 69–148.
12. Marron J: Cycloplegia and mydriasis by use of atropine, scopolamine, and homatropine-paradrine. Arch Ophthalmol 1940:23:340–350.
13. Gettes BD, Leopold IH: Evaluation of five new cycloplegic drugs. Arch Ophthalmol 1953;49:24–27.
14. Abraham SU: A new mydriatic and cycloplegic drug: compound 75 GT. Am J Ophthalmol 1953;36:69–73.
15. Nussenblatt RB, Palestine AG: Uveitis, Fundamentals and Clinical Practice. Chicago: Year Book Medical Publishers, 1989;137–138.
16. Tsai E, Till JO, Marak GE: Effects of mydriatic agents on neutrophil migration. Ophthalmic Res 1988;20:14–19.
17. Gettes BD: Tropicamide, a new cycloplegic mydriatic. Arch Ophthalmol 1961;65:48–52.
18. Dillon JR, Tyburst CW, Yolton RL: The mydriatic effect of tropicamide on light and dark irides. J Am Optom Assoc 1977;48:653–658.
19. Pollack SL, Hunt JS, Polse KA: Dose-response effects of tropicamide HC1. Am J Optom Physiol Opt 1981;58:361–366.
20. Gambill HD, Ogle KN, Kearns TP: Mydriatic effect of four drugs determined by pupillograph. Arch Ophthalmol 1967;77:740–746.
21. Doughty MJ, Lyle W, Trevino R, et al: A study of mydriasis produced by topical phenylephrine 2.5% in young adults. Can J Optom 1988; 50:40–60.
22. Haddad NJ, Moyer NJ, Riley FC: Mydriatic effect of phenylephrine hydrochloride. Am J Ophthalmol 1970;70:729–733.
23. Smith RB, Read S, Oczypik PM: Mydriatic effect of phenylephrine. Eye Ear Nose Throat Monthly 1976;55:133–134.
24. Neuhaus RW, Helper RS. Mydriatic effect of phenylephrine 10% vs. phenylephrine 2.5% (aq.). Ann Ophthal 1980;12:1159–1160.
25. Fraunfelder FT. Drug-induced Ocular Side Effects and Drug Interactions, 3rd ed. Philadelphia, Lea & Febiger, 1989.
26. Lee PF: The influence of epinephrine and phenylephrine on intraocular pressure. Arch Ophthalmol 1958;60:863–867.
27. Apt L, Henrick A: Pupillary dilatation with single eyedrop mydriatic combinations. Am J Ophthalmol 1980;89:553–559.
28. Sinclair SH, Pelham V, Giovanoni R, Regan CD: Mydriatic solution

for outpatient indirect ophthalmoscopy. Arch Ophthalmol 1980;98:1572–1574.

29. Jaurequi MJ, Poise KA: Mydriatic effect using phenylephrine and proparacaine. Am J Optom Physiol Opt 1974;51:545–549.

30. Marr WG, Wood R, Senterfit L, Sigelman S: Effect of topical anesthetics on regeneration of corneal epithelium. Am J Ophthalmol 1957; 43:606–610.

31. Zimmerman TJ, Kooner KS, Kandarakis AS, Fiegler LP: Improving the therapeutic index of topically applied ocular drugs. Arch Ophthalmol 1984;102:551–553.

32. Janes RC, Stiles JF: The penetration of C14 labeled atropine into the eye. Arch Ophthalmol 1959;62:69–74.

33. Hoffman BB, Lefkowitz RJ: Catecholamines and sympathomimetic drugs. In: Gilman AG, Rail TW, Nies AS, Taylor P, eds. Goodman and Gilman's The Pharmacological Basis of therapeutics. New York, Pergamon Press, 1990, pp 187–220.

34. Steinman WC, Millstein ME, Sinclair SH: Pupillary dilation with tropicamide 1% for funduscopic screening. A study of duration of action. Ann Intern Med 1987;107:181–184.

35. Huber MSE, Smith SA, Smith SE. Mydriatic drug for diabetic patients. Br J Ophthalmol 1985,69:425–427.

36. AMA Drug Evaluation. Chicago: American Medical Association, 1994;2123–2136.

37. Smith RE, Nozik RA. Uveitis, a Clinical Approach to Diagnosis and Management. Baltimore, Williams & Wilkins, 1989, pp 51–72.

38. Heath P, Geiter CW: Use of phenylephrine hydrochloride (neosynephrine) in ophthalmology. Arch Ophthalmol 1949;41:172–177.

39. Potter DE: Drugs that alter the autonomic nervous system function. In: Lamberts DW, Potter DE, eds: Clinical Ophthalmic Pharmacology. Boston, Little, Brown, 1987, pp 297–334.

40. Shaw BR, Lewis RA: Intraocular pressure elevation after pupillary dilation in open angle glaucoma. Arch Ophthalmol 1986;104:1185–1188.

41. Freund M, Merin S: Toxic effect of scopolamine eyedrops. Am J Ophthalmol 1970;70:637–639.

42. Hoefnagel D: Toxic effects of atropine and homatropine eyedrops in children. N Engl J Med 1961;264:168–17 1.

43. Cramp J: Reported cases of reactions and side effects of the drugs which optometrists use. Aust J Optom 1976;59:13–25.

44. Binkhorst RD, Weinstein GW, Baretz RM, Glahane MS: Psychotic reaction induced by cyclopentolate. Am J Ophthalmol 1963;56:1243–1245.

45. Kennerdel JS, Wucher FP: Cyclopentolate associated with two cases of grand mal seizure. Arch Ophthalmol 1972;87:634–635.

46. Isenberg SJ, Abrams C, Hyman PE: Effects of cyclopentolate eyedrops on gastric secretary function in pre-term infants. Ophthalmology 1985;92:698–700.

47. Wahl JW: Systemic reactions to tropicamide. Arch Ophthalmol 1969;82:320–321.

48. Meyer SM, Fraunfelder FT: Phenylephrine hydrochloride. Ophthalmology 1980;87:1177–1880.

49. Geyer O, Lazar M. Allergic blepharoconjunctivitis due to phenylephrine. J Ocul Pharmacol 1988;4:123–126.

50. Mitsui Y, Takagi Y. Nature of aqueous floaters due to sympathomimetic mydriatics. Arch Ophthalmol 1961;65:626–631.

51. Edelhauser HF, Hine JE, Pederson H, et al: The effect of phenylephrine on the comea. Arch Ophthalmol 1979;97:937–947.

52. Brown MM, Brown GC, Spaeth GL: Lack of side effects from topically administered 10% phenylephrine eyedrops. A controlled study. Arch Ophthalmol 1980;98:487–489.

53. Lynch MG, Brown RH, Goode SM, et al: Reduction of phenylephrine drop size in infants achieves equal dilation with decreased systemic absorption. Arch Ophthalmol 1987;105:1364–1365.

54. Isenberg S, Everett S, Parethoff E: A comparison of mydriatic eye drops in low-weight infants. Ophthalmology 1984;91:278–279.

55. Eggers HM: Toxicity of drugs used in the diagnosis and treatment of strabismus. In: Srinivasan DB, ed: Ocular Therapeutics. New York, Masson, 1980, pp 115–122.

56. Fraunfelder FT, Scafidi AF: Possible adverse effects from topical ocular 10% phenylephrine. Am J Ophthalmol 1978;85:862–868.

57. Kim JM, Stevenson CE, Mathewson HS: Hypertensive reactions to phenylephrine eyedrops in patients with sympathetic denervation. Am J Ophthalmol 1978;85:862–868.

58. Robertson D: Contraindication to the use of ocular phenylephrine in idiopathic orthostatic hypotension. Am J Ophthalmol 1979;87:819–822.

59. Kumar V, Schoenwald RD, Barcelios WA, et al: Aqueous vs. viscous phenylephrine. 1. Systemic absorption and cardiovascular effects. Arch Ophthalmol 1986;104:1189–1191.

60. Myers MG: Beta adrenoceptor antagonism and pressor response to phenylephrine. Clin Pharmacol Ther 1984;36:57–63.

61. Heinonen OP, Slone D, Shapiro S: Birth Defects and Drugs in Pregnancy. Littleton, Publishing Sciences Group, 1977, pp 297–313, 345–356.

62. Smith NT, Corgascio AN: The use and misuse of pressor agents. Anesthesiology 1970;33:58–101.

63. Ayrumlooi J, Tobias M, Berg P: The effects of scopolamine and ancillary analgesics on the fetal heart rate recording. J Reprod Med 1980;25:323–326.

64. Samples JR, Meyer SM: Use of ophthalmic medications in pregnant and nursing women. Am J Ophthalmol 1988;106:616–623.

65. Chiri NB, Gold AA, Breinin G: Iris cysts and miotics. Arch Ophthalmol 1964;71:611–616.

NONSTEROIDAL ANTI-INFLAMMATORY DRUGS

Albert T. Vitale and C. Stephen Foster

INTRODUCTION, HISTORY, AND SOURCE

In the last 20 years, we have witnessed the development of a family of clinically useful aspirin-like, nonsteroidal anti-inflammatory drugs (NSAIDs), which are among the most widely prescribed agents in general medicine for the treatment of inflammation associated with rheumatic diseases and which have recently become commercially available worldwide as ophthalmic eye drops.[1] In ophthalmic practice, these agents are used principally in the prevention and treatment of cystoid macular edema (CME), intraoperative miosis, and postoperative inflammation associated with cataract surgery. In addition, NSAID therapy, especially in conjunction with topical, periocular, or systemic steroids, constitutes an important facet of our approach to the management of patients with uveitis. Specifically, these agents are steroid sparing and are useful in prevention of disease relapse and macular edema recurrence associated with intraocular inflammation.

Before the emergence of corticosteroids, nonsteroidal agents, such as aspirin, were used in treatment of severe intraocular inflammation.[2] With the demonstration in the early 1970s of the inhibitory effect of aspirin on the synthesis of prostaglandins[3] (potent inflammatory mediators), other NSAIDs were developed in an effort to provide effective anti-inflammatory activity while obviating the dose-limiting side effects associated with corticosteroids. Today, several chemical classes of synthetic NSAIDs exist and have anti-inflammatory, antipyretic, and analgesic properties similar to those of aspirin (Table 11–1) by virtue of their common pharmacodynamics. At the time of this writing, four nonsteroidal solutions have been approved by the Food and Drug Administration (FDA) for ophthalmic use in the United States (Table 11–2), whereas in Europe and in other parts of the world, NSAIDs have been more widely used in treatment of intraocular inflammation and its sequelae (CME).

OFFICIAL DRUG NAME AND CHEMISTRY

The more commonly prescribed systemic NSAIDs are shown according to chemical class, along with their nonproprietary name, the manufacturer, the trade name, and the typical daily adult dosage in Table 11–1. The currently available topical preparations are similarly shown in Table 11–2. Representative structural formulas from each chemical class of NSAID are shown in Figure 11–1. Although

TABLE 11–1. SYSTEMIC NONSTEROIDAL ANTI-INFLAMMATORY AGENTS

| DRUG CLASS | DRUG | | SUPPLIED (mg) | TYPICAL ADULT DAILY DOSE (mg) |
	Generic	Trade Name		
Salicylates	Aspirin	Multiple	325–925	650 every 4 hr
	Diflunisal	Dolobid (MSD, West Point, PA)	250, 500	250–500 bid
Fenamates	Mefenamate	Pronstel (Parke-Davis, Morris Plains, NJ)	250	250 qid
	Meclofenamate	Meclomen (Parke-Davis)	50, 100	50–100 qid
Indoles	Indomethacin	Indocin (MSD)	25, 50, 75(SR)	25–50 tid-qid, 75 bid
	Sulindac	Clinoril (MSD)	150, 200	150–200 bid
	Tolmetrin	Tolectin (McNeil, Raritan, NJ)	200, 400, 600	400 tid
Phenylacetic acids	Diclofenac	Voltaren (Geigy, Summit, NJ)	25, 50, 75	50–75 bid
Phenylalkanoic acids	Fenoprofen	Nalfon (Lilly, Indianapolis, IN)	200, 300, 600	300–600 tid
	Ketoprofen	Oridus (Wyeth, Philadelphia, PA)	25, 50, 75	75 tid–50 qid
	Piroxicam	Feldene (Pfizer, New York, NY)	10, 20	10 bid, 20 qd
	Flurbiprofen	Ansaid (Upjohn, Kalamazoo, MI)	50, 100	100 tid
	Ketorolac	Toradol (Syntex, Nutley, NJ)	10	10 qid
	Naproxen	Naprosyn (Syntex)	250, 375, 500	250–500 bid
		Anaprox (Syntex)	275, 550	275–550 bid
	Ibuprofen	Motrin (Upjohn)	200, 300, 400, 600, 800	400–800 tid
		Rufen (Boots, Whippany, NJ)		
		Advil (Whitehall, Madison, NJ)		
		Nuprin (Bristol Meyers, Princeton, NJ)		
Pyrazolons	Phenylbutazone	Butazolidin (Geigy)	100	100 tid–qid
		Azolid (USV, Westborough, MA)		
	Oxyphenylbutazone	Tendearil (Geigy)	100	100 tid–qid
		Osalid (USV)		
Para-aminophenols	Acetaminophen	Multiple	80, 325, 500, 650	650 every 4 hr
Cox-2 inhibitors	Celecoxib	Celebrex (Pharmacia, Peapack, NJ)	100, 200	100 bid, 200 bid
	Rofecoxib	Vioxx (Merck & Co., Whitehouse Station, NJ)	12.5, 25, 50	12.5 qd, 2 5qd, 50 qd

bid, twice daily; tid, three times daily; qid, four times daily; qd, daily; hr, hours.

TABLE 11–2. TOPICAL NONSTEROIDAL ANTI-INFLAMMATORY AGENTS

DRUG			
Generic	Trade Name	SUPPLIED	TYPICAL DOSES
Flurbiprofen[*,†]	Ocufen (Allergan, Irvine, CA)	0.03% Solution	One drop every 30 min, 2 hr preoperatively (total dose 4 drops)
Suprofen[*,†]	Profenal (Alcon, Fort Worth, TX)	1.0% Solution	Two drops at 1, 2, and 3 hr preoperatively or every 4 hr while awake on the day of surgery
Diclofenal[*]	Voltaren (Ciba Vision, Duluth, GA)	0.1% Solution	qid
Ketorolac[*]	Acular (Syntex, Nutley, NJ)	0.5% Solution	tid
Indomethacin	Indocid (MSD, West Point, PA)	0.5%–1% Suspension	qid

[*]Approved by the Food and Drug Administration for ophthalmic use.
[†]Approved for intraoperative miosis only.

these compounds are heterogeneous, their unifying and defining feature is the absence of a steroid nucleus in their chemical structure (as compared with the chemical structure of hydrocortisone). Of the chemical classes enumerated, the salicylates, fenarnates, and pyrazolone derivatives are either unstable in solution or too toxic for ocular applications.[4] In contrast, the phenylalkanoic acids are water soluble, allowing the formulation of flurbiprofen and suprofen as Ocufen 0.03% (Allergan, Irvine, CA) and Profenal 1% (Alcon, Fort Worth, TX) ophthalmic solutions respectively. These preparations have been approved by the FDA for inhibition of intraoperative miosis during cataract surgery.[5, 6] Most recently, ketorolac tromethamine 0.5% (Acular, Allergan) has become available as a topical agent for treatment of allergic conjunctivitis.[4] Likewise, diclofenac 0.1% (Voltaren, Ciba Vision, Duluth, GA), a water-soluble phenylacetic acid derivative, has been approved for treatment of inflammation after cataract surgery.[7]

PHARMACOLOGY

The mechanism by which all NSAIDs mediate their pharmacologic effects is related in part to the inhibition of cyclooxygenase, the enzyme responsible for conversion of arachidonic acid (AA) to cyclic endoperoxidases (PGG_2, PGH_2), the precursors of prostaglandins, in ocular and

nonocular tissues (Fig. 11–2).[8] Plasma membrane–bound AA is released from phospholipid through the action of phospholipase-A and generates substrate for the cyclooxygenase and lipoxygenase catabolic pathways, with subsequent prostaglandin and leukotriene (LT) generation. Cyclooxygenase inhibition is the specific action of the NSAIDs, although lipoxygenase activity may be affected to some degree by diclofenac. Theoretically, specific inhibition of cyclooxygenase could indirectly enhance the production of LTs by shunting more AA to be metabolized by lipoxygenase. In contrast, corticosteroids, which retard the release of AA by inhibiting phospholipase-A, inhibit both the cyclooxygenase and lipoxygenase pathway products.[9] This phenomenon may explain the superior anti-inflammatory potency of corticosteroids as compared with that of NSAIDs and may provide the basis for therapeutic synergism when these agents are used together.

The pharmacologic actions of NSAIDs are probably more complex than was previously appreciated, involving more than sole inhibition of cyclogenase.[1] There appears to be a correlation between the anti-inflammatory potency of NSAIDs with the degree of albumin binding, as well as a relationship between anti-inflammatory activity, NSAID acidity, and the efficacy of inhibition of prostaglandin synthesis. Evidence also shows that NSAIDs have

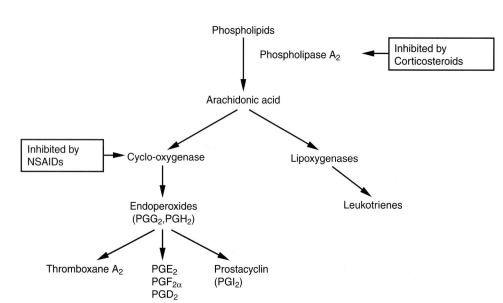

FIGURE 11–1. Chemical structures of representative nonsteroidal anti-inflammatory drugs. *A*, Aspirin (salicylates). *B*, Mefenemerate (tenemates). *C*, Indomethacin (indoles). *D*, Diclofenal (phenylacetic acids). *E*, Flurbiprofen (phenylalkanoic acids). *F*, Phenylbutazone (pyrazolones). *G*, Acetaminophen (*para*-aminophenols).

A. ASPIRIN

B. MEFENAMIC ACID

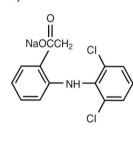

C. INDOMETHACIN
[Indocin]

D. DICLOFENAC SODIUM
[Voltaren]

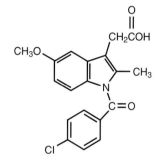

FIGURE 11–2. Arachidonic metabolic pathways.

E. FLURBIPROFEN
[Ansaid]

F. PHENYLBUTAZONE

G. ACETAMINOPHEN

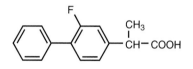

free radical scavenger activity,[10] as well as antichemotactic activity, which modulates humoral and cellular events during inflammatory reactions.[11]

CLINICAL PHARMACOLOGY

All NSAIDs share, to some degree, anti-inflammatory, antipyretic, and analgesic properties; however, there are important differences among individual agents with respect to these activities. For example, acetaminophen is commonly prescribed to reduce fever and mild pain but is only weakly anti-inflammatory and has no effect on platelets and bleeding time. Although the reasons for these differences are poorly defined, they may relate to differential enzyme inhibition in the target tissues.[8] Furthermore, the diversity of NSAID pharmacologic activity is directly related to the multifaceted biologic effects of prostaglandins, whose biosynthesis they inhibit.

Prostaglandins are 20 carbon, unsaturated fatty acid derivatives with a cyclopentane ring, present in nearly every organ, including the eye. In addition to their well-known role in the inflammatory response, prostaglandins are believed to play important roles in the control of pain, body temperature, blood coagulation, intraocular pressure (IOP), lipid and carbohydrate metabolism, and cardiovascular and renal physiology.[8]

The link between prostaglandins and the eye dates back to the isolation of a substance termed irin from extracts of rabbit iris tissue nearly 45 years ago.[12] This substance, which produced pupillary constriction when injected into the anterior chamber of animal eyes, was later shown to contain prostaglandins.[13] In addition to inducing miosis, prostaglandins have a diverse spectrum of action in the eye, increasing inflammation,[14] enhancing vascular permeability of blood-ocular barriers,[15] and producing conjunctival hyperemia, and changes in IOP[16] (Table 11–3). Furthermore, increased levels of prostaglandins have been detected in the aqueous humor after trauma,[15] cataract surgery,[17] and laser iridotomy.[18]

TABLE 11–3. OCULAR EFFECTS OF PROSTAGLANDINS

PGD_2	Vasodilation and chemosis
PGE, PGE_2	Vasodilation and miosis, increase IOP, capillary permeability, and inflammation
PGE_2	Decreased IOP, minimal effect on inflammation or miosis

The precise mechanism of prostaglandin action is not known. Some prostaglandins display differential effects on various tissues, whereas others behave antagonistically with one another.[7] These factors notwithstanding, it is the NSAID-mediated cyclooxygenase inhibition of prostaglandin biosynthesis that is responsible for their therapeutic effects in ophthalmology: the prevention and treatment of CME, intraoperative miosis, and intraocular inflammation associated with cataract surgery and uveitis.

PHARMACEUTICS

The dosage sizes and typical frequency of administration for adults of the more commonly prescribed systemic NSAIDs are shown in Table 11–1. Currently available topical preparations are shown in Table 11–2. All systemic NSAIDs should be taken with food, milk, or antacid.

PHARMACOKINETICS

All orally administered NSAIDs are readily absorbed from the gastrointestinal (GI) tract, reaching peak serum concentrations in 0.5 to 5 hours.[19] A correlation between plasma concentration and therapeutic efficacy has been demonstrated for aspirin and naproxen; however, this relationship has not been established for other NSAIDs.[20]

All NSAIDs are highly protein bound (90% to 99%), especially to albumin and at ocular tissues, and have a small volume of distribution.[4] These characteristics may increase the risk of potential adverse interactions with drugs that share a similar high avidity for plasma proteins (e.g., oral hypoglycemic agents and anticoagulants).[20]

The liver is the major site of NSAID metabolism, with the unchanged drug and its metabolites excreted primarily by the kidneys and secondarily in the feces. The plasma elimination half-lives (t1/2) of different NSAIDs vary greatly, which probably relates to enterohepatic circulation.[4] Therefore, patients with compromised renal or hepatic function are at risk of development of toxic side effects of NSAIDs, even at recommended doses.

Topically applied NSAIDs are distributed throughout the ocular tissues, including the cornea, conjunctiva, sclera, iris, ciliary body, lens, retina, choroid, vitreous, and aqueous humor[21] and provide adequate levels in the latter to inhibit prostaglandin synthesis in animal studies.[5, 22] Although good ocular penetration is achieved after systemic administration of NSAIDs, topically applied drug appears to provide superior bioavailability in the anterior chamber.[23]

Finally, a significant percentage of topically applied NSAID drugs may gain access to the systemic circulation through the nasolacrimal duct.[21, 24] Although only a small quantity of drug is ultimately absorbed systemically after topical instillation, as is attested by the paucity of systemic side effects associated with this route versus that of oral administration, we should not assume that the topical route is completely devoid of such toxicity.[4]

THERAPEUTIC USE

Prevention of Intraoperative Miosis

The single most important risk factor for vitreous loss and zonular breaks during extracapsular cataract surgery with intraocular lens (IOL) implantation is decreasing pupil size.[25] Surgical trauma is believed to stimulate production of certain prostaglandins that mediate miosis independently of cholinergic mechanisms.[26] Two topical NSAIDs, flurbiprofen 0.03% and suprofen 1%, have been approved by the FDA for use in the United States to ameliorate this problem. Flurbiprofen 0.03%, administered every 30 minutes, beginning 2 hours before surgery, was shown in two double-masked, placebo-controlled, randomized studies to limit intraoperative miosis during anterior segment surgery.[5, 27] A similarly designed multicenter trial of topical suprofen 1% showed pupillary constriction to be reduced during cataract surgery when two drops were administered every 4 hours on the day before surgery and every hour for three doses immediately before surgery.[28] Preoperative treatment is crucial because topically applied NSAIDs block the synthesis of prostaglandins rather than their effects on the iris once the prostaglandins are formed. Although these studies clearly show a statistically significant inhibitory effect on intraoperative miosis, the use of topical NSAIDs routinely by all surgeons may not be associated with a clinically significant inhibitory effect.[4] The changes in pupil size observed in these studies are small, vary considerably from one surgeon to the next, and significant changes in pupil size in control eyes are larger, in several instances, than in NSAID-treated eyes.[1] These findings suggest that surgical miosis may be mediated in part by as yet unidentified endogenous factors independent of surgical technique or prostaglandin pharmacodynamics.[4]

Postsurgical Inflammation

Many well-controlled clinical studies provide evidence that NSAIDs topically applied before and immediately after cataract surgery are useful in the management of postoperative inflammation.[1] Such treatment might serve to obviate the potential untoward side effects of secondary glaucoma, increased risk of infection, and impaired wound healing associated with topical steroid use (see Chapter 9, Corticosteroids, Side Effects and Toxicity).

Postoperative inflammation, as measure directly (slit-lamp examination) or indirectly (fluorophotometry in detecting perturbation in the blood-aqueous barrier) appears to be reduced by several topical NSAIDs, including indocin 1.0%,[29] flurbiprofen 0.03%,[30] ketorolac 0.5%,[31, 32] and diclofenac 0.1%[7] in randomized, double-masked, placebo-controlled comparisons. The treatment effect was observed after both intracapsular and extracapsular surgery, irrespective of IOL implantation and whether corticosteroids were administered concurrently or postoperatively. A good correlation between slit-lamp and anterior ocular fluorophotometry observations was noted and was confirmed by more recent studies in which a laser cell flare meter method was used.[4]

Ketorolac 0.5% versus dexamethasone 0.1%[33] and diclofenac 0.1%, 0.5%, and 0.01% versus prednisolone 1%[34] have been compared in randomized, controlled, double-masked studies. These two treatment arms were not statistically different in reducing postoperative inflammation, as judged by slit-lamp examinations for cells, flare, and chemosis; however, topical NSAIDs were superior to topical steroids in reducing the breakdown of the blood-aqueous barrier, as measured by fluorophotometry.[4]

These studies suggest that topical NSAIDs may serve as possible substitutes for corticosteroids in the management of postoperative inflammation. However, at present, only diclofenac 0.1%, one drop four times daily, beginning 24 hours after cataract surgery, has been approved by the FDA for this purpose.

Prophylaxis and Treatment of Cystoid Macular Edema

Common to all disease entities associated with CME is the disruption of the inner or outer blood-retinal barrier.[35] Free radicals generated by ultraviolet light, vitreous traction, and inflammation have all been implicated in its pathogenesis and undoubtedly play a central role in the evolution of CME after cataract surgery or that associated with uveitis. The many well-designed clinical studies that have demonstrated a beneficial effect of both topical and systemic NSAID therapy for prevention of angiographic CME and the treatment of chronic symptomatic CME after cataract surgery have been thoughtfully and comprehensively reviewed elsewhere.[1, 36, 37] In the assessment of the therapeutic efficacy of NSAIDs in treatment of CME, the following have been consistently emphasized: (1) the importance of double-masked, randomized, placebo-controlled comparisons in an entity whose natural history is marked by spontaneous remission and recurrences; (2) the differentiation between angiographic and clinically significant CME; and (3) the separation of prophylactic treatment from therapy for established CME.

Of the most frequently cited controlled studies establishing the efficacy of topical NSAIDs in the prophylaxis of angiographic CME after cataract extraction,[38-40] only one has demonstrated a statistically significant improvement in Snellen visual acuity,[38] an effect that was not sustained longer than 3 months. The use of non-Snellen parameters of visual function and the benefit of prophylactic therapy for more than 1 year have not yet been evaluated. Furthermore, in these studies, corticosteroids were administered concurrently in the postoperative period, introducing the potential for therapeutic synergism between the two drugs and thus rendering conclusions with regard to NSAID monotherapy difficult. A recent double-masked, placebo-controlled study demonstrated a statistically significant reduction in postoperative angiographic CME, however, although with no significant improvement in visual acuity, after prophylactic treatment with topical ketorolac 0.5%, one drop three times daily, initiated 1 day preoperatively and continued for 19 days postoperatively, without concurrent use of corticosteroids.[41]

Finally, two double-masked, placebo-controlled, randomized studies have provided evidence that topical ketorolac 0.5% may improve vision in some patients with CME that has been present for 6 months or more after cataract extraction.[42, 43] One regimen for the treatment of established CME begins with intensive topical steroids (eight times daily) and topical NSAIDs (four to six times daily) for 2 weeks. If no significant improvement or worsening of CME is observed, systemic NSAIDs are instituted and topical NSAIDs are discontinued.[44]

Uveitis

NSAID therapy is an important adjunct in our therapeutic approach to patients with uveitis, particularly when it is used in conjunction with topical, periocular, and systemic steroids. Not only have these medicines been shown to decrease intraocular inflammation after cataract extraction and to be useful in prophylaxis and treatment of CME, but they may also be steroid sparing, reducing the total amount of corticosteroid required to eliminate inflammation. Such is true of topical NSAID therapy; we believe that these agents do not produce a clinically profound reduction in intraocular inflammation per se, but instead obviate steroid-induced side effects in patients with chronic uveitis by allowing a reduction in the effective dose of steroid. Indeed, 5.0% tolmetin versus 0.5% prednisolone versus saline was compared in a double-masked, randomized, controlled clinical trial of 100 patients with acute nongranulomatous anterior uveitis. No statistically significant difference in "cure" rate was demonstrated at the end of the 3-week study.[45] Similarly, 49 patients with acute anterior uveitis randomized to a masked comparison between 1% indomethacin and 0.1% dexamethasone applied six times daily manifested a more marked reduction in inflammation in the steroid group by day 7, with no difference between the two groups at 2 weeks.[46]

Similarly, little evidence supports the use of systemic NSAIDs as the sole agent during an episode of acute anterior uveitis. However, in our experience, oral NSAIDs are particularly useful in long-term management of recurrent anterior uveitis, substantially reducing the amount of corticosteroid required to achieve inflammatory quiescence and enabling patients, in many cases, to maintain a steady course without inflammatory exacerbations once steroids have been discontinued. Adjunctive therapy with systemic NSAIDs was shown to reduce the inflammatory activity and allow a reduction in the dose of corticosteroids in a group of children with chronic iridocyclitis[47] and to prevent further attacks of juvenile rheumatoid arthritis–associated iridocyclitis.[48]

In cases of posterior uveitis and secondary vasculitis, we find oral NSAID agents to be effective in eliminating macular edema and preventing its recurrence. Typically, we initially treat patients with a combination of transseptal steroid (Kenalog 40 mg) and an oral NSAID (Voltaren 75 mg twice daily). In some instances, systemic oral prednisone (1 mg/kg/day) is administered every morning for 7 to 14 days, depending on the severity of intraocular inflammation. Steroids are tapered and discontinued once the macular edema has been eliminated and the uveitis controlled; however, the NSAID is continued for 6 to 12 months, barring the occurrence of drug-induced toxicity. Primary retinal vasculitis does not appear to be amenable to oral NSAID therapy. We consider steroids and cytotoxic agents necessary in such cases.

Finally, the safety and efficacy of systemic NSAIDs has been evaluated in a nonrandomized, uncontrolled fashion in a large uveitis population at the Massachusetts Eye and Ear Infirmary in the past 10 years. At the time of this writing, diclofenac (Voltaren) and diflunisal (Dolobid) are the safest and most effective agents, with indomethacin (Indocin SR) and naproxen (Naprosyn) ranking close seconds. Piroxicam (Feldene), sulindac (Clinoril), and ibuprofen (Motrin) have been the least effective for therapy of intraocular inflammatory disease and associated macular edema (see Table 11–1). Cyclooxygenase has been determined to be composed of two isoenzymes, COX-1 and COX-2, each with nearly identical tertiary structures of the active binding site with but a single amino acid difference. But that single amino acid difference confers extraordinary functional differences to these two isoenzymes. The COX-1 isoenzyme catalyzes two different types of reactions, a peroxidase reaction and a cyclooxygenase one, with clear evidence that COX-1 has virtually no effect on inflammatory and on analgesia, but rather functions widely in homeostatic roles in the kidney, gut, and elsewhere. One of its primary functions in the gut involves the production of mucin, a protectant for the epithelial lining of the gut; inhibition of this function by nonsteroidal anti-inflammatory agents that inhibit COX-1 reduce this protecticve mechanism, leaving the luminal lining of the gut more susceptible to damage from acidic gastric secretions. In contrast, inhibition of COX-2 has little effect on COX-1 derived prostaglandin E_2 production in the gastric mucosa, and so has little effect on mucin production by that mucosa.[49] But COX-2 inhibition potently inhibits production of COX-2 derived prostaglandin E_2 in several different models of inflammation, whereas selective inhibition of COX-1 does not.[49] These selective differences in COX-1 and COX-2 inhibition led to the development of highly selective inhibitors of COX-2 in the quest for potent inhibition of one inflammatory pathway (cyclooxygeanse generation of prostaglandins) without one of the more limiting side effects of nonselective cyclooxygenase inhibition, namely development of peptic ulcer disease. Two such COX-2 selective inhibitors have reached the United States market at the time of this writing, celecoxib (Celebrex) and refocoxib (Vioxx), both receiving approval of the United States Food and Drug Administration for sale for the treatment of osteoarthritis and or rheumatoid arthritis. Both have now been used by us in the care of patients with ocular inflammatory disease, including uveitis and the cystoid macular edema associated with it. Our clinical impressions are that these COX-2 selective inhibitors are safer than the nonselective ones, and that chronic use of them can prevent relapse of uveitis in approximately 70% of patients who have had repeated recurrences of non-granulomatous anterior uveitis, particulary HLA-B 27-associated uveitis. The COX-2 selective inhibitors have been shown to be effective in the care of patients with osteoarthritis and with rheumatoid arthritis,[50, 51] and the rate of endoscopically documented gastrointestinal mucosal erosions in patients receiving COX-2 selective inhibitors is less than half that of patients receiving the non-selective

cyclooxygenase inbibitor naproxen.[51] Additionally, the COX-2 selective inhibitors do not inhibit platelet activity, nor do they prolong bleeding time. They do interact with lithium and with fluconazole but not with methotrexate or warfarin.[52] The COX-2 selective inhibitor nonsteroidal anti-inflammatory agents (NSAIDs) currently available in the United States at the time of this writing are shown separate from the nonselective NSAIDs in Table 11–2.

Just as a variation exists in individual responsiveness to any given NSAID in the treatment of rheumatic disease, so, too, an apparent differential effectiveness exists between one NSAID and another in management of uveitis. We will try three different NSAIDs before declaring that any given patient is unlikely to benefit from this form of therapy.

Other Therapeutic Uses

Oral NSAIDs are the agent of choice for the treatment of episcleritis and for most cases of simple, diffuse, and nodular scleritis, although, as is true of adjunctive therapy in uveitis, sequential trials of several NSAIDs may be required before one that is completely effective is found.[53] Topical NSAIDs do not appear to be effective in management of episcleritis,[54] and topical steroids prolong the overall duration of the patient's problem, with a greater number of recurrences after discontinuation of therapy, unnecessarily exposing the patient to the potential side effects of such treatment. The treatment of scleritis associated with collagen vascular or connective tissue diseases is more complex, frequently requiring more potent therapy in addition to NSAIDs. For patients with scleritis, in whom a diagnosis of Wegener's granulomatosis or polyarteritis nodosa has been made, or for individuals with necrotizing scleritis associated with rheumatoid arthritis or relapsing polychondritis, immunosuppressive chemotherapy is mandatory.[53]

Finally, topical NSAIDs may be useful in management of ocular allergic disorders. Topical flurbiprofen 0.03% and suprofen 1% have been reported to be superior to placebo in treatment of allergic conjunctivitis[55] and vernal conjunctivitis,[56] respectively, and ketorolac 0.5% reduces the pruritus frequently associated with seasonal allergic conjunctivitis.[4]

SIDE EFFECTS AND TOXICITY

Topical Administration

The most common side effects after topical NSAID administration are transient burning, stinging, and conjunctival hyperemia.[4] Despite modifications in the formulation of NSAIDs in an effort to minimize ocular irritation, burning and stinging may still occur, presenting a potential compliance problem. In addition, postoperative atopic mydriasis has been reported in patients receiving topical NSAIDs before cataract surgery.[1] The pharmacologic mechanism mediating this phenomenon is poorly defined,[57] and its relationship to a similar adverse event after uncomplicated cataract surgery in patients not receiving preoperative NSAIDs has not been evaluated.[58, 59]

Topical NSAIDs are contraindicated in patients with active dendritic or geographic herpes keratitis.[60] Although preliminary studies have not demonstrated an adverse effect of topical NSAIDs on either fungal[61] or bacterial[62] ocular infections, it would be imprudent to assume that such therapy is completely risk free.

Systemic Administration

Oral NSAIDs have been associated with a wide variety of adverse reactions; those most severe and clinically significant are GI, central nervous system (CNS), hematologic, renal, hepatic, dermatologic, and immunologic. GI irritation is the most common side effect, ranging from nausea, vomiting, and cramps to gastric and intestinal ulceration, with a potential for significant bleeding and anemia.[20] The relative risk of developing a clinically significant peptic ulcer is three to eight times greater among patients receiving oral NSAID therapy, particularly among the elderly and anyone with a prior history of gastroduodenal ulcer or GI bleeding, and the risk is compounded by the concomitant use of oral corticosteroids, alcohol, anticoagulants and tobacco.[63] Ten to twenty percent of patients taking NSAIDs become dyspeptic, and 5% to 15% discontinue NSAID therapy because of this complication. Sadly, dyspepsia *is not* a good proxy monitor for serious NSAID-induced gastric mucosal ulceration, and 13 of every 1000 rheumatoid arthritis patients taking NSAIDs for 1 year have a *serious* gastrointestinal complication. For those hospitalized for such problems, 5% to 10% die from the NSAID complication. Thus, 16,000 or more patients with rheumatoid arthritis or osteoarthritis die annually in the United States as a consequence of NSAID side effects. NSAIDs are believed to inhibit locally protective prostaglandins (PGE_2, PGI_2) responsible for gastric mucin production, thus potentiating the possibility of GI erosion.[8] Consequently, antacids and H_2-blocking agents *do not* prevent NSAID-induced ulcers,[64] whereas misoprostol (Cytotec), a prostaglandin analogue, may offer some protection in patients at risk of developing this complication.[65]

CNS side effects of NSAIDs include somnolence, dizziness, lightheadedness, confusion, fatigue, anxiety, depression, psychotic episodes, and headache. Headache is a well-known side effect of indomethacin and is reported in more than 10% of patients treated with this drug.[20]

Hematologic toxicity is manifested clinically by a prolonged bleeding time. All NSAIDs inhibit platelet production of thromboxane A_2, a potent platelet aggregator.[66] Aplastic anemia, agranulocytosis, and related blood dyscrasias have been reported but are exceedingly rare.[20]

NSAIDs have little effect on renal function in healthy persons; however, they may decrease renal blood flow and glomerular filtration in patients with congestive heart failure, chronic renal failure, cirrhosis with ascites, or hypovolemia of any etiology and thus precipitate acute renal failure. In such clinical conditions, renal perfusion is maintained by the vasodilatory effects of locally produced prostaglandin against reflex pressor effects.[8] NSAIDs abrogate this prostaglandin-mediated autoregulatory phenomenon.[67]

Hepatic reactions occur occasionally, and include hepatitis and abnormal results of liver function tests. Predisposing factors to acute liver injury include impaired renal clearance, large doses, prolonged therapy, intercurrent viral illness, and advanced age.[68]

Dermatologic reactions to systemic NSAID therapy commonly include urticaria, exanthema, photosensitivity, and pruritus. More important, potentially serious entities such as toxic epidermal necrolysis, erythema multiforme, and anaphylactoid reactions have been induced by these agents.[69]

Metabolic changes, including fluid retention, edema, weight gain, and hypersensitivity reactions, have been reported with all NSAIDs.[20] A history of the latter, or allergic reaction to aspirin, to which NSAIDs may exhibit cross-sensitivity, constitutes a definitive contraindication to their use. In addition, patients with the syndrome of nasal polyps, angioedema, and bronchospastic reactivity to aspirin should not be treated with NSAIDs.[70]

Overdose

Overdose of NSAIDs, other than salicylates and phenylbutazone, rarely presents a serious problem.[71] In general, significant symptoms of NSAID overdose occur after ingestion of 5 to 10 times the average therapeutic dose. Presenting signs and symptoms range from GI upset, nystagmus, drowsiness, tinnitus, and disorientation to seizures, acute renal failure, cardiopulmonary arrest, and coma. The diagnosis is based largely on a history of NSAID ingestion because signs and symptoms are nonspecific and specific serum levels of drug are usually unavailable. Therapy consists of emergency and supportive measures (maintenance of an airway, fluid volume, and treatment of seizures) and decontamination procedures, including induction of emesis, gastric lavage, and administration of activated charcoal and cathartics. Although no specific antidote to NSAID poisoning exists, vitamin K may be used in patients with prolonged prothrombin times. Because NSAIDs are highly protein bound and extensively metabolized, hemodialysis, peritoneal dialysis, and forced diuresis are not likely to be effective.[72] In contrast, hemodialysis is very effective in rapidly removing salicylates and correcting acid-base and fluid abnormalities arising as a consequence of aspirin overdose. In addition, sodium bicarbonate is frequently administered to treat the metabolic acidosis and enhance salicylate clearance by the kidneys. Supportive and decontamination measures are similarly critical to management of salicylate overdose.

HIGH-RISK GROUPS

All patients should be educated concerning the signs and symptoms of serious GI toxicity and the measures by which they might be diminished (smoking and ethanol cessation and ingestion of medication with food). Patients at greatest risk of these complications include those with a history of peptic ulcer disease, those treated concomitantly with oral corticosteroids, and elderly patients.[63]

The risk of NSAID-induced acute renal failure is increased in patients with underlying chronic renal failure, atherosclerosis, hepatic sclerosis (especially with ascites), and volume depletion. Such patients require vigilant monitoring of blood urea nitrogen (BUN), creatinine level, and urinary sediment.[8] Elderly patients, whose renal function usually is reduced, should also be monitored closely.[73] Furthermore, persons with impaired renal function are at risk of developing hepatotoxicity. Early signs of hepatotoxicity in an otherwise healthy patient are heralded by abnormalities in the liver function tests, especially the alanine aminotransferase (ALT) level.

Patients with underlying bleeding disorders should use NSAIDs cautiously because NSAIDs impair platelet aggregation and prolong bleeding time. Patients undergoing surgical procedures should discontinue oral NSAIDs 24 to 48 hours preoperatively, whereas with aspirin treatment, 7 to 10 hours are required for recovery of platelet functional activity.[20]

The choice of NSAID in children is limited and should be restricted to the drugs that have been tested extensively in this age group, that is, aspirin, naproxen, and tolmetin.[8] Of particular note, administration of aspirin to a child in the setting of a viral febrile illness is contraindicated, because of its association with Reye's syndrome.

No evidence suggests that salicylates have teratogenic effects on the human fetus.[74] Although fewer human data are available, other NSAIDs have not been associated with teratogenicity in animal studies.[20] Despite these findings, NSAIDs are generally not recommended during pregnancy unless they are absolutely necessary, in which case aspirin at low doses is probably the safest treatment. Administration of aspirin or any other NSAID during the last 6 months of pregnancy may prolong gestation and labor, increase the risk of postpartum hemorrhage, and promote intrauterine closure of the ductus arteriosus.[8] Side effects produced by NSAID therapy during breast feeding are uncommon; however, metabolic acidosis in infants of mothers receiving salicylates has been reported.[20]

The development of cyclooxygenase-2 (COX-2)–selective NSAIDs represents a significant advance, because COX-2 and not COX-1 (the cyclooxygenase responsible for the production of gastric mucin) is the primary therapeutic NSAID target. Preliminary data indicate that the prevalence of NSAID-induced endoscopically detectable gastric mucosal ulcerations and erosions is significantly less in those patients treated with the highly selective COX-2 NSAIDs, compared with those patients treated with nonselective NSAIDs.

Prophylactic use of prostanoids (misoprostol) or proton pump inhibitors (omeprazole) but not H-2 receptor antagonists or mucosal protective agents (sucralfate) does offer significant protection against NSAID-induced gastric mucosal erosions and ulceration.

DRUG INTERACTIONS

NSAIDs are highly bound to plasma proteins and therefore may displace certain other concomitantly administered drugs from a common binding site, potentiating these actions and producing significant adverse effects. Such is the case with concurrent therapy with warfarin, sulfonylurea hypoglycemic agents, and methotrexate; dosage must be adjusted to prevent potential untoward effects.[8] This is particularly important in patients treated with warfarin, because of the intrinsic antiplatelet activity of NSAIDs.

Both NSAIDs and lithium are excreted by the proximal convoluted tubule in the kidney. Their concomitant administration, especially with diclofenac, has resulted in reduced lithium clearance and lithium toxicity.[20] Proben-

ecid, which also acts at the proximal convoluted tubule, may also impair NSAID metabolism and excretion.

Concomitant administration of NSAIDs and cyclosporine may produce synergistic nephrotoxicity by reducing renal blood flow. A transient but significant increase in serum creatinine has been observed after combined therapy with these agents.[75]

MAJOR CLINICAL TRIALS

A summary and discussion of the major clinical trials with regard to the therapeutic efficacy of NSAIDs in ophthalmology appears in the superb therapeutic review article by Flach.[1] Many of these studies, as well as others relevant to NSAID therapy in uveitis, are cited and discussed in the Therapeutic Use section.

References

1. Flach AJ: Cyclo-oxygenase inhibitors in ophthalmology. Surv Ophthalmol 1992;36:259–284.
2. Gifford H: On the treatment of sympathetic ophthalmia by large doses of salicylate of sodium aspirin or other salicylate compounds. Ophthalmoscope 1910;8:257–258.
3. Vane JR: Inhibition of prostaglandin synthesis as a mechanism of action for aspirin-like drugs. Nature 1971;231:232–235.
4. Flach AJ: Nonsteroidal anti-inflammatory drugs in ophthalmology. Int Ophthalmol Clin 1993;33:1–7.
5. Summary basis of approval for Ocufen (Allergan's Flurbiprofen) subsequent to new drug application. Washington, DC, Department of Health and Human Services, Food and Drug Administration, 1987, pp 19–404.
6. Summary basis of approval for Profenal (Alcon's Suprofen) subsequent to new drug application. Washington, DC, Department of Health and Human Services, Food and Drug Administration, 1989, pp 19–387.
7. Vickers FF, McGuigan LJB, Ford C, et al: The effect of diclofenal sodium ophthalmic on the treatment of postoperative inflammation. Invest Ophthalmol Vis Sci (ARVO Suppl) 1991;32:793.
8. Insel PA: Analgesic-antidiuretics and antiinflammatory agents: Drugs employed in the treatment of rheumatoid arthritis and gout. In: Gilman AG, Rail TW, Nies AS, Taylor P, eds: Goodman and Gilman's The Pharmacological Basis of Therapeutics. New York, Pergamon Press, 1990, pp 638–681.
9. Haynes RC: Adrenocorticotropic hormone; adrenocorticosteroids and their synthetic analogs; inhibitors of the synthesis and actions of adrenocorticotropic hormones. In: Gilman AG, Rail TW, Nies AS, Taylor P, eds: Goodman and Gilman's The Pharmacological Basis of Therapeutics. New York, Pergamon Press, 1990, pp 1431–1462.
10. Burne K, Glatt M, Graf P: Minireview: Mechanisms of action of anti-inflammatory drugs. Gen Pharmacol 1976;7:27–33.
11. Abramson SB, Weissmann G: The mechanism of action of nonsteroidal antiinflammatory drugs. Arthritis Rheum 1989;32:1–9.
12. Ambache N: Irin, a smooth muscle contracting substance present in rabbit iris. J Physiol (Lond) 1955;29:65–66.
13. Bito LZ: Prostaglandins, other eicosanoids and their derivatives as potential antiglaucoma agents. In: Drance SM, Neufeld AH, eds: Applied Pharmacology in Medical Treatments of Glaucoma. New York, Grune & Stratton, 1984, Ch. 20.
14. Bhattacherjer P: Prostaglandin and inflammatory reactions in the eye. Methods Find Eye Clin Pharmacol 1980;2:17–31.
15. Eakins KE: Prostaglandins and non-prostaglandin-mediated breakdown of the blood-aqueous barrier. Exp Eye Res 1977; 80(Suppl): 483–498.
16. Abelson MB, Butrus SI, Kliman GH, et al: Topical arachidonic acid: A model for screening anti-inflammatory agents. J Ocul Pharmacol Ther 1987;3:63–75.
17. Miyake K, Sugiyama S, Norismatsu I, Ozawa T: Prevention of cystoid macular edema after lens extraction by topical indomethacin: III. Radioimmunoassay measurement of prostaglandins in the aqueous during and after lens extraction procedures. Graefes Arch Clin Exp Ophthalmol 1978;209:83–88.
18. Unger WG, Bass MS: Prostaglandin and nerve mediated response of

the rabbit eye to argon laser irradiation of the iris. Ophthalmologica 1977;175:153–158.

19. Porter RS: Factors determining efficacy of NSAIDs. Drug Intelligence and Clinical Pharmacology 1984;18:42–51.

20. AMA Drug Evaluations. Chicago, American Medical Association. 1994, pp 1814–1833.

21. Ling TL, Combs OL: Ocular bioavailability and tissue distribution of ketorolac tromethamine in rabbits. J Pharm Sci 1987;76:289–294.

22. Anderson JA, Chen CC, Vita JB: Disposition of topical flurbiprofen in normal and aphakic rabbit eyes. Arch Ophthalmol 1982;100:642–645.

23. Sanders DR, Goldstick B, Kraff C, et al: Aqueous penetration of oral and topical indomethacin in humans. Arch Ophthalmol 1983;101:1614–1616.

24. Tang-Lui DD, Liu SS, Weinkam RJ: Ocular and systemic bioavailability of ophthalmic flurbiprofen. J Pharmacokinet Biopharm 1984;12:611–626.

25. Guzek JP, Holm M, Cotter JB, et al: Risk factors for intraoperative complications in 1000 extracapsular cases. Ophthalmology 1983:94: 461–466.

26. Cole DF, Unger WG: Prostaglandins as mediators for the responses of the eye due to trauma. Exp Eye Res 1973;17:357–368.

27. Keates RH, McGowan KA: Clinical trial of flurbiprofen to maintain pupillary dilation during cataract surgery. Ann Ophthalmol 1984;16:919–921.

28. Stark WJ, Fagadu WR, Stewart RH: Reduction of pupillary constriction during cataract surgery using suprofen. Arch Ophthalmol 1986;104:364–366.

29. Sanders DR, Kraff ML: Steroidal and nonsteroidal anti-inflammatory agents. Effects on postsurgical inflammation and blood-aqueous barrier breakdown. Arch Ophthalmol 1984;102:1453–1456.

30. Sabiston ME, Tessler D, Sumersk H, et al: Reduction of inflammation following cataract surgery by flurbiprofen. Ophthalmol Surg 1987;18:873–877.

31. Flach AJ, Graham J, Kruger LP, et al: Quantitative assessment of postsurgical breakdown of the blood-aqueous barrier following administration of ketorolac tromethamine solution, A double-masked, paired comparison with vehicle-placebo solution study. Arch Ophthalmol 1988;106:344–347.

32. Flach AJ, Lavelle CL, Olander KW, et al: The effect of ketorolac 0.5% solution in reducing postsurgical inflammation following ECCE with IOL. Double-masked, parallel comparison with vehicle. Ophthalmology 1988;75:1279–1284.

33. Flach AJ, Kraff MC, Sanders DR, Tanenbaum L: The quantitative effect of 0.5% ketorolac tromethamine solution and dexamethasone phosphate 0.1% solution on postsurgical blood-aqueous barrier. Arch Ophthalmol 1988;106:480–483.

34. Kraff MC, Sanders DR, McGuigan L, et al: Inhibition of blood-aqueous humor barrier breakdown with diclofenac. A fluorophotometric study. Arch Ophthalmol 1990;108:380–383.

35. Jampol LM, Po SM. Macular edema. In: Ryan SJ, ed: Retina, Vol 2. St. Louis, CV Mosby, 1994, pp 999–1008.

36. Jampol LM: Pharmacologic therapy of aphakic cystoid macular edema: A review. Ophthalmology 1982;89:891–897.

37. Jampol LM: Pharmacologic therapy of aphakic and pseudophakic cystoid macular edema: 1985 update. Ophthalmology 1985;92:807–810.

38. Miyake K, Sakamura S, Miura H: Long-term follow-up study of the prevention of aphakic cystoid macular edema by topical indomethacin. Br J Ophthalmol 1980:64:324–328.

39. Yannuzzi LA, Landau AN, Turtz AL: Incidence of aphakic cystoid macular edema with the use of topical indomethacin. Ophthalmology 1981;88:947–954.

40. Kraff MC, Sanders DR, Jampol LM, et al: Prophylaxis of pseudophakic cystoid macular edema with topical indomethacin. Ophthalmology 1982;89:885–890.

41. Flach Al, Stegman RC, Graham J: Prophylaxis of aphakic cystoid macular edema without corticosteroids. Ophthalmology 1940; 97:1253–1258.

42. Flach AJ, Jampol LM, Yannuzzi LA, et al: Improvement in visual acuity in chronic aphakic and pseudophakic cystoid macular edema after treatment with topical 0.5% ketorolac ophthalmic solution. Am J Ophthalmol 1991;112:514–519.

43. Flach AJ, Dolan BJ, Irvine AR: Effectiveness of ketorolac 0.5% solution for chronic aphakic and pseudophakic cystoid macular edema. Am J Ophthalmol 1987;103:479–486.

44. To K, Abelson ME, Neufeld A: Nonsteroidal antiinflammatory drugs. In: Albert DM, Jakobiec FA, eds: Principles and Practice of Ophthalmology: Basic Sciences. Philadelphia, W.B. Saunders Company, 1994, pp 1022–1027.

45. Young BJ, Cunningham WF, Akingbehin T: Double-masked, controlled clinical trial of 5% tolmetin versus 0.5% prednisolone versus 0.9% saline in acute endogenous nongranulomatous anterior uveitis. Br J Ophthalmol 1981;26:389–391.

46. Sind BB, Krogh L: Topical indomethacin, a prostaglandin inhibitor, in acute anterior uveitis. A controlled clinical trial of non-steroid versus steroid anti-inflammatory treatment. Acta Ophthalmol 1991;69:145–148.

47. Olsen NY, Lindsley CB, Godfrey WA: Nonsteroidal anti-inflammatory drug therapy in chronic childhood iridocyclitis. Am J Dis Child 1998;142:1289–1292.

48. Giordano M: Long-term prophylaxis of recurring spondylitic iridocyclitis with antimalarials and non-steroidal antiphlogistics [German]. Z Rheumatol 1982;41:105–106.

49. Evolution in Arthritis Management. Focus on Celecoxib. Washington Crossing, PA, Scientific Frontiers, Inc, 1999.

50. Hubbard R, Gein GS, Woods E, Yu S, Zhao W: Efficcacy, tolerability and safety of celecoxib, a specific COX-2 inhibitor, in osteoarthritis. Arthritis Rheum 1998;41(Suppl):S196. Abstract 982.

51. Geis GS, Hubbard R, Callison D, Yu S, Zhao W: Safety and efficacy of celecoxib, a specific COX-2 inhibitor, in patients with rheumatoid arthritis. Arthritis Rheum 1998;41(Suppl):S364. Abstract 1990.

52. Karim A, Tolbert D, Piergies A, et al. Celecoxib, a specific COX-2 inhibitor, lacks significant drug-drug interactions with methotrexate or warfarin. Arthritis Rheum 1998;41(Suppl):S315. Abstract 1698.

53. Foster CS, Sainz de la Maza M: The sclera. New York, Springer-Verlag, 1993, pp 299–307.

54. Lyons CJ, Hakin KN, Watson PG: Topical flurbiprofen: An effective treatment for episcleritis? Eye 1990;4:521–525.

55. Bishop K, Abelson M, Cheetham J, et al: Evaluation of flurbiprofen in the treatment of antigen-induced allergic conjunctivitis. Invest Ophthalmol Vis Sci (A RVO Suppl) 1990;31:487.

56. Buckley DC, Caldwell DR, Reaves TA. Treatment of vernal conjunctivitis with suprofen, topical non-steroidal anti-inflammatory agent. Invest Ophthalmol Vis Sci (ARVO Suppl) 1986;27:29.

57. Eakins KE, Whitelock RAF, Bennett A, Martenet AL: Prostaglandin-like activity in ocular inflammation. Br Med J 1972;3:452–453.

58. Lam S, Beck RW, Han D, Creighton JB: Atonic pupil after cataract surgery. Ophthalmology 1989;96:589–590.

59. Percival SPB: Results after intracapsular extraction: The atonic pupil. Ophthalmic Surg 1977;8:138–143.

60. Physician's Desk Reference for Ophthalmology. Montvale, NJ, Medical Economics Data, 1993, p 236.

61. Fraser-Smith EB, Matthews TR: Effect of ketorolac on *Candida albicans* ocular infection in rabbits. Arch Ophthalmol 1987;105:264–267.

62. Fraser-Smith EB, Matthews TR: Effect of ketorolac on *Pseudomonas aeruginosa* ocular infection in rabbits. J Ocul Pharm 1988;4:101–109.

63. Griffin MR, Piper JM, Daugherty JR, et al: Non-steroidal antiflammatory drug use and increased risk for peptic ulcer disease in elderly persons. Ann Intern Med 1991;114:257–263.

64. Soil AH, Weinstein WM, Kurata J, McCarthy D: Nonsteroidal anti-inflammatory drugs and peptic ulcer disease. Ann Intern Med 1991;114: 307–319.

65. Graham DY, Agrawal NM, Roth SH: Prevention of NSAID-induced gastric ulcer with misoprostol, multicentre, double-blind, placebo-controlled trial. Lancet 1988;2:1277–1280.

66. Hamburg M, Svensson J, Samuelsson B: Thromboxane: A new group of biologically active compounds derived from prostaglandin endoperoxides. Proc Natl Acad Sci USA 1975;72:2994–2998.

67. Clive DM, Stoff JS: Renal syndromes associated with nonsteroidal antiinflammatory drugs. N Engl J Med 1984;310:563–572.

68. Rodriguez LAG: The role of nonsteroidal antiinflammatory drugs in acute liver injury. Br Med J 1992;305:865–868.

69. Davis LS: New uses for old drugs. In: Wolverton SE, Wilkins JK, eds: Systemic Drugs for Skin Diseases. Philadelphia: W.B. Saunders Company, 1991, pp 375–376.

70. Foster CS: Nonsteroidal anti-inflammatory and immunosuppressive agents. In: Lamberts DW, Potter DE, eds. Clinical ophthalmic pharmacology. Boston: Little, Brown, 1987;179–181.

71. Meredith TI, Vale JA: Non-narcotic analgesics; problems of overdosage. Drugs 1986;32(suppl 4):177–205.

72. Kim S: Salicylates. In: Olsen KR, ed. Poisoning and drug overdose. Norwalk, CT: Appleton and Lange, 1990;261–264.

73. Gurwitz JH, Avorn J, Ross-Degnan D, Lipsitz LA: Nonsteroidal anti-inflammatory drug-associated azotemia in the very old. JAMA 1990;264–471.

74. Byron MA:. Treatment of rheumatic diseases. RMJ 1987;294:236–238.

75. Harris KFI, Jenkins D, Walls J: Nonsteroidal antiinflammatory drugs and cyclosporine. A potentially serious adverse interaction. Transplantation 1988;46:598–599.

12 — IMMUNOSUPPRESSIVE CHEMOTHERAPY

C. Stephen Foster and Albert T. Vitale

GENERAL CONSIDERATIONS

Although the use of immunosuppressive and biologic agents to inhibit immune reactions is at least half a century old,[1] in the past decade, we have witnessed the development of several new modalities and effective treatment strategies for the management of inflammatory and immunologic ocular disease. This evolution has been possible largely because we have achieved better insight into the pathophysiology of inflammation and an improved understanding of the immune system's role in the genesis of localized ocular disease as well as the secondary ocular manifestations of systemic diseases and because more potent and selective immunomodulating drugs have been developed. The goal of therapy is suppression of the immune inflammatory response, whether it is due to trauma, surgery, infection, or response to foreign or self-antigens, so that the integrity of ocular structures critical to good visual function is preserved.

Immunosuppressive agents, by definition, suppress development of at least one type of immune reaction: They modify the specific immune sensitization of lymphoid cells.[1] However, the precise mechanisms by which these agents achieve their effects remain to be elucidated, because it is often difficult to distinguish between drug-mediated suppression of the immune response itself and suppression of the inflammatory expression thereof. A common feature of this family of drugs is their ability to interfere with the synthesis of nucleic acids or proteins, or both (Fig. 12–1). Although these actions are commonly invoked as the major immunosuppressive mechanism because of the exquisite sensitivity of lymphoid proliferation and cytokine elaboration after antigenic stimulation to this type of interference, the effect of immunosuppressive agents cannot be explained by this notion alone.[1] This is not surprising, given the extraordinary complexity and interdependence of various immunoregulatory networks.

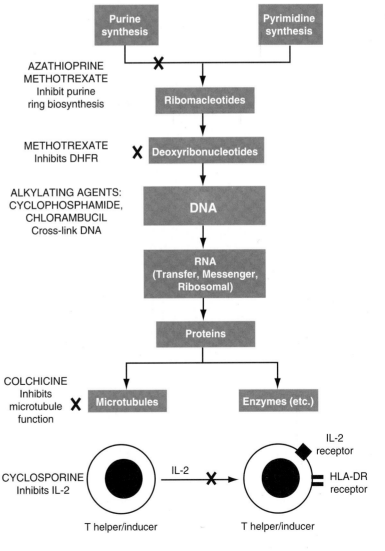

FIGURE 12–1. Mechanism of action of immunosuppressive agents used in the treatment of uveitis. (Adapted from Calabresi P, Chabner BA: Chemotherapy of neoplastic diseases. In: Gilman AG, Rall TW, Nies AS, Taylor P, eds: Goodman and Gilman's The Pharmacological Basis of Therapeutics. New York, Pergamon Press, 1990, p 1208.)

TABLE 12–1. IMMUNOSUPPRESSIVE DRUGS: CLASS, DOSAGE, AND ROUTE OF ADMINISTRATION

CLASS/DRUG	DOSE AND ROUTE
Alkylating agents	
Cyclophosphamide	1–3.0 mg-kg/day, PO, IV
Chlorambucil	0.1 mg/kg/day, PO
Antimetabolites	
Azathioprine	1–3.0 mg/kg/day, PO
Methotrexate	0.15 mg/kg once weekly, PO, subcutaneous, IM
Antibiotics	
Cyclosporine	2.5–5.0 mg/kg/day, PO
FK 506	0.1–0.15 mg/kg/day, PO
Rapamycin	
Dapsone	25–50 mg, 2–3 times daily, PO
Adjuvants	
Bromocriptine	2.5 mg, 3–4 times daily, PO
Ketoconazole	200 mg/1–2 times daily, PO
Colchicine	0.5–0.6 mg, 2–3 times daily, PO

The immunosuppressive drugs for which sufficient experience and information exists to warrant their use in the treatment of ocular inflammatory conditions are shown in Table 12–1 according to drug class and include the following: the alkylating agents (cyclophosphamide and chlorambucil), antimetabolites (azathioprine, methotrexate, leflunomide, and mycophenolate mofetil), antibiotics (cyclosporine-A, FK 506, sirolimus [rapamycin], and dapsone), receptor antagonists (etanercept and daclizumab [Zenapax] and immune-related adjuvants (bromocriptine, ketoconazole, and colchicine).

Because of concerns regarding their low therapeutic index, immunosuppressive agents were, until recently, reserved for treatment of severe, sight-threatening, steroid-resistant uveitis or for use in patients who had developed unacceptable steroid-induced adverse effects. Now, instead of being regarded as merely steroid sparing, these drugs are often used as first-line agents for a variety of diseases with destructive ocular sequelae such as Wegener's granulomatosis and Adamantiades-Behçet disease (ABD), for which long-term remission or cure may be achieved. We consider the concurrence of ocular inflammatory disease and polyarteritis nodosa, relapsing polychondritis (especially with renal involvement), or necrotizing scleritis in association with rheumatoid arthritis to be absolute indications for institution of immunosuppressive chemotherapy. The International Uveitis Study Group recommendations include sympathetic ophthalmia and Vogt-Koyanagi-Harada syndrome (VKH) in this category,[2] and we have expanded the list of entities that constitute absolute indications for use of immunosuppressive therapies (Table 12–2). The patients must be adequately immunosuppressed yet be spared the potentially serious consequences of drug toxicity (Table 12–3). In the hands of physicians trained in their use and monitoring, the administration of immunosuppressive agents appears to produce fewer serious adverse effects than does chronic use of systemic steroids. Immunosuppressive agents represent the final rung in our stepladder approach to the medical treatment of ocular inflammatory disease. The safe use of these drugs begins with exclusion

TABLE 12–2. GENERAL CATEGORIZATION OF INDICATIONS FOR IMMUNOSUPPRESSIVE CHEMOTHERAPY

Absolute
  Adamantiades-Behçet disease with retinal involvement
  Sympathetic ophthalmia
  Vogt-Koyanagi-Harada syndrome
  Rheumatoid necrotizing scleritis and/or peripheral ulcerative keratitis
  Wegener's granulomatosis
  Polyarteritis nodosa
  Relapsing polychondritis with scleritis
  Juvenile rheumatoid arthritis associated iridocyclitis unresponsive to conventional therapy
  Ocular cicatricial pemphigoid
  Bilateral Mooren's ulcer
Relative
  Intermediate uveitis
  Retinal vasculitis with central vascular leakage
  Severe chronic iridocyclitis
Questionable
  Intermediate uveitis in children
  Sarcoid-associated uveitis inadequately responsive to steroid
  Keratoplasty with multiple rejections

of infectious, mechanical, or other treatable causes of ocular inflammation. Diagnostic studies are then obtained, both based on a careful review of systems and from the physical findings. Whenever possible, biopsy and histologic examination of inflamed tissue are performed (e.g., conjunctival biopsy in patients with ocular cicatricial pemphigoid), because they provide the most reliable guide to the nature of an underlying immunopathologic process. Collaboration with a laboratory expert in the processing and interpretation of such material is essential. The diagnosis, based on the available data and modified as new information is obtained, serves to guide the therapeutic approach. Immunosuppressive chemotherapy

TABLE 12–3. MAJOR ADVERSE REACTIONS OF IMMUNOSUPPRESSIVE DRUGS

DRUG	ADVERSE REACTION
Cyclophosphamide	Sterile hemorrhagic cystitis, myelosuppression, reversible alopecia, secondary malignancies, transient blurring of vision
Chlorambucil	Myelosuppression (moderate but rapid), gonadal dysfunction, secondary malignancies
Methotrexate	Hepatotoxicity, ulcerative stomatitis, bone marrow suppression, diarrhea
Azathioprine	Bone marrow suppression (leukopenia), nausea, secondary infections
Cyclosporine	Nephrotoxicity, hypertension, hyperuricemia, hyperglycemia, hepatotoxicity, nausea, and vomiting
FK 506	Similar to cyclosporine; neurotoxicity
Sirolimus (rapamycin)	Unknown
Dapsone	Hemolytic anemia, methemoglobinemia, nausea, mononucleosis-like syndrome, blurred vision
Bromocriptine	Postural hypotension, nausea, vomiting
Ketoconazole	Hepatotoxicity, endocrine abnormalities, gastrointestinal upset
Colchicine	Nausea, vomiting, diarrhea, bone marrow suppression

is instituted as first-line therapy only when there is an absolute indication for its use. It is rarely necessary for most cases of uveitis.

Informed consent is obtained and documented, and the patient is given an explanation of the potential risks and benefits involved in any therapeutic modality (periocular or systemic steroids, nonsteroidal anti-inflammatory drugs [NSAIDs], or immunosuppressive agents) used in the management of patients with progressive, vision-threatening, destructive ocular inflammatory disease. We begin with steroids, use them aggressively in the maximally tolerated doses, and administer them by all possible routes (topical, periocular injection, systemic). If, despite this approach, the patient's disease is chronic or subject to frequent relapses, we add an oral NSAID to the treatment regimen. If this combination fails to achieve the goal of total quiescence of all ocular inflammation or produces adverse side effects that are unacceptable to either the patient or the physician, the patient is offered the alternative of a systemic immunosuppressive chemotherapeutic drug.

The choice of the immunosuppressive agent is individualized for each patient and depends on a variety of considerations, including the underlying disease, the patient's age, sex, and medical status (Table 12–4). Patients are carefully screened for risk factors that might preclude the use of certain immunosuppressive agents (i.e., hepatic disease for methotrexate and renal disease for cyclosporine). Patients are also informed of the proper dosing and intake, potential adverse reactions, and alternatives to immunosuppressive therapy. For example, adequate hydration with oral use of cyclophosphamide substantially reduces the risk of hemorrhagic cystitis, whereas sperm banking is advisable for young patients who are to receive therapy with chlorambucil.

The responsibility for the details of the management of patients requiring immunosuppressive chemotherapy must lie with a clinician, who, by virtue of training and experience, is truly expert in the use of these agents and in the recognition and treatment of potentially serious side effects that may arise. A "hand-in-glove" collaboration between the ophthalmologist and the chemotherapist—usually, in our experience, an oncologist or hematologist—works most effectively for patients requiring such medications.

In contrast to our approach with corticosteroids, with immunosuppressive agents we start with a low dose of drug and titrate it according to the patient's clinical condition. An adequate therapeutic response and the identification and management of adverse effects are best achieved by careful ocular examination and review of systems at specified intervals to detect subtle changes rather than by exclusive reliance on laboratory results.

Notwithstanding, periodic complete hemograms, including differential and platelet values, should be obtained in all patients before therapy is initiated and again at 1- to 4-week intervals to monitor for myelosuppression. We avoid depressing the leukocyte count below 3500 cells/μl or the neutrophil count below 1500 cells/μl, and avoid thrombocytopenia less than 75,000 platelets/μl.[3] In addition, liver function tests, urinalysis, blood urea nitrogen (BUN), and serum creatinine should be obtained before initiation of therapy and at intervals of 1 to 4 months, depending on the medication. The frequency of this schedule will depend on the particular agent used and its major potential toxicity, with more frequent monitoring at the initiation of therapy, during changes in drug dosage, and during episodes of drug toxicity management.

If an adequate clinical response is not observed after a minimum of 3 months of treatment at the maximal tolerable dosage or if toxicity precludes continuation of therapy, the medication should be discontinued and consideration given to substituting an alternative immunosuppressive agent. If, instead, a good clinical response is obtained and the patient is free of cellular inflammatory activity in the eye, the drug may be tapered and discontinued in most patients after 2 years of therapy if their disease does not recur.

We have successfully treated a wide variety of uveitic and other ocular inflammatory disorders with immunosuppressive chemotherapy using this stepladder paradigm over the past 25 years. Details of the pharmacology of the individual immunosuppressive agents used in this strategy follow.

TABLE 12–4. MAJOR INDICATIONS FOR SPECIFIC IMMUNOSUPPRESSIVE DRUGS

DRUG	INDICATION
Cyclophosphamide	Wegener's granulomatosis, polyarteritis nodosa, necrotizing scleritis associated with rheumatoid arthritis or relapsing polychondritis, Mooren's ulcer, cicatricial pemphigoid, sympathetic ophthalmia, Adamantiades-Behçet disease
Chlorambucil	Adamantiades-Behçet disease, sympathetic ophthalmia, juvenile rheumatoid arthritis (JRA)–associated iridocyclitis
Methotrexate	Sympathetic ophthalmia, scleritis, JRA-associated iridocyclitis
Azathioprine	Adamantiades-Behçet disease, Wegener's granulomatosis, systemic lupus erythematosus, scleritis, cicatricial pemphigoid, JRA-associated iridocyclitis
Cyclosporine	Adamantiades-Behçet disease, birdshot retinochoroidopathy, sarcoidosis, pars planitis, Vogt-Koyanagi-Harada syndrome, sympathetic ophthalmia, idiopathic posterior uveitis, corneal graft rejection
FK 506	Adamantiades-Behçet disease, idiopathic posterior uveitis
Sirolimus (rapamycin)	Unknown, adjunct to cyclosporine
Dapsone	Cicatricial pemphigoid, relapsing polychondritis
Bromocriptine	Adjunct to cyclosporine, iridocyclitis, thyroid ophthalmopathy
Ketoconazole	Adjunct to cyclosporine
Colchicine	Adamantiades-Behçet disease

CYTOTOXIC IMMUNOSUPPRESSIVE DRUGS

The alkylating agents, primarily cyclophosphamide and chlorambucil, and the antimetabolites methotrexate, azathioprine, leflunomide, and mycophenolate mofetil constitute the two major categories of cytotoxic drugs used in management of ocular inflammatory disease. As a group, the alkylators are more potent agents and consequently are more apt to produce toxic adverse effects.

Alkylating Agents

Cyclophosphamide

HISTORY AND SOURCE

Cyclophosphamide belongs to the nitrogen mustard family of alkylating agents and is one of the most widely used immunosuppressive chemotherapeutic agents in the treatment of autoimmune inflammatory disease. The profound leukopenia and aplasia of lymphoid tissue induced by these agents was first reported in 1919 after sulfur mustard was used as a chemical weapon in World War I.[4] The potentially beneficial application of those agents to human disease was first appreciated in the 1940s, when nitrogen mustard was administered to patients with lymphoma.[5] In the early 1950s, Roda-Perez[5] first reported use of cyclophosphamide for treatment of uveitis of unknown etiology, almost predating the introduction of corticosteroids into ophthalmic practice.[6, 7] Today, cyclophosphamide plays a primary role in treatment of several potentially lethal systemic vasculitides with destructive ocular involvement (Wegener's granulomatosis and polyarteritis nodosa), as well as several other forms of extraocular and intraocular inflammatory diseases that are poorly responsive to corticosteroids (see Table 12–4).

OFFICIAL DRUG NAME AND CHEMISTRY

Cyclophosphamide (Cytoxan, Neosar) is 2-*bis*[(2-chloroethyl)amino]tetrahydro-2H-1,3,2-oxazophosphorine 2-oxide monohydrate and has a molecular weight of 279.1. It is a cyclic oxazophosphorine (Fig. 12–2) derived from mechlorethamine with the molecular formula of $C_7H_{15}C_{12}N_2O_2PH_2O$. The biologic activity of this compound is based on the presence of the *bis*-(chloroethyl)amino group attached to the phosphorus of oxazophosphorine, and its cyclic structure enhances its chemical stability.[8]

PHARMACOLOGY

Cyclophosphamide, like many other immunosuppressive agents, is a prodrug and must be converted in vivo by the hepatic microsomal cytochrome P-450 mixed function oxidase system into its active metabolites, phosphoramide mustard and 4-hydroxycyclophosphamide.[9] These products act through nucleophilic substitution reactions resulting in formation of covalent cross linkages (alkylation) with DNA, thereby mediating their major immunosuppressive activity (see Fig. 12–1). By targeting the 7-nitrogen atom of guanine, cyclophosphamide promotes guanidine-thymidine linkages with resultant DNA miscoding, breaks in single-stranded DNA, and formation

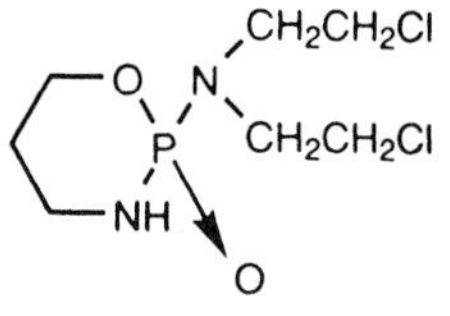

FIGURE 12–2. Chemical structure of cyclophosphamide.

of phosphodiester bonds after repair of those breaks, with resultant defective cell function.[8] Cross-linkages occur not only between DNA strands but also between DNA and RNA and between these molecules and cellular proteins, with consequent cytotoxicity.[10] The actions of cyclophosphamide are cell cycle nonspecific.

CLINICAL PHARMACOLOGY

In doses used clinically, cyclophosphamide has a profound effect on lymphoid cells. Both B- and T-cell function are depressed, although with acute administration of high doses of drug, B cells appear to be more affected.[11] In lower doses, or with chronic administration, however, it is likely that cyclophosphamide depresses B- and T-cell populations equally.[12, 13] The inhibitory effect on the humoral immune system results in suppression of both primary and secondary antibody responses.[11, 14, 15] Cyclophosphamide is also effective in inhibiting cell-mediated immunity, such as the delayed-type skin hypersensitivity (DTH) reaction in both humans and animals.[5] It is the only immunosuppressive agent that can induce immunologic tolerance to a particulate antigen.[10] Development of such tolerance entails complex kinetics and pharmacokinetics, because the drug must be given 24 to 48 hours after antigen priming.[16] Although the mechanism of such tolerance is likely to involve the activity of suppressor T cells that develop after antigen priming, low doses of cyclophosphamide in animal models have been shown to enhance immunoreactivity paradoxically by preferentially depressing suppressor T cells, resulting in release from tolerance and the expression of DTH. Higher doses of drug suppressed both T-helper and suppressor T-cell subsets, with consequent blunting of T-cell–mediated humoral and DTH responses.[17–19] Therefore, the dosage and timing of cyclophosphamide administration apparently are critical to its effect on lymphocyte subsets, which complicates judgments with respect to its clinical use in new applications.[10] Although cyclophosphamide has little effect on fully developed macrophages, it does inhibit development of monocyte precursors. Finally, cyclophosphamide has been shown to prevent development of autoimmune disease in the NZB/NZW F mouse model of systemic lupus erythematosus.[20]

PHARMACEUTICS

Cyclophosphamide (Cytoxan, Bristol-Myers Squibb) is supplied as 25- and 50-mg tablets and as a powder in 100-, 200-, and 500-mg and 1- and 3-g vials (Neosar, Adria, and Cytoxan, Bristol-Myers Squibb) for injection. The drug may be administered orally, intramuscularly, intravenously, intrapleurally, or intraperitoneally. Use with benzyl alcohol–preserved diluents should be avoided.

PHARMACOKINETICS AND METABOLISM

Approximately 75% of an oral dose of cyclophosphamide is absorbed from the gastrointestinal (GI) tract, reaching peak plasma levels approximately 1 hour after ingestion, and is widely distributed throughout the body, including the brain.[21] The drug undergoes metabolic conversion in the liver into its cytotoxic metabolites, which are approximately 50% bound to serum albumin. The plasma half-life ($t_{1/2}$) of cyclophosphamide is 4 to 6 hours, with 10%

to 20% of the native drug, which itself is unbound to plasma proteins, being excreted unchanged in the urine.[22] Although the metabolites of cyclophosphamide are oxidized further into inactive products, the acrolein metabolite is believed to play a central role in bladder toxicity.[21]

THERAPEUTIC USE

Cyclophosphamide is the treatment of choice for any patient with ocular manifestations of Wegener's granulomatosis or polyarteritis nodosa. Cyclophosphamide, used alone or in combination with systemic steroids, is superior to corticosteroids alone in treating the necrotizing scleritis of Wegener's granulomatosis; with combination therapy, it produces dramatic improvement in patient survival in both disease entities.[23–26]

Cyclophosphamide is also the most effective treatment for patients with highly destructive forms of ocular inflammation (peripheral ulcerative keratitis) associated with rheumatoid arthritis. Its use correlates positively with survival of those with active systemic and necrotizing ocular disease.[28, 29]

Although the extraocular manifestations of relapsing polychondritis commonly respond to systemic therapy with dapsone, the necrotizing scleritis and peripheral ulcerative keratitis observed in some of these patients is often more refractory to immunomodulatory therapy than is that associated with Wegener's granulomatosis, polyarteritis nodosa, or rheumatoid arthritis.[30, 31] In such intransigent cases, we have found that cyclophosphamide, with or without systemic steroid and NSAID therapy, is efficacious.[32]

Bilateral Mooren's ulcer, although rare, is similarly recalcitrant to conventional therapy, resulting in progressive, relentless corneal destruction. Foster[33] and Brown and Mondino[34] reported excellent recovery rates and improved prognoses, respectively, in such cases when cyclophosphamide was used. In patients with active, progressive, ocular cicatricial pemphigoid, cyclophosphamide may be used as first-line treatment. Foster,[35] in a randomized, double-masked, clinical trial, demonstrated that cyclophosphamide, in combination with prednisone, is superior to steroid alone. Typically, the duration of cyclophosphamide therapy is 1 year, with a relapse rate of approximately 20% after discontinuation of therapy.[36]

ABD, affecting the retina or visceral structures, requires immunosuppressive chemotherapy. Either cyclophosphamide or chlorambucil is an appropriate choice for treatment of the posterior uveitis or retinal vasculitis manifestations of this entity. Cyclophosphamide was shown to be superior to steroids in suppressing ocular inflammation in patients with ABD.[37] Similarly, oral cyclophosphamide produced ocular and systemic improvement in a patient with Adamantiades-Behçet disease who had been previously unresponsive to systemic corticosteroids.[38] Although chlorambucil may be the single most efficacious agent in management of ABD, capable of inducing long-term disease remission, intravenous pulse therapy with cyclophosphamide may be a highly effective alternative.[39] We and other researchers[40] have shown both agents to be superior to cyclosporine (cyclosporine A [CSA]) in management of the posterior segment manifestations of ABD.

Using our stepladder approach, we have successfully treated many other forms of posterior uveitis with cytotoxic agents, including cyclophosphamide, in patients who have been unresponsive to conventional therapy or who have developed unacceptable steroid-induced side effects (see Table 12–4). Buckley and Gills[41] reported that oral cyclophosphamide was effective in the management of nine patients with pars planitis. Similarly, Wong[42] reported a favorable treatment effect in a small number of patients treated with intravenous cyclophosphamide. More recently, Martenet[43] described a 21-year experience in treating 268 patients with uveitis of various etiologies, including sympathetic ophthalmia, with cytotoxic medication, predominantly cyclophosphamide in combination with procarbazine; visual acuity improved in approximately half of the patients and stabilized in the remainder, with very few treatment failures. The major cause for reduced visual acuity during the study period, even in successful cases, was chronic macular edema and cataract formation. Other than a few isolated cases of azoospermia, no important systemic or hematologic complications were observed.

DOSAGE AND ROUTE

The recommended dose of cyclophosphamide for the treatment of ocular disease is 1 to 2 mg/kg/day, administered orally (see Table 12–1). We prefer that patients take their total daily dose in the morning, instructing them to maintain adequate oral fluids throughout the rest of the day, in an effort to induce frequent voiding. In this way, the risk of hemorrhagic cystitis from prolonged contact of the bladder mucosa with cyclophosphamide metabolites is minimized. Intravenous administration of cyclophosphamide offers certain advantages over oral administration and is useful in the following clinical situations: (1) It permits rapid induction in patients with severe ocular inflammatory involvement (i.e., fulminant retinal vasculitis in association with ABD); (2) it avoids prolonged bladder exposure, allowing larger doses, yet less frequent dosing in patients with hemorrhagic cystitis induced from oral intake; and (3) it induces only transient neutropenia, making intercurrent infections less likely.

We administer 1 g/m^2 body surface area of cyclophosphamide intravenously in 250 ml normal saline, piggybacked onto the second half of 1 L 0.5% dextrose in water, infused in a 2-hour period. These infusions are repeated every 3 to 4 weeks, depending on the clinical response and the nadir of the leukocyte count.

Complete hemograms, including platelet levels and leukocyte differentials, and urinalysis must be obtained before initiation of therapy and then again on a weekly basis until the drug dosage, disease activity, and hematologic parameters have stabilized.[16] Our goal is to maintain a mild leukopenia: Unlike with many immunosuppressive agents, the level of leukopenia achieved with cyclophosphamide is a reasonable monitor of the adequacy of immunosuppression. We try, however, to avoid a leukocyte count less than 3500 cells/μl, a neutrophil count less than 1500 cells/μl, and a platelet count less than 75,000 cells/μl.[3] Thereafter, performing hematologic monitoring every 2 weeks and obtaining a monthly serum chemistry profile are appropriate.

SIDE EFFECTS AND TOXICITY

A wide variety of toxic effects has been observed (see Table 12–3). As many as 70% of patients experience anorexia, nausea, vomiting, or stomatitis, effects that apparently are dose related.[22] We emphasize that for doses we use in the care of our patients with ocular inflammation, the incidence of such side effects is much lower. Five to thirty percent of patients receiving intensive or prolonged therapy experience alopecia, which is usually reversible.[21]

The most common dose-limiting toxicity of cyclophosphamide is bone marrow depression, the leukocytes being more significantly affected than the platelets. The nadir of leukopenia usually occurs within 1 to 2 weeks after intravenous therapy is initiated; recovery is observed within 10 days of the last dose.[44]

A relatively common and well-recognized dose-limiting adverse effect is sterile hemorrhagic cystitis, which results from high concentrations of active metabolites (e.g., acrolein) in the bladder.[8] The onset of this complication is variable, occurring as early as 24 hours after initiation of therapy to as late as several weeks after drug discontinuation.[44] Should this complication arise, patients must undergo cystoscopy, so that other causes of microscopic hematuria, such as nephritis associated with Wegener's granulomatosis, can be excluded. In addition, the patient's dosing schedule and routine for fluid intake in the afternoon and evening should be carefully reviewed. If hemorrhagic cystitis is confirmed, the bleeding is usually self-limited, with most patients responding to drug cessation, high fluid intake, and bed rest. In severe cases, however, supravesical urinary diversion may be necessary.[45] With morning dosing, adequate hydration (2 to 3 L fluid during the day), and frequent voiding, the incidence and severity of this complication may be significantly reduced.[35, 41]

Cyclophosphamide has been associated with development of secondary malignancies, most commonly acute myelocytic leukemia and bladder carcinoma, in patients with intercurrent neoplastic, rheumatologic, or renal disease who have received cumulative doses in excess of 76 g.[46] It has been recommended that patients who have received daily doses in excess of 50 mg cyclophosphamide for more than 2 years or who have experienced multiple episodes of hemorrhagic cystitis undergo routine screening, including yearly urine cytology.[47] If suspicious or malignant cells are present, biopsy of abnormal areas is mandatory.

Gonadal dysfunction, including azoospermia and amenorrhea, has been observed in 60% of patients after 6 months of treatment with cyclophosphamide.[48] Because this effect may be irreversible, sperm banking is advisable before initiation of therapy, particularly if protracted therapy is anticipated.

Ocular side effects have been reported, including dry eyes in as many as 50% of patients treated, blurred vision, and increased intraocular pressure (IOP).[49] The mechanism underlying those adverse effects or a causal link to cyclophosphamide therapy itself is poorly defined.[16]

Other less common adverse effects include cardiac myopathy (usually occurring with large doses), hepatic dysfunction, irreversible pulmonary fibrosis, impaired renal clearance of water with resultant hyponatremia, and anaphylaxis.[22]

OVERDOSE

Signs and symptoms of cyclophosphamide overdose are identical to the toxic effects previously discussed herein. No specific antidote exists. Management is generally supportive, with appropriate treatment of concurrent infection, myelosuppression, or cardiac toxicity as indicated.

Recently, a human granulocyte colony-stimulating factor (G-CSF) has become available through recombinant DNA technology. Filgrastim (Neupogen, Amgen) has been shown to be safe and effective in accelerating recovery of neutrophil counts after the administration of a variety of chemotherapeutic regimens, and thus decreases the risk of systemic infection.[22] Filgrastim may be administered subcutaneously or intravenously at an initial dose of 5 μg/kg/day, as a single daily injection, for neutrophil counts less than 500 μl. The drug should not be initiated until 24 hours after a given dose of chemotherapy and should be discontinued 24 hours before the next cycle of chemotherapy. The dose may be increased by 5 μg/kg/day after 5 to 7 days, with daily administration of filgrastim until the neutrophil count returns to normal levels (i.e., more than 10,000 μl).[22]

HIGH-RISK GROUPS

Clinicians must be vigilant in detecting untoward toxicity or the development of opportunistic infections in any patient treated with cyclophosphamide who is concurrently receiving immunosuppression for an independent reason: previous radiation therapy, tumor cell infiltration of the bone marrow, or previous therapy with cytotoxic agents. Viral infections, especially herpes zoster, tend to occur more readily in neutropenic patients receiving cyclophosphamide.[50] Cytotoxic therapy, in general, is contraindicated in patients with focal chorioretinitis, herpes simplex, herpes zoster, cytomegalovirus (CMV), acquired immunodeficiency syndrome (AIDS) retinopathy, toxoplasmosis, tuberculosis, and fungal infections.[51]

Because the major routes of metabolism and excretion for cyclophosphamide are hepatic and renal, dosage reductions have been recommended for patients with hepatic and renal dysfunction. However, anephric patients treated with full doses of cyclophosphamide failed to exhibit increased hematologic or other toxic side effects.[52]

Because cyclophosphamide is a teratogen, causing central nervous system (CNS) and skeletal abnormalities in the fetus, contraception is advisable during cyclophosphamide therapy. Nursing mothers should be cautioned that the drug is excreted in the breast milk and may exert toxic effects in their infants.[50]

The use of cytotoxic drugs (cyclophosphamide, chlorambucil, azathioprine, or methotrexate) in children for treatment of non–life-threatening inflammatory disease is less controversial today than even 5 years ago, due in large measure to the pioneering work of rheumatologists treating children with juvenile rheumatoid arthritis

(JRA). Although there is little question about the efficacy of such therapy in children with, for example, JRA-associated iridocyclitis that is unresponsive to steroids and other conventional treatments, the potential risks of delayed malignancy or sterility associated with the treatment must be seriously considered, especially with regard to alkylating agent therapy, because of the age of the patients. We explore the merits and drawbacks of the various treatment options with both the patient and the parents, making the decision of whether or not to use cytotoxic agents on an individual basis. It is hoped that prospective comparative trials in this patient group will clarify the relative risks and benefits of systemic immunosuppressive chemotherapy early in the course of chronic inflammation associated with JRA.[10]

CONTRAINDICATIONS
Cyclophosphamide is contraindicated in patients with severely depressed bone marrow function and in those with a history of hypersensitivity to the drug.

DRUG INTERACTIONS
The metabolism of cyclophosphamide is affected by drugs that induce (phenobarbital) or inhibit (allopurinol) the hepatic microsomal mixed function oxidase system.[22] Consequently, concurrent administration of allopurinol prolongs the serum $t\frac{1}{2}$ of cyclophosphamide, and chronic administration of high doses of phenobarbital increases its metabolism and leukopenic activity. Chloramphenicol and corticosteroids may inhibit microsomal enzyme metabolism of cyclophosphamide and thus blunt its action, and the effects of agents such as halothane, nitrous oxide, and succinylcholine are enhanced by cyclophosphamide.[44] In addition, cyclophosphamide increases the myocardial toxicity of doxorubicin.[21] Finally, other immunosuppressive agents may have synergistic immunosuppressive and carcinogenic effects.

MAJOR CLINICAL TRIALS
Clinical studies of importance with respect to the efficacy of each of the individual immunosuppressive agents for treatment of noninfectious inflammatory ocular disease are cited and discussed in the Therapeutic Use section.

Chlorambucil
Chlorambucil was first synthesized in the early 1950s and was subsequently introduced into the clinical world primarily for the treatment of malignant lymphoma.[5] Today, it is the treatment of choice for chronic lymphocytic leukemia and primary (Waldenström's) macroglobulinemia and is sometimes used to treat the vasculitic complications of rheumatoid arthritis, autoimmune hemolytic anemias associated with cold agglutinins, and Hodgkin's disease.[22] Chlorambucil was introduced into ophthalmic practice in 1970 when Mamo and Azzam[53] first reported its efficacy in the treatment of Adamantiades-Behçet disease and today remains the most frequently used immunosuppressive agent in its management.

OFFICIAL DRUG NAME AND CHEMISTRY
Chlorambucil (Leukeran) is 2-[*bis*(chloroethyl)amino]-benzenebutanoic acid with a molecular weight of 304.21.

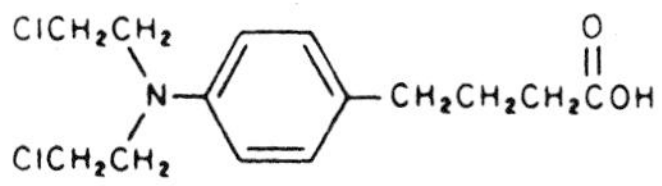

FIGURE 12–3. Chemical structure of chlorambucil.

Its structure (Fig. 12–3) as an aromatic derivative of mechlorethamine renders it essentially inert, making it suitable for oral administration.[5]

PHARMACOLOGY
Chlorambucil, like cyclophosphamide, is a nitrogen mustard derivative; the two share many similar pharmacologic properties, including a common mechanism of action (see Fig. 12–1). As an alkylating agent, chlorambucil interferes with DNA replication and RNA transcription, ultimately resulting in disruption of nucleic acid function. These actions are cell cycle nonspecific.

CLINICAL PHARMACOLOGY
Chlorambucil has immunosuppressive properties, exerting its action principally through suppression of B lymphocytes. It is the slowest acting nitrogen mustard derivative in clinical use, requiring 2 weeks to have an effect.[50] Its cytotoxic effects on the bone marrow, lymphoid organs, and epithelial tissues are similar to those of other agents in this class of drugs.[8]

PHARMACEUTICS
Chlorambucil (Leukeran, Glaxo-Wellcome, Research Triangle Park, NC) is available in 2-mg sugar-coated tablets for oral use. The drug should be stored at 59° to 77°F in a dry place.

PHARMACOKINETICS AND METABOLISM
Chlorambucil is readily absorbed after oral administration, reaching peak plasma levels in 1 hour and is distributed throughout the tissues in a fairly homogeneous fashion.[44] As an unmetabolized prodrug, chlorambucil is extensively bound to plasma and tissue proteins, with a plasma $t\frac{1}{2}$ of 1 to 5 hours. It is extensively metabolized in the liver to the active principal phenylacetic acid mustard, which itself retains a $t\frac{1}{2}$ of approximately 2.5 hours.[22] Renal excretion is the major route of elimination for this and other metabolites; very little drug is excreted unchanged in the urine or feces.

THERAPEUTIC USE
The efficacy of chlorambucil in the management of ocular or neuro–Adamantiades-Behçet disease has been confirmed by numerous investigators[54–58] since its introduction by Mamo and Azzam.[53] Although Tabbara[59] questioned the use of this agent because of concerns about its effect on spermatogenesis, long-term remissions and cures have been reported with chlorambucil in patients with Adamantiades-Behçet disease.[60, 61] In managing Adamantiades-Behçet disease, we treated 8 of 29 patients with chlorambucil, effecting long-term inflammatory control in all but one.[69] Although cyclosporine, when used at high doses (10 mg/kg/day), has been reported to produce dramatic and prompt responses in patients with

Adamantiades-Behçet disease,[62] this dose is now clearly contraindicated because of its nephrotoxicity. At more acceptable, less nephrotoxic doses (5 to 7 mg/kg/day), cyclosporine may not induce long-standing drug-free remissions and is, in our experience and that of other investigators,[63] distinctly inferior to chlorambucil, cyclophosphamide, and azathioprine in the care of the ocular complications of Adamantiades-Behçet disease.

Chlorambucil has also been used successfully in the treatment of various other forms of uveitis that are recalcitrant to conventional therapy (see Table 12–4). Godfrey and colleagues[64] reported that 10 of 31 patients with intractable idiopathic uveitis improved with chlorambucil. Andrasch and associates[65] conducted a trial in which 25 patients were treated with either azathioprine in combination with low-dose steroids or chlorambucil. All 13 patients with severe chronic uveitis responded to chlorambucil, whereas 10 of them were either intolerant of or failed to respond to azathioprine. Jennings and Tessler[66] have presented data confirming the observations of previous investigators[43, 64] that suggest that chlorambucil may be effective in treatment of sympathetic ophthalmia.

Finally, several investigators[64, 67, 68] have shown intractable JRA-associated iridocyclitis to be responsive to chlorambucil. Although Godfrey and coworkers[64] reported equivocal results in one patient, Kanski[67] described favorable responses in five of six patients with ocular inflammation associated with JRA who were treated with chlorambucil. Foster and Barrett[68] achieved complete inflammatory control in three patients with JRA-associated iridocyclitis, one of whom had been unresponsive to systemic and topical corticosteroids, NSAIDs, and methotrexate.

DOSAGE AND ROUTE OF ADMINISTRATION

Several dosage regimens have been suggested for oral administration of chlorambucil. Godfrey and associates[64] advocate an initial dose of 2 mg/day, increased by an additional 2 mg/day for a maximal dose of 10 to 12 mg/day or until a favorable clinical response is observed. We prefer to begin with a dose of 0.1 mg/kg/day, titrating the dose based on the clinical response and drug tolerance every 3 weeks, for a maximum daily dose of 18 mg/day (see Table 12–1). Such high doses are used only in cases of severe sight-threatening inflammation in patients who display no untoward reaction to the drug. All patients receiving chlorambucil require vigilant monitoring for potential adverse reactions, particularly myelosuppression, because this complication increases significantly at doses greater than 10 mg/day. Hematologic monitoring is performed, as previously described for cyclophosphamide, with similar target parameters for leukocyte, neutrophil, and platelet counts. We advocate increased vigilance in monitoring at approximately 3 months of treatment. A dose-accumulation effect on the bone marrow is common, and the dosage must be reduced progressively in the ensuing 3 to 6 months. Liver function tests should be repeated every 3 to 4 months.

SIDE EFFECTS AND TOXICITY

Hematologic toxicity is the most prominent adverse effect of chlorambucil therapy (see Table 12–3). Myelosuppression is usually moderate, gradual, and reversible.[69] However, abrupt and profound leukopenia, sometimes persisting for months after discontinuation of chlorambucil, may occur, particularly when high doses (10 mg/day) are administered for prolonged times. If leukocyte or platelet counts fall below the target level, the dose of chlorambucil should be reduced. If profound depression occurs, the drug must be discontinued.

Chlorambucil may produce significant gonadal dysfunction. In a group of 10 patients reported by Tabbara,[59] 7 developed oligospermia and 3 acquired azoospermia when a dose of 0.2 mg/kg was used. We do not recommend this dose. This effect may or may not be reversible after therapy is discontinued. As with cyclophosphamide, before initiation of therapy with chlorambucil, sperm banking should be recommended to adolescent men and adults who are still planning a family. In women, potentially irreversible ovarian dysfunction resulting in a medication-induced menopause may arise with prolonged therapy.[70]

Malignancies, mostly acute leukemia, have been reported in patients with polycythemia vera receiving daily doses greater than 4 mg[71] and in patients with breast cancer who are receiving protracted therapy with chlorambucil.[72] Other, less commonly encountered toxicities include GI distress, pulmonary fibrosis, hepatitis, rash, and CNS stimulation,[44] including seizures in adults and children.[73]

OVERDOSE

There is no specific antidote for overdosage with chlorambucil, the signs and symptoms of which mirror its toxicity. As with cyclophosphamide, management is supportive, with appropriate treatment of concurrent infections and myelosuppression with G-CSF as indicated.

HIGH-RISK GROUPS

Chlorambucil is a potential teratogen and has been reported to cause urogenital abnormalities in the offspring of mothers receiving this drug during the first trimester of pregnancy.[74] Although no well-controlled studies have been performed in pregnant women, those of childbearing age should avoid becoming pregnant, and those who become pregnant while receiving chlorambucil should be advised of the potential hazard to the fetus. Whether the drug is excreted in the breast milk is not known.

As with cyclophosphamide, the safety and effectiveness of chlorambucil for the treatment of sight-threatening ocular inflammatory disease in the pediatric age group is controversial and is best considered on a case-by-case basis.

CONTRAINDICATIONS

Chlorambucil is contraindicated in patients who have demonstrated either previous resistance or hypersensitivity to it.

DRUG INTERACTIONS

There are no known drug-drug interactions with chlorambucil, although other immunosuppressive agents undoubtedly have an additive effect.

MAJOR CHEMICAL TRIALS

Major clinical trials are described in the Therapeutic Use section.

Antimetabolites

Methotrexate

HISTORY AND SOURCE

In 1948, inhibitors of the vitamin folic acid were first reported to produce striking, although temporary, remissions in acute leukemia in children.[75] Subsequently, in 1963, the curative potential of chemotherapy in human cancer was demonstrated when methotrexate was shown to produce long-term, complete remissions of trophoblastic choriocarcinoma in women.[76] Today, methotrexate is the agent of choice (in combination with mercaptopurine) in the maintenance therapy of acute lymphocytic leukemia[22] and is effective in treatment of a variety of systemic inflammatory conditions, including psoriasis, rheumatoid arthritis refractory to conventional therapy, JRA, Reiter's disease, polymyositis and, in rare cases, sarcoidosis.[10, 77, 78] The use of methotrexate in the management of ocular inflammatory disease has been reported rarely, with the first citation by Wong and Hersh[79] appearing in 1965. Experience with this agent in treatment of non–life-threatening systemic inflammatory disease has grown, and methotrexate is now frequently the first immunosuppressive agent considered for use in cases of pediatric uveitis refractory to more conventional therapy.

OFFICIAL DRUG NAME AND CHEMISTRY

Methotrexate (Folex, Mexate, Rheumatrex) is 4-amino-N^{10}-methylpteroylglutamic acid, with a molecular weight of 454.5. Its structure (Fig. 12–4) is analogous to that of folic acid, differing only in two areas: the amino group in the 4-carbon position is substituted for a hydroxyl group, and a methyl group at the N^{10} position appears instead of a hydrogen atom.[80]

PHARMACOLOGY

Methotrexate prevents the conversion of dihydrofolate to tetrahydrofolate by competitively and irreversibly binding to the enzyme dihydrofolate reductase (DHFR).[8] Tetrahydrofolate is an essential cofactor in the production of 1-carbon units critical to synthesis of purine nucleotides and thymidylate. In addition, a less rapid, partially reversible competitive inhibition of thymidylate synthetase also occurs within 24 hours after methotrexate administration.[8] The net effect is inhibition of DNA synthesis, repair, RNA synthesis, and cell division in a cell cycle–specific (S phase) fashion (Fig. 12–5).

The blockage of DHFR can be bypassed clinically by

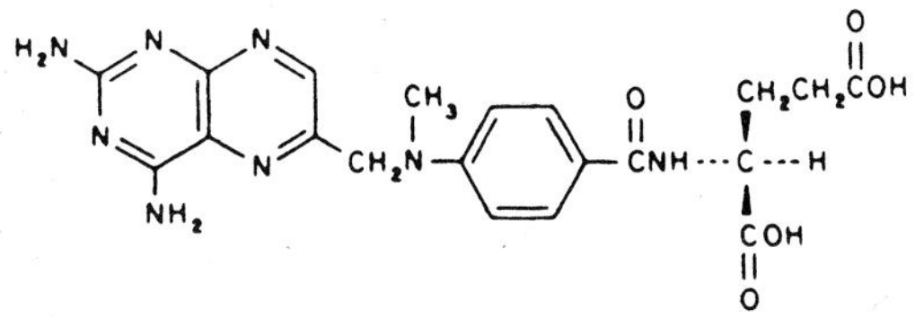

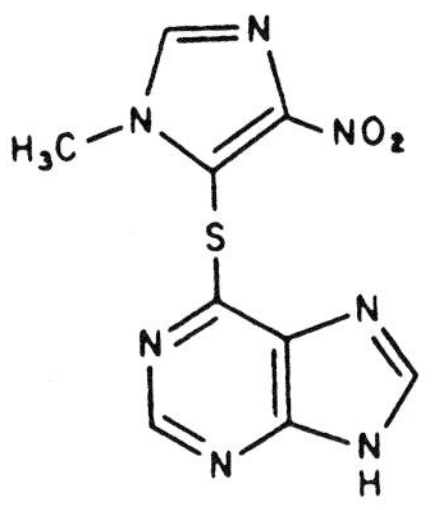

FIGURE 12–5. Chemical structure of azathioprine.

use of leucovorin calcium (N^5-formyltetrahydrofolate, folinic acid, citrovorum factor), a fully functional folate coenzyme.[8] So-called leucovorin rescue is achieved, allowing recovery of normal tissues and permitting use of larger doses of methotrexate.

CLINICAL PHARMACOLOGY

Methotrexate has little effect on resting cells; instead, it exerts its cytotoxic actions in actively proliferating tissues such as malignant cells, fetal cells, cells of the GI tract, urinary bladder, buccal mucosa, and bone marrow. By inhibiting DNA synthesis in immunologically competent cells, methotrexate has some activity as an immunosuppressive agent. Both B and T cells are affected,[81] and the primary and secondary antibody responses can be suppressed when administered during antigen encounter.[82, 83] Apparently, it has no significant effect on cell-mediated immunity. Low-dose methotrexate has been shown to depress acute-phase reactants while leaving cellular parameters unaltered.[84, 85] These observations have led some investigators to suggest that, at these doses, methotrexate acts more as an antiinflammatory agent than as an immunosuppressive agent, possibly explaining its reduced effectiveness in treatment of chronic uveitis and retinal vasculitis as compared with that in treatment of scleritis and orbital myositis.[86]

PHARMACEUTICS

Methotrexate (Lederle, Philadelphia) is available in 2.5-mg tablets and as preparations for injection (intravenous, intramuscular, intrathecal) as follows: methotrexate (Lederle) solution, 2.5 and 25 mg/ml; (methotrexate LPF) powder, 20, 50, 100, 250 mg and 1 g; and Folex (Adria) solution, 25 mg/ml.

PHARMACOKINETICS AND METABOLISM

Orally administered methotrexate is readily absorbed through a dose-dependent, saturable active transport system, with peak plasma concentrations attained in 1 to 4 hours. The peak plasma concentration after intramuscular injection is 30 minutes to 2 hours. Once absorbed, the plasma concentration of methotrexate undergoes a triphasic reduction: The first phase is the fastest (0.75 hours) and reflects drug distribution throughout the body; the second occurs over 2 to 4 hours and represents renal excretion; the third phase, varying between 10 and 27 hours, is the terminal $t\frac{1}{2}$ of the drug and is believed to reflect the slow release of DHFR bound to methotrexate from the tissues.[87]

Approximately 50% of methotrexate is bound to

FIGURE 12–4. Chemical structure of methotrexate.

plasma proteins, with the remaining unbound fraction mediating its cytotoxic effects.[8] Drug concentrations and duration of cellular exposure are important determinants of these effects and are influenced by factors that might increase the unbound portion (displacement from plasma proteins by other drugs) or prolong drug elimination (renal insufficiency). Methotrexate is transported into cells by carrier-mediated active transport systems and stored intracellularly in the form of polyglutamate conjugates, which may be important determinants of the site and duration of action.[22] Methotrexate is believed to be minimally metabolized, with 50% to 90% excreted unchanged in the urine by a combination of glomerular filtration and active tubular secretion.[8] The drug does accumulate in the liver and kidney, however, particularly after high doses, prolonged administration, or both. Retention of the drug as polyglutamates for long periods is postulated to play a key role in methotrexate toxicity.[80]

THERAPEUTIC USE

Concern regarding the adverse effects of methotrexate may have limited its use in management of ocular inflammatory disease (see Table 12–4). In their initial reports, Wong and Hersh[79, 88] reported favorable responses in 9 of 10 patients with steroid-resistant cyclitis who were treated with high-dose (25 mg/m²) intravenous methotrexate every 4 hours for 6 weeks. Although few serious adverse reactions occurred, inflammatory symptoms recurred in more than half of the patients when therapy was discontinued. Wong[89] successfully used a similar strategy in treating a patient with sympathetic ophthalmia recalcitrant to conventional therapy. Lazar and colleagues[90] obtained similarly encouraging results in 14 of 17 patients with various steroid-resistant uveitis, including four with sympathetic ophthalmia, who were treated with intravenous methotrexate. However, this success was associated with significant drug-induced toxicity, including GI complications, secondary infections, and laboratory evidence of liver damage.

The reduced frequency and severity of adverse reactions reported with oral or intramuscular low-dose, pulsed (weekly) methotrexate therapy in the dermatologic and rheumatologic literature[92] have been exploited in management of a variety of ocular inflammatory disorders. Methotrexate may be sufficient to control scleritis associated with collagen vascular diseases such as Reiter's syndrome and rheumatoid arthritis, but not in collagen diseases complicated by relapsing polychondritis.[32] Uveitic entities, for which once-weekly oral or intramuscular methotrexate may be particularly well-suited, include those associated with Reiter's syndrome, ankylosing spondylitis, inflammatory bowel disease, psoriatic arthritis, and JRA.[10, 68] In retrospective study, 56% of 12 patients with chronic uveitis-vitritis and retinal vasculitis responded to oral low-dose, pulsed methotrexate in combination with corticosteroids.[86] In the same study, 9 of 10 patients with inflammatory pseudotumor, orbital myositis, and scleritis showed improvement, with 5 (50%) achieving disease remission. Most recently, Dev and associates[93] reported that low-dose methotrexate was effective in controlling previously uncontrolled inflammation in 20 eyes of 11 patients with sarcoid-associated panuveitis with preserved

or improved visual acuity in 90% of patients, allowing elimination of corticosteroids in certain patients and permitting successful cataract surgery in those in whom it had been previously impossible.

DOSAGE AND ROUTE OF ADMINISTRATION

We initiate methotrexate therapy with a weekly dose of 2.5 mg to 10 mg administered orally, intramuscularly, or intravenously, as either a single or divided dose, in a 36- to 48-hour period (see Table 12–1). The dose is escalated gradually as dictated by the clinical response to a maximum of 50 mg/week.

Methotrexate has a delayed onset of action, requiring 3 to 6 weeks to take effect.[50] Complete hemograms, with platelet and differential values, should be obtained before the onset of therapy and at intervals of 1 to 4 weeks. Similarly, pretreatment liver function tests, urinalysis, BUN, and serum creatinine should be obtained, and tests should be repeated every 3 to 6 weeks.

SIDE EFFECTS AND TOXICITY

Myelosuppression is the major dose-limiting toxicity of methotrexate (see Table 12–3). Leukopenia and thrombocytopenia appear in the first 2 weeks after a bolus dose or short-term infusion, usually with rapid recovery. Although more prolonged and severe myelosuppression is more commonly associated with higher doses, or occurs in patients with compromised renal, liver, or bone marrow function, pancytopenia has been reported with low-dose methotrexate therapy.[94] Leucovorin is given in such cases to rescue the bone marrow, optimally in 6 to 8 hours after methotrexate administration, and is continued for 72 hours thereafter.[87] Doses equal to or greater than the last dose of methotrexate are administered either intravenously, generally ranging from 10 to 15 mg/m², or orally at doses not in excess of 25 mg, every 6 hours. Depending on the serum methotrexate levels at 24 and 72 hours after dosing, leucovorin rescue should be continued until the levels of methotrexate decrease to less than 10^{-8} M.[95] Although leucovorin effectively counteracts the toxic side effects of folic acid antagonists such as methotrexate, it also impairs its therapeutic efficacy.

Considerable attention has been focused on methotrexate-induced hepatotoxicity, which may develop after short- and long-term use. Acute liver toxicity, manifested by a transient increase in serum transaminases may be evident within a few days of high-dose methotrexate administration. Chronic, low-dose methotrexate therapy, as is commonly used in management of some patients with psoriasis or rheumatoid arthritis, may lead to hepatic fibrosis and, occasionally, to cirrhosis.[80] Liver function tests are not reliable indices of the development of hepatic fibrosis; liver biopsy is the definitive diagnostic procedure. Current guidelines suggest a biopsy before administration of methotrexate in patients at high risk of development of hepatotoxicity (those with obesity, alcoholism, or intercurrent liver or kidney disease) and in all patients receiving a cumulative dose of 1.5 g if further treatment with methotrexate is anticipated.[95] The role of routine liver biopsy in the follow-up of patients receiving low-dose methotrexate has been challenged, especially in light of the small numbers of patients who develop clinical, laboratory, and histopathologic evidence of liver disease while being treated with this regimen.[92, 96] Therefore, the clinician must decide, on a case-by-case basis, whether the cost and risk of the procedure outweigh the possibility that biopsy results will dictate a change in the patient's management. We do not treat patients who are at increased risk of development of hepatotoxicity with methotrexate, and we do not monitor patients whom we do treat with liver biopsy.

Pulmonary toxicity, including acute pneumonitis and pulmonary fibrosis, has been reported with both low- and high-dose methotrexate therapy. Pneumonitis presents with a dry nonproductive cough with dyspnea, high fever, and hypoxemia, and probably represents either an idiosyncratic reaction or hypersensitivity.[97] It usually responds to discontinuation of methotrexate and brief systemic steroid therapy.

GI toxicities include nausea, ulcerative mucositis, and diarrhea, all of which may respond to dosage reduction.[98] Alopecia, dermatitis, and acute renal failure due to precipitation of drug in the renal tubules may occur with high-dose regimens.[80] To date, no controlled data in humans or animals indicate that methotrexate is carcinogenic.[99–101] Finally, ocular side effects are not uncommon; they include irritation, photophobia, aggravation of seborrheic blepharitis, and epiphora in 25% of patients.[49] These signs and symptoms usually abate with time and do not necessitate discontinuation of drug.

OVERDOSE

The signs and symptoms of methotrexate overdosage parallel its toxic side effects. Leucovorin should be administered as promptly as possible to diminish these effects. General supportive measures, as in management of any drug overdose, should be instituted.

HIGH-RISK GROUPS

Methotrexate is a known teratogen and abortifacient, and may cause oligospermia.[87] Women of childbearing age treated with this medication must use reliable contraception. In addition, owing to concerns regarding the mutagenic potential of methotrexate, both men and women should allow at least a 12-week period to elapse between discontinuation of therapy and attempt at conception. Methotrexate therapy is also ill advised in nursing mothers because of the potential serious adverse reactions from this drug in breast-fed infants. The safety and effectiveness of methotrexate in the pediatric age group has not been established; however, one study indicates that this agent is well-tolerated in children with JRA.[102]

The risk of developing serious liver disease from treatment with low-dose methotrexate increases with age and other factors.[92] Decreasing renal and hepatic reserves in the elderly contributes significantly to this problem; therefore, clinicians should use extreme caution in administering methotrexate in this age group. Callen and Kulp-Shorten[80] suggest performing a creatinine clearance in any patient older than 50 years for whom methotrexate treatment is considered and that a value less than 50 ml/ minute constitutes a contraindication to its use.

CONTRAINDICATIONS

Groups in whom methotrexate therapy is contraindicated include pregnant or nursing women; patients with known alcoholism, alcoholic liver disease, or chronic liver disease of any etiology; patients with immunodeficiency states, irrespective of cause; patients with pre-existing blood dyscrasias or bone marrow suppression, and any patient with a known hypersensitivity to the drug.

DRUG INTERACTIONS

Concomitant consumption of salicylates, sulfonamides, chloramphenicol, or tetracycline may increase the fraction of unbound serum methotrexate through displacement from plasma proteins, thereby potentiating the risk of methotrexate-induced adverse effects. Similarly, concurrent treatment with drugs such as NSAIDs or probenecid, which impair renal blood flow or tubular secretion, may delay drug excretion and lead to severe toxicity.[22]

MAJOR CLINICAL TRIALS

Major clinical trials are described in the Therapeutic Use section.

Azathioprine

HISTORY AND SOURCE

Azathioprine was introduced and developed in the early 1960s as a derivative of 6-mercaptopurine (6-MP) in an effort to produce a drug with similar immunosuppressive action but a more prolonged duration of activity.[21] Today, 6-MP is rarely used; however, azathioprine remains a mainstay in organ transplant surgery and is one of the most widely used agents in treatment of dermatologic and autoimmune diseases; it is approved by the Food and Drug Administration (FDA) for use in patients with rheumatoid arthritis. 6-MP and azathioprine were introduced into ophthalmic practice by Newell and coworkers in 1966[103] and 1967[104] and were among the first immunosuppressants used for treatment of ocular immune-mediated disorders.

OFFICIAL DRUG NAME AND CHEMISTRY

Chemically, azathioprine (Imuran, Glaxo-Wellcome, Research Triangle Park, NC) is 6[(1-methyl-4-nitroimidazole-5-yl)thio]purine with a molecular weight of 277.29 (see Fig. 12–5). It is an imidazolyl derivative of 6-MP and, therefore, is classified as a purine analogue. Both drugs are structurally similar to hypoxanthine, an important precursor in purine metabolism.[8]

PHARMACOLOGY

Azathioprine is a prodrug that is quickly metabolized in the liver to its active form, 6-MP, which, in turn, interferes with purine metabolism and ultimately with DNA, RNA, and protein synthesis (see Fig. 12–1). Specifically, 6-MP, through its conversion to thioinosine-5-phosphate, a purine analogue, provides a false precursor, thereby impairing adenine and guanine nucleotide formation.[8] DNA metabolism is inhibited in a cell cycle–specific (S phase) manner.

CLINICAL PHARMACOLOGY

Although the immunosuppressive effects of azathioprine probably relate to the disruption of DNA synthesis in immunocompetent lymphoid cells, its action is incompletely understood and cannot be explained by this mechanism alone. The humoral immune response is relatively unaffected by azathioprine when administered in therapeutic, nontoxic doses of 2 to 3 mg/kg/day. However, variable alterations in antibody production can occur when large doses of thiopurine are administered within 48 hours of antigen priming and may induce temporary tolerance when administered in conjunction with large doses of antigen.[1]

Azathioprine has been shown to suppress both B and T lymphocytes, the effect of which is relatively more selective for the latter cellular subset.[105] In addition, thiopurines suppress the mixed lymphocyte reaction in vivo, depress recirculating T lymphocytes that are in the process of homing, and suppress the development of monocyte precursors and thus the participation of K cells (which themselves are derived from monocyte precursors) in antibody-dependent cytotoxicity reactions.[10] Although thiopurines inhibit delayed-type hypersensitivity reactions and prolong renal, skin, and cardiac allografts, they do not affect development of autoimmune disease in New Zealand black mice. which is mainly antibody mediated.[20]

PHARMACEUTICS

Azathioprine (Imuran, Glaxo-Wellcome, Research Triangle Park, NC) is available as 50-mg tablets for oral administration or as a lyophilized powder equivalent to 100 mg drug for intravenous use. This medication should be stored in a dry place at 59° to 77°F and should be protected from light.

PHARMACOKINETICS AND METABOLISM

After oral administration, approximately 50% of azathioprine is absorbed within 2 hours.[21] It is rapidly metabolized in erythrocytes and in the liver, where it is cleaved to mercaptopurine and then catabolized to various methylated derivatives. Specifically, xanthine oxidase catalyzes the formation of 6-thiouric acid, the principal metabolite, whereas approximately 10% of azathioprine is cleaved to form 1-methyl-4-nitro-5-thioimidizole.[8] Proportionate variation in these metabolites may explain the differences in the magnitude and duration of drug effects among individual patients.

Approximately 30% of both azathioprine and 6-MP are bound to serum protein. Renal clearance accounts for less than 2% of its excretions and neither drug is detectable in the urine after 8 hours.[22] Typical doses of azathioprine produce blood levels of less than 1 μg/ml; however, because both the magnitude and duration of its clinical effects correlate with the level of thiopurine nucleotide in the target tissues, blood levels of azathioprine or 6-MP are of little value in guiding therapy.[21] Cytotoxicity is enhanced in patients with renal insufficiency because effects may persist long after drug clearance is complete.

THERAPEUTIC USE

Many reports in the ophthalmic literature describe successful control of various corticosteroid-resistant ocular inflammatory diseases and uveitic syndromes with azathioprine, alone or in combination with corticosteroids or other immunosuppressive agents (see Table 12–4). Azathioprine has been effective in treatment of scleritis associated with relapsing polychondritis (RP)[32] and as an adjunctive, second-line agent in control of progressive conjunctival inflammation in ocular cicatricial pemphigoid.[35]

Reports of the efficacy of azathioprine in various uveitic syndromes have been variable. Newell and associates[104] treated 20 patients with uveitis of different etiologies and found that azathioprine was most effective in those with pars planitis. Andrash and coworkers[65] reported that azathioprine, in combination with corticosteroids, was effective in 12 of 22 patients with chronic uveitis. However, azathioprine was discontinued in four patients who failed to respond and in six with GI distress. In contradistinction, Mathews and colleagues[106] showed that azathioprine, compared with placebo in a controlled, double-masked trial, was no more effective than placebo in reducing the inflammatory activity of 19 patients with chronic iridocyclitis. Whereas Moore,[107] using a combination of azathioprine and corticosteroids, reported successful treatment of sympathetic ophthalmia in a child in 1968, subsequent work by Newell and Krill[104] and Martenet[43] failed to duplicate this experience. In our practice,[108] azathioprine has been effective in treatment of JRA-associated iridocyclitis unresponsive to conventional steroid therapy.

In treatment of Adamantiades-Behçet disease, a 2-year, double-masked, randomized, controlled study demonstrated that azathioprine (2.5 mg/kg/day) prevented development of new eye lesions and reduced the frequency and intensity of recurrent inflammation in patients with established ocular or systemic disease.[109] No serious adverse effects were reported among the 37 treated patients. Foster and coworkers[39] reported more equivocal results among eight patients with Adamantiades-Behçet disease. Inflammatory control was achieved in one patient treated with a combination of azathioprine and corticosteroids and in two patients receiving azathioprine and cyclosporine; however, therapy had to be discontinued in one patient who developed severe leukopenia.[39] We do not consider azathioprine the most effective drug for treatment of Adamantiades-Behçet disease.

Frequently, we use azathioprine as a steroid-sparing drug, allowing systemic steroids to be tapered to an acceptable level, with eventual discontinuation. Entities for which we have found this approach valuable include multifocal choroiditis with panuveitis, sympathetic ophthalmia, VKH, sarcoidosis, pars planitis, and Reiter's syndrome–associated iridocyclitis.

DOSAGE AND ROUTE OF ADMINISTRATION

A single or divided oral dose of azathioprine administered as 2 to 3 mg/kg/day is suggested (see Table 12–1). This amount should be reduced by 25% if allopurinol is administered concomitantly, because allopurinol interferes with the metabolism of 6-MP[8] (described in Drug Interactions section). The clinical response and laboratory parameters should be monitored in the same way suggested for chlorambucil and cyclophosphamide.

SIDE EFFECTS AND TOXICITY

The frequency and severity of adverse effects of azathioprine depend on the dose, duration of therapy, and on the nature of any underlying disease (renal, hepatic) that might potentiate toxicity (see Table 12–3). Although reports in the ophthalmic literature suggest that azathioprine is well tolerated, vigilant hematologic monitoring is crucial, because bone marrow suppression with leukopenia and thrombocytopenia are common.[44] Typically, myelosuppression is delayed, appearing 1 to 2 weeks after initiation of therapy, and may persist for days to weeks after the drug has been discontinued. Prompt dosage reduction or withdrawal of azathioprine may be necessary if myelosuppression is severe.

Symptomatic GI discomfort (nausea, vomiting, and diarrhea) is the most common side effect and the principal reason for discontinuation of azathioprine therapy.[109] Other adverse effects include interstitial pneumonitis, hepatocellular necrosis, pancreatitis, stomatitis, alopecia, and rarely, secondary infections.[51, 110]

Azathioprine has been implicated in potentiating the risk of neoplasia, especially leukemia and lymphomas, in transplant patients.[111] However, several studies have demonstrated no difference in the overall frequency of malignancy in the general population from that observed in patients with rheumatoid arthritis receiving conventional doses of azathioprine.[112, 113]

OVERDOSE

Ingestion of very large doses of azathioprine may lead to bone marrow hypoplasia, bleeding, infection, and death. In the single case report of a renal transplant patient who ingested a dose of 7500 mg of azathioprine, the immediate toxic reactions were nausea, vomiting, and diarrhea, followed by leukopenia, and mild abnormalities of liver function.[114] All laboratory values had returned to normal 6 days after the overdose. In addition to general supportive measures, including induction of emesis and gastric lavage, hemodialysis has been shown to remove 45% of drug in an 8-hour period.[115]

HIGH-RISK GROUPS

The administration of azathioprine should be avoided whenever possible in pregnant women because it has been shown to be mutagenic and teratogenic in laboratory animals and to cross the placenta in humans.[22] Conception should also be avoided for a period of not less than 12 weeks after discontinuation of therapy. Likewise, use of azathioprine in nursing mothers is not recommended because the drug or its metabolites are transferred at low levels in the breast milk.[116] The safety and efficacy of azathioprine in the pediatric age group have not been established. Patients with impaired renal function, especially the elderly or in patients who have just undergone kidney transplantation, may have delayed clearance of azathioprine and its metabolites and require dosage adjustments to avoid toxic sequelae.

CONTRAINDICATIONS

Azathioprine is contraindicated in patients with a history of hypersensitivity to the drug or in those who are immunosuppressed and in patients with rheumatoid arthritis

previously treated with alkylating agents in whom the risk of neoplasia is potentially high.[117]

DRUG INTERACTIONS

Because allopurinol inhibits xanthine oxidase, thereby impairing the conversion of azathioprine to its metabolites, the dosage of azathioprine should be reduced by 25% in patients treated concomitantly with these medications. Severe leukopenia associated with use of angiotensin-converting enzyme inhibitors in patients receiving azathioprine has been reported.[118] The clearance of azathioprine may be affected by drugs that inhibit (ketoconazole, erythromycin) or induce (phenatoin, rifampin, phenobarbital) the hepatic microsomal enzyme system.[22]

MAJOR CLINICAL TRIALS

Major clinical trials are described in the Therapeutic Use section.

Leflunomide

HISTORY AND SOURCE

Leflunomide (Arava) is a pyrimidine synthesis inhibitor approved by the FDA in 1998 for the treatment of rheumatoid arthritis.

OFFICIAL DRUG NAME AND CHEMISTRY

Leflunomide's chemical name is N-(4′-trifluoromethyl-phenyl)-s-methylosoxazole-4-carboxamide. Its empirical formula is $C_{12}H_9F_3N_2O_2$, molecular weight 270.2.

PHARMACOLOGY

Leflunomide is a prodrug, metabolized to its active metabolite, A77 1126 (M1). M1 is responsible for all of leflunomide's in vivo immunomodulatory activity through inhibition of dihydro-orotate dehydrogenase, an enzyme involved in de novo pyrimidine synthesis.

CLINICAL PHARMACOLOGY

Leflunomide is superior to placebo in reducing the signs and symptoms of rheumatoid arthritis, and is at least equivalent to methotrexate and to sulfasalazine in masked comparison trials in the care of such patients.

PHARMACEUTICS

Leflunomide (Arava, Hoechst Marion Roussel) is supplied as 10-, 20-, and 100-mg tablets for oral administration.

PHARMACOKINETICS AND METABOLISM

Following oral administration approximately 80% of the dose is bioavailable, and the active metabolite, M1, is highly albumin bound (79.3%). Both liver and GI tract cells are involved in the metabolism, and M1 is eliminated through the metabolic breakdown and excretion by kidneys and biliary tract. Peak plasma levels of M1 occur 6 to 12 hours after oral administration, and elimination is slow, with an M1 t½ of approximately 2 weeks, owing to biliary recycling.

THERAPEUTIC USE

Leflunomide is FDA approved for the treatment of adults with rheumatoid arthritis. A loading dose of 100 mg is given for 3 days to facilitate rapid attainment of steady-state levels of M1. Daily maintenance therapy therein follows at 20 mg/day. The dose may be reduced to 10 mg/day if mild hepatotoxicity, as judged by rising hepatic enzymes, is encountered. Leflunomide has been used concomitantly with oral NSAIDs, steroids, and methotrexate, with only the latter increasing the frequency of liver toxicity. Coadministration with rifampin is not advisable, since plasma M1 levels steadily rise with this drug combination.

Leflunomide compared favorably with methotrexate in randomized, masked premarketing trials, leading to the FDA approval of this immunomodulator for the treatment of rheumatoid arthritis. Its use in ophthalmology, to our knowledge, thus far has been (in our clinic) restricted to patients with uveitis who have been intolerant of or unresponsive to methotrexate.

SIDE EFFECTS AND TOXICITY
Leflunomide's most common side effect is diarrhea. Alopecia, rash, and hepatotoxicity are the other side effects occurring at a notable incidence greater than in a placebo treatment group. It has not been associated with sterility or with an increased risk of malignancy.

HIGH-RISK GROUPS
Leflunomide is contraindicated in patients with known hypersensitivity to it, in patients with liver or renal disease, and in women who are or who may become pregnant (it is teratogenic). It is also not recommended for patients who are already immunosuppressed or who are infected.

DRUG INTERACTIONS
M1 causes increased free plasma levels of most NSAIDs tested (e.g., diclofenac, ibuprofen), probably by inhibiting Cyp450 2C9, which is responsible for the metabolism of many NSAIDs. Rifampin significantly increases serum levels of Arava.

Mycophenolate Mofetil

HISTORY AND SOURCE
Mycophenolate mofetil (CellCept, Roche Laboratories) is an immunosuppressive agent developed and marketed by Hoffman LaRoche, gaining FDA approval for use in prevention of solid organ transplant rejection in 1995.

OFFICIAL DRUG NAME AND CHEMISTRY
Mycophenolate mofetil (CellCept) is the z-morpholinoethyl ester of mycophenolic acid, which is immunosuppressive. The clinical name of mycophenolate mofetil is 2-morpholinoethyl (E)-6-(1,3-dihydro-4-hydroxy-6-methoxy-7-methyl-3-oxo-5-isobenzofuranyl)-4-methyl-4-hexenoate. The empirical formula is $C_{23}H_{31}NO_7$, and the molecular weight is 433.50. Its structural formula is shown later in the chapter in Figure 12–9.

PHARMACOLOGY
Mycophenolate mofetil is a potent, selective, uncompetitive, reversible inhibitor of inosine monophosphate dehydrogenase and, therefore, inhibits de novo purine synthesis. This results in selective inhibitory effects on rapidly dividing cells, such as activated lymphocytes. Additionally, mycophenolate mofetil suppresses antibody formation and interferes with lymphocyte-vascular endothelial cell interactions.

CLINICAL PHARMACOLOGY
Mycophenolate mofetil prolongs solid organ allogeneic transplants (heart, liver, kidney) in animals, and even reverses established transplant rejection in model systems of cardiac allografts. It also inhibits animal models of immune-mediated inflammation. It is a potent, selective, uncompetitive but reversible inhibitor of inosine monophosphate dehydrogenase, and so inhibits the de novo pathway of guanosine synthesis. Unlike most cell types, which can use salvage pathways for purine synthesis, T and B cells cannot, and so are highly dependent on the de novo pathway for growth and proliferation. Mycophenolic acid inhibits T- and B-cell proliferative responses to mitogenic and allospecific stimuli, suppresses antibody production, and inhibits lymphocyte recruitment to sites of inflammation.

PHARMACEUTICS
Mycophenolate mofetil (CellCept, Roche Laboratories, Nutley, NJ) is available as 250-mg capsules and as 500-mg tablets for oral administration. It should be stored at 59° to 86°F and shielded from light.

PHARMACOKINETICS AND METABOLISM
Mycophenolate mofetil is rapidly absorbed after oral administration and is metabolized to the active immunosuppressive moiety mycophenolate acid. It is 97% bound to plasma albumin. Further metabolism to inactive products is followed by (primarily) renal excretion.

THERAPEUTIC USE
Mycophenolate mofetil is marketed for prevention of solid organ transplant rejection. We have had extensive experience with it in the "off-label" use of treating patients with noninfectious, autoimmune inflammatory eye disease (scleritis and uveitis). The typical dose is 1 g twice daily; higher doses may be used but are associated with considerably greater toxicity.

SIDE EFFECTS AND TOXICITY
Secondary infection, renal and liver toxicity, increased risk of malignancy, impotence, anorexia, alopecia, nausea, and leukopenia are the primary toxicity concerns, and appropriate discussion with patients of the relative risks and benefits and probability of a serious side effect is obviously critical.

HIGH-RISK GROUPS
Patients who are immunocompromised before mycophenolate mofetil therapy and those with renal impairment represent the primary high-risk groups of patients.

DRUG INTERACTIONS
Acyclovir, gancyclovir, and mycophenolate metabolic products may compete for renal tubular secretion. Mycophenolate absorption is reduced by the concomitant use

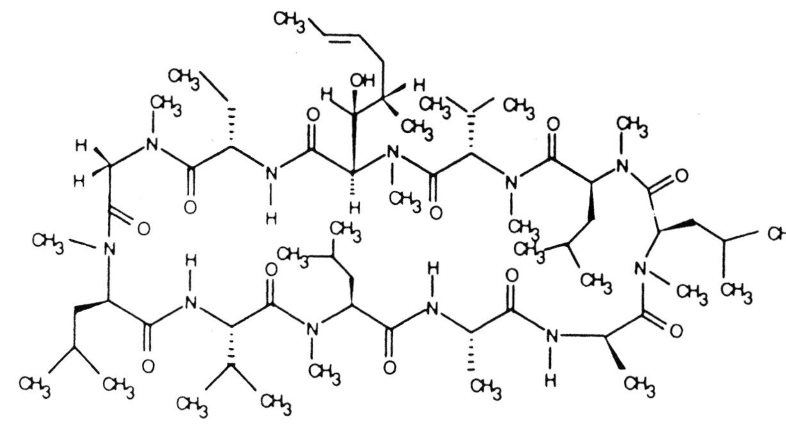

FIGURE 12–6. Chemical structure of cyclosporin A.

of antacids. Cholestyramine decreases plasma levels of mycophenolic acid by 40% after administration of mycophenolate mofetil.

NONCYTOTOXIC IMMUNOSUPPRESSIVE DRUGS

The role of noncytotoxic agents in control of immune-related ocular inflammation has grown in importance and in scope with the development of drugs that mediate immunosuppression by selectively and reversibly targeting cellular subsets in the immune system without producing undue myelosuppression. Cyclosporine is the prototypical example of such an agent; however, several other naturally occurring and synthetic antibiotics (FK 506 and sirolimus [rapamycin]) show great promise in their capacity to suppress autoimmune uveitis, Other antibiotics, such as dapsone, have been explored for their anti-inflammatory effects in treatment of inflammatory and immune diseases with potentially destructive ocular sequelae. Finally, several drugs have been used primarily as adjuvants to immunosuppressive agents, either as a dosage-lowering strategy (bromocriptine or ketoconazole with cyclosporine) or in the prophylaxis of recurrent inflammatory disease (colchicine for Adamantiades-Behçet disease).

Antibiotics

Cyclosporine

HISTORY AND SOURCE
Cyclosporin A, also known as CSA, is a fungal metabolite that was discovered by Borel at Sandoz Laboratories (1969–1970).[119] Although the drug was originally isolated from cultures of *Tolypocladium inflatum* Gams and *Clindrocarpon lucidum* as part of a screening program for new antifungal agents, its profound and specific immunosuppressive properties became readily apparent.[120] CSA was first shown to be effective in suppressing autoimmune uveitis by Nussenblatt and coworkers[121, 122] and was subsequently applied to treatment of a variety of rheumatic diseases. CSA, and the emergence of similar immune-selective agents, has revolutionized the arena of organ transplantation and holds the promise of more effective and specific treatment of destructive systemic and ocular autoimmune disease. Three excellent reviews of the phar-

macology, immunology, and clinical uses of CSA have been published.[123–125]

OFFICIAL DRUG NAME AND CHEMISTRY
Cyclosporine (Sandoz, East Hanover, NJ) is a neutral, hydrophobic, cyclic endecapeptide (molecular weight 1203 daltons) consisting of 11 amino acids, one of which, the 9-carbon residue at position 1, is unique (Fig. 12–6).[126] The amino acids at positions 1, 2, 3, 10, and 11 form a hydrophilic active site, with the biologic action of the molecule being very sensitive to changes in stereochemical configurations at these positions.[124, 126]

PHARMACOLOGY
The mechanism by which CSA reversibly inhibits T-cell–mediated (particularly helper T cell) alloimmune and autoimmune responses is not completely understood, attesting to the enormous complexity underlying T-cell activation (see Fig. 12–1). Before being activated, T cells are primed by virtue of specific immunorecognition with antigen presented by antigen-presenting cells (APCs) to express receptors for certain lymphokines (e.g., interleukin-1, IL-1) on their cell surface, which act to promote cellular maturation. Activation takes place through a second series of T-cell recognition events, which result in the synthesis of other lymphokines (e.g., IL-2), which promote clonal expansion and cytoaggressive potential.[125] The best evidence obtained thus far indicates that CSA disrupts the transmission of signals from the T-cell receptor (TCR) to genes that encode for multiple lymphokines and enzymes necessary for activation of resting T cells and cytoaggression, while leaving the T-cell priming reaction unaffected.[126] FK 506 (Fig. 12–7), although structurally distinct from CSA, is believed to act through a similar molecular mechanism, resulting in the inhibition of T-helper cell activation, lymphokine production, and lymphocyte proliferation. In contrast, sirolimus (rapamycin) (Fig. 12–8), although it is a closely related structural analogue of FK 506, exhibits a distinct mode of action, affecting the T-cell activation-proliferation pathway at a later stage, and is discussed separately.

CLINICAL PHARMACOLOGY
After engagement of the TCR with antigen complexed with class I or II major histocompatibility (MHC)-associated peptides on the cell surface, activation of the

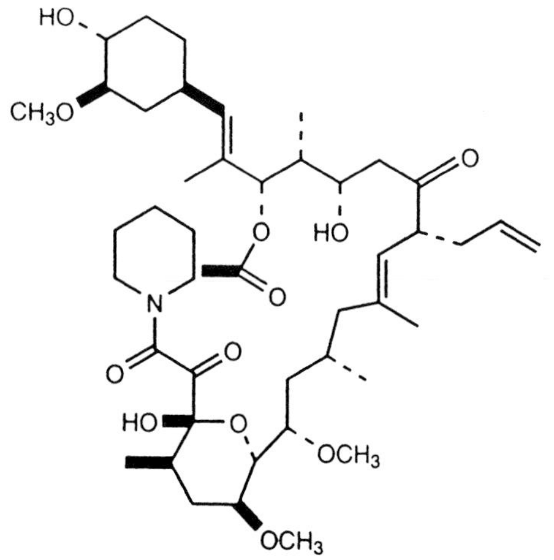

FIGURE 12–7. Chemical structure of FK 506.

TCR signal transmission pathway proceeds through the cytoplasm through calcium (Ca^{2+})-dependent or Ca^{2+}-independent pathways.[127] Ca^{2+}-independent pathways are initiated through protein kinase C (PKC)–triggered reactions. Ca^{2+}-dependent activation eventuates in promotion of specific nuclear transcription factors, such as nuclear factor of activated T cells (NF-AT), which regulate the transcription of genes involved in T-cell activation, such as that for IL-2 (Fig. 12–9). NF-AT itself consists of two subunits: a cytoplasmic component (NF-ATc), which is translocated into the nucleus under the influence of TCR activation pathways, and a newly synthesized nuclear subunit (NF-ATn). Both components are necessary for the binding of NF-AT to DNA and transcriptional activation of, for example, the IL-2 gene.[127]

CSA binds to cyclophilin, a 17-kDa cytosolic protein belonging to a family of proteins termed immunophilins, and is concentrated intracellularly. Similarly, FK 506–binding protein, another immunophilin, binds both FK 506 and sirolimus (rapamycin). These binding proteins, isoforms of which are present in most mammalian cells, have been shown to have peptidyl proline *cis-trans* isomerase (PPIase) activity, enzymes that participate in the

unfolding of cytoplasmic proteins, exposing their functional conformation.[128]

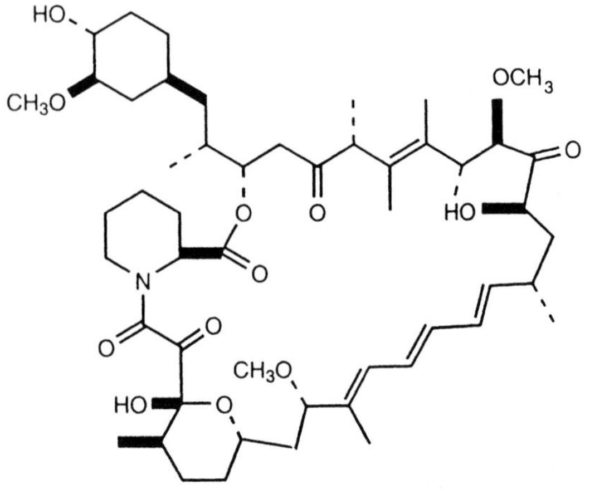

When bound to their respective immunophilins, CSA and FK 506 form a ternary complex with calcineurin, inhibiting calmodulin binding together with the Ca^{2+}-activated phosphatase activity of calcineurin (see Fig. 12–9).[129] This results in inhibition of dephosphorylation of the cytoplasmic subunit of NF-AT and thus inhibits its translocation into the nucleus and subsequent activation of transcription of the IL-2 gene (among others).[130] Neither CSA nor FK 506 has impact on the cascade of events that follow T-cell cytokine gene activation.

Therefore, CSA and FK 506 halt the progression of Ca^{2+}-dependent T-cell activation early in the cell cycle (from Go to G), and thus suppress the synthesis of IL-2, IL-3, IL-4, IL-5, TNF-α, and interferon-γ (IFN-γ), all important cellular immune signals.[131, 132] In addition, both drugs inhibit expression of the IL-2 receptor and may also inhibit IL-1 release from APCs such as monocytes.[10]

The actions of CSA and FK 506 are selective, affecting T helper-inducer and cytotoxic subsets preferentially while leaving T-suppressor cells relatively uninhibited, thereby setting the stage for suppression of immune responses. These drugs markedly decrease antibody production to T-cell–dependent antigens, inhibit cytotoxic activity generated in mixed leukocyte reactions, and prolong the viability of skin, kidney, liver, heart, and pancreas allografts in experimental animals and in humans.[51] They may also mitigate graft-versus-host disease (GVHD) and prolong the life of other transplanted tissues such as the cornea.

PHARMACEUTICS

Cyclosporine (Sandimmune, Neoral, Sandoz, East Hanover, NJ) is available for oral administration as a solution containing 100 mg/ml vehicle (12.5% ethanol in olive oil), which is mixed with milk or orange juice immediately before ingestion. It is also formulated as 25- and 100-mg (12.7% ethanol) soft gelatin capsules.

For intravenous use, CSA is formulated as a solution containing 50 mg drug and 1 ml vehicle (33% ethanol in polyoxethylated castor oil) and is diluted with 0.9% sodium chloride or 5% dextrose immediately before infusion. CSA for topical use is not commercially available; however, 1% to 2% CSA eye drops may be easily prepared using the oral formulation, a procedure that is described in detail by de Smet and Nussenblatt.[125]

PHARMACOKINETICS AND METABOLISM

Absorption of CSA from the GI tract is slow and incomplete, the bioavailability varying from 20% to 50%, with a mean value of 30% of the oral dose.[128] Peak plasma levels are achieved within 3 to 4 hours of ingestion. Administration of CSA with food increases the peak and trough blood concentrations, whereas malabsorption of the drug is common after orthotopic liver transplantation or biliary diversion or in association with inflammatory bowel disease, reduced gastric emptying, and GI motility.[22]

The volume of distribution ranges from less than 1 L/kg to 13 L/kg, with most drug being distributed outside

FIGURE 12–8. Chemical structure of sirolimus (rapamycin).

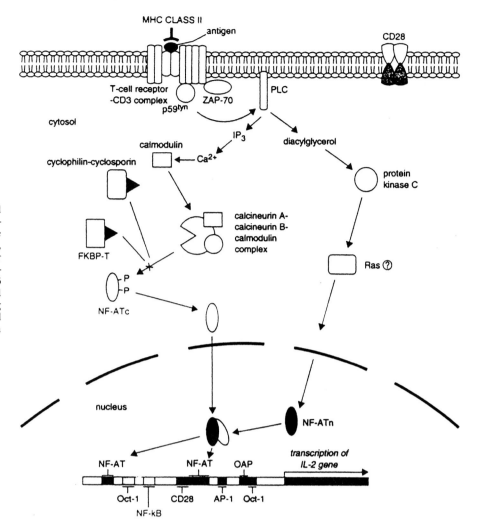

FIGURE 12–9. The T-cell receptor signal transduction pathway leading to interleukin-2 (IL-2) transcription. PLC, phospholipidase C; IP3, inositol 1,4,5-triphosphate; NF-ATc, the cytoplasmic component of the nuclear factor of activated T cells; NF-ATn, the nuclear component of NF-AT; FKBP, FK 506 binding protein. (From Liu J: FK 506 and cyclosporin, molecular probes for studying intracellular signal transduction. Immunol Today 1993;14:293, with permission from Elsevier Science.)

the blood volume. Distribution within whole blood is concentration dependent, with approximately 60% to 75% of drug contained in erythrocytes and 10% to 20% concentrated in leukocytes, apparently reflecting the content of cyclophilin in the latter.[128] Uptake by both erythrocytes and leukocytes becomes saturated at high concentrations. Approximately 90% of CSA in the circulation is bound to plasma proteins, primarily lipoproteins. Although some drug circulates "free" in the plasma, this fraction does not correlate with the total blood level of CSA or with adverse side effects.[133]

The extent of tissue deposition varies among patients, with fat having the highest concentration of drug, approximately 10 times that in plasma.[123] However, because there is apparently no connection between obesity and the volume of distribution, factors other than the lipophilic nature of CSA, such as the tissue content of cytoplasmic binding proteins, which themselves may accumulate drug for months after discontinuation of therapy, are probably involved.[124] High concentrations of CSA are also detected in the liver, kidney, pancreas, adrenal, and lymphoid tissue, whereas very low levels occur in the brain.[123]

Ocular bioavailability depends on the route of administration and the integrity of the blood-ocular barriers.[125]

After systemic administration of CSA in patients with chronic flare, the concentration of drug in the aqueous has been shown to be 40% that of the plasma concentration,[134] whereas in experimental animals with uninflamed ocular tissues, very poor ocular penetration was achieved.[135] Furthermore, in animal models, CSA appears to be concentrated in ocular pigment, and thus might influence intraocular drug concentration.[136]

Topically applied CSA penetrates the cornea poorly and fails to achieve therapeutically efficacious concentrations when the epithelium is intact.[137, 138] However, using collagen shields containing CSA, Chen reported cornea and aqueous concentrations on the order of 10 times that obtained with drops.[139] The use of an α-cyclodextrin vehicle was reported to achieve similar concentrations.[140] Periocular or intracameral administration of CSA has not been used in humans.[141]

CSA is extensively metabolized in the liver by cytochrome P-450, undergoing hydroxylation or demethylation.[142] Enterohepatic recirculation occurs, with most of the drug being excreted in the bile and only 6% appearing in the urine. The median t½ is 6.7 to 8.7 hours.[124] CSA clearance varies in individuals with concomitant administration of drugs that have impact on cytochrome P-450 activity (described in the Drug Interactions section), in patients with hepatic impairment, in the elderly, and in children (described in the High-Risk Groups section).

THERAPEUTIC USE

CSA has been used to treat a wide variety of ocular immune-mediated disorders. It appears to be particularly useful in patients with bilateral, sight-threatening uveitis of a noninfectious etiology when both the retina and choroid are involved, who have either become dependent on systemic corticosteroids for the control of intraocular inflammation, or who have become intolerant of conventional therapy with this medication (see Table 12–4).

Nussenblatt and associates of the National Eye Institute were first to report the efficacy of CSA at doses of 10 mg/kg/day in patients with intractable uveitis of various etiologies (including Adamantiades-Behçet disease, birdshot retinochoroidopathy, sarcoidosis, pars planitis, VKH, multiple sclerosis, sympathetic ophthalmia, and idiopathic vitritis) refractory to corticosteroid and cytotoxic agents.[62, 121, 122, 143, 144] These observations were subsequently corroborated by other investigators in two uncontrolled, nonrandomized trials[145, 146] and in treatment of birdshot retinochoroidopathy,[147] Adamantiades-Behçet disease,[148] and VKH.[149] In a recent randomized, double-masked study, Nussenblatt and coworkers[150] demonstrated that CSA, when used as monotherapy, was effective in controlling intraocular inflammation in 46% of 56 patients who were intolerant of steroids; another 35% of patients in the study responded to combined CSA and systemic steroid therapy. In these studies and in two additional double-masked trials,[151, 152] demonstrating the clinical efficacy of CSA for various forms of noninfectious uveitis, a dose of 10 mg/kg/day was used, a dose now known to be associated with a 100% incidence of untoward nephrotoxic and hypertensive effects. Low-dose CSA therapy (mean maintenance dose 4.0 ± 1.1 mg/kg/day) alone[153] or in combination with corticosteroids,[154] has been used successfully in the management of noninfectious uveitis, with resultant improvement or stabilization of visual acuity in 85% of patients and a reduction or stabilization of vitreous inflammation in 97% of eyes monitored for as long as 2 years.[154, 155] Nephrotoxic and hypertensive side effects were less frequent but not completely avoided; nephrotoxicity in older patients with underlying systemic hypertension was particularly troublesome.[155] Low-dose CSA therapy (2.5 to 5.0 mg/kg/day) has also been successfully used, either alone or in combination with other immunosuppressive agents, in the treatment of birdshot retinochoroidopathy with resultant improvement or stabilization of visual acuity in most patients and few drug-induced side effects.[156]

In the management of Adamantiades-Behçet disease, initial reports clearly demonstrated the superiority of CSA to colchicine[151] or to the combination of cytotoxic agents and steroids[157] in the prevention of ocular inflammatory recurrence when dosage schedules of 10 mg/kg/day were used. However, such high-dose regimens produce unacceptable nephrotoxic side effects, and less toxic doses of 5 to 7 mg/kg/day, in our experience[39] and in that of other investigators,[63] are distinctly inferior to cytotoxic agents (azathioprine, cyclophosphamide, and chlorambucil) in the management of the posterior segment manifes-

tations and inflammatory recurrences in patients with Adamantiades-Behçet disease.

A recent retrospective study of a small number of patients with severe ocular Adamantiades-Behçet disease[158] showed a trend toward therapeutic success and diminished nephrotoxicity in those treated with a combination of CSA (mean dosage 6.2 mg/kg/day) and prednisone (mean dosage 29.4 mg/day) as compared with treatment with CSA alone (mean dosage 8.6 mg/kg/day). The definitive efficacy and long-term outcome of combined CSA regimens with prednisone and other immunosuppressive agents (e.g., azathioprine) in Adamantiades-Behçet disease and other uveitic entities await critical evaluation in prospective, randomized trials.

Several uncontrolled studies involving small numbers of patients support the efficacy of systemic CSA for treatment of corneal ulceration with or without scleral melting[123, 159, 160] and for peripheral ulcerative keratitis associated with Wegener's granulomatosis.[161, 162] Use of systemic CSA was also successful in preventing corneal transplant rejection in high-risk eyes; the overall success rate during the follow-up period was impressive.[163, 164]

Despite its poor penetration into the eye, topical CSA has been successfully used in treatment of a variety of immune-mediated ocular surface phenomena, including ligneous conjunctivitis,[165, 166] vernal conjunctivitis,[167–169] and high-risk corneal grafts.[170, 171] Its efficacy for the latter indication should be clarified by the long-awaited results of a multicenter clinical trial, and the usefulness of topical CSA for other oculocutaneous disorders, such as Sjögren's syndrome and atopic keratoconjunctivitis, is under investigation.

DOSAGE AND ROUTE OF ADMINISTRATION

Our philosophy regarding the care of patients with uveitis in general has been one of complete intolerance of even low-grade inflammation and a limited tolerance of steroid use in patients for whom alternative anti-inflammatory medication is a reasonable option, in an effort to limit permanent structural damage to vital ocular structures. For these reasons, in patients in whom conventional therapy has failed and in whom a reasonable chance for visual rehabilitation exists, we rely on the degree of vitreal and retinal inflammation rather than on visual acuity as the parameters determining the threshold for initiation of CSA therapy, subsequent dosage adjustments, and the addition of other steroid-sparing agents. Provided that no contraindication to its use exists (uncontrolled systemic hypertension, abnormal renal or liver function tests, pregnancy, or drug hypersensitivity), we initiate CSA therapy at 2.5 mg/kg/day, once daily, with dosage increments of 50 mg to a maximum of 5 mg/kg/day and titrated to the clinical response (see Table 12–1). If no response is observed at this dosage after 1 month, we occasionally increase the dosage to 7.5 mg/kg/day for no more than 4 weeks and taper it to 5 mg/kg/day once inflammation has been controlled. If no response is evident after 3 months of treatment, the medication is discontinued. If, on the other hand, a favorable response is achieved, we attempt to taper systemic steroids and maintain the lowest possible dose of CSA that provides an adequate therapeutic effect, while minimizing toxicity, for at least 1 year.

In our experience and that of other investigators,[145, 146] recurrent inflammation is most often associated with attempted reductions of CSA dosage, necessitating a compensatory upward dosage adjustment or addition of a steroid-sparing agent such as azathioprine.

Nussenblatt and colleagues advocate initial therapy with combined low-dose CSA (2.5 mg/kg/day twice daily) and reduced-dose prednisone (0.2 to 0.5 mg/kg/day) for 2 to 3 months, with subsequent taper of either CSA or steroid, depending on the clinical response and the needs of the patient.[125] Not only has this strategy proved effective,[150, 154, 158] but combination therapy with other adjunctive agents such as bromocriptine[172] and ketoconazole[173] has also been advocated to reduce the dosage of CSA necessary to achieve inflammatory control and thus decrease both the risk of untoward toxicity and the cost of therapy (described in section on Adjuvants to Immunosuppressive Therapy).

Ben Ezra and associates[174] have proposed guidelines for use of low-dose CSA in Adamantiades-Behçet disease, the fundamental principles of which have been extended and are shared by most investigators in caring for patients with noninfectious bilateral, intermediate, or posterior uveitis. This entails evaluation and treatment of patients for evidence of untoward renal or hypertensive effects before and during therapy, with vigilant attention paid to increases in the serum creatinine levels more than 30% above baseline and to physical parameters (sustained systolic blood pressure [BP] more than 140 mm Hg or diastolic BP more than 90 mm Hg), which might require dosage reduction or cessation of therapy. Correspondingly, a complete hemogram with differential, serum creatinine, and BUN determinations, as well as urinalysis, and liver function tests should be obtained before therapy is initiated and they should be repeated periodically, together with determination of creatinine clearance, to monitor potential CSA-induced toxic effects.

Although adjusting the dose of CSA according to trough levels may result in a more favorable clinical course than will a fixed dose regimen,[124] routine sampling of the trough level is probably not necessary with lower initial drug doses (2.5 to 5 mg/kg/day) if renal function is carefully monitored. In circumstances in which blood monitoring might be judicious (hepatic dysfunction or patient noncompliance), the trough level should be obtained 12 hours after the last dose. More accurate measurements are obtained from whole blood than from serum levels[175, 176] and with daily doses of CSA greater than 3 mg/kg/day. Although acceptable trough values for kidney and bone marrow recipients range from 100 to 250 mg/ml,[177, 178] corresponding values for low-dose regimens used in ocular disease have not been definitively established. Furthermore, reference ranges vary depending on the measurement method used.

SIDE EFFECTS AND TOXICITY

Most of the toxic side effects of CSA therapy described in the literature were reported in association with high-dose (10 mg/kg/day) schedules in organ transplant recipients. Although current low-dose regimens (5 mg/kg/day) produce fewer adverse reactions, nephrotoxicity and hypertension are the most common and worrisome

events encountered by ophthalmologists, particularly with the chronic administration of CSA (see Table 12–3).

Nephrotoxicity is manifested clinically by increased serum creatinine with a disproportionate increase in BUN, preserved urine output and sodium reabsorption, decreased creatinine clearance, and in the extreme, systemic hypertension.[179] Dose-dependent CSA alterations in renal hemodynamics, including vasoconstriction of the afferent glomerular arteriole with subsequent decrease in renal blood flow, are believed to produce a reduction in glomerular filtration rate (GFR).[148] Initially, CSA-induced nephrotoxicity is reversible by dose reduction; however, chronic, irreversible, interstitial fibrosis and renal tubular atrophy can occur, particularly in patients treated with high doses or in whom the serum creatinine is allowed to remain at persistently increased levels. Indeed, initial studies with high-dose CSA indicated that nephrotoxicity, as demonstrated by renal biopsy, may precede an increase in serum creatinine, suggesting that serum creatinine underestimates the potential for renal damage and should not be used as the sole marker of renal toxicity.[180] Subsequent work has shown that minimal pathologic changes, as evidenced by renal biopsy, are produced when lower starting doses (7.5 mg/kg/day or less) are used.[181, 182]

Nevertheless, functional changes are still observed, as manifested by an increase in serum creatinine levels and the frequent occurrence of systemic hypertension during the first 12 months of low-dose CSA (mean maintenance 4.0 ± 1.1 mg/kg/day) therapy, either alone or in combination with systemic steroids.[153–155] Clinicopathologic data from a recent large series of patients with autoimmune or inflammatory disease treated with a maintenance dose of CSA 5 mg/kg/day or less suggest, however, that their functional perturbations are not likely to translate into permanent renal damage provided that the serum creatinine remains within 30% of its baseline value.[183] Furthermore, these data indicate that CSA-associated nephropathy may be related more to the maximal dose administered rather than to the cumulative effects of smaller doses. We[156] and other investigators[184] have shown that the potential for serious renal complications may be reduced if initial doses of 2.5 or 5 mg/kg daily are used rather than 7.5 or 10 mg/kg daily and if vigilant attention is paid to renal functional indexes.

Hypertension develops, or is exacerbated, in a dose-dependent reversible fashion in approximately 15% to 25% of patients within the first few weeks of initiation of CSA therapy.[185] Hypertension is more common in patients treated with the combination of CSA and steroids than in patients treated with CSA alone[186] and in those with impaired renal function.[50] An abrupt increase in systemic BP after prolonged CSA therapy, particularly in obese patients, may signal imminent renal toxicity and should prompt the clinician to obtain a trough CSA level and check the serum creatinine.[125] Systemic hypertension promptly responds to dosage reduction in most cases, and its presence, before or during therapy, does not constitute a contraindication to use of CSA, provided that it is aggressively controlled.

Although CSA does not induce leukopenia, it is associated with a normochromic, normocytic anemia in 25% of patients, an increased sedimentation rate in 40% of patients,[187] and a mild, dose-dependent increase in the serum transaminases and bilirubin levels.[124] Hyperuricemia and gouty arthritis[188] are common among transplant recipients, and increases in total serum cholesterol due to an increased low-density lipoprotein fraction have also been reported in such patients treated with CSA.[189]

Lymphoproliferative disease has developed in patients receiving CSA; however, these neoplasms do not appear to be due to the drug itself but rather to immunosuppression in general. The incidence of lymphoma was no greater in patients receiving CSA than in those treated with other immunosuppressive agents in a large clinical series of 5000 transplant recipients who were monitored for 5 years.[123] Whereas CSA is known to increase serum prolactin levels, causing gynecomastia in men and promoting the growth of benign breast adenomas in women, no definitive association between breast carcinoma and CSA has been demonstrated to date.[125]

Other common adverse reactions include paresthesias and temperature hypersensitivity, which develops within days of initiation of CSA therapy, as well as nausea and vomiting, none of which usually require discontinuation of therapy.[110] Hirsutism of mild to moderate degree may develop in 50% of patients during the first few months of therapy, as well as gingival hyperplasia, exacerbated by poor oral hygiene, in as many as 25% of patients.[123] Neurotoxicity, as manifested by a fine hand tremor that usually abates during therapy, and a reversible myopathy have been detected in patients after liver transplantation.[16, 50] An increased risk of opportunistic infections with herpesviruses, *Candida,* and *Pneumocystis* is a potential complication of immunosuppression with CSA.[51]

Ocular side effects due to systemic use of CSA include decreased vision, lid erythema and nonspecific conjunctivitis, visual hallucinations, and conjunctival and retinal hemorrhages secondary to anemia. Topically applied CSA is reasonably well tolerated, although eyelid irritation and burning sensation may occur.[49]

OVERDOSE

Experience with overdosage with CSA is minimal. Transient hepatotoxicity and nephrotoxicity, together with hypertension, dysesthesias, flushing, and GI upset, may occur, lasting no more than a few days.[114] General supportive measures and symptomatic treatment should be instituted, as in all cases of drug overdosage.

HIGH-RISK GROUPS

CSA readily crosses the placenta to the fetus. Although it has been shown to be embryotoxic and fetotoxic in experimental animals, it is not an animal teratogen, and the limited experience in women thus far indicates that it is unlikely to be a human teratogen.[190] Successful pregnancies have been reported in patients receiving CSA, with growth retardation being the most common problem in infants exposed to the drug in utero.[190] Nevertheless, CSA should be used during pregnancy only when the potential benefit justifies the risk to the fetus. Because the drug is excreted in the human milk, it is to be avoided in nursing mothers.

Although no well-controlled studies have been conducted in the pediatric age group, CSA has been used successfully in children without undue adverse effects. Higher doses of drug are necessary in children, because the clearance rate in children is 45% higher than in adults.[175] The converse is true in the elderly and in patients with hepatic disease in whom drug clearance is slower; therefore, they are at increased risk of development of toxic side effects.

CONTRAINDICATIONS

Contraindications to the use of CSA include uncontrolled systemic hypertension, hepatic disease, renal insufficiency, pregnancy, and a history of hypersensitivity to the drug.

DRUG INTERACTIONS

There are many important drug interactions associated with CSA. Synergistic nephrotoxicity may occur with concomitant use of aminoglycosides, amphotericin B, ketoconazole, vancomycin, melphalan, cimetidine, ranitidine, trimethoprim with sulfamethoxazole, ciprofloxacin, and NSAIDs.[22] By inhibiting the local prostaglandin production, NSAIDs potentiate CSA nephrotoxicity by further compromising renal blood flow.[50] NSAIDs have been shown to produce a transient yet significant increase in serum creatinine when used with CSA,[191] an effect that may prove particularly problematic because of the widespread availability of these drugs.

Because CSA is extensively metabolized by the hepatic microsomal enzyme system, drugs that affect cytochrome P-450 will alter blood levels of the drug. Medications that have been reported to inhibit these enzymes and thus increase CSA levels include verapamil, diltiazem, ketoconazole, fluconazole, itraconazole, danazol, bromocriptine, metoclopramide, erythromycin, and methylprednisolone.[22] Drugs that induce cytochrome P-450, thereby reducing the level of CSA, include rifampin, phenytoin, phenobarbital, and carbamazepine.[22]

Other drug interactions include digitalis toxicity resulting from an apparent reduction in the volume of distribution of digitalis when it is administered with CSA,[50] convulsions with concomitant administration of large doses of methylprednisolone, and reversible myopathy with rhabdomyolysis with combined lovastatin and CSA therapy.[22]

MAJOR CLINICAL TRIALS

Major clinical trials are described in the Therapeutic Use section.

FK 506 and Sirolimus (Rapamycin)

FK 506 and sirolimus (rapamycin) are among the more promising immunosuppressive agents that resemble CSA in their effects without producing cytotoxicity. FK 506, now known as tacrolimus (Prograf, Fujisawa, Deerfield, IL), was recently approved by the FDA for prophylaxis of organ rejection for patients undergoing allogenic liver transplantation. For the sake of simplicity and to avoid confusion, we refer to this drug by its original investigational name, FK 506, because it is referenced as such in the literature.

FK 506 is a macrolide antibiotic that was discovered in 1984 at the Fujisawa Pharmaceutical Company during a routine screening for naturally occurring immunosuppressive agents; it was extracted from the fermentation broth of a strain of soil fungus, *Streptomyces tsukubaensis*, found in the Tsukuba region of Japan.[192] This compound was shown to have a spectrum of activity similar to that of CSA in experimental models of transplantation and autoimmunity. Clinical trials with FK 506 were initiated in February 1989 at the University of Pittsburgh, primarily involving liver transplantation and subsequently extended to heart, kidney, and small bowel transplantation. Its early success in this arena, with the demonstration that steroids could be tapered more rapidly with FK 506 than with CSA, suggested that FK 506 might be applicable to other clinical conditions as monotherapy.[126] Mochizuki and associates[193] were the first to establish the efficacy of FK 506 in the treatment of uveitis, both in experimental animals and in patients.

Sirolimus (rapamycin) is also a macrolide antibiotic that was discovered as an antifungal agent produced by *Streptomyces hygroscopicus* and isolated from a soil sample collected from Easter Island (RAPA Nui).[194] Despite its structural similarity to FK 506 and its similar immunosuppressive effectiveness in experimental transplant models, sirolimus was discovered to have a mechanism of action distinct from those of FK 506 and CSA. Likewise, because its toxicity may be caused by distinct mechanisms, sirolimus may prove useful as the sole agent or provide a strategy for combination therapy with CSA that maximizes immunosuppression and mitigates drug toxicity.[126] No information regarding use of sirolimus in humans is available at present because the drug is presently undergoing phase I trials. One report, however, indicated that sirolimus is useful in treatment of autoimmune uveitis in rats.[195]

OFFICIAL DRUG NAME AND CHEMISTRY
FK 506, now known as tacrolimus (Prograf, Fujisawa), is a 822-kDa molecule ($C_{44}H_{69}NO_{12} \cdot H_2O$) (see Fig. 12–7). It is insoluble in water, but readily dissolves in organic solvents such as methanol, ethanol, and acetone.[196]

Sirolimus (rapamycin) ($C_{51}H_{79}NO_{13}$) has a molecular weight of 914.2 kDa and shares the unusual hemiketal masked α, β-diketo amide moiety with FK 506 yet has a larger ring structure and a unique triene segment (see Fig. 12–8).[197]

PHARMACOLOGY
FK 506 and CSA, although structurally distinct, share many pharmacologic properties, including a similar mechanism of action (see Fig. 12–9). In essence, both FK 506 and CSA, complexed with their respective binding proteins, suppress cell-mediated immunity in a synergistic fashion by inhibiting DNA translation of specific lymphokines (IL-2, IL-3, IL-4, and IFN-8) and the expression of the IL-2 receptor on activated T cells. FK 506, however, is at least 10 times more potent than CSA, both in vitro and in vivo.[127] Sirolimus, on the other hand, blunts the response of T cells and B cells to specific lymphokines rather than inhibiting their production.[131, 132]

CLINICAL PHARMACOLOGY
Although sirolimus and FK 506 share similar immunosuppressive potencies and structural characteristics and even

bind to the same immunophilin (FK binding position), they affect immune cells in vitro quite differently. Although it is not cytotoxic, sirolimus differs from FK 506 in that protein synthesis in resting lymphocytes and constitutive DNA synthesis in transformed cells is inhibited.[126] Whereas FK 506 and CSA inhibit Ca^{2+}-dependent T-cell activation, thereby preventing transcription of early-phase lymphokine genes, sirolimus blocks both Ca^{2+}-dependent and independent T-cell activation without preventing the expression of these genes.[131, 133, 198, 199] In contrast to FK 506 and CSA, sirolimus has no effect on the expression of the IL-2 receptor. In addition, sirolimus blocks Ca^{2+}-dependent T-cell division at a later stage in the cell cycle than does FK 506 or CSA by preventing the advancement of cells into S phase by acting in late G (FK 506), as opposed to blocking cell division at the G_0-G_1 interface (CSA).[198] As a consequence, sirolimus inhibits the proliferation of activated T cells even when added 12 hours after stimulation, whereas FK 506 and CSA are effective only if added in the first few hours after T-cell stimulation.[128]

On a molecular level, whereas the sirolimus-FK–binding protein complex is necessary for its inhibitory action, the precise target analogous to calcineurin for FK 506 and CSA has yet to be identified. Sirolimus does not affect NF-AT translocation, but is believed to inhibit T cell activation in G_1 instead by inhibiting the activity of phosphatase enzymes.[199] Whatever the ultimate putative target might be, the common sirolimus/FK 506-immunophilin complex interacts with other molecules to create functionally different complexes that mediate the particular suppressive effects for each drug.[198]

In essence, sirolimus, unlike FK 506 or CSA, does not consistently inhibit the synthesis of IL-2, its receptor, or other lymphokines but instead acts like a functional antagonist to cytokine action, inhibiting the proliferation of T cells in response to IL-2 and IL-4. Because of their differential actions throughout the cell cycle, FK 506 and CSA exert their action on resting T cells and are unlikely to have an immunosuppressive effect once T cells have been fully activated, whereas the antiproliferative effects of sirolimus are independent of the commitment step in T-cell activation.[131, 132]

Finally, all three agents are immune selective, with the thrust of immunosuppression resulting from inhibition of helper T-cell activities. In addition, FK 506 may selectively prevent maturation of helper T cells in the thymus,[198] whereas sirolimus suppresses a wider spectrum of both T- and B-cell activation pathways.[131, 132]

The powerful immunosuppressive properties of FK 506 in vivo are manifested by its ability to prolong the survival of a variety of organ and skin grafts in rodents, dogs, nonhuman primates, and humans.[196] Moreover, the demonstration that FK 506 can reverse ongoing acute or early chronic liver rejection distinguishes it from CSA.[200] Its apparent hepatotropic properties, as compared with those of other agents, are poorly understood but may explain its early success in liver transplantation. Sirolimus has also been shown to suppress acute rejection of organ and skin allografts in rodents and in nonhuman primates as well as to mitigate GVH and host-versus-graft (HVG) reactions.[198]

PHARMACEUTICS

FK 506, which is marketed as tacrolimus (Prograf, Fujisawa), is available for oral administration as capsules containing 1 mg or 5 mg anhydrous drug or as a sterile solution for intravenous injection. The intravenous injection contains the equivalent of 5 mg anhydrous FK 506 in 1 ml polyoxyl 60 hydrogenated castor oil and dehydrated alcohol. It is supplied as an ampule, which is diluted in either 0.9% sodium chloride or 5% dextrose in water before use.

Sirolimus is an investigational agent, and attempts to create a single formulation suitable for all routes of administration have not been successful. Because sirolimus is extremely insoluble in aqueous physiologic buffers, attempts to deliver the drug orally in a 0.2% carboxymethylcellulose suspension or parenterally in a Cremophor EL–based vehicle have resulted in variable drug bioavailability in experimental animals.[197] To date, sirolimus solubilized in a polysorbate/polyethylene glycol (PEG)–based solution, delivered by continuous intravenous infusion, affords the best opportunity to study the intrinsic properties of the drug.[197, 198]

PHARMACOKINETICS AND METABOLISM

FK 506 is variably and poorly absorbed from the GI tract after oral administration. The absolute oral bioavailability may range from 5% to 67% (mean 27%) in transplant patients with various degrees of hepatic function.[22] A peak plasma concentration of 0.5 to 5.6 mg/L (as measured by enzyme-linked immunosorbent assay [ELISA] using a monoclonal anti-FK 506 antibody) was observed within 0.5 to 8 hours of a single oral dose of 0.15 mg/kg, whereas the concentration detected after intravenous infusion of a similar dose of drug administered in 2 hours ranged from 10 to 24 mg/L.[201] Although trough plasma concentrations have been reported to correlate poorly with the dose, apparently a close correlation exists between the area under the FK 506 concentration-time curve and the concentrations of drug in whole blood and plasma.[201] Unlike that of cyclosporine, FK 506 absorption is not dependent on the availability of bile in the gut; however, the presence of food may decrease its absorption.[22]

FK 506 is widely distributed throughout the bodily tissues, with a large volume of distribution (1300 L), conferred largely by its highly lipophilic nature.[201] In the vascular compartment, the drug is highly bound to erythrocytes, with a mean blood plasma trough concentration of 10:1.[22] The differential plasma-erythrocyte distribution of FK 506 is influenced by the drug concentration, hematocrit, and temperature. Plasma concentrations at 37°C are approximately twice those at 24°C; therefore, the plasma and whole blood concentrations of drug are nonlinearly related.[201] In plasma, FK 506 is highly bound (88%) to plasma proteins, chiefly albumin.

FK 506 is extensively metabolized in the liver by N-demethylation and hydroxylation, with less than 1% of the parent compound being excreted unchanged in the bile, feces, or urine in a 48-hour period.[202] Two of the nine metabolites of FK 506 have been shown to retain immunosuppressive activity in vitro.[201] The plasma elimi-nation t½, varies, from 3.5 to 40.5 hours (mean 8.7 hours).[22]

Like CSA, FK 506 has a dose-dependent effect on different components of the hepatic mixed function oxidate system, with consequent alterations in its own metabolism induced by drugs that either induce or inhibit cytochrome P-450. Similarly, because of its extensive hepatic metabolism, the plasma concentration, t½, and clearance of FK 506 are increased in patients with liver disease, whereas patients with renal impairment are not expected to show similar alterations in these parameters.[201]

The pharmacokinetics of sirolimus remain unknown, due largely to the limited sensitivity of most readily available assays for detection of picogram quantities of drug in the bodily fluids. The development of an ELISA with monoclonal antibodies of sufficient sensitivity may obviate this problem and provide a practical method for routine screening of drug levels.[191]

THERAPEUTIC USE

FK 506. Although the therapeutic efficacy and benefits of FK 506 in prevention and reversal of organ transplantation, particularly hepatic, are implicit given its approval by the FDA for this purpose, the application of this drug for treatment of other autoimmune phenomena is now under investigation in both animal models and in humans (see Table 12–4). FK 506 has been shown to prevent the development of experimental collagen-induced arthritis,[203] insulin-dependent diabetes,[204] autoimmune glomerulonephritis,[205] and experimental allergic encephalomyelitis (EAE)[206] in rats, and to reduce proteinuria significantly and prolong survival in a mouse model (New Zealand black/white [NZB/W] hybrid) of systemic lupus erythematosus.[207] Kawashima and colleagues[208, 209] demonstrated that FK 506 suppresses development of experimental autoimmune uveitis (EAU) in rats at doses 10 to 30 times lower than CSA doses when administered from 0 to 14 days postimmunization with uveitogenic antigen.[208, 209] Subsequent work has shown the effectiveness of FK 506 in suppressing induction of EAU in primates.[210]

Although experience with FK 506 in human autoimmune disease has been limited, both the efficacy and therapeutic potential of this agent have been demonstrated in several entities, including psoriasis,[211] nephrotic syndrome,[212] and noninfectious uveitis.[213] With regard to the latter, Mochizuki and coworkers[213] reported favorable results in an open, multicentered study in which FK 506 was used as monotherapy in the treatment of 53 patients (41 with Adamantiades-Behçet disease) with refractory uveitis. The majority (76.5%) were judged to have disease reduction, after dosage adjustments, during the 12-week trial. Visual acuity remained stable or improved in 72.9% of 96 treated eyes, and the number of recurrent ocular inflammatory episodes in Adamantiades-Behçet disease patients was markedly reduced. Furthermore, for reasons that are not clear, FK 506 therapy was effective in 7 of 11 patients who had been refractory to prior treatment with CSA.[213]

DOSAGE AND ROUTE OF ADMINISTRATION

In the study of Mochizuki and colleagues,[213] the therapeutic efficacy of FK 506 administered orally for refractory noninfectious uveitis was dosage dependent. A daily dose of 0.05 mg/kg/day orally was inadequate in most patients, whereas a daily dose of 0.1 to 0.15 mg/kg/day proved efficacious, with little associated toxicity, and this dose was suggested for appropriate maintenance[213] (see Table 12–1). Higher doses (0.15 and 2.0 mg/kg/day), although more effective than 0.1 mg/kg/day, produced various undesirable side effects, requiring careful monitoring. In addition, it was recommended that FK 506 trough levels be maintained between 15 and 25 mg/ml, because these levels correlate with both therapeutic efficacy and the incidence of adverse side effects. Finally, as with CSA, a complete hemogram, liver function tests, and serum BUN and creatinine determinations performed before the initiation of therapy, as well as determination of creatinine clearance, repeated periodically (every 3 to 4 months), are necessary.

Sirolimus (Rapamycin). In addition to its beneficial effects on experimental organ allografts, sirolimus, like FK 506, has been shown to be effective treatment for autoimmune disease in experimental animals.[130, 195, 214] Roberge and colleagues[195] have demonstrated the efficacy of sirolimus in preventing development of EAU in rats, dose dependently, when administered for 14 days by continuous intravenous (IV) infusion, whether initiated on the day of, or 1 week after, disease induction. At doses of 0.1 and 0.5 mg/kg IV, sirolimus prevented EAU in 12 of 14 rats in each dose group, whereas at a dose of 1 mg/kg, sirolimus completely suppressed disease development.[195]

The synergistic effect between sirolimus and CSA observed in vitro and in rodent and canine models of organ transplantation[129, 197] has also been demonstrated in a rat model of EAU[215]; in this study, intramuscular (IM) injection of CSA (2 mg/kg) prevented the onset of disease in only 3 of the 15 animals, whereas in combination with sirolimus (0.01 mg/kg IV), it prevented development of EAU completely. These observations, together with sirolimus's unique immunosuppressive profile, indicate its high clinical potential, particularly in combination with CSA or other immunosuppressive agents, in the treatment of autoimmune uveitis. Such combination strategies might provide maximal therapeutic efficacy at the lowest possible dose of either agent and thereby limit the potential toxic consequences of treatment.[216]

SIDE EFFECTS AND TOXICITY

FK 506. FK 506 and CSA share similar major side effect profiles (nephrotoxicity, hypertension, neurotoxicity, and hyperglycemia); however, hirsutism, gingival hyperplasia, and coarsening of facial features have not been reported in patients treated with FK 506[215] (see Table 12–3). The major dose-limiting side effect is chronic nephrotoxicity, the overall incidence, clinical presentation, and pathophysiology of which are essentially the same as those of CSA. Although the GFR appears to be less adversely affected by FK 506 in the long term, its effect on renal structural integrity with prolonged use requires further study.[201] Renal impairment developed in 28.3% of 53 patients treated with FK 506 for refractory uveitis, and although this side effect was dose dependent, transient, and mild in most patients, it was severe enough to require discontinuation of therapy in 3.[213]

Neurologic side effects reported in transplant patients most often occur after intravenous administration and range in severity from minor reactions (headache, paresthesias, tremors, and sleep disturbances) in approximately 20% of patients to major neurotoxicity (expressive aphasia, seizures, akinetic mutism, encephalopathy, and coma), reported in less than 10%.[201] In the FK 506 uveitis study, neurologic symptoms, including a meningitis-like clinical picture, developed dose dependently after oral administration in 12 of 53 patients and resolved with dosage reduction or discontinuation of therapy.[213]

Other adverse reactions reported by Mochizuki and colleagues[213] in their FK 506 uveitis study included GI symptoms (18.9% of 53 patients) and transient hyperglycemia (13.2% of 53 patients). Among transplant patients, transient hyperglycemia commonly occurs in the perioperative period, with as many as 20% of patients requiring insulin therapy at 6 months; at 1 year, as few as 5.5% are still insulin dependent.[201]

Opportunistic bacterial, viral, and fungal infections are potential complications of immunosuppression with either FK 506 or CSA. Although 20% of FK 506–treated transplant patients developed CMV infections at the University of Pittsburgh Medical Center, no patient treated with this agent for nontransplant indications developed such an infection.[217] The incidence of post-transplant lymphoproliferative disorders at the same institution in association with FK 506 was reported to be 1.6%.[218]

Whereas systemic hypertension may occur with either CSA or FK 506, its incidence is less frequent[217] and discontinuation of antihypertensive therapy is more common with FK 506.[201] In addition, both drugs have been associated with the rare occurrence of hemolytic anemia; however, unlike with CSA, with FK 506 hypercholesterolemia is not a complication of therapy.[201]

OVERDOSE

There is little experience with FK 506 overdose. It produces no unique reactions other than the toxic side effects previously described, and treatment consists of general supportive measures, as in any case of drug overdosage.[219] Owing to the extensive plasma protein and erythrocyte binding of FK 506, it is unlikely that hemodialysis would be an effective intervention.

Sirolimus (Rapamycin). Although it may be tempting to extend conclusions regarding drug toxicity in animal models to humans, such an approach is often confounded by significant inconsistencies, as experience with both CSA and FK 506 has shown. For example, the major dose-limiting toxicity of both agents in clinical practice is nephrotoxicity, whereas in animal models therapeutic doses of CSA were relatively nontoxic.[197] Although it produces severe anorexia and widespread vasculitis in dogs, FK 506 is well tolerated in rodents[216] and has a favorable therapeutic index in humans despite intercurrent neurotoxicity and nephrotoxicity.[220] Nevertheless, sirolimus apparently is not nephrotoxic in animals. Continuous intravenous infusion of drug for 14 days in hypertensive rats produced little alteration in the clinical indices of renal function (urine output, plasma creatinine, and creatinine clearance), and histologic examination of the kidneys showed significant pathologic changes.[197] Sirolimus administered in a similar manner produced an initial body weight loss in rats during the first week of treatment, with normal weight gain thereafter.[195] In a murine model of CMV infection, sirolimus produced less susceptibility to primary CMV infection than CSA, and combined CSA-sirolimus regimens did not increase the morbidity of hosts carrying latent virus.[197]

HIGH-RISK GROUPS

Because of its extensive metabolism by the liver, blood levels of FK 506 may be significantly increased in patients with hepatic impairment, placing them at risk of development of neurotoxicity and nephrotoxicity.[216] Likewise, patients with underlying renal disease may require dosage adjustments and risk further compromise in their kidney function as a consequence of FK 506-induced nephrotoxicity. Elderly patients, who may have both reduced renal and hepatic reserves, should be carefully monitored for development of toxic side effects. Because of its hyperglycemic and hypertensive effects, patients with diabetes mellitus and systemic hypertension also require vigilant monitoring and medical control if FK 506 is to be implemented.

FK 506 does not exhibit mutagenic activity in vivo or in vitro. Fetotoxicity has been demonstrated in animals, and teratogenic effects have been observed.[127] FK 506 crosses the placenta. Although no well-controlled studies of pregnant women have been conducted, FK 506 during pregnancy has been associated with neonatal hyperkalemia and renal dysfunction.[219] Therefore, its use during pregnancy should be reserved for circumstances in which the potential benefit to the mother justifies the risk to the fetus. Because FK 506 is excreted in human milk, it should be avoided during nursing.

Children have undergone successful liver transplantation with FK 506 immunosuppression.[201] As with CSA, pediatric patients receiving FK 506 generally require higher doses to maintain adequate blood trough levels.

CONTRAINDICATIONS

Anaphylactic reactions have occurred with use of FK 506, most often in patients receiving injectable preparations of FK 506 containing castor oil derivatives.[219] Therefore, FK 506 is contraindicated in patients with a known hypersensitivity to the drug or vehicle. It is further recommended that patients receiving intravenous therapy receive oral drug instead as soon as it can be tolerated.

DRUG INTERACTIONS

The same potential for synergistic nephrotoxicity previously described for CSA (described in CSA, Drug Interactions section) exists with coadministration of FK 506 and agents with known renal toxic effects. For this reason, CSA and FK 506 should not be used simultaneously.[201]

FK 506, like CSA, is metabolized by cytochrome P-450; therefore, drugs that either potentiate or inhibit these enzymes are expected to produce corresponding changes in FK 506 metabolism, with respective decreased or increased blood levels of FK 506 during concomitant administration. Those drugs producing either increased or decreased blood levels of FK 506 because of their effects on the hepatic microsomal enzymes are identical to those

previously described for CSA (CSA, Drug Interactions section).[201]

As during treatment with other immunosuppressive agents. vaccinations may be less effective during treatment with FK 506. Use of live vaccines should be avoided.[219]

MAJOR CLINICAL TRIALS

Major clinical trials are described in the Therapeutic Use section.

Etanercept

HISTORY AND SOURCE

Etanercept is a fusion protein created and developed by Immunex Corporation and receiving FDA approval for the treatment of patients with rheumatoid arthritis who had not responded adequately to one or more other disease-modifying antirheumatic drugs in 1999. It is composed of soluble TNF receptor and a human IgG Fc fragment. The concept of developing such an agent that would compete for TNF occupancy derived from the discovery of TNF as an important cytokine involved in the immunopathology of rheumatoid arthritis.

OFFICIAL DRUG NAME AND CHEMISTRY

Etanercept (Enbrel, Immunex Corporation) is a fusion protein composed of dimeric soluble p75 TNF receptor and human IgG Fc fragment.

PHARMACOLOGY

Etanercept inhibits TNF-α activity in vitro, and suppresses inflammation in animal models. Collagen-induced arthritis in mice is suppressed by etanercept therapy. Etanercept inhibits binding of both TNF-α and TNF-β to cell surface TNF receptors, rendering TNF biologically inactive. Therefore, it is capable of modulating biologic responses that are induced or regulated by TNF. Such responses include expression of adhesion molecules responsible for leukocyte migration, synthesis of inflammatory cytokines, and synthesis of matrix metalloproteinases.

CLINICAL PHARMACOLOGY

The safety and efficacy of Enbrel has been assessed in multiple randomized, double-masked clinical trials, both comparing the agent with placebo and with other disease-modifying antirheumatic drugs. It has been studied as an "add-on" drug, as well as a replacement drug. Its proven safety and efficacy prompted the United States Food and Drug Administration to approve its sale for treatment of rheumatoid arthritis in 1999. The drug is clearly efficacious, both as monotherapy and as an adjunctive therapy added to another disease-modifying agent in the care of patients with rheumatoid disease. Clinical response generally occurs between 1 and 2 weeks after the initiation of therapy, and a response always has occurred, if it is going to occur, by 3 months of therapy. In the trial of patients with juvenile rheumatoid arthritis, patients aged 4 to 17 with moderate to severe JRA that was refractory to (or the patient had been intolerant to) methotrexate were studied, while the patients continued to take a stable dose of a single NSAID or prednisone. Seventy-four percent of these children demonstrated a clear-cut clinical response, and these children were then randomized either to continue Enbrel or to be switched to a placebo. Twenty-four percent of the patients remaining on Enbrel experienced a flare of JRA disease activity over the ensuing 4 months, a strikingly lower number than those who had been switched to placebo (77%).

PHARMACEUTICS
Etanercept (Enbrel, Immunex Corporation, Seattle, WA) is supplied as a sterile, white, preservative-free powder for reconstitution with 1 ml of sterile bacteriostatic water for subsequent parenteral administration. The solution is clear and colorless, with a pH of 7.4. The lyophilized powder is supplied in single-use vials containing 25 mg of etanercept, 40 mg of mannitol, 10 mg of sucrose, and 1.2 mg of tromethamine.

PHARMACOKINETICS
The median t½ of etanercept after administration of 25 mg subcutaneously is 98 to 300 hours (median 115 hours). The maximum serum concentration is approximately 1.2 µg/ml. Serum levels increase with repeated dosing, and after 6 months of 25 mg subcutaneous administration twice weekly, serum levels reach a median of 3.0 µg/ml. Pediatric patients with juvenile rheumatoid arthritis (ages 4–17 years) administered 0.4 mg/kg of etanercept for up to 18 weeks achieved average serum concentrations of 2.1 µg/ml (range 0.7 to 4.3).

THERAPEUTIC USE
Etanercept is administered subcutaneously, 25 mg, twice weekly in the care of patients with adult or juvenile rheumatoid arthritis that is incompletely responsive to one or more other disease modifying agents. Its use as an adjunctive anti-inflammatory agent for ocular inflammatory disease is under study at the time of this writing.

SIDE EFFECTS AND TOXICITY
Because TNF plays an important role in inflammatory responses, including those in defense from infectious agents, inhibition of TNF may increase the risk of uncontrolled infection. Premarketing experience suggested that this might be the case, with 29% of patients receiving etanercept developing upper respiratory infections, compared with 16% of placebo-treated patients. Data from a sepsis clinical trial suggested that etanercept may increase the risk of death in patients who develop sepsis.

HIGH-RISK GROUPS
Patients with rheumatoid arthritis are at increased risk of infection-related death (2% to 7%) anyway, and this is further increased with immunosuppressive therapy (steroids, methotrexate, azathioprine). Adjunctive therapy with etanercept may increase this risk.

DRUG INTERACTIONS
Specific drug-interaction studies have, to date, been performed with etanercept.

Daclizumab

HISTORY AND SOURCE
Daclizumab (Zenapax, Hoffman-LaRoche, Inc.) was developed for treatment and prevention of solid organ transplant rejection. It is a "humanized" monoclonal antibody directed against the CD25 molecule (IL-2 receptor), which is dramatically upregulated on the surface of activated lymphocytes. It gained FDA approval in 1998.

OFFICIAL DRUG NAME AND CHEMISTRY
Daclizumab (Zenapax) is a humanized IgG$_1$ monoclonal antibody directed against the alpha chain of the CD25 molecule.

PHARMACOLOGY
Daclizumab binds to the alpha chain of CD25 or interleukin 2 receptor (IL-2r) and blocks IL-2–mediated responses.

CLINICAL PHARMACOLOGY
The safety and efficacy of Zenapax for the prophylaxis of acute organ transplant rejection in adult patients receiving their first cadaveric kidney transplant has been assessed in two randomized double-masked placebo-controlled multicenter trials,[221a] comparing a dose of 1.0 mg/kg body weight of Zenapax with placebo when each agent was administered as part of a standard immunosuppressive regimen containing either cyclosporin and corticosteroids or cyclosporin, corticosteroids, and azathioprine to prevent acute renal allograft rejection. Zenapax dosing was initiated within 24 hours before transplantation and subsequently was given every 14 days for a total of five doses. Zenapax significantly reduced the incidence of biopsy-proven acute renal allograft rejections, both at the 6-month and at the 12-month assessment periods. No difference in patient survival was observed. In a separate study, which was randomized and double masked, in which Zenapax or placebo was added to an immunosuppressive regimen of cyclosporin, mycophenolate mofetil, and steroids to assess tolerability, pharmacokinetics, and drug interactions, the addition of Zenapax to the immunosuppressive regimen did not result in an increased incidence of adverse events. The incidence of transplant rejection events was 12% in the group receiving Zenapax and was 20% in those patients who had placebo added to their cyclosporin, steroid, and mycophenolate mofetil immunosuppressive regimen.

PHARMACEUTICS
Zenapax 25 mg/5 ml is supplied as a clear, sterile, colorless concentrate for further dilution and intravenous administration. Each milliliter of Zenapax contains 5 mg of daclizumab.

PHARMACOKINETICS AND METABOLISM
Daclizumab has an in vivo t½ of 20 days, with complete saturation of the IL-2rα chain on circulating lymphocytes after dosing of 1 mg/kg once every 2 weeks. Estimated concentrations of daclizumab of 4 µg/ml for at least 3 months after initial dosing is in the appropriate therapeutic range for blocking IL-2–mediated responses.

THERAPEUTIC USE

The efficacy and safety of daclizumab have been tested in multicenter trials of reduction in the incidence of biopsy-proven acute renal allograft rejection. Daclizumab or placebo were added to the typical immunosuppressive regimen (e.g., prednisone, cyclosporin, and azathioprine). Patient survival was significantly greater at 1 year following transplantation in the daclizumab-treated group, as was allograft survival. Similar results were obtained in later trials in which mycophenolate mofetil, prednisone, and cyclosporine formed the basic immunosuppressive regimen.

SIDE EFFECTS AND TOXICITY

The incidence and types of adverse events observed in the pre-marketing studies were similar in both placebo-treated and in Zenapax-treated patients. All patients, of course, were already receiving a polypharmacologic immunosuppressive chemotherapeutic regimen of cyclosporine and corticosteroids with or without another immunosuppressant. The incidence of malignancy 1 year after treatment was 2.7% in the placebo group and 1.5% in the Zenapax group, and the overall incidence of infectious episodes was not higher in the Zenapax-treated patients compared with the placebo-treated patients.

HIGH-RISK GROUPS

The main high risk group consists of patients with known hypersensitivity to daclizumab.

DRUG INTERACTIONS

The following medications have been administered in clinical trials with Zenapax with limited experience in the delineation of drug interactions: cyclosporine, prednisone, mycophenolate mofetil, azathioprine, gancyclovir, acyclovir, tacrolimus, antithymocyte globulin, antilymphocyte globulin, and muromonab-CD3.

Dapsone

HISTORY AND SOURCE

Dapsone was first synthesized in 1908 by Fromm and Wittmann; however, it was not until the 1940s that the drug gained prominence as the first truly effective therapy for leprosy.[221] Today, dapsone is the mainstay of therapy for leprosy for more than 2 million people. In addition, it produces dramatic clinical effects in treatment of both dermatitis herpetiformis and bullous pemphigoid.[221] Person and Roger,[222] in the late 1970s, and Rogers and colleagues,[223] in the early 1980s, showed dapsone to be effective in controlling both the systemic and ocular inflammatory activity of cicatricial pemphigoid, a potentially blinding and fatal disease.

OFFICIAL DRUG NAME AND CHEMISTRY

Dapsone, 4,4'-diaminodiphenyl sulfone (DDS), molecular weight 248.3, is a synthetic sulfone. Its structural formula is shown in Figure 12–10.

PHARMACOLOGY

Dapsone has both antimicrobial and anti-inflammatory activity, although the mechanisms by which it influences the inflammatory and immune systems are not clear.

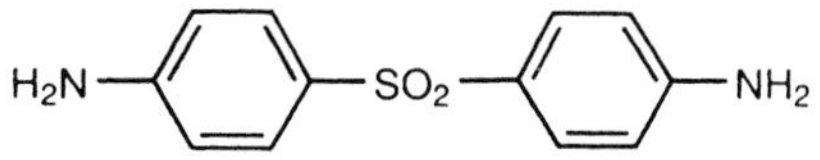

FIGURE 12–10. Chemical structure of dapsone.

CLINICAL PHARMACOLOGY

Antimicrobial Activity. Dapsone has both bactericidal and bacteriostatic activity against *Mycobacterium leprae*, readily penetrating bacterial cells. The mechanism of action is the same as that of the sulfonamides[224]; that is, dapsone competitively inhibits *p*-aminobenzoic acid (PABA) in the microorganism, thereby interrupting purine and, ultimately, nucleic acid biosynthesis. This inhibition is reversible when the sulfonamide is displaced by excess PABA.

Dapsone is also effective against plasmodia throughout its life cycle and retains full activity against plasmodia that have developed resistance to 4-aminoquinolone antimalarials.[225] This factor may explain the low prevalence of malaria in patients with leprosy who are treated with dapsone.[221] In addition, the antibiotic spectrum of dapsone has been expanded to include *Pneumocystis carinii* infection in patients with AIDS and cutaneous leishmaniasis.[226]

Anti-inflammatory Activity. Dapsone is believed to mediate its anti-inflammatory effects in dermatitis herpetiformis and pemphigoid by a variety of mechanisms. Evidence suggests that dapsone stabilizes lysosomal membranes, decreasing the release of their contents,[227, 228] and interferes with the myeloperoxidase-H_2O_2-halide–mediated cytotoxic system of neutrophils.[228, 229] In addition, dapsone has been shown to inhibit the Arthus reaction and adjuvant-induced arthritis in a manner similar to that of corticosteroids and indomethacin.[228]

PHARMACEUTICS

Dapsone (DDS, Jacobus, Princeton, NJ) is supplied as either 25- or 100-mg tablets. The drug may be stored at room temperature but should be protected from light.

PHARMACOKINETICS AND METABOLISM

Dapsone is slowly, yet almost completely, absorbed from the GI tract, reaching peak plasma levels within 4 to 6 hours of ingestion, and achieves steady-state serum levels in 1 week.[226] For inexplicable reasons, higher dapsone blood levels are achieved in women than in men.[230]

Dapsone is distributed throughout the total body water and in all tissues; however, it tends to be retained by the skin, liver, kidneys, and muscles[224] but penetrates ocular tissues poorly.[226] Dapsone undergoes extensive enterohepatic recirculation and tends to remain in the circulation for a long time, with a mean elimination t½ of 22 hours.[224]

Approximately 70% of dapsone is protein-bound and undergoes acetylation in the liver, the rate of which is genetically determined. Acetylation rate (slow versus fast) has no impact on the clinical efficacy of the drug or its associated adverse effects.[228] Dapsone and its metabolites are conjugated with glucuronic acid in the liver and excreted by the kidneys. Of a single 100-mg oral dose, 90% is eliminated in 9 days, with approximately 90% of the drug excreted in the urine and 10% excreted in the bile.[226]

THERAPEUTIC USE

Nonophthalmic uses of dapsone include treatment of leprosy, malaria, dermatitis, herpetiformis, bullous pemphigoid, cicatricial pemphigoid, pemphigus vulgaris, relapsing polychondritis, *P. carinii* infection in patients with AIDS, and cutaneous leishmaniasis.

Ophthalmic uses of dapsone include cicatricial pemphigoid affecting the conjunctiva (OCP) and scleritis associated with RP (see Table 12–4). Foster[35] confirmed the initial favorable outcomes reported by Person and Rogers[222] and Rogers and colleagues[223] in their use of dapsone for treatment of more than 130 patients with OCP: The progression of fibrosis was halted in 70% of cases. Dapsone is recommended as the first-line agent for treatment of OCP if the inflammatory activity is not severe, the disease is not rapidly progressive, and the patient is not glucose-6-phosphate dehydrogenase (G6-PD)–deficient.[16] A response is usually observed within 4 weeks of initiation of therapy.

Dapsone has also been shown to be useful in the treatment of the extraocular manifestations of RP[231, 232]; however, its efficacy with regard to the ocular manifestations of this disease is uncertain.[233] Using dapsone alone or in combination with NSAIDs or systemic corticosteroids, Hoang-Xuan and associates[32] reported a favorable response in 6 of 11 patients with simple or nodular scleritis associated with RP. Dapsone is ineffective in treatment of necrotizing scleritis associated with RP, because this entity is among the most recalcitrant ocular inflammatory diseases to even the most aggressive chemotherapeutic strategies.[30]

DOSAGE AND ROUTE OF ADMINISTRATION

Dapsone treatment is initiated at 25 mg, administered twice daily for 1 week (see Table 12–1). The dose is increased to 50 mg twice daily, with further adjustments depending on the clinical response and drug tolerance, to a maximum of 150 mg/day.[35] Slow dosage tapering to a maintenance level should begin once the inflammatory process is brought under control. Average dose reduction time is 8 months (range 4 months to 2.5 years).[51] Depending on the disease process, patients with OCP in whom dapsone therapy has failed or who exhibit severe progressive inflammatory disease usually respond to cyclophosphamide (described in Cyclophosphamide, Therapeutic Use section).

Patients with simple or nodular scleritis associated with RP in whom a combination of NSAID and dapsone has failed have systemic steroids added to their therapeutic regimen—typically 1 mg/kg/day with a rapid taper once the scleritis has completely resolved, with substitution of an alternate-day schedule once the 20-mg/day level has been reached. Steroids are then tapered as previously described (see Chapter 69, Corticosteroids, Therapeutic Use section). If the scleritis fails to respond to this combination, we add low-dose methotrexate (7.5 to 15 mg/wk) or daily azathioprine (2 mg/kg/day).[30] For necrotizing scleritis associated with RP, we most commonly use the combination of high-dose systemic corticosteroids and cyclophosphamide, resorting in some patients to once-weekly pulse therapy with the latter agent.[30]

Before therapy is initiated, baseline laboratory studies should be obtained, including a complete hemogram with differential and reticulocyte count, a chemistry profile including serum creatinine and BUN determinations, and liver function tests, urinalysis, and a G6-PD level. Because most patients receiving dapsone experience low-grade hemolysis, and because of its hepatotoxic potential, monitoring the hemogram and reticulocyte count early in the course of therapy, together with the liver function tests, is helpful in assessing whether a slow escalation in the dose is acceptable. We typically monitor the hemogram and reticulocyte count every 2 weeks for the first 3 months of therapy and every 6 weeks thereafter. Renal and hepatic function are monitored monthly during the first 3 months of therapy and then periodically every 3 to 4 months. Methemoglobin levels should be obtained only as clinically indicated (in patients with cardiopulmonary disease or methemoglobin reductase deficiency).[226]

SIDE EFFECTS AND TOXICITY

Dose-related hemolysis and methemoglobinemia are the most frequent adverse effects associated with dapsone therapy (see Table 12–3), the latter occurring in most patients receiving 200 mg or more of drug daily, irrespective of G6-PD levels.[234] In normal patients, anemia is usually not apparent until 3 to 4 weeks after initiation of therapy and rarely necessitates drug discontinuation. In contrast, hemolysis is more common and more severe and occurs at reduced dosages and earlier in the course of therapy in patients with G6-PD deficiency.[228] Dapsone is believed to mediate this reaction in G6-PD–deficient patients by oxidizing glutathione, the reduced form of which is essential to the protection of erythrocytes from hemolysis. Therefore, determining baseline G6-PD levels is mandatory in all patients for whom dapsone therapy is contemplated. Death resulting from agranulocytosis, aplastic anemia, and other blood dyscrasias has been reported in association with dapsone treatment.[235]

Other possible adverse effects of dapsone treatment include a reversible peripheral neuropathy, toxic hepatitis and cholestatic jaundice, GI intolerance, cutaneous hypersensitivity reactions, and a potentially fatal mononucleosis-like syndrome.[228, 234] The latter occurs rarely and is believed to be a hypersensitivity reaction characterized by fever, malaise, exfoliative dermatitis, methemoglobinemia, anemia. lymphadenopathy, and hepatomegaly with jaundice. Eosinophilia and an increased number of atypical lymphocytes are generally present.[226] The condition improves with dapsone discontinuation and institution of corticosteroid therapy.

OVERDOSE

Signs and symptoms of acute dapsone overdosage, appearing minutes to 24 hours after ingestion, include hyperexcitability, nausea, and vomiting.[114] Supportive measures, especially emesis induction and gastric lavage, should be instituted. Methemoglobinemia-induced depression, seizures, and severe cyanosis require immediate treatment with methylene blue (MB), 1 to 2 mg/kg IV, irrespective of the patient's methemoglobin reductase status.[236] If methemoglobin reaccumulates, the dose of MB may be repeated in 30 minutes. For nonemergent therapy, MB may be administered orally in doses of 3 to 5 mg/kg every 4 to 6 hours. Because MB reduction is dependent on G6-PD, it is contraindicated in G6-PD–deficient patients.[114]

HIGH-RISK GROUPS
Dapsone should be used with extreme caution in patients with G6-PD deficiency or methemoglobin reductase deficiency, leukopenia, severe anemia, liver disease, and renal insufficiency.[126] Elderly patients, who may have compromised hepatic and renal reserves, should likewise be monitored closely.

Dapsone readily crosses the placenta. Although it has been shown to be carcinogenic in laboratory rodents, no teratogenic or fetal abnormalities have been reported in humans.[22] Nevertheless, use of this medication in pregnant women has not been adequately studied, and one should not assume that it poses no risk to the fetus. Because dapsone is excreted in the breast milk in significant quantities, it should be avoided in nursing mothers to protect the neonate from potential hemolytic reactions. Dapsone may be safely used in the pediatric age group, in a schedule similar to that used for adults, but in reduced doses.[114]

CONTRAINDICATIONS
Dapsone is contraindicated in patients with a history of hypersensitivity to the drug or its derivatives, including sulfonamides.

DRUG INTERACTIONS
Probenecid may prolong the serum $t\frac{1}{2}$ of dapsone by reducing its renal excretion. Concurrent use with rifampin, on the other hand, may reduce the serum concentration of dapsone by as much as 10-fold, because it induces hepatic microsomal enzyme activity and thus dapsone metabolism.[22] Concomitant use of dapsone with drugs that can also cause anemia or leukopenia, such as folic acid antagonists and trimethoprim, requires vigilant hematologic monitoring.[226]

MAJOR CLINICAL TRIALS
Major clinical trials are described in the Therapeutic Use section.

Adjuvants to Immunosuppressive Therapy
Several agents have been used primarily as adjuvants to immunosuppressive drugs: bromocriptine or ketoconazole in combination with CSA as a dosage-lowering strategy and colchicine as a prophylactic agent in management of inflammatory recurrences in Adamantiades-Behçet disease.

Bromocriptine

HISTORY AND SOURCE
Bromocriptine, a semisynthetic ergot alkaloid, was initially developed in 1967 as an inhibitor of prolactin secretion and was subsequently shown to stimulate directly and compete with specific binding to dopaminergic receptors

in various tissues throughout the body.[236] Today, bromocriptine is widely used in the management of Parkinson's disease and in a wide range of conditions associated with hyperprolactinemia, including amenorrhea and galactorrhea, female infertility, postpartum lactation, and pituitary adenoma. With the demonstration of prolactin's powerful immunomodulatory properties, bromocriptine has been applied as an adjunctive agent in management of noninfectious ocular inflammatory disease in both animal models and in humans.[110]

OFFICIAL DRUG NAME AND CHEMISTRY
Bromocriptine mesylate (Parlodel, Sandoz), molecular weight 654.62, is an ergot derivative of lysergic acid. The addition of the bromine atom to this alkaloid confers its potent dopaminergic activity (Fig. 12–11).[237]

PHARMACOLOGY
The pharmacologic action of bromocriptine is directly related to its stimulation of dopamine receptors in the CNS, the cardiovascular system, the GI system, and the hypophysis-pituitary axis (HPA).[237] In the HPA, secretion of prolactin from the anterior pituitary is modulated by dopamine (prolactin inhibitory factor), which is synthesized in the hypothalmus and transported to its target by the hypothalamohypophyseal portal capillary system.[236] Bromocriptine, as a dopamine agonist, thereby inhibits prolactin secretion.

CLINICAL PHARMACOLOGY
Prolactin has potent effects on the immune system. Experimental studies in rats, in which prolactin levels were reduced either by hypophysectomy or bromocriptine administration, resulted in a marked decrease in both the humoral and cellular immune responses.[238, 239] In addition, prolactin stimulates lymphocyte activation, binds to receptors on B cells, and competes with cyclosporine for receptors on T cells.[240–242] Palestine and associates[243] demonstrated an enhanced effect of low-dose CSA used in combination with bromocriptine in treatment of experimental autoimmune uveitis. This effect was most pronounced in female animals with high prolactin levels, suggesting that the efficacy of a given dose of CSA is enhanced by bromocriptine's inhibition of prolactin secretion.

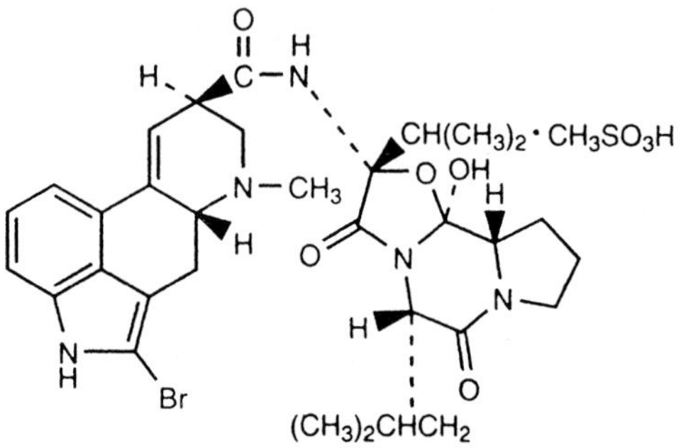

FIGURE 12–11. Chemical structure of bromocriptine.

PHARMACEUTICS

Bromocriptine (Parlodel, Sandoz) is formulated as 5-mg capsules and 2.5-mg tablets for oral use. It should be stored below 75°F in a light-resistant container.

PHARMACOKINETICS AND METABOLISM

Bromocriptine is rapidly absorbed after oral administration, achieving peak plasma levels in 1 to 3 hours, with a positive linear relationship between dose and peak plasma level over a wide range of doses.[236] First-pass metabolism of the absorbed dose is greater than 90%, with the majority (98%) being excreted in the feces and only 2% excreted in the urine.[22] The plasma t½ is 3 hours, and serum prolactin levels remain suppressed for as long as 14 hours after a single dose.[236]

THERAPEUTIC USE

No definitive indications for the use of bromocriptine in uveitis have been formulated (see Table 12–4). Bromocriptine alone was reported to be efficacious in the treatment of steroid-dependent, recurrent anterior uveitis in four patients with associated Parkinson's disease or hyperprolactinemia.[244] However, a similar effect was not observed in a small, randomized, double-masked study in which all subjects had pretreatment prolactin levels at the lower border of normal.[245] This study suggested that the use of bromocriptine in recurrent anterior uveitis may be limited to patients with concomitantly abnormal dopamine or prolactin levels.

The effective use of bromocriptine combined with low-dose CSA (4 mg/kg/day) as a dosage-lowering strategy was demonstrated by Palestine and colleagues in their treatment of 14 patients with bilateral, sight-threatening uveitis of various etiologies (eight with intermediate uveitis, three with Adamantiades-Behçet disease, two with sarcoidosis, and one with idiopathic disease).[172] Not only was vision significantly improved in 8 of 14 patients, but nephrotoxicity was also curtailed, with no increase in serum creatinine during the 6-month follow-up period. However, the long-term efficacy of this particular therapeutic combination is, according to the same group of investigators, inferior to that of orally administered steroid and CSA.[141]

Finally, bromocriptine was reported to be effective in the treatment of thyroid ophthalmopathy.[246–248] Increased pretreatment thyroid-stimulating hormone and prolactin levels were associated with clinical improvement after bromocriptine therapy in many, but not all, cases.

DOSAGE AND ROUTE OF ADMINISTRATION

To minimize early adverse side effects, low-dose bromocriptine (1.25 mg) is administered orally, with food, at bedtime. The dose is then gradually increased to 2.5 mg, three or four times daily (see Table 12–1).[16, 236]

SIDE EFFECTS AND TOXICITY

Early adverse effects, including nausea, vomiting, and postural hypotension, are common with initiation of bromocriptine therapy and may be minimized by ingestion of the medication with food or at bedtime (see Table 12–3).[22] Although tolerance to nausea and orthostatic lightheadedness may develop in 3 to 4 days, rarely, a first-dose syncopal phenomenon can occur.[236] Other, less common effects observed in patients treated with larger doses include headache, dyspepsia, constipation, nasal congestion, dryness of the mouth, nocturnal leg cramps, depression, impaired concentration, nightmares, peripheral digital vasospasm on exposure to cold, and pleural thickening.[22] Dry eye symptoms associated with bromocriptine have also been reported.[249]

OVERDOSE

Bromocriptine overdosage may produce nausea, vomiting, and severe hypotension. Treatment consists of supportive measures, especially gastric lavage and administration of intravenous fluids to treat hypotension.[250]

HIGH-RISK GROUPS

Teratogenicity and other adverse effects to the mother or fetus have not been associated with the use of bromocriptine for induction of ovulation or during pregnancy.[236] Nevertheless, because bromocriptine crosses the placenta and may suppress fetal prolactin levels, the drug should be avoided during pregnancy unless indicated. Mothers who choose to breast-feed their infants should avoid bromocriptine since it suppresses lactation. The safety and efficacy of this agent have not been established in the pediatric age range. Continued surveillance is necessary for development of any late-appearing adverse effects in the pediatric age group and among children born to mothers treated with bromocriptine during a portion of their pregnancy.

The safety and efficacy of bromocriptine in elderly patients, or in those with renal or hepatic disease, have not been established. Caution must be exercised in administering bromocriptine concurrently with any antihypertensive medication.

CONTRAINDICATIONS

Bromocriptine should not be administered to patients with uncontrolled systemic hypertension, toxemia of pregnancy, or a history of hypersensitivity to ergot alkaloids.[114]

DRUG INTERACTIONS

The hepatic clearance of bromocriptine may be reduced by the concomitant administration of erythromycin.[22] In addition, the efficacy of bromocriptine may be diminished in patients who are also receiving agents that exhibit clopamine antagonism (i.e., phenothiazines).[114]

MAJOR CLINICAL TRIALS

Major clinical trials are described in the Therapeutic Use section.

Ketoconazole

HISTORY AND SOURCE

The development of ketoconazole marks an important breakthrough in antifungal therapy, because it was the first synthetic, orally effective, broad-spectrum antimycotic agent.[251] The clinical experience with this drug and its congeners is now extensive. In fact, a clinically significant drug interaction between ketoconazole and systemi-

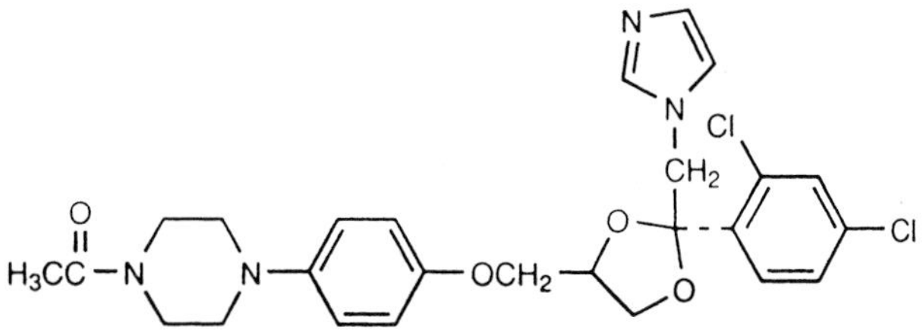

FIGURE 12–12. Chemical structure of ketoconazole.

cally administered CSA has been exploited in an attempt to minimize the effective dose, toxicity, and cost associated with CSA in the therapy of both renal allograft rejection[251] and noninfectious endogenous uveitis.[173]

OFFICIAL DRUG NAME AND CHEMISTRY

Ketoconazole (Nizoral, Janssen, Titusville, NJ), molecular weight 531.44, is an imidazole drug. Modifications of its basic imidazole structure (Fig. 12–12) have spawned multiple antifungal agents (e.g., clotrimazole, econazole, miconazole, and itraconazole), with each substitution providing drugs with different physical characteristics.[252]

PHARMACOLOGY

The primary mechanism of action of all imidazoles is inhibition of sterol metabolism. Specifically, ketoconazole prevents ergosterol synthesis by inhibiting the cytochrome P-450 enzyme system that catalyzes the C14-demethylation of lanosterol, the precursor of ergosterol.[253] This effect produces changes in the fungal cell membrane phospholipid composition, altering its permeability characteristics and impairing membrane-bound enzyme systems necessary for growth.[224] The inhibition of ergosterol biosynthesis in fungi is much more pronounced than that of cholesterol formation in mammalian cells, explaining the differential toxicity of ketoconazole in humans versus fungi.[252]

CLINICAL PHARMACOLOGY

Ketoconazole is fungistatic at low concentrations and fungicidal at high concentrations. It is active against candidiasis, pityrosporosis, dermatophytosis, blastomycosis, coccidioidomycosis, cryptococcosis, and histoplasmosis.[252]

The inhibitory action of this drug on the cytochrome P-450 system has additional important clinical implications, especially with respect to clinically significant drug interactions, both adverse and potentially therapeutic. Specifically, concomitant administration of ketoconazole with CSA, which is also extensively metabolized by the hepatic cytochrome P-450 enzymes,[142] results in increased blood concentrations of CSA that may become toxic if the dose is not adjusted.[254, 255] Therefore, this interaction provides the rationale for a combined drug strategy, allowing reduced yet effective doses of CSA while minimizing the risk of potential drug toxicity.

PHARMACEUTICS

Ketoconazole (Nizoral, Janssen) is available as 200-mg tablets for oral use and as a 2% topical cream.

PHARMACOKINETICS AND METABOLISM

The absorption of ketoconazole is variable among patients and depends mainly on gastric acidity. Because the optimal solubility of ketoconazole in water requires a pH lower than 3, bioavailability is markedly reduced in patients with achlorhydria (especially in the elderly and in patients with AIDS), and in those treated with antacids, H2 receptor antagonists, anticholinergics, and antiparkinsonian agents.[251, 253] Suboptimal absorption may be minimized by the administration of ketoconazole 2 hours before these latter agents are administered to patients who require them.

After oral doses of 200, 400, and 800 mg of ketoconazole, respective peak plasma concentrations of 4, 8, and 20 mg/ml are achieved in approximately 2 hours.[224, 256] The plasma $t\frac{1}{2}$ appears to be dose-dependent, varying from 1 to 2 hours to as long as 8 hours with a dose of 800 mg.[224, 257]

Ketoconazole is extensively metabolized by the hepatic cytochrome P-450 enzyme system, with the inactive metabolites being excreted by the biliary system and appearing in the feces.[253] Very little active drug is excreted in the urine. Approximately 84% of ketoconazole is bound to plasma proteins (mostly albumin), 15% to erythrocytes, and 1% is free.[258] Therefore, renal insufficiency, hemodialysis, or peritoneal dialysis has little effect on drug metabolism, whereas pre-existing liver disease warrants careful laboratory monitoring, given ketoconazole's inherent potential for hepatotoxicity.[252] However, even with moderate hepatic dysfunction, preliminary studies have shown no effect on the concentration of ketoconazole in the blood.[224]

Ketoconazole has wide tissue distribution, achieving effective concentrations in keratinocytes, saliva, and vaginal fluid.[252] However, concentrations in the CSF are only 1% to 4% of those in the serum at usual therapeutic doses in patients with fungal meningitis.[22]

THERAPEUTIC USE

For nonophthalmic purposes, ketoconazole is the drug of choice for treatment of nonmeningeal blastomycosis, histoplasmosis, coccidioidomycosis, pseudallescheriasis, and paracoccidioidomycosis in otherwise healthy, immunocompetent patients.[259] It is also the preferred treatment for chronic mucocutaneous candidiasis and is effective in the control of severe oral and esophageal candidiasis, as well as in severe recalcitrant dermatophyte infections.[252]

The combined use of ketoconazole with CSA was initially reported in a group of 18 patients undergoing renal transplantation in whom a reduction of 30% in their usual maintenance CSA dose of 8 mg/kg/day was achieved.[251] None of the patients developed CSA-associated adverse events during the 13-month follow-up period.

DeSmet and associates[173] of the National Eye Institute have demonstrated the efficacy of combination therapy with ketoconazole (200 mg/day) and low-dose CSA (5 mg/kg/day), together with prednisone (0 to 0.5 mg/kg/day) in maintaining inflammatory remission in a double-masked, placebo-controlled study of 10 patients with endogenous uveitis (see Tables 12–1 and 12–4). These patients, who were all in clinical remission while being treated with combined low-dose CSA and prednisone therapy, had their CSA dose initially reduced by 70% in a 3-day period. Four of six (66%) control subjects experienced recurrent inflammatory episodes, whereas none of the four patients treated with the ketoconazole combination had a relapse of uveitis during the 3-month follow-up period. Furthermore, some patients treated with this combination continued to show improvement in their visual acuity, suggesting that the sustained drug levels of CSA afforded by the addition of ketoconazole are more effective in maintaining remission than are the more dramatic fluctuations in drug concentration produced by the usual treatment schedule.[173]

Not only was a much smaller volume of CSA necessary to control inflammation in the ketoconazole-treated group, but toxicity was also limited to a transient decrease in GFR in two patients, at 1 month, which promptly returned to a normal rate after further reduction in the CSA dose.[173] The researchers suggested that when ketoconazole is added to the therapeutic regimen, the dose of CSA should initially be decreased by 30% of its baseline value and continued at this reduced dose for a minimum of four CSA t½ (several days), after which time a whole blood CSA level should be obtained.[125, 173] Further CSA dosage reductions may be indicated if this level remains increased. Initial careful monitoring of the serum creatinine and for clinical signs of acute CSA toxicity is necessary. Maintenance of the whole blood levels of CSA within the lower range of normal (500 to 1000 ng/L) minimizes CSA-associated toxicity.[173]

SIDE EFFECTS AND TOXICITY

The most important adverse effects of ketoconazole therapy are hepatotoxicity and those arising from its influence on steroid biosynthesis (see Table 12–3).

Hepatotoxicity. Ketoconazole-induced hepatotoxicity is believed to be due to a metabolic idiosyncracy in susceptible patients.[251] The abrupt onset of potentially fatal hepatic dysfunction resembling viral hepatitis occurs in approximately 1 in 15,000 exposed patients, especially middle-aged women, between days 11 and 68 of ketoconazole therapy.[260] Both the physician and the patient should have a heightened awareness of this potential complication. Asymptomatic and reversible elevations in the alanine and aspartate aminotransferase levels occur in 2% to 5% of patients.[22]

Steroid Synthesis. Although the ketoconazole-mediated inhibition of steroid biosynthesis with regard to cytochrome P-450 enzymes is more pronounced in fungi than in humans, several endocrinologic abnormalities are known to occur in patients treated with this medication. Approximately 10% of women experience menstrual irregularity, and a variable number of men report gynecomastia, decreased libido and potency, and oligospermia.[224] Doses of ketoconazole as low as 400 mg/day may cause a reversible reduction in free testosterone and estradiol plasma levels, whereas higher doses (600 to 800 mg/day) may transiently inhibit adrenal steroidogenesis by blocking the 11-hydroxylation step of synthesis.[22] Hypoadrenalism has been reported, especially with high doses of ketoconazole: therefore, this drug should be avoided in

patients undergoing major surgery or in those exposed to other significant stressful conditions.[224]

Other less severe but more common side effects include dose-related GI upset (nausea and vomiting), occurring in approximately 50% of patients receiving 800 mg daily.[22] An allergic rash occurs in approximately 4% of patients and pruritus without rash occurs in about 2% of individuals.[224]

OVERDOSE

General supportive measures, together with gastric lavage with sodium bicarbonate, should be instituted in the event of accidental overdosage of ketoconazole.

HIGH-RISK GROUPS

Ketoconazole has been shown to be teratogenic in animal models, producing syndactyly and oligodactyly in the offspring of rats when given at doses of 80 mg/kg/day (10 times the human dose).[22] Because data are insufficient to allow evaluation of the safety of the drug in pregnant women, it should be avoided during pregnancy unless the potential benefit to the mother outweighs the risk to the fetus. Because ketoconazole is excreted in the breast milk, mothers treated with the drug should not breast feed.

Likewise, the use of ketoconazole has not been studied systematically in the pediatric age group. Indeed, no information is available on use of this medication in children younger than 2 years of age.[114]

The absence of gastric acidity compromises the absorption of ketoconazole. Therefore, reduced bioavailability of drug may complicate therapy in the elderly and in patients with AIDS, both of whom frequently have achlorhydria.

CONTRAINDICATIONS

Concomitant administration of ketoconazole with terfenadine or astemizole inhibits their metabolism and increases the plasma levels of both drugs and the active metabolite of the latter, placing the patient at risk of potentially fatal cardiac arrhythmias.[114] Ketoconazole is also contraindicated in any patient with a known hypersensitivity to it or any other imidazole drug.

DRUG INTERACTIONS

Concomitant administration of ketoconazole with coumarin-like agents enhances the anticoagulant effect of the coumarin-like agents.[252] The blood level of CSA is increased by ketoconazole. In addition, ketoconazole reduces the clearance of chlordiazepoxide, theophylline, and methylprednisolone.[22]

Conversely, concurrent use of ketoconazole with rifampin, isoniazid, or both results in decreased ketoconazole concentrations.[114] Coadministration of phenytoin and ketoconazole produces alterations in the levels of one or both of these drugs.[252]

MAJOR CLINICAL TRIALS

Major clinical trials are described in the Therapeutic Use section.

Colchicine

HISTORY AND SOURCE

Colchicine, an alkaloid derived from the autumn crocus *Colchicum autumnale*, has been used for treatment of acute gout since the 6th century AD.[261] Colchicine was isolated from *Colchicum* in 1820 and first synthesized in 1965.[262] Although its anti-inflammatory properties are best known in management of gout, colchicine is the drug of choice for treatment of familial Mediterranean fever and is effective in a variety of dermatologic and systemic diseases, such as psoriasis and Adamantiades-Behçet disease, which are characterized by neutrophil participation in the lesions.[263–265] It is in the prophylaxis of the recurrent ocular and systemic inflammatory manifestations of Adamantiades-Behçet disease that ophthalmologists find colchicine most useful.

OFFICIAL DRUG NAME AND CHEMISTRY

Colchicine, a phenanthrene derivative, is acetyltrimethyl colchicinic acid (Fig. 12–13). It has a molecular weight of 399.44; the empirical formula is $C_{22}H_{25}NO_6$.

PHARMACOLOGY

Colchicine exhibits both anti-inflammatory and antimitotic properties, mediated mainly through its inhibition of microtubular formation (see Fig. 12–1).[261]

CLINICAL PHARMACOLOGY

Colchicine's anti-inflammatory characteristics are poorly understood and chiefly involve depression of neutrophil motility, adhesiveness, chemotaxis, and lysosomal degranulation.[262] The drug is concentrated extremely well in leukocytes, where it binds to dimers of tubulin, thus preventing the assembly of tubulin subunits. This disrupts the function of the spindle apparatus, arresting mitosis in metaphase, and causes the depolymerization and disappearance of fibrillar microtubules in granulocytes and other motile cells.[265–267] In this way, the migration of granulocytes to the site of inflammation, together with release of lactic acid and proinflammatory lysosomal enzymes, is inhibited, thereby breaking the cycle leading to the inflammatory response.[261]

Colchicine has also been shown to inhibit release of histamine from mast cell granules in vitro, secretion of insulin and parathormone, and movement of melanin granules in melanophores.[263, 264] These effects are believed to be due to colchicine's inhibition of granule translocation by the microtubular system.[261]

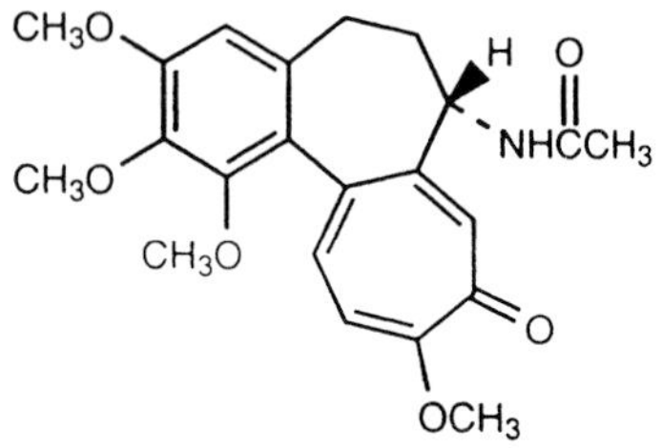

FIGURE 12–13. Chemical structure of colchicine.

PHARMACEUTICS

Colchicine (generic) is available as 0.5-mg and 0.6-mg tablets for oral use and as a sterile solution (0.5 mg/ml) for injection. It should be shielded from ultraviolet light exposure to prevent its degradation into inactive products.[261]

PHARMACOKINETICS AND METABOLISM

Colchicine is rapidly absorbed after oral administration, reaching peak plasma concentrations between 30 and 120 minutes after ingestion.[263] After intravenous injection of a 1-mg bolus in normal subjects, the mean elimination t½ is 601 ± 155 ml/min and the apparent volume of distribution is 2 L/kg.[22] Protein binding is minimal.

Large amounts of colchicine enter the intestinal tract in the bile and intestinal secretions, with high concentrations also occurring in the kidney, liver, and spleen. However, the drug is largely excluded from the brain, heart, and skeletal muscle.[261] Colchicine can also be detected in peripheral leukocytes for at least 9 days after a single intravenous dose.[261]

The drug undergoes hepatic metabolism, most being eliminated in the feces, with 10% to 20% excreted in the urine.[263] In patients with hepatic dysfunction, a greater fraction of colchicine is shunted from the liver and excreted in the urine.[261]

THERAPEUTIC USE

Colchicine has been proved effective, alone or in combination with other immunosuppressive agents, in controlling the ocular and systemic manifestations of Adamantiades-Behçet disease (see Table 12–4). [264, 268–275] In a series of 131 patients with Adamantiades-Behçet disease reported by Mizushima and associates,[274] 105 patients responded to colchicine. Foster and colleagues[39] used colchicine to treat 19 patients with Adamantiades-Behçet disease, successfully preventing inflammatory flare-ups in three patients with mild disease; 15 others required concomitant immunosuppressive therapy. Colchicine was discontinued in one patient because of diarrhea.

Because enhanced neutrophil migration is a characteristic feature of Adamantiades-Behçet disease, colchicine is most useful in prophylaxis of recurrent inflammatory episodes (rather than in treatment of active disease) or in the rare patient with mild, unilateral involvement in whom the clinician wishes to defer immunosuppressive therapy.[110] In countries where the incidence of Adamantiades-Behçet disease is high, there is no consensus regarding its utility; colchicine therapy is more popular in Japan than in Turkey and is of equivocal value in whites.

DOSAGE AND ROUTE OF ADMINISTRATION

The recommended dose is 0.5 to 0.6 mg orally two to three times daily (see Table 12–1).[16, 272, 274, 275]

SIDE EFFECTS AND TOXICITY

The most common adverse effect of colchicine therapy is GI upset (see Table 12–3). Although the drug is well tolerated in moderate dosages, the function of the rapidly proliferating epithelial cells in the GI tract is altered such that nausea, vomiting, abdominal cramping, hyperperistalsis, and watery diarrhea can occur at therapeutic doses, especially with 0.6 mg administered three times a day.[263] Drugs to control vomiting and diarrhea may be useful, but to avoid more serious toxicity, colchicine should be discontinued once symptoms of intolerance occur. The intravenous route obviates these GI side effects and produces a faster therapeutic effect; however, extravasation produces inflammation and necrosis of skin and soft tissues.[261]

Chronic administration of colchicine can produce leukopenia, aplastic anemia, thrombocytopenia, myopathy, and alopecia.[262] Azoospermia and megaloblastic anemia secondary to vitamin B_{12} malabsorption have also been described.[263] Complete hemogram and platelet counts, together with serum chemistries and urinalyses should be performed before the initiation of therapy and periodically (every 3 to 4 months) thereafter.

Overdose

The fatal oral dose of colchicine in adults is approximately 20 mg.[22] Signs and symptoms of acute poisoning include fever, hemorrhagic gastroenteritis, extensive vascular damage, nephrotoxicity, muscular depression, and an ascending paralysis of the CNS.[261] In addition, a cholera-like syndrome with severe fluid and electrolyte disturbances may ensue, together with respiratory distress syndrome, disseminated intravascular coagulation, bone marrow failure, and ultimately shock.[262]

Management of acute intoxication is symptomatic and includes general supportive measures; repeated doses of activated charcoal orally with gastric lavage; maintenance of fluid volume; treatment of hypothermia; administration of vitamin K, fresh frozen plasma, or platelets as indicated for coagulopathy; parenteral nutrition; correction of electrolyte disturbances and intravenous administration of benzodiazepines if generalized seizures occur.[22] Reversible alopecia and rebound leukocytosis are common in patients who survive serious colchicine intoxication.[22, 263]

High-Risk Groups

Colchicine should be administered with great caution in the elderly, especially those with renal, hepatic, GI, or cardiovascular disease.[261] Oral colchicine often causes diarrhea before relieving gout in elderly patients.[22] Furthermore, diminished hepatic and renal reserves in these patients increase the plasma levels of colchicine, placing them at increased risk of development of chronic toxicity.

Colchicine has been reported to be teratogenic in humans[276] and should not be used during pregnancy.[262] Whether the drug is excreted in the breast milk is not known; therefore, caution must be exercised when colchicine is administered to nursing mothers. Its safety and efficacy have yet to be established in children.

Colchicine is contraindicated in patients with severe GI, renal, hepatic, or cardiac disorders, especially in the presence of combined kidney and liver disease.[114] A hypersensitivity reaction to the drug also constitutes a contraindication to its use.

Drug Interactions

Colchicine has been reported to induce a reversible malabsorption of vitamin B_{12}, with resultant megaloblastic anemia, presumably by altering the function of the ileal mucosa.[263]

Major Clinical Trials

Major clinical trials are described in the Therapeutic Use section.

References

1. Bach JH: The mode of action of immunosuppressive drugs. Amsterdam, Elsevier North Holland, 1975.
2. Biswas J, Rao NA: Management of intraocular inflammation. In: Ryan SJ, ed: Retina, vol. 2. St. Louis: Mosby–Year Book, 1994, pp 1061–1069.
3. Foster CS, Wilson SA, Ekins MB: Immunosuppressive therapy for ocular cicatricial pemphigoid. Ophthalmology 1982;99:340–353.
4. Krumbhaar EB, Krumbhaar HD: The blood and bone marrow in yellow cross gas (mustard gas) poisoning: Changes produced in the bone marrow of fatal cases. J Med Res 1919;40:497–507.
5. Gery I, Nussenblatt RB: Immunosuppressive drugs. In: Sears ML, ed: Pharmacology of the eye. Berlin, Springer-Verlag, 1984, pp 586–609.
6. Roda-Perez E: Sobre un case se uveitis de etiologia ignota tratado con mostaza introgenada. Rev Clin Esp 1951;40:265–267.
7. Roda-Perez E: El tratamiento de las uveitis de etiologia ignota con mostaza nitrogenada. Arch Soc Ofial Hisp Am 1952;12:131–151.
8. Calabresi P, Chabner BA: Chemotherapy of neoplastic diseases. In: Gilman AG, Rall TW, Nies AS, Taylor P, eds. Goodman and Gilman's the Pharmacological Basis of Therapeutics. New York, Pergamon Press, 1990, pp 1202–1263.
9. Brock N: Oxazaphosphorine cytostatics: Past-present-future: Seventh Cain Memorial Award Lecture. Cancer Res 1989;49:1–7.
10. Foster CS: Pharmacologic treatment of immune disorders. In: Albert DM, Jakobiec FA, eds: Principles and Practice of Ophthalmology, Basic Sciences. Philadelphia, WB Saunders, 1994, pp 1076–1084.
11. Stockman GP, Heim LR, South MA, Trentin JJ: Differential effects of cyclophosphamide on the B and T cell compartments of adult mice. J Immunol 1973;110:277–282.
12. Clements PJ, Yu DTY, Levy J, Paulus HE, Barnett EU: Effects of cyclophosphamide on B and T lymphocytes in rheumatoid arthritis. Arthritis Rheum 1974;17:347–353.
13. Fauci AS, Date DC, Wolff SM: Cyclophosphamide and lymphocyte subpopulations in Wegener's granulomatosis. Arthritis Rheum 1974;17:355–361.
14. Lerman SP, Weidanz WP: The effect of cyclophosphamide on the ontogeny of the humoral immune response in chickens. J Immunol 1970;105:614–619.
15. Hemady R, Tauber J, Foster CS: Immunosuppressive drugs in immune and inflammatory disease. Surv Ophthalmol 1991;35:359–385.
16. Foster CS: Nonsteroidal anti-inflammatory and immunosuppressive agents. In: Lamberts DW, Potter DE, eds: Clinical Ophthalmic Pharmacology. Boston, Little, Brown, 1987, pp 181–192.
17. Askenase PQ, Hayden BJ, Gershon RK: Augmentation of delayed type hypersensitivity by doses of cyclophosphamide which do not affect antibody responses. J Exp Med 1975;141:697–702.
18. Shand FL, Liew FY: Differential sensitivity to cyclophosphamide of helper T cells for humoral responses and suppressor T cells for delayed-type hypersensitivity. Eur J Immunol 1980;10:480–483.
19. Tabor DK, Kiel DP, Jacobs RF: Cyclophosphamide-sensitive activity of suppressor T cells during treponemal infection. Immunology 1987;62:127–132.
20. Lemmel E, Hurd ER, Ziff M: Differential effects of 6 mercaptopurine and cyclophosphamide on autoimmune phenomena in NZB mice. Clin Exp Immunol 1971;8:355–362.
21. Rapini RP, Jordan RE, Wolverton SE: Cytotoxic agents. In: Wolverton SE, Wilkins JK, eds: Systemic Drugs for Skin Diseases. Philadelphia, WB Saunders, 1991, pp 125–151.
22. AMA drug evaluations. Chicago: American Medical Association, 1991, pp 396, 1059, 1654–1655, 1671–1672, 1843–1844, 1972–1973, 1891–1913, 2009–2034, 2140–2141, 2351–2353.
23. Brubaker R, Font RL, Shepero EM: Granulomatous sclerouveitis, regression of ocular lesions with cyclophosphamide and prednisone. Arch Ophthalmol 1971;86:517–524.

24. Foster CS: Immunosuppressive therapy for external ocular inflammatory disease. Ophthalmology 1980;87:140–150.

25. Jampol LM, West C, Goldberg MF: Therapy of scleritis with cytotoxic agents, Am J Ophthalmol 1978;86:266–271.

26. Fauci AS, Haynes BF, Katz P, Wolff SM: Wegener's granulomatosis: Prospective clinical and therapeutic experience with 85 patients for 21 years. Ann Intern Med 1983;98:75–85.

27. Fauci AS, Duppman JZ, Wolff SM: Cyclophosphamide induced remissions in advanced polyarteritis nodosa. Am J Med 1978;64:890–894.

28. Fosdick WM, Parsons JL, Hill DF: Long-term cyclophosphamide therapy in rheumatoid arthritis. Arthritis Rheum 1968;9:151–161.

29. Foster CS, Forstot SL, Wilson LA: Mortality rate in rheumatoid arthritis patients developing necrotizing scleritis or peripheral ulcerative keratitis, effects of systemic immunosuppression. Ophthalmology 1984;91:1253–1263.

30. Foster CS, Sainz de la Maza M: The Sclera. New York, Springer-Verlag, 1993, pp 299–307.

31. Watson PG, Hazleman BL: The Sclera and Systemic Disorders. Philadelphia, WB Saunders, 1976, pp 90–154.

32. Huang-Xuan T, Foster CS, Rice BA: Scleritis in relapsing polychondritis: Response to therapy. Ophthalmology 1990;97:892–898.

33. Foster CS: Systemic immunosuppressive therapy for progressive bilateral Mooren's ulcer. Ophthalmology 1985;92:1436–1439.

34. Brown SI, Mondino BJ: Therapy of Mooren's ulcer. Am J Ophthalmol 1984;98:1–6.

35. Foster CS: Cicatricial pemphigoid. Trans Am Ophthalmol Soc 1986;84:527–663.

36. Neumann R, Tauber J, Foster CS: Remission and recurrence after withdrawal of therapy for ocular cicatricial pemphigoid. Ophthalmology 1991;98:858–862.

37. Oniki S, Kurakazu K, Kawata K: Immunosuppressive treatment of Behçet's disease with cyclophosphamide. Jpn J Ophthalmol 1976;20:32–40.

38. Gills JP, Buckley CE: Cyclophosphamide therapy of Behçet's disease. Ann Ophthalmol 1970;2:399–405.

39. Foster CS, Baer JC, Raizman MB: Therapeutic responses to systemic immunosuppressive chemotherapy agents in patients with Behçet's syndrome affecting the eyes. In: O'Duffy JD, Kokmen E, eds: Behçet's Disease: Basic and Clinical Aspects. New York, Marcel Dekker, 1991, pp 581–588.

40. Fain O, Du LTH, Wechsler B: Pulse cyclophosphamide in Behçet's disease. In: O'Duffy JD, Kokmen E, eds: Behçet's Disease: Basic and Clinical Aspects. New York, Marcel Dekker, 1991, pp 569–573.

41. Buckley CE, Durham NC, Gills JP: Cyclophosphamide therapy of peripheral uveitis. Arch Intern Med 1969;124:29–35.

42. Wong VG: Immunosuppressive therapy of ocular inflammatory diseases. Arch Ophthalmol 1969,81:628–637.

43. Martenet AC: Immunosuppressive therapy of uveitis: mid- and long-term follow up after classical cytostatic treatment. In: Usui M, Ohno S, Aoki K, eds: Ocular Immunology Today. New York, Excerpta Medica, 1990, pp 443–446.

44. Dorr RT, Fritz WL: Cancer Chemotherapy Handbook. New York, Elsevier/North Holland, 1980.

45. Berkson BM, Come LG, Shapiro I: Severe cystitis induced by cyclophosphamide, role of surgical management. JAMA 1973;225:605–606.

46. Puri HC, Campbell RA: Cyclophosphamide and malignancy. Lancet 1977,1:1306.

47. Levine CA, Richie JP: Urological complications of cyclophosphamide. J Urol 1989;141:1063–1069.

48. Fairley KF, Barrie JV, Johnson W: Sterility and testicular atrophy related to cyclophosphamide therapy. Lancet 1972;1:568–569.

49. Fraunfelder FT, Meyer SM: Ocular toxicity from antineoplastic agents. Ophthalmology 1983;90:1–3.

50. Rubin B, Palestine AG: Complications of corticosteroids and immunosuppressive drugs. Int Ophthalmol Clin 1989;29:159–169.

51. Pavan-Langston D, Dunkel EC: Handbook of Ocular Drug Therapy and Ocular Side Effects of Systemic Drugs. Boston, Little, Brown, 1991, pp 203–213.

52. Colvin M, Chabner BA: Alkylating agents. In: Chabner BA, Collins JM, eds: Cancer Chemotherapy: Principles and Practice. Philadelphia, JB Lippincott, 1990, pp 276–313.

53. Mamo JG, Azzam SA: Treatment of Behçet's disease with chlorambucil. Arch Ophthalmol 1970;84:446–450.

54. Ben Ezra D, Cohen E: Treatment and visual prognosis in Behçet's disease. Br J Ophthalmol 1986;70:589–592.

55. Bietti GB, Ceruili L, Pivetti-Pezzi P: Behçet's disease and immunosuppressive treatment. Mod Probl Ophthalmol 1976;16:314–323.

56. O'Duffy JD, Robertson DM, Goldstein NP: Chlorambucil in the treatment of uveitis and meningoencephalitis of Behçet's disease. Am J Med 1984;76:75–84.

57. Pezzi PD, Gaspani U, DeLiso P, Catarinelli G: Prognosis in Behçet's disease. Ann Ophthalmol 1985;17:20–25.

58. Tricoulis D: Treatment of Behçet's disease with chlorambucil. Br J Ophthalmol 1976;60:55–57.

59. Tabbara KF: Chlorambucil in Behçet's disease, a reappraisal. Ophthalmology 1983;90:906–908.

60. Abdalla MI, Bahgat N: Long-lasting remission of Behçet's disease after chlorambucil therapy. Br J Ophthalmol 1993;57:706–710.

61. Elliot JH, Ballinger WH: Behçet's syndrome. Treatment with chlorambucil. Trans Am Ophthalmol Soc 1984;82:264–281.

62. Nussenblatt RB, Palestine AG: Chan CC, Ochizuki M, Yancey K: Effectiveness of cyclosporine therapy for Behçet's disease. Arthritis Rheum 1985;28:671–679.

63. Chavis PS, Antonios SR, Tabbara KF: Cyclosporine effects on optic nerve and retinal vasculitis in Behçet's disease. Doc Ophthalmol 1992;80:133–142.

64. Godfrey WA, Epstein WV, O'Connor GR, et al: The use of chlorambucil in intractable idiopathic uveitis. Am J Ophthalmol 1974;78:415–428.

65. Andrasch RH, Profsky B, Burns RP: Immunosuppressive therapy for severe chronic uveitis. Arch Ophthalmol 1978;96:247–251.

66. Jennings T, Tessler HH: Twenty cases of sympathetic ophthalmia. Br J Ophthalmol 1989;73:140–145.

67. Kanski JJ: Anterior uveitis in juvenile rheumatoid arthritis. Arch Ophthalmol 1977;95:1794–1797.

68. Foster CS, Barrett F: Cataract development and cataract surgery in patients with juvenile rheumatoid arthritis–associated iridocyclitis. Ophthalmology 1993;100:809–817.

69. Clements PJ, Davis J: Cytotoxic drugs: Their clinical application to the rheumatic diseases. Semin Arthritis Rheum 1986;15:231–254.

70. Sobrinho LG, Levine RA, DeConti RL: Amenorrhea in patients with Hodgkin's disease treated with antineoplastic agents. Am J Obstet Gynecol 1971;109:135–139.

71. Berk PA, Goldberg JD, Silverman MN, et al: Increased incidence of acute leukemia in polycythemia vera associated with chlorambucil therapy. N Engl J Med 1981;304:441–447.

72. Lemer HJ: Acute myelogenous leukemia in students receiving chlorambucil as long-term adjuvant chemotherapy for stage II breast cancer. Cancer Treat Rep 1978;62:1135–1138.

73. Williams SA, Makker SP, Grupe WE: Seizures, a significant side effect of chlorambucil therapy in children. J Pediatr 1978;93:510–518.

74. Shotton D, Monic IW: Possible teratogenic effect of chlorambucil on a human fetus. JAMA 1963;186:74–75.

75. Farber S, Diamond LK, Mercer RD, et al: Temporary remissions in acute leukemia in children produced by folic antagonist 4-amethopteroylglutamic acid (aminopterin). N Engl J Med 1948;238:787–793.

76. Hertz R: Folic acid antagonists. Effects on the cell and patient. Clinical staff conference at NIH. Ann Intern Med 1963;59:931–956.

77. Weinblatt ME, Kremer JM: Methotrexate in rheumatoid arthritis. J Am Acad Dermatol 1988;19:126–128.

78. Lally EV, Ho G: A review of methotrexate therapy in Reiter's syndrome. Semin Arthritis Rheum 1985;15:139–145.

79. Wong VG, Hersh EM: Methotrexate in the therapy of cyclitis. Trans Am Acad Ophthalmol Otolaryngol 1965;69:279–293.

80. Callen JP, Kulp-Shorten CL: Methotrexate. In: Wolverton SE, Wilkins JK, eds: Systemic Drugs for Skin Diseases. Philadelphia, WB Saunders, 1991, pp 152–166.

81. Werkheiser W: The biochemical, cellular, and pharmacologic action and effects of the folic acid antagonists. Cancer Res 1963;23:1277–1285.

82. Hersh EM, Carbone PP, Wong VG, Greireich EJ: Inhibition of primary immune response in man by antimetabolites. Cancer Res 1965;25:1997–2001.

83. Mitchell MS, Wade ME, DeConti RC, et al: Immune suppressive effects of cytosine arabinoside and methotrexate in man. Ann Intern Med 1969;70:535–547.

84. Andersen PA, West SG, O'Dell JR, et al: Weekly pulse methotrexate in rheumatoid arthritis. Clinical and immunologic effects in a randomized, double-blind study. Ann Intern Med 1985;103:489–496.

85. Weinblatt ME, Coblyn JS, Fox DA, et al: Efficacy of low-dose methotrexate in rheumatoid arthritis. N Engl J Med 1985;312:818–822.

86. Shah SS, Lowder CY, Schmidt MA, et al: Low-dose methotrexate therapy for ocular inflammatory disease. Ophthalmology 1992;99:1419–1423.

87. Olsen EA: The pharmacology of methotrexate. J Am Acad Dermatol 1991;25:306–317.

88. Wong VG: Methotrexate treatment of uveal disease. Am J Med Sci 1966;251:239–241.

89. Wong VG, Hersh EM, McMaster PRB: Treatment of a presumed case of sympathetic ophthalmia with methotrexate. Arch Ophthalmol 1966;76:66–76.

90. Lazar M, Weiner MJ, Leopold IH: Treatment of uveitis with methotrexate. Am I Ophthalmol 1969;67:383–387.

91. Weinstein G, Roenigk HH, Mailbach H, et al: Psoriasis-liver-methotrexate interactions. Arch Dermatol 1973:108:36–42.

92. Walker AM, Funch D, Dreyer NA, et al: Determinants of serious liver disease among patients receiving low-dose methotrexate for rheumatoid arthritis. Arthritis Rheum 1993;36:329–335.

93. Dev S, McCallum RM, Jaffee GJ: Methotrexate treatment for sarcoid-associated panuveitis. Ophthalmology 1999;106:111.

94. Shupack JL, Webster OF: Pancytopenia following low-dose oral methotrexate therapy for psoriasis. JAMA 1988;259:3594–3596.

95. Roenigk HH, Auerbach R, Maibach HI, Weinstein GD: Methotrexate in psoriasis: revised guidelines. J Am Acad Dermatol 1988;19:145–156.

96. Phillips CA, Cera PJ, Mangan TF, Newman ED: Clinical liver disease in patients with rheumatoid arthritis taking methotrexate. J Rheumatol 1989;16:487–493.

97. Ridley MG, Wolfe CS, Mathews JH: Life-threatening acute pneumonitis during low-dose methotrexate treatment for rheumatoid arthritis: A case report and review of the literature. Ann Rheum Dis 1988;47:784–788.

98. Schein PS, Winokur SH: Immunosuppressive and cytotoxic chemotherapy: long-term complications. Ann Intern Med 1975;82:94–95.

99. Balin PL, Tindall JP, Roenigk HH: Is methotrexate therapy for psoriasis carcinogenic? A modified retrospective-prospective analysis. JAMA 1975;232:359–362.

100. Rustin GJ, Rustin F, Dent J, et al: No increase in second tumors after cytotoxic chemotherapy for gestational trophoblastic tumors. N Engl J Med 1983:308:473–476.

101. Nyfors A, Jensen H: Frequency of malignant neoplasms in 248 long-term methotrexate-treated psoriatics: A preliminary study. Dermatologica 1983;167:260–261.

102. Giannini EH, Brewer EJ, Kuzmina N, et al: Methotrexate in resistant juvenile rheumatoid arthritis. N Engl J Med 1992;326:1043–1049.

103. Newell FW, Krill AE: Treatment of uveitis with azathioprine (Imuran). Trans Ophthalmol Soc UK 1967;87:499–511.

104. Newell FW, Krill AE, Thompson A: The treatment of uveitis with six-mercaptopurine. Am J Ophthalmol 1966;61:1250–1255.

105. Rollingshoff M, Schrader J, Wagner H: Effect of azathioprine and cytosine arabinoside on humoral and cellular immunity in vitro. Clin Exp Immunol 1973;15:261–269.

106. Mathews JD, Crawford BA, Bignell JL, Mackay IR: Azathioprine in active iridocyclitis, a double blind controlled trial. Br J Ophthalmol 1969;53:327–330.

107. Moore EE: Sympathetic ophthalmia treated with azathioprine. Br J Ophthalmol 1968;52:688–690.

108. Hemady R, Baer JC, Foster CS: Immunosuppressive drugs in the management of progressive, corticosteroid-resistant uveitis associated with juvenile rheumatoid arthritis. Int Ophthalmol Clin 1992;32:241–252.

109. Yazici H, Pazarli H, Bames CG, et al: A controlled trial of azathioprine in Behçet's syndrome. N Engl J Med 1990;322:281–285.

110. Nussenblatt RB, Palestine AG: Uveitis, Fundamentals and Clinical Practice. Chicago, Year Book Medical Publishers, 1989, pp 116–144.

111. Penn I: Malignancies associated with immunosuppressive or cytotoxic therapy. Surgery 1978;83:492–502.

112. Singh G, Fries IF, Spitz P, Williams CA: Toxic effects of azathioprine in rheumatoid arthritis. Arthritis Rheum 1989;32:837–843.

113. Castor WC, Bull FE: Review of United States data on neoplasms in rheumatoid arthritis. Am J Med 1985;78(Suppl 1A):133–138.

114. Physicians' Desk Reference. Montvale, NJ, Medical Economics Data, 1994, pp 703–704, 1081, 1096, 2067, 2071–2074, 2114.

115. Schusziarra V, Zickursch V, Schlamp R, Siemensen HC: Pharmacokinetics of azathioprine under haemodialysis. Int J Clin Pharmacol Biopharm 1976;14:298–302.

116. Coulam CB, Moyer TP, Jiang NS, Zincke H: Breast-feeding after renal transplantation. Transplant Proc 1982;14:605–609.

117. Hoover R, Fraumeni JF: Drug-induced cancer. Cancer 1981;47:1071–1080.

118. Kirchertz EJ, Gröne HJ, Rieger J, et al: Successful low dose captopril rechallenge following drug-induced leukopenia. Lancet 1981;1:1362–1363.

119. Borel JF: The history of cyclosporin A and its significance. In: White DJG, ed: Cyclosporin A. New York, Elsevier Biomedical Press, 1982, pp 5–17.

120. Borel JF, Feurer C, Magnee C, Stabelin H: Effects of the new anti-lymphocyte peptide cyclosporin A in animals. Immunology 1977;32:1017–1025.

121. Nussenblatt RB, Palestine AG, Rook AH, et al: Treatment of intraocular inflammation with cyclosporin A. Lancet 1983;1:235–238.

122. Nussenblatt RB, Palestine AG, Chan CC: Cyclosporine A therapy in the treatment of intraocular inflammatory disease resistant to systemic corticosteroids and cytotoxic agents. Am J Ophthalmol 1983;96:275–282.

123. Nussenblatt RB, Palestine AG: Cyclosporine: Immunology, pharmacology and therapeutic uses. Surv Ophthalmol 1986;31:159–169.

124. Kahan BD: Cyclosporine. N Engl J Med 1989;321:1725–1738.

125. deSmet MD, Nussenblatt RB: Clinical use of cyclosporine in ocular disease. Int Ophthalmol Clin 1993;33:31–45.

126. Sigal NH, Dumont FJ: Cyclosporin A, FK-506, and rapamycin: Pharmacologic probes of lymphocyte signal transduction. Annu Rev Immunol 1992;10:519–560.

127. Thompson AW, Starzi TE: FK 506 and autoimmune disease: Perspective and prospects. Autoimmunity 1992;12:303–313.

128. Handschumacher RE: Immunosuppressive agents. In: Gilman AC, Rail TW, Nies AS, Taylor P, eds: Goodman and Gilman's The Pharmacological Basis of Therapeutics. New York, Pergamon Press, 1990, pp 1264–1276.

129. Liu J: FK 506 and cyclosporin, molecular probes for studying intracellular signal transduction. Immunol Today 1993;14:290–295.

130. Sigal SN: Immunosuppressive profile of rapamycin. Ann N Y Acad Sci 1993;685:1–8.

131. Chang JY, Sehgal SN: Pharmacology of rapamycin: A new immunosuppressive agent. B J Rheumatol 1991;30(Suppl 2):62–65.

132. Chang JY, Sehgal SN, Bansbach CC: FK 506 and rapamycin: Novel pharmacological probes of the immune response. Trends Pharmacol Sci 1991;12:218–223.

133. Ryffel B, Foxwell BM, Mihatsch MJ, et al: Biologic significance of cyclosporine metabolites. Transplant 1988;20(Suppl 2):575–584.

134. Palestine AG, Nussenblatt RE, Chan CC: Cyclosporine penetration into the anterior chamber and cerebrospinal fluid. Am J Ophthalmol 1985;99:210–211.

135. Ben Ezra D, Maftzir G: Ocular penetration of cyclosporine A in the rat eye. Arch Ophthalmol 1990;108:584–587.

136. Tabbara KF, Al Sayyed Y: Ocular bioavailability of cyclosporin after oral administration. Transplant Proc 1988;20(Suppl 2):656–659.

137. Diaz-Llopis M, Menezo JL: Penetration of 2% cyclosporin eyedrops into the aqueous humour. Br J Ophthalmol 1989;73:600–603.

138. Ben Ezra D, Maftizir G, deCourten C, Timonen P: Ocular penetration of cyclosporin A. III. The human eye. Br J Ophthalmol 1990;74:350–352.

139. Reidy JJ, Gebhardt BM, Kaufman HE: The collagen shield. A new vehicle for the delivery of cyclosporin A to the eye. Cornea 1990;9:196–199.

140. Kanai A, Alba RM, Takano T, et al: The effect on the cornea of alpha cyclodextrin vehicle for cyclosporin eye drops. Transplant Proc 1989;21:3150–3152.

141. Nussenblatt RB: The expanding use of immunosuppression in the treatment of noninfectious ocular disease. J Autoimmun 1992;5 247–257.

142. Beveridge T: Pharmacokinetics and metabolism of cyclosporin A. In: White DJG, ed: Cyclosporin A. New York, Elsevier Biomedical Press, 1982, pp 35–44.

143. Nussenblatt RB, Palestine AG, Chan CC, et al. Improvement of uveitis and optic nerve disease by cyclosporine in a patient with multiple sclerosis. Am J Ophthalmol 1984;97:790–791.

144. Nussenblatt RB, Palestine AG, Chan CC: Cyclosporine therapy for uveitis: Long-term follow up. J Ocul Pharmacol 1985;1:369–382.

145. Graham EM, Sanders MD, James DG, et al: Cyclosporin A in the treatment of posterior uveitis. Trans Ophthalmol Soc UK 1985;104:146–151.

146. Wakefield D, McCluskey P: Cyclosporine: A therapy in inflammatory eye disease. J Ocul Pharmacol 1991;7:221–226.

147. LeHoang P, Girard B, Deray G, et al: Cyclosporine in the treatment of birdshot retinochoroidopathy. Transplant Proc 1988;20(Suppl 4):128–130.

148. Binder AI, Graham EM, Sanders MD, et al: Cyclosporin A in the treatment of severe Behçet's uveitis. Br J Rheumatol 1987;76:285–291.

149. Wakefield D, McCluskey P, Reece G: Cyclosporin therapy in Vogt-Koyanagi-Harada disease. Aust N Z J Ophthalmol 1990;18:137–142.

150. Nussenblatt RB, Palestine AG, Chan CC, et al: Randomized, double-masked study of cyclosporine compared to prednisolone in the treatment of endogenous uveitis. Am J Ophthalmol 1991;112:38–146.

151. Masuda K, Nakajima A, Urayama A, et al: Double-masked trial of cyclosporin versus colchicine and long-term open study of cyclosporin in Behçet's disease. Lancet 1989;1:1093–1096.

152. deVries J, Baarsma GS, Zaai MJW, et al: Cyclosporin in the treatment of severe chronic idiopathic uveitis. Br J Ophthalmol 1990;74:344–349.

153. Towler HMA, Cliffe AM, Whiting PH, Forrester JV: Low dose cyclosporin A therapy in chronic posterior uveitis. Eye 1989;3:282–287.

154. Towler HMA, Whiting PH, Forrester JV: Combination low dose cyclosporin A and steroid therapy in chronic intraocular inflammation. Eye 1990;4:514–520.

155. Towler HMA, Lightman SL, Forrester JV: Low-dose cyclosporin therapy of ocular inflammation: Preliminary report of a long-term follow-up study. J Autoimmun 1992;5(Suppl A):259–264.

156. Vitale AT, Rodriguez A, Foster CS: Low-dose cyclosporine therapy in the treatment of birdshot retinochoroidopathy. Ophthalmology 1994;101:782–831.

157. Ben Ezra DE, Cohen E, Chajek T, et al: Evaluation of conventional therapy versus cyclosporine A in Behçet's syndrome. Transplant Proc 1988;20(Suppl 4):143–146.

158. Whitcup SM, Salvo EC, Nussenblatt RB: Combined cyclosporine and corticosteroid therapy for sight-threatening uveitis in Behçet's disease. Am J Ophthalmol 1994;118:39–45.

159. Hoffman F, Widerholt M: Local treatment of necrotizing scleritis with cyclosporin A. Cornea 1985;4:3–7.

160. Wiebking WJ, Mehlfed T: Local treatment of corneal ulcers and scleromalacias with cyclosporin A. Fortschr Ophthalmol 1986;83:345–347.

161. Kruit PJ, VanBalen AT, Stilma JS: Cyclosporin A treatment in two cases of corneal peripheral melting syndromes. Doc Ophthalmol 1985;59:33–39.

162. Kruit PJ: Cyclosporine A treatment in four cases with corneal melting syndrome. Transplant Proc 1988;90(Suppl):170–172.

163. Hill JC: The use of cyclosporine in high-risk keratoplasty. Am J Ophthalmol 1989;107:506–510.

164. Miller K, Huber C, Niederwieser D, Gottinger W: Successful engraftment of high-risk corneal allografts with short-term immunosuppression with cyclosporine. Transplantation 1988;45:651–653.

165. Holland EJ, Chan CC, Kuwabara T, et al: Immunohistological findings and results of treatment with cyclosporine in ligneous conjunctivitis. Am J Ophthalmol 1989;107:160–166.

166. Rubin BI, Holland EJ, deSmet MD, et al: Response of reactivated ligneous conjunctivitis to topical cyclosporine. Am J Ophthalmol 1991;112:95–96.

167. Ben Ezra D, Peter J, Brodsky M, Cohen E: Cyclosporine eyedrops for the treatment of severe vernal keratoconjunctivitis. Am J Ophthalmol 1986;101:278–282.

168. Bleik PH, Tabbara KF. Topical cyclosporine in vernal keratoconjunctivitis. Ophthalmology 1991;98:1679–1684.

169. Secchi AG, Tognon MS, Leonardi A: Topical use of cyclosporine in the treatment of vernal keratoconjunctivitis. Am J Ophthalmol 1990;110:641–645.

170. Goichot-Bonnat L, De Beauregard C, Saragoossi JJ, Pouloquen Y: Usage de la cyclosporine A collyre dans la prévention du reject de greffe de corne chez l'homme: I. Evolution préopératoire de 4 yeux atteints de kératite métaherpetique. J Fr Ophthalmol 1987;10:207–211.

171. Belin MW, Bouchard CS, Frantz S, Chmielinska J: Topical cyclosporine in high-risk corneal transplants. Ophthalmology 1989;96:1144–1150.

172. Palestine AG, Nussenblatt RB, Gelato M: Therapy of human autoimmune uveitis with low-dose cyclosporine plus bromocriptine. Transplant Proc 1988;20(Suppl):131–135.

173. deSmet MD, Rubin BJ, Whitcup SM, et al: Combined use of cyclosporine and ketoconazole in the treatment of endogenous uveitis. Am J Ophthalmol 1992;113:687–690.

174. Ben Ezra D, Nussenblatt RB, Timchen P: Optimal Use of Sandimmune in Endogenous Uveitis. Berlin, Springer-Verlag, 1988.

175. Vine W, Bowers LD: Cyclosporine structure, pharmacokinetics, and therapeutic drug monitoring. Crit Rev Clin Lab Sci 1987;25:275–311.

176. Masri MA: Cyclosporine blood level monitoring by three special methods: RIA H3, RIA I125 and fluorescence polarization: Comparison of accuracy, cost, reproducibility and percent recovery. Transplant Proc 1992;24:1716–1717.

177. Ball PE, Munzer H, Keller HP, et al: Specific 3H radioimmunoassay with a monoclonal antibody for monitoring cyclosporine in blood. Clin Chem 1988;34:257–260.

178. Kahan BD, Wideman CA, Reid M, et al: The value of serial trough cyclosporine levels in human renal transplantation. Transplant Proc 1984;16:1195–1199.

179. Kahan BD: Cyclosporine nephrotoxicity: Pathogenesis, prophylaxis, therapy and prognosis. Am J Kidney Dis 1986;8:323–331.

180. Palestine AG, Austin HA, Balow JE, et al: Renal histopathologic alterations in patients treated with cyclosporine for uveitis. N Engl J Med 1986;314:1293–1298.

181. Mihatsch MJ, Steiner K, Abeywickrama KH, et al: Risk factors for the development of chronic cyclosporine-nephrotoxicity. Clin Nephrol 1988;29:165–175.

182. Miescher PA, Favre H, Chatelanat F, Mihatsch MJ: Combined steroid-cyclosporine treatment of chronic autoimmune diseases. Clinical results and assessment of nephrotoxicity by renal biopsy. Klin Wochenschr 1987;65:727–736.

183. Feutren G, Mihatsch MJ: Risk factors for cyclosporine-induced nephrotoxicity in patients with autoimmune diseases. N Engl J Med 1992;326:1654–1660.

184. Nussenblatt RB, de Smet MD, Rubin B, et al: A masked, randomized, dose-response study between cyclosporine A and G in the treatment of sight-threatening uveitis of noninfectious origin. Am J Ophthalmol 1993;115:583–591.

185. de Groen PL: Cyclosporine. A review and its specific use in liver transplantation. Mayo Clin Proc 1989;64:680–689.

186. Loughran TP, Deeg HJ, Dahlberg S, et al: Incidence of hypertension after marrow transplantation among 112 patients randomized to either cyclosporine or methotrexate as graft-vs-host disease prophylaxis. Br J Haematol 1985;59:547–553.

187. Palestine AG, Nussenblatt RB, Chan CC: Side effects of systemic cyclosporine in patients not undergoing transplantation. Am J Med 1984;77:652–656.

188. Lin HY, Rocher LL, McQuillan MA, et al: Cyclosporine-induced hyperuricemia and gout. N Engl J Med 1989;321:287–292.

189. Ballantyne CM, Podet EJ, Patsch WP, et al: Effects of cyclosporine therapy on plasma lipoprotein levels. JAMA 1989;262:53–56.

190. Briggs GG, Freeman RK, Yaffe SJ: Drugs Used in Pregnancy and Lactation. Baltimore, Williams & Wilkins, 1990, pp 174–176.

191. Harris KP, Jenkins D, Walls J: Nonsteroidal antiinflammatory drugs and cyclosporine. A potentially serious adverse interaction. Transplantation 1988;46:598–599.

192. Kino T, Hatanaka H, Hashimoto M, et al: FK-506, a novel immunosuppressant isolated from Streptomyces. I. Fermentation isolation. Physico-chemical and biological characteristics. J Antibiot 1987;40:1249–1255.

193. Mocizuki M, Masuda K, Sakane T, et al: A multicenter clinical open trial of FK 506 in refractory uveitis, including Behçet's disease. Transplant Proc 1991;23:3343–3346.

194. Sehgal S, Baker H, Vezina C: Rapamycin (AY-22, 989), a new antifungal antibiotic. II. Fermentation, isolation and characterization. J Antibiot 1975;28:727–732.

195. Roberge FG, Xu D, Chan CC, et al: Treatment of autoimmune neuroretinitis in the rat with rapamycin, an inhibitor of lymphocyte growth factor signal transduction. Curr Eye Res 1993;12:197–203.

196. Thompson AW: FK-506—how much potential? Immunol Today 1999;10:6–9.

197. Kahan BD, Chang JY, Sehgal S: Preclinical evaluation of a new potent immunosuppressive agent, rapamycin. Transplantation 1991;52:185–191.

198. Morris RE. Rapamycin: FK 506's fraternal twin or distant cousin? Immunol Today 1991;12:137–140.

199. Morris RE: In vivo immunopharmacology of the macrolides FK 506 and rapamycin: Toward the era of rational immunosuppressive drug discovery, development. and use. Transplant Proc 1991;23:2722–2724.

200. Thompson AW: The immunosuppressive macrolides FK-506 and rapamycin. Immunol Lett 1991;29:105–111.

201. Peters DH, Fitton A, Plosker GL, Faulds D: Tacrolimus: A review of its pharmacology and therapeutic potential in hepatic and renal transplantation. Drugs 1993;46:746–794.

202. Venkataramanan R, Jain A, Cadoff E, et al: Pharmacokinetics of FK 506: Preclinical and clinical studies. Transplant Proc 1990;22:52–56.

203. Arita C, Hotokebuchi T, Miyahaka H, et al: Inhibition by FK 506 of established lesions of collagen-induced arthritis in rats. Clin Exp Immunol 1990;82:456–461.

204. Murase N, Lieberman I, Nalesnik M, et al: Prevention of spontaneous diabetes in BB rats with FK 506. Lancet 1990;336:373–374.

205. Okuba Y, Tukada Y, Marzawa A, et al: FK 506, a novel immunosuppressive agent, induces antigen-specific immunotolerance in active Heymann's nephritis and in the autologous phase of Masugi nephritis. Clin Exp Immunol 1990;82:450–455.

206. Inamura N, Hashimoto M, Nakahara K, et al: Immunosuppressive effect of FK 506 on experimental allergic encephalomyelitis in rats. Int J Immunopharmacol 1988;10:991–995.

207. Takabayashi K, Koike T, Kurasawa K, et al: Effects of FK 506, a novel immunosuppressive drug on murine systemic lupus erythematosus. Clin Immunol Immunopathol 1989;51:110–117.

208. Kawashima H, Fujino Y. Mochizuki M: Effects of a new immunosuppressive agent. FK 506, on experimental autoimmune uveoretinitis in rats. Invest Ophthalmol Vis Sci 1988;29:1265–1271.

209. Kawashima H, Fujino Y, Mochizuki M: Antigen-specific suppressor cells induced by FK 506 in experimental autoimmune uveoretinitis in the rat. Invest Ophthalmol Vis Sci 1990;31:31–38.

210. Fujino Y, Chan CC, deSmet MD, et al: FK 506 treatment of experimental autoimmune uveoretinitis in primates. Transplant Proc 1991;23:3335–3338.

211. Jegasothy B, Ackerman CD, Todo S, et al: FK 506—a new therapeutic agent for severe, recalcitrant psoriasis. Arch Dermatol 1992;128:781–785.

212. McCauley J, Shapiro R, Scantlebury V, et al: FK 506 in the management of transplant-related nephrotic syndrome and steroid-resistant nephrotic syndrome. Transplant Proc 1991;23:3354–3356.

213. Mochizuki M. Masuda K, Tuyoshi S, et al: A clinical trial of FK 506 in refractory uveitis. Am J Ophthalmol 1993;115:763–769.

214. Martel RR, Klicius J, Galet S: Inhibition of the immune response by rapamycin. A new antifungal antibiotic. Can J Physiol Pharmacol 1977;55:48–51.

215. Martin DF, DeBarge LR, Nussenblatt RB, et al: Synergistic effect of rapamycin and cyclosporine A on the inhibition of experimental autoimmune uveoretinitis. Invest Ophthalmol Vis Sci 1993;34(Suppl):1476.

216. Macleod AM. Thompson AW: FK 506: An immunosuppressant for the 1990s? Lancet 1991;337:25–27.

217. Fung JJ, Alessiani M, Abu-Elmagd K, et al: Adverse effects associated with the use of FK 506. Transplant Proc 1991;23:3105–3108.

218. Reyes J, Tzakis A, Green M, et al: Post-transplant lymphoproliferative disorders occurring under primary FK 506 immunosuppression. Transplant Proc 1991;23:3044–3046.

219. Product Information Package Insert. PrografTM. Deerfield, IL, Fujisawa, USA, Inc., 1994.

220. Shapiro R, Fung JJ, Jain AB, et al: The side effects of FK 506 in humans. Transplant Proc 1990;22:35–36.

221. Wozel G: The story of sulfones in tropical medicine and dermatology, Int J Dermatol 1989;28:17–21.

221a. Ekberg H, Backman L, Tufveson G, Tyden G: Zenapax (daclizumab) reduces the incidence of acute rejection episodes and improves patient survival following renal transplantation. No. 14874 and No. 14393 Zenapax Study Groups. Transplant Proc 1999;31:267–268.

222. Person JR, Rogers RS: Bullous pemphigoid responding to sulfapyridine and the sulfones. Arch Dermatol 1977;113:610–615.

223. Rogers RS, Seehafer JR, Perry HO: Treatment of cicatricial (benign mucous membrane) pemphigoid with dapsone. J Am Acad Dermatol 1982;6:215–223.

224. Mandell GL, Sande MA: Antimicrobial agents: Drugs used in the chemotherapy of tuberculosis and leprosy. In: Gilman AG, Rall TW, Nies AS, Taylor P, eds: Goodman and Gilman's The Pharmacological Basis of Therapeutics. New York, Pergamon Press, 1990, pp 1159–1164, 1169–1171.

225. Wozel G, Barth J: Current aspects of modes of action of dapsone. Int J Dermatol 1988;27:547–552.

226. Geer KE: Dapsone and sulfapyridine. In: Wolverton SE, Wilkin JK, eds: Systemic Drugs for Skin Diseases. Philadelphia, WB Saunders, 1991, pp 247–264.

227. Barranco VP: Inhibition of lysosomal enzymes by dapsone. Arch Dermatol 1974;110:563–566.

228. Lang PG: Sulfones and sulfonamides in dermatology today. J Am Acad Dermatol 1979;1:479–492.

229. Stendahl O, Molin L, Dahlgren C: The inhibition of polymorphonuclear leukocyte cytotoxicity by dapsone, a possible mechanism in the treatment of dermatitis herpetiformis. J Clin Invest 1978;62:214–220.

230. Pieters FA, Zuidema J: The pharmacokinetics of dapsone after oral administration to healthy volunteers. Br J Clin Pharmacol 1986;22:491–494.

231. Barranco VP, Minor DB, Solomon H: Treatment of relapsing polychondritis with dapsone. Arch Dermatol 1976:112:1286–1288.

232. Martin J, Roenigk HH, Lynch W, Tingwald FR: Relapsing polychondritis treated with dapsone. Arch Dermatol 1976;112:1272–1274.

233. Matoba A, Plager S, Barber J, McCulley JP: Keratitis in relapsing polychondritis. Ann Ophthalmol 1984;16:367–370.

234. DeGowin RL: A review of therapeutic and hemolytic effects of dapsone. Arch Intern Med 1967;120:242–248.

235. Potter MN, Yates P, Slade R, Kennedy CT: Agranulocytosis caused by dapsone therapy for granuloma annulare. J Am Acad Dermatol 1989;30:87–88.

236. Vance ML, Evans WS, Thomer WO: Bromocriptine. Ann Intern Med 1984;100:78–91.

237. Cedarbaum JM, Schleifer LS: Drugs for Parkinson's disease, spasticity, and acute muscle spasma. In: Gilman AG, Rall TW, Nies AS, Taylor P, eds: Goodman and Gilman's The Pharmacological Basis of Therapeutics. New York, Pergamon Press, 1990, pp 474–475.

238. Berczi I, Nazy E, Asa SC, Kovacs K: Pituitary hormones and contact sensitivity in rats. Allergy 1983;38:325–330.

239. Berczi I, Nagy E, Asa SL, Kovacs K: The influence of pituitary hormones on adjuvant arthritis. Arthritis Rheum 1984;27:682–688.

240. Russell DH, Matrisian L, Kibler R, et al: Prolactin receptors on human lymphocytes and their modulation by cyclosporine. Biochem Biophys Res Commun 1984;121:899–906.

241. Russell DH, Kibler R, Matfisian L, et al: Prolactin receptors on human T and B lymphocytes: Antagonism of prolactin binding by cyclosporine. J Immunol 1985;134:3027–3031.

242. Russell DH, Larson DF: Prolactin induced polyamine biosynthesis in spleen and thymus: specific inhibition by cyclosporine. Immunopharmacology 1985;9:165–174.

243. Palestine AG, Muellenberg-Coulombre CB, Kim MK, et al: Bromocriptine and low dose cyclosporine in the treatment of experimental autoimmune uveitis in rats. J Clin Invest 1987;79:1078–1081.

244. Hedner LP, Bynke G: Endogenous iridocyclitis relieved during treatment with bromocriptine. Am J Ophthalmol 1985;100:618–619.

245. Palestine AG, Nussenblatt RB: The effect of bromocriptine on anterior uveitis. Am J Ophthalmol 1988;106:488–489.

246. Lopatynsky MD, Krohel GB: Bromocriptine therapy for thyroid ophthalmology. Am J Ophthalmol 1989;107:680–681.

247. Kazeen KN, Zinkevich IV, Karaseva JI, Kostareva LN: Short-term results of parlodel treatment of patients with diffuse goiter complicated by endocrine ophthalmopathy. Probl Endocrinol 1987;33:3–5.

248. Kolodziej-Maciejewska H, Reterski Z: Positive effect of bromocriptine treatment in Graves' disease orbitopathy. Exp Clin Endocrinol 1985;86:241–242.

249. Frey WH, Nelson ID, Frick ML, Elde RR: Prolactin immunoreactivity in human tears and lacrimal gland: possible implications for tear production. In: Holly FJ, Lamberts DE, MacKenn DL, eds: The Periocular Tear Film in Health, Disease, and Contact Lens Wear. Lubbock, TX, Dry Eye Institute, 1986, pp 798–807.

250. American hospital formulary service drug information. Bethesda, MD, Board of Directors of the American Society of Hospital Pharmacists, 1994, pp 2431–2435.

251. First MR, Schroeder TJ, Weiskittel P, et al: Concomitant administration of cyclosporine and ketoconazole in renal transplant recipients. Lancet 1989;2:1198–1201.

252. Millikan LE, Schrum JP: Antifungal agents. In: Wolverton SE, Wilkin JK, eds: Systemic Drugs for Skin Diseases. Philadelphia, WB Saunders, 1991, pp 29–36.

253. Van Tyle JH: Ketoconazole. Pharmacotherapy 1984;4:343–373.

254. Gumbleton M, Brown JE, Hawksworth G, Whiting PH: The possible relationship between hepatic drug metabolism and ketoconazole enhancement of cyclosporine nephrotoxicity. Transplantation 1985;40:454–455.

255. Anderson JE, Morris RE, Blaschke TF: Pharmacodynamics of cyclosporine-ketoconazole interaction in mice. Combined therapy potentiates cyclosporine immunosuppression and toxicity. Transplantation 1987;43:529–533.

256. Daneshmend TK, Warnock EL, Turner A, Roberts CL: Pharmacokinetics of ketoconazole in normal subjects. J Antimicrob Chemother 1981;8:299–304.

257. Huang YC, Colaizzi JL, Bierman RH, et al: Pharmacokinetics and dose proportionality of ketoconazole in normal volunteers. Antimicrob Agents Chemother 1986;30:206–210.

258. Heel RC, Brogden RN, Carmine A, et al: Ketoconazole: A review of its therapeutic efficacy in superficial and systemic fungal infections. Drugs 1982;23:1–36.

259. NSAID Mycoses Study Group: Treatment of blastomycosis and histoplasmosis with ketoconazole. Ann Intern Med 1985;103:861–892.

260. Lewis JH, Zimmerman HI, Benson GD, Ishak KG: Hepatic injury associated with ketoconazole therapy. Analysis of 33 cases. Gastroenterology 1984;86:502–513.

261. Insel PA: Analgesic-antipyretics and antiinflammatory agents: Drugs employed in the treatment of rheumatoid arthritis and gout. In: Gilman AG, Rail TW, Nies AS, Taylor P, eds: Goodman and Gilman's The Pharmacological Basis of Therapeutics. New York, Pergamon Press, 1990, pp 674–676.

262. Davis LS: New uses for old drugs. In: Wilverton SE, Wilkin JK, eds: Systemic Drugs for Skin Diseases. Philadelphia, WB Saunders, 1991, pp 364–367.

263. Famary JP: Colchicine in therapy, state of the art and nonperspectives for an old drug. Clin Exp Rheumatol 1988;6:305–317.

264. Harper RM, Allen BS: Use of colchicine in the treatment of Behçet's disease. Int J Dermatol 1992;21:551–554.

265. Ehrenfeld M, Levy M, Bareli M, et al: Effect of colchicine on polymorphonuclear leukocyte chemotaxis in human volunteers. Br J Clin Pharmacol 1980;10:297–300.

266. Malawista SE: The action of colchicine in acute gouty arthritis. Arthritis Rheum 1975;19(Suppl):835–846.

267. Pesanti EL, Ayline SG: Colchicine effects on lysosomal enzyme induction and intracellular degradation in the cultivated macrophage. J Exp Med 1975;141:1030–1046.

268. Sander HM, Randle HW: Use of colchicine in Behçet's syndrome. Cutis 1986;37:344–348.

269. Jorizzo JL, Hudson RD, Schmalstieg FC, et al: Behçet's syndrome immune regulation, circulating immune complexes, neutrophil migration, and colchicine therapy. J Am Acad Dermatol 1994;10:205–214.

270. Gatot A, Tovi F: Colchicine therapy in recurrent oral ulcers [letter]. Arch Dermatol 1984;120:994.

271. Ruah CB, Stram JR, Chasin WD: Treatment of severe recurrent aphthous stomatitis with colchicine. Arch Otolaryngol Head Neck Surg 1988;114:671–675.

272. Frayha RA: Arthropathy of Behçet's disease with marked synovial pleocytosis responsive to colchicine. Arthritis Rheum 1982;25:235–236.

273. Hijikata K, Masuda K: Visual prognosis in Behçet's disease: Effects of cyclophosphamide and colchicine. Jpn J Ophthalmol 1978;22:506–519.

274. Mizushima Y, Matsumura N, Mori M, et al: Colchicine in Behçet's disease. Lancet 1977;2:1037.

275. Raynor A, Askari AD: Behçet's disease and treatment with colchicine. J Am Acad Dermatol 1980;2:396–450.

276. Ferreira NR, Buonicotti A: Trisomy after colchicine therapy. Lancet 1968;2:1304.

13 ─ DIAGNOSTIC SURGERY

E. Mitchel Opremcak and C. Stephen Foster

INTRODUCTION

Uveitis is generally considered a medical subspecialty within ophthalmology; yet surgery is required in the care of many patients who have uveitis. The surgery is diverse and may be indicated both for diagnostic and for therapeutic purposes. Diagnostic surgery in the care of patients with uveitis is, quite frankly, probably underutilized.

Because the surgery that may be indicated in the diagnostic and therapeutic care of patients with uveitis is diverse, a fully trained uveitis specialist who has had perhaps more than one type of subspecialty fellowship training may be capable of personally performing all surgery that may be required, from cornea to retina. However, most often the uveitis specialist must collaborate closely with other subspecialists in accomplishing all that is needed to provide total care for such patients.

This chapter is devoted to diagnostic surgical procedures that may be indicated in the pursuit of the underlying diagnosis of uveitis. Such procedures are generally undertaken only after all reasonable noninvasive studies have been performed and have failed to disclose the underlying cause of the patient's uveitis. The chapter that follows this one addresses therapeutic surgery in the care of patients with uveitis.

PARACENTESIS

Anterior chamber paracentesis for harvesting aqueous for diagnostic purposes has been used much more extensively over the past 50 years in Europe than in the United States. The reason for this dichotomy in practice patterns is unclear, but it may derive from the belief in North America that the data obtained from the predominant type of analysis performed on harvested aqueous humor, specifically, measurement of antibody levels in an effort to determine whether or not an infectious agent is causing the uveitis, are insufficiently convincing to warrant the effort to make the special arrangements necessary for analyzing the aqueous humor for putative antibodies. Indeed, almost no one in North America has systematically employed the Goldmann-Witmer or the Dernouchamps antibody coefficient test, as many Europeans have done over the past 50 years, when the possibility of an infectious cause of uveitis came to mind. The coefficient is calculated as shown in Figure 13–1.

The total amount of immunoglobulin in aqueous humor and in serum, as well as the specific amount of immunoglobulin antibody directed against the suspected microbe, must be measured; higher than normal levels of protein, immunoglobulin, and antibody directed against some particular microbe will be found in the aqueous humor of a patient with an inflamed eye, which is a consequence of blood-eye barrier breakdown. Hence, simply finding a higher than expected level of anti–herpes simplex virus (HSV) antibody in the aqueous humor might lead one to falsely conclude that the patient's uveitis was secondary to herpes simplex virus (with local manufacturing of anti-herpes antibody by B cells and plasma cells residing in the iris) when, in fact, the patient has simply had antibodies directed against herpes in the serum passively leak through iris vasculature into the aqueous humor. Simultaneous measurement of both protein (e.g., immunoglobulin) and specific anti-herpes antibody in both aqueous humor and serum allows one to control for the possibility of simple passive diffusion. Using the "cut-off" coefficient values recommended by Witmer, one can then reasonably conclude that plasma cells and B lymphocytes in the eye locally produce antibody directed against herpes simplex virus, if one finds a coefficient of 4 or greater. This would then prompt one to conclude that the patient's uveitis is secondary to herpes simplex virus; long-term therapy with oral acyclovir to suppress chronic or recurrent HSV reactivation from latency may then add additional circumstantial evidence to the notion of recurrent HSV uveitis.

Paracentesis may also be confirmatory in the instance of suspected phacoantigenic uveitis. Paracentesis with harvesting of aqueous and preparation of a cytospin preparation on a glass slide, followed by staining and microscopy, would disclose large numbers of macrophages, many with engulfed lens material, and would complete a picture that is virtually pathognomonic of phacogenic uveitis.

Finally, polymerase chain reaction (PCR) technology has revolutionized our ability to definitively diagnose infectious causes of uveitis. Obtaining ample material from the eye to ensure an inoculum of sufficient concentration to result in positive cultures in instances of infectious uveitis is quite difficult. It takes, after all, a certain quantum of microbes that will survive and grow to the point of being detectable in the laboratory to establish a nidus in culture conditions; many instances exist in which the number of microbes available for harvesting is so small as to result in negative cultures after such harvesting. Theoretically, however, one could begin with but a single copy of DNA from the microbe and still, through PCR technology, amplify that genetic material to quantities sufficient to be detectable through conventional laboratory techniques. Thus, PCR amplification of gene sequences from microbes present in minute quantities in aqueous humor, vitreous, and biopsy specimens has enabled clinicians to definitively diagnose infectious causes of uveitis. Of course, one must have a limited number of putative microbial causes of uveitis in mind in order to amplify the harvested genetic material with the appropriate oligonucleotide primer pairs, each specific for the microbial contenders under study.

The PCR technique is highly sophisticated and complex, and is subject to both misperformance and misinterpretation. More and more commercial diagnostic PCR laboratories have become available over the past 5 years,

215

$$\frac{\text{Titer of antibody in aqueous}}{\text{Titer of antibody in serum}} \times \frac{\text{Concentration of serum globulins}}{\text{Concentration of aqueous globulins}}$$

Results: 0.5 to 2   no intraocular antibody production
2 to 4   suggestive of intraocular antibody production
≥ 4 diagnostic of intraocular antibody production

FIGURE 13–1. The Goldmann-Witmer coefficient.

however, that meet licensing and stringency requirements to safeguard against false-positive results; they undergo periodic testing to ensure appropriate detection of positive samples and accurate identification of negative samples that do not contain microbial DNA. Thus, the ability of ophthalmologists to easily request and receive such analyses of harvested intraocular material in patients with uveitis is steadily increasing. We believe this technology not only will change the landscape of our care of large numbers of patients with uveitis, but also may shed new light on some of the syndromes heretofore typically considered "idiopathic."

VITRECTOMY

Diagnostic vitreoretinal surgery should be considered when other noninvasive methods of diagnosis have failed to establish a pathoetiologic mechanism. Patients who have a severe, sight-threatening form of uveitis (and in whom empirical medical treatment has failed to control the intraocular inflammation) should be considered for diagnostic surgical procedures. The goals of ocular biopsy should be to acquire microbiologic, cytologic, histologic, immunologic, and genetic information for modifying and directing medical treatments. Patients with acute or chronic postoperative inflammation may have bacterial or fungal endophthalmitis; patients with chronic inflammation that has failed to fully respond to anti-inflammatory medication may have endogenous infectious endophthalmitis or intraocular malignancy. Diagnostic vitrectomy is the critical diagnostic step in determining the cause of inflammation in these instances (Fig. 13–2).

Pars plana vitrectomy can be performed to obtain both diluted and undiluted vitreous humor for analysis. A modified, three-port vitrectomy can be performed using an infusion saline solution to control the level of intraocular pressure during the procedure. Control of the pressure in a closed system can minimize the complications of intraoperative hypotony, as well as choroidal detachments and expulsive hemorrhage, all of which are more common in eyes with uveitis. The infusion line should be placed and secured in the inferior temporal quadrant and inspected for proper location within the vitreous cavity. Patients with intraocular inflammation often have scleral thickening, choroidal edema, and exudative retinal detachments. Infusion cannulas of standard length may not gain free access to the vitreous cavity. Infusion of saline in such an instance, when the cannula tip is under the retina or within the choroid, can result in disastrous iatrogenic complications, including subretinal hemorrhage, choroidal detachment, and separation of the retina. Longer infusion cannulas (4 to 6 millimeters) are often required to reach the vitreous cavity of patients with uveitis, and one must directly visualize the cannula prior to beginning the infusion.

In contrast to therapeutic vitrectomies, the initial specimen in diagnostic cases should be obtained undiluted, before the infusion port is turned on. A small amount of vitreous (0.5 to 1 ml) should be obtained directly from the vitrectomy handpiece tubing through an in-line stopcock attached to a syringe. The latter method of obtaining an undiluted vitreous specimen reduces the risk of vitreoreti-

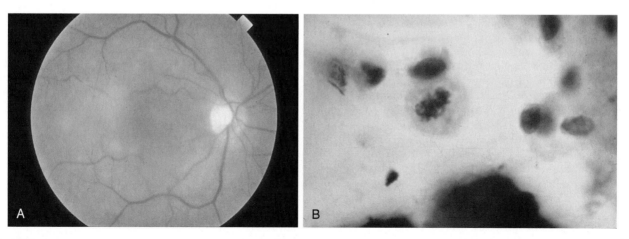

FIGURE 13–2. *A,* Fundus photograph of a 65-year-old patient with chronic, medically unresponsive vitritis and multifocal, subretinal infiltrates. *B,* Photomicrograph of a vitreous biopsy showing neoplastic cells with mitotic figures establishing a diagnosis of intraocular, non-Hodgkin's lymphoma. See color insert.

nal traction and retinal detachment that is associated with straight needle aspiration because the vitreous cutter ensures that no vitreous still attached to retina is aspirated. The infusion line is then opened, and a standard vitrectomy performed.

Patients with uveitis can present intraoperative challenges due to media opacification. Band keratopathy, posterior synechiae, cyclitic membranes, and cataract often need to be addressed before the actual vitrectomy is performed to improve visualization of the posterior segment. Surgical approaches to these conditions are presented elsewhere.

Both the vitreous washings and the undiluted vitreous aspirate should be immediately delivered for microbiologic and cytologic analysis.[1-3] A portion of the sample should be sent for viral, fungal, and both aerobic and anaerobic bacterial culture. The laboratory should be instructed to keep the bacterial cultures longer than the standard 3 to 5 days because chronic anaerobic endophthalmitis is caused by a slow-growing, anaerobic bacterium.

Propionibacterium may require 5 to 14 days to grow (Fig. 13–3).[4] Millipore filtration should be performed on the vitreous washings to concentrate any microorganisms and cellular elements. The filter can be sterilely cut in the laboratory for microbiologic culture. The washings can be processed for immunohistochemical staining, or cells in cellular specimens can be sorted for monoclonality and cell subtyping. This information may establish the malignant nature of the "inflammatory" cells in patients with lymphoma. Newer genetic assays can be performed in certain settings to discover the DNA of specific microbes that are difficult to culture. Polymerase chain reaction and cDNA probes can be employed to detect DNA from many viruses such as herpes simplex virus, varicella zoster virus, and cytomegalovirus, as well as protozoal DNA, such as in *Toxoplasma gondii*.

RETINAL BIOPSY

In certain conditions, the inflammatory process is localized primarily to sensory retina or retinal pigment epithelium. *Toxoplasma gondii*, herpes simplex virus, varicella zoster virus, and cytomegalovirus are common intracellular pathogens that spread by cell-to-cell contact within the retina.[5] The vitreous may harbor few or none of the responsible microorganisms (Fig. 13–4). Certain bacteria and fungi, such as *Mycobacterium* and *Candida*, may also produce retinitis. Sarcoidosis or other idiopathic syndromes that have a poorly understood disease mechanism, such as serpiginous choroiditis, can primarily involve the retina and may be sight-threatening. In these patients, a diagnostic vitrectomy would yield very little information. Retinal biopsy can be performed to better understand the disease process and to help establish a diagnosis.

Before a retinal biopsy is performed, the location of the tissue to be sampled must be carefully considered. The biopsy site should be chosen carefully to minimize both intraoperative and postoperative complications.[5, 6] Injury to the optic nerve, macula, and major vessels should be avoided. The site should be located away from any major vascular arcades. A location in the superior retina is preferred, if possible, to allow for postoperative gas tamponade repair of the iatrogenic retinal opening. A superior nasal location is ideal in that any unexpected hemorrhage will not involve the macula. Further, the lesion should be located behind the equator of the eye. Anterior lesions are difficult to access using handheld vitrectomy instruments. Also of importance is the need to select an area of active disease. A biopsy of normal retina or inactive, atrophic, or "burned out" retinal disease will not provide useful information. Instead, the biopsy site should be at the border of normal retina and active retinal disease.[5, 7]

A vitrectomy is performed to gain access to the retina, clear the media, and allow for gas tamponade. The site is identified and surrounded with a double or triple row of laser photocoagulation; the endolaser probe is used to seal the retinal hole and assist with intraoperative hemostasis. If the retina is already detached, internal diathermy can be substituted. In cases in which the retina is attached, a cannula is used to inject saline under the sensory retina to create a small bleb. An incision is then made in the retina using a needle knife, and intraocular

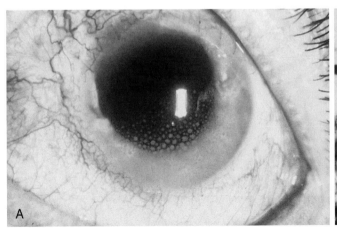
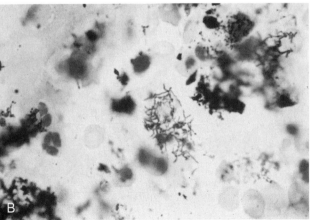

FIGURE 13–3. *A,* Anterior segment photograph from a patient with low-grade uveitis, 4 weeks following cataract surgery, showing "dirty" keratic precipitates. *B,* Photomicrograph of a Gram's stain of a vitreous aspirate from the same patient showing gram-positive, pleomorphic bacilli. Anaerobic cultures grew *Propionibacterium granulosa* after an 8-day incubation. See color insert.

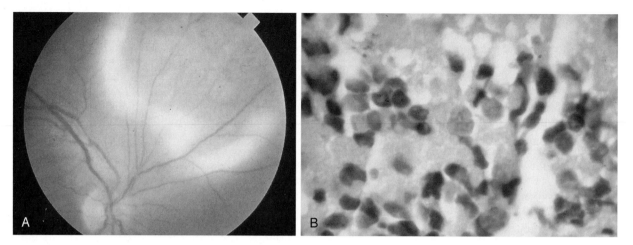

FIGURE 13–4. *A,* Fundus photograph from an immunosuppressed patient with a progressive, brushfire-like retinitis of unknown etiology that was unresponsive to antiviral therapy. *B,* Photomicrograph of a retinal biopsy showing toxoplasmosis of organisms and tissue cysts. The vitreous specimen did not show toxoplasmosis organisms. See color insert.

scissors are used to complete the sensory retinectomy. Forceps are then used to grasp the specimen and remove it from the eye. Care should be taken not to lose the retinal biopsy sample as the forceps leave the eye at the sclerotomy site. The retina is then reattached via pneumatic air-fluid exchange techniques. The patient should be examined for other retinal breaks, which should be treated with laser or retinal cryopexy. The eye is then closed and a long-acting, nonexpansile concentration of perfluoropropane (15%) and sulfahexafluoride (20%) is exchanged with the air.

Subretinal lesions such as helminthic disease, cysticercosis, and ophthalmomyiasis or disease of the retinal pigment epithelium such as serpiginous choroiditis can be biopsied using similar surgical techniques (Fig. 13–5).[5, 7] The overlying sensory retina is not excised, but the area of disease beneath the retina is grasped with subretinal forceps and removed. Bleeding can be controlled by increasing the intraocular pressure via raising the infusion bottle height. Laser or internal diathermy

can then be used to obtain further hemostasis and seal the break. Air or a long-acting gas tamponade is then employed to flatten the sensory retina.

The retinal specimen can be sectioned into three pieces with a needle knife under the operating microscope.[8] One sample should be frozen in cryostat compound for immunopathology, the second piece fixed with 4% glutaraldehyde for light and electronmicroscopic study, and the third piece sent for microbiologic studies (culture and PCR). In most cases of suspected infectious retinitis, viral cultures are of critical importance and should take priority over bacterial or fungal culture if the specimen quantity is limited.

CHORIORETINAL BIOPSY

Chorioretinal biopsy should be considered in patients who have an unidentified, medically unresponsive, bilateral, sight-threatening inflammatory process that involves either the choroid or both the retina and choroid.[7, 9, 10] The information obtained should help establish whether

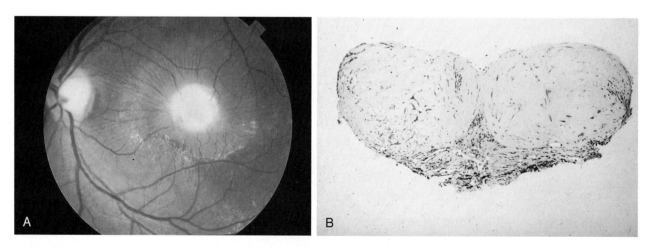

FIGURE 13–5. *A,* Fundus photograph of a submacular lesion in a 24-year-old patient with vitritis and a subretinal lesion who was referred for ocular cysticercosis. *B,* Photomicrograph of the submacular lesion showing a fibrovascular scar. *Cysticercus* sp. was not found in serial sections and the etiology of the inflammatory scar was unknown. See color insert.

the process is infectious, immunologic, malignant, or degenerative. In many cases, chorioretinal biopsy has established a specific diagnosis or disease mechanism and resulted in specific treatment strategies (Figs. 13–6 and 13–7).

Prior to performance of a chorioretinal biopsy, the location of the biopsy should be carefully selected. As was explained in the discussion on retinal biopsy, major vessels should be avoided. A location in the upper half of the fundus should be picked to allow postoperative gas tamponade and repair of the chorioretinal defect. This site should be at the border of the normal retina and the active chorioretinal disease process. Unlike retinal biopsy, these lesions should be anterior to the equator for purposes of surgical access. It is difficult to perform an eye wall biopsy for lesions posterior to the equator of the eye.

A standard vitrectomy is performed and the biopsy site is carefully identified via indirect ophthalmoscopy. The area is then localized on the surface of the eye via scleral depression and marked with a surgical pen. With the laser indirect ophthalmoscope, a double or triple row of retinal photocoagulation is placed surrounding the biopsy site to minimize bleeding and the risk of retinal detachment. The eye is filled with air, and a partial-thickness scleral flap (6 × 6 mm) is dissected over the marked area (Fig. 13–8). The edges of the bed are treated with diathermy, and a needle knife is used to incise the sclera, choroid, and retina. Small retinal or Vannas scissors are then used to cut a 3.5- to 4-mm square specimen. The edge of the biopsy specimen is carefully grasped and removed. The scleral flap is sutured closed with nylon suture, and the eye is filled with a nonexpansile concentration of sulfahexafluoride or perfluoropropane gas. The specimen is then processed as described for a retinal biopsy.

The risk of chorioretinal biopsy include intraoperative hypotony, choroidal detachment, and vitreous hemorrhage.[7, 9, 10] Postoperative complications include retinal detachment, hypotony, choroidal hemorrhage, vitreous hemorrhage, endophthalmitis, and cataract. Late-onset complications include a greater risk for proliferative vitreoretinopathy (PVR), and even loss of the eye. These

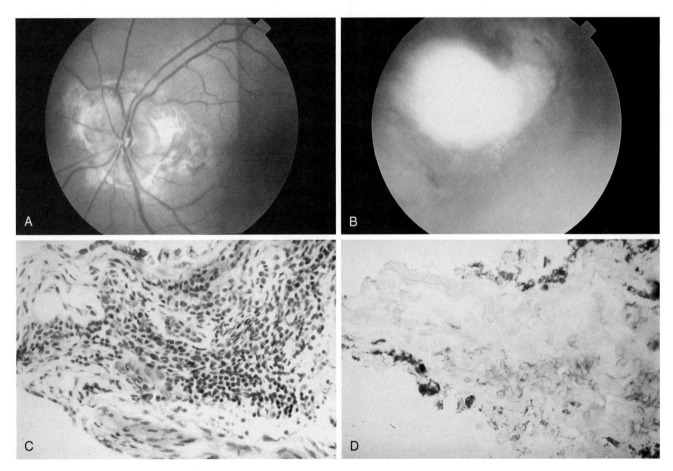

FIGURE 13–6. *A,* Fundus photograph of a patient with a 15-year history of multifocal choroiditis and panuveitis (MCP) of unknown etiology. The patient was intolerant of corticosteroid agents. The right eye was NLP and the left eye had active MCP and a progressive, macula threatening lesion. *B,* Fundus photograph of the superior chorioretinal biopsy site showing the underlying sclera. The retina remained attached following surgery. *C,* Photomicrograph of a chorioretinal biopsy specimen showing choroidal infiltration with epithelioid cells, plasma cells, eosinophils, and a Dalen-Fuchs nodule, which support a diagnosis of sympathetic ophthalmia. Infectious organisms were not identified. Following the operation, the patient recalled traumatic, strabismus surgery as a child that may have been the original trauma inducing the uveitis. *D,* Immunohistochemical staining of the same biopsy specimen showing activated CD4+, helper T cells (red-stained mononuclear cells) supporting an active, cellular immune response. See color insert.

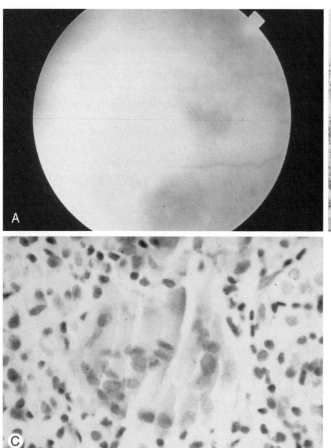

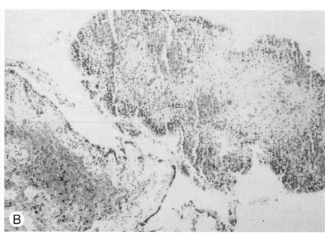

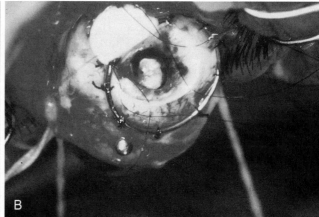

FIGURE 13–7. *A,* Fundus photograph of a patient with bilateral, progressive, sight-threatening retinitis and a negative diagnostic work-up. *B,* Chorioretinal biopsy specimen showing a full-thickness retinitis and a mild mononuclear infiltration of the choroid. *C,* High-magnification of the retina, showing noncaseating, granuloma, and primary retinal sarcoidosis. Extensive laboratory and radiologic examination failed to demonstrate evidence of systemic disease. See color insert.

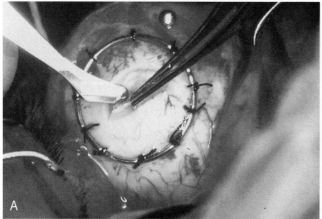

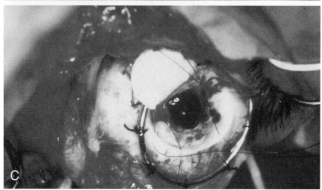

FIGURE 13–8. *A,* Chorioretinal biopsy—partial-thickness scleral flap dissection. *B,* Chorioretinal biopsy—chorioretinal sample, cut from the scleral bed. Note the diathermy marks at the margins and the preplaced, nylon sutures. *C,* Chorioretinal biopsy—remaining cortical vitreous at the chorioretinal biopsy site; the specimen has been removed.

diagnostic surgical procedures should be performed only in patients with severe, unresponsive, and sight-threatening forms of uveitis and are an alternative to diagnostic enucleation.

References

1. Green WR: Diagnostic cytopathology of ocular fluid specimens. Ophthalmology 1984;91:726–749.
2. Davis JL, Solomon D, Nussenblatt RB, et al: Immunocytochemical staining of vitreous cells. Ophthalmology 1992;99:250–256.
3. Stulting RD, Leif RC, Clarkson JG, et al: Centrifugal cytology of ocular fluids. Arch Ophthalmol 1992;100:822–825.
4. Bishop KB, Orosz CG: Limiting dilution analysis for alloreactive TCGF-secretory T cells: Two related LDA methods that can discriminate between unstimulated precursor T cells and in vivo alloactivated T cells. Transplantation 1989;47:671–677.
5. Freeman WR, Henderly DE, Wan WL, et al: Prevalence, pathophysiology, and treatment of rhegmatogenous retinal detachment in treated cytomegalovirus retinitis. Am J Ophthalmol 1987;103:527–536.
6. Nussenblatt RB, Whitcup SM, Palestine AG: Surgical treatment in uveitis. In: Uveitis: Fundamentals and Clinical Practice, 2nd ed. St. Louis, Missouri, Mosby, 1996, p 148.
7. Freeman WR: Application of vitreoretinal surgery to inflammatory and infectious disease of the posterior segment. Int Ophthalmol Clin 1992;32:15–33.
8. Clarkson JG, Blumenkranz MS, Culbertson WW, et al: Retinal detachment following the acute retinal necrosis syndrome. Ophthalmology 1984;91:1665–1668.
9. Martin DF, Chan CC, de Smet MD, et al: The role of chorioretinal biopsy in the management of posterior uveitis. Ophthalmology 1993;100:705–714.
10. Peyman GA, Juarez CP, Raichand M: Full-thickness eye wall biopsy: Long term results in 9 patients. Br J Ophthalmol 1981;65:723–726.

14 THERAPEUTIC SURGERY: CORNEA, IRIS, CATARACT, GLAUCOMA, VITREOUS, RETINAL

C. Stephen Foster and E. Mitchel Opremcak

The preceding chapter addressed the various diagnostic surgical procedures that may be indicated in the care of patients with uveitis. This chapter discusses various therapeutic surgical procedures that may be required in the care of such patients. And whereas it is undoubtedly true that most well-trained ophthalmologists may be technically capable of performing many of the procedures, we would caution that operating on an eye that has been repeatedly or chronically inflamed is very different from operating on one that has not been inflamed. History has shown that some of the damage done from chronic inflammation is commonly permanent, so that even if the eye appears clinically quiet, it responds to surgery violently, with abnormal, excessive bleeding; exuberant inflammation; and unexpected postoperative pressure responses (hypertension or hypotony). Cataracta complicata, the cataract of the uveitis patient, got its well-deserved name through the many years of frustrated experience of ophthalmologists who operated on such cataracts. Exuberant inflammation with resultant proliferative vitreoretinopathy is an all-too-familiar phenomenon to vitreoretinal surgeons who have experience in the posterior segment surgical care of patients with uveitis.

Consequently, we would emphasize two essential points at this juncture:

1. Prevention is preferable to any surgery. Care of patients with uveitis through therapies that stop the inflammation and allow the patient to remain in remission off steroids can prevent cataract, glaucoma, and maculopathy development.
2. Surgery for the complications of uveitis is best done after active inflammation has been quiet for as long as is practicable, and even then, adjunctive supplemental steroid therapy should be generously used perioperatively and intraoperatively: topically, by regional injection, and systemically.

CORNEA

Patients with chronic uveitis (most particularly those who have the onset of uveitis in childhood) may develop calcium deposition at the level of the corneal epithelial basement membrane zone and Bowman's membrane. This problem typically begins in the corneal periphery (Fig. 14–1) but may advance sufficiently into the central part of the cornea as to obscure the ophthalmologist's ability to assess the patient's intraocular features adequately, or to obscure the surgeon's view in other aspects of surgical care of the patient with uveitis. Such calcium deposition can be removed either by phototherapeutic keratectomy or by ethylenediaminetetraacetic acid (EDTA) chelation and superficial keratectomy. Phototherapeutic keratectomy carries with it the disadvantage

of progressive removal of corneal substance, if, as is so often the case, multiple recurrences of band keratopathy occur; hence, this section is restricted to a description of EDTA chelation and superficial keratectomy in the treatment of band keratopathy.

Breinin first described this procedure in 1954, employing 0.01 and 0.05 molar concentrations of (disodium) EDTA.[1] We have had considerable experience with this procedure over the past 25 years on the Ocular Immunology & Uveitis Service of the Massachusetts Eye and Ear Infirmary, and it is our technique of choice in dealing with patients with band keratopathy. The procedure is performed as follows.

Under general, regional injection, or topical anesthesia (depending on the personality and age of the patient), the epithelium overlying the calcium deposition is gently removed with a #15 Bard-Parker blade or a Desmarres scarifier (Greishaber #68108), employing a technique of wiping the epithelium off, ensuring that no cuts are made in Bowman's membrane. Once the epithelium has been removed, a plastic, glass, cardboard, or steel well of some sort is positioned over the affected area. Care is taken to ensure survival of sufficient numbers of limbal stem cells to repopulate the denuded cornea with corneally derived epithelium. An example of the well we typically employ is shown in Figure 14–2, which is fashioned from a 3-ml plastic syringe. A solution of 0.35% EDTA is placed into the well, and the well is held in position for 5 minutes. The well is then removed, and the surface of the eye is vigorously irrigated with balanced salt solution. The surgical knife is then used to scrape the loosened flakes of

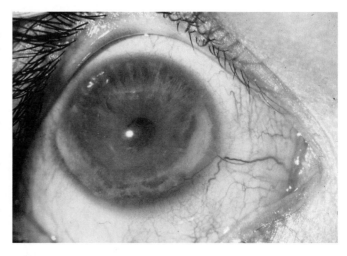

FIGURE 14–1. Classic band keratopathy in a patient with juvenile rheumatoid arthritis–associated recurrent iridocyclitis. Note that, thus far, the band keratopathy is limited to the corneal periphery, and, therefore, is visually insignificant.

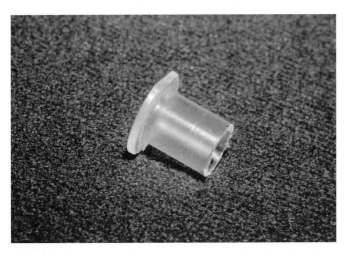

FIGURE 14–2. A plastic well created by cutting a plastic syringe. This well is placed, hub down, onto the cornea to create a watertight well into which EDTA can be placed, remaining for 5 minutes, to chelate calcium in a patient with band keratopathy.

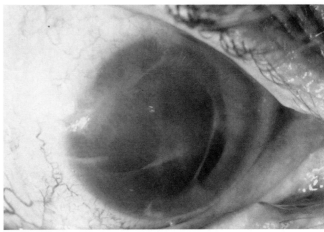

FIGURE 14–4. Postoperative EDTA chelation, same patient (and eye) as shown in Figure 14–3.

calcium, and the procedure is repeated as many times as is required to achieve complete removal of the calcium. Overly vigorous scraping and cutting should be avoided. Cycloplegic and antibiotic medication is then instilled, and a continuous-wear bandage soft lens is applied. The eye is patched, and the patient is evaluated the next day in the outpatient clinic. With the use of the soft contact lens and cycloplegia, pain control is generally straightforward with simple oral analgesics. The epithelium generally has repopulated the corneal surface within 1 week following surgery, and the bandage soft lens may or may not then be removed, depending on the patient's preference. Topical antibiotic and steroid is typically employed by us throughout the healing course. Figures 14–3 and 14–4 illustrate preoperative and postoperative examples of this procedure.

IRIS

Patients with uveitis may develop posterior synechiae sufficient to produce pupillary block and iris bombé, with acute glaucoma. Ordinarily, in a patient with nonuveitic

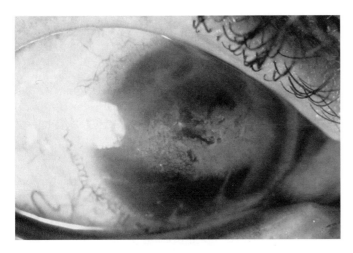

FIGURE 14–3. Preoperative EDTA chelation of a patient's cornea with band keratopathy.

pupillary block glaucoma, laser iridotomy is the most straightforward technique for abrogating this problem. However, in the inflamed eye, even if one is successful in achieving an iridotomy through laser surgery, closure of the iridotomy commonly occurs, particularly if the patient's iris is significantly pigmented. Patients with blue irides may be sufficiently treated with laser iridotomy, but patients with brown irides rarely are.

Laser Iridotomy

We prefer a preparatory treatment with argon laser at two sites in the iris periphery, typically 10 to 20 applications per site, at a power of 200 milliwatts, 0.1-second duration, 50-micron spot size. We then perform the definitive iridotomy with yttrium aluminum garnet (YAG) laser, in the middle of the two foci that have previously been prepared with the argon laser. The amount of energy required to achieve the iridotomy is approximately 4 millijoules. Sometimes only one application is required; rarely are more than three applications required.

Surgical Iridectomy

This is our procedure of choice for any patient with brown irides and uveitis who develops pupillary seclusion and iris bombé. A 1 clock hour peritomy is created, and a precisely vertical incision at the posterior surgical limbus is fashioned, 2 mm in length, with attention to ensuring that the internal length of the wound is equal to the external length of the wound, down to but not including perforation into the anterior chamber. Then, with one stroke, from one side of the wound to the other, Descemet's membrane is incised, allowing instant prolapse of a "knuckle" of peripheral iris, thereby avoiding the necessity to invade the anterior chamber. If such spontaneous prolapse does not occur, pressure on the sclera posterior to the incision typically will result in such spontaneous prolapse. The prolapsed "knuckle" of iris is then excised, and the cornea, which is anterior to the incision, is stroked with a smooth instrument, from wound to central cornea, multiple times, an action which results, more often than not, in spontaneous regression of the cut edges of the iridectomy back into the eye, again avoiding

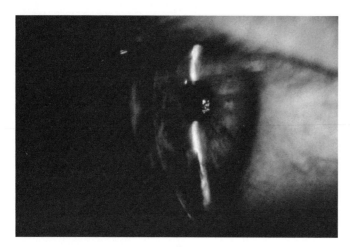

FIGURE 14–5. Preoperative slit-lamp photograph of a patient with uveitis and iris bombé.

the need for instrumentation of the anterior chamber. The wound is closed with a single 10-0 nylon suture, whose knot is buried. Depending on the case, we may perform two such iridectomies in two separate locations. Subconjunctival dexamethasone sodium phosphate and triamcinolone acetonide are injected under the conjunctiva, antibiotic and steroid medications are applied to the eye, and the eye is patched. Figures 14–5 and 14–6 illustrate preoperative and postoperative examples of this procedure.

CATARACT

Cataract surgery in the patient with a history of uveitis is more difficult than cataract surgery in the patient without such a history. Cataracta complicata deservedly earned its name as a consequence of the special challenges posed to the surgeon due to alterations in tissue and in biology of the eye after multiple episodes of recurrent uveitis. Damage to ocular structures before the surgery may preclude a good visual outcome, no matter how "elegant" the technical aspects of the surgery might be. For example, allowing persistence of even low-grade inflammation

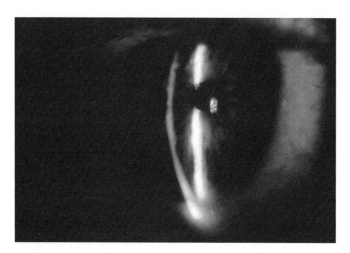

FIGURE 14–6. Postoperative photograph of the same patient shown in Figure 14–5 following peripheral iridectomy.

can produce maculopathy, chronic macular edema, epiretinal membrane, optic neuropathy, glaucoma, and glaucomatous optic neuropathy or cyclitic membrane and associated hypotony with progressive phthisis. The complicated uveitic cataract is also challenging from the standpoint of iris pathology, which frequently accompanies such cataract: posterior synechia, delicacy of the iris vasculature, pupillary membranes, and the permanent breakdown of the blood and aqueous barrier, with a propensity for very exuberant outpouring of protein and inflammatory cells following even the most gentle cataract operation.

The traditional reported success rate of cataract surgery for the uveitic cataract, as a consequence of these special challenges, has historically been considerably less than that for patients without a past history of uveitis.[2-5] Happily, however, substantial progress has occurred over the past 20 years, and not just as a result of improved microsurgical techniques and surgical materials (e.g., viscoelastics) but most notably because of the increasing unwillingness of large numbers of ophthalmologists to allow patients with uveitis to continue to experience chronic inflammation or multiple recurrences of inflammation. It is the increasing intolerance of ophthalmologists around the world for such inflammation, we believe, that has set the stage for increasingly successful cataract operations in patients who develop a cataract in the background context of a history of uveitis.[6-9]

The indications for cataract surgery in a patient with uveitic cataract include visual rehabilitation, enhancing the ophthalmologist's visualization of the posterior segment for ongoing assessment, and removal of a protein-leaking lens in the patient with phacogenic uveitis. Except in the removal of a protein leaking lens, we believe that one of the essential elements for success in surgery of the uveitic cataract is complete abolition of all active inflammation for a substantial period before surgery (e.g., 3 months), and ongoing, longitudinal control of inflammation following surgery. The decision making can be complex, beginning with the diagnostic pursuit and the preoperative medications. For example, failure to diagnose that a patient's recurrent uveitis is a result of infection with herpes simplex virus (HSV) will surely result in imperfect decisions about preoperative medications (HSV uveitis would be treated with chronic oral acyclovir and with perioperative topical steroids), and a higher likelihood of an imperfect outcome than if the appropriate diagnostic work had been studiously pursued ahead of time. Similarly, the decision of whether or not to incorporate adjunctive surgery into the cataract operation (for example, glaucoma-filtering surgery or pars plana vitrectomy) can also be complex. Therefore, we would advocate vigorous efforts to establish a definitive diagnosis, vigorous therapy to deal definitively with the established diagnosis and to control all inflammation before cataract surgery, and the administration of perioperative supplementary anti-inflammatory therapy, unless contraindicated, in the form of 1 mg/kg/day of prednisone, a drop of 1% prednisolone acetate eight times a day beginning 2 days before surgery, and an oral nonsteroidal anti-inflammatory agent, such as celecoxib, 100 mg po bid, and a topical nonsteroidal anti-inflammatory agent such as flurbiprofen (Ocufen) qid.

The decision to implant an intraocular lens (IOL) into the eye of a patient who has previously suffered from uveitis and who has developed cataract can be incredibly complex, and sometimes even the best efforts to "get it right" fail. Although there still exist today a few ophthalmic surgeons who believe that, because of their special surgical skills, they can do cataract surgery that is so elegant and atraumatic that they can get away with IOL implantation into virtually any eye with an excellent long-term postoperative result, most ophthalmic surgeons recognize that there are, in fact, some patients with a history of uveitis who are extremely poor risk candidates for long-term tolerance of an IOL implant. Sequential deposition of cells and fibrin onto the IOL, formation of a perilenticular membrane, and stimulation of persistent inflammation can result in such individuals in progressive membrane formation, contraction of which can result in ciliary body dysfunction and/or frank ciliary body detachment, ocular hypotony, chronic macular edema, and eventually fixed macular pathology that precludes the patient ever achieving good vision. Indeed, we recently reported on 19 such eyes, which ultimately required explanation of the lens implant in order to simply salvage the globe. The surgery was associated with preservation and restoration of vision in some cases, but some patients were never able to see well with the affected eye.[10] Sadly, three of the 19 cases were patients in whom we had made the decision to implant the lens implant using our admittedly conservative criteria for making that judgment. And despite our conservatism, these patients did not tolerate the presence of the IOL and ultimately had to have the IOL removed. The major risk factors that we identified in this reported series included inflammation concentrated at the intermediate zone of the eye (e.g., pars planitis) and cases in which the inflammation involved all areas of the eye (panuveitis). Additionally, those patients with a chronic disease, such as sarcoidosis, which was unlikely to "burnout" or to be amenable to remission induction through medication were also at high risk. The highest risk group of patients were those with juvenile rheumatoid arthritis, who were still young, and in whom periodic flare-ups of uveitis were still occurring.

The surgical technique that we employ in the straightforward cataract surgery includes four paracentesis wounds in the four quadrants of the peripheral cornea in preparation for the use of iris hooks after lysis of synechia, for pupillary expansion (Fig. 14–7) and a clear corneal incision for performance of capsulorrhexis and phacoemulsification. A peripheral iridectomy may be performed, depending on the past history of the patient and the violence of the past episodes of uveitis. The capsular fornices are directly inspected after removal of all of the cortex, in an effort to ensure that cortex, which can stimulate excessive postoperative inflammation, is not left in the eye. A foldable posterior lens implant is placed into the capsular bag, provided the patient is a good candidate for receiving a lens implant (Fig. 14–8). Intraocular dexamethasone phosphate, 400 µg, is instilled into the anterior chamber after the wound is closed, and the

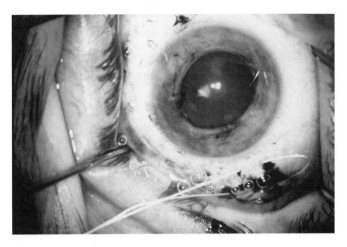

FIGURE 14–7. Pupillary expansion at the time of cataract surgery in a patient with chronic uveitis. Note that, in this photograph, the pupil has been expanded by a papillary expander that fits over the papillary sphincter.

preoperative adjunctive anti-inflammatory medications are continued, although tapered, for 1 month after surgery.

It is common, in our practice, for pars plana vitrectomy to be combined with the aforementioned operation, because so many of the patients whom we see have had uveitis that has involved the posterior segment, and therefore significant vitreal or vitreoretinal pathology, or both, has developed. In such an instance, we typically perform the cataract extraction, close the wound, create the three sclerostomy sites for the vitrectomy (Fig. 14–9), proceed to near total vitrectomy (with aggressive indentation through scleral depression), and then the closure of the sclerostomies and implantation of the IOL. Performing the surgery in this way simply obviates the need to work with the impediments of the variation between pseudophakic optics and aphakic optics during the vitrectomy.

In 1989, we published the first results of a series of patients with complicated uveitic cataract who underwent

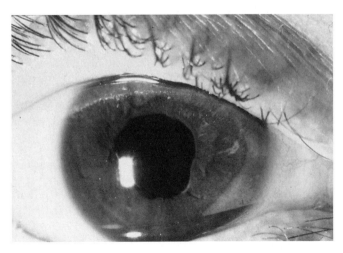

FIGURE 14–8. Foldable posterior chamber lens implant in place in the capsular bag of a patient with a history of uveitis. Photograph has been taken 1 month following phacoemulsification and posterior chamber lens implantation.

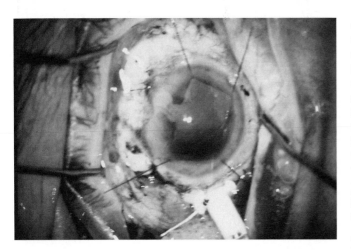

FIGURE 14–9. Ancillary surgical sites have been prepared in this patient whose pupil has been expanded with iris hooks. Note the three sclerostomy sites, including the one for the infusion canulla in preparation for the pars plana vitrectomy, which is now to follow the removal of the cataract.

cataract extraction with posterior lens implantation, examining the question of whether or not a patient with past history of uveitis would tolerate a lens implant following cataract removal.[6] The patients were specially selected, excluding from consideration all patients with a past history of juvenile rheumatoid arthritis, and all patients with a history of difficult-to-control panuveitis. The results indicated that with proper selection, the incorporation of a posterior lens implant into the surgical plan of a patient with uveitic cataract was a reasonable option, with visual outcomes equal to or better than those noted with simple removal of the cataract and subsequent aphakic contact lens or spectacle correction of vision.[6] Additional studies of this sort were performed, with more homogenous patients groups, including patients with pars planitis,[11] patients with sarcoidosis and patients with juvenile rheumatoid arthritis (JRA).[13]

In the latter group (patients with JRA) the results were particularly gratifying, because historically the rehabilitation success rate in this patient population had been so abysmal. For example, Key and Kimura had found that only 15% of their patients were successfully rehabilitated following cataract surgery.[3] Smiley and colleagues[4] published similar results, and Kanski and Shun-Shin,[5] in 1984, published the results of such surgery in 162 eyes suffering JRA-associated uveitis, finding that only 30% of those eyes saw 20/40 or better, and sadly, fully 65% were legally blind. The features that precluded good vision after successful cataract surgery in these series were permanent anatomic alterations that had developed as the result of many years of chronic, low-grade inflammation, not surgical misadventures and complications. Our success rate was significantly better than those reported in these earlier reports, but we, too, were frustrated by the findings, in all-too-many of the eyes, of fixed macular and/or optic nerve pathology as a consequence of chronic inflammation that could have been (indeed, should have been) controlled years earlier. Seventy-six percent of our patients were rehabilitated to the 20/40 or better vision level following combined phacoemulsifi-

cation and pars plana vitrectomy, without incorporation of a lens implant into the surgical plan. One more note of substantial interest is the fact that of the 60 patients studied, 10 (17%) required escalation of medical therapy to the level of systemic immunomodulatory agents to achieve total abolition of all active inflammation. Furthermore, 72 of the 100 eyes in the 60 patients followed by us were phakic, with clear lenses, at the onset of our involvement in their care. Only 13 eyes in 12 patients in this group developed cataract under our care, a very loud testament to the prophylactic benefits of a therapeutic philosophy that embraces an intolerance to even low-grade inflammation, as well as an intolerance to chronic steroid use.

We conclude that prevention of cataract through earlier, more aggressive systemic therapy is one of the keys to long-term progress in this area. Furthermore, we believe that a more aggressive philosophy with respect to systemic therapy is the key to the prevention of fixed macular, optic nerve, trabecular meshwork, and ciliary body pathology as well. Successful visual rehabilitation through cataract surgery of the uveitic cataract is much more possible today than it was just 20 years ago, and we attribute the progress that has been made in this area to the increasing willingness of ophthalmologists around the world to consider alternatives to steroids in their care of patients with uveitis.

GLAUCOMA

The problem of uveitic glaucoma is very common, indeed, much more common than is generally appreciated in the ophthalmic community. It is an additional vision-robbing contributor in 10% to 20% of patients with most forms of uveitis,[14] and in approximately 40% of patients with JRA-associated uveitis.[15] And it is incredibly challenging, because of the inflammatory component to it, because of the young age of many of the patients, and because of the steroid contribution to elevations in intraocular pressure in some of the patients requiring steroid treatment for their uveitis.

For angle-closure glaucoma, peripheral iridectomy or iridotomy is obviously required, and we still will offer laser iridotomy to our patients with blue irides. We no longer offer this option to our patients with brown irides, because our experience has been that such iridotomies almost always close within 2 to 3 months of the iridotomy having been performed. For these patients, we perform a straightforward surgical peripheral iridectomy.

Synechiolysis and chamber deepening may also be indicated in the selected uveitic glaucoma patient with pupillary block who has peripheral anterior synechia. The problems with both of these procedures typically are those of postoperative inflammation, truly recurrent episodes of uveitis, and sabotage of the intended result from the operation. This is also the case after standard filtration procedures. Indeed, the long-term success rate of trabeculectomy in patients with uveitic glaucoma is quite poor. Although Hoskins reported a 67% success rate at 1 year,[16] and although Hill[17] and Stavrou[18] reported 81% and 73%, and 92% and 83% 1- and 2- year success rates after trabeculectomy without antimetabolite therapy, Towler showed that the success rate fell off rather dramat-

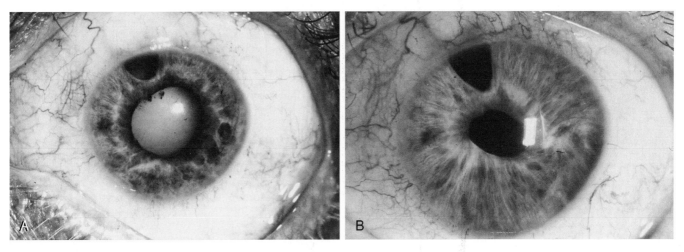

FIGURE 14–10. *A,* Preoperative photograph in a patient with the "complicated" uveitic cataract and glaucoma, status post-glaucoma filtering surgery. *B,* Same patient as shown in *A* following phacoemulsification following an inferior access entry point, with a posterior chamber lens implant in place.

ically with increasing years; his 2-year success rate was 80%, but the 5-year success rate of control was only 30%.[19] With the incorporation of antimetabolites in the surgery, Towler showed a 2-year success rate of 90%, but regrettably, only 50% of the patients were still controlled at 5 years.[19] Patitsas reported a 71% 2-year success rate in trabeculectomies with mitomycin C for uveitic glaucoma,[20] and Jampel reported that none of his patients, at 5 years following surgery, were controlled[21] (Fig. 14–10).

The use of tube or valve shunts has had a similarly checkered past, with Hill and associates reporting a 79% success rate with 2-year follow-up[17] and Gil-Carrasco reporting a 57% success rate at 1 year with the Ahmed valve.[22]

We studied 21 eyes of 19 patients with uveitic glaucoma uncontrolled on maximum medical therapy who had systemic immunomodulatory therapy for maintenance of control of inflammation and who had Ahmed valve implantation surgery for their uncontrolled glaucoma. The follow-up (average 36.4 months) ranged from 18 to 58 months, and the mean reduction of intraocular pressure was 25 mm (average 23.7), with a mean reduction of antiglaucoma medications from three preoperatively to 0.6 postoperatively; 67% of the patients were on no glaucoma medications at all.[23] No eye lost a single line of Snellen acuity, and 43% had improved vision as the result of adjunctive cataract or vitrectomy surgery. One eye required blood injection and tube ligation for persistent hypotony, and one of the valves failed and had to be replaced.

Our technique for Ahmed valve implantation includes the perioperative use of immunomodulatory therapy as required for control of the uveitis, adjunctive prednisone at 1 mg/kg/day, starting 3 days before surgery, and perioperatively eight times a day topical prednisolone acetate 1%. We have used the model S-2, 185-mm Ahmed valve, with the leading edge placed 9 mm posterior to the limbus, and the tube placed either through the limbus or through the pars plana; we strongly prefer the latter in vitrectomized eyes of aphakic patients, because so many of these patients are young and will be better suited for contact lens fitting following surgery (Fig. 14–11).

We would emphasize that uveitic glaucoma is a very important, additional vision-robbing problem in uveitis patients that is very difficult to treat. Medical therapy is important but is often insufficient. We strongly believe that control of inflammation, preoperatively and postoperatively, and especially prevention of all uveitis recurrences over the long term, is critical for enhanced likelihood of glaucoma surgery success in caring for patients with uveitic glaucoma. Filtration surgery for uveitic glaucoma has a checkered record, with late failures common, and we believe that recurrent inflammation contributes to this filter failure. The same undoubtedly will be true for valve/tube shunt procedures as well, and hence our strong recommendation, that just as in cataract surgery, aggressive efforts be made to abolish all active inflammation longitudinally.

VITREOUS

With its many complex and delicate intraocular structures the eye has low tolerance for inflammation. The physio-

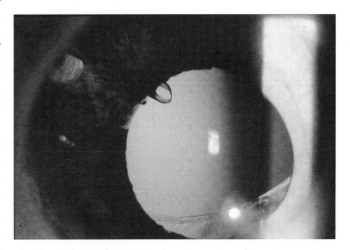

FIGURE 14–11. Patient with uveitic glaucoma, status post cataract surgery and total pars plana vitrectomy, followed by placement of an Ahmed glaucoma tube valve. Note that the tube of the valve has been placed through the pars plana into the vitrectomized vitreous cavity.

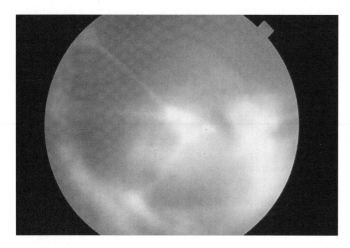

FIGURE 14–12. Fundus photograph of a patient with acute retinal necrosis (ARN). The severe vitritis resulted in vitreoretinal traction on the macula and optic nerve.

logic milieu of the eye needs to maintain multiple, clear tissues, including the cornea, lens, vitreous, and retina, for visual function. Intraocular inflammation can result in destruction of these structures, and therefore, all forms of uveitis are potentially vision threatening. Vitreous opacification, vitreoretinal traction, persistent cystoid macular edema, medically unresponsive vitritis, and lens-induced uveitis can be treated surgically via vitrectomy techniques (Fig. 14–12).

Control of perioperative inflammation is essential for all therapeutic surgical cases. Efforts to establish a patheoetiologic mechanism and the design of medical regimens to control or eliminate the intraocular inflammation before elective surgery is required for a successful outcome. In certain circumstances, this dictum cannot be realized. Endophthalmitis, lens-induced uveitis, and vitreous surgery designed to control medically unresponsive uveitis, by definition, must be performed while the eye is still inflamed. Surgery under these circumstances (in the presence of active intraocular inflammation) carries a much higher potential for surgical complications.

Vitreous surgery is performed using a standard three-port vitrectomy procedure. A longer infusion tip is often required in uveitis patients to accommodate scleral thickening, choroidal edema, or retinal separation that is frequently encountered in an eye with uveitis. Special care should be taken to ensure proper location of the infusion canula within the vitreous cavity before turning on the infusion in these patients. A bimanual technique of vitrectomy, membranectomy, or lensectomy can be performed to remove vitreous cells and debris, epiretinal membranes, neovascular tissue, or lens material.

Patients with intermediate or diffuse uveitis may benefit from vitrectomy simply as a result of the removal of the media opacities and vitreous debris.[24] A clear vitreous cavity also facilitates the ophthalmologist in conducting the necessary postoperative fundus examinations and in detecting cystoid macular edema (CME). The débridement of inflammatory cells and mediators is also believed to have a curative or moderating effect on the clinical course in patients with pars planitis, juvenile rheumatoid arthritis, and sarcoidosis (Fig. 14–13).[25–29] In addition to removing inflammatory cells, it is possible that vitrectomy removes any inciting foreign or autologous antigenic material. Type II collagen is an autoantigen found only in the vitreous cavity and in joints.[30] It is an immunoreactive protein that can produce arthritis and uveitis in animal models. Patients with several uveitis syndromes have T cells in their blood that are reactive to type II collagen.[31] Vitrectomy removes this "autoantigen," and much like removing lens proteins in a phacogenic uveitis patient, may thereby moderate the inflammation. Vitrectomy may also remove autoreactive helper T cells from the eye that are recruiting other nonspecific inflammatory cells. Transplantation research has shown that graft rejection is mediated by only a few antigen specific helper T cells found at the rejection site.[32] These cells are responsible for recruiting other nonspecific inflammatory cells into the foreign tissue, resulting in graft rejection. Vitrectomy may therefore remove these isolated, helper T-cell populations responsible for promoting and maintaining the uveitis. Finally, vitrectomy and lensectomy alters the immunologic milieu of the eye. Converting the eye to a

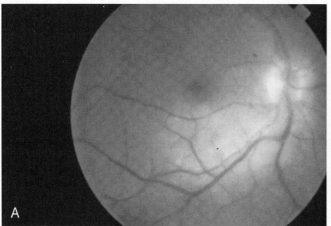
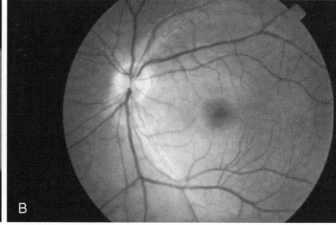

FIGURE 14–13. *A,* Fundus photograph of the right eye from a 17-year-old girl with chronic, medically unresponsive, pars planitis and CME receiving maximal medical therapy and visual acuity of 20/200. *B,* Fundus photograph of the left eye from the same patient showing clear media, and resolution of the vitritis and cystoid macular edema (CME) following therapeutic vitrectomy. Vision returned to 20/20 and remained quiet for 7 years. The right eye continued to have recurrent uveitis and ultimately required vitrectomy surgery.

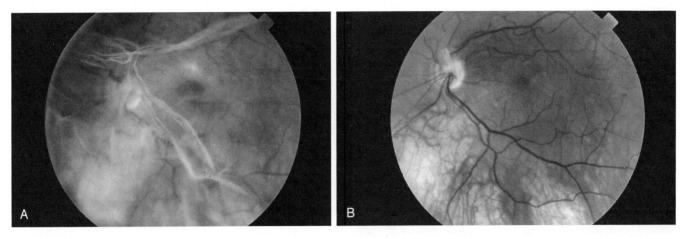

FIGURE 14–14. *A,* Fundus photograph of a 39-year-old woman with persistent, nonclearing inflammatory membranes in the vitreous and a traction macular detachment following retinal toxoplasmosis. Visual acuity is 20/400. *B,* Fundus photograph of the same patient following therapeutic vitrectomy and membranectomy showing successful removal of the membranes and return of 20/20 visual acuity.

unicameral state may allow for a more immunologically tolerant environment to be established.[33] Each of these postulated mechanisms may play a role in lessening the uveitis, and by that, reduce the severity of CME. The beneficial effects of vitrectomy, however, are not universal for all patients with uveitis.[34, 35] Patients with intermediate forms of uveitis may respond better than those with predominantly anterior or posterior uveitis.[25–29]

Membrane removal can be done at the same time as the vitrectomy to repair many of the complications of uveitis.[34] Intraocular picks, spatulas, scissors, needle knifes, and various forceps can be used to remove inflammatory membranes from the retina and ciliary body (Fig. 14–14). Anteroposterior, vitreomacular tractions from an inflamed vitreous body may play a role in maintaining chronic CME or create a shallow macular detachment. Eliminating this traction through vitrectomy and membranectomy surgery may improve macular function. Epiretinal membrane (ERM) formation frequently occurs in eyes with uveitis. Tangential traction caused by epiretinal membranes cause decreased vision via wrinkling of the macula and secondary CME. These membranes can be successfully removed at the time of the vitrectomy via delamination or en bloc techniques.

One of the mechanisms for hypotony in patients with uveitis is the formation of a cyclitic membrane. Chronic traction of the ciliary body results in ciliary body detachment and reduced aqueous humor formation. Vitrectomy and cyclitic membrane removal can be performed to reattach the ciliary body. A skilled assistant is required to assist in scleral depression in the region of the ciliary body, so that the surgeon can dissect and remove the inflammatory membrane or surgically segment it to reduce traction.

Lens-induced uveitis occurs when lens material is retained in the eye following cataract surgery or ocular trauma. If a significant amount of nuclear material is dropped into the vitreous cavity during cataract surgery, a lens-induced uveitis is likely (Fig. 14–15). Vitrectomy combined with pars plana lensectomy should be performed to remove inciting autoantigenic lens material. Following a standard vitrectomy, a fragmentation handpiece is used to phacoemulsify the retained lens material.

Care should be taken not to injure the macula during the fragmentation process.

At the end of any vitreoretinal surgery, the eye should be inspected for any iatrogenic retinal breaks; if breaks are present, they should be treated with retinal laser or cryopexy. Unless contraindicated, all uveitic vitrectomized eyes receive 400 μg of dexamethasone in the vitreous cavity and 40 mg of triamcinolone in the sub-Tenon space. This greatly assists in controlling excessive postoperative inflammation and fibrin formation. Regional and intraocular corticosteroids are contraindicated or are to be used with extreme caution in a patient with a possible infectious etiology (e.g., toxoplasmosis or viral diseases). A rapid and severe retinal necrosis can occur as a result of the potent immunosuppressive effect of these drugs (Fig. 14–16). Appropriate antimicrobial agents need to be used in conjunction with corticosteroid drug delivery in these settings.

RETINAL

Retinal detachment, ischemia, necrosis, and subretinal neovascular membrane formation are common complica-

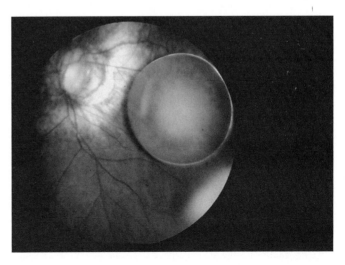

FIGURE 14–15. Fundus photograph of a patient with Marfan's syndrome showing mild vitritis and a lens that became dislocated during cataract surgery. Vitrectomy and pars plana lensectomy was successful at removing the dislocated lens and controlling the lens-induced uveitis.

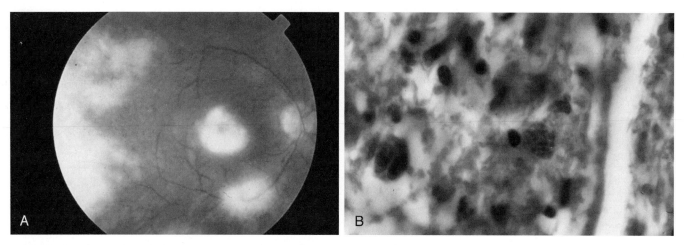

FIGURE 14–16. *A,* Fundus photograph of a patient with a rapidly progressing, multifocal, necrotizing retinitis following a sub-Tenon's injection of 40 mg triamcinolone. *B,* Retinal biopsy shows toxoplasma organisms in the areas of retinal necrosis. The infectious retinitis was facilitated by the profound, immunosuppressive effects of regional corticosteroids.

tions of uveitis.[35–39] Many of these sequelae can be addressed by laser, retinal cryopexy or retinal surgical techniques. As with other surgical endeavors, control of perioperative inflammation is an important goal prior to elective retinal surgery. These patients frequently have cataract, posterior synechiae and vitreous opacification that need to be addressed either prior to, or at the time of the vitreoretinal surgery.

Retinal detachment can occur in uveitis patients through various mechanisms. Retinal tears may occur unrelated to the uveitis or as a result of the intraocular inflammation. Often these tears can be treated with standard retinal laser or cryopexy. Inflammatory membranes create traction on the retina and result in retinal tears and detachment. Cytomegalovirus, varicella zoster virus, and toxoplasmosis can cause retinal necrosis and create multiple, posterior retinal breaks.[37, 38] Prophylactic laser photocoagulation can be performed at the boundary of healthy retina and the areas of retinal necrosis to reduce the risk for retinal detachment (Fig. 14–17). Toxocariasis, cyclitic membranes in juvenile rheumatoid arthritis and

anterior vitreous scarring in pars planitis can produce giant retinal tears and detachment.[35, 39] Myopic patients who develop exudative retinal detachment from syphilis or Vogt-Koyanagi-Harada syndrome (VKH) may have a rhegmatogenous component that needs to be addressed for successful retinal repair.

Regardless of the mechanism, the principles of the repair are the same: (1) relieve vitreous tractions, (2) seal the breaks, and (3) attach the sensory retina to the underlying retinal pigment epithelium (RPE). Although standard scleral buckle surgery or pneumatic retinopexy can accomplish these goals in simple detachments associated with uveitis (Fig. 14–18), many patients have more complex detachments that cannot be repaired by scleral buckle alone. Diseases such as acute retinal necrosis/ bilateral acute retinal necrosis (ARN/BARN) or cytomegalovirus retinitis produce multiple and posterior breaks that cannot be sealed by scleral buckles (Fig. 14–19). Instead, internal repair is required through vitrectomy and long-acting gas or silicon oil tamponade.[37, 38] Vitrectomy can more efficiently remove complex, multilaminar

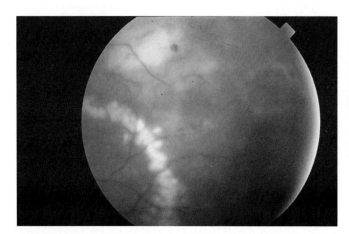

FIGURE 14–17. Fundus photograph of a patient with resolving acute retinal necrosis (ARN) and peripheral retinal necrosis. Prophylactic laser retinopexy was performed in healthy non-necrotic retina to prevent retinal detachment. Note the areas of peripheral retinal necrosis.

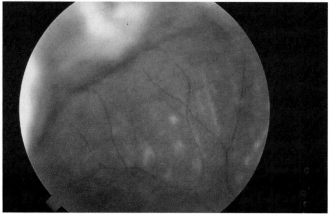

FIGURE 14–18. Fundus photograph of a patient with birdshot chorioretinitis and a rhegmatogenous retinal detachment repaired via scleral buckle surgery. Note the cream-colored retinal lesions and the attached retina on the buckle.

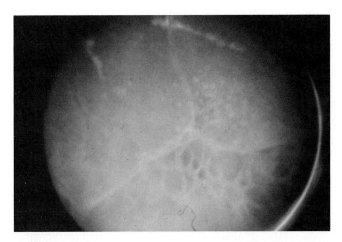

FIGURE 14–19. Fundus photograph of a patient with multiple, posterior, retinal breaks following resolution of bilateral acute retinal necrosis (BARN).

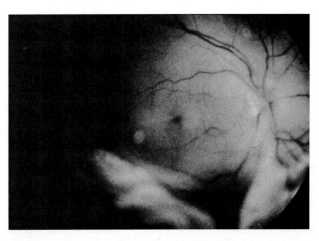

FIGURE 14–21. Fundus photograph of a patient with both a rhegmatogenous and exudative retinal detachment from syphilitic uveitis and high myopia. The retina was repaired by both scleral buckle and medical therapy, including penicillin and oral prednisone.

tractional membranes that are often present in pars planitis, sarcoidosis, and ARN/BARN. Posterior tears can be sealed through endolaser photocoagulation more effectively than through external cryopexy. Multiple tears can be supported more efficiently through the surface tension created by gas or silicon oil tamponade (Fig. 14–20). Therefore, internal repair is more often used to repair the retina in uveitis than in patients with routine rhegmatogenous detachments.

Retinal detachment in patients with uveitis can have an exudative component. Both the rhegmatogenous component and the exudative aspect of the detachment need to be addressed simultaneously. Repair of a retinal break in a patient with high myopia and a bilateral syphilitic exudative retinal detachment without controlling the uveitis will not be successful (Fig. 14–21). Likewise, an exudative retinal detachment from posterior scleritis or VKH syndrome will not respond to medical therapy if there is an undetected retinal break.

Anatomic and visual success are greatly influenced by the underlying uveitis syndrome and the health of the

optic nerve and macula. Choroidal thickening and retinal edema may lessen the effect of cryopexy and laser in creating a permanent adhesion at the site of the retinal tear. Both laser and retinal cryopexy are destructive procedures and may incite aggressive postoperative inflammation. Post-operative fibrin formation may be enhanced in eyes with uveitis and fibrin formation may promote cyclitic membrane formation and proliferative vitreoretinopathy (PVR). In patients with excessive postoperative fibrin, tissue plasminogen activator (tPA) can be injected into the eye to assist in clearing of the fibrin and prevent these complications (Fig. 14–22). Ultimately, visual prognosis is predicated on whether the macula was detached and on the pre-existing maculopathy. Final visual acuity will be greatly influenced by presence of fixed macular cysts, macular scarring, subfoveal neovascularization, ischemia, CME, or retinal necrosis. Finally, patients have a better visual prognosis if the macula is not involved than those who present with a macula-off detachment.

Many forms of posterior uveitis are associated with retinal or subretinal neovascular membranes.[40] Patients with Adamantiades-Behçet disease, systemic lupus erythematosus (SLE), and sarcoidosis may develop large areas of retinal capillary nonperfusion and secondary retinal neovascularization (Fig. 14–23). Fluorescein angiography can define the areas of ischemia and help direct panretinal laser photocoagulation when indicated (Fig. 14–24). Efforts to control the underlying disease and halt the progressive microvascular disease should be attempted. Retinal neovascularization may progress in patients with sarcoidosis by medical therapy alone (Fig. 14–25). Persistent ischemia and retinal neovascularization can be treated with panretinal photocoagulation to the areas of ischemia. Successful laser can reduce the risk of recurrent vitreous hemorrhages.

Patients with ocular histoplasmosis, punctate inner choroiditis, serpiginous choroiditis, VKH, birdshot chorioretinitis, sympathetic ophthalmia, and many other forms of posterior uveitis may develop subretinal neovascular membranes (SRNVMs), resulting in loss of macular function due to serous or hemorrhagic exudation. If

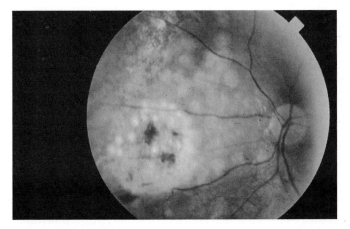

FIGURE 14–20. Fundus photograph of a patient with cytomegalovirus retinitis and a silicon oil-filled eye, following internal repair of a retinal detachment. Note the inactive viral retinitis and the laser reaction surrounding the posterior retinal breaks.

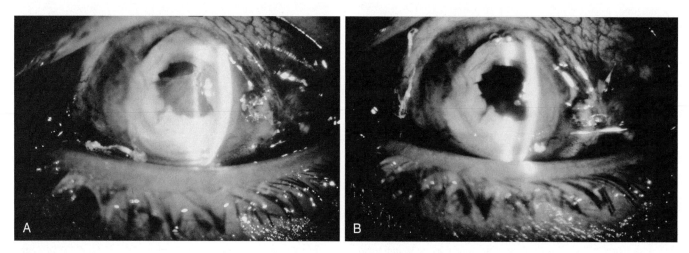

FIGURE 14–22. *A,* Anterior segment photograph of a patient 24 hours following Molteno tube implantation for glaucoma in an eye with severe uveitis. Note the pupillary fibrin membrane. *B,* Photograph of the same eye 5 minutes following the injection of 10 μg of tPA into the anterior chamber. Note the complete resolution of the fibrin in the anterior chamber. The eye remained quiet without worsening uveitis or additional fibrin formation.

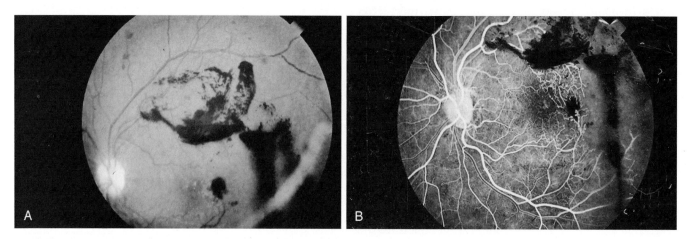

FIGURE 14–23. *A,* Fundus photograph of a patient with systemic lupus erythematosus showing vitreous hemorrhage, preretinal hemorrhage, and retinal arteriolitis. *B,* Fluorescein angiogram of the same patient showing areas of capillary nonperfusion, retinal ischemia, and retinal neovascularization.

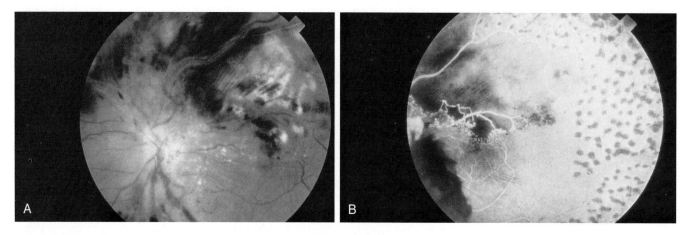

FIGURE 14–24. *A,* Fundus photograph of a patient with Adamantiades-Behçet disease and retinal vasculitis, hemorrhage, and cotton-wool spots. *B,* Fluorescein angiogram of the same patient showing laser photocoagulation to the areas of retinal ischemia.

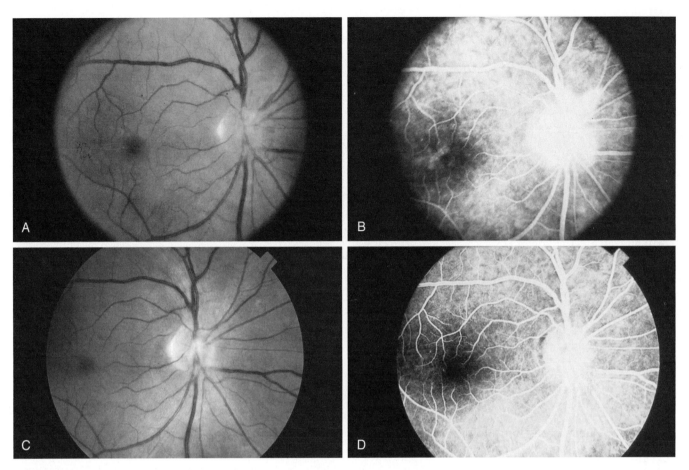

FIGURE 14–25. *A*, Fundus photograph from a patient with sarcoidosis and vitritis with neovascularization of the disc (NVD). Visual acuity was 20/100. *B*, Fluorescein angiogram of the same patient showing cystoid macular edema (CME) and NVD. *C*, Fundus photograph of the same patient 6 weeks following oral corticosteroid therapy and control of the uveitis. Note the resolution of the NVD. Vision improved to 20/20. *D*, Fluorescein angiogram of the same patient showing resolution of the CME and NVD.

these are extrafoveal (200 to 2500 μm from the fovea) or juxtafoveal (1 to 200 μm from the center of the fovea) laser photocoagulation can reduce the risk of visual loss. The multicenter Macular Photocoagulation Study Group demonstrated a six line loss of vision in 50% of untreated patients over a 24-month period as compared with a 22% loss of 6 lines in the laser-treated group in patients with

ocular histoplasmosis syndrome. The membrane is typically outlined with laser using 100 μm spots for 0.1 second. The power is determined by observing the tissue reaction and obtaining the desired whitish yellow burn. The lesion is then filled in with 200 μm laser spot for 0.2 second and then overlapped by 200 to 500 μm burns for 0.5 second (Fig. 14–26). The underlying choroiditis may

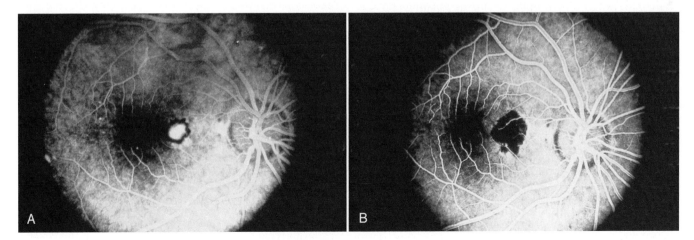

FIGURE 14–26. *A*, Fluorescein angiogram from a patient with juxtafoveal subretinal neovascular membrane (SRNVM) from presumed ocular histoplasmosis syndrome (POHS) with vision of 20/400. *B*, Fluorescein angiogram from the same patient following laser photocoagulation of the SRNVM and return of 20/25 vision. Note the destruction of the neovascular membrane.

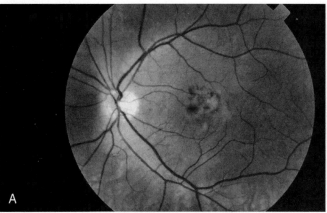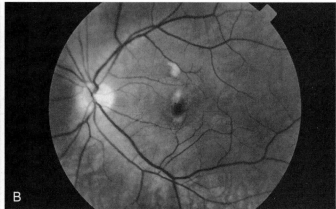

FIGURE 14–27. *A,* Fundus photograph of a patient with subfoveal SRNVM and 20/400 visual acuity. Note the subfoveal serous fluid hemorrhage. *B,* Fundus photograph of the same patient following submacular surgery and surgical removal of the SRNVM. Note the resolution of the subretinal fluid and hemorrhage. Vision improved to 20/20 following removal of the neovascular complex.

be aggravated by laser photocoagulation, thereby promoting further neovascularization. Control of the underlying uveitis is recommended before laser treatment to prevent this complication. Oral or regional corticosteroids should be considered before laser surgery in patients with an inflammatory etiology for the subretinal neovascularization.

If the neovascularization membrane is in a subfoveal location (less than 1 μm from the foveal center), laser photocoagulation may reduce vision by destruction of the foveal photoreceptors. Submacular surgery can be performed to excise these lesions surgically. A vitrectomy is performed and a needle knife is used to perform a retinotomy adjacent to the SRNVM. The membrane is mobilized and subretinal forceps are then used to grasp the membrane and remove it through the small retinotomy (Fig. 14–27). The vitreous cavity is filled with air. Laser photocoagulation is not typically required. Postoperative visual acuity can stabilize or improve in 83% of all eyes, but recurrent neovascularization may occur in 30% to 50% of patients.

Retinal cryopexy has been advocated for the treatment of peripheral retinal neovascularization in patients with pars planitis. Laser photocoagulation of the peripheral retina can accomplish similar results by ablating the retina and causing involution of vitreous base neovascularization. Such treatment can reduce the frequency of vitreous hemorrhage and may reduce the severity of the intermediate uveitis and moderate CME. Although the mechanism of this form of therapy is unknown, cryopexy may destroy the helper T cells in the vitreous gel that are responsible for recruiting other inflammatory cells into the vitreous cavity. Alternatively, it may re-establish the blood-eye barrier or ablate ischemic tissues. A double freeze-thaw cycle is delivered to the area of inflammatory debris.

References

1. Breinin GM, DeVoe AG: Chelation of calcium with edathamil calcium-disodium in band keratopathy and corneal calcium affections. Arch Ophthalmol 1954;52:840–851.
2. Ridley H: Cataract surgery in chronic uveitis. Trans Ophthalmol Soc UK 1965;85:519–525.
3. Key SN III, Kimura SJ: Iridocyclitis associated with juvenile rheumatoid arthritis. Am J Ophthalmol 1975;80:425–429.
4. Smiley WK: The eye in juvenile rheumatoid arthritis. Trans Ophthalmol Soc UK 1974;94:817–829.
5. Kanski JJ, Shun-Shin GA: Systemic uveitis syndromes in childhood: an analysis of 340 cases. Ophthalmology 1984;91:1247–1252.
6. Foster CS, Fong LP, Singh G: Cataract surgery and intraocular lens implantation in patients with uveitis. Ophthalmology 1989;96:281–288.
7. Tabbara K, Chavis P: Cataract extraction in patients with chronic postoperative uveitis. Int Ophthalmol Clin 1995;35:121–131.
8. O'Neill D, Murray P, Patel B, Hamilton A: Extracapsular cataract surgery with and without intraocular lens implantation in Fuchs' heterochromic iridocyclitis. Ophthalmology 1995;102:1362–1368.
9. Foster RE, Lowder CY, Meisler DM, Zakov ZN: Extracapsular cataract extraction and posterior chamber intraocular lens implantation in uveitis patients. Ophthalmology 1992;99:1234–1241.
10. Foster CS, Stavrou P, Zafirakis P, et al: Intraocular lens explantation in patients with uveitis. Am J Ophthalmol 1999;128:31–37.
11. Foster CS: Cataract surgery and intraocular lens implantation in patients with pars planitis. Recent Advances in Uveitis. Proceedings of the Third International Symposium on Uveitis. Brussels, Belgium, Kugler Publishers, 1993, pp 593–595.
12. Akova YA, Foster CS: Cataract surgery in patients with sarcoidosis-associated uveitis. Ophthalmology 1994;101:473–479.
13. Foster CS, Barrett F: Cataract development and cataract surgery in patients with juvenile rheumatoid arthritis associated iridocyclitis. Ophthalmology 1993;100:809–817.
14. Panek WC, Holland GN, Lee DA, Christensen RE: Glaucoma in patients with uveitis. Br J Ophthalmol 1990;74:223–227.
15. Foster CS, Havrilikova K, Tugal-Tutkun I, et al: Secondary glaucoma in patients with juvenile rheumatoid arthritis. Acta Ophthalmol 2000;78:576.
16. Hoskins HD Jr, Hetherington J Jr, Shaffer RN: Surgical management of the inflammatory glaucomas. Perspect Ophthalmol 1977;1:173–181.
17. Hill RA, Nguyen QH, Baerveldt G, et al: Trabeculectomy and Molteno implantation for glaucomas associated with uveitis. Ophthalmology 1993;100:903–908.
18. Stavrou P, Mission GP, Rowson NJ, Murray PI: Trabeculectomy in uveitis. Oc Immunol Inflamm 1995;3:209–215.
19. Towler HMA, Bates AK, Broadway DC, Lightman S: Primary trabeculectomy with 5-fluorouracil for glaucoma secondary to uveitis. Oc Immunol Inflamm 1995;3:163–170.
20. Patitsas C, Rockwood EJ, Meisler DM, Lowder CY: Glaucoma filtering surgery with postoperative 5-fluorouracil in patients with intraocular inflammatory disease. Ophthalmology 1992;99:594–599.
21. Jampel HD, Jabs DA, Quigley HA: Trabeculectomy with 5-fluorouracil for adult inflammatory glaucoma. Am J Ophthalmol 1990;109:168–173.
22. Gil-Carrasco F, Salinas-VanOrman E, Recillas-Gispert C, et al:

Ahmed valve implant for uncontrolled uveitic glaucoma. Oc Immunol Inflamm 1998;6:27–37.

23. DaMata A, Burk SE, Netland PA, et al: Management of uveitic glaucoma with Ahmed Glaucoma Valve implantation. Ophthalmology 1999;106:2168–2172.

24. Fitzgerald CR: Pars plana vitrectomy for vitreous opacity secondary to presumed toxoplasmosis. Arch Ophthalmol 1980;98:321–323.

25. Algvere P, Alanko H, Dickhoff K, et al: Pars plana vitrectomy in the management of intraocular inflammation. Acta Ophthalmol 1981;59:727–736.

26. Diamond JG, Kaplan HJ: Uveitic effect of vitrectomy combined with lensectomy. Ophthalmology 1979;86:1320–1329.

27. Diamond JG, Kaplan HJ: Lensectomy and vitrectomy for complicated cataract secondary to uveitis. Arch Ophthalmol 1978;96:1798–1804.

28. Bacskulin A, Eckardt C: Results of pars plana vitrectomy in chronic uveitis in children. Ophthalmologie 1993;90:434–439.

29. Kaplan HJ: Surgical treatment of intermediate uveitis. In: Boke WRF, Manthey KF, Nussenblatt RB, eds: Intermediate uveitis, Vol 23. Basel, Karger Basel, 1992, pp 185–189.

30. Stuart JM, Cremer MA, Dixit SN, et al: Collagen-induced arthritis in rats. Comparison of vitreous and cartilage derived collagens. Arhritis Rheum 1979;22:347–352.

31. Opremcak EM, Scales DK, Cowans AB. Cell mediated autoimmune mechanisms in uveitis. Association for Research in Vision and Ophthalmology 1993;34/4:1104.

32. Bishop KB, Orosz CG: Limiting dilution analysis for alloreactive TCGF-secretory T cells: Two related LDA methods that can discriminate between unstimulated precursor T cells and in vivo alloactivated T cells. Transplantation 1989;47:671–677.

33. Michels RG: Vitrectomy for macular pucker. Ophthalmology 1984;91:54–61.

34. Streilein JW: Anterior chamber associated immune deviation: the privilege of immunity in the eye. Surv Ophthalmol 1990;35:67–73.

35. Michelson JB, Nozik RA: Inflammatory retinal detachment. In: Michelson JB, Nozik RA, eds: Surgical Treatment of Ocular Inflammatory Disease. Philadelphia, JB Lippincott, 1988.

36. Smith RE, Nozik RA: Retinal detachment in uveitis. In: Smith RE, Nozik RA: Uveitis: A Clinical Approach to Diagnosis and Management, 2nd ed. Baltimore, Williams & Wilkins, 1998.

37. Clarkson JG, Blumenkranz MS, Culbertson WW, et al: Retinal detachment following the acute retinal necrosis syndrome. Ophthalmology 1984;91:1665–1668.

38. Jabs DA, Enger C, Haller L, et al: Retinal detachments in patients with cytomegalovirus retinitis. Arch Ophthalmol 1991;109:794–799.

39. Kreiger AE: Management of combined inflammatory and rhegmatogenous retinal detachments (AIDS and ARN). In: Ryan SJ, ed: Retina, 2nd ed, Vol III. St. Louis, Mosby, 1994, p 2489.

40. Nussenblatt RB, Whitcup SM, Palestine AG: Surgical treatment in uveitis. In: Uveitis: Fundamentals and Clinical Practice, 2nd ed. St Louis, Mosby, 1996, p 148.

Part III

THE UVEITIS SYNDROMES: Infectious

15 ── SYPHILIS

C. Michael Samson and C. Stephen Foster

DEFINITION

Syphilis is an infection by the spirochete bacterium *Treponema pallidum*. It is a sexually transmitted disease, entering the body through the genitals, mouth, or tiny breaks in the skin. If the condition is left untreated, it will progress through four stages, with the potential to cause morbidity to any of the major body organs. It can persist in the infected individual for an entire lifetime and reveal itself in various manifestations, its symptoms capable of mimicking a great variety of diseases. Because of this, it has been called the Great Imitator, and despite increased public awareness, sensitive laboratory tests, and effective treatment, it remains in the differential of many diseases to this day.

HISTORY

The disease acquired its name from the work of the Italian poet Hiero Fracastor. The title of his poem, *Syphilis, sive Morbo Gallico*, referred not only to the disease but also to the main character, Syphilis, a shepherd who carried the affliction. Although the poem was written in 1530, the disease did not become widely known as syphilis until many years thereafter. Previous to this, it was known as the "French Pox," a name given to it (by Italians) owing to its spread through Europe accompanying the armies of King Charles VII of France, whose ranks included infected Spanish mercenaries recently returned from ventures to the New World. It struck many soldiers in King Charles' camps during his siege of Naples and allowed the French the opportunity to coin a name they found less offensive: "the Neapolitan Pox."[1]

In 1905, Schaudin and Hoffman isolated the spirochete *T. pallidum* from skin lesions of infected patients.[2] Soon afterward, studies revealed that patients infected with syphilis created antibodies against extracts of normal mammalian tissues, like cardiolipin.[3] This allowed for the development of a blood test that could detect infected individuals, and Wasserman introduced a test to detect these antibodies in 1910.[4] This test became an essential tool in diagnosing the disease. Despite the ability to detect infected individuals, successful treatment of syphilis did not come until 1943, with the discovery of penicillin, which has been the mainstay of treatment to this day.[5]

EPIDEMIOLOGY

The most common presentation of syphilis in the eye is uveitis. Before the 1940s, syphilis was considered one of the leading causes of all cases of uveitis, second only to tuberculosis. In current times, it is considered a rare cause of uveitis. This apparent decrease in uveitis cases attributed to the spirochetal infection is most likely a result of two factors. First, the discovery of penicillin gave physicians an effective treatment. Especially when treated during the initial stages, antibiotic treatment allows for a reliable cure with little risk to the patient; previously, the mainstay treatment consisted of arsenic derivatives, which caused significant morbidity to individuals owing to its toxicity, and its effectiveness in treating syphilis was questionable. Since the introduction of penicillin, cases of syphilis dropped worldwide, especially in industrialized countries.

The second reason syphilis was seen less often as a cause of uveitis was the discovery of tests for other entities that could also cause uveitis. Blood tests for toxoplasmosis and histoplasmosis became available, with a concomitant increase in uveitis diagnosed secondary to these entities. Sarcoidosis was also found to be associated with ocular inflammation. In conjunction with reliable tests for syphilis, it was found that many cases of uveitis were in fact caused by these newer entities, whereas decades earlier, they would have been attributed to "the Great Imitator."

Syphilis is believed to currently comprise less than 1% to 2% of all uveitis cases.[6] It is the authors' belief that there is little importance in establishing the incidence of syphilis among the causes of uveitis for several reasons. First, there are very specific and sensitive serologic tests that are universally available that can easily establish the diagnosis. Second, it is one of the few uveitic entities for which a treatment exists that can exact a long-term cure. Third, one of every three untreated patients with latent stage syphilis will progress to tertiary stage syphilis, resulting in significant risk of neurologic or cardiologic morbidity. Finally, one can never rule out syphilis as a cause of uveitis based solely on clinical presentation. Most reported case series state that the majority of patients in whom syphilitic uveitis is diagnosed were patients in whom the ocular disease was the only manifestation of syphilis infection. Schlaegel wrote in the 1970s that he had "never seen a case of uveitis in secondary syphilis—most cases were picked up on routine FTA testing."[6] We believe that it is unethical not to rule out syphilis in almost all cases of uveitis, or in any case of unexplained ocular inflammation.

CLINICAL PRESENTATION

Syphilis

Because syphilis had been described for 500 years before a successful treatment was available, much is known about

TABLE 15–1. THE STAGES OF UNTREATED SYPHILIS

STAGE	MANIFESTATIONS	DOES UVEITIS PRESENT?
Primary	Chancre	No
Secondary	Rash, lymphadenopathy	Yes
Latent	No evident systemic disease	Yes, most common
Tertiary	Cardiovascular syphilis, neurosyphilis, benign tertiary	Yes

its natural history. Surprisingly, detailed descriptions of its signs and clinical course are not different from our experiences to this day, with the exception that late manifestations of syphilis are becoming rarer. The progression of untreated syphilis has been categorized into four stages (Table 15–1).

The first stage, primary syphilis, is characterized by the chancre, which initiates at the inoculation site. Chancres usually appear about 3 weeks after infection, although this period can range from 2 to 6 weeks. They usually develop in the genitalia but have been reported to initially occur in the mouth or skin. They have also been reported to present on the conjunctiva or the lids. These lesions are painless papules, which eventually ulcerate. They are filled with numerous spirochetes and usually resolve without treatment roughly 4 weeks after their appearance.

If the condition is left untreated, patients progress to secondary syphilis 4 to 10 weeks after the initial manifestation of the disease. Secondary syphilis denotes the stage during which spirochetes are disseminated in the blood. The symptoms are characterized by generalized rash and lymphadenopathy. The rash is maculopapular, and may appear quite prominent on the palms and soles. Other symptoms may include fever, malaise, headache, nausea, anorexia, hair loss, mouth ulcers, and joint pains. Many different organs can be involved during secondary syphilis, including the liver, kidneys, and the gastrointestinal tract. The eyes are affected in approximately 10% of cases.[7] Eye involvement, including uveitis, usually presents much later than the other systemic manifestations, up to 6 months after initial infection. Like the primary stage, these symptoms are transient, and usually resolve spontaneously over several weeks.

The following stage is called the latent stage, a time in which clinical disease is not detectable, nor is the infection contagious. This stage can last for the individuals' entire lifetime. The latent stage is divided into early latent (up to 1 year after initial infection) and late latent (after 1 year) periods. One third of patients progress to tertiary syphilis.

Tertiary syphilis represents an obliterative endarteritis that can affect most body systems. It is divided into three major groups: benign tertiary syphilis, cardiovascular syphilis, and neurosyphilis. The characteristic lesion of benign tertiary syphilis is the gumma. Histologically, the gumma is a granuloma. This lesion is usually found in the skin and mucous membranes but can occur anywhere in the body, and it has been found in the choroid and iris. Cardiovascular syphilis includes aortitis, aortic aneurysms, aortic valve insufficiency, and narrowing of the coronary

ostia. Neurosyphilis includes meningovascular syphilis, parenchymatous neurosyphilis, and tabes dorsalis. Unlike benign tertiary syphilis, cardiovascular and neurosyphilis carry severe risks of morbidity and mortality.

Syphilitic Anterior Uveitis

Syphilitic uveitis can occur as soon as 6 weeks after infection. Presentation during secondary syphilis is usually delayed and can appear approximately 6 months after other secondary signs (e.g., generalized rash) have resolved. Syphilitic uveitis may also first manifest in late latent syphilis, many years after initial infection. This is probably characteristic of most patients who develop syphilitic uveitis, since in the majority of reported cases, affected patients present without systemic signs of syphilis at or near the time of initial presentations. This delay may allow clinicians to overlook syphilis as a potential cause of uveitis if the patient is not specifically questioned. Alternatively, patients may not recall having been infected or may not recall if or what kind of treatment they received in the past.

Syphilitic uveitis may affect the anterior segment, posterior segment, or both. Anterior uveitis may present with an associated vitritis, or remain confined to the anterior segment only (Table 15–2). Recent case series suggest that anterior uveitis with vitritis is more common than isolated anterior inflammation.[1] It may present unilaterally or bilaterally, with bilateral disease reported in 44% to 71% of cases.[1, 2, 8] Additionally, syphilitic uveitis is one of the few types of uveitis that commonly presents as granulomatous inflammation[9] and can present with iris nodules similar in appearance to those seen in other granulomatous diseases. Barile and Flynn[2] reported that 67% of cases in their series of syphilitic anterior uveitis were granulomatous in nature.

Another finding in syphilitic uveitis involving the anterior chamber is roseolae of the iris.[6] These roseolae result from engorgement of the superficial vessels of the iris, usually in the middle third of the iris. They usually occur in secondary stage, around 6 weeks after initial infection. According to Duke-Elder[10], they are very rare but may present without other signs of ocular inflammation and may represent the first eye finding in syphilis infection. Schwartz and O'Connor reported a patient with syphilitic uveitis who presented with roseolae, who later had areas evolving into iris papules.[11] Iris angiogram revealed leakage of the dilated vessels, and those in the region of the papules. Leakage persisted even after the papules and roseolae resolved.

Interstitial keratitis, posterior synechiae, lens disloca-

TABLE 15–2. CLINICAL CHARACTERISTICS OR SIGNS OF SYPHILITIC ANTERIOR UVEITIS

Unilateral or bilateral
Granulomatous or nongranulomatous
Iris nodules
Anterior with or without anterior vitritis
Interstitial keratitis
Dilated iris vessels (roseolae of the iris)
Lens dislocation
Iris atrophy

tion, and iris atrophy are other signs that can be seen in the anterior segment in association with syphilitic uveitis.

Syphilitic Posterior Uveitis

Syphilis can affect the posterior segment (Table 15–3). In the series of patients with ocular syphilis reported from our center, 65% had involvement of the posterior segment. Barile and Flynn[2] found posterior involvement in only 36% of their patients. The posterior involvement can take on many different forms.

The most common posterior segment involvement is chorioretinitis. The fundus initially displays several active lesions, which are typically grayish yellow in color. These lesions can number from a few to numerous, and they can be seen anywhere in the fundus, although there is a preference for the posterior pole or near the equator. The lesions are small, perhaps from one half to a full disk diameter in size but can coalesce to become confluent. Serous retinal detachment (SRD), disk edema, and vasculitis are occasional associated signs. The amount of vitreal cells varies, although most case series report a significant degree of vitreal involvement.

Syphilis can present as a focal chorioretinitis.[12] There are several case reports describing acute central chorioretinitis as an initial manifestation of syphilis. Initially, the patient complains of blurred vision or a central scotoma. There is neurosensory detachment of the retina, which is associated with small retinal hemorrhages and exudate. Deep chorioretinal lesions are localized under the area of detachment. An uncommon presentation is that of a macular pseudohypopyon: Ouano and colleagues[13] described a case that presented as a vitritis with SRD of the macula. In their patient, there was turbid yellow fluid in the inferior one third of the SRD, appearing with a meniscus level, and hence the name "pseudohypopyon."[13]

Retinitis without choroidal involvement is yet another potential clinical presentation of syphilis in the posterior segment.[14, 15] Syphilitic neuroretinitis presents with focal areas of retinal edema, usually in the posterior pole, and an associated papillitis with retinal edema around the optic disk. Vasculitis is commonly associated, and vitritis is often present, while anterior inflammation is mild or absent. Fluorescein angiography shows intraretinal lesions in the areas of retinitis, disk leakage, and vessel wall staining.

Another variation of posterior segment involvement is a process localized at the level of the retinal pigment epithelium (RPE).[16] In 1990, Gass coined the term "syphilitic posterior placoid chorioretinitis," and he described six patients with secondary syphilis who showed one or more macular or juxtapapillary placoid lesions at the level of the RPE. According to the authors, the biomicroscopic and fluorescein angiographic findings of those localized placoid lesions of syphilitic chorioretinitis may represent one of the most specific findings in secondary syphilis described to date.

Syphilis can present as a necrotizing retinitis.[17] Clinically, this form presents with patches of retinitis in the midperiphery and peripheral retina, which can become confluent. These lesions may be accompanied by vasculitis and vascular occlusions. Clinically, it can be indistinguishable from acute retinal necrosis (ARN), herpes simplex retinitis, or cytomegalovirus retinitis. However, it differs by its dramatic response to intravenous penicillin and can have a good visual outcome without the complications associated with the aforementioned entities.[17]

Isolated retinal vasculitis has also been associated with syphilis infection.[18–20] One such entity, retinal arteriolitis, presents with yellow exudates adjacent to the artery. These exudates may present diffusely or focally, resembling emboli or plaques as seen in central or branch retinal artery occlusion. However, fluorescein angiography demonstrates no filling defects, and the lesions are stable over time, suggesting they are focal areas of perivascular exudate.[7] Other forms of vasculitis can affect the larger arterial branches, the venous branches[13], or both. The clinical appearance depends on the severity of the disease process, ranging from increased vessel girth and tortuosity to extensive perivascular exudate and fibrosis with obliteration of the small peripheral vessels. Focal venous vasculitis can masquerade as branch vein occlusion.[17, 20]

Syphilis is in the differential diagnosis of intermediate uveitis.[1] As mentioned earlier, intraocular inflammation of the anterior segment in syphilitic disease is often associated with a vitreal reaction. If the vitreal involvement is more prominent than anterior segment inflammation, it will resemble the picture of intermediate uveitis as seen in other entities (e.g., Lyme disease or sarcoidosis). Associated signs that are typically seen in intermediate uveitis due to other entities, like macular edema, peripheral vasculitis, and disk edema, may also be present. A true pars plana exudate usually is not present.

Finally, patients can present with a true panuveitis.[9] In Barile and Flynn's series,[2] 27% of their patients presented with panuveitis, and Tamesis and Foster[1] found that almost half of their patients presented with ocular inflammation in both anterior and posterior segments. Papillitis,[9] vitritis,[1, 8, 15] serous retinal detachment,[8, 21] disciform macular detachment,[22] subretinal fibrosis,[22] and uveal effusion[21] are other described signs of syphilitic posterior segment involvement.

PATHOLOGY AND PATHOGENESIS

Damage and destruction of ocular tissue is secondary to the host inflammatory response directed against invading spirochetes. Reports in the literature of the isolation of spirochetes from eye pathologic specimens are uncommon.[23–25] However, examination of aqueous humor samples in patients with syphilitic uveitis have revealed treponemes in the eye.[9] In the 1960s, several authors reported on finding treponeme-like forms from aqueous samples obtained by diagnostic paracentesis (a common practice in the United States at that time, and a commonly prac-

TABLE 15–3. THE MANIFESTATIONS OF SYPHILITIC POSTERIOR UVEITIS

DIFFUSE CHORIORETINITIS	NECROTIZING RETINITIS
Focal chorioretinitis	Retinal vasculitis
Retinitis/neuroretinitis	Intermediate uveitis
"Posterior placoid chorioretinitis"	Panuveitis

ticed procedure in Europe and other areas of the world today) or during cataract surgery. In some of the studies, the spiral forms could be successfully labeled with anti–*T. pallidum* globulin. Although there was concern of false-positive findings from mouth treponemes, which are part of the normal human flora, passive transfer studies of these spiral forms into laboratory animals resulted in seroconversion to a Venereal Disease Research Laboratory (VDRL)– and fluorescent treponemal antibody (FTA)–reactive state, suggestive more of *T. pallidum* rather than nonpathogenic commensal organisms.[25, 26]

The role of the host immune response in syphilitic infection is still being investigated. One important fact is that long-term immunity against syphilis is not conferred after initial infection: A treated individual may be reinfected on subsequent exposures. The other interesting point is the chronicity of syphilis infection, which can last for a host's entire lifespan. One mechanism proposed to play a role in chronic infections is a switch from a Th1-mediated process to that of a Th2-mediated type. Most acute infections are resolved by the Th1 pathway, which eventually leads to cure and long-term immunity. Evidence shows that in leishmaniasis, another cause of chronic infection, organism components preferentially activate Th2 lymphocytes, leading to minimization of Th1 effects and predisposing one to chronic infection. It has also been shown that administration of factors that induce switching from Th2 to Th1 (e.g., interferon gamma) can reverse this effect. Some evidence suggests that syphilis may also work in this manner, but additional studies are necessary to explore this theory further.

There is evidence to support the idea that syphilis may induce autoimmune disease in infected individuals. In the course of mapping the genome of *T. pallidum*, researchers identified a coding region that resembles one found in sequences coding for mammalian fibronectins. Animals immunized with such molecules were found to have modified responses when challenged with viable *T. pallidum*, and also developed classic Arthus reaction when injected intradermally, suggesting that antifibronectin antibodies may play a role in immune complex formation.

Indeed, immune complexes have been shown to play an important part in the pathogenesis of certain syphilitic entities in vivo.[27] Solling and colleagues[28] showed that C1q-binding immune complexes are elevated in patients with secondary syphilis but not in those with primary syphilis; not enough data were available to examine latent or tertiary stages. Gamble and colleagues[29] were able to isolate antitreponemal antibodies within the glomerular deposits in a patient with nephrotic syndrome secondary to syphilis. Tourville and associates[30] showed that such glomerular deposits also contain treponemal antigens. It is possible that such antigen-antibody complexes may play a role in ocular inflammation.

The complete genome of *T. pallidum* has been determined, consisting of 1.1 million base pairs containing 1041 open reading frames.[4] The difficulty in culturing *T. pallidum* in vivo has frustrated scientists' ability to study the pathogenic mechanisms of the microbe. Knowledge of the genomic structure will allow investigators to study the organism's protein products, permitting greater understanding of their role as biologic and pathogenic factors. The potential future benefits include a greater un-derstanding of the virulence factors of the organism, as well as the development of a method of culture, more specific and sensitive diagnostic tests, and a vaccine.

DIAGNOSTIC TESTS

There is no standard method of culturing *T. pallidum* at this time. Diagnosis of syphilis as the causative agent in a patient with uveitis usually relies on serologic tests in association with the clinical picture. There are two groups of serologic tests commonly used: nonspecific tests and specific tests (Table 15–4).

Nonspecific tests quantify the amount of serum antibody directed against particular host antigens. These antigens are typically incorporated by the infecting spirochete; the host is then stimulated to produce nonspecific antibodies against these antigens. The main antigen of this type is cardiolipin, which is a phospholipid produced by the liver.

The most commonly used nonspecific tests are the rapid plasma reagin (RPR) test, and the VDRL test. These tests quantify the amount of anticardiolipin antibody present in serum. Results are reported as reactive, weakly reactive, borderline, and nonreactive. The sensitivity and specificity depend on the stage of syphilis and status of treatment. Titers generally are high during active infection, like secondary syphilis, but drop when spirochetes are not active, such as in latent syphilis or after completion of successful treatment. Serum titers do not correlate with the disease severity.[31, 32]

Specific tests quantify the amount of serum antibody directed against treponemal antigens. The most commonly used test today is the fluorescent treponemal antigen absorption (FTA-ABS) test. FTA-ABS tests become positive during secondary stage and remain positive for the patient's lifetime, regardless of treatment status. FTA-ABS testing is much more sensitive than nonspecific serologic tests during latent stage, the stage in which most uveitic patients will present.

Another diagnostic tool is the direct demonstration of spirochetes. Treponemes can be visualized by incubating body fluid containing the infective organisms with fluorescent-tagged antibody and visualizing it under darkfield microscopy.[25] One limitation to the test is that it requires obtaining infected body fluid, which is usually only possible in patients with primary syphilis (i.e., from the initial chancre) or secondary syphilis, when an open pustule on the skin is present. Another limitation is that antibodies may cross-react with other species of treponemes, including nonpathogenic commensal treponemes harbored in the oral cavity, for example. However, several series have described the use of testing aqueous humor for spirochetes with this technique in patients with clinical evi-

TABLE 15–4. DIAGNOSTIC TESTS FOR SYPHILIS

Nonspecific tests: rapid plasma reagin (RPR), Venereal Disease Research Laboratory (VDRL)
Specific tests: Fluorescent treponemal antibody absorption test (FTA-ABS), Microhemagglutination assay for *T. pallidum* (MHA-TP)
T. pallidum immobilization test (TPI)
T. pallidum particle agglutination (TP-PA)
Darkfield microscopy
Polymerase chain reaction (PCR)

dence or suspicion of syphilis. Treponemes were recovered from aqueous in many cases, and treatment was associated with disappearance of these organisms. Unfortunately, these studies are small, uncontrolled case series, and no definitive conclusions can safely be made.

Polymerase chain reaction (PCR) testing for syphilis is now possible. Several different PCR assays are available, and with the complete mapping of the *T. pallidum* genome, more will become available. Currently targeted regions include a 366 bp region of the 16S rRNA, and the 5′ and 3′ flanking regions of the 15-kDa lipoprotein gene (tpp15), which can aid in the differentiation of different subspecies of *T. pallidum*. In vivo studies of PCR testing for syphilis show that positive specimens may persist even after treatment, owing to the slow elimination of the organisms from the body by macrophages. The DNA of dead organisms injected into rabbits may persist for up to 30 days.

However, the clinical usefulness of PCR testing in syphilitic uveitis is still yet to be determined. Theoretically, it would be useful in circumstances when FTA-ABS testing was not reliable. Such circumstances are difficult to imagine but conceivably would include those patients who concomitantly had a disease associated with false-positive FTA-ABS results (e.g., systemic lupus erythematosus), or in the 2% of patients whose FTA-ABS returns as falsely negative during latent or late syphilis. Realistically, PCR will aid most in research studies, because it will help determine whether spirochetes (or their antigens) are present in late lesions in which live treponemes are difficult to harvest (e.g., late skin manifestations), and may help in our understanding of immunity to syphilis.

Perils in Serology Interpretation

An understanding of the limitations of serologic testing in syphilis is essential to the investigating physician. Misinterpretation of the tests may lead to unwarranted anxiety by the patient and the patient's sexual partners, and the possibility of overlooking another serious disease process.

False-positive results in RPR and VDRL testing have been described in a variety of medical conditions. Transient false-positive results, persisting for no longer than 6 months, have been associated with atypical pneumonia, malaria, and vaccinations. Persistent false-positive RPR and VDRL results are seen in systemic lupus erythematosus, leprosy, and advanced age. Falsely positive VDRL tests have been reported in narcotic addicts.

False-positive results have also been described in FTA-ABS testing. These disorders include systemic lupus erythematosus, rheumatoid arthritis, and biliary cirrhosis. Advanced age has also been associated with false-positive FTA-ABS results. These false-positive results tend to persist for the patients' lifetime, most likely representing antibodies that coincidentally cross-react with antibody against treponemal antigens. Intravenous fluorescein testing does not have any effect on FTA-ABS testing.[33] The microhemagglutination assay for *T. pallidum* (MHA-TP) was commonly used as a second, confirmatory test in an effort to reduce the likelihood of basing therapy on a falsely positive FTA-ABS; it is no longer commercially available. The *T. pallidum* particle agglutination test (TP-PA) shows 97% agreement with the MHA-TP, and it is

this test and Western blotting (the gold standard) that are now most appropriate for confirming a positive FTA-ABS.

Sensitivity of FTA-ABS Testing

VDRL and FTA-ABS testing are comparable in primary and secondary disease, the sensitivity increasing from 70% and 85% to 99% and 100%, as the anticardiolipin antibodies increase. However, most patients diagnosed with ocular syphilis described in the literature fall under the category of latent syphilis. In this population, VDRL testing is falsely negative in 30% of these patients, whereas FTA-ABS testing is falsely negative in only 1% to 2% of these patients. But the false-positive rate can be as high as 10% in patients with AIDS.

Examination of the cerebrospinal fluid (CSF) for syphilis is warranted in every case of syphilis found in patients with uveitis. It is necessary in staging, because neurosyphilis has its own associated morbidity and mortality separate from ocular disease. Also, one cannot clinically assess which uveitic patients will also have neurosyphilis.[34] Disk edema is not a reliable indicator of a positive yield from CSF studies; nor is the absence of disk edema an assurance of a normal spinal tap.[34] It should be noted, however, that most case reports of syphilitic uveitis patients have found a low prevalence of positive results from CSF analysis among patients tested.[2, 8]

TREATMENT

Penicillin has been the mainstay of treatment for syphilis since its introduction in the 1940s. There are two regimens used in syphilitic uveitis as reported in the literature. Some authors use the Centers for Disease Control and Prevention (CDC) recommendation for latent syphilis, which consists of intramuscular injections of penicillin once weekly for 3 weeks. Other authors consider ocular syphilis a form of neurosyphilis and use the treatment recommendations for this: intravenous penicillin daily for 10 to 14 days.

There is substantial evidence favoring the use of the neurosyphilis regimen for the treatment of syphilitic uveitis, the least of which are the multiple reports in the literature describing treatment failures with intramuscular penicillin. To underscore this belief, in Barile and Flynn's study,[2] 34% of their patients had already undergone treatment for syphilis before the onset of uveitis, although they do state that the previous treatment was poorly documented, poorly recalled, and appeared incomplete in many cases.

T. pallidum divides only once every 30 hours.[6] Because of this factor, sustained levels of penicillin in the aqueous must be maintained in order to exert its bactericidal effect. It has been shown that a single intramuscular injection of 2.5 million units of penicillin yields adequately bactericidal levels in the aqueous. However, the levels drop below the minimum inhibitory concentration (MIC) to kill *T. pallidum* in less than 2 hours. It has been shown that the addition of probenecid sustains the penicillin levels in the aqueous, presumably by competing with the transport of penicillin across the ciliary body. Still, this is yet more theoretic support that a regimen of weekly intramuscular injections is inadequate in the treatment of intraocular syphilis, and that intravenous therapy should be considered the standard of care for these patients.

The CDC recommendations for the neurosyphilis regimen in the average adult is infusion of intravenous penicillin G 18 to 24 million units per day for 10 to 14 days.[35] Patients can then be supplemented with intramuscular benzathine penicillin G at a dose of 2.4 million units weekly for 3 weeks (Table 15–5).

There are reports of "relapse" of syphilis in patients who had previously received treatment. Several case reports indicate that many of these relapses probably represent inadequate treatment due to poor patient compliance.[2] Another possibility is the inadequacy of intramuscular penicillin therapy in the treatment of all intraocular syphilis infections.[31] Finally, another explanation is the possibility of L-forms of the spirochete: Without cell walls, L-forms would be resistant to the action of penicillin. This last mechanism is only speculative and requires further study. Reinfection is also possible.

Penicillin allergy requires alternative medication (see Table 15–5). Traditionally, tetracycline or doxycycline have been the alternative treatments. Doxycycline is given at 200 mg orally once daily, whereas tetracycline is given at 500 mg orally four times daily. The treatment regimen for these medications is administered for 30 days. Macrolides (e.g., clarithromycin) are other alternatives, and some initial reports using ceftriaxone are encouraging, although the treating clinician is reminded of the cross-reactivity of cephalosporins and penicillins.[31, 36] Chloramphenicol has also been reported to have been used with success.[37] Another approach is penicillin desensitization. Increasing dosages of penicillin are given, orally or intravenously, with careful monitoring. Chisholm and colleagues reported on 16 successful desensitization procedures performed on pregnant women infected with syphilis.[38]

SYPHILIS IN PATIENTS WITH HUMAN IMMUNODEFICIENCY VIRUS INFECTION

The incidence of syphilitic uveitis in patients with human immunodeficiency virus (HIV) infection is probably not greater than that in non–HIV-positive population. Some reports find syphilis as an etiology of only 1% of cases of uveitis in patients with HIV, similar to series of non–HIV-infected patients with syphilitic uveitis.[31] This finding is also supported by the fact that ocular syphilis in patients with HIV-1 does not seem to be correlated with decreased absolute T4 cell counts.[31, 32] The natural course of syphilis is altered by HIV infection: It tends to run a more severe course and requires longer treatment for adequate cure.[34, 39, 40]

Manifestations of ocular syphilis in HIV-positive individuals are similar to those in immunocompetent individuals, and include iridocyclitis,[31] intermediate uveitis,[31] panuveitis,[40] papillitis,[31, 32, 41, 42] optic perineuritis, branch retinal vein occlusion, neuroretinitis, chorioretinitis,[37, 43] dense vitritis,[44] retinitis,[31, 32, 41] and serous and rhegmatogenous retinal detachment.[31, 32, 37, 42, 45] As in non-HIV patients, iritis is the most common manifestation of ocular syphilis in HIV-positive individuals, accounting for up to 70% of cases.[42] Ocular syphilis may be the presenting sign of HIV infection and neurosyphilis.[32] Coexisting syphilitic uveitis and HIV infection has been reported to masquerade as Crohn's disease.[43]

HIV-infected patients have been shown to have relapses of syphilis infection despite the administration of high-dose intravenous penicillin therapy.[32, 46] It is possible that prolonged treatment is necessary in this group of patients. Deschnese and colleagues recommend treating HIV-infected patients with ocular syphilis for a full 14-day neurosyphilis course with the supplemental weekly penicillin intramuscular injections.[47]

Monitoring of successful treatment by serologic testing is not accurate in HIV-infected patients, because they are slower to seroconvert from a positive to a negative RPR status despite treatment. However, a randomized trial showed that these patients were not at higher risk for treatment failure and probably represent another facet of their altered immune response. Additionally, one study showed that at 1-year follow-up of HIV-infected individuals after treatment for syphilis, 9% of patients showed reversion to a negative FTA-ABS status. Immunoblotting studies of serum of HIV-infected individuals who are FTA negative reveal positive antibodies reactive against *T. pallidum* antigens: RPR reactivity in these individuals were overlooked in light of their negative FTA status and history of intravenous (IV) drug abuse. This further supports that HIV infection may alter the response to serologic testing for syphilis to make such testing unreliable in certain individuals.

COMPLICATIONS

Complications from syphilitic uveitis are no different from those from other types of uveitis. Cataracts and glaucoma can occur as a result of inflammation or topical steroids. Macular edema and epiretinal membranes are major causes of significant visual loss. Retinal detachments are usually exudative in nature and resolve with appropriate medical therapy without the need for surgical intervention. However, rhegmatogenous retinal detachments have also been observed and are related to the development of proliferative vitreoretinopathy, leading to retinal traction and the development of a tear.

Choroidal neovascular membrane is a rare complication of syphilitic uveitis. Chorioretinitis leads to changes in retinal pigment epithelium and breaks in Bruch's membrane. These breaks may predispose the patient to the development of neovascular membranes. Because cases are so rare, it is unclear whether laser photocoagulation has a poor or favorable effect in the treatment of these membranes. However, medical treatment aimed at eliminating syphilis and controlling intraocular inflammation is warranted, because such treatment has been known to cause remission of neovascular membranes in other uveitis entities.

Complications can occur secondary to treatment. Un-

TABLE 15–5. TREATMENT FOR SYPHILITIC UVEITIS

Intravenous penicillin G 18 to 24 million units daily for 10 to 14 days
For penicillin-allergic patients:
Tetracycline hydrochloride 500 mg PO QID for 30 days *or*
Doxycycline 100 mg PO BID for 14 days
Consider penicillin desensitization in certain individuals

recognized penicillin allergy requires switching to an alternative antibiotic such as doxycycline. Even in the absence of a drug allergy, patients should be monitored for the Jarisch-Herxheimer reaction. This occurs as the result of a hypersensitivity reaction of the host to treponemal antigens, which are released in large numbers as spirochetes are killed during the initial infusions.[48] Patients present with fever, myalgia, headache, and malaise. There may be a concomitant increase in the severity of the ocular manifestations.[9, 17] Although nonsteroidal anti-inflammatory drugs may alleviate the systemic symptoms, increased local steroids and the use of systemic corticosteroids may become necessary to control severe inflammation. However, supportive care and observation are usually all that is necessary in the majority of cases.

PROGNOSIS

If the condition is recognized early and treated appropriately, the majority of cases of syphilis infection can result in a cure.[1, 2, 8] In untreated cases, approximately one third of patients progress to tertiary syphilis, with potentially serious morbidity and mortality if cardiovascular syphilis or neurosyphilis develop. Unfortunately, several reports confirm that ophthalmologists are often guilty of overlooking syphilis as a potential cause of ocular inflammation.[1, 2]

CONCLUSIONS

Syphilis is one of the few treatable causes of uveitis. Its ability to present in a wide variety of uveitic forms is reflective of its status as "the Great Imitator" in its systemic manifestations. Because of this, it is not suggested by any particular clinical presentation, and requires the appropriate blood testing in all patients with uveitis, or any ocular inflammation of unknown etiology. The ophthalmologist who appropriately screens and treats this disease may not only save patients' vision but may also prevent morbidity and death.

References

1. Tamesis R, Foster CS: Ocular syphilis. Ophthalmology 1990; 97:1281–1287.
2. Barile GR, Flynn H: Syphilis exposure in patients with uveitis. Ophthalmology 1997;104:1605–1609.
3. Margo C, Hamed, L: Ocular syphilis. Surv Ophthalmol 1992;37:203–220.
4. Fraser C, Norris SJ, Weinstock GM, et al: Complete genome sequence of *Treponema pallidum*, the syphilis spirochete. Science 1998;281:375–388.
5. Greene R: History of Medicine. New York, Institute for Research in History/Haworth Press, 1988.
6. Schlaegel TF, O'Connor GR: Metastatic nonsuppurative uveitis. Int Ophthalmol Clin 1977;17:87–108.
7. Crouch ER, Goldberg MF: Retinal periarteritis secondary to syphilis. Arch Ophthalmol 1975;93:384–387.
8. Deschenes J, Seamone CD, Baines MG: Acquired ocular syphilis: Diagnosis and treatment. Ann Ophthalmol 1992;24:134–138.
9. Belin MW, Baltch AL, Hay PB: Secondary syphilitic uveitis. Am J Ophthalmol 1981;92:210–214.
10. Duke-Elder S. Perkins ES: Diseases of the ureal tract. In: Duke-Elder S, ed: System of Ophthalmology, vol 9. London, Kingston, 1966.
11. Schwartz LK, O'Connor GR: Secondary syphilis with iris papules. Am J Ophthalmol 1980;90:380–384.
12. de Souza EC, Jalkh AE, Trempe CL, et al: Unusual central chorioretinitis as the first manifestation of early secondary syphilis. Am J Ophthalmol 1988;105:271–276.
13. Ouano DP, Brucker AJ, Saran BR: Macular pseudohypopyon from secondary syphilis. Am J Ophthalmol 1995;119:372–374.
14. Savir H, Kurz O: Fluorescein angiography in syphilitic retinal vasculitis. Ann Ophthalmology 1976;8:713–716.
15. Stoumbos VD, Klein ML: Syphilitic retinitis in a patient with acquired immunodeficiency syndrome–related complex. Am J Ophthalmol 1987;103:103–104.
16. Gass JDM, Braunstein RA, Chenoweth RG: Acute syphilitic posterior placoid Chorioretinitis. Ophthalmology 1990;97:1288–1297.
17. Mendelsohn AD, Jampol LM: Syphilitic retinitis. Retina 1984;4:221–224.
18. Regan CDJ, Foster CS: Retinal vascular diseases: Clinical presentation and diagnosis. Int Ophthalmol Clin 1986;26:25–53.
19. Halperin LS, Berger AS, Grand MG: Syphilitic disc edema and periphlebitis. Retina 1990;10:223–225.
20. Lobes LA, Folk JC: Syphilitic phlebitis simulating branch vein occlusion. Ann Ophthalmol 1981;13:825–827.
21. DeLuise VP et al. Syphilitic retinal detachment and uveal effusion. Am J Ophthalmol 94:757–761, 1982.
22. Saari M: Disciform detachment of the macula. Acta Ophthalmol 1978;56:510–517.
23. Montenegro ENR, Israel CW, Nicol WG, Smith JL: Histopathologic demonstration of spirochetes in the human eye. Am J Ophthalmol 1969;67:335–345.
24. Blodi FC, Hervouet F: Syphilitic Chorioretinitis. Arch Ophthalmol 1968;79:294–296.
25. Smith JL, Israel CW: Treponemes in aqueous humor in late seronegative syphilis. Transactions of the American Academy of Ophthalmology and Otolaryngology 1968;72:63–74.
26. Golden B, Thompson HS: Implications of spiral form in the eye. Surv Ophthalmol 1969;14:179–183.
27. Wozniczko-Orlowska G, Milgrom F: Immune complexes in syphilis sera. J Immunol 1981;127:1048–1051.
28. Solling J, From E, Mogensen CE: The role of immune complexes in early syphilis and in the Jarisch-Herxheimer reaction. Acta Derm 1982;62:325–329.
29. Gamble CN, Reardan JB: Immunopathogenesis of syphilitic glomerulonephritis. Elution of antitreponem antibody from glomerular immune-complex deposits. N Engl J Med 1975;202:449–454.
30. Tourville DR, Byrd LH, Kim DU, et al: Treponemal antigen in immunopathogenesis of syphilitic glomerulonephritis. Am J Pathol 1976;82:479.
31. Shalaby IA, Dunn JP, Semba RD, Jabs DA: Syphilitic uveitis in human immunodeficiency virus-infected patients. Arch Ophthalmol 1997;115:469–473.
32. McLeish WM, Pulido JS, Holland S, et al: The ocular manifestations of syphilis in the human immunodeficiency virus type 1–infected host. Ophthalmology 1990;97:196–203.
33. Jost BF, Olk RJ, Spirner MH, et al: Effect of intravenous fluorescein on fluorescent treponemal antibody testing. Am J Ophthalmol 1986;102:278–279.
34. Katz DA, Berger JR, Duncan RC: Neurosyphilis. Arch Neurol 1993;50:243–249.
35. Beary CD, Hooton TM, Collier AC, Lukehart SA: Neurologic relapse after benzathine penicillin therapy for secondary syphilis in a patient with HIV infection. N Engl J Med 1987;316:1587–1589.
36. Dowell ME, et al: Response of latent syphilis or neurosyphilis to ceftriaxone therapy in persons infected with human immunodeficiency virus. Am J Med 1992;93:481–487.
37. Passo MS, Rosenbaum JT: Ocular Syphilis in patients with human immunodeficiency virus infection. Am J Ophthalmol 1988;106:1–6.
38. Chisholm CA, Katz VL, McDonald TL, Bowes WA: Penicillin desensitization in the treatment of syphilis during pregnancy. Am J Perinatol 1997;14:553–554.
39. Johns DR, Tierney M, Felsenstein D: Alteration in the natural history of neurosyphilis by concurrent infection with the human immunodeficiency virus. N Engl J Med 1987;316:1569–1572.
40. Hodge WG, Seiff SR, Margolis TP: Ocular opportunistic infection incidences among patients who are HIV positive compared to patients who are HIV negative. Ophthalmology 1998;105:895–900.
41. Levy JH, Liss RA, Maguire AM: Neurosyphilis and ocular syphilis in patients with concurrent human immunodeficiency virus infection. Retina 1989;9:175–180.
42. Becerra LI, Ksiazek SM, Savino PJ, et al. Syphilitic uveitis in human immunodeficiency virus–infected and noninfected patients. Ophthalmology 1989;96:1727–1730.
43. Kleiner RC, Najarian L, Levenson J, Kaplan HJ: AIDS complicated by syphilis can mimic uveitis and Crohn's disease. Arch Ophthalmol 1987;105:1486–1487.

44. Kuo IC, Kapusta MA, Rao NA: Vitritis as the primary manifestation of ocular syphilis in patients with HIV infection. Am J Ophthalmol 1998;125:306–311.
45. Williams JK, Kirsch LS, Russack V, Freeman WR: Rhegmatogenous retinal detachments in HIV-positive patients with ocular syphilis. Ophthalmic Surg Lasers 1996;27:699–705.
46. Gordon SM, Eaton ME, George R, et al: The response of symptomatic neurosyphilis to high-dose intravenous penicillin G in patients with human immunodeficiency virus infection. N Engl J Med 1994;331:1469–1473.
47. Deschenes J, Seamone CD, Baines MG: Acquired ocular syphilis: Diagnosis and treatment. Am Ophthalmol 1992;24:134–138.
48. Solling J, Solling K, Jacobsen KU, et al: Circulating immune complexes in syphilis. Acta Derm Venereol 1978;58:263–267.

John C. Baer

LYME BORRELIOSIS

Definition

Lyme borreliosis is a multisystem disorder caused by *Borrelia burgdorferi* infection and its sequelae. This spirochete is transmitted by a tick vector. Diagnosis is based on clinical history and examination with support from laboratory data.

History

In 1975, a cluster of children was identified in Old Lyme, Connecticut, with a syndrome mimicking juvenile rheumatoid arthritis.[1, 2] Erythema migrans, and neurologic and cardiac manifestations were subsequently recognized as part of the syndrome, which became known as Lyme disease or Lyme borreliosis.[3]

Erythema migrans had been recognized in European reports earlier in the century and attributed to bites by *Ixodes ricinus* ticks.[4, 5] The epidemiologic studies of Lyme patients also suggested a vector-borne disease transmitted by Ixodes ticks.[6] In 1982, a previously unidentified spirochete, *B. burgdorferi*, was isolated from Ixodes ticks[7, 8] and in patients with Lyme disease,[8] confirming it as the causative agent.

Since the identification of *B. burgdorferi*, it has been recognized that there are several distinct genospecies. The group has become known collectively as *B. burgdorferi* sensu lato. At least three genospecies cause disease in Europe: *B. burgdorferi* sensu stricto, *B. afzelii*, and *B. garinii*.[9, 10] In the United States, only *B. burgdorferi* sensu stricto has been implicated. Other genospecies, for example, *B. valaisiana*, *B. lusitaniae*, and *B. japonica*, have been identified, but their role in human disease is not established.[9, 11]

Epidemiology

Since its recognition in 1975, Lyme borreliosis has been reported in North America, Europe, and Asia. There have been isolated reports from Australia, Africa, and South America, although these are not generally considered to be endemic regions for Lyme borreliosis.

In the United States, the Centers for Disease Control and Prevention has received reports of Lyme borreliosis from 48 of the 50 states and from the District of Columbia. However, cases are highly concentrated in the Northeast, Mid-Atlantic and upper Midwest regions. A focal "hot spot" has also been identified in the Pacific Northwest.

In 1996, the overall annual incidence in the United States was 6.2 cases per 100,000.[12] Eight states had an incidence that exceeded the national average, and these eight accounted for 91% of the reported 16,461 cases (Table 16–1). Incidence exceeded 100 cases per 100,000 population in 18 counties and reached 1247.5 cases per 100,000 population in Nantucket County, Massachusetts, the highest county-specific incidence in 1996.[12]

The number of cases reported to the Centers for Disease Control and Prevention increased annually through 1996, with a moderate decline in 1997. The steadily increasing incidence probably represents a combination of increased tick density in endemic areas and better reporting.[13]

Incidence data from Europe is less comprehensive because of variation in reporting practices among countries. Reporting of Lyme borreliosis cases is mandatory only in Slovenia and Scotland.[14] Only neuroborreliosis is reportable in Denmark. Estimates of incidence in other European countries depend on published scientific studies, and indirect methods such as tick counts and prevalence of seropositivity in the population.[9]

The incidence appears to be higher in Eastern Europe than in Western Europe. In Austria and Slovenia, incidence exceeds 100 cases per 100,000 population per year (Table 16–2), with a peak incidence of 350 per 100,000 in some states of eastern and southern Austria.[9] Focal areas of higher incidence occur in regions of Northern Europe, where overall incidence is low.[15] This usually occurs in areas where there is a larger deer population to support the tick vector.[14] A similar pattern is seen in the Far East.[16]

Persons of all ages are affected by Lyme borreliosis. The incidence is highest in children younger than 15[9, 17] and adults aged 30 to 59 years.[17] The incidence of clinical manifestations varies with age[9] with cranial neuropathy more common and chronic disease manifestations less common in children than adults.[18]

The incidence is somewhat higher in men than women.[9, 12] Although the majority of cases are believed to arise from exposure around domestic residences, occupational and recreational exposures are also important and may help explain the gender difference. Because of the nature of the vector transmission, the onset of first signs and symptoms most often occurs during warmer weather.[19]

TABLE 16–1. ANNUAL INCIDENCE OF LYME BORRELIOSIS IN THE UNITED STATES BY STATE IN 1996[12]

STATE	ANNUAL INCIDENCE PER 100,000 POPULATION
Connecticut	94.8
Rhode Island	53.9
New York	29.2
New Jersey	27.4
Delaware	23.9
Pennsylvania	23.3
Maryland	8.8
Wisconsin	7.7
Minnesota	5.4
Massachusetts	5.3
Maine	4.9
Vermont	4.4
New Hampshire	4
37 states and Washington, DC	1.4 or less

TABLE 16–2. ESTIMATED INCIDENCE OF LYME BORRELIOSIS IN EUROPE[9]

COUNTRY	ANNUAL INCIDENCE PER 100,000 POPULATION
United Kingdom	0.3
Ireland	0.6
France	16.0
Germany	25.0
Switzerland	30.4
Czech Republic	39.0
Bulgaria	55.0
Sweden (south)	69.0
Slovenia	120.0
Austria	130.0

Clinical Characteristics of Systemic Disease

Lyme borreliosis is a multisystem disorder whose most prominent manifestations affect the skin, nervous system, musculoskeletal system, and heart. A wide spectrum of eye involvement has been described. The clinical course has been divided into early, disseminated, and persistent (or late) stages (Table 16–3). Patients may not exhibit all stages.

Early Disease

Erythema migrans is the characteristic rash of early disease. A red macular lesion forms at the site of the tick bite 2 to 28 days after the bite.[20] Because of the size of the tick, most patients do not remember the bite. As the lesion enlarges and becomes papular, the paracentral area may clear, forming a "bull's eye" or target shape with the site of the bite at the center (Fig. 16–1). The lesion may itch or be painful but is often asymptomatic.

The rate of expansion of erythema migrans lesions is about 1 cm per day to a maximum size of 20 to 30 cm diameter.[20, 21] Constitutional symptoms including fever, malaise, fatigue, myalgias, and arthralgias often accompany the rash. According to one standard surveillance definition of erythema migrans, a skin lesion must have a delayed onset and expand to a diameter exceeding 5

TABLE 16–3. SYSTEMIC MANIFESTATIONS OF LYME BORRELIOSIS

EARLY STAGE
Erythema migrans

DISSEMINATED STAGE
Erythema chronica migrans
Borrelial lymphocytoma
Arthritis
Meningitis
Cranial neuropathy
Motor and sensory radiculitis
Encephalitis/myelitis

PERSISTENT STAGE
Acrodermatitis chronica atrophicans
Arthritis
Encephalopathy
Sensory neuropathy

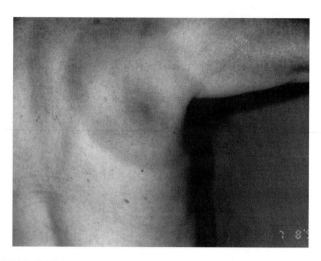

FIGURE 16–1. Erythema migrans is a target-shaped skin lesion centered around the site of the tick bite. (Courtesy of the Centers for Disease Control and Prevention, Division of Vector-Borne Infectious Diseases.)

cm in an individual known to have been exposed to a potential tick habitat in the previous 30 days.[22] These criteria help avoid confusion with tick or insect bite hypersensitivity reactions, which have an onset within hours, are smaller in size, and are of shorter duration. Bites from other ticks and insects, cellulitis, hyperkeratotic disorders, contact dermatitis, tinea, and granuloma annulare may also be confused with erythema migrans.[21] In Missouri, an area with a low incidence of Lyme borreliosis, a study of patients with rashes mimicking erythema migrans failed to identify borrelia in biopsy specimens but showed a possible association to tick bite by *Amblyomma americanum*.[23]

When erythema migrans is positively identified, it is diagnostic of Lyme borreliosis. However, as many as 20% to 40% of patients never develop a rash.[22, 24]

Disseminated Disease

SKIN MANIFESTATIONS
Several weeks after exposure, hematogenous dissemination occurs with potential involvement of the skin, nervous system, joints, heart, and eyes. Secondary erythema migrans lesions may occur at sites remote from the tick bite (known as erythema chronicum migrans). *Borrelia* lymphocytoma (also known as lymphocytoma benigna cutis) is a bluish red lesion with a predilection for the ear lobes of children and the nipple region of adults.[20] This manifestation is more commonly reported in European patients than in the United States.

JOINT MANIFESTATIONS
Up to 80% of untreated erythema migrans patients in the United States develop joint manifestations.[25] While joint involvement is less common in Europe, the clinical presentation is similar to that in North American patients.[25] The arthritis is typically monoarthritis or oligoarthritis of large joints most commonly involving the knee. The process may be chronic, or recurrent, with each episode resolving over days to months. Tendons and

small joints, especially the temporomandibular joint, may be affected.[25] Especially in children, joint manifestations may be the only clinical feature of Lyme borreliosis.[25]

NEUROLOGIC MANIFESTATIONS

Neurologic involvement occurs in the disseminated and persistent stages of Lyme borreliosis, and can affect both the central and peripheral nervous systems. In the central nervous system (CNS), meningeal signs, cranial neuropathy, and radiculitis are accompanied by pleocytic lymphocytosis in the cerebrospinal fluid (CSF).[26, 27] Meningeal involvement may present with headache, nausea, photophobia, and vomiting. Cranial nerve palsy may be unilateral or bilateral, and most often affects the facial nerve. Both sensory and motor radiculopathy occurs. Neurologic involvement more commonly presents with meningeal signs in the United States, whereas painful radiculitis is more common in Europe.[26] Symptoms of encephalitis such as alterations in mood, behavior, and mental capacity suggest direct brain involvement.

CARDIAC MANIFESTATIONS

Cardiac involvement occurs in fewer than 5% of treated patients.[28] The most common manifestation is atrioventricular block of varying degree.[29] Other conduction system defects, arrhythmias, myocarditis, and pericarditis also occur.[29]

Persistent Disease

The skin, nervous system, and joints are most often affected in late disease. Acrodermatitis chronica atrophicans is a bluish red lesion usually found on the extremities, predominately in women between 40 and 70 years old.[20] Fibrous bands and nodules may form. In its late stages, the lesion becomes atrophic and wrinkled. This lesion is much more commonly reported in European patients than in the United States.

Late neurologic involvement manifests as subacute or chronic encephalopathy with subtle memory and cognitive dysfunction, progressive encephalomyelitis with white matter lesions, and peripheral neuropathy.[26–28] In late joint disease, the duration of acute attacks of arthritis may become longer, and intermittent arthritis may become chronic.[2, 25]

Some patients with so-called atypical clinical manifestations of Lyme borreliosis may actually be coinfected with other tick-borne pathogens, for example, the parasite *Babesia microti* or the *Ehrlichia* species, which causes human granulocytic ehrlichiosis. Coinfection is discussed further in the section titled "Coinfection."

Clinical Characteristics of Ocular Disease

As with systemic findings, the ocular findings of Lyme borreliosis differ with the stage of disease (Table 16–4), and patients may not present with clinical manifestations from each stage. Most descriptions of eye findings in the literature consist of case reports and case series. These reports provide excellent insight into the spectrum of eye manifestations, but caution is appropriate given the limitations of Lyme serologic testing and the tendency to overdiagnose Lyme borreliosis.[28, 30]

TABLE 16–4. OCULAR MANIFESTATIONS OF LYME BORRELIOSIS

EARLY STAGE
Conjunctivitis
Episcleritis

DISSEMINATED STAGE
Cranial neuropathy
Papillitis
Papilledema
Optic atrophy
Pupillary abnormalities
Anterior, intermediate, and posterior uveitis
Neuroretinitis
Retinitis
Retinal vasculitis
Choroiditis
Panuveitis

PERSISTENT STAGE
Chronic intraocular inflammation
Keratitis
Episcleritis

Early Disease

CONJUNCTIVITIS

Following a tick bite, in the early stages of disease, photophobia and conjunctivitis may accompany the constitutional symptoms.[31] Conjunctivitis is present in approximately 11% of patients.[1, 32] Because the eye signs and symptoms are generally mild and self-limited, the patient often is not seen by an ophthalmologist. Case reports in the ophthalmic literature have described follicular conjunctivitis with positive Lyme serology.[31, 33]

EPISCLERITIS

Episcleritis may accompany the conjunctivitis and erythema migrans during the local phase or early disseminated phases.[15] It has also been reported during the late, persistent phase of the disease, described later.

Disseminated Disease

NEURO-OPHTHALMIC MANIFESTATIONS

In the disseminated phase of the disease, neuro-ophthalmic manifestations accompany the neurologic involvement. Cranial neuropathy and optic nerve involvement are the most common.

CRANIAL NEUROPATHY

Seventh cranial nerve palsy (Bell's palsy) is the most common cranial neuropathy.[34, 35] In one series, 10% of Lyme borreliosis patients had seventh nerve palsies.[36] As many as 25% of new-onset Bell's palsy cases may be attributed to Lyme borreliosis in endemic areas.[36] The palsy is bilateral in up to one-third of patients.[34, 37]

Involvement of the sixth cranial nerve may be unilateral or bilateral.[34, 38] Third, fourth, and fifth cranial neuropathies also occur, but less frequently.[39, 40] Multiple cranial nerves may be affected in the same patient. Cranial neuropathies result from direct infection or inflammation

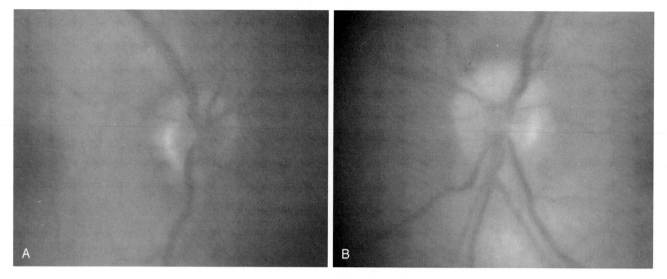

FIGURE 16–2. A young woman complaining of bilateral floaters was noted to have bilateral vitritis and papillitis. Visual acuity was 20/20 OU. Lyme serology was positive. The vitritis and papillitis cleared promptly after antibiotic treatment. Convalescent titer confirmed the diagnosis.

of the nerve, or indirectly as a result of meningitis, autoimmune process, or increased intracranial pressure.[34, 38, 39, 41] Cranial neuropathies often resolve without sequelae over weeks to months but may recur even after treatment.[38, 42]

OPTIC NERVE INVOLVEMENT

Optic nerve findings include optic neuritis, papilledema, and papillitis. Isolated optic nerve involvement has been reported.[43] Papilledema occurs in association with meningitis and increased intracranial pressure[38, 44] and may present as transient visual obscurations. Optic nerve inflammation may result in optic atrophy.[43–47]

Papillitis often occurs in association with Lyme uveitis[15] (Fig. 16–2). Optic nerve swelling in patients with positive Lyme serology has been described as optic neuritis or ischemic optic neuropathy. This has led to speculation about borreliosis as a cause of multiple sclerosis and temporal arteritis. As reviewed elsewhere, these associations have not been confirmed and probably represent overdiagnosis or coincidence.[39]

PUPILLARY INVOLVEMENT

Horner's syndrome has been described early in the clinical course in several patients.[39, 48] Tonic pupil[44] and mydriasis[15] have also been described.

INTRAOCULAR INFLAMMATION

Anterior uveitis, intermediate uveitis, neuroretinitis, retinal vasculitis, choroiditis, and panuveitis have all been reported as a result of infection with *B. burgdorferi* sensu lato.[15, 45, 49–56] These protean presentations are similar to those described for syphilis, caused by another spirochete, *Treponema pallidum*.

In the author's experience, and that of others,[15, 42, 45, 52, 53, 57] intermediate uveitis is one of the most common intraocular presentations (Figs. 16–2 and 16–3). The vitritis is frequently severe (Fig. 16–4). It may be accompanied by a granulomatous anterior chamber reaction, papillitis, neurosensory retinitis, choroiditis, or panuveitis[15, 45] (see Fig. 16–3).

Lyme choroiditis, especially if it is long standing, leads to clumping and atrophy of the retinal pigment epithelium, and may be confused with other syndromes.[15, 51] Filling of choriocapillaris is delayed or uneven with areas of choroidal hyperfluorescence and blockage by pigmentary clumping. Retinal vasculitis may affect the disc, posterior pole, or periphery. Fluorescein angiography demonstrates late filling of retinal vessels with perivasculitis or occlusion.

ORBITAL INFLAMMATION

One case of orbital inflammation in a child has been reported, with pain, proptosis, and diplopia.[58] Enlargement of the extraocular muscles was confirmed radiographically. Although systemic myositis occurs in Lyme

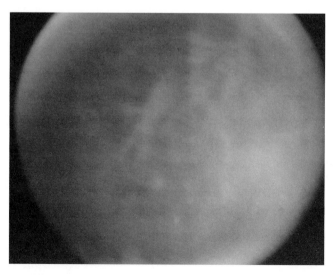

FIGURE 16–3. Vitreous "snowballs" are present in the inferior vitreous cavity of a patient with Lyme borreliosis. (Courtesy of William W. Culbertson, M.D.)

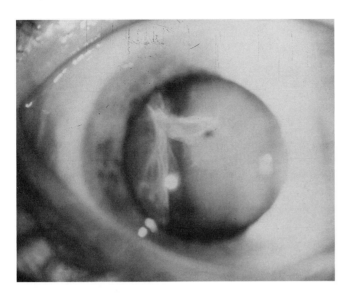

FIGURE 16–4. Severe vitritis in a patient with Lyme borreliosis and intraocular involvement. (Courtesy of William W. Culbertson, M.D.)

borreliosis, the diagnosis of Lyme borreliosis in this case has been questioned.[27, 39]

Persistent Disease

KERATITIS

Keratitis occurs months to years after onset of infection. Patients complain of mild blurring of vision and photophobia. On clinical examination, keratitis presents as a patchy or nebular subepithelial and stromal infiltration, usually bilateral.[31, 42, 59–62] The infiltrates have indistinct borders, may be peripheral or diffuse, and may involve both superficial and deep stroma. Keratic precipitates may underlie the infiltrates.[31] Neovascularization is minimal or absent. Episcleritis may accompany the keratitis or reappear as an isolated late manifestation.[31, 62] Because keratitis responds to topical steroids alone, it has been speculated that it is an autoimmune rather than an infectious process.

PATHOGENESIS

Ecology

In the Northeast, Mid-Atlantic, and Mid-West regions of the United States, *Ixodes scapularis* (commonly known as the black-footed tick, the deer tick, or the bear tick) is the vector for Lyme borreliosis. The literature first associated Lyme borreliosis with the vector *I. dammini*, a new species of Ixodes tick. Separate species status has since been rejected for this tick, and it is now recognized as a northern variant of *I. scapularis*.[63]

I. scapularis has a 2-year life cycle.[42] After the tick egg hatches in the spring, the larva-stage tick attaches to a passing small mammal for a blood meal. The preferred host is the white-footed mouse, *Peromyscus leucopus*. After the blood meal, the larva is dormant over the winter until it molts into a nymph. The following spring, the nymph stage takes a blood meal for 3 to 4 days. Again, the preferred host is the white-footed mouse, although birds and other mammals including humans may serve as host.

The nymph molts into an adult, and in late summer or fall, the adult takes a third blood meal. The adult's preferred host is the white-tailed deer. After the blood meal, the ticks mate, and the adult female tick drops to the ground to lay her eggs and restart the cycle.

During their blood meals, the larval-stage and nymph-stage ticks become infected with *B. burgdorferi* by feeding on an infected mouse. After molting to the nymph or adult stage respectively, the infected tick can infect the subsequent host during the next blood meal. Because the nymph population feeds earlier in the season than the following year's larvae, there is a reservoir of infection in the white-footed mouse population to infect the new larvae and perpetuate the cycle. Unlike white-footed mice, white-tailed deer are not competent reservoirs for borrelia infection.

An average of 25% of nymphs become infected as larvae.[63] An average of 50% of adults become infected in the larval or nymph stage but before their adult meal. Despite the higher infection rate in adults, most human infection is attributed to a bite by a nymph-stage tick because nymphs are more aggressive feeders, are more numerous than adults, and feed during the warm months, when human encounters are more likely. Nymphs are also smaller in size and are less likely to be noted and removed before transmission of infection (Fig. 16–5). Transmission of borreliosis is less likely early in the blood meal.[64]

In the Western United States, *I. pacificus*, the Western black-footed tick, has been identified as the vector for Lyme borreliosis. This tick feeds on lizards as its preferred host. Lizards, like white-tailed deer, are incompetent reservoirs of infection. Occasionally, however, *I. pacificus* will feed on a secondary host, for example, a rodent or human. There is a reservoir of infection in rodents maintained by a second tick, *I. neotomae*. *I. neotomae* is host specific and, therefore, not a vector for human infection.[63] However, when *I. pacificus* feeds on an infected rodent, then takes a subsequent blood meal from a human, borrelia infection can be transmitted.

In Europe, *I. ricinus* is the primary tick vector. Other possible tick vectors, *I. hexagonus* and *I. uriae*, have also been described.[63] Competent reservoir hosts include mice (*Apodermus flavicollis* and *A. sylvaticus*) and voles (*Clethrionomys glariolus*). In Asia, *I. persulcatus* and *I. ovatis* are the tick vectors.[16]

Genospecies

Several genospecies of *B. burgdorferi* sensu lato have been identified.[10] Although each genospecies is clearly capable of causing a broad range of clinical manifestations, individual clinical manifestations of Lyme borreliosis have been associated with particular genospecies.[65, 66]

B. burgdorferi sensu stricto is the genospecies implicated in North American Lyme borreliosis but only in a portion of European disease. Patients with Lyme disease in North America were first identified as a cluster of patients with oligoarthritis,[1] and arthritis is more common in American patients with Lyme disease than European patients.[25] It has since been recognized that patients infected with *B. burgdorferi* sensu stricto are more likely to experience joint symptoms and arthritis.

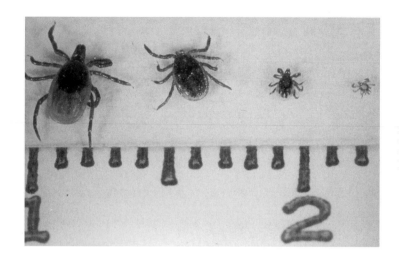

FIGURE 16–5. *Ixodes scapularis* ticks are shown above a centimeter ruler. From left, they are an adult female, an adult male, a nymph, and a larva. (Courtesy of the Centers for Disease Control and Prevention, Division of Vector-Borne Infectious Diseases.)

B. afzelii is associated with acrodermatitis chronicum atrophicans, and *B. garinii* has been associated with increased risk of neurologic symptoms. These two genospecies have been identified as infectious agents in Europe, where acrodermatitis and neurologic symptoms are more commonly recognized than in the United States.

It has been postulated that some cases of broad organ system involvement in Europe may represent infection with more than one genospecies, either from multiple tick bites or from a bite by a tick simultaneously infected with more than one genospecies.[67]

Host Sensitivity

Differences in human host response may also be responsible for some differences in clinical manifestations. In North American patients, chronic arthritis has been associated with HLA-DR4 and HLA-DR2.[68] Patients who are HLA-DR4 positive also have a poorer response to antibiotic treatment.[68] European studies have been contradictory on these associations.[69, 70, 71]

An association has been identified between risk of developing chronic arthritis and increased humoral response to the borrelia outer surface proteins (Osp).[72] However, this association has not been identified for other chronic Lyme manifestations, for example, chronic neuroborreliosis.

Immunopathogenesis

The interaction between the spirochete, tick, and human host is complex. During the tick's blood meal, *B. burgdorferi* uses the plasminogen and plasminogen activators from the host's blood to enhance dissemination of spirochetes in the tick and to increase the number of spirochetes in the tick's salivary glands.[73] Plasminogen may also enhance the efficiency of spread of organism in the host's skin and tissues.[73, 74]

Tick saliva down-regulates the host immune response and may promote spirochete infection and persistence. The down-regulation by saliva persists throughout the duration of the blood meal.[74]

At the time of the blood meal, the presence of the borrelia's outer surface protein A (OspA) is down-regulated, while OspC is up-regulated. Because OspA is highly immunogenic, this may be a way to evade or adapt to host defenses.[74] The host humoral response to OspA occurs only late in the course of disease possibly after there is an adaptation to host response.[72, 74]

After invasion, *B. burgdorferi* is capable of attaching to human cell receptors and may use this process to facilitate migration across vascular endothelium. Once it is established in the host, the organism resides predominantly in the extracellular compartment but has been identified intracellularly. It has been postulated that the intracellular location may contribute to protection of the organism from effective treatment with some antibiotics and contribute to persistent disease.[74]

Once disseminated infection occurs, the organism is capable of persisting despite an intense inflammatory response by the host. In vitro studies have demonstrated that *B. burgdorferi* is a potent stimulator of interleukin-1 (IL-1), tumor necrosis factor α (TNF-α), and other inflammatory factors in macrophages and monocytes.[74, 75] The outer surface protein OspA stimulates production of the cytokines IL-6, IL-8, and other chemokines by endothelial cells and fibroblasts,[76, 77] and stimulates the production of the cell adhesion molecules E-selectin, P-selectin, ICAM-1, and VCAM by endothelial cells.[76–78] Other spirochete components also seem to cause up-regulation of adhesion molecules.[79] The up-regulation of the adhesion molecules may result in migration of neutrophils into the perivascular space as part of the pathogenesis of Lyme-associated tissue damage.[80]

During the humoral response, both immunoglobulin (IgM) and IgG are produced against multiple borrelia antigens. The start of IgM production and the switch to IgG production occur at different times for different antigens. Animal studies suggest that humoral immunity is an effective protection against infection with *B. burgdorferi* if immunity is present before infection or shortly after infection.[74] It has been postulated that pre-existing antibody protection may be effective in part because ingestion of antibody during the blood meal kills spirochetes in the tick gut before host infection.[74] A recombinant lipidated OspA vaccine for *B. burgdorferi* sensu stricto recently has been marketed for human use.[81]

Animals immunized later after infection tended to

progress to chronic disease. In humans with persistent disease, infection has been demonstrated despite detectable levels of Lyme-specific antibodies.

Cell-mediated immunity also appears to play a role in modulating the severity of infection. In mouse models, CD4+ helper cells of the Th1 subset increase the joint inflammation, but Th2 cells appear to be preventive.[82, 83] In humans, a subset of CD4+ cells that produces the same pattern of lymphokines as murine Th1 cells is selectively activated by *B. burgdorferi*.[84]

Late in the course of Lyme borreliosis, chronic inflammatory manifestations sometimes occur in the absence of active infection. An autoimmune response may account for this in some cases. Molecular mimicry has been proposed as one possible autoimmune mechanism.[85] Patients with neurologic involvement have antiaxonal antibodies in their serum,[86] and there are cross-reactive epitopes between human axons and borrelia flagella.[87] This factor may contribute to Lyme peripheral neuropathy during the late stage of the disease.

Diagnosis

Clinical Diagnosis

The diagnosis of Lyme borreliosis is primarily based on clinical presentation with support from laboratory data.[24, 88, 89] The Centers for Disease Control and Prevention has established a set of diagnostic criteria for disease surveillance.[22] These criteria have been adopted for clinical use[24, 89] and are presented in Table 16–5.

Erythema migrans is the best clinical marker for Lyme borreliosis and is present in 60% to 80% of patients. In cases of erythema migrans, serologic testing is not routinely recommended, does not greatly increase the likelihood of a correct diagnosis,[89] and may be misleading because of the time lag until seroconversion.

Clinical diagnosis in the disseminated and persistent stages of disease is based on the musculoskeletal, neurologic, and cardiovascular manifestations outlined in Table 16–5, with confirmation by laboratory testing.

Another diagnostic system proposes assigning point values to signs, symptoms, and laboratory results. Based on the point score, patients are classified as unlikely, possible, or highly likely to have Lyme borreliosis (per Joseph J. Burrascano, Jr, M.D., http://www2.lymenet.org/domino/file.nsf/UID/guidelines).

Laboratory Testing

CULTURE

The gold standard for laboratory diagnosis of infection is culture of the organism from a tissue or fluid specimen. Unfortunately, except for skin biopsies, *B. burgdorferi* is difficult to culture from tissue and bodily fluids.[71, 89]

Culture of a skin punch biopsy from erythema migrans is positive in 60% to 80% of verified cases and may be helpful in atypical cases.[89–91] As already discussed, erythema migrans can be confused with other annular rashes.[21, 23] A positive culture from a punch biopsy of the leading edge of a skin lesion is diagnostic of Lyme borreliosis, but a negative result does not rule out the diagnosis.

TABLE 16–5. DIAGNOSIS OF LYME BORRELIOSIS[22, 86, 87]

CONFIRMED CASE:

Erythema migrans or
At least one late manifestation that is laboratory confirmed

LATE MANIFESTATIONS:

Musculoskeletal system—Recurrent, brief attacks (weeks or months) of objective joint swelling in one or a few joints, sometimes followed by chronic arthritis in one or a few joints. Manifestations not considered as criteria for diagnosis include chronic progressive arthritis not preceded by brief attacks and chronic symmetrical polyarthritis. Additionally, arthralgia, myalgia, or fibromyalgia syndromes alone are not criteria for musculoskeletal involvement.
Nervous system—Any of the following, alone or in combination: lymphocytic meningitis; cranial neuritis; particularly facial palsy (may be bilateral); radiculoneuropathy; or, rarely, encephalomyelitis. Encephalomyelitis must be confirmed by demonstration of antibody production against *Borrelia burgdorferi* in the cerebrospinal fluid (CSF), evidenced by a higher titer of antibody in CSF than in serum. Headache, fatigue, paresthesia, or mildly stiff neck alone are not criteria for neurologic involvement.
Cardiovascular system—Acute onset of high-grade (second degree or third degree) atrioventricular conduction defects that resolve in days to weeks and are sometimes associated with myocarditis. Palpitations, bradycardia, bundle branch block, or myocarditis alone are not criteria for cardiovascular involvement.

LABORATORY CONFIRMATION:

Isolation of *B. burgdorferi* from a clinical specimen or
Demonstration of diagnostic immunoglobulin M (IgM) or immunoglobulin G (IgG) antibodies to *B. burgdorferi* in serum or CSF. A two-test approach using a sensitive enzyme immunoassay or immunofluorescence antibody followed by Western blot is recommended.
Significant change in IgM or IgG antibody response to *B. burgdorferi* in paired acute- and convalescent-phase serum samples.

SEROLOGY

Serology, usually by enzyme-linked immunosorbent assay (ELISA), is the most commonly used diagnostic test in the clinical setting. The indirect immunofluorescence assay can also be used, but it requires more expertise in interpretation and is more difficult to automate. Unfortunately, there is great inter-test variability and poor agreement among commercially available test kits.[92] Even among reference laboratories, the accuracy and precision of results has been variable.[93]

The ELISA method uses a colorimetric measure to assess the binding of immunoglobulin in the serum specimen to Lyme antigen that has been applied to the ELISA plate. The result of ELISA testing comes in the form of an optical density. The level at which a measurement is positive has not been standardized for Lyme borreliosis, but it has been recommended that the optical density be at least three standard deviations above the mean reading for negative controls.[89] Optical density readings are taken on progressively diluted aliquots of the serum specimen to determine the highest "titer" at which the specimen is positive for Lyme-specific IgM, for IgG, or for IgM and IgG combined. ELISA results are classified as negative, equivocal, and positive, depending on the titer. Again, recommendations have been made regarding the titers at which results become equivocal and positive, but no universal standard has been adopted.[89] The variation in testing method suggests that the clinician may wish to question the laboratory about the Lyme antigen used, ask whether IgM and IgG were tested separately or together, and request that titers be reported.

There is general agreement that Western blotting should be used to confirm equivocal serologic tests.[89, 93–95] Some also advocate confirming all positive tests as well.[89, 94, 95] If there are cross-reacting antibodies (e.g., other spirochete infections, ehrlichia, rickettsia, HIV) or polyclonal B-cell activation (e.g., Epstein-Barr virus infection or systemic lupus erythematosus),[11] the immunoblot can correctly identify equivocal or false-positive ELISA results as truly negative. It also confirms equivocal and weakly reactive ELISA tests as true positive results.[15] Western blotting has been recommended for both IgM and IgG if the illness has lasted for less than 1 month and for IgG only if the disease has lasted for longer than 1 month.[95]

The Western blot technique separates proteins by weight using gel electrophoresis. After blotting the proteins onto nitrocellulose paper, the paper is reacted with a serum specimen, then checked for antigen-antibody complexes. If antibodies specific for borrelia protein antigens are present in the serum, they are detected adhering to the bands of protein on the blot. For Lyme borreliosis, guidelines have been proposed about which pattern of Lyme-specific protein bands must be present to consider the blot positive.[95] These guidelines improve the specificity of Western blotting, but it has been suggested that they may be so restrictive as to decrease sensitivity.[11]

False-negative results from serologic tests also occur. Because seroconversion has a lag time of 4 weeks or longer after initial infection, and depending on the particular antigen tested, patients with early infection may have negative serologic results.[96] It has been proposed that a false-negative result may also occur after incomplete antibiotic treatment early in the disease course. The treatment may blunt or delay the antibody response while still permitting persistence of *B. burgdorferi* infection. Patients with detectable borrelia-specific antibodies present in the form of immune complexes may also be classified as seronegative.[96] A false-negative ELISA test may also result if the lower threshold for equivocal results is set too high and Western blot confirmation is not performed.[15] In general, when rigorously performed serologic testing is negative late in the disease process, alternate diagnoses should be considered.[15, 21] Seronegative patients with probable Lyme-associated intraocular inflammation have been reported, but the details of the serologic testing method are not given.[55]

The sensitivity of serologic testing increases with the length of borrelia infection. In one study of a two-step test protocol (ELISA followed by Western blot), the sensitivity in patients with erythema migrans (57% to 76%) or early neurologic involvement (63% to 75%) was lower than in patients with arthritis (89% to 95%) or late neurologic findings (91% to 100%).[93] In a combined analysis of two other studies, the sensitivity was 59% for erythema migrans and 95% after several weeks of infection,[89] and the specificity was 93% for erythema migrans and 81% in later disease. Sensitivity and specificity in patients with early or late eye findings have not been well defined.

The predictive value of a positive or negative test changes with the pretest likelihood of having the disease (e.g., the prevalence of the disease in the population studied). In Lyme borreliosis, great care must be taken in interpreting a positive test in a patient who has a pretest probability of less than 20% of having the disease (e.g., vague symptoms or no history of exposure to an endemic area for Lyme borreliosis). In these patients, a positive result is more likely to represent a false-positive result than a true positive result.[89, 97–99] For this reason, it has been recommended that Lyme titers should not routinely be included in the screening work-up of uveitis in patients in a nonendemic area for Lyme borreliosis.[97] Likewise, in the cases in which the pretest probability of Lyme borreliosis is high (greater than 80%) based on clinical presentation, positive serologic testing does not add substantially to the already high probability that Lyme is the correct diagnosis.[89] Therefore, it is recommended that patients with typical erythema migrans should not routinely undergo serologic testing.[22, 24, 89]

Serologic testing can also be used to determine Lyme-specific antibody levels within infected body compartments. In infected compartments that are sequestered from the systemic circulation (e.g., the CNS, joints, and eye), the antibody level in compartmental fluid may be higher than in the serum. Paired samples of compartmental fluid and serum are measured by ELISA for specific antibody after diluting the specimens to achieve equal total immunoglobulin levels.[89] A higher antibody titer in the compartment compared with the serum is suggestive of local antibody production in the compartment in response to active borrelia infection. An alternative method is to measure the levels of total and specific antibodies in each specimen, then to calculate an antibody–to–total immunoglobulin ratio for the compartment and the serum. A higher ratio in the compartment suggests local antibody production and active infection.

HISTOPATHOLOGY

Histopathologic examination using silver stain can identify spirochetes in tissue specimens. While identification of spirochetes in tissue is suggestive, it is not diagnostic for *B. burgdorferi* sensu lato because other spirochetes may have a similar histologic appearance. Connective tissue fibers or artifacts may be misinterpreted as organisms.[28] Similar concerns arise when staining tissue with monoclonal antibodies. Spirochetes have been identified histologically in the vitreous compartment.[47, 55]

POLYMERASE CHAIN REACTION

Polymerase chain reaction (PCR) has been used to amplify both genomic and plasmid *B. burgdorferi* DNA. Because standardized guidelines for PCR use are not yet defined, the procedure is not in routine clinical use. PCR has been applied to skin, urine, serum, and cerebrospinal, synovial, and ocular fluids,[100] with the highest yield from skin specimens.[11]

As in all circumstances with PCR, the specificity of the primers used and the risk of contamination must be considered.[28] The fact that detection of *B. burgdorferi* DNA may not indicate the presence of viable organisms is also a theoretical consideration.[11, 28]

T-cell proliferation assay may be helpful in distinguishing persistent infection from inflammation in patients with chronic neurologic or joint symptoms.[89, 101] Further confirmation of the test's usefulness is needed.

Prevention

Because Ixodes ticks are transferred to a host when the host comes in contact with low-growing vegetation, prevention strategies for Lyme borreliosis in humans focus on limiting access to body surfaces by the tick. Tucking or taping the cuff of pant legs, wearing light-colored clothes so that ticks are more visible, use of insect repellent, and careful inspection for and removal of ticks after outdoor activities reduce the risk of tick contact. Even after a tick bite, early removal of the tick reduces the risk of spirochete transmission because a blood meal of several hours duration is required for efficient transmission of spirochetes.[64]

A vaccine for Lyme borreliosis has become available.[81] The vaccine is a lipidated recombinant outer surface protein A (OspA) from *B. burgdorferi* sensu stricto. In a multicenter clinical trial in the United States, the efficacy in preventing asymptomatic seroconversion was 83% after two doses and 100% after three doses. The efficacy in preventing Lyme borreliosis was 50% after two doses and 78% after three doses. The duration of protection is unknown. Because patients with successfully treated Lyme borreliosis may become reinfected, the duration of vaccine protection is probably limited.[85] The vaccine may act by reducing the number of viable spirochetes inside the tick when antibody is ingested during the blood meal.[85] In the United States, the vaccine is recommended for those with frequent or prolonged exposure to ticks in areas that are endemic for Lyme borreliosis.[81]

Treatment

β-lactam and tetracycline antibiotics are effective against *B. burgdorferi* sensu lato. As in other spirochetal diseases, 15% of patients may experience a Jarisch-Herxheimer reaction within hours of treatment.[102] Patients may experience constitutional symptoms, fever, tachycardia, vasodilation, and an increased white blood cell count. Prophylactic measures with anti-inflammatory agents should be considered and an infectious disease consultation may be helpful prior to treatment.

The usefulness of prophylactic antibiotic treatment for Lyme borreliosis after tick bite but before the onset of symptoms has not been proved.[103] The risk of developing clinical disease after untreated deer tick bite is between 1% and 2%.[18, 103] Careful observation for signs and symptoms of Lyme borreliosis before initiation of testing and treatment appears to be safe, because early treatment has a high success rate with low morbidity.[102, 104] This approach also appears to be more cost effective.[105]

If erythema migrans does develop, it can be treated with oral antibiotics alone.[102, 104] The current recommendation for adults is 2 to 3 weeks of treatment with doxycycline 100 mg bid, or amoxicillin 500 mg qid (with or without probenecid), or cefuroxime 500 mg bid.[21, 28, 104] Treatment regimens for children, pregnant women, and those with beta lactam allergy have also been developed.[28]

For Lyme arthritis, oral antibiotic therapy with doxycycline, amoxicillin, or cefuroxime for 1 to 2 months is first-line therapy, with a response rate of 80% to 90%.[106]

Intravenous therapy with ceftriaxone (2 g IV qd in adults) is a more costly alternative.[21, 106, 107]

Intravenous therapy is recommended for neuroborreliosis with CNS involvement and for all but the mildest cardiac manifestations.[21, 29] A regimen of ceftriaxone 2 g qd or cefotaxime 2 g q8h for 2 to 4 weeks has been recommended. In cases of isolated facial nerve palsy without CNS involvement, oral treatment may be adequate.[21, 26, 28] However, it is important to recognize any subtle CNS involvement, because treatment with oral antibiotics, and especially with amoxicillin and probenecid, may be counterproductive.[28, 106]

Treatment of ocular manifestations is based largely on case reports and case series. The mild conjunctivitis that occurs during the early stages of infection is self-limited and requires no specific ocular therapy. As already described, the accompanying systemic manifestations of early disease should be treated with oral antibiotics.

For intraocular involvement, the route and duration of antibiotic treatment has not been well defined.[42, 45, 108] It is probably most appropriate to consider intraocular involvement as a possible manifestation of neuroborreliosis. A detailed neurologic evaluation and a lumbar puncture are recommended. Confirmation of accompanying CNS involvement is an indication for intravenous antibiotic therapy, as in other cases of neuroborreliosis with CNS involvement. In the absence of CNS involvement, oral antibiotic treatment may be curative.[42, 45] However, in some cases of intraocular involvement, oral therapy has been reported to suppress the signs and symptoms with relapse occurring when the antibiotic is stopped.[45] If the response to oral therapy is not rapid and complete, intravenous therapy should be considered.[108]

After systemic antibiotic treatment has been initiated, residual intraocular inflammation may be treated with topical corticosteroids and mydriatics. Lyme keratitis, a late manifestation, is also treated with topical corticosteroids.[59, 60] The use of systemic corticosteroids has been described as part of the management of Lyme borreliosis.[35, 45] However, this is controversial because systemic corticosteroid treatment has been associated with an increased risk of antibiotic treatment failure.[45, 109]

The ocular response to systemic antibiotic therapy can be used as a guide to planning further therapy. As in all cases of intermediate and posterior uveitis, resolution of the cells in the vitreous cavity is a gradual process. If there is appropriate response of other ocular signs and symptoms, incomplete resolution of inflammatory cells in the vitreous should not be mistakenly regarded as a treatment failure.[108] As in systemic Lyme borreliosis, treatment failure in cases of intraocular disease should prompt a reconsideration of the diagnosis.[28]

Prognosis

Natural history studies show that during the early and disseminated stages of Lyme borreliosis, clinical disease is often self-limited even without treatment. Erythema migrans and the early constitutional signs resolve without treatment after several weeks.[110] After dissemination, there may be a period of months or years when Lyme borreliosis is clinically silent before symptoms of nervous system, joint, heart, eye, or other organ system involvement becomes apparent. Many untreated patients will not exhibit late manifestations, and of those who do, some may experience spontaneous resolution.[25, 39, 111]

When the condition is left untreated, neurologic manifestations often follow an intermittent, relapsing course.[37, 38] Arthritis also has a relapsing and remitting course with prolonged remissions in some untreated patients.[2, 25] Intraocular inflammation and neuro-ophthalmic manifestations may be intermittent or chronic.[45, 48, 108]

Chronic inflammation is more common during the late phase of disease. Symptoms of chronic arthritis,[2, 25] chronic neurologic findings (i.e., encephalopathy and sensory neuropathy), and chronic skin involvement (e.g., acrodermatitis chronica atrophicans) may be persistent or even progressive.

With early diagnosis, appropriate antibiotic therapy is curative with no long-term sequelae in a majority of cases. Untreated patients who do have long-standing disease manifestations also usually respond to antibiotic therapy.[74] However, additional long-term morbidity is associated with later treatment.[112]

In a minority of patients, chronic neurologic and joint manifestations persist or reappear despite antibiotic treatment. This chronic course has been attributed to persistent spirochete infection, immune response to persistent infection, immune response to spirochete antigen in the absence of active infection, and molecular mimicry.[85] Advanced tissue destruction may explain the persistence of symptoms in some patients in the absence of persistent infection or inflammation.[113] Despite prior antibiotic treatment, retreatment can produce temporary or permanent improvement in some chronic neurologic manifestations.[110] Cases of intraocular involvement with a chronic or relapsing course have been described.[45, 108] As in neurologic involvement, additional treatment with intravenous antibiotics should be considered.

COMPLICATIONS

The term post-Lyme syndrome has been used to describe a subset of patients with complaints of arthralgias, soft tissue pain, fatigue, memory impairment, difficulty concentrating, confusion, headache, malaise, and depression. These symptoms do not respond to continued antibiotic therapy. Unfortunately, there is a tendency to use the term chronic Lyme disease to refer both to these patients with subjective complaints and to patients with late stage Lyme borreliosis who have objective signs of persistent or recurrent joint inflammation or neurologic dysfunction.

Great effort should be made to document any objective evidence to support subjective reports. In particular, the mild progressive encephalopathy of late Lyme borreliosis is easily missed and can be documented by psychometric testing and CSF abnormalities.[114] Patients with this late manifestation may respond to further antibiotic treatment, while those with subjective symptoms alone generally do not.[113, 114]

Cases of post-Lyme syndrome can often be attributed to another disease process, even in patients in whom the diagnosis of Lyme borreliosis has previously been confirmed.[30] The differential diagnosis includes a number of syndromes in which subjective symptoms are prominent: fibromyalgia, chronic fatigue syndrome, and de-

pression. As discussed later, coinfection with a second vector-borne disease should also be considered.

Fibromyalgia, in particular, has been mistaken for or attributed to Lyme borreliosis. It has been identified soon after rigorously diagnosed borrelia infection, raising the possibility that it may be triggered by the infection.[30, 110] However, fibromyalgia can follow other infectious processes,[28] does not respond to antibiotics,[28] and is clinically distinct from the rheumatic presentation of Lyme borreliosis.[110] It should not be regarded as a form of chronic Lyme borreliosis.

Other neurologic and psychiatric illnesses should also be considered. Alzheimer's, multiple sclerosis, amyotrophic lateral sclerosis, and demyelinating disease have all been mistakenly attributed to Lyme borreliosis.[28, 30] In patients with depressed mental function without CNS abnormalities, reactive depression may provide the explanation.[114]

Most patients with long-standing *B. burgdorferi* infection are strongly seropositive.[21] Confirmed seronegativity in a patient who carries the diagnosis of chronic Lyme disease or "post-Lyme syndrome" should prompt a diligent search for an alternate diagnosis.[21]

Coinfection

Several infectious diseases other than borrelia are transmitted by Ixodes ticks. These ticks are the vector for the parasite which causes human babesiosis, for *Ehrlichia* which causes human granulocytic ehrlichiosis, and possibly for viruses known to cause encephalitis.[28]

Human babesiosis is caused by an intraerythrocytic parasite, *B. microti*. *B. microti* is endemic in many of the same areas where *B. burgdorferi* is found. The illness presents with fever, chills, sweats, arthralgias, headache, and fatigue.[85, 115] Eye findings are rare, but retinal nerve fiber layer infarcts have been reported.[116, 117] A positive blood smear is diagnostic, but false-negative results are frequent. Serology and PCR may assist in the diagnosis. Conventional treatment is with clindamycin and quinine. Without treatment, there may be prolongation of symptoms and persistence of babesia in the blood.[118] Even with treatment, recrudescent disease may occur years later.

Simultaneous Lyme borreliosis and babesiosis has been well documented.[115, 119] Coinfection may alter the clinical course of Lyme borreliosis. In one study, 11% of those with clinical Lyme disease were simultaneously infected with babesia.[115] In these patients, fatigue, headache, nausea, sweats, anorexia, chills, emotional lability, conjunctivitis, and splenomegaly were more frequent than in patients who had Lyme disease alone. Patients with coinfection had more signs and symptoms, had longer duration of their symptoms, and spirochetemia persisted longer. Coinfection was characterized by persistent and debilitating fatigue lasting for more than 6 months in 35% of coinfected patients.

Human granulocytic ehrlichiosis has been recognized as an emerging vector-borne disease.[120] The organism causing this disorder is similar to *Ehrlichia equi* and *E. phagocytophilia*, which cause disease in animals, and the three organisms may represent different strains of a single species.[120] The organism has been identified over a broad geographic region in the United States and in Europe, and because of the shared Ixodes vector, there is geographic overlap with the endemic areas for babesiosis and Lyme borreliosis.[120]

Human granulocytic ehrlichiosis presents as a flulike illness with fever, chills, malaise, headaches, nausea, and vomiting.[121] Leukopenia, thrombocytopenia, and hepatic involvement are typically present on laboratory testing. The condition may be fatal, especially in the elderly. In one retrospective study, two of 41 patients died.[121] Eye findings have not yet been identified in human granulocytic ehrlichiosis, but they occasionally occur with other human ehrlichioses,[122, 123] and in animals.[124] Diagnosis is made by a positive smear of the buffy coat, but a negative smear does not rule out the diagnosis.[125] Serology and PCR can also be used to assist in the diagnosis. The infection is treated with tetracyclines.

Concurrence of Lyme borreliosis and human granulocytic ehrlichiosis has been reported.[125–127] Coinfection may alter the clinical presentation of borreliosis and the response to treatment.[28] Because ehrlichiosis may cause immunosuppression, simultaneous infection with *Ehrlichia* and *B. burgdorferi* may cause a more refractory or severe presentation of Lyme borreliosis.

Even in the absence of coinfection, human granulocytic ehrlichiosis can cause a false-positive result for Lyme ELISA and immunoblot tests.[127] This may lead to the incorrect diagnosis of atypical Lyme disease. When a patient presents with a new-onset febrile illness following Ixodes tick exposure, associated with constitutional signs and positive Lyme serology, but without erythema migrans, one should consider human granulocytic ehrlichiosis.[128] If empirical antibiotic therapy is to be given, a tetracycline should be considered instead of a β-lactam because the tetracycline will cover both infectious agents.[128]

Coinfection probably accounts for some cases of post-Lyme syndrome. Because simultaneous infection with *Babesia, Ehrlichia,* or other yet-to-be-identified tick-borne diseases may alter the clinical presentation of Lyme borreliosis, patients with Lyme disease who demonstrate atypical symptoms, a severe or prolonged clinical course, or who are refractory to appropriate treatment should be evaluated for other concurrent infectious disease.

Summary

Lyme borreliosis is a spirochetal infection commonly affecting the skin, joints, and nervous system. A minority of patients have ocular involvement. A self-limiting conjunctivitis may accompany early infection. With dissemination, neuro-ophthalmic signs and intraocular inflammation occur. Anterior uveitis, intermediate uveitis, neuroretinitis, retinal vasculitis, choroiditis, papillitis, and panuveitis have been described. Keratitis and episcleritis occur during the late stages of disease.

The diagnosis is made by careful history and thorough physical examination. Confirmation by laboratory testing is indicated in some cases. Early treatment with appropriate antibiotic therapy is curative. Late sequelae involving the skin, joints, and nervous system can occur.

RELAPSING FEVER

Definition

Relapsing fever is an acute borrelia infection that is characterized clinically by fever, followed by an afebrile period, then recurrence of the fever. Several species of borrelia have been implicated. Disease transmission has two vector patterns: louse borne and tick borne.

Epidemiology

Louse-borne disease is transmitted by the body louse *Pediculus humanus.* When the human host scratches the site of infestation, lice infected with *Borrelia recurrentis* are crushed, and the infected material is rubbed into the abraded skin. The cycle is perpetuated by lice that feed on an infected host, become infected, then transfer to an uninfected host, and are crushed. There does not appear to be an animal reservoir.

The distribution of louse-borne disease is worldwide and is more dependent on living conditions than geography. The last large epidemic occurred during and after World War II, when millions of people were infected in the Mediterranean basin, North Africa, and the Middle East. Because of famine and poor social conditions, endemic patterns of disease have been identified in East Africa, and in parts of South America and the Far East.

Tick-borne relapsing fever is transmitted by several species of *Ornithodoros* tick, each of which is associated with a corresponding borrelia species.[129] When all tick-vector combinations are considered, the geographic distribution of tick-borne disease includes portions of North and Central America, Southeastern Europe, and portions of Africa, Asia, and the Middle and Far East.

In the United States, *Ornithodoros hermsi* and *Ornithodoros turicata* ticks infected with *B. hermsii* and *B. turicatae* respectively inhabit the burrows or nests of rodents who serve as asymptomatic hosts for the infection.[130] Each summer and fall, sporadic cases of tick-borne relapsing fever are reported throughout the Western and Southwestern United States, from Texas to the state of Washington.[130] Common-source epidemics occur when humans interrupt the natural infection cycle and become incidental hosts.[95, 130–133] These epidemics are associated with having stayed in wilderness cabins or caves that harbor the borrows or nests of infected rodents. Symptoms may not develop until the patient has returned to his or her home, which may be outside the endemic area for relapsing fever.

Clinical Characteristics

The manifestation for which the disease is named is the recurrent intermittent episodes of fever. After an incubation period lasting days to weeks, fever, constitutional symptoms, and photophobia begin. A period of defervescence is followed by an afebrile period of relative well-being, then recurrence of the fever. This cycle may be repeated many times.

Patients with louse-borne disease are generally sicker. In severe cases, cardiac involvement, hepatitis with secondary jaundice, and splenic enlargement may occur. Bleeding is common, presenting as petechiae, ecchymoses, hematuria, and epistaxis. Infrequently, massive hemorrhage occurs. Meningismus and headache are commonly reported, but CSF abnormalities are not.[134] Intracranial bleeding may cause these symptoms in some patients. Encephalopathy and depressed mental status may occur. Eye involvement has not been reported.[134]

In tick-borne disease, patients may be unaware of having been exposed because *Ornithodoros* ticks are night feeders whose bite often goes unnoticed.[130] An eschar may develop at the site of the bite. After the incubation period, the first episode of fever occurs. As the fever abates, petechial, macular, or papular rash may present in up to half of patients. In untreated patients, an afebrile period of about 1 week is typically followed by 2 to 4 subsequent recurrences of fever, each less severe than the previous. This pattern is quite variable. Other clinical features include hepatomegaly and splenomegaly.

Some species of borrelia causing tick-borne relapsing fever are neurotropic: *B. turicatae* in the Southwestern United States, and *B. duttonii* in Sub-Saharan Africa.[134] In untreated patients, neurologic manifestations similar to those of Lyme borreliosis may occur after several recurrences of fever. These include radiculopathy, neuropsychiatric changes, and cranial neuritis, especially Bell's palsy.[134]

Ocular involvement in tick-borne relapsing fever is associated with the neurotrophic borrelia species and, to a lesser extent, with *B. hispanica*, endemic in Northern Africa.[134] As with neurologic disease, ocular manifestations present after 3 to 4 febrile episodes. Anterior uveitis, vitritis, choroiditis, and optic neuropathy have been described.[134-137] Ocular involvement occurs in 10% to 15% of patients.

Pathogenesis

The pathogenesis of the relapsing course of fever is attributed to continuous variation in the borrelia outer surface protein antigens. Fever accompanies the spirochetemia with each new antigenic variant until the organisms are cleared and the cycle repeats itself.[138]

Diagnosis

During febrile periods, a peripheral blood smear can be examined for spirochetes. The presence of spirochetes is diagnostic for relapsing fever. A thick smear[135] or fluorescence microscopy after staining with acridine orange may increase the sensitivity.[135, 139] Smears are negative when the patient is afebrile. Culture of borrelia from blood is possible but requires special medium and is not widely available clinically.[140]

Serologic testing for relapsing fever has not been standardized. ELISA has a high degree of cross-reactivity with *B. burgdorferi*, but Western blot testing for *B. burgdorferi* is negative. Because Lyme serology testing is widely available clinically, some have suggested that a positive Lyme ELISA and a negative Lyme Western blot could be used as a screening serologic test for relapsing fever until a standardized test is available. This combination of tests could aid in the diagnosis of relapsing fever during an afebrile period or when the peripheral blood smear is negative. In the United States, Western blot testing for at least one tick-borne species, *B. hermsii*, is available through the Centers for Disease Control and Prevention.

In the United States, the endemic areas for tick-borne relapsing fever and Lyme borreliosis are beginning to overlap. This may cause a diagnostic dilemma in patients with neurologic or ocular involvement, because manifestations of the two conditions may be similar.[134, 141]

Treatment

Oral tetracyclines are the most commonly used treatment for both tick-borne and louse-borne disease. β-lactam antibiotics are also effective. As in Lyme borreliosis, neurologic disease is treated with intravenous therapy, for example, ceftriaxone. Intraocular involvement should prompt a work-up for evidence of neurologic involvement.

Summary

Relapsing fever is an acute borrelial infection that is transmitted by tick and louse vectors. Neurologic and ocular manifestations of tick-borne disease have some similarity to those of Lyme borreliosis.

Acknowledgement

The author wishes to thank medical librarians Vicky Spitalniak and Dianne Deck for their assistance in the preparation of this manuscript.

References

1. Steere AC, Malawista SE, Hardin JA, et al: Lyme arthritis: An epidemic of oligoarticular arthritis in children and adults in three Connecticut communities. Arthritis Rheum 1977;20:7.
2. Steere AC: Diagnosis and treatment of Lyme arthritis. Med Clin North Am 1977; 81:179–194.
3. Steere AC, Malawista SE, Hardin JA, et al: Erythema chronicum migrans and Lyme arthritis: The enlarging spectrum. Ann Intern Med 1977;86:685.
4. Lipschutz B. Uber eine seltene Erythemform (Erythema chronicum migrans). Arch Dermatol Syph 1913:118:349.
5. Afzelius A: Erythema chronicum migrans. Acta Derm Venereol (Stockh) 1921;2:120.
6. Steere AC, Broderick TF, Malawista SE: Erythema chronicum migrans and Lyme arthritis: Epidemiologic evidence for a tick vector. Am J Epidemiol 1978;108:312.
7. Burgdorfer W, Barbour AG, Hayes SF, et al: Lyme disease—a tick-borne spirochetosis? Science 1982;216:1317.
8. Steere AC, Grodzicki RL, Kornblatt AN, et al: The spirochetal etiology of Lyme disease. N Engl J Med 1983;308:733–740.
9. O'Connell S, Granstrom M, Gray JS, et al: Epidemiology of European Lyme borreliosis. Zentralbl Bakteriol 1998;287:229–240.
10. Musser JM: Molecular population genetic analysis of emerging bacterial pathogens: Selected insights. Emerg Infect Dis 1996;2:1–17.
11. Coyle PK: *Borrelia burgdorferi* infection: Clinical diagnostic techniques. Immunol Invest 1997;26:117–128.
12. Centers for Disease Control and Prevention. Lyme disease—United States, 1996. MMWR 1997;46:531–535.
13. Centers for Disease Control and Prevention: Summary of notifiable diseases—United States, 1996. MMWR 1997;45:1–87.
14. Handysides S: Surveillance of Lyme disease in Europe. Eurosurveillance Weekly 1998;2:4–5.
15. Karma A, Seppälä I, Mikkilä, et al: Diagnosis and clinical characteristics of ocular Lyme borreliosis. Am J Ophthalmol 1995;119:127–135.
16. Isogai E, Isogai H, Kotake S, et al: Detection of antibodies against *Borrelia burgdorferi* in patients with uveitis. Am J Ophthalmol 1991;112:23–30.
17. Centers for Disease Control and Prevention: Notice to readers of availability of Lyme disease vaccine. MMWR 1999;48:35–36.
18. Shapiro ED, Gerber MA, Holabird NB, et al: A controlled trial of antimicrobial prophylaxis for Lyme disease after deer-tick bites. N Engl J Med 1992;327:1769–1773.
19. Centers for Disease Control and Prevention: Lyme disease: Connecticut. MMWR 1988;37:1–3.
20. Berger BW, Johnson RC, Kodner C, et al: Cultivation of *Borrelia burgdorferi* from erythema migrans lesions and perilesional skin. J Clin Microbiol 1992;30:359–361.
21. Rahn DW, Felz MW: Lyme disease update: Current approach to

early, disseminated, and late disease. Postgrad Med 1998;103:51–70.

22. Centers for Disease Control and Prevention: Case definitions for infectious conditions under public health surveillance. MMWR 1997;46(RR–10):20–21.

23. Campbell GL, Paul WS, Schriefer ME, et al: Epidemiologic and diagnostic studies of patients with suspected early Lyme disease, Missouri, 1990–1993. J Infect Dis 1995;172:470–480.

24. American College of Physicians: Guidelines for laboratory evaluation in the diagnosis of Lyme disease. Ann Intern Med 1997;127:1106–1108.

25. Steere AC, Schoen RT, Taylor E: The clinical evolution of Lyme arthritis. Ann Intern Med 1987;107:725–731.

26. Haass A: Lyme neuroborreliosis. Curr Opin Neurol 1998;11:253–258.

27. Winterkorn JMS: Lyme disease: Neurologic and ophthalmic manifestations. Surv Ophthalmol 1990;35:191–204.

28. Nadelman RB, Wormser GP: Lyme borreliosis. Lancet 1998;352:557–565.

29. Paparone PW: Cardiovascular manifestations of Lyme disease. J Am Osteopath Assoc 1997;97:156–161.

30. Steere AC, Taylor E, McHugh GL, et al: The overdiagnosis of Lyme disease. JAMA 1993;269:1812–1816.

31. Flach AJ, Lavoie PE: Episcleritis, conjunctivitis, and keratitis as other manifestations of Lyme disease. Ophthalmology 1990;97:973–975.

32. Steere AC: Medical progress—Lyme disease. N Engl J Med 1989;321:586–596.

33. Mombaerts IM, Maudgal PC, Knockaert DC: Bilateral follicular conjunctivitis as a manifestation of Lyme disease. Am J Ophthalmol 1991;112:96–97.

34. Pacher AR, Steere AC: The triad of neurologic manifestations in Lyme disease: Meningitis, cranial neuritis, and radiculoneuritis. Neurology 1985;35:47–53.

35. Steere AC: Lyme disease. N Engl J Med 1989;321:586–596.

36. Halpern JJ, Golightly M: Long Island Neuroborreliosis Collaborative Study Group. Lyme borreliosis in Bell's palsy. Neurology 1992;42:1268–1270.

37. Clark JR, Carlson RD, Sasaki CT, et al: Facial paralysis in Lyme disease. Laryngoscope 1985;95:1341–1345.

38. Lesser RL, Kornmehl EW, Pachner AR, et al. Neuro-ophthalmic manifestations of Lyme disease. Ophthalmology 1990;97:699–706.

39. Balcer LJ, Winterkorn JMS, Galetta SL: Neuro-ophthalmic manifestations of Lyme disease. J Neuro-Ophthal 1997;17(2):108–121.

40. Savas R, Sommer A, Gueckel F, Georgi M: Isolated oculomotor nerve paralysis in Lyme disease: MRI. Neuroradiology 1997;39(2):139–141.

41. Lesser RL. Ocular manifestations of Lyme disease. Am J Med 1995;98(Suppl 4A):60–62.

42. Zaidman GW: The ocular manifestations of Lyme disease. Int Ophthalmol Clin 1997;37:13–28.

43. Jacobson DM, Marx JJ, Dlesk A: Frequency and clinical significance of Lyme seropositivity in patients with isolated optic neuritis. Neurology 1991;41(5):706–711.

44. Reik L, Burgdorfer W, Donaldson JO: Neurologic abnormalities in Lyme disease without erythema chronicum migrans. Am J Med 1986;81:73–78.

45. Winward KE, Smith JL, Culbertson WW, et al: Ocular Lyme borreliosis. Am J Ophthalmol 1989;108:651–657.

46. Kauffmann DJH, Wormser GP: Ocular Lyme disease: Case report and review of the literature. Br J Ophthalmol 1990;74:325–327.

47. Halpern JJ, Luft BJ, Anand AK, et al: Lyme neuroborreliosis: Central nervous system manifestations. Neurology 1989;29:753–759.

48. Glauser TA, Brennan PJ, Galetta SL: Reversible Horner's syndrome and Lyme disease. J Clin Neuroophthalmol 1989;9:225–228.

49. Steere AC, Duray PH, Kauffmann DJ, et al: Unilateral blindness caused by infection with the Lyme disease spirochete, Borrelia burgdorferi. Ann Intern Med 1985;103:382–384.

50. Aaberg TM: The expanding ophthalmologic spectrum of Lyme disease. Am J Ophthalmol 1989;107:77–80.

51. Bialasiewicz AA, Ruprecht KW, Naumann GOH, et al: Bilateral diffuse choroiditis and exudative retinal detachments with evidence of Lyme disease. Am J Ophthalmol 1988;105:419–420.

52. Copeland RA, Nozik RA, Shimokaji G: Uveitis in Lyme disease. Ophthalmology 1989;107(Suppl):127.

53. Scholes GN, Teske M: Lyme disease and pars planitis. Ophthalmology 1989;107(Suppl):126.

54. Zierhut M, Kreissig F, Pickert A: Panuveitis with positive serological tests for syphilis and Lyme disease. J Clin Neuroophthalmol 1989;9:71–75.

55. Schubert HD, Greenebaum E, Neu H: Cytologically proven seronegative Lyme choroiditis and vitritis. Retina 1994;14:39–42.

56. Karma A, Stenborg T, Summanen P, et al: Long-term follow-up of chronic Lyme neuroretinitis. Retina 1996;16:505–509.

57. Breeveld J, Rothova A, Kuiper H: Intermediate uveitis and Lyme borreliosis. Br J Ophthalmol 1992;76:181–182.

58. Seidenberg KB, Leib ML: Orbital myositis with Lyme disease. Am J Ophthalmol 1990;109:13–16.

59. Baum J, Barza M, Weinstein P, et al: Bilateral keratitis as a manifestation of Lyme disease. Am J Ophthalmol 1988;105:75–77.

60. Kornmehl EW, Lesser RL, Jaros P, et al: Bilateral keratitis in Lyme disease. Ophthalmology 1989;96:1194–1197.

61. Orlin SE, Lauffer JL: Lyme disease keratitis. Am J Ophthalmol 1989;107:678–680.

62. Zaidman GW: Episcleritis and symblepharon associated with Lyme keratitis. Am J Ophthalmol 1990;109:487–488.

63. Barbour AG, Fish D: The biological and social phenomenon of Lyme disease. Science 1993;260:1610–1616.

64. Piesman J, Mather TN, Sinsky RJ, et al: Duration of tick attachment and Borrelia burgdorferi transmission. J Clin Microbiol 1987;25:557–558.

65. van Dam AP, Kuiper H, Vos K, et al: Different genospecies of Borrelia burgdorferi are associated with different species of Borrelia burgdorferi sensu lato. Clin Infect Dis 1993;17:708–717.

66. Balmelli T, Piffaretti J-C: Association between different clinical manifestations of Lyme disease and different species of Borrelia burgdorferi sensu lato. Res Microbiol 1995;146:329–340.

67. Pichon B, Godfroid E, Hoyois B, et al: Simultaneous infection of Ixodes ricinus nymphs by two Borrelia burgdorferi sensu lato species: Possible implications for clinical manifestations. Emerg Infect Dis 1995;1:89–90.

68. Steere AC, Dwyer E, Winchester R: Association of chronic Lyme arthritis with HLA-DR4 and HLA-DR2 alleles. N Engl J Med 1990;323:219–223.

69. Majsky A, Bojar M, Jirous J: Lyme disease and HLA-DR antigens. Tissue Antigens 1987;30:188–189.

70. Pfluger KH, Reimers CD, Neubert U, et al: Lyme borreliosis and possible association with HLA-antigens. Tissue Antigens 1989;33:375–381.

71. Preac-Mursic V, Pfister HW, Spiegel H, et al: First isolation of Borrelia burgdorferi from an iris biopsy. J Clin Neuroophthalmol 1993;13:155–161.

72. Kalish RA, Leong JM, Steere AC: Association of treatment-resistant chronic Lyme arthritis with HLA-DR4 and antibody reactivity to OspA and OspB of Borrelia burgdorferi. Infect Immun 1993;61:2774–2779.

73. Coleman JL, Gebbia JA, Piesman J, et al: Plasminogen is required for efficient dissemination of B. burgdorferi in ticks and for enhancement of spirochetemia in mice. Cell 1997;89:1111–1119.

74. Hu LT, Klempner MS: Host-pathogen interactions in the immunopathogenesis of Lyme disease. J Clin Immunol 1997;17:354–365.

75. Sprenger H, Krause A, Kaufmann A, et al: Borrelia burgdorferi induces chemokines in human monocytes. Infect Immun 1997;65:4384–4388.

76. Wooten RM, Modur VR, McIntyre TM, et al: Borrelia burgdorferi outer membrane protein A induces nuclear translocation of nuclear factor–kappa B and inflammatory activation in human endothelial cells. J Immunol 1996;157:4584–4590.

77. Ebnet K, Brown KD, Siebenlist UK, et al: Borrelia burgdorferi activates nuclear factor–kappa B and is a potent inducer of chemokine and adhesion molecule gene expression in endothelial cells and fibroblasts. J Immunol 1997;158:3285–3892.

78. Boggemeyer E, Stehle T, Schaible UE, et al: Borrelia burgdorferi upregulates the adhesion molecules E-selectin, P-selectin, ICAM-1 and VCAM1 on mouse endothelioma cells in vitro. Cell Adhes Commun 1994;2(2):145–157.

79. Sellati TJ, Abrescia LD, Radolf JD, et al: Outer surface lipoproteins of Borrelia burgdorferi activate vascular endothelium in vitro. Infect Immun 1996;64:3180–3187.

80. Sellati TJ, Burns MJ, Ficazzola MA, et al: *Borrelia burgdorferi* upregulates expression of adhesion molecules on endothelial cells and promotes transendothelial migration of neutrophils in vitro. Infect Immun 1995;63:4439–4447.

81. Centers for Disease Control and Prevention: Notice to readers: Availability of Lyme disease vaccine. MMWR 1999;48:35–36, 43.

82. Keane-Myers A, Nickell SP: T cell subset–dependent modulation of immunity to *Borrelia burgdorferi* in mice. J Immunol 1995; 154:1770–1776.

83. Keane-Myers A, Nickell SP: Role of IL-4 and IFN-gamma in modulation of immunity of *Borrelia burgdorferi* in mice. J Immunol 1995;155:2020–2028.

84. Yssel H, Shanafelt MC, Soderberg C, et al: *Borrelia burgdorferi* activates a T helper type 1–like T cell subset in Lyme arthritis. J Exp Med 1991;174:593–601.

85. Evans J: Lyme disease. Curr Opin Rheumatol 1998;10:339–346.

86. Sigal L, Tatum A: Lyme disease patients' serum contains IgM antibodies to *Borrelia burgdorferi* that cross-react with neuronal antigens. Neurology 1988;38:1439–1442.

87. Sigal LH, Tatum AH: Lyme disease patients' serum contains IgM antibodies to *Borrelia burgdorferi* that cross-react with neuronal antigens. Neurology 1988;38:1439–1442.

88. Nightingale SL: Public health advisory: Limitations, uses, and interpretation of assays for supporting clinical diagnosis of Lyme disease. JAMA 1997;278:805.

89. Tugwell P, Dennis DT, Weinstein A, et al: Laboratory evaluation in the diagnosis of Lyme disease. Ann Intern Med 1997;127:1109–1123.

90. Wormser GP, Forseter G, Cooper D, et al: Use of a novel technique of cutaneous lavage for diagnosis of Lyme disease associated with erythema migrans. JAMA 1992;268:1311–1313.

91. Berger BW, Lesser RL: Lyme disease. Dermatol Clin 1992;10:763–775.

92. Quan TJ, Wilmoth BA, Carter LG, Bailey RE: A comparison of some commercially available serodiagnostic kits for Lyme disease. In: Proceedings of the First National Conference on Lyme Disease Testing (Dearborn, Michigan). Washington DC: Association of State and Territorial Public Health Laboratory Directors, 1991, pp 61–73.

93. Craven RB, Quan TJ, Bailey RE, et al: Improved serodiagnostic testing for Lyme disease: Results of a multicenter serologic evaluation. Emerg Infect Dis 1996;2:136.

94. Johnson BJ, Robbins KE, Bailey RE, et al: Serodiagnosis of Lyme disease: Accuracy of a two-step approach using a flagella-based ELISA and immunoblotting. J Infect Dis 1996;174:346–353.

95. Centers for Disease Control and Prevention: Recommendation for test performance and interpretation from the Second National Conference on Serologic Diagnosis of Lyme Disease. MMWR 1995;44:590–591.

96. Schutzer SE, Coyle PK, Dunn JJ, et al: Early and specific antibody response to OspA in Lyme disease. J Clin Invest 1994;94:454–457.

97. Rosenbaum JT: Prevalence of Lyme disease among patients with uveitis. Am J Ophthalmol 1991;112:462–463.

98. Mikkila H, Seppala I, Leirisalo-Repo M, et al: The significance of serum anti-Borrelia antibodies in the diagnostic work-up of uveitis. Eur J Ophthalmol 1997;7:251–255.

99. Breeveld J, Kuiper H, Spanjaard L, et al: Uveitis and Lyme borreliosis. Br J Ophthalmol 1993;77:480–481.

100. Hilton E, Smith C, Sood S: Ocular Lyme borreliosis diagnosed by polymerase chain reaction on vitreous fluid. Ann Intern Med 1996;1125:424–425.

101. Dressler F, Yoshinari NH, Steere AC: The T-cell proliferative assay in the diagnosis of Lyme disease. Ann Intern Med 1991;115:533–539

102. Nadelman RB, Luger SW, Frank E, et al: Comparison of cefuroxime axetil and doxycycline in the treatment of early Lyme disease. Ann Intern Med 1992;117:273–280.

103. Warshafsky S, Nowakowski J, Nadelman RB, et al: Efficacy of antibiotic prophylaxis for prevention of Lyme disease. J Gen Intern Med 1996;11:329–333.

104. Dattwyler RJ, Volkman DJ, Conaty SM, et al: Amoxicillin plus probenecid versus doxycycline for treatment of erythema migrans borreliosis. Lancet 1990;336:1404–1406.

105. Fix AD, Strickland GT, Grant J: Tick bites and Lyme disease in an endemic setting: Problematic use of serologic testing and prophylactic antibiotic therapy. JAMA 1998;279:206–210.

106. Steere AC, Levin RE, Molloy PJ, et al: Treatment of Lyme arthritis. Arthritis Rheum 1994;37:878–888.

107. Eckman MH, Steere AC, Kalish RA, et al: Cost effectiveness of oral as compared with intravenous antibiotic therapy for patients with early Lyme disease or Lyme arthritis. N Engl J Med 1997;337:357–363.

108. Suttorp-Schulten MSA, Kuiper H, Kijlstra A, et al: Long-term effects of ceftriaxone treatment on intraocular lyme borreliosis. Am J Ophthalmol 1993;116:571–575.

109. Dattwyler RJ, Halpern JJ, Volkman DJ, et al: Treatment of late Lyme borreliosis—randomised comparison of ceftriaxone and penicillin. Lancet 1988;1:1191–1194.

110. Rahn DW: Natural history of Lyme disease. In: Rahn DW, Evans J (eds): Lyme disease. Philadelphia, American College of Physicians, 1998, p 35.

111. Szer IS, Taylor E, Steere AC: The long-term course of children with Lyme arthritis. N Engl J Med 1991;325:159–163.

112. Shadick NA, Phillips CB, Logigian EL, et al: The long-term clinical outcomes of Lyme disease. A population-based retrospective cohort study. Ann Intern Med 1994;121:560–567.

113. Logigian EL, Kaplan RF, Steere AC: Chronic neurologic manifestations of Lyme disease. N Engl J Med 1990;323:1438–1444.

114. Kaplan RF, Jones-Woodward L: Lyme encephalopathy: A neuropsychological perspective. Semin Neurol 1997;17:31–37.

115. Krause PJ, Telford SR 3rd, Spielman A, et al: Concurrent Lyme disease and babesiosis: Evidence for increased severity and duration of illness. JAMA 1996;275:1657–1660.

116. Zweifach PH, Shovlin J: Retinal nerve fiber layer infarct in a patient with babesiosis. Am J Ophthalmol 1991;112:597–598.

117. Ortiz JM, Eagle RC Jr: Ocular findings in human babesiosis (Nantucket fever). Am J Ophthalmol 1982;93:307–311.

118. Krause PJ, Spielman A, Telford SR 3rd, et al: Persistent parasitemia after acute babesiosis. N Engl J Med 1998;339:160–165.

119. Sweeney CJ, Ghassemi M, Agger WA, et al: Co-infection with *Babesia microti* and *Borrelia burgdorferi* in a western Wisconsin resident. Mayo Clin Proc 1998;73:338–341.

120. Walker DH, Barbour AG, Oliver JH, et al. Emerging bacterial zoonotic and vector-borne diseases: Ecological and epidemiological factors. JAMA 1996;275:463–469.

121. Bakken JS, Krueth J, Wilson-Nordskog C, et al: Clinical and laboratory characteristics of human granulocytic ehrlichiosis. JAMA 1996;275:199–205.

122. Carter N, Miller NR: Fourth nerve palsy caused by *Ehrlichia chaffeensis*. J Neuroophthalmol 1997;17:47–50.

123. Petersen LR, Sawyer LA, Fishbein DB, et al: An outbreak of ehrlichiosis in members of an Army Reserve unit exposed to ticks. J Infect Dis 1989;159:562–568.

124. Goodhead AD: Uveitis in dogs and cats: Guidelines for the practitioner. J S Afr Vet Assoc 1996;67:12–19.

125. Nadelman RB, Horowitz HW, Hsieh TC, et al: Simultaneous human granulocytic ehrlichiosis and Lyme borreliosis. N Engl J Med 1997;337:27–30.

126. Barton LL, Luisiri A, Dawson JE, et al: Simultaneous infection with an *Ehrlichia* and *Borrelia burgdorferi* in a child. Ann N Y Acad Sci 1990;590:68–69.

127. Paparone PW, Glenn WB: Lyme disease with concurrent ehrlichiosis. J Am Osteopath Assoc 1994 Jul;94:568–570, 573, 577.

128. Wormser GP, Horowitz HW, Dumler JS, et al: False-positive Lyme disease serology in human granulocytic ehrlichiosis. Lancet 1996;347(9006):981–982.

129. Barbour A, Fish D: Biology of Borrelia species. Microbiol Rev 1986;50:381–400.

130. Centers for Disease Control and Prevention: Common source of outbreak of relapsing fever—California. MMWR 1990;39:579–586.

131. Meader CN: Five cases of relapsing fever originating in Colorado, with positive blood findings in two. Colo Med 1915;12:365–369.

132. Thompson RS, Burgdorfer W, Russell R, et al: Outbreak of tick-borne relapsing fever in Spokane County, Washington. JAMA 1969;210:1045–1050.

133. Boyer KM, Munford RS, Maupin GO, et al: Tick-borne relapsing fever: An interstate outbreak originating at Grand Canyon National Park. Am J Epidemiol 1977;105:469–479.

134. Cadavid D, Barbour AG: Neuroborreliosis during relapsing fever: Review of the clinical manifestations, pathology, and treatment of infections in humans and experimental animals. Clin Infect Dis 1998;26:151–164.

135. Horton JM, Blaser MJ: The spectrum of relapsing fever in the Rocky Mountains. Arch Intern Med 1985;145:871–875.
136. Southern PM, Sanford JP: Relapsing fever: A clinical and microbiological review. Medicine 1969;48:129–149.
137. Hamilton JB: Ocular complication in relapsing fever. Br J Ophthalmol 1943;27:68–80.
138. Barbour AG: Antigenic variation of a relapsing fever Borrelia species. Annu Rev Microbiol 1990;44:155–71.
139. Sciotto CG, Lauer BA, White WL, et al: Detection of Borrelia in acridine orange-stained blood smears by fluorescence microscopy. Arch Pathol Lab Med 1983;107:384–386.
140. Spach DH, Liles WC, Campbell Gl, et al: Tick-borne diseases in the United States. N Engl J Med 1993;329:936–947.
141. Rawlings JA. An overview of tick-borne relapsing fever with emphasis on outbreaks in Texas. Tex Med 1995;91:56–59.

DEFINITION

There are currently 11 recognized species of the genus *Bartonella.* Four are recognized as human pathogens: *B. bacilliformis* (bartonellosis or Carrión's disease), *B. quintana* (trench fever), *B. elizabethae* (endocarditis), and *B. henselae.* Members of the genus *Bartonella* are classified within the alpha subdivision of the Proteobacteria. They are gram-negative, oxidase-negative, fastidious, and aerobic bacilli. Their growth on blood agar is slow, usually requiring at least 12 to 14 days. *B. henselae* is the bacterial pathogen associated with the clinical entity commonly known as cat-scratch disease (CSD). *B. henselae* (formerly *Rochalimaea henselae*) is an emerging pathogen that has only recently been positively identified as a cause of neuroretinitis. Our understanding of the numerous clinical manifestations of CSD and their appropriate treatment are evolving.

HISTORY

Human *Bartonella* infection was first recognized in 1909 by Alberto Barton, who noted infected erythrocytes in patients with bartonellosis (Carrión's disease).[1] The first recorded observation of CSD is thought to have been made by Parinaud in 1889 when he associated conjunctivitis and enlarged regional lymph nodes with exposure to animals.[2] The condition was termed Parinaud's oculoglandular syndrome. Debré was the first to associate the disease with cats when he encountered a 10-year-old boy with suppurative adenopathy.[2] The boy, who played and slept with cats, was initially thought to have tuberculosis, but the disease remitted spontaneously. The term *cat-scratch fever* was coined by Foshay in 1932.[3] Presme and Marchland associated CSD with Parinaud's oculoglandular syndrome in 1950, whereas Sweeny and Drance associated CSD with intraocular inflammation in 1970.[4] Leber first described a case of stellate neuroretinitis characterized by optic disc edema and a macular star. The condition became known as Leber's idiopathic stellate neuroretinitis (LISN). Gass suggested that LISN represents a primary optic neuropathy with macular manifestations.[5] Gass later hypothesized that *B. henselae* is a causative agent of LISN,[6] but positive identification of its role as the pathogen of CSD and CSD-associated neuroretinitis was later demonstrated by serologic testing, blood and tissue cultures, histopathologic examination, and immunologic testing.[7-10]

EPIDEMIOLOGY

CSD occurs in immunocompetent individuals of all ages worldwide and is the leading cause of regional lymphadenopathy in children and young adults. CSD is more common in children and adolescents, possibly because they are more likely to provoke a cat to scratch or bite. There is no known sex or ethnic predilection toward CSD.

The prevalence of CSD in the United States is approximately 22,000 cases per year.[11] The disease is most prevalent in the southern states, California, and Hawaii, which reflects the distribution of cat fleas, *B. henselae* antibodies, and positive blood cultures in cats.[12] In the San Francisco area, *B. henselae* was isolated from the blood of 41% of pet, pound, and stray cats.[13] Pet cats reside in nearly one third of U.S. homes and provide a vast reservoir from which human *B. henselae* infection may be acquired.[14] The infection is not known to be transmitted from human to human. CSD follows a seasonal pattern, with peaks in the fall and winter months, although cases have been reported at all times of the year.[15, 16] Daniels and MacMurray report that 30% of patients are under 10 years and two thirds are under 30 years of age.[17] They report a positive history of contact with cats in 92% of cases and a history of associated trauma such as a bite or scratch in 76% of those cases. Although the incidence of ocular involvement in cases of CSD is not known with certainty, studies by Margileth estimate that between 5% and 10% of CSD patients develop conjunctivitis, and 30 of 2006 cases of CSD developed neuroretinitis.[18, 19]

CLINICAL FEATURES

B. henselae infection is associated with a wide range of systemic and ocular symptoms and findings. Primary inoculation often results in a systemic infection. The eye is rarely the primary site of inoculation. More commonly, a scratch or bite occurs on the hands, arms, or neck. Systemic signs and symptoms usually precede ocular manifestations and are of importance in establishing the diagnosis. Three to 10 days after inoculation, a small erythematous papule forms on the skin at the site of inoculation. Seven to 14 days after exposure, conjunctival injection, chemosis, and watery discharge may follow. Follicular conjunctivitis may affect the bulbar and palpebral conjunctiva, and if the conjunctiva is the site of inoculation, a conjunctival granuloma may be present at the inoculation site. Two to 3 weeks after the scratch, regional lymphadenopathy occurs and is often accompanied by myalgias, malaise, fatigue, and low-grade fever. The skin papule may have faded by this time. Most patients experience localized disease with mild systemic symptoms that resolve within several months. The presence of conjunctivitis accompanied by regional lymphadenopathy defines the clinical entity known as Parinaud's oculoglandular syndrome.

The most common complaint in CSD neuroretinitis is decreased vision.[20] The onset of visual symptoms usually follows the inoculation by approximately 1 month, and it follows the onset of constitutional symptoms by approximately 2 to 3 weeks.[21] The visual acuity usually ranges from 20/25 to 20/200 but may be worse in some cases. The condition is usually unilateral but may be bilateral in both immunocompetent and immunocompromised patients.[22, 23] When the condition is bilateral, one eye is often affected more than the fellow eye. A relative afferent pupillary defect is usually present. Most patients pre-

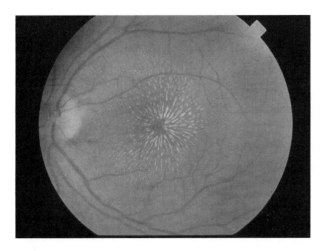

FIGURE 17–1. A macular star accompanied by an intraretinal hemorrhage near the optic disc.

sent to the ophthalmologist with the striking clinical features of optic disc edema and a macular star. The optic disc is the primary target of the neuroretinitis.[5] The inflammatory process leads to leakage from the optic disc and retinal microvasculature with accumulation of intraretinal lipids in the pattern of a macular star (Fig. 17–1). The macular star may be partial or complete. When a partial star pattern is seen, it is usually present in the nasal macula. In severe cases, lipid exudates can be seen well outside the macula and maculopapillary bundle or nasal to the optic disc.[24] The macular star resolves in approximately 8 to 12 weeks (Fig. 17–2). There may be one or more white areas of inner retinitis or chorioretinitis, which some authors have found to be more common than a macular star.[20, 25, 26] A neurosensory detachment of the macula or inferior retina as well as a few posterior vitreous cells may be noted.[23, 27] When present, intraretinal hemorrhages and cotton-wool spots reflect the involvement of the retinal microvasculature. Less commonly, branch retinal arteriolar occlusion or branch retinal venous occlusion may be associated with an area of focal retinitis.[20]

CSD may occasionally present with a large focal in-

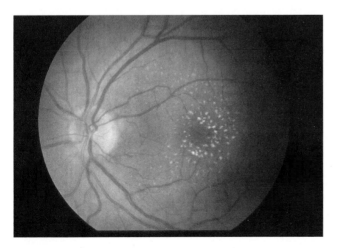

FIGURE 17–2. Partial resolution of the macular star 6 weeks later.

flammatory mass in the posterior pole. Cunningham and colleagues reported two cases of an inflammatory mass of the optic nerve head,[24] while Pollock and Kristinsson documented a choroidal inflammatory lesion associated with CSD.[28] Occasionally, the inflammatory lesion is highly vascular, resembling the lesions seen in bacillary angiomatosis, a condition characterized by multiple vascular skin and mucous membrane lesions associated with *B. henselae* infection in patients with acquired immunodeficiency syndrome (AIDS).[26, 29, 30]

Fluorescein angiography demonstrates early peripapillary telangiectasis with progressive leakage from the disc and vessels. Formal visual field testing often demonstrates a cecocentral scotoma, a paracentral scotoma, or an enlarged physiologic blind spot.[21, 23]

Other forms of ocular inflammation associated with CSD include intermediate uveitis,[31] anterior uveitis,[23] conjunctivitis, and orbital abscess.[32] Conjunctivitis is associated with Parinaud's oculoglandular syndrome. The conjunctiva is thought to become involved either by direct inoculation by a cat or by indirect inoculation with contaminated hands.[15]

The prognosis is very good, because most patients with CSD neuroretinitis recover excellent visual acuity.[6, 26] There may be mild residual color vision abnormalities. The average visually evoked potential (VEP) is reduced when compared to an unaffected fellow eye, but the electroretinogram (ERG) remains normal.[16] Mild optic nerve dysfunction is the most common cause of residual visual loss.

In patients with AIDS, *B. henselae* is known to cause bacillary angiomatosis, a disease characterized by the presence of any number of vascular lesions involving one or more organ systems. Nearly any organ system may be affected, either singly or in combination with other organ systems. The skin is frequently involved, and the lesions may be easily mistaken for Kaposi's sarcoma.[33] One case of bacillary angiomatosis of the conjunctiva has been reported.[30]

PATHOGENESIS AND IMMUNOLOGY

In human disease, *B. henselae* was initially characterized by Relman and colleagues in the tissue of patients with bacillary angiomatosis of AIDS.[10] Subsequently, Regnery described *B. henselae* antibodies in 86% of patients with CSD, compared with 6% of healthy controls.[7] Further histopathologic, serologic, and molecular biologic analyses have confirmed this agent as the cause of both entities.

Current evidence would suggest that the predominant mode of transmission of *B. henselae* is through a cat scratch or bite. Polymerase chain reaction (PCR) assays have detected *B. henselae* in fleas from infected cats,[13] and experimental transmission from cat to cat via the cat flea (*Ctenocephalides felis*) has been demonstrated.[34] There are no data to confirm that arthropods play a role in the pathogenesis of human disease, but cat fleas are often not specific with regard to host, biting both cats and humans. It has been proposed that they may act as a vector of transmission of *B. henselae* from cat to human.[13] Most cases are acquired from cats less than 1 year old.

The exact etiology of CSD-associated neuroretinitis is

not understood. It is unknown whether fundus changes are the direct result of optic nerve or intraocular infection, or both, by *Bartonella* or if the ocular findings represent a parainfectious inflammatory response. *B. henselae* has been isolated from a focus of retinitis in a patient with human immunodeficiency virus (HIV),[35] and *B. bacilliformis* has been shown to invade vascular endothelium.[36]

Western blot analysis is being used as a means to determine the important antigens that trigger the immunologic response of the host.[8, 37] Identification of such antigens may lead to the development of a human vaccine for CSD.

DIAGNOSIS

The diagnosis of CSD is currently based on clinical features supported by laboratory testing to detect genetic material from *B. henselae* or the host's immunologic response to the organism. The earliest tests for CSD took the form of skin tests with antigens prepared from lymph node aspirates of CSD patients.[38] A positive skin test is likely to remain positive for life.[15] The Warthin-Starry silver impregnation stain applied to a lymph node or conjunctival biopsy may demonstrate bacilli in the tissue. The organism can be identified by culture on blood-enriched agar or cocultivation in cell culture, but it may require 12 to 45 days before colonies become apparent.[39] With the development of serologic testing for *B. henselae*, the diagnosis is no longer made by exclusion. An indirect fluorescent antibody (IFA) test was developed to detect the humoral response to the organism and was found to be 88% sensitive and 94% specific.[7] Titers greater than 1:64 are considered positive. Enzyme immunoassay (EIA) and Western blot procedures were later developed, and EIA was shown to have IgG sensitivity of 86% to 95% and specificity of 96% compared with IFA.[8, 9] More recently, PCR assays have been employed for diagnostic purposes. Relman and colleagues developed the first primers for the specific detection of *Bartonella* DNA.[10] PCR is able to determine the presence of *B. henselae* in a very small sample of serum or other body fluids by detecting and amplifying a small fragment of the bacterial 16S rRNA gene.

TREATMENT

There are no guidelines for the treatment of CSD or its ocular complications, because randomized controlled trials have not been performed. Consequently, there is disagreement regarding the efficacy of antibiotic treatment for CSD in the immunocompetent individual. Although *B. henselae* is sensitive to a number of antibiotics in vitro,[40] only aminoglycosides have been shown to have bactericidal activity against the bartonellae.[41] Many physicians do not treat mild to moderate systemic CSD, but those who do often use a 10- to 14-day course of doxycycline, erythromycin, trimethoprim-sulfamethoxazole, rifampin, or intramuscular gentamicin.[42, 43] The effect of oral steroids on the course of the disease is unknown. Overall, the response to treatment is usually unimpressive.[43]

Golnik and colleagues noted improvement in visual acuity in three patients with intraocular inflammation treated with oral ciprofloxacin 500 mg twice daily.[23] Two of the three were treated with oral prednisone 40 mg/day after beginning ciprofloxacin. They treated another patient with oral doxycycline 250 mg four times daily and also noted prompt improvement in visual acuity with less optic disc edema and fewer vitreous cells. It is noteworthy that one of the patients who responded favorably to ciprofloxacin and another who responded favorably to doxycycline first experienced their initial visual loss while taking cephalexin 250 mg four times daily and dicloxacillin 250 mg four times daily, respectively. Both of these patients began antibiotic treatment earlier in the course of their disease. Because the natural history of *Bartonella*-associated neuroretinitis has not been well defined, it is not apparent whether antibiotics hasten visual recovery or the recovery is expected at that point in the natural course of the disease. Other investigators report favorable responses to treatment with oral antibiotics.[16, 25, 31] The safety of ciprofloxacin in individuals younger than 18 years of age has not been established, and the use of doxycycline in those younger than 9 years of age is contraindicated because of the risk of permanent discoloration of the teeth.[44]

One case of bacillary angiomatosis of the conjunctiva was successfully treated with topical gentamicin and systemic erythromycin, which brought about resolution of the lesion in 8 weeks.[30]

The prevention of CSD may be possible with the future development of vaccines for both cats and humans.[45] For the time being, common sense would dictate immediate cleansing and disinfection of any cat scratch or bite as well as avoiding contact with stray felines.

DIFFERENTIAL DIAGNOSIS

Parinaud's oculoglandular syndrome is a clinical entity with numerous other etiologies. Additional causes of conjunctivitis with regional lymphadenopathy include tularemia (*Francisella tularensis*; necrotizing conjunctivitis with lymphadenopathy), sporotrichosis (*Sporotrichum schenckii*; ulcerative nodules on eyelids with lymphadenopathy), tuberculosis, syphilis, infectious mononucleosis, coccidioidomycosis, lymphogranuloma venereum, leprosy, and *Yersinia*.[46, 47] A number of infectious and inflammatory conditions have been identified as causes of neuroretinitis, including tuberculosis, toxoplasmosis, syphilis, Lyme disease, toxocariasis, leptospirosis, mumps, varicella, and herpes simplex.[6] A macular star accompanied by vitritis has been specifically reported in association with toxoplasmosis.[48] Other causes of a macular star include vascular disorders such as acute systemic hypertension,[49] increased intracranial pressure,[50] and anterior ischemic optic neuropathy.[6] By inflammatory or ischemic mechanisms, or both, each of these conditions may compromise the microvasculature of the optic disc, resulting in leakage of serum and lipids with subsequent macular star formation.

CONCLUSION

When a patient presents with conjunctivitis and a history of feline exposure, or with neuroretinitis, retinitis, chorioretinitis, papillitis, or intermediate uveitis, a detailed history must be taken with attention to the systemic manifestations of CSD. Treatment guidelines for CSD-associated neuroretinitis are poorly defined. If antibiotic treatment is considered, oral ciprofloxacin 500 mg twice daily or doxycycline 250 mg four times daily are appropriate choices. The effect of oral steroids on the course of disease is unknown. Our understanding of CSD and its ocular complications has expanded exponentially over the past 10 years. We can hope that current and future research will bring a deeper understanding of the etiology of CSD-associated neuroretinitis, as well as guidelines for treatment.

References

1. Maurin M, Birtles R, Raoult D: Current knowledge of Bartonella species. Eur J Clin Microbiol Infect Dis 1997;16:487–506.
2. Jerris RJ, Regnery RL: Will the real agent of cat scratch disease please stand up? Ann Rev Microbiol 1996;50:707–725.
3. Henry M: Leptothricosis conjunctivae (Parinaud's conjunctivitis). Trans Pacific Coast Oto-ophthalmol Soc 1952;33:173–196.
4. Sweeny VP, Drance SN: Optic neuritis and comprehensive neuropathy associated with cat scratch disease. Can Med Assoc J 1970;103:1380–1381.
5. Gass JD: Diseases of the optic nerve that may simulate macular disease. Trans Am Acad Ophthalmol Otolaryngol 1977;83:766.
6. Dreyer RF, Hopen G, Gass JDM, Smith JL: Leber's idiopathic stellate neuroretinitis. Arch Ophthalmol 1984;102:1140–1145.
7. Regnery RJ, Olson JG, Perkins BA, Bibb W: Serological response to *Rochalimaea henselae* antigen in suspected cat scratch disease. Lancet 1992;339:1443–1445.
8. Litwin CM, Martins TB, Hill HR: Immunologic response to *Bartonella henselae* as determined by enzyme immunoassay and Western blot analysis. Am J Clin Pathol 1997;108:202–209.
9. Barka NE, Hadfield T, Patnaik M, et al: EIA for detection of *Rochalimaea henselae*-reactive IgG, IgM, and IgA antibodies in patients with suspected cat scratch disease. J Infect Dis 1993;167:1503–1504.
10. Relman DA, Loutit JS, Schmidt TM, et al: The agent of bacillary angiomatosis: An approach to the identification of uncultured pathogens. N Engl J Med 1990;323:1573.
11. Jackson LA, Perkins BA, Wenger JD: Cat scratch disease in the United States: An analysis of three national databases. Am J Public Health 1993;83:1707–1711.
12. Jameson P, Green C, Regnery R, et al: Prevalence of *Bartonella henselae* antibodies in pet cats throughout regions of North America. J Infect Dis 1995;172:1145–1149.
13. Koehler JE, Glasor CA, Tappero JW: *Rochalimaea henselae* infection: A new zoonosis with the domestic cat as reservoir. JAMA 1994;271:531–535.
14. Wise JK, Yang JJ: Veterinary service market for companion animals. Part I: Companion animal ownership and demographics. J Am Vet Med Assoc 1992;201:990–992.
15. Carithers HA: Cat scratch disease: An overview based on a study of 1200 patients. Am J Dis Child 1985;139:1124–1133.
16. Reed JB, Scales DK, Wong MT, et al: *Bartonella henselae* neuroretinitis in cat scratch disease. Ophthalmology 1998;105:459–466.
17. Daniels WB, MacMurray FG: Cat scratch disease: Report of one hundred sixty cases. JAMA 1954;154:1247–1251.
18. Margileth AM, Hadfield T: Cat scratch disease: Etiology, pathogenesis, diagnosis, and management. American Society of Clinical Pathologists Teleconference Series, Chicago, IL, April 21, 1994.
19. Margileth AM: Cat scratch disease. In: Aronoff, SC, ed: Advances in Pediatric Infectious Diseases, vol 8. St. Louis, MO, Mosby, 1993, pp 1–21.
20. Solley WA, Martin DF, Newman NJ, et al: Cat scratch disease: Posterior segment manifestations. Ophthalmology 1999;106:1546–1553.
21. Newson RW, Martin TJ, Wasilauskas B: Cat-scratch disease diagnosed serologically using an enzyme immunoassay in a patient with neuroretinitis. Arch Ophthalmol 1996;114:493–494.
22. Schlossberg D, Morad Y, Krouse TB, et al: Culture-proved disseminated cat-scratch disease in acquired immunodeficiency syndrome. Arch Intern Med 1989;149:1437–1439.
23. Golnik KC, Marotto ME, Maher MF, et al: Ophthalmic manifestations of *Rochalimaea* species. Am J Ophthalmol 1994;118:145–151.
24. Cunningham ET, McDonald HR, Schatz H, et al: Inflammatory mass of the optic nerve head associated with systemic *Bartonella henselae* infection. Arch Ophthalmol 1997;115:1596–1597.
25. Ormerod LD, Skolnick KA, Menosky MM, et al: Retinal and choroidal manifestations of cat-scratch disease. Ophthalmology 1998;105:1024–1031.
26. Gass JDM: Stereoscopic Atlas of Macular Diseases: Diagnosis and Treatment, 4th ed. St. Louis, MO, Mosby, 1997, pp 604–606.
27. Zacchei AC, Newman NJ, Sternberg P: Serous retinal detachment of the macula associated with cat-scratch disease. Am J Ophthalmol 1995;120:796–797.
28. Pollock SC, Kristinsson J: Cat-scratch disease manifesting as unifocal helioid choroiditis. Arch Ophthalmol 1998;116:1249–1251.
29. Fish RH, Hogan RN, Nightingale SD, et al: Peripapillary angiomatosis associated with cat-scratch neuroretinitis. Arch Ophthalmol 1992;110:323.
30. Lee WR, Chawla JC, Reid R: Bacillary angiomatosis of the conjunctiva. Am J Ophthalmol 1994;118:152–157.
31. Soheilian M, Markomichelakis N, Foster CS: Intermediate uveitis and retinal vasculitis as manifestations of cat scratch disease. Am J Ophthalmol 1996;122:582–584.
32. Gaebler JW, Burgett RA, Caldmeyer KS: Subacute orbital abscess in a four-year-old girl with a new kitten. Pediatr Infect Dis J 1998;17:844–846.
33. LeBoit PE, Berger TG, Egbert BM, et al: Epithelioid haemangioma-like vascular proliferation in AIDS: Manifestation of cat scratch disease bacillus infection? Lancet 1988;1(8592):960–963.
34. Chomel BB, Kasten RW, Floyd-Hawkins K, et al: Experimental transmission of *Bartonella henselae* by the cat flea. J Clin Microbiol 1996;34:1952–1956.
35. Warren K, Golstein E, Hung VS, et al: Use of retinal biopsy to diagnose *Bartonella* (formerly *Rochalimaea*) *henselae* retinitis in an HIV-infected patient. Arch Ophthalmol 1998;116:937–940.
36. Garcia FU, Wojita J, Hoover RL: Interactions between live *Bartonella bacilliformis* and endothelial cells. J Infect Dis 1992;165:1138–1141.
37. McGill SL, Regnery RL, Karem KL: Characterization of human immunoglobulin (Ig) isotype and IgG subclass response to *Bartonella henselae* infection. Infect Immun 1998;66:5916–5920.
38. Moriarity RA: Cat scratch disease. Infect Dis Clin North Am 1987;1:575–590.
39. Maurin M, Birtles R, Raoult D: Current knowledge of *Bartonella* species. Eur J Clin Microbiol Infect Dis 1997;16:487–506.
40. Lucey D, Dolan MJ, Moss CW, et al: Relapsing illness due to *Rochalimaea henselae* in immunocompetent hosts: Implication for therapy and new epidemiological associations. Clin Infect Dis 1992;14:683–688.
41. Musso D, Drancourt M, Raoult D: Lack of bactericidal effect of antibiotics except aminoglycosides on *Bartonella* (*Rochalimaea*) *henselae*. J Antimicrob Chemother 1995;36:101–108.
42. Margileth AM: Antibiotic therapy for cat-scratch disease: Clinical study of therapeutic outcome in 268 patients and a review of the literature. Pediatr Infect Dis J 1992;11:474–478.
43. Spach DH, Koehler JE: *Bartonella*-associated infections. Infect Dis Clin North Am 1998;12:137–155.
44. Physician's Desk Reference, 53rd ed. Montvale, NJ, Medical Economics, 1999, pp 641–646, 2427–2430.
45. Olsen CW: Vaccination of cats against emerging and reemerging zoonotic pathogens. Adv Vet Med 1999;41:333–346.
46. Chandler JW, Sugar J, Edelhauser HF: Textbook of Ophthalmology, vol 8. St. Louis, MO, Mosby. 1994, pp 2–26.
47. Chin GN, Hyndiuk RA: Parinaud's Oculoglandular Conjunctivitis. In: Tasman W, Jaeger EA, eds: Duane's Clinical Ophthalmology, vol 4. Philadelphia, Lippincott, 1992, pp 1–6.
48. Burnett AJ, Shortt SG, Isaac-Renton J, et al: Multiple cases of acquired toxoplasmosis retinitis presenting in an outbreak. Ophthalmology 1998;105:1032–1037.
49. Noble KG. Hypertensive retinopathy simulating Leber idiopathic stellate neuroretinitis. Arch Ophthalmol 1997;115:1594–1595.
50. Maitland CG, Miller NR: Neuroretinitis. Arch Ophthalmol 1984;102:1146–1150.

TUBERCULOSIS

C. Michael Samson and C. Stephen Foster

DEFINITION

Tuberculosis (TB) is an airborne communicable disease caused by *Mycobacterium tuberculosis* or by one of three other closely related mycobacterial species (*M. bovis*, *M. africanum*, and *M. microti*). The term tuberculosis implies active disease: Only 10% of infected individuals become symptomatic; 90% remain infected for the rest of their lives without manifesting disease.

Ocular tuberculosis encompasses any infection by *M. tuberculosis* in the eye, around the eye, or on its surface. Classically, ocular tuberculosis has been divided into two types: primary and secondary. Primary ocular TB implies that the eye is the initial port of entry; this type includes conjunctival, corneal, and scleral disease. Secondary disease implies that organisms spread to the eye hematogenously; this type includes tuberculous uveitis. These ocular definitions should not be confused with the definitions of primary and secondary systemic tuberculosis, which differentiate between disease from recent infection as opposed to reactivation of old disease.

HISTORY

Tuberculosis has caused suffering in humans since ancient times: Egyptian mummies dated back to 2400 BC show pathologic evidence of tuberculous spondylitis.[1] The disease has been called by many names, including phthisis, consumption, and the "white plague." Robert Koch developed a staining technique that could demonstrate *M. tuberculosis*, and in 1882, he proved that these bacilli were the cause of the various TB lesions in animal experiments, the same experiments that helped him formulate his now-famous postulates.[2] The first report of a case of tuberculous disease of the eye is attributed to Maitre-Jan, who in 1711 described a case of an iris nodule that led to corneal perforation.[3] The first description of histopathologically proven tuberculosis of the eye was by Von Michel in 1883.[4]

Robert Koch developed the use of injections of "old" tuberculosis (heat-killed mycobacteria) as a potential remedy, not as a diagnostic test. Less than two decades later, von Pirquet developed a scratch test; soon after, Mantoux introduced the intradermal tuberculin skin test. It was not until the late 1940s that the purified protein derivative (PPD) test became available.[2] The other diagnostic aid in the fight against TB was the x-ray, first developed by Wilhelm Konrad von Röntgen in 1895.[1] The x-ray provided physicians with a tool by which they could objectively monitor the progress of TB patients.

The most important advance in the history of TB was the discovery of curative antibiotics. In 1943, streptomycin was shown to cure *M. tuberculosis* infection in animals, with little associated systemic toxicity. The following year, streptomycin was used to successfully cure an infected human patient. Isoniazid, pyrazinamide, and cycloserine therapy followed in the 1950s, and ethambutol and rifampin in the 1960s.

EPIDEMIOLOGY

There has been a decline in the prevalence of uveitis cases attributed to TB since the beginning of the 20th century. In Woods' series of uveitis patients reported in 1944, just over half were thought to be due to *M. tuberculosis*, whereas in Schlaegel's series 25 years later, only 0.28% of cases were attributed to the mycobacterium. In 1996, Biswas reported only five cases of microbiologically proven tuberculous uveitis in 1273 patients (0.60%) seen over 2 years at a uveitis referral clinic in India, a country in which TB is endemic. This trend has been attributed to the decline of TB, the discovery of other entities capable of causing granulomatous inflammation, and the diminished emphasis placed on TB by ophthalmologists.[5]

The overall decrease of the incidence of TB in developed countries commenced in the 19th century, attributed to improved living conditions.[6] With the discovery of effective antibiotics, deaths due to TB continued to fall. In the United States, there was an average annual decline of 5.6% of reported cases from the 1940s to 1984. From 1985 to 1993, however, annual TB began to rise, increasing 14% over that short period. This was in part attributed to the acquired inmmunodeficiency syndrome (AIDS) epidemic, but increased immigration from countries where TB is endemic, transmission of TB in congregate settings (health care facilities, correctional facilities, and homeless shelters), and a deterioration of the healthcare infrastructure were also contributing factors.[1] Recently, TB in developed countries seems to be on the decline again, most likely due to the institution of direct observed therapy and the initial benefits from the new protease inhibitors in the human immunodeficiency virus (HIV)–infected population.[7] Worldwide, however, it remains a significant problem, with some estimates as high as one third of the world's population being infected.[9]

Even when ocular TB was believed to be a major cause of uveitis, ophthalmologists of the time agreed that eye disease in patients with active systemic TB was uncommon. In 1967, Donahue reported ocular morbidity of only 1.4% in a TB sanatorium.[10] In a recent study, Biswas and Badrinath prospectively examined 1005 consecutive mycobacteria-infected patients in India and likewise found a very small percentage of eye disease: only 14 patients, or 1.39%.[11] A recent survey of autopsy eyes found only 0.4% of AIDS patients with ocular involvement affected by *M. tuberculosis*.[11a] These findings support the contention of past ophthalmologists that the eye is somewhat protected against infection by *M. tuberculosis*.

Known risk factors for TB infection include close contact with infected individuals and HIV infection. In addition, individuals from countries in which TB is endemic are at risk; these countries include Haiti, India, Mexico, the People's Republic of China, the Philippines, and Vietnam.

CLINICAL PRESENTATION

The main difficulty in the accurate collection of authentic cases of ocular TB is that diagnosis is often presumptive[12];

histopathologic confirmation from ocular specimens is uncommon. Some ophthalmologists extend diagnostic criteria to include patients presenting with ocular manifestations known to be caused by *M. tuberculosis* if there is histopathologically confirmed systemic infection. Another extension of the diagnostic criteria includes cases that manifest findings typical of TB that subsequently respond to empiric antimycobacterial therapy. Ocular involvement in these cases, in the strictest sense, is still presumptive. Analysis of these cases is helpful in attempting to understand intraocular TB and its manifestations, but one must keep in mind that cases without histopathologic confirmation may actually represent nontuberculous disease.

Uveitis is the most common ocular manifestation of TB. Scleritis may present concomitantly with uveitis. Lid lesions,[13] orbital involvement, conjunctival involvement,[14, 15] and keratitis are other ocular manifestations and usually do not present in association with uveitis. External disease is presumed to be primary ocular TB, whereas uveitis is thought to occur by hematogenous spread from distant foci of infection.

The most common presentation of tuberculous uveitis is of disseminated choroiditis.[16–18] The discrete lesions may number from five to several hundred. The lesions range from 0.5 to 3.0 mm in diameter, and may vary in size and elevation within the same eye.[18] They are deep, in the choroid; appear yellow, white, or gray; and are fairly well circumscribed. In the vast majority of cases, the lesions present in the posterior pole. Right eyes may be more affected than left eyes. Disc edema with nerve fiber layer hemorrhages can also be seen.[18] An associated anterior uveitis may be severe, mild, or absent.

After uveitis, the next most common clinical presentation is a single tubercle, also termed focal choroiditis.[19] In these cases, a single choroidal mass is the characteristic feature on presentation, although a few adjacent satellite lesions may also be seen. A large tubercle may measure up to 4.0 mm in diameter; however, reports of choroidal masses up to 14 mm in diameter have been reported.[20] The mass is typically elevated, and may be accompanied by an overlying serous retinal detachment.[19, 21] A macular star may develop.[19, 21] Other posterior manifestations include subretinal abscess, retinal detachment, retinal vasculitis,[22] and optic neuritis.

Anterior tuberculous uveitis is typically granulomatous with extensive granulomatous keratic precipitates.[22] Iris nodules can also be seen.[22] An accompanying vitritis is not uncommon, and can be so dense as to obscure fundus details.[22] Intraocular pressure may be normal or elevated.[22] Other anterior presentations include an exudative mass in the anterior chamber, and an associated scleritis with spontaneous perforation.[23]

TB is typically considered in the differential diagnosis of chronic anterior granulomatous uveitis without posterior segment involvement. Cases that fit this clinical picture with microbiologic confirmation of mycobacterium infection, however, are rare. A total of 46 cases of intraocular TB confirmed by histopathologic or microbiologic specimens from the eye exists in the literature[23–25]; only six describe anterior uveitis without posterior involvement. On closer inspection, one of the six cases represented a post-traumatic infection, and in two others, the posterior segment was not visualized, one of which was eventually shown to have diffuse choroidal involvement on pathologic examination.[26]

Uveitis due to *M. tuberculosis* may present as a panophthalmitis. Similar in presentation to acute onset endophthalmitis, inflammation can be severe and unrelenting; the eye can be lost in a matter of days, even with the initiation of appropriate therapy.[24, 27] Sometimes, an epibulbar mass can be seen[27] and can be a sign of spontaneous scleral perforation due to massive caseating necrosis.

It would be useful for the ophthalmologist to know if ocular TB is more or less likely to present in patients with signs of active or past systemic TB infection, but review of the literature is not helpful in this regard. Many case reports represent "presumptive ocular tuberculosis." The clinician should keep in mind that histopathologically proven intraocular TB has been shown to occur in patients without systemic signs or symptoms of TB infection other than reactive skin testing: Hence, the absence of clinically evident systemic TB does not rule out the possibility of ocular TB.

Although TB may manifest in the eye without these signs, the ophthalmologist should include questions directed toward the possibility of systemic TB infection in the review of systems of patients with uveitis. Most clinicians are familiar with the symptoms and signs of pulmonary TB, but the possibility of extrapulmonary disease, often accompanied by headache, change in mental status, localized back pain, increased abdominal girth, or abdominal pain, must not be ignored. Fever, sweats, and weight loss are present in both pulmonary and extrapulmonary infections, and are often present in systemic tuberculosis.

PATHOLOGY

The chronicity of tuberculosis is the main reason that it has remained one of the most important diseases in the history of humanity, even in modern times. Its ability to remain dormant in its host for years explains how it was able to spread to all the continents.[28] Therefore, it is critical to understand how *M. tuberculosis* accomplishes this, in order to help guide our therapeutic approach.

Most understanding of the pathogenesis of TB comes from study of lesions in the lung. Many pathologic characteristics of these lesions are probably applicable to disease in the eye. In an active lesion, one can classify the different populations of mycobacterial organisms based on their activity.[29] The "actively multiplying group" resides extracellularly in an open area of necrosis and represents the majority of organisms within the lesion. The "slow-growing group" can be found either in closed necrotic lesions or intracellularly within macrophages.

Detailed reports of pathologic eye specimens from recent cases of intraocular TB are uncommon. This is in part due to the success and effectiveness of modern treatment of the disease, resulting in less need for enucleation. Furthermore, diagnostic procedures to obtain aqueous or vitreous samples for the purpose of microbiologic and histopathologic examinations are considered risky by most clinicians, who are more likely to start treatment based on presumptive evidence of infection when other clinical noninvasive testing (positive PPD, history of previously treated tuberculosis) is available.

Ocular TB pathology reports vary depending on the prevalence of TB; reports from developed countries tend to be from older literature and more recent reports are from countries where TB is endemic. Many of the cases represent panophthalmitis, followed by blind painful eye, requiring enucleation.[27]

Typically, the choroid is the site with the most severe involvement, demonstrating multiple tubercles with surrounding necrosis, and extension to the overlying retina. Caseating necrosis is specific but not always present.[20] Lymphocytes, plasma cells, and giant cells accompany the essential epithelioid cells as the major infiltrating inflammatory cells. The iris and ciliary body usually also demonstrate inflammatory cells, granulomas, and caseation necrosis. Occasionally, a cyclitic membrane is present. Corneal findings may range from little involvement to marked thinning and diffuse inflammation with stromal neovascularization. The sclera is usually uninvolved; if affected, it may show a focal area of necrosis or, occasionally, spontaneous perforation. The optic nerve usually shows inflammation and may contain granulomas. Appropriate staining will reveal disseminated acid-fast bacilli.

PATHOGENESIS

The reaction of the immune system to *M. tuberculosis* serves as the model for what is now known as type IV hypersensitivity and is the basis for the mechanism behind tuberculin skin testing. Interestingly, Koch's original use of heat-killed (or "old") tuberculin in patients was intended as a cure for TB. This was based on the well-known fact of the time that animals injected with large amounts of attenuated mycobacteria became immunized against the disease. Although Koch did not meet with the great success he had hoped for, the idea was reborn as the bacille Calmette-Guérin (BCG) vaccination, which used a live, nonvirulent strain of bovine mycobacterium.[2]

As with other infections, the immunopathologic process of infection with *M. tuberculosis* is a struggle between two forces: the bacteria and its virulence factors, and the host's immune response. The fact that only 10% of infected individuals eventually develop disease suggests that an adequate immune response can mount an effective defense against the organism, and that factors deleteriously affecting the immune system may allow the disease to develop. Laboratory studies using murine models and human cell cultures have helped provide a better understanding of the immunology behind TB infection.

The ability to replicate within cells, specifically macrophages and monocytes, is critical to the ability of *M. tuberculosis* to cause disease. Interferon gamma (IFN-γ) has been shown to be capable of modifying macrophage capabilities with regard to immunity against TB. Mice resistant to TB infection carry a specific gene known as the *bcg* locus; macrophages of these mice demonstrate high respiratory burst activity. Such mycobacteria-killing activity is enhanced by IFN-γ, which is a macrophage activating factor. Inhibition of IFN-γ in these mice leads to increased susceptibility to TB. Evidence from human studies seems to support the positive effect of IFN-γ on macrophage activity. Swaminathan and coauthors found

that peripheral blood mononuclear cells (PBMCs) in children with active TB had lower IFN-γ production than did PBMCs of children who were PPD reactive but without systemic infection.[30] Furthermore, cytotoxic T lymphocytes able to recognize *M. tuberculosis* antigens have been isolated from human serum; these cells are capable of recognizing and lysing monocytes acutely infected with *M. tuberculosis*.[31]

Another critical protective immune response is the ability to form granulomas. Granuloma formation is also probably dependent on relative concentrations of particular cytokines, with interleukin-1β (IL-1β) and tumor necrosis factor α (TNF-α) having been implicated as important factors. If BCG-resistant mice are treated with anti-TNF-α antibody before challenge with BCG, they fail to form granulomas and they develop lethal BCG infection. Although these studies do not have any direct clinical applications, it is clear that a patient's ability to limit tissue destruction and organism replication might be modifiable with cytokine-directed therapy, therapy already available in clinical practice.

The emergence of multidrug-resistant (MDR) TB led to the increased interest in research aimed at discovering the mechanism of antituberculous medications and the mechanisms behind antimicrobial resistance. Various gene mutations can result in different mechanisms of loss of susceptibilities to drugs, including decreased interaction with drug, impaired conversion of the drug to the active form, and overcoming the antimicrobial therapy by a "superphysiologic" state. Other mutations exist in which resistance is confirmed, but the exact mechanisms are unknown.[32]

DIAGNOSTIC TESTS

Fluorescein Angiogram

Fluorescein angiogram testing may be helpful in cases in which a single or prominent choroidal mass is present. Typically, the choroidal mass exhibits diffuse fluorescence in the early arterial phase, which evolves into intense diffuse hyperfluorescence by the venous phase. Large vessels are typically not present within the choroidal lesion. These findings may aid the clinician in suspecting TB over other entities such as choroidal melanoma or metastasis. Careful examination of fluorescein angiogram findings may reveal data that are clearly not consistent with choroidal melanoma, thus avoiding unnecessary enucleation.[20]

Tuberculin Skin Testing

The first test in the investigation of a patient in whom TB is suspected is usually tuberculin skin testing. Tuberculin comprises killed *M. tuberculosis*. The standard PPD is known as PPD-S. A positive response in most individuals is an area of induration equal to or greater than 10 mm, but in certain high-risk groups, a reaction of 5 mm or greater is sufficient to indicate exposure. Abrams and Schlaegel found that 11 of 18 patients in a tuberculous uveitis series would have been falsely read as nonresponders if a 10-mm cutoff had been used, but notably their series consisted of patients in whom diagnosis was presumptive.[12] False-positive results may occur with prior

BCG vaccination or infection with nontuberculous myco-bacteria.[33]

Certain basic facts must be kept in mind when using and interpreting these diagnostic tests. First, tuberculin skin testing is not a diagnostic test for tuberculosis disease: it determines only whether an individual has been infected by mycobacteria, and only 10% of such people are believed to go on to active disease. In patients from areas in which TB is endemic, it not uncommon to have positive tuberculin skin test incidence as high as 35% to 40%, most of whom never get the disease. PPD testing cannot distinguish between past and active disease.[33] Furthermore, it is not completely reliable; patients in whom cellular immunity is depressed (e.g., HIV infection) often show nonreactive skin tests.[20] Likewise, the immune response lessens in certain individuals and may require a booster shot 1 to 2 weeks after the initial injection. Finally, not all patients with active tuberculosis respond to tuberculin skin testing: Studies report 10% to 25% of active TB patients as nonresponders.[33]

Knowledge of BCG vaccination is also important in the interpretation of a positive PPD. BCG is a vaccine consisting of a live mycobacterium, a species not able to cause disease. BCG vaccination is most commonly used in developing countries in which TB is endemic. Its usefulness is controversial. Beliefs vary about the length of time one is positive to BCG. According to the American Thoracic Society (ATS), a single BCG vaccination during the first year of life rarely remains positive. A single BCG vaccination during childhood or adulthood remains positive for about 5 years. Multiple BCG vaccinations probably result in lifelong reactivity.

It has not been confirmed that worsening of the uveitis following PPD testing is a reliable diagnostic sign of a tuberculous etiology. In fact, it has been shown that uveitis may be triggered by PPD testing in the absence of evidence of systemic TB infection and without prior history of uveitis.[34]

Isolation of Mycobacteria—Acid-Fast Staining and Culture

The next step in TB diagnosis is isolation of organisms from systemically infected sites. This process usually consists of sputum testing, but collection of urine, gastric aspirates, or cervical lymph node biopsy are relatively benign procedures. Acid-fast staining and culture are both used to identify the causative organisms.

Most ophthalmologists attribute ocular disease to *M. tuberculosis* if a known ocular manifestation occurs in conjunction with isolation of mycobacteria from other body sites, either concurrently or in the recent past. However, when documented systemic disease occurred in the patient's distant past, it is more difficult to attribute ocular involvement as the only site of reactivation. If such a patient also has a history of having completed adequate treatment for TB, another dilemma arises, the possibility of drug-resistant TB. This poses significant risks for both treating and withholding treatment, and direct diagnostic methods may be required for the ophthalmologist to be comfortable with instituting therapy with potential systemic toxicity.

There are two general approaches to diagnosing TB localized to the eye. The first method is acquiring intraocular fluid. Both anterior chamber taps and pars plana vitrectomy, known methods for diagnosing intraocular infection from other causes (endogenous bacterial and fungal endophthalmitis, for example), have also been used to identify mycobacteria.[24] These fluids can be sent for acid-fast staining and culture. Acid-fast staining is rapid but is neither sensitive nor specific. There is some evidence that fluorescence microscopy may be a more sensitive test for visualizing tubercle bacilli.[20] Culture is extremely specific and sensitive and provides information on susceptibility, but is limited by delay in obtaining results. It is the gold standard to which other tests are compared in clinical and laboratory studies.

Isolation of Mycobacteria—Nucleic Acid Amplification

Ocular specimens may also be tested using nucleic acid amplification techniques. This is especially useful in anterior chamber taps, in which the small amount of harvested material is unlikely to yield useful information when analyzed by standard methods. Two general nucleic acid amplification methods are available: transcription-mediated amplification (TMA), which targets unique *M. tuberculosis* rRNA sequences (specifically, the 16S rRNA), and polymerase chain reaction (PCR), which targets unique *M. tuberculosis* DNA sequences. The *M. tuberculosis* direct test (MTD) is a commercially available assay based on TMA; there are also several commercial assays based on PCR. Each method can furnish a result in less than 7 hours.[33, 35]

Clinical studies have used both MTD and PCR, with most data obtained from studies of pulmonary disease (i.e., sputum samples). Both methods yield high specificity and sensitivity when used in conjunction with acid-fast bacillus smears. PCR-based methods with a sensitivity as high as 100% have been reported, but some studies show a specificity as low as 70%.[33] False-positive results are an unfortunate consequence of extremely sensitive tests.[36] Theoretically, MTD carries certain advantages over PCR. MTD might yield fewer false-positive results because RNA degrades easily outside of the reaction tube. In addition, MTD should result in higher sensitivity, because there are 2000 rRNA copies per mycobacterium versus 10 to 16 copies of DNA targets.[37] However, studies comparing PCR and MTD testing on sputum specimens revealed similar results.[33, 37] Other clinical uses of MTD and PCR have included examination of gastric aspirates and tissue samples.[38] Because these tests are new, their exact role in the diagnosis of systemic tuberculosis has not yet been defined.[33]

Nucleic acid amplification techniques have been used to diagnose intraocular TB in uveitis cases.[36, 38-40] Five cases were diagnosed by anterior chamber tap, and one case used PCR applied to an ocular pathologic specimen. However, specificity and sensitivity from ocular specimens are not known. Clinical studies lack sufficient numbers, and to our knowledge, laboratory studies have not been performed. It is possible that biologic fluids from different organ sites may require different preparation techniques from those used to prepare sputum samples. For example, use of MTD in cerebrospinal fluid seemed to give better results when a 500-μl sample was used (instead of the 50 μl required from respiratory specimens) if specimens were pretreated with sodium dodecyl sulfate and amplification time was increased to 3 hours.[33] Similar special preparation techniques may need to be applied to ocular specimens for optimal results.

Additionally, it is of concern that among the six patients reported in the literature who had a positive PCR for *M. tuberculosis*, only one had histologic confirmation of TB infection, which was by cervical lymph node biopsy. Only two of the six patients had other objective signs suggestive of TB infection: one had a history of pulmonary TB, and one other had a strongly positive PPD; the other four had no other clinical data suggesting TB infection. Although others believe that positive rapid diagnostic tests in the absence of positive acid-fast smears or culture may warrant initiation of antituberculous therapy, ophthalmologists are well advised to proceed with caution when using and interpreting these tests until more reliable data come to light.[37, 39]

The second approach to achieving a diagnosis of *M. tuberculosis* infection in isolated eye disease is chorioretinal biopsy.[17] This procedure entails more risks to the patient. However, it is used in patients in whom the clinical evidence also suggests other infectious causes that may present as a mass (sarcoid, fungal) when different diagnostic entities call for radically different therapies. Nucleic acid amplification techniques used in addition to histologic examination may be useful.

The last and most dramatic approach is enucleation. This is usually reserved for patients presenting with a blind painful eye, or with aggressive bilateral panophthalmitis with one eye salvageable and one eye lost. In cytomegalovirus retinitis, acute retinal necrosis, and endogenous bacterial and fungal endophthalmitis, enucleation is performed in an attempt to establish a definitive diagnosis to save the remaining eye. Ocular TB is reported to occur bilaterally and has been known to present as a fulminant panophthalmitis.[26, 27]

The last relevant aspect in the diagnosis of intraocular TB is that of drug susceptibility. The importance of establishing susceptibilities in a time when MDR strains are modifying Centers for Disease Control and Prevention (CDCP) therapy recommendations may suggest that ophthalmologists take more aggressive steps toward obtaining ocular specimens for culture than has been done in the past. "Presumed" ocular TB may not be an engaging diagnosis for the patient or the physician when it requires numerous medications on a daily basis for a minimum of 6 months.

Although standard methods of determining antimicrobial resistance have been successfully used for years, these methods carry the same disadvantage as culture identification of *M. tuberculosis*: The tests take time, from weeks to months. Increased knowledge of the cell biology and genetics of *M. tuberculosis* has led to the development of PCR tests capable of detecting genes associated with antimicrobial resistance. Similar techniques have been used to detect point mutations associated with resistance to antituberculous medications. These methods have the advantages of rapid acquisition of the desired information (as little as 24 hours), and increased safety for microbiology technicians by decreasing risk of infection as compared with standard culture techniques. These tests include PCR restriction fragment length polymorphism (RFLP) analysis, PCR single-strand conformation polymorphism (SSCP), universal heteroduplex generator analysis, and DNA oligonucleotide arrays on silica microchips.[41]

Therapeutic Trial

Schlaegel and associates conducted a study examining the effectiveness of antituberculous therapy in uveitis patients without evidence of systemic TB.[42] Their results led to the recommendation that a therapeutic trial of isoniazid at 300 mg daily for 3 weeks be attempted in these patients; a favorable clinical response was considered indicative of a tuberculous etiology of the uveitis, and warranted proceeding to a complete regimen. Randomized double-blind trials, however, show no difference between isoniazid (INH) and placebo, suggesting that the approach described earlier is probably invalid. Additionally, single-dose therapy in a patient with suspected TB does not meet with current recommendations for prophylaxis in most regions.

TREATMENT

It is important for the ophthalmologist to be familiar with current guidelines for TB treatment, even if the treatment specifics are deferred to the internist or other specialist. First, the ophthalmologist can prepare the patient for the difficult regimen that must be followed. Nonadherence to the program can sabotage a condition that could have been cured, and even strict compliance can still lead to loss of vision, owing to the virulence of this organism. Second, these medications have potential toxicities, including eye-related adverse effects; the ophthalmologist has an ethical and medicolegal obligation to monitor for the relevant symptoms of these possibilities on follow-up examinations. Last, TB is an epidemic with evidence suggesting that it continues to cause significant morbidity and mortality worldwide. It will certainly be a condition most physicians will encounter during their career in the 21st century.

The drugs that make up first-line treatment of TB are INH, rifampin, pyrazinamide (PZA), streptomycin, and ethambutol. They are first-line drugs because they are bactericidal (although ethambutol requires a higher starting dose for this to be true). Isoniazid and rifampin each are bactericidal for both actively dividing extracellular and slow-dividing intracellular mycobacteria; used in combination, they are very effective in susceptible populations.[28] PZA is the only other first-line therapy capable of targeting slow-growing intracellular organisms; this probably explains its excellent efficacy in early treatment.[28] Streptomycin and ethambutol are effective mainly against actively dividing organisms.[28]

Current CDC recommendations use INH and rifampin combined therapy as the core of treatment for a minimum of 6 months. Because of the evolution of MDR strains, PZA has been added to the starting regimen and is used in conjunction with the two main drugs for the first 2 months of treatment. In areas in which prevalence of INH resistance exceeds 4%, streptomycin or ethambutol is added as the fourth drug. The "added" drugs are discontinued when susceptibility testing shows that the organisms are susceptible to both INH and rifampin.

When resistance to antimicrobial agents is detected, treatment is more complex. Isolated resistance to INH or rifampin requires continuation of the supplemental first-line agents. Discontinuation of the drug to which there is resistance is not routine, because some clinicians believe that there is benefit to continuation if the resistance level is low. When MDR is present (resistance to at least INH and rifampin), authorities recommend treatment with three or four drugs to which the mycobacterium is susceptible and prolongation of therapy.[43] Some evidence supports the efficacy of quinolones, and second-line agents, such as cycloserine and para-aminosalicylic acid, have been known to be effective, albeit less so than first-line drugs, and with increased risk of drug toxicity.[41] Consultation with an infectious disease expert or other knowledgeable authority is recommended in cases of MDR TB.

Direct observed therapy (DOT) is the process of receiving treatment under the direct supervision of a health-care worker. It plays a critical role in TB therapy because compliance with long-term treatment is essential for cure. First instituted in 1979 as a method of targeting patients identified as noncompliant, it has since been promoted to the standard of care in the treatment of tuberculosis.[44] This came as a result not only of the obvious effectiveness in improving patient compliance, but because of the newer problems of emerging MDR strains in the HIV epidemic. Furthermore, studies demonstrated that degree of noncompliance did not vary with any demographic variables; there are no good methods to reliably predict which patients will adhere to treatment.[44]

DOT has generally been enforced in large urban centers. Up to one third of new TB cases in these regions are thought to be contracted by recent transmission and not by reactivation of old disease.[45] Major cities around the United States have each implemented their unique DOT legislation and programs.[44, 46–49] In New York City in 1993, the Commissioner of Health was given the power to use legal action to ensure treatment of patients infected with TB. A study of the first 2 years of the program showed an incredible 96% rate of treatment completion among patients legally required to undergo treatment; ultimately, new cases decreased by 55% and MDR disease decreased by 87.3% between 1992 and 1997.[50]

These recent actions have opened debate about the differences in public opinion concerning the conflict posed by DOT: the rights of the individual versus the benefits to society.[7, 45] Because of the debate, proponents of legal action must tread lightly in cases in which danger to society is not obvious, and health department policies typically institute detention only when all less restrictive approaches fail to work.[7] This will generally work against the ophthalmologist, because intraocular TB is often encountered in patients with no concurrent sign of active systemic disease. Convincing a legal authority that it is to the public's benefit to detain a patient with isolated ocular disease would be extremely difficult. However, current legal doctrine also allows detention of a patient to perform diagnostic tests if TB infection is suspected. An ophthalmologist who reveals evidence of potential systemic disease during a review of systems may be able to justify invoking legal action to ensure diagnosis (or absence of disease), and subsequently ensure compliance to treatment.[50] This touchy issue will most likely spur more research to find therapies that work as effectively as the currently available medications without the necessity of long-term treatment.

COMPLICATIONS

Many of the complications of tuberculous uveitis are also commonly seen in uveitis from other causes; these include posterior synechiae, retinal detachment, and neovascular glaucoma. Some complications are more specific—subretinal abscesses, for example. There are also a few case reports of spontaneous scleral rupture. Retinal neovascularization can be seen,[22, 51] with one report noting a good response to sector ablation with argon laser photocoagulation while the patient was on antimycobacterial treatment.[52]

Unfortunately, enucleation or evisceration of a blind and painful eye is not a rare consequence of tuberculous uveitis.[20, 24, 27, 53] These cases tend to present as uncontrolled panophthalmitis, which can progress unremittingly even when the patient is on antimycobacterial treatment.

Complications can occur from the antimycobacterial therapy itself. Isoniazid toxicity includes neurologic toxicity, which includes peripheral neuritis, insomnia, increased agitation, urinary retention, and seizures. These effects are thought to occur from a relative pyridoxine deficiency and can be minimized with the administration of pyridoxine. INH is also associated with hepatotoxicity, and associated fatalities have been reported. Rifampin has been associated with thrombocytopenia, nephritis, and liver toxicity. Pyrazinamide has also been associated with liver toxicity. Ethambutol has been associated with optic neuritis that can regress with discontinuation of the drug. Streptomycin is associated with eighth nerve toxicity. INH can increase blood levels of phenytoin, and rifampin induces microsomal enzymes and can affect metabolism of microsome-dependent drugs (e.g., warfarin).

TUBERCULOSIS AND HIV

HIV disease is a contributing factor in the re-emergence of TB in recent times. Because of impaired cell-mediated immunity in HIV-infected individuals, one would expect to see increased susceptibility and increased severity of TB when compared with TB infection in patients with intact immune systems. This is, in fact, what is observed: patients with AIDS have nearly 500 times the risk of contracting TB than those in the general population.[10]

Most reported cases of TB uveitis in HIV-infected individuals occur in the context of chorioretinitis presenting in association with active systemic TB or while on treatment for proven systemic infection[54–56] (Table 18–1). Sometimes, choroidal tubercles are noted on routine ophthalmic examination in the absence of ocular complaints. Tuberculous eye lesions undergo resolution paralleling the systemic course.[54, 56] One case report described a patient whose autopsy revealed disseminated miliary TB, which had not been suspected clinically.[25] Ophthalmologic examination of the patient had revealed two

TABLE 18–1. CASE REPORTS ON HIV-INFECTED PATIENTS WITH TB UVEITIS

AUTHORS	PATIENT CHARACTERISTIC	EYE	METHOD OF DIAGNOSIS	SYSTEMIC SIGNS OF TB?	TYPE OF UVEITIS
Croxatto JO et al, 1986[25]	32 yo m	OU	Biopsy (postmortem)	Yes	Focal chorioretinitis OD; cotton-wool spots OU
Blodi BA et al, 1989[55]	34 yo m	OD	Presumed (positive sputum culture)	Yes	Granulomatous anterior uveitis, disseminated chorioretinitis OD
Blazques EP et al, 1994[54]	31 yo m	OD	Presumed (tests positive for systemic)	Yes	Focal chorioretinitis OD
	28 yo m	OU	Presumed (tests positive for systemic)	Yes (systemic + meningitis)	Focal chorioretinitis OU
	35 yo m	OD	Presumed (tests positive for systemic)	Yes	Focal chorioretinitis OD
	19 yo m	OU	Presumed (tests positive for systemic)	Yes	Disseminated chorioretinitis OU
Muccioli C et al, 1996[56]	35 yo w	OU	Presumed (AFB-positive sputum)	Yes	Focal chorioretinitis OD; vitritis OU
Recillas-Gispert C et al, 1997[40]	29 yo w	OS	PCR from aqueous specimen	Yes	Anterior uveitis, vitritis, vasculitis OS

AFB, Acid-fast bacilli; PCR, polymerase chain reaction.

choroidal nodules in the right eye, illustrating that routine ophthalmologic examination may aid the internist in formulating a differential diagnosis in an HIV-infected patient with an undiagnosed systemic illness.

The treatment of TB in HIV-infected individuals is also problematic. Patients with AIDS often have decreased gastrointestinal absorption, resulting in inadequate serum levels of the antimycobacterial drugs. The CDC recommends extending the duration of TB treatment in HIV-infected individuals.

PROGNOSIS

If TB is diagnosed and treated promptly, in most cases, a cure follows. With appropriate monitoring and adherence to current treatment guidelines, medications are safe and well tolerated. Reports in the ophthalmic literature support the fact that current antituberculous medications are extremely effective, and failures in treating ocular disease have been attributed to delayed diagnosis, a rapid and aggressive course, death of the patient to systemic infection, or noncompliance.

The most common reason cited for treatment failure among patients with pulmonary TB is nonadherence to the therapeutic regimen. In New York City in 1991, a study showed that 89% of 189 patients failed to complete therapy, and 80% of those brought back failed a second time.[44] Resistance to isoniazid or rifampin in 1991 was 23%, the high number most likely related to the number of patients who stopped treatment before eradicating the organism from their body. It is for this reason DOT is now recommended by the CDC as a routine part of treatment.

Failures in DOT cases have led investigators to realize that other aspects of the disease process and therapy are still not well understood. One such aspect is therapeutic drug monitoring (TDM),[57] the process of adjusting drug doses based on serum concentration. Bioassays demonstrate that bioavailability of the drug can vary greatly among individuals and may account for failures in which compliance is not an issue.[58]

SUMMARY

Mycobacterium tuberculosis is one of the few causes of uveitis for which we have a definitive, highly effective treatment. Its most common manifestation is disseminated or focal chorioretinitis, which may be associated with vitritis or anterior uveitis. It can occur both in patients with active TB infection and in patients without signs or symptoms of systemic TB. Definitive diagnosis is often difficult; treatment is often instituted if other contributory objective data strongly support the diagnosis. Prognosis is excellent if an appropriate drug regimen is prescribed and patient compliance can be ensured.

References

1. Silverstein AM: Changing trends in the etiologic diagnosis of uveitis. Doc Ophthalmol 1997;94:25–37.
2. Beutner EH: Tuberculosis of the skin: Historical perspectives on tuberculin and Bacille Calmette Guerin. J Dermatol 1997;36:73–77.
3. Maitre-Jan A: Trate des maladies des yeux. Troyes, 1711, p 456. (Cited in: Duke-Elder S: System of Ophthalmology: Diseases of the Uveal Tract, vol 9. St. Louis, CV Mosby, 1966, p 248.
4. Von Michel J: Ueber iris und iritis. Albrecht v Grafes Arch Ophthalmol 1881;27:171–282. (Cited in: Helm CJ, Holland GN: Ocular tuberculosis. Surv Ophthalmol 1993;38:3, 229–256).
5. Abrams J, Schlaegel TF: The role of the isoniazid therapeutic test in tuberculous uveitis. Am J Ophthalmol 1982;94:511–515.
6. McDermott LJ, Glassroth J: Natural history and epidemiology. Dis Mon 1997;43:131–155.
7. Lerner BH: Catching patients: Tuberculosis and detention in the 1990s. Chest 1999;115:346–341.
8. McCray E, Weinbaum CM, Braden CR, Onorato IM: The epidemiology of tuberculosis in the United States. Clin Chest 1997;18:1, 99–113.
9. Snider GL: Tuberculosis then and now: A personal perspective on the last 50 years. Ann Intern Med 1997;126:237–243.
10. Donahue HC: Ophthalmologic experience in a tuberculosis sanatorium. Am J Ophthalmol 1967;64:742–748.
11. Biswas J, Badrinath S: Ocular morbidity in patients with active systemic tuberculosis. Int Ophthalmol 1996;19:293–298.
11a. Morinelli EN, Dugal PU, Riffenburgh R, Rao NA: Infectious multifocal choroiditis in patients with acquired immune deficiency syndrome. Ophthalmology 1993;100:1014–1021.
12. Abrams J, Schlaegel TF: The tuberculin skin test in the diagnosis of tuberculous uveitis. Am J Ophthalmol 1983;96:295–298.
13. Zoric LD, Zoric DL, Zoric DM: Bilateral tuberculous abscesses on

the face (eyelids) of a child [letter]. Am J Ophthalmol 1996; 121:717–718.

14. Cameron JA, Nasr AM, Chavis P: Epibulbar and ocular tuberculosis. Arch Ophthalmol 1996;114:770–771.

15. Anhalt EF, Zavell S, Chang G, Byron HM: Conjunctival tuberculosis. Am J Ophthalmol 1960;50:265–269.

16. Grewal A, Kim RY, Cunningham ET: Miliary tuberculosis. Arch Ophthalmol 1998;116:953–954.

17. Barondes MJ, Sponsel WE, Stevens TS, Plotnik RD: Tuberculous choroiditis diagnosed by chorioretinal endobiopsy. Am J Ophthalmol 1991;112:460–461.

18. Mansour AM, Haymond R: Choroidal tuberculomas without evidence of extraocular tuberculosis. Graefe's Arch Clin Exp Ophthalmol 1990;228:382–385.

19. Cangemi FE, Freidman AH, Josephberg R: Tuberculoma of the choroid. Ophthalmology 1980;87:252–258.

20. Lyon CE, Grimson BS, Pfeiffer RLL, et al: Clinicopathological correlation of a solitary choroidal tuberculoma. Ophthalmol 1985; 92:845–850.

21. Berinstein DM, Gentile RC, McCormick SA, Walsh JB: Primary choroidal tuberculoma. Arch Ophthalmol 1997;115:430–431.

22. Rosen PH, Spalton DJ, Graham EM: Intraocular tuberculosis. Eye 1990;4:486–492.

23. Biswas J, Narain S, Das D, Ganesh SK: Pattern of uveitis in a referral uveitis clinic in India. Int Ophthalmol 1996;20:223–228.

24. Biswas J, Madhavan HN, Gopal L, Badrinath SS: Intraocular tuberculosis. Clinicopathologic study of five case. Retina 1995;15:461–468.

25. Croxatto JO, Mestre C, Puente S, Gonzalez G: Nonreactive tuberculosis in a patient with acquired immune deficiency syndrome [letter]. Am J Ophthalmol 1986;102:659–660.

26. Dvorak-Theobald G: Acute tuberculous endophthalmitis. Am J Ophthalmol 1958;45:403–407.

27. Ni C, Papale JJ, Robinson NL, Wu BF: Uveal tuberculosis. Int Ophthalmol Clin 1982;22:103–124.

28. Stead WW: The origin and erratic global spread of tuberculosis. Clin Chest 1997;18:65–78.

29. Dutt AK, Stead W: The treatment of tuberculosis. Dis Mon 1997;43:247–271.

30. Swaminathan S, Gong J, Zhang M, et al: Cytokine production in children with tuberculosis infection and disease. Clin Infect Dis 1999;28:1290–1293.

31. Mohaghehhpour N, Gammon D, Kawamura LM, et al: CTL Response to *Mycobacterium tuberculosis*: Identification of an immunogenic epitope in the 19-kDa lipoprotein. J Immunol 1998;161:2400–2406.

32. Telenti A: Genetics of drug resistance in tuberculosis. Clin Chest 1997;18:55–64.

33. LoBue PA, Catanzaro A: The diagnosis of tuberculosis. Dis Mon 1997;43:185–219.

34. Burgoyne CF, Verstraeten TC, Friberg TR: Tuberculin skin-test induced uveitis in the absence of tuberculosis. Graefes Arch Clin Exp Ophthalmol 1991;229:232–236.

35. Jonas V, Longiaru M: Detection of *Mycobacterium tuberculosis* by molecular methods. Clin Lab Med 1997;17:119–128.

36. Kotake S, Kimura K, Yoshikawa K, et al: Polymerase chain reaction for the detection of *Mycobacterium tuberculosis* in ocular tuberculosis [letter]. Am J Ophthalmol 1994;117:805–806.

37. Gladwin MT, Plorde JJ, Martin TR: Clinical application of the *Mycobacterium tuberculosis* direct test. Chest 1998;114:317–323.

38. Sarvanantahn N, Wiselka M, Bibby K: Intraocular tuberculosis without detectable systemic infection. Arch Ophthalmol 1998;116:1386–1388.

39. Bowyer JD Gormley PO, Seth R, et al: Choroidal tuberculosis diagnosed by polymerase chain reaction. Ophthalmol 1999;106:290–294.

40. Recillas-Gispert C, Ortega-Larrocea G, Arellanes-Garcia L, et al: Chorioretinitis secondary to *Mycobacterium tuberculosis* in acquired immune deficiency syndrome. Retina 1997;17:437–439.

41. Cokerill FR: Conventional and genetic laboratory tests used to guide antimicrobial therapy. Mayo Clin Proc 1998;73:1007–1021.

42. Schlaegel TF Jr, Webber JC: Double-blind therapeutic trial of isoniazid in 344 patients with uveitis. Br J Ophthalmol 1969;52:425–427.

43. Bradford WZ, Daley CL: Multiple drug-resistant tuberculosis. Infect Dis Clin North A 1998; 12:157–172.

44. Fujiwara PI, Larkin C, Frieden TR: Directly observed therapy in New York City. Clin Chest 1997;18:135–148.

45. Campion EW: Liberty and the control of tuberculosis. N Engl J Med 1999;340:385–386.

46. Chaluk CP, Pope DS: The Baltimore city health department program of directly observed therapy for tuberculosis. Clin Chest 1997;18:149–154.

47. Weis SE: Universal directly observed therapy. Clin Chest 1997;18:155–163.

48. Schecter GF: Supervised therapy in San Francisco. Clin Chest 1997;18:165–168.

49. Sbarbaro JA: Directly observed therapy. Clin Chest 1997;8:131–133.

50. Gasner MR, Maw KL, Fledman GE, et al: The use of legal action in New York City to ensure treatment of tuberculosis. N Engl J Med 1999;340:359–365.

51. Chung YM, Yeh TS, Sheu SJ, Liu JH: Macular subretinal neovascularization in choroidal tuberculosis: Ann Ophthalmol 1989;21:225–229.

52. Gur S, Silverstone BZ, Zylberman R, Berson D: Chorioretinitis and extrapulmonary tuberculosis. Ann Ophthalmol 1987;19:112–115.

53. Darrel RW: Acute tuberculous panophthalmitis. Arch Ophthalmol 1967;78:51–54.

54. Blazques EP, Rodriguez MM, Mendes Ramos MJ: Tuberculous choroiditis and acquired immunodeficiency syndrome. Ann Ophthalmol 1994;26:50–54.

55. Blodi BA, Johnson MW, McLeish WM, Gass JD: Presumed choroidal tuberculosis in a human immunodeficiency virus infected host. Am J Ophthalmol 1989;108:605–606.

56. Muccioli C, Belfort R: Presumed ocular and central nervous system tuberculosis in a patient with the acquired immunodeficiency syndrome [letter]. Am J Ophthalmol 1996; 121:217–219.

57. Peloquin CA: Using therapeutic drug monitoring to dose the antimycobacterial drugs. Clin Chest 1997;18:79–87.

58. Heifets L: Mycobacterial laboratory. Clin Chest 1997;18:35–53.

59. Helm CJ, Holland GN: Ocular tuberculosis. Surv Ophthalmol 1993;38:229–256.

19 — LEPTOSPIROSIS

M. Reza Dana

DEFINITION AND HISTORY

Leptospirosis is a zoonotic infection caused by the gram-negative helical spirochete *Leptospira interrogans*. The infection, which has a worldwide distribution, is most common in warmer climates. The reservoir for leptospirosis is animals, often rodents and cattle, which excrete leptospires in their urine as a result of chronic infection. The disease is usually contracted by humans exposed to contaminated soil or surface water. It is characterized by an acute short phase of 7 to 10 days, followed by an immune phase that may last for many months. Ophthalmic complications of systemic leptospirosis were first reported by Adolf Weil in 1886.[1, 2] Inflammatory ophthalmic disease, which typically occurs several months after the onset of the acute systemic disease, can vary greatly in presentation and severity. However, leptospiral uveitis generally has a favorable prognosis if diagnosed and treated appropriately.

EPIDEMIOLOGY

Leptospirosis is one of the most common zoonoses in the world.[3] Although the distribution is worldwide, it occurs most frequently in the tropical and subtropical areas of the globe, and in developing nations where contact with infected animals, or water or soil contaminated with their urine, is most likely to occur.[4, 5] The natural hosts of leptospira are rodents, dogs, pigs, and cattle, which may transmit the disease to humans.[6] Maternal-fetal transmission may occur but is thought to be uncommon. The most common sources of infection include urine of infected animals, and contaminated surface water or mud harboring infectious leptospira from animal excretions. Infection occurs via direct contact with animal blood or urine (e.g., farmers and abattoir workers) or, more commonly, via indirect contact with contaminated water, as may happen with farmers in rice paddies, sewer workers, or swimmers in contaminated waters.[5, 7] Leptospires usually enter the body through mucous membranes or skin abrasions.[5] Because of these epidemiologic characteristics of disease transmission, the majority of infected patients are young men and boys in the lower socioeconomic strata of the population.

Because the disease occurs primarily in less developed areas of the globe, the true incidence remains largely unknown. It is believed, however, that the prevalence of leptospirosis is underreported, even in the United States, where many cases eventually related to leptospirosis are initially misdiagnosed.[8, 9] In countries where leptospirosis is endemic, it is often confused with malaria, tuberculosis, viral hepatitis, typhoid, aseptic meningitis, influenza, or other infections, because these diseases themselves are so common in these areas.[10, 11] In the United States, where approximately 100 cases are reported annually to the Centers for Disease Control and Prevention in Atlanta, leptospirosis is most common in Hawaii.[5] This disease is considered an important occupational hazard of taro farming, which involves wading in shallow water.

CLINICAL CHARACTERISTICS

Nonocular Disease

The spectrum of human disease caused by leptospira species is extremely wide, ranging from subclinical infection to a fatal syndrome (Weil's syndrome), characterized by multisystem hemorrhage, renal failure, jaundice, and cardiac shock.[10] Accordingly, mortality can vary greatly from nearly zero to over 30%, depending on multiple variables including the serovar of the infecting organism.[10, 12] Generally, the disease is biphasic.[11] It begins acutely with the abrupt onset of fever, headache, fatigue, and myalgia. Some patients develop significant abdominal pain and associated nausea and vomiting, or diarrhea. These symptoms herald the onset of the *spirochetemic* phase of the illness, during which spirochetes can be found in the blood, cerebrospinal fluid, kidneys, and other organs.[13] Although a variety of rashes can accompany other stigmata of the disease, there is no consistent pattern to the rashes.[14] Occurrence of leptospirosis in pregnancy carries a high risk of intrauterine infection and fetal death.[6]

The spirochetemic phase can vary from 2 to 3 days of mild disease to 7 to 10 days of severe multisystem symptoms in some patients. The septicemic stage of leptospirosis is followed by the *spirocheturic* (or immune) phase of the disease. This occurs as a result of the immune response to the infection; however, the kidneys and ocular compartments can harbor live leptospira for a longer period.[5, 10] There is often a quiescent period between the two stages of the illness before the immune phase becomes clinically apparent. The subsequent course of the illness depends largely on which of the two clinical syndromes develops: *anicteric* leptospirosis (90% of cases), or *icteric* leptospirosis (10% of cases), according to the degree of hepatic involvement. Many patients with anicteric disease have a mild course characterized by a self-limited condition that can resolve with no serious sequelae. The most important features of the immune stage are meningitis and leptospiruria. Fever is generally not a prominent sign. Other symptoms may develop such as nonmeningitic neurologic manifestations, nerve palsies, myelitis, or uveitis, which can occur many months after the acute stage of the illness. Commonly, patients with anicteric disease seek medical attention without a clear preceding illness.[5] On the other hand, some patients with very mild septicemic disease do not develop any clinical disease during the immune phase of the disease.

Unlike the mild course of anicteric leptospirosis, icteric disease, which is characterized by jaundice and azotemia, can lead to a mortality rate of over 10% to 30%. In fact, the illness in some individuals is so severe that it obscures the biphasic nature of the disease.[5] In Weil's syndrome, patients may progress rapidly to multisystem failure with a high chance of mortality unless they receive early (e.g., in the first 4 days) antimicrobial and supportive treatment (see later) for their illness.

Ocular Disease

The incidence of ocular disease in leptospirosis remains unknown. Given that systemic leptospirosis is underdiagnosed[9] and leptospiral uveitis often occurs many months after the onset of the systemic disease, there is little doubt that the burden of eye disease due to leptospirosis is underestimated. The earliest and most common sign of ocular leptospirosis is conjunctival hyperemia or hemorrhage,[6, 15, 16] but this finding does not lead to visual disability. In contrast, the most serious ocular complication of leptospirosis is the development of uveitis. It is estimated that uveitis occurs in 2% to 10% of patients suffering from leptospirosis.[12] This syndrome, which was first described by Weil,[2] has been reported to occur either early, or as late as several years after the onset of the systemic disease.[15, 16]

Two distinct categories of leptospiral uveitis have been described. One form involves patients who develop anterior uveitis with photophobia, blurred vision, and pain. Leptospiral anterior uveitis, which is thought to be largely benign,[17, 18] is believed to be the most common form of uveitis in leptospirosis by a number of investigators.[1, 15, 17] A second group of patients are those who develop posterior segment involvement including vitritis, choroiditis, papillitis, or panuveitis.[1, 19] In a study of leptospiral and nonleptospiral uveitis in India, Chu and colleagues[10] evaluated a number of clinical variables to determine the constellation of findings most suggestive of leptospiral uveitis in an endemic area. These investigators concluded that *in comparison* to other forms of uveitis, leptospirosis has a higher propensity for posterior uveitis, vasculitis, papillitis, and vitritis. The potential development of posterior findings including vitreal membranes, retinal exudates, and optic neuritis in leptospirosis is well documented.[1, 19–21] However, it remains unclear whether generalizations regarding disease manifestations in one geographic region can be validly applied to other endemic areas. Disparities in data regarding the ocular presentation of leptospirosis most likely occur because the clinical presentation of infectious disease depends both on the virulence of the infecting organism and on the genotype of the host (which dictates the immune response to the infectious agent). Because of significant variations in both these parameters between different geographic locales, leptospiral uveitis may present very differently from one endemic area to another.

Two recent case series have evaluated the ocular manifestations of leptospirosis. Martins and coworkers reported on 21 patients, 20 men and one woman, presenting with acute systemic leptospirosis in Brazil.[16] They reported conjunctival hyperemia among 86%, increased retinal venous caliber among 57%, optic nerve head hyperemia among 57%, subconjunctival hemorrhage among 19%, optic disk edema among 5%, and retinal vasculitis and hemorrhage among 5%. The visual acuity of affected patients ranged from 20/20 to light perception. Interestingly, they did not observe a single case of anterior segment inflammation, underscoring the fact that

uveitis tends to occur in the late immune phase of leptospirosis.

In the other recent series, Rathinam and coinvestigators reported on cases of uveitis seen in Madurai, India, after heavy rainfall and unexpected flooding led to an epidemic outbreak of leptospirosis.[4] In 73 consecutive patients with leptospiral uveitis associated with this epidemic, 111 eyes were examined. As in the group in Brazil, the vast majority (82%) of patients were young men (mean age, 35), and 78% were classified as having "low socioeconomic status," emphasizing the group at highest risk for this zoonosis. Of the 73 patients, 52% had bilateral involvement. Among the 111 eyes with uveitis, panuveitis was seen in 95%, anterior uveitis alone in 3%, and vitritis alone in 2%. Typical anterior segment findings among these patients included nongranulomatous reaction (92%), posterior synechiae (24%), and hypopyon (13%). Typical posterior segment findings included vitreous inflammation and debris (89%), and intermittent periphlebitis (51%). Notably, macular edema, epiretinal membrane formation, and intermediate uveitis were distinctly rare complications, occurring in less than 2% to 3% of affected eyes. Interestingly, in spite of the frequency of posterior findings and panuveitis, final visual acuity was 20/20 in 52% of eyes; another 16% showed improvement in acuity following treatment, but not to the level of 20/20. The authors of this study concluded that the prognosis of leptospiral uveitis is generally favorable even when the ocular inflammation is severe and the involvement is posterior.[4]

PATHOGENESIS

Leptospirosis is a zoonotic infection caused by the gram-negative helical spirochete *Leptospira*. Spirochetes are grouped together on the basis of their common structural features and motility characteristics.[11] Within the order Spirochaetales are two families: Spirochaetales and Leptospiraceae. Four genera belong to the former, and two to the latter. Of the six genera, three—*Treponema*, *Borrelia*, and *Leptospira*—contain organisms that cause human disease. The leptospira can be divided into those that are pathogenic (i.e., *L. interrogans*) and those that are saprophytic (i.e., *L. biflexa*).[5] The saprophytes can be differentiated from the pathogens by their ability to grow at lower temperatures. Among the pathogenic species *L. interrogans* are over 200 serovars. *Serovars* that are closely related because they share common antigenic epitopes are grouped into *serogroups.*

These organisms have a short incubation period, and as early as the first week after infection the host IgM response can be detected. This peaks during the next 2 to 4 weeks and may remain positive for significantly longer. The exact immunopathogenesis of leptospiral uveitis is not completely understood. It has been proposed that uveitis occurs because antileptospiral antibodies are slow to migrate into the anterior chamber but are rapidly cleared, allowing the organism to flourish.[22] It has been speculated that the clinical disease in leptospirosis is both a reflection of bacterial toxins or enzymes released by the infecting organisms that can cause direct tissue injury,[15, 23] and an immune vasculopathy related to activation of complement and deposition of immune complexes. This microangiopathy can lead to neutrophil margination to the vascular endothelium—thereby allowing tissue injury after transendothelial migration of activated leukocytes.[24]

LABORATORY DIAGNOSIS

Diagnosis of human leptospiral infection relies on either isolation of the causative organism, or its DNA, from body fluids, or demonstration of a rise in specific serum antibodies.[25] Detection of leptospires in body fluids by darkfield microscopy is limited because of proteinaceous filaments (pseudoleptospires) that can be present.[26] The isolation of leptospira is best done during the early spirochetemic phase of the infection—typically during the first week of infection. During this period, leptospira may be isolated from blood and cerebrospinal fluid (CSF), although the yield is higher from the blood.[11] Recovery can be optimized if samples are obtained daily, preferably before antibiotic therapy, although delay in treatment in an attempt to increase diagnostic yield is generally ill-advised, as other diagnostic measures may be employed (see later). Usually, only one to two drops of blood are inoculated in medium (bovine serum albumin–Tween 80, semisolid [0.2% agar]), because larger inocula are paradoxically associated with growth inhibition.[11, 27] One method of increasing the yield of the infecting organism is to inject the specimen derived from the patient into hamsters or guinea pigs, and then to isolate the leptospires from moribund animals. Isolation media are incubated at 30°C and examined weekly. Growth is usually detectable after 2 weeks of incubation, but it may require longer than 6 weeks. After the first 1 to 2 weeks of disease, when leptospirosis enters its spirocheturic phase, leptospires may be detected in urine, where they are shed for 1 month or longer. Because the organism has a short half-life in acidic urine, specimens should be cultured as soon as possible—usually within the hour.[11]

Isolation of leptospira, as has been described, is difficult and very resource intensive. Moreover, because of the time lag between culture and diagnosis, isolation techniques for spirochetal disease are not always useful from an acute patient management standpoint. Over the years, the microscopic agglutination test (MAT) has become the reference test for diagnosis of leptospiral disease. This test, which can detect antibodies to many different serovars, is complex and needs maintenance of stock cultures of different leptospiral serovars; hence, it is best performed in specialized reference laboratories such as those of the World Health Organization or the Centers for Disease Control and Prevention.[4, 10, 25] Generally, serum samples from suspected patients are collected and diluted at 1:50 to 1:100 and tested against a pool of several dozen pathogenic serovars of *L. interrogans*. Reactive sera are then subjected to serial twofold dilutions and reacted against each serovar to determine the end-point titer.[4, 10] Because there is cross-reactivity to different serovars, standard practice dictates that the serovar reacting at the highest titer is presumed to be the one responsible for the infection.

The MAT requires a specialized laboratory and personnel.[25] For this reason, practical diagnosis of leptospirosis is becoming increasingly based on enzyme-linked immu-

nosorbent assays (ELISA) for leptospiral-specific antibodies. ELISA offers a rapid, sensitive, and specific assay for detecting immunity to leptospiral antigens, and it is less susceptible to subjective interpretation of laboratory personnel than MAT.[9, 25, 28, 29] ELISA kits are commercially available and have been shown to have a 100% sensitivity when tested to known infected sera. ELISA titers can be positive for sera from patients with *Brucella*, Epstein-Barr virus, cytomegalovirus, mycoplasma, Q fever, toxoplasma, and several other diseases, but the reactive titers in these cases are almost universally low. Moreover, the persistence of high IgM titers in leptospirosis for as long as 48 *months* after infection, which has been reported by multiple investigators,[25] makes assaying for IgM a sensitive and good initial screen for leptospirosis. High titers can then be confirmed by MAT in a specialized reference laboratory.

More recently, polymerase chain reaction (PCR) has been used to amplify leptospiral DNA.[10, 30, 31] PCR can be used to detect leptospiral DNA in aqueous humor of individuals with suspected leptospiral uveitis.[18] The capacity of PCR to profoundly amplify low copy numbers of DNA theoretically provides for a highly sensitive assay.[10] In a recent study in India, 28% of aqueous humor PCR-positive leptospiral uveitis patients did not demonstrate serum antileptospiral antibodies.[10] Hence, it remains unknown whether leptospiral uveitis correlates well with serum antibody titers. It has been postulated that because uveitis typically occurs months after the acute illness and seroconversion, systemic antibody levels may not be sensitive indicators of disease. However, because concerns regarding false-positive and false-negative results with PCR persist, it is strongly advisable to use this diagnostic modality primarily in cases when the diagnosis is uncertain and as an adjunct to ELISA and MAT.

DIFFERENTIAL DIAGNOSIS

The diagnosis of leptospiral disease is primarily based on clinical and laboratory criteria. Because none of the ocular findings are specific or pathognomonic, definitive diagnosis requires laboratory confirmation. However, because timely treatment can have significant extraocular ramifications, it is important to consider and discuss the differential diagnosis.

Although leptospiral uveitis may present with profound anterior chamber inflammation and hypopyon, it may be differentiated from HLA-B27-associated uveitis by the high prevalence of bilaterality, vitreal inflammation, and vasculitis. These features, although possible in seronegative spondyloarthropathies, are uncommon. Moreover, the nonocular clinical presentation in HLA-B27-associated disease is very different from that seen in leptospirosis. Leptospiral uveitis may be differentiated from idiopathic pars planitis by the preponderance of cystoid macular edema in idiopathic pars planitis, and intense anterior chamber inflammation in the former. Occasionally, leptospiral disease can be confused with Adamantiades-Behçet's disease (ABD), especially because ABD can also cause panuveitis, retinitis, and central nervous system stigmata. However, the pattern of vasculitis varies between these entities. ABD patients often have occlusive vasculitis as opposed to the intermittent periphlebitis seen in leptospirosis. Moreover, ABD is associated with HLA-B5/51, whereas such an association is not present in leptospirosis. Similarly, patients with Eales' disease have peripheral vasculitis and neovascularization, whereas severe vitritis and panuveitis are uncommon. Finally, because mycobacterial and spirochetal diseases often coexist with a similar epidemiology, it is important to consider ocular tuberculosis (TB) in the differential diagnosis. Patients with the ocular TB are purified-protein-derivative (PPD) positive, and they often have positive chest x-ray findings suggestive of granulomata. Ocular TB is among the great masqueraders, but there is often a choroidal tubercle and the uveitis is typically granulomatous in type, as opposed to the overwhelmingly nongranulomatous disease in leptospiral uveitis.

TREATMENT

There is some controversy about the treatment of leptospirosis.[32] First, it is important to recognize that results of in vitro susceptibility testing for leptospires cannot be automatically extrapolated to the clinical setting.[11] In vitro susceptibility studies suggest that pathogenic leptospiral serovars are susceptible to all of the commonly used antibiotics except chloramphenicol. However, whereas the minimal inhibitory concentration (MIC) for penicillin G is generally low, penicillin appears to have inadequate leptospiricidal activity in vivo.[33] Hence, although penicillin G is highly effective against some spirochetes (e.g., treponemes), it should not be assumed that it is the drug of choice for leptospirosis. At present, doxycycline at the adult dose of 100 mg twice daily for 10 to 14 days is the standard antimicrobial treatment,[34, 35] although many alternatives including cephalosporins may be used instead.[36, 37] A critical facet of systemic treatment is that it should be instituted, whenever possible, during the first 4 days of illness to shorten the duration and decrease the severity of the disease. Significant controversy exists concerning the effectiveness of antimicrobial therapy later in the course of the disease.[4, 11] Most authors believe that treatment late in the course of the disease is of limited value. However, because others have argued that pathogenic leptospira can survive and multiply in the blood and anterior chamber for a long time,[38] we agree with the recommendations of Rathinam and colleagues,[4] who propose systemic antibiotic treatment for eye disease even months after onset of the acute systemic illness.

In addition to instituting appropriate systemic antimicrobial treatment, the care of the patient with leptospiral uveitis involves judicious use of local (topical and periocular depot injections) corticosteroids to suppress ocular inflammation. Anticholinergic mydriatics can relax the iris sphincter and provide some relief to patients with ocular pain. Moreover, anticholinergics can help with the resolution of anterior uveitis by promoting restoration of the blood-ocular barrier. Most uveitic cases are brought under rapid control with adoption of these standard anti-inflammatory measures. There is no place for immunosuppressive chemotherapy in the care of patients with leptospiral disease.

PROGNOSIS

Most of the available data suggest that the visual prognosis of leptospiral uveitis is quite favorable.[4, 16] Attention to fundamentals of good ophthalmologic care of uveitis patients, namely suppression of ocular inflammation and treatment of comorbidities such as ocular hypertension and macular edema, is imperative. Because leptospirosis is an infectious disease, it is important (particularly in the acute phase) to institute proper systemic antibacterial treatment before intensive anti-inflammatory strategies are employed, as the latter can suppress innate and acquired immune responses to pathogenic leptospira.

The most critical prognosticator for the patient with leptospirosis is the severity of the systemic illness as detailed in the preceding sections. Patients with multisystem disease (Weil syndrome) and impending renal failure need life-saving dialysis,[16] and those with hemorrhagic disease need intensive intravenous fluids to prevent cardiac shock. Often, with appropriate and timely treatment, even the most severe cases of leptospiral infection can be successfully treated with little to no functional deficits.

CONCLUSIONS

Leptospirosis is a common zoonosis, particularly among patients from low socioeconomic strata of developing nations. Leptospiral uveitis can have a wide range of presentations during both the acute and chronic phases of the illness. Most patients have a favorable visual prognosis with appropriate therapy, even when the ocular involvement is extensive and severe. Timely diagnosis of leptospirosis is critical not only for maximizing visual potential but also for appropriate systemic monitoring and treatment of extraocular involvement in this potentially fatal condition. Ultimately, effective public health and sanitation measures in endemic areas are imperative for optimal protection of farmers and other laborers against exposure to infecting leptospira.

References

1. Duke-Elder S, Perkins ES: Diseases of the uveal tract. In: Duke-Elder S, ed: System of Ophthalmology, vol. 9. London, Henry Kimpton, 1966, p 322.
2. Weil A: Uber eine Eigentumliche mit Tumor, Icterus, und Nephritis Einhergehende Akute Infektionskrankheit (English summary). Dtsh Arch Klin Med 1886;39:209.
3. Letocart M, Baranton G, Perolat P: Rapid identification of pathogenic *Leptospira* species (*Leptospira interrogans.*, *L. borgpetersenii*, and *L. kirsneri*) with species-specific DNA probes produced by arbitrarily primed PCR. J. Clin Microbiol 1997;35:248.
4. Rathinam SR, Rathinam S, Selvaraj S, et al: Uveitis associated with an epidemic outbreak of leptospirosis. Am J Ophthalmol 1997;124:71.
5. Terpstra WJ, Ligthart GS, Schoone GJ: ELISA for the detection of specific IgM and IgG in human leptospirosis. J Gen Microbiol 1985;131:377.
6. Faine S: *Leptospira* and Leptospirosis. Boca Raton, FL, CRC Press, 1994.
7. Waitkins SA: Update on leptospirosis. 1985;290:1502.
8. Heath CW Jr., Alexander AD, Galton MM: Leptospirosis in the United States. N Engl J Med 1965;273:857.
9. Petchclai B, Kunakorn M, Hiranris S, et al: Enzyme-linked immunoabsorbent assay for leptospirosis immunoglobulin M specific antibody using surface antigen from a pathogenic *Leptospira*: A comparison with indirect hemagglutination and microagglutination tests. J Med Assoc Thai 1992;75:203.
10. Chu KM, Rathinam R, Namperumalsamy P, Dean D: Identification of *Leptospira* species in the pathogenesis of uveitis and determination of clinical ocular characteristics in South India. J Infect Dis 1998;177:1314.
11. Johnson RC, Harris VG: Differentiation of pathogenic and sapro-

phytic leptospires. I. Growth at low temperatures. J Bacteriol 1967;94:27.

12. Johnson RC: Isolation techniques for spirochetes and their sensitivity to antibiotics in vitro and in vivo. Rev Infect Dis 1989;II(S):S1505.

13. Feigin RD, Anderson DC: Human leptospirosis. Crit Rev Clin Lab Sci 1975;5:413.

14. Schmid GP, Steere AC, Kornblatt AN, et al: Newly recognized species (*"Leptospira inadai"* serovar *lyme*) isolated from human skin. J Clin Microbiol 1986;24:484.

15. Farr RW: Leptospirosis. Clin Infect Dis 1995;21:1.

16. Martins MG, Matos KTF, da Silva MV, de Abreu MT: Ocular manifestations in the acute phase of leptospirosis. Ocul Immunol Inflamm 1998;6:75.

17. Barkay S, Garzozi H: Leptospirosis and uveitis. Ann Ophthalmol 1984;16:164.

18. Merien R, Perolat P, Mancel E, et al: Detection of *Leptospira* DNA by polymerase chain reaction in aqueous humor of a patient with unilateral uveitis. J Infect Dis 1993;168:1335.

19. Levin N, Ngyuyen-Khoa JL, Charpentier D, et al: Panuveitis with papillitis in leptospirosis. Am J Ophthalmol 1994;117:118.

20. Whitcup SM, Raizman MB: Spirochetal infections and the eye. In: Albert DM, Jakobiec AF, eds: Principles and Practice of Ophthalmology, vol 5. Philadelphia, W.B. Saunders, 1994, p 3089.

21. Woods AC: Granulomatous uveitis. In: Endogenous Inflammations of the Uveal Tract. Baltimore, Williams and Wilkins, 1961, p 76.

22. Austoni M, Moro F: L'uveite quale manifestazione della sindrome oculoinflammatoria della leptospirosi, con particolare riguarelo ad una forma di ciclite sierosa silente in pazienti clinicamente guariti. G Mal Infett Parassit 1952;4:339; summary in Exerpta Med [sect 12} Opthalmol 1954;8:353.

23. Watt, G: Leptospirosis. In: Strickland GT, ed: Hunter's Tropical Medicine. Philadelphia, W.B. Saunders, 1991, p 317.

24. Dobrina A, Nardon E, Vecile E, et al: *Leptospira icterohemorrhagiae* and *Leptospire peptidoglycans* induce endothelial cell adhesiveness for polymorphonuclear leukocytes. Infect Immun 1995;63:2995.

25. Winslow WE, Merry DJ, Pirc ML, Devine P: Evaluation of a commercial enzyme-linked immunosorbent assay for detection of immuno-globulin M antibody in diagnosis of human leptospiral infection. J Clin Microbiol 1997;35:1938.

26. Faine S, Alder B: Leptospirosis. In: Hartwig N, ed: Clinical Microbiology Update Program, no 24. Department of Microbiology, Monash University, Melbourne, Victoria, Australia, 1984, pp 7–19.

27. Johnson RC: Leptospirosis. In: Strickland GT, ed: Hunter's Tropical and Geographic Medicine. Philadelphia, W.B. Saunders, 1990, p 889.

28. Cinco M, Balanzin D, Banfi E: Evaluation of an immunoenzymatic test (ELISA) for the diagnosis of leptospirosis in Italy. Eur J Epidemiol 1992;8:677.

29. da Silva MV, Camargo ED, Vaz AJ, Batista L: Immunodiagnosis of human leptospirosis using saliva. Trans R Soc Trop Med Hyg. 1992;86:560.

30. Bal AE, Gravekamp C, Hartskeerl RA, et al: Detection of leptospires in urine by PCR for early diagnosis of leptospirosis. J Clin Microbiol 1994;32:1894.

31. Brown PD, Gravekamp C, Carrington DG, et al: Evaluation of the polymerase chain reaction for early diagnosis of leptospirosis. J Med Microbiol 1995;43:110.

32. Stoenner HG: Treatment and control of leptospirosis. In: Johnson RC, ed: The Biology of Parasitic Spirochetes. New York, Academic Press, 1976, p 375.

33. Cook AR, Thompson RE: The effects of oleandomycin, erythromycin, carbomycin, and penicillin G on *Leptospira icterohaemorrhagiae* in vitro and in experimental animals. Antibiot Chemother 1957;7:425.

34. McClain JBL, Ballou WR, Harrison SM, Steinweg DL: Doxycycline therapy for leptospirosis. Ann Intern Med 1984;100:696.

35. Takafuji ET, Kirkpatrick JW, Miller RN, et al: An efficacy trial of doxycycline chemoprophylaxis against leptospirosis. N Engl J Med 1984;310:497.

36. Alexander AD, Rule PL: Penicillins, cephalosporins, and tetracyclines in treatment of hamsters with fatal leptospirosis. Antimicrob Agents Chemother 1986;30:835.

37. Oie S, Hironaga K, Koshiro A, et al: In vitro susceptibilities of five *Leptospira* strains to 16 antimicrobial agents. Antimicrob Agents Chemother 1983;24:905.

38. Gollop JH, Katz AR, Rudov RC, Sasaki DM: Rat bite leptospirosis. West J Med 1993;159:76.

Albert T. Vitale

DEFINITION

Brucellosis is a zoonotic disorder caused by infection with *Brucella* spp. and remains a major source of disease in domesticated animals and in humans in many parts of the world. Its clinical manifestations in humans include a broad spectrum of multisystemic and ocular findings, with uveitis being the most common ophthalmic presentation. Diagnosis requires a high degree of suspicion within the appropriate clinical context and may be confirmed by serologic testing and by isolation and culture of the causative organism. Timely recognition of this disease is highly desirable, because therapy with specific antimicrobial agents may be curative.

HISTORY

Following the capture of Malta from the French in 1799, many British soldiers were afflicted by a febrile illness known as *Malta fever*, a disease that had been prevalent in the Mediterranean region for centuries.[1] Its etiology was elucidated by the army surgeon, Sir David Bruce, who recovered the organism (which he called *Micrococcus melitensis*) from the spleens of 19 fatal cases in 1887, and for whom the disease is named.[2] Other names for this malady have included *undulant fever, melitensis fever, Mediterranean fever,* and *Bang's disease* following the isolation of a similar organism *(Brucella abortus)* from cows in Denmark in 1897.[1]

Ocular brucellosis was first recognized in domestic animals by Fabyan in 1912,[3] whereas that in humans was initially reported by Lemaire,[4] who in 1924 described bilateral optic neuritis complicating a case of brucellar meningitis. Since that time, numerous case series and individual reports of ophthalmic brucellosis involving multiple ocular structures, especially the uvea, have appeared in the literature.[5–15]

ETIOLOGY

Brucellosis is caused by small aerobic, nonmotile, non–spore-forming, gram-negative coccobacilli, of which seven species with multiple biotypes have been identified: *Brucella melitensis* (three biovars), *B. abortus* (seven biovars), *B. suis* (five biovars), *B. neotomae, B. ovis, B. canis,* and most recently, a type affecting marine mammals, tentatively named *B. maris*.[16, 17] Each species may have one or more hosts; the principal host or hosts of *B. melitensis* are sheep, goats, camels, and some cattle, while that of *B. abortus* is cattle, *B. suis* is swine, *B. neotomae* is the rat, *B. ovis* is sheep, and *B. canis* is the dog. *B. abortus* is the most widespread form among animals, whereas in humans, *B. abortus, B. suis, B. canis,* and *B. melitensis* may produce disease, with *B. melitensis* being the most pathogenic and clinically apparent.

EPIDEMIOLOGY

Brucellosis is distributed worldwide, infecting an estimated one-half million individuals annually, and remains a significant economic problem with respect to disease among domesticated animals and livestock.[17] Although mandatory pasteurization of dairy products and veterinary control measures (livestock slaughter, quarantine, and vaccination) have dramatically reduced the incidence of human brucellosis to less than 0.5 cases per 100,000 population in the United States,[18] it remains prevalent in the developing world, especially in the Mediterranean basin, the Arab Gulf countries, India, and in certain regions of Central and South America. Since 1980, fewer than 200 cases have been reported annually in the United States, with more than half of these being from four states (Texas, California, Virginia, and Florida). In Saudi Arabia, where the disease is endemic, the prevalence of brucellosis has been estimated to range between 8.8% and 38%.[19–21]

In domesticated animals, *Brucella* spp. infection manifests as a chronic genitourinary tract infection, eventuating in abortions, retained placentas, epididymitis, and chronic interstitial mastitis.[17, 22] Erythritol, a growth factor for *Brucella*, has been demonstrated in the seminal vesicles and placentas of sheep, goats, swine, and cattle but not in human tissues.[17, 22, 23] Recently, the *ery* gene has been reported to have undergone a 7.2-kbp deletion in the *B. abortus* strain, possibly explaining this strain's erythritol sensitivity, and its attenuation.[16, 24]

Human disease may follow consumption of contaminated meat, unpasteurized milk or cheese, or through occupational contact with infected animals and their products.[16, 25] Transmission may occur directly through abraded skin or mucous membranes, by aerosolization,[26] and even from cosmetics prepared from bovine placental extracts.[27] High-risk groups include abattoir workers, meat inspectors, animal handlers, veterinarians, laboratory workers handling the organism,[27–30] and travelers to endemic areas.[31] Although human-to-human transmission has been reported through tissue transplantation or sexual contact, such incidences are exceedingly rare.[32]

Brucellosis in children comprises 3% to 10% of all reported cases and is often a mild and self-limited process.[33] However, the diagnosis must be considered in any child residing in an endemic area who presents with a febrile illness and a history of animal exposure.[34]

MOLECULAR GENETICS, PATHOLOGY, AND IMMUNOLOGY

Over the past decade, substantial progress has been made in the characterization of the molecular genetics of *Brucella*, as is superbly reviewed by Corbel.[16] *Brucella* is classified as a monospecific genus, with all its members demonstrating greater than 95% homology in DNA-pairing studies,[35] with the average molecular complexity of the genome being 2.37×10^9 daltons and the molar G+C being 58% to 59%.[36] Natural plasmids have not been detected in *Brucella*, with the genome being comprised of two chromosomes (2.1 and 1.5 mbp respectively), which encode all essential metabolic and replicative functions.[37, 38] Ribosomal RNA sequencing has identified a phylogenetic relationship to *Agrobacterium, Phyllobacterium, Ochrobacterium, Rhizobium,* and the *Bartonella* group.[39–42]

The susceptibility and magnitude of infection with *Brucella* are dependent on multiple factors, including the route and size of the inoculum, the nutritional and immune status of the host, and the species itself, with *B. melitensis* and *B. suis* being the most virulent in humans, followed by *B. abortus* and *B. canis.*[17, 25] The principal determinant of both the antibody response and of virulence is the cell wall lipopolysaccharide (LPS) complex, which contains two major surface antigens (A and M).[16, 17] The structure of the LPS of smooth-phase strains (S-LPS) is essentially the same as that of nonsmooth strains (R-LPS), except for minor differences in the O-specific side chains, with the specificity of the R-LPS being conferred largely by the core polysaccharide.[16] Virulence and resistance to intracellular killing by polymorphonuclear leukocytes (PMNs) appear to be associated with S-LPS strains.[25]

Having invaded the body through the portal of entry (skin, mucous membranes, lungs, or gastrointestinal tract), *brucellae* are phagocytized by PMNs and macrophages. These microorganisms are capable of surviving within phagocytic cells for prolonged periods of time, having evolved a number of mechanisms to evade intracellular killing. Survival within PMNs appears to involve a potent superoxide dismutase system.[43] The production of adenine and guanine monophosphate, which inhibit phagolysozome fusion, degranulation of peroxidase-positive granules in PMNs, and thus the myeloperoxidase-H_2O_2-halide antibacterial system, is thought to promote intracellular survival,[44] and may be responsible for the greater virulence of *B. melitensis.*[45]

Organisms capable of evading killing by PMNs migrate to regional lymph notes, the systemic circulation, and the organs of the reticuloendothelial system (RES), most notably the spleen, where they may survive and multiply within monocytes and macrophages. Survival within macrophages is promoted by the production of specific stress-induced proteins.[16, 46] Macrophage activation is associated with intracellular killing of the organism and the release of endotoxin from the bacterial cell wall, the latter being at least partially responsible for some of the signs and symptoms of acute brucellosis.[17, 47, 48]

Both humoral and cell-mediated immune responses arise in response to brucellosis infection and to immunization with live-attenuated vaccines. Antibodies to *Brucella* are detectable within 1 to 2 weeks following exposure.[25] IgM rises first and begins to decline within 3 months from the onset of the infection. The switch to the IgG isotype occurs by the second week and may remain elevated for at least a year in untreated patients.[49] IgG levels are undetectable or fall to very low levels within 6 months in adequately treated individuals. IgA antibodies are detectable weeks after the appearance of IgG.[17] Reinfection or disease recrudescence may be heralded by elevated IgG and possibly IgM anti-*Brucella* antibody titers.[49] A recent study suggests, however, that IgG and not IgM antibody levels become elevated in relapsing brucellosis.[50] Undoubtedly, specific antibodies opsonize *Brucellae,* promoting uptake by phagocytic cells and reducing the num-

ber of organisms in the liver and spleen, and appear to play a role in resistance.[51–53] However, the elimination of intracellular microorganisms requires the activation of macrophages and the development of Th1-type cell-mediated immunity.[25] Studies in experimental animals have demonstrated the presence of lymphokines and cytokines (IL-1, IL-2, IFN-γ, TNF-α) 7 to 10 days following infection, produced by specifically sensitized T lymphocytes, which activate macrophages and enhance the elimination of intracellular bacteria.[17, 25, 54, 55] Coincident with the development of cellular immunity, granulomata may form in the liver and spleen, together with dermal hypersensitivity to various *Brucella* antigens.[17, 25]

Clinical manifestations of acute brucellosis are thought to be the direct consequence of infection with the microorganism itself; however, immune complex–mediated disease has been described.[17, 56] In addition, autoantibodies (rheumatoid factor and antinuclear antibodies) have been reported in patients with active disease, suggesting a putative pathogenetic role.[57]

The pathogenesis of ocular disease, which may manifest during either the acute or chronic phase of systemic brucellosis, is largely unknown. Because systemic infection is necessary for the production of disease, it is quite conceivable that some of the ocular manifestations are due to direct bacterial invasion, at least during the acute phase of disease. With respect to the pathogenesis of uveitis, which may evolve well after adequate systemic therapy for the acute disease, a combination of synergistic mechanisms, including initial direct invasion of the microorganism with subsequent hypersensitivity to bacterial products or the development of autoimmunity, are likely to be operative.

CLINICAL FEATURES

Systemic Disease

Systemic brucellosis may involve any organ system in the body with protean nonspecific signs and symptoms, the nature and severity of which are related to the immune status of the host, the presence or absence of underlying disease, and the species and strain of the offending organism. More severe disease and subsequent complications involving multiple organ systems are more often associated with infection by *B. melitensis,* and, to a lesser extent, *B. suis,* than that with *B. abortus* or *B. canis.*[58] Clinically, brucellosis may be divided into subclinical disease, acute or subacute illness, localized disease and complications, relapsing infection, and chronic disease.

Subclinical Disease

The incubation period for brucellosis is variable, ranging from 1 week to several months, with symptoms generally appearing within 2 to 3 weeks of inoculation.[17, 25] Subclinical disease is most often diagnosed serologically among high-risk individuals (e.g., veterinarians, abattoir workers) and manifests as a mild flulike illness, usually without sequela. Subclinical cases are common among children from endemic areas and are thought to outnumber clinically apparent brucellosis by 12:1.[33]

Acute and Subacute Illness

In approximately 50% of patients, acute brucellosis may present as an acute, toxic illness arising over a period of days (especially with *B. melitensis* infection), whereas in the remainder, the onset is insidious. Acute disease is characterized by multiple somatic complaints, of which fever, drenching sweats, chills, and weakness are present in over 90% of cases.[59-61] Fever, which occurs in all patients at some point during the illness, tends to peak in the afternoon, whereas an undulating or intermittent pattern, once thought to be characteristic of the disease, is distinctly unusual.[10, 60, 61] Other common symptoms include malaise, headache, anorexia, weight loss, myalgias, arthralgias, and back pain. Mild lymphadenopathy, involving predominantly the cervical and inguinal chains, together with splenomegaly, may occur in up to 21% and 30% of patients, respectively.[60]

Localized Disease and Complications

Almost any organ or organ system may become involved with, and develop complications arising from, *Brucella* infection, particularly those containing elements of the reticuloendothelial system. In such instances, the disease is said to be localized, more commonly involving bone, central nervous system (CNS), heart, lungs, hepatobiliary system, testes, and skin. Localized disease may arise with either acute or chronic infection.

Osteoarticular involvement is most frequent, occurring in approximately 40% of cases in some series.[62] Sacroiliitis, arthritis involving the knee and hip joints, spondylitis, tenosynovitis, osteomyelitis, and bursitis have all been reported. The sacroiliac joint is most commonly involved in regions where infection with *B. melitensis* is predominant.[63] Spondylitis, which has been reported to occur in 5% of cases,[64] usually develops in elderly patients, presenting as pain over the involved vertebral bodies, and may be complicated by the development of paraspinal abscesses requiring surgical drainage.[17] In contrast to tuberculous spondylitis, spinal brucellosis more frequently involves the lumbar vertebrae.[25]

Gastrointestinal and hepatobiliary complications are not uncommon, with between 30% and 60% of patients exhibiting mildly abnormal liver function tests and a smaller percentage developing hepatomegaly.[59] A broad spectrum of hepatic lesions has been described in cases of *B. melitensis* infection, with a notable paucity of granuloma formation,[65] whereas those caused by *B. abortus* characteristically produce noncaseating epithelioid granulomata similar to those seen in sarcoidosis.[66] Localized infection by *B. suis* is commonly associated with hepatic abscesses and chronic suppurative lesions of the liver and spleen.[67] Whereas these hepatic lesions may be extensive, they usually respond to treatment, with the incidence of cirrhosis being extremely rare.[25, 67]

Pulmonary symptoms may arise following inhalation of infected aerosols, with cough and dyspnea being reported in up to 15% of cases.[68] Hilar adenopathy, interstitial infiltrates, lung nodules, abscesses, emphysema, and pneumothorax have also been described.[17]

Genitourinary involvement is uncommon, with unilateral acute orchitis or epididymo-orchitis being the most frequent manifestation.[17] Renal involvement is rare; however, caseating granulomata and calcifications resembling renal tuberculosis have been reported.[69]

It is well established that brucellosis may produce abortions in animals. Whether infection with *Brucella* per se increases the risk of abortion in humans, as compared with that of other bacteremic infections occurring during pregnancy, has not been properly evaluated in case-controlled studies.[17, 25]

Frank CNS involvement is rare, occurring in less than 2% of cases, with acute or chronic meningitis being the most common manifestation.[70, 71] On the other hand, depression and mental fatigue are commonly observed among patients with brucellosis.[25] Examination of the cerebrospinal fluid (CSF) usually reveals a lymphocytic pleocytosis with an elevated protein and a reduced glucose level.[71] Except in cases of acute meningitis, the organism is rarely cultured from the CSF; however, *Brucella*-specific antibodies are usually present in the CSF, providing specific confirmation for the diagnosis of neurobrucellosis.[17, 71]

The most common cause of death among patients with brucellosis is endocarditis, occurring in less than 2% of cases.[72] Treatment usually involves both the administration of systemic antibiotics and surgical replacement of the involved (usually the aortic) valve[73]; however, successful conservative treatment of *Brucella* endocarditis, with antibiotics alone, has been described.[74]

Cutaneous manifestations of brucellosis are often transient and nonspecific, occurring in approximately 5% of patients.[60] Erythema nodosum, papules, a variety of rashes (eczematous, rubeliform, scarlatinoform), petechiae, purpura, and cutaneous granulomatous vasculitis have all been reported.[17]

Relapsing Infection

Relapsing disease occurs in up to 10% of patients with brucellosis,[33] usually within weeks to months after the completion of antibiotic therapy.[25] The cause of disease relapse is thought to relate to the intracellular location of the organism and its ability to evade phagocytosis, particularly when sequestered in a localized site requiring surgical drainage, together with an inadequate or abbreviated course of antibiotic therapy. Although antibiotic-resistant strains have been isolated,[75] they are not thought to be responsible for the vast majority of relapses.

Chronic Disease

Chronic brucellosis, by definition, is disease that persists for more than 1 year. Many of these patients manifest objective signs of infection and are found, on thorough examination, to have actually relapsing disease due to inadequate antibiotic treatment or to sequestered localized infection.[76] A subset of these patients with no objective signs of infection complain of fatigue, malaise, and depression, benefitting little from retreatment with antibiotics. The question of whether these patients may suffer from a form of psychoneurosis, or whether their delayed convalescence, despite adequate treatment, may be a variant of the chronic fatigue syndrome, is a matter for further study.[77]

The Immunocompromised Host

An increased incidence of brucellosis has been observed in patients with Hodgkin's disease and other lymphomas.[33] In contrast, human immunodeficiency virus (HIV) infection did not seem to increase the incidence of brucellosis in one series of 12 HIV-infected patients diagnosed with brucellosis.[78] Conversely, the evolution of HIV did not appear to be influenced by the presence of brucellosis The clinical presentation, diagnosis, response to therapy, and outcome were similar to those observed in non–HIV-infected patients.

Vaccine-Related Disease

In recent years, cases of brucellosis among veterinarians accidentally inoculated with vaccines derived from strains with attenuated virulence for immunization of animals (*B. abortus* strain 19 and *B. melitensis* strain Rev-1) have been reported.[79, 80] Percutaneous needle sticks, conjunctival splashes, or ingestion are the common modes of exposure. Veterinarians previously exposed to *Brucella* are at less risk of acquiring the disease by virtue of pre-existing antibodies but frequently develop severe inflammation at the site of the inoculation. The absence of pre-existing antibodies to *Brucella* and exposure through the conjunctival route (larger inoculum size) are associated with a greater risk of acquiring the disease. In general, vaccine-associated disease is milder than the natural disease.

Ocular Manifestations

Eye disease in systemic brucellosis is uncommon but may involve a wide variety of ocular structures. Although 20% of patients reported by Spink had visual symptoms, only 2% manifested ocular findings.[60] Of 100 consecutive cases of systemic brucellosis seen in Saudi Arabia, the prevalence of ophthalmic disease was found to be 3%.[81] The array of ocular disease includes (Table 20–1) nummular keratitis, corneal ulceration, scleritis, granulomatous or nongranulomatous iridocyclitis, vitritis, panuveitis, endophthalmitis, multifocal choroiditis, retinitis, retinal vasculitis, cystoid macular edema (CME), retinal detachment, papilledema, retrobulbar optic neuritis, chiasmal arachnoiditis, and optic atrophy.[5–15, 81, 82]

Uveitis is thought to be the most common ocular manifestation of brucellosis,[1, 5, 12, 13, 81, 82] developing in one or both eyes, usually during the acute phase of systemic infection. However, it may persist as chronic, smoldering, recurrent intraocular inflammation, either after initial treatment with systemic antibiotics[82] or in cases in which the diagnosis was not suspected.[13]

Anterior uveitis may be either granulomatous or nongranulomatous, ranging in severity from mild inflammation with typical "mutton-fat" keratic precipitates to severe inflammation with the development of hypopyon, metastatic endophthalmitis, and phthisis bulbi.[1, 11] Chronic iridocyclitis may produce thickening of the iris with the formation of Koeppe's nodules, posterior synechiae, lenticular opacities, and secondary glaucoma.

Multifocal choroiditis, either in a geographic pattern[12] or associated with circumscribed nodular exudates with little surrounding retinal edema or inflammation,[1] is thought to be characteristic of posterior segment disease. Well-circumscribed choroidal lesions in the retinal periphery have also been recently described.[82] Although the choroidal exudates usually resolve, leaving hyperpigmented scars in their wake, they may recur.[1]

Vitritis of varying degrees is quite common. Cystoid macular edema, retinal vasculitis,[12, 81] and retinal detachment[9] may also complicate brucellar uveitis.

Optic nerve involvement, usually as a direct extension of leptomeningeal infection, may manifest as papilledema, retrobulbar optic neuritis, optic atrophy, or arachnoiditis of the chiasm, with accompanying enlargement of the blind spots, bilateral visual field constriction, and in some cases, profound visual loss.[8, 14] In the series reported by Puig-Solanes and coworkers,[8] 44 of 413 (10.7%) patients were observed to have optic nerve involvement, whereas only eight had uveitis.

Uncommon ocular manifestations of brucellosis include nummular subepithelial corneal infiltrates or ulcers with accompanying iritis, as reported by Woods[6] among five patients with serologic or allergic evidence of *Brucella* exposure. Conjunctivitis and scleritis, of either the diffuse or nodular variety, have also been described.[12]

DIAGNOSIS

The diagnosis of both systemic and ocular brucellosis cannot be made on clinical grounds alone, because most patients present with nonspecific signs and symptoms shared by many other infectious diseases. However, a history of fever, chills, arthralgias and night sweats, together with that of occupational exposure, travel to endemic areas, or the ingestion of unpasteurized milk or dairy products, raises brucellosis as a diagnostic possibility. The definitive diagnosis of brucellosis relies on the isolation and culture of the organism from the blood, bone marrow, or other tissues, including the ocular fluids. Routine laboratory tests are generally uninformative, except that there may be a mild leukocytopenia, or abnormal liver function tests. A presumptive diagnosis is suggested by elevated or rising titers of specific anti-*Brucella* antibodies. Overall, blood cultures are positive in 10% to 30% of cases of acute brucellosis,[33] with a much higher yield on blood and bone marrow specimens (70% and 90%, respectively) in patients infected with *B. melitensis*.[17] Among individuals with meningitis, the CSF is culture positive in 45% of cases.[33] Isolation of the organism in subacute cases of *B. melitensis* and chronic infection with all other species is typically unrewarding. Because the organisms are slow growing, cultures should be main-

TABLE 20–1. OPHTHALMIC FINDINGS IN BRUCELLOSIS

Nummular keratitis	Endophthalmitis
Corneal ulcer	Multifocal choroiditis
	Retinitis
Scleritis	Retinal vasculitis
Diffuse	Cystoid macular edema
Nodular	Retinal detachment
Uveitis	**Optic nerve involvement**
Iridocyclitis	Papilledema
Granulomatous	Retrobulbar optic neuritis
Nongranulomatous	Arachnoiditis of the chiasm
Vitritis	Optic atrophy
Panuveitis	

tained for between 4 and 6 weeks. A commonly employed method uses the Casteñeda system; however, radiometric detection systems and lysis concentration have shortened the incubation time to a matter of days.[83] Although brucellae have not been cultured or demonstrated histopathologically from the cornea in patients with keratitis, *B. melitensis* biotype 3 was successfully cultured in a 17-year-old patient found to have *Brucella*-induced endophthalmitis.[11] In another patient with uveitis, the organism was isolated from a paravertebral abscess.[13]

A variety of serologic techniques have been applied in the presumptive diagnosis of brucellosis, the most common of which is the serum agglutination test (SAT). This test, which uses an antigen prepared from *B. abortus* strain 119, detects antibodies against *B. abortus*, *B. melitensis*, and *B. suis* but not *B. canis*.[25] Infection with *B. canis* requires specific *B. canis* agglutination tests or an enzyme-linked immunosorbent assay (ELISA), which uses an antigen prepared from the outer membrane proteins of *B. melitensis*.[84] The SAT, which measures the total quantity of agglutinating antibody (i.e., both IgG and IgM), is considered significant with titers in excess of 1:160 in patients with acute or recently acquired infection. However, these titers may persist for more than 1 year, even after appropriate antibiotic therapy, obfuscating the differentiation between relapsing and chronic disease. The quantity of specific IgG antibody may be determined by the addition of 0.05 M 2-mercaptoethanol (2-ME) to the SAT, which inactivates IgM antibodies.[85] Although no single value is uniformly diagnostic, a 2-ME *Brucella* titer of 1:160 or greater is indicative of ongoing infection, whereas a titer of less than 1:160 argues against chronic disease if it is obtained a year or more following the onset of the illness.[85, 86]

In cases of ocular brucellosis, calculation of the Witmer coefficient of ocular and systemic antibodies may be diagnostically valuable.[87] Akduman and colleagues[15] reported a case of brucellar uveitis that presented 3 months following systemic antibiotic therapy in which the agglutination titer in the vitreous specimen (1:640) far exceeded that of the aqueous humor (1:40) and the serum (1:20).

A false-negative SAT may occur due to the presence of blocking antibodies in the patient's serum.[25] This effect may be obviated by diluting the serum beyond 1:320 and repeating the SAT in patients with initially negative results yet clinically suspected of having brucellosis. In addition, the *Brucella* SAT may cross-react with antibodies in patients infected with *Francisella tularensis*, *Yersinia enterocolitica*, or *Vibrio cholerae*.[17]

Among the newer available serologic tests, the ELISA appears to be the most sensitive. In a prospective study of 400 cases of brucellosis in Kuwait, ELISA readily detected *Brucella*-specific immunoglobulins IgG, IgM, and IgA in the CSF and allowed the differentiation, based on serum immunoglobulin profiles, of patients with chronic (elevated IgG and IgA) from acute (elevated IgM alone or IgG, IgM, or IgA) disease.[10] More experience with ELISA is necessary before it replaces the SAT, because the SAT remains the serologic "gold standard."

Polymerase chain reaction (PCR), using random or

TABLE 20–2. DIFFERENTIAL DIAGNOSIS OF OCULAR BRUCELLOSIS

Infectious
  Tuberculosis
  Syphilis
  Lyme disease
  Outer retinal toxoplasmosis
  Diffuse unilateral subacute neuroretinitis (DUSN)
  Septic choroiditis
  Viral retinitis (cytomegalovirus, herpes simplex, herpes zoster)
  Presumed ocular histoplasmosis syndrome (POHS)
Noninfectious
  Sarcoidosis
  Multifocal choroiditis and panuveitis (MCP)
  Subretinal fibrosis and uveitis (SFU)
  Vogt-Koyanagi-Harada syndrome (VKH)
  Birdshot retinochoroidopathy (BSRC)
  Acute posterior multifocal placoid pigment epitheliopathy (APMPPE)
  Multiple evanescent white dot syndrome (MEWDS)
  Punctate inner choroidopathy (PIC)
  Sympathetic ophthalmia
  Masquerade syndrome (large-cell lymphoma)
  Collagen vascular disease
  HLA-B27–associated iridocyclitis

selected oligonucleotide primers, is a promising diagnostic technique.[88, 89] Likewise, Western blotting against selected cytoplasmic proteins may prove to be a useful screening modality for the differentiation between acute and subclinical infection.[16, 90] Finally, although dermal hypersensitivity reactions are common among patients with brucellosis, skin testing is neither standardized nor employed for diagnostic purposes.[25]

The differential diagnosis of ocular brucellosis is broad and requires the systematic exclusion of other infectious and noninfectious causes of uveitis, especially those producing multifocal choroiditis (Table 20–2). Among the infectious entities to be considered, the most important are tuberculosis and syphilis, because their antimicrobial therapy is specific and different from that of brucellosis. Other infectious diseases would include Lyme disease, outer retinal toxoplasmosis, diffuse unilateral subacute neuroretinitis (DUSN), septic choroiditis, viral retinitis (cytomegalovirus, herpes simplex, herpes zoster), and presumed ocular histoplasmosis syndrome (POHS).

Among the noninfectious uveitides simulating brucellar multifocal choroiditis, sarcoidosis is the most important differential, followed by those entities listed in Table 20–2. Because some patients with ocular brucellosis may present with iridocyclitis, with or without posterior uveitis, together with the not infrequent occurrence of osteoarticular involvement, HLA-B27–associated ocular inflammatory disease, as well as that associated with collagen vascular diseases, should be considered in the differential diagnosis.

TREATMENT

Effective antibiotic therapy for brucellosis requires good intracellular penetration because the organisms are facultative intracellular pathogens, a prolonged course to prevent relapse, and bactericidal drugs for the treatment of endocarditis and CNS disease. Moreover, monotherapy with agents such as tetracycline, streptomycin, rifampin, or trimethoprim-sulfamethoxazole (TMP-SMZ) result in an unacceptably high (10% to 40%) rate of relapse.[59, 91] Although it is generally agreed that combination therapy is indicated, there is no consensus as to which regimen is optimal for the treatment of systemic brucellosis.

The combination of tetracycline 2 g/day orally for 6 weeks plus streptomycin 1 g/day intramuscularly for 3 weeks has been widely employed for the treatment of acute brucellosis in the absence of endocarditis or CNS involvement and is associated with a less than 5% relapse rate.[25, 92] Doxycycline has replaced tetracycline owing to its longer half-life and the need for less frequent dosing. Gentamicin, although equally effective and less toxic than streptomycin, has been used as a second agent, but both drugs require parenteral administration.[93]

The regimen currently recommended by the World Health Organization is doxycycline 200 mg/day orally plus rifampin 600 to 900 mg/day orally for a 6-week period.[54] Rifampin has excellent intracellular penetration, crosses the blood-brain barrier well, and is the drug of choice for pregnant women.[54] Similar efficacy has been demonstrated in studies comparing the doxycycline-rifampin and the doxycycline-streptomycin regimens, although the latter may be more effective for the treatment of complications such as spondylitis.[94, 95]

Whereas monotherapy with TMP-SMZ is associated with an unacceptably high rate of relapse in adults,[91] it may be used as an alternative to rifampin during pregnancy and is the preferred drug for the treatment of children younger than 6 years of age with acute brucellosis for whom tetracyclines are contraindicated.[25] The drug is administered four times daily orally for 6 weeks, with some experts advocating the concomitant use of gentamicin for the first 5 days to prevent relapse.[96]

As with other drugs that demonstrate good in vitro activity against *Brucella*, the fluoroquinolones, specifically ofloxacin, were associated with high relapse rates when used alone. However, the combination of ofloxacin 400 mg plus rifampin 600 mg daily compared favorably with the doxycycline (200 mg)-rifampin (600-mg) regimen when administered for 6 weeks.[97]

The treatment of endocarditis and CNS complications arising from systemic brucellosis infection is similar to that described for acute disease, except that longer courses of therapy are recommended, usually between 6 and 9 months.[25] In addition to prolonged antibiotic therapy, endocarditis frequently requires cardiac surgery to replace the infected valve.[72, 73] Brucellar meningitis has responded to triple therapy with doxycycline, rifampin, and TMP-SMZ.[71] However, some authorities have suggested that a combination of rifampin and a third-generation cephalosporin, such as ceftriaxone or ceftizoxime, be employed in these patients, because both drugs achieve good CSF levels.[98, 99]

Therapy for uveitis associated with brucellosis mandates adequate initial treatment of the underlying infectious disease, as outlined earlier. As with treatment of CNS complications, there is a rationale for the use of rifampin and a third-generation cephalosporin for eyes with uveitis in which intraocular pathogens are demonstrated, because these agents also achieve good intraocular drug levels. However, many cases of brucellar uveitis may appear after adequate initial antibiotic therapy, supporting the notion that, at least in some cases, the ocular manifestations are due to a noninfectious immune response. Treatment in such cases would then consist of nonspecific anti-inflammatory therapy with topical or systemic steroids, titrated to the degree and location of the intraocular inflammation, provided the systemic disease has been adequately controlled with antibiotic therapy.

PROGNOSIS

With the prompt institution of appropriate antimicrobial therapy, most cases of acute brucellosis are curable. Prolonged antibiotic therapy reduces the risk of localized and chronic disease. Most patients develop immunity to reinfection following the initial infection with *Brucella*.[33] Endocarditis associated with severe congestive heart failure is the leading cause of mortality, occurring in less than 2% of patients.[72]

Similarly, the visual prognosis with ocular disease depends on timely diagnosis and treatment. Tabbara and Al-Kassini reported a case of a young woman with chronic, recurrent uveitis in which the diagnosis of ocular brucellosis was missed for a period of 9 years.[13] With appropriate antibiotic therapy, the patient's symptoms improved dramatically, with a reduction of the intraocular inflammation and a marked improvement in visual acuity. Secondary complications arising from inappropriately treated chronic, smoldering intraocular inflammation (cataract, glaucoma, cystic macula, optic neuropathy and vitreous condensation with fibrosis and tractional retinal detachment) may produce irreversible damage to ocular structures critical for good vision. Patients with optic nerve involvement[8, 14] or choroiditis involving the fovea may experience profound visual loss.

PREVENTION

The elimination of brucellosis among domesticated animals and livestock is the principal means for the prevention of human disease. Surveillance and eradication programs for the identification and elimination of infected animals and the use of *B. abortus* strain 119 vaccine in cattle and *B. melitensis* strain Rev-1 vaccine in sheep and goats has virtually eliminated the disease in these animals in the United States.[18, 25] The implementation, execution, and funding of such programs in the developing world remains problematic. Nevertheless, pasteurizing or heating milk to 60°C for 10 minutes kills *Brucella* in dairy products.[81]

Both live attenuated vaccines[100] and a variety of killed Brucella fractions[101] have been used to immunize humans at high risk of contracting the disease; however, these strategies are not without the risk of producing disease itself or are of heretofore unproven benefit. Hence, universal precautions should be exercised by individuals at high risk for contracting the disease, and travelers to endemic regions should be educated as to the potential avenues of exposure.

CONCLUSION

Although brucellosis among animals and humans is uncommon in developed countries, it remains a significant economic and public health problem in many parts of the developing world, especially where it is endemic. A heightened degree of clinical suspicion in patients with an exposure history, together with supporting serologic testing, isolation, and culture of the organism, are essential to making the diagnosis. Early institution of specific multiagent antimicrobial therapy may be curative, reduce morbidity, and is an essential first step in the treatment of associated ocular disease. Uveitis is the most common ophthalmic manifestation, although virtually any ocular structure may be involved. The precise pathogenesis of intraocular inflammation is unknown but may involve direct invasion of the microorganism, a noninfectious immune response, or both. As with systemic infection, prompt recognition and timely treatment of intraocular inflammation is vital for the preservation of vision.

References

1. Duke-Elder S, Perkins ES: Disease of the uveal tract. In: Duke-Elder S, ed: System of Ophthalmology, vol 9. London, Kimpton, 1966, pp 236–242.
2. Bruce D: Note on the discovery of microorganism in Malta fever. Practitioner 1887;39:161–170.
3. Fabyan M: A contribution to the pathogenesis of *B. abortus*, Bang.-II. J Med Res 1912;21:441–487.
4. Lemaire MG: Méningite a mélitocoques altérations importantes du liquide céphalo-rachidien. Bulletins et Mémoires de la Société Médecin de l'Hôpital de Paris 1924;48:1636–1652.
5. Green J: Ocular manifestations in brucellosis (undulant fever). Arch Ophthalmol 1939;21:51–67.
6. Woods AC: Nummular keratitis and ocular brucellosis. Arch Ophthalmol 1946;35;490–508.
7. Foggit KD: Ocular disease due to brucellosis. Br J Ophthalmol 1953;38:273.
8. Puig-Solanes M, Heatley J, Arenas F, et al: Ocular complications in brucellosis. Am J Ophthalmol 1953;36:675–689.
9. Rolando I, Carbone A, Haro D, et al: Retinal detachment in chronic brucellosis. Am J Ophthalmol 1985;99:733–734.
10. Lulu AR, Arah GF, Khateeb MI, et al: Human brucellosis in Kuwait: A prospective study of 400 cases. Q J Med 1988;66:39–54.
11. Al-Faran MF: *Brucella melitensis* endogenous endophthalmitis. Ophthalmologica 1990;201:19–22.
12. Tabbara KF: Brucellosis and nonsyphilitic treponemal uveitis. Int Ophthalmol Clin 1990;30:294–296.
13. Tabbara KF, Al-Kassini H: Ocular brucellosis. Br J Ophthalmol 1990;74:249–250.
14. Abd Elrazak M: *Brucella* optic neuritis. Arch Intern Med 1991;151:776–778.
15. Akduman L, Or M, Hasenreisoglu B, et al: A case of ocular brucellosis: Importance of ocular specimen. Acta Ophthalmol 1993;71;130–132.
16. Corbel MJ: Brucellosis: An overview. Emerg Infect Dis 1997;3:213–221.
17. Mikolich DJ, Boyce JM: *Brucella* species. In: Mandell GL, Douglas RG, Bennett JE, eds: Principles and Practices of Infectious Diseases, 3rd ed. New York, Churchill Livingstone, 1990, pp 1735–1742.
18. Centers for Disease Control: Disease Information, Division of Bacterial and Mycotic Diseases. Brucellosis. Atlanta, Centers for Disease Control, December, 1999.
19. Talukder MA, Moaz A, Al-Admawy O, et al: Brucellosis: Experiences in Saudi Arabia. Dev Biol Stand 1984;56:597–599.
20. Arrighi HM: Brucellosis surveillance in Saudi Arabia's Eastern Province. Ann Saudi Med 1986;6(Suppl 5):5–10.
21. Talukder MA, Abomelha MS, Higham RH: Brucellosis in a farming community in Saudi Arabia. Dev Biol Stand 1984;56:593–595.
22. Evans LS, Tessler HH: Brucellosis. In: Gold DH, Weingeist TA, eds: The Eye in Systemic Disease. Philadelphia, Lippincott, 1990, pp 159–161.
23. Al-Kaff AS: Ocular brucellosis. Int Ophthalmol Clin 1995;35:139–145.
24. Sangari FJ, García-Lobo JM, Aguero J: The *Brucella abortus* vaccine strain B19 carries a deletion in the erythritol catabolic genes. FEMS Microbiol Lett 1994;121:337–342.
25. Young EJ: An overview of human brucellosis. Clin Infect Dis 1995;21:283–290.
26. Kaufmann AF: Airborne spread of brucellosis. Ann N Y Acad Sci 1980;353:105–114.
27. Grave W, Sturm AW: Brucellosis associated with a beauty parlour. Lancet 1983;1:1326–1327.
28. Al-Aska AK: Laboratory acquired brucellosis. J Hosp Infec 1989;14:69–71.
29. Kiel FW: Brucellosis among hospital employees in Saudi Arabia. Infect Control Hosp Epidemiol 1993;14:268–272.
30. Mazuelos-Martin E: Outbreak of *Brucella melitensis* among microbiology laboratory workers. J Clin Microbiol 1994;32:2035–2036.
31. Steffen R: Antacids—a risk factor in travelers' brucellosis. Scand J Infect Dis 1977;9:311–312.
32. Mantur BG, Mangalgi SS, Mulimani B: *Brucella melitensis*—a sexually transmissible agent. Lancet 1996;347:1763.
33. Salata RA: Brucellosis. In: Wyngarden JB, Smith LH, Bennett JC, eds: Cecil Textbook of Medicine, ed. 19, vol. II. Philadelphia, WB Saunders, 1992, pp 1727–1729.
34. Benjamin B: Childhood brucellosis in Southwestern Saudi Arabia: A 5-year experience. J Trop Pediatr 1992;38:167–172.
35. Verger JM, Grimont F, Grimont PAD, et al: *Brucella*, a monospecific genus as shown by deoxyribonucleic acid hybridization. Int J Syst Bacteriol 1985;35:292–295.
36. De Ley J, Mannheim W, Segers P, et al: Ribosomal ribonucleic acid cistron similarities and taxonomic neighbourhood of *Brucella* and CDC Group Vd. Int J Syst Bacteriol 1987;37:35–42.
37. Michaux S, Paillisson J, Carles-Nurit MJ, et al: Presence of two independent chromosomes in the *Brucella melitensis* 16 M genome. J Bacteriol 1993;175:701–705.
38. Jumas-Bitlak E, Maugard C, Michaux-Charachon S, et al: Study of the organization of *Escherichia coli*, *Brucella melitensis*, and *Argobacterium tumefaciens* by insertion of a unique restriction site. Microbiology 1995;141:2425–2432.
39. Cieslak TJ, Robb ML, Drabick CJ, et al: Catheter-associated sepsis caused by *Onchrobactrum anthropi*: A report of a case and review of related non-fermentative bacteria. Clin Infect Dis 1992;14:902–907.
40. Da Costa M, Guillou J-P, Garin-Bastuji B, et al: Specificity of six gene sequences for the detection of the genus *Brucella* by DNA amplification. J Appl Bacteriol 1996;81:267–275.
41. Minnick MF, Stiegler GL: Nucleotide sequence and comparison of the 5S ribosomal genes of *Rochalimaea henselae*, *R. quintana*, and *Brucella abortus*. Nucleic Acids Res 1993;21:2518.
42. Relman DA, Lepp PW, Sadler KN, et al: Phylogenetic relationships among the agent of bacillary angiomatosis, *Bartonella bacilliformis*, and other alpha-proteobacteria. Mol Microbiol 1992;6:1801–1807.
43. Bricker BJ, Tabatabai LB, Jurge BA, et al: Cloning, expression and occurrence of the *Brucella* Cu-Zn dismutase. Infect Immun 1990;58:2933–2939.
44. Canning PC, Roth JA, Deyoe BL: Release of 5'-guanosine monophosphate and adenine by *Brucella abortus* and their role in the intracellular survival of the bacteria. J Infect Dis 1986;154:464–470.
45. Young EJ, Borchert M, Kretzer FL, et al: Phagocytosis and killing of *Brucella* by human polymorphonuclear leukocytes. J Infect Dis 1985;151:682–690.
46. Lin J, Ficht TA: Protein synthesis in *Brucella abortus* induced during macrophage infection. Infect Immun 1995;63:1409–1414.
47. Abernathy RS, Spink WW: Studies with *Brucella* endotoxin in humans: The significance and susceptibility to endotoxin in the pathogenesis of brucellosis. J Clin Invest 1958;37:219–231.
48. Spink WW: Host-parasite relationship in brucellosis. Lancet 1964;2:161–164.
49. White RG: Immunoglobulin profiles of the chronic antibody response: Discussion in relation to *Brucella* infection. Postgrad Med J 1998;54:595–601.
50. Pellicer J, Ariza J, Fox A: Specific antibodies detected during relapse of human brucellosis. J Infect Dis 1998;157:918–924.
51. Guerra H, Deter AL, Williams RP: Infection at the subcellular level. II. Distribution and fate of intravenously injected *Brucellae* within phagocytic cells of guinea pigs. Infect Immun 1973;8:694–699.
52. Sulitzeanu D: Mechanism of immunity against *Brucella*. Nature 1965;205:1086–1088.

53. Plommet M, Plommet AM: Immune serum-mediated effects of brucellosis evolution in mice. Infect Immun 1983;41:97–105.

54. Joint FAO/WHO Expert Committee on Brucellosis: Geneva, World Health Organization, 1986.

55. Meyer ME: Brucellosis. In: Samter M, ed: Immunological Diseases. Boston, Little Brown, 1978, pp 651–659.

56. Hodinka L, Gomor B, Meretey K: HLA-B27–associated spondylarthritis in chronic brucellosis. Lancet 1978;1:499.

57. Gotuzzo E, Bocanegra JS, Alacron GS, et al: Humoral immune abnormalities in human brucellosis. Allergol Immunopathol (Madr) 1985;13:417–424.

58. Braude AI: Studies in the pathology and pathogenesis of experimental brucellosis I. A comparison of the pathogenicity of *Brucella abortus, Brucella melitensis,* and *Brucella suis* for guinea pigs. J Infect Dis 1951;89:76–82.

59. Buchanan TM, Faber LC, Feldman RA: Brucellosis in the United States, 1960–1972. An abattoir-associated disease. Part I, clinical features and therapy. Medicine 1974;53:403–413.

60. Spink WW: The Nature of Brucellosis. Minneapolis, University of Minnesota Press, 1956.

61. Dalrymple-Champneyes W: *Brucella* Infection and Undulant Fever in Man. London, Oxford University Press, 1960.

62. Mousa ARM, Muhtaseb SA, Almudallal DS, et al: Osteoarticular complications of brucellosis: A study of 169 cases. Rev Infect Dis 1987;9:531–543.

63. Ariza J, Pujol M, Valverde J, et al: Brucellar sacroiliitis: Findings in 63 episodes and current relevance. Clin Infect Dis 1993;16:761–765.

64. Ariza J, Gudiol F, Valverde J, et al: Brucellar spondylitis: A detailed analysis based on current findings. Rev Infect Dis 1985;7:656–664.

65. Young EJ: *Brucella melitensis* hepatitis: The absence of granulomas. Ann Intern Med 1979;91:414–415.

66. Spink WW, Hoffbauer FW, Walker WW, et al: Histopathology of the liver in human brucellosis. J Lab Clin Med 1949;34:40–58.

67. Williams RK, Crossley K: Acute and chronic hepatic involvement of brucellosis. Gastroenterology 1982;83:455–458.

68. Lubani MM, Lulu AR, Araj GF, et al: Pulmonary brucellosis. Q J Med 1989;71:319–324.

69. Kelalis PP, Greene LF, Weed LA: Brucellosis of the urogenital tract. A mimic of tuberculosis. J Urol 1962;88:347–353.

70. Bouza E, García de la Torre M, Parras E, et al: Brucellar meningitis. Rev Infect Dis 1987;9:810–822.

71. McLean DR, Russell N, Khan MY: Neurobrucellosis: Clinical and therapeutic features. Clin Infect Dis 1992;15:582–590.

72. Al-Harthi SS: The morbidity and mortality pattern of *Brucella* endocarditis. Int J Cardiol 1989;25:321–324.

73. Jacobs F, Abramowicz D, Vereerstiaeten P, et al: *Brucella* endocarditis: The role of combined medical and surgical treatment. Rev Infect Dis 1990;12:740–744.

74. Cohen N, Golik A, Alon I, et al: Conservative treatment for *Brucella* endocarditis. Clin Cardiol 1997;20:291–294.

75. de Raotlin de la Roy YM, Grignon B, Grollier G, et al: Rifampicin resistance in a strain of *Brucella melitensis* after treatment with doxycycline and rifampicin [letter]. J Antimicrob Chemother 1986;18:648–649.

76. Spink WW: What is chronic brucellosis? Ann Intern Med 1951;35:358–374.

77. Cluff LE: Medical aspects of delayed convalescence. Rev Infect Dis 1991;13(Suppl 1):S138–S140.

78. Moreno S, Ariza J, Espinosa D, et al: Brucellosis in patients infected with the human immunodeficiency virus. Eur J Clin Microbiol Infect Dis 1998;17:319–326.

79. Spink WN, Thompson H: Human brucellosis caused by *Brucella abortus* strain 19. JAMA 1953;153:1162–1165.

80. Blasco JM, Diaz R: *Brucella melitensis* Rev-1 vaccine as a cause of human brucellosis [letter]. Lancet 1993;342:805.

81. Tabbara KF: Brucellosis. In: Pepose JS, Holland GN, Wilhelmus KR, eds: Ocular Infection and Immunity. St. Louis, Mosby–Year Book, 1996, pp 1249–1251.

82. Walker J, Sharma OP, Rao NA: Brucellosis and uveitis. Am J Ophthalmol 1992;114:374–375.

83. Kolman S, Maayan MC, Gotesman G, et al: Comparison of the Bactec and lysis concentration methods for recovering *Brucella* species from clinical specimens. Eur J Clin Microbiol Infect Dis 1991;10:647–648.

84. Hunter SB, Bibb WF, Shah CN, et al: Enzyme-linked immunosorbent assay with outer membrane proteins of *Brucella melitensis* to measure immune response to *Brucella* species. J Clin Microbiol 1986;24:566–572.

85. Young EJ: Serologic diagnosis of human brucellosis: Analysis of 214 cases by agglutination tests and review of the literature. Rev Infect Dis 1991;13:359–372.

86. Buchanan TM, Faber LC: 2 Mercaptoethanol *Brucella* agglutination test: Usefulness for predicting recovery from brucellosis. J Clin Microbiol 1980;11:691–693.

87. Renoux GM, Larmande A, Poletti JA: Le diagnostic biologique de la brucellose ocularies. Arch Ophthalmol 1977;37:767–770.

88. Matar FM, Khreissir IA, Abdonoor AM: Rapid laboratory confirmation of human brucellosis by PCR analysis of a target sequence on the 31-kilodalton *Brucella* antigen DNA. J Clin Microbiol 1996;34:477–478.

89. Herman L, De Ridder H: Identification of *Brucella* spp by using the polymerase chain reaction. Appl Environ Microbiol 1992;58:2099–2101.

90. Goldbaum FA, Leoni J, Walach JC, et al: Characterisation of an 18 kilodalton *Brucella* cytoplasmic protein which appears to be a serological marker of active infection of both human and bovine brucellosis. J Clin Microbiol 1993;31:2141–2145.

91. Ariza J, Gudiol F, Pallares R, et al: Comparative trial of co-trimoxazole versus tetracycline-streptomycin in treating human brucellosis. J Infect Dis 1985;152:1358–1359.

92. Elberg SS: A Guide to the Diagnosis, Treatment and Prevention of Human Brucellosis, WHO Document VPH/81.31. Geneva, World Health Organization, 1981.

93. Rubenstein E, Lang R, Shasha B, et al: In vitro susceptibility of *Brucella melitensis* to antibiotics. Antimicrob Agents Chemother 1991;35:1925–1927.

94. Ariza J, Gudiol F, Pallares R, et al: Comparative trial of rifampin-doxycycline versus tetracycline-streptomycin in the therapy of human brucellosis. Antimicrob Agents Chemother 1985;28:548–551.

95. Ariza J, Gudiol F, Pallares R, et al: Treatment of human brucellosis with doxycycline plus rifampin or doxycycline plus streptomycin: a randomized, double-blind study. Ann Intern Med 1992;117:25–30.

96. Hall WH: Modern chemotherapy in brucellosis in humans. Rev Infect Dis 1990;12:1060–1069.

97. Akova M, Uzun O, Akalin N, et al: Quinolones in treatment of human brucellosis: A comparative trial of ofloxacin-rifampin versus doxycycline-rifampin. Antimicrob Agents Chemother 1993; 37:1831–1834.

98. Young ES: Human brucellosis. Rev Infect Dis 1983;5:821–842.

99. Palenque E, Otero JR, Noriega AR: In vitro susceptibility of *Brucella melitensis* to new cephalosporins crossing the blood-brain barrier. Antimicrob Agents Chemother 1986;29:182–183.

100. Vershilova PA: The use of live vaccine for vaccination of human beings against brucellosis in the USSR. Bull World Health Organ 1961;24:85–89.

101. Roux J: Les vaccinations dans les brucelloses humaines et animales. Bull Inst Pasteur 1972;70:145–202.

OCULAR WHIPPLE'S DISEASE

Roxanne Chan and C. Stephen Foster

Whipple's disease is a rare chronic bacterial infection with multiorgan manifestations. Primary involvement is of the gastrointestinal tract and its lymphatic drainage.[1, 2] Other common sites of disease include the lungs, heart, central nervous system (CNS), kidneys, and eyes. Whipple's disease is often difficult to diagnose and treat, especially when there is eye involvement, which was first reported by Jones and Paulley in 1949.[3] The fatality rate is high if the disease is left untreated by antibiotics; therefore, the bacterial infection must be recognized so that timely management is initiated.

Three important developments concerning Whipple's disease occurred in the last 15 years: A probable pathognomonic disorder was described and named oculomasticatory myorrhythmia (OMM)[4]; polymerase chain reaction (PCR) analysis confirmed the bacterial nature of Whipple's disease with greater sensitivity and specificity than either light microscopy (LM) or electron microscopy (EM); and the emergence of acquired immunodeficiency syndrome (AIDS) in the mid 1980s, with its concomitant opportunistic infections, introduced a challenging differential diagnosis and has heretofore unknown effects on the disease process and mechanism of Whipple's disease. This chapter will review Whipple's disease, including a discussion of the aforementioned new developments.

DEFINITION

Whipple's disease is defined on the basis of clinical features and LM, EM, or PCR of biopsy specimen findings. The presence of periodic acid–Schiff (PAS)-positive macrophages on LM of the small intestine, or the presence of characteristic bacilli on EM, or a diagnostic amplified DNA sequence on PCR in affected tissues is required to confirm clinical suspicions.

HISTORY

Perhaps Allchin and Hebb described the first Whipple's disease case in 1895[5]; however, if so, they apparently did not realize their patient had a new disease.[6] George Hoyt Whipple described in 1907 a patient "characterized by a gradual loss of weight and strength, stools consisting chiefly of neutral fat and fatty acids, indefinite abdominal signs, and a peculiar multiple arthritis," and he is given credit today for his recognition of this as a new disease.[1] The first case of ocular Whipple's disease (OWD) was reported by Jones and Paulley in 1949.[3]

EPIDEMIOLOGY

Since Whipple's description, there were 617 more systemic cases reported up to 1986. The prevalence and death rate are unknown because of the low incidence rate of 18 to 30 systemic cases per year per 100,000 people. OWD is even more unusual, occurring in 19 of 696 patients with systemic Whipple's disease.[6]

Although both the systemic and the ocular forms of Whipple's disease are rare, they are well described. Whip-ple's disease usually affects middle-aged Caucasian men in the United States and continental Europe. There may possibly be an increased incidence in farmers.[7] The peak age for systemic disease is 40 to 49 years, with a range from 3 months to 81 years.[2] Eighty-eight percent of patients are in their fifth decade.[8, 9] This disease is not familial but may be associated with HLA-B27.

Eye manifestations are present in the 76 cases we have collected between 1907 and 1999 (Table 21–1). These, including four new cases of ours, are consistent with the well-known but unexplained middle-aged white male predominance (Table 21–2). Patient age and sex are presented in Table 21–3. There are more patients older than 49 years among those with uveitis only (50%) than among those with neurophthalmologic manifestations (33.3%). In this review, 76.3% of patients were male and 22.4% female. The most common age group, 40 to 49 years (38.2%), is consistent with that reported for systemic Whipple's disease. The age range in our four patients is 26 to 69 years.

ETIOLOGY

Direct transmission from one person to another has not been established, nor has the reproducibility of the disease in laboratory animals, either as origin or vector.[10] The mechanism of dissemination is also unclear. Robert Koch's postulates have not been satisfied because the bacterium causing Whipple's disease has not been cultured. Therefore, the presumed bacterial etiology of Whipple's disease has been studied with methods such as LM and EM. The Whipple's bacterium was characterized in 1991 by its 16S rRNA.[11]

After PCR showed that the Whipple's disease bacterium was not closely related to any known genus, the name *Tropheryma whippelii* was proposed.[12] This name describes an actinomycete (a high guanine-plus-cytosine [G + C], Gram-positive bacillus) most closely related to the nocardioform *Rhodobacter equi*.[13] If *T. whippelii* is a soil bacterium like its phylogenetic neighbors, then an explanation for the large proportion of farmers with Whipple's disease may be possible if its place in normal human flora can safely be excluded.[7] Although seemingly more common in patients who are farmers or who are otherwise exposed to dirt, as in Case 1, inciting factors or vectors are still unknown.[6]

PATHOLOGY

Light microscopy of intestinal mucosa reveals PAS positive and diastase-resistant bacilli within foamy macrophages. There are three pathologic lesions described in the eye.[14] LM of brain or spinal cord shows multifocal nodules of inflammation, which have a predilection for the gray matter of the hypothalamus, cingulate gyrus, basal ganglia, insular cortex, and cerebellum. Subependymal nodules found in periventricular and periaqueductal areas that resemble tumors may be difficult for antibiotics to penetrate.[15]

TABLE 21-1. OPHTHALMIC WHIPPLE'S DISEASE CASES IN THE LITERATURE

GROUP 1 Central (CNS)	O	G	A	GROUP 2 Central & Peripheral	O	G	A	GROUP 3 Peripheral (Eye)	O	G	A
PRE-1984											
Jones & Paulley (1949)[54]				Smith et al. (1965)[54]				Dybkaer (1965)[54]			
Tracey & Brolsma (1950)[54]				Switz et al. (1969)[54]				Knox et al. (1968)[54]			
Hendrix et al. (1950)[54]				Feurle et al. (1976)[54]				Vazquez Rodriguez et al. (1972)[54]			
Ritama & Haapanen (1953)[54]				Knox et al. (1976)[54]				Leland & Chambers (1978)[54]			
Kruke & Stochdorph (1962)[54]				Font (1978)/Finelli (1977)/Johnson (1979)[54]				Selsky et al. (1984)[97]			
Lampert et al. (1962)[54]				Canoso et al. (1978)[54]				Durant (1984) a[98]			
Enziger & Helwig (1963)[54]				Schliep et al. (1979)[54]				Durant (1984) b[98]			
Badenoch et al. (1963)[54]				Gartner (1980)[54]				Avila (1984) a[54]			
Stoupal et al. (1969)[54]				Schmitt et al. (1981)/Clancy (1975)[14, 96]				Avila (1984) b[54]			
Henry et al. (1974)[54]											
Knox et al. (1976) a[54]											
Knox et al. (1976) b[54]											
Knox et al. (1976) c[54]											
Masson et al. (1976)[54]											
Silbert et al. (1976)[54]											
Feurle et al. (1976) a[54]											
Feurle et al. (1976) b[54]											
Finelli et al. (1977)[54, 94]											
DeJonghe, et al. (1979)/ vanBogaert (1963)[54]	1										
Fernandez Pascual et al. (1979)[54]											
Welcker et al. (1981) a[54]											
Welcker et al. (1981) b[54]											
Malamud and Harrington[55]											
Romanul (1977)[61]											
Halperin (1982)[95]											
POST-1984											
Schwartz et al. (1986) a[4]	1	0	1	Knox et al. (1995)[14]	1	0	PM	Rickman et al. (1995)[12]	0	0	1
Schwartz et al. (1986) b[4]	1	PM	PM	Riskind (new)	0	0	1	Wechsler et al. (1995)*[35]	0	0	1
Robson (1990)[40]		1	NS					Hollerbach et al. (1995)*[36]	0	0	1
Amarenco (1991)[15]	1	0	0					Schrenk et al. (1994)[37]	0	0	1
Adler (1989)[28]	1	0	1					Disdier (1991)[41]	0	1	1
Grotta (1987)[29]	1	0	1					Playford (1992)[18]	0	1	1
Adams (1987)[42]	0	0	0					Foster (new)	0	1	1
Tison (1992)[30]	1	0	1					Foster (new)	0	1	1
Hausser (1988)[31]	1	1	0					Yannuzzi (new)	0	1	1
Simpson (1995)[43]	1	1	1					Williams (1998)[38]	0	1	1
Jankovic (1986)/Nath (1987)[44, 47]	1	1	0					Nishimura (1998)[39]	0	0	1
Brown (1990)[45]	0	1	0								
Fleming et al. (1988)[48]	0	NS	0								
Louis (1997)/Lynch (1997) a[32, 49]	1	1	0								
Louis (1997)/Lynch (1997) b[32, 49]	1	0	0								
Louis (1997)/Lynch (1997) c[32, 49]	1	1	LF								
Rajput (1997)[33]	0	1	0								
Verhagen (1997)[34]	0	1	1								
Cooper et al. (1994)[19]	0	1	1								
Wroe et al. (1991)[46]	0	0	1								
TOTAL											
45				11				19			

0 = no significant improvement, 1 = significant improvement, NS = not specified, LF = lost follow-up, PM = postmortem, O = oculomasticatory myorhythmia (OMM), G = gastrointestinal symptoms, A = antibiotics, a = Case a, b = Case b, c = Case c.

*Classified by abstract only.

TABLE 21–2. WHIPPLE'S DISEASE WITH OCULAR INFLAMMATION

CASE	AGE (YR)/ SEX	PRESENTING SIGNS AND SYMPTOMS	OCULAR MANIFESTATIONS	PRINCIPAL METHOD OF DIAGNOSIS
1	53/F	Floaters, decreased vision	Keratic precipitates, multiple 200 to 400 μm white choroidal lesions, macular edema, vitreous strands	PCR (vitreous)
2	34/M	Decreased vision	Papillitis, multifocal chorioretinitis	PAS-positive (duodenum)
3	69/M	Floaters	Circumferential inflammatory debris accumulation and diffuse vitreous infiltrate, epiretinal membrane, cotton-wool spot, macular edema	PAS-positive (jejunum)
4	44/F	Progressive memory loss, onset of diplopia and ataxia, oligomenorrhea	Filamentary keratitis	PAS-positive (hypothalamus), classical neurophthalmologic findings

PCR, polymerase chain reaction; PAS, periodic acid–Schiff.

Electronic microscopy reveals characteristic "bacillary bodies" with a trilaminar outer cell membrane.[16]

IMMUNOLOGY

The immunopathology of Whipple's disease is still unclear. An altered host response is proposed to explain the predisposition of certain individuals for direct bacterial invasion or proliferation. Evidence of direct damage is seen in the identification of rod-shaped bacteria in the retina.[17] Therefore, protection from, or ability to eliminate, infection in these individuals may be impaired. Immune system defects may be cell mediated (decreased T-cell function) or humoral (decreased immunoglobulin A response), or there may be macrophage defects (difficulties phagocytosing intracellular gram-positive bacteria), leading to altered cytokine profile (gamma interferon, interleukin 12, CD11b, and decreased CD4/CD8 ratio). On the other hand, hypersensitivity phenomena (erythema nodosum, arthralgias, fever, and contact dermatitis), supported by identified circulating rhamnose-binding antibodies against organisms and the presence of circulating immune complexes, are also possible.[18]

Patients with cell-mediated deficiencies may be predisposed to relapse. These include those treated with methotrexate (MTX)[19] and corticosteroids,[20] or those who are immunocompromised, such as by AIDS[21] and leukopenia.[20] As in AIDS patients, there are signs of impaired cellular immunity with decreased T-helper cells (decreased CD4/CD8 ratio) during active Whipple's disease.[7, 22] There is one PCR-confirmed AIDS patient with

Whipple's disease.[21] This 56-year-old man is the first reported confirmed case, with the same deletion of cytosine at position 1160 of Whipple's-specific DNA sequence as another patient.[23] Although the clinical symptoms of patients with AIDS and Whipple's disease are very similar, the PAS-positive macrophages on LM were not as prominent and did not resemble the sickle-form particle-containing cells characteristic of Whipple's disease, and so the case had to be diagnosed with PCR. The coexistence of AIDS and Whipple's disease may be coincidental, or *T. whippelii* may have acted as an opportunistic pathogen. Prior to the use of PCR in 1992, there was confusion because of the LM resemblance of Whipple's disease to opportunistic infections such as those caused by the *Mycobacterium avium-intracellulare* complex (MAC) and *R. equis*.[24, 25] Whipple's disease has coexisted with opportunistic diseases.[23, 26, 27]

CLINICAL CHARACTERISTICS

Extraocular

Whipple's disease is a chronic, relapsing, multiorgan disease. Extraintestinal signs and symptoms, which may be minimal, as in Case 1 (Table 21–2, Figs. 21–1 and 21–2), include, most commonly, arthralgias, often months to years before diagnosis. Fever, weight loss, pericarditis, and pleural effusions (Case 2 and see Table 21–2) also occur. The patient shown in Case 3 (see Table 21–2; Figs. 21–3 to 21–5) had had one episode of abdominal pain.

TABLE 21–3. AGE AND SEX DISTRIBUTION

GROUP:	1		2		3		TOTAL	TOTAL %
Male	36		7		15		58	76.3
Female	8		4		5		17	22.4
Not specified	1		0		0		1	1.3
Total	45		11		20		76	100
	M	**F**	**M**	**F**	**M**	**F**	**Total**	**Total %**
<40 years	7	2	1	2	4	2	18	23.7
40–49 years	18	2	3	2	4	0	29	38.2
>49 years	11	4	3	0	7	3	28	36.8
Not specified	1	0	0	0	0	0	1	1.3
Total	37	8	7	4	15	5	76	100
Male range	31–65		32–65		34–69		32–69	
Female range	28–69		26–44		33–59		26–69	

Patients older than 49 years (Group 1: 15/45 = 33.3%; Group 3: 10/20 = 50%).

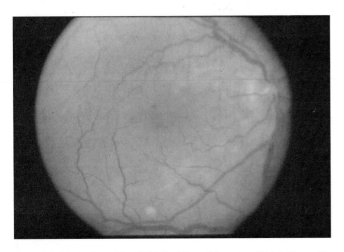

FIGURE 21–1. Case #1: Multiple faint, white choroidal lesions. (See color insert.)

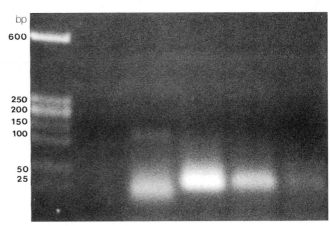

FIGURE 21–2. Case #1: Agarose gel showing band specific for *Tropheryma whippelii*. (See color insert.)

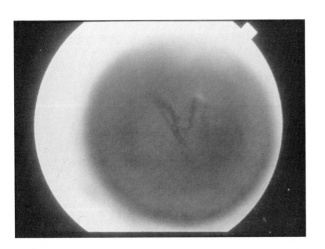

FIGURE 21–3. Case #3: Vitreous strands. (See color insert.)

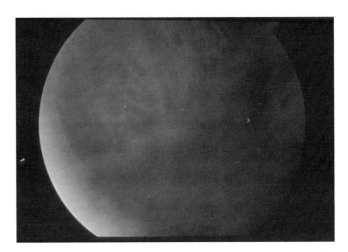

FIGURE 21–4. Case #3: Diffuse, fluffy, white infiltrate. (See color insert.)

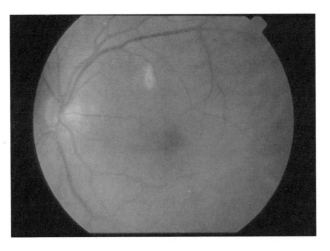

FIGURE 21–5. Case #3: Cotton-wool spot in superior macula. (See color insert.)

TABLE 21–4. PRESENTING SYMPTOMS IN 32 CASES PUBLISHED AFTER 1984

GROUP:	1 (REF)	NUMBER	2 (REF)	NUMBER	3 (REF)	NUMBER	TOTAL	%
Gastrointestinal	10, 24, 26	3	Case 4	1	35, 38, 39, Case 3	4	8	25
Arthralgias/arthritis[a]	9(2), 12, 13, 15, 16, 22(2), 24, 25, 26	11			4, 35, 36, 37, Case 1, Case 2, 40, 41	8	19	59.4
Central nervous system ocular	11, 14, 17, 18, 20, 22, 27	7	Case 4, 32	2		0	9	28.1
		0		0	40, 41	2	2	6.3

One case did not specify presenting symptoms.[21]
[a]Migratory polyarthralgias are most specific.[4, 9(2), 16, 22, 24, 25, 36, 37, Case 2]

The most common presenting manifestations of Whipple's disease are gastrointestinal (weight loss, malabsorption, abdominal pain) and polyarthralgias (migratory, nondeforming, and seronegative) (Table 21–4).[4, 12, 19, 28–39] Others presented with gastrointestinal tract, CNS, and ocular symptoms.[14, 15, 18, 19, 32, 33, 35, 38–46] Late terminal-phase gastrointestinal disease may include fever, weight loss, diarrhea, and steatorrhea.[31, 33, 34, 37, 40, 41, 43, 44, 47–49] Arthralgias usually appear about 1 year before the malabsorption syndrome, especially if there is also fever or persistent lymphadenopathy.

Sarcoid-like disturbances, which may include symptoms and signs such as migratory nondeforming arthralgias, abdominal pain, increased skin pigmentation, lymphadenopathy, chronic nonproductive cough, pleural effusion, mediastinal widening from adenopathy, and chest pain from pleurisy can also occur. Extraintestinal involvement includes primarily the CNS, heart, and sometimes the lungs, but the involvement of these sites plus the eyes is unusual. CNS manifestations, in order of descending frequency, are dementia, supranuclear ophthalmoplegia, myoclonus, and hypothalamic signs such as insomnia, hyperphagia, and polydipsia.[50]

Ocular

Uveitis

Ocular inflammation caused by Whipple's disease often occurs late in the course of disease, leading to vision impairment (Table 21–5). Concomitant gastrointestinal, neurologic, or other systemic manifestations are possible, but ocular findings may be solely CNS or intraocular.[51, 52]

Common primary intraocular involvement of this group includes keratitis, inflammatory vitreous opacities (vitritis), vitreous hemorrhage, retinal hemorrhage, retinitis, choroiditis, chorioretinitis, optic atrophy, papilledema, and cotton-wool spots.[12] Also reported are retrobulbar neuritis, glaucoma, bilateral central scotomas, chemosis, fibrovascular pannus, epiphora, and superficial punctate keratitis. Iris nodules and greasy keratic precipitates, like those of sarcoidosis, have also been reported. Cases 1 to 3 in our series had abdominal manifestations prior to visual change with or without floaters, indicative of posterior uveitis. These findings may be superimposed upon the neurologic findings of ophthalmoplegia, supranuclear gaze palsy, nystagmus, myoclonus, and ptosis.

Neurophthalmology

Central nervous system involvement is diagnosed by clinical presentation in about 10% of all patients with Whipple's disease.[53] Some authors believe that as many as 43% to 100% of patients have CNS colonization with *T. whippelii* without neurologic signs. The CNS is a repository for bacteria that cause CNS relapse, the most common, often late, and devastating complication of Whipple's disease.[6, 48] Probably all patients have CNS involvement; however, all are not clinically obvious.[15] Generally, there is concomitant gastrointestinal involvement.

Neurophthalmologic disease usually causes ophthalmoplegia (primarily supranuclear, with occasional progression to total, without response to head or caloric stimulation), gaze palsy, and/or nystagmus. Myoclonus may be independent or associated with cranial musculature, eyes, jaws, and face involvement. Headaches, ptosis, seizures, and ataxia also occur.

Another neurophthalmologic manifestation is oculomasticatory myorhythmia (OMM), named since the last OWD review[54] when researchers collected two cases of what was then probably a newly described disorder.[4] Perhaps Knox's case is the first documented OMM case.[55] OMM consists of pendular vergent oscillations (PVOs) or smooth vergent nystagmus associated with tongue and mandibular myoclonus, not be confused with oculopalatal myoclonus. These patients generally have gaze paralysis, hypersomnia, and arthralgias without early magnetic resonance imaging (MRI) or gastrointestinal findings. The fundamental characteristics of OMM are high ampli-

TABLE 21–5. OCULAR INFLAMMATION COMPARED TO CNS CASES

GROUP:	1	%	2	%	3	%	TOTAL
Before 1984	25	58.1	9	20.9	9	20.9	43
After 1984	20	60.1	2	6.1	11	33.3	33
Total	45		11		20		76

tude (5° to 25°), low frequency (0.5 to 1.6 Hz), smooth continuous oscillations in the z-axis without palatal movement. The oscillations in OMM are unrelated to those in Parinaud's syndrome, and unrelated to saccadic effort, visual stimuli, or sleep. There is no palatal myoclonus, nor olivary pseudohypertrophy, one of the hallmarks of oculopalatal myoclonus. The case described by DeJonghe and coworkers[56] resembles spinal segmental myoclonus but seems to be of brain stem origin instead. The remaining differential diagnoses are the other disorders with pendular nystagmus. The lesion(s) responsible for these abnormal movements have not been found.[4, 28] The suggestion of cerebral atrophy has been made because a prominent feature is dementia, which, along with myoclonus, may be attributed to diffuse cerebral cortical disease, but this does not explain the more specific lesion of a supranuclear palsy.[14, 57]

Since Schwartz's first observations, 14 additional OMM cases have been described (see Table 21–1).[4, 9, 14, 28–32, 43, 44, 54, 56] CNS and intraocular involvement can also occur together.

DIAGNOSIS

Whipple's disease is typically difficult to diagnose because of its diverse clinical signs and symptoms, especially in patients with minimal or no gastrointestinal manifestations. In 1907, Whipple used Levaditi silver stain to reveal rod-shaped organisms.[1] Hendrix diagnosed 23 cases via clinical descriptions in 1950.[59] Analysis of tissue samples by LM, EM, and/or PCR is required to confirm clinical suspicions because *T. whippelii* has not been cultured[58] (Table 21–6).

McManus developed the PAS stain in 1946. In 1949, Black-Shaffer was the first to show PAS-positive inclusions within the lamina propria of the small intestine and lymph nodes of patients with Whipple's disease.[60] These inclusions were also diastase resistant; they corresponded to foamy macrophages, which contained fragmented bacteria and large numbers of phagocytosed intact bacteria.[7] Hendrix then confirmed 4 of his 23 clinically described cases by LM in 1950.[59] Jejunal biopsy (Case 3, see Table 21–2), the gastrointestinal diagnostic procedure of choice, reveals clubbed villi and a lamina propria infiltrated with PAS-positive bacteria both within and outside of foamy macrophages. However, patchy or submucosal disease (Case 2) may result in negative biopsies. We found PAS-positive "foamy" macrophages in both the duodenum and vitreous aspirates in Case 2, in the jejunum in Case 3, and in the hypothalamus in Case 4.

Electron microscopy or PCR, in addition to PAS stain-ing, is required in extraintestinal sites whenever diagnosis has not been established on the basis of gastrointestinal pathology. Yardley and Hendrix first confirmed the LM findings by EM in 1961.[16] The "bacillary bodies" have a characteristic trilaminar outer cell membrane on EM. Delicate intracellular and extracellular rodlike bacillary structures detected with both silver and PAS staining were confirmed with EM.

Although late diagnosis may be made with the pathognomonic neurologic findings of OMM, a potential tool for definitive diagnosis is now possible with PCR,[13] which allows identification of early or difficult-to-diagnose systemic disease because of its greater sensitivity. This technique may simplify diagnosis of nonintestinal specimens and show the disease to be more common than suspected.[50]

It is unfortunate that there is no single diagnostic test for Whipple's disease. Pitfalls abound in the available methods. PAS also stains gastric lipophages, colonic muciphages, brain, and lymph node macrophages, and it does not stain macrophages in granulomas.[16] Laboratory findings may include increased white blood cells and mononuclear cells in the vitreous. Brain biopsy, when there is high suspicion of CNS disease, is possible, but lesions are frequently inaccessible and high false negatives may occur because of the focal nature of the lesions.[42, 57, 62, 63] MRI may show high signal intensity[42] but may not be able to detect focal lesions.[64] Computed tomography scans usually do not show abnormalities.[65]

Diagnosis is often late because the nonspecific presenting signs and symptoms and the extensive differential diagnosis delay the initiation of investigation. Most biopsies are performed later in the clinical course. A survey of presenting signs and symptoms published after 1984 reveals that 59.4% of patients first exhibit arthralgias or arthritis (migratory polyarthralgia is most specific, 27%) and only 6.3% demonstrated ocular findings (see Table 21–4).

One of 4 new and 2 of 72 published OWD cases were diagnosed by PCR on vitreous samples and subsequently treated successfully with antibiotics without devastating CNS sequelae.[12, 38] Case 1 is the third reported case in which PCR was used to detect the *T. whippelii* 16sRNA in a vitreous sample. This patient responded to the prompt institution of appropriate antibiotic therapy.

Laboratory Technique

Probably the most sensitive indicator of persistent organisms is PCR when used on vitreous samples. This method requires rigorous and well-controlled experimental proce-

TABLE 21–6. DIAGNOSIS OF WHIPPLE'S DISEASE

DIAGNOSTIC METHOD	FIRST DESCRIBED FOR WD	YEARS
Clinical	G. H. Whipple: first case report	1907–1949
Light microscopy	Non-PAS staining	1949 to present
	Black-Shaffer[60]: PAS+ in lamina propria of small intestine and lymph nodes pathognomonic	
Electron microscopy	Yardley and Hendrix (16): bacillary bodies	1961 to present
Polymerase chain reaction	Rickman[61]	1992 to present

PAS, periodic acid–Schiff.

dures to ensure validity of results.[7] Rickman described a 57-year-old woman in whom a mononuclear cell infiltrate composed of foamy macrophages was found in vitreous samples.[12, 61]

Oligonucleotide primers were used to amplify a universally conserved 1321-base sequence to identify the bacillus.[12]

The PCR technique was used to detect the 16S ribosomal RNA (rRNA) gene from *T. whippelii* isolated from the vitreous of Case 1 reported from the Ocular Immunology & Uveitis Service of the Massachusetts Eye and Ear Infirmary. Briefly, DNA in 300 microliters (μl) of undiluted vitreous from our Case 1 was extracted in an equal volume of phenol/chloroform/isoamyl alcohol (25:24:1), mixed vigorously for 30 sec, and then microcentrifuged for 15 sec at 13,000 rpm (room temperature). The top aqueous phase and organic interface (about 250 μl) containing DNA was removed to a new Eppendorf tube. Twenty-five microliters of 3M sodium acetate, pH 5.2, was added, followed by the addition of 825 μl ice-cold 100% ethanol. After mixing, the sample was stored at −70°C overnight. It was then centrifuged for 5 min at 13,000 rpm at room temperature. The pellet was dried and resuspended in 20 μl TE buffer (10 mM Tris-HCl and 1 mM EDTA, pH 8.0) at room temperature and stored at −20°C for PCR analysis.

The *T. whippelii* 16S rRNA primer, W4RB (5'CGG GAT CCT GTG AGT CCC CGC CAT TAC GC) was obtained from Ransom Hill Bioscience (Ramona, CA) and used to amplify a 154-base-pair (bp) internal portion of the *T. whippelii* 16S rRNA gene. PCR was performed with the DNA mixture in a 20 μl reaction volume containing 20 mM Tris-HCl (pH 8.3), 50 mM KCl, 1.5 mM MgCl$_2$, 100 μM each dNTP, 2 mg/ml bovine serum albumin, specific 5' and 3' primers, and 0.2 units (5 units/μl) of Taq DNA polymerase (Boehringer Mannheim, IN). The optimal concentration for each primer set (4 μl sense and antisense) was as follows: positive control, negative control, *T. whippelii*, varicella zoster (VZV), herpes simplex (HSV), cytomegalovirus (CMV), *Borrelia burgdorferi* (Lyme) disease, toxoplasmosis, and *Mycobacterium tuberculosis* (TB) (5 pmol/μl each). Thirty-five cycles were used for all samples. Amplification was performed in a thermocycler model 9600 Perkin Elmer Cetus (Norwalk, CT) programmed for denaturation at 94°C for 10 seconds, annealing at 55°C for 1 min, and extension at 72°C for 7 min. PCR products were electrophoretically fractionated on a 1.5% agarose gel, stained with ethidium bromide, visualized by ultraviolet light, and photodocumented using Polaroid photography. The observed PCR products corresponded to their expected molecular weights (HSV = 327 bp, VZV = 203 bp, CMV = 361 bp, TB = 240 bp, *Toxoplasma* = 193 bp, Lyme = 248 bp, and *T. whippelii* = 154 bp).

DIFFERENTIAL DIAGNOSIS

Whipple's disease is a great mimic that bears similarities to gastrointestinal, neurologic, and other diseases that affect multiple organs and have protean manifestations. Patients with uveitis may have a choroiditis-like picture, similar to that of presumed ocular histoplasmosis, multifocal choroiditis and panuveitis, sarcoidosis, malig-

nancy (i.e., primary intraocular lymphoma), MAC, amyloidosis, tuberculosis, and/or retinal vasculitis (as in collagen vascular diseases, or Lyme disease). Patients with histoplasmosis usually have maculopathy, peripapillary pigment changes, and a clear vitreous.

Mycobacterium avium-intracellulare complex is a systemic opportunistic infection that often involves immunocompromised patients; the organism is acid fast, easily cultured, and causes 50- to 100-μm choroidal lesions without visual changes.[21] Immunologic defects predispose AIDS patients to entities such as MAC, which also have PAS-positive granular macrophages. However, since they are also acid fast, they are unlike those found in Whipple's disease. Concomitant MAC and Whipple's disease has been reported by several authors.[3, 24, 25] Other illnesses resembling Whipple's disease, but not necessarily AIDS related, include *M. paratuberculosis* and *R. equi*.[13]

The deep yellow choroidal granulomas of sarcoidosis may look like those of histoplasmosis, but vitreal inflammatory cells are typically present in sarcoid uveitis. Patients with Whipple's disease may have iris nodules and greasy keratic precipitates like those found in sarcoidosis.[66–69] These clinical resemblances may be the result of antigenic and structural similarities.[70, 71]

Adamantiades-Behçet's disease is a multisystemic disorder that presents with not only recurrent aphthous and genital ulcerations, but also eye involvement similar to OWD. Eye disease may be rapidly progressive and is usually present at the onset of the disease. Patients with Adamantiades-Behçet's disease may have iritis, posterior uveitis, retinal vascular occlusions, and optic neuritis. Rarely, the hallmark hypopyon uveitis is seen. CNS manifestations, more common in northern Europe and the United States, include benign intracranial hypertension, a multiple sclerosis–like picture, pyramidal involvement, and psychiatric disturbances. Other systemic manifestations are nondeforming arthritis, mucosal ulcerations of the gut, skin problems, and thrombosis or vasculitis.

The patients in Cases 1 to 3 had a nonspecific uveitis similar to that of the reported cases, whereas the patient in Case 4 developed filamentary keratitis.

TREATMENT

Medical

Whipple's disease was invariably fatal prior to the discovery of the bacterial etiology and subsequent availability and use of antibiotics.[72] Before 1957, the diagnosis of Whipple's disease had the same significance as end-stage AIDS does today. Steroids and adrenocorticotropic hormone (ACTH), employed for treatment in the mid 1950s, achieved clinical remissions of short duration.[73] Radiation therapy was apparently not successful.

After the first accidental and successful antibiotic treatment for Whipple's disease with chloramphenicol, other antibiotics, such as tetracycline (Case 1 initially, and Case 2), penicillin, and streptomycin have been employed.[74] Nevertheless, steroids remained a controversial adjunct to antibiotics[16, 73, 75] until Davis[20] compared steroids and antibiotics in 15 patients (on steroids, 2 of 7 died, 5 of 7 did poorly; on antibiotics, 8 of 8 did well). Since then, many antibiotics were used, with some prompt responses.

Tetracycline is most commonly used, with a 43% relapse rate.[72]

Successfully treated cases include both mono- and multidrug systemic regimens such as 1.2 million units procaine penicillin and 1 g streptomycin for 10 to 14 days followed by PO tetracycline for 10 to 12 months[9] or intravenous (IV) chloramphenicol for 10 days then para-aminosalicylic acid and INH.[76] Chloramphenicol,[74] IV and PO penicillin,[77] PO ampicillin,[78] trimethoprim-sulfamethoxazole (TMP-SMX),[52, 79, 80] and rarely salicylazosulfapyridine,[9] chlortetracycline,[9] and doxycyline[81] have all been used.

All patients may have CNS involvement,[51] but probably only 10% to 20% present clinically.[82] Treatment after CNS relapse is generally not successful except to halt progression.[57] Antibiotic effectiveness is unclear for intraocular and CNS Whipple's disease, even though antibiotic therapy achieves good results with gastrointestinal involvement. The blood–brain and blood–retina barriers are challenges for drug penetration.

Neurologic relapse even after systemic improvement is still the most common and most serious complication.[83] Of the 672 patients reviewed by Dobbins, 179 died of Whipple's disease, with 68 deaths since 1961 and 16 deaths between 1980 and 1986.[6] Based on empirical observations, Ryser and Keinath suggested the current drug of choice, TMP-SMX (Bactrim, Septra) (Cases 1, 3, and 4) for improved CNS penetration.[72, 84] Optimal duration of antibiotic therapy has yet to be determined, but 1 year of double-strength TMP-SMX (960 mg) twice a day after 2 weeks of IV therapy is the current empirically recommended treatment.[72, 83] Various combinations of initial IV therapy have been proposed: (1) ceftriaxone 2 g twice daily and streptomycin 1 g daily for 2 weeks, (2) TMP-SMX 960 mg twice daily for 1 to 2 weeks, or (3) penicillin 1.2 million units and streptomycin 1 g daily for 10 to 14 days.[72, 83]

Drugs that penetrate the blood–brain barrier and blood–retina barrier are TMP-SMX, IV penicillin, chloramphenicol, IV ceftriaxone, and PO cefixime, but these are still inadequate. TMP-SMX remains the recommended first-line therapy.[72, 84] The signs most amenable to treatment may be gaze palsies and nystagmus.

Although they may eradicate Whipple's disease from the gut, PO tetracycline and PO penicillin are no longer recommended as monotherapies because neither penetrates uninflamed meninges.[72] The CNS becomes a reservoir of bacteria for future relapse if the CNS concentration is not high enough. Tetracycline predisposes to CNS relapse in otherwise asymptomatic patients[55, 75, 84] and in those with residual nonprogressive neurologic problems.[55, 77, 86] PO penicillin has similar problems, with CNS relapse despite good systemic response.[28] Relapse is as high as 43%, compared to 23% for other monotherapies.[72] Chloramphenicol and TMP-SMX may be successful[72] and some recommend it for all cases of Whipple's disease.[84]

After treatment with systemic antibiotics is begun, fever dissipates in the first few days and the patient experiences rapid clinical improvement. Upper gastrointestinal series show improvement after 4 months and return to normal after 12 months,[85] supporting the recommended 1-year

systemic antibiotic plan. However, there is still a need for improved or alternative therapies, especially for TMP-SMX-intolerant,[12] granulocytopenic,[42] or resistant patients. Ceftriaxone resolved some of the neurologic sequelae in one patient.[28] Another patient relapsed while on TMP-SMX and MTX and was treated successfully with cefixime.[19] Perfloxacin, a quinolone that crosses the blood–brain barrier readily, has produced moderate neurologic improvement.

Others suggest prophylactic treatment of patients with supranuclear palsies and uveitis.[87] However, if relapse still occurs, accessory regimens such as IV chloramphenicol and IV penicillin or ampicillin for 2 to 4 weeks may be needed.[77, 81, 86] Treating all patients with IV penicillin and streptomycin followed by PO TMP-SMX,[88] erythromycin,[28] or PO cotrimoxazole for 1 year[82] has also been suggested.[72]

Even with antibiotic treatment, the bacillary bodies remain in macrophages causing little or no cellular injury for up to a year.[7] Although antibiotics are effective, no one antibiotic is wholly curative and there is often relapse (especially CNS), even with TMP-SMX. Studies of drug treatment in OWD that need to be done include comparison of antibiotic effectiveness and toxicity for systemic and intraocular disease, trial of the new fluoroquinolones (e.g., ciprofloxacin),[89–91] experimental drug delivery methods such as liposomes,[92] and whether the best treatments for CNS ocular disease and intraocular Whipple's disease are the same.

Surgical
Therapeutic vitrectomy is performed if there are marked vitreous opacities. The vitreous aspirate can be diagnostic.

CONCLUSION
Since George Hoyt Whipple's 1907 case report, advances in basic science, immunology, and molecular genetics and their clinical applications have provided a better understanding of the pathogenetic role of bacteria in Whipple's disease and have led to improved methods of diagnosis and treatment. Although this broader understanding of human pathobiology has been forged, the process by which *T. whippelii* induces disease is still not fully understood.

High clinical suspicion should be maintained for Whipple's disease in patients with uveitis or classical neurophthalmologic findings. PCR may be used on tissue samples, including vitreous, from patients with uveitis and suspected ophthalmic Whipple's disease for earlier definitive diagnosis, when the disease may be more amenable to antibiotic treatment than later. The reports in the literature of patients with ophthalmic manifestations of Whipple's disease suggest that current antibiotics are not always effective once late manifestations occur. Recognition of migratory polyarthralgias, the most common and specific presenting manifestation, will also facilitate an earlier diagnosis.

References
1. Whipple GH: A hitherto undescribed disease characterized anatomically by deposits of fat and fatty acids in the intestinal and mesenteric lymphatic tissues. Johns Hopkins Hosp Bull 1907;18:382–391.

2. Comer GM, Brandt LJ, Abissi CJ: Whipple's disease: A review. Am J Gastroenterol 1983;78:107–114.
3. Jones FA, Paulley JW: Intestinal lipodystrophy (Whipple's disease). Lancet 1949;1:214–216.
4. Schwartz MA, Selhorst JB, Ochs Al, et al: Oculomasticatory myorhythmia: A unique movement disorder occurring in Whipple's disease. Ann Neurol 1986;20:677–683.
5. Allchin WH, Hebb RG: Lymphangiectasis intestini. Trans Path Soc Lond 1895;46:221–223.
6. Dobbins WO: Whipple's Disease. Springfield, IL, Charles C. Thomas, 1987.
7. Donaldson RM Jr: Whipple's disease—Rare malady with uncommon potential. N Engl J Med 1992;327:346–348.
8. Chears WC Jr, Hargrove MD Jr, Verner JV Jr, et al: Whipple's disease: A review of 12 patients from one service. Am J Med 1961;30:226–234.
9. Maizel H, Ruggin JM, Dobbins WO III: Whipple's disease: A review of 19 patients from one hospital and a review of the literature since 1950. Medicine 1970;49:175–120.
10. Dobbins WO III: Whipple's disease: An historical perspective. Q J Med 1985;56:523–531.
11. Wilson KH, Blitchington R, Frothingham R, Wilson JA: Phylogeny of the Whipple's-disease-associated bacterium. Lancet 1991; 338:474–475.
12. Rickman LS, Freeman WR, Green WR, et al: Uveitis caused by *Tropheryma whippelii* (Whipple's bacillus) [brief report]. N Engl J Med 1995;332:363–366.
13. Relman DA, Schmidt TM, MacDermott RP, Falkow S: Identification of the uncultured bacillus of Whipple's disease. N Engl J Med 1992;327:293–301.
14. Knox DL, Green WR, Troncoso JC, et al: Cerebral ocular Whipple's disease: A 62-year odyssey from death to diagnosis. Neurology 1995;45:617–625.
15. Amarenco P, Roullet E, Hannoun L, Marteau R: Progressive supranuclear palsy as the sole manifestation of systemic Whipple's disease treated with perfloxacin. J Neurol Neurosurg Psychiatry 1991;54:1121–1122.
16. Yardley JH, Hendrix TR: Combined electron and light microscopy in Whipple's disease: Demonstration of "bacillary bodies" in the intestine. Johns Hopkins Med J 1961;109:80–98.
17. Font RL, Rao NA, Issarescu S, et al: Ocular involvement in Whipple's disease: Light and electron microscopic observations. Arch Ophthalmol 1978;96:1431–1436.
18. Playford RJ, Schulenburg E, Herrington CS, Hodgson HJF: Whipple's disease complicated by a retinal Jarisch Herxheimer reaction: A case report. Gut 1992;33:132.
19. Cooper GS, Blades EW, Remler BF, et al: Central nervous system Whipple's disease: Relapse during therapy with trimethoprim-sulfamethoxazole and remission with cefixime. Gastroenterology 1994;106:782–786.
20. Davis TD Jr, McBee JW, Borland JL Jr, et al: The effect of antibiotic and steroid therapy in Whipple's disease. Gastroenterology 1963;44:112–116.
21. Maiwald M, Meier-Willerson HJ, Hartmann M, von Herbay A: Detection of *Tropheryma whippelii* DNA in a patient with AIDS. J Clin Microbiol 1995;33:1354–1356.
22. Marth T, Roux M, von Herbay, et al: Persistent reduction of complement receptor 3 alpha-chain expressing mononuclear blood cells and transient inhibitory serum factors in Whipple's disease. Clin Immunol Immunopathol 1994;72:217–226.
23. Meier-Willerson HJ, Maiwald M, von Herbay A: Whipple's disease associated with opportunistic infections. Dtsch Med Wochenschr 1993;118:854–860.
24. Gillin JS, Urmacher C, West R, Shike M: Disseminated *Mycobacterium avium-intracellulare* infection in acquired immunodeficiency syndrome mimicking Whipple's disease. Gastroenterology 1983; 85:1187–1191.
25. Wang HH, Tollerud D, Danar D, et al: Another Whipple-like disease in AIDS? N Engl J Med 1986;314:1577–1578.
26. Bassotti G, Pelli MA, Ribacchi R, et al: *Giardia lamblia* infestation reveals underlying Whipple's disease in a patient with long-standing constipation. Am J Gastroenterol 1991;86:371–374.
27. Maliha GM, Hepps KS, Maia DM. Whipple's disease can mimic chronic AIDS enteropathy. Am J Gastroenterol 1991;86:79–81.
28. Adler CH, Galetta SL. Oculo-facial-skeletal myorhythmia in Whipple's disease: Treatment with ceftriaxone. Ann Intern Med 1990;112:467–469.
29. Grotta JC, Petigrew LC, Schmidt WA, et al: Oculomasticatory myorhythmia. Ann Neurol 1987;22:395–396.
30. Tison F, Louvet-Giendaj C, Henry P, et al: Permanent bruxism as a manifestation of the oculo-facial syndrome related to systemic Whipple's disease. Mov Disord 1992;7:82–85.
31. Hausser-Hauw C, Roullet E, Robert R, Marteau R: Oculo-facial-skeletal myorhythmia as a cerebral complication of systemic Whipple's disease. Mov Disord 1988;3:179–184.
32. Louis ED, Lynch T, Kaufmann P, et al: Diagnostic guidelines in central nervous system Whipple's disease. Ann Neurol 1996;40:561–568.
33. Rajput AH, McHattie JD: Ophthalmoplegia and leg myorhythmia in Whipple's disease: Report of a case. Mov Disord 1997;12:111–114.
34. Verhagen WI, Huygen PL, Dalman JE, Schuurmans MM: Whipple's disease and the central nervous system. A case report and a review of the literature. Clin Neurol Neurosurg 1996;98:299–304.
35. Wechsler B, Fior R, Reux I, et al: Uveitis: Late complications of undiagnosed Whipple's disease. Rev Med Interne 1995;16:687–690.
36. Hollerbach S, Holstege A, Muscholl M, et al: Masked course of Whipple's disease with uveitis, infection, endocardial involvement and abdominal lymphomas—case report and review of the literature. Z Gastroenterol 1995;33:362–367.
37. Schrenk M, Metz K, Heiligenhaus A, et al: Ocular involvement in Whipple's disease. Klin Monatsbl Augenheilkd 1994;204:538–541.
38. Williams JG, Edward DP, Tessler HH, et al: Ocular manifestations of Whipple's disease: An atypical presentation. Arch Ophthalmol 1998;116:1232–1234.
39. Nishimura JK, Cook BE, Pach JM: Whipple's disease presenting as posterior uveitis without prominent gastrointestinal symptoms. Am J Ophthalmol 1998;126:130–132.
40. Robson DK, Faraj BB, Hamal PB, Ironside JW: Whipple's disease with cerebral involvement. Postgrad Med J 1990;66:724–726.
41. Disdier P, Harle J-R, Morris-Vidal D, et al: Chemosis associated with Whipple's disease. Am J Ophthalmol 1991;112:217–219.
42. Adams M, Rhyner PA, Day J, et al: Whipple's disease confined to the central nervous system. Ann Neurol 1987;21:104–108.
43. Simpson DA, Wishnow R, Gargulinski RB, Pawlak AM: Oculofacial-skeletal myorhythmia in central nervous system Whipple's disease: Additional case and review of the literature. Mov Disord 1995;10:195–200.
44. Jankovic J, Pardo R: Segmental myoclonus: Clinical and pharmacologic study. Arch Neurol 1986;43:1025–1031.
45. Brown AP, Lane JC, Murayama S, Vollmer DG: Whipple's disease presenting with isolated neurological symptoms. J Neurosurg 1990;73:623–627.
46. Wroe SJ, Pires M, Harding B, Shorvon S: Whipple's disease confined to the CNS presenting with multiple intracerebral mass lesions. J Neurol Neurosurg Psychiatry 1991;54:989–992.
47. Nath A, Jankovic J, Pettigrew LC: Movement disorders and AIDS. Neurology 1987;37:37–41.
48. Fleming JL, Wiesner RH, Shorter RG: Whipple's disease: Clinical, biochemical, and histopathologic features and assessment of treatment in 29 patients. Mayo Clin Proc 1988;63:539–551.
49. Lynch T, Fahn S: Oculofacial-skeletal myorhythmia in Whipple's disease. Mov Disord 1997;12:625–626.
50. Dobbins WO III. The diagnosis of Whipple's disease. N Engl J Med 1995;332:390–392.
51. Powers JM, Rawe SE: A neuropathologic study of Whipple's disease. Acta Neuropathol 1979;48:223–226.
52. Sieracki JC, Fine G, Horn RC Jr, et al: Central nervous system involvement in Whipple's disease. J Neuropathol Exp Neurol 1960;19:70–75.
53. Schliep G, Muller W, Schaefer HE, et al: Morbus Whipple. Fortschr Neurol Psychiatr 1979;47:167–208.
54. Avila MP, Jalkh AE, Feldman E, et al: Manifestations of Whipple's disease in the posterior segment of the eye. Arch Ophthalmol 1984;102:384–390.
55. Knox DL, Bayless TM, Pittman FE: Neurologic disease in patients with treated Whipple's disease. Medicine (Baltimore) 1976;55:467–476.
56. DeJonghe P, Martin JJ, Budka H, Ceuterick C: Cerebral manifestations of disease. Acta Neurol Belg 1979;79:305–313.
57. Pollock S, Lewis PD, Kendall B: Whipple's disease confined to the nervous system. J Neurol Neurosurg Psychiatry 1981;44:1104–1109.

58. Fredricks DM, Relman DA: Cultivation of Whipple's bacillus: The irony and the ecstasy. Lancet 1997;350:1262–1263.

59. Hendrix JP, Black-Schaffer B, Withers RW, et al: Whipple's intestinal lipodystrophy: Report of four cases and discussion of possible pathogenic factors. Arch Intern Med 1950;85:91–131.

60. Black-Shaffer B: Tinctoral demonstration of glycoprotein in Whipple's disease. Proc Soc Exp Biol Med 1949;72:225–227.

61. Rickman LS, Freeman WR, Green WR, et al: Brief report: Uveitis caused by *Tropheryma whippelii*. N Engl J Med 1995;332:363–366.

62. Romanul FCA, Radvany J, Rosales RK: Whipple's disease confined to the brain: A case studied clinically and pathologically. J Neurol Neurosurg Psychiatry 1977;40:901–909.

63. Feurle GE, Volk B, Waldherr R: Cerebral Whipple's disease and negative jejunal histology. N Engl J Med 1979;300:907–908.

64. Robson DK, Faraj BB, Hamal PB, Ironside JW: Whipple's disease with cerebral involvement. Postgrad Med J 1990;66:724–726.

65. Grossman RI, Davis KR, Halperin J: Cranial computed tomography in Whipple's disease. J Comput Assist Tomogr 1981;5:246–248.

66. Cho C, Linscheer WG, Hirschkorn MA, Ashutosh K: Sarcoid-like granulomas as an early manifestation of Whipple's disease. Gastroenterology 1984;87:941–947.

67. Mansbach CM 2d, Whelburne JD, Steven RD, Dobbins WO 3d: Lymph-node bacilliform bodies resembling those of Whipple's disease in a patient without intestinal involvement. Ann Intern Med 1978;89:64–66.

68. Southern JF, Moscicki RA, Magro C, et al: Lymphedema, lymphocytic myocarditis, and sarcoid-like granulomatosis. Manifestations of Whipple's disease. JAMA 1989;261:1467–1470.

69. Spapen HD, Segers O, De Wit N, et al: Electron microscopic detection of Whipple's bacillus in sarcoid-like periodic acid-Schiff-negative granulomas. Dig Dis Sci 1989;34:640–643.

70. Relman DA: The identification of uncultured microbial pathogens. J Infect Dis 1993;168:1–8.

71. Rook GA, Stanford JL: Slow bacterial infections or autoimmunity? Immunol Today 1992;13:160–164.

72. Keinath RD, Merrell DE, Vlietstra R, Dobbins WO: Antibiotic treatment and relapse in Whipple's disease. Gastroenterology 1985; 88:1867–1873.

73. Bayless TM: Whipple's disease: Newer concepts of therapy. Adv Intern Med 1970;16:171–189.

74. Paulley JW: A case of Whipple's disease (intestinal lipodystrophy). Gastroenterology 1952;22:128–133.

75. Thompson P, Ledingham JM, Howard AJ, Brown CL: Meningitis in Whipple's disease. Br Med J 1978;2:14–15.

76. Maxwell JD, Ferguson A, McKay AM, et al: Lymphocytes in Whipple's disease. Lancet 1968;1:887–889.

77. Schmitt BP, Richardson H, Smith E, et al: Encephalopathy complicates Whipple's disease: Failure to respond to antibiotics. Ann Intern Med 1981;94:51–52.

78. Hawkins CF, Farr M, Morris CJ, et al: Detection by electron microscope of rod-shaped organisms in synovial membrane from a patient with the arthritis of Whipple's disease. Ann Rheum Dis 1976;35:502–509.

79. Elsborg L, Gravgaard E, Jacobsen NO: Treatment of Whipple's disease with sulphamethoxazole-trimethoprim. Acta Med Scand 1975;204:423–427.

80. Tauris P, Moesner J: Whipple's disease—clinical and histopathological changes during treatment with sulphamethoxazole-trimethoprim. Acta Med Scand 1978;204:423–427.

81. Feurle GE, Dorken B, Schopf E, Lenhard V: HLA-B27 and defects in the T-cell system in Whipple's disease. Eur J Clin Invest 1979;9:385–389.

82. Dobbins WO 3rd: Whipple's disease. Mayo Clin Proc 1988;63:623–624.

83. Schnider PJ, Reisinger EC, Berger T, et al: Treatment guidelines in central nervous system Whipple's disease [letter]. Ann Neurol 1997; 41:561–562.

84. Ryser RJ, Locksley RM, Eng SC, et al: Reversal of dementia associated with Whipple's disease by trimethoprim-sulfamethoxazole, drugs that penetrate the blood-brain barrier. Gastroenterology 1984;86:745–752.

85. Phillips RL, Carlson HS: The roentgenographic and clinical findings in Whipple's disease. A review of 8 patients. Am J Roentgenol 1975;124:268–273.

86. Feldman M, Hendler RS, Morrison EB: Acute meningoencephalitis after withdrawal of antibiotics in Whipple's disease. Ann Intern Med 1980;93:709–711.

87. Finelli PF, McEntree WJ, Lessell S, et al: Whipple's disease with predominantly neuroophthalmic manifestations. Ann Neurol 1977;1:247–252.

88. Alba D, Molina F, Vazquez JJ: Neurologic manifestations of Whipple disease. An Med Interna 1995;12:508–512.

89. El Baba FZ, Trousdale MD, Gauderman WJ, et al: Intravitreal penetration of oral ciprofloxacin in humans. Ophthalmology 1992; 99:483–486.

90. Cokingtin CD, Hyndiuk RA: Insights from experimental data on ciprofloxacin in the treatment of bacterial keratitis and ocular infections. Am J Ophthalmol 1991;112(suppl):25S–28S.

91. Serdarevic ON: Role of the fluoroquinolones in ophthalmology. Int Ophthalmol Clin 1993;33:163–178.

92. Niesman MR: The use of liposomes as drug carriers in ophthalmology. Crit Rev Ther Drug Carrier Syst 1992;9:1–38.

22 — RICKETTSIAL DISEASES

Richard Bazin

DEFINITION

Tick-Borne Diseases

Rickettsial agents are first characterized by the fact that most of them are transmitted by tick bites. Tick-borne diseases in the United States are caused by disparate types of microbes, including spirochetes (*Borrelia burgdorferi*, the agent of Lyme disease, and other *Borrelia* species, agents of tick-borne relapsing fever), pleomorphic bacteria (*Francisella tularensis*, the agent of tularemia), rickettsia (*Rickettsia rickettsii*, the agent of Rocky Mountain spotted fever [RMSF], and *Ehrlichia chaffeensis*, the agent of ehrlichiosis), viruses (*Coltivirus* species, agents of Colorado tick fever), and protozoa (*Babesia* species, agents of babesiosis). There is also a toxin that causes tick paralysis.[1]

Ticks are obligate blood-sucking members of the class Arachnida, a group of arthropods also including scorpions, spiders, and mites. Ticks are grouped into three different families, two of which, the Ixodidae and the Argasidae, are known to infest humans by transmitting microbes through bites.

The Ixodidae (hard ticks) are characterized by a hard dorsal sclerotized shield, the scutum. The life cycle of most hard ticks takes 2 years for completion and includes the egg, larva, immature nymph, and mature adult. At each stage after the egg, a blood meal is required for morphogenesis. While it is feeding, the hard tick may stay attached to the host for hours to days, and evidence of a bite should be looked for when a tick-borne disease is suspected. Hard ticks are responsible for transmitting Lyme disease, tularemia, RMSF, ehrlichiosis, Colorado tick fever, babesiosis, and tick paralysis.[1]

The Argasidae (soft ticks) lack the scutum and can be identified by their leathery integument. Their life cycle may go through several nymphal stages, and they may take many blood meals lasting less than 30 minutes at each stage. They can survive many years without feeding. Soft ticks are known for transmitting relapsing fever[1] but not rickettsiosis.

Microbiologic Characteristics

Rickettsiae are obligate intracellular organisms. They can survive in nature through a cycle involving mammalian reservoirs and insect vectors. Usually, humans are only incidental hosts, with the tick transmitting the disease during feeding. Humans do not seem to be useful in propagating rickettsiae in nature.[2] Many rickettsial agents share the life of their insect vectors in a commensal fashion. On the other hand, *Rickettsia prowazekii* (louse-borne typhus) will kill its vector in 1 to 3 weeks. Three organisms (*R. rickettsii* [RMSF], *Rickettsia tsutsugamushi* [scrub typhus], and *Rickettsia akari* [rickettsialpox]) are transmitted transovarially to their vector's eggs. When the infected larval, nymph, or adult form of the arthropod feeds on small mammals or livestock, it infects them with the bacteria, creating zoonotic reservoirs capable of reinfecting naïve ticks that will feed on their blood.[2]

Rickettsiae are fastidious gram-negative bacteria. They are small pleomorphic coccobacilli measuring 0.3 μm in diameter for the coccal form, and 0.3 by 1.0 to 2.0 μm in the bacillary form.[3] The cell wall possesses the ultrastructural appearance of a gram-negative bacterium and contains lipopolysaccharide (LPS). However, rickettsiae are difficult to stain with the Gram stain. Giemsa, Gimenez, or acridine orange stains might be more suitable to visualize these bacteria.[2, 4]

Rickettsia species include two major, antigenically defined groups: the spotted fever and the typhus group, and a third group that includes other more disparate bacteria types. The first two groups are closely related genetically but differ in their surface-exposed proteins and LPS. Their outer membrane proteins contain cross-reactive antigens and surface-exposed epitopes that are species specific.[3] Cell wall LPS is also responsible for the cross-reactivity of rickettsiae with *Legionella* and *Proteus vulgaris*, which is the basis of the Weil-Felix agglutination test.[4] In this rather insensitive and nonspecific test, immune serum from infected patients has been shown to cause agglutination of the OX-19 and OX-2 strains of *P. vulgaris*.[3] Usually, gram-negative bacterial endotoxins are related to the LPS in their cell walls. Interestingly, *Coxiella burnetii* (Q fever) LPS is rather nontoxic compared to the LPS from other gram-negative bacteria, since even at doses over 80 μg per embryo, toxic reactions are not detected. In comparison, *Salmonella typhimurium* LPS is toxic in nanogram amounts.[4]

Spores and plasmids have been described in *C. burnetii*. Spores may account for the fact that this bacterium, as opposed to other rickettsiae, can survive outside the intracellular environment for months. It is also resistant to relative dehydration and chemical disinfection. Fortunately, Lysol 1% and 5% hydrogen peroxide can destroy it. Three different plasmids have been described for *C. burnetii*, and there seems to be a correlation between the plasmid content and the virulence of the bacteria.[4]

Rickettsiae contain both RNA and DNA, possess synthetic and energy-producing enzymes, and multiply by binary fission. They are able to synthesize adenosine triphosphate (ATP) via the metabolism of glutamate. *R. prowazekii* (epidemic typhus) has a sophisticated transport mechanism exchanging ATP from the host's cytosol for its own energy-depleted ADP. Many rickettsiae also have different transport mechanisms to obtain vital substances like amino acids from their host. The most extreme example of adaptation is *C. burnetii*, which can survive and proliferate in the harsh, inhospitable environment of phagolysosomes.[3] Because of all these adaptations and independent metabolic activities, it is believed that rickettsiae are not degenerate forms of bacteria but rather a successfully evolved form of intracellular microorganisms.

Since rickettsiae are obligate intracellular organisms, they cannot be grown on agar plates or in broth. Eukaryotic cells are necessary for their growth (cell culture, embryonated eggs, susceptible animals),[3] but because of non-negligible hazards for laboratory workers, especially with *C. burnetii*, which resists desiccation and many disinfectants and requires only 10 viable organisms to cause infection in humans, such cultures are often not desirable.[5]

Classification

Rickettsial diseases are classified into three major categories: the spotted fever group, the typhus group, and the other diseases group (e.g., those caused by *Ehrlichia* and *Coxiella*) (Table 22–1).

The genus *Bartonella* (*B. quintana* [trench fever], *B. henselae* [cat scratch disease], *B. bacilliformis* [Oroya fever]), formerly known as *Rochalimaea* and once thought to be closely related to rickettsiae, is now, after recent phylogenetic analyses, considered to be more closely related to the *Brucella* and *Agrobacterium* genera.[3, 6]

HISTORY

In the past, humanity has been plagued by disastrous epidemics because of poor sanitary conditions, during famines, or after major armed conflicts. Malaria, yellow fever, cholera, bubonic plague, and epidemic and murine typhus, to name a few, claimed millions of lives during these epidemics.

Although typhus, as we see it today, has a low death rate even if left untreated, it used to be a highly fatal disease in its epidemic form, the spread of the disease being promoted by poor hygiene and overcrowded condi-

tions. Napoleon's Russian campaign in the early 1800s is famous for the terrible toll typhus took.[7] One sergeant in Napoleon's army related how he could not get to sleep because he was covered by lice. Despite the fact that he tried to get rid of them by burning his clothes, lice would continuously come back for 2 months. Many soldiers swarmed with lice developed spotted fever (typhus) after they were bitten. When they returned home, they caused epidemics in many major cities in Europe.[8] Famous typhus epidemics took place in Philadelphia in 1837, and there were epidemics of typhoid, scarlet fever, and yellow fever in Philadelphia, New York, Boston, New Orleans, Baltimore, Memphis, and Washington D.C. in the aftermath of the civil war in the mid 1860s.[9] During and immediately after World War I, 30 million persons suffered epidemic typhus. Three million deaths resulted.[2]

The microbial agent responsible for RMSF was identified by Howard Taylor Ricketts[10–12] in the early 1900s; the disease was originally described in the late 19th century following outbreaks in the Bitter Root and Snake Valleys of Montana and Idaho. Not only did Ricketts identify the etiologic agent that bears his name, but he also characterized its vector and route of transmission, as well as the protective role of immune serum, which was a remarkable task at that time.[13] In 1919, Wolbach identified the rickettsial pathogen within endothelial cells.[14]

In 1935, Derrick, a medical officer of health in Queensland, Australia, conducted a query about an outbreak of febrile illness affecting 20 of the 800 employees of a Brisbane meat works. He coined the term Q (for

TABLE 22–1. RICKETTSIA CLASSIFICATION

DISEASE	ORGANISM	GEOGRAPHIC DISTRIBUTION	RESERVOIR	TRANSMISSION TO HUMAN
SPOTTED FEVER GROUP				
Rocky Mountain spotted fever	*Rickettsia rickettsii*	United States	Ticks	Tick bite
Mediterranean spotted fever (boutonneuse fever)	*Rickettsia conorii*	Mediterranean basin, Africa, India	Ticks	Tick bite
African tick-bite fever	*Rickettsia africae*	Africa	Cattle	Tick bite
Queensland tick typhus	*Rickettsia australis*	Australia	Ticks	Tick bite
Siberian tick typhus	*Rickettsia sibirica*	Russia, China, Mongolia, Pakistan	Ticks	Tick bite
Oriental spotted fever	*Rickettsia japonica*	Japan	Unknown	Arthropod bite
Rickettsialpox	*Rickettsia akari*	North America, Europe, Korea	Mites	Mite bite
TYPHUS GROUP				
Epidemic typhus	*Rickettsia prowazekii*	Africa, United States, Asia	Humans, flying squirrels	Louse feces
Murine typhus (endemic typhus)	*Rickettsia typhi*	Worldwide	Fleas, rats	Flea feces
Scrub typhus	*Rickettsia tsutsugamushi*	Asia, Australia, South Pacific	Trombiculid mite	Larva (chigger) of trombiculid mite
OTHER DISEASES				
Q Fever	*Coxiella burnetii*	Worldwide	Ticks, ungulates	Aerosol from infected birth products
Sennetsu fever	*Ehrlichia sennetsu*	Japan	Unknown	Unknown
Human monocytic ehrlichiosis	*Ehrlichia chaffeensis*	Europe, Africa, North America	Tick?, dog?	Tick bite
Human granulocytic ehrlichiosis	*Ehrlichia* species	North America	Deer?, tick?	Tick bite

query) fever to name this new disease. Burnet and Freeman demonstrated later that Q fever was indeed caused by rickettsial bacteria.[4]

Canine ehrlichiosis was first described in 1935, and until 1987, when the first human case (monocytic ehrlichiosis from *E. chaffeensis*) was described,[15] it was mainly considered a veterinary disease. In 1994, human granulocytic ehrlichiosis was described in a small outbreak of a tick-fever disease in Minnesota and Wisconsin related to a different species of *Ehrlichia*.[16]

EPIDEMIOLOGY

Rickettsioses are zoonoses. Most of them are transmitted to humans by the bite of contaminated arthropods (tick, mite, flea, louse, chigger). Hence, their geographic distribution is closely related to that of their insect vectors, which is, most of the time, also the reservoir host (see Table 22–1). Q fever is the exception; it is distributed worldwide and is transmitted to humans by aerosol from contaminated products (especially during parturition) of cattle, sheep, goats, and also cats. It is more likely to occur in rural areas or among abattoir workers.[3]

Although Lyme disease is the leading vector-borne disease in the United States, with an incidence of 9600 reported cases in 1992, RMSF is the most frequently reported rickettsial disease, with an annual incidence of about 600 to 1200 reported cases.[1] Its causative agent, *R. rickettsii*, is inoculated through the skin by the bite of *Dermacentor andersoni*, the wood tick.[13]

Ironically, in the United States, the prevalence of RMSF between 1981 and 1991 was higher in the southern Atlantic states and in the west-south-central region than in the Rocky Mountain states. The local prevalence in highly endemic areas such as North Carolina could be as high as 14.59 per 100,000 inhabitants.[4] In a survey of 262 confirmed or highly probable cases of RMSF between 1977 and 1980 from six states where it was endemic, 99% of the cases were diagnosed between April 1 and September 30. The incidence of RMSF was highest among children, with a median age of 15 years. Males accounted for 55% and whites for 85% of the cases. Clinical complications ranging from psychiatric problems to organ failure occurred in 9% of the cases. The death rate was 4%.[17]

Rickettsialpox is caused by *R. akari*, which is transmitted among mice by mouse ectoparasites and to humans by bloodsucking mites. It was first described in 1946 following an outbreak originating in a mouse- and mite-infested apartment house in New York. The disease produced blister-like rashes resembling those of chickenpox, hence the name rickettsialpox. Since 1946, about 800 cases have been reported. More than half occurred in the 3 years following the initial episode.[18, 19]

Other rickettsial spotted fevers are mostly encountered in continents other than North America. Rarely do we have the opportunity to see the active diseases unless they are brought back by travelers returning from specific endemic areas. Most of those diseases resemble RMSF in their epidemiology and mode of transmission, except for African tick-bite fever (*Rickettsia africae*), with cattle as the natural reservoir for the bacteria (see Table 22–1).[20]

Epidemic or louse-borne typhus is caused by *R. prowazekii*. The natural reservoir for the bacteria is an infected human. The cycle begins when a louse feeds on a rickettsemic human. The bacteria infect the louse alimentary tract, and within 1 week, abundant rickettsial organisms are found in its feces. When the infected louse is allowed to infest another person, rickettsial bacteria can be transmitted to the victim. When the louse takes a blood meal, it defecates. The irritation causes the person to scratch, and the louse feces then infect the bite wound. Inoculation through mucous membranes by contaminated louse feces is also possible. The louse dies within 3 weeks of the rickettsial infection, which is not passed to its offspring. A person suffering from the recrudescent form of epidemic typhus, the Brill-Zinsser disease, can, indeed, transmit the bacteria to infesting lice. The southern flying squirrel distributed over most of the eastern states of the United States could also be a reservoir for *R. prowazekii*. The bacteria is probably transmitted among these rodents by squirrel lice and/or fleas.[21]

Louse-borne typhus is usually found in areas of crowded population with poor hygiene conditions, as occur during wars or natural disasters, especially in winter months. The disease is then responsible for an elevated number of casualties. Although similar conditions are found in some developing countries, the death rate is lower because of the availability of even minimal medical facilities. A survey of 3759 cases in Ethiopia in 1984 reported 3.8% fatalities.[22]

Murine typhus is caused by *Rickettsia typhi*, which is found worldwide in warm-climate countries near ports and where rat populations are high and flea vectors are available. Other associations have also been reported with opossums and cat fleas. The flea vector is infected by transovarian transmission from its mother or by blood-feeding on a rickettsemic animal. Humans acquire the infection via flea feces by scratching a pruritic flea-bite wound or by direct contamination of the conjunctiva or the respiratory tract. The widespread use of insecticides has considerably lowered the incidence of murine typhus in developed countries. Fatality rates are between 1% and 4%.[3, 23]

R. tsutsugamushi is the organism causing scrub typhus, a zoonosis found in the Far East. It gets its name from the secondary vegetation in transitional terrain between forest and clearings where the vector lives. The rickettsia is transmitted to humans by the bite of infected larval-stage trombiculid mites (chiggers). That mites are probably the major reservoir for the bacteria has been deduced from its transovarial transmission, and from the facts that most chiggers feed only once and that they spend their whole life within several meters of where they hatch. Mortality rates of 0% to 30% have been reported.[24]

Q fever, caused by *C. burnetii*, is found worldwide; its principal animal reservoirs are cattle, sheep, goats, ticks, and cats. The natural cycle of transmission probably involves ticks or arthropods infecting domestic ungulates or small mammals, but not humans. Infected animals remain asymptomatic until parturition, when the heavily infected placenta contaminates the environment. Air samples can be positive for up to 2 weeks after parturition, and viable organisms can be found in the soil for up to

150 days. Humans get the disease through lung infection after they have inhaled contaminated aerosols. Q fever is mostly an occupational disease affecting farmers, abattoir workers, and veterinarians. Contamination can also result from exposure to infected milk or parturient cats or when skinning wild rabbits, as well as from contact with contaminated manure, straw, or dust. Laboratory personnel are also at risk.[25, 26]

Human monocytic and human granulocytic ehrlichioses are caused by E. chaffeensis and by other Ehrlichia species, respectively. Since they have been described only recently, not much is known about their epidemiology. Exposures are mostly during the early summer months and in rural areas. Reservoirs for the bacteria are suspected to be rodents or dogs because of their ability to remain persistently infected.[3, 27] Although the disease can be quite severe, the death rate fortunately seems low. There were no deaths in a recent report on 18 patients with human granulocytic ehrlichiosis.[28]

Interestingly, a prospective study demonstrated that under conditions of intense tick exposure, there could be a high rate of seroconversion for rickettsiae without clinical evidence of the disease.[29]

PATHOPHYSIOLOGY, IMMUNOLOGY, PATHOLOGY, AND PATHOGENESIS

Rickettsial organisms can invade their human victims in three ways. They can directly access the blood stream from a portal of entry in the skin, following the bite of an infected tick, arthropod, mite, or chigger. The spotted fever disease group, the ehrlichioses, and scrub typhus are transmitted this way.

Second, the organism can contaminate a person who scratches the bite, contaminating the wound with infected louse feces. This is how epidemic and murine typhus are spread to humans.

Finally, Q fever is transmitted to the respiratory system of the victim when he inhales aerosols from contaminated products of an infected animal. The microorganisms proliferate in the lung macrophages and finally gain access to the blood stream, where they can spread to distant organs.

For most of the organisms of the spotted fever and typhus groups, the target cells are the endothelial cells of the blood vessels and their vascular smooth muscle cells. After they have been phagocytized and have entered the cells, the organisms leave the phagosomes and proliferate intracellularly. Severe damage to the small arteries, veins, and capillaries of many organs results in disseminated vasculitis. The possible mechanisms for cellular damage include activation of rickettsial phospholipase or protease, or free-radical peroxidation of host cell membranes. Rickettsial LPS toxin is relatively nontoxic and does not seem to be involved in tissue injury.[2, 3]

Because of multifocal areas of endothelial injury, there is loss of intravascular fluid into the interstitial space, with resulting edema, low blood volume, reduced perfusion to the organs, and, eventually, damaged blood vessels and altered function of tissues and organs (e.g., hemorrhagic rash, encephalitis, pneumonitis, and hepatitis). Attempted plugging of the injured vessels results in platelet consumption and relative secondary thrombocytopenia.

Cutaneous necrosis caused by obliteration of infected blood vessels at the site of the tick bite is responsible for the eschar, or tache noire, described for many of the rickettsioses.[3]

The membrane LPS of the spotted fever group of rickettsiae is strongly immunogenic, with known cross-reactivity with other members of the group as well as with Proteus and Legionella species. Unfortunately, antibodies directed against rickettsial LPS do not afford much protection against infection in the animal model. T lymphocytes, interferon-γ (IFN-γ), and tumor necrosis factor-α (TNF-α) seem to play important roles in immune defense against rickettsiosis.[2]

The target cells for C. burnetii are macrophages of the lungs, then of liver, bone marrow, spleen, heart valves, and other organs. The organisms are phagocytized, but they have the rare ability to proliferate inside the harsh environment of the host cells' phagolysosomes. The LPS of C. burnetii is also relatively nonendotoxic. T-lymphocyte–mediated granuloma formation seems to be one of the important immune defense mechanisms against this disease.[3] Liver and bone marrow biopsies and autopsy material disclose a characteristic granuloma for Q fever infection: It has a clear central space surrounded by inflammatory cells and a fibrin ring (doughnut lesion).[25]

The target cells for the genus Ehrlichia bacteria are cells of the hematopoietic and lymphoreticular systems. The organisms make characteristic clusters, called morulae, within membrane-bound cytoplasmic vacuoles of monocytes and macrophages (human monocytic ehrlichiosis) or neutrophils (human granulocytic ehrlichiosis). Findings in bone marrow biopsies may include granulomas, myeloid hyperplasia, and megakaryocytosis. Although endothelial injury and thrombosis have not been described, perivasculitis with lymphohistiocytic infiltrates of the brain, kidneys, heart, and lungs is commonly seen. Defense mechanisms against Ehrlichia species might include opsonization of macrophages and INF-γ–stimulated macrophage killing.[3, 27]

CLINICAL CHARACTERISTICS

General

A rickettsial disease should be suspected when, during spring or summer, a patient presents with the classic triad of high fever, headache, and rash. A history of outdoor activities, occupational exposure, or tick attachment is frequent. Some of the distinctive clinical characteristics of the rickettsioses are summarized in Table 22–2.

Systemic

The initial clinical presentation of most of the diseases in the spotted fever group includes high fever, myalgia, and headaches. A tache noire develops at the site of the arthropod bite. Gastrointestinal involvement with nausea, vomiting, and abdominal tenderness is frequent. Neurologic signs ranging from small focal deficits to major neuropsychiatric disturbances have been reported. The maculopapular rash may be present at the time of presentation or in the following days. In RMSF, it typically starts around the wrists and ankles and eventually spreads to the trunk. Involvement of the palms and soles is consid-

TABLE 22–2. CLINICAL CHARACTERISTICS OF RICKETTSIOSES

DISEASE	ORGANISM (INCUBATION PERIOD, DAYS)	RASH DISTRIBUTION	TACHE NOIRE-ESCHAR	OTHER FEATURES
SPOTTED FEVER GROUP				
Rocky Mountain spotted fever	*Rickettsia rickettsii* (2–14)	Extremities to trunk (palms & soles)	No	Neuropsychiatric symptoms
Mediterranean spotted fever	*Rickettsia conorii*	Trunk, extremities	Yes	—
African tick-bite fever	*Rickettsia africae* (within 7)	Weak or absent	Multiple	Lymphadenopathy, lymphangitis
Queensland tick typhus	*Rickettsia australis*	Trunk, extremities	Yes	—
Siberian tick typhus	*Rickettsia sibirica*	Trunk, extremities	Yes	—
Rickettsialpox	*Rickettsia akari* (9–14)	Vesicular: trunk, extremities	Yes	Lymphadenopathy
TYPHUS GROUP				
Epidemic typhus	*Rickettsia prowazekii* (7)	Trunk + axilla to extremities	No	Brill-Zinsser disease = recurrent form
Murine typhus	*Rickettsia typhi* (7–14)	Trunk to extremities	No	—
Scrub typhus	*Rickettsia tsutsugamushi* (6–18)	Trunk to extremities	Yes	Lymphadenopathy
OTHER DISEASES				
Q fever	*Coxiella burnetii* (14–39)	Rare	No	Pneumonia, chronic endocarditis
Sennetsu fever	*Ehrlichia sennetsu* (14)	Very rare	No	Lymphadenopathy
Human monocytic ehrlichiosis	*Ehrlichia chaffeensis* (7)	Maculopapular	No	Lymphadenopathy
Human granulocytic ehrlichiosis	*Ehrlichia* species (1–14)	Rare	No	—

ered characteristic. In other spotted fever rickettsioses, the rash instead starts over the trunk and later spreads centrifugally to the extremities. Skin necrosis or gangrene secondary to vasculitic complications has been reported in 4% of cases.[3, 4]

In rickettsialpox, the initial lesion that develops at the site of a mite bite is papulovesicular. It evolves to form an eschar with local lymphadenopathy. High fever begins abruptly about 1 week later, and a few days afterward red macules, papules, and papulovesicles resembling chickenpox develop.[19]

In African tick-bite fever, multiple taches noires with lymphadenopathy and lymphangitis have been described.[20]

The initial clinical presentation for the typhus group of rickettsioses is similar to that of the spotted fever group, with high fever, myalgia, and rash. In epidemic typhus, lung and potentially severe neurologic involvement have been reported. A recurrent form of the disorder, the Brill-Zinsser disease, may develop years after the initial infection, following stress or decreased immunity.[3, 21] In murine typhus, neurologic symptoms are found in up to 45% of the patients and may include confusion, seizures, and ataxia.[23]

Patients affected by Q fever also present with high fever, headache, malaise, and myalgia, but a rash is not found. Pneumonia is present in up to 90% of patients; it is characterized by patchy infiltrates on chest radiographs. Hepatitis with minimal elevation of the transaminase enzymes is found in 85% of patients. Jaundice is uncommon. Endocarditis is a rare but serious complication of Q fever because it can be lethal. When endocarditis develops, there is usually concomitant hepatic involvement.[25, 26]

Patients with ehrlichiosis present with fever, myalgia, or arthralgia. Less than 50% develop a maculopapular rash; this is seen more frequently in children. A finding of abnormal liver enzymes is common. Rare complications include respiratory and renal insufficiency, neurologic abnormalities, and gastrointestinal hemorrhage.[27, 28]

Ocular Involvement

Ocular involvement in rickettsioses is not reported frequently. Since it can be mild, it is probably overlooked much of the time. I am not aware of a prospective study that has systematically addressed this issue.

Contamination of the conjunctiva by a spurt of tick blood has been implicated as the apparent portal of entry for *R. rickettsii* systemic infection.[13] Conjunctivitis was reported in 30% of the cases in a retrospective study including 262 patients suffering from confirmed or highly probable RMSF between 1977 and 1980 in the United States.[17] Conjunctival petechiae and subconjunctival hemorrhages have also been described.[30]

Rare descriptions of keratitis or corneal ulcerations are found in the literature.[30] A well-documented case of Mediterranean spotted fever keratitis was reported in 1992. The authors believed that the corneal infection was probably secondary to contamination from the tears during systemic rickettsiosis in a 69-year-old man with chronic alcoholism. The lesion consisted of an ameboid type of ulceration similar to herpetic epithelial keratitis.

Corneal scrapings were positive for *R. rickettsii* antigens with direct immunofluorescence studies and negative to herpes simplex immunologic and cytopathic tests. It responded readily to the use of topical tetracycline ointment.[31]

Mild to moderate nongranulomatous anterior uveitis has been described with rickettsioses.[32] It usually resolves with topical corticosteroids and mydriatic treatment, or when the infectious disease subsides after appropriate systemic antibiotic treatment.

An iris nodule, similar to the typhus nodule reported at autopsy of the central nervous system following typhus rickettsioses, was reported by Duffey and Hammer in 1987.[33]

A case of endogenous endophthalmitis caused by *Rickettsia conorii* and apparently proved by serologic and vitreous direct and indirect immunofluorescence was reported by Mendivil and Cuarto in 1998.[34] A 50-year-old man presented with a leg tick-bite eschar, fever, arthromyalgia, and fatigue of 6-day duration. He developed unilateral loss of vision with relative afferent pupillary defect and hypopyon. Vitreous cultures remained negative, but the ocular condition cleared after intravitreal chloramphenicol injection and systemic doxycycline.

Since the physiopathologic basis for rickettsial infectious diseases is vasculitic, most of the ocular inflammatory lesions involve the retinal or optic nerve vasculature. They can include optic nerve head edema; intraretinal hemorrhages; cotton-wool spots; dilated, tortuous retinal veins; vasculitis; and retinal vessel occlusion.[35–37] Fluorescein angiography of the retina of a 9-year-old girl with RMSF demonstrated focal areas of capillary nonperfusion with cotton-wool spots and perivascular staining in the infarcted areas. Late-phase photographs showed hyperfluorescence of the optic disk.[35]

There are reports of multiple small retinal white spots or small retinal infiltrates during rickettsioses. Moderate vitreous inflammation can be found, and white retinal infiltrates are seen localized in the neurosensory retina (Fig. 22–1). A blocking effect is produced by these lesions on fluorescein angiography. The lesions usually resolve without clinical and angiographic scarring in a few weeks following appropriate systemic antibiotic treatment.[37–39] These multiple white dots might be similar to those seen in multiple evanescent white dot syndrome (MEWDS), an acute, multifocal, self-limiting disease affecting young adults after a flulike syndrome.[38]

DIAGNOSIS

There are no rapid laboratory tests for rickettsioses. The best early diagnostic tool is the physician's high index of suspicion in the presence of high fever, general malaise, headache, and a rash in a patient living in or traveling back from a region endemic for rickettsioses. Occupational contact with infected birth products of farm animals should also be inquired about.

A complete and careful physical exam is essential. The physician should first look for the presence of the insect vector (louse, flea, or tick). The hard ticks can stay attached for days on their victims and can be overlooked if located on the back or in the axillary or inguinal region. Rash can be very subtle. Tick bites that later develop tache noire should be searched for.

The diagnosis of rickettsioses is confirmed when positive serologic tests are found in a patient with a compatible clinical presentation. Positive serologic criteria usually include either initial high antibody titer or a fourfold rise of the titer in the convalescent serum. Serologic tests may include complement-fixing antibody, enzyme immunoassay, indirect fluorescent antibody, indirect hemagglutination, and latex agglutination.[3] The relatively nonspecific and insensitive Weil-Felix test has become obsolete.[17] Case confirmation with serology might take 2 to 3 weeks. Furthermore, early antibiotic treatment tends to blunt and delay the antibody response to the bacteria.[18]

Another interesting test has been described in Europe for the diagnosis of rickettsioses. Endothelial cells are isolated from blood samples with the use of immunomagnetic beads coated with endothelial cell–specific IgG1 monoclonal antibodies. The presence of rickettsiae can then be determined using either specific immunofluorescent staining or amplification by polymerase chain reaction.[20]

Direct fluorescent antibody testing on paraffin-embedded biopsy specimens from eschars or papulovesicles has been reported in rickettsialpox.[19]

When ehrlichiosis is suspected, a search should be made for morulae in blood buffy-coat smears stained with Wright's stain. The test is positive in up to 80% of cases as early as the day of initial presentation.[28, 40]

Because rickettsiae are both fastidious and hazardous organisms, many microbiology laboratories are reluctant to undertake their isolation and identification.[3] Nonspecific laboratory changes during rickettsemia may include anemia, leukocytosis, leukopenia, thrombocytopenia, hyponatremia, hypoalbuminemia, liver function abnormalities, renal function impairment, coagulation disturbances, and cerebrospinal fluid abnormalities with leukocytosis and hypoglycorrhachia.[13, 25, 41]

TREATMENT

Prevention is the best approach for rickettsial diseases. Good sanitary habits and special attention to tick bites in endemic areas are recommended. An attached tick is

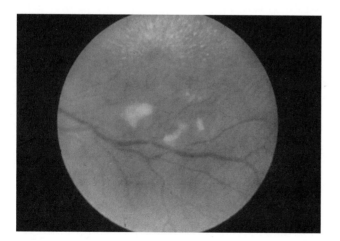

FIGURE 22–1. Retinal involvement in Rickettsioses. Note the periarteritis, the macular star exudate, and the retinal infiltrates. (Courtesy of C. Stephen Foster, M.D.) (See color insert.)

best removed with a pair of forceps, trying to keep the arthropod intact. The wound should then be cleansed.[4]

Except for epidemic typhus (*R. prowazekii*) and possibly soon for Q fever (*C. burnetii*), human vaccine is not currently available for the rickettsioses. Vaccination is recommended for individuals who are at high risk of becoming infected: scientific investigators, laboratory personnel, people working or traveling in endemic areas, and medical personnel providing care where typhus is found.[4, 18, 21, 23, 24, 26, 27]

Anterior uveitis can be treated with topical steroids and mydriatic drops. Retinal lesions usually respond to systemic antibiotic treatment.

Rickettsemia is best treated with oral tetracyclines (25–50 mg/kg/day) or chloramphenicol (50–75 mg/kg/day) in four divided doses. Doxycycline (100 mg every 12 h) is also very effective, and quinolones (ciprofloxacin [1.5 g/day], and ofloxacin) have been recently described as valuable alternatives. The drugs can be administered orally or intravenously. Because of the effect of tetracyclines on developing bones and teeth, chloramphenicol or quinolones are preferred in pregnant women and in young children.[4, 18, 21, 23, 24]

Chloramphenicol is not effective in ehrlichiosis, where tetracycline or doxycycline is the treatment of choice. Rifampin was shown to have in vitro ehrlichicidal properties, but its clinical effectiveness has not been evaluated.[27]

The treatment of choice for acute Q fever is also tetracycline. Chloramphenicol and quinolones may also be used. Although generally quite effective in treating any form of atypical pneumonia, erythromycin might be relatively ineffective for the most severe cases of Q fever pneumonia, unless rifampin (300 mg by mouth twice daily) is added.[25, 26] There is usually a consensus about using a combination of antibiotics for many months to treat Q fever endocarditis, a chronic, potentially lethal form of *C. burnetii* infection. The therapeutic regimen might include doxycycline with trimethoprim-sulfamethoxazole or rifampin, doxycycline with fluoroquinolones, or doxycycline with chloroquine or amantadine for months to 2 years. Antibody titers should be monitored regularly. Successful therapy is usually accompanied by normalization of the erythrocyte sedimentation rate, the anemia, and the hyperglobulinemia. Valve replacement may be necessary.[26]

COMPLICATIONS

When appropriate therapy is initiated promptly, most patients recover rapidly and without complications from rickettsioses. Many are fortunate to recover without systemic treatment. Unfortunately, however, rickettsial agents have the potential to cause important systemic complications, including death.

The possible systemic complications for rickettsial disease include hemolytic anemia, coagulopathies, focal neurologic deficits, seizures, severe psychiatric disturbances and coma, hepatitis, skin necrosis, renal insufficiency, chronic endocarditis, and osteomyelitis.

Fortunately, unless the disease has caused irreversible damage from obstructed blood vessels, most rickettsial ocular lesions resolve without residual visual impairment. This is especially so if systemic antibiotics are used.

PROGNOSIS

The sooner the clinical diagnosis of rickettsial infection is made and appropriate treatment is begun, the better the prognosis. Where medical facilities are easily obtainable, the mortality rate for RMSF is less than 4%, but it can reach 20% to 25% if treatment is delayed or inappropriate.[3]

Better overall sanitary conditions also favorably affect the prognosis of the epidemic forms of rickettsioses such as murine or epidemic typhus. In the aftermath of war or natural disasters, the casualties among people living in overcrowded areas with poor hygiene can reach the thousands, whereas with better sanitary conditions, even in developing countries where medical facilities are limited, the fatality rate is about 4%.[22]

CONCLUSIONS

Rickettsial diseases are characterized by the triad of high fever, headache and general malaise, and skin rash. Occupational hazard (abattoir workers or contact with contaminated birth products of farm animals), living in or traveling back from an endemic area for rickettsioses, or a history of tick bites is usually found when interviewing the patient.

The early diagnosis relies entirely on a high index of suspicion and keen clinical acumen, and the sooner the appropriate antibiotic regimen is initiated, the better the prognosis. Although following a tick bite, there is a significant percentage of seroconversion without clinical disease and of spontaneous remission without treatment, rickettsioses are severe, potentially lethal diseases and should be treated accordingly.

There is hope that with better sanitary conditions including the control of rat reservoirs and of flea or lice vectors the incidence of the epidemic forms of rickettsioses (murine and epidemic typhus) could be lowered in the areas where it is now endemic.

Finally, the development of new, more rapid diagnostic tools needs to be encouraged. In the search for specific rickettsial antigens, the use of immunomagnetic beads to isolate endothelial cells from blood samples[20] may become a gold standard in early detection of the disease. If this test is proved to be reliable, it should improve the prognosis for rickettsioses.

References

1. Spach DH, Liles WC, Campbell GL, et al: Tick-borne diseases in the United States. N Engl J Med 1993;329:936–947.
2. Saah AJ: Rickettsiosis: Introduction. In: Mandell GL, Douglas JE, and Bennett R, eds: Principles and Practice of Infectious Diseases. New York, Churchill Livingstone, 1995, pp 1719–1720.
3. Walker DH: Rickettsiae. In: Baron A, ed: Medical Microbiology. Galveston, TX, The University of Texas Medical Branch at Galveston, 1996, pp 487–501.
4. Walker DH, Raoult D: *Rickettsia rickettsii* and other spotted fever group rickettsiae (Rocky Mountain spotted fever and other spotted fevers). In: Mandell GL, Douglas JE, and Bennett R, eds: Principles and Practice of Infectious Diseases. New York, Churchill Livingstone, 1995, pp 1721–1727.
5. CDC and NIH: Rickettsial agents. In: Biosafety in Microbiological and Biomedical Laboratories. 1993. Washington, DC, Centers for Disease Control and Prevention and the National Institutes of Health.
6. Slater NL, Welch DF: *Rochalimaea* species (recently renamed *Bartonella*). In: Mandell GL, Douglas JE, and Bennett R, eds: Principles

and Practice of Infectious Diseases. New York, Churchill Livingstone, 1995, pp 1741–1747.

7. Pfeiffer CJ: The Art and Practice of Western Medicine in the Early Nineteenth Century. Jefferson, NC, McFarland, 1985.

8. Major RH: Disease and Destiny. Logan Clendening. Lawrence, KS, University of Kansas Press, 1958.

9. American epidemics. Ohio Network of American History and Research Center. www.infinet.com/~dzimmerm/ohionet.html.

10. Ricketts HT: A summary of investigations of the nature and means of transmission of Rocky Mountain spotted fever. Trans Chicago Pathol Soc 1906;7:73–82.

11. Ricketts HT: The study of Rocky Mountain spotted fever (tick fever?) by means of animal inoculations. A preliminary communication. JAMA 1906;47:33–36.

12. Ricketts HT: Some aspects of Rocky Mountain spotted fever as shown by recent investigations. Med Record 1909;76:843–855.

13. Kirk JL, Fine DP, Sexton DJ, Muchmore HG: Rocky Mountain spotted fever. A clinical review based on 48 confirmed cases. Medicine 1990;69:35–45.

14. Wolbach SB: Studies on Rocky Mountain spotted fever. J Med Res 1919;41:2–197.

15. Maeda K, Markowitz N, Hawley RC, et al: Human infection with *Ehrlichia canis*, a leucocytic rickettsia. N Engl J Med 1987;316:853–856.

16. Chen SM, Dumler JS, Bakken JS, et al: Identification of a granulocytotropic *Ehrlichia* species as the etiologic agent of human disease. J Clin Microbiol 1994;32:589–595.

17. Helmick CG, Bernard KW, D'Angelo LJ: Rocky Mountain spotted fever: Clinical, laboratory, and epidemiological features of 262 cases. J Infect Dis 1984;150:480–488.

18. Saah AJ: *Rickettsia akari* (rickettsialpox). In: Mandell GL, Douglas JE, and Bennett R, eds: Principles and Practice of Infectious Diseases. New York, Churchill Livingstone, 1995, p 1727.

19. Kass EM, Szaniawski WK, Levy H, et al: Rickettsialpox in a New York City hospital, 1980 to 1989. N Engl J Med 1994;331:1612–1617.

20. Brouqui P, Harle JR, Delmont J, et al: African tick-bite fever. An imported spotless rickettsiosis. Arch Intern Med 1997;157:119–124.

21. Saah AJ: *Rickettsia prowazekii* (epidemic or louse-borne typhus). In: Mandell GL, Douglas JE, and Bennett R, eds: Principles and Practice of Infectious Diseases. New York, Churchill Livingstone, 1995, pp 1735–1737.

22. World Health Organization: Louse-borne typhus: 1983–1984. Weekly Epidemiol Rec 1984;57:45–46.

23. Dumler JS, Walker DH: Murine typhus. In: Mandell GL, Douglas JE, and Bennett R, eds: Principles and Practice of Infectious Diseases. New York, Churchill Livingstone, 1995, pp 1737–1739.

24. Saah AJ: *Rickettsia tsutsugamuchi* (scrub typhus). In Mandell GL, Douglas JE, and Bennett R, eds: Principles and Practice of Infectious Diseases. New York, Churchill Livingstone, 1995, pp 1740–1741.

25. Sawyer LA, Fishbein DB, McDade J: Q fever: Current concepts. Rev Infect Dis 1987;9:935–946.

26. Marrie TJ: *Coxiella burnetii* (Q fever). In: Mandell GL, Douglas JE, and Bennett R, eds: Principles and Practice of Infectious Diseases. New York, Churchill Livingstone, 1995, pp 1727–1735.

27. Walker DH, Dumler JS: *Ehrlichia chaffeensis* (human ehrlichiosis) and other ehrlichiae. In: Mandell GL, Douglas JE, and Bennett R, eds: Principles and Practice of Infectious Diseases. New York, Churchill Livingstone, 1995, pp 1747–1752.

28. Aguero-Rosenfeld ME, Horowitz HW, Wormser GP, et al: Human granulocytic ehrlichiosis: A case series from a medical center in New York State. Ann Intern Med 1996;125:904–908.

29. Sanchez JL, Chandler WH, Fishbein DB, et al: A cluster of tick-borne infections: Association with military training and asymptomatic infections due to *Rickettsia rickettsii*. Trans R Soc Trop Med Hyg 1992;86:321–325.

30. François J: Rickettsiae in ophthalmology. Ophtalmologica 1968;156:459–472.

31. Alio J, Ruiz-Beltran R, Herrera I, et al: Rickettsial keratitis in a case of Mediterranean spotted fever. Eur J Ophthalmol 1992;2:41–43.

32. Cherubini TD, Spaeth GL: Anterior nongranulomatous uveitis associated with Rocky Mountain spotted fever. First report of a case. Arch Ophthalmol 1969;81:363–365.

33. Duffey RJ, Hammer ME: The ocular manifestations of Rocky Mountain spotted fever. Ann Ophthalmol 1987;19:301–303.

34. Mendivil A, Cuarto V: Endogenous endophthalmitis caused by *Rickettsia conorii*. Acta Ophthalmol Scand 1998;76:121–122.

35. Smith TW, Burton TC: The retinal manifestations of Rocky Mountain spotted fever. Am J Ophthalmol 1977;84:259–262.

36. Sulewski ME, Green WR: Ocular histopathologic features of a presumed case of Rocky Mountain spotted fever. Retina 1986;6:125–130.

37. Hudson HL, Thach AB, Lopez PF: Retinal manifestations of acute murine typhus. Int Ophthalmol 1997;21:121–126.

38. Lu TM, Kuo BI, Chung YM, Liu CY: Murine typhus presenting with multiple white dots in the retina. Scand J Infect Dis 1997;29:632–633.

39. Lukas JR, Egger S, Parschalk B, Stur M: Bilateral small retinal infiltrates during rickettsial infection. Br J Ophthalmol 1998;82:1217–1218.

40. Bakken JS, Krueth J, Wilson-Nordskog C, et al: Clinical and laboratory characteristics of human granulocytic ehrlichiosis. JAMA 1996;275:199–205.

41. Dumler JS, Taylor JP, Walker DH: Clinical and laboratory features of murine typhus in South Texas, 1980 through 1987. JAMA 1991;266:1365–1370.

Elisabeth M. Messmer

DEFINITION

Leprosy (Hansen's disease) is a chronic granulomatous infectious disease caused by *Mycobacterium leprae*. It mainly involves skin, peripheral nerves, mucous membranes, and ocular structures. According to the World Health Organization (WHO), a "case of leprosy" is defined as a person having one or more of the following features, and who has yet to complete a full course of treatment:[1]

- Hypopigmented or reddish skin lesion(s) with definite loss of sensation
- Involvement of the peripheral nerves, as demonstrated by definite thickening with loss of sensation
- Skin-smear positive for acid-fast bacilli

Unfortunately, the WHO considers as "leprosy patients" only those who are untreated or on active treatment. This may be misleading in treated cases of leprosy with ongoing eye disease or leprosy-related visual disability.

Depending on the resistance to infection, leprosy may present as tuberculoid (TT), borderline (TB, BB, BL), or lepromatous (LL) leprosy on a continuous disease spectrum.[2, 3] Leprosy patients may be classified as having multibacillary or paucibacillary leprosy according to the degree of skin-smear positivity.[4, 5] Because services for processing skin smears are not always available and their reliability is often doubtful, patients are increasingly being classified on clinical grounds. The assumption is that the protective immunity is inversely correlated with the number of skin lesions. The WHO therefore proposes the following classification, which has an important impact on therapeutic decisions:

- Paucibacillary single-lesion leprosy (one skin lesion)
- Paucibacillary leprosy (two to five skin lesions)
- Multibacillary leprosy (more than five skin lesions)[1]

According to the U.S. Department of Health and Human Services, Centers for Disease Control, leprosy belongs to the group of "Notifiable Diseases."[6]

HISTORY

References to leprosy can be found in the ancient Indian literature (Sushruta Samhita, 600 BC), described as kushtha (kushnati = to gnaw or sashtha = bad, evil) and in the ancient Chinese medical literature as Da Feng (circa 400 BC).[7, 8] It is generally doubted that leprosy is mentioned in the Bible as tsara'ath, because there is no description of associated nerve damage.[7]

In the Western world, no identifiable clinical descriptions of leprosy are known prior to the third century BC, when the lepromatous type came to be known to the physicians of Alexandria under the name elephantiasis. What Hippocrates and other ancient scholars called lepra was an ill-defined and nonspecific eruption of the skin.[7] Wars and crusades caused an epidemic spread of leprosy, which peaked in Europe between the 10th and 14th centuries AD. Contradicting the traditional view that leprosy was overdiagnosed in the Middle Ages, approximately 80% of the skeletal remains of persons buried in medieval leprosaria reveal the bone changes of leprosy.[9] Central and South America were probably free from leprosy before the Spaniards and Portuguese introduced it in the 16th century and thereafter. Similarly, leprosy was probably unknown in North America until introduced by successive waves of western European immigrants and slaves from Africa.[7]

Probably the most important scientific event in the history of leprosy took place in 1873 in Bergen, Norway, where Hansen observed rod-shaped bodies in unstained fluid from skin lesions of leprosy patients. He announced them as the cause of the disease in 1874.[10] As early as 1873, Bull and Hansen[11] drew attention to leprous eye complications, which may present in up to 100% of patients with longstanding disease.

In more recent years, important breakthroughs in leprosy management and research were reported: the introduction of sulphones for chemotherapy (1943),[12] the recognition of selective growth of *M. leprae* in cool parts of the body (1956),[13] the development of the mouse footpad model (1960),[14] the identification of the nine-banded armadillo as an experimental model of leprosy (1971),[15] the purification of antigens of *M. leprae* (1980),[16] and the establishment of genomic libraries of *M. leprae* (1985).[17, 18]

EPIDEMIOLOGY

Considerable progress has been made in the fight against leprosy during the past 10 to 15 years, following the introduction of multidrug therapy (MDT) regimens. Current estimates indicate that there are about 1.15 million cases of leprosy in the world, compared with 10 to 12 million cases in the mid 1980s.[1] During the past 12 years, the number of registered cases in the world has fallen by about 85% in almost all countries and regions where leprosy is endemic.[1] The highest prevalence of leprosy is in central Africa, the Middle East, and Southeast Asia, including India and Indonesia.[19] Although leprosy is regarded primarily as a tropical disease, 122 new cases were reported in the United States in 1997. The number of reported cases in the United States peaked in 1985 with 361 newly diagnosed leprosy patients, but it has remained stable since 1988.[6]

Imported rather than indigenous cases are responsible for the growing incidence of leprosy in the United States, reflecting the increase in numbers of refugees and immigrants, as well as increased world travel and work abroad by American citizens.[20] Indigenous areas continue to exist in Hawaii, Texas, and California.[6, 20, 21]

Although humans are considered the major host and reservoir of *M. leprae*, other animals, including the armadillo, chimpanzee, and mangabey monkey, have also been incriminated as reservoirs of infection.[1] The epidemiologic significance of these findings is unknown, but is likely to be very limited.[1] There is no evidence to suggest an association between HIV infection and leprosy.[22] However, previous infection with tuberculosis has been implicated in the resistance to leprosy, and protection against leprosy by bacillus Calmette-Guérin (BCG) vaccination was demonstrated in five large field trials conducted in India, Malawi, Myanmar, Papua New Guinea, and Uganda. The protective effect, however, varied from 20% to 80%. The addition of killed *M. leprae* did not improve the protection afforded by BCG vaccination alone in either of the trials.[1]

The risk of becoming infected with *M. leprae* remains a controversial issue. A view still prevalent is that subjects become infected only after close and prolonged contact with an infectious patient. However, Godal and colleagues reported that an immune response to *M. leprae*, indicated by a reactive lymphocyte transformation assay, is present in 50% of contacts of tuberculoid or treated lepromatous patients and in more than 50% of individuals with occupational contact of leprosy for more than 1 year.[23] It seems that leprosy is more highly infectious than indicated by the prevalence of the disease, and that subclinical infections are common but are eliminated by an appropriate cellular immune response.[1, 23, 24] Airborne spread from the infected upper respiratory tract and discharges from ulcerative skin lesions are considered the major routes of transmission of viable leprosy bacilli. Leprous infection from mother to child may occur by transplacental transmission[25] and by infected breast milk. Insects have been incriminated as carriers of *M. leprae*, but the epidemiology of leprosy is not consistent with a primarily vector-borne transmission. Insect bites may favor the penetration of *M. leprae* deposited on the skin.[7, 26]

Factors that influence susceptibility to leprosy infection include age (bimodal age distribution, with the first peak in childhood and a plateau between 30 and 60 years), male sex, and low socioeconomic background.[7, 21] Not only may genetic factors influence the pathogenesis of leprosy as seen in identical twins,[7] but genetic markers such as human leukocytic antigens (HLA) may also control the type of leprosy that develops.[24, 27] There is striking geographic variation in the prevalence of the lepromatous form of leprosy, from below 5% in Burkina Faso to over 60% in Malaysia. Lucio leprosy, a distinct form of lepromatous leprosy, appears to be confined to Latin America.[21]

There are few, if any, true incidence data to predict ocular involvement in leprosy. Depending on the investigator, prevalence of ocular leprosy ranges from 0.8% to 100%.[28] Many investigators believe that ocular involvement would develop in all leprosy patients with longstanding, untreated disease.[29-32]

Approximately 2 million people currently have disabilities related to leprosy. Blindness due to leprosy was seen in 3.2% of the patients, whereas 7.1% of leprosy patients had severe visual impairment (visual acuity less than 20/200) in a study of 4772 leprosy patients reported by ffytche.[33] The three major causes of visual disability and blindness in leprosy patients are corneal involvement, uveal disease, and cataract formation.[34] Excess mortality with a 4.8-fold risk of death associated with blindness was reported in leprosy patients.[35]

CLINICAL CHARACTERISTICS

Systemic Findings

Leprosy ranges from single, selfhealing, symptomless macules to relentless progressive disease. Anesthetic skin lesions, enlarged peripheral nerves, and acid-fast bacilli in skin smears are the main systemic findings in leprosy. The signs and symptoms of the disease result from three interrelated processes: (1) the growth and dissemination of *M. leprae*, (2) the host immune response, and (3) damage to nerves.[21]

Typically, the earliest sign of leprosy is a macule that is slightly hypoesthetic and erythematous or hypopigmented (indeterminate leprosy).

Skin lesions of lepromatous (LL) leprosy vary from poorly defined macules to papules, nodules, plaques, or diffuse infiltrations. They tend to be numerous and symmetrically distributed. Sensory disturbances develop later in the course of the disease and are not as distinct as in tuberculoid leprosy. In tuberculoid (TT) leprosy, early macular lesions are sharply defined and hypopigmented or erythematous, with distinct sensory impairment. Typically, there is a single, well-defined lesion, or only a few, which are asymmetrically distributed. Borderline (BT, BB, BL) leprosy spans the spectrum between TT and LL. Damage to peripheral nerves is often pronounced.[21]

The clinical course of leprosy is often exacerbated by acute episodes called leprosy reactions. These reactions fall into two groups: (1) type I reactions, with increased cell-mediated immunity (reversal reactions) or decreased cell-mediated immunity (downgrading reactions), and (2) type II reactions (erythema nodosum leprosum [ENL]), with decreased cell-mediated and altered humoral immunity with deposition of immune complexes in the lesions.[21, 36] In both type I reactions, skin lesions become erythematous and edematous, and acute neuritis is common. In ENL, leprosy patients typically develop tender subcutaneous nodules, fever, lymphadenopathy, arthralgias, and vasculitis. Type I and type II reactions carry an increased risk for ocular complications.[21, 37-39]

Ocular Lesions

Ocular involvement in leprosy varies depending on many factors, including the form of leprosy, the duration of the disease, and the previous systemic and local treatment. Ocular lesions may occur by four mechanisms: (1) spread of leprous lesions from adjacent skin or nasal mucosa, (2) neuritis with infranuclear facial nerve palsy or trigeminal nerve involvement and subsequent corneal damage, (3) direct intraocular infection with *M. leprae*, and (4) allergic reaction to *M. leprae* antigen. Lepromatous leprosy tends to be associated with more severe intraocular involvement, whereas patients with tuberculoid leprosy typically present with early involvement of the motor and sensory nerves with resulting corneal problems.[40]

Lids, Cornea, and Conjunctiva

Brow hair loss and loss of lashes (madarosis) are perhaps the most common manifestations of leprosy.[40] It does not have any functional relevance, but it represents a stigma for the patient. Lagophthalmos caused by seventh nerve paralysis, often accompanied by ectropion, occurs in about 20% of leprosy patients independent of the type of disease.[41] Lagophthalmos is mostly bilateral and a late complication in multibacillary cases, whereas it occurs unilaterally and early in the course of the disease in paucibacillary patients, often associated with leprosy reactions.[42] Lagophthalmos resulted in corneal disease (exposure keratitis, ulcer, or opacity) in 87% of afflicted leprosy patients in a recent study in China.[43] Trigeminal nerve involvement, causing corneal hypesthesia, frequently accompanies facial nerve palsy in leprosy, and the effect of this combination is catastrophic, with a high risk for sight-threatening corneal complications.[44, 45] Furthermore, leprosy causes denervation of the lacrimal gland and infiltration of the meibomian glands of the lids, resulting in tear film abnormalities that contribute to corneal morbidity.[46, 47]

Focally enlarged corneal nerves, resembling beads on a string, are pathognomonic of leprosy. Frequently, patients with leprosy exhibit an asymptomatic, avascular, punctate keratitis in the superior quadrant of the cornea caused by direct bacterial invasion. Less frequently, an interstitial keratitis may develop. Classic leprous pannus with microlepromata within the network of newly formed blood vessels occurs late in the course of the disease. Frank corneal lepromas are a rare manifestation of leprosy.

Pterygium formation associated with lepromatous granuloma of the conjunctiva has been reported to occur in leprosy patients.[48]

Sclera

Nodular episcleritis and scleritis usually consist of a focal leproma and an inflammatory response. Diffuse episcleritis and scleritis may also occur as an immunologically driven disease with immune complex deposition without direct bacillary invasion. It is typically observed during leprosy reactions and is often associated with keratitis or iridocyclitis. Chronic or recurrent scleritis may lead to scleral necrosis, scleral "melt," and staphyloma formation.[49]

Iris, Ciliary Body

Uveal tract involvement is primarily seen in lepromatous leprosy, and its incidence is directly proportional to disease duration. In a recent worldwide study on the ocular complications of leprosy in 4772 patients, iris involvement occurred in at least one eye in 7.2% of patients, with variation between centers ranging from 0.5% to 23.8%.[34] Iridocyclitis and sequelae were responsible for blindness in at least 5.4% of eyes.[34]

Lepromatous iridocyclitis may be (1) caused by direct invasion of *M. leprae* into ocular structures, hematogenously or by way of ciliary nerves, (2) neuroparalytic, the result of an early involvement of iris sympathetic nerves,[50] or (3) a uveal hypersensitivity to *M. leprae* antigen in association with a leprosy reaction.[40, 50, 51] *M. leprae* has been isolated from the iris of normal-appearing eyes,[52] and it has been suggested that the iris is a site in which *M. leprae* might survive long after skin smears have become negative.[53]

Early subtle signs of iris and ciliary body involvement are autonomic dysfunction, including diminished pupil-

lary reactions[54, 55] with denervation hypersensitivity to adrenergic agents,[50, 56] and reduced accomodation[57] with early presbyopia.[58] Iris involvement can be divided into four main groups: acute iridocyclitis, chronic iridocyclitis, miliary iris lepromas, and nodular iris lepromas.

ACUTE, DIFFUSE, PLASTIC IRIDOCYCLITIS

Acute nongranulomatous iridocyclitis is a common, often bilateral, accompaniment of the type II (ENL) reaction. Its clinical presentation does not differ from other forms of acute nonleprous iritis. The course of the disease is often fulminant, with a sudden painful onset, conjunctival hyperemia, keratic precipitates, aqueous cells, and flare, often with hypopyon formation, posterior synechiae, and secondary glaucoma.[50] Spontaneous hyphema may also occur as a result of the fragility of the iris vasculature.[40]

CHRONIC IRIDOCYCLITIS

The more common chronic iridocyclitis is less dramatic but potentially blinding. It is a low-grade, granulomatous or nongranulomatous iridocyclitis common in lepromatous leprosy but also seen in the tuberculoid form. It is characterized by a lack of symptoms and overt signs, although slit-lamp examination may show aqueous cells and flare with fine or mutton-fat keratic precipitates scattered all over the corneal endothelium[50] (Fig. 23–1). However, its chronic course eventually leads to severe iris atrophy and polycoria. Iris adhesions slowly progress to seclude and occlude the pupil. Small, nonreacting pupils, caused by the involvement of sympathetic iris nerves, exaggerate the visual impairment created by developing lens changes and corneal opacities.[50]

MILIARY IRIS LEPROMAS (IRIS PEARLS)

Equally asymptomatic is the development of miliary iris lepromas (iris pearls) in the early stages of the disease. These small, glistening, white lesions are pathognomonic for leprosy (Fig. 23–2) and have been shown to represent aggregates of tightly packed living and dead bacilli lying within mononuclear cells (foam or lepra cells). Iris pearls usually develop within a year or two of the commencement of iritis, with little accompanying inflammation or

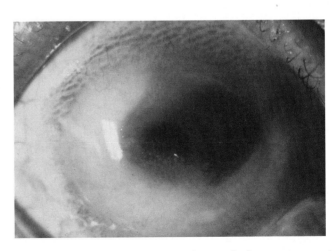

FIGURE 23–1. Lepromatous uveitis with corneal edema, retrocorneal fibrovascular membrane formation, mutton-fat keratic precipitates, 3+ anterior chamber inflammation, and secluded pupil. (See color insert.)

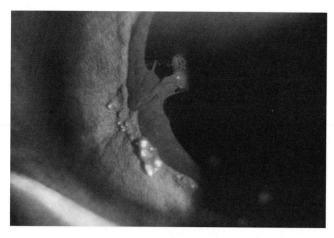

FIGURE 23–2. Iris granuloma formation (so-called iris pearls) in lepromatous uveitis. (From Messmer EM, Raizman MB, Foster CS: Lepromatous uveitis diagnosed by iris biopsy. Graefes Arch Clin Exp Ophthalmol 1998;236:717–719. Copyright © 1998 Springer-Verlag.) (See color insert.)

foreign body reaction.[59, 60] Iris pearls are situated mainly at the pupil margin around the collarette, resembling a necklace[59] or the beads of a rosary.[61] Pearls may also develop deep in the iris stroma and occasionally at the iris periphery. Typically, iris pearls slowly increase in size and tend to aggregate.[50, 62] They may become pedunculated and eventually drop off into the anterior chamber, where they are well tolerated and produce no inflammatory reaction. They are a transient phenomenon and are rarely responsible for any visual impairment.

NODULAR IRIS LEPROMAS

Bacterial invasion of the iris may also give rise to the formation of a nodular leproma. Nodular iris lepromas are yellow, globular, polymorphic masses that occur less commonly than iris pearls. They may occur in clinically uninflamed eyes.[63] Rarely, they disrupt the iris architecture and interfere with vision.[50]

Posterior Segment Lesions

Uveitis in leprosy usually involves the iris and ciliary body, but it spares the choroid because of the organism's predilection for cooler parts of the body.[64, 65] Rarely, leprosy "pearls" have been described in the anterior choroid[66–68] or as retinal pearls situated near the posterior pole of the eye, thus affecting vision.[66–68]

Choroidal involvement described in the literature includes proliferation of retinal pigment epithelium (RPE),[69] hypopigmented patches in the fundus,[70] peripheral nonspecific choroiditis,[69] and disseminated choroiditis,[71] as well as "colloid degeneration" in the area of the macula.[72] However, these chorioretinal manifestations are thought to be nonspecific and the result of reaction to the sensitized uveal tract.[72]

Ocular Changes During Leprosy Reactions

The great majority of type I reactions occur either before treatment or during the first 6 months of treatment, especially in borderline-tuberculoid (BT) patients. Lagophthalmos often develops as a result of a type I reaction,

especially when associated with an erythematous facial skin lesion.[73]

Type II reactions (ENL) may develop in multibacillary patients with longstanding untreated disease, but up to 50% of patients develop ENL within the first year of antileprosy treatment.[74] BL and LL leprosy patients are, in particular, at risk of acute iridocyclitis and (epi-)scleritis during treatment and early follow-up. However, once an eye has had acute iridocyclitis, it seems more prone to recurrent uveitis, without generalized signs of type II reaction.

Ocular Complications

Ocular Hypotony and Glaucoma

Decreased intraocular pressures are typically found in the majority of patients with leprous iridocyclitis.[75–77] Chronic uveitis is thought to affect the secretory epithelium of the ciliary body and prevent its proper functioning. Moreover, low intraocular pressures might be related to abnormalities in the autonomic innervation of the anterior segment of the eye, with large postural changes in intraocular pressure seen in these patients.[78] Interestingly, low intraocular pressures were also observed in household contacts of patients with leprosy, suggesting that these persons suffered from a subclinical infection with early autonomic nervous system or early ciliary body involvement.[79] Profound ocular hypotension may eventually lead to a phthisical eye.[80]

Glaucoma is considered to be an uncommon, but often unrecognized and untreated, complication of leprosy, with a reported average prevalence of 3.9%[81] to 12%.[82, 83] At the GWL Hansen's Disease Centre, Carville, LA, however, 20.5% of leprosy patients are followed as glaucoma patients or as glaucoma suspects.[84] Secondary open angle glaucoma with a history of chronic uveitis and chronic angle closure after intraocular inflammation are the most prominent types, but primary open angle glaucoma and acute angle closure glaucoma caused by iris bombé also occur.[82]

Cataract

Primary or secondary cataract formation was responsible for nearly half of the blindness in a recent study examining ocular complications of leprosy.[34] Direct invasion of the lens by *M. leprae* has never been demonstrated, and many authors deny the existence of a true leprosy cataract. A possible cause for cataract formation in leprosy patients was suggested by Prabhakaran, who noted that the reaction of *M. leprae* with dopa produces high local concentrations of quinones, which are known to be cataractogenic.[85]

Cataract may be secondary to anterior segment damage, particularly iridocyclitis,[50, 72, 86] but in most regions where leprosy is endemic, cataract is the most common cause of blindness in the general community, and its association with leprosy is often coincidental.[80] However, multibacillary leprosy patients completing multidrug therapy have a high prevalence of cataract, and social stigmata of the disease often exclude these patients from receiving surgery.[87]

OCULAR HISTOPATHOLOGY

Eyes of armadillos and immunocompetent mice infected with leprosy showed early infiltration of the anterior angle region, ciliary body, iris root, and limbal area with lymphocytes, plasma cells, and macrophages.[88, 89] In virtually all ocular tissues except the lens, retina, optic nerve, and aqueous and vitreous humor, M. leprae could be isolated in the armadillo, whereas only immune-deficient mice showed considerable numbers of M. leprae in the iris and ciliary body.[88, 89] A mangabey monkey, infected with leprosy 46 months earlier, showed early ocular involvement of the cornea with a subepithelial limbal infiltrate, the location of acid-fast bacilli in limbal nerves and blood vessels, and markedly damaged keratocytes by electron microscopy.[90]

Tissue reactions in humans vary from the intense delayed-type hypersensitivity granulomas of tuberculoid leprosy, to diffuse lymphohistiocytic dermal infiltrates with large vacuolated macrophages (lepra or foam cells) in lepromatous leprosy.[21] Histopathologic studies of human eyes have mainly been limited to those with extensive advanced leprosy. Conjunctival biopsies performed in leprosy patients revealed decreased goblet cells, evidence of chronic inflammation,[47] and, rarely, M. leprae.[91] Iris specimens obtained during cataract surgery disclosed chronic inflammatory reactions of patients with clinically quiet eyes. Moreover, smooth muscle disruption and destruction, a cause of the miotic pupil in leprosy, was demonstrated. M. leprae was found in the iris tissue of patients whose skin smears were negative and who had completed dapsone or multidrug therapy.[92, 93] Lepra cells containing globi composed of closely packed M. leprae, coalesce to form clinically visible miliary iris lepromata (iris pearls).[60]

In enucleated eyes following intractable uveitis or painful phthisis in patients with untreated leprosy, granulomatous infiltration of the peripheral iris and cornea with lepra cells, lymphocytes, and plasma cells was observed. Large numbers of M. leprae were present, within lepra cells and extracellularly. Strands of inflammatory cells extended from the ciliary process through the vitreous, with acid-fast bacilli in some of the cell clumps. Several retinal vessels revealed an intense perivascular infiltrate, predominately composed of lymphocytes.[94, 95] Sometimes small granulomas may be seen in the retina associated with local destruction of the RPE.[95]

PATHOGENESIS AND IMMUNOLOGY

The great variety of clinically established leprosy is mainly the result of the ability of the individual to mount a cell-mediated immune response adequate to localize, and possibly to lyse and evacuate, M. leprae. There is a continuous spectrum from the almost completely refractory to the almost completely susceptible patient, from the paucibacillary to the multibacillary form of the disease.

M. leprae

M. leprae is an obligate intracellular bacterium measuring 0.5 by 3.0 to 8.0 μm. Mycolic acids in the cell wall are probably responsible for the acid-fastness. In tissues, viable organisms stain solidly with the Fite-Faraco acid-fast stain. M. leprae has probably the longest generation time

(11 to 13 days) of any known bacterium pathogenic for humans; it has resisted all attempts at in vitro cultivation.[21] M. leprae is known to invade and multiply in the cooler regions of the body, and that property seems to be the main reason for the selective involvement of the anterior segment of the eye.[96] The invading organism may show minimal strain variations, but the response of the patient varies within the widest possible limits.

Immunology

In tuberculoid leprosy, cellular immunity is intact, as indicated by tubercle formation, intact delayed cutaneous hypersensitivity, well-developed paracortical areas in lymph nodes, and lymphocyte transformation in the presence of M. leprae in vitro. Antibodies to M. leprae antigen can be detected in the sera of less than 10% of patients with tuberculoid leprosy.[97]

In lepromatous leprosy, cellular immunity is decreased, with diffuse leproma formation, poorly developed paracortical areas in lymph nodes, negative lymphocyte transformation assay, depression of delayed-type hypersensitivity reaction, and slow rejection of skin grafts.[7, 97, 98] The humoral immune system is intact, with high titers of antibody to M. leprae antigen in most lepromatous patients. Moreover, many autoantibodies including cryoglobulins, rheumatoid factor, thyroglobulin antibodies, antinuclear antibodies, antismooth muscle antibodies, antineural antibodies, and myelin basic protein antibodies are produced.[51, 99–101] Antibodies do not seem to have any protective or useful role in leprosy. On the contrary, antigen–antibody complexes are involved in the pathogenesis of type II leprosy reactions. Cytokines appear to play an important role in the modulation of the immune response, with interferon gamma (IFN-γ), tumor necrosis factor alpha (TNF-α), interleukin (IL)-2, and IL-6 conferring protective immunity to M. leprae.[102–104] Serum IL-1β levels may have a prognostic value for the susceptibility of leprosy patients to the development of reactions.[105]

Leprosy patients may move their position on the clinical and immunologic spectrum toward the lepromatous pole if untreated, or toward the tuberculoid pole if treated. This observation indicates that the presence of M. leprae itself specifically depresses cellular immunity.[106]

Reversal upgrading reactions represent abrupt increases in cell-mediated immunity. Increases in available mycobacterial antigen (e.g., after starting antileprosy treatment) trigger a type IV immune reaction. The pathogenesis of type II reactions (ENL) includes a typical immune complex disease (type III Arthus immune reaction) accompanied by decreases in the number and function of suppressor T cells and an increase in IL-2 production.[36, 107]

In acute lepromatous uveitis during a type II leprosy reaction, suppressor T cells were reduced during the acute attack and returned to normal after inflammation had subsided.[51] Unchecked T-helper cell activity may result in an overproduction of serum autoantibodies, raised serum immunoglobulins, and an immune-complex-mediated inflammation. In support of this notion, vasculitis or perivasculitis has been observed in iris specimens of patients with inactive lepromatous uveitis.[51]

Additionally, immunogenetic factors probably play a

role in the development of uveitis in leprosy patients. In the Japanese population, HLA-DR2 contributes to the susceptibility to uveitis in leprosy.[108]

DIAGNOSIS

The diagnosis of leprosy is based mainly on clinical signs and symptoms including skin manifestations and nerve involvement.[1] Sites of predilection for peripheral nerve damage are, in order of decreasing frequency, the ulnar nerve, the posterior tibial nerve, and the external popliteal nerve.[7] The diagnosis is confirmed by demonstration of the typical acid- and alcohol-fast organisms in material obtained by the slit-smear method from the skin or nasal mucosa. Sometimes, confirmation of the diagnosis must rest on a histologic examination of involved skin, nerve, or ocular tissue.[7, 62, 63, 91, 109] However, the quality of skin smears and of microscopy in countries endemic for leprosy is often insufficient.[1] Nevertheless, despite the great variety of clinical presentations, most leprosy patients can be diagnosed on the clinical findings, given an adequate familiarity with the disease.

The lepromin reaction is still used as an indicator of the ability of the host to mount a cell-mediated immune response to *M. leprae.* However, its usefulness in diagnosis and classification and as a marker of protective immunity is very limited. The WHO recommended that the use of lepromin should be restricted to research purposes.[1]

In cases of ocular leprosy, meticulous history taking and a high index of suspicion on the part of the physician are the key factors to obtaining a correct diagnosis. *M. leprae* may be isolated from conjunctival tissue,[91] scleral nodules,[63] aqueous humor,[63, 109] and iris tissue.[62] (Fig. 23–3).

DIFFERENTIAL DIAGNOSIS

The conditions with which leprosy may be confused are varied. Skin lesions may be modified by factors like pigmentation, nutrition, insulation, and hyperkeratosis. The differential diagnosis for macular skin lesions includes

birthmarks, vitiligo, leukoderma, mycotic lesions, nutritional dyschromias, granuloma multiforme, seborrheic dermatitis, and erythema multiforme. Raised skin lesions may be confused with conditions such as psoriasis, dermatitis, lichen planus, lupus vulgaris, lupus erythematosus, and cutaneous sarcoidosis. Nodular skin lesions resemble lesions in histoplasmosis, Kaposi's sarcomatosis, or von Recklinghausen's neurofibromatosis. Peripheral nerve lesions are, of course, not confined to leprosy, but the combination of peripheral nerve damage with enlargement, hardness, and tenderness of these nerves at sites of predilection is practically diagnostic.[7]

Acute lepromatous iridocyclitis in and of itself is not distinct from, and may be confused with, any other acute nonleprous uveitis. The differential diagnosis of chronic granulomatous iritis includes uveitis associated with sarcoidosis, tuberculosis, Lyme disease, syphilis, toxoplasmosis, herpes simplex, and varicella-zoster infection. Iris pearls in chronic iridocyclitis are readily distinguished from Gilbert-Koeppe nodules in that they arise deep in the stroma of the iris, and they become superficial or migratory only after many months to years. Whereas iris pearls are opaque, dense, creamy-yellow, and firm, Gilbert-Koeppe nodules are grayish, semitranslucent, and soft in appearance.[60]

TREATMENT

Systemic Disease

Dapsone has been the standard treatment for leprosy, but drug resistance in *M. leprae* was reported in 1964 for dapsone[110] and in 1976 for rifampicin[111] (both have been used with success as monotherapy for leprosy). To prevent drug resistance resulting from the selection of resistant mutants present in multibacillary leprosy, the WHO recommended MDT regimens in 1982.[112] For multibacillary cases, the standard MDT regimen includes rifampicin (600 mg once monthly), dapsone (100 mg/d), and clofazimine (300 mg once monthly and 50 mg/d) for 24 months. Paucibacillary leprosy should be treated with rifampicin (600 mg once monthly) and dapsone (100 mg/d) for 6 months. However, potent new drugs, such as ofloxacin, minocycline, and clarithromycin, offer the potential to increase the effectiveness and possibly to shorten the duration of antileprosy chemotherapy. For single-lesion paucibacillary leprosy, a single-dose drug regimen (called ROM) consisting of rifampicin (600 mg), ofloxacin (400 mg), and minocycline (100 mg) is recommended.[1]

Dapsone

The antimicrobial effect of dapsone is the result of its inhibition of folic acid production, which results in the suppression of DNA and RNA synthesis. Dapsone is inexpensive and relatively nontoxic in the doses used, although mild hemolytic anemia is common and occasional cases of delayed hypersensitivity reactions and agranulocytosis have been reported. When given at a dosage of 100 mg/d, dapsone is weakly bactericidal against *M. leprae.* In combination with clofazimine, it killed more than 99.9% of viable *M. leprae* in nude mice after 12 weeks.[113]

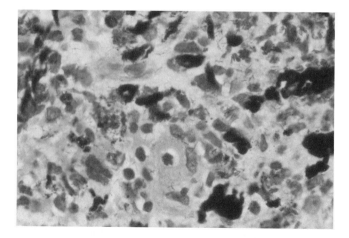

FIGURE 23–3. Iris biopsy in patient with lepromatous uveitis disclosed abundant Wade-Fite–positive intra-cellular and extracellular organisms consistent with *Mycobacterium leprae* (Wate-Fite stain, ×330). (From Messmer EM, Raizman MB, Foster CS: Lepromatous uveitis diagnosed by iris biopsy. Graefes Arch Clin Exp Ophthalmol 1998;236:717–719. Copyright © 1998 Springer-Verlag.) (See color insert.)

Rifampicin

Rifampicin is by far the most effective antileprosy drug. It inhibits bacterial RNA polymerase and suppresses chain formation in RNA synthesis. Given at a monthly dose of 600 mg, it is highly bactericidal against *M. leprae*. Rifampicin is relatively nontoxic, although occasional cases of renal failure, thrombocytopenia, influenza-like syndrome, and hepatitis have been reported.[1]

Clofazimine

The active ingredient of clofazimine is a substituted iminophenazine dye. The precise mode of action is not completely understood. In the standard MDT regimen, clofazimine is given 300 mg once monthly, plus 50 mg/d. Clofazimine is virtually nontoxic. Pigmentation of the skin is common, but it clears completely after treatment is discontinued.[1] Polychromatic corneal and conjunctival crystals were observed after therapy with clofazimine, but they resolved within several weeks of discontinuation of the drug.[114]

Ofloxacin/Sparfloxacin/Pefloxacin

Several fluoroquinolones have been reported to be effective in the treatment of leprosy.[115–119] The optimal dosage for ofloxacin seems to be 400 mg/d.[117] Although a single dose of ofloxacin displayed a modest bactericidal effect against *M. leprae*, 22 doses killed 99.9% of the viable *M. leprae* in patients with lepromatous leprosy. Side effects include gastrointestinal and central nervous system complaints, including insomnia, headaches, dizziness, and hallucinations.[1] Multidrug resistance to dapsone, rifampicin, and ofloxacin in *M. leprae* has been reported.[120]

Minocycline

Minocycline, a member of the tetracyclines, has significant bactericidal activity against *M. leprae*. The standard dose of 100 mg/d has been shown to be effective clinically when administered to patients with lepromatous leprosy.[121–123] Side effects include discoloration of teeth in children, occasional pigmentation of the skin, gastrointestinal symptoms, and central nervous complaints. It should not be given to children or during pregnancy.[1]

Clarithromycin

Clarithromycin is a member of the macrolide antibiotics family and displays significant bactericidal activity against *M. leprae* in mice[124] and in humans.[125] In patients with lepromatous leprosy, daily administration of 500 mg/d killed 99% of viable *M. leprae* within 28 days. Side effects are mainly gastrointestinal complaints.

Immunotherapy

The rationale for immunotherapy is to boost cell-mediated immunity. Relatively small, unblinded trials showed encouraging results.[126, 127] But in the absence of any long-term follow-up, and because of an apparent increase in type I reactions, immunotherapy should not be recommended for routine clinical practice.[1, 128]

Management of Reactions

The drug of choice for type I reactions and severe type II reactions (ENL) is prednisolone at a dosage of 40 to 60 mg (up to 1 mg/kg). Mild type II reactions can be managed with analgesic or antipyretic drugs. Thalidomide (100 mg three times a day) is also effective for the treatment of severe ENL.[74, 129] Clofazimine (300 mg/d) may be given in type II reactions while withdrawing steroids.[1, 129] Cyclosporin A can induce remissions in types I and II leprosy reactions.[130, 131]

Management of Ocular Complications

After the introduction of dapsone treatment in leprosy, a reduction in the occurrence and progression of eye lesions[132–134] and a decline in the prevalence of blindness in leprosy was reported.[135] The ocular status remained normal or unaltered in leprosy patients treated with MDT regimens. Lesions such as (epi-)scleritis, iritis, and lepromas subsided on MDT. New complications were usually minor and were related to reactions and the duration of disease.[136] Therefore, the mainstay in the management of ocular complications in leprosy is the continuation of systemic treatment to halt progression of infiltration and thus limit ocular damage.

Lid deformities must be repaired promptly, especially if facial and trigeminal nerve palsy coexist, to protect the cornea. In lagophthalmos of recent onset associated with a leprosy reaction, systemic steroid treatment is effective.[137]

Management of iridocyclitis includes topical corticosteroids, mydriatics, and, in severe cases, the addition of subconjunctival/peribulbar or oral steroids. Oral clofazimine (100 mg three times a day) is a useful adjuvant in the treatment of leprous uveitis, as are topical and oral nonsteroidal anti-inflammatory agents.[138] Secondary glaucoma must be treated appropriately.

CONCLUSIONS

As a result of ignorance and the social stigma that still exists throughout the world, many leprosy patients are without therapy until late in the course of the disease. Ocular leprosy, however, is the archetypal preventable disease, and simple treatment at an early stage will usually avoid major irreversible damage later. The recognition and treatment of chronic iridocyclitis represents one of the greatest challenges in the care of leprosy patients. Unfortunately, patients are dismissed from leprosy control programs and are considered "cures" by the WHO after completing MDT regimens. However, 21.3% of patients showed potentially sight-threatening lesions after being discharged from care,[80] and the eyes of patients with lepromatous leprosy may harbor living organisms or antigen long after the skin is bacteriologically negative. Completion of systemic leprosy therapy should not be regarded as a guarantee that the eyes are safe, and regular ophthalmologic examinations should be continued long after the patient has been classified as "cured."[80]

References

1. WHO: WHO Expert Committee on Leprosy: Seventh report. WHO Tech Rep Ser 874. Geneva, 1998.
2. Ridley DS, Jopling WH: Classification of leprosy according to immunity. A five-group system. Int J Lepr 1966;34:255–273.
3. Leiker DL: Classification of leprosy. Lepr Rev 1966;37:7–15.
4. WHO Study Group: Chemotherapy of leprosy for control programmes. WHO Tech Rep Ser 675. Geneva, 1982.

5. Flageul B: Quelle place reste-t-il à la classification de Ridley et Jopling en 1997? (Editorial). Acta Lepr 1997;10:187.
6. Summary of notifiable diseases, United States, 1997. MMWR Morb Mortal Wkly Rep 1998;46:3–87.
7. Browne SG: Leprosy. In: Acta Clinica, 3rd ed. Basle, Switzerland, Ciba-Geigy Ltd, 1984, pp 12–14.
8. Thangaraj RH, Yawalkar SJ: Leprosy for medical practitioners and paramedical workers. Basle, Switzerland, Ciba-Geigy Ltd, 1986.
9. Ell SR: Plague and leprosy in the Middle Ages: A paradoxical cross-immunity? Int J Lepr 1987;55:345–350.
10. Harboe M: Armauer Hansen: The man and his work. Int J Lepr 1973;41:417–424.
11. Bull OB, Hansen GA: The Leprous Diseases of the Eye (Reprinted). London, Lewis, 1873.
12. Faget GH, Pogge RC, Johansen FA, et al: The Promin treatment of leprosy: A progress report. Publ Health Rep 1943;58:1729–1741.
13. Binford CH: Comprehensive program for inoculation of human leprosy into laboratory animals. Publ Health Rep 1956;71:955–956.
14. Shepard CC: The experimental disease that follows the injection of human leprosy bacilli into footpads of mice. J Exp Med 1960;112:445–454.
15. Storrs EE: The nine-banded armadillo: A model for leprosy and other biomedical research. Int J Lepr 1971;39:703–714.
16. Brennan PJ, Barrow WW: Evidence for species-specific lipid antigens in Mycobacterium leprae. Int J Lepr 1980;48:382–387.
17. Clark-Curtiss JE, Jacobs WR, Docherty MA, et al: Molecular analysis of DNA and construction of genomic libraries of Mycobacterium leprae. J Bacteriol 1985;161:1093–1102.
18. Young RA, Mehra V, Sweetser D, et al: Genes for the major protein antigens of Mycobacterium leprae. Nature 1985;316:450–452.
19. Noordeen SK: A look at world leprosy. Lepr Rev 1990;62:72–86.
20. Neill MA, Hightower AW, Broome CV: Leprosy in the United States, 1971–1981. J Infect Dis 1985;152:1064–1069.
21. Meyers WM, Marty AM: Current concepts in the pathogenesis of leprosy. Drugs 1991;41:832–856.
22. Lucas S: Human immunodeficiency virus and leprosy (Editorial). Lepr Rev 1993;64:97–103.
23. Godal T, Negassi K: Subclinical infection in leprosy. Br Med J 1973;3:557–559.
24. Dethlefs R: Editorial: Leprosy. Aust N Z J Ophthalmol 1989;17:211–213.
25. Duncan ME, Melsom R, Pearson JM, et al: A clinical and immunological study of four babies of mothers with lepromatous leprosy, two of whom developed leprosy in infancy. Int J Lepr Other Mycobact Dis 1983;51:7–17.
26. Geater JG: The fly as potential vector in the transmission of leprosy. Lepr Rev 1975;46:279–286.
27. Vries de RRP, Eden van W, Rood van JJ: HLA-linked control of leprosy type. Int J Lepr 1984;52S:693.
28. Renard G, Dhermy P, Harter P, et al: Les atteintes du globe oculaire au cours de la lepre. Arch Ophtal (Paris) 1963;23:249–252.
29. Choyce DP: Discussions on ocular leprosy. Trans R Soc Trop Med Hyg 1970;64:43–45.
30. Hobbs HE: The blinding lesions of leprosy. Lepr Rev 1971;42:131–137.
31. Kirwan EW: The ocular complications of common tropical diseases. Trop Dis Bull 1956;53:693–695.
32. Harley RD: Ocular leprosy in Panama. Am J Ophthalmol 1946;29:295–316.
33. ffytche TJ: The prevalence of disabling ocular complications of leprosy: A global study. Indian J Lepr 1998;70:49–59.
34. Courtright P: The epidemiology of ocular complications of leprosy. Indian J Lepr 1998;70:33–37.
35. Courtright P, Kim SH, Lee HS, Lewallen S: Excess mortality associated with blindness in leprosy patients in Korea. Lepr Rev 1997;68:326–330.
36. Modlin RL, Mehra V, Jordan R, et al: In situ and in vitro characterization of the cellular immune response in erythema nodosum leprosum. J Immunol 1986;136:883–886.
37. Shorey P, Krishnan MM, Dhawan S, Garg BR: Ocular changes in reactions in leprosy. Lepr Rev 1989;60:102–108.
38. Hogeweg M, Faber WR: Progression of eye lesions in leprosy: Ten year follow-up study in the Netherlands. Int J Lepr Other Mycobact Dis 1991;59:392–397.
39. Rajan MA: Longitudinal follow-up of eyes in leprosy. Indian J Lepr 1998;70:109–114.
40. Schwab IR: Ocular leprosy. Infect Dis Clin North Am 1992;6:953–961.
41. Daniel E: Lagophthalmos in leprosy. Indian J Lepr 1998;70:39–47.
42. Yan LB, Chang GC, Li WZ, et al: Analysis of 2114 cases of lagophthalmos in leprosy. China Lepr J 1993;9:6–8.
43. Courtright P, Lewallen S, Le HY, et al: Lagophthalmos in a multibacillary population under multidrug therapy in the People's Republic of China. Lepr Rev 1995;66:214–219.
44. Karacorlu MA, Cakmer T, Saylan T: Corneal sensitivity and correlations between decreased sensitivity and anterior segment pathology in ocular leprosy. Br J Ophthalmol 1991;75:117–119.
45. Hieselaar LC, Hogeweg M, Vries de CL: Corneal sensitivity in patients with leprosy and in controls. Br J Ophthalmol 1995;79:993–995.
46. Hodges EJ, Ostler HB, Courtright P, Gelber RH: Keratoconjunctivitis sicca in leprosy. Lepr Rev 1987;58:413–417.
47. Lamba PA, Rohatgi J, Bose S: Factors influencing corneal involvement in leprosy. Int J Lepr 1987;55:667–671.
48. Daniel E, Thompson K, Ebenezer GJ, et al: Pterygium in lepromatous leprosy. Int J Lepr 1996;64:428–432.
49. Poon A, MacLean H, McKelvie P: Recurrent scleritis in lepromatous leprosy. Aust N Z J Ophthalmol 1998;26:51–55.
50. ffytche TF: Role of iris changes as a cause of blindness in lepromatous leprosy. Br J Ophthalmol 1981;65:231–239.
51. Murray PI, Kerr Muir MG, Rahi AHS: Immunopathogenesis of acute lepromatous uveitis: A case report. Lepr Rev 1986;57:163–168.
52. Fuchs A: Ophthalmologisches und Medizinisches aus den Tropen. Klin Monatsbl Augenheilkd 1935;94:244–249.
53. ffytche TF: Editorial: Importance of early diagnosis in ocular leprosy. Br J Ophthalmol 1989;73:939.
54. Karacorlu M, Sürel Z, Cakiner T, et al: Pupil cycle time and early autonomic involvement in ocular leprosy. Br J Ophthalmol 1991;75:45–48.
55. Daniel E, Rao PSS: Pupil cycle time in leprosy patients without clinically apparent ocular pathology. Int J Lepr 1995;63:529–534.
56. Swift TR, Bauschard FD: Pupillary reactions in lepromatous leprosy. Int J Lepr 1972;40:142–148.
57. Lewallen S, Courtright P, Lee HS: Ocular autonomic dysfunction and intraocular pressure in leprosy. Br J Ophthalmol 1989;73:946–949.
58. Johnstone PAS, George AD, Meyers WA: Ocular lesions in leprosy. Ann Ophthalmol 1991;23:297–303.
59. Barros de M: A clinical study of leprous iritis. Int J Lepr 1940;8:353–360.
60. Allen JH: The pathology of ocular leprosy. II: Miliary lepromas of iris. Am J Ophthalmol 1966;61:987–992.
61. Ebenezer R: Symposium on uveitis. Iritis in leprosy. Proc All-India Ophthalmol Soc 1963;19:183–188.
62. Messmer EM, Raizman MB, Foster CS: Lepromatous uveitis diagnosed by iris biopsy. Graefes Arch Clin Exp Ophthalmol 1998;236:717–719.
63. Michelson JB, Roth AM, Waring GO: Lepromatous iridocyclitis diagnosed by anterior chamber paracentesis. Am J Ophthalmol 1979;88:674–679.
64. Allen JH, Brand M: Ocular leprosy. In: Locatcher-Khorazo D, Seegal BC, eds: Microbiology of the Eye, St. Louis, Mosby, 1972, pp 131–154.
65. Drutz DJ, Chen TS, Lu WH: The continuous bacteriemia of lepromatous leprosy. N Engl J Med 1972;287:159–164.
66. Moneiro LG, Campos WR, Oréfice F, Grossi MAF: Study of ocular changes in leprosy patients. Indian J Lepr 1998;70:197–202.
67. Somerset EJ, Sen NR: Leprosy lesions of the fundus oculi. Br J Ophthalmol 1956;40:167–172.
68. Elliot DC: A report of leprosy lesions of the fundus. Int J Lepr 1948;16:347–348.
69. Ticho V, Ben Sira I. Ocular leprosy in Malawi. Br J Ophthalmol 1970;54:107–112.
70. Chatterjee S, Chaudhury S: Hypopigmented patches in fundus in leprosy. Lepr Rev 1964;35:88–90.
71. Duke-Elder, Leigh AG: Leprosy. In: Duke Elder S, ed: System of Ophthalmology. London, Henry Kimpton, 1965, pp 844–852.
72. Weerekoon L: Ocular leprosy in West Malaysia: Search for a posterior segment lesion. Br J Ophthalmol 1972;56:106–113.

73. Hogeweg MK, Kiran KU, Suneetha S: The significance of facial patches and type I reaction for the development of facial nerve damage in leprosy. A retrospective study among 1226 paucibacillary leprosy patients. Lepr Rev 1991;62:143–149.

74. Meyerson MS: Erythema nosodum leprosum. Int J Dermatol 1996;35:389–392.

75. Brandt F, Malla OK, Anten JGF: Influence of untreated chronic plastic iridocyclitis on intraocular pressure in leprous patients. Br J Ophthalmol 1981;65:240–242.

76. Karacorlu MA, Cakiner T, Saylan T: Influence of untreated chronic plastic iridocyclitis on intraocular pressure in leprosy patients. Br J Ophthalmol 1991;75:120–122.

77. Slem G: Clinical studies of ocular leprosy. Am J Ophthalmol 1971;71:431–434.

78. Lewallen S, Hussein N, Courtright P, et al: Intraocular pressure and iris denervation in Hansen's disease. Int J Lepr 1990;58:39–43.

79. Hussein N, Chiang T, Ehsan Q, Hussain R: Intraocular pressure decrease in household contacts of patients with Hansen's disease and endemic control subjects. Am J Ophthalmol 1992;114:479–483.

80. ffytche TF. Residual sight-threatening lesions in leprosy patients completing multidrug therapy and sulphone therapy. Lepr Rev 1991;62:35–43.

81. Spaide R, Nattis R, Lipka A, D'Amico R: Ocular findings in leprosy in the United States. Am J Ophthalmol 1985;100:411–416.

82. Walton RC, Ball SF, Joffrion VC: Glaucoma in Hansen's disease. Br J Ophthalmol 1991;75:270–272.

83. Shields JA, Waring GO 3d, Monte LG: Ocular findings in leprosy. Am J Ophthalmol 1974;77:880–890.

84. Joffrion VC: Eye lesions in leprosy—Glaucoma and tension. Lepr Rev 1989;60:328.

85. Prabhakaran K: Cataract in leprosy: A biochemical approach. Lepr Rev 1971;42:11–13.

86. Brandt F, Kampik A, Malla OK, et al: Blindness from cataract formation in leprosy. Dev Ophthalmol 1983;7:1–12.

87. ffytche TF: The continuing challenge of ocular leprosy. Br J Ophthalmol 1991;75:123–124.

88. Hobbs HE, Harman DJ, Rees RJW, McDougall AC: Ocular histopathology in animals experimentally infected with Mycobacterium leprae and M. lepraemurium. Br J Ophthalmol 1978;62:516–524.

89. Brandt F, Zhou HM, Shi ZR, et al: The pathology of the eye in armadillos experimentally infected with Mycobacterium leprae. Lepr Rev 1990;61:112–131.

90. Malaty R, Meyers WM, Walsh GP, et al: Histopathological changes in the eyes of mangabey monkeys with lepromatous leprosy. Int J Lepr 1988;56:443–448.

91. Campos WB, Oréfice F, Sucena MA, Rodrigues CAF: Conjunctival biopsy in patients with leprosy. Indian J Lepr 1998;70:291–294.

92. Brandt F, Zhou HM, Shi ZR, et al: Histopathological findings in the iris of dapsone treated leprosy patients. Br J Ophthalmol 1990;74:14–18.

93. Daniel E, Ebenezer GJ, Job CK: Pathology of iris in leprosy. Br J Ophthalmol 1997;81:490–492.

94. Robertson I, Weiner JM, Finkelstein E: Untreated Hansen's disease of the eye: A clinicopathological report. Aust J Ophthalmol 1984;12:335–339.

95. Hui-Min Z, Zhen-Rong S, Job CK: Unusual histological lesions in the eye of a leprosy patient. Int J Lepr 1987;55:507–509.

96. Job CK, Ebenezer GJ, Thompson K, Daniel E: Pathology of eye in leprosy. Indian J Lepr 1998;70:79–91.

97. Bryceson A, Pfaltzgraff RE: Leprosy, 2nd ed. Edinburgh, 1979.

98. Turk JL, Waters MFR: Cell-mediated immunity in patients with leprosy. Lancet 1969;2:243–246.

99. Shwe T: Clinical significance of autoimmune antibodies in leprosy. Trans R Soc Trop Med Hyg 1972;66:749–753.

100. Park JY, Cho SN, Youn JK, et al: Detection of antibodies to human nerve antigens in sera from leprosy patients by ELISA. Clin Exp Immunol 1992;87:368–372.

101. Córsico B, Croce MV, Mukherjee R, Segal-Eiras A: Identification of myelin basic proteins in circulating immune complexes associated with lepromatous leprosy. Clin Immunol Immunopathol 1994;71:38–43.

102. Champsi JH, Bermudez LE, Young LS: The role of cytokines in mycobacterial infection. Biotherapy 1994;7:187–193.

103. Sugita Y, Miyamoto M, Koseki M, et al: Suppression of tumour necrosis factor-α expression in leprosy skin lesions during treatment for leprosy. Br J Dermatol 1997;136:393–397.

104. Barnes PF, Chatterjee D, Brennan PJ, et al: Tumor necrosis factor production in patients with leprosy. Infect Immun 1992;60:1441–1446.

105. Moubasher AEA, Kamel NA, Zedan H, Raheem DEA: Cytokines in leprosy, II. Effect of treatment on serum cytokines in leprosy. Int J Dermatol 1998;37:741–746.

106. Mohagheghpour N, Gelber RR, Engleman EG: T-cell defect in lepromatous leprosy is reversible in vitro in the absence of exogenous growth factors. J Immunol 1986;138:570–574.

107. Mshana RN: Hypothesis: Erythema nodosum leprosum is precipitated by an imbalance of T lymphocytes. Lepr Rev 1982;53:1–7.

108. Joko S, Nugama J, Fujino Y, et al: Nippon-Ganka-Gakkai-Zasshi 1995;99:1181–1185.

109. Campos WR, Oréfice F, Sucena MA, Rodrigues CAF: Bilateral iridocyclitis caused by Mycobacterium leprae diagnosed through paracentesis. Indian J Lepr 1998;70:27–31.

110. Pettit JHS, Rees RJW: Sulphone resistance in leprosy. Lancet 1964;1:673–674.

111. Jacobson RR, Hastings RC: Rifampicin-resistant leprosy. Lancet 1976;2:1304–1305.

112. WHO: Chemotherapy of leprosy for control programmes. Report of a WHO Study Group. Tech Rep Ser 675, Geng, 1982.

113. Ji B, Perani EG, Petinom C, Grosset JH: Bactericidal activities of combinations of new drugs against Mycobacterium leprae in nude mice. Antimicro Agents Chemother 1996;40:393–399.

114. Font RL, Sobol W, Matoba A: Polychromatic corneal and conjunctival crystals secondary to Clofazimine therapy in a leper. Ophthalmology 1989;96:311–315.

115. Saito H, Tomioka H, Nagashima K: In vitro and in vivo activities of ofloxacin against Mycobacterium leprae infection induced in mice. Int J Lepr Other Mycobact Dis 1986;54:560–562.

116. Ji B, Perani EG, Petinom C, Grosset JH: Bactericidal activities of single or multiple doses of various combinations of new antileprosy drugs and/or rifampin against M. leprae in mice. Int J Lepr 1992;60:556–561.

117. Ji B, Perani EG, Petinom C, et al: Clinical trial of ofloxacin alone and in combination with dapsone plus clofazimine for treatment of lepromatous leprosy. Antimicrob Agents Chemother 1994;38:662–667.

118. Mochizuki Y, Oishi M, Nishiyama C, Iida T: Active leprosy treated effectively with ofloxacin. Intern Med 1996;35:749–751.

119. Chan GP, Garcia-Ignacio BY, Chavez VE, et al: Clinical trial of sparfloxacin for lepromatous leprosy. Antimicrob Agents Chemother 1994;38:61–65.

120. Cambau E, Perani E, Guillemin I, et al: Multidrug-resistance to dapsone, rifampicin, and ofloxacin in Mycobacterium leprae. Lancet 1997;349:103–104.

121. Ji B, Jamet P, Perani E, et al: Powerful bactericidal activities of clarithromycin and minocycline against Mycobacterium leprae in lepromatous leprosy. J Infect Dis 1993;168:188–190.

122. Gelber RH, Fukuda K, Byrd S, et al: A clinical trial of minocycline in lepromatous leprosy. Br Med J 1992;304:91–92.

123. Ji B, Jamet P, Perani EG, et al: Bactericidal activity of single dose of clarithromycin plus minocycline, with or without ofloxacin, against Mycobacterium leprae in patients. Antimicrob Agents Chemother 1996;40:2137–2141.

124. Ji B, Perani EG, Grosset JH: Effectiveness of clarithromycin and minocycline alone and in combination against experimental Mycobacterium leprae infection in mice. Antimicrob Agents Chemother 1991;35:579–581.

125. Gelber RH: Successful treatment of a lepromatous patient with clarithromycin. Int J Lepr Other Mycobact Dis 1995;63:113–115.

126. Majumder V, Mukerjee A, Hajra SK, et al: Immunotherapy of far-advanced lepromatous leprosy patients with low-dose Convit vaccine along with multidrug therapy (Calcutta trial). Int J Lepr 1996;64:26–36.

127. Talwar GP, Zaheer SA, Mukherjee R, et al: Immunotherapeutic effects of a vaccine based on a saprophytic cultivable mycobacterium, Mycobacterium W in multibacillary leprosy patients. Vaccine 1990;8:121–129.

128. Whitty C: Editorial: Mycobacterium W immunotherapy in leprosy. Lepr Rev 1998;69:222–224.

129. Jakeman P, Smith WCS: Thalidomide in leprosy reactions. Lancet 1994;343:432–433.

130. Uyemura K, Dixon FP, Wong L, et al: Effect of cyclosporine A in erythema nodosum leprosum. J Immunol 1986;137:3620–3623.

131. Miller RA, Shen JY, Rea TH, Harnish JP: Treatment of chronic erythema nodosum leprosum with cyclosporine A produces clinical and immunohistologic remission. Int J Lepr 1987;55:441–449.

132. Amendola F: Ocular and otolaryngological leprosy before and since sulfone therapy. Int J Lepr 1955;23:280–283.

133. Brandt F, Kist P, Wos J: Augenbefunde bei Lepra. Ergebnisse einer Studie im Green-Pastures-Leprosy Hospital Pokhara/Nepal. Klin Monatsbl Augenheilkd 1981;178:55–58.

134. Ticho U, Sira IB: Ocular leprosy in Malawi. Clinical and therapeutic survey of 8,325 leprosy patients. Br J Ophthalmol 1970;54:107–112.

135. Emiru VP: Ocular leprosy in Uganda. Br J Ophthalmol 1970;54:740–743.

136. Rajan MA: Eye in multi-drug therapy. Indian J Lepr 1990;62:33–38.

137. Thompson K, Daniel E: Management of ocular problems in leprosy. Indian J Lepr 1998;70:295–315.

138. Brand ME: Care of eye in Hansen's disease, 3rd ed. Gillis W Long Hansen's Disease Centre, Carville, LA, 1993.

24 — HERPESVIRUSES

Arnd Heiligenhaus, Horst Helbig,
and Melanie Fiedler

HERPES SIMPLEX VIRUS AND VARICELLA ZOSTER VIRUS

Virology

The term "herpes" stems from the Greek word "herpein," which means "to spread." Herpesviruses are widely disseminated in nature and can be found in nearly all animal species. About 100 different herpesviruses have been described so far, and eight of them are found in humans: herpes simplex virus 1 (HSV-1), herpes simplex virus 2 (HSV-2), varicella zoster virus (VZV), human cytomegalovirus (CMV), Epstein-Barr virus (EBV), and human herpesviruses 6, 7, and 8 (HHV-6, HHV-7, HHV-8).[1–3]

The members of the family herpesviridae share a characteristic architecture. The core contains linear double-stranded DNA and is surrounded by the icosahedral capsid consisting of 162 capsomeres, the tegument, an amorphous material, and the envelope. The envelope is derived from the core membrane of the infected cells and consists of lipids with inserted viral glycoprotein spikes. The lipid content of the envelope is responsible for the sensitivity of herpesviruses to lipid solvents and detergents.[3, 4]

Specific receptors of the glycoproteins of the viral envelope that recognize complementary receptors on the host target cell membrane and bind to them (adsorption) are a prerequisite for the viral infection. The envelope of the herpesvirus and the cell membrane fuse, and the nucleocapsid of the virus then penetrates into the cell. The viral proteins are typically produced in a cascade. First, the immediate early proteins are produced, then the early proteins, followed by the late proteins.[5] In the diagnosis of CMV infections, using cell culture to detect an immediate early antigen and of early antigen, the pp65 antigen in peripheral blood mononuclear cells (PBMCs) has become an important method (Figs. 24–1 and 24–2).

All herpesviruses share certain biologic properties. They all have a large number of enzymes that are involved in nucleic acid metabolism, DNA synthesis, and possibly the procession of proteins. The synthesis of DNA and the assembly of the capsid take place in the nucleus. The production of infectious virus particles in the cytoplasm leads to the destruction of the infected cell. All known herpesviruses establish latent or clinically silent infection in their natural hosts.[3]

The status of latency is restricted to a small range of susceptible cells that vary among the different members of the herpesvirus family. During latency, the herpesvirus genomes form closed circular molecules, and only a small number of viral proteins is expressed, with no mature virus produced. There is evidence that selected regulatory genes are active and may maintain latency, but neither the mechanisms to keep the status of latency nor the factors that cause reactivation to mature viral assembly and replication are completely understood so far.

After reactivation from latency, infectious viruses are transported to peripheral tissues, for example, by axonal transport. It depends on the immune response of the host as to whether reactivation takes a symptomatic or asymptomatic course.[3, 6]

The family of herpesviridae can be divided into three subfamilies according to differences in host range, reproduction rate, and cell tropism. HSV-1, HSV-2, VZV, and

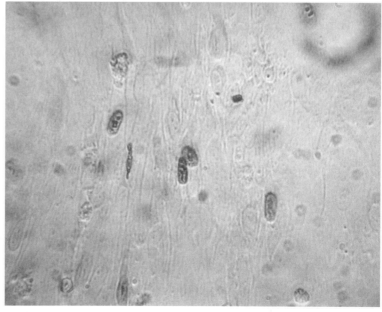

FIGURE 24–I. Detection of a CMV immediate early antigen in CMV-infected fibroblasts 36 hours after inoculation by an enzyme immunoassay.

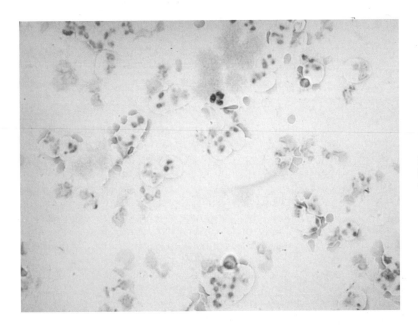

FIGURE 24–2. Detection of a CMV early antigen (pp65) in peripheral blood mononuclear cells of a patient by an enzyme immunoassay.

HHV-8 belong to the subfamily of alpha herpesviruses; CMV and probably HHV-6 and HHV-7 to the beta herpesviruses; and EBV is in the family of gamma herpesviruses.[3] Table 24–1 summarizes the clinical characteristics of herpesviruses that are infectious for humans.

The two types of herpes simplex viruses described are HSV-1 and HSV-2. HSV-1 and HSV-2 are transmitted during close personal contact. HSV-1 causes labial infections (e.g., via transmission from mother to child), and HSV-2 is normally transmitted via sexual contact. The primary infection with HSV-1 is mostly asymptomatic but may occur as gingivostomatitis or, less commonly, as conjunctivitis or keratitis. In most cases, infections with HSV-2 are acquired after infections with HSV-1 and can therefore be regarded as reinfections. This infection by HSV-2 remains asymptomatic in most cases because of the partial specific immune response already present. In contrast to this, primary infections with HSV-2 without previous contact with HSV-1 may cause apparent local and systemic symptoms.

The primary infection with HSV typically involves the mucosa. The virus replicates intracellularly and infects other cells in the mucosa per continuitatem. Lymphogenous-hematogenous spread is rarely found. The virus penetrates in the nerve ends in the mucosa and is transported retrograde via the axon into sensory ganglia. After a period of productive infection, replication decreases and a persistent and latent infection is established. A wide range of factors, for example, exposure to ultraviolet (UV) light, fever, and stress, can cause a new period of

TABLE 24–I. SOME IMPORTANT CHARACTERISTICS OF HERPESVIRUSES THAT ARE INFECTIOUS IN HUMANS*

HERPESVIRUS		SUBFAMILY[1]	SITE OF LATENCY	PRIMARY INFECTION	SYMPTOMATIC REACTIVATION
Human herpesvirus 1	HSV-1	α	Sensory ganglia	Gingivostomatitis, keratoconjunctivitis, skin infection, genital disease, encephalitis	Herpes labialis, keratoconjunctivitis, skin infection, encephalitis
Human herpesvirus 2	HSV-2	α	Sensory ganglia	Genital disease, gingivostomatitis, encephalitis, neonatal infection	Genital disease, skin infection
Human herpesvirus 3	VZV	α	Sensory ganglia	Varicella	Zoster
Human herpesvirus 4	CMV	β	Lymphoreticular cells, probably kidney and other tissues	Mononucleosis, hepatitis, neonatal infection	Pneumonia, retinitis, colitis
Human herpesvirus 5	EBV	γ	Oropharyngeal epithelial sites, B-lymphocytes, lymphoid tissues	Mononucleosis, hepatitis	Cofactor for "post-transplant" lymphomas
Human herpesvirus 6	HHV-6	β/γ	Peripheral blood leukocytes?	Exanthem subitum, lymphadenopathy	Post-tranplant complications, dimensions not clear so far
Human herpesvirus 7	HHV-7	β		No clear evidence for disease	
Human herpesvirus 8	HHV-8	γ		Associated with Kaposi's sarcoma	

*This table includes only a partial listing.

viral replication, a reactivation. This new period of viral replication can be asymptomatic or cause symptoms (e.g., orolabial lesions or the various ocular manifestations).

VZV causes two distinct diseases. Varicella, or chickenpox, is seen in primary infection. It is usually a mild, self-limited infection in children. Zoster occurs after reactivation of the persistent latent VZV infection in sensory ganglia.

Typical clinical pictures of intraocular inflammation induced by alpha herpesviruses include endotheliitis, trabeculitis, iridocyclitis, acute retinal necrosis (ARN), and variants of necrotizing herpes retinopathy.[7] The clinical pictures of the various forms of intraocular inflammation caused by alpha herpesviruses share many similarities, so in individual cases, it is often not possible to differentiate HSV from VZV. Nevertheless, the case history and clinical signs can sometimes point to the causative virus. In a few patients, HSV-1 forms typical blister-like skin eruptions,[8, 9] or zoster dermatitis may be present.[10, 11]

History

Iritis and glaucoma secondary to herpesvirus infections of the anterior uvea were characterized in the late 1970s.[12, 13] The clinical picture of ARN was first described by Urayama and coworkers in 1971.[14] The disease has been characterized by a combination of peripheral, confluent, necrotizing retinitis, retinal arteritis, and intraocular inflammation. The pathogenetic connection with the herpesviruses was proved by Culbertson and associates in 1982.[15]

Epidemiology

Iritis frequently occurs concomitantly with HSV keratitis but may also develop without it. Previously, it has been shown that iritis presents in up to 40% of the patients with acute herpes zoster ophthalmicus.[16]

Necrotizing retinitis from HSV or VZV is a rare disease. The susceptibility for development of herpes retinitis is probably influenced by genetic factors, but HLA associations have differed greatly between the populations studied.[17, 18] The individual immune status seems to be of special importance. The disease is more common in patients with an impairment of the cellular immune responses, for example, in the elderly population or in patients under immunosuppressive therapy, with acquired immunodeficiency syndrome (AIDS), or malignancies.[11, 19–21] ARN shows a two-peak age distribution, with the first peak at 20 years of age and the second at about 50 years of age. HSV infections manifest themselves in early adulthood and are presumably responsible for the first peak. Zoster dermatitis most likely attacks the older population, which may explain the second peak.[22]

HSV or VZV retinitis may be seen in certain clinical settings. Congenital varicella zoster retinitis may be observed in the first or second trimester of pregnancy in connection with chickenpox or zoster dermatitis. Retinitis has also been seen in association with chickenpox in adulthood or after the manifestation of HSV encephalitis.[23–25] Although it has been suggested that the diagnosis of ARN should only be used in otherwise healthy patients, this syndrome has also been described in immunocompromised patients.[20, 26] In comparison to retinitis from CMV and toxoplasmosis, retinitis from HSV or VZV in AIDS patients is rare.

Clinical Characteristics

Iridocyclitis and Trabeculitis

Iritis or trabeculitis may appear with and without corneal HSV lesions. It has been pointed out that iritis in an eye with a known history of herpetic keratitis should be considered herpetic until proved otherwise by the clinical findings or by laboratory testing.[27] Patients suffer from redness, photophobia, pain, and visual impairment. Involvement of the anterior uvea is characterized by typical clinical findings, including ciliary flush, fine or mutton fat keratic precipitates and various degrees of cellular reaction in the anterior chamber. Iritis commonly occurs concurrently with HSV stromal keratitis or endotheliitis. The anterior chamber reaction in these patients is often minimal. Generally, herpesvirus iritis may be focal or diffuse. In focal iritis, iris hyperemia and posterior synechiae are circumscribed and typically leave defects of the pigment epithelium. The diffuse form of HSV iritis is much more common. It is characterized by circumferential iris edema, severe cell and flare reaction in the aqueous humor, and is frequently complicated by fulminant fibrin deposition, hypopyon, complete synechiae formation, or secondary glaucoma. Iris masses have been seen that were masquerading as an iris melanoma.[28, 29] The inflammation may involve the trabecular meshwork endothelium, which has been termed "trabeculitis." Clinically, trabeculitis is characterized by a sudden increase of the intraocular pressure and is associated with decompensation of the corneal endothelium.[12, 30] The glaucomatous episodes may be temporary, but in some individuals, glaucomatous damage of the optic nerve follows.

Iridocyclitis is the commonest finding from zoster ophthalmicus and usually presents within the first week of acute disease, but exacerbations have also been seen months after acute herpes zoster. The diagnosis of VZV uveitis may be particularly difficult in cases without a previous zoster dermatitis ("sine herpete"). The course of the iridocyclitis may be mild with few anterior chamber cells and flare, or severe with pain, blurred vision, ciliary hyperemia, miosis, keratic precipitates, and iris hyperemia. Fibrinous exudation into the anterior chamber may be followed by synechia formation. Additional typical findings are iris sector atrophy and sphincter damage. Hypopyon, hyphema, hypotony, and, very rarely, phthisis bulbi have occurred.[16] A series of patients with acute fulminant granulomatous iridocyclitis without known skin eruptions has been reported, in which it was emphasized that herpes zoster sine herpete should be suspected as a potential diagnosis in certain clinical conditions.[31] Glaucoma has been noted in 10% of the patients.

Acute Retinal Necrosis

The most frequent complaints include irritation, slight pain, reddening of the eye, photophobia, tearing, blurring in the facial field, and various grades of visual impairment. ARN begins with sharply demarcated retinal necrosis in the periphery, which rapidly spreads. This is accompanied by occluding vasculitis and severe inflammation in the anterior chamber and vitreous body.[7, 32]

ARN begins with an anterior uveitis. The patient's symptoms may be minimal, and examination of the anterior segment may only reveal fine or speckled keratic precipitates.[33, 34] The retinal lesions tend to be round, polymorphous, and yellowish white, and are located at the level of the retinal pigment epithelium or the deep layers of the retina.[35] These lesions are described as retinal exudate, retinitis, white or yellowish white retinal infiltrates, or as a white, swollen retina. They are mostly found between the middle periphery and the ora serrata, the borders of which have a scalloped appearance.[36] Retinal vasculitis and optic nerve head swelling may develop simultaneously.[32]

Over the ensuing 3 to 21 days, the retinal necrosis spreads quickly peripherally, posteriorly, and circumferentially.[7] It may involve several quadrants, to the vascular arcades, or may involve the whole retinal circumference. The macula itself is often spared. The affected retinal area is homogeneously white and thickened, and the posterior border is sharply demarcated (Fig. 24–3). Sometimes the lesions inside a quadrant show a triangular form, the point of which points to the optic nerve. Vascular sheathing and attenuation of retinal arterioles develop. The sheathing of the venules is clearly less pronounced. Often, all of the vessels between the optic nerve and the periphery are affected; in other cases, only segments are conspicuously involved. Frequently, vascular nonperfusion can be found, particularly in the periphery, which may result in retinal neovascularization. Simultaneously, dense vitritis develops. Further progression is mostly characterized by the development of multiple, small or perivascular intraretinal hemorrhages in the affected area. Only in exceptional cases do larger subretinal or epiretinal hemorrhages arise.

The regression of ARN begins at the outer peripheral edge, in particular next to the venules, whereby the affected area takes on a Swiss cheese–like pattern.[33] It ends in retinal atrophy. The white retinal coloration recedes, followed by a salt-and-pepper pigmentation with a sharp line of demarcation between the normal and affected retina (Fig. 24–4). Simultaneously, the cellular infiltration

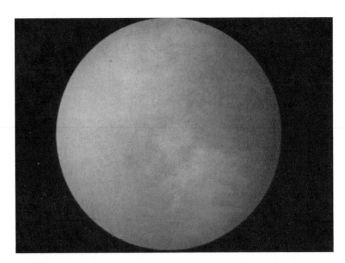

FIGURE 24–4. Regression of acute retinal necrosis with "Swiss cheese–like pattern" and retinal atrophy. (See color insert.)

of the vitreous body usually progresses considerably. Membranes develop, with posterior vitreous detachment, and frequently, proliferative vitreoretinopathy develops.[33] In untreated patients, the inflammation usually heals in 6 to 12 weeks.[33]

A distinctive course of necrotizing herpetic retinopathy in patients with advanced AIDS has been described and is called "progressive outer retinal necrosis syndrome" (PORN). Deep retinal infiltration with a multifocal distribution and involvement of the macula are frequently present initially. Inflammatory spots spread very rapidly to confluence, leaving large areas of necrosis in their wake. The outer retinal layers are principally involved, with little involvement of the retinal vessels, giving the characteristic cracked mud appearance of the fundus. On the other hand, there is a conspicuous discrepancy from the rest of the accompanying inflammation. When low CD4 cell counts are present, the retinal necrosis is accompanied only by a slight vitritis, minimal vasculitis and neuritis (15% to 20%), and minimal inflammation of the anterior chamber.[37, 38] Varicella zoster virus retrobulbar optic neuritis preceding retinitis has been described in patients with AIDS.[39]

Other Retinopathies

Twenty-five percent of the children affected from congenital varicella zoster infections show cataracts, and in 37%, pigmented, mostly unilateral chorioretinal scarring can be found. The spectrum of changes also includes optic disc atrophy and microphthalmos, often in combination with generalized malformation.[40–42]

The retinal changes in chickenpox-associated retinitis commonly develop when the skin lesions are healing.[43, 44] Most of those affected are immunocompromised.[45] In addition to focal retinitis, mild retinal vasculitis and vitritis are observed, and occasionally also choroiditis and exudative retinal detachments. The inflammation typically resolves within a few weeks without consequences.[43, 44] Only in a few individual cases is ARN observed.[45]

In congenital HSV infections in the first or second

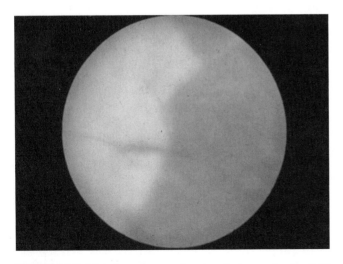

FIGURE 24–3. Clinical appearance of acute retinal necrosis with vitritis, yellowish white retinal infiltrates, and vasculitis. (See color insert.)

trimester, salt-and-pepper pigmentation or circumscribed retinal scarring can be observed, and rarely also optic disc atrophy, vitritis, and microphthalmus. Generalized malformation is often found. The course of neonatal HSV retinitis, which in most cases is acquired in the birth canal (HSV-2), varies considerably. The disease can become manifest in a third of the infected infants and mostly develops 4 to 12 days after birth. After conjunctivitis and keratitis, retinitis is the third most common form of ocular involvement. Retinitis is often observed in connection with HSV encephalitis, herpes skin lesions, and keratitis. Often, only a sharply demarcated retinal area is affected, and 28% of the cases later show chorioretinal scarring and changes in the retinal pigment epithelium. Rarely, a fulminant course has been described, which resulted in complete retinal necrosis, retinal detachment, and optic disc atrophy in both eyes. Recurrences later in life have been noted.[46–54]

The necrotizing retinitis associated with HSV encephalitis manifests itself in both eyes with rapid progression to complete retinal detachment.[25, 55, 56]

Pathogenesis

Iridocyclitis and Trabeculitis

The etiology of these forms of HSV disease are not well established. Intact virus particles have been isolated from the aqueous humor, but there is significant evidence for an important role of immune reactions.[12, 57] Histopathologically, the iris stroma is primarily infiltrated with lymphocytic cells.

HSV has been isolated from aqueous aspirates in eyes with endotheliitis and trabeculitis.[12] It has been suggested that the HSV infection of the trabecular meshwork cells leaves swelling and obstruction of the trabecular meshwork by inflammatory debris, and eventually scars develop. Because herpes simplex virus has also been detected in the aqueous humor from patients with Posner-Schlossman syndrome, it has been speculated that it may play a role in the origin of this disease.[58] Furthermore, polymerase chain reaction (PCR) evidence suggests that HSV DNA is present in the corneal specimens from patients with iridocorneal endothelial syndrome, which implies that this entity has an HSV origin.[59]

The histologic reports on VZV uveitis have disclosed perineuritis and perivasculitis with a chronic inflammatory cell infiltration mainly consisting of plasma cells and lymphocytes. Chronic uveitis from VZV is believed to represent an immune response against persistent inactivated viral antigens in the eye or continuing low-grade viral replication.[60, 61] There is evidence that occlusive vasculitis plays an important role in zoster uveitis, and that focal or sectorial iris atrophy is a result of the ischemic necrosis.[62] Ocular hypotony may occur from necrosis of the ciliary body. It has been speculated that the trabecular meshwork may be clogged with inflammatory cell debris.

Acute Retinal Necrosis

The acute stage of ARN is characterized by necrotizing retinitis of all retinal layers. The retinal vessels in the diseased area show fibrinoid necrosis of the vessel wall and vascular occlusion. The retinal pigment epithelium shows focal necrosis and is occasionally separated from Bruch's membrane. The necrotic retinal cells reach the overlying vitreous body, where inflammatory cells surround it. The necrotic retina is sharply demarcated adjacent to the intact retina. Histologically, there are intranuclear inclusions present at these junctional areas; and by electron microscopy, virus particles can be detected in the retinal cells.[25, 56, 63] The bordering choroid shows severe choroiditis with vascular occlusions. At the same time, optic nerve neuritis and papillitis arise. Inflammatory cells infiltrate the aqueous humor and the anterior chamber angle. The iris and ciliary body show nongranulomatous and granulomatous cell infiltration and perivasculitis.[15, 62, 64] In the healing phase, the process leads to complete disintegration of the retina and optic nerve with reactive metaplasia of the retinal pigment epithelium.[48, 65]

The histopathologic picture of necrotizing retinitis in patients with advanced AIDS (PORN) has a few peculiarities. Initially, there is multifocal retinal necrosis of the outer or all retinal layers. Only minimal intraocular inflammatory signs are found, which include vasculitis and optic neuritis. In a recent study performed on a transscleral eye wall biopsy in a patient with AIDS and PORN, intranuclear inclusion bodies have also been detected in the choroidal cells.[66]

There is experimental evidence that ARN is caused by alpha herpesviruses (VZV and HSV). Herpesvirus can be demonstrated in the retinal lesions and vitreous body in retinitis patients by culture methods, histology or electron microscopy, immunohistochemistry, and PCR methods.[8, 15, 27, 38, 64, 67]

The etiology of ARN remains elusive. After a primary infection or reactivation of the herpesviruses from latency, virus replication follows. From animal experiments[68] it is known that viruses migrate through the parasympathetic fibers of the oculomotor nerve that serves the iris and ciliary bodies in the central nervous system (CNS) from the infected eye. The viral replication within the CNS is fairly well limited to the nucleus of the visual system and the suprachiasmatic area of the hypothalamus. Viruses migrate from the brain to the retina via retrograde axonal transport through the optic nerve, along the endocrine-optic path between the retina and the suprachiasmatic nucleus of the hypothalamus.[69] From this site, the viral invasion can spread out to the contralateral regions, which may explain the involvement of the fellow eye in patients with bilateral acute retinal necrosis (BARN). Along the optic nerve, the viruses can reach the ganglion cells of the retina.[70]

The retinal pathology represents viral-induced cytopathology.[71, 72] However, the accompanying immune reactions are responsible for the further inflammatory process that finally results in the development of retinal necrosis.[71, 73] Local as well as systemic factors come into effect.[73] It has been shown that the retinal HSV infection is under the control of T lymphocytes,[74] and a contribution of T lymphocytes to the pathogenesis of ARN has been suggested.[75] The severe vascular occlusions lead to ischemia of the retina and choroid, and promote the development of necrosis. The massive breakdown of the blood-retinal barrier, with the resulting increase in protein content of the vitreous, is associated with a proliferative and chemoactive effect on the pigment epithelium and the fibroblasts, which, in turn, promotes the development of proliferative vitreoretinopathy (PVR). The widespread retinal necrosis produces multiple posteriorly located retinal holes; and this, together with the development of vitreous traction and PVR, results in the frequent occurrence of retinal detachment.

Diagnosis

Iridocyclitis and Trabeculitis

The medical history is sometimes positive for episodes of HSV keratitis. Even in the absence of such a history or corneal scarring, however, one may find that the corneal sensation is depressed relative to the unaffected cornea. The diagnosis is based on the typical clinical appearance, including the pattern of keratic precipitates, mild flare and cells in the anterior chamber, focal or diffuse iris hyperemia, fulminant inflammatory episodes with high intraocular pressures and (especially) foci of iris atrophy (Fig. 24–5). Endotheliitis may be present in a white eye. Profound redness of the eye, markedly elevated intraocular pressure, corneal haziness from endothelial decompensation, and keratic precipitates are typical for trabeculitis.[30]

In herpes zoster ophthalmicus, fluorescein angiography discloses that the iris vessels at the sites of atrophy are occluded. This is in contrast to the findings in HSV disease that typically has intact iris circulation in the atrophic areas.[76] Aqueous humor aspirates may be analyzed for antibodies directed against HSV or VZV by the enzyme-linked immunosorbent assay (ELISA) method. Detecting viral DNA in the aqueous humor using PCR technology may be very useful in cases of zoster "sine herpete" or in cases without the typical HSV corneal

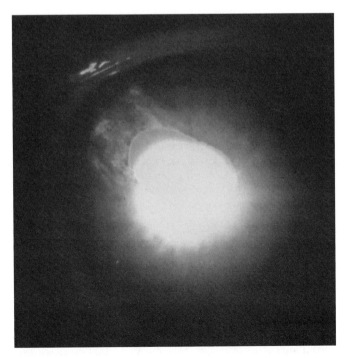

FIGURE 24–5. Iris atrophy in a patient with HSV. (See color insert.)

lesions.[77] Despite its high sensitivity, even the PCR method yielded positive results in only 30% of the patients with anterior uveitis in a recent study.[78] Although some authors have previously shown that herpesviruses can be isolated from aqueous humor obtained from patients with HSV iritis, trabeculitis, and secondary glaucoma,[12] others have concluded that viral growth is rarely detected in culture and that this method is not particularly useful for the diagnosis.

Acute Retinal Necrosis and Other Retinopathies

ARN and variants of necrotizing herpetic retinopathy in general are diagnosed on the basis of the characteristic clinical picture and the course of the infection.[7] The diagnosis can be substantiated by the clinical signs of a systemic herpes infection. In atypical cases, various laboratory investigations are extremely helpful (see later).

Fluorescein Angiography

The fluorescence angiographic findings in the acute stage of ARN include dye leakage from the retinal venules, arterioles, and capillaries. Often, leakage is observed from the optic disc. In the affected peripheral retinal areas, vascular occlusions arise, primarily of the retinal arterioles and capillaries. Retinal neovascularization may be seen. In addition, spotted choroidal ischemia is conspicuous.[32]

Typical fluorescein angiographic findings in the healing stage of ARN are characterized by atrophy of the retinal pigment epithelium, destruction of the choriocapillaris, and retinal nonperfusion.

Laboratory Investigations

In patients with an atypical clinical presentation, and with rapid progression of the retinal inflammation, laboratory tests on aspirates from the aqueous humor and vitreous body can be useful. Negative test results do not rule out the disease complex, however. In doubtful cases, a chorioretinal biopsy may be indicated.[79] The detection of herpesvirus by culture methods is regarded as proof of a viral genesis of the retinitis,[8] although the large time interval until the results are available is a distinct disadvantage. Another argument against these test methods is that the cultures were occasionally negative, even when a large number of viruses could be demonstrated by electron microscopy[8]; but it is technically simple, as is immunofluorescence staining with virus-specific antibodies[8, 80] or in situ hybridization.[65] In the initial stages, immunofluorescence, culture methods, and electron microscopy can be recommended.[81] The PCR technique also permits detection of virus particles even in minimal amounts in the aqueous humor or vitreous fluid.[38, 82–84] In a recent study, PCR analysis from intraocular fluid has been able to detect the inciting virus in all patients with ARN.[85] In the later stages, determination of intraocularly produced antibodies can be helpful,[85, 89a] whereas antibody titers[80] or the immune complexes in the serum often remain negative and the specific antibodies in the cerebrospinal fluid can only occasionally be demonstrated.[24, 46]

Differential Diagnosis of Acute Retinal Necrosis

CMV retinitis mostly affects immunocompromised patients, especially those with AIDS. In the classic case, granular, hemorrhagic retinal lesions arise with centrifugal spread, yellowish white perivascular infiltration, and retinal edema, with or without vascular sheathing. In the healing stage, atrophy of the retina and pigment epithelium develops with fibrosis of the affected retina. Behçet's disease is a systemic disease characterized by typical oral and genital aphthous ulcers, hypopyon, panuveitis, arthritis, cutaneous lesions, CNS involvement, and necrotizing angiitis. The course is typified by periods of acute exacerbation and remission, with occlusive retinal vasculitis and typical retinal infiltrates and hemorrhages. Bacterial, mycotic, or parasitic endophthalmitis can be ruled out in most cases by the medical history and clinical signs. Intravenous drug abuse, a history of trauma, abdominal operations, or immunosuppression should bring to mind an infectious etiology. In toxoplasmic retinochoroiditis, lesions are typically white and focal, with overlying vitreous inflammatory infiltration. The old chorioretinal scars are demarcated from the area of recurrent disease. Intraocular lymphoma can manifest as subretinal material with retinal elevations and can mimic intermediate uveitis. The course is not as rapid as in ARN. In doubtful cases, intraocular lymphoma can be ruled out with cytologic investigations from cells in the vitreous body and lack of focal intracranial lesions. Sarcoidosis is characterized by intravitreous, preretinal, intraretinal and uveal granulomata, and periphlebitis and the typical signs of systemic disease. Periphlebitis or (less often) periarteritis, tubercles and tuberculomata, and a positive PPD are typical for tuberculosis.

Treatment

Iridocyclitis and Trabeculitis

Topical antiviral therapy has little or no effect on the course of disease. In a recently published controlled clinical trial, oral acyclovir proved to be therapeutically useful. However, there is still disagreement on whether or not oral acyclovir actually has a preventive effect on ophthalmic complications after zoster ophthalmicus.[90] The inflammation usually responds promptly to topical corticosteroids. However, the dosages and length of corticosteroid treatment differ considerably, and must be evaluated on an individual basis according to the inflammatory activity. Steroids must be tapered gradually when inflammation is under control. Some patients must be continued on topical low-dose or low-potency corticosteroid medication. Cycloplegics should be given to all patients. Long-term acyclovir prophylaxis may be important to prevent additional episodes.[91]

Elevated intraocular pressure is an indication for the use of antiglaucomatous medication. In eyes with progressive glaucomatous damage of the optic disc, trabeculectomies with or without mitomycin C, seton placement, or cyclophotocoagulation may be warranted.

Acute Retinal Necrosis

Antiviral agents

The major treatment of alpha herpesvirus retinitis consists of antiviral agents; acyclovir is the most commonly used drug; it is very effective against HSV and VZV. In 2 days after the beginning of therapy, the existing lesions from ARN start to regress and formation of further lesions is hindered.[92] Treatment with acyclovir reduces infection of the fellow eye from 70% to 13% in the first year.[93] Nevertheless, the density of the vitreous usually increases, because this represents a secondary inflammatory reaction to the retinal necrosis and not a cytopathologic viral effect. Although retinitis generally responds well to acyclovir in otherwise healthy patients, in patients with AIDS, there is mostly no positive change in the course, and the visual prognosis is not improved.[38] Because absorption from the gastrointestinal tract is only 10% to 20%, the initial application should be intravenous. The dosage is 15 mg/kg body weight in three doses for 7 to 21 days.[92] Then 2 to 4 g daily is recommended for a further 4 to 6 weeks.[94] The effectiveness of intravitreal acyclovir or ganciclovir (DHPG) injections, which have been given in individual cases with ARN or PORN,[95, 96] is undefined.

In patients with AIDS or other immunodeficiencies with retinal necrosis, DHPG, foscarnet, bromovinyldeoxyuridine, or sorivudine appeared to be more effective than acyclovir.[34, 37, 79, 97, 98] Long-term maintenance doses of acyclovir are used in AIDS patients to avoid later recurrences,[37, 99] but when the medication is changed, recurrences may occur.[7, 100, 101] Because prolonged acyclovir treatment increases the chance that the virus will become resistant, therapy may be switched to foscarnet or vidarabine. Retinitis associated with multiple viruses may indicate modifications in the therapy.

Anti-Inflammatory Therapy

Whereas the application of antiviral drugs is undisputed in alpha herpesvirus retinitis, treatment with systemic corticosteroids is controversial. The fact that the immune reaction plays a central role in the evolution of retinal necrosis and vitreous infiltration speaks in favor of the use of corticosteroids. High-dose prednisone not only suppresses the intraocular inflammation but also helps resolve the vitreous infiltration and opacity.[33, 92] However, because virus replication can be promoted through corticosteroids, steroids should only be applied in combination with antiviral drugs and only after the beginning of antiviral therapy.[64] Medication may be initiated at 1 to 2 mg/kg. In contrast, the topical application of steroids to eliminate inflammation in the anterior chamber is uniformly recommended.

Although in animal experiments an improvement in herpetic necrotizing chorioretinitis has been observed with immunoglobulins,[102] the clinical effect of this approach is not clear. Despite its high price, perhaps immunoglobulin should be used in cases with rapid progression.

The occlusive vasculopathy and vasculitis associated with herpetic retinitis do not respond sufficiently to therapy. The effect of anticoagulants, aspirin, and corticosteroids is unclear.[64] Photocoagulation has been advocated for the treatment of retinal neovascularization. In individual patients with optic neuropathy, corticosteroids or anticoagulants were administered, but their influence on the course of the disease is not clear. In selected cases with profound enlargement of the optic nerve, optic nerve sheath decompression has been performed.[103]

Retinal Detachment in Acute Retinal Necrosis

Retinal Detachment Surgery. Late retinal detachment is a serious and frequent complication of ARN, occurring in more than 75% of untreated cases within 6 to 12 weeks from the onset of retinitis.[104–108] The combination of large, multiple, and posteriorly localized retinal tears typical for necrotizing herpetic retinitis, with severe vitreous infiltration, and the association with proliferative vitreoretinopathy make pars plana vitrectomy the operative method most often selected to treat retinal detachment in these cases.[22, 104] Use of long-term internal tamponades, e.g., silicon oil, often allows good anatomic results,[81, 92, 105, 106] although several surgical procedures are frequently necessary. Nevertheless, less than half of the eyes operated upon have a postoperative visual acuity of 20/200 or better.[81, 106]

Detachment Prophylaxis. Because photocoagulation creates firm chorioretinal adhesions at the areas that could develop tears, it has been suggested as an effective prophylaxis against retinal detachment in alpha herpesvirus retinitis. A series of uncontrolled clinical studies indicates that it may be possible to reduce the rate of retinal detachments by prophylactic photocoagulation.[107, 108] However, we must also consider that the good success rate in these studies might also be based on the milder form of retinitis or on simultaneous treatment with acyclovir and steroids. In another study, 93% of the AIDS patients with severe necrotizing retinitis developed retinal detachment despite laser photocoagulation.[37] In general, laser photocoagulation should be applied early before the increasing infiltration of the vitreous makes it impossible to perform the procedure.

Whether or not early vitrectomy actually reduces the rate of retinal detachments is unclear. Surgical removal of the vitreous scaffold and of the infiltrating inflammatory material may inhibit the development of tractional retinal detachment. Indeed, vitrectomy has been effective in several cases in preventing the development of retinal detachment with good visual results.[94, 95]

Complications

During the course of iridocyclitis, a wide range of complications may develop, including iris atrophy, posterior synechiae, secondary glaucoma, cataract formation, hypotony and phthisis bulbi. The most common typical complication resulting from endotheliitis or trabeculitis is secondary glaucoma.

In up to 75% of the patients with ARN, retinal detachment develops.[33, 92, 105] Typically, the detachment does not arise during the active inflammatory phase, but during the retinal atrophy process, that is, with an interval of 1 to several months after the onset of symptoms. The retinal detachments develop from retinal tears that have typical patterns and localization. The retinal tears are usually centrally localized at the border between the affected and healthy retina or in the necrotic, disintegrated retina. The tears commonly are very large, grouped, and localized in different quandrants.[105] Vitreous body traction

and proliferative vitreoretinopathy are further complicating factors. Generally, the risk of a later retinal detachment rises with the extension of the necrosis, formation of retinal tears, and the severity of the proliferative vitreoretinopathy.[109]

Occlusion of the large vessels in the clinical context of arterial occlusion or venous thrombosis may be observed. Often, compromised vascular perfusion of the retina and choroidal circulation may serve to decrease vision. In the acute inflammatory phase, exudative retinal detachments occasionally arise.[32]

Progressive optic neuropathy, both primary and secondary to global retinal necrosis, may result in optic atrophy. It has been speculated that inflammation and ischemia of the optic nerve may be the primary causes for optic atrophy that finally occurs in some patients.[15, 103]

Prognosis

Visual prognosis is largely dependent on the presence of retinal detachment, vascular occlusion, and optic neuritis.[110–112] If the condition is left untreated, in about 35% of the cases, the disease attacks the fellow eye as well; hence, the acronym BARN. After an interval of 5 days to 30 years, the second eye can be affected.[9, 24, 33, 113–115] Initial reports demonstrated that more than 60% of patients with ARN had a final visual acuity of 20/50 or worse.[32, 33] When treated with antiviral drugs and steroids, however, 30% to 60% of patients did not suffer such severe visual loss.[92, 116] Similarly, early reports regarding retinal reattachment surgery in ARN demonstrated a 63% successful reattachment rate, with 56% of these eyes seeing 20/200 or better.[104] Five years later, the same group of investigators reported a 95% reattachment rate using more sophisticated vitreoretinal techniques; however, only 40% of these anatomically reattached eyes saw better than 20/200.[117]

The prognosis of alpha herpesvirus retinitis in AIDS patients is very poor. In 90% of these patients, the disease is bilateral (BARN). Various complications develop rapidly, and 70% of the diseased eyes become blind within 4 weeks.[37] The rate of rhegmatogenous retinal detachment is even higher than in the remaining healthy individuals,[81] probably because in AIDS patients, the retinitis responds poorly to antiviral drug therapy and there is a tendency toward recurrence.[81, 100] Mixed infections of necrotizing retinitis with CMV retinitis and toxoplasmosis chorioretinitis have also been reported.

EPSTEIN-BARR VIRUS

Definition

EBV belongs to the group of gamma herpesviruses.[118] It contains a double-strand DNA and is surrounded by a complex capsid and envelope. Morphologically, EBV cannot be distinguished from the other herpesviruses.

Epidemiology

EBV is widespread. About 90% of the population are seroconverted by the time they reach their thirties. Transmission occurs primarily via the saliva, but it can also happen through blood transfusions. The fact that 15% to 25% of all seropositive healthy individuals shed the virus in their saliva is regarded as the main reason for its broad distribution. The primary infection with a clinical picture of infectious mononucleosis mostly affects the age group of 14 to 18 year olds.[119] EBV is also reported to have a pathogenic role in the development of nasopharyngeal carcinoma and Burkitt's lymphoma. In addition, associations have been found between mononucleosis that has run its course and the later appearance of Sjögren's syndrome.[120]

Clinical Characteristics

Ocular involvement in EBV infections occurs mostly in primary infections in the context of infectious mononucleosis. Intraocular inflammation may develop several months after the onset of acute infectious mononucleosis. The ocular manifestation of EBV infection encompasses a wide range of anterior segment or neurophthalmic features. Follicular conjunctivitis is seen most often.[121] Also, stromal keratitis and episcleritis can appear. Severe bilateral iritis and iridocyclitis have been seen in other patients.[122] Almost all structures of the posterior ocular segments can be affected. Macular edema, retinal hemorrhages, and punctate outer retinitis[123] or multifocal choroiditis have been seen.[124–126] Secondary subretinal neovascularization and progressive subretinal fibrosis and uveitis syndrome[127] may occur. In individual cases, disc edema or optic neuritis has been described as the main finding, which completely regressed with restitution.[128] In the retinal pigment epithelium, fine scars and pigmentary changes may remain. The retinal vessels are generally unaffected. In the context of severe panuveitis, dense vitritis has been noted.[89, 129]

Pathogenesis

EBV shows B-cell tropism. Healing occurs from neutralizing antibodies and the T-cell response, but the pathogenetic role of EBV in intraocular inflammation is undefined. There is no biopsy-proven evidence that the replicating virus is a direct cause of the posterior uveitis.

Diagnosis

Depending on the time after transmission, antibodies directed against EBV-specific capsid antigens can prove EBV disease. The antibodies directed against nuclear antigen (EBNA) are positive after 6 to 8 weeks; antibodies against "diffuse/restricted antigens" (EA-D/R) can be detected after 3 to 4 weeks.[130]

A similar variety of clinical changes in the posterior segment of the eye can be caused by sarcoidosis, tuberculosis, or syphilis. The clinical appearance of retinal and choroidal infiltrations can be confused with the acute phase of toxoplasmosis, histoplasmosis, or idiopathic white-dot syndromes.

Therapy

Because the ocular disease is mostly self-limited, no treatment is indicated. Occasionally, the iritis necessitates the topical application of corticosteroids and cycloplegic drops, and occasionally, a systemic course of corticosteroids may be indicated.[89]

Complications

The prognosis concerning vision may be poor in cases with chorioretinitis and panuveitis complicated by subretinal neovascularization or cystoid macular edema. Recalcitrant, chronic, smoldering focal or diffuse chorioretinitis is occasionally complicated by the development of secondary cataract formation.

CYTOMEGALOVIRUS

Definition

CMV belongs to the group of herpesviruses. It is a ubiquitous pathogen in the general population but rarely causes clinically apparent disease in an immunocompetent individual. In immunosuppressed patients, CMV can be pathogenic and cause gastrointestinal, CNS, and pulmonary disease. The most common manifestation, however, is CMV retinitis, which is the most frequent cause of blindness in patients with AIDS.

History

"Cytomegalia" was described in 1921 by Goodpasture[131] as the histopathologic finding of large mononuclear inclusions in various organs of a child. The virus responsible for this disease was visualized by electron microscopy,[132] isolated, and grown in culture[133] in the 1950s.

CMV eye disease was described in a newborn child in 1947[134] and in an adult under chemotherapy in 1964.[135] In the pre-AIDS era, CMV retinitis was a rare disease that was found in adults under medical immunosuppression.[35] In the 1980s with the AIDS pandemic, CMV retinitis became the most common form of posterior uveitis in urban populations.[136] With the introduction of highly active antiretroviral therapy (HAART) in AIDS patients, the incidence of CMV retinitis has declined significantly.[137, 138]

Epidemiology

In about half of a normal population, antibodies against CMV can be detected. In homosexual men, nearly 100% are infected.[139] In the vast majority, CMV infection in immunocompetent hosts does not produce symptomatic disease. Only a small percentage may develop infectious mononucleosis–like symptoms.[140]

Primary infection of pregnant women with CMV is the most common cause for intrauterine infection in Western countries. Fortunately, only about 10% of the babies have neonatal disease.[141] There is a 20% mortality rate associated with congenital CMV disease, 90% of the affected survivors develop CNS disease,[142] and in 15% of the babies, retinitis is found.[141]

The mode of transmission probably requires close contact with body fluids containing the virus. Sexual contact may be an important source of infection in homosexual men. CMV reaches the eye via infected cells in the blood stream, and the risk for retinitis in immunosuppressed patients can be assessed by the CMV DNA burden in the blood.[143] Owing to systemic viremia, bilateral retinitis and an association of retinitis with extraocular CMV disease are commonly found.

In patients with AIDS, CMV is one of the most common[144, 145] and most expensive[146] opportunistic infections and is the major cause of blindness.[147] Although the definition of the Centers for Disease Control and Prevention in Atlanta includes CMV retinitis as one of the diseases that defines the diagnosis of AIDS, it is rarely the first manifestation of AIDS and usually presents in an advanced disease stage.[148] The risk for developing CMV retinitis strongly depends on the immune status of the patient, which can be assessed by the number of CD4+ cells in the blood. Almost all cases of CMV retinitis occur in patients with a CD4+ count below 50 cells/mm³ and only rarely with a CD4+ count of more than 100 cells/mm³.[149, 150] Altogether, CMV retinitis occurs in developed countries in about 20% of AIDS patients.[136, 151, 152] In African AIDS patients, CMV retinitis is rare.[153]

With the introduction of HAART, the picture is changing. The incidence of opportunistic infections including CMV retinitis in patients with AIDS dropped by more than 80% from 1994 to 1997.[138] CMV retinitis, however, is not going to disappear. Failure of anti-HIV therapy to improve the immune status sufficiently, CMV retinitis in patients not receiving antiretroviral therapy, and the development of HIV drug resistance are all still challenging problems.

Clinical Characteristics

CMV retinitis commonly begins in the peripheral retina. Symptoms of the early disease may therefore be minimal or initially even absent. Blurring and floaters may be experienced, as well as unspecific visual disturbances. Symptomatic scotomas are usually noticed only if more central parts of the retina are involved. In patients at risk with CD4+ cells below 50 cells/mm³ or if other organs have CMV disease, ophthalmologic screening with dilated pupils every 3 to 4 months is recommended.[149] It should be noted, however, that CMV retinitis may occur in patients under HAART who have CD4 counts of more than 100 cells/mm³.[154] Patients should be educated to pay attention to the symptoms and seek ophthalmologic care after the onset of visual disturbances. In selected motivated patients, entoptic perimetry can be helpful as a screening test for CMV retinitis.[150]

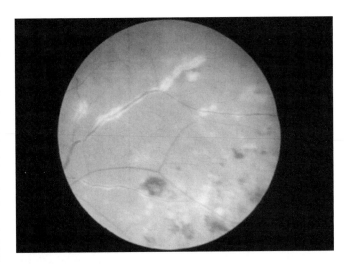

FIGURE 24–7. Clinical appearance of CMV retinitis: frosted branch angiitis. (See color insert.)

Early CMV retinitis begins with a small, white retinal infiltrate. At this stage, it may be difficult to differentiate from a cotton-wool spot that is commonly present in HIV-related microvasculopathy. Large and atypical cotton-wool spots in patients with AIDS should therefore be regarded as suspect. Two distinct types of clinical appearances may be seen that represent the ends of a continuous spectrum with intermediate forms commonly occurring. The first form is characterized by fluffy, dense, white confluent opacifications of the retina with no atrophic zone in the center of the lesion (Fig. 24–6). This type commonly has multiple retinal hemorrhages, with perivascular location and perivasculitis and is more commonly found closer to the posterior pole, with an arcuate distribution following the nerve fiber layer. In selected patients, perivasculitis may be predominant, with a clinical picture resembling "frosted branch angiitis" (Fig. 24–7).[155] The second form has more granular, less opaque-appearing lesions and shows a central atrophic zone, fewer hemorrhages, and less vascular sheathing (Fig. 24–8).

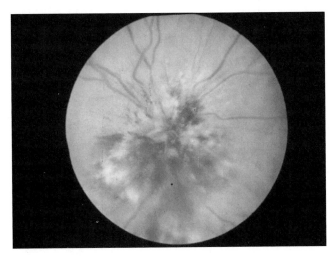

FIGURE 24–6. Clinical appearance of CMV retinitis: fluffy, dense, white confluent retinal infiltrations, multiple retinal hemorrhages, and perivasculitis. (See color insert.)

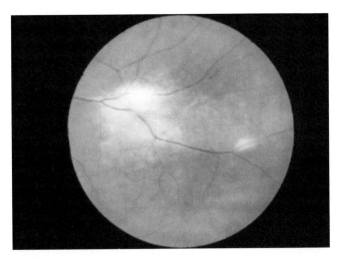

FIGURE 24–8. Clinical appearance of CMV retinitis: granular, less-opaque lesions. (See color insert.)

In both forms, there are no sharply defined edges of the involved retina. The affected area commonly has irregular borders and is surrounded by satellite infiltrates. The optic disc can be infiltrated as retinitis progresses toward the posterior pole. Primary involvement of the optic disc is less common. There is mostly a low-grade vitritis. Only a mild anterior chamber inflammatory reaction may be present.

Fulminant courses with rapid progression rarely occur. Progression of the retinal infiltration without therapy usually is slow, at about 0.2 mm per week, leading to complete destruction of the entire retina in about 3 to 6 months.[156] The clinical course is probably dependent on the immune status of the patient. Complete necrosis of the involved retina develops and atrophic zones with stippling of the underlying retinal pigment epithelium are usually left behind in the center of the lesion as the active lesions resolve. Only the active edges are edematous and opaque.

With anti-CMV treatment, the active lesions also become atrophic and the infiltration at the edges becomes less opaque. Remaining opacities do not necessarily represent active inflammation. If they do not progress, they can be caused by fibrosis or necrotic debris that has not cleared. Progression under maintenance therapy is mostly slow and with only mild opacification of the edges of the lesion. Serial photographs are much more sensitive than funduscopy or fundus drawings for the detection of relapsing CMV retinitis. Monthly follow-up of inactive lesions is recommended.

Rarely, CMV infections of the retina may present as ARN in immunocompetent[157] and immunocompromised patients.[158] CMV has been detected in selected cases of conjunctivitis, iridocyclitis or keratitis, but a causal relationship for CMV with ocular diseases other than retinitis is probably very rare.

Pathophysiology, Immunology, Pathology, and Pathogenesis

After primary infection, CMV is disseminated by the blood stream, and replication can be found in multiple organ tissues, in polymorphonuclear leukocytes, monocytes, and T lymphocytes. Despite the fact that primary CMV infection is a systemic infection, healthy individuals commonly are without apparent symptoms. This suggests that the CMV-specific immune response must be protective. Both the humoral and cellular immune response, especially the T-cell response, contribute to this observation.[159] After primary infection, CMV remains in its host, establishing a latent infection typical for all herpesviruses. The viruses persist in latency in a large variety of tissues, in lymphoreticular cells, and in the secretory glands.[3] In patients with AIDS, CMV infection is one of the most important opportunistic infections. Ninety percent of these patients develop CMV infections,[160] generally representing reactivation from latency.

In most cases, the retina is infected via hematogenous spread during an episode of systemic CMV replication. An infection via the optic nerve by extension from the CNS or CMV papillitis is less common. There is experimental evidence that an impaired antiviral T-cell response is of particular importance for the development of the

retinitis.[161, 162] The microangiopathy caused by HIV infection of capillary endothelial cells probably facilitates the passage of CMV-infected cells from the blood stream to the retina. The higher incidence of CMV retinitis in patients with AIDS in comparison to other patients under immunosuppression may be facilitated by this endothelial tropism.[163]

Histopathologic examinations have revealed that CMV infects all layers of the retina, including the pigmented epithelium, but without choroidal involvement. It has been demonstrated that HIV accelerates the CMV replication in coinfected retinal cells. Nerve fiber infarcts, retinal hemorrhages, opacifications, and perivascular sheathing can be found.[164]

Diagnosis

The diagnosis of CMV retinitis is usually based on clinical criteria with the typical ophthalmoscopic picture in an immunosuppressed individual. Serum antibodies can be detected in the majority of the normal population and do not have significant diagnostic value. Elevated or rising CMV DNA blood levels appear to be associated with the development of CMV organ disease[165] and may be helpful in selected cases. Additional diagnostic tools usually require tests on intraocular fluid or tissue.

Antibody levels from vitreous and aqueous humor compared with the serum levels (using the Goldmann-Witmer coefficient) can support the diagnosis in difficult cases,[166] but polyclonal stimulation and reduced antibody formation in immunosuppressed individuals may render interpretation of the results difficult. Virus culture and PCR from ocular tissue or fluid can directly demonstrate the presence of viral DNA,[167] but because CMV can persist in the tissue without causing disease, these laboratory tests are helpful only together with the clinical picture. Especially in the differentiation of active and inactive disease, the clinical findings are vastly more important than laboratory tests.

The differential diagnosis of early CMV retinitis must include mainly cotton-wool spots. In more advanced cases, retinitis caused by herpes simplex or varicella zoster virus (ARN and PORN), syphilitic retinitis, toxoplasmic retinochoroiditis, fungal infections, and intraocular lymphomas are the most important diseases that have to be differentiated from CMV retinitis.[168]

Treatment

The treatment of patients with CMV retinitis is complex and demanding, and requires close collaboration between the ophthalmologist and the treating physician. The drugs used have considerable side effects and interactions. In most cases, therapy is inconvenient (IV or intraocular). The therapeutic plan must be individualized depending on the immune status, concomitant medications, individual tolerance, and the patient's personal preferences concerning the effectiveness and risks of the treatment, as well as restrictions and impact they might have on the quality of life.

Anti-CMV drugs are, in general, virostatic and cannot completely eliminate the viral DNA from the retinal cells. Therefore, if immunosuppression persists and anti-CMV treatment is stopped, progression of the disease is inevitable if the follow-up is long enough. Without therapy, progression of CMV occurs within 2 to 3 weeks.[145] Life-long maintenance therapy is therefore required. Even under maintenance therapy, relapses occur after several months, probably because resistant strains of the virus develop or the immune function of the patient declines. With the introduction of potent antiretroviral therapy (HAART), however, this concept of life-long maintenance therapy is challenged.

Improving the Immune Status

In patients under medical immunosuppression, discontinuation or reduction of the dose of the chemotherapy may be sufficient to restore immunocompetence and effectively stop CMV retinitis.[169] In AIDS patients, improving the immune status has only recently been made possible with the introduction of HAART, a regimen that combines two reverse transcriptase inhibitors and one antiprotease medication. This drug combination reduces HIV-1 replication, increases CD4+ cell counts (immune reconstruction), and decreases levels of activation markers.[170] As a result, this therapy has changed the present evolution of AIDS.[137] It improves the function of the immune system and increases survival.[171] Early introduction of potent antiretroviral therapy is now recommended for patients with HIV infections.[172] With this treatment, a dramatic decline in the incidence of opportunistic infections, including CMV retinitis, has been observed.[138]

HAART is not only beneficial for prevention but also for treating patients who are already suffering from CMV retinitis. In selected patients, regression of CMV retinitis associated with protease-inhibitor treatment has been observed without additional specific anti-CMV medications.[173–175] However, it is difficult to predict whether the immune system will recover sufficiently to control CMV retinitis without additional anti-CMV treatment and if it does, when this will occur. For immediate, effective treatment and to preserve as much of the retina as possible, especially in patients with sight-threatening retinitis involving the posterior pole, anti-CMV treatment is still mandatory. Patients presenting with CMV retinitis who have not previously received antiretroviral therapy commonly have limited access to medical care, and this fact also (or poor compliance) must be taken into consideration in the therapeutic plan.

For patients with inactive CMV retinitis, life-long anti-CMV therapy was necessary before HAART. If CD4 increases after HAART, a beneficial effect on CMV recurrences has been observed.[176] Most patients with quiescent CMV retinitis after HAART have demonstrated strong CMV-specific CD4+ lymphocyte responses, indicating that the loss of CMV-specific CD4+ lymphocyte responses in individuals infected with HIV-1 who have active CMV disease may be restored.[177] In selected patients with immune reconstitution after initiation of HAART, with elevated CD4+ counts above 100 cells/μl, prolonged relapse-free intervals during the reconstitution period before CD4+ counts rise above 100 cells/μl, and completely inactive retinitis, anti-CMV therapy can be discontinued at least temporarily. Reduced risks of drug toxicity and drug-resistant organisms are potential benefits. Patients who are able to stop daily IV maintenance therapy

definitely experience an improved quality of life. However, close observation for evidence of recurrent retinitis is indicated. Longer follow-up of these patients is needed to determine how long such therapy may be interrupted and when anti-CMV therapy has to be reinstituted.[178–180] Some patients respond to antiretroviral therapy with an increase to 500 cells/μl, but retinitis still showed reactivation, indicating that immunologic deficits to specific pathogens may persist despite an overall improvement in the immune system, and that the CD4 cell count is not an absolutely reliable indicator.[181]

Systemic Anti-Cytomegalovirus Virostatic Treatment

DHPG, foscarnet, and cidofovir are the most commonly used drugs in the treatment of CMV retinitis. Active CMV disease is treated with an induction therapy of 2 to 3 weeks' duration, followed by maintenance therapy.[182] In the preprotease inhibitor era, maintenance therapy did not absolutely prevent the occurrence of retinitis, but the time until a relapse occurred increased considerably. In patients receiving maintenance therapy, survival is also longer, probably because CMV had a direct impact on mortality.[183] First relapses of retinitis can be treated with a reinduction with the same drug. A shortening of the intervals between subsequent relapses is commonly observed. In cases of repeated relapses and disease refractory to therapy, the drug should be changed or local application chosen.

DHPG was the first effective anti-CMV drug introduced in 1984.[184] The main side effect of DHPG is neutropenia and thrombopenia, but neutrophil counts can be elevated by concomitantly using granulocyte colony–stimulating factor (G-CSF).[185] Induction therapy requires IV infusions twice daily, followed by maintenance therapy with daily IV infusion. Alternatively, DHPG maintenance therapy can be administered orally, but the bioavailability of the orally administered drug is poor and the patient has to swallow 12 to 24 pills daily, and at least in lower dosages, the effectiveness appears less than with IV application.[186]

Foscarnet is the least convenient anti-CMV therapy because it requires 2-hour IV infusion and concomitant hydration twice daily during the induction phase. Its main side effect is nephrotoxicity. Intravenous DHPG or foscarnet are equivalent in controlling CMV retinitis.[187] Foscarnet, however, is associated with a slightly reduced mortality compared with DHPG, possibly owing to its inherent antiretroviral activity, but patients may not tolerate foscarnet as well as DHPG.[188] In relapsed CMV retinitis with poor therapeutic effect of one drug, a combination of DHPG and foscarnet may be synergistic.[189]

Intravenous DHPG or foscarnet is an inconvenient and costly treatment. Both require an indwelling central venous catheter, which carries a risk of a sepsis in about two cases per 1000 catheter days.[190]

Cidofovir has a prolonged antiviral activity and can be administered IV weekly during the induction phase and biweekly thereafter. Therefore, it, does not require an indwelling central venous catheter. It is, however, nephrotoxic, and concomitant use of probenecid and hydration is necessary. Ocular side effects are anterior uveitis and hypotony.[191–193] DHPG and cidofovir have a synergistic effect in inhibiting CMV replication. Combination therapy with intravenous cidofovir and oral DHPG (a regimen that does not require indwelling central venous catheter access) might enhance clinical efficacy.[194]

Local Anti-Cytomegalovirus Virostatic Treatment

In patients who cannot tolerate high-dose IV therapy, local intraocular application of anti-CMV medication is an alternative approach, but this does not prevent extraocular CMV disease and contralateral eye disease. Therefore, local therapy should be combined with systemic therapy (e.g., oral DHPG) whenever possible.[195]

Intravitreal injections of DHPG[196] or foscarnet[197] can be performed two to three times weekly for the induction phase and weekly for maintenance. Intravitreous injections of cidofovir are effective if repeated in 5- to 6-week intervals, but uveitis and hypotony are serious complications.[198]

The DHPG intraocular implant is a sustained-release device that provides consistently high intraocular levels of the drug and appears to be the drug of choice in immediately sight-threatening retinitis cases involving the posterior pole because the implant has clinically the most rapid therapeutic effect (Fig. 24–9).[182] This therapeutic approach requires a surgical intervention with the risk of complications such as vitreous hemorrhage, endophthalmitis, and retinal detachment.[114] Progression of the retinitis occurs with the implant after 221 days versus 71 days with intravenous DHPG. Thus, the sustained-release DHPG implant is more effective than intravenous DHPG.[199] Depletion of the drug occurs after 5 to 8 months, and the device has to be replaced. In patients with recurrent CMV retinitis treated with the DHPG implant, concomitant antiretroviral therapy improves the outcome.[200] With increased patient survival and the potential for CMV retinitis to be controlled by effective antiretroviral therapy, the indications for the DHPG intraocular implant are changing.[201]

Fomivirsen provides a new and interesting therapeutic concept. It is an antisense oligonucleotide that specifically inhibits the replication of human CMV by binding to complementary sequences of messenger RNA of the virus. For treatment of CMV retinitis, it has to be injected intravitreally.[202, 203]

Complications

Loss of vision in patients with CMV retinitis is due to either involvement of the macula or optic disc or retinal detachment. With the introduction of effective antiviral treatment, the incidence of progression of retinitis and macular involvement decreases, but retinal detachment may develop with active as well as inactive CMV retinitis in 20% to 30% of eyes within 6 months. Vitreous traction on the atrophic retina can cause multiple, large, and commonly posteriorly located retinal holes. Risk factors for retinal detachment in CMV retinitis are involvement of large areas of the peripheral retina and active retinitis.[204] Bilateral detachment is common.[81] Laser treatment may delay but not prevent progression of rhegmatogenous retinal detachment in CMV retinitis.[181, 205] Scleral buckling is only effective in cases with peripheral holes. The best treatment available for most cases of CMV retinitis and retinal detachment is probably vitrectomy with silicone oil tamponade.[200, 206, 207] This procedure has a high success rate but generates important side effects, such as a hyperopia of about 6 diopters in phakic eyes. The inevitable development of lens opacifications in silicone-filled eyes becomes a growing problem with the increasing life expectancy of these patients.

A new clinical syndrome has been observed after introduction of HAART in patients with CMV retinitis. With the recovery of the immune system, the intraocular immune response to the virus creates an inflammatory response in a previously quiet eye with inactive CMV retinitis. Enhanced inflammatory activity has also been observed in other organs after treatment with protease inhibitors.[208] So-called immune recovery vitritis develops in more than 50% of patients with inactive CMV retinitis who responded to HAART with an increase of CD4 cell counts of more than 60 cells/mm[3].[209] This inflammation may be accompanied by papillitis, cystoid macular edema,[210] or vitreomacular traction syndrome.[211] Therapy with oral or sub-Tenon's injections of corticosteroids may influence this condition positively.

Prognosis

The prognosis for vision and survival in patients with CMV retinitis is mutually dependent. The longer the life expectancy, the more demanding the task for the ophthalmologist to preserve vision for longer time periods. With improved antiretroviral therapy, the mortality rate in patients with AIDS dropped by 80% from 1995 to 1998.[212] The mean survival after the diagnosis of CMV retinitis was 224 days in patients who took no further antiretroviral therapy, and 914 days in those who took a protease inhibitor. In the early 1990s, central vision could be preserved with systemic anti-CMV drugs in the majority of CMV retinitis patients for a limited time period, but about 10% of the patients had a vision of less than 20/40 in the better eye after 6 months.[187] Median time to loss of vision below 20/200 in the better eye was 21 months.[213] Since that time, new antiretroviral and anti-

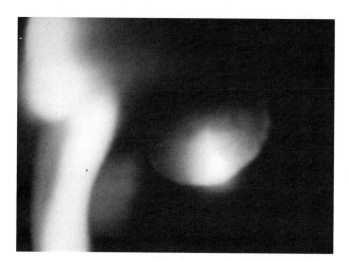

FIGURE 24–9. Slit-lamp appearance of a sustained-release ganciclovir implant.

CMV treatment modalities have been introduced. Retinal detachment can be repaired more successfully with silicone oil.[214] However, the fruition of this progress in positively changing the epidemiology of blindness in patients with AIDS still needs to be evaluated.

CONCLUSIONS

The situation for patients with CMV retinitis and AIDS has dramatically changed within a very short time. In the early 1980s, it was an untreatable blinding disease in patients with a life expectancy limited to several months. In the late 1990s, several effective therapeutic modalities are available to prevent and treat CMV retinitis; but in many cases, current treatment options are still unsatisfactory, and further progress awaits the development of new pharmacologic and surgical strategies for the treatment and prevention of disease.

References

1. Chang Y, Moore PS: Kaposi's sarcoma (KS)–associated herpesvirus and its role in KS. Infect Agents Dis 1996;5:215.
2. Moore PS, Chang Y: Kaposi's sarcoma–associated herpesvirus. In: Richman DD, Whitley RJ, Hayden FG, eds: Clinical Virology. New York, Churchill Livingston, 1997.
3. Roizman B: Herpesviridae. In: Fields BN, Knipe DM, Howley PM, eds: Virology, 3rd ed. Philadelphia, Lippincott-Raven, 1996.
4. Spring SB, Roizman B: Herpes simplex virus products in productive and abortive infection. III. Differentiation of infectious virus derived from nucleus and cytoplasm with respect to stability and size. J Virol 1968;2:979.
5. Straus SE: Introduction to herpesviridae. In: Mandell GL, Bennett JE, Dolin R, eds: Principles and Practice of Infectious Disease, 4th ed. New York, Churchill Livingstone, 1995.
6. Roizman B, Sears A: Herpes simplex viruses and their replication. In: Fields BN, Knipe DM, Howley PM, eds: Virology, 3rd ed. Philadelphia, Lippincott-Raven, 1996.
7. Holland GN, and the Executive Committee of the American Uveitis Society: Standard diagnostic criteria for the acute retinal necrosis syndrome. Am J Ophthalmol 1994;117:663.
8. Lewis ML, Culbertson WW, Post JD, et al: Herpes simplex virus type 1. A cause of the acute retinal necrosis syndrome. Ophthalmology 1989;96:875.
9. Ludwig IH, Zegarra H, Zakov N: The acute retinal necrosis syndrome. Possible herpes simplex retinitis. Ophthalmology 1984;91:1659.
10. Jensen J: A case of herpes zoster ophthalmicus complicated with neuroretinitis. Acta Ophthalmol 1948;26:551.
11. Partamian LG, Morse PH, Klein HZ: Herpes simplex type 1 retinitis in an adult with systemic herpes zoster. Am J Ophthalmol 1981;92:215.
12. Sundmacher R, Neumann-Haefelin D: Herpes simplex virus isolation from the aqueous of patients suffering from focal iritis, endotheliitis, and prolonged disciform keratitis with glaucoma. Klin Montatsbl Augenheilkd 1979;104:488.
13. Robin J, Stergner J, Kaufman H: Progressive herpetic corneal endotheliitis. Am J Ophthalmol 1985;100:336.
14. Urayama A, Yamada N, Sasaki T, et al: Unilateral acute uveitis with periarteritis and detachment. Jpn J Clin Ophthalmol 1971;25:607.
15. Culbertson WM, Blumenkranz MS, Haines H, et al: The acute retinal necrosis syndrome. Part 2: Histopathology and etiology. Ophthalmology 1982;89:1317.
16. Womack L, Liesegang T: Complications of herpes zoster ophthalmicus. Arch Ophthalmol 1983;101:42.
17. Holland GN, Cornell PJ, Park MS, et al: An association between acute retinal necrosis syndrome and HLA-DQw7 and phenotype Bw62, DR4. Am J Ophthalmol 1989;108:370.
18. Ichikaw T, Sakai J, Usui M, et al: HLA antigens of patients with Kirisawa's uveitis and herpetic keratitis. J Eye (Atarashii Ganka) 1989;6:107–114.
19. Chambers RB, Derick RJ, Davidorf FH, et al: Varicella-zoster retinitis in human immunodeficiency virus infection. Arch Ophthalmol 1989;107:960.
20. Jabs DA, Schachat AP, Liss R, et al: Presumed varicella zoster retinitis in immunocompromised patients. Retina 1987;7:9.
21. Uninsky E, Jampol LM, Kaufman S, et al: Disseminated herpes simplex infection with retinitis in a renal allograft recipient. Ophthalmology 1983;90:175.
22. Duker JS, Blumenkranz MS: Diagnosis and management of the acute retinal necrosis (ARN) syndrome. Surv Ophthalmol 1991;35:327.
23. Bloom JN, Katz JI, Kaufman HE: Herpes simplex retinitis and encephalitis in an adult. Arch Ophthalmol 1977;95:1798.
24. Gartry DS, Spalton DJ, Tilzey A, Hykin PG: Acute retinal necrosis syndrome. Br J Ophthalmol 1991;75:292.
25. Minckler DS, McLean EB, Shaw CM, et al: Herpesvirus hominis encephalitis and retinitis. Arch Ophthalmol 1976;94:89.
26. Frieberg TR, Jost BF: Acute retinal necrosis in an immunosuppressed patient. Am J Ophthalmol 1984;98:515.
27. Pavan-Langston D, Dunkel EC: Ocular varicella-zoster virus infection in the guinea pig. A new in vivo model. Arch Ophthalmol 1989;107:1068.
28. Gupta K, Hoepner J, Streeten B: Pseudomelanoma of the iris in herpes simplex keratouveitis. Ophthalmology 1986;93:1524.
29. Liesegang TJ: Classification of herpes simplex virus keratitis and anterior uveitis. Cornea 1999;18:127.
30. Sundmacher R: A clinico-virologic classification of herpetic anterior segment disease with special reference to intraocular herpes. In: Sundmacher R, ed: Herpetische Augenerkrankungen. Bergmann, München, 1981, p 203.
31. Schwab IR: Herpes zoster sine herpete. A potential cause of iridoplegic granulomatous iridocyclitis. Ophthalmology 1997;194:1421.
32. Hayreh SS: So-called acute retinal necrosis syndrome, an acute ocular panvasculitis syndrome. Dev Ophthalmol 1985;10:40.
33. Fisher JP, Lewis ML, Blumenkranz M, et al: The acute retinal necrosis syndrome. Part 1: Clinical manifestations. Ophthalmology 1982;89:1309.
34. Safrin S, Berger TG, Wolfe PR, et al: Foscarnet therapy in five patients with AIDS and acyclovir-resistant varicella-zoster virus infection. Ann Intern Med 1991;115:19.
35. Okinamin S, Tsukahara I: Acute severe uveitis with retinal vasculitis and retinal detachment. Ophthalmologica 1979;179:276.
36. Margolis T, Irvine AR, Hoyt WF, et al: Acute retinal necrosis syndrome presenting with papillitis and arcuate neuroretinitis. Ophthalmology 1988;95:937.
37. Engstrom RE, Holland GN, Margolis TP, et al: The progressive outer retinal necrosis syndrome. A variant of necrotizing herpetic retinopathy in patients with AIDS. Ophthalmology 1994;101:1488.
38. Forster DJ, Dugel PU, Frangieh GT, et al: Rapidly progressive outer retinal necrosis in the acquired immunodeficiency syndrome. Am J Ophthalmol 1990;110:341.
39. Lee MS, Cooney EL, Stoessel KM, Gariano RF: Varicella zoster virus retrobulbar optic neuritis preceding retinitis in patients with acquired immune deficiency syndrome. Ophthalmology 1998;105:467.
40. Charles NC, Bennett TW, Margolis S: Ocular pathology of the congenital varicella syndrome. Arch Ophthalmol 1977;95:2034.
41. DeNicola LK, Hanshaw JB: Congenital and neonatal varicella. J Pediatrics 1979;94:175.
42. Duehr PA: Herpes zoster as a cause of congenital cataract. Am J Ophthalmol 1955;39:157.
43. Copenhaver RM: Chickenpox with retinopathy. Arch Ophthalmol 1966;75:199.
44. Culbertson WW, Brod RD, Flynn HW, et al: Chickenpox-associated acute retinal necrosis syndrome. Ophthalmology 1991;98:1641.
45. Matsuo T, Koyama M, Matsuo N: Acute retinal necrosis as a novel complication of chickenpox in adults. Br J Ophthalmol 1990;74:443.
46. Azazi, M, Samuelsson A, Linde A, et al: Intrathecal antibody production against viruses of the herpesvirus family in acute retinal necrosis syndrome. Am J Ophthalmol 1991;112:76.
47. Cibis GW: Neonatal herpes simplex retinitis. Graefe's Arch Clin Exp Ohthalmol 1975;196:39.
48. Cogan DG, Kuwabara T, Young GF, et al: Herpes simplex retinopathy in an infant. Arch Ophthalmol 1964;72:641.
49. Hagler WS, Walters PV, Nahmias AJ: Ocular involvement in neonatal herpes simplex virus infection. Arch Ophthalmol 1969;82:169.

50. Nahmias AJ, Visintine AM, Caldwell DR, et al: Eye infections with herpes simplex viruses in neonates. Surv Ophthalmol 1976;21:100.

51. Reersted P, Hansen B: Chorioretinitis of the newborn with herpes simplex type 1. Report of a case. Acta Ophthalmol 1979;57:1096.

52. Reynolds JD, Griebel M, Mallory S, et al: Congenital herpes simplex retinitis. Am J Ophthalmol 1986;102:33.

53. Whitley RJ, Nahmias AJ, Visintine AM, et al: The natural history of herpes simplex virus infection of mother and newborn. Pediatrics 1980;66:489.

54. Yanoff M, Allman MI, Fine BS: Congenital herpes simplex virus, type 2, bilateral endophthalmitis. Trans Am Ophthalmol Soc 1977;575:325.

55. Bloom SM, Snady-McCoy L: Multifocal choroiditis uveitis occurring after herpes zoster ophthalmicus. Am J Ophthalmol 1989;108:733.

56. Cibis GW, Flynn JT, Davis B: Herpes simplex retinitis. Arch Ophthalmol 1978;96:299.

57. Pavan Langston D, Brockhurst R. Herpes simplex panuveitis: A clinical report. Arch Ophthalmol 1969;81:783.

58. Yamamoto S, Pavan-Langston D, Tada R, et al: Possible role of herpes simplex virus in the origin of Posner-Schlossman syndrome. Am J Ophthalmol 1995;119:796.

59. Alvarado JA, Underwood JL, Green R, et al: Detection of herpes simplex viral DNA in the iridocorneal endothelial syndrome. Arch Ophthalmol 1994;112:1601.

60. Wenkel H, Rummelt V, Fleckenstein B, et al: Detection of varicella zoster virus DNA and viral antigen in human eyes after herpes zoster ophthalmicus. Ophthalmology 1998;105:1323.

61. Zaal MJW, Maudgal PC, Rietveld PC, et al: Chronic ocular zoster. Curr Eye Res 1991;10(Suppl):125.

62. Naumann GOH, Gass J, Font R: Histopathology of herpes zoster ophthalmicus. Am J Ophthalmol 1968;65:533.

63. Johnson BL, Wisotzkey HM: Neuroretinitis associated with herpes simplex encephalitis in an adult. Am J Ophthalmol 1977;83:481.

64. Culbertson WW, Blumenkranz MS, Pepose JS, et al: Varicella zoster virus is a cause of the acute retinal necrosis syndrome. Ophthalmology 1986;93:559.

65. Rummelt V, Wenkel H, Rummelt C, et al: Detection of varicella zoster virus DNA and viral antigen in the late stage of bilateral acute retinal necrosis syndrome. Arch Ophthalmol 1992;110:1132.

66. Greven CM, Ford J, Stanton C, et al: Progressive outer retinal necrosis secondary to varicella zoster virus in acquired immune deficiency syndrome. Retina 1995;15:14.

67. Pepose JS, Kreiger AE, Tomiyasu U, et al: Immunocytologic localization of herpes simplex type 1 viral antigens in herpetic retinitis and encephalitis in an adult. Ophthalmology 1985;92:160.

68. Szily von A: Ein Beitrag zur Erforschung der sympathischen Ophthalmie und zur Pathogenese des hämatogenen Herpes corneae. Klin Monatsbl Augenheilkd 1924;75:593.

69. Vann VR, Atherton SS: Neural spread of herpes simplex virus after anterior chamber inoculation. Invest Ophthalmol Vis Sci 1991;32:2462.

70. Pettit TH, Kimura SJ, Uchida Y, et al: Herpes simplex uveitis: An experimental study with the fluorescein-labeled antibody technique. Invest Ophthalmol Vis Sci 1965;4:349.

71. Holland GN, Togni BI, Briones OC, et al: A microscopic study of herpes simplex virus retinopathy in mice. Invest Ophthalmol Vis Sci 1987;28:1181.

72. Whittum-Hudson JA, Pepose JS: Immunologic modulation of virus-induced pathology in a murine model of acute herpetic retinal necrosis. Invest Ophthalmol Vis Sci 1987;28:1541.

73. Whittum JA, McCulley JP, Niederkorn JY, Streilein W: Ocular disease induced in mice by anterior chamber inoculation of herpes simplex virus. Invest Ophthalmol Vis Sci 1984;25:1065.

74. Whittum-Hudson J, Farazdaghi M, Prendergast RA: A role for T lymphocytes in preventing experimental herpes simplex virus type 1–induced retinitis. Invest Ophthalmol Vis Sci 1985;26:1524.

75. Verjans GM, Feron EJ, Dings ME, et al: T cells specific for the triggering virus infiltrate the eye in patients with herpes simplex virus–mediated acute retinal necrosis. J Infect Dis 1998;178:27.

76. Marsh R, Easty D, Jones B: Iritis and iris atrophy in herpes zoster ophthalmicus. Am J Ophthalmol 1974;78:255.

77. Yamamoto S, Tada R, Shimomura Y, et al: Detecting varicella zoster virus DNA in iridocyclitis using polymerase chain reaction: A case of zoster sine herpete. Arch Ophthalmol 1995b;113:1358.

78. Schacher S, Garweg JG, Russ C, et al: Die Diagnostik der herpetischen Uveitis and Keratouveitis. Klin Monatsbl Augenheilkd 1998;212:359.

79. Freeman WR, Thomas EL, Rao N, et al: Demonstration of herpes group virus in acute retinal necrosis syndrome. Am J Ophthalmol 1986;102:701.

80. Soushi S, Ozawa H, Matsuhashi M, et al: Demonstration of varicella-zoster virus antigens in the vitreous aspirates of patients with acute retinal necrosis syndrome. Ophthalmology 1988;95:1394.

81. Sidikaro Y, Silver L, Holland GN, et al: Rhegmatogenous retinal detachments in patients with AIDS and necrotizing retinal infections. Ophthalmology 1991;98:129.

82. Helbig H, Bornfeld N, Bechrakis NE, et al: Varicella-zoster-Virus-Infektionen der Netzhaut bei Patienten mit und ohne Immunsuppression. Klin Monatsbl Augenheilkd 1994;205:103.

83. Nishi M, Hanashiro R, Mori S, et al: Polymerase chain reaction for the detection of the varicella-zoster genome in ocular samples from patients with acute retinal necrosis. Am J Ophthalmol 1992;114:603.

84. Yamamoto S, Pavan-Langston D, Kinoshita S, et al: Detecting herpesvirus DNA in uveitis using the polymerase chain reaction. Br J Ophthalmol 1996;80:469.

85. De Boer JH, Verhagen C, Bruinenberg M, et al: Serologic and polymerase chain reaction analysis of intraocular fluids in the diagnosis of infectious uveitis. Am J Ophthalmol 1996;121:650.

86. Goldmann H, Witmer R: Antikörper im Kammerwasser. Ophthalmologica 1954;127:323.

87. Pepose JS, Flowers B, Stewart JA: Herpesvirus antibody levels in the etiologic diagnosis of the acute retinal necrosis syndrome. Am J Ophthalmol 1992;113:248.

88. Sarkies N, Gregor Z, Forsey T, Darougar S: Antibodies to herpes simplex virus type 1 in intraocular fluids of patients with acute retinal necrosis. Br J Ophthalmol 1986;70:81.

89. Witmer R: Clinical implications of aqueous humor studies in uveitis. Am J Ophthalmol 1978;86:39.

89a. Wong KW, D'Amico DJ, Hedges TR, et al: Ocular involvement with chronic Epstein-Barr virus disease. Arch Ophthalmol 1987;105:788.

90. Aylward GW, Claoue MP, March RJ, et al: Influence of oral acyclovir on ocular complications of herpes zoster ophthalmicus. Eye 1994;8:70.

91. Herpetic Eye Disease Study Group: Acyclovir for the prevention of recurrent herpes simplex virus eye disease. N Engl J Med 1998;339:300.

92. Blumenkranz MS, Culbertson WW, Clarkson JG, et al: Treatment of the acute retinal necrosis syndrome with intravenous acyclovir. Ophthalmology 1986;93:296.

93. Paylay DA, Sternberg P, Davis J, et al: Decrease in the risk of bilateral acute retinal necrosis by acyclovir therapy. Am J Ophthalmol 1991;112:250.

94. Carney MD, Peyman GA, Goldberg MF, et al: Acute retinal necrosis. Retina 1986;6:85.

95. Peyman GA, Goldberg MF, Uninsky E, et al: Vitrectomy and intravitreal antiviral drug therapy in acute retinal necrosis syndrome. Report of two cases. Arch Ophthalmol 1984;102:618.

96. Meffert SA, Kertes PJ, Lim PL, et al: Successful treatment of progressive outer retinal necrosis using high-dose intravitreal ganciclovir. Retina 1997;17:560.

97. Dullert H, Maudgal PC, Leys A, et al: Bromovinyldeoxyuridine treatment of outer retinal necrosis due to varicella-zoster virus; a case-report. Bull Soc Belge Ophtalmol 1996;262:107.

98. Moorthy RS, Weinberg DV, Teich SA, et al: Management of varicella zoster virus retinitis in AIDS. Br J Ophthalmol 1997;81:189.

99. Sellitti TP, Huang AJW, Schiffman J, et al: Association of herpes zoster ophthalmicus with acquired immunodeficiency syndrome and acute retinal necrosis. Am J Ophthalmol 1993;116:297.

100. Johnston WH, Holland GN, Engstrom RE, et al: Recurrence of presumed varicella-zoster retinopathy in patients with acquired immunodeficiency syndrome. Am J Ophthalmol 1993;116:42.

101. Pavesio CE, Mitchell SM, Barton K, et al: Progressive outer retinal necrosis (PORN) in AIDS patients: A different appearance of varicella-zoster retinitis. Eye 1995;9:271.

102. Merchant A, Fletcher J, Medina CA, et al: Pharmacomanipulation of HSV-1 induced chorioretinitis in mice. Eye 1997;11:504.

103. Sergott RC, Belmont JB, Savino PJ, et al: Optic nerve involvement

in the acute retinal necrosis syndrome. Arch Ophthalmol 1985;103:1160.

104. Clarkson JG, Blumenkranz MS, Culbertson WW, et al: Retinal detachment following the acute retinal necrosis syndrome. Ophthalmology 1984;91:1665.

105. Anand, R, DH Fischer: Silicone oil in the management of retinal detachment with acute retinal necrosis. In: Freeman HM, Tolentino FI, eds: Proliferative vitreoretinopathy. New York, Springer, 1989, pp 99–115.

106. Weinberg DV, Lyon AT: Repair of retinal detachments due to herpes varicella-zoster virus retinitis in patients with acquired immune deficiency syndrome. Ophthalmology 1997;104:279.

107. Han DP, Lewis H, Williams GA, et al: Laser photocoagulation in the acute retinal necrosis syndrome. Arch Ophthalmol 1987;105:1051.

108. Sternberg P Jr, Han DP, Yeo JH, et al: Photocoagulation to prevent retinal detachment in acute retinal necrosis. Ophthalmology 1988;95:1389.

109. Saari KM, Böke W, Manthey KF, et al: Bilateral acute retinal necrosis. Am J Ophthalmol 1982;93:403.

110. Sternberg P, Knox DL, Finkelstein D, et al: Acute retinal necrosis syndrome. Retina 1982;2:145.

111. Willerson D, Aaberg TM, Reeser FH: Necrotizing vaso-occlusive retinitis. Am J Ophthalmol 1977;84:209.

112. Matsuo T, Nakayama T, Koyama T, et al: A proposed mild type of acute retinal necrosis syndrome. Am J Ophthalmol 1988;105:579.

113. Ezra E, Pearson RV, Etchells DE, Gregor ZJ: Delayed fellow eye involvement in acute retinal necrosis syndrome. Am J Ophthalmol 1995;120:115.

114. Martinez J, Lambert HM, Capone A, et al: Delayed bilateral involvement in the acute retinal necrosis syndrome. Am J Ophthalmol 1992;113:103.

115. Price FW, Schlaegel TF: Bilateral acute retinal necrosis. Am J Ophthalmol 1980;89:419.

116. Matsuo T, Morimoto K, Matsuo N: Factors associated with poor visual outcome in acute retinal necrosis. Br J Ophthalmol 1991;75:450.

117. Blumenkranz MS, Clarkson J, Culbertson WW, et al: Visual results and complications after retinal reattachment in the acute retinal necrosis syndrome. Retina 1989;9:170–174.

118. Schooley RT, Dolin R: Epstein-Barr virus (infectious mononucleosis). In: Mandell GL, Douglas RG, Bennett JE, eds: Principles and Practice of Infectious Diseases, Vol III. New York, Churchill Livingstone, 1990, p 1172.

119. Henle W, Henle G: Epstein-Barr virus and infectious mononucleosis. N Engl J Med 1973;288:263.

120. Pflugfelder SC, Roussel TJ, Culbertson WW: Primary Sjögren's syndrome after infectious mononucleosis. JAMA 1987;257:1049.

121. Gardner BP, Margolis TP, Mondino BJ: Conjunctival lymphocytic nodule associated with Epstein-Barr virus. Am J Ophthalmol 1991;112:567.

122. Morishima N, Miyakawa S, Akazawa Y, et al: A case of uveitis associated with chronic active Epstein-Barr virus infection. Ophthalmologica 1996;210:186.

123. Raymond LA, Wilson CA, Linnemann CC: Punctate outer retinitis in acute EBV infection. Am J Ophthalmol 1987;104:424.

124. Blaustein A, Caccavo A: Infectious mononucleosis complicated by bilateral papilloretinal edema. Arch Ophthalmol 1950;43:853.

125. Tiedeman JS: Epstein-Barr viral antibodies in multifocal choroiditis and panuveitis. Am J Ophthalmol 1987;104:659.

126. Spaide RF, Sugin S, Yanuzzi LA, et al: Epstein-Barr virus antibodies in multifocal choroiditis and panuveitis. Am J Ophthalmol 1991;112:410.

127. Palestine AG, Nussenblatt RB, Chan CC, et al: Histopathology of subretinal fibrosis and uveitis syndrome. Ophthalmology 1985;92:838.

128. Boynge TW, von Hagen KO: Severe optic neuritis in infectious mononucleosis: Report of a case. JAMA 1952;148:933.

129. Karpe G, Wising P: Retinal changes with acute reduction of vision as initial symptoms of infectious mononucleosis. Acta Ophthalmol 1948;26:19.

130. Yoser SL, Forster DJ, Rao NA: Systemic viral infections and their retinal and choroidal manifestations (major review). Surv Ophthalmol 1993;37:313.

131. Goodpasture EM, Talbot FB: Concerning the nature of protozoan-like cells in certain lesions of infancy. Am J Dis Child 1921;21:415.

132. Minders WH: Die Aetiologie der Cytomegalia infantum. Schweiz Med Wochenschr 1953;83:1180.

133. Weller TH, McCauley MC, Craig JM: Isolation of intranuclear producing agents from infants with illnesses resembling cytomegalovirus inclusion disease. Proc Cos Exp Biol Med 1957;94:4.

134. Kalfayan B: Inclusion disease in infancy. Arch Pathol 1947;44:467.

135. Smith ME: Retinal involvement in adult cytomegalic inclusion disease. Arch Ophthalmol 1966;72:44.

136. Freeman WR, Lerner CW, Mines JA, et al: A prospective study of the ophthalmologic findings in the acquired immune deficiency syndrome. Am J Ophthalmol 1984;97:133.

137. Guex-Crosier Y: Diagnosis and treatment of ocular viral infections in AIDS patients. Rev Med Suisse Romande 1998;118:941.

138. Palella FJ Jr, Delaney KM, Moorman AC, et al: Declining morbidity and mortality among patients with advanced human immunodeficiency virus infection. HIV Outpatient Study Investigators. N Engl J Med 1998;338:853.

139. Drew WL, Mintz L, Miner RC, et al: Prevalence of cytomegalovirus infection in homosexual men. J Infect Dis 1981;143:188.

140. Klemola E, Stenstrom R, Essen RV: Pneumonia as a clinical manifestation of cytomegalovirus infection in previously healthy adults. Scand J Infect Dis 1972;4:7.

141. Dobbins JG, Stewart JA, Demmler GJ: Surveillance of congenital cytomegalovirus disease, 1990–1991. Collaborating Registry Group. MMWR CDC Surveill Summ 1992;41:35.

142. Pass RF, Stagno S, Myers GJ, et al: Outcome of symptomatic congenital cytomegalovirus infection: Results of long-term longitudinal follow-up. Pediatrics 1980;66:758.

143. Rasmussen L, Zipeto D, Wolitz RA, et al: Risk for retinitis in patients with AIDS can be assessed by quantitation of threshold levels of cytomegalovirus DNA burden in blood. J Infect Dis 1997;176:1146.

144. Holland GN, Gottlieb MS, Yee RD, et al: Ocular disorders associated with a new severe acquired cellular immunodeficiency syndrome. Am J Ophthalmol 1982;93:393.

145. Jabs DA, Enger C, Bartlett JG: Cytomegalovirus retinitis and acquired immunodeficiency syndrome. Arch Ophthalmol 1989;107:75.

146. Moore RD, Chaisson RE: Cost-utility analysis of prophylactic treatment with oral ganciclovir for cytomegalovirus retinitis. J Acquir Immune Defic Syndr Hum Retrovirol 1997;16:15.

147. Hoover DR, Peng Y, Saah A, et al: Occurrence of cytomegalovirus retinitis after human immunodeficiency virus immunosuppression. Arch Ophthalmol 1996;114:821.

148. Sison RF, Holland GN, MacArthur LJ, et al: Cytomegalovirus retinopathy as the initial manifestation of the acquired immunodeficiency syndrome. Am J Ophthalmol 1991;112:243.

149. Kuppermann BD, Petty JG, Richman DD, et al: Correlation between CD4+ counts and prevalence of cytomegalovirus retinitis and human immunodeficiency virus–related noninfectious retinal vasculopathy in patients with acquired immunodeficiency syndrome. Am J Ophthalmol 1993;115:575.

150. Pertel P, Hirschtick R, Phair J, et al.: Risk of developing cytomegalovirus retinitis in persons infected with the human immunodeficiency virus. J Acquir Immune Defic Syndr 1992;5:1069.

151. Jabs DA, Green WR, Fox R, et al: Ocular manifestations of acquired immune deficiency syndrome. Ophthalmology 1989;96:1092.

152. Pepose JS, Holland GN, Nestor MS, et al: Acquired immune deficiency syndrome. Pathogenic mechanisms of ocular disease. Ophthalmology 1985;92:472.

153. Kestelyn P, Van de Perre P, Rouvroy D, et al: A prospective study of the ophthalmologic findings in the acquired immune deficiency syndrome in Africa. Am J Ophthalmol 1985;100:230.

154. Jacobson MA, Zegans M, Pavan PR, et al: Cytomegalovirus retinitis after initiation of highly active antiretroviral therapy. Lancet 1997;349:1443.

155. Spaide RF, Vitale AT, Toth IR, et al: Frosted branch angiitis associated with cytomegalovirus retinitis. Am J Ophthalmol 1992;113:522.

156. Holland GN, Shuler JD: Progression rates of cytomegalovirus retinopathy in ganciclovir-treated and untreated patients. Arch Ophthalmol 1992;110:1435.

157. Schwoerer J, Othenin-Girard P, Herbort CP: Acute retinal necrosis: A new pathophysiological hypothesis. Ophthalmologica 1991;203:172.

158. Akpek EK, Kent C, Jakobiec F, et al: Bilateral acute retinal necrosis caused by cytomegalovirus in an immunocompromised patient. Am J Ophthalmol 1999;127:93.

159. Britt WJ, Alford CA: Cytomegalovirus. In: Fields BN, Knipe DM, Howley PM, eds: Virology, 3rd ed. Philadelphia, Lippincott-Raven, 1996, pp 1146–1178.

160. Gallant JE, Moore RD, Richman DD, et al: Incidence and natural history of cytomegalovirus disease in patients with advanced human immunodeficiency virus disease treated with zidovudine. J Infect Dis 1992;166:1223.

161. Atherton SS, Newell CK, Kanter MY, et al: T cell depletion increases susceptibility to murine cytomegalovirus retinitis. Invest Ophthalmol Vis Sci 1992;33:3353.

162. Bale JF, O'Neil ME, Folberg R: Murine cytomegalovirus ocular infection in immunocompetent and cyclophosphamide-treated mice: Potentiation of ocular infection by cyclophosphamide. Invest Ophthalmol Vis Sci 1991;32:1749.

163. Skolnik PR, Pomerantz RJ, de la Monte SM, et al: Dual infection of retina with human immunodeficiency virus type 1 and cytomegalovirus. Am J Ophthalmol 1989;107:361.

164. D'Amico DJ: Diseases of the retina. N Engl J Med 1994;331:95.

165. Tufail A, Moe AA, Miller MJ, et al: Quantitative cytomegalovirus DNA level in the blood and its relationship to cytomegalovirus retinitis in patients with acquired immune deficiency syndrome. Ophthalmology 1999;106:133.

166. Davis JL, Feuer W, Culbertson WW, et al: Interpretation of intraocular and serum antibody levels in necrotizing retinitis. Retina 1995;15:233.

167. Knox CM, Chandler D, Short GA, et al: Polymerase chain reaction-based assays of vitreous samples for the diagnosis of viral retinitis. Use in diagnostic dilemmas. Ophthalmology 1998;105:37.

168. Holland GN, Tufail A, Jordan MC: Cytomegalovirus diseases. In: Pepose JC, Holland GN, Wilhelmus KR, eds: Ocular infection and immunity. St. Louis, Mosby, 1996, p 1088.

169. Pollard RB, Egbert PR, Gallagher JG, et al: Cytomegalovirus retinitis in immunosuppressed hosts. I. Natural history and effects of treatment with adenine arabinoside. Ann Intern Med 1980;93:655.

170. Collier AC, Coombs RW, Schoenfeld DA, et al: Treatment of human immunodeficiency virus infection with saquinavir, zidovudine, and zalcitabine. AIDS Clinical Trials Group. N Engl J Med 1996;334:1011.

171. Cameron DW, Heath-Chiozzi M, Danner S, et al: Randomised placebo-controlled trial of ritonavir in advanced HIV-1 disease. The Advanced HIV Disease Ritonavir Study Group. Lancet 1998;351:543.

172. Carpenter CC, Fischl MA, Hammer SM, et al: Antiretroviral therapy for HIV infection in 1998: Updated recommendations of the International AIDS Society-USA Panel. JAMA 1998;280:78.

173. Reed JB, Schwab IR, Gordon J, et al: Regression of cytomegalovirus retinitis associated with protease-inhibitor treatment in patients with AIDS. Am J Ophthalmol 1997;124:199.

174. Whitcup SM, Cunningham ET, Jr, Polis MA, et al: Spontaneous and sustained resolution of CMV retinitis in patients receiving highly active antiretroviral therapy. Br J Ophthalmol 1998;82:845.

175. Whitcup SM, Fortin E, Nussenblatt RB, et al: Therapeutic effect of combination antiretroviral therapy on cytomegalovirus retinitis. JAMA 1997;277:1519.

176. van den Horn GJ, Meenken C, Danner SA, et al: Effects of protease inhibitors on the course of CMV retinitis in relation to CD4+ lymphocyte responses in HIV+ patients. Br J Ophthalmol 1998;82:988.

177. Komanduri KV, Viswanathan MN, Wieder ED, et al: Restoration of cytomegalovirus-specific CD4+ T-lymphocyte responses after ganciclovir and highly active antiretroviral therapy in individuals infected with HIV-1. Nat Med 1998;4:953.

178. Jabs DA, Bolton SG, Dunn JP, et al: Discontinuing anticytomegalovirus therapy in patients with immune reconstitution after combination antiretroviral therapy. Am J Ophthalmol 1998;126:817.

179. Macdonald JC, Torriani FJ, Morse LS, et al: Lack of reactivation of cytomegalovirus (CMV) retinitis after stopping CMV maintenance therapy in AIDS patients with sustained elevations in CD4 T cells in response to highly active antiretroviral therapy. J Infect Dis 1998;177:1182.

180. Vrabec TR, Baldassano VF, Whitcup SM: Discontinuation of maintenance therapy in patients with quiescent cytomegalovirus retinitis and elevated CD4+ counts. Ophthalmology 1998;105:1259.

181. Frame RD, Hutchins RK, Shakan KJ, et al: Progression of cytomegaloviral retinitis in a patient responding to highly active antiretroviral therapy. Invest Ophthalmol Vis Sci 1999;40:873.

182. Whitley RJ, Jacobson MA, Friedberg DN, et al: Guidelines for the treatment of cytomegalovirus diseases in patients with AIDS in the era of potent antiretroviral therapy: Recommendations of an international panel. International AIDS Society-USA. Arch Intern Med 1998;158:957.

183. Verbraak FD, van den Horn GJ, van der Meer JT, et al: Risk of developing CMV retinitis following non-ocular CMV end organ disease in AIDS patients. Br J Ophthalmol 1998;82:748.

184. Felsenstein D, D'Amico DJ, Hirsch MS, et al: Treatment of cytomegalovirus retinitis with 9-[2-hydroxy-1-(hydroxymethyl)ethoxymethyl]guanine. Ann Intern Med 1985;103:377.

185. Hardy WD: Combined ganciclovir and recombinant human granulocyte-macrophage colony-stimulating factor in the treatment of cytomegalovirus retinitis in AIDS patients. J Acquir Immune Defic Syndr 1991;4(Suppl):22.

186. Drew WL, Ives D, Lalezari JP, et al: Oral ganciclovir as maintenance treatment for cytomegalovirus retinitis in patients with AIDS. Syntex Cooperative Oral Ganciclovir Study Group. N Engl J Med 1995;333:615.

187. Studies of Ocular Complications of AIDS Research Group in Collaboration with the AIDS Clinical Trials Group: Foscarnet-Ganciclovir Cytomegalovirus Retinitis Trial. 4. Visual outcomes. Ophthalmology 1994;101:1250.

188. Studies of Ocular Complications of AIDS Research Group in Collaboration with the AIDS Clinical Trials Group: Mortality in patients with the acquired immunodeficiency syndrome treated with either foscarnet or ganciclovir for cytomegalovirus retinitis. N Engl J Med 1992;326:213.

189. Studies of Ocular Complications of AIDS Research Group in Collaboration with the AIDS Clinical Trials Group: Combination Foscarnet and ganciclovir therapy vs. monotherapy for the treatment of relapsed cytomegalovirus retinitis in patients with AIDS. The Cytomegalovirus Retreatment Trial. Arch Ophthalmol 1996;114:23.

190. Skoutelis AT, Murphy RL, MacDonell KB, et al: Indwelling central venous catheter infections in patients with acquired immune deficiency syndrome. J Acquir Immune Defic Syndr 1990;3:335.

191. Davis JL, Taskintuna I, Freeman WR, et al: Iritis and hypotony after treatment with intravenous cidofovir for cytomegalovirus retinitis. Arch Ophthalmol 1997;115:733.

192. Lalezari JP, Stagg RJ, Kuppermann BD, et al: Intravenous cidofovir for peripheral cytomegalovirus retinitis in patients with AIDS. A randomized, controlled trial. Ann Intern Med 1997;126:257.

193. Studies of Ocular Complications of AIDS Research Group in Collaboration with the AIDS Clinical Trials Group: Parenteral cidofovir for cytomegalovirus retinitis in patients with AIDS: The HPMPC peripheral cytomegalovirus retinitis trial. A randomized, controlled trial. Ann Intern Med 1997;126:264.

194. Jacobson MA, Wilson S, Stanley H, et al: Phase I study of combination therapy with intravenous cidofovir and oral ganciclovir for cytomegalovirus retinitis in patients with AIDS. Clin Infect Dis 1999;28:528.

195. Martin DF, Kuppermann BD, Wolitz RA, et al: Oral ganciclovir for patients with cytomegalovirus retinitis treated with a ganciclovir implant. Roche Ganciclovir Study Group. N Engl J Med 1999;340:1063.

196. Cochereau-Massin I, Lehoang P, Lautier-Frau M, et al: Efficacy and tolerance of intravitreal ganciclovir in cytomegalovirus retinitis in acquired immune deficiency syndrome. Ophthalmology 1991;98:1348.

197. Diaz-Llopis M, Espana E, Munoz G, et al: High dose intravitreal foscarnet in the treatment of cytomegalovirus retinitis in AIDS. Br J Ophthalmol 1994;78:120.

198. Taskintuna I, Rahhal FM, Rao NA, et al: Adverse events and autopsy findings after intravitreous cidofovir (HPMPC) therapy in patients with acquired immune deficiency syndrome (AIDS). Ophthalmology 1997;104:1827.

199. Musch DC, Martin DF, Gordon JF, et al: Treatment of cytomegalovirus retinitis with a sustained-release ganciclovir implant. The Ganciclovir Implant Study Group. N Engl J Med 1997;337:83.

200. Davis JL, Tabandeh H, Feuer WJ, et al: Effect of potent antiretroviral therapy on recurrent cytomegalovirus retinitis treated with the ganciclovir implant. Am J Ophthalmol 1999;127:283.

201. Martin DF, Dunn JP, Davis JL et al: Use of the ganciclovir implant for the treatment of cytomegalovirus retinitis in the era of potent antiretroviral therapy: Recommendations of the International AIDS Society-USA panel [see comments]. Am J Ophthalmol 1999;127:329.

202. Perry CM, Balfour JA: Fomivirsen. Drugs 1999;57:375.

203. Piascik P: Fomiversen sodium approved to treat CMV retinitis. J Am Pharm Assoc 1999;39:84.

204. Freeman WR, Friedberg DN, Berry C, et al: Risk factors for development of rhegmatogenous retinal detachment in patients with cytomegalovirus retinitis. Am J Ophthalmol 1993;116:713.

205. Davis JL, Hummer J, Feuer WJ: Laser photocoagulation for retinal detachments and retinal tears in cytomegalovirus retinitis. Ophthalmology 1997;104:2053.

206. Azen SP, Scott IU, Flynn HW, Jr, et al: Silicone oil in the repair of complex retinal detachments. A prospective observational multicenter study. Ophthalmology 1998;105:1587.

207. Nasemann JE, Mutsch A, Wiltfang R, et al: Early pars plana vitrectomy without buckling procedure in cytomegalovirus retinitis–induced retinal detachment. Retina 1995;15:111.

208. Carr A, Cooper DA: Restoration of immunity to chronic hepatitis B infection in HIV-infected patient on protease inhibitor. Lancet 1997;349:995.

209. Karavellas MP, Plummer DJ, Macdonald JC, et al: Incidence of immune recovery vitritis in cytomegalovirus retinitis patients following institution of successful highly active antiretroviral therapy. J Infect Dis 1999;179:697.

210. Welzl-Hinterkorner E, Tholen H, Sturmer J, et al: Bilateral cystoid macular edema following successful treatment of AIDS-associated CMV retinitis. Ophthalmologe 1999;96:87.

211. Canzano JC, Reed JB, Morse LS: Vitreomacular traction syndrome following highly active antiretroviral therapy in AIDS patients with cytomegalovirus retinitis. Retina 1998;18:443.

212. Mocroft A, Vella S, Benfield TL, et al: Changing patterns of mortality across Europe in patients infected with HIV-1. EuroSIDA Study Group. Lancet 1998;352:1725.

213. Jabs DA: Ocular manifestations of HIV infection. Trans Am Ophthalmol Soc 1995;93:623.

214. Davis JL, Serfass MS, Lai MY, et al: Silicone oil in repair of retinal detachments caused by necrotizing retinitis in HIV infection. Arch Ophthalmol 1995;113:1401.

Aaron L. Sobol and Ramzi K. Hemady

DEFINITION

Rift Valley fever (RVF) is an epizootic acute febrile illness primarily affecting domesticated cattle. It is caused by an arthropod-borne plebovirus in the family Bunyaviridae. The virus can also infect humans, causing a spectrum of disease ranging from a mild constitutional illness to fatal complications including hemorrhagic fever and meningoencephalitis.[1] Reports of ocular manifestations in human outbreaks are well recognized as a significant cause of morbidity.

HISTORY

The virus was first described in 1931 following an outbreak in cattle and humans in the Rift Valley in East Africa.[2] Since then, there have been sporadic outbreaks in at least 25 African countries, usually associated with periods of heavy rainfall, most recently in Kenya in 1998.[3] Until fairly recently, these outbreaks were thought to cause mortality in cattle and only a flulike illness in humans. During a South African outbreak in 1950 there were an estimated 20,000 human infections but few deaths despite 100,000 sheep and cattle fatalities during the same period. However, the epidemic in South Africa in 1974 to 1975 produced at least 70 human deaths, and the epidemic in Egypt in 1977 to 1978 produced 598 fatalities, highlighting the potentially fatal nature of this infection in humans.[4]

Freed[5] and Schrire[6] first characterized ophthalmic complications from RVF virus in 1951. Since then, many reports have been published describing a macular or paramacular syndrome of edema with exudative-type lesions and hemorrhage.

EPIDEMIOLOGY

The Great Rift Valley is a geological depression extending more than 4830 km from Syria in southwestern Asia along the eastern African coast to Mozambique in southeastern Africa. Although the disease was first noted in this region of East Africa, outbreaks have been seen throughout the continent. RVF has not been reported in cattle outside of Africa and was localized to sub-Saharan Africa until the 1977 outbreak in Egypt. There is a report of an international traveler in Canada diagnosed with RVF in 1979.[7]

PATHOGENESIS

The virus is transmitted by numerous species of mosquitoes, with the genera Culex and Aedes playing dominant roles in the viral cycle (Fig. 25–1). Culex spread the virus to humans and animals through blood meals. The cattle serve as a repository for amplification of the virus as uninfected mosquitoes that bite viremic vertebrates may become infected. The Aedes has been implicated in maintaining the epizootic outbreaks by depositing virus-laden eggs in soil that hatch when ground pools form during heavy rains.[8, 9]

In past outbreaks, the majority of the human infections were in farmers, farm laborers, and veterinary surgeons that handled the carcasses of infected cattle. A Senegali study showed that individuals in endemic areas who worked with livestock had a five- to six-fold risk of having positive RVF viral IgG over individuals who did not handle livestock.[8] A Kenyan task force found that contact with livestock was significantly associated with serologic evidence of acute infection with RVF virus.[3]

It appears that RVF is primarily spread to animals by mosquitoes; the method of transmission to humans is less clear. Besides arthropod vectors, there are indications that inhalation can be a route of transmission. Infection in humans exposed to aerosol contamination during animal slaughter or to infection by contact during meat preparation is well recognized. The virus has been experimentally transmitted through contaminated blood, and several laboratory workers have contracted the disease. The meat of affected animals is not infectious, and neither person-to-person nor nosocomial transmission have been documented.[1, 10]

CLINICAL CHARACTERISTICS

Typical signs in animals include fever, weakness, anorexia, and evidence of abdominal pain. Lambs and calves are more susceptible to the fatal form of RVF than adults. Abortion may reach 100% and accounts for one of the major economic impacts of the outbreaks.

The incubation periods in humans is generally from 3 to 7 days, followed by one of four clinical syndromes, the most common of which is an uncomplicated febrile illness with constitutional symptoms. This is characterized by abrupt onset of fever with a biphasic temperature curve, mimicking dengue fever. The main symptoms are headache, arthralgias, "back-breaking" myalgias, and gastrointestinal disturbances. The fever subsides in 12 to 36 hours, and the other symptoms are relieved within 4 days. Several authors have noted that conjunctivitis and photophobia are common early symptoms, although anterior uveitis is relatively uncommon.[11]

Ocular, hematologic, and neurologic involvement characterize the other three clinical syndromes, respectively. The ocular syndrome has been reported to be present in 1% to 20% of RVF infections, and the hematologic and neurologic forms have been reported in 0.2% to 2% of RVF infections.[1, 3, 4, 8, 12]

Ocular involvement typically follows a brief febrile illness. Decreased visual acuity usually begins from 2 to 7 days after onset of fever.[13] Siam described the largest series of serologically proven RVF with ocular manifestations during the 1977 epidemic in Egypt.[11] The most common findings were bilateral macular and paramacular exudative-like lesions with retinal edema and hemorrhage. Some cases were associated with anterior inflammation or vitritis. Other findings included retinal vasculitis, ranging from sheathing of the arterioles in the area of the exudative lesions to a diffuse vasculitis.

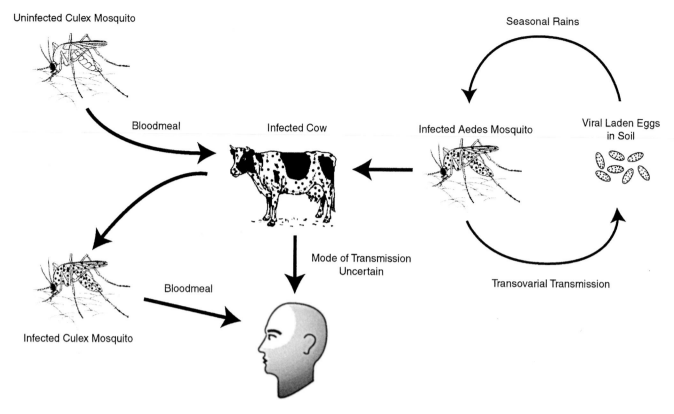

Uninfected Culex Mosquito

Seasonal Rains

Bloodmeal

Infected Cow

Infected Aedes Mosquito

Viral Laden Eggs
in Soil

Mode of Transmission
Uncertain

Bloodmeal

Transovarial Transmission

Infected Culex Mosquito

FIGURE 25–1. Rift Valley fever virus life cycle.

The visual deficit appears to be related to the size and degree of vascular involvement, ranging from slight impairment to light perception. Although small case studies suggested that permanent visual deficit was unusual, larger studies have noted a 40% to 50% persistence of deficits despite resolution of retinal edema.[4, 12]

Fluorescein angiography typically showed delayed filling of both the retinal and choroidal circulation, although one small case series suggested sparing of the choroidal circulation.[5] There is obscured choroidal fluorescence in the area corresponding to the lesion and delayed peripapillary choroidal filling in the arteriovenous phase. Macular and paramacular leakage may be seen. Angiography following convalescence may show residual delay in peripapillary filling and loss of macular vessels.[14]

Deutman and Klomp described a patient with severe macular lesions and serologic evidence suggestive of RVF, as well as bilateral optic nerve pallor.[15] The electroretinogram was almost unrecordable in one eye and somewhat better in the other. The visual-evoked potentials (VEP) were not recordable in one and only minimally recordable in the other. The electro-oculogram (EOG) was flat in both eyes and did not show any change in light adaptation.

The hematologic complications consist of a generalized hemorrhagic state, including epistaxis, hematemesis, and melena. These complications usually occur within 2 to 4 days of an acute febrile illness. Liver function tests in affected patients have shown elevated serum transaminases, hyperbilirubinemia, and a prolonged prothrombin time. Shock and hepatic insufficiency contribute to the high mortality rate.[13]

Meningoencephalitis is well recognized and typically presents 5 to 10 days following a febrile illness. Presentation includes changes in mental status, meningismus, and vertigo. Evaluation of cerebrospinal fluid shows pleocytosis with lymphocyte predominance and normal glucose and protein concentrations.[4, 13]

PATHOLOGY

The RVF virus is a hepatotropic virus, and the most characteristic microscopic lesion is a diffuse focal hepatic necrosis. Eosinophilic granules may occur in the hepatocytes. Autopsies have shown diffuse petechial and ecchymotic hemorrhages in all organ systems.[4] There are no published reports describing ocular pathology.

DIAGNOSIS

Diagnosis should be considered in the presence of animal outbreaks of RVF. Selective involvement of lambs and calves, high abortion rates, and characteristic liver lesions provide presumptive evidence but virus isolation is necessary to confirm the diagnosis. In Kenya in 1998, diagnostic confirmation was made by detection of IgM antibodies, virus isolation, reverse-transcriptase polymerase chain reaction for viral nucleic acid, or immunohistochemistry.[3]

A fourfold or greater rise in hemagglutination-inhibition or complement fixation antibody titers to RVF virus was seen in six of eight patients with uncomplicated RVF and in five of five patients with meningoencephalitis.[13]

DIFFERENTIAL DIAGNOSIS

The differential diagnosis for RVF retinitis includes other viral entities such as measles, rubella, and influenza. These diseases can be differentiated from RVF by clinical history and serologic testing. Rickettsial infections have been reported to cause retinitis; a history of tick bites and antibody titers can aid in the diagnosis. Lyme disease can mimic RVF and can be ruled out with antibody titers.[6]

Other hemorrhagic fever viruses have been reported to have ocular involvement. The hemorrhagic fever with renal syndrome is associated with two major causative viruses, the Hantaan virus and the Puumala virus. Hantaan disease has been associated with anterior uveitis during the acute febrile phase.[16] Marburg and Ebola viruses, of the family Filoviridae, have been implicated in multiple epidemics of hemorrhagic fever in sub-Saharan Africa and in a primate import quarantine facility in Reston, Virginia.[16] About one half of the patients had conjunctivitis in the early febrile stage and late sequelae have included anterior uveitis. Marburg virus has been isolated from the anterior chamber nearly 3 months following disease onset.[16] Hemorrhagic fever in the United States is noted in the Hantavirus pulmonary syndrome, which has not been reported to have ocular complications.[16]

TREATMENT

No specific effective treatment has been demonstrated for the hemorrhagic or encephalitic complications of RVF. Ribavirin, an antiviral agent, and polyriboinosinic-polyribocytidylic acid, an interferon inducer, have shown encouraging results in experimental studies in animals, as has passive antibody transfusion.[17] No treatment has yet been evaluated in a clinical setting, however. Epidemic disease is best prevented with vaccination of livestock. Live-attenuated and inactivated vaccines are available in Africa for veterinary use. A single dose of the live-attenuated RVF MP-12 vaccine is immunogenic, nonabortogenic, and protective of the animal and fetus against experimental challenge with virulent virus. The duration of the protective response is unknown, and the vaccine is being tested for use in humans. An inactivated vaccine produced for the U.S. Army is available and recommended for exposed laboratory workers and veterinarians working in sub-Saharan Africa.[18] There are no reported treatments for the ocular complications.

CONCLUSIONS

Ocular complications occur in approximately 20% of cases of RVF, a viral epidemic illness predominantly distributed in sub-Saharan Africa. The typical presentation includes unilateral or bilateral macular and paramacular exudates with edema, retinal hemorrhages, and vascular sheathing and occlusion. Anterior uveitis has been noted, and conjunctivitis and photophobia may be common presenting symptoms. Diagnosis is based on serologic testing. No specific effective treatment exists.

References

1. House JA, Turell MJ, Mebus CA: Rift Valley fever: Present status and risk to the western hemisphere. Ann N Y Acad Sci 1992;653:233–242.
2. Daubney R, Hudson JR, Garnham PC: Enzootic hepatitis or Rift Valley fever: An undescribed virus of sheep, cattle, and man from East Africa. J Pathol 1931;34:545–549.
3. Centers for Disease Control: Rift Valley fever—East Africa, 1997–1998. MMWR 1998;47:261–264.
4. McIntosh BM, Russell D, Dos Santos I, Gear JHS: Rift Valley fever in humans in South Africa. South African Medical Journal 1980;58:803–806.
5. Freed I, Rift Valley fever in man, complicated by retinal changes and loss of vision. S Afr Med J 1951;25:930–932.
6. Schrire L: Macular changes in Rift Valley fever. S Afr Med J 1951;25:926–929.
7. Centers for Disease Control and Prevention: Rift Valley fever with retinopathy—Canada. MMWR 1980;28:607–608.
8. Wilson ML, Chapman LE, Hall DB, et al: Rift Valley fever in rural northern Senegal: Human risk factors and potential vectors. Am J Trop Med Hyg 1994;50:663–675.
9. Wilson ML: Rift Valley fever virus ecology and the epidemiology of disease emergence. Ann N Y Acad Sci 1994;740:169–180.
10. Ghoneim NH, Woods GT, Rift Valley fever in its epidemiology in Egypt: A review. J Med 1983;14:55–75.
11. Siam AL, Meegan JM, Gharbawi KF: Rift Valley fever ocular manifestations: Observations during the 1977 epidemic in Egypt. Br J Ophthalmol 1980;64:366–374.
12. Arthur RR, El-Sharkawy MS, Cope SE, et al: Recurrence of Rift Valley fever in Egypt. Lancet 1993;342:1149–1150.
13. Laughlin LW, Meegan JM, Straubgaugh LJ, et al: Epidemic Rift Valley fever in Egypt: Observations of the spectrum of human illness. Trans R Soc Trop Med Hyg 1979;73:630–633.
14. Yoser SL, Forster, DJ, Rao, NA: Systemic viral infections and their retinal and choroidal manifestations. Surv Ophthalmol 1993;37:313–352.
15. Deutman AF, Klomp HJ: Rift Valley Fever retinitis. Am J Ophthal 1981;92:38–42.
16. Peters CJ: Harrison's Principles of Internal Medicine, 14th ed. New York, McGraw Hill, 1998, pp 1142–1147.
17. Peters CJ, Reynolds JA, Slone TW, et al: Prophylaxis of Rift Valley fever with antiviral drugs, immune serum, an interferon inducer, and a macrophage activator. Antiviral Res 1986;6:285–297.
18. Morrill, JC, Mebus, CA, Peters, CJ: Safety and efficacy of a mutagen-attenuated Rift Valley fever virus vaccine in cattle. Am J Vet Res 1997;58:1104–1109.

26 MEASLES

Erik Letko and C. Stephen Foster

DEFINITION

Measles (rubeola) is an acute, highly contagious viral disease. The definition of "probable measles" proposed by the Centers for Disease Control and Prevention includes the following clinical signs and symptoms: (1) a generalized rash lasting 3 or more days, (2) a temperature greater than 101°F, and (3) cough, coryza, or conjunctivitis.[1]

HISTORY

From antiquity until the beginning of the 17th century, measles and smallpox were frequently confused. The first written record of measles comes from the 10th century by the Persian physician Rhazes.[2] But even Rhazes referred to the description of the disease by a famous Hebrew physician, El Yahudi, who lived 300 years earlier. Repeated epidemics of measles in Europe were reported in the 17th century.[3] The first report on measles in America described an epidemic in Boston in 1657.[4] From that time onward, the reduction of epidemic intervals in Europe was noted as a consequence of rapid immigration to North America.

The first epidemiologic data were reported in 1846 by Panum,[5] who noticed that the incubation period for the disease was 14 days, that lifelong immunity followed recovery from the infection, and that spread was through human-to-human contagion via the respiratory route. It is evident that Shakespeare was aware of the latter in *Coriolanus*.[2] The first attempt to immunize against measles was performed by Home in 1758.[6] The pathognomonic exanthem for measles was precisely described by Koplik at the end of the 19th century.[7–9] In 1954, measles agents were isolated in human and simian renal cell cultures,[10] and in 1963, the first inactivated and attenuated measles vaccines became available.[11] A nationwide immunization program was begun in the United States in 1965.

CONGENITAL MEASLES

Epidemiology

During the pre-vaccine era, most persons contracted measles before reaching adulthood. Therefore, only four to six pregnancies per 100,000 were complicated by measles during this time period.[12] In the postvaccine era, the proportion of measles in pregnancy is larger.[13] Because of the low incidence of measles infection in adults, congenital measles is rare compared with acquired infection. Nevertheless, maternal measles can result in fetal death or congenital anomalies.[14, 15] The majority of women who contract measles during pregnancy do not have a history of vaccination against the virus.[14]

Clinical Characteristics

Infection during the third trimester of pregnancy causes spontaneous abortion in about 20% of women and may also result in premature birth. Newborns with congenital measles infection may present with the following anomalies: cardiopathy, pyloric stenosis, genu valgum, deafness, mongolism, vertebral anomalies, cleft lip, cleft palate, or rudimentary ear. Ocular manifestations of congenital measles include dacryostenosis, cataract, and pigmentary retinopathy. Ophthalmoscopy reveals optic nerve head drusen and bilateral diffuse scattered pigmentary retinopathy with involvement of both the posterior pole and the retinal periphery.[16] The retinopathy may be associated with retinal edema, macular star formation, and arteriolar attenuation.[17]

Pathophysiology, Immunology, Pathology, and Pathogenesis

Congenital and acquired measles infection is caused by a single-stranded RNA virus belonging to the genus *Morbillivirus* in the Paramyxoviridae family. The virion is circular or oval in shape and enveloped, and has a diameter of 120 to 250 nm.[18, 19] Humans and monkeys are the only natural hosts of the measles virus. Congenital measles infection is transmitted through the placenta and may result in fetal demise or serious congenital anomalies.

Diagnosis

Diagnosis of congenital measles infection is made by history of maternal measles and the presence of congenital anomalies. The electroretinogram does not show any abnormalities; however, an enlarged blind spot in visual field may appear as a consequence of drusen of the optic disc.[16]

Treatment

Congenital measles is a self-limiting disease, and no specific treatment is available.

Prognosis

The prognosis for patients with congenital measles depends on the extent and nature of congenital anomalies. Interestingly, the visual acuities in reported patients with congenital rubeola retinopathy have been normal.[16, 17]

ACQUIRED MEASLES

Epidemiology

Before the introduction of the measles vaccine, 95% of Americans were infected with measles by the age of 15 years.[20, 21] As a consequence of nationwide vaccination, there has been a marked decrease in the incidence of the disease, with a shift in the age of presentation from children to adolescents and young adults.[21–23] Despite the availability of measles vaccine in the United States, however, there are still large numbers of Americans who are susceptible to the disease. Complete eradication of the disease has not been achieved owing to several factors, including primary vaccine failure reported in 5% to 8%, lack of vaccination (i.e., parental apathy, contraindications based on existing medical conditions, or religious convictions), and importation of measles from other countries.[18, 24]

Clinical Characteristics

The mucosal involvement consists of a catarrhal reaction of the conjunctiva and respiratory mucosa, as well as petechial lesions of the palate and pharynx. One to two days before the onset of the rash, Koplik's spots appear. These are small, bluish-white dots surrounded by a red areola, typically localized on the buccal mucosa opposite the lower molars, but their presence on the conjunctiva, caruncle, vagina, rectum, and intestinal mucosa has been observed as well.[25] The Koplik spots disappear by the second day following the skin eruption. The characteristic skin eruption starts as pink macules (discrete, irregular, and erythematous) behind the ear, on the forehead, and on the neck. They rapidly become maculopapular in nature and spread downward during the next 3 days to involve the face, trunk, arms, and legs.[18, 19, 26, 27]

Conjunctivitis, together with cough and coryza, are considered the classic triad in measles. However, conjunctivitis need not be clinically present in all affected patients.[28] It is usually mild, catarrhal, papillary, and nonpurulent. Pseudomembranes may occur,[29] and in debilitated patients, severe, true conjunctival membranes may develop.[26] An associated epithelial keratitis, presenting in 76% of patients,[30] is the most common ocular manifestation in acquired measles infection.[28–31] It is usually mild and bilateral. Keratitis begins at the limbus, progresses centrally to the cornea, and usually does not affect the Bowman layer. The keratitis develops in the prodromal phase or at the time of the onset of the rash and resolves several days afterward. However, in some patients, it may persist as long as 4 months.[28, 29, 31] Corneal sensation is unaffected, and the corneal lesions resolve without scarring.[32]

Other, less common ocular findings include Koplik's spots, which may occur on the caruncle and on the conjunctiva, where they are also called Hirschberg's spots.[19, 26] Stimon's line is a sharply demarcated transverse linear injection of the lower lid margin present at the onset of conjunctivitis.[19] Blepharitis and gangrene of the eyelids are rare.[26]

Rubeola retinopathy may occur either in presence or in absence of encephalitis, complicating acquired measles infection.[33] Patients may present with a sudden decreased vision bilaterally 6 to 12 days after the appearance of measles exanthem.[26, 33] Acquired measles retinitis has been described and is characterized by clear media, blurry disc margins, diffuse retinal edema, attenuated arterioles, scattered retinal hemorrhages, and a star-shaped macular edema.

The following retinal findings were observed after the resolution of acute measles retinopathy: pale optic disc, parapapillary vascular sheathing, mild attenuation of arterioles, and secondary pigmentary retinopathy with a "bone corpuscle" or "salt-and-pepper" pattern.[33] A retinopathy described as pigmented paravenous retinochoroidal atrophy with abnormal visual field and electroretinogram might develop several years after acute measles infection as a consequence of measles retinopathy.[34]

Pathophysiology, Immunology, Pathology, and Pathogenesis

The measles virus is highly contagious. Transmission of the virus in acquired disease occurs by the transfer of nasopharyngeal secretions directly or in airborne droplets from an infected individual to the mucous membranes of the upper respiratory tract or conjunctiva of a susceptible individual.[18, 19] Infected individuals may transmit the virus from 5 days after exposure to 5 days following the skin rash, which may appear 14 days after initial exposure. The prodromal period, 9 to 10 days after exposure, is the most contagious.[18, 19]

The first contact with the highly infective virus is at the mucous membrane of the respiratory tract. The conjunctiva also might act as a portal of entry for the measles infection.[30] If it is not inactivated by mucus or specific secretory immunoglobulin A antibodies, the virus enters the ciliated columnar epithelium.[35] During the primary viremia, 2 to 6 days after the infection, the virus is transported intracellularly within the formed elements of the blood. An extensive proliferation of virus follows in the reticuloendothelial system in the tonsils, spleen, liver, bone marrow, and other lymphoid tissues. The second viremia starts 10 days after the infection, with proliferation of the virus inside the leukocytes. Neutralizing antibodies appear 14 days after infection, at the time of the appearance of the rash. The rash is an expression of immunologic defense, and in patients with severely impaired cell-mediated immunity, a measles infection may run its course without the presence of rash.[36, 37] A more severe clinical course with higher incidence of complications such as pneumonitis and encephalitis has been observed in immunocompromised patients.[38]

A single episode of infection with measles virus and successful vaccination with live attenuated measles vaccine confers lifelong immunity. The use of live attenuated measles vaccine induces active immunity in about 95% of susceptible individuals and should be provided for all individuals older than 12 months of age, because younger infants might still have circulating maternal neutralizing antibodies to measles.[18, 19, 39, 40]

Histopathologically, Koplik's spots represent necrosis of the epithelium, and the skin rash shows multinucleated giant cells, parakeratosis, and dyskeratosis.[25]

Multinucleated giant cells with eosinophilic cytoplasmic inclusion bodies appear not only in the epithelium but also in lymphoid tissues. Inclusion bodies may become visible 16 to 20 hours after infection in the cytoplasm and 96 to 120 hours after infection inside the nucleus.[36] In electron microscopic studies, inclusion bodies are visible as granular masses, with the characteristic measurements of the RNA helix.

Diagnosis

Diagnosis of measles is made by observation of the sequence of clinical symptoms. The measles virus can be recovered from the nasopharynx, conjunctiva, lymphoid tissues, respiratory mucous membranes, urine, and blood for a few days before skin eruption and 1 or 2 days afterward.[18, 19] Virus isolation in cell cultures has been achieved in monkey and dog kidney tissue, and chick embryo chorioallantoic membranes. Serum immuno-globulin M antibodies can be detected within 1 or 2 days after the onset of the skin rash.[18, 19] Peak titers of serum antibodies occur in 2 to 4 weeks. The complement-fixing antibodies may diminish gradually over a period of years. Virus-neutralizing and hemagglutination-inhibiting (HI) antibodies show an initial decrease in concentration for 2 to 6 months after the attainment of maximum titers but persist indefinitely thereafter.[18, 19]

During the prodromal phase and early eruptive phase of measles, multinucleated giant cells with eosinophilic inclusions in both the nuclei and cytoplasm can be identi-fied in sputum, nasal secretions, and urine.[18, 19]

The diagnosis of measles retinopathy is made by the history of recent measles infection and ophthalmoscopic findings. Fluorescein angiography of the fundus in pa-tients with measles retinopathy reveals a generalized in-creased transmission of background choroidal fluores-cence due to widespread pigment epithelial disturbance with characteristic salt and pepper pattern. Visual field was reported to be constricted and the ERG may reveal either normal or low activity.[33]

Retinal findings similar to macular star formation and pigmentary changes of the retina may be observed in patients with other viral infections such as mumps or influenza A. Measles retinitis may be distinguished from Leber's stellate idiopathic neuroretinitis and central se-rous chorioretinopathy by the absence of systemic symp-toms.

Treatment

Uncomplicated measles infection is usually a self-limiting disease, and supportive treatment is usually sufficient. However, in high-risk patients such as pregnant women, children younger than 1 year of age, and immunosup-pressed patients, the course of measles infection can be altered by treatment with gamma-globulin 0.25 ml/kg of body weight if therapy is begun 6 days after exposure.[18, 19, 39] In patients with vitamin A deficiency, oral administra-tion of vitamin A results in decreased mortality rate.[41]

Treatment of the ocular manifestations is symptomatic, with the use of topical antiviral or antibiotics to prevent secondary infections in patients with keratitis or conjunc-tivitis. A combination of systemic corticosteroids and anti-biotics has been successfully used in treatment of measles retinopathy in one case.[33]

Complications

Systemic complications of measles infection include en-cephalitis, acute glomerulonephritis, disseminated intra-vascular coagulation, otitis media, laryngotracheitis, pneumonia, appendicitis, and myocarditis.[42]

Keratitis in patients with secondary bacterial infections or in debilitated patients can become ulcerative with consequent corneal neovascularization, or it may become purulent, with progression to corneal perforation, pan-ophthalmitis, and phthisis bulbi.[26, 27] These severe corneal ulcer complications are most frequent in developing countries as a consequence of malnutrition, vitamin A deficiency, protein deficiencies, and racial, geographic, and cellular immunity factors.[43, 44]

Other uncommon ocular findings may be associated with the central nervous system complications of rubeola such as optic atrophy, optic neuritis, papilledema, central retinal vein occlusion, neuroretinitis, chorioretinitis, ex-traocular muscle palsies, nystagmus, abnormal eye move-ments, and cortical blindness.[19]

Prognosis

In developing countries approximately 1% of children with measles develop permanent ocular damage.[45] Ac-cording to one study, 43.7% of students in blind school institutions in a developing country were blind as a conse-quence of measles infection.[46] The term postmeasles blindness (PMB) is restricted to the corneal complica-tions of the disease.[30] Concomitant HSV infection, folk remedies, confluence of keratitis, and vitamin A defi-ciency are associated with poor visual prognosis.[47]

In cases of measles retinitis the long-term prognosis is good. After an initial period of decreased visual acuity, the vision improves in subsequent weeks to months. How-ever, the visual fields remain constricted and the ERG may not regain full activity.

SUBACUTE SCLEROSING PANENCEPHALITIS

Epidemiology

Subacute sclerosing panencephalitis (SSPE), first de-scribed by Dawson in 1933, is a chronic degenerative disease of the central nervous system complicating mea-sles virus infection.[48] Its prevalence has been estimated at 3.5 cases per 10 million persons younger than 20 years.[49] The occurrence of SSPE in boys is approximately two times greater than that in girls,[50, 51] with male-to-female ratio of 1.8:1.[50] The onset of SSPE is usually 6 to 7 years after acute measles, but later onset has been reported as well.[52] Individuals who had measles before the age of 2 years are at higher risk of developing SSPE. The majority of patients manifest neurologic signs before the age of 20 years.

Clinical Characteristics

The typical clinical picture of SSPE has three stages. Behavioral changes and intellectual deterioration are present in the first stage. The second stage is character-ized by extrapyramidal signs and cortical blindness. De-mentia develops in the third stage, with death within 1 to 3 years of disease onset.

Approximately 50% of patients develop ocular symp-toms.[53–56] Ocular symptoms may precede neurologic man-ifestations by several weeks to 2 years.[57] Maculopathy con-sisting of pigment epithelial changes and focal retinitis in 36% of patients is the most typical ocular finding[55, 57–63] (Fig. 26–1; see also color insert). The retinitis can spread within several days from the macula to the posterior pole and peripheral retina.[52, 54, 64–67] Other ocular findings include disc edema, papillitis, optic nerve edema and pallor, retinitis, serous retinal detachment, retinal hemor-rhage, chorioretinitis, vasculitis, preretinal membrane, retinal folds, macular hole, cortical blindness, hemianop-sia, horizontal nystagmus, and ptosis.[53–56, 58, 61, 62, 65, 66, 68] Characteristically, there is little or no vitreous inflamma-

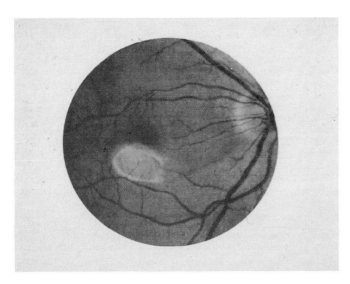

FIGURE 26–1. Ophthalmoscopic photograph, right macula. Note the well circumscribed, deep retinal opacification inferior to the fovea, with faint nerve fiber layer swelling extending from the lesion to the optic disk. (From Park DW, Boldt HC, Massicotte SJ, et al: Subacute sclerosing panencephalitis manifesting as viral retinitis: Clinical and histopathologic findings. Am J Ophthalmol 1997;123:533–543. With permission from Elsevier Science.) (See Color insert.)

tion.[52, 54–56, 58, 60, 64, 65, 68] The retinitis resolves, leaving retinal pigment epithelium mottling and scarring.[52, 54, 59, 61, 62, 67, 68]

Pathophysiology, Immunology, Pathology, and Pathogenesis

The classic measles virus replicates by budding and fusion. Subacute sclerosing panencephalitis is caused by measles virus, so-called "slow virus," deficient of certain virion polypeptides, such as matrix (M), hemagglutinin (H), and fusion (F) proteins. These proteins are necessary for alignment of the virus along the host-cell plasma membrane and subsequent budding and release of the virus from the host cell. Defects in these proteins, particularly in M protein, allow the virus to stay in its intracellular form and to spread by cell-to-cell contact.[69–72] The disease is a true panencephalitis, affecting both gray and white matter.

Immunohistochemical studies of brain tissue of SSPE patients has revealed increased expression of interleukin-1 (IL-1), IL-6, tumor necrosis factor-α (TNF-α), interferon-γ (IFN-γ), IL-2, and lymphotoxin.[73] Interestingly, only IL-1 and intercellular adhesion molecule 1 (ICAM-1) were elevated in cerebrospinal fluid.[74] The way in which these cytokines reached the cerebrospinal fluid is not known.

IFN appears to play an important role in the pathogenesis of SSPE. The intracellular virus can revert to the productive form in vitro on removal of IFN.[75] And abnormally low IFN-α and IFN-β levels were found in cerebrospinal fluid of patients with SSPE,[76, 77] and their peripheral mononuclear cells failed to produce IFN in vitro.[78] However, an in vitro resistance of SSPE virus to IFN has been observed as well.[79]

The virus in patients with SSPE is thought to reach the eye by hematogenous dissemination.[61] In the eye, the virus primarily affects the retina, with secondary involvement of the retinal pigment epithelium and choroid.[58, 62] Histopathology shows necrotizing retinopathy with eosinophilic inclusion bodies in both the cytoplasm and nucleus of neuronal glial and pigment epithelial cells. In addition, depigmentation and proliferation of the pigment epithelium with or without lymphocytic infiltration in choroids is observed.[48, 58, 60, 62, 66] Immunohistology reveals the measles virus antigen on nucleocapsids of the nuclear and cytoplasmic inclusions.[66] On electron microscopy, filamentous microtubular structures representing measles virus nucleocapsids of characteristic size are present in the retinal lesions, similar to those in the CNS.[60, 62]

Diagnosis

Diagnosis requires a high degree of suspicion and should be suspected in school-age children who exhibit unexplained, slowly progressive, cognitive, emotional, or neurologic dysfunction.

The diagnosis is made by the presence of three of five criteria, which include (1) clinical course, (2) biopsy or necropsy results, (3) EEG pattern, (4) elevated globulin levels in cerebrospinal fluid, and (5) elevated levels of IgG measles antibodies in serum and cerebrospinal fluid.[50, 80] Absence of IgM measles antibodies provides evidence against a new, acute-onset infection. Ophthalmoscopic signs may appear before the development of the neurologic disease and do not necessarily correspond to a particular stage of neurologic impairment.

Fluorescein angiography (FA) typically shows optic nerve staining, and precapillary arteriole and postcapillary venous occlusion with staining of the retinal lesions in the area of acute retinitis.[52, 59] The retinal lesions may resolve, leaving retinal pigment epithelial window defects on FA.[52]

Ocular findings similar to those seen in SSPE might be observed in patients with multiple sclerosis (MS) or in patients with unexplained optic atrophy and retinitis. Differentiating features between MS and SSPE include the fact that MS is not a panencephalitis, and MRI in patients with MS usually reveals focal lesions of white matter. In addition, cystoid macular edema (CME) is common in patients with MS but has not been seen in patients with SSPE.

Treatment

There is no definitive treatment for SSPE. However, intracameral IFN-α[82–84] may induce remission or stabilize the clinical course. Potential resistance to IFN-α might be overcome by higher doses administered for a longer period of time.[82]

Inosiplex, a 1:3 molar complex of inosine with dimethylaminoisopropanol-p-acetamidobenzoate, is a drug with both direct antiviral and immunomodulatory properties.[84] Early oral administration of inosiplex may delay the neurologic progression of the disease, with prolonged survival.[81, 84]

Treatment with a combination of intravenous IgG and inosiplex has been reported in one case as well.[85] The clinical symptoms rapidly improved after the treatment; however, the high titer of antibodies persisted. The efficacy and mechanism of action of this therapy remain unclear.

Prognosis

SSPE is generally considered to be a progressive fatal disease within 1 to 3 years of first clinical signs and symptoms.[50, 51] In addition to this classic clinical presentation, a chronic slowly progressive form, a fulminant form leading to death within several weeks, and a "stuttering" form with remissions and relapses have been reported.[50, 86] Spontaneous remission may occur in approximately 5% of patients.[87]

CONCLUSION

Measles infection can affect multiple ocular structures and produce devastating neurologic disease. Keratitis, the most common ocular sign, is benign in developed countries. However, in less developed countries it represents a common cause of blindness. Moreover, over a million children die each year as a result of measles in underdeveloped countries. Vaccination provided by the World Health Organization may reduce this morbidity and mortality.

SSPE, the late manifestation of measles infection, is a rare, fatal disease with high incidence of necrotizing retinitis. Regrettably, there is no definitive treatment for SSPE thus far, and the disease is almost universally fatal.

References

1. Centers for Disease Control and Prevention: Case definitions for public health surveillance. MMWR 1990;39(no. RR-13):1–43.
2. Wilson GS: Measles as a universal disease. Am J Dis Child 1962;103:219–223.
3. Katz SL, Enders JF: Measles virus. In: Horsfall FL Jr, Tamm T, eds: Viral and Rickettsial Infections of Man. Philadelphia, J.B. Lippincott, 1965, pp 784–801.
4. Caulfield E: Early measles epidemics in America. Yale J Biol Med 1943;15:531–536.
5. Panum PL: Observations made during the epidemic of measles on Faroe Island in the year 1846. Med Classics 1939;3:829–886.
6. Home F: Medical facts and experiments. London, A. Millar, 1759.
7. Koplik H: The diagnosis of the invasion of measles from a study of the exanthema as it appears on the buccal mucous membrane. Arch Pediatr 1896;13:918.
8. Koplik H: A new diagnostic sign of measles. Med Rec 1898;53:505.
9. Koplik H: The new diagnostic spots of measles on the buccal mucosa and labial mucous membrane. Med News 1899;74:673.
10. Enders JF, Peebles TC: Propagation in tissue cultures of cytopathogenic agents from patients with measles. Proc Soc Exp Biol Med 1954;86:277–286.
11. Krugman S: Present status of measles and rubella immunization in the United States: A medical progress report. J Pediatr 1971;78:1–16.
12. Gershon AA: Chickenpox, measles, and mumps. In: Remington JS, Klein JO, eds: Infectious diseases of the fetus and newborn infant. Philadelphia, WB Saunders, 1990, pp 395–445.
13. Centers for Disease Control. Measles—United States, 1990. MMWR 1991;40:369–372.
14. Eberhart-Phillips JE, Frederick PD, Baron RC, Mascola L: Measles in pregnancy: A descriptive study of 58 cases. Obstet Gynecol 1993;82:797–801.
15. Siegel M: Congenital malformations following chickenpox, measles, mumps, and hepatitis. Results of a cohort study. JAMA 1973;226:1521.
16. Metz HS, Harkey ME: Pigmentary retinopathy following maternal measles (morbilli) infection. Am J Ophthalmol 1968;66:1107.
17. Guzzinati GC: Sulla possibilità di lesioni oculari congenita da morbillo e da epatite epidemica. Boll Ocul (Italia) 1954;12:833–841.
18. Ray CG: Measles (rubeola). In: Thorn GW, et al, eds: Harrison's Principles of Internal Medicine, 8th ed, vol. I. New York, McGraw-Hill Company, 1977.
19. Katz SL: Measles. In: Rudolph AM, Barnett HL, Einhord AH, eds: Pediatrics, 16th ed. New York, Appleton-Century-Crofts, 1977.
20. Collins SD, Wheeler RE, Shannon RD: Occurrence of whooping cough, chickenpox, mumps, measles, and German measles in 200,000 survey families in 28 large cities. Bethesda, Maryland, National Institute of Health, 1943.
21. Hinman AR, Brandling-Bennett AD, Nieburg PI: The opportunity and obligation to eliminate measles from the United States. JAMA 1979;242:1157–1162.
22. Hinman AR, Brandling-Bennett AD, Bernier RH, et al: Current features of measles in the United States. Epidemiol Rev 1980;2:153.
23. Measles—United States, 1977–1980. MMWR 1980;29:598–599.
24. Hinman AR, Eddings DL, Kirby CD, et al: Progress in measles elimination. JAMA 1982;247:1592–1595.
25. Bergstrom TJ: Measles infection of the eye. In Darrell RW (ed): Viral Diseases of the Eye. Philadelphia, Lea & Febiger, 1985, p 233.
26. Fedukowicz HB: Measles. In: External Infections of the Eye. 2nd ed. New York, Appleton-Century-Crofts, 1978, pp 214–216.
27. Hiles DA, Cignetti FE: Measles. In: Harley RD, ed: Pediatric Ophthalmology. Philadelphia, W.B. Saunders Company, 1975, p 683.
28. Deckard PS, Bergstrom TJ: Rubeola keratitis. Ophthalmology 1981;88:812–813.
29. Thygeson P: Ocular viral diseases. Med Clin North Am 1959;43:1419–1440.
30. Dekkers NWHM: The cornea in measles. In: Darrell RW (ed): Viral Diseases of the Eye. Philadelphia, Lea & Febiger, 1985, p 239.
31. Florman AL, Agatston HJ: Keratoconjunctivitis as a diagnostic aid in measles. JAMA 1962;179:568–570.
32. Doggart JG: Superficial punctate keratitis. Br J Ophthalmol 1933;17:65–82.
33. Scheie HG, Morse PH: Rubeola retinopathy. Arch Ophthalmol 1972;88:341–344.
34. Foxman SG, Heckenlively JR, Sinclair SH: Rubeola retinopathy and pigmented paravenous retinochoroidal atrophy. Am J Ophthalmol 1985;99:605–606.
35. Dawson CR: How does the external eye resist infection? (Editorial.) Invest Ophthalmol 1976;15:971–974.
36. Morgan EM, Papp F: Measles virus and its associated diseases. Bacteriol Rev 1977;41:636–666.
37. Scheifele DW, Forbes CE: The biology of measles in African children. East Afr Med J 1973;50:169–173.
38. Kaplan LJ, Daum RS, Smaron M: Severe measles in immunocompromised patient. JAMA 1992;267:1237–1241.
39. Immunization Practices Advisory Committee: Measles prevention. MMWR 1982;31:217–224, 229–231.
40. Krugman RD, Rosenberg R, McIntosh K, et al: Further attenuated live measles vaccines: The need for revised recommendations. J Pediatr 1977;91:766–767.
41. Barclay AJ, Foster A, Sommer A: Vitamin A supplements and mortality related to measles: randomized clinical trial. Br Med J 1987;294:294–296.
42. Cherry JD: Measles. In Feigin RD, Cherry JD, eds: Textbook of pediatric infectious diseases, Vol II. Philadelphia, W.B. Saunders Co, 1992, p 1591.
43. Frederique G, Howard RO, Boniuk V: Corneal ulcers in rubeola. Am J Ophthalmol 1969;68:996–1003.
44. Sandorf-Smith JH, Whittle HC: Corneal ulceration following measles in Nigerian children. Br J Ophthalmol 1979;63:720–724.
45. Morley D: Severe measles in the tropics. Br Med J 1969;1:297.
46. Chirambo MC, Benezra D: Causes of blindness in students in blind school institutions in a developing country. Br J Ophthalmol 1976;60:665.
47. Foster A, Sommer A: Corneal ulceration, measles, and childhood blindness in Tanzania. Br J Ophthalmol 1987;71:331.
48. Dawson JR Jr: Cellular inclusions in cerebral lesions of lethargic encephalitis. Am J Pathol 1933;9:7.
49. Modlin JF, Halsey NA, Eddins DL, et al: Epidemiology of subacute sclerosing panencephalitis. J Pediatr 1979;94:231.
50. Dyken PR: Subacute sclerosing panencephalitis. Neurol Clin 1985;3:179.
51. Sussman J, Compston DAS: Subacute sclerosing panencephalitis in Wales. Q J Med 1994;87:23.
52. Park DW, Boldt C, Massicotte SJ, et al: Subacute sclerosing panencephalitis manifesting as viral retinitis: clinical and histopathologic findings. Am J Ophthalmol 1997;123:533.
53. Salmon JF, Pan EL, Murray AND: Visual loss with dancing extremities and mental disturbances. Surv Ophthalmol 1991;35:299.

54. Morgan B, Cohen DN, Rothner AD, et al: Ocular manifestations of subacute sclerosing panencephalitis. Am J Dis Child 1976;130:1019.

55. Robb RM, Watters GV: Ophthalmic manifestation of subacute sclerosing panencephalitis. Arch Ophthalmol 1970;83:426.

56. Hiatt RL, Grizzard HT, McNeer P, Jabbour JT: Ophthalmologic manifestations of subacute sclerosing panencephalitis (Dawson encephalitis). Trans Am Acad Ophthalmol Otolaryngol 1971;75:344.

57. Zagami AS, Lethlean AK: Chorioretinitis as a possible very early manifestation of subacute sclerosing panencephalitis. Aust N Z J Med 1991;21:350.

58. DeLaey JJ, Hanssens M, Colette P, et al: Subacute sclerosing panencephalitis: Fundus changes and histopathologic correlations. Doc Ophthalmol 1983;56:11.

59. Kovacs B, Vastag O: Fluoroangiographic picture of the acute stage of the retinal lesion in subacute sclerosing panencephalitis. Ophthalmologica 1978;177:264.

60. Landers MB, Klintworth GK: Subacute sclerosing panencephalitis (SSPE). Arch Ophthalmol 1971;86:156.

61. Meyers E, Mailin M, Zonis S: Subacute sclerosing panencephalitis: Clinicopathological study of the eyes. J Pediatr Ophthalmol Strabismus 1978;15:19.

62. Nelson DA, Weiner A, Yanoff M, et al: Retinal lesions in subacute sclerosing panencephalitis. Arch Ophthalmol 1970;84:613.

63. Otradovec J: Chorioretinitis centralis bei leucoencephalitis subacuta sclerotisans Van Bogaert. Ophthalmologica 1963;146:65.

64. Brudet-Wickel CLM, Hogweg M, DeWolf-Rouendaal D: Subacute sclerosing panencephalitis (SSPE). Doc Ophthalmol 1982;52:241.

65. Grayina RF, Nakarishi AS, Faden A: Subacute sclerosing panencephalitis. Am J Ophthalmol 1978;86:106.

66. Font RL, Jenis EH, Truck KD: Measles maculopathy associated with subacute sclerosing panencephalitis. Arch Pathol 1973;96:168.

67. LaPiana FG, Tso MOM, Jenis EH: The retinal lesions of subacute sclerosing panencephalitis. Ann Ophthalmol 1974;6:603.

68. Raymond LA, Kerstine RS, Shelburne SA: Praeretinal vitreous membrane in subacute sclerosing panencephalitis. Arch Ophthalmol 1976;94:1412.

69. Cattaneo R, Schmid A, Rebmann G, et al: Accumulated measles virus mutations in a case of subacute sclerosing panencephalitis: Interrupted matrix protein reading frame and transcription alteration. Virology 1986;154:97.

70. Choppin PW: Measles virus and chronic neurological diseases. Ann Neurol 1981;9:17.

71. Hall WW, Lamb RA, Choppin PW: Measles and SSPE virus protein: Lack of antibodies to the M protein in patients with subacute sclerosing panencephalitis. Proc Natl Acad Sci U S A 1979;76:2047.

72. Johnson KP, Norrby E, Swoveland P, et al: Experimental subacute sclerosing panencephalitis: Selective disappearance of measles virus matrix protein from the central nervous system. J Infect Dis 1981;144:161.

73. Nagano I, Nakamura S, Yoshioka M, et al: Expression of cytokines in brain lesions in subacute sclerosing panencephalitis. Neurology 1994;44:710.

74. Mehta PD, Kulczycki J, Mehta SP, et al: Increased levels of interleukin-1β and soluble intercellular adhesion molecule-1 in cerebrospinal fluid of patients with subacute sclerosing panencephalitis. J Infect Dis 1997;175:689.

75. Carrigan DR, Kabacoff CM: Identification of a nonproductive, cell-associated form of measles virus by its resistance to inhibition by recombinant human interferon. J Virol 1987;61:1919.

76. Dussaix E, Lebon P, Ponsot G, et al: Intrathecal synthesis of different interferons in patients with various neurological diseases. Acta Neurol Scand 1985;71:504.

77. Lebon P, Boutin B, Dulac O, et al: Interferon in acute and subacute panencephalitis. Br J Med 1988;296:9.

78. Gadoth N, Kott E, Levin S, et al: The interferon system in subacute sclerosing panencephalitis and its response to isoprinosine. Brain Dev 1989;11:308.

79. Crespi M, Chin MN, Schoub BD, et al: Effects of interferon on Vero cells persistently infected with SSPE virus and lytically infected with measles virus. Arch Virol 1986;90:87.

80. Sever JL, Krebs H, Ley A, et al: Diagnosis of subacute sclerosing panencephalitis: The value and availability of measles antibody determination. JAMA 1974;228:604.

81. Yalaz K, Anlar B, Oktem F, et al: Intraventricular interferon and oral inosiplex in the treatment of subacute sclerosing panencephalitis. Neurology 1992;42:488.

82. Kuroki S, Tsutsui T, Yoshioka M, et al: The effect of intraventricular interferon on subacute sclerosing panencephalitis. Brain Dev 1989;11:65.

83. Anlar B, Yalaz K, Oktem F, et al: Long-term follow-up of patients with subacute sclerosing panencephalitis treated with intraventricular α-interferon. Neurology 1997;48:526.

84. Jones CE, Dyken PR, Huttenlocher PR, et al: Inosiplex therapy in subacute sclerosing panencephalitis. Lancet 1982;8:1034.

85. Gurer YK, Kukner S, Sarica B: Intravenous γ-globulin treatment in a patient with subacute sclerosing panencephalitis. Pediatr Neurol 1996;14:72.

86. Risk WS, Haddad FS: The variable natural history of subacute sclerosing panencephalitis: A study of 118 cases from the Middle East. Arch Neurol 1979;56:610.

87. Risk WS, Haddad FS, Chemali R: Substantial spontaneous long-term improvement in subacute sclerosing panencephalitis: Six cases from the Middle East and a review of the literature. Arch Neurol 1978;35:494–502.

27 | RUBELLA

Erik Letko and C. Stephen Foster

DEFINITION

Rubella is an acute, contagious, exanthematous disease caused by rubella virus.

HISTORY

Two German physicians, De Bergen (in 1752),[1] and Orlow (in 1758),[2] provided the first clinical descriptions of rubella, calling the disorder Rotheln. The disease became known as German Measles in English speaking countries. A Scottish physician, Veale, used the name rubella for the first time in 1866.[3] In 1941, an Australian ophthalmologist, Gregg, noticed congenital defects in babies of mothers who contracted rubella during pregnancy.[4] However, Gregg cited Mitchell, who first observed retinopathy in congenital rubella. Hiro and Tasaka in 1938 showed that rubella was caused by a virus.[5] The isolation of the virus in 1962 by Weller and Neva[6] enabled vaccine development. Since 1969, live attenuated rubella vaccine has been available in the United States.[7]

CONGENITAL RUBELLA

Epidemiology

Epidemiologic data on congenital rubella had not been reported until 1966 when The National Register for Congenital Rubella was established. It is clear that the incidence rate depends on the month of the mother's pregnancy in which maternal infection occurs, as well as on the presence or absence of epidemics in each year. Thirty-six percent of maternal rubella between the 1st and 8th week of pregnancy ended in abortion or stillbirth, and 25% had gross fetal anomalies.[8] Fifty-two percent of the instances of maternal rubella occurring between 9th and 12th week resulted in the birth of babies with congenital defects, whereas the rate fell to 16% if the mother had become infected between 13 and 20 weeks of gestation. There were no such congenital defects reported if the maternal infection occurred after week 20 of pregnancy.[8] In another study, a risk of 3% malformations and 4% stillbirth has been estimated if maternal rubella infection is contracted after 12 weeks of pregnancy.[9]

Clinical Characteristics

The classic features of congenital rubella syndrome are manifested by hearing, ocular, and cardiac defects.[4, 10] However, anomalies may be present in other organ systems.[11] Congenital malformations, including ocular anomalies associated with congenital rubella syndrome, can be present at birth, shortly after birth, or later in life.[12, 13] The overall incidence of ocular anomalies is 30% to 78% (Table 27–1). Bilateral or unilateral deafness, the most common symptom, is present in 80% to 90% of infants with congenital rubella. Cataracts and microphthalmia are the most frequent cause of poor visual acuity.[14] Patients with congenital rubella are at higher risk for developing diabetes and subsequent diabetic retinopathy.[15]

Pigmentary retinopathy, described as "salt and pepper," is one of the most common ocular manifestations of congenital rubella (Fig. 27–1). It usually remains stable throughout life, but in some patients, the retinopathy may become progressive and cause continual tissue destruction and scarring (Fig. 27–2).[16] Moreover, some eyes may develop pigmentary retinopathy later in life.[17] The visual acuity in eyes with congenital rubella pigmentary retinopathy in the absence of other ocular symptoms is usually but not always good, with visual acuity as poor as 20/200 having been reported.[16] Subretinal neovascularization in the absence of a rupture of Bruch's membrane is a complication of pigmentary retinopathy. The neovascularization develops later in life and can cause either sudden loss of vision as a consequence of subretinal hemorrhage or gradual vision impairment due to disciform scarring in the macula.[18–21] The electroretinogram (ERG) in such eyes remains normal.[22]

Keratic precipitates are reported in eyes with cataracts after either cataract extraction or cataract resorption. Patients with congenital cataracts associated with congenital rubella syndrome may have an increased inflammatory response after cataract surgery, probably as a consequence of the virus persistence in the cataractous lens.[23]

Pathophysiology, Immunology, Pathology, and Pathogenesis

Fetal infection can develop by the ascending route from cervix as well as by primary placental infection.[24, 25] Only newborns with congenital rubella syndrome who had ex-

TABLE 27–1. OCULAR MANIFESTATIONS OF CONGENITAL RUBELLA

SYMPTOM	INCIDENCE (%)	REFERENCE
Retinopathy	9–88	38, 62, 64, 68
Cataract	16–85	38, 69
Strabismus	9–60	61, 69
Nystagmus	13–44	38, 64
Microphthalmia	10–63	38, 69
Amblyopia	1–16	14, 38
Glaucoma	2–25	60
Buphthalmos	11	38
Lid defects	10	38
Persistent hyaloid artery	9	38
Iris coloboma	1–5	14, 64
Iris atrophy	7	38
Optic atrophy	4–9	14, 38
Corneal haze	1–25	38, 64
Phthisis bulbi	7	38
Dacryostenosis	2–5	14, 38, 64
Keratoconus	rare	59
Keratic precipitates	rare	23
Aphakia	rare	67, 72
Any eye disease	30–78	14, 60, 65

Adapted from Givens KT, Lee DA, Jones T, Ilstrup DM: Congenital rubella syndrome: Ophthalmic manifestations and associated systemic disorders. Br J Ophthalmol 1993;77:358–363.

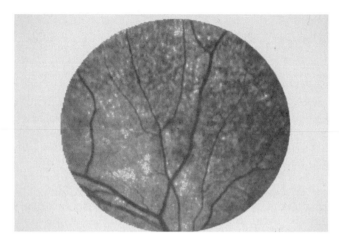

FIGURE 27–1. A typical "salt-and-pepper" pigmentary mottling in congenital rubella. (Reprinted from Orth DH, Fishman GA, Segall M, et al: Rubella maculopathy. Br J Ophthalmol 1980;64:201–205, Fig. 3a, with permission of the editor.)

perienced rubella infection during the first 12 weeks of gestation showed significantly reduced levels of antibodies directed to both the E1 and E2 rubella virus epitopes. Asymptomatic newborns infected later than week 10 of gestation have normal levels of antibodies.[26] Rubella virus can persist in infants with congenital rubella as long as 4.5 years after their birth.[27] Defects in congenital rubella result from both specific cell damage and generalized vascular damage resulting in mitotic arrest and reduction; that is, cellular necrosis and cellular deficiency with reduction in number of cells in organs. Disturbance of organogenesis, particularly in the first 16 weeks of pregnancy, and tissue destruction and scarring are the consequences of fetal rubella infection.[28–30] Termination of susceptibility in the second trimester is consistent with development of the fetal immune response and increased transfer of maternal IgG.[30] The pathogenesis of rubella embryopathy has not been elucidated on a cellular level, but it is thought that the virus inhibits the cellular multiplication together with the establishment of persistent infection during organogenesis. Multiple organ damage is manifested shortly after the birth, but delayed manifestations several months or years later in life are reported as well.[24] A spectrum of delayed manifestations of congenital rubella is described in the literature.[23, 29] Chronic persistence of the virus with extension of the infection, growth of the virus resulting in reduced growth rate and shortened lifespan of body cells, autoimmune response, genetic susceptibility, vascular damage by virus, and reactive hypervascularization are hypothesized to explain this phenomenon as well.[24, 30] At autopsy, rubella virus has been isolated from clear lens of infants with congenital rubella syndrome[31] and from cataractous lens as late as 35 months of age.[32]

Focal necrosis of the ciliary epithelium, pars plicata, and pars plana is considered to be characteristic of ocular rubella.[33] The histopathology of the iris stroma reveals atrophy, hypoplasia or absence of the dilator muscle and hypoplasia of the sphincter muscle of the iris, and vacuolization and focal necrosis of the pigment epithelium of the iris and ciliary body.[33, 34] The absence of inflammatory

response suggests that these changes occur before the development of an immune response in the fetus.

However, the presence of a nongranulomatous uveitis with lymphocytic infiltration of the anterior uvea, plasma cells, and histiocytes suggests that such changes must occur in later fetal life or in the early neonatal period.[35–36] The presence of pigment on the anterior lens capsule may further support this hypothesis.[20] A clinical correlation of active iritis has been described in one report.[37]

Pigmentary retinopathy is indeed confined to the pigment epithelium and does not involve the neurosensory retina or underlying choroids capillaries. At histopathology, it is present as an uneven distribution of pigment in the cells of the retinal pigment epithelium. However, in later fetal life and in infancy, the underlying choroid may be infiltrated with lymphocytes, suggesting an inflammatory response.[38]

Diagnosis

The diagnosis of congenital rubella is made by the presence of maternal rubella infection and congenital anomalies. Detection of serum IgM antibodies to rubella is a useful diagnostic tool in children with anomalies from uneventful pregnancies.[39] Viral isolation from the nose, throat, urine, buffy coat of the blood, or cerebrospinal fluid is the best method to prove congenital rubella. Monitoring the IgM antibodies after the birth can be helpful in questionable cases. If the level of IgM antibodies does not drop four- to eightfold by the age of 3 months and continues to fall to nondetectable levels, congenital rubella can be confirmed.

Fluorescein angiography of the retina in patients with pigmentary retinopathy associated with congenital rubella reveals both hyperfluorescent and hypofluorescent areas due to the diffuse pigment epithelial mottling. The early venous stage of the fluorescein angiogram may show new vessels replete with discrete hyperfluorescence in the presence of subretinal neovascularization with subsequent leakage in the later phase of the study. Accumulation of fluorescein is seen beneath pigment epithelium

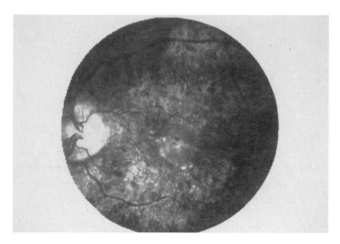

FIGURE 27–2. Congenital rubella. Diffuse pigment epithelial mottling with "salt-and-pepper" appearance, and a yellowish disciform scar. (Reprinted from Orth DH, Fishman GA, Segall M, et al: Rubella maculopathy. Br J Ophthalmol 1980;64:201–205, Fig. 2a, with permission of the editor.)

in cases of hemorrhage pigment epithelial detachment complicating subretinal neovascularization. In the presence of a disciform scar, the early phase of fluorescein angiography shows a pigment epithelial window defect secondary to the fibrotic tissue, whereas the late phase reveals an increased hyperfluorescence due to staining of the scar.[18–21]

The ERG in patients with pigmentary retinopathy is normal. Slight abnormalities may be present if subretinal hemorrhage develops.[18]

Treatment

Immune globulin given to women susceptible to rubella infection in the first 20 weeks of pregnancy or within 72 hours after the exposure may prevent both maternal and congenital infection. Most infants with congenital rubella are actively infected at the time of birth, that is, they are contagious and, therefore, must be placed in isolation until the viral cultures become negative. The treatment of congenital anomalies is symptomatic. It is obviously important to examine "normal" children born to mothers with maternal rubella infection during the first several years after birth because of a possible late manifestation of congenital rubella. Increased inflammation after cataract surgery typically responds well to topical steroid therapy.[23] Photocoagulation should be considered in patients with subretinal neovascularization.

Prognosis

The prognosis depends on the severity of congenital malformations and potential progression later in life. If the subretinal neovascularization, particularly with subretinal hemorrhage develops, the patients usually suffer from permanent decrease of vision because of the subsequent disciform scarring in the macula. However, involution of subretinal hemorrhage without disciform scarring with full restoration of visual acuity has been also reported.[40]

ACQUIRED RUBELLA

Epidemiology

Before the initiation of widespread vaccination programs, rubella epidemics occurred in 6- to 9-year intervals, with each cycle over a 3- to 4-year period.[41] After the introduction of rubella vaccine in the United States, there has been no nationwide epidemic of rubella reported. In closed populations such as families, military training centers, and institutions for the mentally handicapped, the infection will occur in 100% of susceptible individuals.[42] The highest attack rate occurred in the 5- to 9-year-old children in the prevaccine era. However, in the postvaccine era, 50% of rubella infection was reported in persons older than 19 years of age. The vaccination programs focus on children to prevent epidemics and on young women of childbearing age to prevent maternal and congenital rubella, respectively.[43, 44] Rubella is usually a winter and spring disease, but sporadic infections occur throughout the year in large urban areas.[45]

Clinical Characteristics

The incubation period for acquired infection is 14 to 21 days. Skin rash is the first sign of rubella infection in children. Prodromes can occur in adolescents and adults 1 to 5 days before the onset of the rash.[46] The rubella exanthem appears first on the face and then spreads toward the hands and feet. The erythematous and maculopapular exanthem involves the whole body in 24 hours and disappears by the third day. In some individuals, the skin rash is not present. Lymphadenopathy is a major clinical manifestation of rubella. The occurrence of fever is variable.

Arthritis, encephalitis, and thrombocytopenic or nonthrombocytopenic purpura can complicate the course of acquired rubella infection.

Ocular manifestations of acquired rubella include conjunctivitis, epithelial keratitis, and retinitis. Conjunctivitis, the most common ocular finding in acquired rubella, is present in 70% of patients. Epithelial keratitis, reported in 7.6% of patients, resolves without sequelae within one week.[47, 34] Retinitis is a rare complication of acquired rubella.[48, 49] Decreased vision is the major symptom. On examination, optic media are clear, but cells in the anterior chamber may be present. The retinal findings include dark gray atrophic lesions of the retinal pigment epithelium, flat detachment of the retinal neuroepithelium at the posterior pole, and bullous and diffuse detachment of the retina. A case of bilateral optic neuritis diagnosed 3 weeks after measles, mumps, and rubella vaccination is described in the literature as well.[50]

Pathophysiology, Immunology, Pathology, and Pathogenesis

Rubella infection is caused by rubella virus from the Rubivirus genus of the family Togaviridae.[31] Humans are the only known vertebrate hosts, although animals can be experimentally infected.[51] The rubella virion is spherical, with a diameter of 60 to 70 nm. The virion contains three major polypeptides—E1, E2, and C.[52] E1 and E2 are located on the viral surface membrane, and C is located in the nucleocapsid along with the genomic RNA.[52] Specific viral antigens can be identified by hemagglutination-inhibition, complement-fixation, neutralization, immunofluorescence, radioimmunoassay, precipitation, platelet aggregation, latex agglutination, and passive hemagglutination.[11] Rubella infection is characterized by the appearance of IgM, IgG, and IgA antibodies in the serum. The IgM antibodies persist no longer than 8 weeks after the onset of the infection. The IgA antibodies are elevated in the case of natural rubella infection or nasal immunization.[53] Cellular immune response and circulating virus-antibody immune complexes are believed to cause skin rash and arthritis. Life-long persistence of cell-mediated immunity without reinfection is reported.[54] The rubella-specific response is suppressed during pregnancy.[55]

The infection is spread by the respiratory route.[56, 57] Respiratory epithelium of the nasopharynx is the primary site of inoculation. The virus then spreads to the regional lymph nodes. Replication occurs in both respiratory epithelium and in lymph nodes, followed by viremia. Rubella virus has been isolated from lymph nodes, urine, cerebrospinal fluid, conjunctiva, breast milk, synovial fluid, lung, and skin at sites where rash was both present and absent.[11]

Diagnosis

The diagnosis of rubella can be difficult, because in some cases, there is a lack of pathognomonic findings. However, rubella usually occurs in epidemics, which makes the diagnosis easier. The rubella infection can be definitely confirmed by virus isolation or by serologic tests in uncertain cases.

Fluorescein angiogram in patients with retinitis associated with acquired rubella infection shows hyperfluorescent areas with no leakage from the retinal vessels.

Treatment

Treatment in patients with uncomplicated acquired rubella infection is symptomatic. The rubella retinitis and postvaccination optic neuritis respond well to systemic steroids.[49, 50]

Complications

The course of acquired rubella can be complicated by arthritis, encephalitis, and thrombocytopenic purpura.[11] Persistent scotoma following optic neuritis after measles, mumps, and rubella vaccination is described in the literature.[50]

Prognosis

The prognosis in acquired rubella is excellent unless encephalitis or thrombocytopenic purpura develop. The retinitis typically resolves, leaving retinal pigment epithelial damage. The visual acuity usually improves but does not always return to normal in each eye.[48, 49] Rapid improvement of visual acuities is reported after optic neuritis following measles, mumps, and rubella vaccination.[50]

CONCLUSIONS

Maternal rubella is likely to cause damage to the fetus. Ocular manifestation and hearing loss are the most common manifestations of congenital rubella. Because of a potential progression or development of new symptoms, congenital rubella should be considered as a chronic disease capable of progressive damage, and patients with the disorder should be monitored regularly.

Acquired rubella is usually harmless to the eye, although retinitis (rare), may affect vision. The diagnosis should be considered in patients with recent rubella infection who develop uveitis.

References

1. Griffith JPC: Rubella (Rotheln: German measles). With a report of one hundred and fifty cases. Medical Record 1887;32:11–41.
2. Wesselhoeft C: Rubella (German measles). N Engl J Med 1947;236:943–950, 978–988.
3. Veale H: History of an epidemic of Rotheln, with observations on this pathology. Edinb Med J 1866;12:404–414.
4. Gregg NM: Congenital cataract following German measles in the mother. Transactions of the Ophthalmological Society of Austria 1941;3:35–46.
5. Hiro VY, Tasaka S: Die Rotheln sind eine Viruskrankenheit. Monatsschr Kinderheilk 1938;76:328–332.
6. Weller TH, Neva F: Propagation in tissue culture of cytopathic agents from patients with rubella-like illness. Proc Soc Exp Biol Med 1962;111:215–225.
7. Meyer HM, Hopps HE, Parkman PD, et al: Control of measles and rubella through use of attenuated vaccines. Am J Clin Pathol 1978;70:128.
8. Sallomi SJ: Rubella in pregnancy. A review of prospective studies from the literature. Obstet Gynecol 1966;27:252–256.
9. Cockburn WC: World aspects of the epidemiology of rubella. Am J Dis Child 1969;118:112.
10. Gregg NM: Further observations on congenital defects in infants following maternal rubella. Transactions of the Ophthalmological Society of Austria 1944; 4:119–125.
11. Cherry JD: Rubella virus. In: Feigin RD, Cherry JD, eds: Textbook of Pediatric Infectious Diseases, Vol II. Philadelphia, W.B. Saunders, 1992, pp 1922–1949.
12. Hancock MT, Huntley CC, Sever JL: Congenital rubella syndrome with immunoglobulin disorder. J Pediatr 1968;72:636–645.
13. Murphy AM, Reid RR, Pollard I, et al: Rubella cataracts. Further clinical and virologic observations. Am J Ophthalmol 1967;64:1109–1119.
14. Givens KT, Lee DA, Jones T, Ilstrup DM: Congenital rubella syndrome: Ophthalmic manifestations and associated systemic disorders. Br J Ophthalmol 1993;77:358–363.
15. Menser MA, Dods L, Harley JD: A twenty-five year follow-up of congenital rubella. Lancet 1967;ii:1347–1350.
16. Collis WJ, Cohen DN: Rubella retinopathy: A progressive disorder. Arch Ophthalmol 1970;84:33–35.
17. Wolff SM: Ocular aspects of congenital rubella. In: Ryan SJ, Smith RE, eds: Selective Topics on the Eye in Systemic Disease. New York, Grune and Stratton, 1974, p 205.
18. Deutman AF, Grizzard WS: Rubella retinopathy and subretinal neovascularization. Am J Ophthalmol 1978;85:82.
19. Frank KE, Purnell EW: Subretinal neovascularization following rubella retinopathy. Am J Ophthalmol 1978;86:462.
20. Orth DH, Fishman GA, Segall M, et al: Rubella maculopathy. Br J Ophthalmol 1980;64:201–205.
21. Slusher MM, Tyler ME: Rubella retinopathy and subretinal neovascularization. Am J Ophthalmol 1982;14:292.
22. Krill AE: The retinal disease of rubella. Arch Ophthalmol 1967;77:445–449.
23. Boger WP: Late ocular manifestation in congenital rubella syndrome. Ophthalmology 1980;87:1244–1252.
24. Sever JL, South MA, Shaver KA: Delayed manifestations of congenital rubella. Rev Infect Dis 1985;7:S164.
25. Vaheri A, Vesikari T, Oker-Blom N, et al: Isolation of attenuated rubella-vaccine virus from human products of conception and uterine cervix. N Engl J Med 1972;286:1071–1074.
26. Meitsch K, Enders G, Wolinsky JS, et al: The role of rubella-immunoblot and rubella-peptide-EIA for the diagnosis of the congenital rubella syndrome during the prenatal and newborn periods. J Med Virol 1997;51:280.
27. Shewmon DA, Cherry JD, Kirby SE: Shedding of rubella virus in a 4 1/2-year-old boy with congenital rubella syndrome. Pediatr Infect Dis 1982;Sep–Oct:342–343.
28. Atreya CD, Lee NS, Forng RY: The rubella virus putative replicase interacts with the retinoblastoma tumor suppressor protein. Virus Genes 1998;16:177.
29. South MA, Sever JL: Teratogen update: The congenital rubella syndrome. Teratology 1985;31:297–307.
30. Webster WS: Teratogen update: Congenital rubella. Teratology 1998;58:13.
31. Bellanti JA, Artenstein MS, Olson LC, et al: Congenital rubella: Clinicopathologic, virologic and immunologic studies. Am J Dis Child 1965;110:464.
32. Menser MA, Harley JD, Hertzberg R, et al: Persistence of virus in lens for three years after prenatal rubella. Lancet 1967;2:387–388.
33. Boniuk M, Zimmerman LE: Ocular pathology in the rubella syndrome. Arch Ophthalmol 1967;77:455.
34. Zimmerman LE: Histopathologic basis for ocular manifestations of congenital rubella syndrome. Am J Ophthalmol 1968;65:837.
35. Yanoff M, Schaefer DB, Scheie HG: Rubella ocular syndrome: Clinical significance of viral and pathological studies. Transactions of the American Academy of Ophthalmology and Otolaryngology 1968;122:1049.
36. Zimmerman LE, Font RL: Congenital malformations of the eye: Some recent advances in the knowledge of the pathogenesis and histopathological characteristics. JAMA 1966;196:684.
37. Krause AC: Congenital cataracts following rubella in pregnancy. Ann Surg 1945;122:1049.
38. Wolff SM: The ocular manifestations of congenital rubella. A pro-

spective study of 328 cases of congenital rubella. J Pediatr Ophthalmol 1973;10:101–141.

39. Stiehm ER, Ammann AJ, Cherry JD: Elevated cord macroglobulins in the diagnosis of intrauterine infections. N Engl J Med 1966;275:971–977.

40. Bonomo PP: Involution without disciform scarring of subretinal neovascularization in presumed rubella retinopathy. A case report. Acta Ophthalmol 1982;60:141.

41. Horstman DM: Rubella. In: Evans AS, ed: Viral Infections of Humans: Epidemiology and Control, 3rd ed. New York, Plenum Medical Book Company, 1990, pp 617–631.

42. Horstman DM, Liebhaber H, LeBouvier GL, et al: Rubella: Reinfection of vaccinated and naturally immune persons exposed in an epidemic. N Engl J Med 1970;283:771–778.

43. National Communicable Disease Center: Rubella Surveillance. Atlanta, GA, Centers for Disease Control, 1969.

44. Hambling MH: Effect of a vaccination programme on the distribution of rubella antibodies in women of childbearing age. Lancet 1975;1:1130–1138.

45. Communicable Disease Center: Provisional Information in Selected Notifiable Diseases in the United States and on Deaths in Selected Cities for Week Ended September 3, 1964. MMWR 1964;13:349–360.

46. Gross PA, Portnoy B, Mathies AW Jr, et al: A rubella outbreak among adolescent boys. Am J Dis Child 1970;119:326.

47. Matoba A: Ocular viral infections. Pediatr Infect Dis 1984;3:358–368.

48. Gerstle C, Zim KM: Rubella-associated retinitis in adult. Report of a case. Mt Sinai J Med 1976;43:303.

49. Hayashi M, Yoshimura N, Kondo T: Acute rubella retinal pigment epithelitis in an adult. Am J Ophthalmol 1982;93:285–288.

50. Kazarian EL, Gager WE: Optic neuritis complicating measles, mumps, and rubella vaccination. Am J Ophthalmol 1978;86:544–547.

51. Plotkin SA: Rubella virus. In: Lenette EH, Schmidt JH, eds: Diagnostic Procedures for Viral and Rickettsial Infections. New York, American Public Health Association, 1969, p 364.

52. Pettersen RF, Oker-Blom C, Kalkkinen N, et al: Molecular and antigenic characteristics and synthesis of rubella virus structural proteins. Rev Infect Dis 1985;7:S140.

53. Ogra PL, Kerr-Grant D, Umana G, et al: Antibody response in serum and nasopharynx after naturally acquired and vaccine-induced infection with rubella virus. N Engl J Med 1971;285:1333.

54. Rossier E, Phipps PH, Weber JM, et al: Persistence of humoral and cell-mediated immunity to rubella virus in cloistered nuns and in schoolteachers. J Infect Dis 1981;144:137.

55. Thong YH, Steele RW, Vincent MM, et al: Impaired *in vitro* cell-mediated immunity to rubella virus during pregnancy. N Engl J Med 1973;289:604.

56. Green RH, Balsamo MR, Gilles JP, et al: Studies of the natural history and prevention of rubella. Am J Dis Child 1965;110:348–365.

57. Heggie AD, Robins FC: Natural rubella acquired after birth. Clinical features and complications. Am J Dis Child 1969;118:12–17.

58. Arnold JJ, McIntosh EDG, Martin FJ, Menser MA: A fifty-year follow-up of ocular defects in congenital rubella: Late ocular manifestations. Aust N Z J Ophyhalmol 1994;22:1.

59. Boger WP, Petersen RA, Robb RM: Keratoconus and acute hydrops in mentally retarded patients with congenital rubella syndrome. Am J Opthalmol 1981;91:213–223.

60. Boniuk M: Glaucoma in the congenital rubella syndrome. Int Ophthalmol Clin 1972;12:121.

61. Boniuk V: Systemic and ocular manifestations of the rubella syndrome. Int Ophthalmol Clin 1972;12:67.

62. Boniuk V: Rubella. Int Ophthalmol Clin 1975;15:229.

63. Fenner F: Classification and nomenclature of viruses. Second report of the International Committee on Taxonomy of Viruses. Intervirology 1976;7:1–115.

64. Geltzer AI, Guber D, Sears ML: Ocular manifestations of the 1964–1965 rubella epidemic. Am J Ophthalmol 1967;63:221.

65. Harley RD: Discussion comments in: Boniuk V, Boniuk M. The prevalence of phthisis bulbi as a complication of cataract surgery in the congenital rubella syndrome. Transactions of the American Academy of Ophthalmology and Otolaryngology 1970;74:360.

66. Heggie AD: Pathogenesis of the rubella exanthem: Distribution of rubella virus in the skin during rubella with and without rash. J Infect Dis 1978;134:74–77.

67. Johnson BL, Cheng KP: Congenital aphakia: A clinicopathologic report of three cases. J Pediatr Ophthalmol Strabismus 1997;34:35.

68. Krill AE: Retinopathy secondary to rubella. Int Ophthalmol Clin 1972;12:89.

69. O'Neill JF: Strabismus in congenital rubella. Arch Ophthalmol 1967;77:450.

70. Seppala M, Vaheri A: Natural rubella infection of the female genital tract. Lancet 1974;1:46–47.

71. Wolter JR, Insel PA, Arbor A, et al: Eye pathology following maternal rubella. J Pediatr Ophthalmol 1966; 3:29.

72. Wolter JR, Hall RC, Masson GL: Unilateral primary congenital aphakia. Am J Ophthalmol 1964; 58:1011.

28 | PRESUMED OCULAR HISTOPLASMOSIS SYNDROME

Gurinder Singh

DEFINITION

An ocular syndrome of macular scar, peripheral punched-out chorioretinal scars ("histo spots"), and pigmented peripapillary degeneration with clear vitreous is *presumed* to be associated with the fungus *Histoplasma capsulatum*, thereby its name, presumed ocular histoplasmosis syndrome (POHS). Accruing epidemiologic and immunologic evidence has supported the association of these ocular manifestations with systemic infection by this fungus. Still, the definite pathogenesis has eluded scientists. It appears to result from a complex and ill-defined interaction of the fungal pathogen and the body's immune reaction to it, presenting in a specific pattern in certain endemic areas in the United States. Systemic fungal infection by *H. capsulatum* is seen worldwide, but the ocular presentation in the form of POHS was thought to be a phenomenon seen only in certain parts of the United States. More recently, POHS has been reported in England and in Europe, where it is clinically indistinguishable from that seen in the United States, albeit with negative skin testing.

POHS, also called presumed ocular histoplasmosis or simply ocular histoplasmosis, is a distinct entity, distinguished from the exudative/productive *H. capsulatum* infection of ocular tissues that is part of disseminated histoplasmosis.

The latter is a rare disease of infants with immature immune systems, of immunosuppressed adults, and, even more rarely, of adults without any known immune deficiency.[1, 2] Systemic disseminated histoplasmosis can manifest in three major forms: (1) mild influenza-like respiratory symptoms with fever, malaise, and fatigue; (2) acute progressive life-threatening disease; and (3) chronic granulomatous disease mimicking tuberculosis. The ocular manifestations in systemic disseminated histoplasmosis can include retinitis, optic neuritis, and uveitis.[3] It can present as panuveitis, vitritis, iritis, focal retinitis, and severe endophthalmitis.[4] It may even occur as an exogenous infection after intraocular surgery.[5] *H. capsulatum* has been cultured and identified histopathologically from ocular tissue of patients with ocular involvement in disseminated histoplasmosis[6–9] but not in POHS[10] (as discussed later). This chapter will be limited to POHS without further elaboration on the ocular manifestations of disseminated systemic histoplasmosis.

HISTORY

The first to identify an *H. capsulatum* infection was Darling, at the autopsy of a patient in 1906.[11, 12] In 1942, Reid and colleagues[13] published the ocular findings in a patient dying of acute disseminated histoplasmosis. In 1951, Krause and Hopkins[14] reported a case of hemorrhagic retinitis and exudative chorioretinitis, which flared up with the histoplasmin skin test. On reviewing this case

report, Schlaegel[15] hypothesized that the choroiditis was probably associated with histoplasmosis. However, Woods and Wahlen[16] were the first to describe an ocular syndrome of disciform macular detachment and peripheral chorioretinal scars in otherwise healthy adults. Schlaegel and Kenney[17] added peripapillary atrophy and pigment changes to the features described by Woods and Wahlen, completing the classic triad of what we now know as POHS.

MYCOLOGY

The causative organism *H. capsulatum* is a dimorphic fungus belonging to the class Ascomycetes.[18] It grows in the soil in the mycelial (mold) phase and inside animals or birds in the yeast phase. Primary histoplasmosis infection occurs typically by inhaling either microconidia (small spores), macroconidia (large spores), or mycelial (hyphae) fragments. These fragments penetrate the lungs but get entrapped in reticuloendothelial cells. An inflammatory reaction heals the infection and leaves small calcified lesions in lungs, liver, spleen, and lymph nodes that can be seen on radiologic examination.[19]

EPIDEMIOLOGY

Geographic Distribution

Systemic histoplasmosis is a worldwide phenomenon occuring between 45° north and 45° south of the equator. The mycelial form of this fungus grows in the upper 2 inches of the soil, fertilized by droppings of birds, chicken, and bats, along the rivers of central and southeastern United States, Central and South America, Asia, Italy, Turkey, Israel, England, Australia, Japan, and Puerto Rico.[20] However, POHS has been described primarily in the endemic areas of the valleys of the Ohio and Mississippi rivers (including Indiana, Ohio, Illinois, Kentucky, Tennessee, and Mississippi), in mid-Atlantic states such as Maryland, and in the San Joaquin Valley of California.[21] Ocular findings mimicking POHS have been reported in England, Europe, and the Northwestern United States where histoplasmosis is not endemic.[22–25]

Prevalence

The prevalence of POHS in the United States has been reported to be 1.6% in Ohio[26] and 2.6% in western Maryland.[21] In a study done in Ohio[26] (in an institutionalized population of 1417 adults, including whites and blacks, men and women), the prevalence of ocular histoplasmosis was 1.6%. Over 50% of this population reacted positively to a histoplasmin skin test. All of those who had signs of ocular histoplasmosis either reacted positively to the skin test or had radiographic findings consistent with systemic histoplasmosis infection. Twenty-two of 842 residents of Walkersville, Maryland,[21] had ocular histo spots, giving a prevalence rate of 2.6%. Davidorf and Anderson found the prevalence to be as high as 12.9% in an "Earth Day epidemic" in an endemic area.[27] POHS has a prevalence of 0.5% among the blind in endemic areas of Tennessee.[28]

Incidence

Little is known about the overall incidence of ocular histoplasmosis, even in endemic areas in the United States, because most of the lesions are asymptomatic. POHS causes significant central visual impairment in at least 2000 young and middle-aged adults in the United States each year.[29] It is estimated that 1 adult in 40,000 in Tennessee will become legally blind from untreated POHS-related maculopathy.[28] In this endemic area, POHS has an annual incidence of 2.8% among the blind.[28]

Age

Vision-threatening disciform ocular histoplasmosis is a disease of young adults in their thirties and forties, significantly more common in the population from 30 to 39 years of age. It is thought that asymptomatic ocular involvement by histoplasmosis in the form of atrophic chorioretinal scars occurs in early life but remains undetected until it becomes symptomatic or is detected on a routine eye examination. The median age of 36 is considered the most reliable estimate.[30]

Hawkins and Ganley,[31] in an epidemiologic study conducted in Washington County, Maryland, determined that the 15-year risk of visual impairment and blindness appears to be higher among adults aged 30 years and older who have only peripheral atrophic scars of POHS than among individuals living in the same endemic community but without such scars.

Sex and Race

Ocular histoplasmosis presenting as atrophic peripheral and/or monocular macular scars is seen equally in men and women and in blacks and whites. But the disciform macular type of histoplasmosis is more commonly seen in whites, and considerably less commonly in blacks,[32, 33] and bilateral macular involvement is seen more frequently in men than in women.[34]

Involvement of the Second Eye

The incidence of the development of a symptomatic disciform lesion in the second eye is considerable. The reported annual incidence of ocular histoplasmosis in the second eye varies from 1.7%,[35] to 2%,[36] to 12%,[37] based on 40, 25, and 105 patients followed for a mean of 13, 10, and 2 years, respectively, in young adults. Older adults who already have a disciform lesion in one eye because of POHS are at low risk of developing a disciform lesion in the fellow eye later in life.[31]

Histocompatibility Antigens

Histocompatibility antigen analysis in POHS patients suggests a potential immunogenetic predisposition for development of histo spots and disciform macular lesions. Godfrey and colleagues[38] and Braley and associates[39] found an association of human leukocyte antigen (HLA)-B7 with macular histoplasmosis lesions, with a relative risk of 11.8. There is no association of this antigen with peripheral histo spots. Another antigen, HLA-DRw2, has been found to have some apparent association with disciform macular lesions[40] as well as in patients with exclusively peripheral histo spots.[41] Both B7[38, 39] and DRw2[40] are two to four times more common among patients with macular disciform lesions, and DRw2[40] is twice as common among patients with only peripheral histo spots than among control populations. It is hypothesized that expression of both the B7 and the DRw2 alleles may predispose patients to exudative maculopathy and macular scarring. Another interesting observation is that POHS in black patients with disciform lesions shows no B7 association but a strong correlation with DRw2 when compared with control populations.[32]

In a recent study, immunophenotyping in POHS-like retinopathy has revealed no significant preferential expression.[42] Analysis of the T-cell receptor variable region and HLA typing have failed to reveal any links. All lymphocyte markers were unremarkable, with the exception of CD38, which was significantly raised compared with controls.[42] A type of multifocal choroiditis with panuveitis mimics POHS[25, 43] and occurs in nonendemic areas of the United States.[25] The clinical features of this entity resemble those of POHS, but the immunologic responses to histoplasma antigen do not.[25] These findings suggest that POHS seen in endemic areas and POHS-like retinopathy seen in nonendemic areas probably have different etiologic origins and are two different entities.[22–25]

CLINICAL CHARACTERISTICS

A triad of disseminated choroiditis (histo spots), maculopathy (macular chorioretinal or disciform scar), and peripapillary chorioretinal degenerative changes (atrophic and pigmentary changes) constitutes the classic syndrome of presumed ocular histoplasmosis. Another characteristic finding of "clear vitreous" has been added to the syndrome; that is, the disorder is not accompanied by inflammation resulting in inflammatory cells in the vitreous. This constellation of clinical findings that identifies POHS has remained essentially unchanged since its original description. At present, the clinical appearance of POHS includes multiple, small, atrophic, punched-out chorioretinal scars in the mid periphery and posterior pole (the histo spots), linear peripheral atrophic tracks or streaks of such scars, and peripapillary chorioretinal degeneration with or without choroidal neovascularization (CNV) in the macula. These discrete focal lesions occur frequently in both eyes without anterior segment or vitreous inflammation. These findings in a white, 20 to 50 years of age, who has lived in or visited the histoplasmosis endemic areas of the United States, and who may be HLA-B7 positive (for macular disease) further support the diagnosis of POHS.[44]

Disseminated Choroiditis

Disseminated choroiditis usually goes undetected because of its asymptomatic peripheral lesions. It manifests as mild choroidal inflammation that is self-limiting, and as it heals it leaves behind histo spots. Rarely, choroiditis can cause photopsia by irritating the contiguous rods and cones. In the active acute stage, choroiditis lesions appear as small, yellowish gray, raised spots, scattered in the periequatorial region or posterior to the equator. The overlying retina may have a slight ground-glass–like haze from tissue swelling. These lesions resemble, and should be differentiated from, the nodules of miliary tuberculosis, sarcoidosis, nocardiosis, coccidioidomycosis, and cryptococcosis.

Histo Spots

Disseminated choroiditis produces the typical histo spots. These are small, circular, depigmented, and atrophic chorioretinal scars, measuring about 0.2 to 0.7 disc diameter in size, and they may have a pigment clump in the center.[30] On average, these number between four to eight per eye, but the range is from 0 to 70. In two thirds of the cases, these spots are bilateral and randomly distributed throughout the mid periphery and posterior to the equator of all quadrants of the fundus (Fig. 28–1*A,B*). This might suggest hematogenous dissemination of the fungus or its antigen to the eye, because the greater number of scars occurs in areas of greater blood supply.[30] In the acute stage, a slight yellowish swelling of the choroid and overlying retina gives a ground-glass–like haze to the retina and produces ill-defined edges to the spots (Fig. 28–1*C*). In the atrophic stage, the spots look punched-out, with sharp edges, round or oval in shape, and with slight depression of the retinal pigment epithelium and choroid (Fig. 28–1*D*). The atrophic changes make the underlying choroidal vessels infrequently visualized

through these spots. Similar-looking lesions have been reproduced in animal models after intravenous injection of *H. capsulatum*.[45]

Based on their clinical photographic appearance, the histo spots have been classified as typical or atypical.[46] Typical histo spots are atrophic lesions, representing the inactive scar lesion, that have distinct borders, a punched-out appearance, and a uniformly flat or excavated bottom (Fig. 28–1*A* and *D*). Atypical histo spots, representing the acute active lesions, are creamy yellow lesions (Fig. 28–1*C*) that are hyperfluorescent on fluorescein angiograms, with less distinct borders and a slightly elevated rather than an excavated appearance.[46] It has been suggested that atypical histo spots in the macula may be more likely sites of development of subsequent CNV than are typical punched-out atrophic scars.[46]

Linear Streaks

In 5% of POHS patients, histo spots occur in the equatorial ocular region arranged in a linear pattern, or streaks, running parallel to the ora serrata.[47, 48] This finding is a fourth sign of the syndrome. These streaks consist of hypopigmented and hyperpigmented, circumlinear, peripheral chorioretinal scars, which are clumps of histo spots arranged in linear fashion (Fig. 28–2). These streaks have also been seen in the multifocal choroiditis and panuveitis syndrome that can in some respects mimic POHS,[43] and in pathologic myopia.[22, 49]

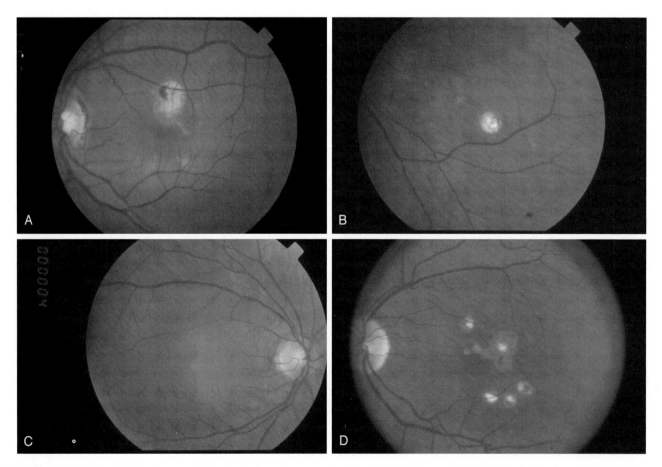

FIGURE 28–1. *A*, Color fundus photograph illustrating juxtafoveal punched-out typical "histo spot." *B*, Peripheral "histo spot" in the same eye. *C*, Ground-glass–like macular "atypical histo spot" with ill-defined edges. *D*, Multiple macular "histo spots" in another patient. (See Color insert.)

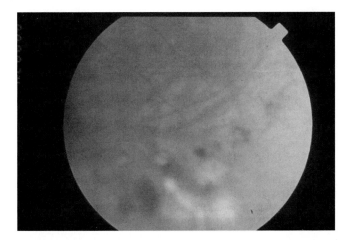

FIGURE 28-2. Color fundus photograph illustrating a clump of histo spots arranged in linear fashion in peripheral retina to constitute linear streaks. (See Color insert.)

Peripapillary Chorioretinal Degeneration/Choroiditis/Atrophic Scarring/Pigment Changes

Peripapillary chorioretinal degeneration, pigment changes, and atrophic scarring, presumably caused by an underlying choroiditis, are frequent diagnostic findings in the majority of patients with POHS. An atrophic depigmented area surrounds a pigmented crescent around the optic nerve head (Fig. 28–3A to C). These are asymptomatic lesions that appear as enlarged blind spots on perimetry. Rarely, these lesions appear to be nodular and can harbor subretinal neovascular membranes. The subretinal CNV can spontaneously bleed (Fig. 28–3D). Resultant hemorrhagic episodes because of CNV make these lesions symptomatic in 11% of POHS patients. The hemorrhage surrounds the disc in most cases. Occasionally, it is limited to the nasal or temporal side. Subretinal hemorrhage leads to a detachment of the sensory retina that may extend into the macula and cause loss of vision (Fig. 28–3D). Peripapillary chorioretinal degeneration is seen in both eyes in about 70% of patients who have associated macular disease, and in an additional 15% of patients in only one eye.[50] Peripapillary degenerative and atrophic pigment changes are seen in only 18% to 28% of patients who have just the peripheral histo spots and no macular involvement.[30]

Clear Vitreous

Presumed ocular histoplasmosis does not cause associated vitreous inflammation. Clear vitreous is an important and integral part of the clinical appearance of POHS.[51] Only rarely are cells ever seen in either the anterior chamber or the vitreous humor. When vitreous cells are seen, other entities, such as multifocal choroiditis and panuveitis syndrome, should be considered.

Maculopathy

Most patients with POHS are diagnosed incidentally and are asymptomatic. Although usually a benign syndrome, POHS becomes symptomatic because of recurrence or reactivation of macular lesions. The symptoms include waviness or distortion of linear contours, metamorphopsia, macropsia, and micropsia. The symptoms are similar to those of age-related macular degeneration, ocular migraine, and central serous choroidopathy. Patients with POHS often can tell when a recurrence or reactivation is beginning, before the signs become manifest enough for the ophthalmologist to see them.

CNV in the macula can cause a sudden, abrupt decrease in central vision if the underlying CNV pushes the retina upward because of blood, fluid, or lipid deposits, giving the retina a gray-green, ground-glass appearance. Before the introduction of fluorescein angiography, CNV could not be differentiated from retinal pigment epithelial detachment and central serous choroidopathy. Probably for that reason, retinal pigment epithelial (RPE) detachment and central serous choroidopathy were reported in 7% and more frequent hemorrhagic macular lesions were reported in 63% of patients.[52] Rarely, it may have associated vitreous hemorrhage.[53] In POHS eyes, the patients with macular histo spots have a 1 in 4 chance of recurrence in the macula over the ensuing 3 years. However, if no macular histo spots are present, then the chances of recurrence in the macula are only about 1 in 50.[54] It seems that atypical histo spots are more prone to develop CNV than regular atrophic typical histo spots.[46] Recurrence or reactivation of macular lesion leads to severe visual impairment in 60% of the involved eyes, and only 10% to 15% of eyes maintain 20/20 vision after a 2-year period.

An asymptomatic macular lesion in POHS may occur as an atrophic punched-out pigmented scar similar to the regular histo spot (see Fig. 28–1A). But the more commonly seen lesion that causes debilitating visual loss is a raised, heaped-up fibrovascular scar, referred to as a disciform macular scar (Fig. 28–4). It develops as a result of hemorrhagic retinal detachment and CNV. At times, CNV is difficult to diagnose on biomicroscopic exam alone because of absence of hemorrhage or pigmentation.[55] Rarely, subretinal neovascularization leading to disciform scar has been seen in the absence of previous pigmentary changes. This denotes a nidus of activity[56] and invisible foci of choroidal inflammation in this disorder.[57]

The active disciform lesions appear to arise at the edge of old lesions,[33] producing recurrence or the reactivation of the old atrophic scars. Therefore, the development of a disciform macular lesion in the second eye depends on whether there are old atrophic macular histo scars or not. In the absence of macular scars, the risk of a symptomatic lesion in the fellow eye is less than 1% per year of follow-up.[36, 58]

Submacular neovascularization in POHS leads to exudative maculopathy and macular detachment or swelling that heals with disciform scarring in the macular area. Visual loss is secondary to these macular changes. It is estimated that 1 in 1000 adults in an endemic area has disciform macular scarring in one eye,[21, 54] and 1 in 10 affected patients has bilateral macular scarring[54] from POHS. One third of the patients diagnosed as having POHS develop bilateral CNV or disciform lesions within 1 to 7 years of follow-up.[59] According to one estimate, POHS causes significant visual impairment in at least 2000 young and middle-aged adults in the United States

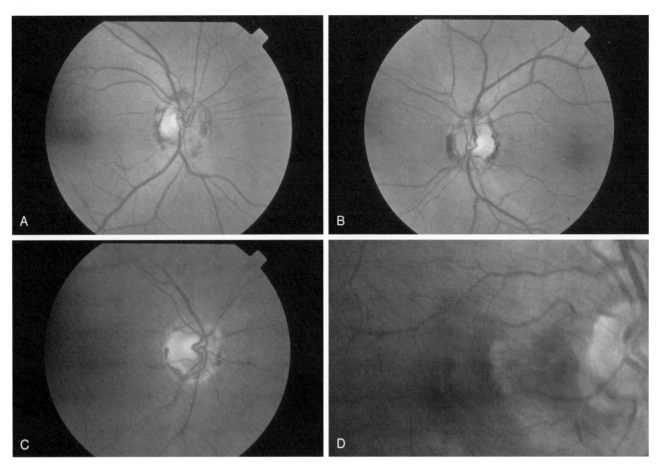

FIGURE 28–3. *A,* and *B,* Color fundus photographs illustrating bilateral peripapillary chorioretinal degeneration in POHS. *C,* Peripapillary chorioretinal degeneration in another patient. *D,* Peripapillary CNV causing subretinal hemorrhage extending into the macular area. (See Color insert.)

each year.[60] Untreated subretinal CNV within the foveal avascular zone leads to a final visual acuity of less than or equal to 20/200 in two thirds of patients.[61]

The risk of developing a disciform macular lesion has been reported to be as high as 25% when the atrophic scars are present in the macular region. This risk is reported to be only 1 in 50 if no macular scars are noted in POHS.[59] It has been well documented that 50% to

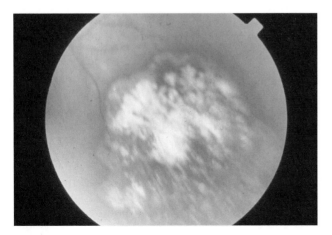

FIGURE 28–4. Color fundus photograph illustrating disciform macular scar in POHS. (See Color insert.)

70% of untreated eyes have significant central visual loss (i.e., a final visual acuity of 20/200 or worse).[29, 62] About 10% to 16% of patients with macular CNV, who are under 30 years of age, who have small submacular membranes with small involvement of the foveal avascular zone, and who have no vision loss in the other eye retain good functional vision (i.e., 20/40 or better).[29, 62]

Overall, the eyes with POHS carry excellent visual prognosis, except for the ones with macular lesions. Asymptomatic eyes without any ophthalmoscopic or angiographic evidence of focal macular or paramacular chorioretinal scars carry an excellent visual prognosis in patient with POHS.[33] The high risk of developing a neovascular membrane in the contralateral eye, at the rate of 8% to 24% over a 3-year period,[63, 64] justifies periodic examination and Amsler grid testing in patients with macular POHS lesions. De novo CNV can develop in areas without preexisting atrophic histo spots or pigmentary lesions.[56, 65–70] Even patients without pre-existing macular lesions have a certain risk of developing CNV.[10]

Spontaneous Improvement of Visual Acuity

An interesting phenomenon of spontaneous improvement of visual acuity in 10 of 700 patients with POHS has been reported[71] and may follow active exudation.[72–75] Eleven of 12 patients who developed reactivation of inflammatory lesions had resolution of the foci, documented by fluorescein angiography, with lessening of symptoms and improvement of visual acuity,[76] despite the presence of CNV[72] and macular scarring secondary to the CNV.[29, 77, 78] This appears to be related to spontaneous involution of CNV. Visual recovery may also occur by development of eccentric fixation[79] or by reversal of an organic amblyopia with disappearance of central scotoma.[71] Visual improvement has been seen in response to corticosteroid treatment,[58, 80] laser photocoagulation[46, 48, 63, 64, 73–75, 81–90] and submacular surgery.[91–95]

According to one study, 14% of eyes with active CNV, including some with foveal membranes, retained a visual acuity of 20/40 or better over a follow-up period that ranged from 12 to 109 months.[62] A pigment ring forms around the fibrovascular membrane and changes the leaking membrane to one that stains with fluorescein but does not leak.[72] The pigment ring and fibrosis contain the hemorrhaging and leaking vessels, and the subretinal fluid resolves with time, thereby producing spontaneous visual improvement.

It is well documented that 7% of patients with subfoveal, subretinal neovascularization in POHS eyes have spontaneous visual improvement without any treatment.[91] As stated, it has also been documented that in many cases there is spontaneous involution of the subretinal CNV and excellent visual recovery without any treatment.[72] Patients who are young, who have good initial visual acuity at the time of ocular involvement, who have less than 50% of the foveal avascular zone involved in the process, and in whom the membrane extends less than 200 μm beyond the center of the foveal avascular zone have a good visual prognosis.[29]

Disappearing Lesions

The histo spots have been observed to enlarge in size and increase in number over a period of time. Similarly, the spots have been observed to decrease in size and even disappear. In a prospective clinical study, 12 patients developed active inflammatory lesions; 11 had spontaneous resolution of the foci with lessening of symptoms and improvement in visual acuity and fluorescein angiographic findings.[76] One of these 12 patients developed typical CNV about 8 months after the onset of symptoms.[76] The phenomenon of disappearing lesions has been well documented by both clinical and fluorescein angiographic examinations in animal models.[10, 96]

PATHOGENESIS/PATHOPHYSIOLOGY/ IMMUNOLOGY/PATHOLOGY

It is not known with certainty when and how the primary infection with *H. capsulatum* occurs in human beings. Indeed, it is not even certain that all cases with the clinical characteristics of POHS were ever even exposed to the microbe. One might logically speculate that exposure to other microbes could provoke the identical clinical response in a genetically susceptible individual, hence the appearance of the POHS picture in patients in England, Holland, and elsewhere.[22–25, 48] It is believed that primary infection is acquired early in life, probably during childhood to adolescence, through inhalation of microconidia (small spores) and/or macroconidia (large

spores). It begins as asymptomatic, systemic infection with the organism in the overwhelming majority of cases. Some patients develop a mild upper respiratory infection.

The spore form of the fungus changes to its yeast phase within lung tissue. It spreads to other parts of the body via the blood stream. The organisms are entrapped in the reticuloendothelial tissues; dead or latent *H. capsulatum* cells are found in numerous organs at autopsy or as calcified spots on radiologic examinations.[68] Ocular histoplasmosis, however, does not become apparent until 10 to 30 years later.[97] POHS rarely follows disseminated infection with *H. capsulatum* or chronic pulmonary histoplasmosis. The foci with dead or latent organisms later become sources themselves of subsequent asymptomatic transient episodes of *H. capsulatum* fungemia. Such episodes of fungemia may eventually seed the choroid to produce a multifocal granulomatous chorioretinitis that heals as atrophic histo scars as the host response rapidly destroys the organism.[98–101]

Hematogenous spread of *H. capsulatum* to the eye could explain its frequent bilaterality, the number and random distribution of histo spots throughout the fundus,[30, 33] and the changing pattern of peripheral atrophic histo spots over many years.[66–68, 102] Inflammatory injury caused by *H. capsulatum*–induced chorioretinitis leads to damage to Bruch's membrane, RPE, and choriocapillaris. That may result in an atrophic scar, CNV formation, or exudative retinal detachment. The development of subretinal hemorrhage from either CNV or direct damage to the RPE or choriocapillaris persists for a while but eventually heals as a fibrovascular scar. The findings in animal models have been observed clinically in the development of disciform maculopathy contiguous to atrophic scars in individuals with POHS.[33, 100]

The reasons for abnormal vascular proliferation in the macular region are still unknown. It may be the unique anatomic characteristics of the macular tissue that induce a unique wound-healing response to injury caused by *H. capsulatum*. Also, as mentioned, based on the histocompatibility data, there seems to be a certain predisposition to develop atrophic scars (histo spots) rather than disciform lesions in the macula. HLA-B7–positive individuals are more predisposed to develop macular disciform lesions than peripheral atrophic chorioretinal scars.[39] HLA-DRw2–positive patients are more predisposed to have macular disciform or only peripheral lesions.[41] Similarly, the initial response to primary fungal infection is different from the reactivation or re-exposure to the histoplasma antigens. Initially, the lesions are small and, most of the time, subclinical. However, re-exposure to histoplasma antigens induces vascular proliferation and symptomatic disciform lesions surrounding an atrophic scar.[33]

Other hypotheses proposed to explain the ocular response in POHS have included (1) larger initial inoculum of the fungus,[103, 104] (2) reinfection,[16, 105] (3) hypersensitivity,[16, 97] and (4) the presence of other risk factors that compromise the vascular system[106, 107] or the immune system.[108]

Animal Studies

Much effort has been devoted to develop an adequate animal model of POHS in producing ocular lesions comparable to those seen in humans. Histoplasmosis occurs naturally as choroiditis in cats and as retinitis in dogs.[109] Initial animal experiments met with disappointment because intraocular inoculation of *H. capsulatum* in animals generally produced acute anterior segment inflammation, extensive vitreous clouding, or some other features that were not characteristic of human POHS.[110] Success was achieved only by the use of intravenous or intracarotid inoculations of *H. capsulatum* to produce acute choroiditis lesions that spontaneously and relatively rapidly resolved into lesions typical of human POHS, including peripapillary scarring, RPE defects, and punched-out atrophic histo spots, as well as "disappearing lesion," and minimal inflammatory reaction.[99] Hemorrhagic maculopathy has not been produced in animal models.[110] Subretinal neovascularization was observed in one eye of a nonhuman primate 1 year after injection with the organism.[111] This lesion was not seen with fluorescein angiography, presumably because of the presence of tight junctions and therefore no leakage.[111]

It is important to understand that the organisms have not been demonstrated by culture or special stains in lesions present for longer than 6 weeks.[99] A feature common to all eyes studied, including those whose lesions were clinically inactive or had clinically disappeared, was the persistence of small foci of lymphocytes in the choroid. Damage to Bruch's membrane was observed in some specimens. It is postulated that these occult foci of lymphocytes appear beneath an intact and normal-appearing RPE–Bruch's membrane complex and retina, in areas where clinically disappearing lesions had been. They provide the potential site and source for reactivation of the so-called de novo lesions that can appear to arise from normal retina in humans with POHS.[99] The persistence of these chronic inflammatory cells and foci, and not the organisms, throughout the choroid of apparently healed eyes leads to "new" lesions and subretinal CNV.[99, 110]

DIAGNOSIS

The diagnosis of POHS is essentially a clinical one, depending on the clinical appearance of characteristic punched-out histo spots in one or both eyes, peripapillary degeneration, pigment changes and histo scars, and linear tracks and streaks in the equatorial region, with or without macular atrophic or disciform scar. The syndrome has not fulfilled the requirements of Koch's postulates, and the dimorphic fungal organism has never been cultured from an individual with POHS or isolated from an eye with classical lesions of POHS. Instead, epidemiologic and skin testing evidence has been used to implicate this fungus as the etiologic agent of POHS. The definite etiology of POHS remains unproven.[2] Ocular lesions identical to POHS have been seen in patients in the United Kingdom, Europe, and elsewhere where *H. capsulatum* is not endemic and patients do not have any other signs of systemic infection.[22–25]

Two tests that were done in the past to diagnose POHS but are not performed any more are the histoplasmin skin test and the histoplasma complement fixation test. The histoplasmin skin test is diagnostic of POHS. The reactivity to histoplasmin antigen usually appears early after exposure to the fungus and persists for a lifetime. It is negative in 11% of patients who have clinically typical POHS. At one time, it was considered the most valuable measure for the laboratory diagnosis of ocular histoplasmosis, but it is not performed today because of the risk of flare-up of a maculopathy, seen in 7% of patients who may have visible or invisible previous macular lesions. The complement fixation test for circulating antibodies against histoplasmin antigen has not been of much value in supporting the diagnosis because of its poor seropositivity. It is seropositive in only one third of patients with typical histoplasmosis choroiditis.[48]

The following tests may help to support the diagnosis of POHS.

Chest X-Ray

X-ray examination of the chest may show calcified lesions because of primary disseminated histoplasmosis infection. These findings in the presence of typical ocular signs of POHS in the eye(s) confirm the diagnosis. Similar calcific lesions are seen also in pulmonary tuberculosis, sarcoidosis, and some fungal infections.

HLA Typing

As mentioned previously, the prevalence of histocompatibility antigens HLA-B7 and HLA-DRw2 among cases of POHS suggests a genetic predisposition for the development of peripheral histo spots and disciform macular scarring. Immunophenotyping in POHS-like retinopathy has revealed no significant preferential expression,[42] and these analyses might be of help in differentiating POHS from POHS-like retinopathy. Similar observations have been reported from the nonendemic northwestern United States.[25]

DIFFERENTIAL DIAGNOSIS

The confluent type of circumpapillary choroiditis, white dots, pigment changes, scarring, and macular lesions may be confused with the following manifestations:

Myopic Crescent. A myopic crescent is a pale crescent outside the scleral ring, usually on the temporal side, but it may become annular. It is usually bilateral. The thin pigment rim lies on its outer edge and not inside the crescent. Foster-Fuchs spots are degenerative macular lesions that could progress to disciform detachment. The atrophic scars are whiter, more punched out or scalloped, and located only near the posterior pole (unlike histo spots). The macular involvement occurs around age 30 to 50 years, and the eyes are myopic between −3D to −25D.

Senile Halo. A senile halo usually forms a yellow-red or pale red crescent on the temporal side of the optic nerve head in the elderly as an aging change, and it is usually bilateral.

Inferior Crescent. An inferior crescent is a white or yellow-white lesion, has a uniform border, is often slightly raised over the surrounding tissue, and has a thin rim of pigment on the outer rim beyond which the choroid itself is thinned.

Peripapillary Choroidal Coloboma. An atypical, minimal, peripapillary choroidal coloboma can rarely lead to retinal detachment and can mimic findings of active histoplasmosis choroiditis. Coloboma can be distinguished from histo lesions by stereoscopic fundus photography and fluorescein angiography.[112]

Optic Nerve Drusen. Drusen of the optic nerve head are usually bilateral, glistening, raised lesions occurring over the disc surface and not on the disc margin, seen in younger patients in their teens and twenties, and there is usually a family history of drusen. The clinical appearance of drusen may simulate that of papillitis or papilledema. Drusen of the optic nerve may cause nerve fiber bundle defect on visual field examination. Rarely, drusen may cause hemorrhagic retinal detachment that may spread from nerve head to the macular area,[113] and it becomes even harder to distinguish drusen from peripapillary histo scars. Usually, other histo spots do not accompany drusen, except in endemic areas coincidentally.

Multifocal Choroiditis and Panuveitis (MCP). MCP presents initially with small and discrete inflammatory lesions at the level of the choroid and RPE, along with little or no vitreous inflammation. Within weeks or a few months, patients with multifocal choroiditis routinely develop new spots on follow-up, have prominent vitreous inflammation, and often have progressive visual loss. There could be acute antibody production to Epstein-Barr virus in patients with multifocal choroiditis.

Multiple Evanescent White Dot Syndrome (MEWDS). MEWDS has widely scattered, active gray-white lesions, early punctate and an often wreath-shaped pattern of hyperfluorescence in the area of activity, and a decrease in the electroretinogram α-wave. The fundus and visual functions return to normal in 7 to 10 weeks.

Acute Posterior Multifocal Placoid Pigment Epitheliopathy (APMPPE). APMPPE presents as acute loss of vision occurring in one or both eyes of young people of either sex, with spontaneous recovery in a few weeks. Classically, circumscribed yellow-white lesions occur in the fundus at the level of the RPE. Initially, these lesions are hypofluorescent on fluorescein angiography; later they hyperfluoresce. There is a wide spectrum of presentation and clinical features of APMPPE.

Punctate Inner Choroidopathy (PIC). PIC is a disease that affects the choroid and RPE and is most common in young women. The acute lesions are small (100 to 300 μm), yellow, and moderately well defined. The lesions gradually become more atrophic and form deep cylindrical and discrete scars. Pigmented tissue occasionally fills the center of the cylindrical scar, making it appear less deep. There could be associated shallow serous retinal detachments over the PIC lesions without neovascularization, and these detachments gradually resolve. Patients with PIC have acute symptoms of blurred vision, flickering lights, and scotomas. In the acute phases of the disease, the patients can often outline scotomas that correspond to individual lesions. These acute lesions are hyperfluorescent in the early phase and then gradually leak in the late phase.

Angioid Streaks. Angioid streaks are fundus findings in collagen tissue disorders such as pseudoxanthoma elasticum, senile elastosis, osteitis deformans, and Ehlers-Denlos syndrome. Peau d'orange skin changes precede fundus changes of angioid streaks in these conditions. The salmon-colored spots very closely resemble histo spots and may also have disciform macular detachment.

Rarely, drusen of the optic nerve may also be associated findings, along with angioid streaks.

Granulomatous Fundus Lesions. Ocular presentations of toxoplasmosis, tuberculosis, coccidioidomycosis, syphilis, sarcoidosis, and toxocariasis may mimic granulomas and scarring seen in POHS. Clear vitreous without any signs of inflammation such as keratic precipitates, flare and cells, vitreous cells, and cotton-balls in vitreous distinguish POHS from the other granulomatous fundus conditions.

TREATMENT

Laser Photocoagulation

Maumenee and Ryan[87] and Watzke and Leaverton[90] were the first to suggest the use of laser photocoagulation to treat POHS using xenon-arc photocoagulation.[88, 90, 113] In 1979, the Macular Photocoagulation Study (MPS) group, sponsored by the National Eye Institute, initiated its first prospective randomized multicenter controlled clinical trial, called the Ocular Histoplasmosis Study (OHS). The purpose of this trial was to determine whether argon laser photocoagulation was beneficial in preventing severe visual acuity loss in eyes with CNV secondary to POHS. The data from this study demonstrated definite effectiveness of argon laser photocoagulation in treating such membranes.[73] After an 18-month follow-up, it was demonstrated that only 9.4% of laser-treated eyes (11 of 117) had lost six lines or more of visual acuity from the baseline as compared with 34.2% of untreated eyes (39 of 114).[73] Based on these encouraging results from the OHS, the MPS group recommended laser photocoagulation to be the treatment of choice in treating subretinal CNV.[73]

For better selection of patients undergoing laser treatment, the subretinal neovascular membranes are classified[29, 73] according to their location as follows:

1. Subfoveal membranes are the well-defined subretinal neovascular membranes that have fluorescein angiographic evidence of neovascularization extending under the center of the foveal avascular zone (FAZ), with or without a pigment ring, blocked fluorescence, or blood (Fig. 28–5*A* and *B*).
2. Juxtafoveal membranes are the well-defined subretinal neovascular membranes that have fluorescein angiographic evidence of neovascularization extending to 1 to 200 μm from the center of the FAZ, with or without pigment ring, blocked fluorescence, or blood extending closer or through the center of the fovea: The term also refers to a neovascular membrane more than 200 μm from the center of the FAZ and a pigment ring, blocked fluorescence, or blood extending up to 200 μm from the FAZ.
3. Extrafoveal choroidal neovascularization membranes (CNV) are the neovascular membranes that have the fluorescein angiographic evidence of the neovascularization extending more than 200 μm from the center of the membrane and no continuous pigment ring, blocked fluorescence, or blood.

Extrafoveal Laser Photocoagulation

The eligibility criteria for the patients in the OHS included well-defined extrafoveal CNV that had a foveal or

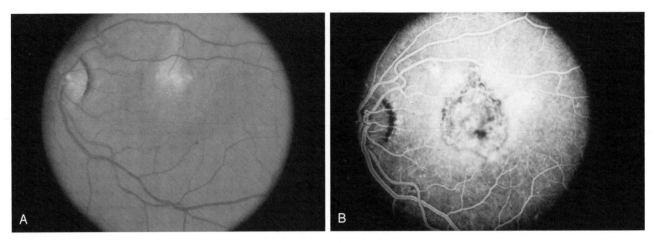

FIGURE 28–5. *A*, Color photograph illustrating macular choroidal neovascularization (CNV) in POHS. *B*, Fluorescein angiogram of the same eye to show CNV. (See Color insert.)

posterior edge more than 200 μm and up to 2500 μm away from the center of the FAZ, and a visual acuity in the affected eye of at least 20/100 or better. Other signs of POHS were also present in the affected eyes. The visual symptoms of subretinal CNV were decreased visual acuity, distortion on Amsler grid chart, uniocular diplopia, or metamorphopsia. Eligible eyes were randomized to argon laser treatment or to no treatment (the control group). After laser treatment, the eyes were re-examined twice a year to check visual acuity and to take colored photographs. Each eye had fluorescein angiography performed preoperatively, 6 and 12 months postoperatively, and annually thereafter.

About 4 years after initiating this study, it was concluded by the MPS Data and Safety Monitoring Committee that argon laser photocoagulation was beneficial in preventing or delaying loss of visual acuity secondary to POHS, and no further patients were enrolled. The data gathered by the MPS group from 242 subjects (and 245 eyes) enrolled over a 4-year period demonstrated that the untreated eyes with extrafoveal CNV due to POHS had a 2.3 times greater risk of losing six or more lines of visual acuity when compared with laser-treated eyes.[73] On the MPS chart, a loss of six lines of visual acuity from the initial baseline (rather than final visual acuity) was equivalent to a fourfold increase in the minimal angle of resolution or visual angle.

These encouraging results met with some pessimism when a large percentage (26%) of treated eyes developed recurrent neovascularization; 31 of the 40 recurrences were contiguous to a previously treated area. Also, new areas of CNV not contiguous to the laser scars developed in another 7% of laser-treated eyes.[75] Most recurrences were seen early, about 22% occurring within 6 months, the figure increasing to only about 28% 2 years after treatment.[63] Despite these recurrences, the laser-treated eyes had significantly improved visual outcome compared with the untreated eyes. Long-term follow-up of 3 years revealed that the eyes with recurrences had an average visual acuity of 20/60. These results were far superior to the natural course of the disease, and reinforced the beneficial effect of argon laser photocoagulation.

In 1991, the MPS group reported its 5-year results of

laser photocoagulation treatment for extrafoveal CNV secondary to POHS.[75] The group upheld its earlier recommendation that laser photocoagulation was beneficial in preventing severe visual loss from POHS. Untreated eyes had 3.6 times the risk of severe visual loss that laser-treated eyes had. Only 12% of laser-treated eyes demonstrated a decrease in visual acuity of six lines or more from baseline visual acuity, compared with 42% of untreated eyes.[75]

Juxtafoveal Laser Photocoagulation

The second trial by the MPS group was initiated in 1981 to evaluate the efficacy of krypton red laser photocoagulation in treating juxtafoveal neovascular disciform lesions secondary to POHS. Krypton laser treatment of POHS-related CNV had been found effective in previous studies.[114–116] The eligibility criteria for this study included patients who had neovascular lesions of POHS with the foveal or posterior edge inside the FAZ but still not subfoveal. Precisely, it meant that the foveal-edge CNV was 1 to 199 μm from the center of the foveal avascular zone, or 200 μm or more from the center of the FAZ with blood and/or blocked fluorescence within 200 μm of the center of the FAZ. These eyes were randomized for either krypton laser treatment or no laser treatment (the control group).

One-year follow-up showed that only 6.6% of laser-treated eyes (8 of 121) had lost six or more lines of visual acuity as compared with 24.8% of untreated eyes (31 of 125). By 3 years after randomization, the corresponding values were 4.6% (3 of 64) and 24.6% (15 of 61). Based on these results, after a 4-year period in 1986, the MPS Data and Safety Monitoring Committee intervened, concluding from the accumulated data from 289 eyes enrolled that krypton laser–treated eyes were significantly less likely to lose visual acuity than were untreated eyes.[74] The 5-year follow-up revealed that only 12% of laser-treated versus 28% of untreated eyes had lost six or more lines from the baseline visual acuity.[83] The problem of persistent CNV contiguous with the laser-treated scar was again observed in a large percent (33%) of laser-treated eyes. New, noncontiguous areas of CNV developed in an additional 2% of eyes.[83]

Summarizing the findings from three randomized clinical trials of krypton laser treatment of juxtafoveal neovascular lesions revealed that untreated eyes with POHS had 2.6 times higher unadjusted estimated relative risk of losing 6 lines of visual acuity than laser-treated eyes from the 1-year through the 5-year examination period.[83] Accurate and complete krypton laser treatment of juxtafoveal CNV, particularly close to the foveal center, was found to lessen persistent CNV[81] and was required for the patient to have the best chance of avoiding further severe visual acuity loss.[85, 87]

The Canadian Ophthalmology Study group,[89] in a multicenter, randomized, controlled clinical trial, found krypton red laser photocoagulation to be *no* better than argon laser when treating well-defined extrafoveal CNV. Nevertheless, in a nonrandomized retrospective analysis over an average follow-up of 9.6 years, it was found that laser photocoagulation of POHS-related juxtafoveal and extrafoveal CNV had long-term benefits in preventing severe visual loss.[117] The results of this study revealed that the visual acuity of 20/40 or better was obtained in 71% of eyes laser-treated for extrafoveal CNV and 68% of eyes laser-treated for juxtafoveal CNV. Recurrent CNV was observed in 23% of laser-treated eyes during the mean follow-up of 9.6 years.[117]

Peripapillary Laser Photocoagulation

Results of laser treatment of extrafoveal or juxtafoveal peripapillary CNV, or CNV that was located nasal to the fovea, demonstrated beneficial effects after 3 years of follow-up.[85] After a 3-year follow-up of laser-treated and untreated eyes with CNV nasal to the fovea or in the peripapillary area, 11% of the laser-treated eyes (6 of 54) versus 41% of the untreated eyes (21 of 51) had lost six or more lines of visual acuity. Among eyes with peripapillary CNV lesions, 14% of the treated eyes (3/22) versus 26% of the untreated eyes (6/23) had lost six or more lines of visual acuity after a 3-year follow-up. Among the eyes with nasal CNV lesions, 9% of the treated eyes (3/32) versus 54% of the untreated eyes (15/28) had lost six or more lines of visual acuity after 3 years of follow-up.

Thermal damage to the optic disc and papillomacular nerve bundle is a serious potential risk of laser treatment of peripapillary CNV and CNV lesions nasal to the fovea, respectively. However, based on these results, the MPS group recommended laser treatment for peripapillary CNV and CNV nasal to the fovea, because the risks of treatment were outweighed by the potential loss of vision caused by growth and extension of the membrane into the fovea.[85]

Subfoveal Laser Photocoagulation

Encouraged by these results, a pilot study was undertaken to evaluate the effectiveness of laser photocoagulation in treating subfoveal CNV.[118] However, there was difficulty in recruiting patients for this study because most of the eyes had already been treated before they could get to the advanced stage of subfoveal membranes. It was hypothesized that most of the CNV originated outside the fovea as extrafoveal or juxtafoveal membranes and were treated before they could grow into the subfoveal region. Only 25 patients were enrolled in this study, and they had a fairly short follow-up. Laser treatment of subfoveal CNV offers little benefit when compared to the natural history of the disease without treatment. Investigators were initially encouraged by the results of the MPS study for subfoveal treatment of age-related macular degeneration. The data from this study demonstrated that laser photocoagulation of subfoveal membranes neither caused marked decrease nor significant increase in vision in the eyes evaluated.[118] Nevertheless, laser treatment of subfoveal CNV would sacrifice central vision in 14% to 23% of eyes with POHS that, according to natural history studies, may retain vision of 20/40 or better.[118]

At present, laser photocoagulation is the treatment of choice in managing macular CNV.[73] Laser photocoagulation is performed to destroy the entire net of CNV (Fig 28–6A and B). Various studies have demonstrated that photocoagulation does not prevent recurrences of CNV, but it helps to dry up the active primary or recurrent lesions. CNV is suspected from a pigment ring, retinal detachment, and subretinal or retinal hemorrhage. The CNV is confirmed with fluorescein angiography before laser treatment. A recent angiogram is needed to localize the treatment area before performing the laser photocoagulation, because the CNV does change with time.[73]

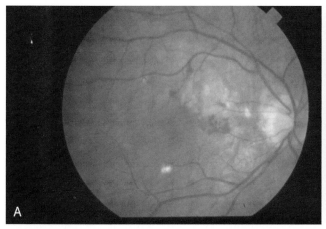 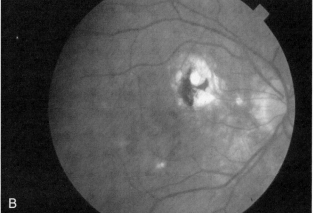

FIGURE 28–6. *A,* Macular CNV causing foveal/subfoveal hemorrhage. *B,* Same eye six months after laser photocoagulation treatment to extrafoveal CNV with persistent CNV inferotemporal to the foveal center.

Long burns achieve more effective closure of the neovascular membranes but are a higher risk to the fovea. The end point is a uniformly white ring of coagulation around the membrane to enclose it.[48, 73]

Laser Photocoagulation for Persistent or Recurrent CNV

Evaluation of MPS results indicated that additional laser treatment was required if fluorescein angiography revealed leakage from persisting or new vessels along or within the margin of the treatment scar.[73] Symptomatically, the laser photocoagulation may cause worsening of vision during the first week after treatment because of retinal swelling, which resolves with time. However, if the vision starts to worsen again, there is concern that the CNV has not been completely destroyed. Re-evaluation to make sure that all the CNV is destroyed is therefore essential. Immediately after laser treatment, the tissue coagulation blocks adequate assessment of CNV. Also, the extent of CNV is difficult to assess under retinal or choroidal hemorrhage. Therefore, it is recommended that all the area of hemorrhage be treated to ensure full treatment of the underlying CNV. The subretinal CNV that cannot be fully treated by photocoagulation carries a poor prognosis.[48]

Partial photocoagulation of subretinal CNV was thought to worsen the visual outcome because of stimulating the remaining CNV to proliferate and cause hemorrhaging.[119] Schlaegel[88] has refuted this observation. Even partial treatment of a CNV complex within 3 months of its start helps to reduce the size of retinal detachment and decrease the size of related scotoma, and the vision improves.[88]

Various protocols for the treatment of CNV associated with POHS have been suggested. Schlaegel advocated laser photocoagulation to begin at the end of the CNV distant from the fovea to determine the correct dosage of photocoagulation before moving around to the fovea side. The foveal edge of the CNV was treated with 0.2 seconds exposure time and 100-μm–sized severe burns. The rest of the CNV was treated with 0.5 seconds exposure time and 200-μm–sized burns.[48]

Laser Photocoagulation Protocol Used by the MPS Group

In the MPS study,[73] photocoagulation of CNV was performed using the argon blue-green laser. Fluorescein angiogram was obtained within 72 hours before treatment in each patient. Retrobulbar anesthesia was given to ensure immobility of the eyeball during treatment. The goal of treatment was to obliterate the neovascular complex. The treatment was begun by placing a noncontiguous row of 100-μm light-intensity burns 100 μm to 125 μm beyond the neovascular complex at durations of 0.1 to 0.2 seconds. The CNV complex included the hyperfluorescent new vessels and any adjacent blood, pigment, or blocked fluorescence. Once the CNV complex had been outlined, the foveal edge was treated with overlapping 200-μm burns at duration of 0.2 seconds. Treatment was continued by placing overlapping 200-μm burns along the entire perimeter of the complex. Treatment was completed by placing overlapping 200-μm to 500-μm lesions at duration of 0.5 seconds over the entire CNV complex. The final appearance was an intense white lesion.[73]

There were two important exceptions to this protocol. First, when the foveal edge of the CNV complex was within 350 μm of the center of the FAZ, the edge could be treated with overlapping 100-μm burns instead of 200-μm burns. Second, when the new vessel complex was 200 μm to 300 μm from the center of the FAZ, the intense lesion did not have to be extended a full 100 μm beyond the CNV complex. However, it was required that the entire complex be covered with intense coagulation.[73]

Additional laser treatment was performed when fluorescein leakage indicated new vessels along or within the margin of the treatment scar. It was not performed when new vessels recurred within 200 μm of the center of FAZ.[73]

Complications of Laser Photocoagulation

Laser photocoagulation is not a complication-free treatment for CNV in POHS. Scars from juxtafoveal laser photocoagulation have a tendency to expand and enlarge over time and involve the center of FAZ.[120] Argon laser–induced scars have been observed to expand toward the foveal avascular zone at a rate of 152 μm per year for the first 2 years after laser treatment and 22 μm per year thereafter.[120] After 10 years of follow-up, it has been found that the average scar was 3.23 times larger than the original treatment area. Argon laser has caused a macular hole formation in a patient with POHS.[120] Persistent or recurrent CNV contiguous with the laser treatment scar has been reported in 33% of laser-treated eyes,[82] and an additional 2% of eyes developed new noncontiguous areas of CNV.[82] Thermal damage to the disc and papillomacular bundle is an additional potential complication of laser photocoagulation of peripapillary CNV and CNV nasal to the fovea.[85]

Corticosteroids

Inactive and scarred lesions in POHS do not need any treatment until signs of reactivation. The use of systemic or periocular corticosteroids is advocated in patients with subfoveal neovascular membranes or CNV and reactivation of macular lesions. It has been recommended that high-dose oral corticosteroids be used immediately upon finding symptoms of macular lesions, with continuation until laser photocoagulation is administered.[122, 123]

The rationale for using systemic or periocular corticosteroids is based on the presence of lymphocytic infiltrates in POHS lesions[41, 65] and the persistent foci of lymphocytes in the choroid. These lesions represent persistent low-grade inflammatory foci and probably reactivate the previously inactive histo spots and de novo lesions. Anti-inflammatory agents probably limit the inciting stimulus as well as reduce the resulting reparative process that leads to scarring. Sub-Tenon injection of corticosteroids should be considered if symptomatic macular disease is present and no CNV can be detected, or, if it is detected, it is not treatable by laser because of its proximity to fovea or being subfoveal.[10]

On one hand, corticosteroids have been demonstrated in the past to have a beneficial effect in treating acute macular lesions and their reactivation, which can cause a sudden drop in visual acuity.[51] Prednisone 40 to 100 mg per day[80] to 50 to 120 mg every other day, by mouth, and long-acting steroid injections (40 mg of methylprednisolone acetate)[48] were started at the earliest signs that histo scar reactivation was threatening macular and central vision. On the other hand, it is felt that the final visual outcome is not affected by high-dose long-term steroid therapy once the CNV encroaches upon the foveal and juxtafoveal region.[29] In one study, with an average follow-up of 39 months, 81% of eyes treated with corticosteroids had visual acuity worse than 20/40 (6/12), and almost 70% of these were 20/200 (6/60) or worse.[29]

The beneficial role of corticosteroids has never been proven with controlled clinical trials. Corticosteroids do have a beneficial role in treating eyes that have POHS and CNV in the extrafoveal[73] and juxtafoveal[74] regions. Since the introduction of laser photocoagulation in managing extrafoveal and juxtafoveal lesions in POHS, the role of corticosteroids has diminished, and steroids are given only while preparing the patient for laser photocoagulation[51] or to patients who cannot have the laser treatment because of the proximity of CNV to fovea or when it is subfoveal.

Complications of Corticosteroids

Long-term use of oral corticosteroids carries its own side effects and complications. Repeated injections to the sub-Tenon carry risks of orbital infection, blepharoptosis, baggy eyelids, scleral melt, steroid-induced glaucoma, and posterior subcapsular cataract formation.[48]

Submacular/Subretinal Surgery

Surgical removal of CNV is now possible. Subretinal surgery was first performed in 1980 by Machemer,[92] but its application for removing CNV was introduced by Thomas and Kaplan in 1991.[95] Two patients with CNV caused by POHS (and resultant visual acuity of 20/400) were operated on successfully. After a short follow-up of 3 to 7 months, one patient recovered visual acuity to 20/20 and the second to 20/40.[95] This dramatic improvement in visual acuity has not been reported subsequently. Visual improvement by just two Snellen lines 1 week to 6 months after surgical removal of subfoveal CNV has been reported in 8 of 15 patients.[91] Also, recurrent neovascularization developed in 2 of the 15 eyes.[91]

Subretinal membranes have been classified as type I, in which the predominance of the CNV resides below the RPE, and type II, in which the CNV resides between the neurosensory retina and the RPE.[124] It is the latter type of CNV that appears most amenable to surgical extraction.[124] Thomas and coworkers have suggested two types of procedures on patients who have subfoveal CNV complex secondary to POHS.[94] Either the choroidal circulation to the neovascular membranes could be disconnected, or the choroidal neovascular complex could be extracted through the retinotomy site after performing vitrectomy.[94] Visual improvement by at least two Snellen lines was observed in 6 of 16 eyes followed 1 to 8 months and operated on by extraction of the CNV complex. None of the four eyes that had the membranes' choroidal circulation disconnected demonstrated any visual improvement.[123]

More recently, in a nonrandomized, uncontrolled, retrospective study with an average follow-up of 10.5 months, about 31% of 67 eyes with POHS-related subfoveal CNV achieved a visual acuity of 20/40 or better after undergoing subretinal surgery.[93] Eyes with better preoperative vision (>20/100) had significantly better final visual acuity than the eyes with poor preoperative vision (<20/200).[93] Recurrences of CNV were successfully treated with laser photocoagulation and thereby did not affect the final visual outcome.

Similarly, a retrospective review of 67 eyes that had surgical removal of subfoveal CNV caused by POHS demonstrated that the ingrowth site of subfoveal CNV could be identified in the majority of eyes, and that a significant number of eyes with subfoveal CNV have an extrafoveal ingrowth site. The eyes with an extrafoveal ingrowth site have a favorable visual prognosis after surgical removal of CNV. If the ingrowth site is subfoveal or not identifiable, the visual prognosis after surgery is guarded.[125]

In another retrospective study, visual recovery after submacular surgery in POHS was associated with postoperative perfusion of the subfoveal choriocapillaris.[126] The best-corrected visual acuity was an improvement of at least two Snellen lines in 71% of the perfused and 14% of nonperfused eyes. It remains to be seen if the development of techniques to maintain or re-establish perfusion of the subfoveal choriocapillaris after surgery could improve visual outcome in these eyes.[126] Another retrospective study demonstrated that the ingrowth site of subfoveal CNV was a predictor of visual outcome after submacular surgical excision of CNV.[125] If the ingrowth site of subfoveal CNV was extrafoveal, the surgical removal of CNV was favorable, but if the ingrowth site of CNV was subfoveal or not identifiable, the visual prognosis was guarded.[125]

Subretinal microsurgery is still in its infancy and going through its developmental stages. Initial encouraging results have not been consistently reproduced. Appropriate case selection and surgical timing of intervention to maximize visual benefits from submacular surgery still need to be defined. Several points need to be considered before deciding on subretinal or subfoveal surgery to remove CNV in POHS. First, all surgeons have stressed the importance of choosing the prospective patients very carefully. Submacular surgery is not for all patients with POHS, or perhaps even for most. Initial results of surgical removal of CNV in age-related maculopathy have not been impressive.[51] Patients may need replacement of their nonfunctioning or barely functioning RPE cells along with removal of subfoveal neovascular membrane. Second, surgical removal of subretinal or subfoveal neovascular membranes is followed by a high recurrence rate and the results do not outweigh the results of other therapeutic modalities, especially laser photocoagulation.[51] Third, and finally, a confounding point is the spontaneous regression of neovascular membranes in some patients with POHS, particularly in the young who happen to be good candidates for surgery.[51]

A randomized, controlled, prospective, multicenter trial, the Submacular Study Trial (SST) was organized to evaluate subfoveal surgery for POHS. Specifically, this study evaluates subfoveal surgery and compares it to observation for the treatment of eyes with POHS and subfoveal CNV.

Histopathologic and ultrastructural findings of surgically excised CNV from patients who had undergone submacular surgery demonstrated fibrovascular tissue, fibrocellular tissue, or hemorrhage in all cases. Vascular endothelium and RPE were the most common constituents of the CNV.[61, 127–129]

Complications of Submacular/Subretinal Surgery

CNV secondary to POHS often arises from focal defects in Bruch's membrane and proliferates anterior to the RPE.[124] This type of membrane may be removed with preservation of the underlying RPE and choriocapillaris requisite to restoring visual function.[130] Submacular surgery carries all the risks of vitrectomy surgery. Retinal detachment, retinal tears without detachment, endophthalmitis, subretinal hemorrhage, cataract formation, and premacular fibrosis have been reported as complications of submacular surgery.[130]

Recurrent neovascularization after subretinal surgery is a common problem. Recurrence should be differentiated from persistence of CNV because of incomplete removal of CNV membranes. Early recognition of persistent or recurrent CNV may allow laser photocoagulation in CNV away from the fovea for better visual prognosis.[131] Subfoveal recurrence is the most difficult to manage, making it an ideal clinical model for testing antiangiogenic agents[131] because laser treatment of subfoveal CNV destroys the fovea and is not recommended.[132]

Younger patient age and the absence of previous laser photocoagulation are factors associated with a favorable visual prognosis after submacular surgery to remove subfoveal CNV.[133] As discussed previously, the ingrowth site of subfoveal CNV in POHS has been associated with visual prognosis after submacular surgical removal of CNV. Eyes with an extrafoveal ingrowth site have a favorable visual prognosis after the surgical removal of the CNV. If the ingrowth site is subfoveal or not identifiable, the visual prognosis after submacular surgery is guarded.[125] Despite good results, the appropriate management of patients with POHS and subfoveal CNV remains controversial.

Amphotericin B

It is presumed that the ocular histoplasmosis syndrome is caused by previous exposure to the fungus *H. capsulatum*. Because no organisms have been identified in human histopathologic specimens and none are found in the animal model 6 weeks after infection,[10] the use of antifungal amphotericin B has *no role* in the treatment of POHS or reactivated macular lesions.

CONCLUSIONS

Although many questions remain unanswered concerning the cause of ocular histoplasmosis, the epidemiologic, immunologic, experimental, and histopathologic data and evidence make a fairly compelling case that the fungus *H. capsulatum* is the causative agent for the constellation of ocular lesions that is clinically recognized as POHS. On the basis of these data and evidence, it has been proposed to call the entity *ocular histoplasmosis* and

drop the term presumed. Nevertheless, the syndrome of ocular lesions is still called presumed ocular histoplasmosis syndrome.

Since the efficacy of laser photocoagulation in treating extrafoveal and juxtafoveal CNV lesions is proven in controlled clinical trials, there is some hope for the patients suffering from POHS. The high-risk patients who have lost vision in one eye are encouraged to self-monitor their reading vision and regularly use an Amsler grid chart with each eye independently. This is recommended to detect new patches of neovascularization that may arise, either in the eye already affected or in the fellow good eye. Laser treatment is then recommended.

Further research is needed to better understand the pathophysiologic process that results in CNV and to develop animal models to explore potential antiangiogenic drugs to intervene in that process.

References

1. Cohen PR, Grossman ME, Silvers DN: Disseminated histoplasmosis and human immunodeficiency virus. Int J Dermatol 1991;30:614–622.
2. Katz BJ, Scott WE, Folk JC: Acute histoplasmosis choroiditis in 2 immunocompetent brothers. Arch Ophthalmol 1997;115:1470–1472.
3. Specht CS, Mitchell KT, Bauman AE, et al: Ocular histoplasmosis with retinitis in a patient with acquired immune deficiency syndrome. Ophthalmology 1991;98:1356–1359.
4. Weingeist TA, Watzke RC: Ocular involvement by *Histoplasma capsulatum*. Int Ophthalmol Clin 1983;23:33–47.
5. Pulido JS, Folberg R, Carter KD, et al: *Histoplasma capsulatum* endophthalmitis after cataract extraction. Ophthalmology 1990;97:217–220.
6. Craig EL, Suie T: *Histoplasma capsulatum* in human ocular tissue. Arch Ophthalmol 1974;91:285–289.
7. Goldstein BG, Buettner H: Histoplasmic endophthalmitis: A clinico-pathologic correlation. Arch Ophthalmol 1983;101:774–777.
8. Hoefnagels KL, Pijpers PM: *Histoplasma capsulatum* in a human eye. Am J Ophthalmol 1967;63:715–723.
9. Klintworth GK, Hollingsworth AS, Lusman PA, Bradford WD: Granulomatous choroiditis in a case of disseminated histoplasmosis: Histologic demonstration of *Histoplasma capsulatum* in choroidal lesions. Arch Ophthalmol 1973;90:45–48.
10. Brown DM, Weingeist TA, Smith RE: Histoplasmosis. In: Pepose JS, Holland GN, Wilhelmus KR, eds: Ocular Infection and Immunity. St Louis, Mosby Year-Book, 1996, pp 1252–1261.
11. Darling ST: A protozoan general infection producing pseudo tubercles in the lungs and focal necrosis in the liver, spleen, and lymph nodes. JAMA 1906;46:1283.
12. Darling ST: Histoplasmosis: A fatal infectious disease resembling kala-azar found among natives of tropical America. Arch Intern Med 1908;2:107–123.
13. Reid JD, Scherer JH, Herbut PA, et al: Systemic histoplasmosis diagnosed before death and produced experimentally in guinea pigs. J Lab Clin Med 1942;27:419–434.
14. Krause AC, Hopkins WG: Ocular manifestations of histoplasmosis. Am J Ophthalmol 1951;34:564–566.
15. Schlaegel TF: Granulomatous uveitis: An etiologic survey of 100 cases. Trans Am Acad Ophthalmol Otolaryngol 1958;62:813–824.
16. Woods AC, Wahlen HE: The probable role of benign histoplasmosis in the etiology of granulomatous uveitis. Trans Am Ophthalmol Soc 1959;57:318–343.
17. Schlaegel TF, Kenney D: Changes around the optic nerve-head in presumed ocular histoplasmosis. Am J Ophthalmol 1966;62:454–458.
18. Schwartz J: Histoplasmosis. New York, Praeger, 1981.
19. Baker RD: Histoplasmosis in routine autopsies. Am J Clin Pathol 1964;41:457–470.
20. Furcolow ML: Histoplasmosis. Clin Notes Resp Dis 1967;6:3.
21. Smith RE, Ganley JP: An epidemiological study of presumed ocular histoplasmosis. Trans Am Acad Ophthalmol Otolaryngol 1971;75:994–1005.

22. Bottoni FG, Deutman AF, Aandekerk AL: Presumed ocular histoplasmosis syndrome and linear streak lesions. Br J Ophthalmol 1989; 73:528–535.

23. Braunstein RA, Rosen DA, Bird AC: Ocular histoplasmosis syndrome in the United Kingdom. Br J Ophthalmol 1974;58:893–898.

24. Suttorp-Schulten MS, Bollemeijer JG, Bos PJ, Rothova A: Presumed ocular histoplasmosis in the Netherlands- an area without histoplasmosis. Br J Ophthalmol 1997;81:7–11.

25. Watzke RC, Klein ML, Wener MH: Histoplasmosis-like choroiditis in a nonendemic area: The northwest United States. Retina 1998;18:204–212.

26. Asbury T: The status of presumed ocular histoplasmosis: Including a report of a survey. Trans Am Ophthalmol Soc 1966;64:371–400.

27. Davidorf FH, Anderson JD: Ocular lesions in the Earth Day 1970 histoplasmosis epidemic. Int Ophthalmol Clin 1975;15:51–60.

28. Olk RJ, Burgess DB, McCormick PA: Subfoveal and juxtafoveal subretinal neovascularization in the presumed ocular histoplasmosis syndrome. Visual prognosis. Ophthalmology 1984;91:1592–1602.

29. Feman SS, Podgorski SF, Penn MK: Blindness from presumed ocular histoplasmosis in Tennessee. Ophthalmology 1982;89:1295–1298.

30. Smith RE, Ganley JP, Knox DL: Presumed ocular histoplasmosis. II. Patterns of peripheral and peripapillary scarring in persons with nonmacular disease. Arch Ophthalmol 1972;87:251–257.

31. Hawkins BS, Ganley JP, for the Washington County Follow-up Eye Study Group: Risk of visual impairment attributable to ocular histoplasmosis. Arch Ophthalmol 1994;112:655–666.

32. Baskin MA, Jampol LM, Huamonte FU, et al: Macular lesions in blacks with the presumed ocular histoplasmosis syndrome. Am J Ophthalmol 1980;89:77–83.

33. Gass JDM, Wilkinson CP: Follow-up study of presumed ocular histoplasmosis. Trans Am Acad Ophthalmol Otolaryngol 1972;76:672–693.

34. Schlaegel TF, Weber JC: Follow-up study of presumed histoplasmic choroiditis. Am J Ophthalmol 1971;71:1192–1195.

35. Watzke RC, Claussen RW: The long-term course of multifocal choroiditis (presumed ocular histoplasmosis). Am J Ophthalmol 1981;91:750–760.

36. Lewis ML, Schiffman JC: Long-term follow-up of the second eye in ocular histoplasmosis. Int Ophthalmol Clin 1983;23:125–135.

37. Sawelson H, Goldberg RE, Annesley WH, Tomer TL: Presumed ocular histoplasmosis: The fellow eye. Arch Ophthalmol 1976;94:221–224.

38. Godfrey WA, Sabates R, Cross DE: Association of presumed ocular histoplasmosis with HLA-B7. Am J Ophthalmol 1978;85:854–858.

39. Braley RE, Meredith TA, Aaberg TM, et al: The prevalence of HLA-B7 in presumed ocular histoplasmosis. Am J Ophthalmol 1978;85:859–861.

40. Meredith TA, Smith RE, Duquesnoy RJ: Association of HLA-DRw2 antigen with presumed ocular histoplasmosis. Am J Ophthalmol 1980;89:70–76.

41. Meredith TA, Green WR, Key SN, et al: Ocular histoplasmosis: Clinicopathologic correlation of 3 cases. Surv Ophthalmol 1977;22:189–205.

42. Hodgkins PR, Lane AC, Chisholm IM, et al: Immunophenotyping in presumed ocular histoplasmosis-like retinopathy. Eye 1995;9:56–63.

43. Dreyer RF, Gass JDM: Multifocal choroiditis and panuveitis. A syndrome that mimics ocular histoplasmosis. Arch Ophthalmol 1984;102:1776–1784.

44. Hawkins BS, Alexander J, Schachat AP: Ocular histoplasmosis. In: Schachat AP, Murphy RB, Ryan SJ, eds: Retina, 2nd ed. St Louis, Mosby Year-Book, 1994, pp 1661–1675.

45. Wong VG: Focal choroidopathy in experimental ocular histoplasmosis. Trans Am Ophthalmol Soc 1972;70:615–630.

46. Macular Photocoagulation Study Group: Five-year follow-up of fellow eyes of individuals with ocular histoplasmosis and unilateral extrafoveal or juxtafoveal choroidal neovascularization. Arch Ophthalmol 1996;114:667–688.

47. Fountain JA, Schlaegel TF: Linear streaks of the equator in presumed ocular histoplasmosis syndrome. Arch Ophthalmol 1981;99:246.

48. Schlaegel TF: Presumed ocular histoplasmosis. In: Tasman W, Jaeger EA, eds: Duane's Clinical Ophthalmology. Philadelphia, J.B. Lippincott, 1989, vol 4, chapter 48.

49. Spaide RF, Yannuzzi LA, Freund KB: Linear streaks in multifocal choroiditis and panuveitis. Retina 1991;11:229–231.

50. Schlaegel TF, Weber JC, Helveston E, Kennedy D: Presumed histoplasmosis choroiditis. Am J Ophthalmol 1967;63:919–925.

51. Nussenblatt RB, Whitcup SM, Palestine AG: Ocular histoplasmosis. In: Nussenblatt RB, Whitcup SM, Palestine AG, eds: Uveitis: Fundamentals and Clinical Practice, 2nd ed. St Louis, Mosby Year-Book, 1996, pp 229–237.

52. Walma D, Schlaegel TF: Presumed histoplasmic choroiditis. Am J Ophthalmol 1964;57:107–110.

53. Kranias G: Vitreous hemorrhage secondary to presumed ocular histoplasmosis syndrome. Ann Ophthalmol 1985;17:295–298.

54. Schlaegel TF: Ocular Histoplasmosis. New York, Grune & Stratton, 1977.

55. Rivers MB, Pulido JS, Folk JC: Ill-defined choroidal neovascularization within ocular histoplasmosis scars. Retina 1992;12:90–95.

56. Ryan SJ: De novo subretinal neovascularization in the histoplasmosis syndrome. Arch Ophthalmol 1976;94:321–327.

57. Schlaegel TF: The concept of invisible choroiditis in the ocular histoplasmosis syndrome. Int Ophthalmol Clin 1983;23:55–63.

58. Schlaegel TF: In discussion of Gass JDM and Wilkinson CP: Follow-up study of presumed ocular histoplasmosis. Trans Am Acad Ophthalmol Otolaryngol 1972;76:693–694.

59. Martin DF, Whitcup SM: Syndromes of possible infectious origin. In: Tabbara KF, Hyndiuk RA, eds: Infections of the Eye. Boston, Little, Brown, 1996, pp 595–597.

60. Meredith TA, Smith RE, Braley RE, et al: The prevalence of HLA-B7 in presumed ocular histoplasmosis in patients with peripheral atrophic scars. Am J Ophthalmol 1978;86:325–328.

61. Grossniklaus HE, Hutchinson AK, Capone AJ, et al: Clinical pathologic features of surgically excised choroidal neovascular membranes. Ophthalmology 1994;101:1099–1111.

62. Kleiner RC, Ratner CM, Enger C, et al: Subfoveal neovascularization in the ocular histoplasmosis syndrome: A natural history study. Retina 1988;8:225–229.

63. Macular Photocoagulation Study Group: Recurrent choroidal neovascularization after argon laser photocoagulation for neovascular maculopathy. Arch Ophthalmol 1986;104:503–512.

64. Macular Photocoagulation Study Group: Argon laser photocoagulation for neovascular maculopathy: Three-year results from randomized clinical trials. Arch Ophthalmol 1986;104:694–701.

65. Irvine AR, Spencer WH, Hogan MJ, et al: Presumed chronic ocular histoplasmosis syndrome: A clinical-pathologic case report. Trans Am Ophthalmol Soc 1976;94:91.

66. Krill AE, Christi MI, Klien BA, et al: Multifocal inner choroiditis. Trans Am Acad Ophthalmol Otolaryngol 1969;73:222–245.

67. Lewis ML, Van Newkirk MR, Gass JD: Follow-up study of presumed ocular histoplasmosis syndrome. Ophthalmology 1980;87:390–399.

68. Schlaegel TF: The natural history of histo spots in the disc and macular area. Int Ophthalmol Clin 1975;15:19–28.

69. Smith RE, Ganley JP: The natural history of non-disciform ocular histoplasmosis. Can J Ophthalmol 1977;12:114–120.

70. Watzke RC: Presumed histoplasmosis syndrome. Trans New Orleans Acad Ophthalmol 1983;31:89–96.

71. Jost BF, Olk RJ, Burgess DB: Factors related to spontaneous visual recovery in the ocular histoplasmosis syndrome. Retina 1987;7:1–8.

72. Campochiaro PA, Morgan KM, Conway BP, Stathos J: Spontaneous involution of subfoveal neovascularization. Am J Ophthalmol 1990;109:668–675.

73. Macular Photocoagulation Study Group: Argon laser photocoagulation for ocular histoplasmosis: Results of a randomized clinical trial. Arch Ophthalmol 1983;101:1347–1357.

74. Macular Photocoagulation Study Group: Krypton laser photocoagulation for neovascular lesions of ocular histoplasmosis: Results of a randomized clinical trial. Arch Ophthalmol 1987;105:1499–1507.

75. Macular Photocoagulation Study Group: Argon laser photocoagulation for neovascular maculopathy: Five-year results from randomized clinical trials. Arch Ophthalmol 1991;109:1109–1114.

76. Callanan D, Fish GE, Anand R: Reactivation of inflammatory lesions in ocular histoplasmosis. Arch Ophthalmol 1998;116:470–474.

77. Orlando RG, Davidorf EH: Spontaneous recovery phenomenon in the presumed ocular histoplasmosis syndrome. Int Ophthalmol Clin 1983;23:137–149.

78. Singerman LJ, Wong BA, Smith S: Spontaneous visual improve-

ment in the first affected eye of patients with bilateral disciform scars. Retina 1985;5:135.

79. Harris MJ, Robbins D, Dieter JM: Eccentric visual acuity in patients with macular disease. Ophthalmology 1985;92:1550.

80. Gass JDM: Stereoscopic Atlas of Macular Diseases: Diagnosis and Treatment, 3rd ed. St Louis, CV Mosby, 1978, pp 112–128.

81. Macular Photocoagulation Study Group: Persistent and recurrent neovascularization after krypton laser photocoagulation for neovascular lesions of ocular histoplasmosis. Arch Ophthalmol 1989;107:344–352.

82. Macular Photocoagulation Study Group. Krypton laser photocoagulation for idiopathic neovascular lesions: Results of a randomized clinical trial. Arch Ophthalmol 1990;108:832–837.

83. Macular Photocoagulation Study Group: Laser photocoagulation for juxtafoveal choroidal neovascularization. Arch Ophthalmol 1994;112:500–509.

84. Macular Photocoagulation Study Group: Evaluation of argon green vs krypton red laser for photocoagulation of subfoveal choroidal neovascularization in the Macular Photocoagulation Study. Arch Ophthalmol 1994;112:1176–1184.

85. Macular Photocoagulation Study Group: Laser photocoagulation for neovascular lesions nasal to the fovea: Results from clinical trials for lesions secondary to ocular histoplasmosis or idiopathic causes. Arch Ophthalmol 1995;113:56–61.

86. Macular Photocoagulation Study Group: The influence of treatment extent on the visual acuity of eyes treated with krypton laser for juxtafoveal choroidal neovascularization. Arch Ophthalmol 1995;113:190–194.

87. Maumenee AE, Ryan SJ: Photocoagulation of disciform macular lesions in the ocular histoplasmosis syndrome. Am J Ophthalmol 1973;75:13.

88. Schlaegel TF: Partial photocoagulation in the presumed ocular histoplasmosis syndrome. Perspect Ophthalmol 1977;1:25.

89. The Canadian Ophthalmology Study Group: Argon green vs krypton red laser photocoagulation for extrafoveal choroidal neovascularization: One-year results in ocular histoplasmosis. Arch Ophthalmol 1994;112:1166–1173.

90. Watzke RC, Leaverton PE: Light coagulation in presumed histoplasmic choroiditis. Arch Ophthalmol 1971;86:127.

91. Berger AS, Kaplan HJ: Clinical experience with the surgical removal of subfoveal neovascular membranes: Short-term postoperative results. Ophthalmology 1992;99:969–975.

92. Machemer R: Surgical approaches to subretinal strands. Am J Ophthalmol 1980;90:81–85.

93. Thomas MA, Dickinson JD, Melberg NS, et al: Visual results after surgical removal of subfoveal choroidal neovascular membranes. Ophthalmology 1994;101:1384–1396.

94. Thomas MA, Grand MG, Williams DF, et al: Surgical management of subfoveal choroidal neovascularization. Ophthalmology 1992;99:952–968.

95. Thomas MA, Kaplan HJ: Surgical removal of subfoveal neovascularization in the presumed ocular histoplasmosis syndrome. Am J Ophthalmol 1991;111:1–7.

96. Anderson A, Clifford W, Palvolgyi I, et al: Immunopathology of chronic experimental histoplasmic choroiditis in the primate. Invest Ophthalmol Vis Sci 1992;33:1637–1641.

97. Ganley JP: Epidemiologic characteristics of presumed ocular histoplasmosis. Acta Ophthalmol 1973;119(suppl):1–63.

98. Smith RE, Dunn S, Jester JV: Natural history of experimental histoplasmic choroiditis in the primate. I. Clinical features. Invest Ophthalmol Vis Sci 1984;25:801–809.

99. Smith RE, Dunn S, Jester JV: Natural history of experimental histoplasmic choroiditis in the primate. II. Histopathologic features. Invest Ophthalmol Vis Sci 1984;25:810–819.

100. Smith RE, O'Connor GR, Halde CJ, et al: Clinical course in rabbits after experimental induction of ocular histoplasmosis. Am J Ophthalmol 1973;76:284–293.

101. Smith RE, Scalarone M, O'Connor GR, Halde CJ: Detection of *Histoplasma capsulatum* by fluorescent antibody techniques in experimental ocular histoplasmosis. Am J Ophthalmol 1973;76:375–380.

102. Tewari RP, Sharma DK, Mathur A: Significance of thymus-derived lymphocytes in immunity elicited by immunization with ribosomes or live yeast cells of *Histoplasma capsulatum*. J Infect Dis 1978;138:605–613.

103. Davidorf FH: The role of T-lymphocytes in the reactivation of presumed ocular histoplasmosis scars. Int Ophthalmol Clin 1975;15:111–124.

104. Smith RE. Natural history and reactivation studies of experimental ocular histoplasmosis in a primate model. Trans Am Ophthalmol Soc 1982;80:695–757.

105. Smith RE, Macy JI, Parrett C, Irvine J: Variations in acute multifocal histoplasmic choroiditis in the primate. Invest Ophthalmol Vis Sci 1978;17:1005–1018.

106. Aronson SB, Fish MB, Pollycove M, Coon MA: Altered vascular permeability in ocular inflammatory disease. Arch Ophthalmol 1971;85:455–466.

107. Gamble CN, Aronson SB, Brescia FB: Experimental uveitis: 1. The production of recurrent immunologic (Auer) uveitis and its relationship to increased uveal vascular permeability. Arch Ophthalmol 1970;84:321–330.

108. Kaplan HJ, Waldrep JC: Immunologic basis of presumed ocular histoplasmosis. Int Ophthalmol Clin 1983;23:19–31.

109. Gwin RM, Makley TA Jr, Wyman M, et al: Multifocal ocular histoplasmosis in a dog and cat. J Am Vet Med Assoc 1970;176;638–642.

110. Foster CS, Sonntag HG: Essentials of microbiology in uveitis. In: Kraus-Mackiw E, O' Connor GR, eds: Uveitis: Pathophysiology and Therapy, 2nd ed. Stuttgart, Georg Thieme Verlag, 1986, pp 29–46.

111. Jester JV, Smith RE: Subretinal neovascularization after experimental ocular histoplasmosis syndrome. Retina 1987;7:1–8.

112. Hayreh SS, Cullen JF: Atypical minimal peripapillary choroidal colobomata. Br J Ophthalmol 1972;56:86–96.

113. Wise GN, Henkind P, Alterman M: Optic disc drusen and subretinal hemorrhage. Trans Am Acad Ophthalmol Otolaryngol 1974;78:212–219.

114. Bird AC, Grey RHB: Photocoagulation of disciform macular lesions with krypton laser. Br J Ophthalmol 1979;63:669–673.

115. Sabates FN, Lee KY, Ziemianski MC: A comparative study of argon and krypton laser photocoagulation in the treatment of presumed ocular histoplasmosis syndrome. Ophthalmology 1982;89:729–734.

116. Yassur Y, Gilad E, Ben-Sira I: Treatment of macular subretinal neovascularization with the red-light krypton laser in presumed ocular histoplasmosis syndrome. Am J Ophthalmol 1981;91:172–176.

117. Cummings HL, Rehmar AJ, Wood WJ, Isernhagen RD: Long-term results of laser treatment in the ocular histoplasmosis syndrome. Arch Ophthalmol 1995;113:465–468.

118. Fine SL, Wood WJ, Singerman LJ, et al: Laser treatment for subfoveal neovascular membranes in ocular histoplasmosis syndrome: Results of a pilot randomized clinical trial. Arch Ophthalmol 1993;111:19–20.

119. Gass JDM: Choroidal neovascular membranes—Their visualization and treatment. Trans Am Acad Ophthalmol Otolaryngol 1973;77:310–320.

120. Shah SS, Schachat AP, Murphy RP, et al: The evolution of argon laser photocoagulation scars in patients with the ocular histoplasmosis syndrome. Arch Ophthalmol 1988;106:1533–1536.

121. Lim JI, Schachat AP, Conway B: Macular hole formation following laser photocoagulation of choroidal neovascular membranes in a patient with presumed ocular histoplasmosis (letter). Arch Ophthalmol 1991;109:1500–1501.

122. Schlaegel TF: Treatment of the POHS. In: Schlaegel TF, ed. Ocular Histoplasmosis. New York, Raven Press, 1977, pp 209–259.

123. Schlaegel TF: Corticosteroids in the treatment of ocular histoplasmosis. Int Ophthalmol Clin 1983;23:111–123.

124. Gass JDM: Biomicroscopic and histopathologic consideration regarding the feasibility of surgical excision of subfoveal neovascular membranes. Am J Ophthalmol 1994;118:285–298.

125. Melberg NS, Thomas MA, Burgess DB: The surgical removal of subfoveal choroidal neovascularization: Ingrowth site as a predictor of visual outcome. Retina 1996;16:190–195.

126. Akduman L, Del Priore LV, Desai VN, et al: Perfusion of the subfoveal choriocapillaris affects visual recovery after submacular surgery in presumed ocular histoplasmosis syndrome. Am J Ophthalmol 1997;123:90–96.

127. Grossniklaus HE, Green WR: Histopathologic and ultrastructural findings of surgically excised choroidal neovascularization. Submacular surgery trials research group. Arch Ophthalmol 1998; 116:745–749.

128. Makley TA, Craig EL, Worling K: Histopathology of ocular histoplasmosis. Int Ophthalmol Clin 1983;23:1–18.

129. Saxe SJ, Grossniklaus HE, Lopez PF, et al: Ultrastructural features of surgically excised subretinal neovascular membranes in the ocular histoplasmosis syndrome. Arch Ophthalmol 1993;111:88–95.
130. Mann ES, Meredith TA: Ocular Histoplasmosis. In: Guyer DR, Yannuzzi LA, Chang S, et al, eds: Retina-Vitreous-Macula. Philadelphia, W.B. Saunders, 1999, pp 178–188.
131. Melberg NS, Thomas MA, Dickinson JD, Valluri S: Managing recurrent neovascularization after subfoveal surgery in presumed ocular histoplasmosis syndrome. Ophthalmology 1996;103:1064–1067.
132. Campochiaro PA: In discussion: Melberg NS, Thomas MA, Dickinson JD, Valluri S: Managing recurrent neovascularization after subfoveal surgery in presumed ocular histoplasmosis syndrome. Ophthalmology 1996;103:1067–1068.
133. Berger AS, Conway M, Del Priore LV, et al: Submacular surgery for subfoveal choroidal neovascular membranes in patients with presumed ocular histoplasmosis. Arch Ophthalmol 1997;115:991–996.

Acknowledgments

I wish to thank Malika Singh and Mani Singh for their support in completing this chapter.

Elisabeth M. Messmer

DEFINITION

Infectious chorioretinitis/endophthalmitis is defined by the presence of actively replicating organisms within the eye, associated with a variable degree of inflammation. When the organisms are introduced into the eye from outside the body (e.g., at the time of ocular surgery or trauma) the infection is termed exogenous. An infection resulting from septic embolization (from extraocular sources) is termed endogenous. Fungal organisms, such as *Candida* species, are observed in endogenous and, less frequently, in exogenous ocular infections.[1]

Intraocular candidiasis may produce a choroiditis and/or retinitis that may break through to the vitreous and cause endophthalmitis. *Candida* chorioretinitis is defined as the presence of focal, deep, white, infiltrative, chorioretinal lesions with no evidence of direct vitreal involvement except a diffuse vitreous haze. *Candida* endophthalmitis is defined as (1) *Candida* chorioretinitis with extension of the surrounding inflammation into the vitreous, or (2) a vitreous abscess manifesting as intravitreal fluff balls.[2]

HISTORY

In 1877, Grawitz was probably the first author to report ocular candidiasis in animal experiments. He injected *C. albicans* into the vitreous of rabbits, causing vitreous opacities and small, white preretinal "structures."[3] The initial pathologic description of endogenous ocular candidiasis in humans was reported in 1943 by Miale.[4] In 1958, Van Buren published the first clinical report of a patient with multiple myeloma who developed *Candida* chorioretinitis.[5]

Prior to the availability of adequate therapy, treatment for eyes with endophthalmitis was limited to minimizing the cosmetic deformity that resulted as the intravitreal abscess pointed and discharged its liquefied intraocular contents.[1] Almost all eyes with endophthalmitis evolved to complete blindness. Greater awareness of the disease entity, improvement of diagnostic tools, the development of new antifungal agents, alternative routes of antifungal administration, and refined surgical techniques contributed to a better functional outcome. Nevertheless, *Candida* endophthalmitis still carries a grave prognosis for the eye and, in cases of endogenous endophthalmitis, is even a marker for poor patient survival.

EPIDEMIOLOGY

According to the results of the National Nosocomial Infections Surveillance System surveys conducted through 1992, *Candida* has become the fourth most common isolate recovered from blood cultures in the United States.[6] Rates of candidemia have also increased substantially in Europe.[7] Approximately half of all candidal infections occur in surgical intensive care units.[7] It has been reported that the species of *Candida* causing infection have shifted noticeably toward nonalbicans species.[8, 9] DNA typing has verified that transmission occurs from patient to patient and from health care worker to patient.[7]

Among the numerous risk factors for endogenous candidiasis (including *Candida* endophthalmitis) are the use of antibiotics, indwelling catheters, hyperalimentation, cancer therapy, immunosuppressive therapy after organ transplantation, bone marrow transplantation, acquired immunodeficiency syndrome (AIDS), hospitalization in intensive care units, recent intra-abdominal surgery, candiduria, and colonization with *Candida* species.[7, 10–15] Ocular candidiasis has occurred as a complication of spontaneous abortion,[16] as the only initial manifestation of pacemaker endocarditis,[17] and after intravenous anesthesia with propofol.[18] *Candida* endophthalmitis represents one of the most serious and increasingly common ocular complications of intravenous drug abuse.[15, 19–21] Fungal infection may result from contamination of the drug, syringes, needles, or the cotton used to filter the drug before intravenous injection.[20, 21]

Systemic fungal infections, especially candidiasis, have been increasingly encountered among high-risk neonatal patients. *Candida* sepsis was reported to occur in 3% to 4% of premature infants with a birthweight of under 1500 g.[22, 23] Further risk factors include extended antibiotic therapy, prolonged parenteral nutrition or use of fat emulsions, chronic artificial ventilation, and prior surgery.[22, 24–27] In neonates with positive blood, urine, cerebrospinal fluid, or stool cultures of *Candida albicans*, Chen observed candidal meningitis in 55% and *Candida* endophthalmitis in 46% of infants.[28]

Candida endophthalmitis, however, was also reported in otherwise healthy adults.[29, 30] Exact numbers concerning the annual incidence of *Candida* endophthalmitis are not available. Fungal organisms, however, account for more than half of cases of endogenous endophthalmitis, with *Candida albicans* being responsible for 75% to 80% of cases.[31, 32]

Risk factors for exogenous *Candida* endophthalmitis include trauma and ocular surgery, especially cataract extraction with intraocular lens implantion[33–38] and perforating keratoplasty.[39–42]

Fungal endophthalmitis, especially that caused by candidal infection, is a frequent complication reported to occur in 9.9% to 45% of hospitalized patients with candidemia.[10, 11, 43, 44] In a study by Brooks, patient age, sex, underlying diseases, presence of Foley catheters, bacteremia, white blood cell count, use of multiple antibiotics, hyperalimentation, or surgery did not differ between the candidemic patients with and without *Candida* endophthalmitis. Moreover, groups were similar in number of sites colonized with yeast and species of *Candida* recovered.[10] In a prospective multicenter study, Donahue and coworkers examined 118 patients with candidemia adequately treated with antifungal therapy. *Candida* chorioretinitis was seen in only 9% of patients. No patient was shown to progress to *Candida* endophthalmitis.[2]

The presence of *Candida* endophthalmitis in hospitalized patients is an important indicator of systemic candidiasis, as evidenced by the pathologic finding of disseminated candidiasis in 78% of autopsy patients with *Candida* endophthalmitis.[29] The overall mortality of hospitalized patients with candidemia is high (53% to 61%),[12, 13, 45] with almost half the deaths occurring in the first week after candidemia begins. The mortality rate for patients with endogenous *Candida* endophthalmitis is similarly high. Edwards and colleagues reviewed 76 cases of *Candida* endophthalmitis and found an overall mortality of 50%.[46] Menezes and associates reported an overall mortality rate of 77% of severely ill patients with *Candida* endophthalmitis, with an even higher mortality of 80% for intensive care patients.[12] Other authors found mortality rates ranging from 0% to 22% in their patients with *Candida* endophthalmitis who were treated with various antifungal therapies with or without accompanying vitrectomy or intravitreal antifungals.[13, 29, 32, 47]

CLINICAL CHARACTERISTICS

Endogenous *Candida* Chorioretinitis/Endophthalmitis

Ocular symptoms have been reported to be uncommon, especially in patients with peripheral chorioretinal *Candida* lesions or in moribund patients. Brooks noted the complete absence of visual symptoms even in patients with confirmed *Candida* endophthalmitis.[10] Donahue and colleagues reported visual complaints in only 9 of 72 patients with ocular candidiasis.[2] Patients with *Candida* endophthalmitis may complain of mild ocular discomfort, red eye, floaters, and slowly progressing visual loss.[2, 25, 48] *Candida* chorioretinitis, with focal, deep, white, infiltrative, chorioretinal lesions, is mainly bilateral, multiple (often including more than ten lesions), and predominantly observed in the posterior pole.[2, 49] In 13 of 19 eyes with *Candida* chorioretinitis, additional fundus lesions, including nerve-fiber-layer infarcts, intraretinal hemorrhages, and white-centered hemorrhages (Roth spots), were present.[2] Whereas intraretinal hemorrhages are not usually the sole manifestation of intraocular candidiasis, nerve-fiber-layer infarcts and Roth spots are known to occur in hematogenously disseminated ocular infections. Moreover, *Candida* has been isolated from Roth spots,[5, 46] and therefore Roth spots could conceivably represent an early, nonspecific marker of *Candida* infection.[2] Neutropenia may inhibit the formation of typical *Candida* lesions in both animals and humans.[50]

Candida endophthalmitis presents as *Candida* chorioretinitis with extension of the surrounding inflammation into the vitreous, or vitreous abscess manifesting as intravitreal fluff balls. The vitreous opacities may be connected by strands producing a string-of-pearls appearance[15] (Fig. 29–1). Papillitis may be present.[48] *Candida* endophthalmitis follows a more indolent course than that of acute bacterial endophthalmitis.[25]

Anterior segment pathology may include conjunctival hyperemia (only seen in 21% of patients with ocular candidiasis by Donahue[2]) anterior chamber cells, hypopyon, and posterior synechiae formation.[2, 32, 46, 51] Corneal

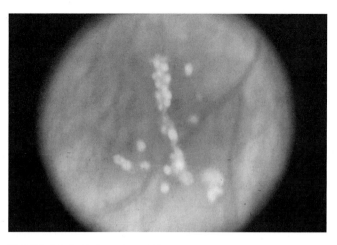

FIGURE 29–1. "String of pearls" appearance to the vitreal exudates in a patient with endogenous *Candida* endophthalmitis. (See Color insert.)

involvement may result in suppurative keratitis with perforation.[26]

Patients with endogenous *Candida* endophthalmitis resulting from intravenous drug abuse may present with no clinical or serologic evidence of systemic candidiasis,[15] suggesting that ocular candidiasis may have been caused by transient candidemia. Anterior uveitis and extensive vitreous involvement are common, and patients do not necessarily show associated retinal lesions.[15, 19] This may result in part from the fact that these patients seek treatment late, when retinal lesions have either resolved or been obscured by pronounced vitreous involvement.[15] Ocular findings in children with endogenous *Candida* endophthalmitis may mimic other ocular disorders. Clinch and associates observed a localized intralenticular candidal abscess presenting as an infantile cataract with associated endophthalmitis in a 6-month-old infant.[25] Shields and coworkers report a systemically healthy 12-month-old boy who developed ocular candidiasis simulating retinoblastoma.[30] Hypopyon formation, synechiae, and the absence of a distinct ocular mass with calcifications on ultrasound and computed tomographic examinations should differentiate endophthalmitis from retinoblastoma in most cases.[30]

Exogenous *Candida* Endophthalmitis

Post-traumatic

Fungal endophthalmitis is a rare but devastating complication of penetrating ocular trauma. Foreign material contaminating the wound, especially wood or other vegetable matter, may harbor fungi.[52, 53] Mycotic endophthalmitis occurring after trauma is often caused by septate filamentous fungi (e.g., *Fusarium solani* and *Aspergillus* species). Yeasts are rarely isolated.[53] The signs of infection frequently are obscured by tissue damage and inflammation as a result of the injury. Therefore, diagnosis and initiation of treatment are often delayed. These factors contribute to the overall poor prognosis associated with traumatic fungal endophthalmitis.[53]

Postoperative

Candida endophthalmitis is a rare complication of intraocular surgery, but it represents a potentially catastrophic event. Endophthalmitis caused by coagulase-negative *Staphylococcus* species and *Propionibacterium acnes* must be included in the differential diagnosis of indolent subacute or chronic cases of postoperative uveitis.

Cataract Surgery. Several cases of non-*Candida*[54–56] and *Candida* endophthalmitis[34, 36, 57] have been reported to have occurred secondary to contaminated solutions. Stern and associates describe a large group of patients who developed *Candida parapsilosis* endophthalmitis 1 to 18 weeks after cataract surgery as a result of contaminated intraocular irrigating solutions. Patients developed indolent inflammation with a fibrinopurulent anterior chamber exudate and vitreous snowball opacities.[34] Discontinuation of topical steroid therapy led to a dramatic increase in intraocular inflammation and ocular discomfort in most patients.[34]

Delayed-onset pseudophakic endophthalmitis caused by *C. parapsilosis* has been reported in three patients 1 to 23 months following cataract extraction with posterior chamber intraocular lens implantation. The patients exhibited keratic precipitates, a white intracapsular plaque thought to contain sequestered organisms within the capsule, stringy white infiltrates in the anterior vitreous adjacent to the capsular remnants, and a mild diffuse vitreitis.[33]

Perforating Keratoplasty. *Candida albicans* endophthalmitis has been reported following penetrating keratoplasty.[39–42] Postkeratoplasty fungal endophthalmitis may originate from the operative site, contaminated solutions, culture media, and contaminated donor tissue. Up to 27% of eyes suitable for corneal transplantation have been found to harbor fungi,[58] and cultures of donor rims as well as corneal storage media were positive for *Candida* species in most of the reported cases of fungal endophthalmitis following perforating keratoplasty.[39–41] Patients with postkeratoplasty *Candida* endophthalmitis typically present with mild to moderate pain, purulent discharge, conjunctival injection, multiple fluffy infiltrates at the graft-host interface, or endothelial plaques associated with vitreitis.[39–41]

COMPLICATIONS

Treated chorioretinal lesions may heal either as a faint gliotic scar, or as a focal defect in the pigment epithelium.[49] However, if left untreated, vitreous invasion with irreversible sequelae may eventuate, producing a vitreoretinal abscess with retinal necrosis, vitreal organization, tractional retinal detachment, cyclitic membrane formation, or phthisis bulbi.[15, 32, 49, 50, 59–61] Even in treated cases, premacular scars may reduce visual acuity permanently.[16, 40, 48, 49] Postinflammatory fibrovascular membranes puckering or tractionally detaching the macula may be surgically removed. McDonald and coworkers report on four eyes undergoing pars plana vitrectomy and membrane peeling after *Candida* endophthalmitis. Postoperative visual acuity ranged from 1/200 to 20/25, depending on the degree of macular pathology and the presence and location of full-thickness retinal scars.[60] In rare cases, choroidal neovascular membranes may develop following endogenous *Candida* endophthalmitis.[62]

PATHOGENESIS/HISTOPATHOLOGY/ IMMUNOLOGY

Candida albicans is normally present as an intestinal saprophyte in 20% to 40% of healthy individuals. Other *Candida* species may also be found in the gastrointestinal tract, although in lower concentrations.[63] In situations of internal environmental change, such as results from chronic use of antibiotics, indwelling catheters, hyperalimentation, immunosuppressive therapy, or recent intraabdominal surgery, *Candida* may become pathogenic.[48] Animal studies[46, 64] and human histopathologic evaluations[46, 64, 65] have demonstrated the ability of *Candida* to spread hematogenously to the choroid and retina. Species of *Candida* other than *C. albicans* that are encountered in human disease include *C. tropicalis, C. parapsilosis, C. krusei, C. stellatoidea, C. guilliermondii, C. lusitaniae, C. glabrata, C. pseudotropicalis,* and *C.rugosa.*[66] Immunocompromised patients with hematologic malignancies are particularly prone to develop non-*albicans* candidal infections.[67]

The relative resistance of the eye to non-*albicans* candidal involvement has been demonstrated in a rabbit model of endophthalmitis by Edward and colleagues.[68] While *C. albicans* caused endophthalmitis at an inoculum of 10^5 colony-forming units (cfu)/ml, 10^8 cfu/ml of *C. tropicalis* and *C. stellatoidea* were necessary to cause chorioretinal lesions. However, these concentrations did not cause endophthalmitis. *C. parapsilosis, C. guilliermondii,* and *C. krusei* were not pathogenic to the eye at the doses studied.[68] In humans, *Candida* species reported to cause endogenous endophthalmitis include *C. albicans, C. tropicalis, C. stellatoides, C. parapsilosis,* and *C. krusei.*[31]

Contradictory data are available in humans with respect to the incidence of endophthalmitis caused by different Candidal species. One study found that disseminated *C. tropicalis* was associated with a higher rate of endophthalmitis than was *C. albicans* (23% versus 6%).[69] Most other studies report the opposite, with the highest rate of endophthalmitis in *C. albicans* fungemia.[2, 10, 32, 43, 51, 66] In patients with intraocular candidiasis, *C. albicans* was the most common species isolated from blood (58%), followed by *C. tropicalis* (14%), *C. (Torulopsis) glabrata* (14%), *C. parapsilosis* (9%), and other species (7%) in a study by Donahue.[2] After infection, *Candida* may persist in ocular tissues for a long time. *C. albicans* was isolated from a rhesus monkey eye 110 days after intravascular inoculation.[70]

The reasons for the susceptibility of the retina to *Candida* infections compared with other organs are unclear. Fungal virulence may relate to the ability of the organism to produce pseudohyphae from blastospores that lodge in the deep capillary plexus of the retina and in the choriocapillaris. The production and localization of various phospholipases in the growing fungal buds suggest that phopholipid-rich tissues such as the retina and choroid may provide a substrate for yeast filamentation.[71] Much of the tissue destruction observed in fungal infection may be not so much the direct consequence of invasion but rather the effect of mediators of inflammation induced by the organisms.[72]

The histopathologic examination of ocular *Candida* lesions may demonstrate a combination of an acute necrotizing process and a chronic granulomatous reaction by histiocytes and round cells occurring primarily in the choroid.[26, 46, 48, 49, 73] Colonies of *Candida*, identified by their characteristic budding pseudohyphae, may be found in the choroid, the retinal pigment epithelium, and Bruch's membrane. Extension into the subretinal space and into the retina occurs secondarily.[48, 49] Retinal involvement is usually accompanied by a macrophage response in the overlying vitreous.[49] The internal limiting membrane of the retina provides no barrier to the spread of *C. albicans*, and if the lesion remains untreated, vitreous invasion may occur.[49] Vitreous lesions are composed largely of neutrophils, macrophages, and epitheloid cells, but they may also harbor *Candida* organisms.[15, 46, 73, 74] In adults, immune responses to *Candida* organisms include monocytic and neutrophilic phagocytosis, along with intracellular killing of fungal organisms.[75] In addition, serum factors and lymphocytic function, particularly T lymphocytes, are important. The patient's immune status and the health of the affected eye modify the immune response to *Candida*. Moreover, the frequent use of corticosteroid eyedrops in the early postoperative period may mitigate signs and symptoms of infection.[40] Newborn infants are probably at higher risk for the development of *Candida* infections because of their normally deficient host immune system and the reduced killing ability of their leukocytes.[76, 77]

DIAGNOSIS

Candida endophthalmitis should be suspected in any patient with one of the known predisposing conditions. The presence of the characteristic white chorioretinal lesions or puff-ball-like vitreous opacities is highly suggestive in the appropriate clinical setting. Because of the lack of clinical or laboratory parameters to distinguish between candidemic patients with and those without endophthalmitis, Brooks recommends early ophthalmoscopic examinations. In his experience, follow-up examinations are often helpful to the clinician in guiding antifungal therapy.[10] Blood, urine, indwelling catheters, and any potential source of infection should be cultured. Additional examinations and tests are helpful in confirming the final diagnosis of ocular candidiasis.

Nonocular Cultures

The significance of candidemia remains problematic. Positive fungal blood cultures may represent skin contamination without candidemia, true but transient candidemia without deep tissue invasion, or candidemia with deep tissue invasion.[43] A presumptive diagnosis of ocular candidiasis may be made if *Candida* is cultured from a source other than the eye (e.g., blood, urine, cerebrospinal fluid) in the presence of typical ocular lesions. Unfortunately, blood cultures are frequently negative in systemic candidiasis.[73, 78]

Antibody Testing

The value of *Candida* antibody testing in serum as an aid in the early diagnosis of disseminated candidiasis remains questionable. Various methods of antibody determination with rather low sensitivity and specificity, including immunodiffusion, counterelectrophoresis, and latex agglutina-

tion (LA), have been employed.[79–82] According to Gentry and colleagues, LA is the most sensitive test for antibody determination.[79] LA titers are, however, rarely of benefit in predicting the presence of endophthalmitis in ocular candidiasis.[43] Mathis and associates observed a significant difference in the local production of specific antibodies in the anterior chamber between patients with *Candida* endophthalmitis and controls. They even report a correlation between the severity of uveitis and antibody titers.[83]

Antigen Testing

Determination of *Candida* antigen titers can offer significant clinical advantages to the treating physician. Some studies have shown relatively high sensitivity and specificity of antigen detection tests for invasive disease caused by *Candida* species.[84] Parke and coworkers demonstrated antigen titers indicative of disseminated disease in three of four patients with endogenous *Candida* endophthalmitis.[43] In a study by Bailey and colleagues, however, all five patients with *Candida* endophthalmitis had a negative LA test for serum antigen.[85] Antigen titers may prove to be more sensitive than antibody titers, especially in immunocompromised patients, who are incapable of mounting an adequate antibody response to *Candida*.

Anterior Chamber Tap and Vitreous Aspiration

Henderson and coworkers confirmed the diagnosis of candidiasis in 62% of eyes with vitreous aspiration, but they found anterior chamber aspiration to be a poor diagnostic technique.[11] Axelrod and Peyman succeeded in culturing *Candida* after aspiration from the vitreous in only one of six untreated rabbit eyes exogenously inoculated with *Candida*, although abundant organisms were demonstrated in all eyes microscopically after enucleation.[87] A random, or even a directed, aspiration can fail to produce positive *Candida* cultures or smears because of the sequestration of the organisms within large-diameter inflammatory nodules.[15] Thus, vitrectomy may be the only procedure that can reliably obtain *Candida* from an infected vitreous.

Pars Plana Vitrectomy

The goal of vitrectomy in eyes with *Candida* endophthalmitis is to confirm the presumptive clinical diagnosis and remove the intravitreal fungal mass and inflammatory debris while delivering safe and therapeutic doses of antibiotics to the infected eye. Diagnostic vitrectomy is especially valuable in a subgroup of patients with presumed localized intraocular infection without clinical or cultural evidence of disseminated disease.[32]

A vitreous infusion suction cutter is necessary to remove formed vitreous for suspected fungal infection. One recommended technique consists of culturing the harvested vitreous specimen under sterile operating room conditions. Samples, diluted by the irrigating solution, are passed through a disposable membrane filter system.[88] Specimens are inoculated onto Sabouraud's agar, blood agar, and liquid brain-heart infusion with gentamicin at room temperature for fungal isolation. For rapid diagnosis, slides are prepared for Gram staining, Giemsa staining, and modified Grocott's methenamine-silver (GMS) stain, and Cellufluor or Calcofluor white techniques for the identification of fungal elements.

If retinoblastoma is a consideration, fine-needle biopsy, rather than vitrectomy, should be performed.[30]

DIFFERENTIAL DIAGNOSIS

The differential diagnosis of *Candida* chorioretinitis includes necrotizing retinopathies caused by herpes viruses such as cytomegalovirus (CMV), herpes simplex virus (HSV), and varicella-zoster virus (VZV), and the acute retinal necrosis syndrome (Table 29–1). Protozoan infections such as toxoplasmic retinochoroiditis or nematode infections (e.g., *Toxocara canis*) may simulate candidal chorioretinitis. Bacterial endophthalmitis and fungal uveitis caused by organisms other than *Candida* (e.g., *Aspergillus* sp., *Cryptococcus neoformans*, *Histoplasma capsulatum*, *Blastomyces dermatitidis*) must be differentiated from ocular candidiasis. Choroidal granulomas (e.g., in ocular sarcoidosis) may mimic candidal chorioretinitis. Retinoblastoma and large cell lymphoma must be included in the differential diagnosis of ocular candidiasis. Even cotton-wool spots may be confused with chorioretinal infection by *Candida*; however, their eventual regression over 5 to 8 weeks, depending on the underlying diagnosis, facilitates their diagnosis.

TREATMENT

Endophthalmitis is a potentially devastating disease that requires aggressive management. Although the incidence of serious infections caused by *Candida* species is rising rapidly, the most appropriate management strategies for such infections remains severely limited because large controlled studies of the various approaches have not been performed.[68]

The mainstay of treatment for *Candida* endophthalmitis has been a combination of systemic and intravitreal amphotericin B with or without pars plana vitrectomy.[18, 49, 51, 61, 68] Newly developed triazole compounds, such as fluconazole, are very promising agents for the therapy of systemic and ocular candidiasis.[89–93] Moreover, the removal of precipitating factors such as intravenous lines is extremely important.

Amphotericin B

Amphotericin B was discovered in 1956[94] and was first used for the treatment of ocular candidiasis in 1960.[95] It acts by binding to cell membrane sterols, resulting in the leakage of cellular constituents and ultimately the death of the organism.[96] It is not absorbed by the gastrointestinal tract and must therefore be given intravenously. The

TABLE 29–1. DIFFERENTIAL DIAGNOSIS OF OCULAR CANDIDIASIS

Bacterial endophthalmitis	Histoplasmosis
Viral retinopathies (CMV, HSV, VZV)	Blastomycosis
Acute retinal necrosis	Sarcoidosis
Toxoplasmic retinochoroiditis	Retinoblastoma
Toxocara canis chorioretinitis	Large cell lymphoma
Aspergillosis	Cotton-wool spots
Cryptococcosis	

CMV, cytomegalovirus; HSV, herpes simplex virus; VZV, varicella-zoster virus.

maximum recommended dose is 0.5 to 1.0 mg/kg/day for an average daily dose of 40 to 50 mg. Therapy should continue until the retinal lesions disappear completely or become small and/or are replaced by fibrous tissue.[32] Although amphotericin B is effective against a wide range of fungal pathogens, its systemic use in treating fungal endophthalmitis is severely limited by poor ocular penetration.[97, 98] Persistent intraocular infection has been reported in spite of an adequate course of treatment when the vitreous is involved.[15, 49] An additional drawback of systemic amphotericin B therapy is the wide spectrum of toxic side effects encountered, ranging from nausea, vomiting, and malaise, to anemia and renal failure. Moreover, a minimum dose of 750 to 1000 mg of amphotericin B is required for cure of candidal endophthalmitis.[15, 46, 89]

Systemically administered antimycotics are important not only to treat endophthalmitis but also in the treatment of systemic infections.[16, 32] If evidence of systemic candidiasis is present, intravenous amphotericin B should be administered. For severe systemic infections, a combination of intravenous amphotericin B and another antifungal drug (e.g., flucytosine) is recommended by some authors because of their synergistic effect.[20, 99] However, the increased risk of bone marrow suppression or diarrhea as a complication of the simultaneous use of these drugs must be weighed against the potential benefit.[99]

The potential toxicity of amphotericin B has led to the development of lipid-associated preparations, including liposomal amphotericin B, amphotericin B colloidal dispersion, and amphotericin B lipid complex. These preparations are less nephrotoxic, but higher systemic doses than those of conventional amphotericin B are needed to achieve the same effect in invasive fungal infections.[100–102] The efficacy of lipid-associated formulations of amphotericin B in the treatment of ocular candidiasis is under investigation.

Studies have shown that amphotericin B can be delivered to the eye in effective concentrations by direct intravitreal injection. Doses of 5 and 10 µg amphotericin B injected intravitreally into eyes of healthy rabbits did not cause retinal toxicity clinically, microscopically, or by electroretinography.[103] The safety of intravitreal injection of amphotericin B in humans has been demonstrated in several case reports in which histopathologic confirmation of a cured infection, absent retinal toxicity, and normal electroretinograms following intravitreal amphotericin B injection are described.[34, 104, 105] A 10-µg dose into a human eye would theoretically provide a concentration of 2.5 µg/ml, which is effective against most fungal pathogens.[103] When there is no extraocular evidence of candidemia or candidiasis, local ocular treatment with intravitreal amphotericin B may be all that is required.[32]

Flucytosine

In an effort to avoid the toxicity of systemic amphotericin B administration, recent studies have evaluated the use of alternate systemic therapy with fluorinated pyrimidine (flucytosine) or imidazole compounds including ketoconazole or fluconazole.[18, 32, 51, 73, 89–93, 99]

Flucytosine is selectively taken up by susceptible fungi and deaminated to 5-fluorouracil, which blocks DNA and RNA synthesis. The suggested oral dose is 50 to 150 mg/

kg/day in four divided doses. It shows excellent oral absorption and ocular penetration, and it is active against *C. albicans*.[73, 106] Systemic administration is relatively risk free, but bone marrow and liver toxicity can occur. Because of a significant incidence of primary resistance during therapy, flucytosine should not be used alone in disseminated disease.[99]

Imidazole derivates

Imidazole derivates act by inhibiting membrane sterols in *C. albicans*; they have good antifungal activity, absorption, and ocular penetration with minimal toxicity.[107, 108] Fluconazole shows improved permeability into the vitreous compared to ketoconazole. It is the only antifungal that penetrates into cerebrospinal fluid. However, candidal resistance was reported in cases treated with imidazole compounds, and a patient developed *Candida* endophthalmitis while receiving fluconazole for the management of candidal pyelonephritis.[109] In a rabbit model, intravenous amphotericin B was superior to intravenous fluconazole in the treatment of *Candida* endophthalmitis.[110] Fluconazole appeared to be efficacious in treating endophthalmitis after 10 to 17 days of therapy, but this salutary treatment effect was lost by day 24, and fluconazole failed to eradicate *C. albicans* from the rabbit eye.[110] Brod and colleagues, however, successfully treated five patients with systemic flucytosine (2 g every 6 hours), or ketoconazole (200 to 400 mg/d) in association with intravitreal amphotericin B injection.[32] They recommend this regimen especially for patients without evidence of disseminated disease.[32] Christmas and Smiddy treated their patients suffering from endogenous *Candida* endophthalmitis with oral fluconazole (200 mg/d) and vitrectomy without intravitreal injection of antifungals. They also report clearance of infection and improvement of visual acuity in all six patients.[92] The successful use of oral fluconazole in a dosage of 200 to 800 mg PO daily for 2 to 4 months as the only treatment for endogenous *Candida* endophthalmitis has also been reported.[18, 73, 89–91]

Other imidazole derivates, such as itraconazole, miconazole, and econazole, are also effective anticandidal substances, and they show good ocular penetration.[111, 112] They are used in the treatment of keratomycosis,[113–117] but therapeutic experience in the management of *Candida* chorioretinitis and endophthalmitis with these drugs is limited and anecdotal.[118]

Corticosteroids

Intraocular and systemic corticosteroids have been suggested as a useful adjunctive treatment in cases of fungal endophthalmitis.[20, 51, 119, 120] However, controversial opinions exist concerning their use in *Candida* endophthalmitis. Steroids may potentiate systemic candidiasis, but they may attenuate the inflammatory response in ocular candidal infection and may prevent vision-threatening sequelae.

Role of Vitrectomy

Pars plana vitrectomy offers several theoretical advantages to the treatment of *Candida* endophthalmitis. In addition to obtaining vitreous biopsy to correctly identify the organism, vitrectomy physically removes a large mass of invading organisms, thereby fulfilling the general surgical criteria of incision and drainage of an abscess. Huang and coworkers demonstrated that intravitreal amphotericin B combined with vitrectomy was more effective in reducing vitreous opacification than was the use of intravitreal amphotericin B alone in a rabbit model of exogenous *Candida* endophthalmitis.[121] In 1976, Snip and Michels reported the successful use of pars plan vitrectomy and intravitreal amphotericin B in the management of endogenous *Candida* endophthalmitis in a patient.[122] Furthermore, it has been shown that infected eyes treated with vitrectomy and intraocular antibiotics have a surprisingly greater number of negative cultures 1 week later than do those treated with intraocular antibiotics alone.[123]

Vitrectomy also removes the scaffold on which fibrotic traction bands might develop, resulting in secondary traction retinal detachment.[124] Moreover, vitreous, as a potential barrier to the diffusion of large molecules such as amphotericin B, is eliminated.[122] Amphotericin clearance and toxicity in vitrectomized versus nonvitrectomized eyes was studied by Doft and coworkers[125] and Baldinger and colleagues.[126] The most rapid decay in amphotericin concentration from the vitreous cavity occurred in aphakic vitrectomized eyes, with a half-life of 1.4 days compared to aphakic normal eyes (4.7 days) and phakic *Candida* infected eyes (8.6 days). Therefore, readministration of intravitreal amphotericin may be necessary 3 to 4 days following vitrectomy if clinically indicated.[32, 125] Toxicity of amphotericin was not increased in vitrectomized eyes.[126]

Pars plana vitrectomy and injection of intravitreal amphotericin B should be considered for moderate to severe vitreous involvement in an eye with presumed ocular candidiasis. Most authors reserve surgery for patients with a visual acuity of 20/400 or less, or when the fundus cannot be visualized due to severe vitreous involvement.[72] The best timing for surgical therapy, however, is still not known. It may well be that early vitrectomy combined with intravitreal injections of amphotericin B offers the best chance for functional improvement.[124]

The role of intraocular lens removal or exchange remains controversial in the management of exogenous *Candida* endophthalmitis following cataract surgery.[34, 35, 37] Successful sterilization of the vitreal cavity does not require routine intraocular lens removal, although recurrences are possible.[34, 35] Stern and colleagues recommend introcular lens explantation only when clinical response to pars plana vitrectomy and intravitreal amphotericin B is inadequate.[34] In cases where white plaque lesions are present at the posterior lens capsule, a large capsulectomy is warranted.[33]

Single case reports have been published on the treatment of *Candida* endophthalmitis in children. In contrast to adults, intravenous infusions with amphotericin B, sometimes combined with flucytosine without vitrectomy, seem to be effective in these cases.[27, 28, 127] Having been treated with systemic antifungals alone, 11 premature infants demonstrated minimal residual ocular pathology.[127] This may be due to the newborns' immature immune system resulting in less vitreous reaction and postinflammatory sequelae.

Prophylaxis

The ultimate goal is to prevent disease. Prophylactic administration of oral nystatin can reduce fungal colonization and infection in very low birthweight infants.[128] The risk of systemic candidiasis can be minimized in patients by following good antibiotic use principles. Indwelling intravascular devices and indwelling bladder catheters should be avoided when possible.[99]

PROGNOSIS

Although rare, spontaneous resolution of endogenous *Candida* endophthalmitis has been reported.[129–131] Usually, the outcome of candidal endophthalmitis is dependent on four main factors: the virulence of the organisms, the duration of the inflammatory response, the prompt diagnosis, and correct management.[39] Moreover, the functional result depends on the extent and site of involvement of the chorioretinal lesions.[25, 27] In recent publications, final visual acuity following endogenous *Candida* endophthalmitis ranged from no light perception and phthisis to 20/15.[19, 20, 32, 73] In five cases with less than 2 months between onset of symptoms and initiation of antifungal therapy, four had a final visual acuity of 20/50 or better, but none of the patients with a delay of more than 2 months had a visual acuity better than 20/80.[32] Another important factor in determining the final visual outcome is the presence of intercurrent complications such as retinal detachments.[32]

Depending on the time to diagnosis and appropriate therapy, visual acuity after postsurgical *Candida* endophthalmitis ranges from 20/25 to phthisis with no light perception. Reasons for bad visual acuity following postsurgical *Candida* endophthalmitis include graft failure, secondary glaucoma, pupillary membrane, and macular scars.[33, 38–41]

Infantile *Candida* endophthalmitis seems to have a good ocular prognosis for children treated promptly with systemic antifungal therapy.[127]

CONCLUSIONS

Ocular candidiasis is one of the infectious causes of uveitis. The presence of *Candida* endophthalmitis is a good indicator of a systemic fungal infection that carries a high mortality in seriously ill patients in intensive care units.[12] Since many of these patients may have negative blood cultures despite extensive visceral involvement, the ophthalmologic examination is an important adjunct in the diagnosis of systemic candidiasis,[12] and serial ophthalmic examinations are an objective measure of therapeutic response.[2] As in any infectious uveitis, steroids can suppress inflammation, but eventually the ocular problem deteriorates. A high index of suspicion is necessary to trigger a decision and to proceed to diagnostic vitrectomy in patients with *Candida* endophthalmitis. A stepladder approach in treatment of ocular candidiasis may be useful. Mild cases of *Candida* chorioretinitis without evidence of systemic disease may be managed with oral azole derivates alone, whereas advanced cases of *Candida* endophthalmitis and patients with candidemia need systemic antifungals and intravitreal amphotericin B injections combined with pars plana vitrectomy.

References

1. Weissgold DB, D'Amico DJ: Rare causes of endophthalmitis. Int Ophthalmol Clin 1996;36:163–177.
2. Donahue SP, Greven CM, Zuravleff JJ, et al: Intraocular candidiasis in patients with candidemia. Clinical implications derived from a prospective multicenter study. Ophthalmology 1994;101:1302–1309.
3. Grawitz P: Beiträge zur systematischen Botanik der pflanzlichen Parasiten mit experimentellen Untersuchungen über die durch sie bedingten Krankheiten. Virchows Arch Path Anat 1877;70:546–588.
4. Miale JB: *Candida albicans* infection confused with tuberculosis. Arch Pathol Lab Med 1943;35:427–437.
5. Van Buren JM: Septic retinitis due to *Candida albicans*. AMA Arch Pathol 1958;65:137–146.
6. Jarvis WR: Epidemiology of nosocomial fungal infections, with emphasis on *Candida* species. Clin Infect Dis 1995;20:1526–1530.
7. Edwards JE: International conference for the development of a consensus on the management and prevention of severe candidal infections. Clin Infect Dis 1997;25:43–59.
8. Wingard JR: Importance of *Candida* species other than *C. albicans* as pathogens in oncology patients. Clin Infect Dis 1995;20:115–125.
9. Pfaller MA: Nosocomial candidiasis: Emerging species, reservoirs, and modes of transmission. Clin Infect Dis 1996;22:S89–94.
10. Brooks RG: Prospective study of *Candida* endophthalmitis in hospitalized patients with candidemia. Arch Intern Med 1989;149:2226–2228.
11. Henderson DK, Edwards JE, Montgomerie JZ: Hematogenous *Candida* endophthalmitis in patients receiving parenteral hyperalimentation fluids. J Infect Dis 1981;143:655–661.
12. Menezes AV, Sigesmund DA, Demajo WA, et al: Mortality of hospitalized patients with *Candida* endophthalmitis. Arch Intern Med 1994;154:2093–2097.
13. Wey SB, Mori M, Pfaller MA, et al.: Hospital-acquired candidemia: The attributable mortality and excess length of stay. Arch Intern Med 1988;148:2642–2645.
14. Coskuncan NM, Jabs DA, Dunn JP, et al: The eye in bone marrow transplantation. VI. Retinal complications. Arch Ophthalmol 1994;112:372–379.
15. Aguilar GL, Blumenkranz MS, Egbert PR, McCulley JP: *Candida* endophthalmitis after intravenous drug abuse. Arch Ophthalmol 1979;97:96–100.
16. Haskjold E, Lippe von der B: Endogenous *Candida* endophthalmitis. Report of two cases. Acta Ophthalmol 1987;65:741–744.
17. Shmuely H, Kremer I, Sagie A, et al: *Candida tropicalis* multifocal endophthalmitis as the only initial manifestion of pacemaker endocarditis. Am J Ophthalmol 1997;123:559–560.
18. Daily MJ, Dickey JB, Packo KH: Endogenous *Candida* endophthalmitis after intravenous anesthesia with propofol. Arch Ophthalmol 1991;109:1081–1084.
19. Sugar HS, Mandell GH, Shalev J: Metastatic endophthalmitis associated with injection of addictive drugs. Am J Ophthalmol 1971;71:1055–1058.
20. Elliott JH, O'Day DM, Gutow GS, et al: Mycotic endophthalmitis in drug abusers. Am J Ophthalmol 1979;88:66–72.
21. Vastine DW, Horsley W, Guth SB, Goldberg MF: Endogenous *Candida* endophthalmitis associated with heroin use. Arch Ophthalmol 1976;94:1805.
22. Baley JE, Kliegman RM, Fanaroff AA: Disseminated fungal infections in very low-birth-weight infants: Clinical manifestations and epidemiology. Pediatrics 1984;73:144–152.
23. Johnson DE, Thompson TR, Green TP, et al: Systemic candidiasis in very low-birth-weight infants (< 1.500 grams). Pediatrics 1984;73:138–143.
24. Weese-Mayer DE, Fondriest DW, Brouillette RT, et al: Risk factors associated with candidemia in the neonatal intensive care unit: A case-control study. Pediatr Infect Dis J 1987;6:190–196.
25. Clinch TE, Duker JS, Eagle RC, et al: Infantile endogenous *Candida* endophthalmitis presenting as cataract. Surv Ophthalmol 1989;34:107–112.
26. Michelson PE, Rupp R, Efthimiadis B: Endogenous *Candida* endophthalmitis leading to bilateral corneal perforation. Am J Ophthalmol 1980;80:800–803.
27. Palmer EA: Endogenous *Candida* endophthalmitis in infants. Am J Ophthalmol 1980;89:388–395.
28. Chen JY: Neonatal candidiasis associated with meningitis and endophthalmitis. Acta Paed Jap 1994;36:261–265.

29. Schmid S, Martenet AC, Oelz O: *Candida* endophthalmitis: Clinical presentation, treatment and outcome in 223 patients. Infection 1991;19:21–24.

30. Shields JA, Shields CL, Eagle RC, et al: Endogenous endophthalmitis simulating retinoblastoma. The 1993 David and Mary Seslen Endowment Lecture. Retina 1995;15:213–219.

31. Wilson FM: Causes and prevention of endophthalmitis. Int Ophthalmol Clin 1987;27:67–73.

32. Brod RD, Flynn HW, Clarkson JG, et al: Endogenous *Candida* endophthalmitis: Management without intravenous amphotericin B. Ophthalmology 1990;97:666–674.

33. Fox GM, Joondeph BC, Flynn HW, et al: Delayed-onset pseudophakic endophthalmitis. Am J Ophthalmol 1991;111:163–173.

34. Stern WA, Tamura E, Jacobs RA, et al: Epidemic postsurgical *Candida* parapsilosis endophthalmitis. Ophthalmology 1985; 92:1701–1709.

35. D'Amico DJ, Noorily SW: Postoperative endophthalmitis. In: Albert DM, Jakobiec FA, eds: Principles and Practice of Ophthalmology, vol 2. Philadelphia, W.B. Saunders, 1994, pp 1159–1169.

36. Wong VKW, Tasman W, Eagle RC, Rodriguez A: Bilateral *Candida* parapsilosis endophthalmitis. Arch Ophthalmol 1997;115:670–672.

37. Kauffman CA, Bradley SF, Vine AK: *Candida* endophthalmitis associated with intraocular lens implantation: Efficacy of fluconazole therapy. Mycoses 1993;36:13–17.

38. Driebe WT, Mandelbaum S, Forster RK, et al: Pseudophakic endophthalmitis: Diagnosis and management. Ophthalmology 1986;93:442–448.

39. Cameron JA, Antonios SR, Cotter JB, et al: Endophthalmitis from contaminated donor corneas following penetrating keratoplasty. Arch Ophthalmol 1991;109:54–59.

40. Insler MS, Urso LF: *Candida albicans* endophthalmitis after penetrating keratoplasty. Am J Ophthalmol 1987;104:57–60.

41. Kloess PM, Stulting RD, Waring III GO, et al: Bacterial and fungal endophthalmitis after penetrating keratoplasty. Am J Ophthalmol 1993;115:309–316.

42. Behrens-Baumann W, Ruechel R, Zimmermann O, Vogel M: *Candida tropicalis* endophthalmitis following penetrating keratoplasty. Br J Ophthalmol 1991;75:565.

43. Parke DW, Jones DB, Gentry LO: Endogenous endophthalmitis among patients with candidemia. Ophthalmology 1982;89:789–796.

44. Bross J, Talbot GH, Maislin G, et al: Risk factors for nosocomial candidemia: A case control study in adults without leukemia. Am J Med 1989;87:614–620.

45. Komshian SV, Uwaydah AK, Sobel JD, et al: Fungemia caused by *Candida* species and *Torulopsis glabrata* in the hospitalized patient: Frequency, characteristics, and evaluation of factors influencing outcome. Rev Infect Dis 1989;11:379–390.

46. Edwards JE, Foos RY, Mongomerie JZ, et al: Ocular manifestations of *Candida* septicemia: A review of seventy-six cases of hematogenous *Candida* endophthalmitis. Medicine 1974;53:47–75.

47. Chignell AH: Endogenous *Candida* endophthalmitis. J R Soc Med 1992;85:721–724.

48. Uliss AE, Walsh JB: *Candida* endophthalmitis. Ophthalmology 1983;90:1378–1379.

49. Griffin JR, Pettit TH, Fishman LS, Foos RY: Blood-borne *Candida* endophthalmitis. A clinical and pathologic study of 21 cases. Arch Ophthalmol 1973;89:450–456.

50. Henderson DK, Hockey LJ, Vukalcic LJ, Edwards JE. Effect of immunosuppression on the development of experimental hematogenous *Candida* endophthalmitis. Infect Immun 1980;27:628–631.

51. Essman TF, Flynn HW, Smiddy WE, et al: Treatment outcomes in a 10-year study of endogenous fungal endophthalmitis. Ophthalmic Surg Lasers 1997;28:185–194.

52. Peyman GA, Carroll CP, Raichand M: Prevention and management of traumatic endophthalmitis. Ophthalmology 1980:87:320–324.

53. Parrish CM, O'Day DM: Traumatic endophthalmitis. Int Ophthalmol Clin 1987;27:112–119.

54. Theodore FH: Etiology and diagnosis of fungal postoperative endophthalmitis. Ophthalmology 1978;85:327–340.

55. Pettit TH, Olson FJ, Foos RY, et al: Fungal endophthalmitis following intraocular lens implantation: A surgical epidemic. Arch Ophthalmol 1980;98:1025–1039.

56. Egerer I, Seehorst W: Histopathologie der exogenen mykotischen Endophthalmitis. Klin Monatsbl Augenheilkd 1976;169:325–331.

57. McCray E, Rampell N, Solomon SL, et al: Outbreak of *Candida* parapsilosis endophthalmitis after cataract extraction and intraocular lens implantation. J Clin Microbiol 1986;24:625–628.

58. White JH: Fungal contamination of donor eyes. Br J Ophthalmol 1969;53:30.

59. Edwards JE, Mongomerie JZ, Foos RY et al: Experimental hematogenous endophthalmitis caused by *Candida albicans*. J Infect Dis 1975;131:647–657.

60. McDonald RH, Bustros de S, Sipperley JO: Vitrectomy for epiretinal membrane with *Candida* chorioretinitis. Ophthalmology 1990;97:466–469.

61. Wolfensberger TJ, Gonvers M: Bilateral endogenous *Candida* endophthalmitis. Retina 1998;18:280–281.

62. Beebe WE, Kirkland C, Price J: A subretinal neovascular membrane as a complication of endogenous *Candida* endophthalmitis. Ann Ophthalmol 1987;19:207–209.

63. Cohen R, Roth FJ, Delgado E, et al: Fungal flora of the normal human small and large intestine. N Engl J Med 1969;280:638–641.

64. Hoffmann DH, Waubke TH: Experimentelle Untersuchungen zur metastatischen Ophthalmie mit *Candida albicans*. Graefes Arch Ophthalmol 1961;164:174–196.

65. Edwards JR, Lehrer RI, Stiehm ER, et al: Severe candidal infections: Clinical perspective, immune defense mechanisms, and current concepts of therapy. Ann Intern Med 1978;89:91–106.

66. Joshi N, Hamory BH: Endophthalmitis caused by non–*albicans* species of *Candida*. Rev Infect Dis 1991;13:281–287.

67. Horn R, Wong B, Kiehn TE, Armstrong D: Fungemia in a cancer hospital: Changing frequency, earlier onset, and results of therapy. Rev Infect Dis 1985;7:646–655.

68. Edwards JE, Mongomerie JZ, Ishida K, et al: Experimental hematogenous endophthalmitis due to *Candida*: Species variation in ocular pathogenicity. J Infect Dis 1977;135:294–297.

69. McDonnell PJ, McDonnell JM, Brown RH, Green WR: Ocular involvement in patients with fungal infections. Ophthalmology 1985;92:706–709.

70. Green MT, Jones DB, Gentry LO: Endogenous *Candida* endophthalmitis in the primate. Invest Ophthalmol Vis Sci 1978;17(s):229.

71. Wilhelmus KR: The pathogenesis of endophthalmitis. Int Ophthalmol Clin 1987;27:74–81.

72. Okada AA, D'Amico DJ: Endogenous endophthalmitis. In: Albert DM, Jakobiec FA, eds: Principles and Practice of Ophthalmology, vol 5. Philadelphia, W.B. Saunders, 1994, pp 3120–3126.

73. Robertson DM, Riley FC, Hermans PE: Endogenous *Candida* oculomycosis. Report of two patients treated with flucytosine. Arch Ophthalmol 1974;91:33–38.

74. Cohen M, Edwards JE, Hensley TJ, Guze LB: Experimental hematogenous *Candida albicans* endophthalmitis: Electron microscopy. Invest Ophthalmol Vis Sci 1977;16:498–511.

75. Baley JE, Annable WL, Kliegman RM: *Candida* endophthalmitis in the premature infant. Pediatrics 1981;98:458–461.

76. Dossett JH: Microbial defenses of the child and man. Deficient host mechanism of the newborn. Pediatr Clin North Am 1972;19:355–372.

77. Xanthou M, Valassi-Adam E, Kintsonidou E, Matsaniotis N: Phagocytosis and killing ability of *Candida albicans* by blood leukocytes of healthy term and preterm babies. Arch Dis Child 1975;50:72–75.

78. Bielsa I, Miro JM, Herrero C, et al: Systemic candidiasis in heroin abusers. Cutaneous findings. Int J Dermatol 1987;26:314–319.

79. Gentry LO McNitt TR, Kaufman L: Use and value of serologic tests for the diagnosis of systemic candidiasis in cancer patients: A prospective study of 146 patients. Curr Microbiol 1978;1:239–242.

80. Meckstroth KL, Reiss E, Keller JW, Kaufman L: Detection of antibodies and antigenemia in leukemic patients with candidiasis by enzyme-linked immunosorbent assay. J Infect Dis 1981;144:24–32.

81. Filice G, Yu B, Armstrong D: Immunodiffusion and agglutination tests for *Candida* in patients with neoplastic disease: Inconsistent correlation of results with invasive infections. J Infect Dis 1977;135:349–357.

82. Stickle D, Kaufman L, Blumer SO, McLaughlin DW: Comparison of a newly developed latex agglutination test and an immunodiffusion test in the diagnosis of systemic candidiasis. Appl Microbiol 1972;23:490–499.

83. Mathis A, Falecaze F, Bessieres MH, et al: Immunological analysis of the aqueous humour in *Candida* endophthalmitis. II: Clinical study. Br J Ophthalmol 1988;72:313–316.

84. Fung JC, Donta ST, Tilton RC: *Candida* detection system (CAND-TEC) to differentiate between *Candida albicans* colonization and disease. J Clin Microbiol 1986;24:542–547.

85. Bailey JW, Sada E, Brass C, Bennett JE: Diagnosis of systemic candidiasis by latex agglutionation for serum antigen. J Clin Microbiol 1985;21:749–752.

86. Henderson DK, Edwards JE, Ishida K, et al: Experimental hematogenous *Candida* endophthalmitis: Diagnostic approaches. Infect Immun 1979;23:858–862.

87. Axelrod AJ, Peyman GA: Intravitreal amphotericin B treatment of experimental fungal endophthalmitis. Am J Ophthalmol 1973;76:584–588.

88. Forster RK, Abbott RL, Gelender H: Management of infectious endophthalmitis. Ophthalmology 1980;87:313–319.

89. Akler ME, Vellend H, Neely DM, et al: Use of fluconazole in the treatment of candidal endophthalmitis. Clin Infect Dis 1995;20:657–664.

90. Laatikainen L, Tuominen M, Dickhoff von K: Treatment of endogenous fungal endophthalmitis with systemic fluconazole with or without vitrectomy. Am J Ophthalmol 1992;113:205–207.

91. Luttrull JK, Wan WL, Kubak BM, et al: Treatment of ocular fungal infection with oral fluconazole. Am J Ophthalmol 1995;119:477–481.

92. Christmas NJ, Smiddy WE: Vitrectomy and systemic fluconazole for treatment of endogenous fungal endophthalmitis. Ophthalmic Surg Lasers 1996;27:1012–1018.

93. Del Palacio A, Cuetara MS, Ferro M, et al: Fluconazole in the management of endophthalmitis in disseminated candidosis of heroin addicts. Mycoses 1993;36:193–199.

94. Gold W, Stout HA, Pagano JF, Donovick R: Amphotericins A and B: Antifungal antibiotics produced by a streptomycete: I. In vitro studies. In: Welch H, Marti-Ibanez F, eds: Antibiotics Annual 1955–1956. New York, Medical Encyclopedia, 1956, p 579.

95. Louria DB, Dineen P: Amphotericin B in the treatment of disseminated moniliasis. JAMA 1960;174:273–279.

96. Medoff G, Kobayashi GS: Strategies in the treatment of systemic fungal infections. N Engl J Med 1980;302:145–155.

97. Green WR, Bennett JE, Goos RD: Ocular penetration of amphotericin B. A report of laboratory studies and a case report of post-surgical cephalosporium endophthalmitis. Arch Ophthalmol 1965;73:769–775.

98. Fisher JF, Taylor AT, Clark J, et al: Penetration of amphotericin B into the human eye. J Infect Dis 1983;147:164.

99. Behlau I, Baker AS: Fungal infections and the eye. In: Albert DM, Jakobiec FA, eds: Principles and Practice of Ophthalmology, vol 5. Philadelphia, W.B. Saunders, 1994, pp 3030–3037.

100. Presterl E, Graninger W: New aspects in the treatment of systemic mycoses. Wien Klin Wochenschr 1998;110:740–750.

101. Ng TT, Denning DW: Liposomal amphotericin B (AmBisome) therapy in invasive fungal infections. Evaluation of United Kingdom compassionate use data. Arch Intern Med 1995;155:1093–1098.

102. Kruger W, Strockschlader M, Russmann B, et al: Experience with liposomal amphotericin B in 60 patients undergoing high-dose therapy and bone marrow or peripheral blood stem cell transplantation. Br J Haematol 1995;91:684–690.

103. Axelrod AJ, Peyman GA, Apple DJ: Toxicity of intravitreal injection of amphotericin B. Am J Ophthalmol 1973;76:578–583.

104. Stern GA, Fetkenhour CL, O'Grady RB: Intravitreal amphotericin B treatment of *Candida* endophthalmitis. Arch Ophthalmol 1977;95:89–93.

105. Ho PC, O'Day DM: *Candida* endophthalmitis and infection of costal cartilages. Br J Ophthalmol 1981;65:333–334.

106. Bennett JE: Chemotherapy of systemic mycoses. N Engl J Med 1974;290:30–32.

107. Debryne D, Ryckelynck J: Pharmacokinetics of fluconazole. Clin Pharmacokinet 1993;24:10–27.

108. O'Day DM, Foulds G, Williams TE, et al: Ocular uptake of fluconazole following oral administration. Arch Ophthalmol 1990;108:1006–1008.

109. Nomura J, Ruskin J: Failure of therapy with fluconazole for candidal endophthalmitis. Clin Infect Dis 1993;17:888–889.

110. Filler SG, Crislip MA, Mayer CL, Edwards JE: Comparison of fluconazole and amphotericin B for treatment of disseminated candidiasis and endophthalmitis in rabbits. Antimicrob Agents Chemother 1991;35:288–292.

111. Savani DV, Perfect JR, Cobo LM, Durack DT: Penetration of new azole compounds into the eye and efficacy in experimental *Candida* endophthalmitis. Antimicrob Agents Chemother 1987;31:6–10.

112. Van Cutsem J: Oral, topical and parenteral antifungal treatment with itraconazole in normal and in immunocompromised animals. Mycoses 1989;32S:14–34.

113. Mohan M, Panda A, Gupta SK: Management of human keratomycosis with miconazole. Aust N Z J Ophthalmol 1989;17:295–297.

114. Ball MA, Rebhun WC, Gaarder JE, Patten V: Evaluation of itraconazole-dimethyl sulfoxide ointment for treatment of keratomycosis in nine horses. J Am Vet Med Assoc 1997;211:199–203.

115. Arocker-Mettinger E, Huber-Spitzy V, Haddad R, Grabner G: Keratomycosis caused by *Candida albicans*. Klin Monatsbl Augenheilkd 1988;193:192–194.

116. Gupta SK: Efficacy of miconazole in experimental keratomycosis. Aust N Z J Ophthalmol 1986;14:373–376.

117. Thomas PA: Mycotic keratitis—an underestimated mycosis. J Med Vet Mycol 1994;32:235–256.

118. Airas KA, Nikoshelainen J: Haematogenous *Candida* endophthalmitis after abdominal surgery. Acta Ophthalmol Copenh 1987;65:450–454.

119. Schulman JA, Peyman GA: Intravitreal corticosteroids as an adjunct in the treatment of bacterial and fungal endophthalmitis. Retina 1992;12:336–340.

120. Coats ML, Peyman GA: Intravitreal corticosteroids in the treatment of exogenous fungal endophthalmitis. Retina 1992;12:46–51.

121. Huang K, Peyman GA, McGetrick J: Vitrectomy in experimental endophthalmitis: I. Fungal infections. Ophthalmic Surg 1979;10:84–86.

122. Snip RC, Michels RG: Pars plana vitrectomy in the management of endogenous *Candida* endophthalmitis. Am J Ophthalmol 1976;82:699–704.

123. Cottingham AJ, Forster RK: Vitrectomy in endophthalmitis. Arch Ophthalmol 1976;94:2078–2081.

124. Barrie T: The place of elective vitrectomy in the management of patients with *Candida* endophthalmitis. Graefes Arch Clin Exp Ophthalmol 1987;225:107–113.

125. Doft BH, Weiskopf J, Nilsson-Ehle I, Wingard LB: Amphotericin clearance in vitrectomized versus nonvitrectomized eyes. Ophthalmology 1985;92:1601–1605.

126. Baldinger J, Doft BH, Burns SA, Johnson B: Retinal toxicity of amphotericin B in vitrectomized versus non-vitrectomized eyes. Br J Ophthalmol 1986;70:657–661.

127. Annable WL, Kachmer ML, DiMarco M, DeSantis D: Long-term follow-up of *Candida* endophthalmitis in the premature infant. J Pediatr Ophthalmol Strabismus 1990;27:103–106.

128. Sims ME, Yoo Y, You H, et al: Prophylactic oral nystatin and fungal infections in very-low-birthweight infants. Am J Perinatol 1988;5:33–36.

129. Horne MJ, Ma MH, Taylor RF, et al: *Candida* endophthalmitis. Med J Aust 1975;1:170–172.

130. Dellon AL, Stark WJ, Chretien PB: Spontaneous resolution of endogenous *Candida* endophthalmitis complicating intravenous hyperalimentation. Am J Ophthalmol 1975;79:648–654.

131. Servant JB, Dutton GN, Ong-Tone L, et al: Candidal endophthalmitis in Glaswegian heroin addicts: Report of an epidemic. Trans Ophthalmol Soc U K 1985;104:297–308.

30 ⊣ COCCIDIOIDOMYCOSIS

Richard R. Tamesis

DEFINITION

Coccidioidomycosis is a disease produced by the soil fungus *Coccidioides immitis*. It is also called the San Joaquin Valley fever or valley fever. *C. immitis* is a dimorphic fungus, which means that it occurs in two forms: (1) growing as a mold with septate hyphae in soil and in culture, and (2) as a nonbudding spherule in host tissue.[1] It is identified by its appearance and by the formation of segmented arthrospores. The fungus grows in the topsoil layers in semiarid areas of the Western Hemisphere. Infection is caused by inhalation of airborne arthrospores that have been dislodged from the soil. The arthrospores form thick-walled spherules inside the host that then rupture and release endospores that spread locally and disseminate.

HISTORY

Coccidioidomycosis affecting the external eye and orbit has been described since 1896, when the disease was first reported in the United States.[2] In 1948, Levitt reported what he believed to be a case of intraocular coccidioidomycosis in a patient with pulmonary coccidioidomycosis.[3] However, it was not until 1967, when Hagele reported a patient with endophthalmitis caused by *C. immitis*, that a case of intraocular coccidioidomycosis was confirmed by histopathology and culture before enucleation or death of the patient.[4]

EPIDEMIOLOGY

C. immitis is endemic in the region known as the lower Sonoran Life Zone, which includes the San Joaquin Valley region of California and the Southwestern United States. The disease also occurs in the arid regions of Mexico, Central America, and parts of South America.

In semiarid climates, winters with heavy rain, followed by hot, dry, dusty periods, favor the rapid multiplication of the arthroconidia. The seasonal occurrence of primary coccidioidomycosis increases during the summer and fall in the Southwestern United States, corresponding to the dusty time of the year. Severe drought followed by heavy rainfall was identified as a factor associated with a 1991–1993 epidemic of coccidioidomycosis in California.[5, 6] Outbreaks have also occurred following earthquakes, dust storms, and archeological excavations.[7–9]

Filipinos, blacks, Native Americans, Mexican Americans, and immunocompromised individuals such as the elderly population, neonates, and those with the acquired immunodeficiency syndrome (AIDS) are at higher risk for developing the disease.[10, 11] Meningitis, lymphadenopathy, and diffuse pulmonary disease are more commonly found in these patients.

CLINICAL CHARACTERISTICS

The lungs, skin, and central nervous system are most commonly affected in patients with coccidioidomycosis. Approximately 40% of infected individuals are symptomatic.[12] The vast majority of symptomatic patients present with a mild upper respiratory tract infection or a pneumonitis characterized by fever, cough, night sweats, and malaise approximately 3 weeks after exposure to the organism. Erythema nodosum or multiforme may appear anywhere from 3 days to 3 weeks after the onset of symptoms. Disseminated infection occurs in less than 1% of patients with pulmonary coccidioidomycosis.[13]

Ocular coccidioidomycosis is rare, even in disseminated disease, and can present as (1) intraocular disease producing iridocyclitis, choroiditis, and chorioretinitis, which can affect one or both eyes; and (2) external disease consisting of blepharitis, keratoconjunctivitis, phlyctenular conjunctivitis, granulomatous conjunctivitis, episcleritis, and scleritis, as well as optic atrophy, extraocular nerve palsies, and orbital infection.[2, 14–16]

Posterior segment involvement can manifest in four different ways: (1) diffuse choroiditis often associated with widely disseminated (and preterminal) systemic disease, (2) large, juxtapapillary choroidal infiltrates with variable involvement of the overlying retina that may be associated with retinal edema and hemorrhage, (3) spherical opacities of the macula or posterior pole at the level of Bruch's membrane and sensory retina associated with macular edema and exudates, and most commonly as (4) small, peripheral chorioretinal scars with central hypopigmentation resembling presumed ocular histoplasmosis scars.[17, 18] Vitreous cells and perivascular sheathing may also be present with posterior segment disease.

About half of all patients present primarily with a granulomatous iridocyclitis without posterior segment involvement. Iris nodules containing the fungus may be seen. Spherules of *C. immitis* can be demonstrated from anterior chamber taps and iris biopsies in these patients.

Although ocular coccidioidomycosis generally occurs in patients with disseminated disease, there are reports of intraocular coccidioidomycosis occurring in otherwise apparently healthy individuals.[19–21]

PATHOPHYSIOLOGY, IMMUNOLOGY, PATHOLOGY, AND PATHOGENESIS

C. immitis produces pyogenic, granulomatous, and mixed reactions.[22] Polymorphonuclear leukocytes suppurate around infecting conidia and inside granulomas when the spherules rupture and release endospores. A granulomatous reaction develops around the developing spherules, which can be found inside foreign body giant cells. Fibrosis, necrosis, and calcification can occur.

Intact cell-mediated immunity serves to limit further extension of these foci and is essential for the host to eliminate this organism. Patients deficient in cell-mediated immunity such as those with AIDS are at risk for developing the chronic and disseminated forms of the disease and may require prolonged therapy. They typically have high titers of complement-fixing anticoccidioidal antibodies with no delayed-type hypersensitivity on skin testing.

373

Distribution of the endospores via the ophthalmic artery to the short posterior ciliary and central retinal arteries can result in miliary retinal and choroidal granulomas. Choroidal granulomas are confined mainly to the middle and large vessel layers.[23] Retinal granulomas are centered in the distribution of the central retinal artery. Anterior segment lesions demonstrate zonal granulomatous inflammation that can involve the uvea and angle structures.

DIAGNOSIS

Patients living in endemic areas who show the characteristic chorioretinal lesions should be suspected of having the disease whether or not they have active intraocular inflammation. Chest x-ray studies may show pneumonitis or characteristic "coin lesions." Biopsy of skin lesions can be especially important in identifying the organism in disseminated coccidioidomycosis.

Confirmation of the diagnosis is generally based on histopathologic, cultural, or molecular evidences of *C. immitis*. The spherules are 30 to 60 μm in size and appear flattened rather than globular.[24] They are refringent on direct examination and stain with periodic acid–Schiff. The endospores are oval in shape. Culturing for the organism can be very dangerous because the mycelial form is highly infectious and requires special handling.

Aqueous and vitreous biopsies can be examined directly for the organism by means of the Papanicolaou stain.[25] Iris biopsies of lesions and nodules can also help establish the diagnosis of ocular coccidioidal infection rapidly.

Immunologic evidence for the diagnosis includes a positive serologic test for anticoccidioidal antibodies in serum, cerebrospinal fluid, vitreous, or aqueous by (1) detection of anticoccidioidal IgM using immunodiffusion, enzyme immunoassay (EIA) latex agglutination, or tube precipitin, or (2) detection of a rising titer of anticoccidioidal IgG by immunodiffusion, EIA, or complement fixation.[26] Serum IgM antibodies appear 1 to 3 weeks after the onset of symptoms in 75% of cases of primary infection and disappear within 4 months.[27] Three months after onset, 50% to 90% of the patients with symptomatic primary infections have complement-fixing serum IgG anticoccidioidal antibody. This antibody may last for 6 to 8 months, although it may occasionally persist longer at low levels even after the infection resolves successfully. A fourfold rising titer is of grave prognostic significance and indicates advanced disease. A falling titer indicates improvement. Negative serologic tests do not exclude the diagnosis of coccidioidomycosis, particularly if chronic pulmonary disease is present.

A valid diagnosis of coccidioidal infection can be made by skin test conversion with the mycelial phase antigen coccidioidin (1:100 dilution) from negative to positive after the onset of clinical signs and symptoms. Spherulin (1:100 dilution), a parasitic phase antigen, may be a more sensitive reagent in detecting delayed hypersensitivity and is just as specific a coccidioidin. The antigen is applied intradermally (0.1 ml). Thirty-six hours is the optimal reaction time, although the readings are usually taken at 24 and 48 hours. Induration greater than 5 mm in diameter is considered a positive reaction. A positive skin test indicates previous exposure or active disease and usually occurs a week after the development of symptoms in about 80% of patients. A negative skin reaction does not rule out coccidioidomycosis. Almost all symptomatic patients are positive a month after the onset of symptoms. Anergy is common in disseminated disease. There is a low degree of cross reactivity with histoplasmosis and blastomycosis.[28] Positive skin tests do not affect serologic testing, although a positive coccidioidin skin test may induce antibodies that cross react with histoplasmin.[29] Skin testing is important primarily in assessing the cellular immunity status of a patient with documented coccidioidal disease and as an epidemiologic tool.

TREATMENT

The cornerstones of therapy for coccidioidomycosis at the present time are amphotericin B and the triazoles fluconazole and itraconazole. The advantages of the triazoles over amphotericin B include oral administration and relative nontoxicity. Fluconazole is effective in treating progressive pulmonary and disseminated coccidioidomycosis.[30] There are, however, no comparative trials comparing amphotericin B to the triazoles in the treatment of coccidioidomycosis, and the triazoles are not currently approved by the U.S. Food and Drug Administration for the treatment of this disease. Miconazole has not been proved to be effective in treating intraocular coccidioidomycosis.[31]

Amphotericin B is the treatment of choice for coccidioidomycosis. It is administered intravenously at a dose of 1 mg/kg body weight per day. A total dose of 500 mg to 1500 mg can be given. Intraocular amphotericin B (5 μg/0.1 ml) is administered during vitrectomy for suspected fungal endophthalmitis. Amphotericin B, however, has poor ocular and central nervous system penetration, retinal toxicity associated with intravitreal injection, and potentially serious dose-limiting systemic side effects.

Fluconazole (Diflucan) is the drug of choice for coccidioidal meningitis. Oral administration results in high concentrations in the cerebrospinal fluid, the aqueous, vitreous, retina, and choroid.[32, 33] It is given orally at a dose of 400 to 800 mg/day. It can be substituted for amphotericin B, but cases of treatment failure have been reported.[34] Intraocular coccidioidomycosis has been successfully treated using fluconazole as the primary agent.[35] The authors of that report believe that amphotericin B should be reserved for patients who fail initial treatment with oral fluconazole.

Itraconazole (Sporanox) has also been used in the treatment of coccidioidomycosis, and it has a response rate of 60% to 80%.[36, 37] It is taken orally at a dose of 200 mg twice daily. Its role in treating ocular coccidioidomycosis is unclear, although it has been used successfully in a uveitis patient with iris-biopsy confirmed coccidioidomycosis.[21]

Acute treatment of progressive pulmonary and extrapulmonary coccidioidomycosis should be followed by long-term maintenance therapy because of a reported high relapse rate after treatment with both amphotericin B and the triazoles.[38, 39] Fluconazole (200 to 400 mg daily), weekly amphotericin B, or itraconazole may be effective. Patients with meningitis and those with the acquired immunodeficiency syndrome with progressive or disseminated coccidioidomycosis should continue with maintenance therapy for life.

COMPLICATIONS

Complications of intraocular coccidioidomycosis include posterior synechiae, cataracts, scleral thinning and staphyloma formation, and secondary glaucoma. The posterior segment lesions can involve the macula and the optic nerve, with devastating consequences to the vision. Epiretinal membranes and serous retinal detachment can occur. Even with aggressive antifungal therapy, the eye can become hypotonous and painful and require enucleation.

PROGNOSIS

Despite systemic antifungal therapy, meningeal involvement carries a grave prognosis.[40–41] In patients with AIDS, less than half respond to treatment, and the mortality rate can climb as high as 70% in those patients with diffuse pulmonary disease.[42]

The prognosis of ocular coccidioidomycosis ultimately depends on the location and severity of the ocular lesions, as well as on prompt diagnosis and treatment of the systemic disease. In general, intravenous and intraocular amphotericin B can sterilize most cases of ocular coccidioidomycosis. However, the prognosis for patients with isolated anterior segment coccidioidomycosis is poor, with the majority requiring enucleation owing to blindness and pain.[21]

CONCLUSIONS

Coccidioidomycosis must be considered in the differential diagnosis of ocular inflammatory disease, especially in patients who have lived in or traveled through endemic areas. The absence of serologic evidence for coccidioidomycosis and lack of systemic manifestations do not rule out the diagnosis of coccidioidal infection. Biopsies of intraocular lesions, including vitreous and aqueous taps, provide rapid diagnosis and may be the most efficient method of facilitating appropriate treatment. Guidelines for therapy have not been clearly established owing to the rarity of the disease. Intravenous amphotericin B is the treatment of choice, although the triazoles such as fluconazole hold promise as a better tolerated form of treatment. The role of intraocular injections of amphotericin B in treating intraocular coccidioidomycosis is unclear, although it is given in suspected cases of fungal endophthalmitis. Patients may require prolonged systemic therapy to prevent relapse and require close collaboration between the ophthalmologist and infectious disease specialists. The prognosis for isolated anterior segment disease is poor, and the majority of these eyes may ultimately require enucleation.

References

1. Bennett JE: Coccidioidomycosis and paracoccidioidomycosis. In: Isselbacher KJ, Braunwald E, Wilson JD, et al (eds): Harrison's Principles of Internal Medicine. New York, McGraw-Hill Book Company, 1994, pp 857–858.
2. Rodenbiker HT, Ganley JP: Ocular coccidioidomycosis. Surv Ophthalmol 1980;24:263–290.
3. Levitt JM: Ocular manifestations in coccidioidomycosis. Am J Ophthalmol 1948;31:1626–1628.
4. Hagele AJ, Evans DJ, Larwood TR: Primary endophthalmic coccidioidomycosis. Report of a case of exogenous primary coccidioidomycosis of the eye diagnosed prior to enucleation. In: Ajello E (ed): Coccidioidomycosis. Tucson, University of Arizona Press, 1967, pp 37–39.
5. CDC: Update: Coccidioidomycosis—California, 1991–1993. MMWR 1994;43:421–423.
6. Pappagianis D: Marked increase in cases of coccidioidomycosis in California: 1991, 1992, and 1993. Clin Infect Dis 1994;19(Suppl 1):S14–18.
7. Schneider E, Hajjeh RA, Spiegel RA, et al: A coccidioidomycosis outbreak following the Northridge, California, earthquake. JAMA 1997;277:904–908.
8. Flynn NM, Hoeprich PD, Kawachi MM, et al: An unusual outbreak of windborne coccidioidomycosis. N Engl J Med 1979;301:358–361.
9. Werner SB, Pappagianis D, Heindl I, et al: An epidemic of coccidioidomycosis among archeology students in Northern California. N Engl J Med 1972;286:507–512.
10. Galgiani JN: Coccidioidomycosis: Changes in clinical expression, serological diagnosis, and therapeutic options. Clin Infect Dis 1992;14(Suppl 1):S100–S105.
11. Granoff DM, Libke RD: Coccidioidomycosis in children. In: Feigin RD, Cherry JD (eds): Textbook of Pediatric Infectious Diseases. Philadelphia, WB Saunders Company, 1981, pp 1488–1500.
12. Drutz DJ, Cadanzaro A: Coccidioidomycosis. Am Rev Resp Dis 1978;117:559–585.
13. Ampel NM, Wieden MA, Galgiani JN: Coccidioidomycosis: Clinic update. Rev Infect Dis 1989;11:897–911.
14. Maguire LJ, Campbell RJ, Edson RS: Coccidioidomycosis with necrotizing granulomatous conjunctivitis. Cornea 1994;13:539–542.
15. Fusaro RM, Bansal S, Records RE: Some unusual periorbital dermatoses. Ann Ophthalmol 1988;20:391–393.
16. Mark AS, Blake P, Atlas SW, et al: Gd-DTPA enhancement of the cisternal portion of the oculomotor nerve on MR imaging. AJNR Am J Neuroradiol 1992;13:1463–1470.
17. Blumenkranz MS, Stevens DA: Endogenous coccidioidal endophthalmitis. Ophthalmology 1980;87:974–984.
18. Lamer L, Paquin F, Lorange G, et al: Macular coccidioidomycosis. Can J Ophthalmol 1982;17:121–123.
19. Zakka KA, Foos RY, Brown WJ. Intraocular coccidioidomycosis. Surv Ophthalmol 1978;22:313–321.
20. Rodenbiker HT, Ganley JP, Galgiani JN, et al: Prevalence of chorioretinal scars associated with coccidioidomycosis. Arch Ophthalmol 1981;99:71–75.
21. Moorthy RS, Rao NA, Sidikaro Y, et al: Coccidioidomycosis iridocyclitis. Ophthalmology 1994;101:1923–1928.
22. Irvine AR Jr: Coccidioidal granuloma of the lid. Trans Am Acad Ophthalmol Otolaryngol 1968;72:751–754.
23. Glasgow BJ, Brown HH, Foos RY: Miliary retinitis in coccidioidomycosis. Am J Ophthalmol 1987;104:24–27.
24. Gori S, Scasso A: Cytologic and differential diagnosis of rhinosporidiosis. Acta Cytologica 1994;38:361–366.
25. Warlick MA, Quan SF, Sobonya RE: Rapid diagnosis of pulmonary coccidioidomycosis. Cytologic vs potassium hydroxide preparations. Arch Intern Med 1983;143:723–725.
26. CDC. Coccidioidomycosis—Arizona, 1990–1995. JAMA 1997;277:104–105.
27. Stevens DA: *Coccidioides immitis.* In: Mandell GL, Douglas RG Jr, Bennett JE (eds): Principles and Practice of Infectious Diseases. New York, John Wiley & Sons, Inc., 1985, pp 1485–1493.
28. Chick EW, Baum GL, Furculow ML, et al: Scientific Assembly statement. The use of skin tests and serologic tests in histoplasmosis, coccidioidomycosis, and blastomycosis, 1973. Am Rev Respir Dis 1973;108:156–159.
29. Pappagianis D, Zimmer BL: Serology of coccidioidomycosis. Clin Microbiol Rev 1990;3:247–268.
30. Catanzaro A, Galgiani JN, Levine BE, et al: Fluconazole in the treatment of chronic pulmonary and nonmeningeal disseminated coccidioidomycosis. Am J Med 1995;98:249–256.
31. Blumenkranz MS, Stevens DA: Therapy of endogenous fungal endophthalmitis. Arch Ophthalmol 1980;98:1216–1220.
32. Tucker RM, Williams PL, Arathoon EG, et al: Pharmacokinetics of fluconazole in cerebrospinal fluid and serum in human coccidioidal meningitis. Antimicrob Agents Chemother 1988;32:369–373.
33. O'Day DM, Foulds G, Williams TE, et al: Ocular uptake of flucona-

zole following oral administration. Arch Ophthalmol 1990;108:1006–1008.

34. Evans TG, Mayer J, Cohen S, et al: Fluconazole failure in the treatment of invasive mycoses. J Infect Dis 1991;164:1232–1235.
35. Luttrull JK, Wan WL, Kubak BM, et al: Treatment of ocular fungal infections with oral fluconazole. Am J Ophthalmol 1995;119:477–481.
36. Graybill JR, Stevens DA, Galgiani JN, et al: Itraconazole treatment of coccidioidomycosis. Am J Med 1990;89:282–290.
37. Tucker RM, Denning DW, Dupont B, et al: Itraconazole therapy for chronic coccidioidal meningitis. Ann Intern Med 1990; 112:108–112.
38. Dewsnup DH, Galgiani JN, Graybill JR, et al: Is it ever safe to stop azole therapy for *Coccidioides immitis* meningitis? Ann Intern Med 1996;125:304–310.
39. Oldgfield EC III, Bone WD, Martin CR, et al: Prediction of relapse after treatment of coccidioidomycosis. Clin Infect Dis 1997;25:1205–1210.
40. Bouza E, Dreyer JS, Hewitt WL, et al: Coccidioidal meningitis: An analysis of thirty-one cases and review of literature. Medicine 1981;60:139–172.
41. Kafka JA, Cataranzo A. Disseminated coccidioidomycosis in children. J Pediatr 1981;98:355–361.
42. Fish DG, Ampel NM, Galciani JN, et al: Coccidioidomycosis during human immunodeficiency virus infection: A review of 77 patients. Medicine (Baltimore) 1990;69:384–391.

31 ┤ CRYPTOCOCCOSIS

Katerina Havrlikova-Dutt

DEFINITION

Cryptococcosis is a systemic infection caused by the saprophytic fungus *Cryptococcus neoformans*. It is known to affect mainly immunocompromised patients, although it can cause disease in an immunocompetent individual as well. Pulmonary and central nervous system (CNS) involvement make up the majority of cases. Cryptococcosis is the most common mycotic infection of the CNS, and ocular involvement occurs in 40% of patients with cryptococcal meningitis.[1]

C. neoformans is a round, encapsulated yeastlike fungus that reproduces by budding. Staining with India ink and Wright's stain shows a large capsule surrounding a cell that has a single bud attached to a narrow bud base.

EPIDEMIOLOGY

C. neoformans is a worldwide saprobe, found in pigeon feces, pigeon nesting places, and contaminated soil.[2] Despite the high concentration of fungus in pigeon feces, the birds are not infected.[3] There is evidence that the disease occurs after the organism is aerosolized and inhaled.[4] Transmission from animals to humans or between humans has not been documented, although a case of cryptococcal endophthalmitis acquired through a corneal transplant from a donor with active cryptococcosis has been reported.[5] There has also been a case report describing *Cryptococcus laurentii* keratitis spread by a rigid gas-permeable contact lens in a patient with onychomycosis.[6]

Cryptococcosis is relatively rare in an immunocompetent host, but in patients with acquired immunodeficiency syndrome (AIDS), it is the fourth most common cause of life-threatening infections.[7] It can also be seen in other immunocompromised patients such as diabetic patients on long-term corticosteroids or individuals with polyarteritis nodosa, lymphoma, systemic lupus erythematosus, Hodgkin's disease, organ transplant recipients, or other systemic diseases treated with immunosuppressive agents.

CLINICAL CHARACTERISTICS

Systemic involvement in cryptococcosis varies widely and includes meningitis, pneumonia, mucocutaneous lesions, multiple skin lesions, pyelonephritis, endocarditis, hepatitis, prostatitis, and ocular infection. In the population of patients with AIDS, *C. neoformans* is an important pathogen producing not only a variety of CNS and neurophthalmic complications (chronic meningitis being the most common) but also devastating disseminated systemic disease.

Ocular manifestations are thought to arise via optic nerve extension from central nervous system involvement[8, 9] but it appears that intraocular involvement can occur via hematogenous spread as well.[10]

Ophthalmic manifestations of cryptococcosis include papilledema, optic neuropathy, chiasmal involvement, optic atrophy, cranial nerve palsies, nystagmus, internuclear ophthalmoplegia, choroiditis, retinis, uveitis, inflammatory iris mass, keratitis, conjunctival granuloma, limbal nodules, phthisis bulbi, periorbital necrotizing fasciitis, orbital infection, exogenous endophthalmitis, and endogenous endophthalmitis.

In most patients ocular involvement is associated with meningitis. Specifically, the ocular involvement usually follows meningitis, but a case of endogenous cryptococcal endophthalmitis without a preceding meningeal infection has been documented. The most common intraocular manifestation is chorioretinitis. The earliest sign is focal or multifocal choroiditis, in which yellowish to white, subretinal, slightly elevated lesions one fifth to one optic disc diameter in size are usually observed. Choroiditis is followed, in rapid succession, by inflammation of the retina, vitreous, and if the condition is left untreated, the anterior segment.

Endogenous cryptococcal endophthalmitis was first reported in 1948,[11] and since then, approximately 15 cases have been reported in the literature.[12–20] The earliest symptom is blurred vision, followed by redness, pain, photophobia, floaters, ocular injection, and profound visual loss. Patients with concomitant cryptococcal meningitis also suffer from headaches and nausea. Ophthalmic findings include injection, anterior chamber cell and flare, mutton fat keratic precipitates, posterior synechiae, yellow or white chorioretinal lesions, retinal perivascular sheathing, subretinal exudate or localized serous retinal detachment, vitreous cells, severe vitreous inflammation with fluffy exudates, preretinal or vitreous abscesses, retinal detachment, and phthisis bulbi.[12–20] The outcome in cryptococcal endophthalmitis is generally rather poor, including blindness or enucleation.

Because cryptococcosis affects mostly immunocompromised patients, the inflammation typical of uveitis in an immunocompetent individual may be lacking. It is important to keep in mind that primary choroidal lesions in patients with AIDS may herald severe systemic disseminated disease. Funduscopic examination may detect disseminated cryptococcal disease before other clinical manifestations, thereby allowing prompt institution of effective therapy.[10]

PATHOGENESIS

C. neoformans is a budding, spore-forming yeast yielding yellow-tan colonies on culture media. Four serotypes (A, B, C, and D) have been identified based on capsular polysaccharide antigen determination with immunofluorescence or agglutination. Types A and D are most commonly pathogenic.[21] Infection occurs via inhalation into the moist environment of the lungs, where the yeast enlarges and starts to bud. A thick polysaccharide capsule forms around each cell. This capsule is immunologically inert and provides protection from phagocytic cells, thus the inflammatory response to infection is variable. Hematogenous spread to the brain leads to cystic clusters of cryptococci associated with minimal inflammatory response. Neutrophils are first to home to the infected area, followed by the monocytes that predominate in the later inflammatory infiltrate.[22] Neutrophils and monocytes can ingest and kill cryptococci in vitro by using the myeloperoxidase-peroxide-halide system[23] or the neutrophil cationic proteins.[24] Encapsulated *C. neoformans* may be sufficiently large to preclude phagocytosis, but they can still be surrounded and killed by "rings" of macrophages.[25] Macrophage activation requires functional, sensitized T cells. Natural killer cells,[26] anticryptococcal antibodies,[27] and T cells may all be involved in the host defense response.

DIAGNOSIS

The diagnosis of cryptococcosis requires a high degree of suspicion and is often presumptive, depending on the clinical context. Definitive diagnosis requires identification of the organism in culture from infected tissue, blood, or body fluids. There are usually no abnormalities in routine blood tests. If signs of meningitis are present, cerebrospinal fluid (CSF) analysis, including cryptococcal antigen testing and fungal culture, should be performed.

When the CNS is involved in immunocompetent patients, the CSF is almost always abnormal with an elevated opening pressure, elevated protein, hypoglycorrhachia at 50%, and 20 to 600 leukocytes/mm^3 with lymphocyte predominance. In severely immunosuppressed patients, there are minimal to no abnormalities of the CSF. India ink smears of the CSF have positive results for cryptococcus in 50% of patients. Solution may be contaminated by nonpathogenic cryptococci; other fungi or artifacts may be mistaken for cryptococci as well.

Centrifuged CSF specimens should be cultured on several different occasions, because negative results do not rule out the disease.

Cryptococcal polysaccharide capsular antigen may be detected in the CSF or serum of 90% of patients with meningoencephalitis.[28] The antigen is detected by latex agglutination; false-positive results may occur in the presence of rheumatoid factor. Anticryptococcal antibodies are also detectable in healthy persons, so culture of cryptococcus remains the definitive diagnostic test.

Cryptococcal serology and fungal cultures of blood, sputum, or urine are often helpful in patients with disseminated disease.[2] If the results of these tests are negative and clinical suspicion still exists, diagnostic vitreous tap, vitrectomy,[24] fine-needle abscess biopsy,[16] or eye wall biopsy[29] can be performed.

DIFFERENTIAL DIAGNOSIS

Multifocal choroiditis due to *Pneumocystis carinii* cannot be distinguished from cryptococcal uveitis by clinical examination alone. A history of *P. carinii* pneumonia and the use of aerosolized pentamidine in patients with AIDS should suggest the former diagnosis. Other opportunistic infections in AIDS patients, including toxoplasmosis, cytomegalovirus, and herpes simplex virus, all of which primarily infect the retina, should be excluded in cases of suspected *C. neoformans* endophthalmitis. Tuberculosis, sarcoidosis, intraocular lymphoma, and uveitis caused by other fungal organisms should also be considered in the differential diagnosis.

TREATMENT

Cryptococcal meningitis is usually fatal without systemic antifungal therapy, and even with treatment, the relapse rate is about 50% in patients with AIDS. Fluconazole (200 to 400 mg/day) has been used as a long-term oral maintenance therapy in an attempt to prevent such recurrences.[22, 29] Combined therapy with oral flucytosine (25 to 35 mg q, 6 h PO) and intravenous amphotericin B (0.4 to 0.6 mg/day) has been recommended as the treatment of choice for patients with disseminated or meningeal cryptococcosis. Oral fluconazole has been successful in some patients with AIDS, as well as others who cannot tolerate the renal toxicity and bone marrow suppression of the combined therapy.[23, 30]

Treatment of endogenous cryptococcal endophthalmitis may require a combination of systemic antifungal agents, intravitreous amphotericin B, and pars plana vitrectomy.

Patients with cryptococcosis should be evaluated every few months for at least 1 year after therapy, even if they are asymptomatic. The CSF, urine, and sputum should be cultured repeatedly.

PROGNOSIS

The outcome for an immunocompetent patient treated for a localized pulmonary infection is usually very good.

The outcome for immunocompromised patients can vary depending on a variety of factors. The mortality rate of immunocompromised patients who do not have AIDS and who have been treated for cryptococcal meningitis is approximately 25%. When predisposing factors such as lymphoreticular malignancy or corticosteroid therapy are present, the mortality rate is 55%. After the initial treatment with amphotericin B, 20% to 25% of patients relapse. Of those cured, 40% suffer significant permanent sequelae, such as visual loss, cranial nerve palsies, motor impairment, personality changes, and decreased mental function.

The prognosis for patients with AIDS is very poor, because these patients are rarely completely cured. The treatment regimen is directed toward suppressing inflammation without interfering with treatment of concomitant diseases.[2]

CONCLUSIONS

Despite its ubiquity throughout the world, *C. neoformans* is an uncommon cause of systemic or ocular disease in the immunocompetent patient. However, in the immunosuppressed host, particularly those individuals afflicted with AIDS, this fungus has become an important pathogen, producing potentially devastating CNS, ocular, and systemic disease. Diagnosis requires a high degree of clinical acumen in the correct clinical context, and despite aggressive treatment with systemic and/or intraocular antifungal agents, the prognosis is guarded. Nevertheless, early diagnosis and treatment of cryptococcosis can not only preserve the patients vision, but may also be life-saving, particularly in the management of patients with AIDS.

References

1. Lesser RL, Simon RM, Leon H, et al: Cryptococcal meningitis and internal ophthalmoplegia. Am J Ophthalmol 1979;87:682.

2. Behlau I, Baker AS: Fungal infections and the eye—cryptococcosis. In: Albert DM, Jakobiec FA, eds: Principles and Practice of Ophthalmology: Clinical Practice, 1st ed, Vol V. Philadelphia, WB Saunders, 1994, p 3045.

3. Littman ML, Walter JE: Cryptococcosis: Current status. Am J Med 1968;45:922.

4. Neilson JB, Fromtling RA, Bulmer GS: Cryptococcus neoformans: Size range of infectious particles from aerosolized soil. Infect Immun 1977;17:634.

5. Beyt BE Jr, Waltman SR: Cryptococcal endophthalmitis after corneal transplantation. N Engl J Med 1978;298:825.

6. Ritterband DC, Seeder JA, Shah MK, et al: A unique case of *Cryptococcus laurentii* keratitis spread by a rigid gas-permeable contact lens in a patient with onychomycosis. Cornea 1998;17:115.

7. Eng RHK, Bishburg E, Smith SM, et al: Cryptococcal infections in patients with the acquired immune deficiency syndrome. Am J Med 1986;81:19.

8. Eng RHK, Bishburg E, Smith SM, et al: Cryptococcal infections in patients with the acquired immune deficiency syndrome. Am J Med 1986;81:19.

9. Ofner S, Baker RS: Visual loss in cryptococcal meningitis. J Clin Neuroophthalmol 1987;7:45.

10. Rostomian K, Dugel PU, Kolahdous-Isfahani A, et al: Presumed multifocal cryptococcal choroidopathy prior to specific systemic manifestation. Int Ophthalmol 1997;21:75.

11. Weiss C, Perry IH, Shevky MC: Infection of the human eye with *Cryptococcus neoformans (Torula histologica; Cryptococcus hominis)*: A clinical and experimental study with a new diagnostic method. Arch Ophthalmol 1948;39:739–751.

12. Denning DW, Armstrong RW, Fishman M, et al: Endophthalmitis in a patient with disseminated cryptococcosis and AIDS who was treated with itraconazole. Rev Infect Dis 1991;13:1126.

13. Grieco MH, Freilich DB, Louria DB: Diagnosis of cryptococcal uveitis with hypertonic media. Am J Ophthalmol 1971;72:171.

14. Henderly DE, Liggett PE, Rao NA: Cryptococcal chorioretinitis and endophthalmitis. Retina 1987;7:75.

15. Hiles DA, Font RL: Bilateral intraocular cryptococcus with unilateral spontaneous regression: Report of a case and review of the literature. Am J Ophthalmol 1968;65:98.

16. Hiss PW, Shields JA, Augsburger JJ: Solitary retrovitreal abscess as the initial manifestation of cryptococcosis. Ophthalmology 1988;95:162.

17. Malton ML, Rinkhoff JS, Doft BS, et al: Cryptococcal endophthalmitis and meningitis associated with acute psychosis and exudative retinal detachment. Am J Ophthalmol 1987;104:438.

18. O'Dowd GJ, Frable WJ: Cryptococcal endophthalmitis: Diagnostic vitreous aspiration cytology. Am J Clin Pathol 1983;79:382.

19. Schields JA, Wright DM, Augsburger JJ, et al: Cryptococcal chorioretinitis. Am J Ophthalmol 1980;89:210.

20. Schulman JA, Leveque C, Coats M, et al: Fatal disseminated cryptococcosis following intraocular involvement. Br J Ophthalmol 1988;72:171.

21. Diamond R: *Cryptococcus neoformans*. In: Mandell GC, Bennett JE, Dolin R, eds: Principles and Practice of Infectious Disease, 4th ed. New York, Churchill-Livingstone, 1995, pp 2331–2340.

22. Gadebush HH: Mechanisms of native and acquired resistance to infection with *Cryptococcus neoformans*. CRC Crit Rev Microbiol 1972;1:311.

23. Diamond RD, Root RK, Bennett JE: Factors influencing killing of *Cryptococcus neoformans* by human leukocytes in vitro. J Infect Dis 1972;125:367.

24. Ganz T, Selsted ME, Szklarek D, et al: Defensins: Natural peptide antibiotics of human neutrophils. J Clin Invest 1985;76:1427.

25. Kalina M, Kletter Y, Aronson M: The interaction of phagocytes and the large-sized parasite, *Cryptococcus neoformans*: Cytochemical and ultrastructural study. Cell Tissue Res 1974;152:165.

26. Hidore MR, Murphy JW: Correlation of natural killer cell activity and clearance of *Cryptococcus neoformans* from mice after adoptive transfer of splenic nylon-wool-nonadherent cells. Infect Immun 1986;51:57.

27. Nabavi N, Murphy JW: Antibody-dependent natural killer cell-mediated growth inhibition of *Cryptococcus neoformans*. Infect Immun 1986;51:556.

28. Benett JE, Bailey JW: Control for rheumatoid factor in the latex test for cryptococcosis. Am J Clin Pathol 1971;56:360.

29. Peyman GA, Juarez CP, Raichand M: Full-thickness eye-wall biopsy: Long-term results in 9 patients. Br J Ophthalmol 1981;65:723.

30. Golnik KC, Newman SA, Wispelway B: Cryptococcal optic neuropathy in the acquired immune deficiency syndrome. J Clin Neuroophthalmol 1991;11:96–103.

Manolette Rangel Roque and C. Stephen Foster

DEFINITION

Sporotrichosis is a chronic infectious disease caused by the filamentous branching fungus *Sporothrix schenckii* (*Sporotrichum schenckii*). It is characterized by subcutaneous, nodular granulomata, which are usually acquired by traumatic implantation through the skin. Ocular involvement ranges from simple conjunctivitis to fulminant endophthalmitis.

HISTORY

The reported literature on sporotrichosis dates back to the turn of the 20th century. In 1809, Link, cited by Gordon,[1] described the genus *Sporotrichum* primarily as a saprophyte on wood. Schenck reported the first described clinical case in 1898.[2] He described a typical lesion occurring on a finger, followed by the formation of a nodular chain. As a result of his research, his name was attached to the organism. The first reported case of *S. schenckii* involving the eye or its adnexa was published in 1907 by Danlos and Blanc.[3] In that same year, DeBeurmann, Gougerot, and Laroche[4] cited a similar case with lid involvement. The first reported case of intraocular *S. schenckii* was published in 1909.[5] Morax then first isolated ocular *S. schenckii* in 1914.[6] In the 1940s, a large outbreak of nearly 3000 cases occurred in South African gold mines as a result of contaminated timber beams.[7] The latest reported case occurred in a patient with acquired immunodeficiency syndrome (AIDS) who had disseminated sporotrichosis with extensive cutaneous involvement.[8]

EPIDEMIOLOGY

Sporothrix schenkii is distributed worldwide but is common in tropical or temperate regions. In the United States, the majority of cases have been found in the Midwestern river valleys, especially those of the Missouri and Missis-sippi rivers. This fungus is common in Mexico and Central America. It is a common saprophyte found in natural vegetation (soil,[9–11] plants, thorns, wood, straw, reeds,[7] etc.). There is a consequent high incidence of infection involving gardeners,[12] forestry workers,[13] agricultural workers, miners, meat packers, and sphagnum moss handlers.[14] Sporotrichosis also can be inoculated by insect stings, animal bites, and cat scratches, or by handling of contaminated fish. Pathogenic sporotricha have also been isolated from the hair of horses and other domestic animals and their excreta.[15]

Mycology

Sporothrix schenckii lives as a saprophyte on plants in many areas of the world. In nature and on culture at room temperature (25°C), the fungus grows as a beige-colored leathery mold that darkens to black with age (Figs. 32–1 and 32–2), but within host tissue or at 37°C on enriched media, it grows as a budding, cigar-shaped yeast (Fig. 32–3). It is identified by its appearance in mold and yeast forms[16, 17] (Figs. 32–4 and 32–5). The hyphae are 2 μm in width; they are segmented and branched and produce oval conidia, which range from 2 to 6 μm in longest diameter.[18]

CLINICAL CHARACTERISTICS

Nonocular Disease

Lymphocutaneous infection is the most common form of sporotrichosis.[9, 10] At the site of entry (usually the hands), a small, painless, pink or purple, verrucous, nodular or ulcerative cutaneous lesion develops anytime from 1 week to several months later. It is a chronic subcutaneous nodular granuloma, usually with spreading lymphatic involvement, following trauma. The nodules may ulcerate and discharge a small amount of serosanguineous exudate.

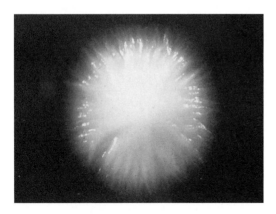

FIGURE 32–1. Young colonies of *Sporothrix schenckii* remain white for some time at 25°C or when incubated at 37°C to induce its yeast phase. (Reprinted from *http://fungusweb.utmb.edu/mycology/sporothrix.html,* with permission from Medical Mycology Research Center, Department of Pathology, University of Texas Medical Branch.) (See color insert.)

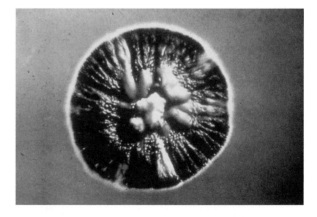

FIGURE 32–2. Older colonies of *Sporothrix schenckii* turn black due to the production of dark conidia that arise directly from the hyphae. (Reprinted from *http://fungusweb.utmb.edu/mycology/sporothrix.html,* with permission from Medical Mycology Research Center, Department of Pathology, University of Texas Medical Branch.) (See color insert.)

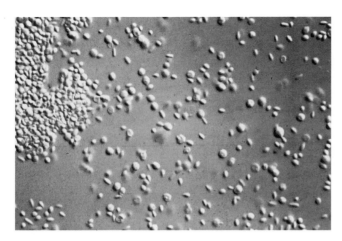

FIGURE 32–3. *Sporothrix schenckii* has a yeast form at 37°C. (Reprinted from *http://fungusweb.utmb.edu/mycology/sporothrix.html,* with permission from Medical Mycology Research Center, Department of Pathology, University of Texas Medical Branch.)

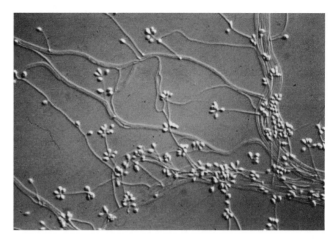

FIGURE 32–4. Conidia arising directly from the hyphae, and conidia arising on denticles from sympodial conidiophores are typical of *Sporothrix schenckii.* (Reprinted from *http://fungusweb.utmb.edu/mycology/sporothrix.html,* with permission from Medical Mycology Research Center, Department of Pathology, University of Texas Medical Branch.)

The primary lesion remains "fixed" in 23% of cases, without lymphatic involvement,[19] originating from the extremities or the face, and persisting for years. These localized cutaneous lesions without lymphatic spread may appear nodular, crusted, weeping, or fungating or may resemble papillomata, folliculitis, or intertrigo. Sporotrichosis may be limited to the site of inoculation (plaque sporotrichosis) and manifests as a nontender, red, maculopapular granuloma, without associated systemic signs and symptoms.

Disseminated sporotrichosis (lesions in more than one organ system) occurs after hematogenous[20, 21] spread from a primary pulmonary or subcutaneous site, in an immunocompromised[22] host. When it occurs, it most commonly affects bones and joints.[9, 10] Reported manifestations of extracutaneous or disseminated sporotrichosis include fungal tendinitis, bursitis, arthritis, osteomyelitis, diffuse skin lesions, meningitis, ocular infection, and vocal cord granulomata. It has been observed in association

with corticosteroid use, sarcoidosis, diabetes mellitus, alcoholism, neoplasia, and AIDS.[8, 22] Multifocal cutaneous sporotrichosis (skin infection beyond a single extremity) is extremely common in cases of dissemination.

Except for a rare primary pulmonary[23] form of infection in which the organism is inhaled in endemic areas or by an immunocompromised host, sporotrichosis most commonly enters the body through the skin, usually in association with some episode of traumatic implantation. Symptoms include the insidious onset of cough, sputum production, malaise, weight loss, low-grade fever, and occasional hemoptysis. A single, chronic, cavitary upper lobe lesion and hilar adenopathy are usually revealed on chest x-ray.[12]

In the rare instance that the central nervous system is involved, focal or diffuse neurologic symptoms and headache and confusion may be present.

An unusual case of lymphocutaneous sporotrichosis was seen in a man who engaged in self-tattooing of his

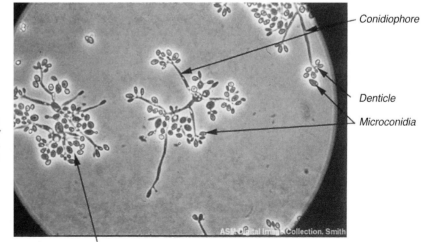

FIGURE 32–5. *Sporothrix schenckii.* (Reprinted from *http://www.asmusa.org/edusrc/library/images/SMITH/Images/IMAGE1-AN.JPG,* with permission from Andrew G. Smith, M.D., and the American Society for Microbiology Instructional Library.)

Conidiophore

Denticle

Microconidia

"Flowerettes", hyphae and conidia, diagnostic of *Sporothrix*

left foot.[24] He admitted to having mowed the lawn wearing only sandals on the same day that he tattooed his foot.

Sporotrichosis can be seen in patients with other systemic illnesses. Three cases of coinfection with *Leishmania* have been described in Columbia.[25] The use of empirical treatments for leishmaniasis, such as poultices or puncturing of the lesion with thorns or wood splinters, was speculated to have caused the introduction of the *Sporothrix*. A woman with Cushing's disease presented with erysipeloid sporotrichosis.[26]

Ocular Disease

In 1966, Alvarez and Lopez-Villegas[27] reported an 11-year-old mestizo boy with primary ocular sporotrichosis. The diagnosis was based on mycologic study of the biopsied left temporal bulbar conjunctiva. Conjunctival sporotrichosis may be a primary infection or may be secondary to involvement of the lid and face. The initial sign of infection in the skin of the eyelid is the appearance of a hard, spherical, movable, nontender nodule that later becomes attached to the skin. It is initially pink, then purple, and finally black and necrotic (sporotrichotic chancre). Multiple subcutaneous nodules appear along the course of the lymphatics draining the area. Numerous soft, yellow, granulomatous nodules, which may ulcerate, develop in the palpebral or bulbar conjunctiva of the involved eye. The conjunctival ulcers usually discharge a small amount of purulent material. Gross enlargement and occasional suppuration of preauricular and submandibular lymph nodes occur.

Most cases of ocular sporotrichosis have an exogenous cause and are acquired through a traumatic injury to the conjunctiva, cornea, or eyelids by a contaminated object. Witherspoon and associates[39] reported a case of exogenous *S. schenckii* endophthalmitis in a 13-year-old boy who was struck in his eye with a stick. They also reviewed previous cases of exogenous and endogenous ocular sporotrichosis, citing older reviews by Gordon in 1947, and Francois and Rysselaere in 1972. Most cases in the 1947 review were exogenous and involved the eyelids, conjunctiva, cornea, lacrimal excretory system, or orbit. But 14 of the 18 cases of intraocular sporotrichosis reported in the 1972 review were endogenous, resulting from disseminated sporotrichosis. The other 4 were cases of postoperative exogenous *S. schenckii* endophthalmitis following cataract surgery.

Presenting symptoms in endogenous *S. schenckii* endophthalmitis include decreased vision, pain, and ocular redness. Most cases have signs of anterior segment inflammation, including granulomatous or nongranulomatous keratic precipitates, iris nodules, and hypopyon. Later sequelae may include posterior synechiae, glaucoma, cataract, and phthisis bulbi. Posterior segment involvement may be manifested by choroiditis, vitritis, or a fluffy white retinal lesion. These latter cases of endogenous sporotrichosis can masquerade as idiopathic panuveitis or posterior uveitis; hence, it is important that the ophthalmologist keep in mind this and other causes of endogenous infectious uveitis.

In 1993, Cartwright and coworkers[28] reported a 24-year-old black male with *S. schenckii* endophthalmitis who presented without a history of trauma or systemic infection and was originally diagnosed with granulomatous uveitis that resulted in scleral perforation. Most patients with endogenous *S. schenckii* endophthalmitis eventually require enucleation. One problem is that it is difficult to culture the organism from blood, urine, or intraocular fluids. Several cases in the Witherspoon study[39] were not accurately diagnosed until enucleation had been performed. In addition, most of the previously reported cases occurred before amphotericin B or modern vitreoretinal surgical techniques were available. A recent case of endogenous *S. schenckii* endophthalmitis involved a 30-year-old man with AIDS and disseminated sporotrichosis. He had a granulomatous uveitis that worsened following topical and subconjunctival corticosteroid therapy. An aqueous aspirate was positive for *S. schenckii*, and the patient received treatment with intravitreous and intravenous amphotericin B. The patient's intraocular inflammation worsened despite negative repeat aqueous and vitreous cultures, and enucleation was eventually required.

PATHOLOGY

Pathogenesis

Traumatic implantation is the main mechanism for infection. Strains that multiply well at 25°C but poorly at 37°C can produce cutaneous lesions. Strains that multiply at both 25°C and 37°C are capable of producing lymphocutaneous or visceral disease. However, inhalation of spores is also known to cause a pulmonary form of disease.

Histopathology

Histopathologic and electronmicroscopic examination of an eye with sporotrichosis reveals suppuration and granulomata, occasionally with caseating necrosis. Organisms morphologically compatible with *S. schenckii* have been demonstrated in the anterior chamber, vitreous cavity,[29] retina,[30] subretinal space, and retinal pigment epithelium.[31] Additional histopathologic findings in other patients with *S. schenckii* endophthalmitis include a granulomatous necrotizing chorioretinitis[31] and intracellular fungi[32] within inflammatory cells. Scattered *S. schenckii* organisms with disrupted protoplasm[30] may occasionally be seen.

Immunology

Historical attempts to demonstrate a positive reaction to the agglutination test have been dispelled by the fact that the spores have been similarly agglutinated by the serum of normal controls. *S. schenckii* can bind to fibronectin, laminin, and type II collagen; the organisms also show differences in binding capacity according to the morphologic form of the fungus.[33] The virulence of *S. schenckii* conidia may be determined by their cell wall composition.[34] Modern research has attempted to give the organism a molecular persona. Cell-mediated immunity is important in determining the extent of disease. *S. schenckii* is processed chiefly by the cellular limb of the immune system; therefore, the relative integrity of the cellular immune system will influence whether the disease remains localized or becomes disseminated.

DIAGNOSIS

The organism is rarely seen on direct examination of tissue. The positive diagnosis of sporotrichosis relies on the identification of the organism.[1] The most reliable means of identification is by culture. It grows well on Sabouraud's glucose agar or blood agar at 25°C. It is resistant to cycloheximide; therefore, Mycosel or Mycobiotic agar may be used for culture. Colony morphology is variable and may be white or pigmented, creamy, or shiny, depending on the strain and specimen type. Animal inoculation may also be performed for specific identification.

S. schenckii can be very difficult to isolate from blood, urine, or ocular fluid, thereby necessitating repeated diagnostic aqueous and vitreous aspiration and culture to isolate the organism. If there is another site of infection, such as a cutaneous lesion or fungal arthritis, biopsy or aspiration of that site with culture may be helpful. Careful examination of Gram's, periodic acid–Schiff, or Gomori methenamine silver stain, as well as immunofluorescence histologic studies of a tissue specimen, may reveal organisms, even when the cultures are negative. Also, specific serologic tests are available to identify antibodies to *S. schenckii* in blood or body fluid. Immunodiffusion, enzyme-linked immunosorbent assay (ELISA), or Western immunoblot testing can be performed on aqueous or vitreous fluid as well. Gallium and bone scans have been helpful in localizing areas of involvement in patients with disseminated sporotrichosis. Despite the well-known difficulties in determining an accurate and timely diagnosis, fine-needle aspiration cytology, later confirmed by tissue biopsy and culture study, was performed and reported in 1999.[35]

DIFFERENTIAL DIAGNOSIS

Before the chain of lesions develops, there is nothing characteristic of the presentation that suggests sporotrichosis. Once the ulcers or chain of nodules appears, sporotrichosis should be suspected. All other causes of granulomatous lesions, however, should be investigated. Syphilis and tuberculosis may be ruled out on the basis of the clinical pictures and the specific lesions seen at biopsy and laboratory testing. Leprosy must also be excluded. In cases of conjunctival involvement, Parinaud's conjunctivitis should be considered and excluded. Other differentials worthy of consideration include causes of severe granulomatous inflammation such as sarcoidosis and fungal endophthalmitis caused by other organisms.

TREATMENT

The approach to treatment of sporotrichosis varies with the disease form. Administration of saturated solution of potassium iodide (SSKI)[1, 36] is the treatment of choice for cutaneous disease. Oral potassium iodide is an effective, inexpensive treatment that has been the standard regimen for decades. Its antifungal effect is not well understood, and it has no direct effect on *S. schenckii*. It is taken orally in milk at an initial dose of 5 drops three times daily, increased by 4 to 5 drops per day up to 12 to 18 ml/day[12] (1 drop equals 50 μl), or until signs of toxicity occur (e.g., lacrimation, salivation, parotid gland swelling, indigestion). When toxicity develops, the therapy should be stopped for a few days and restarted at a lower dose.

Local application of heat to the lesions may be helpful. A pustular, acneiform rash over the face and cape area of the trunk is not an infrequent finding, but it is not an indication to discontinue iodides. To avoid recurrence, iodides should be continued for 4 to 6 weeks after clinical resolution.

Disseminated or extracutaneous sporotrichosis is usually treated with intravenous amphotericin B (0.5 mg/kg/day). Flucytosine[37] has been effective in treating disseminated disease. Itraconazole is also very effective against both *S. schenckii* (in vitro) and disseminated sporotrichosis. Treatment with itraconazole has resulted in response rates of greater than 90%. As a result, itraconazole (200 mg once or twice daily)[17] is likely to become the drug of choice for both disseminated and nondisseminated forms of sporotrichosis, as most patients do not accept oral potassium iodide.[38]

The patient presented by Witherspoon and associates[39] had exogenous *S. schenckii* endophthalmitis, and it was the first case to be successfully treated. The patient underwent pars plana lensectomy and vitrectomy, received topical amphotericin B, and had a repeat vitrectomy with injection of intravitreous amphotericin B. This was the first reported case of *S. schenckii* endophthalmitis treated with vitrectomy. The patient's vision improved from light perception to 20/50. All previous cases of endogenous and exogenous *S. schenckii* endophthalmitis had resulted in enucleation. Successful treatment of endogenous *S. schenckii* endophthalmitis has not been reported.

PROGNOSIS

Sporotrichosis in its cutaneous, lymphocutaneous, and mucocutaneous forms remits and relapses over years without therapy.[12] Spontaneous cure has been reported in plaque sporotrichosis.[40] Most patients with sporotrichosis respond well to treatment, even when the disease has reached a fairly advanced state, provided that the deeper structures of the body are not yet involved. Involvement of the globe is evidence of deep invasion and indicates that the organism has reached the blood stream, unless a history has been elicited of direct perforation by the traumatizing and etiologic agent.[1]

CONCLUSIONS

A high index of suspicion of the clinical entity of sporotrichosis is needed if a properly conducted early laboratory diagnosis is to be achieved. Positive diagnosis of sporotrichosis relies on identification of the organism. The most reliable means of identification is by culture. The treatment of choice for the cutaneous presentation is potassium iodide in its soluble form. For extracutaneous forms, aggressive treatment using systemic antifungal agents (amphotericin B and/or itraconzole), pars plana vitrectomy, and intravitreous amphothericin B is warranted.

References
1. Gordon DM: Ocular sporotrichosis. Arch Ophthalmol 1947;37:56.
2. Schenck BT: On refractory subcutaneous abscesses caused by a fungus, possibly related to the Sporotrochia. Bull Johns Hopkins Hosp 1898;9:286, as cited by Gordon DM: Ocular sporotrichosis. Arch Ophthalmol 1947;37:56.
3. Gordon DM: Ocular sporotrichosis. Arch Ophthalmol 1947;37:56.

4. DeBeurmann CL, Gougerot H, and Laroche: Gomme de la pau-piere. Bull Mem Soc Med Hop Paris 1907;27:1046, as cited by Gordon DM: Ocular sporotrichosis. Arch Ophthalmol 1947;37:56.

5. DeBeurmann CL, Gougerot H: Sporotrichose cachectisante mor-telle. Bull Mem Soc Med Hop Paris 1909;26:1046, as cited in Duanes's Ophthalmology on CD-ROM. Philadelphia, Lippincott-Raven, 1996.

6. Morax V: Uveite sporotrichosique avec gomme sporotrichosique episclerale secondaire: Absence de route autre localization sporotri-chosique decelable. Ann Ocul 1914;152:273, as cited in Duanes's Ophthalmology on CD-ROM. Philadelphia, Lippincott-Raven, 1996.

7. Mackenzie DWR: Subcutaneous mycoses. In: Strickland GT, ed: Hunter's Tropical Medicine, 7th ed. Philadelphia, WB Saunders, 1991, pp 510–515.

8. Ware AJ, Cockerell CJ, Skiest DJ, Kussman HM: Disseminated sporo-trichosis with extensive cutaneous involvement in a patient with AIDS. J Am Acad Dermatol 1999;40(2.2):350–355.

9. Wilson DE, Mann JJ, Bennett JE, Utz JP: Clinical features of extracu-taneous sporotrichosis. Medicine 1967;46:265.

10. Lynch PJ, Voorhees JJ, Harrell ER: Systemic sporotrichosis. Ann Intern Med 1970;73:23.

11. Chang AC, Destouet JM, Murphy WA: Musculoskeletal sporotricho-sis. Skeletal Radiol 1985;12:23.

12. Albert DM, Jakobiec FA, eds: Principles and Practice of Ophthalmol-ogy, on CD-ROM. Philadelphia, WB Saunders, 2000.

13. Powell KE, Talor A, Phillips BJ, et al: Cutaneous sporotrichosis in forestry workers. Epidemic due to contaminated sphagnum moss. JAMA 1978;240:232.

14. Dixon DM, Salkin IF, Duncan RA, et al: Isolation and characteriza-tion of Sporothrix schenckii from clinical and environmental sources associated with the largest U.S. epidemic of sporotrichosis, J Clin Microbiol 1991;29:1106–1113.

15. McGrath H, Singer JI: Ocular sporotrichosis. Am J Ophthalmol 1952;35:102.

16. Pettit TH, Edwards JE Jr, Purdy EP, Bullock JD: Endogenous fungal endophthalmitis. In: Pepose JS, Holland GN, Wilhelmus KR, eds: Ocular Infection and Immunity, 1st ed. Missouri, Mosby, 1996, pp 1278–1281.

17. Bennett JE: Miscellaneous mycoses and prototheca infections. In: Harrison TR, Resnick WR, Wintrobe MM, Thorn GW, et al, eds: Harrison's Principles of Internal Medicine, 14th ed, on CD-ROM. New York, McGraw-Hill, 1998.

18. Rippon JW: The pathogenic fungi and the pathogenic Actinomy-cetes. In: Medical Mycology, 3rd ed. Philadelphia, WB Saunders, 1988.

19. Bennett JE: Sporothrix schenckii. In: Pepoose JS, Holland GN, Wilhel-mus KR, eds: Ocular Infection and Immunity. Missouri, Mosby–Year Book, 1996, p 1278.

20. Satterwhite TK, Kagler WV, Conklin RH, et al: Disseminated sporo-trichosis. JAMA 1978;240:771.

21. Matthay RA, Greene WH: Pulmonary infections in the immunocom-promised patient. Med Clin North Am 1980;64:529.

22. Bibler MR, Luber JH, Glueck HI, Estes SA: Disseminated sporotri-chosis in a patient with HIV infection after treatment for acquired factor VIII inhibitor. JAMA 1986;256:3125.

23. Michelson E: Primary pulmonary sporotrichosis. Ann Thorac Surg 1977;24:83.

24. Bary P, Kuriata MA, Cleaver IJ: Lymphocutaneous sporotrichosis: A case report and unconventional source of infection. Cutis 1999;63(3):173–175.

25. Agudelo SP, Restrepo S, Velez ID: Cutaneous New World leishmaniasis—sporotrichosis coinfection: Report of 3 cases. J Am Acad Dermatol 1999;40(6.1):1002–1004.

26. Kim S, Rusk MH, James WD: Eysipeloid sporotrichosis in a woman with Cushing's disease. J Am Acad Dermatol 1999;40(2.1):272–274.

27. Alvarez RG, Lopez-Villegas A: Primary ocular sporotrichosis. Am J Ophthalmol 1966;62(1):150–151.

28. Cartwright MJ, Promersberger M, Stevens GA: Sporothrix schenckii endophthalmitis presenting as granulomatous uveitis. Br J Ophthal-mol 1993;77:61–62.

29. Cassady JR, Foerster HC: Sporotrichum schenckii endophthalmitis. Arch Ophthalmol 1971;85:71.

30. Kurosawa A, Pollock SC, Collins MP, et al: Sporothrix schenckii en-dophthalmitis in a patient with human immunodeficiency virus infection. Arch Ophthalmol 1988;106:376–380.

31. Font RL, Jakobiec FA: Granulomatous necrotizing retinochoroiditis caused by Sporotrichum schenkii: Report of a case including immuno-fluorescence and electron microscopical studies. Arch Ophthalmol 1976;94:1513.

32. Brod RD, Clarkson JG, Flynn HW Jr, et al: Endogenous fungal endophthalmitis. In: Duane TD, Jaeger EA, eds: Clinical Ophthal-mology, vol 3. Hagerstown, MD, Harper & Row, 1990.

33. Lima OC, Figueiredo CC, Pereira BA, et al: Adhesion of the human pathogen Sporothrix schenckii to several extracellular matrix proteins. Braz J Med Biol Res 1999;32(5):651–657.

34. Fernandes KS, Matthews HL, Lopes Bezerra LM: Differences in virulence of Sporothrix schenckii conidia related to culture conditions and cell-wall components. J Med Microbiol 1999;48(2):195–203.

35. Zaharopoulos P: Fine-needle aspiration cytologic diagnosis of lymphocutaneous sporotrichosis: A case report. Diagn Cytopathol 1999;20(2):74–77.

36. Wescott BL, Nasser A, Jarolim DR: Sporothrix meningitis. Nurse Pract 1999;24(2):90, 93–94, 97–98.

37. Shelley WB, Sica PA JR: Disseminated sporotrichosis of skin and bone cured with 5-fluorocytosine: Photosensitivity as a complication. J Am Acad Dermatol 1983;8:229.

38. Wescott BL, Nasser A, Jarolim DR: Sporothrix meningitis. Nurse Pract 1999;24(2):90, 93–94, 97–98.

39. Witherspoon DC, Kuhn F, Owens D, et al: Endophthalmitis due to Sporothrix schenckii after penetrating ocular injury. Ann Ophthalmol 1990;22:385–388.

40. Bargman HB: Sporotrichosis of the nose with spontaneous cure. Can Med Assoc J 1981;124:1027.

TOXOPLASMOSIS

Andréa Pereira Da Mata and Fernando Oréfice

Toxoplasmosis is caused by the obligate intracellular protozoan *Toxoplasma gondii*. It has a universal distribution and a high serologic prevalence in all countries, but the incidence of *Toxoplasma*-induced disease is much lower. Although it affects humans and animals, the feline species is the only definitive host.

Toxoplasmosis is the most common cause of posterior uveitis in the world,[1-3] accounting for over 80% of the cases in some regions.[4, 5] Recurrence of congenitally acquired toxoplasmosis, once blamed for almost all cases, is still the leading cause of *Toxoplasma* retinochoroiditis, but it is becoming increasingly clear that acquired ocular disease is more common than previously suspected.[6-17] Although active *Toxoplasma* retinochoroiditis usually has a self-limiting course in immunocompetent patients, it can recur and lead to irreversible visual loss should ocular structures critical to good vision (the macula and the optic nerve) be involved. In the immunosuppressed host, *Toxoplasma* infection poses unique diagnostic and therapeutic challenges.

HISTORY

Toxoplasma gondii was discovered independently by two investigators in 1908. Alfonso Splendore in Brazil identified the organism in laboratory rabbits,[18, 19] while Charles Nicolle and Louis Manceaux in Tunis observed the organism in the North African rodent *Ctenodactylus gondii*. Nicolle and Manceaux named the parasite *Toxoplasma gondii*: *Toxoplasma* from the Greek word toxon, meaning arc, describing the small crescent shape of the parasites, and *gondii* from the animal in which it was found.[20, 21] Both papers agreed in most of their observations, but it was Splendore who identified the schizogenous form of reproduction and the formation of true cysts. In the same year, Darling unwittingly described systemic toxoplasmosis at the Gorgas Hospital in Panama. He reported a patient with acute myositis, but misdiagnosed it as sarcosporidiosis. Years later, Chaves-Carballo and Samuel reexamined the biopsy samples and concluded that the parasite was *T. gondii*.[22] Other reports followed, including Castellani (Ceylon, 1914) who attributed a case of fever and splenomegaly to a protozoan, which at the time he named *Toxoplasma pyrogenes*.[23]

The first description of congenital toxoplasmosis with ocular involvement is attributed to Jankû (Prague, 1923), who reported an 11-month-old infant with hydrocephalus, microphthalmia, and a retinal "coloboma" in the macular region. Histopathologically, Jankû identified an oval sporocyst containing numerous dark sporozoites within the outer layer of the choroid in this "colobomatous area."[24] The first photographic documentation of ocular toxoplasmosis was made in Brazil by Belfort Mattos in 1933 (Fig. 33–1). Acquired toxoplasmosis with ocular manifestations was not described until 1940, when Pinkerton and Weinman noted retinal lesions in a young adult with generalized disease.[25] Wilder demonstrated *T. gondii* in stained sections of eyes with "intractable chorioretinitis." This resulted in a shift in the diagnostic mentality of posterior uveitis from tuberculosis being the most common agent to *Toxoplasma* as an important cause of posterior uveitis.[26]

Diagnostic testing for toxoplasmosis was first attempted by Nicolau and Ravelo (1937), who used a complement fixation test to demonstrate the existence of anti-*Toxoplasma* antibodies.[27] However, their test proved to be of low reliability. The introduction of the Sabin-Feldman test in 1948 provided a sensitive and specific method for the detection of antibodies against *T. gondii*, allowing epidemiologic studies to be conducted. By 1960, toxoplasmosis was identified as the most common cause of posterior uveitis in the world.[28] It was not until 1970 that the feline species, primarily the domestic cat, was identified as the definitive host of *T. gondii*.[29, 30]

PATHOGENESIS

The Organism

T. gondii is an obligate intracellular parasite that can be found in the host's tissues and body fluids, such as saliva, milk, semen, urine, and peritoneal fluid. The morphology of the *T. gondii* varies depending on the stage of the life cycle and habitat. It can present in three forms: the tachyzoite, bradyzoite, and sporozoite.

The tachyzoite, also called trophozoite, is the infectious form responsible for the acute phase of the disease. It is approximately 3 by 7 μm in length and 2 to 4 μm in diameter, and it has the shape of a crescent. It was the form first observed by Nicolle and Manceaux that inspired the genus name *Toxoplasma* (Fig. 33–2). The tachyzoite, an obligate intracellular form, may enter the cytoplasmic vacuoles of any nucleated cell. It is mobile and quickly multiplies by endodyogeny until the cell ruptures, releasing more tachyzoites to infect other cells.

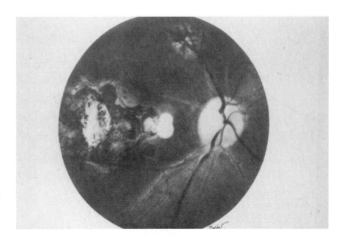

FIGURE 33–1. First photographic documentation of ocular toxoplasmosis. *Taken by* Waldemar Belfort Mattos, Brazil, 1933. (Courtesy of Rubens Belfort Mattus Jr., M.D., Ph.D., UNIFESP, Brazil.)

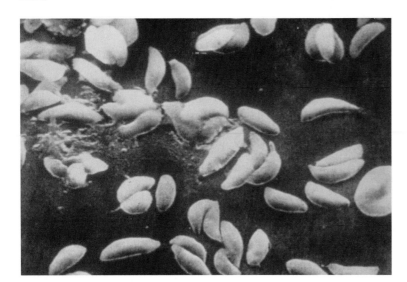

FIGURE 33–2. Scanning electron photomicrograph of *Toxoplasma gondii* tachyzoites. (Courtesy of Rubens Belfort Mattos Jr., M.D., Ph.D., UNIFESP, Brazil.)

The tachyzoite encysts at the first sign of environmental stress such as the host immune response or the presence of antibiotic. The encysted form, known as the bradyzoite, begins to appear as soon as 1 week following infection. Bradyzoites divide slowly inside the cellular vacuole, which eventually becomes part of the cyst's capsule. The wall of a mature cyst is composed of a combination of both host and parasitic components, so the bradyzoites are protected from the host's immune system. The cysts are very resistant and can remain dormant in the host for years without tissue damage.[31] Cysts have a predilection for tissues such as the retina, skeletal muscles, the central nervous system, and the heart, and they persist for the life of the host. They are approximately 10 to 100 μm in size and may contain up to 3000 bradyzoites (Fig. 33–3).[32] For reasons unknown, the cysts may rupture, causing reactivation of the disease and intense inflammation.

Oocysts are produced only in the feline intestinal cells and are excreted in the feces. The oocyst is the most resistant form of the organism and may remain infectious for up to 2 years in warm, moist soil.[32] They are oval and measure 10 to 12 μm in diameter. Within 1 to 21 days after shedding, the oocysts undergo sporulation and become mature, infective oocysts.[33] These mature forms contain two sporocysts, each of which contains four sporozoites. The ingestion of mature oocysts can cause infection in either an intermediate or the definitive host. Sporulation does not occur below 4°C or above 37°C, thus explaining the lower incidence of toxoplasmosis in areas with extreme temperatures.

Life Cycle

The life cycle of *T. gondii* is composed of two distinct phases: the asexual phase, which occurs in all hosts, and the sexual phase that happens only in the intestinal epithelium of the definitive host. Felines, especially domestic cats, are the only definitive host and they sustain both sexual and asexual reproduction. Humans and many other animals, such as cattle, pigs, sheep, and poultry, support asexual reproduction of *T. gondii* and constitute the intermediate host group.

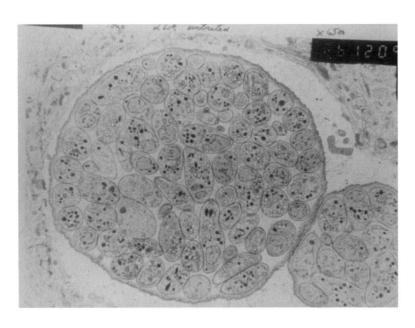

FIGURE 33–3. Transmission electron photomicrograph of *Toxoplasma gondii* tissue cyst in mouse brain. (Courtesy of Fausto Araujo, Ph.D., United States.)

The asexual cycle starts when a susceptible host ingests mature oocysts, tissue cysts contain bradyzoites, or tachyzoites are present in body secretions and raw meat. Tachyzoites that reach the stomach are destroyed by gastric acid, but tachyzoites are very active and may penetrate the oral mucosa. Digestive enzymes break down the walls of both oocysts and tissue cysts, releasing sporozoites and bradyzoites. These organisms then enter cells of the intestinal tract and transform into rapidly multiplying tachyzoites that rupture the cells, releasing free tachyzoites. Extracellular tachyzoites or tachyzoites within leukocytes are transported throughout the body via the lymphatic system and bloodstream, and they can invade any organ or tissue. This initial infection characterizes the acute phase of the disease. Once infected, the host produces specific antibodies, which bind to the extracellular tachyzoites, initiating immune-mediated eradication of the free parasite. However, humoral immunity is ineffective against intracellular parasites and the cellular immune response is called upon to attack the parasitized cells, reducing intracellular multiplication and causing the tachyzoites to encyst.[31] When the immune system has eliminated the tachyzoites, symptoms disappear, and the chronic phase ensues.

The sexual cycle takes place exclusively in the feline intestine, and it is unclear why this phase occurs only in members of the cat family. Cats may initially become infected by eating contaminated meat containing tissue cysts or by ingesting sporulated oocysts. In the cat's intestine, the tachyzoites invade the epithelial cells and start to multiply by schizogony. During this process, gametocytes are formed and fertilized to produce oocysts. The time interval between the infection and the appearance of oocysts in the feces depends on the form of the organism ingested and varies from 3 to 24 days. Excretion continues for up to 20 days, with shedding of as many as 12 million oocysts in a single day. In general, once a cat has cleared the initial infection it will not shed oocysts again. However, if the cat becomes infected with *Isospora felis*, recurrent oocyst shedding may occur.[34]

Transmission

The main mechanism of human infection is by ingestion of tissue cysts in raw or undercooked meat. In the United States, evidence of bradyzoites is seen in approximately 10% to 20% of lamb products and 25% to 35% of pork products, whereas the incidence in beef is only about 1%.[35] Food may also be contaminated with oocysts, especially through dissemination by insects and by food handlers. The second important route of infection is contact with any material contaminated by infected cat feces, such as soil and cat litter. This may result in accidental ingestion or inhalation of oocysts. Infection may also be acquired through ingestion of unpasteurized goat's milk, raw eggs, or unwashed vegetables; transfusion of blood or leukocytes; organ transplantation; and laboratory accidents.[34-38]

Transplacental transmission may occur if a woman is initially infected just before or during pregnancy. Women with positive serology before pregnancy have little or no chance of infecting their fetuses, although on rare occasions, women with chronic latent infection and persistent parasitemia may have one or more affected children.[39, 40] Reactivation of ocular toxoplasmosis during pregnancy does not increase the risk of congenital transmission in an immunocompetent woman.[41]

IMMUNOBIOLOGY

As an obligate intracellular pathogen, *T. gondii*'s reproductive success depends on its ability to penetrate host cells and evade cellular defenses. The tachyzoites actively secrete penetration-enhancing factors (PEFs) that interact with the cellular phospholipid bilayer and allow the organism to invade eukaryotic cells within 5 to 10 seconds.[42-44] During this active penetration, the tachyzoites become enveloped by part of the cell membrane, inducing a new subcellular organelle, the parasitophorous vacuole. The tachyzoites induce molecular and morphologic changes in the parasitophorous vacuole, which prevent acidification and fusion with cellular lysozomes.[42, 45-49] Maintenance of an alkaline pH (7.0 to 8.0) inside the vacuole is one of the main mechanisms that enable survival and replication of the tachyzoites.

The activation of B cells and the humoral immune response is the first step toward control of the *Toxoplasma* infection; this consists of the production of anti–*Toxoplasma*-specific immunoglobulin M (IgM), IgA, IgE, and IgG antibodies. Antibody binding to tachyzoites can result in lysis by the classical complement pathway, but more important, antibody-coated tachyzoites are unable to actively penetrate cells. Instead, these opsonized tachyzoites are recognized by phagocytic cells and are engulfed into phagolysosomes, resulting in destruction of the parasite.[49, 50]

Although the humoral response is important, it is not sufficient to eradicate the intracellular organism. Cell-mediated immunity is the major mechanism involved in the resolution of the active disease.[51] Indeed, a significant feature of the toxoplasmosis infection is the strong and persistent cellular immunity induced by the parasite. Evidence for the importance of cell-mediated immunity comes from immunocompromised patients in whom primary infection or reactivation of chronic *T. gondii* cysts often results in disseminated disease with a high mortality.[52]

The cellular immune response is characterized by activation of macrophages, natural killer (NK) cells, and T cells, and release of their cytokines. Macrophages are activated following phagocytosis of antibody-opsonized *T. gondii,* and they initiate the immune response by producing interleukin 12 (IL-12) and tumor necrosis factor alpha (TNF-α).[53, 54] These monokines stimulate CD8+ T lymphocytes and NK cells to produce interferon-γ (IFN-γ).[55] IFN-γ plays a key role in the immune response to *T. gondii* by enhancing the microbicidal activity of the macrophage.[55, 56] Activated macrophages use toxic oxygen and nitrogen intermediates as well as products of arachidonic acid metabolism to enhance killing intracellular *T. gondii.* Other evidence suggests that IFN-γ may inhibit replication of *Toxoplasma* by tryptophan starvation in retinal pigment epithelial cells.[57] Monokines released by macrophages also stimulate CD4+ Th1 cells to produce IL-2, which in turn activates cytotoxic T cells and NK cells to attack cells infested with *T. gondii* and free tachyzoites.

TABLE 33–1. LIST OF *TOXOPLASMA GONDII* GENES CLONED AND CHARACTERIZED THUS FAR

NAME	OTHER NAMES	LOCALIZATION	KDA (SDS-PAGE)	REFERENCE
SAG1	P30	Surface	30	172–175
SAG2	P22	Surface	22	173, 174, 176
SAG3	P43	Surface	43	173, 174, 177
GRA1	P23, P27	Dense granule	22, 23, 27	178, 180
GRA2	P28	Dense granule	28, 28.5	179, 181–183
GRA3	—	Dense granule	30	180, 184
GRA4	—	Dense granule	40	180, 185
GRA5	P21	Dense granule	21	179, 186
ROP1	PEF	Rhoptry	60, 60.5	183, 187
ROP2	P54, TG34	Rhoptry	54, 55	183, 188
MIC1	—	Micronemes	60	189, 190
TUB1	Alfa-tubulin	Microtubules	—	191
TUB2	Beta-tubulin	Microtubules	—	191
DTS1	DHFR	—	—	192
NTP1	NTPase	Secretory	63	193, 194

Modified from Joiner KA: Cell entry by *Toxoplasma gondii:* All paths do not lead to success. Res Immunol 1993;144:34–38.

Conversely, stimulated CD4+ Th2 cells produce IL-4, IL-5, and IL-10, which modulate the activity of the cell-mediated immune responses to prevent an excessive inflammatory response.[55]

The inflammatory reactions in the eye are generally modified, because the eye is an immunologically privileged site; thus, the local ocular immune response tends to be suppressed to limit tissue damage. In the eye, inflammatory reactions are dominated by CD8+ T cells and CD4+ Th2 cells due to constitutive expression of anti-inflammatory factors such as Fas, Fas ligand, and tumor growth factor beta (TGF-β). *T. gondii*, however, seems to promote the production of factors, such as IFN-γ that abrogate this immune privilege.[55, 58]

The *Toxoplasma* organism has developed another strategy to evade host defenses. When tachyzoites encyst, the tissue cysts become invisible to the immune system, because the cyst wall incorporates cellular components derived from the host and thus is recognized as itself. Cysts may remain dormant for an indefinite period. Factors modulating the reactivation of cysts are poorly understood, but it seems relatively clear that IFN-γ helps to prevent reactivation of chronic toxoplasmosis, possibly by inhibiting cyst rupture.[55, 59] Immunosuppression, however (particularly the depletion of T-helper cells), allows the breakdown of tissue cysts and thus tachyzoite proliferation.

Advances in the field of cellular biology of *T. gondii* have made possible the identification and purification of many cell surface antigens or secreted antigens from the tachyzoites (Table 33–1). The major surface antigen P30, for example, appears to have an important role in both immune and pathogenic mechanisms of the parasite. P30 may be involved in antibody-dependent, complement-mediated lysis of the tachyzoites.[60] Another surface protein, p22, seems to be the target of cellular immune response,[61] and the specific heat shock protein 70 (Hsp-70) may have an important role in the process of bradyzoite–tachyzoite conversion during the reactivation of chronic toxoplasmosis.[62]

EPIDEMIOLOGY AND CLINICAL CHARACTERISTICS

The *T. gondii* infection is one of the most common zoonoses in the world.[63] In all countries, a large percentage of the population has chronic asymptomatic disease. The prevalence varies extensively in different regions, depending on socioeconomic, geographic, and climatic factors. A high prevalence is found in tropical areas close to sea level, and a lower prevalence is found in arid regions, in cold climates, and at high altitudes. These variations are related to environmental influences on the oocysts. In addition, the habit of eating raw meat and the presence of the domestic cat greatly increase the incidence of *Toxoplasma* disease. The prevalence of seroconversion also increases with age. For example, in the United States, 5% to 30% of individuals 10 to 19 years old are seropositive, whereas up to 70% of those over age 50 years show serologic evidence of *T. gondii* exposure.[35] The general prevalence in the United States ranges from 30% to 70%.[64–66] A comparison of positive serology for toxoplasmosis in different populations and geographic regions is shown in Table 33–2.

Congenital Toxoplasmosis

Intrauterine toxoplasmosis infection deserves special attention. Congenital infection has been estimated to affect 3000 infants born in the United States each year.[67, 68] The prevalence of congenital disease parallels the rate of seropositivity (Table 33–3). Approximately 70% of women of child-bearing age in the United States are at risk of

TABLE 33–2. FREQUENCY OF POSITIVE SEROLOGY FOR TOXOPLASMOSIS IN DIFFERENT POPULATIONS

POPULATION	POSITIVITY (%)
Eskimos	0
Navajo Indians	4
England	25
Finland	45
Venezuela	60
Austria	62
Colombia	65
United States	30–70
Brazil	42–83
France	90

Modified from Oréfice F, Bonfioli AA: Toxoplasmose. In: Oréfice F, ed: Uveíte clinica e cirurgica (in prelo). Rio de Janeiro, Brazil, Editora Cultura Medica, 1999; Oréfice F, Belfort R Jr: Toxoplasmose. In: Oréfice F, Belfort R, eds: Uveitis. Sao Paulo, Roca, 1987.

TABLE 33–3. PREVALENCE OF CONGENITAL INFECTION BY *T. GONDII*

POPULATION	REFERENCE	CASES PER 1000 BIRTHS
Alabama	Hunter et al, 1983[195]	0.12
England	Jackson et al, 1987[196]	0.07–0.25
Scotland	Williams et al, 1981[197]	0.46–0.93
United States	Alford, 1982[198]	1
Czech Republic	Palicka, 1982[199]	1.6
Australia	Sfameni et al, 1986[200]	2
Belgium	Foulon et al, 1984[201]	2
Yugoslavia	Logar et al, 1992[202]	3
Switzerland	Bornand, 1991[203]	3.5
Brazil	Camargo Neto, 1978[204]	4
France	Desmonts, 1983[205]	7

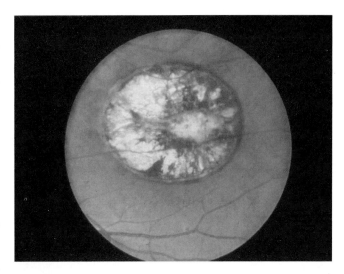

FIGURE 33–4. Typical wagon wheel appearance of a retinochoroidal lesion in congenital toxoplasmosis.

contracting the disease,[32] but the incidence of acquiring toxoplasmosis during pregnancy is only 0.2% to 1%.[35] Among women who first contract toxoplasmosis during pregnancy, the chance of transplacental infection of the fetus is about 40%.[69]

The severity of congenital toxoplasmosis is inversely related to the time of gestational exposure. Vertical transmission is most frequent during the third trimester, when the fetus may be exposed to maternal blood. Fortunately, third-trimester infection usually results in a subclinical form of the disease. If, on the other hand, the infection occurs in the first trimester, it can result in spontaneous abortion or birth of an infant with severe disease. The transplacental infection rate is approximately 10% to 17% in the first trimester, 30% in the second trimester, and 60% to 65% in the third trimester.[34, 41] Most authorities agree that transplacental transmission rates are lower if the mother receives treatment during pregnancy.[70–73] However, a recent study claims that prenatal antibiotic therapy after toxoplasmosis infection during pregnancy has no impact on the fetomaternal transmission rate, but it does reduce the rate and severity of adverse sequelae among the infected infants.[74]

Overall, retinochoroiditis is the most common manifestation of congenital infection, occurring in 70% to 90% of all cases.[64, 67] Most cases of congenital toxoplasmosis present as a subclinical or chronic infection. The newborn may or may not have retinochoroidal scars (Figs. 33–4 and 33–5), intracranial calcifications (Fig. 33–6), or other sequelae of intrauterine infection. After months or even years, these children develop the signs and symptoms of central nervous system involvement, such as hydrocephalus or microcephalus, seizures, psychomotor retardation, development delay, and ocular disease with retinochoroidal lesions, strabismus, and blindness. The identification of subclinical infection is important, because early treatment improves the prognosis.[68]

Some infants with congenital toxoplasmosis are born with clinical signs of active infection. They may present at birth with neurologic involvement or generalized disease, but the former is more frequent. The central nervous system involvement presents as encephalomyelitis, paralysis, meningismus, seizures, respiratory disturbances, hydrocephalus or microcephalus, intracranial calcifications, and failure to thrive. The generalized disease presents with an exanthematous rash, petechiae, ecchymoses, icterus, fever or hypothermia, anemia, lymphadenopathy, hepatosplenomegaly, pneumonitis, vomiting, and diarrhea. This neonatal form is severe and patients frequently develop ocular and neurologic sequelae even with treatment. The most common ocular sequelae are retinochoroidal scars, cataracts, microphthalmia, phthisis bulbi, strabismus, nystagmus, and optic atrophy.

Occasionally, the infant is normal at birth and develops active disease in the first few months of life. This form is more common in premature infants and results in severe disease, but it may also occur in full-term infants, in whom it is less severe.

Acquired Toxoplasmosis

Typically, about 70% of immunocompetent patients who acquire toxoplasmosis are completely symptom free. Even when symptomatic, the disease is usually so mild and nonspecific that the diagnosis is difficult to make, and the condition is frequently unrecognized. The most common

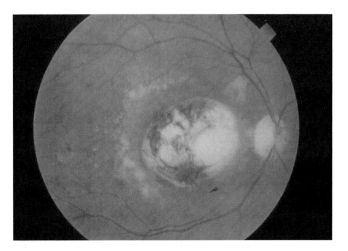

FIGURE 33–5. Classic macular retinochoroidal lesion of congenital toxoplasmosis. (See color insert.)

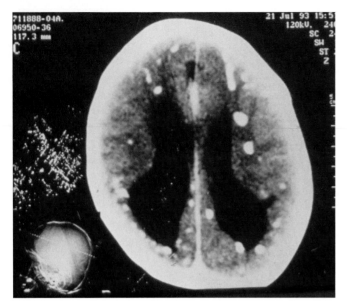

FIGURE 33–6. Contrast-enhanced CT scan demonstrating coarse intracranial calcifications, encephalomalacia and ventriculomegaly in congenital toxoplasmosis.

manifestation of acquired toxoplasmosis is lymphadenopathy affecting one or multiple lymph nodes. Cervical nodes are involved more frequently, followed by suboccipital, supraclavicular, axillary, inguinal, and mediastinal nodes. Involved lymph nodes are usually bilateral, discrete, nontender, and nonsuppurative and they vary in firmness. About 20% to 40% of patients with lymphadenopathy also present with constitutional symptoms resembling a mononucleosis-like illness. The symptoms include headache, malaise, pharyngitis, fatigue, fever, and night sweats. A smaller proportion of symptomatic patients may have a more florid picture including meningismus, meningoencephalitis, myalgias, arthralgias, abdominal pain, and a maculopapular rash that spares palms and soles. Acquired toxoplasmosis in an immunocompetent individual is usually benign and self-limiting, lasting about 2 to 4 weeks. However, malaise and lymphadenopathy may persist or recur in months. Rarely, the clinical manifestations may be very severe and include encephalopathy, pneumonitis, myocarditis, polymyositis, hepatitis, and splenomegaly, resulting in significant morbidity and even mortality.

Acquired ocular toxoplasmosis was once thought to be relatively rare, as it was diagnosed only when the ocular disease occurred following an episode of acute symptomatic systemic disease. Because most acquired *Toxoplasma* disease is asymptomatic, the true incidence of ocular toxoplasmosis in this setting is unclear, but current estimates range from 2% to 20%.[3, 7, 8, 75] Evidence to support the hypothesis that acquired disease may often result in ocular toxoplasmosis comes from epidemiologic studies demonstrating patients with elevated IgM and the frequent occurrence of multiple siblings with ocular disease.[4, 5, 8, 12, 15] When ocular disease occurs as a consequence of acquired toxoplasmosis, it can be simultaneous with the systemic disease or have a delayed onset. The time interval between the systemic disease and ocular

manifestations is variable, and ranges from days to years.[11–14, 17]

Toxoplasmosis in Immunocompromised Patients

Immunocompromised patients are at increased risk for developing acute toxoplasmosis. The disease may be caused by reactivation of a chronic infection, or it may be an acquired infection. *T. gondii* causes a severe, fulminant disease in immunocompromised individuals, including patients with human immunodeficiency virus (HIV), transplant recipients, and, less frequently, lymphoma patients.[76, 77] Toxoplasmosis in these individuals carries a poor prognosis and may be rapidly fatal if untreated. The parasite has an affinity for the central nervous system; consequently, the most common manifestation in patients with acquired immunodeficiency syndrome (AIDS) is intracranial involvement. Patients may present with diffuse neurologic dysfunction, seizures, or even focal neurologic signs due to encephalopathy, meningoencephalitis, and mass lesions. They also may develop multiple organ involvement, especially pneumonitis and myocarditis. *Toxoplasma* pneumonitis may be severe and rapidly progress to acute respiratory failure with hemoptysis, metabolic acidosis, hypotension, and occasionally disseminated intravascular coagulation.

Ocular toxoplasmosis in AIDS patients is relatively uncommon and occurs in only about 1% to 3%,[78–80] and of these cases up to 25% are thought to be the result of a newly acquired infection.[81] When *Toxoplasma* retinochoroiditis occurs in AIDS patients, it is frequently associated with encephalitis. In fact, 25% of AIDS patients with ocular toxoplasmosis also have intracranial involvement. Conversely, 10% to 20% of AIDS patients with intracranial toxoplasmosis also have ocular involvement.[82] One study found that, at autopsy, approximately 40% of all AIDS patients have intracranial *Toxoplasma* abscesses.[83] Thus, all AIDS patients who have ocular toxoplasmosis should undergo a complete neurologic evaluation, including computed tomography (CT) or magnetic resonance imaging (MRI) with contrast, and lumbar puncture.

Unlike the situation in immunocompetent patients, most of the *Toxoplasma* retinal lesions in AIDS patients do not develop adjacent to old retinochoroidal scars. Instead, the lesions occur in a perivascular distribution, which suggests newly acquired infection or dissemination of parasites from other nonocular sites in the body.[80, 81, 84] Retinochoroiditis in AIDS patients may have other atypical features, such as very large areas of severe confluent retinal necrosis,[85] as well as discrete single or multifocal lesions[79, 86] and even bilateral active retinochoroiditis.[87]

Ocular inflammation is variable and depends on the patient's lymphocyte count at the time of active disease. In general, AIDS patients who develop toxoplasmosis are still able to mount enough of a cellular immune response to produce the clinical findings of vascular sheathing, prominent vitritis, and intense anterior uveitis.[81] Ocular toxoplasmosis may follow a devastating course in AIDS patients, with inflammation extending into the orbit, causing orbital cellulitis and panophthalmitis.[88]

The clinical findings of *Toxoplasma* retinochoroiditis in AIDS patients may resemble a wide range of ocular pathologies, and ocular toxoplasmosis should always be suspected. The differential diagnosis may include cytomegalovirus (CMV) retinitis, syphilitic retinitis, and progressive outer retinal necrosis (PORN). However, toxoplasmosis retinochoroiditis does not have the significant retinal hemorrhages seen in CMV retinitis, nor is the retinitis limited to the outer retinal layers, as in PORN.

The utility of serologic testing in the diagnosis of AIDS patients for toxoplasmosis is questionable. IgG titers in AIDS patients are generally nondiagnostic in distinguishing active versus latent *Toxoplasma* retinochoroiditis, as they are not significantly elevated. IgM titers are inconsistently found and are not helpful in diagnosis.

Ocular Toxoplasmosis

The great majority of ocular toxoplasmosis is believed to occur as a consequence of reactivation of congenitally acquired infection. Congenital infection may account for about 80% to 98% of ocular disease. More than 82% of congenitally infected individuals not treated as infants will develop retinal lesions by the time they reach adolescence.[68] Peripheral retinochoroidal scars are the most common ocular finding, occurring in 82% of patients. However, *T. gondii* has a strong predilection for the posterior pole, particularly the macular region; based on comparison of the total retinal area, macular lesions are proportionally much more common, occurring in 76% of patients.[68] The reason for this is unclear, but some authors suggest that the parasites first invade the eye through the posterior ciliary arteries or the optic nerve.[55, 67, 80, 88] Invasion of the eye by way of the optic nerve may give rise to juxtapapillary *Toxoplasma* retinochoroiditis. Some other thoughts as to the macular predilection for *Toxoplasma* include the fact that there is earlier vascularization of the posterior pole than the periphery during development and the fact that the fetal vasculature contains end arterioles. In addition, there may be entrapment of free parasites, or parasites within macrophages, in the terminal capillaries of the fovea.

Ocular toxoplasmosis tends to be a recurrent disease, and two thirds of patients present with relapses. There are many theories as to the cause of recurrent *Toxoplasma* retinochoroiditis. Although it is unknown which mechanism or mechanisms are involved in the recurrence of retinochoroiditis, there are three main scenarios that may account for this phenomenon. The classic teaching has been that recurrence is the result of release of *T. gondii* from cysts. Cysts may rupture and release live organisms that actively invade the retina, or cysts may simply release antigens that stimulate an inflammatory retinochoroiditis. Alternatively, an autoimmune response may develop to retinal antigens such as the retinal S-antigen, which results in retinochoroiditis.[61] Finally, a novel theory suggests that some recurrences may be the result of reinfection. It has been demonstrated that the immunity from a primary *Toxoplasma* infection is not sufficient to prevent reinfection with a new strain of *T. gondii.*[90]

Recurrent lesions frequently develop at the borders of old *Toxoplasma* retinochoroidal scars, so-called satellite lesions (Fig. 33–7). Lesions may also recur in distant sites away from the primary lesion (Fig. 33–8) or in the fellow eye. They are usually single, but they can be multiple. In

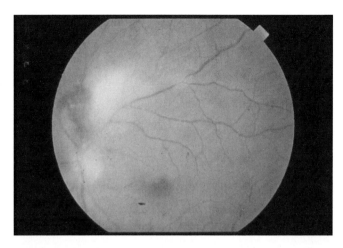

FIGURE 33–7. Active toxoplasma retinitis adjacent to a pigmented juxtapapillary scar. Note also the small, active lesion along the superior branch of the temporal arcade. (See color insert.)

contrast, patients who present with newly acquired ocular toxoplasmosis usually have unilateral, solitary, active lesions without evidence of previous retinochoroidal scarring (Fig. 33–9).

Classically, the initial lesion starts in the superficial retina. As the retinitis progresses, involvement of the full-thickness retina, adjacent choroid, vitreous, and even sclera may occur. Ophthalmoscopically, a yellowish-white or gray exudate is seen, with ill-defined borders caused by surrounding retinal edema (Fig. 33–10). The size of the lesion ranges from 1/10 of a disc diameter to two quadrants of the retina. Slowly, the borders of the lesion become more defined, the exudates and vitritis diminish, and the lesion shows an elevated central area with a whitish-gray to brown discoloration. After a variable time period, pigmentation occurs, particularly in the margins of the lesion. The time required for a retinochoroidal lesion to heal varies, depending on the size of the lesion,

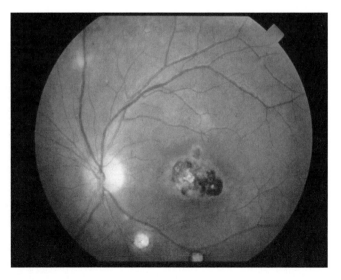

FIGURE 33–8. Recurrent active retinitis distant from the primary pigmented lesion. Note the primary lesion in the macula with evidence of prior recurrences along the inferotemporal arcade, as well as a small, active lesion along the supranasal arcade. (See color insert.)

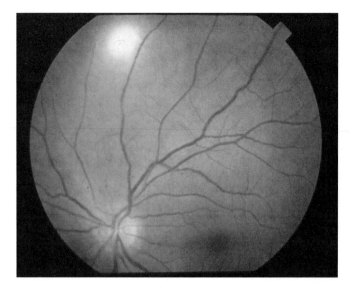

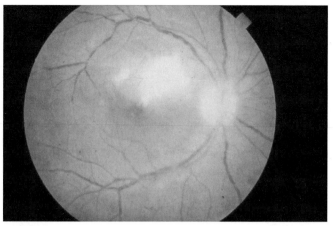

FIGURE 33–10. Active toxoplasma retinitis. Note the yellowish white appearance of the lesion with ill-defined borders due to surrounding retinal edema. There is associated phlebitis of the supratemporal arcade. (See color insert.)

FIGURE 33–9. Unilateral, solitary, active lesion without evidence of chorioretinal scarring typical of acquired toxoplasmosis. (See color insert.)

the treatment delivered, the immunologic condition of the host, and the strain of *T. gondii*.[3, 91, 92]

A healed *Toxoplasma* scar typically has well-defined borders with central retinochoroidal atrophy and peripheral pigment epithelial hyperplasia. In the atrophic central area, either choroidal vessels or bare sclera may be observed. Healing *Toxoplasma* lesions may be complicated by proliferative vitreoretinopathy, retinal gliosis, vascular shunts, and choroidal neovascular membranes (Fig. 33–11*A* and *B*).

The *Toxoplasma* scars themselves have variable appearances. The edges of the scar may present with a lobulated appearance, each lobule corresponding to a healed recurrence. The scar may also vary in depth, resulting from the different layers involved in the necrotizing process. Traction bands are also frequent, and they usually link an old scar to the optic disc (Franceschetti's syndrome) or to a neighboring scar (Fig. 33–12).

Vitritis is usually marked and is present in nearly all cases. When extensive vitritis is present, the active retinal lesion may have the classic ophthalmoscopic appearance of a headlight in the fog (Fig. 33–13). Vitreous involvement may occur as a localized or diffuse exudate, inflammatory cells, pigment, or hemorrhage. Vitreous opacities tend to be slowly reabsorbed and may persist for years after complete resolution of the retinal lesion. When there is severe and prolonged vitreous involvement, vitreous contraction, posterior vitreous detachment, or even retinal detachment may occur.

Vascular involvement, which may occur either in the vicinity of the active lesion or in the distant retina, typically consists of a diffuse or segmental vasculitis produced by antigen–antibody complex deposition in the vessel wall, as well as localized mononuclear cell infiltrates (Fig. 33–14). The vasculitis involves primarily the veins, but arterial involvement is not uncommon. The vasculitis may result in complications such as retinal hemorrhage, vascular obstruction, vascular shunting, and even neovasculari-

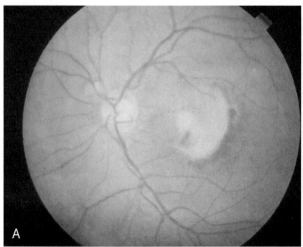

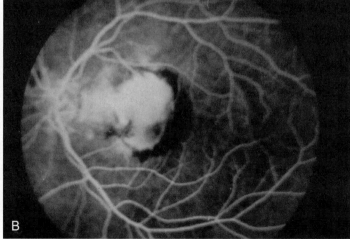

FIGURE 33–11. *A*, Macular toxoplasma scar complicated by a choroidal neovascular membrane. Note the hemorrhage around the neovascular membrane. *B*, Late fluorescein angiogram hyperfluorescence of a choroidal neovascular membrane and blockage by the surrounding hemorrhage. (See color insert.)

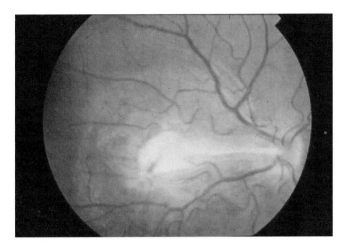

FIGURE 33–12. Franceschetti's syndrome, a traction band from the toxoplasma macular lesion to the optic nerve. (See color insert.)

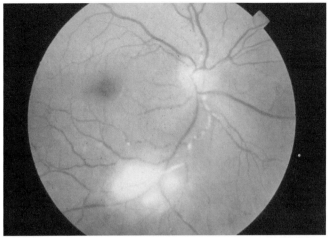

FIGURE 33–14. Segmental arteritis associated with an active toxoplasma lesion in the vicinity of the vessel. The localized perivascular inflammatory accumulations may line up around the vessels and resemble a rosary. (See color insert.)

zation. Kyrieleis arterialitis (the presence of exudates or periarterial plaques not associated with leakage or vascular obstruction) is also observed as an inflammatory response in ocular toxoplasmosis, and its pathogenesis is unknown (Fig. 33–15).[93]

The anterior segment can also be involved with a granulomatous or nongranulomatous inflammatory reaction. This process is believed to develop as a result of a hypersensitivity reaction to *Toxoplasma* antigen, because live *T. gondii* has never been demonstrated in the anterior segment of an immunocompetent patient. The resulting anterior uveitis may be florid, and patients may develop "mutton-fat" keratic precipitates, posterior synechiae, fibrin deposition, and Koeppe and Busacca nodules. Corneal edema may be present even in eyes with normal intraocular pressure due to endothelial dysfunction. The iridocyclitis is usually transient, but prompt therapy is necessary to avoid complications such as pupillary seclusion, rubeosis iridis, secondary glaucoma, and cataracts.

Signs and symptoms of ocular toxoplasmosis vary with age. Children are generally referred to the ophthalmologist with complaints of decreased visual acuity, strabismus,

nystagmus, leukocoria, choroidal coloboma, and microphthalmia. Adolescents and adults typically complain of blurred vision and floaters. If the anterior segment is involved, pain, photophobia, and conjunctival hyperemia may be prominent. The most common cause of visual loss in ocular toxoplasmosis is a macular scar, but other causes for substantial visual loss include dragging of the macula secondary to a peripheral lesion, retinal detachment, macular edema, optic atrophy, cataract, glaucoma, opacified media, amblyopia, and phthisis. Surprisingly, the presence of a large congenital macular scar can be associated with remarkably good vision.[68]

Atypical Forms

PUNCTATE OUTER RETINAL TOXOPLASMOSIS

Punctate outer retinal toxoplasmosis is characterized by small multifocal gray-white lesions that develop in the deep layers of the retina and retinal pigment epithe-

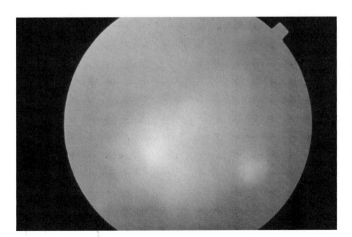

FIGURE 33–13. Active toxoplasma retinitis with marked vitritis producing the classic appearance of a headlight in the fog. (Courtesy of Maria Elenir F. Péret, M.D., COMG, Brazil.) (See color insert.)

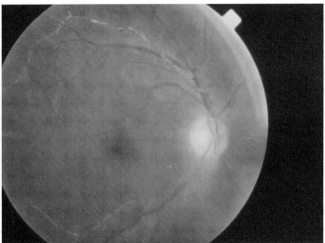

FIGURE 33–15. Toxoplasma periarterial plaques known as kyrieleis arterialitis. (See color insert.)

lium[94, 95] (Fig. 33–16A to D). Acute lesions resolve, leaving behind fine, granular, white scars, but they frequently recur. Because the process is localized to the outer retinal layers, there is little or no overlying vitritis. There is usually significant optic nerve involvement and atrophy associated with the punctate outer retinal lesions. Thus, even without foveal lesions, these patients may suffer significant visual loss as a result of optic neuropathy. However, note that all five cases initially reported by Matthews and Weiter were treated, and all had a final visual acuity of 20/25 or better. In addition, many uveitis experts do not consider treatment for this form of *Toxoplasma* retinochoroiditis.

The punctate outer retinal form occurs most frequently in the first and second decades of life, and it can be congenital or acquired. It is bilateral in a third of the cases, and some patients present with classic *Toxoplasma* retinochoroiditis in one eye and the punctate form in the fellow eye (Fig. 33–17A to D).

The combination of *T. gondii* and host factors that result in the punctate outer retinal form rather than the classical form has not yet been elucidated. Furthermore, the reason a single patient should have the typical form in one eye and the punctate outer retinal form in the other eye is intriguing. Perhaps this form is an immune phenomenon related to exposure of retinal antigens. Indeed, it has been demonstrated that patients with ocular toxoplasmosis develop both cellular and humoral immune responses to retinal antigens.[96–103] However, it is unclear what role, if any, autoimmune sensitization plays in the development of punctate outer retinal lesions. Clearly, this is an area deserving further study.

Occasionally, the punctate outer retinal form is observed in the absence of typical *Toxoplasma* lesions in one or both eyes. If autoimmunity to retinal antigens truly is the cause of this entity, one must suppose a previous subclinical infection that has been overlooked.

NEURORETINITIS

Toxoplasma neuroretinitis, previously known as Jensen's choroiditis, was attributed to tuberculosis. It typically consists of active lesions localized to the juxtapapillary region, aggressively involving the retina and optic nerve (Fig. 33–18). *Toxoplasma* neuroretinitis initially presents as severe papillitis with disc hemorrhages, venous engorgement, and overlying vitritis (Fig. 33–19). Soon after, a juxtapapillary retinochoroiditis and macular star develop (Fig. 33–20). *Toxoplasma* neuroretinitis is an ophthalmic emergency and requires prompt treatment.

NEURITIS

Papillitis in the presence of *Toxoplasma* retinochoroiditis is a relatively frequent finding. In this setting, there is optic nerve involvement associated with a distant retinal lesion (Fig. 33–21A and B). Some authors state that it simply constitutes a reactive edema of the optic disc, but

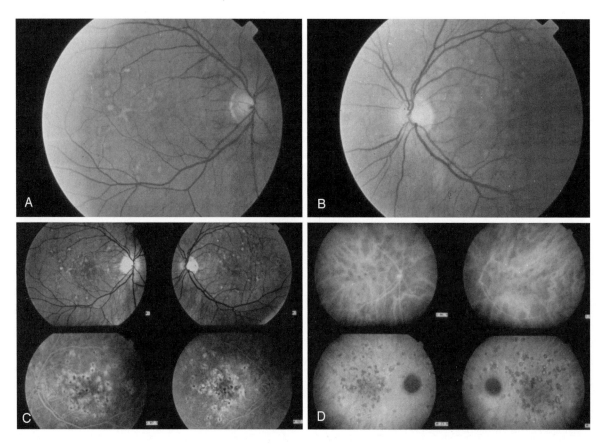

FIGURE 33–16. Right *(A)* and left *(B)* eyes of a patient with the punctate outer retinal form of toxoplasmosis. Note the small, multifocal, gray-white fine, granular scars in the deep layers of the retina and retinal pigment epithelium and the pale optic disc in the left eye. *C,* Red free photographs and fluorescein angiography demonstrating hypofluorescent lesions with hyperfluorescent borders. *D,* Indocyanine green angiography demonstrating hypofluorescence of the lesions throughout the examination with late trace of central staining.

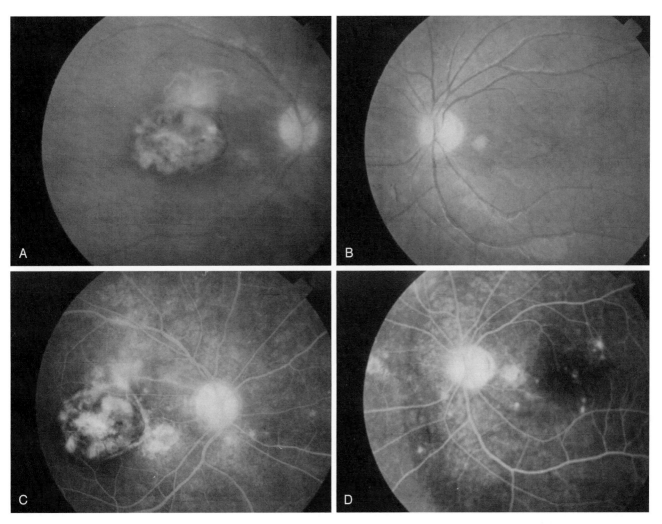

FIGURE 33–17. *A,* Classic toxoplasma retinochoroiditis in the right eye. *B,* Left eye of the same patient demonstrating the punctate outer retinal form. Note the multiple active lesions in the posterior pole and associated temporal optic nerve atrophy. *C,* Late-phase fluorescein angiogram OD showing a mottled appearance of the lesion caused by pigment clumping and atrophy. *D,* Late-phase fluorescein angiogram OS showing multiple hyperfluorescent dots that correspond to the active lesions in the posterior pole.

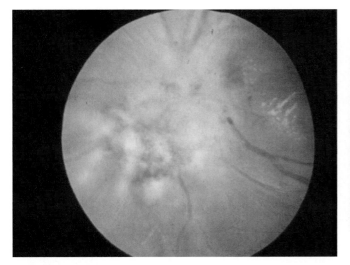

FIGURE 33–18. Juxtapapillary active toxoplasma lesion with severe involvement of the optic nerve. Note the severe papillitis and retinitis with hemorrhages. (See color insert.)

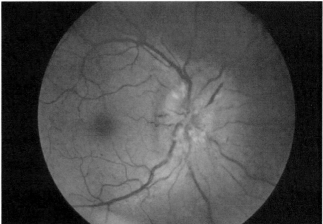

FIGURE 33–19. Initial presentation of toxoplasma neuroretinitis. Note papillitis with disc hemorrhages and venous engorgement prior to the development of retinochoroiditis. (See color insert.)

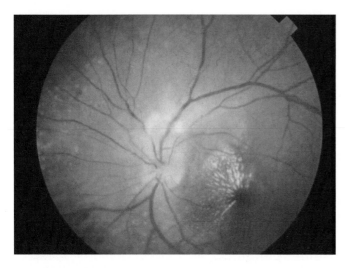

FIGURE 33–20. Toxoplasma neuroretinitis. Note the juxtapapillary active lesion and the deposits of hard exudate around the macula, forming a macular scar.

the markedly decreased visual acuity observed in some patients suggests that it is a true inflammation of the optic nerve. Like neuroretinitis, papillitis demands prompt therapy.

MULTIPLE PSEUDORETINITIS
Multiple pseudoretinitis is characterized by the simultaneous presence of retinal lesions, which appear to be active. However, close observation reveals just a single active *Toxoplasma* lesion accompanied by noncontiguous areas of retinal edema. Once the true active lesion heals, the pseudolesions completely disappear without scarring (Fig. 33–22A and B).

PERIPHERAL LESIONS
Peripheral lesions simulating the snow-banking of pars planitis may be caused by toxoplasmosis. The incidence of these peripheral *Toxoplasma* lesions is probably underestimated because of difficult visualization associated with

cataracts or intense vitritis in severe cases or because of clinical unimportance in asymptomatic or mild cases.

ANTERIOR UVEITIS
A granulomatous iridocyclitis without evidence of retinal toxoplasmosis can develop in both immunocompetent and immunocompromised patients.[16, 104] It is thought that the anterior uveitis is either a hypersensitivity reaction to *Toxoplasma* antigen or a *Toxoplasma* infection in the anterior segment. However, the parasite has never been demonstrated in the anterior segment of immunocompetent patients.

FUCHS' HETEROCHROMIC IRIDOCYCLITIS
Some studies report an association between toxoplasmosis and Fuchs' heterochromic iridocyclitis (FHI), but a cause-and-effect relationship has not been established.[105–108] The incidence of chorioretinal lesions suggestive of toxoplasmosis in patients with FHI is higher than what would be expected from normal population figures and ranges between 8% and 65%.[109] Several mechanisms have been proposed to explain the association between FHI and *Toxoplasma* retinochoroidal lesions. One hypothesis suggests that primary retinochoroidal inflammation results in production of antibodies that cross-react with anterior segment antigens, causing a low-grade anterior uveitis (i.e., FHI).[109] Others posit that there is no statistically significant association between FHI and ocular toxoplasmosis.[110]

UNILATERAL PIGMENTARY RETINOPATHY
Unilateral pigmentary retinopathy, like retinitis pigmentosa, has been reported as a sequela of chronic recurrent ocular toxoplasmosis.[111]

Complications
The most common complication of ocular toxoplasmosis is secondary glaucoma. The glaucoma may be caused by mechanical obstruction of the trabecular meshwork with fibrin, inflammatory cells, or inflammatory debris. In these situations, the intraocular pressure is usually con-

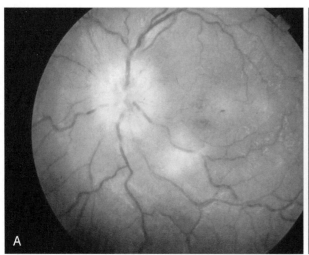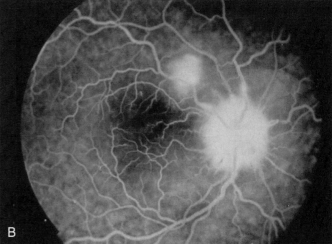

FIGURE 33–21. *A,* Toxoplasma neuritis demonstrating papillitis associated with active retinochoroiditis. *B,* Late-phase fluorescein angiogram demonstrating leakage from the disc as well as the area of retinitis.

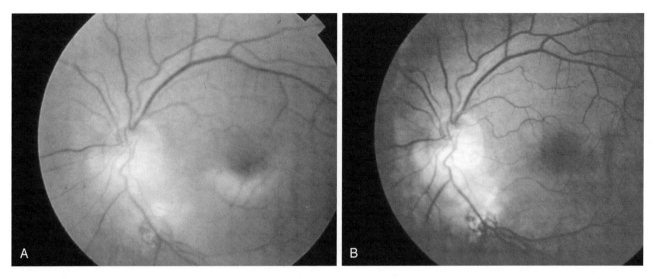

FIGURE 33–22. *A,* Toxoplasma multiple pseudoretinitis. Note the presence of a true active lesion inferior to the optic disc associated with an inferomacular area of retinal edema. *B,* After healing of the retinochoroidal lesion, the pseudolesion completely disappears without scarring. (Courtesy of Professor J. Melamed, UFRGS, Brazil.)

trolled by anti-inflammatory treatment. In cases with intense anterior uveitis, refractory glaucoma may develop as a result of synechial angle closure or seclusio pupillae with iris bombé.

Other complications of ocular toxoplasmosis include cataracts, vitreous hemorrhage, proliferative vitreoretinopathy, retinal detachment, macular dragging, epiretinal membrane, cystoid macular edema, macular hole, retinovascular occlusion, vascular shunts, choroidal neovascular membrane, optic atrophy, and phthisis. Cataracts may result from severe vitreous inflammation or the use of local and systemic corticosteroids. Posterior subcapsular cataract is typical and usually occurs relatively early in the course of the disease.

Vitreous hemorrhage and tractional or rhegmatogenous retinal detachment may result from proliferative vitreoretinopathy and contraction of vitreous bands. Proliferative vitreoretinopathy and tractional bands also may result in macular dragging. In addition, epiretinal membranes may develop, resulting in macular pucker and cystoid macular edema. Cystoid macular edema is also a response to the chronic inflammation. Occasionally, a macular cyst may develop, which, along with tangential traction on the retinal internal limiting membrane and the posterior hyaloid, predisposes to the formation of a macular hole.

Retinal hemorrhages may result from a retinal vein occlusion around or within active lesions. Both branch retinal vein occlusions and branch artery occlusions may occur when a vessel crosses an acute *Toxoplasma* lesion, but venous occlusions are more common. Arteriovenous shunts in the retina and chorioretinal vascular anastomosis may be seen as complications of vascular obstruction in ocular toxoplasmosis. Disruption of Bruch's membrane caused by the necrotizing retinochoroiditis promotes the development of choroidal neovascular membranes, which may develop adjacent to the retinal scar or at a distant location with feeder vessels originating from the scar. Optic nerve atrophy is associated with primary involvement of the optic nerve, peripapillary lesions, or lesions localized in the papillomacular bundle. In addition, punctate outer retinal toxoplasmosis is associated with frequent optic nerve atrophy. Finally, phthisis bulbi is a rare complication in the course of ocular toxoplasmosis, but it may occur in cases with inadequate treatment.

DIFFERENTIAL DIAGNOSIS

Congenital toxoplasmosis of the newborn must be differentiated from the other infectious diseases of the TORCH group (rubella, cytomegalovirus, and herpes simplex virus as well as other congenital infectious diseases that may simulate toxoplasmosis, such as syphilis, tuberculosis, and AIDS). Important ocular entities that may be confused with congenital toxoplasmosis include coloboma, persistent hyperplastic primary vitreous, and retinoblastoma.

Recurrent *Toxoplasma* lesions adjacent to retinochoroidal scars may resemble serpiginous choroiditis. However, in serpiginous choroiditis there is usually a single helicoid chorioretinal scar occurring in the peripapillary area and no significant inflammatory reaction of the anterior segment or vitreous. Other conditions that are important in the differential diagnosis of ocular toxoplasmosis are necrotizing retinitis caused by herpes viridae (cytomegalovirus, herpes simplex, herpes zoster), fungal retinitis (candidiasis, blastomycosis), septic retinitis, ocular toxocariasis, sarcoidosis, syphilis, and tuberculosis.

The atypical forms of ocular toxoplasmosis deserve distinct differential diagnoses. Punctate outer retinal toxoplasmosis must be distinguished from acute posterior multifocal placoid pigment epitheliopathy (APMPPE), punctate inner choroidopathy (PIC), and multifocal choroiditis, as well as diffuse unilateral subacute neuroretinitis (DUSN). In cases of *Toxoplasma* neuroretinitis, other causes of neuroretinitis, such as cat scratch disease and viral syndromes, must be excluded. *Toxoplasma* neuritis should be differentiated from the optic neuritis associated with sarcoidosis and CMV.

HISTOPATHOLOGY

Acute *Toxoplasma* lesions are characterized by cell death and focal necrosis resulting from replicating tachyzoites. There is an intense mononuclear inflammatory response, resulting in the formation of necrotizing granulomas in infected tissues. Tachyzoites are rarely visualized with routine histopathology; however, immunofluorescent techniques using *Toxoplasma*-specific antibodies can often detect the organism. In contrast to the intense inflammation produced by tachyzoites, tissue cysts containing bradyzoites cause little to no inflammation. In fact, it is thought that the bradyzoites are hidden from the immune system by their capsule, and that any inflammation around tissue cysts probably represents destruction of the residual tachyzoite antigens.

Ocular toxoplasmosis may produce an inflammatory response to the invasive parasites, a hypersensitivity reaction to *Toxoplasma* antigens, or both. It is characterized by severe retinitis associated with coagulative necrosis within the retina and frequent secondary involvement of the choroid and even the sclera.[112] Intra- and extracellular tachyzoites, as well as cysts, are found most commonly in the inner retinal layers.[113] The inflammatory response to tachyzoites is largely composed of lymphocytes, plasma cells, macrophages, and epithelioid histiocytes. During the acute retinitis, there may be associated perivasculitis, choroiditis, vitritis, and iridocyclitis.[114] The inflammatory reaction of the iris, ciliary body, and vitreous is mainly composed of mononuclear cells. Studies suggest that anterior uveitis, choroiditis, and vasculitis may be the result of a hypersensitivity reaction.[115–117] This is supported by the fact that the inoculation of dead parasites in eyes of experimental immune animals can produce iridocyclitis, vasculitis, and choroidal inflammation, and *T. gondii* has never been demonstrated in the anterior segment of immunocompetent patients.[115] The retinitis, however, develops only in the presence of active proliferating tachyzoites.[116]

As the inflammation subsides, often all that remains of the retinal and choroidal tissue is an atrophic scar. There is retinal pigment epithelial hyperplasia at the borders of the scar, and this is the usual location of tissue cysts. Tissue cysts can also be seen in distant areas of an unaffected retina with no associated inflammation or scarring.[118] Cysts lie dormant and are immunologically quiescent until they rupture and there is reactivation.

DIAGNOSIS

The definitive diagnosis of toxoplasmosis is made by a direct demonstration of the organism in tissues or body fluids, by in vitro culture, by inoculation and culture in the mouse peritoneum, or by polymerase chain reaction(PCR). Direct demonstration of the parasite is easiest during the acute phase, when the trophozoites can be found in body fluids such as blood, cerebrospinal fluid, urine, and breast milk. The parasite in this phase can be identified microscopically after Giemsa staining. In the chronic phase, tissue cysts may be occasionally identified in biopsy samples by staining with hematoxylin and eosin or silver. Isolation of the parasite can also be accomplished by inoculation of infected secretions or tissues into the peritoneal cavity of mice. There, the parasites multiply and then can be identified in the peritoneal fluid.[119] Alternatively, the mouse's anti-*Toxoplasma* serum titer can be evaluated 4 to 6 weeks after inoculation. Demonstration of the parasite through direct inoculation or through histopathologic identification has great diagnostic value but is generally not practical because it is difficult to grow the parasites in vivo and difficult to detect tachyzoites and tissue cysts histopathologically. Thus, these studies are not used routinely but are reserved for cases where the diagnosis is uncertain.

In practice, the serologic methods are the main tools for confirming exposure to *T. gondii* in cases of suspected toxoplasmosis. Serology alone cannot make the diagnosis. The accuracy of the diagnosis, however, is complicated by the high prevalence of positive *Toxoplasma* titers in the human population. Although serial titers may be important to establish a diagnosis by demonstrating a rising titer, it is not necessary to repeat serologic testing during or after treatment, because serum titers do not correlate with recovery from infection. The serologic tests available for detection of *Toxoplasma*-specific antibodies include the Sabin-Feldman dye test, complement fixation (CF) test, hemagglutination test, immunofluorescence antibody test (IFAT), enzyme-linked immunosorbent assay (ELISA), immunoblotting (IB), and immunosorbent agglutination assay (ISAGA).

Sabin-Feldman Dye Test

The Sabin-Feldman dye test is the standard to which all serologic tests performed to detect anti-*Toxoplasma* antibodies are compared. It is a neutralization test in which the patient's serum is incubated with complement and live *Toxoplasma* organisms, and a dye is employed to quantify the bound antibody. It allows early detection of the infection and has high sensitivity and specificity in both acute and chronic phases, but it is no longer used because it requires maintenance of live virulent parasites in the laboratory, and equally good, safer methods have been developed. Currently, the Sabin-Feldman dye test is restricted to research centers, as a method to standardize new tests.

Complement Fixation Test

The CF test has a good sensitivity only when the level of circulating antibodies is high, which unfortunately delays the diagnosis in early infection. Complement fixation also cannot make the diagnosis in chronic disease (i.e., most cases). Thus, this test is useful only in combination with other tests. It is useful, however, to demonstrate rising titers when IFAT titers are already high. For example, an initially negative CF test becoming positive in the setting of a high, stable IFAT titer is indicative of active infection. CF studies are mainly used for acquired toxoplasmosis.

Hemagglutination Test

The hemagglutination test has good sensitivity and specificity in the acute and chronic phases, but it does not detect early infection. Additionally, it is not accurate for the diagnosis of congenital toxoplasmosis and has large variations in the standard values depending on the laboratory. Therefore, it should be used in combination with other methods.

Immunofluorescence Antibody Test

The immunofluorescence antibody test is a good method for the diagnosis of toxoplasmosis. It is easy to perform, detects early elevations in serum antibodies, and allows quantification of IgM and IgG levels. It has been the most commonly used test in the last two decades, but it has the disadvantage of equivocal results in the presence of cross-reactive antibody.[120] Rheumatoid factor (IgM anti-IgG) may result in a false-positive IgM test, suggesting acute infection, when in reality only IgG anti-*Toxoplasma* antibody is present. This results when anti-*Toxoplasma* IgG antibodies bind to the parasite antigens and rheumatoid factor cross-links these antibodies, producing a false-positive result during IgM anti-*Toxoplasma* testing.[121, 122] Thus, it is essential to remove the rheumatoid factors, or, preferably, anti-IgG antibodies, from the serum in which IgM antibodies will be tested. Additionally, false-positive IgM and IgG titers can occur in the presence of antinuclear antibodies because the immunologic techniques are unable to differentiate some *Toxoplasma* antigens from proteins of human leukocyte nuclei.[122–124] False-positive IgM titers may also result from cross-reactions with antibodies against cytomegalovirus, Epstein-Barr virus, hepatitis A, secondary syphilis, and others. Furthermore, false-negative IgM can result from inhibitory competition when there is excessive anti-*Toxoplasma* IgG.[125]

It is important to note that conventional techniques employed for indirect immunofluorescence begin at a serum dilution of 1:16 to avoid a low specificity. However, ocular disease may well be present and not produce sufficient antibody to be detectable at a dilution of 1:16. Because any titer of antibody is significant for the diagnosis of ocular toxoplasmosis, it is important to test undiluted serum to avoid false-negative results.[126] In cases of suspected ocular toxoplasmosis with negative immunofluorescence titers, the Sabin-Feldman test, the ELISA, or both, should be performed before excluding the diagnosis.

Enzyme-Linked Immunosorbent Assay

The enzyme-linked immunosorbent assay is the test most widely used today. Like the Sabin-Feldman test, it has good sensitivity and specificity.[127] The double-sandwich ELISA is superior to the IFAT with regard to IgM specific-ity because only IgM of the test serum adheres to plates precoated with anti-IgM antiserum. Consequently, rheumatoid factor, antinuclear antibodies, and others do not interfere with the results.[128, 129] The high sensitivity of the ELISA enables detection of IgM antibodies for many months after the acute phase; therefore, it is important to consider the level of IgM, not just the presence of IgM, as a marker of recent infection.[130] The ELISA is also able to determine the affinity of the serum antibodies for the antigen by washing with urea solution. If the infection occurred more than 6 months prior to obtaining the patient's blood for antibody testing, the antibodies are mature and have high affinity for the antigens, whereas serum antibodies present in acute infection tend to have a lower affinity and are more easily dissociated.

Immunosorbent Agglutination Assay

The ISAGA is a method of immunocapture that allows the simultaneous detection of IgA and IgM anti-*Toxoplasma* antibodies. It has good sensitivity and specificity, allowing early diagnosis of congenital toxoplasmosis. In about 10% of cases when the IgM is not detectable in the serum, specific IgA antibodies can be found.[131] Usually, IgA disappears faster than IgM, so it is absent in chronic disease. Therefore, the simultaneous presence of IgA and IgM is useful to confirm acute infection, particularly in cases of suspected primary infection during pregnancy.

Immunoblotting

Immunoblot (a type of western blot) has proven to be of equal or superior sensitivity when compared with the preceding tests, and it allows an earlier diagnosis of congenital toxoplasmosis (Table 33–4).[132] The *Toxoplasma* antigens p16, p32, p40, and p97 have been shown to be specifically recognized by low-affinity antibodies that are produced in early infection.[133]

Interpretation of Serologic Results

In the infant, the diagnosis of toxoplasmosis is determined by a combination of clinical and serologic features. As IgG is passively transmitted to the fetus, its detection does not have diagnostic value. Slowly, maternal IgG decreases in the infant's circulation, and it completely disappears within 18 months. Thus, the follow-up titers may be

TABLE 33–4. SENSITIVITY, SPECIFICITY, POSITIVE PREDICTIVE VALUE OF DIFFERENT TECHNIQUES USED FOR DIAGNOSIS OF CONGENITAL TOXOPLASMOSIS AND CONCORDANCE WITH IMMUNOBLOTTING

TEST	SENSITIVITY	SPECIFICITY	POSITIVE PREDICTIVE VALUE	CONCORDANCE WITH IB (%)
Culture in vitro	40.0	100	100	69.2 (FB) 69.2 (AF)
Inoculation in mice	62.5	100	100	91.7 (FB) 53.8 (AF)
IFAT (IgM)	7.4	97.8	89.6	50.0
ELISA (IgM)	29.6	97.8	97.2	62.5
ISAGA (IgM)	44.4	95.7	93.5	72.9
IB (G + M + A)	92.6	89.1	92.4	100

IFAT, immunofluorescence antibody test; FB, fetal blood; ELISA, enzyme-linked immunosorbent assay; AF, amniotic fluid; ISAGA, immunosorbent agglutination assay; IB, immunoblotting.

Modified from Chumpitazi BFF, Boussaid A, Pelloux H, et al: Diagnosis of congenital toxoplasmosis by immunoblotting and relationship with other methods. J Clin Microbiol 1995;33:1479–1485.

diagnostic. Serum titers that remain constant or increase in value after 1 week of life are diagnostic of fetal infection. However, the best serologic evidence of congenital toxoplasmosis is identification of IgM and IgA.

A recently acquired infection will produce elevated titers of IgM, IgA, and IgE. In addition, the serum titer of IgG may be elevated or rising, but the affinity of these antibodies early in the course of infection is low. By contrast, in chronic cases low titers of high-affinity anti-*Toxoplasma* IgG are present. Because most of the cases of toxoplasmosis are evaluated in the chronic phase, a low IgG titer is expected. However, low IgG titers may also be a sign of recent infection. To differentiate between these two possibilities, serologic testing should be repeated at a time interval of 2 to 4 weeks. A rising titer is indicative of recent infection.

Polymerase Chain Reaction

Recently, PCR has been used to demonstrate parasite DNA, and it has been especially useful in difficult cases.[134] PCR of the amniotic fluid has been used to diagnose intrauterine fetal infection.[135–137] PCR has also been successfully used in the diagnosis of ocular toxoplasmosis using aqueous or vitreous samples.[138, 139] PCR of the cerebrospinal fluid is useful for making the diagnosis of intracranial infection with *Toxoplasma* and may be particularly useful for evaluation of AIDS patients with suspected toxoplasmosis.

Additional Ancillary Evaluations

Other laboratory and ancillary tests may assist in making the diagnosis of toxoplasmosis. Congenital disease can be present with anemia, thrombocytopenia, leukocytosis or leukopenia, atypical lymphocytes, and severe eosinophilia with values up to 30%. Similarly, acquired disease may produce atypical lymphocytes and moderate eosinophilia (5% to 10%). Elevated liver aminotransferases can be present. Evaluation of the cerebrospinal fluid in patients with encephalopathy or meningoencephalitis may demonstrate elevated intracranial pressure, xanthochromia, mononuclear pleocytosis, and elevated protein levels. Imaging studies (CT and MRI) are especially useful to identify cerebral calcifications, which occur in 32% to 87% of patients with congenital toxoplasmosis, and brain lesions in immunocompromised (AIDS) patients.[41, 140]

DIAGNOSIS OF OCULAR TOXOPLASMOSIS

The diagnosis of ocular toxoplasmosis is usually based on clinical findings. Laboratory tests are helpful to support the diagnosis when the ocular manifestations are atypical. The diagnosis should not depend solely on serologic tests, because the antigen load of a small, active lesion in one eye may not be enough to stimulate elevated systemic antibody titers. Indeed, in ocular toxoplasmosis there is a poor correlation between the serum levels of antibody and active disease. It is not unusual to find low or negative IgM and IgG titers in patients with acute symptomatic or recurrent ocular toxoplasmosis. For these reasons, undiluted serum should be used for the detection of anti-*Toxoplasma* antibody in ocular toxoplasmosis.

In patients with atypical lesions, positive serology suggests only a presumptive diagnosis, because there is a high prevalence of anti-*Toxoplasma* antibodies in the human population. It is important to exclude other causes of focal retinochoroiditis, such as syphilis, tuberculosis, sarcoidosis, cytomegalovirus, fungal and viral infections, serpiginous choroiditis, and others. In patients whose diagnosis is unclear, the determination of anti-*Toxoplasma* antibody titers in the aqueous humor can be elucidating. A comparison of serum levels of anti-*Toxoplasma* antibodies with the levels found in aqueous humor may identify intraocular production of antibodies, thus proving active ocular toxoplasmosis. This ratio, corrected for total protein concentration, is known as the coefficient of Witmer-Desmonts (Table 33–5). When the coefficient of Witmer-Desmonts is less than 2 in an immunocompetent patient, there is no active ocular toxoplasmosis. If the ratio is between 2 and 4, it is suggestive of active ocular disease, and when the ratio is 4 or more it is considered diagnostic of active ocular toxoplasmosis.[141] Polyclonal B-cell activation is a possible source of error in this test.

Polymerase Chain Reaction

Recently, PCR has become a powerful tool in making the diagnosis of ocular toxoplasmosis, especially if the serologic tests are equivocal. Aqueous or vitreous samples may be evaluated with high sensitivity and specificity for the presence of *Toxoplasma* DNA sequences using PCR.

Fluorescein Angiogram and Indocyanine Green

In the early stages of toxoplasmosis, a fluorescein angiogram (FA) demonstrates central hypofluorescence because of blockage by the retinal inflammation in active *Toxoplasma* retinochoroiditis. Dye leakage occurs later, expanding from the margins of the lesion. Indocyanine green (ICG) of active lesions may show early hyperfluorescence or hypofluorescence with hyperfluorescence in the late phases (Fig. 33–23A to C).

The retinochoroidal scars in the early phases of the FA may be seen as hypofluorescent due to blockage by retinal pigment epithelium (RPE) hypertrophy or as window defects due to RPE atrophy. Irregular RPE hypertrophy

TABLE 33–5. COEFFICIENT OF WITMER-DESMONTS

$$\frac{\text{Titer of antibody in aqueous humor*}}{\text{Titer of antibody in serum*}} \times \frac{\text{Concentration of serum globulins}}{\text{Concentration of aqueous humor globulins}}$$

RESULTS	
0.5 to 2	No intraocular anti-*Toxoplasma* antibody production
2 to 4	Suggestive of intraocular antibody production
≥4	Diagnostic of intraocular antibody production

*The antibodies are determined by Sabin-Feldman dye test and the immunofluorescence antibody test.

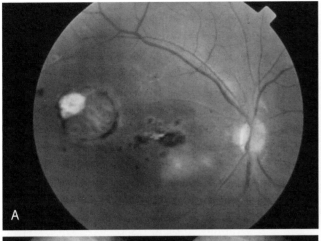
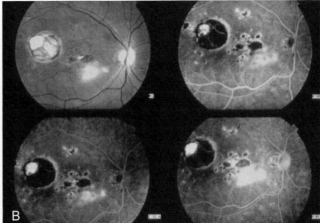
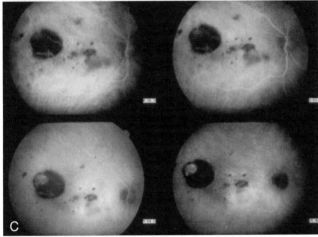

FIGURE 33–23. *A,* Toxoplasma retinochoroiditis demonstrating the varied appearance of several healed scars and an area of active disease inferior to the macula. *B,* Red free photograph and fluorescein angiography demonstrating leakage at the site of active inflammation and blockage with peripheral staining of the scars. *C,* Indocyanine green angiography demonstrating early hypofluorescence with late leakage in the area of active retinitis and blockage with minimal peripheral staining of the scars. Note the area of bare sclera stains with both fluorescein and indocyanine green.

and atrophy may result in a mottled appearance of the lesion. The late phase of the angiogram demonstrates staining of the lesion margins. ICG stains of old lesions are hypofluorescent throughout the exam.

In addition, FA and ICG are useful in the diagnosis of atypical presentations such as the punctate outer retinal form, because they highlight the lesions that follow the same fluorescence pattern as classic *Toxoplasma* lesions. The FA typically shows hyperfluorescence at the margins of the optic disc in patients with *Toxoplasma* neuroretinitis and neuritis. The FA is also helpful in demonstrating associated features such as vasculitis, vascular occlusions, arteriovenous shunts within the retina, and retinochoroidal shunts, as well as macular edema and choroidal neovascular membranes. The ICG angiography is useful for the early diagnosis of recurrent ocular toxoplasmosis because it can identify an area of reactivation not yet detectable by funduscopic exam or FA. FA and ICG are essential for the diagnosis and treatment of complications such as choroidal neovascularization.

THERAPY

Medical Treatment of Toxoplasmosis

Treatment of toxoplasmosis with pyrimethamine, sulfa, and corticosteroid has been employed since it was initially advocated in 1953 by Eyles and Coleman, and this continues to be the most common therapy used throughout the world.[142] In recent years, several new drugs have been

developed that are also effective for the treatment of toxoplasmosis. However, despite advances in research, an ideal therapy that destroys the tissue cysts and prevents recurrence has not been found. Currently, antimicrobial therapy is limited to treatment of active disease (i.e., the tachyzoites).

Antimicrobial therapy is absolutely required for systemic toxoplasmosis in newborns, pregnant women, and immunosuppressed patients, and in acute symptomatic disease. Patients with chronic toxoplasmosis do not require treatment when the disease is inactive, because no treatment is effective at eliminating the tissue cysts. In ocular toxoplasmosis, however, precisely when to apply therapy, for how long, and with what agents remain controversial. Because the active phase of ocular toxoplasmosis is self-limiting, some authorities believe that only vision-threatening lesions require treatment, and their indications for treatment are based on the location and severity of the acute focus. One recent study demonstrated no difference in time to resolution of active ocular lesions with or without pyrimethamine treatment; however, there was a significant reduction in the size of the resulting retinochoroidal scar in patients treated with pyrimethamine.[143]

The generally accepted criteria for treatment include the following:

• A lesion affecting or near the optic nerve (within two disc diameters)

- A lesion within the temporal arcade
- A lesion that threatens a large retinal vessel
- A lesion that has induced a substantial hemorrhage
- A lesion with intense inflammatory reaction
- Extensive chronic exudative lesions regardless of location
- Severe vitreous haze
- Loss of more than two lines in visual acuity
- Persistence of inflammation for more than a month
- Congenital *Toxoplasma* retinochoroiditis in the first year of life
- A newborn diagnosed with congenital toxoplasmosis, regardless of the presence of ocular lesions
- Any lesion in an immunocompromised host

Although these treatment criteria are broad, some authorities believe that all active lesions should be treated. One reason for this recommendation is that active lesions, even those far from the macula, may be associated with decreased visual acuity because of macular edema, macular traction, severe vitritis, or retinal detachment. In addition, active lesions produce tachyzoites that may spread to distant retinal areas and encyst. Treatment of any active lesion reduces the number of tachyzoites and (theoretically) the chances of reactivation in crucial retinal locations.

Specific therapy for toxoplasmosis includes a wide variety of drugs (Table 33–6). Pyrimethamine and sulfonamides are two of the most commonly used anti-*Toxoplasma* agents. They act by inhibiting the synthesis of folic acid, thereby impairing DNA synthesis (*T. gondii* must synthesize folates because the parasite lacks a transmembrane folate-transport system). Because folic acid antagonists act to inhibit DNA synthesis, they only prevent replication of the active parasite.

Pyrimethamine

Pyrimethamine interrupts the metabolic cycle of the parasite by inhibiting the dihydrofolate-reductase enzyme, thereby preventing the conversion of folic acid to folinic acid, which is essential in both DNA and RNA synthesis. Adverse effects of pyrimethamine include dose-related bone marrow suppression (10%) with leukopenia, thrombocytopenia, and megaloblastic anemia, simulating folinic acid deficiency. It is reversible by interruption of treatment or administration of folinic acid. Patients under treatment should be followed by weekly complete blood cell counts, and pyrimethamine should be stopped if the platelet count falls below 100,000/ml or the leukocyte count falls below 4000 cells/µl. Folinic acid should be used simultaneously with pyrimethamine therapy to help prevent these hematologic problems. Pyrimethamine is contraindicated in the first trimester of pregnancy because of potential teratogenicity. Pyrimethamine treatment has been shown to minimize the size of the retinochoroidal scar that forms with resolution of the active lesion.[143] Thus, it is important in the treatment of *Toxoplasma* lesions in the macular area.

Sulfonamides

Sulfonamides are structural analogues and competitive antagonists of paraminobenzoic acid (PABA) and thus prevent normal utilization of PABA for the synthesis of folic acid by the parasites. Sulfonamides and pyrimethamine are synergistic. Sulfonamides are distributed throughout all tissues of the body and readily enter body fluids, including intraocular fluids. The concentration of sulfonamides in the eye reaches 50% to 80% of the simultaneous serum concentration.[144]

Precipitation of sulfonamides in the urine may cause crystalluria, hematuria, and renal damage. Adequate hydration with oral fluids to maintain a urine output of at least 1500 ml/day should avoid the problem. Patients with glucose 6-phosphate dehydrogenase deficiency should not use sulfa medications because of the potential for hemolytic anemia. Other idiosyncratic hematopoietic disorders can occur, including acute hemolytic anemia in 0.05% and agranulocytosis in 0.1% of patients.[144] Hypersensitivity reactions are quite variable and range from photosensitivity to a severe Stevens-Johnson type of reaction involving skin and mucous membranes. The sulfonamides are contraindicated in the third trimester of gestation because they dislodge the fetal bilirubin from serum albumin, causing kernicterus.

Folinic Acid (Leucovorin)

Folinic acid is used as an adjuvant in therapy with antifolate agents such as pyrimethamine. Folinic acid can be utilized by human cells but not by *T. gondii* and prevents bone marrow suppression caused by pyrimethamine and other folinic acid antagonists.

Clindamycin

Clindamycin inhibits ribosomal protein synthesis and acts synergistically with pyrimethamine and sulfonamides. It has good ocular penetration and concentrates in the choroid. Clindamycin has been shown to reduce the number of tissue cysts in experimental animals, but it is unclear if it decreases recurrence.[145, 146] A skin rash occurs in 10% of the patients treated with clindamycin and diarrhea in 2% to 20%. Pseudomembranous colitis can develop in 0.01% to 10% of patients treated with clindamycin, requiring immediate interruption of therapy and administration of vancomycin or metronidazole.

Spiramycin

Spiramycin is an antibiotic structurally similar to azithromycin. It is less effective but also less toxic than the combination of pyrimethamine with sulfadiazine, so it is the drug of choice during pregnancy. It achieves a high concentration in the placenta and has no reported teratogenic effects. Spiramycin may reduce the incidence of congenital transmission. This antibiotic can be obtained only with special permission through the Food and Drug Administration (FDA) in the United States, but it is available in most other countries.

Atovaquone

Atovaquone interferes in the mitochondrial electrical transport chain of *T. gondii*. This drug has potent action against tachyzoites, including those of very virulent strains, and it has been shown to reduce the number of cerebral tissue cysts after acute or chronic infection in the hamster model.[147] Atovaquone has been successfully

TABLE 33–6. DRUGS USED IN THE TREATMENT OF OCULAR TOXOPLASMOSIS

DRUG	DOSAGE	NOTES
Pyrimethamine	Adults: 100 mg loading dose, followed by 25 mg/day for 30–60 days Children: 4 mg/kg loading dose followed by 1 mg/kg/day divided in 2 doses Newborns should be treated daily for the first 6 mo and then 3 times/wk for their first year of life. Dosage: 1 mg/kg/day divided into 2 doses.	Reversible dose-related bone marrow suppression Simultaneous administration of folinic acid Follow weekly with CBC Contraindicated in the first trimester of pregnancy (potential teratogenicity) Minimizes the size of retinochoroidal scar
Sulfadiazine	Adults: 2 g loading dose followed by 1 g every 6 hr for 30–60 days Children: 100 mg/kg/day divided every 6 hr Newborns should be treated daily for their first year of life. Dosage: 100 mg/kg/day divided into 2 doses.	Adverse effects: photosensitivity, Stevens-Johnson syndrome, crystalluria, and hematologic problems Contraindicated in the third trimester of pregnancy (kernicterus) and during breast feeding Hemolytic anemia if G6PD deficient Synergistic with pyrimethamine
Folinic acid	5–20 mg/day during pyrimethamine therapy, depending on neutrophil count	Prevents bone marrow suppression when administered as an adjuvant of pyrimethamine therapy
Clindamycin	300 mg every 6 hours for 30–40 days Children: 16–20 mg/kg/day divided every 6 hr	Adverse effects: skin rashes, diarrhea, and pseudomembranous colitis Synergistic with pyrimethamine and sulfonamides
Spiramycin	Pregnancy: 500 mg every 6 hr for 3 wk; regimen may be repeated after 21 days. Adults: 500–750 mg every 6 hr for 30–40 days Children: 100 mg/kg/day divided every 6 hr	Drug of choice during pregnancy Reduces the incidence of congenital transmission In utero treatment of infected fetus improves visual outcome Not FDA approved
Atovaquone	750 mg every 6 hr for 4–6 wk	Synergistic action with pyrimethamine, sulfadiazine, and clarithromycin No serious adverse effects Take with food to increase bioavailability
Tetracycline	500 mg every 6 hr loading dose, followed by 250 mg every 6 hr for 30–40 days	Contraindicated during pregnancy and in childhood (brown discoloration of the teeth and depression of bone growth)
Minocycline	100–200 mg/day for 30–40 days	Adverse effects: phototoxicity and audiovestibular toxicity
Clarithromycin	1 g every 12 hr loading dose followed by 500 mg every 12 hr for 4 wk	Not FDA approved for children Synergistic action with pyrimethamine, sulfadiazine, and minocycline
Azithromycin	500–1000 mg/day for 3 wk	Synergistic action with pyrimethamine, sulfadiazine, dapsone, and IFNγ
Trimethoprim/ sulfamethoxazole	160/800 mg (one tablet) every 12 hrs for 30–40 days	Significantly less effective than the combination of pyrimethamine and sulfadiazine.
Prednisone	Adults: 40–100 mg/day Children: 1–2 mg/kg/day	Indicated in active disease involving the posterior pole or optic nerve or if there is severe vitreous inflammation. Start at the same time or within 48 hours of initiating antimicrobial therapy, and taper off before discontinuation.

CBC, Complete blood count; G6PD, glucose-6-phosphate dehydrogenase; FDA, U.S. Food and Drug Administration.

applied in the treatment of ocular toxoplasmosis, but unfortunately it has not proven effective for preventing recurrence. There are no reports of seriously adverse effects except for a transient maculopapular rash. Administration with food increases the bioavailability of atovaquone. Atovaquone acts synergistically with pyrimethamine, sulfadiazine, and clarithromycin, and it may be useful in reducing the dose and toxicity of these drugs in the treatment of patients with AIDS and toxoplasmosis.

Tetracyclines

Tetracycline and its derivatives, particularly minocycline, are alternatives in the treatment of toxoplasmosis. They cause phototoxicity and audiovestibular toxicity. Tetracyclines are contraindicated during pregnancy and in childhood because of resultant brown discoloration of the teeth and depression of bone growth. Long-term minocycline therapy has been recommended for massive, chronically active retinochoroidal granulomas.[82]

Clarithromycin

Clarithromycin is a derivative of erythromycin and is effective against *T. gondii*. It works synergistically with pyrimethamine, sulfadiazine, and minocycline. Clarithromycin is not approved by the FDA for children.

Azithromycin

Azithromycin inhibits ribosomal protein synthesis. It is more active against *T. gondii* than the other macrolides, such as roxithromycin and spiramycin. Azithromycin is effective against the encysted forms of the parasite (the bradyzoites) in vitro and is currently being tested clinically.[148, 149] It has synergistic action when associated with pyrimethamine, sulfadiazine, dapsone, and IFN-γ.

Trimethoprim and Sulfamethoxazole

The combination of trimethoprim with sulfamethoxazole (Bactrim) has been used in the treatment of toxoplasmosis in humans. The sulfamethoxazole inhibits the incorporation of PABA in the synthesis of folic acid, whereas trimethoprim prevents reduction from dihydrofolate to tetrahydrofolate. This combination is significantly less active than the combination of pyrimethamine and sulfadiazine but may still be effective in the treatment of toxoplasmosis. Opremcak and colleagues have reported that 16 patients had improvement in vision and resolution of their retinochoroiditis when Bactrim was used, alone or in combination with clindamycin or steroid. Two patients were allergic to the medication.[150]

Trovafloxacin

Trovafloxacin is a new fluoroquinolone with potent activity against *T. gondii*.[151] It acts synergistically with clarithromycin, pyrimethamine, and sulfadiazine.[152] It seems to be a promising agent in the treatment of toxoplasmosis in immunocompromised patients.

Additional Antimicrobial Therapy

Other antibiotics, such as roxithromycin, rifabutin, and rifapentine have shown efficacy in the treatment of toxoplasmosis.[153-155] They have synergistic actions and are useful in combination with other agents, such as pyrimethamine and sulfadiazine. They allow dosage reduction of the drugs, providing significant reduction of adverse effects.

IL-12 has been used with atovaquone and clindamycin to potentiate the effect of these drugs against *T. gondii*. This combination causes a significant increase in the levels of IFN-γ produced by the host.[156] IFN-γ, TNF-α, IL-2, and IL-12 have been proposed for trials in patients with *Toxoplasma* encephalitis.[157] Dideoxyinosine (DDI) is a drug used against HIV, which is active against *T. gondii*. It has been shown to reduce the number of bradyzoites in the brains of chronically infected mice.[158]

Corticosteroids

When there is potential for serious visual impairment due to posterior pole or optic nerve involvement or severe vitreous inflammation, systemic corticosteroids are added to the treatment regimen. The corticosteroids decrease the inflammatory response and therefore reduce the adverse sequelae such as cystoid macular edema, vitritis, retinitis, and vasculitis. The need for a delay in starting systemic steroid therapy is controversial. The introduction of corticosteroids may begin concomitant with antimicrobial therapy or may be delayed by 12 to 48 hours to achieve therapeutic levels of the antimicrobial drugs. Corticosteroids should be tapered off about 2 weeks before discontinuing the anti-*Toxoplasma* therapy. They should not be used without simultaneous antimicrobial cover. Paradoxically, devastating anterior and posterior inflammation can occur following corticosteroid monotherapy.[159, 160] Topical corticosteroids are used for anterior uveitis, but periocular injections are contraindicated to avoid local immunosuppression and uncontrollable disease.[161]

Treatment Failures

Despite adequate treatment, some patients continue to have chronic active retinitis. This may be the result of a particularly virulent strain of *T. gondii*, or it may be be-

cause of a localized immune or even an autoimmune phenomenon. Many studies have demonstrated both a cellular and a humoral immune response to retinal antigens in the setting of ocular toxoplasmosis.[96-103] Although it is unclear what role the immune system plays in chronic active retinitis, immune-mediated disease should be considered if active retinitis persists for more than 4 months on appropriate antibiotics. In addition, evidence of immune sensitization to retinal antigens supports the use of corticosteroid acutely to minimize exposure to and stimulation by retinal antigens. Clinical evidence supporting the role of the immune system in persistent retinitis comes from patients with ocular toxoplasmosis who are corticosteroid dependent. Occasionally, patients with ocular toxoplasmosis respond to treatment including corticosteroid, but when the corticosteroid is withdrawn, active retinitis recurs despite continuous antibiotic administration. Although the reason for this recurrence has not been determined, it may possibly be explained by three different mechanisms. First and most likely, this "reactivation" phenomenon may simply demonstrate immune reactivity to persistent *T. gondii* antigens remaining in the tissues. Second, it may represent a form of localized autoimmunity. Third, the diagnosis of toxoplasmosis may be erroneous.

Surgical Treatment of Ocular Toxoplasmosis

Laser Photocoagulation

Laser photocoagulation in the treatment of ocular toxoplasmosis has a limited role. Although photocoagulation may destroy cysts and tachyzoites and inhibit the spread of infection, its effectiveness is limited. Laser photocoagulation may be considered for recurrences during pregnancy, cases of drug intolerance, lesions associated with choroidal neovascular membranes, and cases that fail to respond or are resistant to medical therapy. Complications of laser photocoagulation are numerous, including retinal and vitreous hemorrhage, epiretinal membrane, and choroidal neovascular membrane formation. Laser photocoagulation is not recommended as prophylaxis because of dubious efficacy and potential complications, and because tissue cysts are often present in a normal-looking retina.

The pattern of photocoagulation employed consists of a triple row of coalescent burns encircling the lesion and confluent burns to the central area (Fig. 33–24A and B). FA should be performed 1 month after laser photocoagulation, and areas of leakage should be retreated. Occasionally, laser photocoagulation cannot be performed because of media opacity. In these cases, cryotherapy has been tried. Cryotherapy, however, is often not able to reach the typical posterior location of the lesions in *Toxoplasma* retinochoroiditis, and it has its own complications.

Pars Plana Vitrectomy

Pars plana vitrectomy may be useful for removal of persistent vitreous opacities or to relieve vitreoretinal traction that may lead to retinal detachment. Epiretinal membrane peeling combined with or without lensectomy may

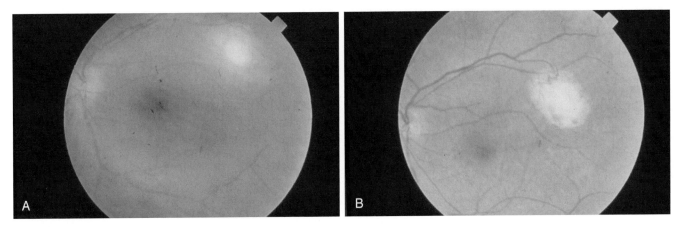

FIGURE 33–24. *A*, Active toxoplasma lesion resistant to prolonged medical therapy. Note that the visual acuity measured 20/70. *B*, The same eye after laser photocoagulation. Note the well-defined, slightly pigmented borders of the lesion. The visual acuity improved to 20/30. (Courtesy of Professor Suel Abujamra, USP, Brazil.) (See color insert.)

be needed to restore visual acuity. Vitrectomy is also believed to remove antigenic proteins, immunoactivating factors, and inflammatory cells from the vitreous. Specific antimicrobial and anti-inflammatory therapy should be administered preoperatively and maintained postoperatively.[113] In the case of choroidal neovascular membranes, surgical removal has been attempted, but whether there was an improvement in visual acuity is questionable.[41]

Therapeutic Regimens

Currently, there are many possible therapeutic options for the treatment of toxoplasmosis, each with its own advantages and disadvantages. We favor the use of pyrimethamine, sulfadiazine, clindamycin, folinic acid, and prednisone for vision-threatening ocular toxoplasmosis in the absence of contravening factors. The optimal duration of specific therapy has not been clearly defined. However, we treat for at least 30 to 60 days in an immunocompetent patient. A positive response to treatment is defined as a sharpening of the borders of the retinochoroidal lesions and improvement of vitreous haze. When therapy is complicated by adverse effects or proves to be ineffective after 4 months, a change in therapy is recommended.

Pregnant women need a special regimen, because the most efficient drugs used for the treatment of toxoplasmosis are potentially harmful to the fetus and the mother. Pyrimethamine is potentially teratogenic and should be avoided, particularly in the first trimester. Sulfadiazine is discouraged in the third trimester because it competes with bilirubin for serum proteins, causing kernicterus. Spiramycin is considered the safest drug during pregnancy and should be combined with sulfadiazine in the first two trimesters and with pyrimethamine in the second and third trimesters. Folinic acid should be added if pyrimethamine is included in the regimen. Spiramycin is not available in the United States but may be acquired from the FDA by special request.

When a pregnant woman acquires toxoplasmosis, spiramycin in combination with pyrimethamine or sulfadiazine may be administered for a 3-week period. If the response is not adequate, the regimen can be repeated after 21 days. Prednisone can be introduced if needed.

Studies demonstrate that antibiotic therapy administered to mothers during pregnancy decreases the percentage of children who will develop retinochoroidal scars during the first and second years of life.[68, 70–72] Close follow-up with an obstetrician is essential.

The newborn with a diagnosis of congenital toxoplasmosis also requires special consideration. Typically, infants present with inactive chorioretinal scars or no lesions at all, but active retinochoroiditis may develop at any time of life. Recent studies demonstrated that the recurrence rate of ocular toxoplasmosis in untreated or undertreated infants is 40% to 67%.[41, 68] Early and prolonged antibiotic therapy throughout the whole first year of life reduces the severity of ocular disease and reduces the recurrence rate to 4% to 13%.[68] These data support the notion that infants with congenital toxoplasmosis should be treated in utero as well as during the entire first year of life regardless of the presence or activity of retinochoroidal lesions.[68, 70–73] The suggested regimen is a combination of pyrimethamine, sulfadiazine, and folinic acid. A new approach to congenital toxoplasmosis is PCR of the amniotic fluid to establish the diagnosis and initiation of treatment in utero for infected fetuses.[162, 163]

In immunocompromised patients, any active retinal lesion deserves treatment because of the high risk of disseminated disease and its complications. A regimen similar to that used for immunocompetent patients may be used for immunosuppressed individuals, with the following modifications. Pyrimethamine may be avoided to prevent further bone marrow suppression and because of its antagonistic action against zidovudine, a retroviral agent often used in the treatment of AIDS.[164] These patients also have a high incidence of allergic reactions, especially to the sulfonamides. Corticosteroids are not recommended, because the immune response is already compromised, and marked inflammation is often not present in HIV-infected individuals. Lifelong maintenance therapy to prevent relapses is required. Lower dosages of pyrimethamine combined with sulfadiazine or clindamycin may be used for this purpose.[165]

PROGNOSIS

The prognosis of ocular toxoplasmosis (that does not involve the optic nerve or the central macula) is favorable in most cases, because the active disease is self-limiting. In some cases, however, sequelae such as a macular retinochoroidal scar, severe vitreous haze, glaucoma, macular edema, epiretinal membrane, choroidal neovascularization, and retinal detachment may cause severe loss of vision. Factors that lead to a worse visual prognosis are large lesions, proximity to the fovea, and a long duration of disease. Early diagnosis and appropriate treatment are essential to minimize complications and loss of vision.

PREVENTION

Measures for the prevention of toxoplasmosis are primarily directed toward prevention of primary infection. Prevention is crucial for seronegative pregnant women and immunocompromised patients. Important measures to prevent infection include the following:

- Meat should be cooked to 60°C (140°F) for at least 15 minutes or frozen to temperatures below −20°C for at least 24 hours to destroy the cysts.
- Any contact with cat feces should be avoided.
- Hands should be washed after touching uncooked meat and after contact with cats or soil that could be contaminated with cat feces.
- Consumption of raw eggs and nonpasteurized milk, particularly goat's milk, should be avoided.
- Fruits and vegetables should be adequately washed before ingestion.
- Daily cleaning of cat litter box removes the oocysts before they become infectious, because they need 1 to 3 days after excretion to undergo sporulation. This duty should be performed only by a nonpregnant individual.
- Blood transfusions and organ transplants from seropositive donors should be avoided if the recipient is seronegative.

Extensive research throughout the world has been aimed toward developing an effective vaccine against toxoplasmosis. Currently, there is a vaccine composed of attenuated tachyzoites that has been used in sheep to prevent abortion due to toxoplasmosis.[166] Vaccination with live tachyzoites, however, is inappropriate in humans. Vaccination with an immunostimulating complex preparation of *T. gondii* antigens has been studied and it seems to induce some immunity in mice.[167] Nearly total protection was observed after immunization with P30 either incorporated into liposomes[168] or in conjunction with QuilA.[169]

Because the most common transmission route of toxoplasmosis is oral, an interesting new approach consists of trials of oral vaccination,[49] which can be combined with adjuvants such as cholera toxin, which is known to enhance the secretory IgA response. Secretory IgA is responsible for a first-line mucosal immunity in the gut and may inhibit organisms before they gain entrance into the circulation. Additionally, oral immunization tends to be both practical and safe in terms of side effects.[170] Other promising work is based on recombinant antigens from different forms of the parasite to produce a vaccine.[171]

CONCLUSION

Toxoplasmosis is a recurrent and progressively destructive ocular and systemic disease, with potentially blinding and even fatal consequences. Fortunately, the mechanisms of disease transmission are well known, allowing the formulation of primary prevention strategies. Once chronic infection has been established and the tissue form has encysted, there is no effective treatment to eradicate the organism. The host immune system plays a vital role in modulating the course of disease. Tissue cysts lie dormant, awaiting the chance to reactivate when immune surveillance falters. Advances in research and treatment continue to be made, improving our ability to prevent, diagnose, and control this disease.

References

1. Henderly DE, Genstler AJ, Smith RE, Rao NA: Changing patterns of uveitis. Am J Ophthalmol 1987;103:131–136.
2. Smith RE, Nozik RA: Uveitis: A Clinical Approach to Diagnosis and Management, 2nd ed. Baltimore, Williams & Wilkins, 1989, pp 128–134.
3. Perkins ES: Ocular toxoplasmosis. Br J Ophthalmol 1973;57:1–17.
4. Fernandes LC, Oréfice F: Aspectos clinicos e epidemiologicos das uveitis em servico de referencia em Belo Horizonte 1970–1993, parte I. Rev Bras Oftal 1996;55:569–578.
5. Fernandes LC, Oréfice F: Aspectos clinicos e epidemiologicos das uveitis em servico de referencia em Belo Horizonte 1970–1993, parte II. Rev Bras Oftal 1996;55:579–592.
6. Silveira CM, Belfort R Jr, Burnier M, Nussenblatt RB: Acquired toxoplasmosis infection as the cause of toxoplasmic retinochoroiditis in families. Am J Ophthalmol 1988;106:362–364.
7. Glasner PD, Silveira C, Kruszon Moran D, et al: An unusually high prevalence of ocular toxoplasmosis in Southern Brazil. Am J Ophthalmol 1992;114:136–144.
8. Pinheiro SRAA, Oréfice F, Andrade GMQ, Caiafa WT: Estudo da toxoplasmose ocular em familias de pacientes portadores de toxolasmose congenita, sistemica e ocular. Arq Bras Oftal 1990;53:4–6.
9. Nussenblatt RB, Belfort R Jr: Ocular toxoplasmosis: An old disease revised. JAMA 1996;71:304–307.
10. Beniz J: Toxoplasmose ocular adquirida (relato de 3 casos). Arq Bras Oftal 1993;56:134–136.
11. Burnett AJ, Shortt SG, Isaac-Renton J, et al: Multiple cases of acquired toxoplasmosis retinitis presenting in an outbreak. Ophthalmology 1998;105:1032–1037.
12. Goncalves ER, Oréfice F, Mendes AG, Pedroso EP: Toxoplasmose adquirida tardia—Relato de 3 casos simultaneos em membros de uma mesma familia. Rev Bras Oftal 1995;54:376–378.
13. Melamed JC: Acquired ocular toxoplasmosis—Late onset. In: Nussenblatt RB, ed: Advances in Ocular Immunology: Proceedings of the 6th International Symposium on the Immunology and Immunopathology of the Eye. New York, Elsevier, 1994, pp 449–452.
14. Montoya JG, Remington JS: Toxoplasmic chorioretinitis in the setting of acute acquired toxoplasmosis. Clin Infect Dis 1996;23:277–282.
15. Silveira C: Estudo da toxoplasmose ocular na regiao de Erechim, RS. Tese de Doutoramento, Sao Paulo, Brazil, 1997; Universidad Federal de Sao Paulo.
16. Oréfice F, Tonelli E: Toxoplasmose adquirida ganglionar associada a uveite anterior granulomatosa sem retinocoroidite. Rev Bras Oftal 1995;54:899–902.
17. Stehling AR, Oréfice F: Toxoplasmose ocular adquirida (relato de 6 casos). Rev Bras Oftal 1996;55:455–465.
18. Splendore A: Un nuovo protozoo parasite del conigli. Rev Soc Sci (Sao Paulo) 1908;3:109–112.
19. Splendore A: Sur un nouveau protozoaire parasite du lapin, deuxieme note preliminaire. Bull Soc Pathol Exot 1909;2:462–465.
20. Nicolle C, Manceaux L: Sur une infection a corps de leishman (ou organismes voisins) du gondii. C R Acad Sci (Paris) 1908;147:763–766.
21. Nicolle C, Manceaux L: Sur un protozoaire nouveau du gondii. Arch Inst Pasteur Tunis 1909;2:97–103.
22. Chaves-Carballo E: Samuel T. Darling and human sarcosporidiosis or toxoplasmosis in Panama. JAMA 1970;211:1687–1689.

23. Castellani A: Protozoa-like bodies in a case of protracted fever with splenomegaly. J Trop Med Hyg (Ceylon) 1914;113.
24. Jankû J: Pathogenesa a pathologicka anatomie tak nazvaneho vrozeneko kolobomu zlute skvmy v oku normalne velikem a mikrophthalmickem nalazem parasitu v sitnici. Casopis Lekaruv Ceskych 1923;62:1021–1027.
25. Pinkerton H, Weinman D: *Toxoplasma* infections in man. Arch Pathol 1940;30:374–392.
26. Wilder HC: *Toxoplasma* chorioretinitis in adults. Arch Ophthalmol 1952;47:425–438.
27. Nicolau S, Ravelo A: La reaction de fixation du complement dans le serum et dans des extraits d'organes d'animaux atteints de toxoplasmose experimentale. Bull Soc Pathol Exot 1937;30:855–859.
28. Sabin AB, Feldman HA: Dyes as microchemical indicators of a new immunity phenomenon affecting a protozoon parasite (*Toxoplasma*). Science 1948;108:660–663.
29. Frenkel JK, Dubey JP, Miller NL: *Toxoplasma gondii* in cats: Fecal stages identified as coccidian oocysts. Science 1970;167:893–896.
30. Hutchison WM, Dunachie JF, Siim JC, Work K: Coccidian-like nature of *Toxoplasma gondii*. Br Med J 1970;1:142–144.
31. Tessler HH: Ocular toxoplasmosis. Int Ophthalmol Clin 1981;21:185–199.
32. Jabs DA: Ocular toxoplasmosis. Int Ophthalmol Clin 1990;30:264–270.
33. Woods AC: Modern concepts of the etiology of uveitis. Am J Ophthalmol 1960;50:1170–1187.
34. McLeod R, Remington JS: Toxoplasmosis. In: Braunwald E, Isselbacher KJ, Petersdorf RG, et al, eds: Harrison's Principles of Internal Medicine, 11th ed. New York, McGraw-Hill, 1987, pp 791–797.
35. Kasper LH: *Toxoplasma* infection. In: Braunwald E, Fauci AS, Isselbacher KJ, et al, eds: Harrison's Principles of Internal Medicine Online. New York: McGraw-Hill, 1999.
36. Siegel SE, Lunde MN, Gelderman AH, et al: Transmission of toxoplasmosis by leukocyte transfusion. Blood 1971;37:388–394.
37. Saari M, Raisanem S: Transmission of acute toxoplasmosis infection: The survival of trophozoites in human tears, saliva, and urine and in cow's milk. Acta Ophthalmol (Kbh) 1974;52:847–852.
38. Pauleikhoff D, Messmer E, Beelen DW, et al: Bone-marrow transplantation and toxoplasmic retinochoroiditis. Graefes Arch Clin Ophthalmol 1987;225:239–243.
39. Lou P, Kazdan J, Basu PK: Ocular toxoplasmosis in three consecutive siblings. Arch Ophthalmol 1978;96:613–614.
40. Stern GA, Romano PE: Congenital ocular toxoplasmosis: Possible occurrence in siblings. Arch Ophthalmol 1978;96:615–617.
41. Oréfice F, Bonfioli AA: Toxoplasmose. In: Oréfice F, ed: Uveite clinica e cirurgica (in prelo). Rio de Janeiro, Brazil, Editora Cultura Medica, 1999.
42. Nichols BA, Chiappino ML, O'Connor GR: Secretion from the rhoptries of *Toxoplasma gondii* during host-cell invasion. J Ultrastruct Res 1983;83:85–98.
43. Schwartzman JD: Inhibition of a penetration enhancing factor of *Toxoplasma gondii* by monoclonal antibodies specific for rhoptries. Infect Immunol 1986;51:760–764.
44. Leriche MA, Dubremetz JF: Characterization of the protein contents of rhoptries and dense granules of *Toxoplasma gondii* tachyzoites by subcellular fractionation and monoclonal antibodies. Mol Biochem Parasitol 1991;45:249–260.
45. Lingelbach K, Joiner KA: The parasitophorous vacuole membrane surrounding plasmodium and toxoplasma: An unusual compartment in infected cells. J Cell Sci 1998;111:1467–1475.
46. Joiner KA, Dubremetz JF: *Toxoplasma gondii*: A protozoan for the nineties. Infect Immunol 1993;61:1169–1172.
47. Sibley LD, Weidner E, Krahenbuhl JL: Phagosome acidification blocked by intracellular *Toxoplasma gondii*. Nature (Lond) 1985;315:416–419.
48. Sibley LD: Interactions between *Toxoplasma gondii* and its mammalian host cells. Semin Cell Biol 1993;4:335–344.
49. Cesbron MF, Dubremetz JF, Sher A: The immunobiology of toxoplasmosis. Res Immunol 1993;144:7–79.
50. Joiner KA, Fuhrman SA, Mietinnen H, et al: *Toxoplasma gondii*: Fusion competence of parasitophorous vacuoles in Fc receptor transfected fibroblasts. Science 1990;249:641–646.
51. Gazzinelli RT, Denkers EY, Sher A: Host resistance to *Toxoplasma gondii*: Model for studying the selective induction of cell-mediated immunity by intracellular parasites. Infect Agents Dis 1993;2:139–149.
52. Gazzinelli RT, Bala S, Stevens R, et al: HIV infection suppresses type 1 lymphokine and IL-12 responses to *Toxoplasma gondii* but fails to inhibit the synthesis of other parasite-induced monokines. J Immunol 1995;155:1565–1574.
53. Hunter CA, Candolfi E, Subauste C, et al: Studies on the role of interleukin-12 in acute murine toxoplasmosis. Immunology 1995;84:16–20.
54. Hunter CA, Chizzonite R, Remington JS: IL-1 beta is required for IL-12 to induce production of IFN-gamma by NK cells: A role for IL-1 beta in the T cell-independent mechanism of resistance against intracellular pathogens. J Immunol 1995;155:4347–4354.
55. Roberts F, McLeod R: Pathogenesis of toxoplasmic retinochoroiditis. Parasitol Today 1999;15:51–57.
56. Denkers EY, Gazzinelli RT: Regulation and function of T-cell-mediated immunity during *Toxoplasma gondii* infection. Clin Microbiol Rev 1998;11:569–588.
57. Nagineni CN, Pardhasaradhi K, Martins MC, et al: Mechanisms of interferon-induced inhibition of *Toxoplasma gondii* replication in human retinal pigment epithelial cells. Infect Immunol 1996;64:4188–4196.
58. Streilein JW, Wilbanks GA, Cousins SW: Immunoregulatory mechanisms of the eye. J Neuroimmunol 1992;39:185–200.
59. Soete M, Dubremetz JF: Kinetics of stage-specific protein expression during tachyzoite-bradyzoite conversion in vitro. Curr Top Immunol 1996;219:76–80.
60. Kasper LH, Crabb JH, Pfefferkon ER: Purification of a major membrane protein of *Toxoplasma gondii* by immunoabsorption with a monoclonal antibody. Infect Immunol 1983;130:2407–2412.
61. Nussenblatt RB, Mittal KK, Fuhrman S, et al: Lymphocyte proliferative responses of patients with toxoplasmosis to parasite and retinal antigens. Am J Ophthalmol 1989;107:632–641.
62. Silva NM, Gazzinelli RT, Silva DA, et al: Expression of *Toxoplasma gondii* during in vivo conversion of bradyzoites to tachyzoites. Infect Immunol 1998;66:3959–3963.
63. Chowdhury MN: Toxoplasmosis: A review. J Med 1986;17:5–6, 373–396.
64. Park SS, To KW, Friedman AH, Jakobiec FA: Infectious causes of posterior uveitis. In: Albert DM, Jakobiec FA, eds: Principles and Practice of Ophthalmology, vol 1. Philadelphia, W.B. Saunders, 1994, pp 460–461.
65. McCabe R, Remington JS: Toxoplasmosis: The time has come. N Engl J Med 1988;318:313–315.
66. Kean BH, Kimball AC, Christenson WN: An epidemic of acute toxoplasmosis. JAMA 1969;208:1002–1006.
67. Roberts T, Frenkel JK: Estimating income losses and other preventable costs caused by congenital toxoplasmosis in people in the United States. JAMA 1990;2:249–256.
68. Mets MB, Holfels E, Boyer KM, et al: Eye manifestations of congenital toxoplasmosis. Am J Ophthalmol 1996;122:309–324.
69. Nussenblatt RB, Palestine AG: Uveitis: Fundamentals and clinical practice. Chicago, Year Book, 1989, pp 336–354.
70. Couvreur J, Desmonts G, Thulliez P: Prophylaxis of congenital toxoplasmosis: Effects of spiramycin on placental infection. J Antimicrob Chemother 1988;22(suppl B):193–200.
71. Hohlfeld P, Daffos F, Thulliez P, et al: Fetal toxoplasmosis: Outcome of pregnancy and infant follow-up after in utero treatment. J Pediatr 1989;115:765–769.
72. Daffos F, Forestier F, Capella-Pavlovsky M: Prenatal management of 746 pregnancies at risk for congenital toxoplasmosis. N Engl J Med 1988;318:271–275.
73. Couvreur J, Thulliez P, Daffos F, et al: Fetal toxoplasmosis: In utero treatment with pyrimethamine sulfamides. Arch Fr Pediatr 1991;48:397–403.
74. Foulon W, Villena I, Stray Pedersen B, et al: Treatment of toxoplasmosis during pregnancy: A multicenter study of impact on fetal transmission and children's sequelae at age 1 year. Am J Obstet Gynecol 1999;180:410–415.
75. Couvreur J, Thulliez P: Toxoplasmosis acquise a localisation oculaire ou neurologique. Presse Med 1996;25:438–442.
76. Cohen SN: Toxoplasmosis in patients receiving immunosuppressive therapy. JAMA 1970;211:657–660.
77. Araujo FG, Remington JS: Toxoplasmosis in immunocompromised patients. Eur J Clin Microbiol 1987;6:1–2.

78. Jabs DA, Green WR, Fox R, et al: Ocular manifestations of acquired immunodeficiency syndrome. Ophthalmology 1989;96:1092–1099.

79. Friedman AH: The retinal lesions of the acquired immune deficiency syndrome. Trans Am Ophthalmol Soc 1984;82:447–491.

80. Tabbara KF: Ocular toxoplasmosis (review). Int Ophthalmol Clin 1990;14:349–351.

81. Holland GN, Engstrom RE, Glasgow BJ, et al: Ocular toxoplasmosis in patients with the acquired immunodeficiency syndrome. Am J Ophthalmol 1988;106:653–667.

82. Khanna A, Goldstein DA, Tessler HH: Protozoal posterior uveitis. In: Yanoff M, Duker JS, eds: Ophthalmology, 1st ed. St. Louis, Mosby, 1999.

83. Hénin D, Duyckaerts C, Chaunu MP, et al: Étude neuropathologique de 31 cas de syndrome d' immuno-dépression acquise. Rev Neurol (Paris) 1987;143:631–642.

84. Moorthy RS, Rao NA: Posterior uveitis. In: Wright KW: Textbook of Ophthalmology on CD-ROM. New York: Williams & Wilkins, 1997.

85. Holland GN: Ocular toxoplasmosis in the immunocompromised host. Int Ophthalmol 1989;13:399–402.

86. Schuman JS, Friedman AH: Retinal manifestations of the acquired immune deficiency syndrome (AIDS): Cytomegalovirus, *Candida albicans, Cryptococcus*, toxoplasmosis and *Pneumocystis carinii*. Trans Ophthalmol Soc UK 1983;103:177–190.

87. Heinemann MH, Gold JMW, Maisel J: Bilateral toxoplasma retinochoroiditis in a patient with acquired immune deficiency syndrome. Retina 1986;6:224–227.

88. Moorthy RS, Smith RE, Rao NA: Progressive Ocular Toxoplasmosis in Patients with Acquired Immunodeficiency Syndrome. Am J Ophthalmol 1993;115:742–747.

89. Manschot WA, Daamen CBF: Connatal Ocular Toxoplasmosis. Arch Ophthalmol 1965;74:48–54.

90. Araujo F, Slifer T, Kim S: Chronic infection with *Toxoplasma gondii* does not prevent acute disease or colonization on the brain with tissue cysts following reinfection with different strains of the parasite. J Parasitol 1997;83:521–522.

91. Rothova A, Meenken C, Buitenhuis HJ, et al: Therapy of ocular toxoplasmosis. Am J Ophthalmol 1993;115:517–523.

92. Ghosh M, Levy PM, Leopold IH: Therapy of toxoplasmosis uveitis. Am J Ophthalmol 1965;59:55.

93. Rodenhäuser JH: Clinical findings and pathogenesis of Kyrieleis' discontinuous reversible arteriopathy in uveitis. Klin Monatsbl Augenheilkd 1969;155:234–243.

94. Doft BH, Gass DM: Punctate outer retinal toxoplasmosis. Arch Ophthalmol 1985;103:1332–1336.

95. Matthews JD, Weiter JJ: Outer retinal toxoplasmosis. Ophthalmology 1988;95:941–946.

96. Nussenblatt RB, Mittal KK, Fuhrman S, et al: Lymphocyte proliferative responses of patients with ocular toxoplasmosis to parasite and retinal antigens. Am J Ophthalmol 1989;107:632–641.

97. Abrahams IW, Gregerson DS: Longitudinal study of serum antibody responses to retinal antigens in acute ocular toxoplasmosis. Am J Ophthalmol 1982;93:224–231.

98. Whittle RM, Wallace GR, Whiston RA, et al: Human antiretinal antibodies in toxoplasma retinochoroiditis. Br J Ophthalmol 1998;82:1017–1021.

99. Kijlstra A, Hoekzema R, Van der Lelij A, et al: Humoral and cellular immune reactions against retinal antigens in clinical disease. Curr Eye Res 1990;9(suppl):85–89.

100. Froebel KS, Armstrong SS, Cliffe AM, et al: An investigation of the general immune status and specific immune responsiveness to retinal (S)-antigen in patients with chronic posterior uveitis. Eye 1989;3:263–270.

101. Gregerson DS, Abrahams IW, Thirkill CE: Serum antibody levels of uveitis patients to bovine retinal antigens. Invest Ophthalmol Vis Sci 1981;21:669–680.

102. Rahi AH, Addison DJ: Autoimmunity and the outer retina. Trans Ophthalmol Soc U K 1983;103:428–437.

103. Abrahams IW, Gregerson DS: Longitudinal study of serum antibody responses to bovine retinal S-antigen in endogenous granulomatous uveitis. Br J Ophthalmol 1983;67:681–684.

104. Rehder JR, Burnier MB Jr, Pavesio CD, et al: Acute unilateral toxoplasmic iridocyclitis in AIDS patients. Am J Ophthalmol 1988;106:740–741.

105. De Abreu MT, Belfort R, Hirata PS: Fuchs' heterochromic cyclitis and ocular toxoplasmosis. Am J Ophthalmol 1982;93:739–744.

106. Arffa RC, Schlaegel TF: Chorioretinal scars in Fuchs' heterochromic iridocyclitis. Arch Ophthalmol 1984;102:1153–1155.

107. Saraux H, Laroche L, Le Hoang P: Secondary Fuchs' heterochromic cyclitis: A new approach to an old disease. Ophthalmologica 1985;190:193–198.

108. Schwab IR: The epidemiologic association of Fuchs' heterochromic iridocyclitis and ocular toxoplasmosis. Am J Ophthalmol 1991;111:356–362.

109. Rutzen AR, Raizman MB: Fuchs' heterochromic iridocyclitis. In: Albert DM, Jakobiec FA, eds: Principles and Practice of Ophthalmology, vol 1. Philadelphia, W.B. Saunders, 1994, pp 503–516.

110. La Hey E, Rothova A, Baarsma GS, et al: Fuchs' heterochromic iridocyclitis is not associated with ocular toxoplasmosis. Arch Ophthalmol 1992;110:806–811.

111. Silveira CM, Belfort R Jr, Nussenblatt R, et al: Unilateral pigmentary retinopathy associated with ocular toxoplasmosis. Am J Ophthalmol 1989;107:682–684.

112. Tabbara KF: Disruption of the choroidoretinal interface by toxoplasma. Eye 1990;4:366–373.

113. Tamesis RR, Foster CS: Toxoplasmosis. In: Albert DM, Jakobiec FA, eds: Principles and Practice of Ophthalmology, vol 2. Philadelphia, W.B. Saunders, 1994, pp 929–933.

114. Zimmerman LE: Ocular pathology of toxoplasmosis. Surv Ophthalmol 1961;6:832–876.

115. Webb RM, Tabbara KF, O'Connor GR: Retinal vasculitis in ocular toxoplasmosis in nonhuman primates. Retina 1984;4:225–231.

116. Newman PE, Ghosheh R, Tabbara KF, et al: The role of hypersensitivity reactions to toxoplasma antigens in experimental ocular toxoplasmosis in nonhuman primates. Am J Ophthalmol 1982;94:159–164.

117. Connor GR: The influence of hypersensitivity on the pathogenesis of ocular toxoplasmosis. Trans Am Ophthalmol Soc 1970;68:501–547.

118. McMenamin PG, Dutton GN, Hay J, Cameron S: The ultrastructural pathology of congenital murine toxoplasmomic retinochoroiditis. Part 1: The localization and morphology of toxoplasma cysts in the retina. Exp Eye Res 1986;43:529–543.

119. Kean BH, Sun T, Ellsworth RM: Color Atlas/Text of Ophthalmic Parasitology. New York, Igaku-Shoin, 1991, pp 9–21.

120. Kelan AE, Ayllon-Leindl L, Labzoffsky NA: Indirect fluorescent antibody method in serodiagnosis of toxoplasmosis. Can J Microbiol 1962;8:545.

121. Fuccillo DA, Madden DL, Tzan N, Sever JL: Difficulties associated with serologic diagnosis of *Toxoplasma gondii* infections. Diagn Clin Immunol 1987;5:8–13.

122. Weiss MJ, Velazquez N, Hofeldt AJ: Serologic tests in the diagnosis of presumed toxoplasmic retinochoroiditis. Am J Ophthalmol 1990;109:407–411.

123. Araujo FG, Barnett EV, Gentry LO, Remington JS: False-positive anti-toxoplasma fluorescent-antibody tests in patients with antinuclear antibodies. Appl Microbiol 1971;22:270–275.

124. Naot Y, Remington JS: An enzyme-linked immunosorbent assay for detection of IgM antibodies to Toxoplasma gondii: Use for diagnosis of acute acquired toxoplasmosis. J Infect Dis 1980;142:757–766.

125. Pyndiah N, Krech U, Price P, Wilhelm J: Simplified chromatographic separation of immunoglobulin M from G and its application to toxoplasma indirect immunofluorescence. J Clin Microbiol 1979;9:170–174.

126. Weiss MJ, Velazquez N, Hofeldt AJ: Serologic tests in the diagnosis of presumed toxoplasmic retinochoroiditis. Am J Ophthalmol 1990;109:407–411.

127. Schlaegel TF Jr: Ocular Toxoplasmosis and Pars Planitis. New York, Grune & Stratton, 1978, pp 138–172.

128. Naot Y, Desmonts G, Remington JS: IgM enzyme-linked immunosorbent assay test for the diagnosis of congenital toxoplasma infection. J Pediatr 1981;98:32–36.

129. Tomasi JP, Schlit AF, Staatbaeder S: Rapid double sandwich enzyme-linked immunosorbent assay for detection of human immunoglobulin anti-*Toxoplasma gondii* antibodies. J Clin Microbiol 1986;24:849–850.

130. Guimaraes O, Oréfice F, Mineo JR, Brandao E: Reacoes de imunofluorescencia indireta e de ELISA na deteccao de anticorpos IgG and IgM no soro de pacientes portadores de retinocoroidite ativa e cicatrizada supostamente toxoplasmica. Rev Bras Oftal 1991;49:241–346.

131. Katina JA, Oréfice F, Mineo JR: Anticorpos IgA específicos no soro e humor aquoso de pacientes com uveíte de provável etiologia toxoplásmica. Rev Bras Oftal 1992;51:209–216.

132. Chumpitazi BFF, Boussaid A, Pelloux H, et al: Diagnosis of congenital toxoplasmosis by immunoblotting and relationship with other methods. J Clin Microbiol 1995;33:1479–1485.

133. Yamamoto YI, Mineo JR, Meneghisse CS, et al: Detection in human sera of IgG, IgM and IgA to excreted/secreted antigens from *Toxoplasma gondii* by use of dot-ELISA and immunoblot assay. Ann Trop Med Parasitol 1998;92:23–30.

134. Brézin AP, Egwuagu CE, Burnier M Jr, et al: Identification of *Toxoplasma gondii* in paraffin-embedded sections by the polymerase chain reaction. Am J Ophthalmol 1990;110:599–604.

135. Hohlfeld P, Daffos F, Costa JM, et al: Prenatal diagnosis of congenital toxoplasmosis with a polymerase-chain-reaction test on amniotic fluid. N Engl J Med 1994;331:695–699.

136. Thulliez P, Daffos F, Forestier F: Diagnosis of toxoplasma infection in the pregnant woman and the unborn child: Current problems. Scand J Infect Dis Suppl 1992;84:18–22.

137. Forestier F, Hohlfeld P, Sole Y, Daffos F: Prenatal diagnosis of congenital toxoplasmosis by PCR: extended experience [letter]. Prenat Diagn 1998;18:407–409.

138. Manners RM, O'Connell S, Gay EC, et al: Use of the polymerase chain reaction in the diagnosis of acquired ocular toxoplasmosis in an immunocompetent adult. Br J Ophthalmol 1994;78:583–584.

139. Aouizerate F, Cazenave J, Poirier L, et al: Detection of *Toxoplasma gondii* in aqueous humor by polymerase chain reaction. Br J Ophthalmol 1993;77:107–110.

140. Couvreur J, Desmonts G: Congenital and maternal toxoplasmosis: A review of 300 congenital cases. Dev Med Child Neurol 1962;4:519.

141. Desmonts G: Definitive serological diagnosis of ocular toxoplasmosis. Arch Ophthalmol 1966;76:839–851.

142. Eyles DE, Coleman N: Synergistic effect of sulphadiazine and daraprin against experimental toxoplasmosis in the mouse. Antibiot Chemother 1953;3:483–490.

143. Rothova A, Meenken C, Buitenhuis HJ, et al: Therapy for ocular toxoplasmosis. Am J Ophthalmol 1993;115:517–523.

144. Mandell GL, Sande MA: Antimicrobial agents. In: Gilman AG, Goodman LS, Ralf TW, Murad F, eds: Goodman and Gilman's The Pharmacological Basis of Therapeutics, 7th ed. New York, Macmillan, 1985, p 1098.

145. Hofflin JM, Remington JS: Clindamycin in a murine model of toxoplasmic encephalitis. Antimicrob Agents Chemother 1987;31:492–496.

146. Tabbara KF, Dy-Liacco J, Nozik RA, et al: Clindamycin in chronic toxoplasmosis: Effect of periocular injections on recoverability of organisms from healed lesions in the rabbit eye. Arch Ophthalmol 1979;97:542–544.

147. Gormley PD, Pavesio CE, Minnasian D, Lightman S: Effects of drug therapy on toxoplasma cysts in an animal model of acute and chronic disease. Invest Ophthalmol Vis Sci 1998;39:1171–1175.

148. Huskinson-Mark J, Araujo FG, Remington JS: Evaluation of the effects of drugs on the cyst form of the *Toxoplasma gondii*. J Infect Dis 1991;164:170–171.

149. Farthing C, Rendel M, Currie B, Seidlin M: Azithromycin for cerebral toxoplasmosis. Lancet 1992;339:437–438.

150. Opremcak EM, Scales DK, Sharpe MR: Trimethoprim-sulfamethoxazole therapy for ocular toxoplasmosis. Ophthalmology 1992;99:920–925.

151. Khan AA, Slifer T, Araujo FG, Remington JS: Trovafloxacin is active against *Toxoplasma gondii*. Antimicrob Agents Chemother 1996;40:1855–1859.

152. Khan AA, Slifer T, Araujo FG, et al: Activity of trovafloxacin in combination with other drugs for treatment of acute murine toxoplasmosis. Antimicrob Agents Chemother 1997;41:893–897.

153. Araujo FG, Khan AA, Remington JS: Rifapentine is active in vitro and in vivo against *Toxoplasma gondii*. Antimicrob Agents Chemother 1996;40:1335–1337.

154. Araujo FG, Slifer T, Remington JS: Rifabutin is active in murine models of toxoplasmosis. Antimicrob Agents Chemother 1994;38:570–575.

155. Araujo FG, Suzuki Y, Remington JS: Use of rifabutin in combination with atovaquone, clindamycin, pyrimethamine, or sulfadiazine for treatment of toxoplasmic encephalitis in mice. Eur J Clin Microbiol Infect Dis 1996;15:394–397.

156. Araujo FG, Hunter CA, Remington JS: Treatment with interleukin 12 in combination with atovaquone or clindamycin significantly increases survival of mice with acute toxoplasmosis. Antimicrob Agents Chemother 1997;41:188–190.

157. Hunter CA, Subauste CS, Remington JS: The role of cytokines in toxoplasmosis. Biotherapy 1994;7:237–247.

158. Sarciron ME, Lawton P, Saccharin C, et al: Effects of 2′, 3′-dideoxyinosine on *Toxoplasma gondii* cysts in mice. Antimicrob Agents Chemother 1997;41:1531–1536.

159. Nicholson DH, Wolchok EB: Ocular toxoplasmosis in an adult receiving long-term corticosteroid therapy. Arch Ophthalmol 1976;94:248–254.

160. Sabates R, Pruett RC, Brockhurst RJ: Fulminary ocular toxoplasmosis. Am J Ophthalmol 1981;92:497–503.

161. O'Connor GR, Frenkel JK: Editorial: Dangers of steroid treatment in toxoplasmosis. Periocular injections and systemic therapy. Arch Ophthalmol 1976;94:213.

162. Couvreur J: Problems of congenital toxoplasmosis. Evolution over four decades. Presse Med 1999;28:753–757.

163. Russo M: Toxoplasmosis in pregnancy. Prevention, diagnosis, and therapy. Recenti Prog Med 1994;85:37–48.

164. Israelsky DM, Tom C, Remington JS: Zidovudine antagonizes the action of pyrimethamine in experimental infection with *Toxoplasma gondii*. Antimicrob Agents Chemother 1989;33:30–34.

165. Morlat P, Leport C: Prevention of toxoplasmosis in immunocompromised patients. Ann Med Interne (Paris) 1997;148:3, 235–239.

166. Dubey JP: Prevention of abortion and neonatal death due to toxoplasmosis by vaccination of goats with the nonpathogenic coccidium *Hammondia hammondi*. Am J Vet Res 1981;42:2155–2157.

167. Uggla A, Araujo FG, Lunden A, et al: Immunizing effects in mice of two *Toxoplasma gondii* ISCOM preparations. J Vet Med 1988;B35:311–314.

168. Bulow R, Boothroyd JC: Protection of mice from fatal *Toxoplasma gondii* infection by immunization with P30 antigen in liposomes. J Immunol 1991;147:3496–3500.

169. Khan IA, Ely KH, Kasper LH: A purified parasite antigen (P30) mediates CD8+ T cell immunity against fatal *Toxoplasma gondii* infection in mice. J Immunol 1991;147:3501–3506.

170. Kraehenbuhl JP, Neutra MR: Molecular and cellular basis of immune protection of mucosal surfaces. Physiol Rev 1992;72:853–879.

171. Alexander J, Jebbari H, Bluethmann H, et al: Immunological control of *Toxoplasma gondii* and appropriate vaccine design. Curr Top Microbiol Immunol 1996;219:183–195.

172. Burg JL, Perelman D, Kasper LH, et al: Molecular analysis of the gene encoding the major surface antigen of *Toxoplasma gondii*. J Immunol 1988;141:3584–3591.

173. Couvreur G, Sadak A, Fortier B, Dubremetz JF: Surface antigens of *Toxoplasma gondii*. Parasitology 1988;97:1–10.

174. Handman E, Goding JW, Dubremetz JF: Detection and characterization of membrane antigens of *Toxoplasma gondii*. J Immunol 1980;124:2578–2583.

175. Tomavo S, Schwarz RT, Dubremetz JF: Evidence for glycosyl-phosphatidylinositol anchoring of *Toxoplasma gondii* major surface antigens. Mol Cell Biol 1989;9:4576–4580.

176. Prince JB, Auer KL, Huskinson J, et al: Cloning, expression, and cDNA sequence of surface antigen P22 from *Toxoplasma gondii*. Mol Biochem Parasitol 1990;43:97–106.

177. Cesbron-Delauw MF, Tomavo S: Unpublished observation.

178. Cesbron-Delauw MF, Guy B, Torpier G, et al: Molecular characterization of a 23-kilodalton major antigen secreted by *Toxoplasma gondii*. Proc Nat Acad Sci 1989;86:7537–7541.

179. Charif H, Darcy F, Torpier G, et al: *Toxoplasma gondii*. Characterization and localization of antigens secreted from taquizoites. Exp Parasitol 1990;71:114–124.

180. Achbarou A, Mercereau-Puijalon O, Sadak A, et al: Differential targeting of dense granule proteins in the parasitophorous vacuole of *Toxoplasma gondii*. Parasitology 1991;103:321–329.

181. Mercier C, Lecordier L, Darcy F, et al: Molecular characterization of a dense granule antigen (GRA2) associated with the network of the parasitophorous vacuole in *Toxoplasma gondii*. Mol Biochem Parasitol 1993;58:71–82.

182. Prince JB, Araujo FG, Remington JS, et al: Cloning of cDNAs encoding a 28-kilodalton antigen of *Toxoplasma gondii*. Mol Biochem Parasitol 1989;34:3–13.

183. Leriche MA, Dubremetz JF: Characterization of the protein contents of rhoptries and dense granules of *Toxoplasma gondii* tachyzoites by subcellular fractionation and monoclonal antibodies. Mol Biochem Parasitol 1991;45:249–260.
184. Bermudes D, Joiner KA: Unpublished observation.
185. Mevelec MN, Chardes T, Mercereau-Puijalon O, et al: Molecular cloning of a gene encoding GRA4, a *Toxoplasma gondii* dense granule protein recognized by mucosal IgA antibodies. Mol Biochem Parasitol 1992;56:227–238.
186. Lecordier L, Mercier C, Torpier G, et al: Molecular structure of a *Toxoplasma gondii* dense granule antigen (GRA5), associated with the parasitophorous vacuole membrane. Mol Biochem Parasitol 1993;59:143–153.
187. Ossorio PN, Schwartzman JD, Boothroyd JC: A *Toxoplasma gondii* rhoptry protein associated with host cell penetration has unusual charge asymmetry. Mol Biochem Parasitol 1992;50:1–16.
188. Saavedra R, Demeuter F, Decourt JL, Herion P: Human T-cell clone identifies a potentially protective 54-kDa protein antigen of *Toxoplasma gondii* cloned and expressed in *Escherichia coli.* J Immunol 1991;147:1975–1982.
189. Achbarou A, Mercereau-Puijalon O, Autheman JM, et al: Characterization of microneme proteins of *Toxoplasma gondii.* Mol Biochem Parasitol 1991;47:223–233.
190. Fourmaux MN, Mercereau-Puijalon O, Dubremetz JF: Unpublished observation.
191. Nagel SD, Boothroyd JC: The α and β tubulins of *Toxoplasma gondii* are encoded by single copy genes containing multiple introns. Mol Biochem Parasitol 1988;29:261–273.
192. Roos D: Unpublished observation.
193. Johnson AM, Illana S, McDonald PJ, Asai T: Cloning, expression and nucleotide sequence of the gene fragment encoding an antigenic portion of the nucleoside triphosphate hydrolase of *Toxoplasma gondii.* Gene 1989;85:215–220.
194. Oréfice F, Belfort R Jr: Toxoplasmose. In: Oréfice F, Belfort R, Roca S, eds: Uveitis. Sao Paulo, 1987.
195. Hunter K, Stagno S, Capps E, Smith RJ: Prenatal screening of pregnant women for infections caused by cytomegalovirus, Epstein-Barr virus, herpesvirus, rubella, and *Toxoplasma gondii.* Am J Obstet Gynecol 1983;145:269–273.
196. Jackson MH, Hutchison WM, Siim JC: A seroepidemiological survey of toxoplasmosis in Scotland and England. Ann Trop Med Parasitol 1987;81:359–365.
197. Williams KA, Scott JM, Macfarlane DE, et al: Congenital toxoplasmosis: A prospective survey in the west of Scotland. J Infect 1981;3:219–229.
198. Alford CA: An epidemiologic overview of intrauterine and perinatal infections of man. Mead Johnson Symp Perinat Dev Med 1982;21:3–11.
199. Palicka P: [Incidence of congenital toxoplasmosis in the Czech population] Cesk Epidemiol Mikrobiol Imunol 1982;31:290–297.
200. Sfameni SF, Skurrie IJ, Gilbert GL: Antenatal screening for congenital infection with rubella, cytomegalovirus and *Toxoplasma.* Aust N Z J Obstet Gynaecol 1986;26:257–260.
201. Foulon W, Naessens A, Volckaert M, et al: Congenital toxoplasmosis: A prospective survey in Brussels. Br J Obstet Gynaecol 1984;91:419–423.
202. Logar J, Novak Antolic Z, Zore A, et al: Incidence of congenital toxoplasmosis in the Republic of Slovenia. Scand J Infect Dis 1992;24:105–108.
203. Bornand JE, Piguet JD: [*Toxoplasma* infestation: Prevalence, risk of congenital infection and development in Geneva from 1973 to 1987.] Schweiz Med Wochenschr 1991;121:21–29.
204. Camargo ME, Leser PG, Kiss MH, Amato Neto V: Serology in early diagnosis of congenital toxoplasmosis. Rev Inst Med Trop Sao Paulo 1978;20:152–160.
205. Desmonts G: [Detection of toxoplasmosis by agglutination of parasites. Value of a very sensitive antigen in the search for specific immunoglobulins G]. Ann Biol Clin (Paris) 1983;41:139–143.

*Jesús Merayo-Lloves, Cindy M. Vredeveld,
and Albert T. Vitale*

DEFINITION

Ocular disease caused by the free-living amebae *Acanthamoeba* and *Naegleria* is an uncommon but severe and progressive, potentially blinding infection. It usually affects the cornea but could also involve the sclera, uveal tract, and other ocular tissues. Early diagnosis is the most important prognostic indicator of successful outcome, so clinical suspicion should be high for patients with painful corneal inflammation of atypical course, whether or not they wear contact lenses, and laboratory confirmation should be sought.

Amebiasis is an intestinal infection caused by *Entamoeba histolytica*. Only 10% of affected individuals demonstrated clinical manifestations (including dysentery and liver abscesses). Ocular infection is rare.

HISTORY AND MICROBIOLOGY

Historical Background

Free-living *Acanthamoeba* (ameba from the Greek αμοιβη, change[1]) was described in 1775 by Von Rosenhof[2] and characterized by an irregular, sluggish, flowing "ameboid motion."[3]

In 1930, Aldo Castellani[4] described the morphological characteristics; Culbertson in 1950 observed brain lesions in mice and monkeys; and Flower reported the first fatal human infection in 1965.[5] The first cases of confirmed *Acanthamoeba* infection of the eye were reported in 1973 by Jones and colleagues[6] at the Ocular Microbiology and Immunology Group meeting, with clinical descriptions of keratitis and uveitis. The first published paper on its morphology appeared in 1975.[7] During the 1980s and 1990s, there was an emergent epidemic of *Acanthamoeba* keratitis[8] in contact lens wearers. Since then, improved education of clinical ophthalmologists has resulted in better prevention, earlier diagnosis, and more aggressive treatment, so the incidence of *Acanthamoeba* keratitis has declined, and the prognosis and visual outcome have improved.[9, 10]

Microbiology

These amebae are pathogenic and opportunistic free-living protozoa that belong to the phylum *Sarcomastigophora*. There are two genera, *Acanthamoeba* and *Naegleria*, and *Acanthamoeba* has five species, *A. castellanii, A. polyphaga, A. culbertsoni, A. rhisodes,* and *A. hatchetti*.[11, 12] The only *Naegleria* species known to cause human infection (meningoencephalitis) is *N. fowleri*.[5] *Acanthamoeba* can cause ocular infection and rare diseases affecting the lungs, skin, and central nervous system,[5, 13] but it is also isolated from nasal and oral mucosae of healthy people.[14] The characteristics of *Acanthamoeba* species have been described,[15] but species differentiation is of limited clinical importance.

Acanthamoeba accounts for the largest population of protozoa. It is ubiquitous, found in virtually every climate,[12] and has been isolated in many water sources, including municipal water supplies and bottled drinking water. *Acanthamoeba* has also been found on contact lenses and in contact lens solutions.[2, 16–18]

Acanthamoeba has a biphasic life cycle. The motile, replicating, infective form (trophozoite) has pseudopodia and spike-shaped projections (acanthopodia) that constitute the locomotor organelles and enable it to attach to surfaces, phagocytizing bacteria and other cells.[16] When environmental conditions are adverse or there are no nutrients,[17] the trophozoites secrete a rich protein outer wall (ectocyst) and a cellulose inner wall (endocyst) and the amebae enter the dormant (cyst) phase[12] by a morphologic change in which both walls meet at various points called ostioles. Cysts are resistant to heat, cold, pH, and medical therapy; they are able to survive the attack of the immune system for months and may become airborne. Under favorable conditions, the trophozoites emerge from the cyst through an ostiole (within 3 days).[13, 14]

Unlike the free-living amebae, the intestinal protozoan *Entamoeba histolytica* causes an infection, amebiasis. Ninety percent of infected individuals are asymptomatic. There is a wide spectrum of clinical manifestations, from dysentery to abscesses in the liver and other organs.[11]

EPIDEMIOLOGY

Healthy individuals are commonly exposed to *Acanthamoeba* species and a high percentage of the population has positive antibodies.[19] All types of water and soil are natural reservoirs,[11] and cysts may be airborne.[14] Humans are the definitive hosts.[11] Keratitis is the most common human disease caused by amebae.[2] The first case was presented in 1973, followed by several case reports with ocular trauma and water exposure in common.[2, 8, 9, 12, 13] In 1984, the first case of *Acanthamoeba* keratitis in a contact lens wearer was reported, and by 1989 more than 250 such cases had been collected by the Centers for Disease Control.[2, 8] Eighty-five percent of infections were in contact lens wearers,[20] with an estimated incidence in this epidemic period from 1.6 to 2.5 per million contact lens wearers in the United States[8] and 1 per 10,000 in the United Kingdom.[9] Interestingly, the increased incidence of *Acanthamoeba* keratitis paralleled that of bacterial keratitis among contact lens wearers.[8, 21] This epidemic has been a lesson to the ophthalmic community: New technologies can be associated with unforeseen complications.[8, 19] Risk factors for *Acanthamoeba* include contact lens wear (specifically, improper contact lens use and hygiene and the use of homemade saline solutions), corneal trauma, and exposure to contaminated water.[2, 9, 13, 22]

About 10% of the world's population is infected with *E. histolytica,* with a high incidence in developing tropical countries. Groups at risk in developed countries include travelers, homosexual men, immigrants, and institutionalized persons.[11] In the reported ocular cases, trauma and fecal-ocular infection were predispositions to infection.[23] Patients with amebic dysentery may develop intermediate uveitis,[32] and examination of stool specimens will disclose the amebae.

PATHOGENESIS AND PATHOLOGY

Pathogenesis

Ocular infection by free-living amebae depends on inoculation with virulent protozoa and the presence of a suitable environment for growth and host response.[12, 13] Amebae can reach the ocular surface through contaminated contact lenses or contact lens material, trauma, and contaminated water. Once the parasite reaches the corneal surface, it must remain in contact and eventually penetrate.[12, 13] Trophozoites bind to corneal epithelium by a mannose-binding protein.[24] Recent articles address the role of lecithin-mediated adhesion and a contact-dependent metalloproteinase in the cytopathogenic mechanism.[25] This union can induce cytolysis or apoptosis of the target cell and may exacerbate the pathogenic cascade by initiating the release of cytolytic factors.[26] Once in the stroma, amebae secrete collagenolytic enzymes that contribute to the dissolution of the stromal matrix.[27]

Although protozoa can penetrate intact corneal epithelium,[21] clinical and experimental data support the association of Acanthamoeba keratitis with epithelial damage and hypoxia, punctate epithelial erosions, and microscopic epithelial breaks[12, 13] related to contact lens wear and trauma. Another possible factor in the pathogenicity of Acanthamoeba is the presence of bacterial colonization of the ocular surface. The coinfection rate with bacteria has been reported to be as high as 58%. In a rat model of Acanthamoeba keratitis, when the cornea is infected with avirulent bacteria an enhancement of the disease develops.[13] Additionally, endosymbiosis has been reported between Acanthamoeba and bacteria.[12] Thus, bacteria may modify the pathogenicity of Acanthamoeba.

Host response is mediated by the humoral and cellular branches of the immune system and by complement activation. Antibodies to this ubiquitous parasite may develop from environmental exposure, and they may act by opsonization, fixation of complement on the amebic membrane, and toxin neutralization.[13] But the role of mucosal immunity seems to be of greater importance. Only topical immunization (which increases local IgA) protects animals from disease, despite high levels of serum antibodies.[10] Mucosal IgA does not affect the viability of Acanthamoeba, but it seems to prevent infection by inhibiting parasite binding to the corneal epithelium.[28]

The cellular response to infection is mainly polymorphonuclear, with a paucity of macrophages and lymphocytes. This response is important in the eradication of trophozoites; however, cysts may resist this assault, survive for long periods of time, and reactivate infection under favorable conditions.

Acanthamoeba is capable of complement activation by the alternative pathway, which may lead to the production of inflammatory mediators,[13] a possible explanation for damage to ocular tissue. The pathogenic form of A. castel-

lanii elaborates plasminogen activator, a substance not detected in the nonpathogenic form. Some authors ascribe a role to plasminogen, with the subsequent activation to plasmin, in the promotion of parasite penetration into the corneal epithelium.[29]

Entamoeba histolytica can affect the eyes through dissemination from systemic amebiasis,[30] or it may be the host immunoresponse that is responsible for ocular disease.[31–33]

Histopathology

Polymorphonuclear leukocytes in the external part of the stroma are the primary immune cells in the first stages of the disease, as in other parasitic infections. Neutrophils are followed by macrophages, with a near absence of lymphocytes. There is necrosis and often a lack of neovascularization.[13] In advanced stages, Wessley's ring results from stromal precipitation of immunocomplex, which is often associated with properdin-mediated activation of the alternative pathway of complement.[12]

Eye adnexa affected by amebiasis show necrosis and abundant E. histolytica.[12]

CLINICAL FEATURES

Acanthamoeba keratitis

Acanthamoeba keratitis begins with an insidious onset of symptoms and signs that may emerge slowly, over several weeks, or worsen rapidly.[13] Patients are typically young, immunocompetent individuals of either sex, with a history of contact lens wear, exposure to contaminated fluids or a foreign body, or minor trauma.[2] However, some patients may demonstrate none of the apparent risk factors, which could delay the diagnosis.[9] Patients typically complain of severe pain and tearing in one eye (rarely bilateral) far out of proportion with clinical observation.[2, 9]

The spectrum of clinical signs ranges from superficial erosions or microcyst edema to full-thickness corneal abscess. Dendritic epitheliopathy is common and could be misdiagnosed as herpes simplex keratitis.[2, 9, 12]

Radial keratoneuritis (perineural infiltrates), when present, is highly suggestive.[13] As the disease progresses Wessley's ring could be present as well as subepithelial infiltrates caused by a delayed immunologic reaction.[12] A distinctive feature is the absence of corneal neovascularization,[13] but vessels may be seen in the final stages covering central leukomas.[9]

Scleritis

Scleritis has been observed in 11%[34] to 40%[35] of cases, usually when the diagnosis was delayed for more than 2 months.[9, 36] Scleral inflammation is characterized by severe ocular pain, deep scleral vascular engorgement, and scleral nodules.[13] After resolution, scleral ectasia may occur.[37] In most cases, scleritis is probably an immunologically driven response rather than a direct infection.[13]

Uveitis

Anterior chamber inflammation occurs in 5% of cases that are diagnosed early, but it rises to 79% when diagnosis is delayed more than 2 months.[9] Hypopyon is present in late stages in 46% of patients.[34] A recent report found a granulomatous reaction involving anterior chamber stroma caused by *Acanthamoeba*.[38]

Chorioretinitis in the contralateral eye of a patient with *Acanthamoeba* keratitis has been reported.[39]

Late Complications

Elevated intraocular pressure and cataracts are occasionally seen in patients with severe and prolonged ocular inflammation.[34] Six percent of patients diagnosed early (in less than 30 days) developed glaucoma, compared with 21% of those diagnosed late (more than 2 months after the onset of symptoms). Similarly, only 3% of patients diagnosed early, compared with 38% of those diagnosed late, developed cataracts.[9] This proves the importance of early recognition and treatment.

Ocular Diseases Associated with Amebiasis

There are only occasional reports of eye infection by *E. histolytica*. Beaver reported a case with amebiasis of the eyelid and conjunctiva that was extended to the orbit. No intraocular disease was present. The risk factors were feco-ocular inoculation and trauma.[30]

Amebiasis has been associated with central serous chorioretinitis.[31] Rodger and colleagues reported an association between dysentery and intermediate uveitis.[32] In cases of dysentery, *Entamoeba* can be found in stool samples, but this is not always true in the case of hepatic cysts.[40]

DIAGNOSIS

Clinical awareness has been heightened by concerted educational efforts during the last decade among ophthalmologists and within the public sector,[8] leading to earlier diagnosis, often before the hallmark signs appear, and reducing the risk of late complications.[8, 12, 13] Physicians should be suspicious of *Acanthamoeba* when a chronic keratitis persists despite adequate topical therapy, even in patients with no risk factors for the infection (10% of ameba keratitis patients are non–contact lens wearers).[9]

Diagnostic tests include in vivo confocal microscopy, corneal cultures, microscopic observation of corneal scrapings, polymerase chain reaction (PCR) of infected samples, and testing of contact lenses and contact lens solutions.

In Vivo Confocal Microscopy

Confocal microscopy is a noninvasive method of magnification with sufficient spatial resolution to reveal trophozoites and cysts from the human cornea in vivo and to detect trophozoites in migration through corneal nerves.[41] Moreover, corneal examination with tandem scanning confocal microscopy has been associated with a marked increase in the detection of *Acanthamoeba*, suggesting that the disease is more prevalent than once suspected.[42]

Laboratory Diagnosis

Several laboratory techniques and protocols have been described.[2, 9, 12, 13, 43, 44] In this chapter, special attention will be given to the Moorfields Eye Hospital protocol.[9, 44]

Before samples are taken, patients should discontinue any previous treatment in order to increase the yield of positive results. Corneal scrapings should be aggressively taken. If there is a high clinical suspicion and cultures are negative, corneal biopsy is indicated. Biopsy can be performed with a 2- to 3-mm trephine from an area of infiltration outside the visual axis.[9, 13] Samples are divided into two parts. One part, to be used for histopathology, is immediately fixed in formaldehyde[9] or methyl alcohol[13] for 3 to 5 minutes. The other part is placed on non-nutrient agar, with or without *Escherichia coli* overlay (*E. coli* may be added later), for culture. If the culture cannot be done immediately, transport in physiologic serum (0.9%) or in ameba transport media. Large volumes of contact lens solution can be filtered with a 5-μm polycarbamate membrane filter, with the filter upside-down for processing. Corneal biopsy may be processed for electron microscopy. All samples should be examined for bacteria, fungi, and virus.[9, 13] A new technique for cytology identification has been described recently by Gardner and associates.[45]

Histopathology

More than 15 stains including Giemsa, periodic acid–Schiff, methylene blue, and calcofluor white may be used to demonstrate *Acanthamoeba*. A solution containing 0.1% calcofluor white (which stains cyst and fungi) with a 0.1% counterstain of Evans blue (which stains trophozoites) is one recommended method.[46] The method employed at the Moorfields Eye Hospital is an immunoperoxidase staining using a polyclonal antibody against *Acanthamoeba*.[9, 44]

Culture

Although *Acanthamoeba* can grow on blood or chocolate agar, cultures should include non-nutrient agar with an *E. coli* overlay. Culture plates should be sealed to prevent evaporation and the loss of the organisms from drying.[13] Plates are incubated at 3°C over 72 hours. If growth is not detected by day 6, plates are moved to 22°C because some amebae grow better at low temperature. Plates are observed for up to 3 weeks if there has been no previous growth.[9] Wavy tracts or irregularly shaped trophozoites may be observed.[9, 13]

Polymerase Chain Reaction and Molecular Biology Techniques

Polymerase chain reaction using primers for *Acanthamoeba* ribosomal RNA is a rapid, sensitive, and specific method for detecting *Acanthamoeba* from epithelial corneal specimens.[47] PCR has the advantage of allowing rapid, sensitive, and specific diagnosis with an extremely low number of parasites. Recently, PCR has been used to confirm confocal microscopic observations of *Acanthamoeba*.[48] PCR and other antibody marker techniques do not differentiate pathogenic from nonpathogenic *Acanthamoeba*, so a differentiation marker based on a colorimeter assay for protease activity is a good complement to these techniques.[49]

Differential Diagnosis

Differential diagnosis should include herpetic, fungal, bacterial, or sterile contact lens–related keratitis.[13] Topical anesthetic-abuse ring keratitis has been misdiagnosed as *Acanthamoeba* keratitis.[50, 51]

TREATMENT

Treatment of ocular infection by *Acanthamoeba* is difficult because the cyst form can be highly resistant to treatment. Resistance to therapy and in vitro activity do not always correlate with in vivo effectiveness.[9] For this reason, most protocols have been established empirically and modified by trial and error. The goals of therapy are to eradicate the parasite, control inflammation, control pain, and treat complications. Surgery can be successful if the eye is free of inflammation. New therapies, such as immunization against *Acanthamoeba* and the induction of protective mucosal IgA, could prove to be successful in the future.[52]

Medical Treatment

Antiamebic Agents

Several agents have been tested for antiamebic effect.[13] Aminoglycosides (neomycin, paromomycin) and imidazoles (miconazole, clotrimazole) probably have limited effectiveness, and aminoglycosides are toxic to epithelium, so they are not recommended.[53] According to the experience of the Moorfields Eye Hospital,[9] a combination of a biguanide and a diamidine, both of which are able to kill cysts, are the drugs of choice. Among the biguanides, 0.02% chlorhexidine and 0.02% polyhexamethyl biguanide (PHMB) are recommended. Diamines available in Europe are propamidine isethionate and hexamidine (Desomedine, Chauvin, France).[9]

Treatment Protocol

Hay and coworkers experienced success with the use of topical propamidine isethionate 0.1% (Brolene, Rhone-Poulenc Roer, Eastbourne, May and Baker, UK) and 0.02% chlorhexidine. Additionally, the combination of polyhexamethylene biguanide 0.02% (Cosmocil, Zeneca Pharmaceuticals, Wilslow, UK) with propamidine (Brolene) is a well-tolerated, nontoxic, and effective treatment.[54]

Both drops are applied hourly day and night for 2 days. On days 3 to 6, medication is given hourly during the daytime only. Propamidine may generate epithelial toxicity, which is reversible with discontinuation of the drops for several days.[54] Therapy is then reestablished on an individual basis with instillation every 3 hours and treatment continuing for 6 to 8 weeks after resolution of the inflammatory signs or after cessation of topical steroid therapy (if used).[55] Some authors recommend maintenance therapy once or twice daily for at least 1 year after the signs of active infection have resolved.[13]

Other treatments include cycloplegia or oral flurbiprofen (50 to 100 mg) up to three times a day for analgesia and for treating scleritis when necessary.[55]

Topical Corticosteroids for Control of Inflammation

Corticosteroids are usually not necessary in cases diagnosed early, as these will usually respond to antiamebic therapy. Fulcher and Dart do not recommend their use until the patient has had 2 weeks with amebicidals.[9] Corti-

costeroids should be maintained until inflammatory activity is abolished. Antiamebic therapy should be continued at least 6 weeks after cessation of steroids.[9] Corticosteroids are effective for controlling pain and anterior chamber inflammation, which, if uncontrolled, eventually results in corneal perforation or secondary glaucoma. Until future studies clarify the role of topical corticosteroids, their use in selected patients is justified.[56]

Treatment of Scleritis, Limbal Inflammation, and Pain

Nonsteroidal anti-inflammatory drugs (NSAIDs; flurbiprofen 50 to 100 mg three times a day) are effective in the treatment of limbal inflammation and scleritis. Scleritis may eventually become a severe complication, and oral steroids or oral cyclosporine A is necessary to control inflammation. In these cases, antiamebic treatment should be complemented with systemic triaconazole.[9]

Pain usually responds to NSAIDs or corticosteroids.[9] For intense discomfort, narcotics may be required, and there are reports of modified retrobulbar injection of alcohol to achieve adequate analgesia.[12]

Surgical Treatment: Keratoplasty and Cryotherapy

Epithelial débridement may enhance the medical therapy for *Acanthamoeba* keratitis. Penetrating keratoplasty is indicated only in patients with vision-impairing corneal scarring once the infection has been resolved and there is no sign of active inflammation.[13, 57] Graft survival is excellent for quiet eyes.[57]

In addition, keratoplasty is indicated when active inflammation and infection are present as a therapeutic effort to preserve eye integrity and to treat corneal perforation.[9, 57] In these cases, cryotherapy should be performed with a freeze-thaw-refreeze of the peripheral host cornea.[58] Medical antiamebic treatment and topical steroids should be maintained.[9] Recurrences are common and typically result in graft failure.[57]

Amebiasis Treatment

Asymptomatic carriers can be treated with luminal agents such as iodoquinol, 650 mg three times a day for 20 days, diloxanide, or paromomycin (500 mg three times a day for 10 days). Acute colitis has a good prognosis when treated with metronidazole (750 mg by mouth for 5 to 10 days) and luminal agents. Liver abscesses can be treated with metronidazole, tinidazole, or ornidazole along with luminal agents.[11]

PREVENTION

Because 85% of *Acanthamoeba* keratitis cases occur in contact lens wearers, preventive measures target these individuals and the eye care practitioners involved in contact lens fitting.[9, 13] Successful prevention depends on the compliance of patients with the proper use and care of contact lenses, including the disposal of single-use lenses after each wearing.[8] Preventive action should be taken in all steps of contact lens use: hand washing, lens cleaning, lens disinfection, rinsing, and storage. Proper cleaning removes debris and bacteria and reduces the risk of amebae adhesion.[13]

Most commercially available solutions, used at appropriate concentrations and times, are effective in killing *Acanthamoeba*,[13] but disinfection with wet heat or hydrogen peroxide in two steps, with 4 hours of disinfection followed by neutralization with a catalytic agent, is recommended.[9] Hydrogen peroxide 3% in one step is *not* enough to kill cysts and trophozoites and chloride solutions kill only bacteria and trophozoites but not cysts, so they are not recommended.[9]

Disinfected contact lenses can be recontaminated if the wearer uses homemade saline solutions that contain tap water or nonpreserving saline solution in a squirt bottle. It is preferable to preserve rinse solution or nonpreserving solution in an aerosol container. In addition, contact lenses can be contaminated by exposure to water while swimming, bathing, or using hot tubs.

Contact lens cases are an important reservoir of *Acanthamoeba* and bacteria. Aggressive cleaning of all surfaces of these cases with very hot water, followed by air drying, can eradicate trophozoites and cysts.[9] Contact lens wearers should consider replacing cases often.

PROGNOSIS

One of the most important causes of poor visual outcome is late diagnosis, causing delay in the delivery of specific therapy.[12] Bacon and colleagues reported that all eyes treated within 1 month of the onset of symptoms had final visual acuity of 20/40 or better, whereas only half of patients who received treatment late in the course of infection achieved visual acuity of 20/40.[9, 12, 59] The chances of treatment success are reduced with inadequate treatment and the use of topical steroids before diagnosis.[9]

Good prognosis after keratoplasty is possible only if the eye is quiet prior to surgery. When inflammation is persistent and remains untreated, cataract and glaucoma are present in 57% of cases and surgical treatment has a poor outcome.[59]

CONCLUSIONS

Acanthamoeba keratitis is a disease that has been observed for the last two decades, and it is now recognized worldwide. Ocular infection remains difficult to diagnose and treat. Preventive actions should be taken by contact lens wearers, who are most commonly affected by the disease. Additionally, ophthalmologists should consider *Acanthamoeba* early in any case of atypical keratitis, because early diagnosis and treatment can greatly improve recovery and visual outcome. Diagnosis can be simplified with the use of confocal microscopy and PCR techniques. Until the discovery of better antibiotic treatments, early and aggressive use of biguanides and management of the associated inflammation should be the standard treatment.

References

1. Diccionario de la Lengua Española. Real Academia Española. Madrid, Espasa-Calpe, 1992.
2. Alizadeh H, Niederkon JY, McCulley JP: Acanthamoebic keratitis. In: Pepose JS, Holand GN, Wilhemus KR, eds: Ocular Infection and Immunity. St. Louis, Mosby, 1996, pp 570, 1062–1071.
3. Sanahan JF, ed: Bailey & Scott's Laboratory Methods for Diagnosis of Parasitic Infections. St. Louis, Mosby–Year Book, 1994, pp 776–861.
4. Castellani A: An amoeba found in cultures of yeast: Preliminary note. J Trop Med Hyg 1930;33:160.
5. Visvesvara GS: Pathogenic and opportunistic free-living amoebae. In: Murray PR, ed: Manual of Clinical Microbiology. Washington, DC, ASM Press, 1995, p 1196.
6. Jones DB, Robinson NR, Visvesvara CS: Paper presented at the Ocular Microbiology and Immunology Group Meeting, Dallas, TX; September 1973. Cited in: Jones DB, Visvesvara GS, Robinson RN: *Acanthamoeba polyphaga* keratitis and *Acanthamoeba uveitis* associated with fatal meningoencephalitis. Trans Ophthalmol Soc UK 1975;95:22.
7. Nagington J, Watson PG, Playfair TJ, et al: Amoebic infection of the eye. Lancet 1974;2:1537–1540.
8. Schaumberg DA, Snow KK, Dana MR: The epidemic of *Acanthamoeba* keratitis. Where do we stand? Cornea 1998;17:3.
9. Fulcher T, Dart JKG: Queratitis por acantomoeba. In: Duran de la Colina J, ed: Complicaciones de las Lentes de Contacto. Madrid, Tecnimedia Editorial, 1998, p 263.
10. McCuley JP, Alizadeh H, Niederhorn JY: *Acanthamoeba* keratitis. CLAO J 1995;21:73.
11. Reed SL: Amoebiasis and infection with free living amoebas. In: Braunwald E, Isselbacher KJ, Petersdorf RG, et al, eds: Harrison's Principles of Internal Medicine. New York, McGraw-Hill, 1994, p 883.
12. Frangie JP, Moore MB: Parasitic infections including *Acanthamoeba*. In: Leibowitz HM, Waring III GO, eds: Corneal Disorders. Clinical Diagnosis and Management. Philadelphia, W.B. Saunders, 1998, p 719.
13. Rutzen AR, Moore MB: Parasitic infections. In: Kaufman HE, Barron BA, McDonald MB, eds: The Cornea. Butterworth-Heinemann, 1998, p 311.
14. Rivera F, Medina F, Ramirez P, et al: Pathogenic and free-living protozoa cultured from the nasopharyngeal and oral region of dental patients. Environ Res 1984;33:428.
15. Byers TJ, Bogler SA, Burianek LL: Analysis of mitochondrial DNA variation as an approach to systematic relationships in the genus *Acanthamoeba*. J Protozoal 1983;30:198.
16. Visvesvara GS: Classification of *Acanthamoeba*. Rev Inf Dis 1992;13:S3691.
17. Badenoch PR: The pathogenesis of *Acanthamoeba* keratitis. Aust N Z J Ophthalmol 1991;19:9.
18. Stapleton F, Seal DV, Dart J: Possible environmental sources of *Acanthamoeba* species that caused keratitis in contact lens wearers. Rev Infect Dis 1991;13:390.
19. Cerva L: *Acanthamoeba culbertsoni* and *Naegleria fowleri*: Occurrence of antibody in man. J Hyg Epidemiol Microbiol Immunol 1989;33:99–103.
20. Stehr-Green JK, Bailey TM, Visvesvara GS: The epidemiology of *Acanthamoeba* keratitis in the United States. Am J Ophthalmol 1989;107:331.
21. Poggio EC, Glymm RJ, Schein OD, et al: The incidence of ulcerative keratitis among users of daily wear and extended wear soft contact lenses. N Engl J Med 1989;321:779.
22. Mathers WD, Sutphin JE, Lane JA, Folberg R: Correlation between surface water contamination with amoeba and the onset of symptoms and diagnosis of amoeba-like keratitis. Br J Ophthalmol 1998;82:1143.
23. Osato MS: Parasitic keratitis and conjunctivitis. In: Smolin G, Thoft RA, eds: The Cornea. Boston, Little, Brown, 1994, p 253.
24. Yang ZT, Cao ZY, Panjwani N. Pathogenicity of *Acanthamoeba* keratitis carbohydrate-mediated host parasite interactions. Infect Immun 1997;65:439.
25. Cao Z, Jefferson DM, Panjwani N. Role of carbohydrate adherence in cytopathogenic mechanisms of *Acanthamoeba*. J Biol Chem 1998;273:15838–15845.
26. Leher H, Silvany R, Alizadeh H, et al: Mannose induces the release of cytopathic factors from *Acanthamoeba*. Infect Immun 1998;66:5–10.
27. He YG, Niederkon JY, McCulley JP, et al: In vivo and in vitro collagenolytic activity of *Acanthamoeba castellanii*. Invest Ophthalmol Vis Sci 1990;31:2235.
28. Leher HF, Alizadeh H, Taylor WM, et al: Role of mucosal IgA in the resistance to *Acanthamoeba* keratitis. Invest Ophth Vis Sci 1998;39:2666.
29. Van Klink F, Alizadeh H, Stewart GL: Characterization and patho-

genic potential of soil isolate and ocular isolate of *Acanthamoeba castellanii* in relation to *Acanthamoeba* keratitis. Curr Eye Res 1992;11:1207.

30. Beaver PC: Cutaneous amoebiasis of the eyelid with extension into the orbit. Am J Trop Med Hyg 1978;27:1133.
31. Braley AE, Hamilton HE: Central serous choroiditis associated with amoebiasis. Arch Ophthalmol 1957;58:1–14.
32. Rodger FC, Chir PK, Hosain ATMM: Night blindness in the tropics. Arch Ophthalmol 1960;63:927.
33. Schlaegel TF, Culbertson C: Experimental *Hartmanella* optic neuritis and uveitis. Ann Ophthalmol 1972;4:103.
34. Bacon AS, Frazer G, Dart JKD, et al: A review of 72 consecutive cases of *Acanthamoeba* keratitis, 1984–1992. Eye 1993;7:719.
35. Manis MJ, Tamaru R, Roth AM, et al: *Acanthamoeba* sclerokeratitis. Determining diagnosis criteria. Arch Ophthalmol 1996;104:1313.
36. Dougherty PJ, Binder PS, Mondino BJ: *Acanthamoeba* sclerokeratitis. Am J Ophthalmol 1994;117:475.
37. Lindquist TD, Fritsche TR, Grutzmacher RD: Scleral ectasia secondary to *Acanthamoeba* keratitis. Cornea 1990;9:74.
38. Mietz H, Font RL: *Acanthamoeba* keratitis with granulomatous reaction involving the stroma and anterior chamber. Arch Ophthalmol 1997;115:259.
39. Johns KJ, O'Day DM, Feman SS: Chorioretinitis in the contralateral eye of a patient with *Acanthamoeba* keratitis. Ophthalmology 1988;95:635.
40. Nussenblatt RB, Whitcup S, Palestine AG: Onchocerciasis and other parasitic infections. In: Nussenblatt RB, Whitcup S, Palestine AG, eds: Uveitis. Fundamentals and Clinical Practice. St. Louis, Mosby, 1996.
41. Ptister DR, Cameron JD, Krachmer JH, Holand EJ: Confocal microscopy findings of *Acanthamoeba* keratitis. Am J Ophthalmol 1996;121:119.
42. Mathers WD, Sutphin JE, Folberg R, et al: Outbreak of keratitis presumed to be caused by *Acanthamoeba*. Am J Ophthalmol 1996;121:129.
43. Isenberg HD, ed: Clinical Microbiology Procedures Handbook, vol 2. Washington, DC, ASM Press, 1992.
44. Allan BDS, Dart JKG: Strategies for the management of microbial keratitis. Br J Ophthalmol 1995;79:777.
45. Gardner LM, Mathers WD, Folberg R: New technique for the cytologic identification of presumed *Acanthamoeba* from corneal epithelial scrapings. Am J Ophthalmol 1999;127:207.
46. Wilhelmus KR, Osato MS, Font RL, et al: Rapid diagnosis of *Acanthamoeba* keratitis using calcofluor white. Arch Ophthalmol 1986;104:1309.
47. Lehmann OJ, Green SM, Morlet N, et al: Polymerase chain reaction analysis of corneal epithelial and tear samples in the diagnosis of *Acanthamoeba* keratitis. Invest Ophthalmol Vis Sci 1998;39:1261.
48. Nelson SE, Mathers R, Folberg R: Confirmation of confocal microscopy diagnosis of *Acanthamoeba* keratitis using polymerase chain reaction analysis. Invest Ophthalmol Vis Sci 1999;40:S263.
49. Khan N, Jarroll EL, Panjwani N, Paget TA: Proteases: A marker for differentiation of pathogenic and nonpathogenic *Acanthamoeba*. Invest Ophthalmol Vis Sci 1999;40:S262.
50. Varga JH, Rubinfield RS, Wolf TC: Topical anesthetic abuse ring keratitis. Report of four cases. Cornea 1997;16:424.
51. Kim JY, Choi YS, Lee JH: Keratitis from corneal anesthetic abuse after photorefractive surgery keratectomy. J Cataract Refract Surg 1997;23:447.
52. Alizadeh H, He Y, McCulley JP, et al: Successful immunization against *Acanthamoeba* keratitis in a pig model. Cornea 1995;14:180.
53. Varga JH, Wolf TC, Jensen HG, et al: Combined treatment with propamidine, neomycin and polyhexamethylene biguanide. Am J Ophthalmol 1993;115:466.
54. Hay S, Kirkness C: Successful medical therapy of *Acanthamoeba* keratitis with topical chlorhexidine and propamidine. Eye 1997;10:413–421.
55. Duguid GM, Dart JKG, Morlet N, et al: Outcome of *Acanthamoeba* keratitis treated with polyhexamethyl biguanide and propamidine. Ophthalmology 1997;104:1587.
56. Park DH, Palay DA, Daya SM, et al: The role of topical corticosteroids in the management of *Acanthamoeba* keratitis. Cornea 1997;16:277.
57. Flicker LA, Kirkness C, Wright P: Prognosis of keratoplasty in *Acanthamoeba* keratitis. Ophthalmology 1993;100:105.
58. Binder PS: Cryotherapy for medically unresponsive *Acanthamoeba* keratitis. Cornea 1989;8:106.
59. Bacon AS, Dart JKG, Fliker LA, et al: *Acanthamoeba* keratitis: The value of early diagnosis. Ophthalmology 1993;100:1238.

Ron Neumann

DEFINITION

Giardiasis is an infection of the small intestine caused by the flagellated protozoan *Giardia lamblia*. It is associated mainly with diarrhea, malabsorption, and weight loss.

EPIDEMIOLOGY

The pathogen is found in all climates and spreads by a variety of routes. Person-to-person spread in day care centers for children and nursing homes has been demonstrated. A common source of spread is contaminated water. Rarely, food contamination after cooking may also be associated with *Giardia* epidemics. Breakdowns of community water filtration systems have been associated with *Giardia* outbreaks in communities, and indeed, *Giardia* is the most frequent cause of waterborne diarrhea in the United States. Animal infections may also contribute to surface water contamination, posing risks for campers who are not mindful of the risk of drinking untreated water.

Giardia is a frequent source of diarrhea in campers returning from endemic areas and travelers to areas where water treatment and hygienic practices are impeded. The incubation period is 7 to 21 days, so it is common for infected travelers to develop symptoms and require medical treatment several weeks after returning home. This longer incubation period serves to distinguish giardiasis from more explosive diarrhea caused by toxigenic *Escherichia coli* and other forms of infectious traveler's diarrhea with shorter incubation periods.[1, 2]

The Organism

The organism may exist as a motile, flagellated, pear-shaped trophozoite, 12 to 15 mm in length, or as a tough-walled oval cyst.

The organism has two nuclei with prominent karyosomes and four pairs of flagella with two ventral suckers. The cyst of the parasite is oval and measures 10 to 20 mm in its longest diameter. Each cyst has four nuclei but no flagella or suckers. On excystation, the organism becomes a trophozoite with two nuclei and starts dividing by binary fission.

In the intestine, the trophozoites may either attach to the microvilli of the intestinal epithelium using an attaching disc or may be free in the mucus layer just above the epithelium. As the trophozoites are carried into the colon, they encyst and pass into the environment. The cysts are protected from many environmental hazards including chlorine concentrations typical to treated municipal water supplies. Ten to twenty-five cysts may be enough to infect a subject drinking contaminated water. The acidic environment of the stomach activates the cysts, which develop into trophozoites that cause active infection. Typically, *Giardia* do not leave the gut and do not penetrate extraintestinal tissues.

PATHOGENICITY

The jejunum is the main site of infection. Infected jejunal mucosa ranges in appearance from normal to marked subtotal mucosal atrophy with submucosal inflammatory cell infiltration, reduced villus height, and elongated crypts. Epithelial cells beneath overlying adherent trophozoites are deformed with blunting of the individual microvilli.

Host humoral and cellular immune responses occur, but their roles in protection as well as pathogenesis are unclear. The increased prevalence of *giardiasis* in persons with immune deficiency syndromes argues for the role of immunity in host defense.

CLINICAL MANIFESTATIONS

Infection can be asymptomatic. Clinical illness, however, is associated with some or all of the following: diarrhea, abdominal cramps, flatulence, nausea, excessive fatigue, bloating, anorexia, and chills. Reversible lactase deficiency and malabsorption of fat and vitamin B_{12} have been documented. The infection is frequently self-limited, but a prolonged, indolent illness with progressive weight loss is possible.

DIAGNOSIS

The diagnosis is established by observing cysts or trophozoites in stools or trophozoites in small bowel contents. The organism may be excreted in stool intermittently, and its identification may therefore be elusive. Repeated negative stool examinations may not rule out the diagnosis. Common practice dictates three stool specimens for a negative conclusion to be drawn. The small bowel contents may be sampled by tube aspiration or by passing a string that will absorb sufficient jejunal fluid for examination. Microscopic examination of a wet preparation of jejunal contents usually reveals motile organisms when infection is present. For extreme cases, small bowel biopsy may be performed. Hematologic values are normal. Occasionally, it may be justified to treat patients when clinical suspicion is high even when laboratory evaluations are repeatedly negative.

TREATMENT

Mepacrine hydrochloride, 100 mg three times per day for 5 to 7 days, or metronidazole, 400 mg three times per day for 5 days, is recommended by the British National Formulary. One course of treatment will suffice for most patients, but some need a second course.

Treatment of infected persons in highly endemic areas is of questionable value because reinfection occurs readily when water supplies are contaminated. All infected persons in nonendemic regions should be treated.[3, 4] (The general information on giardiasis is based on reference 4, which is also recommended for further reading.)

GIARDIA AND THE EYE

Few investigators have suggested the association of *giardiasis* and ocular morbidity, supporting their claim with circumstantial data of simultaneous occurrence of *Giardia* in the stool and ocular disease. The ocular manifestations may be secondary to hypersensitivity reactions to *Giardia* antigen, because the parasite has never been found in extraintestinal tissues.

Anterior uveitis, choroiditis,[5] retinal pigmentary so-called salt-and-pepper alterations[6, 7] and ocular vitelliform macular lesions have been blamed on *Giardia*. Earlier publications associated chorioretinal edema and retinal hemorrhages to *Giardia*.[8] Relating an infectious agent to specific manifestations that occur remote from the infected tissues is extremely difficult. Furthermore it may be impossible when only a minor percentage of the infected population develops these manifestations of a possible hypersensitivity mechanism.

Knox and associates[5] presented three patients with uveitis who did not respond well to corticosteroids. Two patients had hazy vitreous and yellow-white deposits around thickened retinal vessels with sheathing and iridocyclitis. The third patient had evidence of retinal arteritis without vitritis or anterior uveitis. *Giardia lamblia* was found in the stools of these patients. Only one of the three patients improved following combined antiparasitic and corticosteroid therapy. The authors presented a thorough review of the literature, including three French articles that also described various ocular manifestations such as macular edema, anterior uveitis, retinal hemorrhages, neuroretinitis, and vitreous hemorrhage presumed to be secondary giardiasis. One of the authors also described 18 additional patients seen by him with a wide variety of ocular manifestations (e.g., iridocyclitis, toxoplasma-like retinitis, retinal arteritis, pars planitis, keratitis, episcleritis, exudative retinal detachment, amebic choroiditis, chorioretinal atrophy, and nutritional amblyopia) and positive *Giardia* stool tests. A major parameter not mentioned in this article is the prevalence of giardiasis in their population base that did not suffer from ocular manifestations. Also, the prevalence of giardiasis in their overall ophthalmic inflammatory disease patient base was not addressed. It can be argued that their presented data merely reflect widespread giardiasis in their area at the time of their publication with no definitive causative role of the parasite to the ocular disease.

Two large controlled studies of ocular manifestations in *Giardia*-infected children originated in Italy.[6, 7] In the first,[6] ophthalmic evaluation was added to the medical examination of 90 children with symptomatic giardiasis. Ten patients had ocular manifestations. Eight of these children presented with a diffuse salt-and-pepper appearance of the fundus with retinal pigment epithelial involvement in the midperiphery of both eyes. In one of the eight children, atrophic areas of the retinal pigment epithelium were noted, as well as small, hard exudates in one eye. Of the remaining two children, one had evidence of chorioretinitis, and the other had hyperemia of the optic nerve head. After therapy, patients were followed for 1 year. The child with chorioretinitis improved and apparently recovered after additional treatment with systemic corticosteroids. The retinal pigment epithelial changes in the other patients remained the same. None of the additional 200 children with gastrointestinal symptoms unrelated to giardiasis had evidence of salt-and-pepper changes or any other ocular manifestations.

The second, more recent study[7] involved 141 children with active or past giardiasis diagnosed on the basis of microscopic examination of stool specimens or duodenal secretions. Fifty-three children were newly diagnosed and were untreated, 50 had active infections in spite of metronidazole therapy, and 38 had been successfully treated, with negative stool specimens for 1 to 3 years. Salt-and-pepper retinal changes were seen in 28 (19.9%) of the patients (similar distribution of retinal changes was observed in the three patient groups). None of these patients had electroretinographic changes. Five pairs of siblings were found to have retinal changes. In all groups, children who had retinal changes were consistently younger than those with normal retinas. Active choroiditis or other foci of ocular inflammation were not observed in this series. The authors concluded that asymptomatic, nonprogressive retinal lesions are particularly common in younger children with giardiasis. This risk did not seem to be related to the severity of the infection, its duration, or the use of metronidazole but may reflect a genetic predisposition. Of importance is the fact that none of these children had ocular inflammatory manifestations.

These two publications,[6, 7] while clearly associating salt-and-pepper retinal pigmentation to giardiasis, are much less supportive of the association of true ocular inflammation with *Giardia* infection. The pathomechanism of these pigmentary changes is not clear, and the role of inflammation in their evolution is questionable.

The fact that the original observation was repeated only in a few case reports despite the worldwide distribution of *Giardia* infection raises doubt as to the conclusion made in some publications referring to *Giardia* as a causative agent of ocular inflammation. A typical case presented in the Hebrew literature[9] describes a 24-year-old man diagnosed with unilateral acute anterior uveitis that responded poorly to topical and systemic corticosteroid therapy. On admission, examination of the left eye was remarkable for a moderate anterior inflammatory response without structural alterations. The vitreous was clear, but macular edema and partially pigmented nasal choroidal focus of inflammation were observed. Repeated stool tests were notable for the finding of *Giardia* cysts. The authors did not observe any response to systemic and topical steroid therapy until metronidazole was added to the therapeutic regimen. The exact regimen of systemic steroids in the first two weeks of therapy was not specified, and it can be argued that boosting the dose of oral prednisone to 60 mg in the last week resulted in effective anti-inflammatory treatment. Moreover, follow-up was limited to 3 months. These limitations make it difficult to assess the role of the intestinal infection in the development of the uveitis.

Despite these limitations it should be noted that ocular inflammation is common in a variety of intestinal diseases. Uveitis associated with inflammatory bowel syndromes is well known. Also infectious intestinal diseases such as *Shigella*, *Yersinia*, *Klebsiella*, and *Salmonella* may be followed by Reiter's syndrome. The possible alteration of the normal role of the gut in the induction of immune tolerance in chronic intestinal infections may explain extraintestinal hypersensitive responses. Thus, it can be concluded that although theoretical background does exist to support the causative association of *Giardia* intestinal infection and ocular inflammation, actual data to support this point are scarce.

In our view, the current knowledge does not justify the routine testing for *Giardia* cysts in the stool of *all* chronic uveitis patients. It may be justified in those idiopathic cases in which diagnosis does not become apparent despite repeated testing for all other uveitis etiologies relevant for the case and any sort of gastrointestinal symptoms exist. It may also be considered for those patients who do not respond to corticosteroids and for travelers to endemic areas. Duodenal biopsy and culture should be reserved only for those who present with gastrointestinal complaints compatible with the diagnosis of giardiasis. It may also be justified for uveitis patients with idiopathic salt-and-pepper retinal changes. Treatment should be reserved for those patients who are positively diagnosed with the parasite.

References

1. Flanagan PA: *Giardia*—diagnosis, clinical course and epidemiology. Epidemiol Infect 1992;109:1.
2. Hopkins RS, Juranek DD: Acute giardiasis: An improved clinical case definition for epidemiologic studies. Am J Epidemiol 1991;133:402.
3. Sullivan PS, DuPont HL, Arafat RR, et al: Illness and reservoirs associated with *Giardia lamblia* infection in rural Egypt: The case against treatment in developing world environments of high endemicity. Am J Epidemiol 1988;127:1272.
4. Cecil RL, Bennett JC, Plum F: Cecil Textbook of Medicine. Philadelphia, WB Saunders, 1996.
5. Knox DL, King J Jr: Retinal arteritis, iridocyclitis, and giardiasis. Ophthalmology 1982;89:1303.
6. Mantovani PM, Giardino I, Magli A, et al: Intestinal giardiasis associated with ophthalmologic changes. J Pediatr Gastroenterol Nutr 1990;11:196.
7. Corsi A, Nucci C, Knafelz D, et al: Ocular changes associated with *Giardia lamblia* infection in children. Br J Ophthalmol 1998;82:59.
8. Caroll ME, Anast BP, Birch CL: Giardiasis and uveitis. Arch Ophthalmol 1961;65:775.
9. Gelfer S, Scharf J, Zonis S, Mertzbach-D: Acute uveitis associated with *Giardia lamblia* infection. Harefuah 1984;107:75.

36 — TRYPANOSOMIASIS

Tomas Padilla, Jr.

DEFINITION

Trypanosomiasis is a protozoal parasitic infection that includes two varieties: African trypanosomiasis, also called sleeping sickness, and Chagas' disease or American trypanosomiasis. Trypanosomiasis is caused by *Trypanosoma brucei rhodesiense* in tropical East Africa and by *T. brucei gambiense* in West and Central Africa. African trypanosomiasis is transmitted by the bite of an infected tsetse fly found only in that continent. Chagas' disease is caused by *Trypanosoma cruzi* and is spread by blood sucking triatomine insects. Trypanosomiasis is a systemic illness characterized early on by enlargement of the lymph glands and progresses to involve many different organ systems. The end organ most frequently involved in African trypanosomiasis is the central nervous system (CNS), whereas in Chagas' disease, the heart and hollow viscera are most often affected.

HISTORY

African trypanosomiasis has been known in West Africa since records were kept approximately 600 years ago and had been known in the early days of the slave trade.[1] It is believed that the *gambiense* variety is evolutionarily older than the *rhodesiense* subspecies.[2] There are two theories on the evolution of the two subspecies. One holds that *rhodesiense* developed as the *gambiense* variety spread southeastward. Another holds that *T. b. brucei* and *T. b. rhodesiense* developed independently from a common ancestor.[3]

The Brazilian physician Carlos Chagas first reported American trypanosomiasis in 1909, although the disease had also been around for centuries. Chagas' disease was originally an infection of wild animals of the American continent with apparently multiple foci. It became a zoonosis when the reduviid insect vectors adapted to human dwellings.[4] In humans, the disease is present from Chile to the United States.

EPIDEMIOLOGY

African trypanosomiasis is transmitted cyclically by various species of *Glossina* (tsetse fly) and by other blood sucking Diptera during epidemics. Natural populations of *Glossina* are generally resistant to infection by *T. brucei*, and only the parasites that have invaded the salivary glands of Glossina are infective to mammals. Human trypanosomiasis is restricted to the tropics, where annual rainfall exceeds 500 mm. The Western form, caused by *T. brucei gambiense*, has a range that includes the tropical rain forests and surrounding savanna. The other form, caused by *T. b. rhodesiense* is restricted to the eastern third of Africa from the northern boundary of South Africa to Ethiopia. It caused major depopulation in many East African regions early in the 20th century and was practically eliminated during the years 1960 to 1965. From 1970 onward, there occurred a major recrudescence in most of the old foci, and prevalence levels in the mid

1990s were similar to those of the 1930s, especially in countries like Angola and the Democratic Republic of Congo. The number of reported cases in 1995 was 25,000. However, because 55,000,000 people are exposed to the risk of infection and only 4,000,000 are under surveillance, it is estimated that the number of cases is in the vicinity of 300,000 to 500,000.[5] The disease is also epidemic in Sudan and Uganda. It is endemic in Cameroon, the Central African Republic, Chad, Congo, Côte d'Ivoire, Guinea, and Tanzania, where its prevalence is increasing.[6]

Human African trypanosomiasis is focal and rural. Humans are the principal reservoir of infection of *T. b. gambiense*, whereas domestic cattle and wild animals are more important reservoirs of *T. b. rhodesiense*.

It is estimated that 16 to 18 million people are infected with Chagas' disease, and of these, 50,000 die each year. Most *T. cruzi* infections are located in 21 endemic countries of Central and South America, where 100 million people, or 25% of the population, are at risk of contracting the disease.

Chagas' disease is transmitted in several ways in both rural and urban centers. The traditional rural pattern was changed by migration to the cities that occurred in the 1970s and 1980s. Humans and various species of wild and domestic animals constitute the reservoir and the triatomine insects are the vectors. These blood-sucking insects find a favorable habitat in the crevices, walls, and roofs of the houses of the poor in rural areas and urban slums. Another mode of transmission is through the use of unscreened blood for transfusions; the incidence of contamination with *T. cruzi* is between 1.7% and 53.0% in blood banks in some selected cities of Central and South America.[7]

CLINICAL CHARACTERISTICS

African trypanosomiasis begins with the painful bite of a tsetse fly that produces a chancre after 1 to 2 weeks. Several weeks later, other symptoms such as fever, rashes, myalgias and joint pains, headaches, extreme fatigue, and swelling of the hands and periocular areas occur. Winterbottom's sign, prominent supraclavicular or posterior cervical lymphadenopathy, may be seen. As the illness progresses, weight loss is common. In more advanced stages, the parasite invades the central nervous system. When this happens, personality changes, irritability, loss of concentration, dysarthria, gait disturbances, and seizures can occur. Sleep disturbances in the form of insomnia and daytime drowsiness, from which the disease derives its name, are common. If the condition is left untreated, death occurs within several months to years after infection.[8]

Daniels first reported ocular lesions attributed to human African trypanosomiasis in 1915.[9] These lesions consist of a bilateral, diffuse interstitial keratitis accompanied by neovascularization affecting all layers of the cornea, a mild iritis, and periocular congestion. Severe scarring and corneal necrosis may evolve in some cases. They were later noted to be due to other causes such as the toxic effects of trypanocidal drugs or concurrent conditions such as onchocerciasis and trachoma.[10–13] Various animal studies involving dogs, cats, and other domesticated animals demonstrated ocular lesions due to different species of *Trypanosoma* in the form of corneal opacities, blepharitis, conjunctivitis, and keratitis.[14] In his 1974 study, Ikede reported that sheep infected with *T. brucei* developed lesions in the lids, conjunctiva, cornea, retina, optic nerve and extraocular muscles, and he found organisms in the aqueous and interstitial tissues surrounding the eye. The most dramatic clinical change though, was found in five animals 1 to 3 weeks before death. This consisted of bilateral hypopyon visible through an intact cornea. This hypopyon appeared as a milky white exudate that covered the pupil and progressed to fill the entire anterior chamber. This change was associated with lacrimation and photophobia. Similar changes were noted in the anterior chambers of cats infected experimentally with *T. brucei* in a study done by Mortelmans and Neetens in 1975.[15]

Chagas' disease, on the other hand, starts after the bite of a reduviid insect that has become infected following a blood meal from another animal or person already affected by the disease. The victim frequently rubs the site of the bite and smears insect feces containing the parasites into the bite wound, open cuts, the eyes, and other mucous membranes. Often, an insect bite is not necessary to contract the disease. Numerous insects present in the ceilings and rafters of domiciles can drop feces into the mouths and eyes of people who are sleeping or facing upward. Romaña's sign, or local periorbital swelling at and around the site of a bite where insect feces was rubbed into the eye, was first described in Argentina by Cecilio Romaña in 1963.[16] Other routes of transmission include congenital transmission, infection at parturition, ingestion of infected breast milk or uncooked food contaminated with insect feces, or by blood transfusions and organ transplantation.

There are three recognized stages of Chagas' disease.[17] The most recognizable manifestation of the acute stage is Romaña's sign. Other signs and symptoms at this time may include fatigue, fever, loss of appetite and vomiting, rashes, lymphadenopathy, and hepatosplenomegaly. Infants and very young children can develop cerebral edema leading to increased intracranial pressure and death. Symptoms of the acute stage occur in 1% of cases, last for 4 to 8 weeks and disappear, even without treatment. The intermediate stage occurs 8 to 10 weeks after infection, during which time people are asymptomatic but demonstrate antibodies to *T. cruzi* and often the presence of low-level parasitemia. Ten to twenty years after infection, signs and symptoms of the chronic stage may appear in some individuals. Most commonly, these include cardiomyopathy and heart failure or enlargement of the upper and lower digestive tract (megadisease) producing constipation and dysphagia. Köberle in 1974 suggested that the dilatation and elongation of sections of the gastrointestinal tract and cardiomyopathy associated with the chronic stage had a neurogenic origin through denervation from the destruction of sympathetic and parasympathetic ganglia.[18]

The eye is an important portal of entry for *T. cruzi* into the body. However, other than Romaña's sign, there have been few reports of ocular lesions associated with Chagas' disease. In 1997, Fröhlich and colleagues reported, that out of 79 chagasic patients, only six had parafoveal retinal pigment epithelial defects and one case had distinct pigment epithelial atrophy.[19] These lesions did not cause a significant loss of vision. In a follow-up study in 1998, they reported another two patients out of 23 who showed intraocular manifestations. These consisted of one case of fibrae medullares and one case of pigment dispersion. They concluded that the intraocular findings associated with Chagas' disease were rare, harmless postinflammatory changes.[20]

PATHOLOGY

After skin inoculation through the bite of the *Glossina* fly, African trypanosomes multiply in the subcutaneous tissues. From there, they proceed to the blood and lymph nodes, during which time they multiply exponentially for 1 to 3 days. They then disappear from the blood stream but then recover to produce successive waves of parasitemia. This phenomenon is possible because of antigenic variation wherein the parasite is able to evade the immune system of the host by producing different, variable glycoprotein surface antigens during each successive wave of parasitemia.[21] The clinical symptoms accompanying each bout of infestation correspond to malaria-like symptoms and influenza, with fever occurring at the height of the parasitemic wave.[22]

The immune response to trypanosomal antigens is massive, sometimes with detrimental side effects to the host. The most prominent feature is the increased concentration of serum IgM due to the sequential production of early antibodies against the various surface antigens. Circulating IgG-antigen complexes are also found repeatedly during the course of infection resulting in immune lysis of the parasite. A 41- to 46-kDA molecule called trypanosome-released lymphocyte triggering factor may selectively activate CD8$^+$ T cells to produce interferon-gamma that activates macrophages but may concurrently promote parasitic multiplication. Macrophages also bind and destroy parasites in the presence of antibodies. They synthesize large quantities of tumor necrosis factor-α (TNF-α), which promotes parasite destruction but at the same time increases the severity of clinical symptoms. In addition to cytokines and prostaglandins, macrophages also produce antiparasitic nitric acid, which also induces immunosuppression.[23] Other immunologic findings associated with the disease include high levels of rheumatoid factor, heterophile antibody and the presence of many autoantibodies, especially anti-liver and anti-Wassermann antibodies.[22]

One of the effects of macrophage-released substances is the alteration in the permeability of the blood-brain barrier. Trypanosomes and inflammatory cells then invade the meninges through the cerebrospinal fluid to produce a progressive meningoencephalitis with perivascular cuffing with histiocytes, lymphocytes, and plasmocytes. Using magnetic resonance imaging (MRI), the spread can be traced from the meninges to the choroid plexus and periventricular ependymal cells,[24] and the tuberoinfundibula and thalamic-hypothalamic areas. This area of involvement accounts for the disruption in the normal sleep-wake cycle and hence the name, sleeping sickness. Antibodies to CNS components like galactocerebrosides, neurofilaments, and tryptophane are seen in cerebrospinal fluid, and their presence offers a link to the profound demyelination found in the late stages of the disease.[23] Sabbah and associates[24] reported late cortical and subcortical atrophy in one patient but did not mention any visual disturbances.

The pathology caused by *T. cruzi* in Chagas' disease is somewhat different from that caused by *T. brucei*. Lesions in the CNS are not prominent except in infants, young children, and immunodeficient patients, and most can be found in the peripheral nervous system, specifically the ganglia. This process leads to organ dilatation, producing megaviscera and cardiomegaly.[25] Köberle noted that the total number of ganglion cells in the heart, colon, and esophagus of chagasic patients was significantly less than that of nonchagasic patients or chagasic patients whose organs were not involved. He also noted that the organ that is more frequently innervated, the heart, is the one most often involved.[18]

DIAGNOSIS

The preliminary diagnosis of trypanosomiasis may sometimes be made clinically by obtaining a detailed history and physical examination, with special emphasis on travel to or residence in an endemic area and noting any conspicuous lymphadenopathy. Definitive diagnosis is based solely on the presence of trypanosomes through analysis of blood, cerebrospinal fluid, or the biopsy of a chancre, if one is present. In the field, the card agglutination test for trypanosomiasis (CATT) is most often used as an antibody-screening test. This test is performed using a drop of freshly collected heparinized blood.[26] The blood samples that screen positive may then be subjected to further tests such as examination of thick blood films, the use of microhematocrit centrifugation, and miniature anion exchange chromatography and polymerase chain reaction (PCR).[27] Others have suggested that the quantitative buffy coat (QBC) technique, developed for the diagnosis of malaria, may also be another test suitable for in-field screening programs.[28] Lejon and colleagues[29] have proposed the use of a semiquantitative enzyme-linked immunosorbent assay (ELISA), using the variable surface glycoprotein of *T. b. gambiense* as antigen for the detection of antibodies, mostly IgG1, IgG3, and IgM isotypes, in serum and cerebrospinal fluid in determining the clinical stage of sleeping sickness.[29] Also, others have recommended that in poorly equipped laboratories, the diagnosis of CNS involvement can be confirmed by the pleocytosis and elevation of cerebrospinal fluid total protein and IgM levels.[30]

The diagnosis of acute Chagas' disease is achieved in a manner similar to that of sleeping sickness, with direct microscopic examination of anticoagulated blood or a QBC preparation for mottle trypanosomes. History and physical examination are important, especially in the differential diagnosis of organ dilatation in the chronic

stage. Serologic tests such as immunohemagglutination, indirect immunofluorescence assay, and ELISA[31] may be performed to detect the presence of parasite-specific immunoglobulin. Gomes and associates[32] showed that an optimized PCR protocol was very sensitive in detecting the presence of *T. cruzi* in chronic chagasic patients compared with hemoculture and complement mediated lysis. However, because of different end-organ involvement in Chagas' disease as compared with sleeping sickness, the analysis of cerebrospinal fluid is not as crucial.

TREATMENT

There are only a few established drugs today used to treat trypanosomiasis, and most of them were discovered more than 40 years ago. Their mechanism of action is largely unknown except for eflornithine, which is a suicide inhibitor of ornithine decarboxylase. Drawbacks of these drugs include poor oral absorption, systemic toxicity, short duration of action, low efficacy, and the emergence of trypanosomal resistance.[33]

Chemotherapy is one aspect of attempts to control morbidity and mortality in trypanosomiasis. Pentamidine and suramin are most often used for prophylaxis and treatment during the early stages of the disease when the CNS is not involved.[34, 35] Another class of drugs belonging to the melaminyl group, represented by melarsoprol, is useful in treating all stages of trypanosomiasis and is the drug of choice when the CNS is involved. The World Health Organization recommends initial treatment with suramin, followed by three courses of melarsoprol. However, because of melarsoprol toxicity, 5% of treated patients develop arsenical encephalopathy that is often fatal.[23] In some studies, a 7-day intravenous course of eflornithine has been successful following a relapse after melarsoprol treatment failure.[36] Research on alternative trypanocidal drugs continues and some have reported that substrate analogs of 5'-Deoxy-5'(methylthio)adenosine or MTA show promise as novel drugs against trypanosomiasis.[37]

Another front in the struggle for control of trypanosomiasis involves new technology, vector control and public health measures. Conditions that aggravate the problem include war and civil disturbances, economic problems with the dismantling of disease control programs, and reduced health financing owing to lack of funds.[38] Methods other than drugs currently used to help control the spread of the disease include the breeding of trypanosotolerant livestock and vector control through the use of insecticides, traps, targets, and new bait technology. Some have offered the principle of integration as a means of controlling the spread of the disease: existent antitrypanosomal control measures consolidated and integrated with rural development and with control measures for other diseases.[39]

Traditionally, Chagas' disease had no known safe and effective cure for the chronic stage and no drug destroys *T. cruzi* in vivo.[40] Recently, benznidazole was found to be effective in the treatment of the acute and early chronic phase of *T. cruzi* infection. The antitrypanosomal activity of benznidazole stems from its inhibition of ergosterol synthesis. Studies in 1996 confirmed the efficacy of benznidazole treatment at 5 to 8 mg/kg/day for a period of 60 days, which resulted in a 55.8% rate of negative seroconversion of specific antibodies.[41, 42] However, a recent study showed that azole resistance in *T. cruzi* in vitro develops rapidly.[43]

As previously mentioned, African trypanosomiasis, if left untreated, causes meningoencephalitis in which sleep-wake cycle disturbances are prominent. In addition, there is progressive confusion, slurred speech, seizures, and gait disturbances. The parasites may reach the brain parenchyma through the choroid plexus or Virchow-Robin spaces.[25] Other organ systems are also affected, and the patient may show hematologic abnormalities such as anemia, cardiovascular and endocrine disorders, and renal dysfunction. If the condition is allowed to progress, death inevitably results. The most common complication arising from treatment of trypanosomiasis is arsenic encephalopathy or post-therapeutic reactive encephalitis (PTRE). This occurs in 5% to 10% of patients treated with melarsoprol.[24]

Ocular involvement manifesting as a bilateral, diffuse, interstitial keratitis has been described as a rare manifestation of sleeping sickness.[9] Chagas' disease affects primarily the ganglion cells of the upper and lower digestive systems and the heart, resulting in megaviscera and cardiomegaly. Current treatment offers limited success, especially if it is started late in the chronic stage. Most cases of death from Chagas' disease result from heart failure. As mentioned earlier, reports in the literature of ocular involvement other than Romaña's sign are rare; they comprise mostly retinal pigment epithelial defects that have no bearing on visual functioning.

CONCLUSION

Trypanosomiasis is a public health concern of epidemic proportions in certain regions of tropical Africa. It has shown a resurgence during the past 20 years such that its prevalence has reached proportions not seen since the 1930s. It is mostly a meningoencephalitic process that causes large segments of affected populations to become nonproductive members of society; this happens when the parasite reaches the brain and causes the individual to become somnolent and withdrawn—hence, the term African sleeping sickness. Treatment is available and can be effective if given early.

Reports of ocular involvement in humans with trypanosomiasis were made mostly early in the 20th century, although they were later attributed to the effects of trypanocidal drugs or other parasitic infections. However, animal studies have shown that the parasite can invade intraocular structures and cause an intense uveitic reaction.

American trypanosomiasis is caused by *Trypanosoma cruzi* and is most prevalent in sections of Central and South America. People living in thatched, adobe, or mud houses are at greatest risk for contracting the disease because these habitats offer the reduviid insects a favorable place to live and breed. In the eye, retinal pigment epithelial disturbances have been reported in patients with Chagas' disease but these disturbances are not known to contribute to visual impairment. Romaña's sign, characterized by intense periocular soft tissue inflammation at the site of inoculation by insect feces, is the most

visible sign of an acute infection that can still be treated. Unfortunately, not all Chagasic patients manifest this sign, and often, the disease progresses unnoticed until the chronic stage.

In the acute stage, medications such as benznidazole offer some hope of a cure but little except symptomatic relief can be offered to those in the chronic stage.

References

1. Nash TAM: Africa's Bane: The Tsetse Fly. Collins, London, 1969.
2. Baker JR: Speculations on the evolution of the family Trypanosomatidae Doflein. Exp Parasitol 1901; 13:219–233.
3. Baker JR: Epidemiology of African Sleeping Sickness. Symposium on Trypanosomiasis and Leishmaniasis. Venezuelan Academy of Sciences and La Trinidad Medical Center, Caracas, 1974.
4. Zeledón R: Epidemiology, Modes of Transmission, and Reservoir Hosts of Chagas' Disease, Venezuelan Academy of Sciences and La Trinidad Medical Center, Caracas, 1974.
5. World Health Organization Communicable Disease Surveillance and Response. African trypanosomiasis: The Disease (*http://www.who.int/emc/diseases/tryp/trypanodis.htm*). Lyon, France, Department of Communicable Disease Surveillance and Response, World Health Organization, 2000.
6. World Health Organization Communicable Disease Surveillance and Response. African trypanosomiasis: Geographical Distribution (*http://www.who.int/emc/diseases/tryp/trypanogeo.html*). Lyon, France, Department of Communicable Disease and Surveillance, World Health Organization, 2000.
7. World Health Organization Division of Control of Tropical Diseases. Chagas Disease: Burdens and Trends (*http://www.who.int/ctd/chagas/burdens.htm*). Geneva, Switzerland, World Health Organization, 2000.
8. Bryan R, Waskin J, Richards F, et al: African trypanosomiasis in American travelers: A 20-year review. In: Steffen R, Lobel HO, Hayworth J, Bradley DJ, eds: Travel Medicine. Berlin, Springer-Verlag, 1989, pp 384–388.
9. Daniels CW: Eye lesions as a point of importance in directing suspicion to possible trypanosome infection. Ophthalmoscope 1915; 13:595–597.
10. Van den Branden F, Appelmans M: Les troubles visuels au cours du traitement de la trypanosomiase humaine par la tryparsamide (tryponarsyl, trypotan, novatoxyl). Bruxelles Medical 1934; 15:1405–1421.
11. Scott JW: Eye changes in trypanosomiasis. Journal of Tropical Medicine and Hygiene 1944;47:15–17.
12. Ridley H. Ocular lesions in trypanosomiasis. Ann Trop Med Parasitol 1945; 39:66–82.
13. Debeir O: Ocular disturbances and toxic amblyopia in the course of sleeping sickness. Bureau Permanent Interafricain de la Tse-Tse et de la Trypanosomiase No. 200/T 7pp. (Abstracted in Tropical Diseases Bulletin, 1953; 51:150–151).
14. Ikede BO: Ocular lesions in sheep infected with *Trypanosoma brucei*. J Comp Pathol 1974; 84:203–213.
15. Mortelmans J, Neetens A: Ocular lesions in experimental *Trypanosoma brucei* infection in cats. Acta Zool Pathol Antverp 1975; 62:149–172.
16. Romaña, C: Enfermedad de Chagas, Buenos Aires, Lopez Libreros, Argentina, 1963.
17. Centers for Disease Control and Prevention. Chagas Disease—American trypanosomiasis (*http://www.cdc.gov/ncidod/dpd/parasites/chagasdisease/factsht_chagas_disease.htm*). Division of Parasitic Diseases, National Center for Infectious Diseases. Atlanta, Georgia, Centers for Disease Control, 1998.
18. Köberle, F. Pathogenesis of Chagas' disease. Symposium on Trypanosomiasis and Leishmaniasis, Venezuelan Academy of Sciences and La Trinidad Medical Center, Caracas, 1974.
19. Fröhlich SJ, Mino de Kaspar H, Perán R, et al: [Intraocular involvement of Chagas' disease (American trypanosomiasis). Studies in Paraguay/South America.]. Ophthalmologe 1997;94:206–210.
20. Fröhlich SJ, Mino de Kaspar, H, Perán R, et al: [Eye involvement in Chagas disease (American trypanosomiasis). Studies in Paraguay 1996–1997]. Ophthalmologe 1998;95:168–171.
21. Vincendeau P, Okomo-Assoumou MC, Semballa S, et al: Immunol-

ogy and immunopathology of African trypanosomiasis. Med Trop 1996;56:73–78.

22. De Raadt P: Immunity and antigenic variation: Clinical observations suggestive of immune phenomena in African trypanosomiasis. Symposium on Trypanosomiasis and Leishmaniasis, Venezuelan Academy of Sciences and La Trinidad Medical Center, Caracas, 1974.

23. Dumas M, Bouteille B: Human African trypanosomiasis. C R Seances Soc Biol Fil 1996;190:395–408.

24. Sabbah P, Brosset C, Imbert P, et al: Human African trypanosomiasis: MRI. Neuroradiology 1997;39:708–710.

25. Chimelli L, Scarvalli F: Trypanosomiasis. Brain Pathol 1997;7:599–611.

26. Pansaerts R, Van Meirvenne N, Magnus E, et al: Increased sensitivity of the card agglutination test CATT/*Trypanosoma brucei gambiense* by inhibition of complement. Acta Trop 1998;70:349–354.

27. Kanmogne GD, Asonganyi T, Gibson WC: Detection of *Trypanosoma brucei gambiense* in serologically positive but aparasitaemic sleeping-sickness suspects in Cameroon, by PCR. Ann Trop Med Parasitol 1996;90:475–483.

28. Ancelle T, Paugam A, Bourlioux F, et al: Detection of trypanosomes in blood by the Quantitative Buffy Coat (QBC) technique; experimental evaluation. Med Trop 1997;57:245–248.

29. Lejon V, Büscher P, Magnus E, et al: A semi-quantitative ELISA for detection of *Trypanosoma brucei gambiense* specific antibodies in serum and cerebrospinal fluid of sleeping sickness patients. Acta Trop 1998;69:151–164.

30. Miezan TW, Meda HA, Doua F, et al: Assessment of central nervous system involvement in gambiense trypanosomiasis: Value of the cerebro-spinal white cell count. Trop Med Int Health 1998;3:571–575.

31. Vásquez JE, Krusnell J, Orn A, et al: Serological diagnosis of *Trypanosoma rangeli* infected patients. A comparison of different methods and its implications for the diagnosis of Chagas' disease. Scand J Immunol 1997;45:322–330.

32. Gomes ML, Galvao LM, Macedo AM, et al: Chagas disease diagnosis: Comparative analysis of parasitologic, molecular and serologic methods. Am J Trop Med Hyg 1999;60:205–210.

33. Wang CC: Molecular mechanisms and therapeutic approaches to the treatment of African trypanosomiasis. Annu Rev Pharmacol Toxicol 1995;35:93–127.

34. Dumas M, Bouteille B: Current status of trypanosomiasis. Med Trop 1997;57(Supply):56–69.

35. Doua F, Miezan TW, Sanon Singaro JR, et al: The efficacy of pentamidine in the treatment of early-late stage Trypanosoma brucei gambiense trypanosomiasis. Am J Trop Med Hyg 1996;55:586–588.

36. Khonde N, Pépin J, Mpia B: A seven day course of eflornithine for relapsing *Trypanosoma brucei gambiense* sleeping sickness. Trans R Soc Trop Med Hyg 1997;91:212–213.

37. Bacchi CJ, Sanabria K, Spiess AJ, et al: In vivo efficacies of 5'-methylthioadenosine analogs as trypanocides. Antimicrob Agents Chemother 1997;41:2108–2112.

38. Smith DH, Pepin J, Stich AH: Human African trypanosomiasis: An emerging public health crisis. Br Med Bull 1998;54:341–355.

39. Holmes PH: New approaches to the integrated control of trypanosomiasis. Vet Parasitol 1997;71:121–135.

40. Peters W: Drug resistance in trypanosomiasis and leishmaniasis. Symposium on Trypanosomiasis and Leishmaniasis. Venezuelan Academy of Sciences and La Trinidad Medical Center, Caracas 1974.

41. Levi GC, Lobo IM, Kallas EG, et al: Etiological drug treatment of human infection by *Trypanosoma cruzi*. Rev Inst Med Trop Sao Paulo 1996;38:35–38.

42. De Andrade AL, Zicker F, De Oliveira RM, et al: Randomized trial of efficacy of benznidazole in treatment of early *Trypanosoma cruzi* infection. Lancet 1996;348:1407–1413.

43. Buckner FS, Wilson AJ, White TC, et al: Induction of resistance to azole drugs in *Trypanosoma cruzi*. Antimicrob Agents Chemother 1998;42:3245–3250.

Isabelle Cochereau and Thanh Hoang-Xuan

HISTORY/DEFINITION

The first case of histologically proven *Pneumocystis carinii* choroidopathy was reported by Macher and colleagues in 1987 in a patient with the acquired immunodeficiency syndrome (AIDS).[1] The number of new cases reported in patients infected with the human immunodeficiency virus (HIV) has increased but remained low.[2-4] The widespread use of *P. carinii* pneumonia (PCP) prophylaxis with oral trimethoprim-sulfamethoxazole led to a decrease, a few years later, in the incidence of *P. carinii* choroidopathy. The recent advent of highly active antiretroviral therapy (HAART), which restores immunity in HIV-infected patients, induced a sharp drop in the incidence of all AIDS-associated opportunistic infections, particularly PCP. However, it remains crucial not to misdiagnose *P. carinii* choroidopathy, because it is a sign of life-threatening disseminated infection that requires systemic therapy.

EPIDEMIOLOGY

PCP is an opportunistic infection usually limited to the lungs. It occurs in immunodeficient patients, especially subjects infected by HIV. Historically, the huge rise in the incidence of PCP was one of the features that led to the description of the acquired immune deficiency syndrome. PCP is by far the most frequent opportunistic infection in HIV-infected patients, and it is a diagnostic criterion for AIDS.[5] PCP has also been described in HIV-seronegative immunodeficient patients. Patients at risk for PCP are those with lymphocytic leukemia, lymphoma, hypogammaglobulinemia, and allogeneic bone marrow transplantation, and those on high-dose immunosuppressive therapies for cancer, transplantation, or immunologic disorders.[6]

Extrapulmonary *Pneumocystis carinii* infection is located mainly in the lymph nodes and spleen, although cases of liver, bone marrow, gastrointestinal tract, heart, hard palate, thyroid, and choroid involvement have been described. One case of *Pneumocystis carinii* infection of the orbit[7] and one case of infection of the conjunctiva[8] have been reported in patients with AIDS.

Pneumocystis carinii choroidopathy has been reported only in HIV-infected patients, at an estimated incidence of only 1% before the HAART era.[4, 9, 10] Unlike PCP, which occurs at an early stage of the disease when the CD4+ T-lymphocyte count is about 200/mm³, the choroidopathy occurs in patients in the later stages of HIV infection, when the CD4+ T-cell count is less than 50/mm³.[10] The life expectancy of patients with *Pneumocystis carinii* choroidopathy is usually only a few months.[9, 11, 12]

ETIOPATHOGENESIS

In the AIDS setting, *Pneumocystis carinii* choroidopathy occurs mainly in patients who have received primary or secondary PCP prophylaxis with aerosolized pentamidine.[9, 10, 13, 14] As aerosolized pentamidine does not diffuse systemically from the lungs, *Pneumocystis carinii* is able to infect distant organs, in particular the choroid. The incidence of *Pneumocystis carinii* choroidopathy has fallen sharply since the widespread introduction of systemic PCP prophylaxis with oral trimethoprim-sulfamethoxazole.

Pneumocystis carinii is an opportunistic fungus of low virulence, found in the extracellular spaces of infected tissues. As no reliable serologic antigenic test is available, the diagnosis of PCP is based on the detection of the parasite in various specimens, usually bronchoalveolar lavage (BAL) fluid, with special stains (Gomori methenamine silver and Giemsa) or indirect immunofluorescence. BAL examination is occasionally negative in patients receiving prophylaxis with inhaled pentamidine.

PATHOLOGY

Postmortem histopathologic examination of patients with *Pneumocystis carinii* choroidopathy has disclosed choroidal infiltrates containing eosinophilic, acellular, and foamy material.[1, 11, 16] Electron microscopy shows many *Pneumocystis carinii* cysts and trophozoites in choroidal infiltrates.[11]

CLINICAL FEATURES

Pneumocystis carinii choroidopathy is usually discovered incidentally when routine fundus examination discloses one to several yellow-white plaquelike deep lesions (Figs. 37-1 and 37-2) located under the vessels. These are slightly elevated, round or polylobar in shape, they are 0.5 to 6 disc diameters in size,[1, 9, 11, 13] and they become confluent.[16] They are located mainly in the posterior pole up to the equator, but they are never anterior to it.[9] In the absence of treatment, the leading edge of the infiltrate progresses at an estimated 0.5 disc diameter per month.[9] The choroidopathy is bilateral in 76% of patients.[9]

Typically, these choroidal lesions induce no significant visual disturbances, even if they are located beneath the fovea.[9] However, visual acuity may be reduced when they

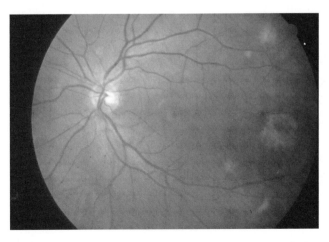

FIGURE 37-1. Choroidal lesions due to *Pneumocystis carinii* infection.

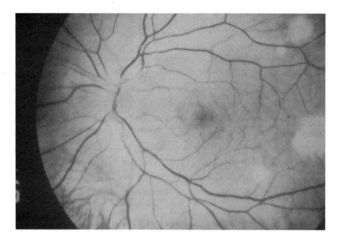

FIGURE 37–2. Pneumocystosis. Red-free photograph.

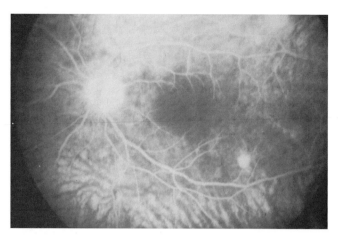

FIGURE 37–4. Pneumocystosis. Late phase of the angiogram. Hyperfluorescence of choroidal lesions.

are associated with serous retinal detachment.[17] Visual field examination discloses a depression corresponding to the choroidal lesions.[9] Inflammation of the anterior chamber and vitreous is usually absent, in part because cell-mediated immunity is severely depressed.

Fluorescein angiography of the lesions shows hypofluorescence in the early phases (Fig. 37–3), and homogenous staining associated with indistinct borders in the later phases (Fig. 37–4).[9, 11, 13, 16]

DIAGNOSIS

The diagnosis of *Pneumocystis carinii* choroidopathy is based on clinical and angiographic signs, a history of progressive PCP or aerosolized prophylaxis, and the efficacy of presumptive therapy. Choroidal biopsy is not performed in patients with suspected *Pneumocystis carinii* choroidopathy, because of the risk of retinal complications.[15] An extensive systemic work-up is mandatory when *Pneumocystis carinii* choroidopathy is suspected, including chest radiographs, liver function tests, arteriolar blood-gas measurements, lactic dehydrogenase assay, computed tomography of the lungs and abdomen, and BAL.

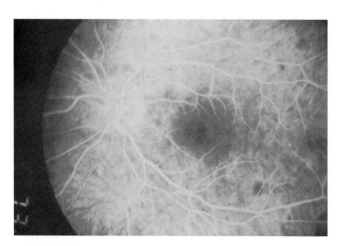

FIGURE 37–3. Pneumocystosis: Early phase of the angiogram. Hypofluorescence of choroidal lesions.

DIFFERENTIAL DIAGNOSIS

The differential diagnoses include tuberculous choroiditis; toxoplasmosis; candidiasis; cryptococcosis; *Mycobacterium avium-intracellulare* infection; lymphoma; histoplasmosis; systemic immunologic diseases such as sarcoidosis, Vogt-Koyanagi-Harada syndrome, and sympathetic ophthalmia; and inflammatory choroidopathies.[12, 15]

Distinguishing *Pneumocystis carinii* choroidopathy from tuberculous choroiditis can be particularly difficult, as tuberculosis and pneumocystosis both occur at an early stage of HIV infection, disseminate to the same distant organs, and induce no inflammation of the aqueous humor or vitreous. However, choroidal tuberculous lesions typically appear as elevated orange masses that can raise the vessels,[18] they are round but not polylobular, and they are often smaller than the lesions caused by *Pneumocystis carinii* choroiditis; in addition, the former tend to increase in size and thickness, whereas the latter increase in surface area only. On the angiogram, late staining of tuberculous foci is less marked and less homogeneous than that of *Pneumocystis carinii* choroidopathy. The isolation of *Mycobacterium tuberculosis* from BAL specimens or other specimens is of value; otherwise, a therapeutic test should be performed.

At the early clinical stage, toxoplasmosis might also be considered in the differential diagnosis. However, later in this disease, the signs rapidly become specific and differ from those of *Pneumocystis carinii* choroidopathy. Fundus examination discloses fluffy borders, satellite vasculitis, vitritis around the focus, and an inflammatory reaction in the vitreous and anterior chamber.[19, 20] The angiograms show hyperfluorescence, starting at the borders of the lesion in the early phases and extending toward the center in the late phase. Concomitant central nervous system toxoplasmosis is frequent, whereas involvement of the lung is uncommon.

Candidiasis is easily distinguished from pneumocystosis by its rapid extension from the lesion into the vitreous, and by inflammation of both the vitreous and the aqueous humor.

The posterior lesions of progressive outer retinal necrosis (PORN) progress more rapidly, become confluent, eventually involve the whole retina, and profoundly compromise vision.[21]

Mycobacterium avium-intracellulare choroidal lesions have not been clearly characterized. The mycobacterium has been identified as a pathogen together with *Pneumocystis carinii* in some lesions.[12, 22]

Choroidal lesions are rare in cryptococcosis. They occur in patients with generalized cryptococcosis or cryptococcal meningitis.

Lymphoma induces lesions that are more yellow, more elevated, and thicker, and that have fluffier borders. The extraocular involvement is also different from that of pneumocystosis.[23]

Histoplasmosis is rare and is found in patients who have lived in areas endemic for histoplasmosis.[24] The lesions are smaller, being less than one disc diameter in size.

Other choroidopathies unrelated to HIV infection can occur, but their incidence is very low, especially in these immunodeficient patients who cannot mount a significant inflammatory reaction.

TREATMENT

Even if the ocular lesions are asymptomatic, *Pneumocystis carinii* choroidopathy necessitates systemic treatment because it is a marker of a disseminated life-threatening infection.

Induction therapy comprises systemic trimethoprim (15 mg/kg daily) and sulfamethoxazole (75 mg/kg daily) or pentamidine (4 mg/kg daily) for at least 3 weeks.[9, 11, 13, 17] The high frequency of systemic adverse reactions to these drugs necessitates careful monitoring. During systemic therapy, the choroidal lesions become paler and disappear very slowly, after several weeks, leaving small pigmentary changes not associated with visual sequelae.[9]

Secondary prophylaxis consists of oral trimethoprim-sulfamethoxazole[25] for as long as the immunodeficiency remains severe. Primary prophylaxis, which is indicated for patients with low CD4+ T-cell counts, also consists of oral trimethoprim-sulfamethoxazole.[26] Aerosolized pentamidine should be used only as adjunctive therapy to prevent pneumocystosis in special cases.

SUMMARY

Prompt recognition of *Pneumocystis carinii* choroidopathy in HIV-infected patients is mandatory, as it is a sign of disseminated life-threatening infection. Its detection requires regular ocular examination because it is usually asymptomatic. The incidence of *Pneumocystis carinii* choroidopathy is now very low because of routine primary pneumocystosis prophylaxis with oral trimethoprim-sulfamethoxazole, and because of the restoration of immunity produced by HAART. However, a further rise in its incidence may occur in the coming years if resistance to HAART increases.

References

1. Macher AM, Bardenstein DS, Zimmerman LE, et al: *Pneumocystis carinii* choroiditis in a male homosexual with AIDS and disseminated pulmonary and extrapulmonary *P. carinii* infection. N Engl J Med 1987;316:1092.

2. Jabs DA: Ocular manifestations of acquired immune deficiency syndrome. Ophthalmology 1989;96:1092–1099.

3. Jabs DA: Ocular manifestations of HIV infections. Trans Am Ophthalmol Soc 1995;93:623–683.

4. Hodge WG, Seiff SR, Margolis TP: Ocular opportunistic infection incidences among patients who are HIV positive compared to patients who are HIV negative. Ophthalmology 1998;105:895–900.

5. Murray JF: NHLBI workshop summary: Pulmonary complications of the acquired immunodeficiency syndrome. Am Rev Respir Dis 1987;135:504–508.

6. Sekpowitz KA: *Pneumocystis carinii* pneumonia in patients without AIDS. Clin Infect Dis 1993;17(suppl 2):S416–422.

7. Friedberg DN, Warren FA, Lee MH, et al: *Pneumocystis carinii* of the orbit. Am J Ophthalmol 1992;113:595–596.

8. Ruggli GM, Weber R, Messmer EP, et al: *Pneumocystis carinii* infection of the conjunctiva in a patient with acquired immune deficiency syndrome. Ophthalmology 1997;104:1853–1856.

9. Shami MJ, Freeman W, Friedberg D, et al: A multicenter study of *Pneumocystis* choroidopathy. Am J Ophthalmol 1991;112:15–22.

10. Sha BE, Benson CA, Deutsch T, et al: *Pneumocystis carinii* choroiditis in patients with AIDS: Clinical features, response to therapy, and outcome. J Acquir Immune Defic Syndr 1992;5:1051–1058.

11. Rao AN, Zimmerman PL, Boyer D, et al: A clinical, histopathologic, and electron microscopic study of *Pneumocystis carinii* choroiditis. Am J Ophthalmol 1989;107:218–228.

12. Morinelli EN, Dugel PU, Riffenburgh R, et al: Infectious multifocal choroiditis in patients with acquired immune deficiency syndrome. Ophthalmology 1993;100:1014–1021.

13. Dugel PU, Rao NA, Forster DJ, et al: *Pneumocystis carinii* choroiditis after long-term aerosolized pentamidine therapy. Am J Ophthalmol 1990;110:113–117.

14. Sneed SR, Blodi CF, Berger BB, et al: *Pneumocystis carinii* choroiditis in patients receiving inhaled pentamidine. N Engl J Med 1990;322:936–937.

15. Freeman WR, Gross JG, Labelle J, et al: *Pneumocystis carinii* choroidopathy. A new clinical entity. Arch Opththalmol 1989;107:863–867.

16. Holland GN, MacArthur LJ, Foos RY: Choroidal PCP. Arch Ophthalmol 1991;109:1454–1455.

17. Foster RE, Lowder CY, Meisler DM, et al: Unifocal presentation, regression with intravenous pentamidine, and choroiditis recurrence. Ophthalmology 1991;98:1360–1365.

18. Muccioli C, Belfort R: Presumed ocular and central nervous system tuberculosis in a patient with the acquired immunodeficiency syndrome. Am J Ophthalmol 1996;212:217–219.

19. Holland GN, Engstrom RE, Glasgow BJ, et al: Ocular toxoplasmosis in patients with the acquired immunodeficiency syndrome. Am J Ophthalmol 1988;106:653–667.

20. Cochereau-Massin I, LeHoang P, Lautier-Frau M, et al: Ocular toxoplasmosis in human immunodeficiency virus-infected patients. Am J Ophthalmol 1992;114:130–135.

21. Forster DJ, Dugel PU, Frangieh GT, et al: Rapidly progressive outer retinal necrosis in the acquired immunodeficiency syndrome. Am J Ophthalmol 1990;110:341–348.

22. Whitcup SM, Fenton RM, Pluda JM, et al: *Pneumocystis carinii* and *Mycobacterium avium-intracellulare* infection of the choroid. Retina 1992;12:331–335.

23. Rivero ME, Kuppermann BD, Wiley CA, et al: Acquired immunodeficiency syndrome-related intraocular B-cell lymphoma. Arch Ophthalmol 1999;117:616–622.

24. Specht CS, Mitchell KT, Bauman AE, et al: Ocular histoplasmosis with retinitis in a patient with acquired immune deficiency syndrome. Ophthalmology 1991;98:1356–1359.

25. Hardy WD, Feinberg J, Finkelstein DD, et al: A controlled trial of trimethoprimsulfamethoxazole or aerosolized pentamidine for secondary prophylaxis of *Pneumocystis carinii* pneumonia in patients with the acquired immunodeficiency syndrome. N Engl J Med 1992;327:1842–1848.

26. Schneider MM, Hoepelman AI, Eeftinck-Sckattenkerk JK, et al: A controlled trial of aerosolized pentamidine or trimethoprim-sulfamethoxazole as primary prophylaxis against *Pneumocystis carinii* pneumonia in patients with human immunodeficiency virus infection. N Engl J Med 1992;327:1836–1841.

OCULAR TOXOCARIASIS

Tatiana Romero-Rangel and C. Stephen Foster

DEFINITION

Toxocariasis is an infectious disease caused by the invasion of tissue by larvae of *Toxocara canis* or *Toxocara cati*, nematode parasites commonly present in the small intestine of dogs or cats, respectively. The infection in humans is most frequently caused by *T. canis*. *Toxocara* larvae are capable of living in many "accidental" hosts, including man, who becomes infected from ingesting the ova from soil contaminated by dogs or cats. *Toxocara* larvae may migrate through the body, invading many different organs. Clinically, human infestation can take three different forms. The two classical expressions are visceral larva migrans (VLM) and ocular toxocariasis. The third clinical manifestation, described more recently, has been called covert toxocariasis. The severity of the disease varies with the number of larvae in the tissues and the immune response of the individual.

ETIOLOGY

The Organism

The biology and morphology of *T. canis* and *T. cati* are similar.[1] Three lips around the mouth, a small intestinal tract, posterior excretory columns, and prominent cervical alae in both sexes are anatomic characteristics that are helpful for making the correct identification and differentiation from other parasites. They are similar to *Ascaris lumbricoides* in appearance but only a quarter to half its size; males are 7 to 9 cm and females are 10 to 17 cm long. Adult worms live in the small intestine of dogs and cats for around 4 months. Adult *T. canis* produces 200,000 eggs per day. Eggs of *Toxocara* are spherical, light brown, and protected by a thick, rough, proteinaceous coat with vitelline membranes. This coat may serve as protection for the larvae, allowing fertilized eggs passed in the feces to survive for months and even years. Development of the second-stage larvae takes 5 to 6 days under favorable conditions of temperature, humidity, and aeration.

Life Cycle in Natural Host

Dogs may acquire the intestinal infection in five different ways: (1) by ingestion of infective embryonated eggs with stage 1 larvae encapsulated inside, (2) by ingestion of infective second-stage larvae infesting the meat of a rodent, (3) by ingestion of advanced-stage larva from the feces or vomit of prenatally infected pups, (4) by transmammary passage of larvae in milk from a lactating bitch to nursing puppies, and (5) by transplacental migration. In cats, transplacental migration has not been proved.[2]

The infective eggs, with first- and second-stage larvae, hatch in the intestine and liberate the third-stage larvae, which penetrate the intestinal wall. Once located in the intestinal wall, the larvae are able to reach the lymphatics and blood vessels, initiating the systemic migration. *Toxocara* larvae pass through the portal circulation and migrate via the liver and heart to alveolar capillaries. The fate of ingested larvae depends on the age and immunity of the host. In puppies, which are more frequently infected, the larvae are able to complete a migratory and developmental cycle. The worms hatch and migrate through the portal system and undergo transtracheal migration. The third-stage larvae are coughed up and aspirated, and they mature into sexually differentiated forms in the small bowel. If the host is an older puppy or an adult dog, particularly with some immunity acquired from past infection, the larvae do not complete the lung migration. They wander through the body, eventually becoming inactive, encysting as second-stage larvae in the tissues. Inactive larvae may be reactivated when a bitch becomes pregnant; they reenter the circulatory system and are carried to the placenta. The larvae pass through the placenta and grow to adult worms in the pups. Most puppies acquire the infection prenatally. However, they generally expel the worms before reaching adulthood. The animal may be asymptomatic or suffer lack of appetite, abdomen enlargement, internal abscess, eosinophilia, and toxocarid pneumonia.[3]

Human Infestation

Humans acquire the infection by eating contaminated soil (geophagia) containing *Toxocara* larvae, or by ingestion of contaminated meat. Children who eat dirt (pica) or who are in close contact with puppies are at particular risk of acquiring the disease. The larvae are not able to complete their normal life cycle in humans because they cannot migrate out of the human lungs to return to the intestine. As the adult worms do not develop in humans, examination of the stool for ova and parasites is unproductive diagnostically.

In the human intestine, the second-stage larvae migrate through the intestinal wall and enter the bloodstream via the portal circulation, traveling then to small vessels of target organs, where they encyst. Once in the tissue, the larvae are encysted by a focal granulomatous reaction, where they can remain alive for months or even years. These granulomas are most commonly found in the brain, liver, lung, and eye.[4]

CLINICAL MANIFESTATIONS

The most frequently recognized clinical manifestation of *Toxocara* invasion is the VLM syndrome. The first case was reported by Beaver and colleagues,[5] who demonstrated the presence of *T. canis*, by liver biopsy, in one child with chronic eosinophilia, cough, pulmonary infiltration, fever, and hepatomegaly. Since this initial study, it has been shown that the VLM is usually caused by the migration of second-stage *T. canis* larvae or, in some cases, by other nematodes.

VLM is typically seen in young children (1 to 4 years of age) with a history of pica.[6] Generally, the course of the disease is subclinical, but it can be symptomatic with various clinical manifestations and levels of severity. Variation in VLM presentations has been suggested to be caused by factors such as patient age, number of larvae ingested, distribution of larvae, and host response. When symptoms are present, general symptoms and clinical signs such as fever, coughing or wheezing, malaise, irritability, weight loss, hepatomegaly, and pruritic eruptions and nodules over the trunk and legs are commonly seen.

During the acute stage, laboratory investigation may reveal leukocytosis from 30,000 to 100,000/mm^3, with 50% to 90% eosinophils. Peripheral eosinophilia has been correlated with the parasitic burden of *Toxocara* larvae and can be seen for months or years after the acute presentation.[7] Therefore, eosinophilia does not implicate, necessarily, an active process. Serum immunoglobulins IgG, IgM, and IgE are usually elevated. Interestingly, anti-A and anti-B titers are positive in some children with VLM. This can be explained, probably, by the presence of *Toxocara* antigens, which stimulate isohemaglutinins.[8] Chest radiographs may show pulmonary infiltrates. However, severe respiratory distress is rare. Central nervous system manifestations such as encephalitis, cerebral eosinophilic granulomata, and seizures (usually of the petit mal type) can be observed.

Since most patients with VLM are asymptomatic, the prognosis is generally excellent. However, clinically manifest cases can leave permanent structural damage to the involved tissues. Additionally, in rare cases, death of patients with severe VLM can occur, usually secondary to central nervous system or myocardial involvement.

Brown[9] summarized 245 reported cases of ocular *T. canis*. He identified ocular toxocariasis as an entity different from VLM, describing the course of the disease and the clinical presentation of each. Cases of ocular toxocariasis differ from classical VLM in that patients are generally older (mean age, 4 to 8 years) and healthy, and they usually have just one eye affected (often infected by one larva). Since inflammation may not be a prominent feature, the lesion is often discovered during an evaluation of leukocoria, strabismus, or decreased vision, or on routine examination. Ocular involvement is usually not present in cases of VLM, and VLM is rarely seen in cases of ocular toxocariasis. However, some cases of ocular toxocariasis have been reported as having symptoms of VLM.[10]

Recently, some cases of irritable bowl syndrome have been attributed to toxocariasis. The diagnosis has been made based on the levels of leukocytes, eosinophils, and enzyme-linked immunosorbent assay (ELISA) titers, and it has been called covert toxocariasis.[11, 12]

HISTORY

Calhoun visualized a nematode larva invading the eye for the first time in 1937.[13] The localization of the larva on the lens allowed a clear identification of the larva as *Ascaris*. The clinical presentation was characterized by severe keratitis and iridocyclitis associated with secondary glaucoma and dislocation of the lens in the right eye of an 8-year-old child. The larva was found to be disintegrating, so an attempt to recover it intact was unsuccessful.

Histopathology of the lesion of ocular toxocariasis was described prior to the recognition of its typical clinical appearance. Wilder, in 1950, observed a common inflammatory pattern characterized by an eosinophilic abscess surrounded by epithelioid and giant cells in 46 eyes, all of which had a similar clinical presentation with a white pupillary reflex.[14] These cases had been previously diagnosed as pseudoglioma, Coats' disease, endophthalmitis, and (in most cases), retinoblastoma. The pathologic findings were of special interest because they appeared similar to those associated with helminth infections elsewhere in the body. Therefore, multiple sections of the tissue were obtained. Nematode larvae or their residual hyaline capsules were found in 24 eyes. The 22 remaining eyes had a similar pathologic appearance, but larval remnants were not found. Wilder named the entity nematode endophthalmitis. At that time, the larvae found in Wilder's series were believed to be a hookworm. It was not until 6 years later that Nichols,[15] while reviewing this series, determined that the larvae present in five eyes were in fact *T. canis*.

Ashton[16] reported the clinical and histopathologic findings of the first four cases of ocular toxocariasis in Great Britain. The eyes had been enucleated because the fundus lesions appeared to be similar to those of retinoblastoma. Ashton described a distinct, second form of the disease characterized by a solitary retinal tumor with slight evidence of inflammation. In one of the cases, in addition to the retinal granuloma, an eosinophilic abscess within the anterior vitreous was detected, as in a previous case reported by Irvine and Irvine.[17] Ashton suggested that the diversity of the clinical picture depended on the site of localization of the larva, the severity of the individual reaction, and the stage at which the eye was examined. He also commented on the importance and necessity of serial sections for histologic diagnosis in any eye of a young person having an unexplained granulomatous reaction, particularly with an eosinophilic component.

Duguid identified *T. canis* larvae in two eyes, and fragments thought to be *T. canis* in four other eyes in histopathologic studies of patients with chronic endophthalmitis.[18, 19] He emphasized the importance of suspicion for *T. canis* as a cause of chronic endophthalmitis in children, along with other known etiologic agents of chronic uveitis. In addition, he discussed the clinical features of the posterior retinal granuloma and chronic endophthalmitis, which were the two most common types of ocular lesions seen in association with ocular toxocariasis in 28 cases described at the Institute of Ophthalmology of London.[20] Subsequently, a variety of clinical presentations were reported.[20, 21]

Wilkinson and Welch[22] reported their experience with 40 patients having presumed or proven intraocular *Toxocara*, in which 17 patients, including one with bilateral involvement, had a peripheral inflammatory mass on clinical presentation. They emphasized the importance of differentiating these lesions from congenital and developmental anomalies, as most of the patients in previous reports and in their series were children.

O'Connor[23] discovered nine patients with peripheral retinal masses joined to the disc by retinal folds while studying 20 uveitis cases. He observed a tubelike structure under the retina, spreading from the disc to the peripheral inflammatory mass, and thought that this clinico-pathologic finding was specific for *Toxocara* infection. Subsequently, other ocular findings such as hemorrhages, exudates, macular lesions, diffuse retinal lesions with associated pigmentary changes, optic atrophy, and narrowing of the retinal arteries have also been described.[24]

EPIDEMIOLOGY

Ocular toxocariasis is a common infectious disease, seen throughout the world. Brown summarized 403 cases of ocular toxocariasis reported in 73 papers from 19 countries.[25] Most papers were reported from the United States (224), Great Britain (144), and Australia (7 cases). In the United States, the population of the southeastern area has been found to be at especially high risk for acquired toxocariasis. It is thought that the actual prevalence of ocular toxocariasis is higher than the reported prevalence in the literature. Factors such as lack of clinical suspicion, subclinical infection in a large number of patients, limited availability of ophthalmic pathologists, and the difficulty in identifying the larvae in pathologic specimens in some cases are among the factors responsible for the underdiagnosis.

Toxocara larvae have been found in both rural and metropolitan areas. It has been reported that 10% to 32% of soil samples collected from parks, playgrounds, and other public places in the United States are contaminated with *Toxocara* eggs. The incidence of infected puppies has been estimated to be from 33% in London to 98% in Columbus, Ohio, to 100% in Brisbane, Australia.[26]

Contact with dogs, especially puppies, is a well-known risk factor for ocular toxocariasis.[6] However, some patients do not have a history of exposure to dogs or cats. It is especially important, therefore, for the ophthalmologist to remember that the most common route of infection is the ingestion of soil contaminated with *Toxocara* larvae. The patient and parents must be questioned about possible geophagia. Although young children (4 to 8 years old) are more commonly affected, cases of adults with ocular toxocariasis have been reported.[27, 28] Studies performed in different populations have shown a varied prevalence of seropositivity for *Toxocara* antibodies. Study of a group of 333 kindergarten children with no ocular or systemic manifestations of toxocariasis disclosed that 106 children (32%) had a positive antibody titer equal to or greater than 1:16 by ELISA assay, and 77 (23%) had titers equal to or greater than 1:32.[29] The large number of healthy children with positive titers for *Toxocara* in this study shows that the presence of a positive titer should be interpreted with caution, particularly in areas where toxocariasis is widely prevalent. For example, an extremely high prevalence was found in a population from Réunion (an island in the Indian Ocean),[30] in which the sera of 387 persons over 15 years old were analyzed by Western blotting using *T. canis* excretory-secretory larval antigens; 92.8% of the sera analyzed demonstrated positive *Toxocara* titers.

Pollard and coworkers[31] found positive ELISA titers in 37 of 41 patients (90%) with suspected ocular toxocariasis. One of these patients, with a 1:16 positive ELISA titer, was found to have retinoblastoma upon enucleation.[32] This case underscores the importance of excluding retinoblastoma in patients who are seropositive for the *Toxocara* parasite, particularly in populations with a high prevalence of toxocariasis. For this reason, it is of extreme importance to perform a complete laboratory investigation, correlating serum ELISA titers with risk factors, clinical findings, and standardized echography, and to obtain aqueous and vitreous ELISA titers, to differentiate between these two entities.

IMMUNOPATHOLOGY

Definitive diagnosis of ocular toxocariasis requires the identification of the larva. Unfortunately, in most specimens the organism has been entirely destroyed. Moreover, if the larva is present, multiple sections of the specimen may be required to find it. This is in part because of the small size of the organism (18 to 21 microns), approximately two to three times the size of a red blood cell. For this reason, a presumptive diagnosis may be made based on the characteristic tissue reaction.[33]

The most common finding in enucleated eyes with ocular toxocariasis is a chronic sclerosing vitritis with a secondary total retinal detachment. Less commonly, *Toxocara* larvae produce a localized retinochoroidal lesion. The underlying retinal pigment epithelium (RPE) is generally involved, with atrophy, hyperplasia, and breaks in Bruch's membrane. The organism induces a focal, necrotizing granulomatous inflammation with varying degrees of intraocular disorganization, characterized by an aggregation of eosinophils, epithelioid cells, multinucleated giant cells, plasma cells, and lymphocytes surrounding the larva or its remnants. Plasma cells are the most common inflammatory cell in the infiltrate (Fig. 38–1).

The presence of inflammation in the absence of the larvae or their remnants has suggested that secreted surface antigens are responsible for the inflammatory reaction.[34] The idea that there is production of localized antibody in ocular toxocariasis has been strongly supported by (1) the observation of higher antibody titers in vitreous and aqueous humor than in the serum, (2) the

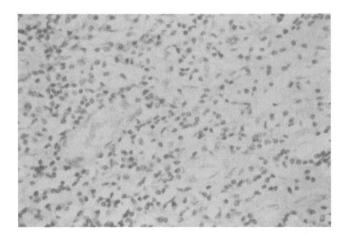

FIGURE 38–1. Histopathology of chorioretinal granuloma in a patient whose eye was enucleated secondary to chronic endophthalmitis and irreparable retinal detachment, ultimately shown to be secondary to toxocariasis. Note the complete loss of choroidal or retinal architecture with the granulomatous inflammatory infiltrate. (See color insert.)

presence of plasma cells in the infiltrate, and (3) a serum *T. canis* antibody detected by ELISA that is fourfold lower in patients with ocular infestation than in patients with systemic VLM. The result may be a local production of small amounts of antibody in the eye, with subsequent lower circulating titers.[35, 36]

In addition, local antibody production has been suggested by the Goldman-Witmer coefficient in patients with ocular toxocariasis. The ratio is considered significant if it is above 4; any ratio less than 1 is considered negative, and between 1 and 4 is considered indeterminant. The Goldman-Witmer coefficient is represented by the following equation, in which AH is aqueous humor and VF is vitreous fluid:

$$\frac{\text{Antibody titer AH or VF}}{\text{Antibody titer serum}} \times \frac{\text{Total IgG AH or VF}}{\text{Total IgG serum}}$$

The Splendore-Hoeppli phenomenon denotes an eosinophilic precipitate that can be observed around the *Toxocara* larva. This phenomenon is not specific to the *Toxocara* organism, as it has been seen around certain other parasites.

Rockey and colleagues[37] studied the interaction in culture of eosinophils and humoral factors from ascarid-infected guinea pig eye with second-stage larvae of *Toxocara canis* and *Ascaris suum*, which are closely related phylogenetically and antigenically. They observed that the eosinophils adhered firmly to the surface of the larvae, to a larval sheath, or to attached eosinophils. Furthermore, they noted the presence of soluble factors in the anterior chamber that had been shown to be important for the adhesion of eosinophils to a parasite surface membrane, and for the cytotoxicity and killing of parasites by eosinophils in tissue culture. These factors include IgG, IgE, eosinophil stimulation promoter, complement, eosinophil chemotactic factor of anaphylaxis, tetrapeptides, histamine, hydrogen peroxide, and superoxide anions. The time of appearance of aqueous humor IgE antibody corresponded to a rapid increase in the intraocular eosinophil infiltrate after a single intraocular infection with second-stage larvae.[37]

A strong hypersensitivity reaction with local IgE production, as well as the presence of eosinophils and antigenic stimulation in *Toxocara* parasitosis, were also found in a clinical study of patients with focal chorioretinitis clinically suggestive of intraocular parasitosis, who had undergone vitrectomy for retinovitreous complications. The values of IgE in two patients with ocular toxocariasis were extremely high (520 and 1074 mg/dl); the corresponding serum titers were 64 and 17, indicating local synthesis of IgE in the vitrectomy fluid. In other ocular parasitic infections, such as toxoplasmosis, high levels of IgE in the vitreous have not been observed. This illustrates that there are different immunologic responses for different parasitic agents in intraocular parasitosis.

CLINICAL VARIATIONS

Intraocular infestation with *T. canis* is typically seen unilaterally in children with a history of contact with dogs or cats, or geophagia. The course of the disease is usually asymptomatic. Impairment of visual acuity is the most common manifestation when symptoms are present. Generally, the youngest children do not report visual changes, even if visual acuity is profoundly affected. Thus, diminished visual acuity is frequently detected in a routine examination. Other clinical manifestations such as strabismus and leukocoria are commonly observed.

Toxocara larvae may involve diverse ocular tissues. The different forms of the ocular disease result from the same pathogenesis. The larvae reach the eye via the bloodstream and become encysted in the ocular tissues. The most commonly affected tissue is the retina, which is frequently affected by a granulomatous reaction located in the posterior pole or in the periphery.[16] Commonly, posterior pole toxocariasis lesions are white or gray, round, and elevated (Fig. 38–2). The diameter is generally one or two disc diameters in size. They may be centered anywhere in the posterior pole, including in juxtapapillary and subfoveal locations. A crescent-shaped dark area, possibly representing a larva, is sometimes seen in the lesions. Depending on the number of larvae and the anatomic location, there may be minimal or massive vitreous inflammation.

The predominance of peripheral granuloma, which appears as a hazy, white, elevated reaction in the peripheral fundus, associated with retinal folds that may extend from the peripheral mass to the optic nerve head, has been observed in some studies (Fig. 38–3). Gillespie and coworkers[38] found a peripheral granuloma to be the most common finding. Wilkinson and Welch[22] described peripheral involvement in 44% of eyes with ocular toxocariasis. The features observed in these cases are similar to those seen in pars planitis.[22, 24, 39, 40] Hogan and coworkers[41] reported a case of a child with a diagnosis of uniocular pars planitis, who had typical snowball exudates over the pars plana and in the vitreous. The child died of unrelated causes, and a microscopic examination of the eye was performed. The histopathologic findings showed eosinophils in the vitreous and a *Toxocara* larva in the periphery of the retina. Based on these observations, it has been suggested that ocular toxocariasis should be excluded in cases of unilateral pars planitis, particularly in children.

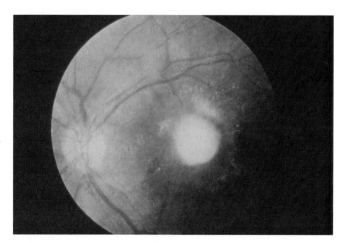

FIGURE 38–2. Posterior granuloma, macular, in a patient with toxocara chorioretinitis. Exuberant vitritis has been controlled with systemic prednisone. (See color insert.)

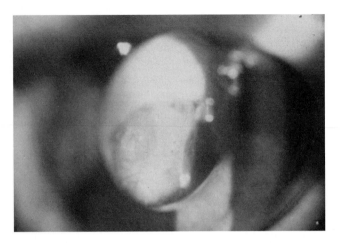

FIGURE 38–3. Peripheral retinitis and retinal detachment in a patient with a peripheral toxocara granuloma. This eye was eventually enucleated and was the source of the histopathology shown in Figure 38–1. (See color insert.)

Another common manifestation of ocular toxocariasis is chronic endophthalmitis.[14, 15] These cases are usually associated with retinal detachment, a low-grade anterior uveitis, posterior synechiae, and a cyclitic membrane between the detached retina and the lens. A hypopyon may develop in severe cases.[42] Papillitis, macular edema, vitreous exudates, and, more rarely, a retrolental mass have been associated findings as well.[18, 19, 42] In children, the most common causes of uveitis involving the posterior pole are *Toxoplasma*, nematodes, and cytomegalovirus.[43] Perkins[20] found toxocariasis to be a presumptive diagnosis in 15 of 150 cases (10%) of children with uveitis. A similar incidence has been found in other studies.[43]

Additionally, scleritis secondary to *Toxocara* larva infestation has been reported.[24, 27, 38, 39] In one study at the Massachusetts Eye and Ear Infirmary, 6 of 130 patients (4.6%) with scleritis had an infectious etiology,[44] including a 70-year-old woman with a history of recurrent nodular scleritis. The diagnosis was presumed to be toxocariasis by the ophthalmoscopic findings, and this was subsequently confirmed by biopsy of the scleral nodule, which disclosed a chronic nongranulomatous inflammation with epithelioid cells in the infiltrate, and by antibody titers, which were positive in a 1:64 dilution. Less frequent presentations such as keratitis, optic neuritis, and motile larva are part of the broad spectrum of clinical manifestations seen in this entity.[24, 39, 45]

COMPLICATIONS

Infestation of the eye by *Toxocara* may result in severely decreased visual acuity as a result of direct retinal injury, by the larva or by secondary effects related to inflammation and scarring.[46] The inflammatory response to the *Toxocara* larva may be intense enough to produce a connective tissue contraction and reduction of the vitreous volume, followed by traction of this tissue on the retina and choroid, often resulting in detachment of these structures. A cyclitic membrane may be formed extending into the anterior portion of the vitreous and along its anterior surface. Contraction of this membrane may result in detachment of the ciliary body and anterior choroid, with subsequent impairment of ciliary body function and hypotony. The major causes of decreased visual acuity that have been reported include vitreous traction band, endophthalmitis, macular lesion, retinal detachment, pars planitis, and papillitis.[47]

In one study, clinical findings such as detached retina, peripheral fibrous mass extending from the optic disc, macular scarring, and changes of the optic disc were seen in asymptomatic patients with positive *Toxocara* titers. The association of these findings and seropositivity for *Toxocara* could be a coincidence; they also could represent the sequelae of ocular toxocariasis in patients who had subclinical inflammation.

Amblyopia may also occur as a complication of toxocariasis, particularly when strabismus is present.[48] Toxocariasis was found to be a common cause of amblyopia in a prospective study in which the etiology of uniocular blindness was analyzed.

DIAGNOSIS
Laboratory Investigations
The diagnosis of ocular toxocariasis is based on the clinical findings and their correlation with serologic tests. Currently, the ELISA, which was introduced by Cypress and colleagues[49] in 1977, is the most accurate available serologic test. A *Toxocara* excretory-secretory or exoantigen product is used as an in vitro test.[50] This test has been shown to be highly specific for *Toxocara* and does not have significant cross-reactivity with other helminthic parasites such as *Ascaris*.

The sensitivity and specificity of the ELISA is approximately 90%. This means that even though 90% of patients with positive results have the disease, 10% of the patients with positive titers do not have ocular toxocariasis. Since cases of retinoblastoma may be included in this 10% of patients with false-positive titers, interpretation of this test has to be correlated with the clinical findings, particularly in areas where *Toxocara* is prevalent.

Pollard and coworkers[31] found an optimal cutoff titer greater than 1:8. However, several patients with ELISA titers as low as the 1:2 dilution, in whom enucleation was performed, had a diagnosis of ocular toxocariasis confirmed by biopsy.[32, 51, 52] Moreover, a long-term follow-up of 20 patients with ocular toxocariasis showed that 85% of these patients had a decrease in serum titer, 10% showed an increase, and 5% were stable.[53] Based on these results, the authors recommend not to exclude the diagnosis of toxocariasis because of a low titer, as the patient may have had a higher titer previously. It has been suggested that any serum titer with clinical correlation could be considered highly significant for *Toxocara*.

More important than serum titer is the detection of antibodies in aqueous humor.[54] In a patient with bilateral panuveitis, *Toxocara* antibodies were detected in the aqueous humor by ELISA assay.[55] A Goldmann-Witmer coefficient of 8.63 was calculated for the right eye, and 8.94 for the left. Cytology of the aqueous or vitreous may be used to support the clinical diagnosis of ocular toxocariasis. If there is evidence of eosinophils in the aqueous or vitreous humor, the diagnosis of parasitic infestation, most likely toxocariasis, is suggested. Recently, cases of ocular toxocariasis due to *T. cati* have been more frequently reported. In some patients with ocular findings of toxocariasis and negative ELISA titers, specific serologic testing for *T. cati* was positive.[56]

Radiologic Evaluation

In addition to the clinical findings and ELISA titers, standardized echography may be useful in helping to establish the diagnosis of ocular toxocariasis. The three most common echographic findings in a group of 11 patients with ocular toxocariasis were (1) a solid, highly reflective peripheral mass (in 91% of the patients the lesion was found in the temporal periphery), (2) vitreous membranes extending between the posterior pole and the mass, and (3) a traction retinal detachment or fold from the posterior pole to the mass.[57]

Although it is useful for detecting the presence of intraocular calcification, computed tomography (CT) cannot absolutely differentiate toxocariasis or other simulating entities from retinoblastoma. In one study, the characteristic findings of toxocariasis on a CT scan have been suggested.[58] Five of 80 pediatric patients with non-rhegmatogenous retinal detachment were diagnosed with ocular toxocariasis.[59] All these patients had pseudomicrophthalmia resulting from a thickened, inflamed sclera that was thought to be a "typical" finding by the authors. None of the patients had evidence of calcification. Furthermore, calcification can occur in any of the simulating conditions, particularly when there is significant ocular disruption or phthisis.

DIFFERENTIAL DIAGNOSIS

The differential diagnosis of toxocariasis is not vast, but it includes retinoblastoma, infectious endophthalmitis, retinopathy of prematurity, persistence of hyperplastic primary vitreous (PHPV), toxoplasmosis, Coats' disease, and familial exudative vitreoretinopathy (FEVR). Differentiation between ocular toxocariasis and retinoblastoma has become less difficult with the development of diagnostic techniques such as ELISA, ultrasonography, and CT. However, ocular toxocariasis is still one of the most frequently recognized, nonmalignant lesions that simulate retinoblastoma.[60] Both entities are seen mostly in children, and leukocoria is a common presentation.

Additionally, the clinical presentation of the solitary retinal mass or diffuse endophthalmitis in toxocariasis may simulate an endophytic retinoblastoma or a unilateral, sporadic retinoblastoma. However, organizing vitreoretinal traction and inflammatory signs that are not commonly associated with retinoblastoma characterize the *Toxocara* lesion.

Of 500 patients referred to the ocular oncology service at Wills Eye Hospital, Philadelphia, with a suspected diagnosis of retinoblastoma, only 288 patients (58%) in fact had it. The other 32% comprised diverse entities such as persistent hyperplastic primary vitreous (28%), Coats' disease (16 %), and presumed ocular toxocariasis (16%). When the distinction between retinoblastoma and toxocariasis is unclear, the *Toxocara* ELISA on aspirated aqueous humor and cytologic examination of the same are justified.

In a study by Felberg and coworkers,[54] five patients with suspected ocular toxocariasis had serum ELISA levels higher than the 1:4 dilution, and aqueous ELISA levels above 1:276. Antibody was not found in the serum or aqueous humor of patients with retinoblastoma, Coats' disease, uveal malignant melanoma, or central retinal artery obstruction.

Finding normal levels of aqueous humor lactate dehydrogenase and phosphoglucose isomerase and the demonstration of eosinophils in vitreous or aqueous aspirates can also facilitate the diagnosis of ocular toxocariasis, and its differentiation from retinoblastoma. Other differentiating features between retinoblastoma (unilateral, sporadic) and toxocariasis include the following:

1. The usual age is 7 to 8 years for ocular toxocariasis but 22 to 24 months for unilateral sporadic retinoblastoma.
2. There is a lack of inflammatory stigmata in retinoblastoma: specifically, no anterior segment scarring, and no secondary cataract, cyclitic membranes, or transvitreal epiretinal membrane formation.
3. Retinoblastoma lesions usually increase in size, whereas those of ocular toxocariasis do not.

Some salient differentiating features between toxocariasis and the other differential entities include the following:

1. Infectious endophthalmitis is distinguished by the history of recent trauma or ocular surgery. Acute signs of external inflammation typical for bacterial endophthalmitis are uncharacteristic in toxocariasis. However, a delayed onset with less virulent bacterial or fungal organisms needs to be differentiated. Vitreous or aqueous sampling for microscopic examination and microbiologic studies should provide a definitive diagnosis in these cases. Endogenous endophthalmitis usually occurs in the setting of immunodeficiency and positive blood cultures.
2. Differentiation between active toxoplasmosis retinitis and toxocariasis may be difficult, particularly when severe vitritis is present. Serologic studies for toxoplasmosis should provide the diagnostic information.
3. Pediatric conditions such as retinopathy of prematurity, FEVR, PHPV, and Coats' disease usually present neonatally or in early infancy and lack the signs of inflammation of the posterior segment. Retinopathy of prematurity is bilateral, encountered in infants with a history of prematurity and low birth weight, and is characterized by proliferative changes in membrane formation involving the retinal periphery. FEVR is bilateral with characteristic retinal vascular abnormalities and membrane formation with an autosomal dominant inheritance pattern. PHPV is congenital, unilateral, and associated with micro-ophthalmia. The characteristic morphology includes that of a fibrovascular stalk from the disc to the posterior lens surface, forming a retrolental fibrovascular mass causing ciliary body traction. Coats' disease is a unilateral condition occurring almost exclusively in young males. This is characterized by a white, fibrotic subretinal mass in the posterior pole. There are typical vascular telangiectasia and lipid exudation with an absence of epiretinal membrane formation.

TREATMENT

Medical

Medical treatment for patients with ocular toxocariasis has been directed toward the inflammatory response that may produce structural damage and decreased vision. The medications that have been used to achieve this goal are steroids, given locally and systemically, alone or in conjunction with systemic antihelmintic agents. As a plan of management, Dinning and colleagues[61] proposed initial treatment with local, periocular, or systemic steroids (prednisolone, 0.5 to 1 mg/kg/day) or surgery in cases where indicated, with the addition of thiabendazole 50 mg/kg/day for 7 days, if the previous treatment failed.

There are reports of clinical improvement of ocular toxocariasis treated with thiabendazole (25 mg/kg twice a day for 5 days, with a maximum of 3 g/day), albendazole (800 mg twice a day for 6 days),[62] and mebendazole (100 to 200 mg twice a day for 5 days). Adequate larvicidal concentrations of thiabendazole given systemically were measured in the aqueous and vitreous humor of a minimally inflamed eye.[63] There are some cases of ocular toxocariasis associated with VLM that have been successfully treated with diethylcarbamazine. Nonspecific medications such as cycloplegic agents are used when the anterior inflammation is present, in order to prevent the development of posterior synechiae and secondary glaucoma.[24]

Surgical

Surgical procedures such as pars plana vitrectomy, cryopexy, and photocoagulation have been used to treat patients with ocular toxocariasis.[64] Pars plana vitrectomy may be beneficial for patients who have not had a satisfactory response to medical treatment, or for those who have marked vitreous fibrosis and tractional complications thereof.[65–67] Belmont and coworkers[65] obtained a dramatic improvement after pars plana vitrectomy in four patients with *Toxocara* endophthalmitis; vitrectomy relieved vitreoretinal traction involving the macula in two of these patients. The employment of pars plana vitrectomy decreased the occurrence of secondary complications due to the progressive inflammation in this study. For this reason, early intervention with this surgical procedure has been recommended.

Small and associates[68] achieved reattachment in 83% of 12 eyes with retinal traction detachments caused by toxocariasis, and vision improved in 7 of the 12 eyes. All had had macular detachment preoperatively; traction folds through the macula preoperatively were associated with a poor visual outcome. Hagler and colleagues[69] reported on 17 patients (eyes) undergoing vitreoretinal procedures for ocular toxocariasis, with improved or stable vision in 15. The final acuity was 20/50 in two eyes, 20/60 to 20/80 in three, and 20/100 to 20/200 in two; eight others had "stabilized" but poor vision, and two eyes deteriorated.

Rodriguez[70] reported on pars plana vitrectomy in 12 eyes affected by chronic ocular toxocariasis endophthalmitis, observing that the anatomic and visual results were better the earlier in the course of the patient's illness the surgery was performed. Six eyes had final visual acuities of 20/20 to 20/40, one was 20/80, one was 20/200, one was 20/400, and three had light perception only. As a result of the surgery, 66% improved visually; one remained unchanged, and three eyes deteriorated. Five of the eyes required multiple surgeries. Abdel-Latif[64] reported three cases of laser photocoagulation therapy for toxocaral chorioretinitis with "satisfactory" results: "The lesion was reduced to a limited flat scar, and the edema around it subsided in a few weeks, with slight improvement of vision." Resolution of inflammation does not guarantee good visual acuity, as antiamblyopia therapy is essential to achieve good vision in the pediatric population.

PROGNOSIS

The final outcome in ocular toxocariasis depends on underlying factors such as the age of the patient, disease duration before diagnosis, structure of the eye involved, degree of inflammation, preexisting amblyopia, and compromise of the macula. The prognosis for improved visual acuity and normal binocular vision is better when the onset of the disease occurs in older patients and the disease is detected early in its course.

CONCLUSIONS

Ocular toxocariasis is a common worldwide ocular infection that affects mostly children. It is found in both rural and metropolitan areas. The most common route of infection is the ingestion of soil contaminated with *Toxocara* larva. In most cases, the course of the disease is mild, but the spectrum of clinical manifestations and severity is broad, and the potential for uniocular blindness due to this entity is well recognized. Consequently, to improve the prognosis, visual acuity screening in daycare centers and in schools may be critical to detect this disease in its early stages.

The diagnosis of toxocariasis is essentially clinical, based on the lesion morphology and supportive laboratory data and imaging studies. Differentiation of ocular toxocariasis from retinoblastoma is critical. To avoid unnecessary enucleation of eyes with ocular toxocariasis, it is imperative to establish an adequate correlation between the clinical findings and diagnostic methods including serum ELISA titers and radiologic evaluation by ultrasound and CT scan. It is of particular importance to perform ELISA *Toxocara* titers on aqueous humor when the clinical diagnosis is not clear or when the serum ELISA is inconclusive.

Treatment is directed at complications arising from intraocular inflammation and vitreous membrane traction. Early vitrectomy may be of value both diagnostically and therapeutically.

Early therapeutic vitrectomy is recommended based on the beneficial results obtained in several patients. If an early vitrectomy is performed, then analysis of ELISA titers and cytology of the vitreous humor should be performed for diagnostic purposes.

References

1. Noble ER, Noble GA: Parasitology. The Biology of Animal Parasites. 5th ed. Philadelphia, Lea & Febiger, 1982.
2. Tabbara KF: Other parasitic infections. In: Tabbara KF, Hyndiuk

RA, eds: Infections of the Eye. Boston, Little Brown & Co, 1985, pp 697–715.

3. Schmidt GD, Roberts LS: Foundations of Parasitology. St. Louis, Times Mirror/Mosby College Publishing, 1985.

4. Park SS, To KW, Fried AH, et al: Infectious causes of posterior uveitis. In: Albert DM, Jakobiec FA: Principles and Practice of Ophthalmology. Clinical Practice. Philadelphia, W.B. Saunders, 1994, pp 450–464.

5. Beaver PC, Snyder CH, Carrera GM, et al: Chronic eosinophilia due to visceral larva migrans. Pediatrics 1952;9:7.

6. Schantz PM, Weis PE, Pollard ZF, et al: Risk factors for toxocaral ocular larva migrans: A case control study. Am J Public health 1980;70:1269.

7. Glickman LT, Schantz PM: Epidemiology and pathogenesis of zoonotic toxocariasis. Epidemiol Rev 1981;3:230–250.

8. Parke DW, Shaver RP: Toxocariasis. In: Pepose JS, Holland GN, Wilhelmus KR: Ocular Infection and Immunity. St. Louis, Mosby, 1996, pp 1225–1235.

9. Brown DH: Ocular *Toxocara canis*: Part II. Clinical review. Pediatr Ophthalmol 1970;7:182.

10. Schimek RA, Perez WA, Carrera GM: Ophthalmic manifestations of visceral larva migrans. Ann Ophthalmol 1979;11:1387.

11. Rasmussen LN, Dirdal M, Birkebaek NH: "Covert toxocariasis" in a child treated with low-dose diethylcarbamazine. Acta Pediatr 1993;82:116.

12. Konate A, Duhamel O, Basset D, et al: Toxocariasis and functional intestinal disorders. Presentation of 4 cases. Gastroenterol Clin Biol 1996;20:909.

13. Calhoun FP: Intraocular invasion by the larva of the ascaris. Arch Ophthalmol 1937;18:963.

14. Wilder HC: Nematode endophthalmitis. Trans Am Acad Ophthalmol Otolaryngol 1950;55:99.

15. Nichols RL: The etiology of visceral larva migrans. I. Diagnostic morphology of infective second stage *Toxocara* larvae. J Parasitol 1956;42:349.

16. Ashton N: Communications: Larval granulomatosis of the retina due to *Toxocara*. Br J Ophthalmol 1960;44:129.

17. Irvine WC, Irvine AR: Nematode endophthalmitis—*Toxocara canis*. Report of a case. Am J Ophthalmol 1959;47:185.

18. Duguid IM: Communications: Chronic endophthalmitis due to *Toxocara*. Br J Ophthalmol 1961;45:705.

19. Duguid IM: Features of ocular infestation by *Toxocara*. Br J Ophthalmol 1961;45:789.

20. Perkins ES: Pattern of uveitis in children. Br J Ophthalmol 1966;50:169.

21. Ferguson EC, Olson LJ: *Toxocara* ocular nematodiasis. Int Ophthalmol Clin 1967;7:583.

22. Wilkinson CP, Welch RB: Intraocular *Toxocara*. Am J Ophthalmol 1971;71:921.

23. O'Connor PR: Visceral larva migrans of the eye. Subretinal tube formation. Arch Ophthalmol 1972;88:526.

24. Shields CL, Shields JA, Barrett J, et al: Vasoproliferative tumors of the ocular fundus. Arch Ophthalmol 1995;113:615.

25. Brown DH: The geography of ocular *Toxocara canis*. Ann Ophthalmol 1974;6:343.

26. Mok CH: Visceral larva migrans. Clin Pediatr 1968;7:565.

27. Raistrick ER, Hart JCD: Ocular toxocariasis in adults. Br J Ophthalmol 1976;60:365.

28. Hart JCD, Raistrick ER: Adult toxocariasis: Uniocular retinal lesion in the 20 to 50-year old group. Trans Ophthalmol Soc U K 1977;97:164.

29. Ellis GS, Pakalnis VA, Worley G, et al: *Toxocara canis* infestation: Clinical and epidemiologic associations with seropositivity in kindergarten children. Ophthalmology 1986;93:1032–1037.

30. Magnaval JF, Michault A, Calon N, et al: Epidemiology of human toxocariasis in la Reunion. Trans R Soc Trop Med Hyg 1994;88:531.

31. Pollard ZF, Jarret WH, Hagler WS, et al: ELISA for diagnosis of ocular toxocariasis. Ophthalmology 1979;86:743.

32. Kielar RA: *Toxocara canis* endophthalmitis with low ELISA titer. Ann Ophthalmol 1983;15:447.

33. Spencer WH: Vitreous. In: Spencer WH, ed: Ophthalmic Pathology. An Atlas and Textbook, 4th ed. Philadelphia, WB Saunders, 1996, pp 623–666.

34. Ghaffoor SYA, Smith HV, Lee WR, et al: Experimental ocular toxocariasis: A mouse model. Br J Ophthalmol 1984;68:89.

35. Liotet S, Bloch-Michel E, Petithory JC, et al: Biological modifica-

tions of the vitreous in intraocular parasitosis: Preliminary study. Int Ophthalmol 1992;16:75.

36. Watzke RC, Oaks JA, Folk JC: *Toxocara canis* infection of the eye: Correlation of clinical observations with developing pathology in the primate model. Arch Ophthalmol 1984;102:282.

37. Rockey JH, John T, Donnelly JJ, et al: In vitro interaction of eosinophils from ascarid-infected eyes with *Ascaris suum* and *Toxocara canis* larvae. Invest Ophthalmol Vis Sci 1983;24:1346.

38. Gillespie SH, Dinning WJ, Voller A, et al: The spectrum of ocular toxocariasis. Eye 1993;7:415.

39. Molk R: Ocular toxocariasis: A review of the literature. Ann Ophthalmol 1983;15:216.

40. Capone A, Aaberg TM: Intermediate uveitis. In: Albert DM, Jakobiec FA: Principles and Practice of Ophthalmology. Clinical Practice. Philadelphia, W.B. Saunders, 1994, pp 423–442.

41. Hogan MJ, Kimura SJ, O'Connor GR: Peripheral retinitis and chronic cyclitis in children. Trans Ophthalmol Soc U K 1966;85:39.

42. Smith PH, Greer CH: Unusual presentation of ocular *Toxocara* infestation. Br J Ophthalmol 1971;55:317.

43. Giles CL: Uveitis in childhood—part III. Posterior. Ann Ophthalmol 1989;21:23.

44. Hemady R, Sainz de la Maza M, Raizman MB, et al: Six cases of scleritis associated with systemic infection. Am J Ophthalmol 1992;114:55.

45. Sorr EM: Meandering ocular toxocariasis. Retina 1984;4:90.

46. Beiran I, Cochavi O, Miller B: "Silent" ocular toxocariasis. Eur J Ophthalmol 1998;8:195.

47. Hagler WS, Jarret H, Chang M: Rhegmatogenous retinal detachment following chorioretinal inflammatory disease. Am J Ophthalmol 1978;86:373.

48. Mulvihill A, Bowell R, Lanigan B, et al: Uniocular childhood blindness: A prospective study. J Pediatr Ophthalmol Strabismus 1997;34:111.

49. Cypress RH, Karol MH, Zidian JL, et al: Larva-specific antibodies in patients with visceral larva migrans. J Infect Dis 1977;135:633.

50. Glickman LT, Grieve RB, Lauria SS, et al: Serodiagnosis of ocular toxocariasis: A comparison of two antigens. J clin Pathol 1985;38:103.

51. Sharkey JA, McKay PS: Ocular toxocariasis in a patient with repeatedly negative ELISA titer to *Toxocara canis*. Br J Ophthalmol 1993;77:253.

52. Searl SS, Moazed K, Albert DM, et al: Ocular toxocariasis presenting as leukocoria in a patient with low ELISA titer to *Toxocara canis*. Ophthalmology 1981;88:1302.

53. Pollard ZF: Long term follow-up in patients with ocular toxocariasis as measured by ELISA titers. Ann Ophthalmol 1987;19:167.

54. Felberg NT, Shields JA, Federman JL: Antibody to *Toxocara canis* in the aqueous humor. Arch Ophthalmol 1981;99:1563.

55. Benitez del Castillo JM, Herreros G, Guillen JL: Bilateral ocular toxocariasis demonstrated by aqueous humor enzyme-linked immunosorbent assay. Am J Ophthalmol 1995;119:514.

56. Sakai R, Kawashima H, Shibui H: *Toxocara cati*-induced ocular toxocariasis. Arch Ophthalmol 1998;116:1686.

57. Wan WL, Cano MR, Pince KJ, et al: Echographic characteristics of ocular toxocariasis. Ophthalmology 1991;98:28.

58. Edwards MG, Pordell GR: Ocular toxocariasis studied by CT scanning. Radiology 1985;157:685.

59. Haik BG, Saint Louis L, Smith ME, et al: Computed tomography of the nonrhegmatogenous retinal detachment in the pediatric patient. Ophthalmology 1985;92:1133.

60. Shields JA, Parsons HM, Shields CL: Lesions simulating retinoblastoma. J Pediatr Ophthalmol Strabismus 1991;28:338.

61. Dinning WJ, Gillespie SH, Cooling RJ, et al: Toxocariasis: A practical approach to management ocular disease. Eye 1988;2:580.

62. Dietrich A, Auer H, Titti M, et al: Ocular toxocariasis in Austria. Dtsch Med Wochenschr 1998;123:626.

63. Maguire AM, Zarbin MA, Connor TB, et al: Ocular penetration of thiabendazole. Arch Ophthalmol 1990;108:1675.

64. Abdel-Latif S: Toxocaral chorioretinitis: Treatment of early cases with photocoagulation. Br J Ophthalmol 1973;57:700.

65. Belmont JB, Irvine A, Benson W, et al: Vitrectomy in ocular toxocariasis. Arch Ophthalmol 1982;100:1912.

66. Grand MG, Roper-Hall G: Pars plana vitrectomy for ocular toxocariasis. Retina 1981;1:258.

67. Werner JC, Ross RD, Green WR, et al: Pars plana vitrectomy and

subretinal surgery for ocular toxocariasis. Arch Ophthalmol 1999;117:532.

68. Small KW, McCuen BW, de Juan E, Machemer R: Surgical management of retinal traction caused by toxocariasis. Am J Ophthalmol 1989;108:10–14.

69. Hagler WS, Pollard ZF, Jarrett WH, Donnelly EH: Results of surgery for ocular *Toxocara canis.* Ophthalmology 1981;88:1081–1086.

70. Rodriguez A: Early pars plana vitrectomy in chronic endophthalmitis of toxocariasis. Graefes Arch Clin Exp Ophthalmol 1986;224:218–220.

39 — ASCARIASIS

Virender S. Sangwan

DEFINITION

Ascariasis is a helminthic infection of humans caused by the nematode *Ascaris lumbricoides*.[1] *A. lumbricoides* is a cosmopolitan parasite and the most prevalent and largest of the human helminths. The normal habitat of the adult worm is the jejunum. The infection is acquired by the ingestion of the embryonated eggs, and the larvae pass through a pulmonary migration phase for maturation.[1]

HISTORY

Ascaris is possibly the earliest recorded human helminth; it is referred to in texts from Mesopotamia, Greece, Rome, and China.[1] The worm was confused with the earthworm and described as such by the Greeks and the Romans. The genus *Ascaris* (from the Greek word "askaris," meaning "worm") was first described by Linnaeus in 1758. Goeze described the roundworm of the pig, *A. sum*, in 1758. Later Davaine (1877), Epstain (1892) and Grassi (1877) showed that *Ascaris* infection occurs by ingestion of the eggs, which mature into adult worms in the intestines.[2]

EPIDEMIOLOGY

In endemic areas, the prevalence of human infestation by *Ascaris* increases sharply during the first 2 to 3 years of age, remains at a maximum between the ages of 4 to 14 years, and declines in adults.[1] The prevalence of ascariasis worldwide is proportional to human population density, standards of education, level of sanitation and agricultural development, regional geoclimatic conditions, and personal and dietary habits of the people. Ascariasis is most prevalent in crowded rural areas. Of course, the lack of sanitary facilities aids fecal contamination of the soil and spread of infection. Primitive agricultural practices using fresh human feces as fertilizer, especially for the production of vegetables, are responsible for the high prevalence of ascariasis in certain regions of the world. Ascariasis is essentially a backyard and household infection primarily propagated by the seeding of the soil immediately around the house with eggs present in the droppings of small children, who, in turn, become reinfected from eggs in the soil during play.[3, 4]

It has been estimated that more than 1.4 billion individuals throughout the world are infected with *A. lumbricoides*.[4] The majority of the infections occur in Asia, with advanced countries having the lowest rates of infection. Ascariasis is highly endemic in China and Southeast Asia, with prevalence rates of 41% to 92%.[5] The prevalence in Japan dropped considerably after World War II: 70% to 80% until 1955, 13% in 1962, and 0.04% in 1992.[1] In the Indian subcontinent, ascariasis is highly endemic in Kashmir (70%), Bangladesh (82%), and Central and Southwest India (20% to 49%).[1] The overall prevalence of the infection in Africa varies from 15% to 27%. The prevalence is also high in Latin America and has not changed over the years.[6] In Europe, the prevalence is low in large cities but can be greater in rural areas, reaching 52% in some areas.[1] Ascariasis is the third most common helminth infection (after hookworm and *Trichuris trichiura* infections) in the United States.[7] Of the 4 million people infected in the United States, a large percentage are immigrants from developing countries, with infection rates of 20% to 60%.[8]

CLINICAL CHARACTERISTICS

Ascaris infects 25% of the world's population; however, most of these infections are without clinical disease. Clinical disease is mostly restricted to subjects with a heavy worm load. Because heavy infections typically occur in a small percentage of individuals, clinical disease is associated with a small minority of the infections. This minority, however, represents an estimated 1.2 to 2.0 million cases of clinical disease worldwide. It is estimated that around 20,000 deaths occur per year as a consequence of ascariasis.[9, 10]

Pulmonary Ascariasis

Pulmonary disease caused by *Ascaris* is due to larvae during their pulmonary migration and maturation. It presents as a self-limiting pneumonia lasting for 2 to 3 weeks and occurs 4 to 16 days after ingestion of the embryonated eggs.[11, 12] The disease is common in endemic zones associated with *Ascaris* infection and reinfection, and it is more severe with reinfections. Children are more susceptible to *Ascaris* pneumonia than adults. Seasonal attacks occur in Saudi Arabia after the onset of spring rains, restarting transmission of *Ascaris*.[13]

The pulmonary disease is caused by larvae in the terminal air spaces and bronchioles, which provoke infiltration with neutrophils, eosinophils, desquamation of epithelium, and exudation of serous fluids, leading to plugging of air spaces and consequent consolidation. The consolidation may affect limited lobules; however, in some cases, it may extend to a single lobe or even multiple lobes.

Ascaris pneumonia is common in children, presenting as sudden onset of fever, frequent spasms of cough and wheezing, dyspnea, and substernal distress. In heavy infection, cough is productive, with hemoptysis. Patients may be in status asthmaticus and require admission to an intensive care unit. An urticarial rash or angioneurotic edema may precede or accompany pulmonary manifestations. Abdominal symptoms, such as right quadrant pain and vomiting, may occur. Physical examination often simulates an atypical pneumonia. X-ray examination of the chest usually shows diffuse mottling and prominence of peribronchial regions. Eosinophilia is typically prominent. The filariform larvae of *A. lumbricoides* can usually be seen on sputum or gastric aspirate examination. Occasionally, there is some biochemical evidence of hepatocellular damage, suggesting larval liver disease.

Intestinal Ascariasis

The adult worm in the upper small bowel usually causes no symptoms and may be discovered through an incidental finding of ascaris eggs on stool examination or when someone presents after passing a worm in stools (or more dramatically through the mouth or nose or any of the body orifices).[14] Worms may appear as linear filling defects on routine barium meal examinations of the small bowel.[11] This is the usual story of a large group of people infected with low worm loads. Vague abdominal symptoms in the form of abdominal pain, distention, nausea, and occasional diarrhea are frequent in children with ascariasis in endemic regions; however, their causal relationship with intestinal ascariasis remains unclear.

Peritoneal Ascariasis

Ascarides may enter the peritoneal cavity through a gangrenous bowel filled to the bursting point with ascarides or through a perforation caused by typhoid, amebic, or tubercular ulcer. In a small percentage, the worms may be seen wandering in the peritoneum with the context of an intact bowel. In either of these conditions, the outcome usually is fatal peritonitis.[15] If patients survive, wandering peritoneal ascarides disintegrate, and a granulomatous reaction is elicited around the disintegrated worm and ascaris eggs. A chronic granulomatous peritonitis with adhesions simulating tubercular peritonitis occurs.[16]

Appendicular Ascariasis

In endemic areas, ascarides may enter the appendix lumen and reach its tip.[1] Acute appendicular colic and development of a gangrenous appendix tip follow, and the worm reaches the peritoneal cavity adjacent to the appendix. Worms may also partially exude through the perforation or lie inside the lumen of the appendix. Examination of such appendices after appendectomy reveals no inflammation of the mucosa of appendix.[14]

Hepatobiliary and Pancreatic Ascariasis

Hepatobiliary and pancreatic ascariasis (HPA) is one of the most common and well-described entities caused by ascaris.[1] Ascarides in the duodenum enter the ampullary orifice and can block it; they can advance further to the bile duct and hepatic ducts. While in the common duct, the cystic duct can be blocked by worms entering its orifice. Less often, worms can reach the gallbladder or enter the pancreatic duct. In HPA, ascarides reach the duodenum, either because of excessive worm load in the jejunum or abnormal mobility after an intestinal infection caused by viruses, bacteria, or other parasites. Ascarides have a great propensity to explore small openings and, while in the duodenum, enter the ampullary orifice. In fact, duodenoscopic examination in HPA often reveals worms moving actively in and out of the bile duct from the duodenum.

Until recently, diagnosis of HPA was made either at laparotomy or at autopsy. The magnitude of the problem of HPA in an endemic area was often underestimated[1] in the reported cases. The worms move actively in and out of the bile duct from the duodenum and usually are not present in the ducts at the time of surgery. In a prospective study, with the use of endoscopic retrograde cholangiopancreatography (ERCP) early in the disease, ascariasis was found as a cause of biliary or pancreatic diseases in 40 of 109 patients.[17, 18] Ascariasis was as common a causative factor as gallstones in biliary disease. From June 1983 to November 1989, 500 cases of HPA were reported from one center.[1] Since then, reports of HPA have increased from number of centers in endemic areas.[19–22]

HPA is more common in women than in men, with a mean age of occurrence around 35.0 years (range 4 to 70 years).[23] Children do suffer from HPA but less often than adults do. This is possibly due to the smaller size of the bile ductal system, making it difficult for the worms to enter.[24] Pregnant women are particularly prone to HPA, and the worm reaches the gallbladder more often than in nonpregnant women.[25] The majority of patients with HPA have had previous surgery on the biliary tree, including cholecystectomy, choledocholithotomy, or sphincteroplasty performed for gallstones. Endoscopic sphincterotomy predispose patients to HPA in endemic areas because of the widened ampullary orifice, which makes it easy for worms to pass into the bile ducts.[26]

Worms usually actively move out of the ductal system into the duodenum. Ultrasound examinations reveal that worms usually move out of the ducts within a week. If worms are present in the duct beyond 10 days and have not changed their position, they are usually dead and can form a nidus for bile duct calculi.

HPA can cause five distinct clinical presentations[27]:

- Biliary colic
- Acalculous cholecystitis
- Acute cholangitis
- Acute pancreatitis
- Hepatic abscess

Ocular Ascariasis

A few cases of ocular ascariasis have been reported.[27–30] Most of these cases represent visceral larva migrans caused by *Toxocara* species rather than by *A. lumbricoides.* In one report, two photographically documented cases showed an active ascaridoid larva in the retinal region, but because neither larva was identified microscopically as *Ascaris* species, it is likely that they belong to the *Toxocara* species.[27, 28] In another report, fragments of a larva obtained from the anterior chamber of the eye of an 8-year-old boy from northern Georgia were identified as *Ascaris,* but the description could not exclude the possibility of a *Toxocara larva.*[29] Similarly the larva obtained from the eye of a 4-year old European girl in Uganda was carefully examined histologically, but it could only be identified as an ascaridoid larva closely related to those of *Toxocaris* and *Baylisascaris.*[30]

In 1956, Kaplan and colleagues[31] reported extraction of an intact young adult *Ascaris* from the nasolacrimal duct of an 18-month-old African girl from Durban. Roche[32] reported a similar case in which an *Ascaris* worm was found in the duct.

Ascaris larvae do not develop in the eye, as was proved by animal experiments with intraocular injection of *Ascaris* ova.[33]

PATHOPHYSIOLOGY, IMMUNOLOGY, PATHOLOGY, AND PATHOGENESIS

Life Cycle

Fertilized eggs passed in the feces require 9 to 13 days for incubation and development of the active, first stage larvae.[34] The larvae undergo two molts. The third stage is the infective form (Fig. 39–1). Under favorable circumstances, eggs may remain viable and capable of infection for a period of months to more than 10 years. Boiling kills the *Ascaris* eggs within minutes.[34] However, eggs are resistant to the usual methods of chemical water purification and can even embryonate in such substances as 2% formalin, potassium dichromate, and 50% solutions of hydrochloric acid, acetic, nitric, or sulfuric acid.

When fully embryonated eggs are swallowed, on reaching the duodenum the larvae erupt from their shells and penetrate the wall to reach the liver by the portal venous system. They proceed from hepatic venules through the right side of the heart to the lungs and, after a delay of several days, break into the alveolar spaces. After increasing in size and molting to the fourth stage, the larvae transit the respiratory tree, pass the gastric barrier and arrive in the jejunum. They mature there and begin producing eggs within 60 to 65 days after being swallowed. The usual life span of an adult ascaris is approximately 1 year, and a single female may lay 200,000 eggs in 1 day.[34]

Immunology

A variety of studies have demonstrated that the capacity to expel nematodes from the intestine is immunologically mediated and, particularly, that $CD4^+$ Th cells are critical for worm expulsion.[35]

Investigation of cytokine production by Th cells during *T. muris* infection has shown that in strains which expel their worms, a predominant Th2 response is generated. This is reflected in the characteristic immune changes controlled by Th2 cytokines, which are associated with worm expulsion: mucosal mastocytosis, intestinal eosinophilia, elevated serum IgE levels, and elevated parasite-specific serum IgGI levels.[36] This is similar to observations made in other models of intestinal nematode infection in which the worms are expelled from the intestine (e.g., *Nippostrongylus brasiliensis, Trichinella spiralis,* and secondary infections by *Heligmosomoides polygyrus*).[35] In contrast, however, analysis of cytokine production in strains of mouse that did not expel *T. muris* showed that a dominant Th1 response became established. This factor was reflected by elevated levels of parasite-specific IgG2a antibody levels in the serum, a subclass controlled by interferon-γ (IFN-γ).

The critical importance of distinct cytokines in controlling worm expulsion and progression to chronic infection was demonstrated by the in vivo administration of cytokine or cytokine receptor–specific neutralizing monoclonal antibodies or recombinant cytokines to *T. muris*–infected animals. The data from these experiments showed that interleukin 4 (IL-4) was critical in host resistance to *T. muris*. Neutralization of its activity in vivo changed an animal from one that would expel the parasite into one that harbored a chronic infection. This was coincident with the suppression of a Th2 response and the induction of a Th1 response. IFN-γ was also shown to be critical for the progression to a chronic infection; injection of anti-IFN-γ antibodies into mice that would normally harbor a chronic infection changed their response status, and the animals then expelled their parasites. This was coincident with the depression of the Th1 response and elevation of a Th2 response.

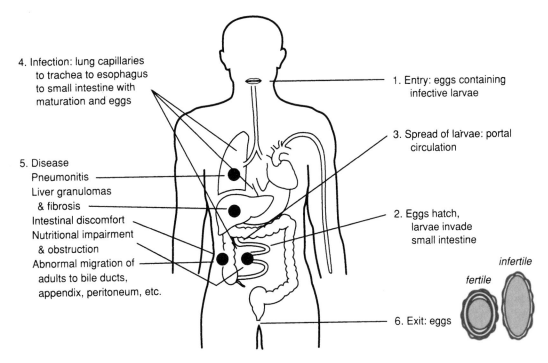

FIGURE 39–1. *Ascaris lumbricoides* life cycle. (From Baron S: Medical Microbiology, 3rd ed. New York, Churchill Livingstone, 1991, p 1113.)

The importance of the kinetics of the response can also be inferred from a series of experiments investigating the cells involved in expulsion of *T. muris*.[35] In these experiments, severe combined immunodeficiency disease mice were reconstituted with high (1×10^7) or low (0.5×10^7) numbers of lymphocytes from normal BALB/c mice. SCID recipients from high cell numbers were able to expel their parasites when infection coincided with the cell transfer. The expulsion of the parasites was associated with a dominant Th2 response.

Pathology

Larval migration often produces important histopathologic changes and symptoms.[34] The worms' passages through the liver rarely give rise to symptoms. If the larvae reach the general circulation, ectopic localization of the larvae in the kidneys, eyes, or central nervous system may rarely give rise to signs and symptoms referable to the parasitized organ. The lung is the site, as a rule, of the greatest damage produced by migrating larvae. Respiratory symptoms develop 26 hours to 5 days after the ingestion of viable eggs. In their passage from the vascular tree to the alveoli, the larvae often produce a bilateral patchy bronchopneumonia known as *Ascaris pneumonia* (Löffler's pneumonia), with edema, eosinophilia, and hemorrhage as the predominating histologic features.[34]

The intestinal mucosa reveals minute hemorrhages at places of larval penetration. Not all the larvae reach the lungs or the liver because they may die in intestinal mucosa. This results in focal areas of inflammation with infiltration of eosinophils and macrophages. In the hepatic sinusoids, mobile larvae do not elicit an inflammatory response. Dead larvae in the liver, however, simulate a granulomatous reaction. Larval migration may involve organs other than liver and lungs. Migration to the kidney, heart, and brain has been observed.

DIAGNOSIS

Gross and microscopic morphology of typical eggs or adult worms in the feces or vomitus are the primary clues to diagnosis.[34] Infertile eggs are not suspended by the zinc sulfate flotation technique, and an occasional case may be missed if this single procedure is used. *Ascaris* eggs first appear in the feces 60 to 75 days after exposure. The eggs may be fertilized or unfertilized.[1] They have a characteristic size and shape, and can be diagnosed easily on a direct smear.[1]

Ascaris pneumonia is confirmed by the radiographic picture of a diffuse, mottled pulmonary infiltrate, together with the identification of third-stage larvae in the sputum. During the stage of pulmonary invasion, high eosinophilia is usually seen. Eosinophilia of 10% or more commonly accompanies ascariasis, but its absence does not rule out the possibility of the infection, particularly when active invasion by larvae has ceased. The easiest and most economical method of investigation is a plain film of the abdomen; in the South African series, this test could confirm the presence of worms in the right hypocondrium in most patients.[37]

On barium-contrast radiographs, ascarids are occasionally discerned in the jejunum or ileum.[34] When they are seen in the intestine, the parasite produces a sharply outlined radioluscency, within which the barium in the worm's intestinal tract appears as a filamentous radiopacity. Worms in the duodenum can be seen entering the ampulla of Vater, the part of the worm within the biliary tree being invisible; this is known as the ampullary cut-off sign.[38]

Ultrasonography and ERCP can help in the diagnosis of HPA. The characteristic sonographic findings of worms in the ducts have been well described.[19, 39] The worms in the gallbladder have much more characteristic appearances and can be identified with ease. The findings of pancreatic ascariasis on ultrasonography are edematous pancreatitis and the four-line sign indicative of the worm and its intestinal tract. Ultrasonography is a highly sensitive and specific method of detection of worms in the biliary tree. However, ultrasonography cannot diagnose duodenal ascariasis; if ultrasonography was used as a screening method, more than half of the patients with HPA would be missed.[23]

ERCP has an advantage as a diagnostic tool in that it permits identification of the worms in the duodenum and those across the papilla. Ascaris in the ducts present as smooth, linear filling defects. ERCP, in addition, has therapeutic potential, facilitating removal of worms from the ducts or the duodenum.[21, 40]

For diagnosis of intraocular disease, a high degree of suspicion is required because it is exceedingly rare. Pars plana vitrectomy may be diagnostic and therapeutic.

TREATMENT

Several drugs are available (Table 39–1) and effective for the treatment of ascariasis. Pyrantel pamoate, mebendazole, and albendazole, however, are drugs of first choice against ascariasis. Parasite immobilization and death of the helminth are slow, and complete clearance of the worm from the gastrointestinal tract may take up to 3 days. Efficacy depends on worm load, strain, pre-existing diarrhea, and gastrointestinal transit time.

In the rare case of ocular involvement, topical anti-inflammatory therapy may be indicated in addition to systemic treatment.

Pyrantel Pamoate

Pyrantel, a cyclic amidine, is a depolarizing neuromuscular blocking agent that results in spastic paralysis of the worm. It also inhibits cholinesterase. It is poorly absorbed, and 50% is excreted in the feces as unchanged drug. Seven percent or less of the dose is found in urine as parent drug and metabolites. It is effective against ascariasis and enterobiasis. The drug is contraindicated

TABLE 39–1. DRUGS USED IN TREATMENT OF ASCARIASIS

DRUGS	DOSE
Pyrantel pamoate	10 mg/kg single dose PO; maximum 1.0 g
Mebendazole	100 mg PO bid × 3 days
Albendazole	400 mg PO (single dose)
Levamisole	120 mg base PO single dose; children 5.0 mg/kg
Piperazine citrate	75 mg/kg qd × 2 days; maximum, 3.5 g

in patients with hepatic disease and during pregnancy. A single dose of 10 mg/kg body weight is taken; purge is advised. Adverse reactions such as anorexia, nausea, vomiting, abdominal cramps, and diarrhea are common. Rarely headache, dizziness, drowsiness, and insomnia may occur. Parasite immobilization and death of the helminth are slow, and complete clearance of the worm from the gastrointestinal tract may take up to 3 days.

Mebendazole
Mebendazole, a benzimidazole carbonate, inhibits the formation of the worm's microtubules and irreversibly blocks glucose uptake by the helminth, thereby depleting the endogenous glycogen stored within the parasite, which it requires for survival and reproduction. Mebendazole has no effect on the glucose level in the host. In addition to ascariasis, mebendazole is effective against *T. trichiura, Enterobius vermicularis, Ancylostoma duodenale,* and *Necator americanus.* In view of its widespread effectiveness, mebendazole is the drug of choice as a broad-spectrum antihelminthic. Mebendazole is embryotoxic and teratogenic in pregnant rats, and it is not recommended for use in pregnant women. Adverse reactions such as transient abdominal pain and diarrhea, with massive infection and expulsion of worms, have occurred in patients. Neutropenia and abnormal liver function tests occur in 5% of patients with intake of large doses. A dose of 100 mg twice daily orally for 3 days is recommended. No special procedure such as fasting or purge is required. If the patient is not cured 3 weeks after treatment, a second course is advised.

Albendazole
Albendazole, methyl 5n-propoxythio-2-benzimidazole carbamate, has an exceptionally broad spectrum of antiparasitic activity. It has the advantage of being effective when given as a single dose for the treatment of *A. lumbricoides.* Therefore, albendazole is ideally suited for mass treatment programs. Periodic treatment with albendazole has been shown to improve the nutritional status of malnourished children with multiple species of intestinal helminths.

Albendazole, like other benzimidazoles, inhibits the assembly of tubulin into microtubules and impairs the uptake of glucose, leading to the depletion of glycogen stores in helminths. It also inhibits helminthic-specific fumarate reductase.

Albendazole is usually well tolerated when given as a single 400-mg dose for the treatment of intestinal nematodes. Diarrhea, abdominal discomfort, or migration of *Ascaris* through the nose or mouth occurs occasionally. High-dose prolonged therapy is occasionally complicated by serum transaminase elevation, bone marrow suppression with neutropenia or thrombocytopenia, or less commonly, alopecia. In view of the potential teratogenicity of benzimidazole compounds, albendazole is contraindicated during pregnancy.

Piperazine
Piperazine derivatives temporarily paralyze the *Ascaris* worms by producing neuromuscular blockage through an anticholinergic action at the myoneural junction; the peristaltic movement of the intestine easily evacuates the paralyzed worms. Piperazine, which has been widely used for more than 25 years for treatment of ascariasis and enterobiasis, is now being withdrawn from the market in developed countries because of sporadic hypersensitive and neurotoxic reactions and because better drugs have been introduced. In developing countries, piperazine is still widely used because it is one of the least expensive drugs available. The daily dose is 75 mg/kg body weight, with a maximum individual dose of 5 g for adults and 2 g for children under 20 kg in weight. The efficacy of a single-dose treatment is 80%, and treatment for 2 consecutive days is effective in more than 90% of ascariasis cases. Patients must not receive concomitant chlorpromazine; convulsions are known to occur, which may occasionally be fatal.

Levamisole
Levamisole, a levorotatory s-isomer of tetramisole, is a potent inhibitor of fumarate reductase activity, which is an enzyme essential in the carbohydrate metabolism of *Ascaris.* Levamisole, which is practically devoid of toxicity for humans, shows nonspecific activation of macrophages and some immunomodulating activities. Used in a single dose of 150 mg for adults and 5 mg/kg in children, it is effective in 96% of patients with ascariasis.

None of the antihelminthics used in treatment of adult worms in the intestinal tract have been proved effective in killing the larvae during their migration phase.

COMPLICATIONS
Systemic complications related to ascariasis include protein-energy malnutrition, retarded growth, intestinal obstruction, perforation, or volvulus. Although ascariasis is a benign condition, migration of worms to extraintestinal sites can be fatal. Migration occurs in response to antihelminthic drugs, purgatives, intercurrent illness, and often without any cause. The propensity for worms to invade the biliary tree is a result of their preference to migrate through small orifices. It may produce biliary colic, acute cholangitis, acute pancreatitis, and hepatic ascariasis (Hong Kong liver).[34]

CONCLUSIONS
Ascariasis is a helminthic infection of global distribution, with more than 1.04 billion persons infected worldwide. The majority of infections occur in the developing countries of Asia and Latin America. Of 4 million people infected in the United States, a large percentage are immigrants from developing countries. *Ascaris*-related clinical disease is restricted to subjects with heavy worm load, and an estimated 1.2 to 2 million such cases, with 20,000 deaths, occurs in endemic areas per year. More often, recurring moderate infection causes stunting of linear growth, causes reduced cognitive function, and aggravates existing malnutrition in children in endemic areas.

References
1. Khroo, MS: Ascariasis. Gastroenterol Clin North Am 1990;25:553–577.
2. Sun T: Ascariasis. In: Sun T, ed: Pathology and Clinical Features of Parasitic Diseases. New York, Masson, 1980, pp 115–120.

3. Ascariasis (Edit). Lancet 1989;1:997.

4. Crompton DWT: The prevalence of ascariasis. Parasitol Today 1988;4:162.

5. Thein H: A profile of ascariasis morbidity in Rangoon Children's Hospital, Burma. J Trop Med Hyg 1987;90:165.

6. Botero D: Epidemiology and public health importance of intestinal nematode infections in Latin America. Prog Drug Res 1975;19:28.

7. Nesse RE, Bratton RL: Ascariasis, an infection to watch for in immigrants. Postgrad Med 1993;93:171.

8. Intestinal protozoan and helminthic infections: Report of WHO Scientific Group. WHO Technical Report Series 666. Geneva, World Health Organization, 1981.

9. Crompton DWT, Nesheim MC, Pawlowski ZS: Ascariasis and Its Public Health Significance. London, Taylor & Francis, 1995.

10. Pawlowski ZS, Davies A: Morbidity and mortality in ascariasis. In: Crompton DWT, Nesheim MC, Pawlowski ZS, eds: Ascariasis and Its Prevention and Control. London, Taylor & Francis, 1989, pp 45–69.

11. Phillis JA, Harrold AJ, Whiteman GV, et al: Pulmonary infiltrates, asthma and eosinophilia due to ascaris sum infestation in man. N Engl J Med 1972;286:965.

12. Spillman RK: Pulmonary ascariasis in tropical communities. Am J Trop Med Hyg 1975;24:791.

13. Gelpi AP, Mustafa A: Seasonal pneumonitis with eosinophilia: A study of larval ascariasis in Saudi Arabia. Am J Trop Med Hyg 1967;6:646.

14. Paul M: The movements of the adult *Ascaris lumbriocoides*. Br J Surg 1972;59:437.

15. Efm SEE: *Ascaris lumbricoides* and intestinal perforation. Br J Surg 1987;74:643.

16. Ochoia B: Surgical complications of ascariasis. World J Surg 1991;15:222.

17. Khuroo MS, Mahajan R, Zargar SA, et al: Prevalence of biliary tract disease in India: A sonographic study in adult population in Kashmir. Gut 1989;30:201.

18. Khuroo MS, Zargar SA: Biliary ascariasis: A common cause of biliary and pancreatic disease in an endemic area. Gastroenterology 1985;88:418.

19. Desai S, Topin K: Biliary ascariasis: Sonographic findings. Am J Roentgenol 1995;164:767.

20. Maddem GJ, Dennison AR, Blumgart LH: Fatal ascaris pancreatitis: An uncommon problem in the West. Gut 1992;33:402.

21. Saraswat VA, Gupta R, Dhiman RK, et al: Biliary ascariasis: Endoscopic extrication of a living worm from the bile duct. Endoscopy 1993;25:553.

22. Schulman A: Intrahepatic biliary stones: Imaging features and a possible relationship with *Ascaris lumbricoides*. Clin Radiol 1993;47:325.

23. Khuroo MS, Zargar SA, Mahajan R: Hepatobiliary and pancreatic ascariasis in India. Lancet 1990;335:1503.

24. Zargar SA, Khuroo MS: Management of biliary ascariasis in children. Ind J Gastroenterol 1990;9:321.

25. Khuroo MS, Zagar SA, Yattoo GN, et al: Sonographic findings in gallbladder ascariasis. J Clin Ultrasound 1990;20:587.

26. Khuroo MS, Dar MY, Yatto GN, et al: Biliary and pancreatic ascariasis: A longterm follow-up. Natl Med J India 1989;2:4.

27. Price AJ Jr, Wadsworth JAC: An intraretinal worm. Arch Ophthalmol 1970;83:768–770.

28. Parson HE: Nematode chorioretinitis: Report of case, with photographs of viable worm. Arch Ophthalmol 1953;47:799–800.

29. Calhoun FP: Intraocular invasion by the larva of the Ascaris. Arch Ophthalmol 1937;18:963–970.

30. Beaver PC, Bowman DD: Ascaridoid larva (nematoda) from the eye of a child in Uganda. Am J Trop Med Hyg 1984;33:1272–1274.

31. Kaplan CS, Freedman L, Elsdon-Dew R: A worm in the eye: A familiar parasite in an unusual situation. S Afr Med J 1956;30:791–792.

32. Roche PJL: Ascaris in the lacrimal duct. Trans R Soc Trop Med Hyg 1971;65:540.

33. Chowdhry AB, Kean BH, Browne HG: Inoculation of helminth eggs into animal eyes. Am J Pathol 1960;36:725–733.

34. Monroe LS: Gastrointestinal parasites. In: Haubrich WS, Schaffner F, eds: Bockus Gastroenterology, 5th ed., Vol 4. Philadelphia, W.B. Saunders, 1995, pp 3113–3196.

35. Grencis RK: T cell and cytokine basis of host variability in response to intestinal nematode infections. Parasitology 1996;112:S31–S37.

36. Else KJ, Grencis RK: Cellular immune response to the nematode parasite *Trichuris muris*. Differential cytokine production during acute or chronic infection. Immunology 1991;72:508–513.

37. Lloyd DA: Hepatobiliary ascariasis in children. Surg Ann 1982;14:277–297.

38. Lloyd DA: Massive hepatobiliary ascariasis in childhood. Br J Surg 1980;68:468–474.

39. Khuroo MS, Zargar SA, Mahajan R, et al: Sonographic appearances in biliary ascariasis. Gastroenterology 1987;93:267.

40. Khuroo MS, Zagar SA, Yattoo GN, et al: Worm extraction and biliary drainage in hepatobiliary and pancreatic ascariasis. Gastrointest Endosc 1993;39:680.

Martin Filipec

DEFINITION

Onchocerciasis is an infectious disease caused by a filarial parasite, *Onchocerca volvulus*. The disease is transmitted by an insect (fly) of the genus *Simulium*. Man is the natural and definitive host of the parasite. The areas of endemic onchocerciasis include equatorial Africa, some regions of Central and South America, and the Eastern Mediterranean, typically in the vicinity of rivers with fast-flowing water, which are breeding sites of the vector flies. Clinical manifestations include characteristic dermatologic involvement, ocular lesions and lymphatic obstruction due to the presence of microfilariae; and subcutaneous nodules caused by adult worms. Blindness is the major disability in onchocerciasis. Approximately 17.7 million individuals are afflicted by this disease—270,000 are blind and another 500,000 have serious visual impairment.

HISTORY

The first description of onchocerciasis was published by John O'Neil[1] in 1875, who described the presence of microfilariae in the skin of Africans living along the Gold Coast (Ghana) who suffered from a disease known locally as "craw-craw."[1] Leuckart, in 1893, described two samples from subcutaneous nodules and named the parasite *Filaria vovulus*.[2] The classification of the *Onchocerca* parasite was made in 1910 with Leuckart's *"Filaria volvulus"* named for the first time, *Onchocerca volvulus*.[3] Pacheco-Luna in 1919[4] and Robles in 1919[5] were the first to associate blindness in America with onchocerciasis and to describe the inflammatory changes in the anterior segment of the eye. Brumpt described the eye disease–causing organism and named the parasite *Onchocerca caecutiens* (blinding).[6] It was demonstrated that *Onchocerca caecutiens* is identical to the previously described *Onchocerca volvulus*.[3] The first description of intraocular microfilariae was made by Juan Luis Torroella, a Mexican ophthalmologist, in 1931.[7] The first report of blindness due to onchocerciasis in Africa was published by Hisette in 1932.[8] He also observed the chorioretinal lesions to be described later by Bryant.[9] A comprehensive description of the ocular manifestations of onchocerciasis, especially those of onchochorioretinitis, was provided in 1945 by Ridley, a British ophthalmologist serving the British army on the Gold Coast of Africa.[10]

In 1902, notions regarding disease transmission were stimulated by Brumpt's suggestion that flies might be responsible for nodule formation.[11] The entomologic description of the blackfly belonging to the genus *Simulium* was reported by Roubaud in 1906.[12] However, it was not until 1926 that Blacklock definitely confirmed *Simulium damnosum* as the vector, with the observation of the development of larval stages of *O. volvulus* in this blackfly.[13]

Up until the 1970s, there were few scientists throughout the world studying onchocerciasis.[14] In 1953, the Expert Committee on Onchocerciasis was established by the World Health Organization (WHO). In its first report in 1954, the Committee attempted to unify terminology and suggested a plan for future research in the field of onchocerciasis and its control.[15] Vector control was shown to be effective in Kenya in 1947 with the use of DDT.[16] With new insights as to the pathogenesis and immunology of this disease, new therapeutic modalities have been developed, providing possible strategies for the control of onchocerciasis. The Onchocerciasis Control Program (OCP) began its operations in 1974 in seven countries in West Africa with extensive larviciding. In 1987, ivermectin, a new, safe, and effective drug suitable for large-scale treatment, became available through a donation by the drug manufacturer Merck and Co., Inc. "for as long as necessary to as many as necessary."

EPIDEMIOLOGY

Onchocerciasis is second to trachoma, the most common infectious cause of blindness worldwide.[17] Ninety-nine percent of all individuals affected by onchocerciasis (and blind because of this disease) live in Africa.[18] The prevalence of the disease has decreased dramatically during the past 20 years in African countries where the OCP operates. On the other hand, in countries outside the OCP and in America, onchocerciasis remains a major public health problem. The epidemiology of onchocerciasis, the distribution of different patterns of the disease, and the type of ocular pathology are dependent on geographic, environmental, and ecologic factors; the type of parasite; the capacity of the vector to transmit the infection; and individual genetic factors and the types of activity within the community.[18] Whenever the blindness rate in the community exceeds 5%, the disease has a deleterious impact, not only on the physical and psychological life of infected individuals, but also on family and community life. The life expectancy of people blinded as the result of onchocerciasis is reduced by approximately 10 to 13 years. The economic life of the whole community deteriorates as entire villages may relocate to areas with a lower risk of infection, but usually with poorer conditions to support subsistence agriculture.[18]

Geographic Distribution

Onchocerciasis is endemic in 34 countries throughout the world. Twenty-eight of these are located in Africa and in the Eastern Mediterranean region (Angola, Benin, Burkina Faso, Burundi, Cameroon, Central African Republic, Chad, Congo, Côte d'Ivoire, Equatorial Guinea, Ethiopia, Gabon, Ghana, Guinea, Guinea-Bissau, Liberia, Malawi, Mali, Niger, Nigeria, Senegal, Sierra Leone, Sudan, Togo, Uganda, Tanzania, Yemen, and Zaire) (Fig. 40–1), and six are in Central and South America (Brazil, Colombia, Ecuador, Guatemala, Mexico, and Venezuela) (Fig. 40–2). The last WHO Report, from 1995,[18] estimates that 122.9 million people worldwide are at risk of infection, 17.7 million are infected, and 270,000 are blind; another 500,000 people are severely visually impaired (Table 40–1). These figures are rough estimates, and

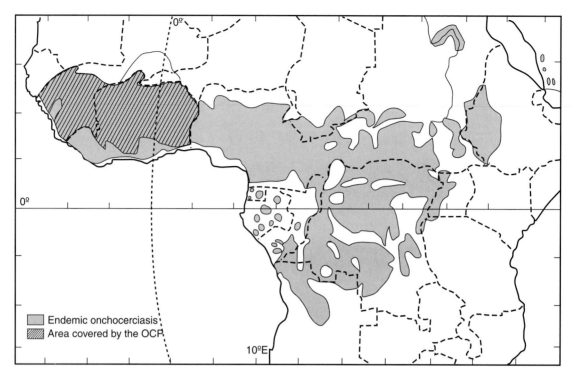

FIGURE 40–I. Geographic distribution of onchocerciasis in Africa and Arabian peninsula. (From Report of a WHO Expert Committee on Onchocerciasis Control. WHO Technical Report Series No 852, p 26, WHO, Geneva, 1995.)

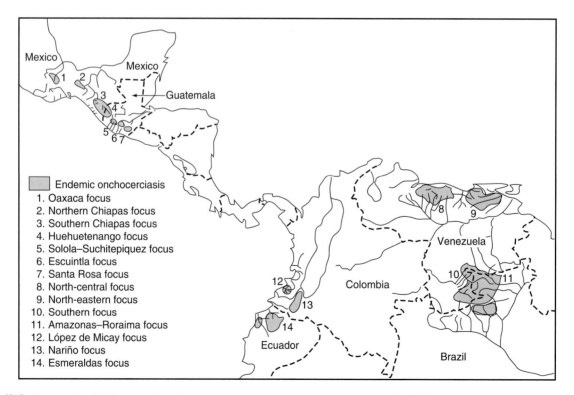

FIGURE 40–2. Geographic distribution of onchocerciasis in the Americas. (From Report of a WHO Expert Committee on Onchocerciasis Control. WHO Technical Report Series No 852, p 27, WHO, Geneva, 1995.)

TABLE 40–1. GLOBAL ESTIMATES OF THE POPULATION AT RISK, INFECTED, AND BLIND BECAUSE OF ONCHOCERCIASIS

REGION	POPULATION AT RISK OF INFECTION (MILLIONS)	POPULATION INFECTED	NUMBER BLIND AS A RESULT OF ONCHOCERCIASIS
Africa			
OCP area:			
Original area	17.6*	10,032	17,650
Extensions	6.0	2,230,000	31,700
non-OCP area:	94.5	15,246,800	217,850
Arabian peninsula	0.1	30,000	0
Americas	4.7	140,455	750
Total	122.9	17,657,287	267,950

OCP = onchocerciasis control program.
*The population given is that which would have been at risk had the OCP not existed.
From Report of a WHO Expert Committee on Onchocerciasis Control. Technical Report Series No 852, p 30. WHO, Geneva, 1995.

comparisons with previous reports are difficult. They are almost certainly an underestimate, as there are no accurate data available from many countries.

Endemicity

To study endemicity and the impact of onchocerciasis on the population, one must evaluate many factors.[19] The most common indicators used in onchocerciasis epidemiology are the prevalence of infection (percentage of active infection in the population), mean microfilaria density (MFD) in skin biopsy specimens, annual transmission potential (ATP), annual biting rate, prevalence of blindness, specific ocular lesions, and demographic data. ATP is the total number of infective L3 larvae that would be transmitted in 1 year to an individual exposed at a capture point for 11 hours per day. The annual biting rate is the total number of bites that would be received in 1 year by an individual exposed at a capture point for 11 hours per day.[18] According to the prevalence of infection, the level of endemicity in the area can be established. Areas with a prevalence of infection lower than 35% are considered hypoendemic. Areas with a prevalence higher than 60% are considered hyperendemic, and mesoendemic areas exhibit a prevalence of between 35% and 60%.[20] Different approaches with varying levels of expense can be used to establish the prevalence of infection in a particular target population. Comparing the use of Small Sample Survey (SSS) on a sample of 390 at-risk persons

and Complete Enumeration Survey (CES) on 1529 people in the same population (using MFD as the target indicator), it was shown that the low-cost SSS gives similar results to the more costly CES.[21]

Demographic Factors

The relatively small number of areas with a high level of endemicity in Central and South America does not correspond to the large density of blackflies in the region. This is probably a consequence of the low population density.[18] The risk for populations from nonendemic areas who migrate to a hyperendemic area is much greater than that for individuals living in long-established onchocerciasis areas.[22] The prevalence of onchocerciasis in this population can be as high as 90%, and the number of ocular complications can reach almost the same level.[23] The first exposure to transmission may be a risk factor for populations from nonendemic areas.[23]

Ecology and Biology of Onchocerciasis

Onchocerciasis occurs typically in areas with a hot climate near the equator. *Onchocerca volvulus* is transmitted by *Simulium* blackflies, and the disease is limited by the requirements of the blackfly for an appropriate breeding habitat, that is, nonpolluted fast-flowing streams and rivers (0.4 to 0.5 m/sec) with highly oxygenated water and submerged vegetation (e.g., tree trunks) and islands that provide support for the eggs and the development of larvae (Fig. 40–3). A hot climate is necessary for *Oncho-*

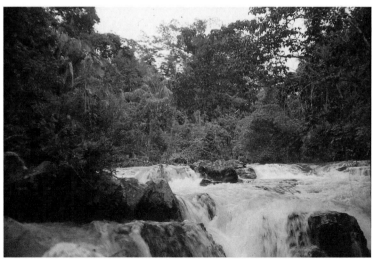

FIGURE 40–3. Typical breeding site of *Simulium* in Upper Ocamo, Venezuela.

TABLE 40–2. CLINICAL NONOCULAR MANIFESTATIONS OF ONCHOCERCIASIS

	GENERALIZED	LOCALIZED
SKIN	Pruritus Papules, macules, urticaria, edema Excoriations, pustules, crusts Scaling ulceration Lichenification ("lizard skin") Atrophy Hyper-, hypopigmentation ("leopard skin")	Acute: people from non-endemic areas Chronic: reactive onchodermatitis ("sowda")
NODULES		
LYMPHATIC	Lymphadenopathy Lymphedema, elephantiasis "Hanging groin," "hottentot apron"	

Adapted from Report of a WHO Expert Committee on Onchocerciasis Control. Technical Report Series No 852, pp 17–18. WHO, Geneva, 1995.

cerca volvulus to quickly develop into L3 stage larvae within the short lifetime of the blackfly host. The intensity of parasite transmission is related to the proportion of blackfly survival after the infective blood meal, the number of infective stage L3 microfilariae per fly, and the biting rate of the fly vector.[24, 25] The altitude may also play an important role in the endemicity status of a particular location. For example, southern Venezuelan communities located below 150 meters above sea level are hypo- or mesoendemic, but those above 150 meters are all hyperendemic. This corresponds to the predominant presence in the more elevated regions of *Simulium guianense* with a high daily biting rate.[26]

CLINICAL FEATURES

The most common clinical manifestations of onchocerciasis involve the skin (Table 40–2) and eye (Table 40–3). Less common are the lesions of the lymphatic draining system associated with hanging groin, hottentot apron, hernias, and elephantiasis (see Table 40–2). An association with other infections and diseases such as lepromatous leprosy,[27] filaria *Mansonella perstans*,[28, 29] epilepsy,[30, 31] and dwarfism (Nakalanga syndrome)[31] has been re-

ported. A matched case-controlled study did not demonstrate a statistically significant relationship between onchocerciasis and epilepsy.[32]

Skin Lesions

Onchocercal dermatitis is the most common manifestation of onchocerciasis. Skin changes are now classified as acute papular onchodermatitis (APOD), chronic papular onchodermatitis (CPOD), lichenified onchodermatitis (LOD), atrophy (ATR), and depigmentation (DPM).[33] Many infected persons are asymptomatic. In some individuals, especially those from nonendemic areas, pruritus may be the only symptom of onchocerciasis.

Acute papular onchodermatitis develops within 6 months to 2 years after infection and is accompanied by very intense itching (gale filarienne). APOD may be accompanied by erythema and skin edema. Secondary infection of these lesions due to scratching is common. Itching and APOD are typical manifestations of infected individuals from nonendemic areas. APOD may disappear quickly or may spread to become vesicular and pustular. The sites of highest predilection are the shoulders, arms, and trunk (Fig. 40–4).

Chronic papular onchodermatitis is characterized by papules, various degrees of itching, and postinflammatory hyperpigmentation (Fig. 40–5). The typical localization of CPOD is on the buttocks, waist area, and shoulders. Involvement of the face ("erispela de la costa") and purplish eruption on the upper body ("mal morado"), described as typical in Central America, are in fact very rare.

Lichenified onchodermatitis is characterized by itching, hyperpigmentation, and hyperkeratosis (lizard skin). LOD is localized preferentially on the limbs and buttocks and is often asymmetric. Atrophy of the skin (presbydermia), localized mostly on buttocks and limbs, is accompanied by loss of elasticity, excessive wrinkling, and scarring (Fig. 40–6).

Depigmentation is typically localized to the pretibial regions when it is described as "leopard skin" (Fig. 40–7). Depigmented areas, together with hyperpigmentation, especially around the hair follicles and normal skin, can be observed.

In the Sudan, Yemen, Guatemala, and Ecuador,[34] a more severe, localized variety of onchodermatitis, known

TABLE 40–3. CLINICAL OCULAR MANIFESTATIONS OF ONCHOCERCIASIS

ANTERIOR SEGMENT	POSTERIOR SEGMENT
Conjunctiva	Retina
Hyperemia	RPE atrophy
Limbitis	Intraretinal deposits
Chemosis	Cotton-wool spots
Nodules	Hemorrhage
Cornea	Hyperpigmentation
Live microfilariae, dead	Choroid
microfilariae	Choriocapillary atrophy
Punctate keratitis, sclerosing	Subretinal fibrosis
keratitis	Pigment hyperplasia,
Anterior chamber, iris	chorioretinitis
Live microfilariae, anterior	Optic nerve
uveitis	Optic neuritis, optic atrophy
Secondary glaucoma	Visual function
Lens	Night blindness, visual field loss
Secondary cataract	Visual impairment, blindness

RPE = retinal pigment epithelium.
Adapted from Report of a WHO Expert Committee on Onchocerciasis Control. Technical Report Series No 852, pp 17–18. WHO, Geneva, 1995.

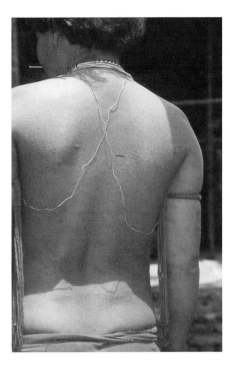

FIGURE 40–4. Acute papular onchodermatitis in an 18-year-old Yano-mami girl, Venezuela. (See color insert.)

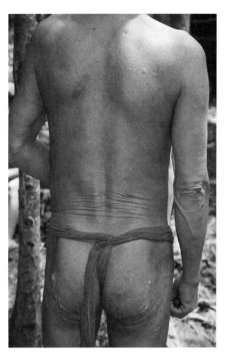

FIGURE 40–6. Atrophic skin with loss of elasticity and excessive wrinkling in a 34-year-old Yanomami man, Venezuela.

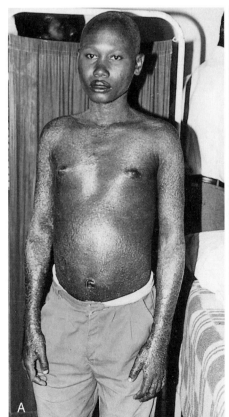

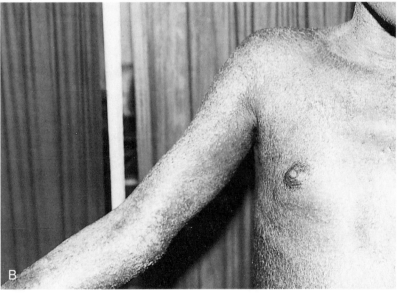

FIGURE 40–5. Chronic papular onchodermatitis (CPOD). (Photo courtesy of E.M. Pedersen.) (See color insert.)

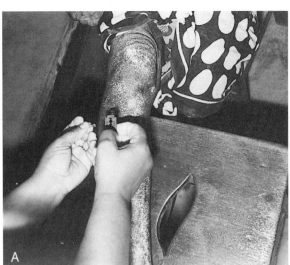
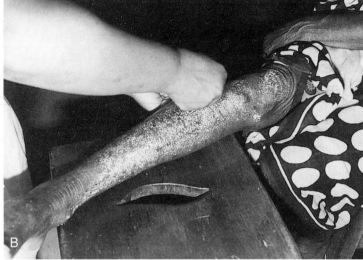

FIGURE 40–7. Pretibial skin depigmentation (leopard skin). (Photo courtesy of P. Magnussen.)

by the Arabic name "sowda" (from the Arabic for "black"), has been described, usually with extensive involvement of one limb. The skin is itchy, swollen, and dark, with scaling papules and pronounced regional lymphadenopathy. The presence of microfilariae in the skin of "sowda" patients is, in comparison with African onchocerciasis, rare.[35]

Nodules (onchocercomata)

Onchocercomata are subcutaneous nodules containing adult worms. They are painless, round to oval lesions that are either movable or fixed to the periosteum or joint capsule. Their size ranges from a few millimeters to several centimeters in diameter. Although most nodules are visible or at least palpable, some are localized deeply and are not easily detectable. New nodules have a tendency to form in the vicinity of old ones. There is variable localization of the nodules in different endemic locations. In Africa, the nodules are most common over bony prominences of the pelvis (iliac crest, coccyx, sacrum, and greater trochanter of the femur). Less common is localization on the knees, abdomen, chest wall (Fig. 40–8), and head. In Central America, the nodules tend to be localized above the waist and around the head. Histologically, the nodules contain a firm fibrous capsule that encases the adult worm. An inflammatory infiltrate of varying intensity (polymorphonuclear to epithelioid cells, macrophages, and giant cells)[34] may form around the worm.

Pathology of the Lymphatic System

Lymph nodes in patients with onchocerciasis may become fibrotic with reduction of germinal centers. Microfilariae, macrophages, plasma cells, eosinophils, and mast cells may be present.[34] Obstruction of lymphatic vessels, with the development of elephantiasis, is not typical for onchocerciasis. Lymphedema can be present in the inguinal or femoral area, producing the phenomenon known as "hanging groin" in males and "hottentot apron" in females.

Ocular Lesions

Ocular signs and symptoms develop primarily because dead microfilariae are present in the eye. Even a high number of living microfilariae are well tolerated in the eye. Observation of microfilariae in the cornea is possible by slit-lamp examination with high magnification or retro-illumination.[36] Dead worms are easily visualized because they are straight and opaque in the cornea. Intraretinal microfilariae can be seen by direct ophthalmoscopy and by three-mirror contact lens examination in which they appear as small reflective opacities with an apple-green tint.[37]

Typical subjective complaints of patients with onchocerciasis include photophobia, tearing, foreign body sensation, pain, and decreased visual acuity.

Conjunctiva

Limbal edema and hyperemia may be present in patients with keratitis punctata. Heavy pigment accumulation close to the areas of corneal involvement has also been

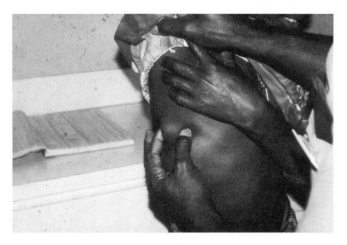

FIGURE 40–8. Subcutaneous nodule (onchocercoma). (Photo courtesy A. Rothova.)

observed.[38] Chronic conjunctivitis with the presence of microfilariae in the conjunctival biopsy specimens of 15 of 25 patients has been described in the Congo. Small, round, 0.5- to 2-mm-diameter nodules may be present in the bulbar conjunctiva.[39] In one case, a microfilaria was found in such a nodule.[40]

Cornea

Punctate keratitis is an early manifestation of corneal involvement in younger patients (average age, 24.6 years).[41] The appearance of corneal changes on slit-lamp examination is characterized by 0.5- to 1.5-mm "snow-flakes" or "fluffy" punctate grayish opacities around dead microfilariae, mainly in the anterior stroma. Up to 50 lesions in one cornea were observed.[42] Punctate keratitis is usually seen after the initiation of microfilaricidal treatment; dead filariae can be observed in the center of the lesion. Opacities are usually transitory with minimal visual impairment.[43] Sclerosing keratitis is associated with long-lasting massive onchocercal infection. The average age of patients with sclerosing keratitis is 41.2 years. The highest density of microfilariae and opacities is found in the corneal periphery nasally and temporally, with a lower density centrally.[41] Prolonged corneal inflammation leads to cicatrization with neovascularization.[42] White corneal opacification usually begins nasally and temporally at the limbus in the interpalpebral fissure (Fig. 40–9), progresses inferiorly (Fig. 40–10), and becomes confluent (Fig. 40–11). When the opacity reaches the optical axis, visual acuity is seriously impaired.

Anterior Uveitis

Living microfilariae may be found in the anterior chamber in one quarter of patients with onchocerciasis.[44, 45] Active anterior uveitis is seen rarely, however, and its severity does not correspond to the number of microfilariae in the anterior chamber. The first sign of anterior uveitis may be the alteration of pupillary reflex to light. Anterior uveitis can vary from chronic, low-grade, non-granulomatous inflammation to severe, turbid, granulomatous uveitis with acute exacerbations accompanied by flare, iris atrophy, anterior and posterior synechiae,

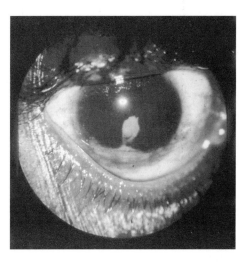

FIGURE 40–10. Sclerosing keratitis: opacification of the inferior cornea with pupillary aperture drawn inferiorly and cataract. (Photo courtesy of A. Rothova.) (See color insert.)

and seclusion and occlusion of the pupillae. The pupil may manifest a characteristic pear-shaped distortion with inferior posterior synechiae (see Fig. 40–10).[46, 47]

Chorioretinitis

Chorioretinal changes in onchocerciasis are usually bilateral and symmetric, and are located temporal to the macula and nasal to the optic nerve. Active inflammation of the retina or choroid is rarely observed.[46, 48] Onchocercal posterior uveitis is slowly progressive. The mildest retinal change in the course of onchocerciasis is retinal pigment epithelium (RPE) atrophy (Fig. 40–12), seen as mottling of fluorescence on fluorescein angiography, sometimes accompanied by atrophy of the choriocapillaris.[46] RPE atrophy can be either diffuse or geographic with distinct borders.[48] Other changes due to chorioretinitis include intraretinal brown and black pigment clumping, intraretinal white and shiny deposits, intraretinal hemorrhages, cotton-wool opacities, and hyperpigmenta-

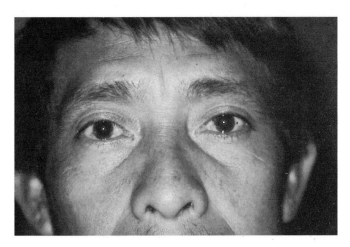

FIGURE 40–9. Incipient sclerosing keratitis: peripheral white corneal opacifications nasally and temporally at the limbus in the interpalpebral fissure of both eyes in a 38-year-old Yanomami man, Ocamo, Venezuela.

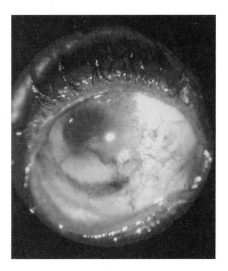

FIGURE 40–11. Advanced sclerosing keratitis with extended opacification of the cornea. (Photo courtesy A. Rothova.) (See color insert.)

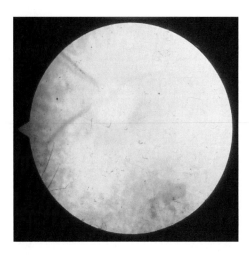

FIGURE 40–12. Fundus changes in onchocerciasis: optic nerve atrophy, diffuse chorioretinal atrophy, and secondary pigmentary changes, pigment clumping in the macular area. (Photo courtesy A. Rothova.) (See color insert.)

tion. Live intraretinal microfilariae anterior to the RPE were observed in 10 of 30 patients examined by Murphy and colleagues.[37] The development of new chorioretinal lesions and the extension of existing lesions are common with or without treatment.[49–52]

Optic Nerve Disease

Optic nerve involvement manifests as either primary or secondary optic atrophy. Optic neuritis, characterized by a congested disc, with or without swelling, is not an uncommon finding, occurring either as a direct result of the disease itself, or as part of the Mazzotti reaction precipitated by therapy with diethylcarbamazine.[18, 46] Optic atrophy may be seen in association with peripapillary hyperpigmentation, scarring, varying degrees of chorioretinal atrophy (see Fig. 40–12), and sheathing of retinal vessels.[18, 46, 48, 53] The prevalence of optic nerve atrophy varies between 1% and 9%.[18] Retinal and optic nerve pathology is often accompanied by serious constriction of the visual field to 5 to 10 degrees and night blindness.[54, 55]

COMPLICATIONS

Chronic inflammation of the anterior segment in onchocerciasis is often associated with complications, the most common being iris atrophy, anterior and posterior synechiae, seclusion of the pupil, secondary glaucoma, and cataract.[54] Glaucoma is usually related to angle closure as a sequela of anterior uveitis. Open-angle glaucoma in patients with a low intensity of infection also occurs.[54] In general, patients with ocular onchocerciasis have lower intraocular pressure.[56, 57] In one study, complicated cataract and secondary glaucoma were found to be the causes of visual loss in 28 of 70 patients with uveitis.[58] In another study, a high prevalence of glaucoma was associated with severe eye infection in young males.[56] Complications related to the therapy are common and are described in the following sections.

ETIOLOGY

Transmission and Life Cycle of *Onchocerca Volvulus*

The female vector ingests microfilariae during a blood meal of an infected human. Microfilariae of *Onchocerca volvulus* migrate through the fly's midgut to the hemocoel, and further to the thoracic muscles. Following several molts, the microfilariae develop into the infective "L3" larval stage over the next 5 to 8 days and are transmitted through the fly's proboscis to the definitive human host during the next blood feeding.

The transmission of microfilariae in utero in humans was shown in Ghana, where microfilariae were found in skin snips and/or in the umbilical cords of newborn children.[59]

Parasite Factors

Onchocerca volvulus, together with *Wuchereria bancrofti*, *Brugia malayi*, *Loa loa*, *Mansonella perstans*, *Mansonella streptocerca*, and *Mansonella ozzardi*, belongs to the group of human filarial parasites. The macrofilariae (adult worms) live in the subcutaneous nodules in man. There are usually three females and one male worm per nodule. Females are 30 to 80 cm × 250 to 450 μm, and they remain for their entire lifetime in one nodule. The male worms are long, 16 to 42 mm × 125 to 200 μm, and they often leave the nodules. The reproductive life of macrofilariae is 9 to 11 years, and their lifespan in total is 13 to 14 years.[60] During their lifetime, females produce millions of microfilariae (Fig. 40–13), which measure 220 to 360 μm × 5 to 9 μm and have a lifespan of 6 to 24 months.[34]

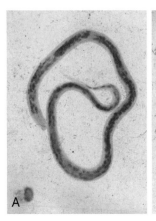
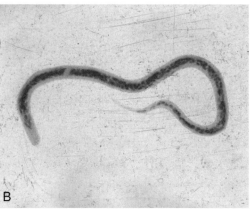

FIGURE 40–13. *Onchocerca volvulus* microfilaria (hematoxylin). It measures 225 × 5 to 7 μm, no sheath, head is slightly enlarged, anterior nuclei are positioned side by side, no nuclei in the end of the tail which is long and pointed. (Photo courtesy of L. Kolárová.)

Microfilariae migrate from the nodules; invade the eye, skin, and lymphatic tissue; and are the cause of most clinical manifestations of onchocerciasis. Serine proteases and metalloproteases produced (especially by "L3" microfilariae) may facilitate their migration and may participate in the tissue destruction.[61] Parasitic nematodes use different strategies to evade the surveillance of the immune system. Nematodes actively produce surface coats that shed antibodies and inflammatory cells.[62] Filarial parasites produce prostaglandins, prostacyclin, and prostaglandin E_2, thereby inhibiting T-cell activation, lymphokine production, and cytotoxicity, and inducing B-cell unresponsiveness.[63]

Biochemical enzyme[64] and genetic[65, 66] studies have demonstrated two different strains of *Onchocerca volvulus*, rain forest and savanna; the savanna strain is associated with a higher rate of blindness (5% to 10%) in comparison with the rain forest strain (1% to 2%). A strong correlation between the classification of rain forest and savanna strains and the epidemiologic pattern of blindness was confirmed by the use of strain-specific DNA probes.[67] There are many other *Onchocerca* strains (e.g., *O. ochengi*, *O. gutturosa*, *O. dukei*, and *O. armillata*) that are transmitted by the same *Simulium* blackfly vectors that transmit *Onchocerca volvulus;* these are not pathogenic in man. The definitive hosts of these species are animals (usually cattle). The use of DNA probes makes it possible to distinguish *Onchocerca volvulus* larvae from those of *Onchocerca ochengi* and other nonhuman parasites of the same species. In North Cameroon, reduced endemicity in an area with a high transmission of *Onchocerca ochengi* through the same vector as *Onchocerca volvulus* was found.[68] This natural inoculation of animal filaria seems to confer cross protection against *Onchocerca volvulus* in humans.[68]

Vector Factors

Onchocerca volvulus is transmitted by a blackfly of the family Simuliidae, genus *Simulium*. The main vectors in Africa and the Arabian peninsula are the *Simulium damnosum* complex and *Simulium neavei* complex. In Central and South America, the most common vectors are the *Simulium ochraceum* and *metallicum* complexes. The adult fly is dark and robust, with short legs that are 2 to 3 mm in length. The lifespan of Simuliidae is, on average, 3 weeks, but in some individuals, survival time may be longer than 4 months.[69] Only females transmit the infection during a blood meal. The bite is painful and usually bleeds, and is surrounded by erythema. There is variable survival of the *Simulium* vector following a blood meal, depending on the microfilarial load and on differential competence in transmission of microfilariae.[70, 71] A study focusing on the transmission of rain forest and savanna strains of *Onchocerca volvulus* by distinct groups of vector flies has shown that there is no preferential transmission in West Africa.[72]

Host Factors

The range of clinical and laboratory manifestations of onchocerciasis varies according to the intensity and type of immune response to the parasite. In general, three groups of individuals exposed to onchocerciasis can be distinguished: (1) generalized pathology or asymptomatic, living in endemic areas, microfilariae-positive, eye pathology common; (2) asymptomatic, living in endemic areas, microfilariae-negative (endemic normal/putatively immune [EN/PI]); (3) local strong skin involvement (sowda), living in endemic areas, few microfilariae, eye pathology rare.[73, 74] The association of different HLA class II haplotypes with the different types of immune and clinical response described earlier was recently demonstrated.[75, 76] Generalized disease is associated with haplotypes DQA1*0101-DQB1*0501 and DQB1*0201; putatively immune individuals (PI) have haplotypes DRB1*1201-DQA1*0501-DQB1*0301-DPA1*02011-DPB1*01011; and localized disease is associated with DPA1*0301-DPB1*0402. The substitution of one amino acid at position 11 of the HLA class II DP alpha 1 chain can be associated either with the disease (methionine) or with the putative immunity (alanine).[77] The important functions of DQ molecules in immune regulation and the types of cytokine response are well established and are probably involved in the pathogenesis of onchocerciasis.[78–80]

Age older than 14 years in individuals living in endemic areas may be associated with significantly greater risk of infection.[81] High intensity of infection with severe ocular pathology is observed to be more prevalent in males[56]; this is usually ascribed to the predominance of outdoor activities in this population. In one study in Ecuador, females were shown to be significantly more frequently putatively immune than males,[82] a finding corresponding to the lower microfilarial densities and reduced clinical manifestations seen in females in the same area.[83]

PATHOGENESIS AND PATHOLOGY

The pathogenesis of onchocerciasis lesions derives directly from the presence of the foreign parasite in human tissue. The living macro- and microfilariae in the human organism provoke, in general, a very low local and systemic host immune response. They travel through the human tissues incredibly easily.[73] The existence of suppressive mechanisms that inhibit the inflammatory response, protecting both the host and the parasite, is in the nature of the phenomenon of parasitism. Most of the pathology that eventually develops is the result of failure of these protective mechanisms due to the host inflammatory response against dying or dead microfilariae. The degree of pathology is directly related to the density of microfilarial infection and the intensity of the inflammatory response. The numbers of microfilariae dying daily in the tissues of infected individuals may range from 10,000 to 500,000, depending on the intensity of infection.[84] The inflammatory response and clinical manifestations depend on the balance between the parasite's ability to evade or suppress host defense mechanisms and the host's ability to regulate its immune response.

Ocular Disease

The lesions in the eye are primarily caused by living, dying, and dead microfilariae. The exact route of entry of microfilariae into the ocular tissues is not completely clear. They may enter the eye by direct invasion from the bulbar conjunctiva[41, 85]; the posterior pole can be invaded by migration along the ciliary vessels and nerves[86]; or they may enter through the retinal and choroidal blood vessels[87] and possibly through the optic nerve via the cerebrospinal fluid.[88] Findings of microfilariae in histologic sections of the sclera suggest the possibility of direct penetration of the parasite.[89] The microfilarial loads in the anterior chamber of the eye correlate significantly with those in the skin.[44, 90, 91] The presence of microfilariae in skin snips from the outer canthus, in the cornea and the anterior chamber, is closely associated with keratitis punctata, sclerosing keratitis, iritis, and optic nerve atrophy.[92, 93] There is no such association with chorioretinitis.[93] Twenty or more microfilariae in the anterior chamber are considered to be a risk factor for blinding onchocerciasis.[94]

There are few data regarding the pathology in the eye because of the lack of specimens for examination. There is no or minimal inflammatory reaction around living microfilariae, and they apparently do not cause substantial damage to the ocular tissues.[53] In the cornea, usually after treatment with diethylcarbamazine, acute inflammation gives rise to transitory snowflake opacities—punctate keratitis. The inflammatory reaction around dying and dead microfilariae is accompanied by edema and infiltration by eosinophils.[53, 57, 95] In sclerosing keratitis, eosinophils, neutrophils, and fibroblasts are observed[53, 57]; these are associated with limbitis.[53] The tendency of the organism to suppress inflammation is supported by immunohistologic studies on the conjunctiva and iris that demonstrate a predominance of CD8+ suppressor T cells among the activated cells, with increased major histocompatability complex (MHC) class II expression[96] and increased expression of interleukin-4 (IL-4) mRNA.[97] Experimental models of onchocercal keratitis have confirmed the greater potential of the savanna strain to produce corneal inflammation[98] and have shown a predominance of CD4+ T cells,[99] with the important participation of eosinophils[100–102] and IgE in the aqueous humor.[101, 103] Upregulation of IL-4 and interleukin-5 (IL-5) mRNA production in the cornea indicates the importance of a Th2-type immune response in the development of onchocercal keratitis in the murine model.[104] In IL-5 gene knockout mice, however, neutrophils were able to mediate keratitis and caused extensive stromal opacification and damage in the absence of eosinophils.[105] An immune response that mediates the development of experimental keratitis does not develop in IL-4 knockout mice.[106] On the other hand, protective immunity, in the absence of IL-4, develops and remains dependent on IL-5 and eosinophils.[107]

The pathogenesis of chorioretinal lesions and optic nerve disease is not very clear. It is difficult to distinguish alterations produced by pathogenic molecules elaborated by the parasite from those resulting from the host immune response.[73] The finding of living microfilariae in the vitreous,[92] in the retina in vivo,[37, 48] and in histologic sections,[53, 86] together with observations that chorioretinal lesions progress within a few days after treatment with diethylcarbamazine,[108, 109] indicates that the direct participation of dying or dead microfilariae and the host inflammatory response play important roles, at least ini-

tially, in the pathogenesis of onchocercal chorioretinitis. A slow progression of pre-existing chorioretinal lesions was also observed after treatment with ivermectin[48, 110] and amocarzine,[51] following a substantial reduction of microfilarial loads in the organism. This observation indicates that the density of microfilariae does not influence the progression of chorioretinitis, and that other factors are probably involved in the etiopathogenesis of chorioretinal lesions. These observations and the finding of antiretinal autoantibodies in the sera and ocular fluids from onchocerciasis patients led to the idea of the possible involvement of autoimmunity in the perpetuation of ocular inflammation. Autoantibodies against retinal S-antigen,[111, 112] interphotoreceptor retinoid-binding protein (IRBP),[111] and inner retinal and retinal photoreceptors[113] were found in the sera and ocular fluids of the patient with onchocerciasis. Immunologic cross-reactivity of recombinant antigen from *Onchocerca volvulus* with the ocular component of the 40,000 M_r in retina, optic nerve, iris, ciliary body, and cornea has been demonstrated, together with the presence of antibodies against this antigen in onchocerciasis patients with posterior segment pathology.[114, 115] In only two studies was there an association between the presence of autoantibodies and the occurrence of chorioretinitis.[112, 115] Two other studies showed no difference in onchocerciasis patients with and without chorioretinitis in the specific cellular lymphoproliferative response to S-antigen, IRBP, or recombinant *Onchocerca volvulus* antigen (Ov39).[116, 117]

Systemic Immune Response

There is clear evidence that immunity against *Onchocerca volvulus* exists, and differences in humoral and cellular responses between putatively immune (PI) individuals and microfiladermic (MF) infected individuals in endemic areas have been studied.[73, 74] Cellular responses to parasite antigens in lymphocyte proliferation tests are usually diminished in MF onchocerciasis patients in comparison to PI individuals.[118–121] The proliferative response can be restored when exogenous IL-2 is added to the culture.[119, 122] The evidence shows a different pattern of cytokine production after stimulation of peripheral blood mononuclear cells (PBMCs) with *Onchocerca volvulus* antigen. A predominant Th2-type response in MF patients and a Th1-type response in PI individuals have been clearly demonstrated.[118, 120, 123] Increased IL-10 production by PBMCs of MF patients without stimulation, in comparison with those from PI individuals, may suppress the Th1-type response and promote the development of the disease.[123]

In one study, the cytokine production was measured by reverse transcription polymerase chain reaction (RT-PCR) with respect to the presence or absence of ocular disease (sclerosing keratitis, uveitis) in MF individuals with both dermal and ocular microfilariae.[124] The expression of IL-4, IL-5, and IL-10 mRNA was significantly higher in persons with ocular disease, but levels of interferon-γ (IFN-γ) were the same in both groups.[124] Repeated treatment of onchocerciasis patients with ivermectin increases cellular immunity and the production of Th1-type cytokines.[120]

The humoral response as measured by production of

specific IgG and IgG subclasses in MF individuals is significantly increased in comparison to that in PI persons.[82, 125–127] Many stage-specific onchocercal antigens are recognized only by sera from PI individuals and sera from mice and chimpanzees immunized by irradiated L3-stage larvae. They are not recognized by sera from infected patients.[128, 129] Increased levels of total and parasite-specific IgE in onchocerciasis patients were also demonstrated.[82, 121] The production of antibodies against tropomyosin isoform (MOv-14) was demonstrated in infected individuals and may play an important role in host protection.[130]

A variety of autoantibodies in onchocerciasis patients have been detected, suggesting a potential role of autoimmunity in the pathogenesis of onchocerciasis. Increased levels of antibodies to calreticulin,[131] an antigen identical to the 46-kD Ro/SS-A human autoantigen,[132] with high (63%) homology to the λRAL-1 antigen of *Onchocerca volvulus*, were detected in patients with onchocerciasis. The anticalreticulin antibodies were significantly increased in patients with ocular pathology.[133] The antibodies to a 2.5-kD antigen identical to human defensins (peptides present in the azurophil granules of neutrophils) have been detected in patients with "sowda."[134]

Both nonspecific and antigen-specific circulating immune complexes have been detected in patients with onchocerciasis.[135–137] The correlation between immune complex levels was found to be positive for skin disease and negative for ocular disease.[138]

DIAGNOSIS

Clinical Diagnosis

A thorough dermatologic and ophthalmic examination can be highly indicative of a diagnosis of onchocerciasis. The observation of characteristic clinical manifestations in endemic areas makes the diagnosis relatively easy. In patients from nonendemic areas, the diagnosis of onchocerciasis should be suspected if there is a history of travel to an endemic area and the patient presents with asymmetric pruritus, acute rash, and swelling of a limb. Definitive diagnosis requires the direct demonstration of the parasite by clinical examination and/or by laboratory investigation.

Examination of cornea, anterior chamber, and iris on slit lamp; study of the vitreous and retina with a three-mirror lens; and the use of direct and indirect ophthalmoscopy are of great importance. The best visualization of live microfilariae in the cornea is attained with high magnification (×25) and retroillumination of the dilated eye. Patients should sit with their heads down on their knees for 2 to 5 minutes to allow free microfilariae to circulate in the aqueous humor before slit-lamp examination of the anterior chamber is performed. For detection of optic nerve involvement, a red-dot card screening test was developed. The time needed to complete the test is 1 to 2 minutes; it records nonperception and desaturation of targets with a sensitivity of 54% and a specificity of 96%.[139] Examination of the visual field by means of perimetry may also be of value.

Laboratory Investigations

Parasitologic Diagnostic Methods

DETECTION OF MICROFILARIAE IN THE SKIN

The classic method for direct demonstration of microfilariae is microscopic, with the use of 0.1 ml of buffer or culture media after an overnight incubation of skin snips at room temperature or 37°C.[140] Two skin snips are prepared by lifting the skin with a needle and making a bloodless cut of the superficial dermis using a corneoscleral trephine or razor blade (Fig. 40–14). Given the geographic differences among skin infection sites in Africa, two skin snips are taken from over each iliac crest, whereas in Central America, the skin is taken from each deltoid or scapular region.[141] This method enables one to determine the prevalence and intensity of the infection. The sensitivity of this method is not great and varies with infection intensity in the area.[142] For this reason, in areas with a low intensity of infection, six skin snips are taken.[141] This diagnostic method is now not well accepted by patients in the areas in which repeated skin snipping was performed. Also, the relatively low sensitivity in the diagnosis of early, light, or preclinical infection led to the development of alternative methods.[143] A new, more sensitive and painless alternative to skin snips is a PCR assay performed with a superficial skin scratch.[144]

DETECTION OF MACROFILARIAE IN NODULES

Ultrasonography may be useful in detecting deep nonpalpable nodules that normally escape clinical detection; it also may help in the differential diagnosis of nodules.[145, 146] Nodule excision with histologic examination of adult worms can help to establish the definitive diagnosis of onchocerciasis. This surgical procedure can be performed under local anesthesia.

Rapid Methods of Diagnosis

These methods are economical, simple, and rapid; they provide tools for evaluating the epidemiologic situation and endemicity within a community. The most common method is an assessment of pretibial skin depigmentation, "leopard skin,"[147, 148] or palpable nodules.[149] The evaluation of subcutaneous nodules by verbal assessment was

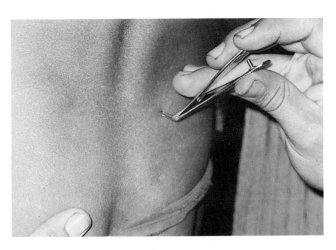

FIGURE 40–14. Skin snip by corneoscleral trephine.

shown to have a sensitivity of 93.5% and a specificity of 83.3%.[150] Alternatively, a rapid community assessment for nodule presence may be achieved with a random sample of 30 men. Once three infectious individuals are identified, the prevalence of infection is likely to be greater than 20%.[149] These methods are not accurate, but they can give a rough estimate of onchocerciasis prevalence.

Immunologic Skin Tests

The Mazzotti test is based on the observation of an adverse reaction after the treatment of onchocerciasis with diethylcarbamazine (DEC).[151] This test may provoke serious complications and is no longer used in the routine diagnosis of onchocerciasis. Use of the Mazzotti test is now acceptable only in patients with suspected onchocerciasis when the parasite is not detectable in the skin or in the eye. The adult patient is given a single dose of 50 mg of DEC per os; 1 to 24 hours later, itching, skin rash, and lymphadenitis are observed as a reaction to the death of microfilariae.[18] The use of topical DEC in a cream, the "Mazzotti patch test,"[152] was considered unreliable and has been abandoned. Because of its low price and relatively good sensitivity (80%) and specificity (97%) when using 10% DEC in Nivea milk, the possibilities for DEC patch test use are now being reevaluated.[143]

Detection of Antibodies

Radioimmunoassay (RIA) and enzyme-linked immunosorbent assay (ELISA) may be used to test for the presence of parasite-specific antibodies. These immunodiagnostic tests are being developed as tools for the detection of preclinical and low-level infections in endemic areas under control. The cardinal problems of low-specificity and sensitivity of these tests were partially solved by the detection of specific *Onchocerca* antigens[153–155] and the cloning of 37 diagnostic specific antigens. Recombinant antigens were tested, and three antigens with high sensitivity to detect early infection (Ov16,[156] Ov71,[157, 158] and Ov11[159]) were selected to form an "antigen tri-cocktail."[160] The data to evaluate the specificity of this potentially very useful test have now been collected.[18] An ELISA assay using a combination of recombinant antigens OC (*Onchocerca* clone) 3.6 and OC 9.3 was shown to be a very sensitive test for detection of new infection.[161]

Detection of Antigen

For a long time there was no satisfactory technique for direct onchocercal antigen detection.[162] New, sensitive, low-cost diagnostic tests to detect *Onchocerca*-specific antigens in tears, urine, and dermal fluid have been recently developed.[163]

DNA Probes

DNA probes specific for *Onchocerca volvulus* have been developed by the differential screening of genomic DNA libraries. These DNA probes have been derived from a single repeated sequence family with a unit length of 150 base pairs, designated as O-150 and present in approximately 2000 copies in the *Onchocerca volvulus* genome.[164] A polymerase chain reaction technique has been developed to recognize different strains (*O. volvulus* and *O. ochengi*) and different forms (rain forest and savanna) of

Onchocerca.[165] This method has been used in the examination of people in endemic areas in Ecuador and Ghana.[166, 167] Positive results have been demonstrated not only in skin snip–positive but also in some skin snip–negative individuals. O-150 PCR techniques allow one to study the transmission of different *Onchocerca* strains and species in fly vectors and in infected individuals.[72, 168] These data are of utmost importance for epidemiologic studies in endemic areas.

DIFFERENTIAL DIAGNOSIS

In the differential diagnosis of the skin symptoms and signs, the following conditions must be excluded: infection with *Mansonella streptocerca*, scabies, insect bites, prickly heat, contact dermatitis, sycosis cruris, post-traumatic and postinflammatory depigmentation, leprosy, tertiary yaws, and superficial mycosis.[169] Subcutaneous nodules, although typical, must be differentiated from lymph nodes, lipomas, fibromas, dermal cysts, and ganglia.[18, 169] Ultrasound examination of nodules may help in this differential diagnosis.[145, 146]

Asymmetric limb edema, isolated or accompanied by pruritus with acute rash, is typical for visitors from nonendemic areas. Blood eosinophilia above 2000/mm³ may be present.[170] There may be some similarity to the eosinophilic cellulitis seen in Well's syndrome.[171] Elevated serum levels of angiotensin-converting enzyme (ACE) have been found in onchocerciasis patients; therefore, the interpretation of ACE activity should be exercised prudently, especially in patients from endemic areas.[172]

Ocular corneal pathology should be distinguished from viral keratitis, exposure keratitis, nutritional keratopathy, phthisis bulbi from other causes,[18] and peripheral keratitis associated with intermediate uveitis. In one report, anterior uveitis with a worm in the cornea of a female from the United States was found to be caused by a zoonotic worm of *Onchocerca* genus (probably *Onchocerca cervicalis* in which the horse is a host).[173] Chorioretinal pathology must be differentiated from other infectious diseases like toxoplasmosis, syphilis, and tuberculosis, which cause similar posterior changes, and from noninfectious ocular diseases such as retinitis pigmentosa.[174]

TREATMENT AND CONTROL

The goals of onchocerciasis treatment are to treat already infected patients in order to prevent debilitating pathologic eye and skin changes, and to break the life cycle of the parasite in order to prevent further transmission of the disease. Two principal strategies exist in the fight against onchocerciasis: (1) treatment by chemotherapy, and (2) control of the blackfly vector. Onchocerciasis can not be eradicated by these means, but a high level of disease control can be reached.[175]

Treatment

In the past, chemotherapy of onchocerciasis was limited to the use of diethylcarbamazine (DEC)[176, 177] and suramin.[176] The use of these two drugs is accompanied by serious systemic adverse effects, like Mazzotti reaction, proteinuria, and an increased serum level of circulating immunocomplexes.[135] Their use can also increase ocular inflammation[109, 135, 178–180] and may be the cause of optic nerve atrophy.[181] DEC is therefore no longer used and suramin is given only with close medical supervision.

Since 1987, a new drug, ivermectin, has become the most widely accepted and used drug in the treatment of onchocerciasis. Ivermectin is a 22,23-dihydro derivative of ivermectin B1, a macrocyclic lactone produced by an actinomycete, *Streptomyces avermitilis*; it is effective against helminthic parasites and arthropods and was first successfully used in veterinary medicine.[182] The efficacy and safety of ivermectin in the treatment of onchocerciasis in humans have been repeatedly demonstrated.[178, 183, 184] The antiparasitic action of ivermectin is not completely understood, but its effect on neurotransmission through stimulation of γ-aminobutyric acid–mediated chloride ion conductance may play a role.[182, 185] The level of resistance to ivermectin has not been described to date.[18]

Ivermectin has a very potent microfilaricidal effect, substantially reducing microfilariae counts within a few days. The maximal effect is reached within a few weeks of treatment and is superior to that of DEC.[178] Twelve months after a repeated 150-μg/kg annual dose of ivermectin treatment for 5 years, reduction of microfilarial loads exceeding 90% have been seen.[186] There is a significantly lower count of microfilariae when the treatment is repeated every 6 months in comparison with an annual treatment schedule at 1 and 2 years after the first treatment, although the difference at 2 years is very small.[187, 188] Another study demonstrated a striking difference in mean microfilarial loads between single-dose treatment and a multiple-dose, 6-month treatment regimen 18 months after the last dose.[189] The loads in the first group were twice as high as those in the second group. The data from this study also suggest that three or more doses of ivermectin given at 6-month intervals significantly slow microfilarial repopulation, probably through a cumulative effect on macrofilariae.[189]

Multiple monthly doses of 150 μg/kg of ivermectin[190] and 6 doses of 100 μg/kg given at 2-week intervals[191] also have some macrofilaricidal effect. At 12 months, 12% of male and 22% of female worms were killed.[190] In a study using 3-month doses, the mortality of female worms at 25th and 34th months was 25.5% and 32.6%, respectively.[192] There was a significantly higher proportion of nodules without male worms, and both the insemination of females and embryogenesis were diminished after the treatment.[190, 191]

Ivermectin also has the ability to decrease the level of transmission through a rapid reduction of vector infectiousness by *Onchocerca volvulus* with individual treatment given as one or two doses of 200 μg/kg of body weight at 6- and 7-month intervals, respectively.[193, 194] Mass treatment given as two annual doses of 150 μg/kg of body weight in a large community of 14,000 people treated in Liberia reduced the number of infected flies (*Simulium yahense*) with developing *Onchocerca volvulus* larvae by 93.4% to 95%.[195] Community-based treatment with ivermectin decreases the transmission of infection as demonstrated by a statistically significant decrease (45% to 77%) in the incidence of new infections in untreated children.[196, 197]

Only a few reports have focused on the effectiveness of ivermectin treatment in the prevention of ocular changes in infected patients and in the improvement of ocular pathology. Most microfilariae disappear from the eyes within a few weeks after the start of treatment with only mild inflammation of the anterior segment; no increased inflammation or other pathology of the posterior pole has been observed.[187, 198, 199] A substantial reduction in the prevalence of punctate keratitis and iridocyclitis after 2 to 6 years of repeated treatment with ivermectin has been described.[187, 200-202] There is either no[202] or a less-marked reduction in the prevalence of sclerosing keratitis.[203] Regression of advanced sclerosing keratitis after repeated multiple-dose treatment was observed,[200] as was reduction or stabilization of optic nerve disease,[200, 203, 204] but no reduction in the prevalence and progression of chorioretinitis was found.[48, 200, 201]

Ivermectin is at the present time the drug of choice for the treatment of onchocerciasis; it is used in a single oral dose of 150 μg/kg of body weight once or twice a year.[205] The dosage schedule used in most large-scale treatment programs is based on a weight-adjusted dose with a target of 150 μg/kg. Standard dosage is 3 mg for 15 to 25 kg, 6 mg for 26 to 44 kg, 9 mg for 45 to 64 kg, and 12 mg for 65 to 85 kg of body weight. The dose range is from 120 to 230 μg/kg. Because of the difficulties of weighing patients and halving the tablets in field conditions, leading to inaccurate doses, a simplified schedule for treatment based on patient height, which can be easily measured, has been suggested.[206] The dose based on height was established as 3 mg for 95 to 124 cm, 6 mg for 125 to 149 cm, and 9 mg for >150 cm. During mass treatment in Nigeria using a standard dosing schedule of 150 μg/kg, 79.6% of patients were underdosed.[207] This led to a new suggested dosing schedule that doubled the standard dose of 150 μg/kg to 300 μg/kg.[208] Ivermectin should not be given to children younger than 5 years of age or weighing less than 15 kg, during pregnancy, to nursing mothers during the first week of their child's life, or to persons with other serious illnesses.[18]

Treatment strategy in expatriates and patients who are visiting or working in endemic areas is not well established. These patients have been successfully treated with the standard dose of 150 μg/kg and were retreated after 1 or 6 months, if necessary. Two reports indicate a higher frequency (61%) of adverse reactions after the first dose of ivermectin in expatriates than in patients living in endemic areas.[208, 209]

Ivermectin is accepted as a safe and powerful drug in individual treatment and also in community-based large-scale treatment programs, having no toxic effects in humans up to a total dose of 1.8 mg/kg of body weight.[18] Most adverse reactions are mild and self-limiting and are observed during the first 2 days after treatment. Most of them are similar to Mazzotti reaction but less severe. The most common reactions are itching, rash, edema of the limbs and face, musculoskeletal pain, painful swelling of lymph nodes, headache, dizziness, weakness, fever, and ocular irritation. Adverse reactions occur in approximately 1.3% to 16% of patients after the first treatment, and in less than 0.5% after the second treatment.[183, 210-213] Severe reactions such as severe symptomatic postural hypotension, dizziness, fever, dyspnea, or pain occurred in 0.24% of a population of 50,929 treated persons.[212] The most common side effect of mass treatment by ivermectin is the passing of intestinal worms like *Ascaris*.[214] In areas with endemic onchocerciasis and loiasis, the development of severe encephalopathy, sometimes with coma, was seen in 0.11% of patients treated with ivermectin.[215] Counts of *Loa loa* microfilariae higher than 8000 microfilariae/ml significantly increase the relative risk of encephalopathy.[215, 216] Before mass treatment, an epidemiologic survey assessing the intensity of *Loa loa* infection should be performed in areas with endemic onchocerciasis and loiasis, as well as close monitoring after the ivermectin treatment.[215, 216] No difference in the rate of major congenital malformations or in the developmental status of 203 children born after inadvertent treatment of their mothers with ivermectin was seen in one study.[217] Mass treatment with ivermectin may decrease the frequency of spontaneous abortion in hyperendemic areas.[218]

Suramin is the only powerful macrofilaricidal drug used for the treatment of onchocerciasis that has good microfilaricidal activity. Because of its high toxicity, it is not used in large-scale treatment programs. The use of suramin is now limited to the treatment of patients leaving an endemic area or patients with uncontrolled onchodermatitis.[18] The total dose of suramin for an adult weighing at least 60 kg should be 4.0 g. If this dose is well tolerated, an additional dose of 1.0 g can be administered.[57] The recommended schedule for treatment with suramin is as follows:

1st week	0.2 g or 3.3 mg/kg
2nd week	0.4 g or 6.7 mg/kg
3rd week	0.6 g or 10.0 mg/kg
4th week	0.8 g or 13.3 mg/kg
5th week	1.0 g or 16.7 mg/kg
6th week	1.0 g or 16.7 mg/kg
Total dose	4.0 g or 66.7 mg/kg

This treatment demonstrated a significant reduction of microfilariae in the skin and in the eye, which lasted for 30 months.[219] The most common serious adverse reactions related to suramin treatment are the Mazzotti reaction, anaphylaxis, nephropathy, skin and mucous membrane exfoliation, icterus, and death.[57] There are concerns about the higher occurrence of optic atrophy and chorioretinitis after treatment with suramin with or without DEC.[176, 219] Suramin treatment is administered intravenously during hospitalization. The patient should be monitored for several weeks after completion of the treatment for the late development of an adverse reaction. Before the administration of subsequent doses of suramin, patients need to have a complete physical examination, as well as urine, hematologic, and ophthalmologic, studies. If all precautions are taken, treatment with suramin is effective and relatively safe.[220]

Early reports of potent microfilaricidal and macrofilaricidal effects of amocarzine, the piperazinyl derivative of amoscanate, from studies in the Americas[221] were not confirmed by further studies in Africa.[222] Treatment of three groups of patients with ivermectin and amocarzine, either separately or in combination, demonstrated an inferior microfilaricidal and macrofilaricidal effect of amocarzine.[222] In addition, amocarzine treatment does not prevent the progression of onchocercal chorioretinopathy.[51]

Local and systemic treatment with corticosteroids and mydriatics also should be considered, together with specific antibiotic therapy with ivermectin for patients with acute ocular inflammation, keratitis, and uveitis.

The possibility of effective local ocular treatment by diethylcarbamazine citrate and levamisole eyedrops was investigated in two studies.[223, 224] Both drugs have the potential for local killing of microfilariae but, because of practical difficulties, this treatment was not studied further.

Nodulectomy

Surgical removal of the source of the microfilariae—adult worms—by nodulectomy would be a logical approach to the treatment of onchocerciasis. The results of vast nodulectomy campaigns in Guatemala and Mexico are, despite some favorable reports, not conclusive.[18] One of the reasons for their poor efficacy is that more than one third of nodules are not palpable and escape examination. A combination of chemotherapy with nodulectomy has been shown to be of some benefit for lesions involving the anterior segment of the eye.[225] Because of improved chemotherapy and the questionable benefit, invasiveness, and technical difficulties associated with surgical procedures (given the geographic areas where onchocerciasis is usually treated), the use of nodulectomy is limited. Because a high concentration of microfilariae in the skin around the eye and in the anterior segment is associated with the presence of a head nodule, consideration should be given to excision of these nodules.[226]

Control

Onchocerciasis represents major health and socioeconomic problems in endemic areas. In hyperendemic areas, high rates of blindness, pruritus, and skin disfiguration lead to instability in community life, the migration of whole villages, the disruption of economic and family life, social stigmatization, and marginalization of infected individuals.[18] The ultimate goal, the eradication of onchocerciasis, is not realistic in the near future; only a high level of disease control is possible.[175] The combination of large-scale treatment with ivermectin and vector control by larviciding seems to be the most powerful strategy for the reduction of onchocerciasis transmission.[227]

The Onchocerciasis Control Program (OCP) was launched by the World Health Organization in 1974 in seven countries in West Africa; later, it was extended to eleven because of an invasion by blackflies from countries outside the OCP.[228] OCP started its operations by extensive larviciding and, beginning in 1989, the use of large-scale treatment with ivermectin. OCP is considered a major success in public health management.[229] It has been estimated that in OCP countries between the years 1974 and 1995, more than 100,000 people were prevented from going blind, 30 million people were protected from ocular and skin lesions, and 10 million children born in this period were not infected and are at no risk of blindness.[18, 230] The introduction of ivermectin and the commitment of its manufacturer, Merck and Company, to a free supply of the drug enabled OCP to add chemotherapy to its program and to develop new programs: the African Program for Onchocerciasis Control (APOC) in 19 African countries not involved in OCP, and the Onchocerciasis Elimination Program in the Americas (OEPA), based mainly on the sustainable delivery of community-directed treatment with Mectizan (ivermectin). The number of treatments provided by the Mectizan Donation Program in Africa and the Americas increased from 1.4 million in 1990 to 19.0 million in 1996.[18, 230]

The elimination of onchocerciasis transmission through vector control is based on the killing of the larvae of the vector (*Simulium* species) in their breeding sites by aerial application of insecticides to rivers. Rotational use of seven insecticides (biologic—*Bacillus thuringiensis;* organophosphates—temephos, phoxim, pyraclofos; synthetic pyrethroids—permethrin, etofenprox; and carbamate—carbosulfan) is the most cost-effective approach; it prevents the development of resistant populations and protects the environment.[231]

A reduction of fly bites can be accomplished by the wearing of clothing that covers most of the body, the use of insect repellents, and the avoidance of breeding sites, especially during the times of peak fly activity (during the morning and in the evening).

Surveillance of the target areas following successful elimination of the parasite reservoir to prevent recrudescence of the transmission is crucial. To evaluate the epidemiologic situation and to predict trends in OCP countries, the computer simulation model ONCHOSIM has been successfully used.[18] For easy determination of the presence of *Onchocerca volvulus* infection in the blackfly pool, PCR may be used.[232, 233]

One of the major limitations in the treatment of onchocerciasis is the lack of safe and effective macrofilaricidal drugs suitable for large-scale treatment. The development of a suitable vaccine would provide yet another avenue for the prevention and control of onchocerciasis.

NATURAL HISTORY AND PROGNOSIS

There is no detailed information concerning the natural history and evolution of onchocerciasis. From a few studies in which the population in endemic areas was followed over the long term, some conclusions can be drawn. The evolution of ocular onchocerciasis is usually slow and protracted, with the period between initial infection and clinical presentation of ocular pathology spanning many years. The skin microfilarial loads have a tendency to increase with age, and the development of eye pathology is closely related to the intensity of infection.[54, 85] The eye disease and blindness are therefore more prevalent in hyperendemic areas; usually only mild ocular involvement is observed in hypoendemic regions.[85] Eye lesions and visual impairment are therefore rare between the ages of 10 and 19 years; they increase during the third decade and reach their zenith after age 40.[85] In areas in which the annual biting rate is lower than 1000 and the ATP is lower than 100, blinding eye lesions should not develop.

In general, anterior segment inflammation is more severe and progressive in disease caused by the savanna strain as compared with the rain forest strain of *Onchocerca volvulus*.[92] Posterior lesions do not exhibit differences among patients from rain forest or savanna areas,[48] but optic neuritis is an important cause of blindness among savanna residents. In hyperendemic areas, the mortality among blind individuals was found to be increased fourfold.[234] In another study, 12 of 16 blind individuals died within a period of 9 years.[52]

CONCLUSIONS

Onchocerciasis is a well-described clinical entity. The wealth of information regarding the pathogenesis and immunobiology of the ocular disease (except posterior segment lesions) has led to the development of sophisticated diagnostic tools, new medications, and effective strategies for the treatment and control of the disease. A major problem in the treatment of onchocerciasis has been the lack of a macrofilaricidal drug. Owing to the major effort of WHO programs and the continual donation of ivermectin by Merck and Company for its treatment, onchocerciasis has ceased to be a major cause of blindness or a major public health problem in OCP countries in West Africa. Unfortunately, this is not true for countries outside the OCP area; thus, onchocerciasis should not be considered a problem solved. Eradication of the disease by the means now available is impossible, and recrudescence of the disease, even in countries in which control has been achieved, is still possible and requires vigilant surveillance.

References

1. O'Neill J: On the presence of a filaria in "craw-craw." Lancet 1875;1:265.
2. Leuckart R: In: Davidson A: Hygiene and Diseases of Warm Climates. Edinburgh, Pentland, 1893, p. 963.
3. Raillet A, Henry A: Les onchocerques; nématodes, parasites du tissu conjonctif. C R Soc Biol Paris 1910;68:248.
4. Pacheco-Luna R: Lésions oculaires au cours d'une épidémie d'érisipele au Guatemala. Bull Soc Pathol Exot 1912;12:461–463.
5. Robles R: Onchocercose humaine au Guatemala produisant la cecité et l'érysipele du littoral. Bull Soc Pathol Exot 1919;12:442.
6. Brumpt E: Une nouvelle filaire pathogene parasite de l'homme (Onchocerca caecutiens n.sp.). Bull Soc Pathol Exot 1919;12:464.
7. Torroella JL: Nota sobre la observación de microfilariae de onchocerca in vivo en el ojo humano. Anal Soc Mex Oftal Oto-Rhino-Lar 1931;9:87–88.
8. Hisette J: Mémoire sur l'Onchocerca volvulus Leuckart et ses manifestations oculaires au Congo Belge. Ann Soc Belge Méd Trop 1932;12:433.
9. Bryant J: Endemic retino-choroiditis in the Anglo-Egyptian Sudan and its possible relationship to *Onchocerca volvulus*. Trans R Soc Trop Med Hyg 1935;28:523.
10. Ridley H: Ocular onchocerciasis including involvement in the Gold Coast. Br J Ophthalmol 1945;10:22–23.
11. Janssens PG: Onchocerques et onchocercoses. Ann Soc Belge Méd Trop 1981;61:155.
12. Roubaud E: Apercus nouveaux, morphologique et biologique, sur les diptères piqueurs du group des simulies. C R Acad Sci (Paris) 1906;143:519.
13. Blacklock DB: The development of *Onchocerca volvulus* in *Simulium damnosum*. Ann Trop Med Parasitol 1926;20:1.
14. Nelson GS: Onchocerciasis. In: Dawes B, ed: Advances in Parasitology, 8th ed. London, New York, Academic Press, 1970, p 173.
15. Organisation Mondiale de la Santé. Comité d'experts de l'onchocercose. Première rapport. Série de Rapports Techniques. Genève, OMS, 1954.
16. Garnham PCC, McMahon JP: The eradication of *Simulium neavei* Roubaud from an onchocerciasis area in Kenya Colony. Bull Entomol Res 1947;37:619.
17. McGavin DDM: Ophthalmology in the tropics and subtropics. In: Cook GC, ed: Manson's Tropical Diseases, 20th ed. London, WB Saunders, 1996, p 223.

18. World Health Organization: Report of a WHO expert committee on onchocerciasis control. Technical Report Series No. 852, WHO: Geneva, 1995.

19. Organisation Mondiale de la Santé. Comité d'experts de l'onchocercose. Série de Rapports Technique No 335. Genève, OMS, 1966.

20. Prost A, Hervouet JP, Thylefors B: Les niveaux d'endémicité dans l'onchocercose. Bull OMS 1979;57:655.

21. Akogun OB, Akoh JI, Okolo A: Comparison of two sample survey methods for hyperendemic onchocerciasis and new focus in Dakka, Nigeria. Rev Biol Trop 1997;45:871.

22. Chippaux JP, Boussinesq M, Ranque S, et al: Occurrence of onchocerciasis in subjects coming from non-endemic areas and migrating to a hyperendemic area. Bull Soc Pathol Exot 1998;91:173.

23. Rolland A: Onchocerciasis in the village of Saint Pierre: An unhappy experience of repopulation in an uncontrolled endemic area. Trans R Soc Trop Med Hyg 1972;66:913.

24. Duke BOL, Anderson J, Fuglsang H: The *Onchocerca volvulus* transmission potentials and associated patterns of onchocerciasis at four Cameroon Sudan-savanna villages. Trop Med Parasitol 1975;26:143.

25. Porter CH, Collins RC, Brandling-Bennett AD: Vector density, parasite prevalence and transmission of *Onchocerca volvulus* in Guatemala. Am J Trop Med Hyg 1988;39:567–574.

26. Vivas-Martínez S, Basáñez MG, Grillet ME, et al: Onchocerciasis in the Amazonian focus of southern Venezuela: Altitude and blackfly species composition as predictors of endemicity to select communities for ivermectin control programmes. Trans R Soc Trop Med Hyg 1998;92:613.

27. Prost A, Nebout M, Rougemont A: Lepromatous leprosy and onchocerciasis. Br Med J 1979;3:589.

28. Gbary AR, Guiguemde TR, Ouedraogo JB, et al: Etude du polyparasitisme filarien en zone de savane au Burkina Faso. Med Trop (Mars) 1987;47:329.

29. Karam M, Weiss N: Seroepidemiological investigations of onchocerciasis in a hyperendemic area of West Africa. Am J Trop Med Hyg 1985;34:907.

30. Kaiser C, Asaba G, Leichsenring M, et al: High incidence of epilepsy related to onchocerciasis in West Uganda. Epilepsy Res 1998;30:247.

31. Newell ED, Vyungimana F, Bradley JE: Epilepsy, retarded growth and onchocerciasis, in two areas of different endemicity of onchocerciasis in Burundi. Trans R Soc Trop Med Hyg 1997;91:525.

32. Druet Cabanac M, Preux PM, Bouteille B, et al: Onchocerciasis and epilepsy: A matched case-control study in the Central African Republic. Am J Epidemiol 1999;149:565.

33. Murdoch ME, Hay RJ, Mackenzie CD, et al: A clinical classification and grading system of the cutaneous changes in onchocerciasis. Br J Dermatol 1993;129:260.

34. Marty AM, Andersen EM: Helminthology. In: Doerr W, Seifert G, eds: Tropical Pathology. Berlin Heidelberg, Springer-Verlag, 1995, p 938.

35. Connor DH, Gibson DW, Neafie RC, et al: Sowda-onchocerciasis in North Yemen: A clinicopathologic study of 18 patients. Am J Trop Med Hyg 1983;32:123.

36. Anderson J, Fuglsang H: Living microfilariae of *Onchocerca volvulus* in the cornea. Br J Ophthalmol 1973;57:712.

37. Murphy RP, Taylor H, Greene BM: Chorioretinal damage in onchocerciasis. Am J Ophthalmol 1984;98:519.

38. von Noorden GK, Buck AA: Ocular onchocerciasis. Arch Ophthalmol 1968;80:26.

39. Weyts EJ: Ocular manifestation in onchocerciasis. Doc Med Geo Trop 1956;8:29.

40. Semba RD, Day SH, Spencer WH: Conjunctival nodules associated with onchocerciasis. Arch Ophthalmol 1985;103:823.

41. Tønjum AM, Thylefors B: Aspects of corneal changes in onchocerciasis. Br J Ophthalmol 1978;62:458.

42. Boussinesq M: L'onchocercose humaine en Afrique. Med Trop 1997;57:389.

43. Garner A: Pathology of ocular onchocerciasis: Human and experimental. Trans R Soc Trop Med Hyg 1976;70:374.

44. Cooper PJ, Proaño R, Beltran C, et al: Onchocerciasis in Ecuador: Ocular findings in *Onchocerca volvulus* infected individuals. Br J Ophthalmol 1995;79:157.

45. Newland HS, White AT, Greene BM, et al: Ocular manifestations of onchocerciasis in a rain forest area of West Africa. Br J Ophthalmol 1991;75:163.

46. Bird AC, Anderson J, Fuglsang H: Morphology of posterior segment lesions of the eye in patients with onchocerciasis. Br J Ophthalmol 1976;60:2.

47. Taylor HR, Nutman TB: Onchocerciasis. In: Pepos JS, Holland GN, Wilhelmus KR, eds: Ocular Infection and Immunity. St. Louis, Mosby–Year Book, 1996, pp 1481–1504.

48. Semba RD, Murphy RP, Newland HS, et al: Longitudinal study of lesions of the posterior segment in onchocerciasis. Ophthalmology 1990;97:1334.

49. Cooper PJ, Guderian RH, Proaño R, et al: The pathogenesis of chorioretinal disease in onchocerciasis. Parasitol Today 1997;13:94.

50. Budden FH: The natural history of ocular onchocerciasis over a period of 14–15 years and the effect on this of a single course of suramin therapy. Trans R Soc Trop Med Hyg 1976;70:484.

51. Cooper PJ, Proaño R, Beltran C, et al: Onchocerciasis in Ecuador: Evolution of chorioretinopathy after amocarzine treatment. Br J Ophthalmol 1996;80:337.

52. Rolland A, Thylefors B, Pairault C: Evolution sur 9 ans de l'onchocercose oculaire dans une communauté villageoise d'Afrique occidentale. Bull World Health Organ 1978;56:805.

53. Rodger FC: Pathogenesis and pathology of ocular onchocerciasis. Part IV. Am J Ophthalmol 1960;49:560.

54. Thylefors B: Ocular onchocerciasis. Bull World Health Organ 1978;56:63.

55. Thylefors B, Tønjum AM: Visual field defects in onchocerciasis. Br J Ophthalmol 1978;62:462.

56. Thylefors B, Duppenthaler JL: Epidemiological aspects of intraocular pressure in an onchocerciasis endemic area. Bull World Health Organ 1979;57:963.

57. World Health Organization: Report of a WHO Expert Committee on Onchocerciasis Control. Technical Report Series No 752. WHO, Geneva, 1987.

58. Ronday MJH, Stilma JS, Barbe RE, et al: Blindness from uveitis in a hospital population in Sierra Leone. Br J Ophthalmol 1994;78:690.

59. Brinkmann UK, Krämer P, Presthus GT, et al: Transmission in utero of microfilariae of *Onchocerca volvulus*. Bull World Health Organ 1976;54:708.

60. Plaisier AP, van Oortmarssen GJ, Remme J, et al: The reproductive life span of *Onchocerca volvulus* in West African savanna. Acta Trop 1991;48:271.

61. Lackey A, James ER, Sakanari JA, et al: Extracellular proteases of onchocerca. Exp Parasitol 1989;68:176.

62. Blaxter ML, Page AP, Rudin W, et al: Nematode surface coats: Actively evading immunity. Parasitol Today 1992;8:243.

63. Liu LX, Weller PF: Arachidonic acid metabolism in filarial parasites. Exp Parasitol 1990;71:496.

64. Flockhart HA, Cibulskis RE, Karam M, et al: *Onchocerca volvulus*: Enzyme polymorphism in relation to the differentiation of the forest and savannah strains of this parasite. Trans R Soc Trop Med Hyg 1986;80:285.

65. Erttmann KD, Meredith SEO, Unnasch TR, et al: Isolation and characterization of form specific DNA sequences of *O. volvulus*. Acta Leiden 1990;59:253.

66. Erttmann KD, Unnasch TR, Greene BM, et al: A DNA sequence specific for forest form *Onchocerca volvulus*. Nature 1987;327:415.

67. Zimmerman PA, Dadzie KY, De Sole G, et al: *Onchocerca volvulus* DNA probe classification correlates with epidemiologic patterns of blindness. J Infect Dis 1992;165:964.

68. Wahl G, Enyong P, Ngosso A, et al: *Onchocerca ochengi*: Epidemiological evidence of cross-protection against Onchocerca volvulus in man. Parasitology 1998;116:349.

69. Naomesi GK: Dry season survival and associated longevity and flight range of *Simulium damnosum* Theobald in Northern Ghana. Ghana Med J 1966;5:95.

70. Basáñez MG, Townson H, Wiliams JR, et al: Density-dependent processes in the transmission of human onchocerciasis: Relationship between microfilarial intake and mortality of the simuliid vector. Parasitology 1996;113:331.

71. Collins RC, Lehmann T, Garcia JCV, et al: Vector competence of *Simulium exiguum* for *Onchocerca volvulus*: Implication for epidemiology of onchocerciasis. Am J Trop Med Hyg 1995;52:213.

72. Toé L, Tang J, Back C, et al: Vector-parasite transmission complexes for onchocersiasis in West Africa. Lancet 1997;349:163.

73. Ottesen EA: Immune responsiveness and the pathogenesis of human onchocerciasis. J Infect Dis 1995;171:659.

74. King CL, Nutman TB: Regulation of the immune response in lymphatic filariasis and onchocerciasis. In: Ash C, Gallagher RB, eds: Immunoparasitology Today. Cambridge, Elsevier Trends Journals, 1991, p A54.
75. Meyer CG, Kremsner PG: Malaria and onchocerciasis: On HLA and related matters. Parasitol Today 1996;12:179.
76. Murdoch ME, Payton A, Abios A, et al: HLA-DQ alleles associate with cutaneous features of onchocerciasis. Hum Immunol 1997;55:46.
77. Meyer CG, Schnittger L, May J: Met-11 of HLA class II DP alpha 1 first domain associated with onchocerciasis. Exp Clin Immunogenet 1996;13:12.
78. Altmann, DM, Sansom D, Marsh SGE: What is the basis for HLA-DQ associations with autoimmune disease? Immunol Today 1991;12:267.
79. Hirayama K, Matsushita S, Kikuchi I, et al: HLA-DQ is epistatic to HLA-DR in controlling the immune response to schistosomal antigen in humans. Nature 1987;327:426.
80. Salgame P, Convit J, Bloom BR: Immunological suppression by human CD8+ T cells is receptor dependent and HLA-DQ restricted. Proc Natl Acad Sci 1991;88:2598.
81. Akogun OB: Filariasis in Gongola state Nigeria I: Clinical and parasitological studies in Mutum-Biyu district. J Hyg Epidemiol Microbiol Immunol 1991;35:383.
82. Elson LH, Guderian RH, Araujo E, et al: Immunity to onchocerciasis: Identification of putatively immune population in a hyperendemic area of Ecuador. J Infect Dis 1994;169:588.
83. Molea J, Guderian RH, Proaño R, et al: Onchocerciasis in Ecuador. IV. Comparative studies of the disease relating to Chachi and Black populations in the province Esmeraldas. Trans R Soc Trop Med Hyg 1984;78:86.
84. Duke BOL: The population dynamics of Onchocerca volvulus in the human host. Trop Med Parasitol 1993;44:61–68.
85. Budden FH: Natural history of onchocerciasis. Br J Ophthalmol 1957;41:214.
86. Neumann E, Gunders AE: Pathogenesis of the posterior segment lesion of ocular onchocerciasis. Am J Ophthalmol 1973;75:82.
87. Fuglsang H, Anderson J: Microfilariae of Onchocerca volvulus in blood and urine before, during and after treatment with diethylcarbamazine. J Helminthol 1974;48:93.
88. Duke BOL, Vincelette J, Moore PJ: Microfilariae in the cerebrospinal fluid, and neurological complications during treatment of onchocerciasis with diethylcarbamazine. Trop Med Parasitol 1976;27:123.
89. Paul EV, Zimmerman LE: Some observations on the ocular pathology of onchocerciasis. Hum Pathol 1977;1:581.
90. Dadzie KY, De Sole G, Remme J: Ocular onchocerciasis and the intensity of infection in the community. 4. The degraded forest of Sierra Leone. Trop Med Parasitol 1992;43:75.
91. Remme J, Dadzie KY, Rolland A, et al: Ocular onchocerciasis and the intensity of infection in the community. 1. West African savanna. Trop Med Parasitol 1989;40:340.
92. Anderson J, Fuglsang H, Hamilton PJS, et al: Study on onchocerciasis in the United Cameroon Republic. II. Comparison of onchocerciasis in the rain-forest and Sudan-savanna. Trans R Soc Trop Med Hyg 1974;68:209.
93. McMahon JE, Sowa SI, Maude GH, et al: Onchocerciasis in Sierra Leone. 3. Relationships between eye lesions and microfilarial prevalence and intensity. Trans R Soc Trop Med Hyg 1988;82:601.
94. World Health Organization: Report of a WHO Expert Committee on Epidemiology of Onchocerciasis. Technical Report Series No. 597. Geneva, WHO, 1976.
95. Mackenzie CD, Williams JF, Sisley BM, et al: Variations in host responses and pathogenesis of human onchocerciasis. Rev Infect Dis 1985;7:802.
96. Chan CC, Ottesen EA, Awadzi K, et al: Immunopathology of ocular onchocerciasis. I. Inflammatory cells infiltrating the anterior segment. Clin Exp Immunol 1989;77:367.
97. Chan CC, Li Q, Brezin AP, et al: Immunopathology of ocular onchocerciasis. III. Th-2 helper cells in the conjunctiva. Ocul Immunol Inflamm 1993;1:71.
98. Duke BOL, Anderson J: A comparison of the lesions produced in the cornea of the rabbit eye by microfilariae of the forest and Sudan-savanna strains of Onchocerca volvulus from Cameroon. I. The clinical picture. Tropenmed Parasitol 1972;23:354.
99. Chakravarti B, Herring TA, Lass JH, et al: Infiltration of CD4+ T cells into cornea during development of Onchocerca volvulus–induced experimental sclerosing keratitis in mice. Cell Immunol 1994;159:306.
100. Donnelly JJ, Rockey JH, Bianco AE, et al: Ocular immunopathologic findings of experimental onchocerciasis. Arch Ophthalmol 1984;102:628.
101. Donnelly JJ, Rockey JH, Taylor HR, et al: Onchocerciasis: Experimental models of ocular disease. Rev Infect Dis 1985;7:820.
102. Pearlman E: Immunopathology of onchocerciasis: A role for eosinophils in onchocercal dermatitis and keratitis. Chem Immunol 1997;66:26.
103. Donnelly JJ, Rockey JH, Bianco AE, et al: Aqueous humor and serum IgE antibody in experimental ocular Onchocerca infection of guinea pigs. Ophthalmic Res 1983;15:61.
104. Chakravarti B, Lagoo Deenadayalan S, Parker JS, et al: In vivo molecular analysis of cytokines in a murine model of ocular onchocerciasis. Up-regulation of IL-4 and IL-5 mRNAs and not IL-2 and INF gamma mRNAs in the cornea due to experimental interstitial keratitis. Immunol Lett 1996;54:59.
105. Pearlman E, Hall LR, Higgins AW, et al: The role of eosinophils and neutrophils in helminth-induced keratitis. Invest Ophthalmol Vis Sci 1998;39:1176.
106. Pearlman E, Lass JH, Bardenstein DS, et al: Interleukin 4 and T helper type 2 cells are required for development of experimental onchocercal keratitis (river blindness). J Exp Med 1995;182:931.
107. Hogarth PJ, Taylor MJ, Bianco AE: IL-5-dependent immunity to microfilariae is independent of IL-4 in a mouse model of onchocerciasis. J Immunol 1998;160:5436.
108. Anderson J, Fuglsang H, Marshall TF: Effects of diethylcarbamazine on ocular onchocerciasis. Tropenmed Parasit 1976;27:263.
109. Bird AC, El Sheikh H, Anderson J, et al: Changes in visual function and in the posterior segment of the eye during treatment of onchocerciasis with diethylcarbamazine citrate. Br J Ophthalmol 1980;64:191.
110. Rothova A, Van der Lelij A, Stilma JS, et al: Ocular involvement in patients with onchocerciasis after repeated treatment with ivermectin. Am J Ophthalmol 1990;110:6.
111. Van der Lelij A, Doekes BS, Hwan BS, et al: Humoral autoimmune response against S-antigen and IRBP in ocular onchocerciasis. Invest Ophthalmol Vis Sci 1990;31:1374.
112. Vingtain P, Thillaye B, Le Hoang P, et al: Sensitivity of patients with ocular onchocerciasis to filarial antigen and retinal autoantigen. 4th International Symposium on the Immunology and Immunopathology of the Eye. 1986, Padova, Italy, p 51.
113. Chan CC, Nussenblatt RB, Kim MK, et al: Immunopathology of ocular onchocerciasis. 2. Anti-retinal autoantibodies in serum and ocular fluids. Ophthalmology 1987;94:439.
114. Braun G, McKechnie NM, Connor V, et al: Immunological cross-reactivity between a cloned antigen of Onchocerca volvulus and a component of the retinal pigment epithelium. J Exp Med 1991;174:169.
115. McKechnie NM, Braun G, Connor V, et al: Immunologic cross-reactivity in the pathogenesis of ocular onchocerciasis. Invest Ophthalmol Vis Sci 1993;34:2888.
116. Van der Lelij A, Rothova A, Stilma JS, et al: Cell-mediated immunity against human retinal extract, s-antigen and interphotoreceptor retinoid-binding protein in onchocercal chorioretinopathy. Invest Ophthalmol Vis Sci 1990;31:2031.
117. Cooper PJ, Guderian RH, Proaño R, et al: Absence of cellular responses to a putative autoantigen in onchocercal chorioretinopathy. Invest Ophthalmol Vis Sci 1996;37:405.
118. Elson LH, Calvopina M, Paredes W, et al: Immunity to onchocerciasis: Putative immune persons produce a Th1-like response to Onchocerca volvulus. J Infect Dis 1995;171:652.
119. Gallin M, Edmonds K, Ellner JJ, et al: Cell-mediated immune responses in human infection with Onchocerca volvulus. J Immunol 1988;140:1999.
120. Soboslay PT, Lüder CGK, Hoffmann WH, et al: Ivermectin-facilitated immunity in onchocerciasis; activation of parasite-specific Th1-type responses with subclinical Onchocerca volvulus infection. Clin Exp Immunol 1994;96:238.
121. Ward DJ, Nutman TB, Zea-Flores G, et al: Onchocerciasis and immunity in humans: Enhanced T cell responsiveness to parasite antigen in putatively immune individuals. J Infect Dis 1988;157:536.

122. Elkhalifa MY, Ghalib HW, Dafa'alla T, et al: Suppression of human lymphocyte responses to specific and non-specific stimuli in human onchocerciasis. Clin Exp Immunol 1991;86:433.

123. Lüder CG, Schulz Key H, Banla M, et al: Immunoregulation in onchocerciasis: Predominance of Th1-type responsiveness to low molecular weight antigens of *Onchocerca volvulus* in exposed individuals without microfilaridermia and clinical disease. Clin Exp Immunol 1996;105:245.

124. Plier DA, Awadzi K, Freedman DO: Immunoregulation in onchocerciasis: Persons with ocular inflammatory disease produce a Th2-like response to *Onchocerca volvulus* antigen. J Infect Dis 1996;174:380.

125. Boyer AE, Tsang VCW, Eberhard ML, et al: Guatemalan human onchocerciasis. II. Evidence for IgG3 involvement in acquired immunity to *Onchocerca volvulus* and identification of possible immune-associated antigens. J Immunol 1991;146:4001.

126. Bratting NW, Krawietz I, Abakar AZ, et al: Strong IgG isotypic antibody response in sowdah type onchocerciasis. J Infect Dis 1994;170:955.

127. Dafa'alla TH, Ghalib HW, Abdelmageed A, et al: The profile of IgG and IgG subclasses of onchocerciasis patients. Clin Exp Immunol 1992;88:258.

128. Irvine M, Johnson EH, Lustigman S: Identification of larval-stage-specific antigens of *Onchocerca volvulus* uniquely recognized by putative immune sera from humans and vaccination sera from animal models. Ann Trop Med Parasitol 1997;91:67.

129. Nutman TB, Steel C, Ward DJ, et al: Immunity to onchocerciasis: Recognition of larval antigens by humans putatively immune to *Onchocerca volvulus* infection. J Infect Dis 1991;163:1128.

130. Jenkins RE, Taylor MJ, Gilvary NJ, et al: Tropomyosin implicated in host protective responses to microfilariae in onchocerciasis. Proc Natl Acad Sci USA 1998;95:7550.

131. Rokeach LA, Haselby J, Meilof JF, et al: Characterization of the autoantigen calreticulin. J Immunol 1991;147:3031.

132. Lux FA, McCauliffe DP, Büttner DW, et al: Serological cross-reactivity between a human Ro/SS-A autoantigen (calreticulin) and the λRAL-1 antigen of *Onchocerca volvulus*. J Clin Invest 1992;89:1945.

133. Meilof JF, Van der Lelij A, Rokeach LA, et al: Autoimmunity and filariasis. Autoantibodies against cytoplasmic cellular proteins in sera of patients with onchocerciasis. J Immunol 1993;10:5800.

134. Gallin MY, Jacobi AB, Büttner DW, et al: Human autoantibody to defensin: Disease association with hyperreactive onchocerciasis (sowda). J Exp Med 1995;182:41.

135. Greene BM, Taylor HR, Brown EJ, et al: Ocular and systemic complications of diethylcarbamazine therapy for onchocerciasis: Association with circulating immune complexes. J Infect Dis 1983;147:890.

136. Paganelli R, Ngu JL, Levinsky RJ: Circulating immune complexes in onchocerciasis. Clin Exp Immunol 1980;39:570.

137. Thambiah G, Whitworth J, Hommel M, et al: Identification and characterization of a parasite antigen in the circulating immune complexes of *Onchocerca volvulus*–infected patients. Trop Med Parasitol 1992;43:271.

138. Sisley BM, Mackenzie CD, Steward MW, et al: Association between clinical disease, circulating antibodies and C1q-binding immune complexes in human onchocerciasis. Parasite Immunol 1987;9:447.

139. Murdoch I, Jones BR, Babalola OE, et al: Red-dot card test of the paracentral field as a screening test for optic nerve disease in onchocerciasis. Bull World Health Organ 1996;74:573.

140. Prost A, Prod'hon J: La diagnostic parasitologique de l'onchocercose. Revue critique des méthodes en usage. Med Trop 1987;38:519.

141. Taylor HR, Muñoz B, Keyvan-Larijani E, et al: Reliability of detection of microfilariae in skin snips in the diagnosis of onchocerciasis. Am J Trop Med 1989;41:467.

142. Taylor HR, Keyvan-Larijani E, Newland HS, et al: Sensitivity of skin snips in the diagnosis of onchocerciasis. Trop Med Parasitol 1987;38:145.

143. Boatin BA, Toé L, Alley ES, et al: Diagnostic in onchocerciasis: Future challenges. Ann Trop Med Parasitol 1998;92(suppl 1):S41.

144. Toé L, Boatim BA, Adjami A, et al: Detection of *Onchocerca volvulus* infection by O–150 polymerase chain reaction analysis of skin scratches. J Infect Dis 1998;178:1.

145. Homeida MA, Mackenzie CD, Williams JF, et al: The detection of onchocercal nodules by ultrasound technique. Trans R Soc Trop Med Hyg 1986;80:570.

146. Leichsenring M, Tröger J, Nelle M, et al: Ultrasonographical investigations of onchocerciasis in Liberia. Am J Trop Med Hyg 1990;43:380.

147. Carme B: Dépistage des foyers d'endemicité filarienne. Méd Trop 1994;54:161.

148. Edungbola LD, Alabi TO, Oni GA, et al: Leopard skin as a rapid diagnostic index for estimating the endemicity of African onchocerciasis. Int J Epidemiol 1987;16:590.

149. Taylor HR, Duke BOL, Muñoz B: The selection of communities for treatment of onchocerciasis with ivermectin. Tropenmed Parasitol 1992;43:267.

150. Law PA, Ngandu ON, Crompton P, et al: Prevalence of *Onchocerca volvulus* nodules in the Sankuru River Valley, Democratic Republic of the Congo, and reliability of verbal assessment as a method for determining prevalence. Am J Trop Med Hyg 1998;59:227.

151. Mazzotti L: Posibilidad de utilizar como medio diagnostico auxiliar en la onchocerciasis, las reacciones alergicas consecutivas a la aministracion del Hetrazan. Mexico City, Revista del Instituto de Salubridad y Enfermedades Tropicales, 1948;9:235.

152. Kilian HD: The use of a topical Mazzotti test in the diagnosis of onchocerciasis. Trop Med Parasitol 1988;39:235.

153. Cabrera Z, Parkhouse RME: Identification of antigens of *Onchocerca volvulus* and *Onchocerca gibsoni* for diagnostic use. Mol Biochem Parasitol 1986;20:225.

154. Lobos E, Weiss N: Identification of non-cross-reacting antigens of *Onchocerca volvulus* with lymphatic filariasis serum pools. Parasitology 1986;93:389.

155. Philipp M, Gómez-Priego A, Parkhouse RME, et al: Identification of an antigen of *Onchocerca volvulus* of possible diagnostic use. Parasitology 1984;89:295.

156. Lobos E, Altmann M, Mengod G, et al: Identification of an *Onchocerca volvulus* cDNA encoding a low-molecular-weight antigen uniquely recognized by onchocerciasis patient sera. Mol Biochem Parasitol 1990;39:135.

157. Lustigman S, Brotman B, Huima T, et al: Molecular cloning and characterisation of Onchocystatin, a cysteine proteinase inhibitor of *Onchocerca volvulus*. J Biol Chem 1992;267:17339.

158. Lustigman S, Brotman B, Johnson ELH: Identification and characterisation of an *Onchocerca volvulus* cDNA clone encoding a microfilarial surface-associated antigen. Mol Biochem Parasitol 1992;50:79.

159. Bradley JE, Helm R, Lahaise M, et al: cDNA clones of *Onchocerca volvulus* low molecular weight antigens provide immunologically specific diagnostic probes. Mol Biochem Parasitol 1991;46:219.

160. Ramachandran CP: Improved immunodiagnostic tests to monitor onchocerciasis control programmes—a multicentre effort. Parasitol Today 1993;9:76.

161. Chandrashekar R, Ogunrinade AF, Weil GJ: Use of recombinant *Onchocerca volvulus* antigens for diagnosis and surveillance of human onchocerciasis. Trop Med Int Health 1996;1:575.

162. Bradley JE, Unnasch TR: Molecular approaches to the diagnosis of onchocerciasis. Adv Parasitol 1996;37:58.

163. Ngu JL, Nkenfou C, Capuli E, et al: Novel, sensitive and low-cost diagnostic tests for "river blindness" detection of specific antigens in tears, urine, and dermal fluid. Trop Med Int Health 1998;3:339.

164. Meredith SE, Unnasch TR, Karam M, et al: Cloning and characterization of an *Onchocerca volvulus* specific DNA sequence. Mol Biochem Parasitol 1989;36:1.

165. Meredith SE, Lando G, Gbakima AA, et al: *Onchocerca volvulus*: Application of the polymerase chain reaction to identification and strain differentiation of the parasite. Exp Parasitol 1991;73:335.

166. Freedman DO, Unnasch TR, Merriweather A, et al: Truly infection-free persons are rare in areas hyperendemic for African onchocerciasis [letter]. J Infect Dis 1994;170:1054.

167. Zimmerman PA, Guderian RH, Araujo E, et al: Polymerase chain reaction–based diagnosis of *Onchocerca volvulus* infection: Improved detection of patients with onchocerciasis. J Infect Dis 1994;169:686.

168. Toé L, Merriweather A, Unnasch TR, et al: DNA probe based classification of the *Simulium damnosum* Theobaldi complex (Diptera: Simuliidae) in the Onchocerciasis Control Programme area in West Africa. Ann Trop Med Parasitol 1994;87:65.

169. McMahon JE, Simonsen PE: Filariasis. In: Cook GC, ed: Manson's

Tropical Diseases, 20th ed. London, WB Saunders, 1996, pp 1345–1346.

170. Nozias JP, Caumes E, Datry A, et al: Apropos of 5 new cases of onchocerciasis edema. Bull Soc Pathol Exot 1997;90:335.

171. Heid E, Friedel J, Koessler A, et al: Onchocercose et syndrome de Wells. Méd Trop 1994;54:423.

172. Ronday MJ, Van der Lelij A, Wienesen M, et al: Elevated serum angiotensin-converting enzyme activity in onchocerciasis. Lung 1996;174:393.

173. Burr WE Jr, Brown MF, Eberhard ML: Zoonotic Onchocerca (Nematoda: Filarioidea) in the cornea of a Colorado resident. Ophthalmology 1988;105:1494.

174. Spadea L, Magni R, Rinaldi G, et al: Unilateral retinitis pigmentosa: Clinical and electrophysiological report of four cases. Ophthalmologica 1998;212:350.

175. Duke BOL: Onchocerciasis (River Blindness)—Can it be eradicated? Parasitol Today 1990;6:82.

176. Anderson J, Fuglsang H: Further studies on the treatment of ocular onchocerciasis with diethylcarbamazine and suramin. Br J Ophthalmol 1978;62:450.

177. Mazzotti L, Hewitt R: Tratamiento de la onchocerciasis por el cloruro del 1-dietilcarbamil-4-metilpiperazine (Hetrazan). Med Mex 1947;28:3.

178. Greene BM, Taylor HR, Cupp EW, et al: Comparison of ivermectin and diethylcarbamazine in the treatment of onchocerciasis. N Engl J Med 1985;313:133.

179. Taylor HR: Recent developments in the treatment of onchocerciasis. Bull World Health Organ 1984;62:509.

180. Taylor HR, Murphy RP, Newland HS, et al: Treatment of onchocerciasis. The ocular effects of ivermectin and diethylcarbamazine. Arch Ophthalmol 1986;104:863.

181. Cousens SN, Yahaya H, Murdoch I, et al: Risk factors for optic nerve disease in communities mesoendemic for savannah onchocerciasis, Kaduna State, Nigeria. Trop Med Int Health 1997;2:89.

182. Campbell WC, Fisher MH, Stapley EO, et al: Ivermectin: A potent new antiparasitic agent. Science 1983;221:823.

183. Aziz MA, Diallo S, Diop IM, et al: Efficacy and tolerance of ivermectin in human onchocerciasis. Lancet 1982;2:171.

184. Pacqué M, Muñoz B, Greene BM, et al: Community-based treatment of onchocerciasis with ivermectin: Safety, efficacy, and acceptability of yearly treatment. J Infect Dis 1991;163:381.

185. Bennett JL, Williams JF, Dave V: Pharmacology of ivermectin. Parasitol Today 1988;4:226.

186. Alley ES, Plaisier AP, Boatin BA, et al: The impact of five years of annual ivermectin treatment on skin microfilarial loads in the onchocerciasis focus of Asubende, Ghana. Trans R Soc Trop Med Hyg 1994;88:581.

187. Greene BM, Dukuly DZ, Munoz B, et al: A comparison of 6-, 12-, and 24-monthly dosing with ivermectin for treatment of onchocerciasis. J Infect Dis 1991;163:376.

188. Vyungimana F, Newell E: Treatment of onchocerciasis with ivermectin (Province of Burundi, Burundi): Parasitologic and clinical evaluation of different periodicities of treatment. Am J Trop Med Hyg 1998;59:828.

189. Whitworth JAG, Downham MD, Lahai G, et al: A community trial of ivermectin for onchocerciasis in Sierra Leone: Compliance and parasitological profiles after three and a half years of intervention. Trop Med Int Health 1996;1:52.

190. Duke BOL, Zea-Flores G, Castro J, et al: Effects of multiple monthly doses of ivermectin on adult Onchocerca volvulus. Am J Trop Med Hyg 1990;43:657.

191. Duke BOL, Pacqué MC, Munoz B, et al: Viability of adult Onchocerca volvulus after six 2-weekly doses of ivermectin. Bull World Health Organ 1991;69:163.

192. Duke BOL, Zea-Flores G, Castro J, et al: Effects of three-month doses of ivermectin on adult Onchocerca volvulus. Am J Trop Med Hyg 1992;46:189.

193. Cupp EW, Bernardo MJ, Kiszewski AE, et al: The effect of ivermectin on transmission of Onchocerca volvulus. Science 1986;231:740.

194. Cupp EW, Ochoa O, Collins RC, et al: The effect of multiple ivermectin treatments on infection of Simulium ochraceum with Onchocerca volvulus. Am J Trop Med Hyg 1989;40:501.

195. Trpis M, Childs JE, Fryauff DJ, et al: Effect of mass treatment of a human population with ivermectin on transmission of Onchocerca volvulus by Simulium yahense in Liberia, West Africa. Am J Trop Med Hyg 1990;42:148.

196. Boussinesq M, Chippaux JP, Ernould JC, et al: Effect of repeated treatments with ivermectin on the incidence of onchocerciasis in northern Cameroon. Am J Trop Med Hyg 1995;3:63.

197. Taylor HR, Pacqué M, Muñoz B, et al: Impact of mass treatment of onchocerciasis with ivermectin on the transmission of infection. Science 1990;250:116.

198. Awadzi K, Dadzie KY, Kläger S, et al: The chemotherapy of onchocerciasis. XIII. Studies with ivermectin in onchocerciasis patients in northern Ghana, a region with long lasting vector control. Trop Med Parasitol 1989;40:361.

199. Dadzie KY, Awadzi K, Bird AC, et al: Ophthalmological results from a placebo controlled comparative 3-dose ivermectin study in the treatment of onchocerciasis. Trop Med Parasitol 1989;40:355.

200. Mabey D, Whitworth JAG, Eckstein M, et al: The effects of multiple doses of ivermectin on ocular onchocerciasis. Ophthalmology 1996;103:1001.

201. Prod'hon J, Boussinesq M, Fobi G, et al: Lutte contre l'onchocercose par ivermectine: Résultats d'une campagne de masse au Nord-Cameroun. Bull World Health Organ 1991;69:443.

202. Whitworth JAG, Gilbert CE, Mabey DM, et al: Effects of repeated doses of ivermectin on ocular onchocerciasis: Community-based trial in Sierra Leone. Lancet 1991;338:1100.

203. Dadzie KY, Remme J, De Sole G: Changes in ocular onchocerciasis after two rounds of community-based ivermectin treatment in a holo-endemic onchocerciasis focus. Trans R Soc Trop Med Hyg 1991;85:267.

204. Abiose A, Jones BR, Cousens SN, et al: Reduction in incidence of optic nerve disease with annual ivermectin to control onchocerciasis. Lancet 1993;341:130.

205. White AT, Newland HS, Taylor HR, et al: Controlled trial and dose-finding study of ivermectin for treatment of onchocerciasis. J Infect Dis 1987;156:463.

206. Taylor HR, Gonzales C, Duke BOL: Simplified dose schedule of ivermectin. Lancet 1993;341:50.

207. Shu EN, Okonkwo PO, Ogbodo SO: An improved schedule for ivermectin as microfilaricidal agent against onchocerciasis. Acta Trop 1997;68:269.

208. Bryan RT, Stokes SL, Spencer HC: Expatriates treated with ivermectin. Lancet 1991;337:304.

209. Davidson RN, Godfrey-Faussett P, Bryceson ADM: Adverse reactions in expatriates treated with ivermectin. Lancet 1990;336:1005.

210. Chijoke CP, Okonkwo PO: Adverse events following mass ivermectin therapy for onchocerciasis. Trans R Soc Trop Med Hyg 1992;86:284.

211. De Sole G, Dadzie KY, Giese J, et al: Lack of adverse reactions in ivermectin treatment of onchocerciasis. Lancet 1990;335:1106.

212. De Sole G, Remme J, Awadzi K, et al: Adverse reactions after large-scale treatment of onchocerciasis with ivermectin: Combined results from eight community trials. Bull World Health Organ 1989;67:707.

213. Pacqué M, Dukuly Z, Greene BM, et al: Community-based treatment of onchocerciasis with ivermectin: Acceptability and early adverse reactions. Bull World Health Organ 1989;67:721.

214. Whitworth JAG, Morgan D, Maude GH, et al: Community-based treatment with ivermectin. Lancet 1988;2:97.

215. Gardon J, Gardon-Wendel N, Demanga-Ngangue, et al: Serious reactions after mass treatment of onchocerciasis with ivermectin in an area endemic for Loa loa infection. Lancet 1997;350:18.

216. Boussinesq M, Gardon J, Gardon-Wendel N, et al: Three probable cases of Loa loa encephalopathy following ivermectin treatment for onchocerciasis. Am J Trop Med Hyg 1998;58:461.

217. Pacqué M, Muñoz B, Poetschke G, et al: Pregnancy outcome after inadvertent ivermectin treatment during community-based distribution. Lancet 1990;336:1486.

218. Guderian RH, Lovato R, Anselmi M, et al: Onchocerciasis and reproductive health in Ecuador. Trans R Soc Trop Med Hyg 1997;91:315.

219. Rougemont A, Thylefors B, Ducam M, et al: Traitement de l'onchocercose par suramine a faible doses progressives dans les collectivités hyperendémiques d'Afrique occidentale. 1. Résultats parasitologiques et surveillance ophtalmologique en zone de transmission non interrompue. Bull OMS 1980;58:917.

220. Chijoke CP, Umeh RE, Mbah AU, et al: Clinical pharmacokinetics of suramin in patients with onchocerciasis. Eur J Clin Pharmacol 1998;54:249.

221. Poltera AA, Zea-Flores G, Guderian R, et al: Onchocercacidal effects of amocarzine (CGP 6140) in Latin America. Lancet 1991;337:583.

222. Awadzi K, Opoku NO, Attah SK, et al: The safety and efficacy of amocarzine in African onchocerciasis and the influence of ivermectin on the clinical and parasitological response to treatment. Ann Trop Med Parasitol 1997;91:281.

223. Jones BR, Anderson J, Fuglsang H: Evaluation of microfilaricidal effects in the cornea from topically applied drugs in ocular onchocerciasis: Trials with levamisole and mebendazole. Br J Ophthalmol 1978;62:440.

224. Jones BR, Anderson J, Fuglsang H: Effects of various concentrations of diethylcarbamazine citrate applied as eye drops in ocular onchocerciasis, and the possibilities of improved therapy from continuous non-pulsed delivery. Br J Ophthalmol 1978;62:428.

225. Fuglsang H, Anderson J: Further observations on the relationship between ocular onchocerciasis and the head nodule, and on the possible benefit of nodulectomy. Br J Ophthalmol 1978;62:445.

226. Anderson J, Fuglsang H, Hamilton PJS, et al: The prognostic value of head nodules and microfilariae in the skin in relation to ocular onchocerciasis. Tropenmed Parasitol 1975;26:191.

227. Guillet P, Sékétéli A, Alley ES, et al: Impact of combined large-scale ivermectin distribution and vector control on transmission of *Onchocerca volvulus* in the Niger basin, Guinea. Bull World Health Organ 1995;73:199.

228. De Sole G, Baker R, Dadzie KY, et al: Onchocerciasis distribution and severity in five West African countries. Bull World Health Organ 1991;69:689.

229. Samba EM: The Onchocerciasis Control Programme in West Africa. Geneva, World Health Organization, 1994.

230. Molyneux DH, Davies JB: Onchocerciasis control: Moving toward the millennium. Parasitol Today 1997;13:417.

231. Hougard JM, Yaméogo L, Sékétéli A, et al: Twenty-two years of blackfly control in the Onchocerciasis Control Programme in West Africa. Parasitol Today 1997;13:425.

232. Davies JB, Oskam L, Luján R, et al: Detection of *Onchocerca volvulus* DNA in pools of wild-caught *Simulium ochraceum* by use of the polymerase chain reaction. Ann Trop Med Parasitol 1998;92:295.

233. Yaméogo L, Toé L, Hougard JM, et al: Pool screen polymerase chain reaction for estimating the prevalence of *Onchocerca volvulus* infection in *Simulium damnosum* sensu lato: Results of a field trial in an area subject to successful vector control. Am J Trop Med Hyg 1999;60:124.

234. Prost A, Vaugelade J: La surmortalité des aveugles en zone de savane ouest-africaine. Bull OMS 1981;59:773.

41 — LOIASIS

Yosuf El-Shabrawi

DEFINITION

Loiasis is a chronic parasitic disease caused by the filarial parasite *Loa loa*. It is characterized by two major features, Calabar swelling (which is localized angioedema) and subconjunctival migration of the filarial worm.[1] Filarial worms such as *Loa loa* are nematodes (roundworms) that dwell in the subcutaneous tissue or lymphatics. Eight nematode species infect humans; of these, four—*Wucheria bancrofti*, *Brugia malayi*, *Onchocerca volvulus*, and *Loa loa*—are responsible for the most serious filarial infections.[2]

HISTORY

Philipp Pigafetta (1533–1603) translated the oral African report of the Portuguese Eduart Lopez into the Italian language. But contrary to the common theory[2a] that *Loa loa* was first noted by Pigafetta, there is no reference to the African eye worm in Pigafetta's work.[2b] The first verified report of a subconjunctival worm was by Mongin. He removed a subconjunctival worm in an African girl in the West Indies in 1770. The name Loa has first noted by a French navy surgeon, Guyot. He frequently found a conjunctivitis caused by worms in natives of Angola, and he described them as *Loa loa*. In 1895, D. Argyll Robertson described the adult worm that he extracted from the eye of a woman who had resided at Old Calabar in West Africa.[3] In 1891, Manson found microfilariae in the blood, naming them "microfilaria diurna." He suggested *Chrysops dimidiata* as the intermediate host, later proven by Leiper in 1913.[3a]

EPIDEMIOLOGY

Loiasis is endemic to the rain forests of Nigeria, Zaire, northwest Angola, the Congo, Chad, the Central African Republic, Gabon, the Cameroon Republic, and southwest Sudan.[4] Up to 13 million people are estimated to be infected. In hyperendemic areas, exposure may approach up to 100%. If *Loa loa* is carried to other parts of the world, as by Africans to America, or European colonists returning home, the worm dies out. The reason is the localization of its intermediate host, the female blood-sucking mangrove flies *Chrysops silacea* and *C. dimidiata*, to the rain forests of Africa. These vectors are day-biting flies that are attracted by people moving through open spaces in the jungle. They usually settle on the ankles, exciting little or no pain, and draw large quantities of blood. These flies are infected by ingesting human blood contaminated with parasitic microfilaria.[4] In Calabar, 3.5% of wild flies that are caught carry *Loa loa*. Monkeys, especially the drill (*Mandrillus leucophaeus*), harbor a form of *Loa*, but the microfilariae of this form are nocturnally periodic and the vectors are the night-biting *Chrysops langi* and *Chrysops centurionis*. Although the two strains have been hybridrized experimentally, it is unlikely that monkeys act as reservoir hosts, because the nocturnal vector species of *Chrysops* do not usually bite humans.

LIFE HISTORY

In the fly, the microfilaria (primarily 250 to 300 μm long by 6 to 8 μm wide)[5] penetrate the intestinal wall and become infectious larvae intracellularly. Within 3 days after ingestion, the larva becomes broad and torpedo shaped; on the fourth and fifth days, the squat form lengthens to 0.8 to 1 mm; on the sixth day, the corkscrew-like appearance is replaced by gentle curves. The development is complete after 10 days, when the microfilariae reach a size of 2 mm by 0.03 mm. Then the larvae congregate in the head of the fly in large numbers. Every time an infected fly feeds, larvae emerge and are deposited on the human skin, from which they disappear rapidly by burrowing into the skin. In the mammalian host, the worms migrate along the interfascial planes, where they develop into adults. In about 4 to 6 months, after mating, the gravid females release microfilariae, which enter the host's circulatory system. After transmission to another fly, a new life cycle is initiated. The microfilariae of *Loa loa* circulate in the blood of humans with a diurnal periodicity whose peak occurs around noon.[4]

MORPHOLOGY

Loa loa is a filiform, cylindrical, whitish, semitransparent worm with numerous round and smooth translucent protuberances and a blunt tail. Males measure 3 to 3.4 cm in length and 0.35 to 0.43 mm in width; females are bigger (5 to 7 cm by 0.5 mm). The cuticle is covered with small bosses, which is helpful in histologically distinguishing *Loa loa* from other filarial parasites.[4] The microfilarial *loa* is similar in size and structure to microfilarial *bancrofti*. In fresh blood, it may be impossible to distinguish them. In dried stained films, *Loa loa* assumes an angular attitude, the tail end giving a corkscrew appearance. Microfilarial *loa* takes up methylene blue (diluted 1:5000) in 10 minutes, as opposed to microfilarial *bancrofti*, which is much slower to do so.[4]

CLINICAL FEATURES

Systemic

The most common pathology associated with *Loa loa* in humans is Calabar swelling,[1, 2] named after the region in Africa where it was first described. Other reported systemic complications include nephropathy,[6] cardiomyopathy,[2] arthritis, lymphangitis, peripheral neuropathy,[7] and encephalopathy.[5, 8, 9] Sites of Calabar swelling[1, 2] are localized areas of erythema and angioedema, often 5 to 10 cm or more in size. They often occur on extremities, typically around joints such as the wrist of knee, and last for about 1 to 3 days before spontaneous regression. If the inflammatory reaction extends to nearby joints or peripheral nerves, corresponding symptoms may emerge. These swellings appear to be caused by hyperemic reactions to adult worms. Calabar swellings are usually found in expatriates and can be totally absent in patients native to areas with high incidences of *Loa loa* infections.[10, 11] They may in some instances occur only during treatment with diethylcarbamazine (DEC). In addition to Calabar swellings, multiple papillomatous erythemas may occur as soon as 1 to 4 weeks after infection.[10, 12] These represent subcutaneous moving larvae.

The nephropathy,[5, 6] generally presenting with proteinuria, appears to be immune-complex mediated. Renal biopsies show signs of chronic glomerulonephritis or membranous glomerulonephropathy. Following DEC treatment, the proteinuria may increase transiently.

Encephalopathy[5, 8, 9] occurred only rarely before treatment with DEC became available, but it has become a feared and increasingly observed complication. The pathogenesis is not yet clear, but two possibilities have been proposed: (1) an allergic reaction to dying microfilaria in association with a pre-existing subacute encephalitis, and (2) a Herxheimer's reaction to released neurotropic endotoxin. The symptoms may range from psychoneurotic complaints such as insomnia, irritability, depression, and headache, to coma and death after treatment with DEC in patients with high concentrations of microfilaremia (over 500 microfilariae per 20 mm³).[1] Microfilariae are often found in the cerebrospinal fluid.[5] Pathologic findings in these patients are (1) a generalized acute cerebral edema, thought to originate as an allergic reaction to the parasite or parasitic "debris" after DEC treatment, or (2) a chronic subacute encephalitis characterized by a necrotizing granulomatous reactions to degenerating microfilariae found not only associated with the cerebral vessels but also extending to the parenchyma. Retinal hemorrhages frequently accompany the encephalitis.

Cardiomyopathy[2, 5] is related to loiasis more circumstantially. Epidemiologic correlations have been found between the distribution of loiasis and endomyocardial fibrosis. Patients present with characteristic cardiac abnormalities, such as fibrosis of the endocardium in one or both ventricles that affects the apex and the inflow tracts. In addition, high levels of peripheral blood eosinophilia and elevated levels of antifilarial titers are found in these patients. Although the relationship between the endomyocardial fibrosis and loiasis is not yet clear, it may be less the filariae themselves and more the eosinophilia that leads to the cardiac damage, because the cardiac lesions found resemble those found in Löffler's fibroblastic parietal endocarditis, an entity characterized by a disorder of eosinophil production known as hypereosinophilic syndrome.[5]

It has become apparent that there are significant differences in clinical manifestations of infections between visitors to endemic regions and natives.[11] In the native population, loiasis is often an asymptomatic infection despite high levels of microfilaremia. Infections may be recognized only after subconjunctival migration of adult worms or manifestations of Calabar swellings. Nephropathy, encephalopathy, and cardiomyopathy are rare. In temporary residents or visitors, allergic symptoms predominate. Calabar swelling tends to be more frequent, microfilaremia is rare, and eosinophilia and increased levels of antifilarial antibodies are characteristic. The lack of microfilaremia sometimes makes the diagnosis difficult.

Ocular Manifestations

The characteristics of ocular involvement by *Loa loa* are listed in Table 41–1.

Lids and Orbit

When the worms appear in the subcutaneous tissues of the lids and orbit, they may induce intense irritation and edema. These swellings may be of considerable size, reaching from the lid margins to the brows, and they may disappear as rapidly as they appear, when the worm burrows into deeper tissues. These sojourns of the worm, leaving the subcutaneous tissues of the lids for the conjunctiva, disappearing into the orbit, flitting over the bridge of the nose to the lids of the other eye or down across the cheek, cause intense irritation to the patient. As a general rule, heat entices the parasite to the surface, whereas cold drives it into deeper tissues.[13, 14]

Conjunctiva

This worm has also been named African eye worm. Subconjunctival migration of the filariae is the most common ocular involvement[16–28] and often the only clinical sign in a patient with loiasis. Their presence under the conjunctiva usually leads to itching, pain, foreign body sensation, irritation, and a mild hyperemia of the conjunctiva. These signs may persist until the worm burrows into deeper tissues or is paralyzed by the instillation of cocaine, bringing instant relief.[13] An acute periorbital angioedema and conjunctival nodules may evolve as the result of the presence of a dead worm.[13] Rarely, the nematode may be encysted in the subconjunctival tissues.[15]

TABLE 41–1. CHARACTERISTICS OF OCULAR INVOLVEMENT BY LOA LOA

Conjunctiva and lids
   Presence of adult worm
   Mild hyperemia
   Periorbital angioedema
   Conjunctival nodules
Anterior segment
   Presence of adult worm
   Edema of the iris and ciliary body
   Fibrous membrane in the chamber angle
   Cells and flare in the anterior chamber
Lens
   Cataract
Choroid
   Chronic perivascular inflammatory infiltrate
   Presence of microfilaria
Retina
   Retinal edema
   Exudative retinal detachment
   Subretinal fluid with the presence of microfilaria
   Large superficial hemorrhagic sheets
   Disseminated yellowish exudates
Retinal vessels
   Obstructed arterioles
   Microaneurysms occluded by microfilaria
   Chronic perivascular inflammatory infiltrate
   Occlusion of the central retinal artery

Anterior Segment

Intracameral migration of *Loa loa* is very rare.[29–31] The worms, if still alive, are usually seen by the patients as moving shadows. Atropine may restrict the movements and kill the worm, but pilocarpine apparently irritates it and makes it burrow deeper into the tissues.[13, 20] The presence of a live worm may in some instances initially cause surprisingly little inflammation.[13, 29, 31] After the worm dies, an eye that has tolerated the living filaria well for a long period may suddenly become inflamed,[13, 31] showing considerable inflammatory response, with signs of extensive iridocyclitis, which is usually associated with some degree of keratitis, a cloudy aqueous, vitreous opacification, and raised intraocular pressure.[13] Apart from these inflammatory signs, however, symptoms may be very mild unless the worms burrow into the ciliary body, in which case the pain may be excrutiating.[31]

Posterior Segment

Reports of posterior segment involvement by *Loa loa* are very limited. As documented by Osuntokun and Olurin[31] and by Toussaint and Danis,[32] the presence of nematodes in the posterior segment is usually associated with massive retinal destruction. In most circumstances, extensive hemorrhagic lesions have been reported, associated with either retinal detachment, retinal neovascularization with vitreous hemorrhage, a subretinal exudate,[31] or the presence of multiple yellowish exudates throughout the retina and the presence of occluded arterioles.[32] Under these circumstances, free microfilariae may be found in the retina and lumina of retinal and choroidal vessels on histologic evaluation. In addition to an inflammatory response, acute retinal ischemia may result from occlusion of the central artery by microfilariae.[33, 34]

Toussaint and Danis[32] described a 38-year-old man who later died of filarial meningoencephalitis. The patient was referred to the hospital because of bilateral reduction of vision with photophobia, increased size of the parotid gland, disseminated petechiae over his whole body, and a mobile worm in the left upper lid. At this stage, the patient was somnolent. Funduscopic examination revealed multiple superficial hemorrhagic lesions, partially covered with a yellowish exudate throughout the retina. In addition, several occluded arterioles were present. The histologic examination showed extensive hemorrhagic sheets, serous exudates, and free microfilariae in the retina. The luminae of several retinal and choroidal vessels were distended by microfilariae and surrounded by chronic inflammatory cells.

Osuntokun and Olurin[31] described two patients with an intraocular *Loa loa*. The first patient, a 22-year-old Nigerian woman, reported to the hospital with a 6-month history of pain, itching, and a sensation of a worm in her right eye. There was no light perception, the cornea was hazy, and, in the anterior chamber, a vigorously moving worm was seen. After enucleation of the eye, a total retinal detachment with gelatinous exudate was seen, with the features of a male *Loa loa* in the anterior chamber. The second patient, a 15-year-old Nigerian girl, was referred to the hospital because of pain and feelings of a worm in her right eye for 5 months. Minimal flare and cells were present in the anterior chamber. The patient was scheduled for surgical removal of the worm 1 week later but did not return until 3 months later, when she complained of further pain. The worm was no longer mobile and was embedded in a thick fibrinous membrane. Because of the development of violent inflammation after removal of the worm, the eye had to be enucleated.

DIAGNOSIS

A definitive diagnosis of loiasis requires the detection of either microfilariae in the peripheral blood, urine, or other body fluid, or the isolation of an adult worm. In practice, the diagnosis must often be based on a characteristic history, clinical presentation, blood eosinophilia, and elevated levels of antifilarial antibodies, particularly in travelers to the endemic regions, who are usually amicrofilaric. Other clinical findings include hypergammaglobulinemia, elevated levels of serum IgE, and elevated leukocytes.[1, 2]

Detection of Microfilaria in Blood

Specimen Collection

Specimens should be collected before treatment is initiated. Since the parasitemia varies with the filarial species, a travel history should be obtained to maximize the best collection time for the species of filaria suspected. The best collection time for *Loa loa* is midday (between 10 AM and 2 PM).

Type of Sample

Venous blood samples provide sufficient material for performing a variety of tests. Earlobe or finger-prick blood may be taken for direct wet, thin, and thick blood smears.

At least two thick smears and two thin smears should be prepared as soon as possible after collection. For increased sensitivity, concentration techniques can be used. These include centrifugation of the blood sample lysed in 2% formalin (Knott's technique), or filtration through a 3-μm Nucleopore membrane. Smears can be stained with Giemsa or hematoxylin and eosin. Filaria may even be detected in the urine or other body fluids of a patient with a high level of microfilaremia or soon after DEC treatment has been initiated.

Pronounced eosinophilia is seen in association with the liberation of microfilariae from the female worm, with corresponding clinical correlates of Calabar swelling and pruritus, thought to be an IgE-mediated allergic response. Typically, the eosinophil count can be from 20,000 to 50,000/mm³.

Microscopy

Loa loa microfilaria are sheathed with a relatively dense nuclear column. The tail tapers and is frequently coiled, and the nuclei extend to the end of the tail.[4]

Molecular Diagnosis

Earlier methods using species-specific radiolabeled probes to target DNA[35] have been replaced by more sensitive and specific polymerase chain reaction–based assays.[36, 37]

Antibody Detection

Diagnosis by the detection of antibodies is of limited value because of substantial cross reactivity between filaria and other helminths. Furthermore, a positive serologic test does not distinguish between past and current infections. For indirect serum immunofluorescence antibody tests[1, 22] or enzyme-linked immunosorbent assays (ELISA),[38] the antigen usually used is from the canine heartworm *Dirofilaria immitis*. Attempts to use a *Loa loa*–specific antigen have been proven sensitive but not adequately specific.[39, 40]

Antigen Detection

Using an immunoassay (e.g., ELISA)[41] for circulating *Loa loa* antigens is a useful approach, especially in cases of low microfilaremia, but its results have to be considered with care because of its high cross reactivity.

TREATMENT

Surgical Removal of the Worm

Adult worms may be removed from under the conjunctiva by first anesthetizing them with either atropine or 10% cocaine. Pilocarpine should not be used, because it is known to irritate the worm, which may then disappear into deeper tissues.[13, 20] The worm should first be firmly immobilized using a forceps and then removed after incising the conjunctiva.

Diethylcarbamazine

DEC has been the therapeutic mainstay for the last 40 years and has proven effective against both the microfilaria and the adult worm. The exact mechanism of action is still not clear. It is thought that DEC leads to a hyperpolarization of the muscle cells of the parasite, inhibiting movement, and that it induces morphologic alterations on the surface layers of the filarial membrane, exposing previously hidden antigenic determinants and stimulating a host inflammatory response.[42–44] The inflammatory response following DEC treatment may take the form of a Mazzotti reaction with dermatologic and neurologic manifestations.

Encephalitis, rarely observed before the introduction of DEC in 1947, has been seen increasingly as a complication of therapy that may lead to death or severe neuropsychiatric sequelae. Persons with microfilaremia (above 500 organisms per 20 mm³ blood) are at highest risk, and a single dose of DEC can precipitate the reaction.[5] Therefore, concomitant treatment with corticosteroids and antihistamines is highly recommended to reduce the risk of allergic reactions caused by the destruction of microfilariae.

The current therapy consists of administering 6 to 8 mg of DEC per kilogram of body weight in three divided doses per day over a 3-week period.[12] Therapy can be initiated with 50 mg three times daily and each dose thereafter is increased by 50 mg until a dose of 6 to 8 mg/kg body weight has been reached. Gradually increasing the dose seems to diminish the adverse side effects caused by the drug. Depending on the microfilaria counts, up to three courses of DEC treatment may be required.[12] In the case of high microfilaremia (500 mi-

crofilariae per 20 mm³ blood), lower starting doses as small as 0.5 mg/kg/day are recommended with additional corticosteroids (40 to 60 mg/day). If the antifilarial treatment does not have any adverse side effects, the prednisone can be rapidly tapered and the DEC dose gradually increased to 6 to 8 mg/kg/day.

Care should be taken to ascertain whether the patient also has onchocerciasis, as DEC can cause severe cutaneous reactions in such patients.[1]

Ivermectin

Ivermectin is a safer drug than DEC and is used in a single dose. Adverse neurologic side effects as seen with DEC have not been described with ivermectin. It has been shown to reduce microfilaremia, but it does not seem to be effective against adult worms.[45, 46] Ivermectin should be given at a dose of 200 to 400 µg/kg body weight. Pretreatment with ivermectin, before the use of DEC, to reduce the chance of neurologic complications seems to be a possible way of treating patients with heavy microfilaremia.

Albendazole

Albendazole, 200 mg twice daily for 3 weeks, is effective only against adult worms.[47] Because of its minimal effect against microfilariae, allergic side effects are very unlikely. The effect of albendazole, based on a continuous slow reduction of microfilaremia, correlates well with the average survival of microfilaria (6 to 14 months).

Mebendazole

Mebendazole, in dosages of 100 to 500 mg 3 times a day over 28 days, has been shown to reduce microfilaremia over 4 to 6 weeks without complications, but it is not known whether it is active against adult worms.[1]

PREVENTION AND CHEMOPROPHYLAXIS

Prevention depends on avoiding places where biting flies are numerous, wearing protective clothing, and using insect repellents. DEC can be used as a chemoprophylactic agent given either at a dose of 300 mg once weekly or 200 mg twice daily over three consecutive days once a month.[48]

References

1. Duke BOL: Loiasis. In: Strickland GT, ed: Hunter's Tropical Medicine, 7th ed. Philadelphia, W.B. Saunders, 1992, pp 727–772.
2. Nutman TB, Weller PF: Harrison's Principles of Internal Medicine, 14th ed. New York, McGraw-Hill, 1998, p 1215.
2a. Belding D: Textbook of Parasitology, 3rd ed. New York, Appleton-Century-Crofts, 1965, p 542.
2b. Gruntzig J: The first description of Loa loa infestation of the eye by Pigafetta: A historical error. Klin Monatsbl Augenheilkd 1976;169:383–386.
3. Lymie S, Bruckner G, Bruckner DA: Diagnostic Medical Parasitology, 3rd ed. Washington, DC, ASM Press, 1997, pp 275–291.
3a. Manson-Bahr: Proc R Soc Med 1939;31:1623.
4. Wilcocks, Manson-Bahr: Manson's Tropical Diseases, 17th ed. Baltimore, Williams and Wilkins, 1972, pp 1051–1054.
5. Ottesen AE, Warren KS, Mahmoud AAF: Tropical and Geographical Medicine, 2nd ed. New York, McGraw-Hill Information Service, 1990, pp 403–405.
6. Pillay VKG, Kirch E, Kurtzman NA: Glomerulonephropathy associated with filarial loiasis. JAMA 1973;225:179.

7. Schofield FD: Two cases of loiasis with peripheral nerve involvement. Trans R Soc Trop Med Hyg 1955;49:588–589.

8. VanBogaert L, Dubois A, Janssen PG: Encephalitis in *Loa loa* filariasis. J Neurol Neurosurg Psychiatry 1955;18:103.

9. Carme B, Boulesteix J, Boutes H, Puruhence MG: Five cases of encephalitis during treatment of loiasis with diethycarbamazine. Am J Trop Med Hyg 1991;44:684–690.

10. Carme B, Mamboueni JP, Copin N, Noireau F: Clinical and biological study of *Loa loa* filariasis in Congolese. Am J Trop Med Hyg 1989;41:331–337.

11. Klion AD, Massougbodji A, Sadeler BC, et al: Loiasis in endemic and nonendemic populations: Immunologically mediated differences in clinical presentation. J Infect Dis 1991;163:1318–1325.

12. Greene BM: Loiasis. In: Gorbach SL, Bratlett NR, Blacklow, eds: Infectious Diseases. Philadelphia: W.B. Saunders, 1992, pp 2012–2013.

13. Duke-Elder WS. Systems of Ophthalmology, 2nd ed. London, Henry Kimpton, 1968, pp 401–405.

14. Fleck BW, MacDonald M: Periocular *Loa loa* in eastern Scotland: A report of two cases. J R Coll Surg Edinb 1987;32:163–165.

15. Carme B, Botaka E, Lehenaff YM: Dead *Loa loa* filaria in a subconjunctival site. Apropos of a case. J Fr Ophthalmol 1988;11:865–867.

16. Reisman J, Krolman GM, Hogg GR: Conjunctival *Loa loa*. Can J Ophthalmol 1974;9:379–380.

17. Johnsons GJ, Axsmith K, Desser SS: The elusive *Loa loa*. A case report of ocular filariasis in Canada. Can J Ophthalmol 1973;8:492–496.

18. Sacks HN, Williams DN, Eifrig DE: Loiasis. Report of a case and review of the literature. Arch Intern Med 1976;136:914–915.

19. Wiesinger EC, Winkler S, Egger S, et al: Afrikanischer Augenwurm als Erstmanifestation einer Loiasis. Dtsch Med Wochenschr 1995;120:1156–1160.

20. Sachs HG, Heep M, Gaberl VP: Chirugische Wurmentfernung bei Loa-Loa Ophthalmie. Klin Monatsbl Augenheilkd 1998;213:367–369.

21. Patel CK, Churchill D, Teimory M, Tabendeh H: Unexplained foreign body sensation: Thinking of loiasis in at risk patients prevents significant morbidity. Eye 1993;7:714–715.

22. Radda TM, Picher O, Egerer I, Gnad HD: Serum immunofluorescence examination in *Loa* ophthalmia. Klin Monatsbl Augenheilkd 1981;178:147–148.

23. Grupp A: A case of Loa-loa filariasis. Klin Monatsbl Augenheilkd 1975;167:70–76.

24. Vey EK: Filaria—Loa-loa: Case report. Ann Ophthalmol 1975;7:389–392.

25. Lee BY, McMillan R: *Loa loa*: Ocular filariasis in an African student in Missouri. Ann Ophthalmol 1984;16:456–458.

26. Clausen M, Roider J, Fuhrmann C, Laqua H: Stabbing pain, conjunctival changes, foreign body sensation and unilateral red eye. Subconjunctival macrofilariasis in systemic *Loa loa* filariasis. Ophthalmology 1998;95:56–57.

27. Farrer WE, Wittner M, Tanowitz HB: African eye worm (*Loa loa*) in a tourist. Ann Ophthalmol 1981;13:1177–1179.

28. Fenton P: *Loa loa*: The African eye worm. Arch Ophthalmol 1966;76:866–867.

29. Carme B, Kaya-Gandaziami G, Pintart D: Localization of the filaria *Loa loa* in the anterior chamber of the eye. Apropos of a case. Acta Trop 1984;41:265–269.

30. Satyavani M, Rao KN: Live male adult *Loa loa* in the anterior chamber of the eye—A case report. Indian J Pathol Microbiol 1993;36:154–157.

31. Osuntokun O, Olurin O: Filarial worm (*Loa loa*) in the anterior chamber. Report of two cases. Br J Ophthalmol 1975;59:166–167.

32. Toussaint D, Danis P: Retinopathy in generalized loa-loa filariasis. A clinicopathological study. Arch Opthalmol 1965;74:470–476.

33. Corrigan M, Hill D: Retinal artery occlusion in loiasis. Br J Ophthalmol 1968;52:477–480.

34. Langlois M: Filarios loa. Thrombose de l'artere centrale de la retine et syndrome cerebellux. Rev Neurol 1962;107:381.

35. Chandrashekar R: Recent advances in diagnosis of filarial infections. Indian J Exp Biol 1997;35:18–26.

36. Toure FS, Kassambra L, Williams T, et al: Human occult loiasis: Improvement in diagnostic sensitivity by the use of a nested polymerase chain reaction. Am J Trop Med Hyg 1998;59:144–149.

37. Singh B: Molecular methods for diagnosis and epidemiological studies of parasitic infections. Int J Parasitol 1997;27:1135–1145.

38. Churchill DR, Morris C, Fakoya A, et al: Clinical and laboratory features in patients with loiasis (*Loa loa* filariasis) in the UK. J Infect 1996;33:103–109.

39. Ogunba E: Serological investigations with *Loa loa* antigens. J Helminthol 1972;46:241–250.

40. Ottesen EA, Weller PF, Lunde MN, Hussein R: Endemic filariasis on a Pacific island. II. Immunologic aspects: Immunoglobulin, complement and specific antifilarial IgG, IgM and IgE antibodies. Am J Trop Med Hyg 1983;31:953–961.

41. Jaoko WG: *Loa loa* antigen detection by ELISA: A new approach to diagnosis. East Afr Med J 1995;72:176–179.

42. Haque A, Capron A, Ouaissi A, et al: Immune unresponsiveness and its possible relation to filarial disease. Contrib Microbiol Immunol 1983;7:9–21.

43. Mackenzie CD, Kron MA: Diethycarbamazine: A review of its action in onchocerciasis, lymphatic filariasis and inflammation. Trop Dis Bull 1985;82:R1.

44. Yazdanbakhsh M, Duym L, Aarden L, Partono F: Serum interleukin-6 levels and adverse reactions to diethycarbamazine in lymphatic filariasis. J Infect Dis 1992;166:453–454.

45. Chippaux JP, Ernould JC, Gardon J, et al: Ivermectin treatment of loiasis. Trans R Soc Trop Med Hyg 1992;86:289.

46. Hovette P, Debonne JM, Touze JE, et al: Efficacy of ivermectin treatment of *Loa loa* filariasis patients without microfilaremia. Ann Trop Med Parasitol 1994;88:93–94.

47. Klion AD, Massoughbodji A, Horton J, et al: Albendazole in human loiasis. Results of double blind, placebo controlled trial. J Infect Dis 1993;168:202–206.

48. Nutman TB, Miller KD, Mulligan M, et al: Diethycarbamazine prophylaxis for human loiasis. Results of a double blind study. N Engl J Med 1988;319:752–756.

42 — CYSTICERCOSIS

Lawrence A. Raymond and Adam H. Kaufman

DEFINITION

Cysticercosis is the most common ocular tapeworm infection. It occurs especially in underdeveloped areas where hygiene is poor. Cysticercosis is usually caused by *Cysticercus cellulosae*, the larval form of the pork tapeworm, *Taenia solium*. Occasionally, cysticercosis in humans is caused by the larvae of the beef tapeworm, *Taenia saginata*.

Humans become infected usually by drinking contaminated water or eating food containing the eggs of *Taenia solium*. If untreated, intraocular cysticercosis usually results in blindness and atrophy of the eye (Fig. 42–1). The best means of cure is surgical removal of the larva, although destruction of the larva can be obtained with diathermy, photocoagulation, or cryogenic applications.

HISTORY

Porcine cysticercosis has been described since antiquity. Cysticercus observed in the anterior chamber of the human eye was first reported by Sömmerring in 1830; the first extraction was by Schott in 1836.[1] Cysticercosis of the posterior segment of the eye was first described by Coccius in 1853.[2] von Graefe was the first surgeon to remove the larva from the vitreous cavity in 1858.[3]

Since 1945, most reports of ocular cysticercosis deal with its treatment. Three of the largest series of cases of ocular cysticercosis were from Brazil and Mexico. Junior[4] collected 111 cases, Santos and colleagues 19 cases,[5, 6] and Cardenas and colleagues 30 cases.[7] These will be reviewed in detail in the sections Treatment and Prognosis. Most other reports since 1945 have been small series of one to three cases.

Hutton and colleagues[8] reported the first successful removal of an intravitreal cysticercus by pars plana vitrectomy in 1976. Postoperative visual acuity was 20/20, but the reported follow-up period was very brief. Later communication with Hutton revealed that there was no further ocular inflammation in his patient after several years.[9]

In 1975, Rodriquez[10] of Bogotá, Columbia, reported at the International Photocoagulation Congress the successful photocoagulation of a small (less than 8 mm), early posterior subretinal cysticercus.

Pavan[11] brought modern vitrectomy instrumentation to a remote area in Peru aboard the Oribus airplane and successfully removed a live submacular cysticercus through a retinotomy in the temporal macula in 1986. This technique avoided making a posterior sclerotomy, which is frequently associated with difficulty in exposure, vitreous hemorrhage, subretinal hemorrhage, uncontrolled vitreous loss, migration of the mobile larva into the vitreous during the surgery, and postoperative anterior segment necrosis after disinsertion of several recti muscles.[2, 11]

EPIDEMIOLOGY

Cysticercosis, the most common ocular tapeworm infection, has a worldwide distribution. Infestation by the pork tapeworm is common in South and Central America, Mexico, the Philippines, India, Eastern Europe, Southeast Asia, and Russia, but it is rare in Great Britain and the United States.[5, 12, 13] Cysticercosis is rare in Jews and Muslims, since these cultures do not generally eat pork. Tapeworm infestation (intestinal taeniasis) is uncommon among religious traditions that eschew pork.[14] However, cysticercosis has no ethnic predilections, being related more frequently to sanitation and poverty than to the ingestion of contaminated pork.

Ocular involvement in cysticercosis occurs in 12.8%[14] to 46%[1] of infected patients. Bilateral ocular involvement[1, 4, 15] and multifocal uniocular involvement[1, 4, 9, 15–17] are very rare.

Ocular cysticercosis seems to be a disorder of the young, often occurring between the ages of 10 and 30 years. There is no sex predilection.[14, 18]

In Poland, Melanowski described an increase (56 cases reported) of ocular cysticercus during World War II.[2] Sixteen years after World War II, there were no cases reported. Improved hygiene was considered the basis for this improvement.[2]

Junior, in 1949, reported 111 cases of ocular cysticercosis from only one hospital in Brazil.[4] Santos and colleagues[5] reported 19 cases of ocular cysticercosis from 1975 to 1978 at one hospital in Mexico. These combined cases outnumber the total of all other cases documented in the recent world literature. The high prevalences in Mexico and Brazil suggest that the patients derive from rural areas and areas with poor sanitation and hygiene.[1]

Ocular cysticercosis has not been a common problem in the Western world since legislation was enacted governing the feeding of human garbage to pigs, disposal of human waste, purification of drinking water, and the enforcement of adequate standards of meat preparation and inspection.[6, 12] With increased international travel to areas where cysticercus is prevalent and endemic, and where inadvertant ingestion of contaminated water and food may occur, this disease may become more frequent in the Western world.[6]

CLINICAL FEATURES

Cysticercosis may affect any portion of the visual pathways from the orbit to the visual cortex; posterior segment involvement seems the most common.[19, 20] The symptoms depend on the location of the ocular involvement. Patients with cysticercosis of the eyelid may have a painless, stationary or slowly enlarging mass.[21] Patients with subconjunctival involvement may be asymptomatic, present with a recurrent conjunctivitis unresponsive to topical antibiotics,[14] or develop a painless or painful swelling of the conjunctiva.[18, 22] Orbital cysticercosis may present as a gradually increasing, painless, nonaxial proptosis.[14] Patients with intraocular cysticercosis may be asymptomatic or present with poor vision, progressive worsening of vision, a single floater, a moving sensation, black spots,

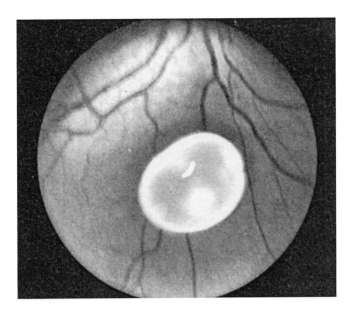

FIGURE 42–1. Cysticercus is pearly white in vitreous. (From Aracena T, Roca F: Macular and peripheral subretinal cysticercosis. Ann Ophthalmol 1981;13:1265.)

ocular discomfort, photophobia, or a red eye.[8, 9, 16, 20, 23] Patients with macular subretinal cysticercosis may describe a sudden central visual loss or a paracentral shadow and moving sensation.[11] Patients with optic nerve involvement may have gradually increasing painless diminution of vision, seizures, or symptoms related to increased intracranial pressure.[14] Epileptiform seizures may occur in cerebral cysticercosis.[24–26] Review of symptoms may reveal a history of epilepsy or previous removal of a tapeworm. About one in 10 patients in Mexico who require brain surgery for the relief of epileptiform seizures is found to have cerebral cysticercosis.[25]

The duration of ocular symptoms before surgical removal varies. Commonly, the patient may have symptoms for a few weeks to months. Intravitreal or subretinal cysticercus without surgical removal of the larva usually leads to blindness within 3 to 5 years.[4, 9, 18]

Visual acuity may be 20/30 in peripheral subretinal cysticercus, or hand motions in submacular cysticercus.[19, 27] The anterior segment examination is variable—evaluation may reveal a quiet eye without conjunctival injection, circumlimbal flush in a patient with two intravitreal cysticerci, or a minimally injected eye with numerous large keratic precipitates and an intense anterior-chamber cellular reaction. A hypopyon may be a presenting sign in intravitreal cysticercosis. The lenses are often clear with an intravitreal cysticercus.[2, 9, 16, 18, 28]

Biomicroscopic examination in intravitreal cysticercosis reveals a variable degree of inflammatory cells in the vitreous body. The vitreous cellular infiltration may be more pronounced during earlier stages of the disorder.[16, 18] With administration of steroid to sub-Tenon's depot and/or orally, the vitreous reaction decreases and a globular translucent cyst in the vitreous becomes visible.[16, 18] With prolonged retention of the live intravitreous cysticercus over a 6-month period, a smoldering 1+ vitritis and iritis may be observed.[16]

While the cysticercus is alive within the eye, it often induces a mild to moderate inflammatory reaction in the anterior chamber and/or vitreous. An intense inflammatory response occurs when the parasite dies. Destruction of a cysticercus 8 mm or larger by diathermy, photocoagulation, or irradiation, without its removal from the eye, usually results in blindness and phthisis, probably resulting from the release of chemical toxins from the parasite and subsequent intraocular inflammation.[4, 8, 29]

Biomicroscopic examination in a case with live submacular cysticercus may reveal minimal or no anterior chamber inflammatory reaction; only the vitreous adjacent to the macula may show inflammatory cells.[19, 28] Edema and hemorrhages in the retina at the posterior pole, subretinal exudate in the macula, retinal vessel sheathing, serous or exudative retinal detachment, retinal pigment epithelial disturbances, and hyperemia and blurring of the optic disc may accompany submacular cysticercus.[2, 23] If the submacular cysticercus emerges into the vitreous leaving a macular break, a chorioretinal scar may develop around the break.[19, 28] In one series of 30 patients in Mexico with intraocular cysticercosis, a high prevalence of retinal detachment (53%) was found in 16 patients at the time of diagnosis.[7] Sometimes a subretinal cysticercus away from the macula or in the peripheral fundus may be accompanied by a focal active necrotizing chorioretinitis[16] or an overlying serous detachment.[30]

The clinical appearance of the parasite in the vitreous or subretinal space is characteristic. It is a globular or spherical, translucent or white cyst with a head, or scolex, that undulates with evagination or invagination in response to the examining light (see Fig. 42–1). The cyst varies in size from about one-fifth to six disc diameters[20, 23, 30] An area of retinal pigment epithelial atrophy is presumed to be the entry site of the cysticercus into the subretinal space.[20]

PATHOGENESIS AND PATHOLOGY

Human cysticercosis is caused by the ingestion of the pork tapeworm, *T. solium*, when contaminated vegetables, fruit, or water is consumed. In this setting, the eggs behave as if they were within the intermediate host—that is, they hatch in the upper intestines in humans. The resulting embryos penetrate the gut, invading lymphatics and the blood stream, and traveling to various organs, including the subcutaneous tissue, brain, heart, and eye. In these various organ tissues, the larvae, known also as larval cysts, grow. Autoinfection can also occur from fecal-oral contamination, with the patient being the definitive host of the adult tapeworm, which releases eggs into the feces. The cycle starts again from the eggs. Sometimes, the patient acquires the parasite by ingestion of undercooked pork containing the larval cysts. In this case, the larval cyst develops in the intestines as the adult tapeworm. Thus, it is possible for the patient to harbor both the larval cyst and the adult tapeworm forms of *T. solium*.[13]

In humans, cysticercosis affects the eye more commonly than any other organ. The cysticercus is capable of invading every ocular tissue. Seventy-two percent of reported cases of ocular cysticercosis involve both retina and vitreous. The parasite has been found more often in the subretinal space (35%) than in the vitreous body (22%).[1, 19] The anterior segment, including ciliary body, iris, and anterior chamber, is a less common site (5%). The lens is rarely a resting site for the parasite, as found by von Graefe in one of 90 cases reported in 1866.[1] A secondary cataract may occur, related to the ocular inflammation associated with the parasite.

In the eye, the embryo develops into a larva, known as a bladder worm or cysticercus. A larva may reach 15 to 18 mm in size over 3 to 4 years.[6] With the larva inside the subretinal space, an exudative retinal detachment may develop. The larva may perforate the retina, causing a retinal break; sometimes the break is self-sealing. Other times the retinal break leads to a rhegmatogenous retinal detachment. The larva can migrate through a retinal break into the vitreous body. If the parasite resides in the macula, macular scarring is likely.[5]

If the larval cyst is untreated, it usually grows until inflammation destroys the eye. Histologically, the necrotic cysticercus is surrounded by a zonal granulomatous inflammatory reaction with an abscess that contains eosinophils.[31, 32] Death of the larva is associated with marked immunologic stimulation[5, 6] and severe endophthalmitis.[5, 31]

The pathogenesis of the common and severe manifestations of ocular infection in untreated intravitreal cysticercosis, leading often to blindness and atrophy of the eye, appears poorly understood. Santos and colleagues[33] developed an experimental animal model using rabbits and *Taenia crassiceps* cysticerci. Group I rabbits were inoculated with a single living cysticercus in the vitreous. Group II rabbits received an intramuscular dose of steroid prior to parasite injection. An intense inflammatory reaction occurred in group I rabbits; group II rabbits had minimal inflammatory changes. Histopathologic studies revealed a severe histiocytic infiltrate with generalized retinal damage in group I and mild inflammatory infiltrate in group II. The ocular lesions in group I rabbits resembled those found in human ocular cysticercosis. These findings suggest that ocular damage in intravitreal cysticercosis might be directly related to inflammatory changes produced by the presence of larval cysticerci.

DIAGNOSIS

The diagnosis of cysticercosis is based on a careful ocular, medical, and epidemiologic history, a review of systems, an ocular examination demonstrating the characteristic larva and associated inflammation (Table 42–1), and a microscopic and histologic examination of the cysticercus. The clinical presence of the motile anterior chamber, intravitreous, or subretinal cysticercus is pathognomonic. Characteristic for the larva of *T. solium* is the translucent, undulating, white cyst with a white head, or scolex. The invaginated scolex appears as a central, dense, white spot and is mobile under bright light within the cystic body (see Fig. 42–1). At other times, the scolex is visible with its hooklets and suckers protruding from the cyst. When exposed to the light of the indirect ophthalmoscope, the scolex returns rapidly to the cyst.[20, 27] Clinically, the scolex may measure approximately 500 by 700 microns in diameter.[11] The cyst may measure between 0.3 and 9 mm.[20, 23, 30]

Ultimately, the diagnosis is established by pathologic

TABLE 42–1. OCULAR CYSTICERCOSIS: DIAGNOSTIC FEATURES

Patient characteristics
  Demographics: Worldwide distribution, but especially in South and Central America, Mexico, India, Eastern Europe and Russia; rare in Jews and Muslims
  Age: 10 to 30 years
  History of ingestion of undercooked, contaminated pork (e.g., scrapple), contaminated vegetables, or water
Ocular symptoms
  Blurred vision
  Ocular discomfort
  Photophobia
  Floaters
  Painful swelling of conjunctiva
  Painless stationary or enlarging mass of eyelid (orbital pseudotumor)
  White mass (leukocoria)
Ocular examination
  Anterior segment
    Variable, from no iritis or mild iritis to intense iritis with hypopyon
    Clear lens
  Posterior Segment
    Variable vitritis, from mild to intense
    Variable posterior vitreous separation
    Cystic larva or larvae
    Retinal break, rhegmatogenous retinal detachment; exudative retinal detachment; chorioretinal scar or atrophy; epimacular membrane
    Optic atrophy, optic disc edema, anterior optic neuritis
Other diagnostic features
  Epileptiform seizures
  Slight fever
  Cysticercus or cysticerci in almost any area within or around the eye

examination with hematoxylin and eosin staining of the surgically removed specimen. Sometimes, a portion of the parasite cannot be identified because of necrosis or its fragmentation.[30] Unlike the larva of the pork tapeworm *T. solium*, the larva of the beef tapeworm has no hooklets.[34, 35]

Fluorescein Angiography

Fluorescein angiography (FA) can be helpful in delineating a clear limit or border for a vessel-spared swelling or cyst of the retina, strengthening the presumption of a larva in the subretinal space.[28] FA may show leakage from retinal vessels near the subretinal larva or on the optic disc.[23] In the early transit phase of FA, the subretinal cysticercus is hypofluorescent. The FA stains the parasite in the recirculation phase.[30]

Ultrasonography

A-scan ultrasonography of subretinal cysticercosis reveals a high-amplitude echo corresponding to the inner cyst wall and overlying retina, which encloses a low-medium amplitude cystic cavity. B-scan ultrasonography reveals a convex curvilinear echo corresponding to the inner cyst wall and the overlying retina and surrounding a smaller round density representing the scolex.[30]

Computerized Axial Tomography and Cerebrospinal Fluid Testing

The potentially life-threatening nature of extraocular cysticercosis is reflected by the 40% mortality of patients with central nervous system involvement.[36] Once the infection is diagnosed, it is important to search for parasites in the central nervous system. Computerized axial tomography (CAT) may reveal intracerebral calcification or hydrocephalus.[36] Testing the cerebrospinal fluid and serum for *T. solium* and *Echinococcus granulosus* antigens may be helpful.

Other Diagnostic Tests

In cysticercosis, anterior chamber paracentesis may reveal a large number of eosinophils.[34] Eosinophilia may be present.[37] If the patient is a definitive host with the adult tapeworm in the gastrointestinal tract, stool examination may reveal the eggs of *T. solium*.[37] Serologically, the cysticercosis diagnosis can be made by the precipitin reaction, complement fixation, or indirect hemagglutination.[20, 37] Radiographs of the calves and thighs may demonstrate the calcifications of cysticercosis.[24] Anticysticercus antibodies have been detected by enzyme-linked immunosorbent assay (ELISA) in approximately 80% of cases with neurocysticercosis and 57% of patients with ocular cysticercosis[7, 38] If at presentation the vitreous is opaque and poorly visualized, investigation to exclude various infections and noninfectious causes of uveitis is important. The tests include ultrasonography of the eye, complete blood count with differential, eosinophil count, erythrocyte sedimentation rate, serum angiotensin-converting enzyme, lysozyme, serologic tests for syphilis, skin testing with purified protein derivative for tuberculosis, and chest radiograph.

DIFFERENTIAL DIAGNOSIS

The diagnosis of intraocular cysticercosis depends on the clarity of the ocular media to view the larva and adequate dilated examination of the eye. The differential diagnosis of intraocular cysticercosis includes conditions that present with a white intraocular spherical mass and cloudy media. When associated with a hazy cornea, cysticercosis may simulate a dislocated lens in the anterior chamber.[39] Preoperative use of steroids cleared the cornea in the case described by Kapoor and colleagues,[39] allowing visibility of the typical undulating movements in the anterior chamber of a free-floating cysticercus, which was extracted. When associated with a hazy vitreous with an intense cellular reaction, cysticercosis may mimic a focal active necrotizing chorioretinitis or retinochoroiditis, such as in toxoplasmosis[16, 31, 40]

Buyck and colleagues[41] reported on 23 children presenting with a retrolental white mass or leukocoria. The underlying disorders were often already much advanced. Six children had retinoblastoma, six had Coats' disease, five had retinopathy of prematurity, four had persistent hyperplastic primary vitreous, one had intraocular cysticercosis, and one had retinal detachment. In differentiating these disorders, study of the vessels in the white mass was the most helpful technique. Ophthalmoscopy, especially with the surgical binocular microscope, resolved the differential diagnosis of each patient with leukocoria even before additional investigation was performed (e.g., ultrasonography or computed tomography [CT] of the skull and orbits as performed for retinoblastoma).

In retinoblastoma, the observation of the vasculature of the retinal tumor is often possible. In Coats' disease, the typical lamp bulb–like vessels are pathognomonic. In persistent hyperplastic primary vitreous, a radial pattern behind the lens is often observed. A retinal tumor in the fellow eye helps to confirm retinoblastoma rather than Coats' disease, which is typically unilateral. Cysticercosis would be very unlikely in a premature infant and should not be confused with the typical findings of retinopathy of prematurity.[41]

Another disorder to be considered in the differential diagnosis of retinal or subretinal cysticercosis includes diffuse unilateral subacute neuroretinitis (DUSN), caused by a motile nematode larva in the retina or subretinal space.[42–44] While both conditions may have unilateral visual loss, vitritis, and a larva moving in response to the examination light, the larva of DUSN is larger and differs in morphology from cysticercus. One of several larvae of DUSN, measuring between 1000 and 2000 microns in length, makes visible subretinal tracks, not observed clinically in cysticercosis.[42–44]

The growth of the larva of cysticercosis over several months leads to a large cystic structure.[14] When located in the subretinal space, cysticercosis may be misdiagnosed as a serous detachment of the retinal pigment epithelium or retina, or as a choroidal tumor.[40]

TREATMENT

Untreated intravitreal or subretinal cysticercus usually leads to blindness and atrophy or phthisis of the eye within 3 to 5 years.[1, 4, 8, 32] Although the live parasite may be tolerated,[20] an intense inflammatory reaction often occurs resulting in destruction of the globe. A few studies advocate photocoagulation of small subretinal cysticerci (less than 8 mm),[5, 10, 19] but most authors report poor results when the dead parasite is allowed to remain in the eye.[1, 4] Junior, reflecting on his experience with 111 cases in one hospital in Brazil, wrote, "To leave the parasite in the eye is to condemn the eye to blindness or total loss."[4]

The management of cysticercosis has taken several forms, depending on the anatomic location of the cyst. Antihelmintic drugs, such as praziquantel and albendazole, have been used in the medical treatment of active neurocysticercosis with viable intraparenchymal parasitic cysts and extraocular cysticercosis.[45, 46] In a randomized, controlled clinical trial of oral albendazole (15 mg/kg once daily for 1 month) compared to a placebo in 24 ultrasonographically diagnosed and ELISA-positive cases of extraocular or orbital cysticerci, marked clinical improvement was seen in all cases in the treatment group at 4 weeks, with collapse of the cyst at 6 weeks (75%) and complete disappearance at 3 months (100%). No clinical or ultrasonographic change was noted in the control group.[46] In a pilot study of oral albendazole (30 mg/kg for 15 days with a low-dose steroid [5 to 10 mg daily]), 20 of 21 patients with orbital myocysticercosis diagnosed by ultrasonography, supported by CT or magnetic resonance imaging, had complete resolution of the cyst. Before treatment, the cysts measured 6.2 to 13.4 mm (mean, 11.4 mm). There was no placebo control group.[47]

Praziquantel and albendazole are usually not effective

in intraocular cysticercosis.[45, 48, 49] The best means of cure is early surgical removal of the larva, although larval destruction by diathermy, cryo treatment, or photocoagulation has sometimes been successful.[5, 10, 50]

Larva in the Anterior Chamber

Junior described a case in which the parasite migrated from the subhyaloid space to the anterior chamber, and the scolex attached itself firmly to the posterior cornea. The parasite was extracted with forceps.[1, 4]

Larva in the Lens

In 1866, von Graefe reported extraction of a cataract, which was complicated by marked iritis. He found in the lens a cysticercus 6 mm in diameter.[1]

Larva in the Vitreous

For the intravitreal cysticercus, pars plana or open-sky vitrectomy has frequently proven successful.[5, 8, 9, 11, 16, 19, 20, 30] The pars plana approach, which utilizes three ports for infusion, endoillumination, and cutting suction techniques, when compared to open-sky vitrectomy, seems to give superior visibility of the larva, unhampered by glare or light scatter from the anterior surface of the vitreous gel, and it less often requires lensectomy.[9] Pavan[11] observed that the scolex jammed in the tip of the 20-gauge tapered needle, preventing aspiration of the larva. If the larva had become disengaged from the needle tip and lodged in the peripheral vitreous skirt, it might have been difficult to retrieve. Fortunately, he released the larva in the vitreous cavity, reapplied a higher suction, and withdrew the extrusion needle with the larva attached to its tip. Alternatively, a larger-gauge extrusion needle may be employed, such as an 18-gauge angiocatheter, as is sometimes used in silicone oil removal, which would allow complete aspiration of the entire cysticercus into the collection bottle.[51]

During removal of the live intravitreal cysticercus, Santos and colleagues[5] and Topilow and colleagues[20] have noted that, although the body of the cyst is usually soft, the head or scolex is hard and sometimes requires a second application to engage or aspirate it from the vitreous cavity. A limited vitrectomy is recommended around the mobile intravitreal parasite to facilitate its capture in the vitreous cavity before performing a subtotal vitrectomy to remove any toxic products released from the cyst. A periocular steroid injection at the conclusion of surgery and then postoperative topical steroid and mydriatics are often required to control the mild subsequent vitritis.

Larva in the Subretinal Space

The classic external approach with a sclerotomy was the initial method of removal of a subretinal cysticercus.[2, 4, 20, 23, 28] The technique required accurate localization as with a retinal break or subretinal metallic foreign body, but during surgery the larva was frequently mobile in the subretinal space or migrated into the vitreous, leading to inadequate localization and failure to remove the parasite.[28, 30] For the more posteriorly situated larva, extensive periocular surgery might be required to achieve adequate exposure and access. A lateral canthotomy and temporary

disinsertion of one or more rectus muscles have frequently been necessary.[2]

Complications of an external approach with a sclerotomy include vitreous hemorrhage,[23] retinal incarceration and vitreous loss,[4] choroidal hemorrhage,[19, 52] failure to remove the larva,[5] anterior segment ischemia after temporary disinsertion of several rectus muscles,[2] retinal detachment,[5, 52] and bacterial endophthalmitis.[5, 27, 52]

Steinmetz and colleagues[30] reported pars plana vitrectomy and retinotomy in the successful removal of a subretinal cysticercus. After removal of the posterior vitreous, a retinotomy was created by endodiathermy over the larva. The suction cutter was inserted through the retinotomy, and the cyst was removed from the subretinal space. Internal drainage of subretinal fluid was followed by endolaser treatment to surround the retinotomy. A gas-fluid exchange was performed, using the long-acting gas 12% perfluoropropane, for tamponade.

Larva in the Submacular Space

Removal of a submacular cysticercus has been achieved by pars plana vitrectomy with retinotomy, followed by gas-fluid exchange and endolaser treatment around the retinotomy, and then postoperative face-down positioning until the air bubble was absorbed.[11]

Larva Attached to the Optic Disc

Zinn and colleagues[9] removed two intravitreous cysticerci from the surface of the optic disc during pars plana vitrectomy. Fibrous or glial-type strands, rather than the suckers or rostella, appeared to be the source of the attachment of the larvae to the surface of the optic disc.

COMPLICATIONS

As previously mentioned, an external approach with a sclerotomy is fraught with many potential complications. Pars plana vitrectomy with retinotomy for surgical removal of subretinal cysticercus minimizes the risk of nonremoval of the larval cyst and improves the visibility of the parasite during surgery. Removal of the posterior hyaloid in cases of subretinal and intravitreal cysticercosis is recommended to prevent the contraction of the vitreous cortex that often leads to a postoperative retinal detachment.[53]

PROGNOSIS

In most cases of untreated intraocular cysticercosis, the parasite will eventually die after 2 to 4 years. The accompanying release of toxins induces an inflammatory reaction that likely will lead to loss of vision and severe intraocular damage.[19, 52] Yet, early removal of the larva from the anterior chamber may allow good vision.[1, 54]

Santos and colleagues[5, 6] treated 19 eyes with intraocular cysticercosis and achieved a successful result in 68% of these patients using various techniques including vitrectomy or sclerotomy to extract the larva from the vitreous or subretinal space or photocoagulation to destroy a small subretinal larva (less than 8 mm in diameter).

Cardenas and colleagues[7] treated 30 eyes with intraocular cysticercus by vitrectomy, sclerotomy, or laser photocoagulation, finding useful vision (20/20 to 20/100) in only 19% and vision of 20/200 or worse in 81%. In their series, there was a high prevalence of retinal detachment (53%) at the time of diagnosis, of subretinal cysticerci in or near the macula (80%), and of dead larvae within 9 of the 12 subretinal cysticerci (75%). A less desirable visual result could be expected with these problems.

CONCLUSIONS

Human cysticercosis is a parasitic infection of the tapeworm *T. solium*. Infection depends on many factors, chiefly hygiene, meat inspection, water treatment, and local or cultural habits. Humans are infected usually by ingesting *T. solium* eggs from contaminated soil, food, or water. For patients in or from endemic areas, it is important to have a high index of suspicion for the diagnosis of cysticercosis. Seizures, subacute proptosis, ocular motility disorders, uveitis, retinal detachment, or optic disc edema may be presenting signs of cysticercosis. Early surgical removal of the larva in the posterior segment by pars plana vitrectomy is advocated, because intraocular parasite death results in marked inflammation and damage to the eye.

References

1. Duke-Elder S, Perkins ES: Diseases of the Uveal Tract. In: Duke-Elder S, ed: System of Ophthalmology, vol 9. St. Louis, CV Mosby, 1966, p 478.
2. Segal P, Mrzyglod S, Smolarz-Dudarewicz J: Subretinal cysticercosis in the macular region. Am J Ophthalmol 1964;57:655.
3. von Graefe A: Cysticercus im Glaskörper durch die Cornea extrahirt. Albrecht von Graefes Arch Ophthalmol 1858;4:171.
4. Junior L: Ocular cysticercosis. Am J Ophthalmol 1949;32:523.
5. Santos R, Dalma A, Ortiz E, et al: Management of subretinal and vitreous cysticercosis—Role of photocoagulation and surgery. Ophthalmology 1979;86:1501.
6. Ganley JP: Discussion of presentation by Santos R, Dalma A, Ortiz E, et al: Management of subretinal and vitreous cysticercosis—Role of photocoagulation and surgery. Ophthalmology 1979;86:1505.
7. Cardenas F, Quiroz H, Plancarte A, et al: *Taenia solium* ocular cysticercosis—Findings in 30 cases. Ann Ophthalmol 1992;24:25.
8. Hutton WL, Vaiser A, Snyder WB: Pars plana vitrectomy for removal of intravitreous cysticercus. Am J Ophthalmol 1976;81:571.
9. Zinn KM, Guillory SL, Friedman AH: Removal of intravitreous cysticerci from the surface of the optic nervehead—A pars plana approach. Arch Ophthalmol 1980;98:714.
10. Rodriquez A: Light coagulation in early posterior subretinal cysticercosis. Presented at the International Photocoagulation Congress, September 28–October 1, 1975.
11. Pavan PR: Submacular cysticercosis. In: Bovino JA, ed: Macular Surgery. Norwalk, Appleton and Lange, 1994, p 165.
12. Franken S: Intraocular cysticercus. Ophthalmologica (Basel) 1975;171:7.
13. King CH: Cestodes (Tapeworms). In: Mandell G, Bennett JE, Dolin R, eds: Principles and Practice of Infectious Diseases, vol 2. New York, Churchill-Livingstone, 1995, p 2544.
14. Malik SRK, Gupta AK, Choudhry S: Ocular cysticercosis. Am J Ophthalmol 1968;66:1168.
15. Kapoor S, Kapoor MS: Ocular cysticercosis. J Pediatr Ophthalmol Strabismus 1978;15:170.
16. Messner KH, Kammerer WS: Intraocular cysticercosis. Arch Ophthalmol 1979;97:1103.
17. Wood TR, Binder PS: Intravitreal and intracameral cysticercosis. Ann Ophthalmol 1979;11:1033.
18. Sen DK, Mohan H: Ocular cysticercosis in India. J Pediatr Ophthalmol Strabismus 1978;15:96.
19. Kruger-Leite E, Jalkh AE, Quiroz H, et al: Intraocular cysticercosis. Am J Ophthalmol 1985;99:252.
20. Topilow HW, Yimoyines DJ, Freeman HM, et al: Bilateral multifocal intraocular cysticercosis. Ophthalmology 1981;88:1166.
21. Perry HD, Font RL: Cysticercosis of the eyelid. Arch Ophthalmol 1978;96:1255.
22. Sen DK, Thomas A: Cysticercus cellulosae causing subconjunctival abscess. Am J Ophthalmol 1969;68:714.
23. Bartholomew RS: Subretinal cysticercosis. Am J Ophthalmol 1975;79:670.
24. Dixon HBF, Hargreaves WH: Cysticercosis (*Taenia solium*)—A further ten years' clinical study, covering 284 cases. Q J Med 1944;13:107.
25. Robbins SL: Textbook of Pathology with Clinical Applications. Philadelphia, W.B. Saunders, 1957, p 381.
26. Stepien L: Cerebral cysticercosis in Poland—Clinical symptoms and operative results in 132 cases. J Neurosurg 1962;19:505.
27. Luger MHA, Stilma JS, Ringens PJ, et al: In-toto removal of a subretinal *Cysticercus cellulosae* by pars plana vitrectomy. Br J Ophthalmol 1991;75:561.
28. Aracena T, Roca F: Macular and peripheral subretinal cysticercosis. Ann Ophthalmol 1981;13:1265.
29. Arciniegas A, Gutierrez F: Our experience in the removal of intravitreal and subretinal cysticerci. Ann Ophthalmol 1988;20:75.
30. Steinmetz RL, Masket S, Sidikaro Y: The successful removal of a subretinal cysticercus by pars plana vitrectomy. Retina 1989;9:276.
31. Hogan MJ, Zimmerman LE: Ophthalmic Pathology—An Atlas and Textbook, 2nd ed. Philadelphia, W.B. Saunders, 1962, pp 25, 488, 566, 644.
32. Yanoff M, Fine BS: Ocular Pathology—A Text and Atlas, 2nd ed. Philadelphia, Harper and Row, 1982, pp 109, 114, 116.
33. Santos A, Paczka JA, Jimenez-Sierra JM, et al: Experimental intravitreous cysticercosis. Graefes Arch Clin Exp Ophthalmol 1996;234:515.
34. Manshot WA: Intraocular cysticercus. Arch Ophthalmol 1968;80:772.
35. Neva FA, Brown HW: The Cestoda, or tapeworms. In: Basic Clinical Parasitology, 6th ed. Norwalk, Appleton and Lange, 1994, p 181.
36. Topilow HW: Cysticercosis. In: Fraunfelder FT, Roy FH, eds: Current Ocular Therapy, 4th ed. Philadelphia, W.B. Saunders, 1995, p 121.
37. Duke-Elder S: Diseases of the Outer Eye (Part 1). In Duke-Elder S, ed: System of Ophthalmology, vol 8. St. Louis, CV Mosby, 1965, p 425.
38. Plancarte A, Espinoza B, Flisser A: Immuno-diagnosis of human neurocysticercosis by enzyme-linked immunosorbent assay. Childs Nerv Syst 1987;3:203.
39. Kapoor S, Sood GC, Aurora AL, et al: Ocular cysticercosis—Report of a free floating cysticercus in the anterior chamber. Acta Ophthalmol 1977;55:927.
40. Gass JD: Stereoscopic Atlas of Macular Diseases: Diagnosis and Treatment, 4th ed, vols 1, 2. St. Louis, Mosby–Year Book, 1997, pp 156, 618.
41. Buyck A, Casteels I, Dralands L, et al: Retrolental white mass. Bull Soc Belge Ophtalmol 1991;241:61.
42. Raymond LA, Gutierrez Y, Strong LE, et al: Living retinal nematode (filarial-like) destroyed with photocoagulation. Ophthalmology 1978;85:944.
43. Kazacos KR, Vestre WA, Kazacos EA, Raymond LA: Diffuse unilateral subacute neuroretinitis syndrome: Probable cause. Arch Ophthalmol 1984;102:967.
44. Kazacos KR, Raymond LA, Kazacos EA, et al: The raccoon ascarid—A probable cause of human ocular larva migrans. Ophthalmology 1985;92:1735.
45. Liu LX, Weller PF: Antiparasitic drugs. N Engl J Med 1996;334:1178.
46. Sihota R, Honavar SG: Oral albendazole in the management of extraocular cysticercosis. Br J Ophthalmol 1994;78:621.
47. Puri P, Grover AK: Medical management of orbital myocysticercosis: A pilot study. Eye 1998;12:795.
48. Kestelyn P, Taelman H: Effect of praziquantel on intraocular cysticercosis—A case report. Br J Ophthalmol 1985;69:788.
49. Santos R, Chavarria M, Aquirre AE: Failure of medical treatment in two cases of intraocular cysticercosis. Am J Ophthalmol 1984;97:249.
50. Michels RG: Indications and results (parasitic endophthalmitis). In: Michel RG: Vitreous Surgery. St. Louis, CV Mosby, 1981, pp 352–353.
51. Wilson CE: Video of removal of intravitreal cysticercus. Presented at Cincinnati Society of Ophthalmology, Cincinnati, OH, March 10, 1998.
52. Gupta A, Gupta R, Pandav SS, et al: Successful surgical removal of encapsulated subretinal cysticercus. Retina 1998;18:563.
53. Quiroz-Mercado H, Santos A: Surgical removal of subretinal cysticercus. Arch Ophthalmol 1998;116:261.
54. Schmidt U, Klauss V, Stefani FH: Unilateral iritis by cysticercal larva in the anterior chamber. Ophthalmologica 1990;200:210.

DIFFUSE UNILATERAL SUBACUTE NEURORETINITIS

Neal P. Barney

DEFINITION

The term diffuse unilateral subacute neuroretinitis (DUSN) was first used by Gass in the February issue of the *Journal of the Royal Society of Medicine* in 1978.[1] He described 29 patients seen with consistent features that included unilateral, insidious loss of vision, usually severe in nature; vitritis; focal and diffuse pigment epithelial (PE) disturbance; retinal vessel narrowing; optic atrophy; retinal circulation time; and subnormal electroretinogram (ERG) findings. This definition was reiterated in the May 1978 issue of *Ophthalmology*.[2] Unique in these series of patients were the observations of the earliest findings of the syndrome. Bascom Palmer Eye Institute had previously noted 13 patients as having unilateral wipe-out syndrome.[3] Gass now added his observations of some early changes in certain patients who subsequently developed the appearance of unilateral wipe-out syndrome.

HISTORY

DUSN is now believed to be caused by a small number of different Nematode larvae. Kuhnt,[4] in 1892, described a motile worm near the macula that proved to be a Nematode on excision. Nayar[5] observed a 2.5-cm worm, likely an adult, that moved from the subretinal space, through the vitreous into the anterior chamber, from where it was extracted. A nematode, resembling onchocerca, was reported protruding through the subretinal space into the vitreous by Barrada.[6] Nematode infestation as a cause of retinal granuloma was first reported in the pathologic review of Wilder.[7] Ashton[8] reported four cases of nematodiasis as a cause of retinal granuloma in children. Parsons[9] found a small, white, motile mass in a patient with severe macular destruction in 1952. Ashton reported four cases of nematodiasis as a cause of retinal granulomas, all in children.[8] It was not until 1968 that Rubin demonstrated findings similar to macular degeneration or healing central serous retinopathy could be attributed to a Nematode infection.[10] Price corroborated these findings but in a patient with a demonstrable motile worm in the left eye.[11] His patient had a previous history of chorioretinitis in the macula of the right eye that is reported as steroid responsive. A worm was never seen in the right eye, only the left. Ten years elapsed before the observations of Gass that connected early changes to the eventual appearance of the unilateral wipe-out syndrome and referral to the syndrome as DUSN. He suggests, at the beginning of his article, a viral etiology, but in an addendum, he indicates the finding of a motile worm in 2 of 12 additional patients.[1]

EPIDEMIOLOGY

Nematode infection in children has long been a concern in the differential diagnosis of intraocular tumors of childhood. Granuloma formation can give a mass effect that could appear as retinoblastoma. The earliest reports by Gass and Raymond contain patients from areas in which nematodiasis is common in animals such as the raccoon. A near-exhaustive search of the literature reveals that 53 cases have been reported in the United States.[3, 8–15]

De Souza,[16] of Brazil, was the first to report two patients outside the United States. He further reported the surgical management of a third case from Brazil.[17] Subsequently, a total of eight patients have been reported in the following countries: Canada, France, Germany, Scotland, and Switzerland.[18–22] The age range in the largest series by Gass is reported as 5 to 22 years with a mean of 12.5 years.[1] The age range in the other reported patients is 4 to 84 years.[8–11, 13–15] In reviewing published papers other than the large Gass series, 17 patients were age 4 through 17 and 22 patients were age 18 through 84.[8–11, 14, 15] The large Gass series contains 10 women and 21 men.[1] Race is difficult to determine from the individual cases. The large Gass series classifies 20 patients as white and five patients as black.[1] The right eye was affected in 13 patients in the large series, and the left eye was affected in 12 patients.[1] The remaining cases totaled 22 right eyes involved and 16 patients with the left eye involved.[8–11, 14, 15]

CLINICAL CHARACTERISTICS

It is now well accepted that the clinical characteristics are manifest in early and late stages. Gass[23] first described the unilateral wipe-out syndrome in patients between 1963 and 1977. His observations in 1978 then led him to conclude that early findings and subsequent progression of DUSN would lead to the clinical appearance of the unilateral wipe-out syndrome.[1]

Typically, patients are young and in good health, with no antecedent illness and no significant past ocular history. In the early stage, symptomatic decrease in visual acuity is reported by the patient in two thirds of cases. Decreased vision in the early stages is discovered during routine examination about one third of the time. Central or paracentral scotoma is the principal complaint of symptomatic patients in the early stage.[1, 2] About one fourth of symptomatic patients with early-stage disease have mild redness and visual obscurations,[24] and a single patient gave a 1-day history of a shifting parafoveal scotoma.[10] One patient gave a 3-week history of transient mild irritation. Photophobia or severe pain is rarely reported.

Three quarters of patients presenting in the late stages have profound vision loss when the condition is first detected. One patient presented with a 2-month history of decreased vision and intermittent micropsia preceded by an 11-year history of nyctalopia.

Visual acuity is profoundly decreased in the majority

of patients who present in the early stages. In a series of 18 patients, 15 of whom presented within 1 month of the onset of decrease of vision, 10 patients had vision worse than 20/200.[12] An afferent pupillary defect is found in nearly every patient regardless of stage of disease. Visual field testing typically reveals a central scotoma with variable peripheral changes in either early or late stages.

Visual acuity is the late stage is profoundly decreased, with 80% or more showing vision of 20/200 or worse.

At present, the most characteristic ocular finding in the early stage is a motile subretinal worm. Gass' series of 25 patients in February of 1978 notes this as an addendum.[1] In his May 1978 series of 36 patients, he notes the presence of a worm in two patients.[2] Many subsequent case reports use the presence of a motile subretinal worm as a defining characteristic of the early stage of the disease. Perhaps more important than the worm, which is very difficult to observe, are the other characteristic early findings noted in Gass' two large series. The eye is typically white externally. The cornea is clear, with only a few patients presenting with anterior chamber cells, flare, and keratic precipitates. Hypopyon is rare. The lens is normally clear. Vitritis is present in all patients and may obscure some details of the fundus. The optic nerve has a blurred margin in just over half of the patients with early-stage disease. The retina has multiple, focal, gray-white to gray-yellow lesions in the deep or outer retinal layer. These vary in size from 1200 to 1500 μm and are found in the peripapillary region and juxtamacular region (Fig. 43–1). It is unusual for lesions to be found in the foveal region. When a motile worm is seen, it seldom overlies a retinal lesion. Occasionally, there is a small serous retinal detachment overlying these lesions. The lesions themselves are evanescent and have the possibility of different outcomes. The lesion may resolve with no pigment epithelial disturbance or residual finding. More commonly, there is mild change in color of the underlying pigment epithelium or focal depigmentation. Rarely, the pigment in the area of the lesion will migrate into the retina near the vessels. The pigment epithelium not affected directly with a lesion often shows a diffuse mot-

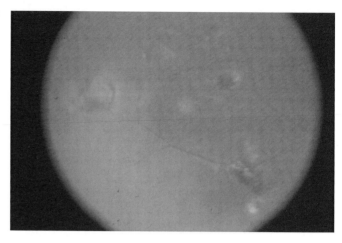

FIGURE 43–2. Late-stage DUSN: Vessel attenuation and chorioretinal scars. (Courtesy of Donald Gass, M.D.) (See color insert.)

tling. Mild retinal arteriole narrowing occurs in one half of eyes in the early stages.

Few comments are found about the anterior segment findings in the late stage other than the lack of cataract development. The presence of optic atrophy and severe retinal arteriole narrowing seems to define the late stage best (Fig. 43–2). Although vitritis may be present, it is found in less than half of patients with late-stage disease. Retinal arteriole sheathing is found in most patients with late-stage disease. Retinal arteriole narrowing may vary by quadrant. The retinal pigment epithelial changes were both focal and diffuse, and were most prominent in the peripapillary and peripheral retina. Focal, atrophic, pigment, and epithelial mottling is also found. Choroidal neovascular membrane is infrequent, but when it is present, it is usually in the periphery. Again, the central macula seems to be spared of most changes seen in the late stages.

PATHOPHYSIOLOGY

The first description of pathologic changes secondary to nematode larva infestation of the eye were presented as findings of granulomas in whole globes.[7] Chorioretinitis as a result of nematode larva was first reported by Parsons in 1952,[9] and then Rubin in 1968.[10] Gass proposes a viral etiology in the body of his first article.[1] As an addendum in this article, he describes twelve additional patients with the same findings, two of which have a motile worm, thought to be toxocariasis. In May of 1978 Gass includes these twelve patients in his series and suggests that more than one etiologic agent can produce DUSN. Since 1978, a heightened awareness of the syndrome, particularly its early stages, almost requires the observation of a motile worm. Attention subsequently focuses on the clinical description of worm size, motility, and species. Three phyla of wormlike animals exist: Annelida (segmented worms), Nemahelminthes (Nematoda or roundworms) and Platyhelminthes (flat worms). There are an estimated 80,000 species of Nematodes that are parasites of vertebrates. Most Nematodes have only one host, the definitive host, and pass through simple or complex life cycles both within and outside of the host. Transmission to a new

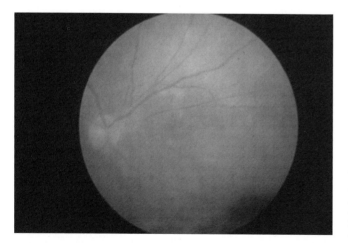

FIGURE 43–1. Early-stage DUSN: vitritis, disc margin swelling, and multiple yellow-white lesions at the level of the retinal pigment epithelium (RPE) and outer retina. (Courtesy of Donald Gass, M.D.) (See color insert.)

host is by ingestion of larva or mature infectious egg, or by transcutaneous passage of the larva. With rare exceptions, Nematodes typically do not multiply in the human host.

Gass described the size of the worm in his initial two cases as 25 to 50 μm in width and 500 μm in length, and tapered at both ends. This is similar to the size reported by Parsons,[9] Rubin,[10] and Price[11] and was believed to be compatible with but not diagnostic of *Toxocara canis.*[2] A review of cases of DUSN in 1983 suggested two endemic areas of the United States, each with a different size worm causing the ocular disease.[12] Four hundred to one thousand microns in length seemed to be the size of the most commonly reported worms in the southern states.[12] The northern states of Kentucky, Illinois, Minnesota, and Nebraska had reports containing worm length of 1500 to 2000 μm. Interestingly, there is a greater likelihood of the longer worm leaving a tract of coarse clumping of pigment epithelium in the wake of its travels.[12] The shorter worm predisposes to leave focal, chorioretinal atrophic scars. In this series, they suggest that the clinical presentation is not consistent with other reports of *Toxocara canis.* Kazacos proposed the raccoon-associated *Baylisascaris* genus as the cause of DUSN, particularly the species *procyonis.*[25] He proposes that the marked zoonotic potential of this larva to cause visceral and ocular larva migraines in a wide variety of mammals and birds makes it an ideal candidate to be a cause of DUSN. Fatal central nervous system disease of two children substantiates the potential for human infection. Experimentally, the larva may be seen in the retina within 3 to 7 days of infection. Additionally, the *Baylisascaris* larvae may grow while they are within the eye and would account for the range of lengths of larvae seen, such as those that are 400 to 2000 μm.[15, 25, 26] Significant morphometric, serologic, and epidemiologic support for *Baylisacaris* as the causative agent was published in a case by Goldberg.[24] Two Brazilian patients were reported to have DUSN, each caused by a worm of 400 to 500 μm in length.[16] The 1500-micron–long worm presenting in a German patient was thought to be consistent with *Baylisascaris* species.[20] Finally, the Trematode, *Alaria mesocercaria,* is suggested as causative of two patients with DUSN by the measure of 500-micron length, but a 150-micron width, which is considerably wider than previously published studies.

The focal pigment epithelial changes seen are easily explained by the location or the travel pattern of the worm. It is speculated that focal chorioretinal white spots are an immune response to a secretion or excretion from the worm.[2] The diffuse pigment epithelial changes are somewhat more difficult to explain except as a toxic reaction. This might be sufficient to account for the outer retinal findings but ERG findings, arterial narrowing, and optic disc pallor are not as easily ascribable to the pigment epithelial changes. Indeed, in one eye with profound vision loss, there were no significant histopathologic correlates.[2] Worms, regardless of species, have been observed in the eye for up to 3 years.

DIAGNOSIS

At present, the diagnosis is made when the clinical characteristics of DUSN are found in conjunction with an intraocular worm. Certainly, the diagnosis may be strongly entertained without the presence of a worm if there is a classic, late-stage appearance. Serologic testing has been variable. Gass found negative *Toxocara* serology in many reported patients.[12] On further inspection, these serology reports need to be evaluated in light of the most likely species and timeliness of the testing. Kazacos points out that three of five of Gass' patients with small worms had positive results on an enzyme-linked immunosorbent assay (ELISA) for *Toxocara* when it was performed when the worm was visible.[26]

Fluorescein angiography findings vary with the stage of disease. In the early stage, there is hypofluorescence of the focal white lesions followed by staining. Mild leakage is commonly seen at the optic disc. Cystoid macular edema is reported but uncommon. Occasionally, there is evidence of peripheral retinal vascular leakage. The late stage of DUSN has delayed appearance of fluorescein in the retinal vessels. Pigmented epithelial alterations cause diffuse, widespread hyperfluorescence. Focal window defects correlate with areas of chorioretinal scar with a loss of pigment epithelium.

Electrodiagnostic testing has been performed on numerous patients. Electroretinographic changes include a mild to moderate decrease in rod and cone function, with the B wave more affected than the A wave. Despite the involvement of the pigment epithelium, there is an abnormal electro-oculogram (EOG) in only about one half of patients. Kelsey believes that the finding of abnormal ERG and normal EOG in some patients strongly implicates the neuroepithelium as diseased in this entity.[27]

The differential diagnosis of the early, multifocal, peripheral lesions includes sarcoid and other entities that cause focal chorioretinitis: toxoplasmosis, histoplasmosis, or multifocal choroiditis and panuveitis. Because the early stage of the disease may produce significant vision loss with apparent direct involvement of the macula, it differs from acute posterior multifocal placoid pigment epitheliopathy (AMPPE) or serpiginous choroiditis. These entities would typically have decreased vision associated with involvement of the macula. The lesions of DUSN usually do not involve the macula. The late stage of DUSN is characterized by optic atrophy, vessel narrowing, and focal and diffuse pigment epithelial abnormalities. These findings may cause confusion with post-traumatic chorioretinopathy, occlusive vascular disease, sarcoid, or a toxic retinopathy.

TREATMENT

Treatment modalities vary with the decade in which the report is made. Parsons[9] used various forms of medication without success. He next planned localized transscleral diathermy under direct visualization, but the worm again moved into the periphery. Photocoagulation is first mentioned as a possible treatment, but it was not carried out by Price.[11]

It is imperative that clear goals be established for any therapeutic attempt with clear temporal windows for judging efficacy. Obviously, the patient with late-stage DUSN, no visible worm, and poor vision is unlikely to benefit from any form of treatment. Early-stage disease with moderate vision loss and confirmation of a visible worm would be parameters suggestive of treatment.

Rubin first employed anthelminthic therapy and corticosteroids.[10] The indications for therapy were a visible worm, 2-day progressive loss of vision from 20/60 to 20/200, and worsening central scotoma. Thiabendazole, 2 g by mouth, for 5 days was started concurrently with prednisone, 40 mg by mouth, for 3 weeks. Chlorpromazine, used to counteract anticipated nausea from thiabendazole use, was discontinued secondary to postural hypotension. Vision returned to 20/60 with some decrease in the size of the scotoma. The worm disappeared from the fundus within 24 to 48 hours after treatment. Concurrent with the disappearance was the development of macular edema and a linear hemorrhage inferior to the macula. Raymond gives the first report of photocoagulation of a worm in October of 1978.[15] Indications for treatment were the presence of a motile worm and a decline in vision to 20/100. Six weeks after symptoms developed, xenon photocoagulation was administered to the worm and adjacent tissues. At the time of treatment, the worm was at the 11:30 position approximately 2.5 disc diameters from the center of the fovea. Vision returned to 20/80. A second patient had argon laser photocoagulation to a worm and maintained 20/20 vision. Several authors have successfully used photocoagulation to eradicate these worms.[12, 16, 20, 28–31] In February 1978, Gass[1] suggests the use of corticosteroids in the early stages. He suggested monitoring improvement of the visual field to judge efficacy. In May 1978, it was clear that the presence of a motile worm should direct one's choice of therapy. Many authors suggest photocoagulation of a worm identified in the periphery.[2]

In this series of 36 patients, two were found to have motile worms. Corticosteroid treatment was initiated with 80 mg of prednisone in both of these 14-year-old boys within 1 month of the onset of symptoms; each patient received a 3- or 4-day course of thiabendazole as 1.5 mg by mouth per day. There was no improvement in vision in either patient. The steroid was tapered to low levels. Gass, regarding thiabendazole treatment in five other patients, found it ineffective as measured by continued motility in three of the five patients.[12] There is no comment regarding the two other patient outcomes. He noted diethylcarbamazine was also ineffective. In each patient in whom anthelmintics failed, photocoagulation or local excision stopped further worm movement.

In 1991, Gass[13] published four cases in which no worm was found and thiabendazole was successfully used. In three of four cases, vitritis was reduced and in two cases, the active lesions resolved without further recurrence. In these two cases, however, one last lesion developed with a resultant chorioretinal scar. This was presumed to be the site of the worm. Transvitreal worm removal has been reported.[17]

At present, treatment of a visible worm with photocoagulation seems to offer the best chance for halting worm motility and resolution of the active gray-white lesions.

COMPLICATIONS

The unilateral nature of this disease is somewhat fortunate given the typically poor visual outcome. Approximately 80% of patients in the late stages will have vision of 20/200 or worse. An afferent pupillary defect is seen in most patients, and visual field changes are remarkable for paracentral scotomas.

There are no reported complications from photocoagulation of the worm. Particularly, there is no evidence that photocoagulation of the worm causes an exuberant inflammatory reaction. Anthelminthic treatment carries with it the risk of toxicity such as nausea, anorexia, dizziness, fatigue, tinnitus, hypotension, and pruritus. Although it is not truly a complication, the risk of resistance is theoretically possible.

PROGNOSIS

DUSN is a unilateral disease with a poor prognosis for vision. Early reports indicate that the disease is present usually for months before diagnosis and treatment. Despite increased awareness and early detection of a worm, in many recent patients, there appears to be significant vision loss.

CONCLUSION

1. Diffuse unilateral neuroretinitis is a multifocal retinochoroiditis.
2. It is reported primarily in North America, but cases have been reported from Europe and South America. It occurs in the first through third decade.
3. A larva of a nematode is implicated as the causative agent
4. Usually, the early stage and certainly the late stage have significant findings suggestive of the disease.
5. Photocoagulation appears to be the treatment of choice.

References

1. Gass JD, Scelfo R: Diffuse unilateral subacute neuroretinitis. J R Soc Med 1978;71:95.
2. Gass JD, Gilbert WR Jr, Guerry R, et al: Diffuse unilateral subacute neuroretinitis. Ophthalmology 1978;85:521.
3. Gass JD: Subretinal migration of a nematode in a patient with diffuse unilateral subacute neuroretinitis. Arch Ophthalmol 1996;114:1526.
4. Kuhnt H: Extraction eines neuen Entozoon aus dem Glaskörper des Menschen. Arch Augenheilk 1892;24:205.
5. Nayar KK, Pillai AK: A case of filariasis oculi. Br J Ophthalmol 1932;16:549.
6. Barrada MA: Filaria in macula. Bull Ophthalmol Soc Egypt 1934;29:63.
7. Wilder HC: Nematode endophthalmitis. Trans Am Acad Ophthalmol Oto 1950; 99–108.
8. Ashton N: Larval granulomatosis of retina due to toxocara. Br J Ophthalmol 1960;44:129.
9. Parsons HE: Nematode chorioretinitis: Report of a case with photographs of viable worm. Arch Ophthalmol 1952;47:799.
10. Rubin ML, Karufman HE, Tierney JP, et al.: An intraretinal nematode (a case report). Trans Am Acad Ophthalmol 1968;72:855.
11. Price JA, Wadsworth JA: An intraretinal worm. Report of a case of macular retinopathy caused by invasion of the retina by a worm. Arch Ophthalmol 1970;83: 68.
12. Gass JD, Braunstein RA: Further observations concerning the diffuse unilateral subacute neuroretinitis syndrome. Arch Ophthalmol 1983;101:1689.
13. Gass JD, Callanan DG, Bowman CB: Successful oral therapy for diffuse unilateral subacute neuroretinitis. Trans Am Ophthalmol Soc 1991;89:97.
14. Deleted.

15. Raymond LA, Gutierrez Y, Strong LE, et al: Living retinal nematode (filarial-like) destroyed with photocoagulation. Ophthalmology 1978;85:944.

16. de Souza EC, da Cunha SL, Gass JD: Diffuse unilateral subacute neuroretinitis in South America. Arch Ophthalmol 1992;110:1261.

17. de Souza EC, Nakashima Y: Diffuse unilateral subacute neuroretinitis. Report of transvitreal surgical removal of a subretinal nematode. Ophthalmology 1995;102:1183.

18. Bernasconi OR, Piguet B: [Unilateral diffuse subacute neuroretinitis]. Klin Monatsbl Augenheilkd 1997;210:327.

19. Kinnear FB, Hay J, Dutton GN, et al: Presumed ocular larva migrans presenting with features of diffuse unilateral subacute neuroretinitis. [Letter.] Br J Ophthalmol 1995;79:1140.

20. Kuchle M, Knorr HL, Medenblik-Frysch S, et al: Diffuse unilateral subacute neuroretinitis syndrome in a German most likely caused by the raccoon roundworm, *Baylisascaris procyonis.* Graefes Arch Clin Exp Ophthalmol 1993;231:48.

21. Salvanet-Bouccara A, Troussier H: [Diffuse unilateral subacute neuroretinitis. Apropos of a case]. J Fr Ophtalmol 1987;10:667.

22. Yuen VH, Chang TS, Hooper PL: Diffuse unilateral subacute neuroretinitis syndrome in Canada. [Letter.] Arch Ophthalmol 1996; 114:1279.

23. Gass JDM, ed: Stereoscopic Atlas of Macular Diseases, ed 2. St. Louis, CV Mosby, 1977, pp 226–227.

24. Goldberg MA, Kazacos KR, Boyce WM, et al: Diffuse unilateral subacute neuroretinitis. Morphometric, serologic, and epidemiologic support for *Baylisascaris* as a causative agent [see comments]. Ophthalmology 1993;100:1695.

25. Kazacos KR, Vestre WA, Kazacos EA, et al: Diffuse unilateral subacute neuroretinitis syndrome: Probable cause. [Letter.] Arch Ophthalmol 1984;102:967.

26. Kazacos KR, Raymond LA, Kazacos EA, et al: The raccoon ascarid. A probable cause of human ocular larva migrans. Ophthalmology 1985;92:1735.

27. Kelsey JH: Diffuse unilateral subacute neuroretinitis. [Letter.] J R Soc Med 1978;71:303.

28. Carney MD, Combs JL: Diffuse unilateral subacute neuroretinitis. Br J Ophthalmol 1991; 75: 633.

29. Casella AM, Farah ME, Belfort R Jr: Antihelminthic drugs in diffuse unilateral subacute neuroretinitis. Am J Ophthalmol 1998;125:109.

30. Matsumoto BT, Adelberg DA, Del Priore LV: Transretinal membrane formation in diffuse unilateral subacute neuroretinitis. Retina 1995;15:146.

31. Sivalingam A, Goldberg RE, Augsburger J, et al: Diffuse unilateral subacute neuroretinitis. Arch Ophthalmol 1991;109:1028.

44 — SCHISTOSOMIASIS (BILHARZIASIS)

Mehran A. Afshari and Nasrin Afshari

DEFINITION

Schistosomiasis or bilharziasis is a parasitic disease of the circulatory system that affects over 200 million people in about 75 countries.[1-3] The disease may cause significant morbidity and mortality in humans. Fortunately, ocular involvement in schistosomiasis is rare. Most of the reported cases of ocular schistosomiasis have granuloma of the conjunctiva.[3, 4] However, adult schistosoma worms have also been found in the anterior chamber and in a branch of the superior ophthalmic vein.[5, 6] Schistosomal choroiditis may occasionally be seen in patients who have hepatosplenic involvement.[7, 8] Other presentations of ocular schistosomiasis include nongranulomatous uveitis, retinal vasculitis, inflammation of the retinal pigment epithelium, dacryoadenitis, orbital pseudotumor, cataract, and optic nerve atrophy.[9-16]

HISTORY

Schistosomiasis is a disease with ancient roots.[3] Calcified Schistosoma eggs have been found in an Egyptian mummy from 1200 BC.[1, 17] In 1851, a German doctor, Theodore Bilharz, discovered the worm responsible for schistosomiasis and named it *Distomum haematobium* (later *Schistosoma haematobium*).[1] Bilharz's name became synonymous with the human disease (bilharziasis). The first effective treatment, tartar emetic, was used by McDonough in 1918.[1]

The first reported case of ophthalmic schistosomiasis was by Sobhy Bey (1928) from Egypt.[18] The patient was an 8-year-old boy with swelling of his tarsal conjunctiva and limbus. Until 1972, only 13 cases of ocular schistosomiasis were reported in the literature.[11] At present, less than 100 cases of ocular schistosomiasis have been reported.

EPIDEMIOLOGY

About 10% of the world population (500 to 600 million people) are exposed to schistosomiasis, and over 200 million people in 75 countries are infected.[1, 2, 19] The disease is endemic in Africa, South America, and Asia.[2] Schistosomiasis is usually seen in areas with fresh water temperature averaging between 25° and 30°C (between 36 degrees north and 34 degrees south latitude).[1] *S. haematobium* is found in Africa and Southwest Asia, *S. japonicum* is present only in the Far East, and *S. mansoni* is found in the Americas, Africa, and Southwest Asia.[20] Unfortunately, because of increased exposure to contaminated water, the number of cases is increasing.[17]

In the United States, more than 400,000 people are infected.[2, 20, 21] Most of these patients are immigrants from the endemic areas (Puerto Rico, Brazil, the Middle East, and the Far East). Because the intermediate host does not exist in the United States, the infection cannot be transmitted in this country.[2]

PARASITOLOGY AND LIFE CYCLE

The three major schistosoma species that infect humans are *S. haematobium*, *S. japonicum*, and *S. mansoni*. Less prevalent species include *S. intercalatum* and *S. mekongi*.[17, 19] All of these species share the same basic life cycle.[19] The most important difference is the location of the adult worms.

Humans are the principal definitive hosts for *S. mansoni* and *S. haematobium*; but *S. japonicum* has a variety of reservoir hosts in addition to humans, including dogs, cats, pigs, cattle, deer, and water buffalo. Humans are infected through contact with water contaminated with the infective stage of the parasite, which is called cercariae.[19, 22] After contact with human skin or the mucous membranes, the microorganisms maintain their position by using their suckers.[20] With the help of secretions from penetration glands, cercariae penetrate the intact skin.[19, 20] Penetration occurs within seconds to 10 minutes after contact by Schistosoma.[20] After entering the human body, the organisms transform into schistosomules or developing schistosomes that have a wormlike appearance.[20] These larva migrate to the lungs and finally to the portal vein, probably through an intravascular route.[19, 20] Schistosomules rapidly mature in the intrahepatic portal vein. The male and female schistosomes pair in the portal vein and then move to the venules of the bladder, ureter, and mesentery based on species of Schistosoma.[19, 20]

Mature *S. haematobium* worms are found in the venous plexus of the bladder and ureter. *S. mansoni* live in the inferior mesenteric veins, and *S. japonicum* worms are in the superior mesenteric veins.[22] Adult worms are about 1 to 2 cm long and are found in pairs.[20, 23] Female worms are carried by the male worms in a groove formed by lateral edges of the male worms.[22] The adult worms migrate in blood vessels without causing local inflammatory response. Fortunately, adult worms do not multiply in the human body, and immunosuppressive medications do not cause an increase in the number of worms.[19] Eggs burrow their way through the blood vessels and into the tissues of the walls of the intestine and bladder, and eventually reach the lumen of the urinary tract or bowel, and then are carried to the outside environment by urine or stool. If the eggs are deposited in fresh water, motile miracidia emerge which infect freshwater snails. These snails, of the genera Biomphalaria, Bulinus, and Oncomelania, are the intermediate hosts. Inside the snails, parasites divide asexually and are released into the water. At this stage, parasites are able to infect humans.[22]

CLINICAL MANIFESTATIONS

Most of the infected individuals are asymptomatic. The clinical manifestations of each type of schistosomiasis depend on the intensity of the infection (i.e., parasitic load) and variation in the host response.[23] Skin penetration by cercaria may or may not cause a pruritic maculopapular rash.[2, 23]

Acute Schistosomiasis (Katayama fever)

Acute schistosomiasis may be seen after infection with *S. mansoni* and *S. japonicum* but is rare in *S. haematobium* infections. Patients report intense transient itching, fever, chills, headache, hives, angioedema, weakness, myalgia, anorexia, weight loss, nonproductive cough, abdominal pain, and diarrhea.[19, 20] Generalized lymphadenopathy, hepatomegaly with tenderness, and splenomegaly are common. Lid edema, urticaria, and purpura may be present.[20] Eosinophilia is almost always present, which may be as high as 90%.[20] Leukocytosis and hyperglobulinemia are also common.[19] Symptoms gradually improve within a few weeks to a few months. The specific diagnosis can be made by testing blood for the antibodies to the adult schistosome gut antigens, by finding the eggs in the stool or urine, or by a rectal biopsy.[19]

Chronic Schistosomiasis

Most of these patients have a low to moderate worm load, and a large number of them are asymptomatic.[23]

The patients with chronic infection caused by *S. mansoni*, *S. japonicum*, or *S. mekongi* may complain of abdominal pain, diarrhea, or dysentery. Blood loss from the gastrointestinal tract may lead to anemia. The eggs may remain in portal circulation, leading to blockage of presinusoidal portal blood flow, resulting in portal hypertension. The earliest clinical sign is hepatomegaly. Later splenomegaly, and hematemesis from esophageal varices may be seen. At the terminal phase, jaundice, ascites, and liver failure develop.[2]

In chronic infection with *S. haematobium*, the worms are located in the veins of the bladder or ureter. Patients complain of micturition frequency, hematuria and dysuria.[2, 22] Urinalysis shows red blood cells, Schistosoma eggs, and occasional leukocytes.[22] The granulomatous reaction to the eggs may lead to obstructive uropathy and irregularities of the urinary bladder wall. Hydroureters, hydronephrosis, and filling defects of the bladder may be seen in imaging studies. In terminal stages, chronic renal failure or bladder cancer may be seen.[2]

Cardiopulmonary Schistosomiasis

Embolization of schistosomal eggs to the lungs is seen frequently at autopsy. In some patients, the eggs cause a significant granulomatous reaction, which leads to pulmonary hypertension and cor pulmonale.[20]

Central Nervous System Schistosomiasis

Brain and spinal cord involvement is rare in schistosomiasis. *S. japonicum* may cause cerebral lesions like granuloma or encephalitis, whereas *S. haematobium* and *S. mansoni* may result in granulomas of the spinal cord.[20]

Ectopic Schistosomiasis

Ectopic lesions in schistosomiasis are not common. Schistosomiasis may involve the uterus, ovary, testis, prostate, spermatic cord, epididymis, pancreas, gall bladder, omentum, stomach, kidney, adrenal gland, globe, and orbit.[3] Ocular schistosomiasis is discussed in detail in the next section.

Ocular Schistosomiasis

Mechanism

The exact route and mechanism by which the schistosomes can reach ectopic sites such as the globe and orbit are not definitely known. The following hypotheses have been postulated.[3–6, 8]

1. Cercariae may penetrate the skin and mucous membrane of various parts of the body, and then develop in nearby local veins. Abboud studied the penetration of cercariae of *S. mansoni* into ocular structures (including eyelids, conjunctiva, sclera, and cornea) of experimental animals.[4] Subconjunctival injection of cercariae and instillation of cercariae on the skin, cornea, and conjunctiva did not cause ocular lesions, but it did produce generalized schistosomiasis. Therefore, the theory supporting the local route of infection through the eye has fallen out of favor.[4]
2. Eggs may reach unusual sites through a patent foramen ovale.
3. Eggs may be deposited by the schistosomes in the gastrointestinal and genitourinary veins and then be filtered through the liver and lung capillary plexus.
4. The worms may migrate and circulate against the blood stream. The presence of worms in a branch of the superior ophthalmic vein supports this theory.
5. Eggs that are free in the portal system may enter the caval system through the enlarged anatomical portocaval collaterals. In portal hypertension, which is common in schistosomiasis, these collaterals are unusually large.

Ocular lesions are caused by *S. haematobium*, and *S. mansoni*. *S. haematobium* is responsible for most of the ocular lesions. Allergic ocular involvement and lid edema may be seen at the time of infestation.[20, 24]

Conjunctival Lesions

The most commonly reported ocular lesion is egg granuloma in the conjunctiva.[5, 16, 25] Conjunctival infection was first reported in Egypt by Sobhey Bey in 1928.[18] These lesions are primarily seen in male patients and are usually unilateral.[15] Conjunctival lesions are small, soft, smooth, and pinkish yellow in color.[15] All of the first nine reported cases occurred in children (seven boys and two girls) from 5 to 12 years of age.[5] Histopathologic examination of most of the cases reveal the presence of schistosomal ova in the granuloma. Badir reported a case in which the worms were observed in situ under the conjunctiva of a 12-year-old boy.[5] The patient had a lesion of the palpebral conjunctiva of the upper eyelid near the medial canthus. The lesion was excised, and a pathologic examination revealed an inflammatory granuloma beneath the epithelium containing a large number of schistosomal eggs. Additionally, in this specimen, a male and a female schistosome were identified in a dilated orbital vein (a branch of the superior ophthalmic vein).[5]

Orbital Schistosomiasis

Jakobiec et al. reported an 11-year-old boy with a mass in his lacrimal gland a year after trauma to his brow (Fig. 44–1). Pathologic examination showed widespread destruction of the lacrimal gland by a granulomatous lesion. Throughout the granuloma, eggs of *S. haematobium* were present.[9] Mortada reported a case of schistosomiasis presented as orbital pseudotumor with eosinophilia. However, neither ova nor worms were found in the biopsy.[26]

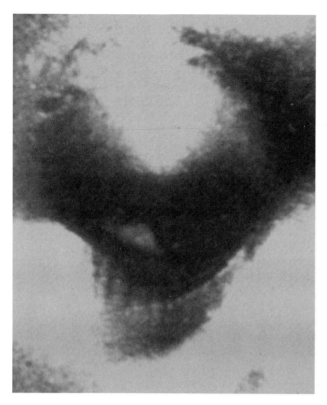

FIGURE 44–1. Schistosomal dacryoadenitis. (From Jakobiec FA, Gess L, Zimmerman LE: Granulomatous dacryoadenitis caused by *Schistosoma haematobium*. Arch Ophthalmol 1977;95:279.)

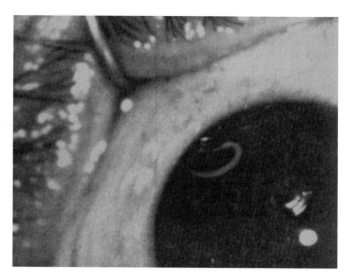

FIGURE 44–2. *S. mansoni* worm in the anterior chamber. (From Newton JC, Kanchanaranya C, Previte LR: Intraocular *Schistosoma mansoni*. Am J Ophthalmol 1968;65:774.)

Intraocular Schistosomiasis

Schistosoma may cause uveitis,[11, 27] choroiditis, chorioretinitis,[7, 8, 27] inflammation of retinal pigment epithelium,[10] maculitis,[11] retinal vasculitis, retinal vascular occlusion, retinal hemorrhage,[4] hyphema,[6] optic nerve swelling,[10] or optic nerve atrophy.[13]

Injection of cercariae of *S. mansoni* into the anterior chamber of experimental animals resulted in aqueous flare, keratic precipitates, and hypopyon.[4] Stein and Char developed an experimental uveitis model in rabbits using intraocular injection of *S. mansoni* eggs.[28] Intraocular inflammation became clinically apparent after five days, and on histologic examination, an eosinophilic infiltrate of the vitreous and choroid were seen. The chorioretinitis caused disruption of the photoreceptor layer. After a month, granuloma developed around the eggs that was similar to schistosomal granuloma in other parts of the body.[28]

Intraocular Worm

A case of *S. mansoni* worm in the anterior chamber has been reported in New York City (Figs. 44–2 and 44–3).[6] The patient was a 19-year-old Hispanic man who presented with hyphema. After absorption of the hyphema, it was noted that a white mobile tubular structure was present in the anterior chamber. The worm was removed surgically, and 3 months later, vision returned to 20/20.[28]

Choroiditis

In a study of 50 patients with hepatosplenic schistosomiasis, five patients were found to have choroiditis.[7] The lesions were yellowish white translucent nodules varying in size and were located in the choroid (Figs. 44–4 and 44–5). An important characteristic of these nodules is their variation in size. The size may correlate with the number of eggs present and with the various phases of their development.[8] In all five cases, the anterior chamber was quiet, but in one patient, there were a small number of cells in the vitreous. These nodules did not interfere with vision if there was no macular nodule.[7] Pittella studied the eyes of two deceased patients with hepatosplenic schistosomiasis.[8] In one patient, three granulomas were found in the choroid. Each granuloma was characterized by *S. mansoni* ova in the choroid, with a slight projection to the retina, surrounded by epithelioid cells in palisade formation, lymphocytes, plasmocytes, and eosinophils (Fig. 44–6).[8]

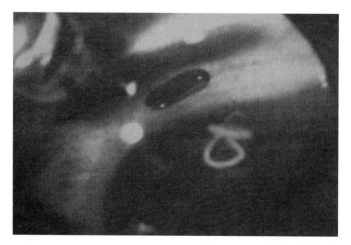

FIGURE 44–3. Gonioscopic view of intraocular *S. mansoni*. (From Newton JC, Kanchanaranya C, Previte LR: Intraocular *Schistosoma mansoni*. Am J Ophthalmol 1968;65:774.)

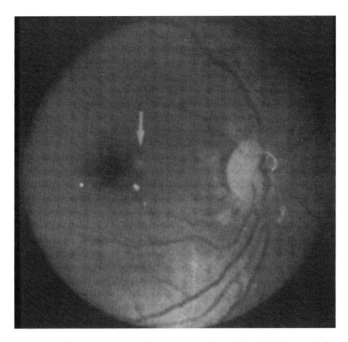

FIGURE 44–4. Medium-sized schistosomal nodules in the posterior pole. (From Orefice F, Simal CJR, Pittella JEH: Schistosomotic choroiditis. I. Funduscopic changes and differential diagnosis. Br J Ophthalmol 1985;69:294.)

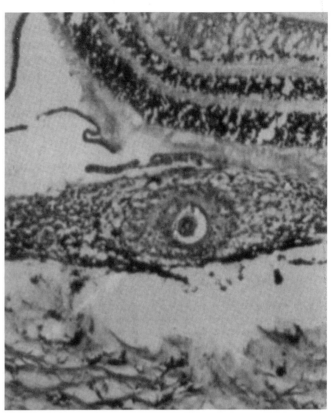

FIGURE 44–6. Schistosomal granuloma in the choroid. (From Pittella JEH and Orefice F: Schistosomotic choroiditis. II. Report of the first case. Br J Ophthalmol 1985;69:300.)

Inflammation of the Retinal Pigment Epithelium

Dickinson reported a 17-year-old man with visual acuity of 20/200, afferent pupillary defect, and iridocyclitis.[10] On funduscopy, optic disc swelling and multiple creamy lesions resembling acute multifocal placoid pigment epitheliopathy were seen. Stool examination revealed *S. mansoni* ova. Six weeks after treatment with praziquantel, the patient's vision returned to normal, the disc swelling resolved, and fundus lesions evolved into chorioretinal scars.[10]

Optic Nerve Involvement

Unilateral optic nerve atrophy and optic nerve swelling may be seen in patients with ocular schistosomiasis.[10, 13] Creed reported a case of optic atrophy in a patient with a history of schistosomiasis.[13] CT scan showed an optic nerve lesion that could be a granuloma encasing an egg.

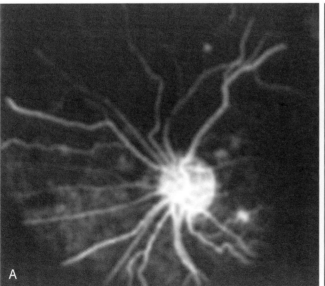

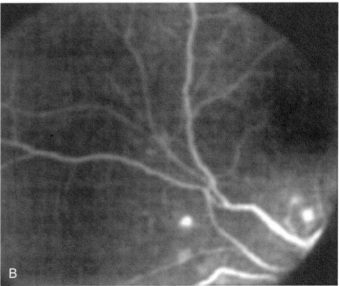

FIGURE 44–5. Fluorescein angiogram showing hyperfluorescent schistosomal nodules. (From Orefice F, Simal CJR, Pittella JEH: Schistosomotic choroiditis. I. Funduscopic changes and differential diagnosis. Br J Ophthalmol 1985;69:294.)

However, there is no histologically proven case of optic nerve involvement in schistosomiasis.

TREATMENT

Systemic

The drug of choice for the treatment of schistosomiasis is praziquantel, which is effective against all types of schistosome species.[2, 19, 22] For patients with *S. haematobium* and *S. mansoni* infections, Praziquantel is prescribed as two oral doses of 20 mg/kg body weight.[2] For treatment of *S. japonicum*, praziquantel is administered as 20 mg/kg body weight in three doses given at four hour intervals.[2, 20]

Ocular

Treatment with praziquantel is usually sufficient except for complicated cases.[24] Topical steroids may be needed to decrease the symptoms of conjunctival schistosomiasis. Excision of periocular nodules is both diagnostic and therapeutic. Uveitis cases may be treated with a combination of systemic antiparasite medications and topical steroids. If a worm is present inside the globe or orbital veins, it can be removed by surgery.[24]

PROGNOSIS

Schistosomal conjunctival granuloma has a good prognosis. However, the prognosis of intraocular schistosomiasis depends on the tissue involved and the extent of involvement.

CONCLUSIONS

Although schistosomiasis is a common systemic disease, its ocular involvement is rare. The most common presentation of ocular schistosomiasis is granuloma of the conjunctiva. However, schistosomiasis may cause uveitis, retinal vasculitis, inflammation of the retinal pigment epithelium, choroiditis, dacryoadenitis, orbital pseudotumor, cataract, and optic nerve atrophy. Praziquantel is the drug of choice for the treatment of schistosomiasis.

References

1. Strickland GT, Abdel-Wahab MF: Schistosomiasis. In: Strickland GT, ed: Hunter's Tropical Medicine, 7th ed. Philadelphia, WB Saunders, 1991, p 781.
2. Mahmoud AAF: Trematodes (schistosomiasis) and other flukes. In: Mandell GL, Bennett JE, Dolin R, eds: Principles and Practice of Infectious Diseases, 4th edition. New York, Churchill Livingstone, 1995, p 2538.
3. Fatt-hi A, Kamel I: Ectopic bilharziasis. J Laryngol Otol 1980; 94:1179.
4. Abboud A, Hanna LS, Ragab HAA: Experimental ocular schistosomiasis. Br J Ophthalmol 1971;55:106.
5. Badir G: Schistosomiasis of the conjunctiva. Br J Ophthalmol 1946;30:215.
6. Newton JC, Kanchanaranya C, Previte LR: Intraocular *Schistosoma mansoni*. Am J Ophthalmol 1968;65:774.
7. Orefice F, Simal CJR, Pittella JEH: Schistosomotic choroiditis. I. Funduscopic changes and differential diagnosis. Br J Ophthalmol 1985;69:294.
8. Pittella JEH, Orefice F: Schistosomotic choroiditis. II. Report of the first case. Br J Ophthalmol 1985;69:300.
9. Jakobiec FA, Gess L, Zimmerman LE: Granulomatous dacryoadenitis caused by *Schistosoma haematobium*. Arch Ophthalmol 1977;95:279.
10. Dickinson AJ, Rosenthal AR, Nicholson KG: Inflammation of the retinal pigment epithelium: A unique presentation of ocular schistosomiasis. Br J Ophthalmol 1990;74:440.
11. Hollwich F, Dieckhues B, Junemann G, et al: Bilharziose des Auges. Klin Mbl Augenheilk 1972;161:430.
12. Tabbara KF, Shoukrey N: Schistosomiasis. In: Gold DH, Weingeist TA, eds: The Eye in Systemic Disease. Philadelphia, JB Lippincott, 1990, p 184.
13. Creed TD: Unilateral optic atrophy presumed secondary to schistosomiasis of the optic nerve. J Am Optom Assoc 1993;64:440.
14. Tabarra KF, Hyndiuk RA, eds: Infections of the Eye, 2nd edition. Boston, Little Brown and Co, 1995, p 191.
15. Duke-Elder SS: System of Ophthalmology. St. Louis, C.V. Mosby, 1976.
16. Kean BH, Sun T, Ellsworth RM, eds: Color Atlas/Text of Ophthalmic Parasitology. New York, Igaku-shoin, 1991.
17. Mahmoud AAF, Wahab MFA: Schistosomiasis. In: Warren KS, Mahmoud AAF, eds: Tropical and Geographical Medicine, 2nd edition. New York, McGraw-Hill, 1990, pp 458–473.
18. Sobhy Bey M: La Bilharziose palpebroconjonctivale. d'Ocul, Tome CLXV 1928;165:675.
19. Nash TE: Schistosomiasis and other trematode infections. In: Fauci AS, Braunwald E, Isselbacher KJ, et al, eds: Harrison's Principles of Internal Medicine, 14th ed. New York, McGraw-Hill, 1998, p 1217.
20. Kline MW, Sullivan TJ: Schistosomiasis. In: Feigin RD, Cherry JD, eds: Textbook of Pediatric Infectious Diseases, 3rd ed. Vol II. Philadelphia, W.B. Saunders, 1992, p 2112.
21. Warren KS: Helminthic diseases endemic in the United States. Am J Trop Med Hyg 1974;23:723.
22. King CH: Schistosomes. In: Behrman RE, Kliegman RM, Arvin AM, eds: Textbook of Pediatrics, 15th ed. Philadelphia, W.B. Saunders, 1996, p 1001.
23. Cheever AW: Schistosomiasis. In: Hoeprich PD, Colin Jordan M, Ronald AR, eds: Infectious Diseases, 5th ed. Philadelphia, J.B. Lippincott Company, 1994, p 864.
24. Fraunfelder FW, Fraunfelder FT: Schistosomiasis. In: Fraunfelder FT, Hampton Roy F, Grove J, eds: Current Ocular Therapy, 4th ed. Philadelphia, W.B. Saunders, 1995, p 134.
25. Abdalla Cairo MI: Schistosomal granulomatosis of the conjunctiva. The Eye, Ear, Nose and Throat Monthly 1967;46:452.
26. Mortada A: Orbital pseudotumors and parasitic infections. Bull Ophthalmol Soc Egypt 1968;61:393.
27. Andrade CDE: Oftalmologica Tropical. Rio de Janeiro, Rodrigues, 1940.
28. Stein PC, Char DH: Intraocular granuloma: A *Schistosoma mansoni* model of ocular inflammation. Invest Ophthalmol Vis Sci 1982;23:479.

45 OPHTHALMOMYIASIS

E. Mitchel Opremcak

DEFINITION

Ophthalmomyiasis is an insect-mediated ocular disorder caused by botfly larvae (order Diptera). Botfly maggots may infest the ocular surface causing ophthalmomyiasis externa or may invade the eye, resulting in a clinical disease termed ophthalmomyiasis interna.

HISTORY

Maggot infestation of necrotic tissue in animals and humans has been a naturally occurring event throughout history. Larvae from the Calliphoridae family of flies are still used to débride and clean medically resistant cases of wound necrosis and severe osteomyelitis.[1, 2] Ocular disease, caused by maggots, was first reported in Austria in 1900.[3] The larva of *Hypoderma bovis* was identified after surgical removal from the eye of a child. Unfortunately, the child died from the complications of chloroform anesthesia. Most of the early reports were in children in the German medical literature and reported a poor visual outcome, often as a result of a purulent chorioretinitis.[4] In 1933, DeBoe published a case of "Dipterous larvae passing from the optic nerve into the vitreous chamber" in the English literature.[5] Anderson reported a case and provided the first review of the literature on ophthalmomyiasis interna in 1934.[6] Since then, several cases have been reported describing the various clinical presentations and evolving treatment strategies, including the use of ophthalmic lasers and vitreoretinal surgical techniques.[2, 7–9]

EPIDEMIOLOGY

Ophthalmomyiasis is an insect-mediated ocular disease caused by the larval stage of several families of flies in the order Diptera.[3, 10, 11] Certain families in this order are obligate parasites and require living tissue to complete their life cycle. The most common cause of ophthalmomyiasis externa is the sheep nasal botfly (*Oestrus ovis*).[12–14] As an obligate parasite, this species requires sheep as the host to complete their developmental cycle. An adult botfly will spray immature larvae into a flock, where they are inhaled into the nasal cavity by the sheep.[4] Once on the mucous membranes, the larvae migrate to the sinuses and develop into mature larvae before leaving the host by falling out the nose. Accidental human infestation has occurred worldwide, in areas endemic to the sheep botfly and in geographic proximity to flocks of sheep. It is postulated that the airborne, immature larvae attach to mucous membranes and conjunctiva of human hosts, resulting in ophthalmomyiasis externa.[15] Rarely, *Oestrus ovis* larvae penetrate the eye to cause ophthalmomyiasis interna.[2]

In contrast, *H. bovis* is an obligate parasite, requiring cattle as the natural host to complete its life cycle.[16–18] This species of botfly lay eggs directly on the skin of a cow, where they hatch. The immature larvae penetrate the skin and migrate through the tissues. Eventually, the mature larvae emerge through the skin again to fall on the ground to pupate. Most of the reported cases of ophthalmomyiasis interna are thought to be caused by this organism. The route of infestation in humans may be via direct deposition of eggs in the conjunctival cul-de-sac, with subsequent penetration of hatched immature larvae into the eye. Alternatively, the maggot may gain access to the eye after migrating through the human host for several months.[9, 18] The mature larva then gains access to the eye by penetrating the sclera, through the optic nerve, or via ciliary vessels. Ophthalmomyiasis interna is often noted in temperate regions that have a significant population of both the host cattle and *H. bovis* botfly.[9]

Other families of flies in the order Diptera have been reported to cause ophthalmomyiasis. Rabbits and rodents are host to *Cuterebra* sp. and larvae from these flies have been reported to cause human disease in North America.[19] Certain flies are facultative parasites (*Calliphora* sp.) and may also cause ophthalmomyiasis. Most cases of orbital myiasis have been associated with the Calliphoridae family of botfly.[3, 20, 21] These flies require decaying organic material for the developmental cycle of the ova, larvae, and adult fly. Opportunistic human infestation by these flies occurs in areas with substandard public health conditions and poor personal hygiene.[9]

CLINICAL CHARACTERISTICS

Ophthalmomyiasis externa is characteristically a unilateral disease of the ocular surface. Patients may complain of tearing, eyelid twitching, ocular irritation, and redness.[11] Visual acuity is typically good but may be slightly impaired. On ocular examination, motile larvae can be seen on the cornea, or in the conjunctival cul-de-sac.[22] Secondary keratitis, conjunctival hyperemia, hemorrhages, and a follicular conjunctivitis can be noted on biomicroscopic examination.

Patients with ophthalmomyiasis interna may be asymptomatic or, early in the course of the disease, may present with unilateral decrease in visual acuity.[6, 23] In the later stages with the death of the maggot, secondary ocular inflammation may result in pain, photophobia, and redness.[24] On biomicroscopic and fundus examination, the observation of a single, motile, white to translucent larva is pathognomonic (Fig. 45–1). The organism is segmented and tapered at both ends. In some instances, the maggot has been reported to move away from the examination light.

Larvae have been observed in the anterior chamber, lens, vitreous, and the subretinal space. They can migrate from the anterior chamber to the vitreous cavity and may leave the eye entirely, leaving behind the characteristic subretinal tracks.[16, 19, 23] In one reported case, a maggot was observed to migrate from the optic nerve head into the vitreous cavity.[5] When under the sensory retina, migration of the maggot results in characteristic, linear scars or "railroad tracks" at the level of the retinal pigment

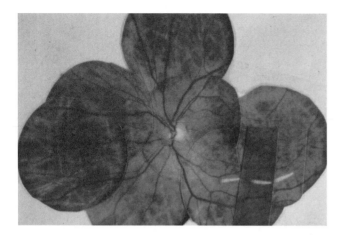

FIGURE 45–1. Composite "collage" fundus photograph demonstrating the etiologic agent of ophthalmomyiasis, the botfly maggot. (From Gass JD: Stereoscopic Atlas of Macular Disease, 3rd ed. St. Louis, CV Mosby, 1987. Courtesy of Constance Fitzgerald, MD, with permission from J. Donald Gass, MD, and Mosby Publishers.) (See color insert.)

epithelium (RPE).[23] (Fig. 45–2) Death of the maggot may result in mild to severe intraocular inflammation. Chorioretinitis, purulent panuveitis, vitreous hemorrhages, and retinal detachment has been reported with the death of a larva in cases of ophthalmomyiasis interna.[17] In most cases, however, death of the larva within the eye has not been associated with significant uveitis.[9]

PATHOGENESIS

Ocular surface disease in ophthalmomyiasis externa is due primarily to mechanical injury caused by the maggot and its mouth hooks and intersegmental spines.[9] Corneal edema, and conjunctival hyperemia and a follicular conjunctivitis are common reactions to the larval infestation and movement. Small conjunctival hemorrhages as a result of tissue damage from the oral hooks and the thorax spines may be observed.

The ocular manifestations and clinical presentation of ophthalmomyiasis interna depends on the route of

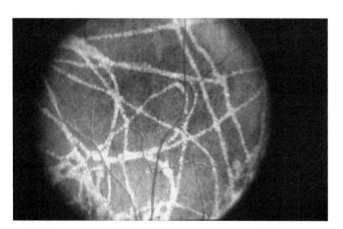

FIGURE 45–2. Fundus photograph of a patient with longstanding ophthalmomyiasis, demonstrating the extensive RPE loss in "track" fashion, evidence of the very extensive amount of migration and travel of the maggot. (From Gass JD: Stereoscopic Atlas of Macular Disease, 3rd ed. St. Louis, CV Mosby, 1987. Courtesy of J. Donald Gass, MD, with permission from Mosby Publishers.) (See color insert.)

migration and location of the organism within the eye. When alive, the mature larva can cause trauma to the delicate intraocular tissues and structures. The subretinal tracks represent such mechanic injury to the RPE. Damage to the optic nerve, secondary macular hemorrhage, and retinal detachment have been reported complications of larval migration through the eye and retina.[17] Uveitis can occur with the death of the larva.[9, 17, 25, 26] In one case in which the maggot was removed surgically, the vitreous contained lymphocytes, eosinophils, plasma cells, and epithelioid cells.[2]

DIAGNOSIS

The diagnosis is made on clinical grounds, by observing the maggot on the ocular surface or within the eye. On fundus examination, the presence of subretinal, crossing, linear tracks are suggestive but not diagnostic for this condition. Although they are characteristic of ophthalmomyiasis, linear scars in the retina have been observed in other helminthic diseases and may be similar in appearance to the linear equatorial streaks in histoplasmosis, angioid streaks, and traumatic choroidal ruptures. Fluorescein angiography may help show the extent of injury to the RPE and macula.[23]

The larva can be specifically identified in cases in which it is surgically removed from the eye. On removal, the maggot should be fixed in formalin and processed for microscopic examination.[9] Characteristic surface structures on the maggot allow classification of the organism to family, genus, and species.[19]

TREATMENT

Treatment for ophthalmomyiasis externa consists of removing the larva from the ocular surface.[11] Topical and regional anesthetics provide both comfort and facilitate the removal process by immobilizing the maggots.[27]

Therapeutic strategies vary for patients with ophthalmomyiasis interna, depending on the location of the maggot and whether the organism is alive or dead.[11] In some case reports, dead larva have been observed within the eye and appear to be well tolerated, with patient retention of good vision and no inflammation.[8, 9] In patients with a dead maggot in the eye and no uveitis, the eye and the larva may be observed without therapy. Such tolerance, however, for a relatively complex organism within the eye would be unexpected. A dead botfly maggot would have multiple unique proteins capable of inciting uveitis unless their antigens are denatured or removed. In most cases, when the maggot is alive, attempts have been made either to kill the organism via laser photocoagulation or surgically to remove it from the eye. Argon laser photocoagulation has been used to kill the larva with some success.[8, 25] In one report, using settings at 10 burns of a 200-μm spot size, at 400 mW, and a 0.1-second duration, laser photocoagulation was successful in killing the maggot without significant intraocular inflammation.[8] It is possible that the photocoagulation denatured the larval antigens and, by that, prevented an inflammatory response. In another patient, photocoagulation was accompanied by a severe, postlaser uveitis.[25] Topical, regional and oral corticosteroids may be used to treat uveitis associated with the death of the larva. In several cases, the larvae was extracted surgically from the eye.[2, 7] Both vitrectomy and subretinal surgical techniques have been employed to remove intraocular maggots. Most of these cases resulted in improved visual acuity following removal of the parasite.

COMPLICATIONS

Complications of ophthalmomyiasis are primarily due to mechanical injury accompanying maggot migration, intraocular inflammation associated with the death of the organism, and trauma from surgical removal.[2, 7, 9, 25] Retinal tears and detachment have been reported in cases of ophthalmomyiasis interna. These problems can be addressed by standard vitreoretinal surgical techniques. Ocular inflammation may occur with the death of the maggot following laser photocoagulation and can be treated with corticosteroid regimens. Vitreoretinal surgical techniques can be complicated by retinal detachment, cataract, hemorrhage, and endophthalmitis. In most cases, these surgical risks are acceptable when compared with the potential injury caused by random, intraocular larval migration and death of the organism.

PROGNOSIS

The prognosis for ophthalmomyiasis externa is good. Removal of the maggots results in return of ocular comfort and resolution of the conjunctival irritation. The visual prognosis for ophthalmomyiasis interna depends on the migration route of the maggot and on whether the death of the larva incites inflammation. A poor visual prognosis can be expected if the path of the maggot involves critical structures such as the optic nerve or the macula. Retinal detachment may be repaired but may be associated with poor central vision if the macula is involved. Laser photocoagulation and death of the maggot may result in uveitis, which can be treated with corticosteroids. Surgical removal of the organism from the vitreous cavity or the subretinal space eliminates this risk and may preserve vision in selected cases.

CONCLUSIONS

Ophthalmomyiasis is a rare, unilateral ocular disease caused by the larvae of the botfly. Several families in the order Diptera can infest human hosts and cause mild ocular surface disorder or a more serious ophthalmomyiasis interna. Surgical removal of the organism may effect a better visual prognosis and reduce the chances of uveitis. Vision may be impaired as a result of mechanical injury to the optic nerve or macula.

References
1. Bunkis J, Gherini S, Walton RL: Maggot therapy revisited. West J Med 1985;142:554.
2. Rapoza PA, Michels RG, Semeraro RJ, et al: Vitrectomy for excision of intraocular larva (*Hypoderma* species). Retina 1986;6:99.
3. Kersten RC, Showkrey NM, Tabbara KF: Orbital myiasis. Ophthalmol 1986;93:128.
4. Hoffman BL, Goldsmid JM: Ophthalmomyiasis caused by *Oestrus ovis* L. (Diptera:Oestridae) in Rhodesia. S Afr Med J 1970;10:644.
5. DeBoe MP: Dipterous larva passing from the optic nerve into the vitreous chamber. Arch Ophthalmol 1933;10:824.
6. Anderson WB: Ophthalmomyiasis interna: Case report and review of the literature. Trans Am Acad Ophthalmol Otolarygol 1934;39:218.
7. Custis PH, Pakalnis VA, Klintworth GK, et al: Posterior internal ophthalmomyiasis: Identification of a surgically removed *Cuterebra larva* by scanning electron microscopy. Ophthalmology 1983;90:1583.
8. Fitzgerald CR, Rubin ML: Intraocular parasite destroyed by photocoagulation. Arch Ophthalmol 1074;91:162.
9. Glasgow BJ: Ophthalmomyiasis. In: Pepose JS, Holland GN, Wilhelmus KR, eds: Ocular Infection and Immunity. St Louis, CV Mosby, 1995, p 1505.
10. Beaver PC, Jung RC, Cupp EW: Clinical Parasitology, 9th ed. Philadelphia, Lea & Febiger, 1984, p 680.
11. Kean BH, Sun T, Ellsworth RM: Ophthalmomyiasis. In: Kean BH, Sun T, Ellsworth RM, eds: Color Atlas/Text of Ophthalmic Parasitology. New York, Igaku-Shoin, 1991, p 105.
12. Cameron JA, Shoukrey NM, Al-Garni AA: Conjunctival ophthalmomyiasis caused by the sheep nasal botfly (*Oestrus ovis*). Am J Ophthalmol 1991;112:331.
13. Harvey JT: Sheep botfly: Ophthalmomyiasis externa. Can J Ophthalmol 1986;21:92.
14. Reingold WJ, Robbin JB, Leipa D, et al: Oestrus ovis ophthalmomyiasis externa. Am J Ophthalmol 1984;97:7.
15. de Vries LAM, van Bijsterveld OP: Ophthalmooestriasis conjuntivitivae. Ophthalmologica 1986;192:193.
16. Mason GI: Bilateral ophthalmomyiasis interna. Am J Ophthalmol 1981;91:65.
17. Edwards KM, Meredith TA, Hagler WS, et al: Ophthalmomyiasis interna causing visual loss. Am J Ophthalmol 1984;97:605.
18. Vine A, Schatz H: Bilateral posterior interior ophthalmomyiasis. Ann Ophthalmol 1981;13:1041.
19. Mathur SP, Makhija JM: Invasion of the orbit by maggots. Br J Ophthalmol 1967;51:406.
20. Glasgow BJ, Maggiano JM: *Cuterbra* ophthalmomyiasis. Am J Ophthalmol 1995;119:512.
21. Wood TR, Slight JR: Bilateral orbital ophthalmomyiasis. Report of a case. Arch Ophthalmol 1970;84:692.
22. Laborde RP, Kaufman HE, Beyer WB: Intracorneal ophthalmomyiasis. Arch Ophthalmol 1988;106:880.
23. Gass JDM, Lewis RA: Subretinal tracks in ophthalmomyiasis. Arch Ophthalmol 1976;94:1500.
24. Slusher MM, Holland WD, Weaver RG, et al: Ophthalmomyiasis interena posterior: Subretinal tracks and intraocular larvae. Arch Ophthalmol 1979;97:885.
25. Forman AR, Cruess AF, Benson WE: Ophthalmomyiasis treated by argon laser photocoagulation. Retina 1984;4:163.
26. Hess C: Severe purulent chorioretinitis with destruction of the retina due to a cause not known up to the present time. Arch Augenh 1913;74:227.
27. Medownick M, Finkelstein E, Lazarus M, et al: Human external ophthalmomyiasis caused by the horse botfly larva (*gastrerophilus* sp.). Aust N Z J Ophthalmol 1985;13:387.

Stefanos Baltatzis

DEFINITION

Ophthalmia nodosa is defined as severe ocular inflammatory reaction precipitated by hairs of certain insect or vegetable material that has come into contact with the eye.

The term "nodosa" is derived from the granulomatous nodule formed on the conjunctiva and in the iris in response to caterpillar hairs or sensory setae.

HISTORY

The dermal reaction to sharp and irritant caterpillar setae (Lepidoptera) was known to the Greeks and the Romans, and was commented upon by Dioscorides and Pliny.[1]

Schon (1861) was the first who described the disease that was later called "pseudotuberculosis" by Wagenwan[2] (1890) and renamed ophthalmia nodosa by Saemich[3] (1904). Gunderson[4] extensively reviewed the disease in 1945.

EPIDEMIOLOGY

The cause of ophthalmia nodosa is region specific, occurring primarily as a result of needles of plants, such as the common burdock, which is found in all the contiguous 48 states of the United States, or urticarial hairs of some caterpillars. According to Watson and associates,[5] only six varieties of caterpillars are known to cause ophthalmia nodosa. Also, hairy spiders commonly called tarantula can cause ophthalmia nodosa, especially in areas where keeping such spiders as pets is fashionable.

Macrothylacia rubi and *Arctia caja* are the caterpillar species found only in British Isles, whereas *Traumetopoea pityocampa* (pine processionary), *Thaumetopoea jordana*, *Isia Isabella,* and *Dedrolimnus pini* may be found in other countries. Two other species have also been associated with ophthalmia nodosa, namely, *Thaumetopoea pinivora*, another pine processionary, and *Thaumetopoea processionary L*, an oak processionary.[5]

Hairy spiders of the family Therapsosidae (commonly called tarantulas) (Fig. 46–1*A* and *B*) possess specialized hairs on the dorsal surface of the abdomen at a density of approximately 10,000/mm,[2] and 0.10 mm in length.[6, 7] When threatened, the spider rapidly vibrates its hind legs across the dorsal abdomen, which is densely covered with barbed hairs. This reaction sprays a cloud of hairs into the path of the perceived threatening predator. Cooke and coworkers[6–8] classified projectile tarantula hairs into four types. Species native to South and Central America, the Caribbean, and Mexico possess the relatively large and sturdy type III hairs, which are known to produce a prolonged and intense urticaria in human tissue. Contact with caterpillar setae occur by direct contact with caterpillars, by contact with the larval cocoon into which setae may be shed and interwoven, by contact with adult Lepidoptera which may carry larval setae on their bodies after emerging from the cocoon, by direct reaction to the adult setae themselves, or by wind-borne spread of setae.

Thus, a definite history of caterpillar contact is not necessary for the diagnosis of the condition. In fact, none of the 103 individuals described by Bishop and Morton[9] (1967) gave a history of direct caterpillar contact.

CLINICAL CHARACTERISTICS

The clinical manifestations of ophthalmia nodosa vary greatly and are classified according to Candera and associates[10] as follows:

Type 1. An acute, anaphylactoid reaction consisting of conjunctival chemosis and inflammation combined with epiphora and foreign body sensation beginning immediately and lasting for weeks. The loose tissues of the eyelid are primarily involved, producing a marked periorbital edema and allergic dermatitis. Shama and colleagues[11] have described an acute toxic or allergic reaction to caterpillar hairs with periorbital edema. Histamine present in the caterpillar hairs has been implicated in this reaction. To date, studies have failed to identify all of the precipitating toxins.

Type 2. Chronic mechanical keratoconjunctivitis caused by hairs lodged in the bulbar or palpebral conjunctiva. The symptoms appear from minutes to days after the hairs reach the eye. The cornea may show linear scratches adjacent to the hair (Fig. 46–2).

Type 3. Formation of one or more gray-yellow conjunctival nodules (granulomas). Setae may be subconjunctival or intracorneal, producing nebulae around them with or without synechiae. The patient may be entirely asymptomatic at this stage.

Type 4. Intense iritis secondary to hair penetration into the anterior chamber (Fig. 46–3). The iritis tends to be severe and is often associated with iris nodules and even with hypopyon. In rare cases, hairs penetrate the lens and cause an intralenticular foreign body reaction.

Type 5. Vitreoretinal involvement (10% to 20%),[12] which may occur relatively early or may develop years after the contact with the hairs (Fig. 46–4). The hairs gain access to the vitreous and subretinal space either by entering the anterior chamber and then penetrating through the iris or lens, or by migrating transclerally from a conjunctival focus. Chorioretinal tracks tend to be pigmented, with a white, inflamed leading edge.

Rare cases of overt endophthalmitis have been reported,[13] but milder forms of vitritis with or without cystoid macular edema or papillitis are more common.

Patients may develop some or all of these features. Although it is possible for each of the five types of reaction to develop sequentially, a patient may manifest only one type even without having a history of contact with caterpillars. Some cases may be due to wind-blown hairs or to forgotten contact with a caterpillar in childhood. The type and severity of the ocular reaction and the ultimate prognosis probably depend on the number of hairs or the amount of foreign material that comes into contact with or gains entry into the eye.

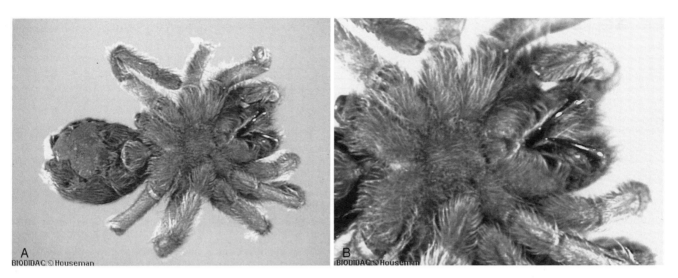

FIGURE 46–1. *A*, Tarantula; ventral surface of the spider, showing tagma, opisthosoma, and prosoma. *B*, Additional, more magnified view of the ventral surface of the tarantula spider showing the fans chelicera. Images courtesy of Antoine Morin and Jon Houseman, from the Biodidac website, URL: http://biodidac.bio.uottawa.ca/.

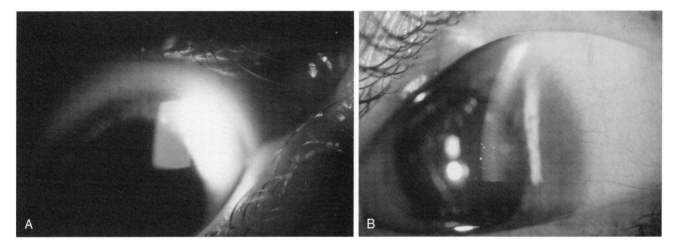

FIGURE 46–2. *A*, Slit-lamp photograph of a patient with ophthalmia nodosa, with keratitis secondary to a tarantula hair. *B*, Ophthalmia nodosa with both keratitis and uveitis. (Courtesy of Dr. E. Mitchel Opremcak.) (See color insert.)

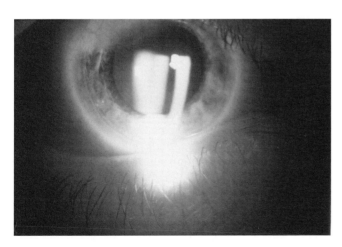

FIGURE 46–3. Ophthalmia nodosa with hypopyon uveitis. (Courtesy of Dr. E. Mitchel Opremcak.) (See color insert.)

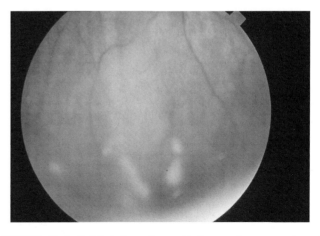

FIGURE 46–4. Ophthalmia nodosa, with intraocular penetration of tarantula hair, with production of posterior uveitis and the formation of vitreal infiltrates, both in the form of snowballs and in the form of a snowman (central figure). (Courtesy of Dr. E. Mitchel Opremcak.) (See color insert.)

PATHOGENESIS AND PATHOLOGY

The pathologic damage caused by setae is a function of their direct toxicity and locomotion. Caterpillar hair toxicity is dependent on the concentration of toxins in the venom gland, which is connected to the hair shaft. The intraocular inflammation is presumably due to both the presence of foreign material and in part to the effect of the urticating toxin.[14] Chemical analysis of the urticating toxin shows a small fraction of water-soluble protein with esterase, protease, and phospholipase activity.[15] The material can also give rise to IgG antibodies in rabbits.[16]

In 1986, Lamy and colleagues[17] identified the urticating protein of the pine processionary caterpillar as thaumeatopoein; there is a similar protein in other urticating caterpillars. Although ophthalmia nodosa has been known for more than a century, the mechanism of caterpillar hair migration into the eye remains controversial. Gunderson and coworkers[12] have suggested that because the setae have no propulsive power of their own, movements of the globe with versions, respirations, and pulse, together with the constant iris movement, propel the spines forward. It can be seen from electron microscopy that the orientation of the spines is vital to facilitation of this forward only movement. Asher[18] proposed that the cellular infiltration around the damaged base of the hair pushes the undamaged tip of the hair toward the direction of least resistance. Whereas the soft conjunctival and episcleral tissues permit the formation of a protruding nodule, the stiffer cornea and sclera do not. As a result, the hair is propelled forward in its same interlamellar space unless the sharp tip happens to enter a neighboring interlamellar space, in which case it will continue to move parallel to the lamellae.

Histopathologically, the granulomatous reaction consists of histiocytes, epithelioid cells, and macrophages surrounding the foreign material.

Occasionally, eosinophils have been observed in the lesion,[2] and in severe cases, there is a perivascular infiltration of chronic inflammatory cells in the retina extending into the scleral channels and the episcleral tissues.

In 1983, Haluska and associates[19] described an experimental model of ophthalmia nodosa in albino rabbits and they found that the lesion produced in the cornea of the animals was similar to that found in the human cornea.

Cross sections of the caterpillar cilia were observed within the cornea surrounded by inflammatory nodules composed of epithelioid and giant cells and mononuclear inflammatory cells. In some sections, giant cells were seen within the center of the fragmented cilia.

DIAGNOSIS

The diagnosis is usually missed, because most physicians are completely unfamiliar with the disease and pay no particular attention to the disorder.

Inspection of the stained cornea under magnification reveals a distinctive pattern of minute linear scratches of the corneal epithelium, which serve to indicate the presence and the location of the cause, in a patient with type II ophthalmia nodosum. These scratches are predominantly vertical, but one may see oblique and horizontal abrasions as well.

Biomicroscopic examination of the everted lid reveals the protruding tip or a minute projecting spicule of caterpillar hair as a dark spot close to the lid margin, surrounded by a small zone of hyperemia, which may be obscured by a tenacious deposit of mucus.

In type 4 and 5 cases, the patient usually presents with an irritable eye, ciliary injection, flare, and cells in the anterior chamber or in the vitreous. Setae can be identified within the corneal stroma embedded in focal exudates; other setae can be found lodged in the iris and adjacent trabecular band.

Fundus examination, which is limited by photophobia, reveals yellow patches of retinochoroiditis with or without vitritis, usually situated at the temporal macular area with the inciting hair lodged at a corresponding point in the vitreous cortex.

TREATMENT

The treatment of reactions to caterpillar hairs or setae depends on the type of ocular involvement.[20]

Type 1 (toxic) reactions should be treated with irrigation and mechanical removal of the visible hairs, followed by administration of antibiotic and steroid drops.

Type 2 reactions (mechanical chronic keratoconjunctivitis) necessitate a meticulous search for minute, often occult fragments of hairs, the removal of which gives immediate relief.

Progression to type 3 reactions (conjunctival, nodules, granulomas, and corneal penetration) is treated with surgical removal of the conjunctival nodule as soon as possible in the hope of preventing intraocular migration of the hairs. Intracorneal hairs can either be removed at the slit lamp, using special forceps, or be observed if the hairs are few and deeply seated. This may be a difficult decision to make. Should there be any evidence of a tendency for movement, which could result in intraocular migration of the hairs, surgical intervention is clearly indicated.

One may consider lamellar or penetrating keratoplasty if the hairs are numerous and located in such a way as to allow their excision within the confines of the trephination.

Type 4 reactions due to penetration into the anterior chamber can be treated with topical steroids. Anterior chamber hairs or iris nodules should be removed, the latter through an iridectomy.

Type 5 reactions (vitritis, vitreoretinal involvement) should be treated with local and systemic steroids, with vitrectomy reserved for resistant cases.

Recently, successful treatment of vitreous reaction by argon laser photocoagulation[21] of the offending hairs has been described. This is based on experimental evidence showing that in vitro either neodymium:yttrium-aluminum-garnet (YAG) laser or argon laser can disrupt the hairs, most importantly by destroying the tip and the reserve barb of the hairs. Raspillar and colleagues have advocated the use of barrier photocoagulation as a strategy to prevent migration of the hair into the macula.[22]

COMPLICATIONS

Allergic dermatitis, nodular conjunctivitis, catarrhal conjunctivitis and marginal keratitis, nummular keratitis, destructive uveitis, nodular iritis (granulomatous response), intralenticular foreign body, severe vitritis and papillitis, subretinal migration of the hairs, and rarely, endophthalmitis and phthisis bulbi necessitating enucleation[13] are among the reported complications of the fulminating type of ophthalmia nodosa.

PROGNOSIS

Although there have been cases reported in the literature in which caterpillar hairs have caused severe damage to the eye,[13] in general, the long-term prognosis of the disease appears to be relatively good, even in the case of intraocular migration of hairs. The uveitis caused by intraocular migration in the majority of cases is responsive to standard steroid management, usually resolving within a few weeks.

CONCLUSIONS

Caterpillar hairs and the American burdock (*Arctium minus*; cocklebur) vegetable needles are responsible for a wide variety of ocular inflammatory reactions, ranging from simple conjunctival, corneal, and anterior chamber involvement to severe vitreous and retinal inflammation.

The treatment depends on the type of location and severity of ocular involvement.

Simple lavage or mechanical removal will suffice for hairs remaining as external foreign bodies. Once they have migrated into the conjunctiva, surgical excision of the foreign bodies is required.

Intracorneal hair may necessitate surgical excision. But if the hairs are deep, simple observation is justified, with further surgical action in cases of progressive migration. Once the hairs enter the anterior chamber, topical steroids usually control the rather intense resultant uveitis. Iris nodules may be excised if they are few in number. Intravitreal hairs may cause vitritis and chorioretinitis, requiring systemic and/or periocular steroid therapy, or even therapeutic vitrectomy.

References

1. Picarelli ZP, Valle JR: In: Buccherl W, Deulofeu V, Buckely EE, eds: Venomous Animals and Their Venoms. New York, Academic Press, 1981.
2. Wagenmann A: Veber Pseudotuberculose Entzundung der Conjunctiva und Iris durch Raupenhaare. Arch Ophthalmol 1890;36:126–134.
3. Saemisch T: Ophthalmia Nodosa, Graefe-Saemisch Handbuch der gesamten Augenheilkunde, 2nd ed, Vol 5, Pt 1. Leipzig, W. Engelman, 1904, pp 548–564.
4. Gunderson T, Heath P, Carron LK: Ophthalmia nodosa. Trans Am Ophthalmol Soc 1945;48:151–167.
5. Watson PG, David S: Ophthalmia nodosa. Br J Ophthalmol 1966;50:209.
6. Berman E: Un cas d' ophtalmia nodosa. Clinique Ophtalmologique 1928. Thése. Université de Lausanne.
7. Cooke JAL, Roth VD, Miller FH: The urticating hairs of the theraphosid spider. Am Museum Noviates 1972, No 2498, p 1.
8. Cooke JAL, Miller FH, Grover RW, Duffy JL: Urticaria caused by tarantula hairs. Am J Trop Med Hyg 1973;22:130.
9. Bishop JW, Morton MR: Caterpillar-hair keratoconjunctivitis. Am J Ophthalmol 1967;64:778–779.
10. Candera W, Pachtman MA, Fountain JA, Wilson FM: Ocular lesions caused by caterpillar hairs (ophthalmia nodosa). Can J Ophthalmol 1984;19:40–44.
11. Shama SK, Etkind PH, Odell TM, et al: Gypsy-moth-caterpillar dermatitis. N Engl J Med 1982;306:1300–1301.
12. Gunderson T, Heath P, Garron LK: Ophthalmia nodosa. Trans Am J Ophthalmol Soc 1945;48:151–167.
13. Steele C, Lucas DR, Ridgway AEA: Endophthalmitis due to caterpillar setae. Br J Ophthalmol 1984;68:284–288.
14. Tyzzer EE: The pathology of the browntail moth dermatitis. J Med Res 1907;16:43–64.
15. DeJong MCJM, Bleumink E: Investigative studies of the dermatitis caused by the larva of the browntail moth III. Chemical analysis of skin-reactive substances. Arch Dermatol Res 1977;259:247–262.
16. Dejong MCJM, Bleumink E IV: Further characterization of skin-reactive substances. Arch Dermatol Res 1977;259:263–281.
17. Lamy M, Pasturead NH, Novak F, et al: Thaumeatopoein: An urticating protein from the hairs and integument of pine processionary caterpillar. Toxicon 1986;24:347–356.
18. Ascher KW: Mechanism of locomotion observed on caterpillar hairs. Am J Ophthalmol 1966;65:354–355.
19. Haluska FG, Puliafito CA, Henriquez A, Albert DM: Experimental gypsy moth (Lymantria dispar) ophthalmia nodosa. Arch Ophthalmol 1983;101:799–801.
20. Fraser SG, Dowd TC, Basanquet RC: Intraocular caterpillar setae. Eye 1994;8:596–598.
21. Marti-Huguet T, Pujol O, Cabiro L, et al: [Endophthalmos caused by intravitreal caterpillar hairs. Treatment by direct photocoagulation with argon laser.] J Fr Ophtalmol 1987;10:559–564.
22. Raspiller A, Lepori JC, George JL: Coriorétinopathie par migration des poils de chenilles. Bull Med Soc Fr Ophtalmol 1984;95:153–156.

HUMAN IMMUNODEFICIENCY VIRUS–ASSOCIATED UVEITIS

Isabelle Cochereau and Thanh Hoang-Xuan

CHANGING PATTERNS OF UVEITIS IN HIV INFECTION

The acquired immunodeficiency syndrome (AIDS) was first recognized in 1981, and human immunodeficiency virus (HIV) was identified as the etiologic agent in 1984. Opportunistic infections are now better diagnosed and their pathogenesis is better known. Progress in the management of HIV-infected patients has led to changes in the profile of the disease.

HIV is a retrovirus that infects CD4+ T lymphocytes, which are pivotal effectors of cell-mediated immunity. HIV integrates the host cell genome, where it induces the synthesis of new virions. The release of the new virions kills the infected cell (Fig. 47–1). The decline in CD4+ T-lymphocyte numbers leads to severe immunodeficiency, permitting the development of opportunistic infections and malignancies. In response to each opportunistic infection, multiplication of the remaining CD4+ T lymphocytes increases the number of circulating virions in a vicious circle. This is why the prevention of opportunistic infections is so important for slowing the progression of HIV disease.

Antiretroviral drugs interfere with various steps of HIV replication (see Fig. 47–1). Reverse-transcriptase inhibitors prevent the transformation of viral RNA into DNA, thereby preventing it from integrating the host cell genome. Protease inhibitors (PIs) prevent the assembly of new viral proteins. The recent advent of highly active antiretroviral therapy (HAART), including at least one PI, has led to a dramatic improvement in the prognosis of HIV infection. HAART induces a marked fall in the frequency of opportunistic infections and malignancies, and a corresponding increase in life expectancy.[1] PIs restore immunity, as reflected by a clinical improvement, an increase in CD4+ T-cell counts,[2] and the decline in HIV viral load. Several PIs are available (Table 47–1) and can be combined in various regimens. However, resistance to PIs is developing, and it is impossible to predict how effective existing drugs will be in a few years' time.

HIV is transmitted by sexual contact (both homosexual and heterosexual), by blood (e.g., contaminated material for intravenous injection, blood products), and from mother to child. In industrialized countries, the main groups at risk are homosexuals with multiple partners, and intravenous drug users, but heterosexual transmission is on the increase. In developing countries, most cases of infection are the result of heterosexual contacts, contaminated blood or materials, and mother to child transmission.

The absolute cumulative number of cases is highest in Africa, followed by the Americas, Asia, and Europe. Treatment and prevention are optimal in the industrialized countries, whereas they are often totally lacking in the developing countries. The World Health Organiza-

tion (WHO) estimates that about 40 million people will be infected worldwide by the year 2000.[3]

The diagnosis of HIV infection is based on the presence of specific antibodies against HIV antigens. Two tests are available: enzyme-linked immunosorbent assay (ELISA) is routinely used for screening, and western blot is used to confirm a positive ELISA. Antibodies usually appear 3 to 6 weeks after primary exposure to HIV, but in some cases they can emerge several months later.

The degree of immunodeficiency is assessed in terms of the CD4+ T-cell count. Most opportunistic infections occur when this count falls below 200 cells/μl, and the most severe complications occur at counts below 50 cells/μl. Syphilis and candidiasis can occur at any CD4+ T-cell count, whereas tuberculosis occurs at around 300 cells/μl, cryptococcal meningitis and toxoplasmosis at around 100 cells/μl, cytomegalovirus (CMV) retinitis, varicella-zoster virus (VZV) retinitis, disseminated *Pneumocystis carinii* pneumonia (PCP), cryptococcosis, and histoplasmosis occur at below 50 cells/μl.

Quantification of plasma HIV RNA (the viral load) reflects the level of HIV replication. The main target of antiretroviral therapies is to drive viral load below the current detection limit. Both CD4+ T-cell counts and viral load are used to adjust antiretroviral therapy and to begin prophylaxis.

The ocular manifestations of HIV infection are many and varied, involving the ocular adnexa, eyeballs, and nerves. Although the most frequent ocular manifestation of AIDS is HIV retinopathy, the main retinal opportunistic infection is CMV retinitis.[4–6] Herpes zoster ophthalmicus, lymphoma, and certain drugs can also cause uveitis.

In industrialized countries, the pattern of ocular involvement in HIV infection has changed over the years.[7] At the beginning of the pandemic, when no treatment was available, CMV retinitis was a sign of approaching death, with a survival time of only a few weeks. Later, the advent of the anti-CMV drugs ganciclovir and foscarnet improved the survival time, especially when maintenance therapy was given routinely. The introduction of the first anti-HIV drugs, followed by routine use of primary prophylaxis for the most common opportunistic infections, led to an increase in life expectancy. However, as more and more patients started to survive for long periods despite severe immunodeficiency, CMV retinitis became increasingly frequent and increasingly resistant to therapy. The frequency of ocular manifestations of HIV infection has further changed since the beginning of the HAART era. Retinitis, especially that induced by CMV, is less frequent. Conversely, inflammatory reactions in the anterior chamber or vitreous are on the increase as a result of immune resconstitution.[8, 9] Patients with healed CMV retinitis can develop vitritis and cystoid macular

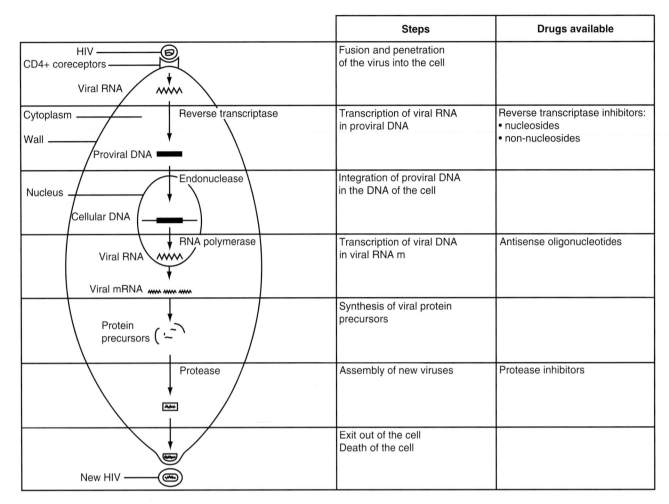

	Steps	Drugs available
	Fusion and penetration of the virus into the cell	
	Transcription of viral RNA in proviral DNA	Reverse transcriptase inhibitors: • nucleosides • non-nucleosides
	Integration of proviral DNA in the DNA of the cell	
	Transcription of viral DNA in viral RNA m	Antisense oligonucleotides
	Synthesis of viral protein precursors	
	Assembly of new viruses	Protease inhibitors
	Exit out of the cell Death of the cell	

FIGURE 47–1. Main steps of HIV infection of the cell.

edema, which alter their visual function despite the fact that the CMV infection itself is controlled. The management of such inflammation in patients recovering from immunodeficiency is a major clinical challenge.

TABLE 47–1. ANTIRETROVIRAL AGENTS CURRENTLY AVAILABLE FOR THE TREATMENT OF HIV INFECTION

Reverse transcriptase inhibitors
   Nucleosides
      Zidovudine (AZT)
      Didanosine (ddI)
      Zalcitabine (ddC)
      Lamivudine (3TC)
      Stavudine (d4T)
      Abacavir
   Non-nucleoside reverse transcriptase inhibitors
      Neviparine
      Delavirdine
      Efavirenz
Protease inhibitors
   Saquinavir
   Ritonavir
   Indinavir
   Nelfinavir
   Amprenavir
   Lopinavir

CHORIORETINAL INVOLVEMENT

As each cause of retinitis is discussed in detail in other sections, only the specificities of AIDS-associated retinitis will be dealt with here.

In HIV infection, ophthalmic involvement often is a sign of a disseminated opportunistic disease. Etiologic diagnosis is crucial, as it can identify a life-threatening infection and enable systemic therapy to be started. The management of these patients requires close collaboration with internists.

Ocular involvement usually requires special monitoring and therapy to preserve visual function. As ocular lesions can be directly observed by fundus examination and photography, they can be used as an indicator of the course of the infection. Indeed, they have been used as a major end point in therapeutic trials, especially those testing systemic anti-CMV drugs.

HIV and the Eye

HIV has been isolated from the cornea, vitreous, and retina. No clinical manifestations seem to be related to its presence in the cornea or vitreous. However, the presence of HIV in the endothelium of the retinal vasculature induces HIV retinopathy, which is the most common form of retinal involvement in HIV-infected patients.

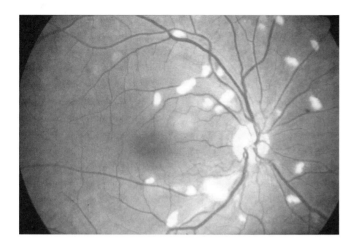

FIGURE 47–2. HIV microangiopathy. (See color insert.)

HIV retinopathy is mainly characterized by cotton-wool spots and scattered intraretinal hemorrhage (Fig. 47–2), both of which are asymptomatic unless they are located in the macular area. Cotton-wool spots have been reported to occur in up to two thirds of patients.[4, 6] They are not specific and are the same as those seen in diabetes mellitus: They consist of fluffy patches in the posterior pole, of different ages, often located along the vessels. Histopathologic examination discloses swollen nerve fibers, which result from disrupted axonal transport caused by ischemia. The etiology of this ischemia is probably multifactorial, including HIV infection of the endothelium of the retinal microvasculature, and deposition of circulating immune complexes. Intraretinal hemorrhages are superficial in the posterior pole and deep in the periphery. HIV retinopathy can occur at any stage of the disease, but its frequency increases with the degree of immunodeficiency.[6, 10, 11]

Isolated perivascular sheathing has been described in the absence of opportunistic retinal infections, mainly in African patients (especially children).[12, 13] The etiology of this perivasculitis is unclear.

Although rare, anterior or posterior uveitis can be related to HIV infection. Systemic antiretroviral drugs such as zidovudine have been reported to be effective on uveitis resistant to corticosteroids[14] and on uveitis associated with small multifocal retinal infiltrates located in the midperiphery or anterior retina.[15]

Opportunistic Chorioretinal Infections

CMV Retinitis

CMV retinitis is by far the most frequent retinal opportunistic infection in HIV-infected patients. It is the only opportunistic eye infection that is a diagnostic criterion for AIDS.[16] Its real frequency is difficult to determine because of recruitment biases in the different published series, but it has changed with the evolution of HIV disease. Early in the pandemic, only a few patients who reached the later stages of immunodeficiency developed CMV retinitis. Later, with increasing life expectancy, the frequency increased. Since the advent of HAART, the incidence of CMV retinitis has been cut by a factor of 6.[17]

CMV retinitis generally occurs when the CD4+ T-cell count falls below $50/\mu l$. The risk of CMV retinitis correlates well with the degree of immunodeficiency.[11, 18] CMV retinitis is more frequent in HIV-infected patients than in HIV-seronegative immunosuppressed patients, probably because the risk factors for HIV infection (sexual contacts and needle sharing) are also risk factors for CMV infection.

CMV retinitis is frequently asymptomatic in HIV-infected patients with severe immunodeficiency, as no cells are present in the anterior chamber or in the vitreous, and as the retinitis has a tendency to affect the periphery before targeting the macula and optic disc. Patients may complain, however, of flashes, floaters, or cloudy vision. Some may even notice loss of peripheral visual field or central vision. The diagnosis of CMV retinitis is based on clinical examination in patients with CD4+ T-cell counts below $50/\mu l$ and those with a suspected systemic opportunistic infection.

The typical course of CMV retinitis is relentless centrifugal extension from the initial lesion toward the entire retina.[19] Typically, the central area of the lesion is healed and atrophic; the borders are edematous, white, and hemorrhagic; and new small patches are scattered throughout the adjacent retina. These patches then coalesce, inducing the advancement of the borders. Without treatment, CMV retinitis destroys the entire retina of patients with severely immunodeficient AIDS.

There are two different clinical appearances of CMV retinitis: the fulminant form, with extensive necrosis and hemorrhage, often located on a vessel in the posterior pole (Fig. 47–3), and the indolent form, with granular borders and no hemorrhage, often located far from a vessel in the periphery (Fig. 47–4).

Several anti-CMV drugs can halt the progression of the retinitis but, being only virustatic, they do not clear CMV from the eye. Maintenance therapy is thus required to prevent relapses of CMV retinitis, for as long as the immunodeficiency persists. The drugs currently available are ganciclovir, foscarnet, cidofovir, and fomivirsen (Table 47–2).

Systemic administration is best, as CMV infection is a systemic disease. However, intravitreous therapy can be of

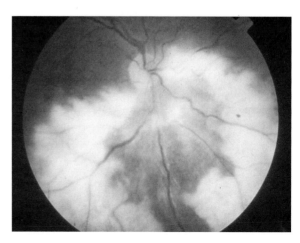

FIGURE 47–3. Fulminant CMV retinitis. (See color insert.)

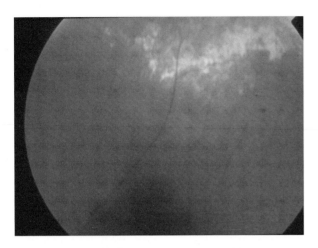

FIGURE 47–4. Indolent CMV retinitis.

value because the retina is the most frequent clinical target of CMV (80%). Local therapy can halt the progression of CMV retinitis, and it is less demanding for the patient relative to systemic therapy. During local therapy alone, contralateral or extraocular CMV infection occurs in 50% and 31% of patients, respectively, at 6 months.[20] Combination with oral ganciclovir may be recommended to prevent further dissemination of CMV during local therapy.[21]

Ganciclovir and foscarnet were the first anti-CMV drugs. After the induction phase (two infusions a day), both drugs induce healing of the lesions within 2 to 4

TABLE 47–2. ANTI-CMV DRUGS CURRENTLY AVAILABLE FOR THE TREATMENT OF CMV RETINITIS

Systemic therapy	
Intravenous ganciclovir	
Induction	5 mg/kg bid.
Maintenance	5 mg/kg once a day
Intravenous foscarnet	
Induction	90 mg/kg bid.
Maintenance	90 mg/kg once a day
Intravenous cidofovir	
Induction	5 mg/kg once a week for 2 weeks
Maintenance	5 mg/kg every 2 weeks
Oral ganciclovir	1 g tid as maintenance therapy only
Intravitreal therapy	
Ganciclovir	2000 μg per injection
Induction	2 injections per week
Maintenance	1 injection per week
Foscarnet	2400 μg per injection
Induction	2 injections per week
Maintenance	1 injection per week
Cidofovir	1 injection of 15 μg every 6 weeks
Fomivirsen	
Naïve patients	165 μg per injection
Induction	3 injections in 3 weeks
Maintenance	1 injection every 2 weeks
Non-naïve patients	330 μg per injection
Induction	2 injections in 4 weeks
Maintenance	1 injection every 4 weeks
Ganciclovir intravitreal device	
Surgical implantation	
Change if relapse (~ 8 months in immunodepressed patients)	

CMV, cytomegalovirus.

weeks. Without maintenance therapy, relapses occurred within 3 weeks.[22] With maintenance therapy (one infusion a day), relapses occur within a mean of 2 months.[23–26] A prospective comparative study of intravenous ganciclovir and foscarnet showed similar times to relapse, 59 and 56 days respectively.[27] However, the patients on foscarnet had a longer survival time, probably in part because of an anti-HIV effect of foscarnet. However, in practice, ganciclovir is the first-line choice because of its better tolerability and simpler administration. Combinations of ganciclovir and foscarnet have been used to overcome resistance to each drug (given at the full dosage to obtain a synergistic effect) or to avoid severe side effects (half-doses of each drug).

Oral ganciclovir is effective as maintenance therapy.[28, 29] The time to relapse is a little shorter than with intravenous ganciclovir, but most patients prefer the oral route despite the large number of tablets to be taken daily.

Intravenous cidofovir has the advantage of being given only once a week during induction therapy, and once every second week during maintenance therapy. On this regimen, the mean time to relapse is 123 days.[30] The main side effects of cidofovir are renal impairment and anterior uveitis.

Initial studies employing a human monoclonal anti-CMV antibody (MSL-109) in patients being treated with standard antiviral regimens demonstrated a delay in progression of CMV retinitis.[31]

Since the advent of HAART, maintenance therapy is discontinued in patients who have a restored immunity.[32–36]

Systemic primary prophylaxis of CMV retinitis with oral ganciclovir halves the relapse rate.[37] The dosages are 1000 mg tid for patients with CD4 + T-cell counts below 50/μl, or up to 100/μl in those with a history of AIDS-defining opportunistic infection.

Valganciclovir, a ganciclovir prodrug, is being assessed in oral induction therapy of CMV retinitis.

Local therapy was initially developed because of the side effects of systemic administration. Ganciclovir has been widely used and has proved to be effective and safe.[38–41] Initially administered at a dose of 200 μg in 0.05 ml per injection, it is now injected into the vitreous at a dose of 2000 μg.[42] Intravitreal foscarnet at a dose of 2.4 mg per injection has shown some efficacy[43] but is probably less potent than intravitreous ganciclovir. Intravitreous injections are still indicated for patients with active CMV retinitis who are starting HAART regimens.

An intraocular ganciclovir implant is the most effective therapy against CMV retinitis, with a time to relapse of 223 days.[20] However, implantation requires surgery, which can precipitate retinal detachment. In case of relapse, the device must be replaced. Intravitreal devices are now mainly used for CMV retinitis resistant to other therapies or in a case of noncompliance with daily treatment.[44–46]

Intravitreal cidofovir was initially promising, with a mean time to relapse of 53 days after a single injection of 20 μg,[47] but its low therapeutic index has restricted its development.[48]

Intravitreal fomivirsen, an antisense drug, is effective on CMV retinitis,[49] but its side effects may restrict its use to last-resort therapy.

The choice of therapy depends on systemic manifestations and individual tolerability. One therapy can be switched to another at any time if necessary. Note that the fall in the incidence of CMV retinitis has slowed down the clinical evaluation of new drugs.

Retinal detachment is a serious complication of CMV retinitis. It occurs in patients with active or healed retinitis, and the risk increases with the area of necrotic retinitis and its extension toward the periphery. Retinal detachment usually necessitates vitrectomy with silicone oil.[50–52] Before the HAART era, the silicone oil was left in the eye; but with the increasing life expectancy of HIV-infected patients the silicone oil should be replaced by gas tamponade after extensive laser barrier therapy.[52] In "macula-on," small, localized retinal detachment, laser photocoagulation delimitation may be successful for a while, but most cases of retinal detachment will break through the laser barrier within weeks to months.[52]

Since the advent of HAART, inflammation of the vitreous has become frequent, affecting up to 60%[53, 54] of eyes in which CMV retinitis remains healed. The vitritis often predominates in the anterior vitreous, with gray flakes responsible for floaters.[55] Anterior inflammation with gray keratic precipitates can occur.[56] Chronic cystoid macular edema can eventually lead to visual deterioration.[57–59] The treatment of these new complications is not clearly defined. Topical anti-inflammatory therapy and oral acetazolamide are ineffective. Systemic steroids have some effect, but they have the disadvantage of increasing the immunodeficiency, with a risk of CMV retinitis recurrence. Tapering is often associated with a relapse of the inflammatory manifestations. Systemic steroids can also increase metabolic disorders such as diabetes mellitus and lipid disturbances, especially in patients on HAART. In patients with unilateral uveitis, injections under Tenon's capsule, are of value despite the risks of elevated intraocular pressure and substantial systemic diffusion leading to systemic side effects.

Ocular Toxoplasmosis

In the United States, ocular toxoplasmosis is estimated to occur in 1% to 2% of patients,[6] and it is more frequent in Europe and the developing countries where the baseline seroprevalence is higher. Ocular toxoplasmosis generally occurs in patients with CD4+ T-cell counts below 150/µl. It can be either acquired or the result of reactivation of a latent infection.[60, 61] In AIDS patients, it can be associated with cerebral toxoplasmosis in up to 40% of patients. It manifests as classical unifocal or multifocal retinitis (Fig. 47–5), or as diffuse necrotizing retinitis in patients with severe immunodeficiency.[62]

An assay for parasitemia can be positive. In contrast to the situation in CMV retinitis, concomitant inflammation of the anterior chamber with posterior synechiae and vitritis are not unusual. Antitoxoplasmic immunoglobulin assay in anterior chamber samples is not of value in AIDS patients because of the major disturbances of immunoglobulin synthesis associated with the disease. Polymerase chain reaction may assist with the diagnosis.

The therapy of ocular toxoplasmosis in HIV-infected patients consists of pyrimethamine plus sulfadiazine or clindamycin. During the induction phase the toxoplasmic

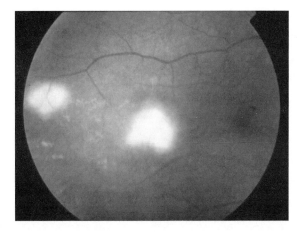

FIGURE 47–5. Ocular toxoplasmosis.

lesions heal within 7 weeks. On maintenance therapy (at half the induction dose), relapses are less frequent than in CMV retinitis, at around 20% after 2 years.[61] The incidence of ocular toxoplasmosis fell drastically after the introduction of primary prophylaxis with oral trimethoprim-sulfamethoxazole, with a further decrease after the advent of HAART.

VZV Retinitis

VZV retinitis is rare, occurring in less than 1% of AIDS patients,[6] but it is a severe retinal infection with a poor prognosis. The most devastating form, called progressive outer retinal necrosis (PORN), is usually reported in patients with profound immunodeficiency (CD4+ T-cell count below 50/µl). PORN is characterized by multifocal deep retinal lesions scattered throughout the fundus. In approximately one third of patients, these outer retinal lesions present in the macular area, with rapid progression to confluence, sometimes giving the appearance of a cherry-red spot (Fig. 47–6). The areas of necrosis are white, and the vessels appear orange by contrast, giving a characteristic "cracked mud" appearance (Fig. 47–7). The advancing borders are preceded by multiple small lesions in the adjacent retina. No inflammation of the anterior chamber or vitreous is noted.

The other form is seen in patients with CD4+ T-cell

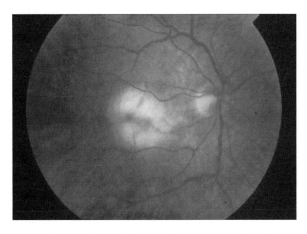

FIGURE 47–6. VZV retinitis: cherry-red spot macula. (See color insert.)

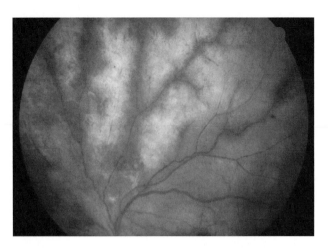

FIGURE 47–7. VZV retinitis: cracked mud appearance. (See color insert.)

counts above 50/μl. It resembles the acute retinal necrosis syndrome described in immunocompetent patients. The necrosis starts from the periphery and extends rapidly toward the posterior pole.[63–65] Inflammation of the anterior chamber is noted, along with vitritis. These two forms are probably two aspects of the same disease occurring at different stages of immunodeficiency. In both varieties, the uniformly poor prognosis is related to the rapidity of lesion extension despite therapy, and the frequency (70%) of retinal detachment, optic nerve involvement, and bilateralization of the retinitis, with 67% of patients in the largest published series to date having a final visual acuity of no light perception.[66] Although some cases of VZV retinitis have responded favorably to acyclovir, the current approach in AIDS patients is to treat very aggressively with intravenous foscarnet combined with intravitreous ganciclovir to obtain kinetic and antiviral synergy.[65]

Pneumocystosis

In contrast with *Pneumocystis carinii* pneumonia, which occurs in patients with CD4+ T-cell counts of 200/μl, *P. carinii* choroidopathy is seen in patients with CD4+ T-cell counts below 50/μl (see Chap. 37). It is a sign of disseminated *P. carinii* infection. It manifests as asymptomatic, plaquelike, yellow-white, round or multilobular foci of the posterior pole (Fig. 47–8), which enhance slowly.[67, 68] No inflammation of the vitreous or anterior chamber is noted. *P. carinii* choroidopathy recedes slowly on systemic trimethoprim-sulfamethoxazole or pentamidine. *P. carinii* choroidopathy has been reported in patients receiving aerosolized pentamidine as primary or secondary prevention of *P. carinii* pneumonia, a form of prophylaxis localized to the lungs, thereby allowing the development of extrapulmonary infection.[69] There have been few recent reports of this entity with the institution of more widespread systemic prophylaxis for *P. carinii*.

Tuberculosis

The choroidal lesions found in disseminated tuberculosis are asymptomatic. They do not induce reactions in the anterior chamber or vitreous. They reflect disseminated tuberculosis and occur in patients with severe immunodeficiency.[70–72] They manifest as either one or a few conspicuous orange lesions with enough relief to raise the vessels (Fig. 47–9), or as miliary lesions scattered through the fundus. Appropriate therapy leads to slow healing.

Cryptococcosis

The most common ocular manifestation of cryptococcosis is papilledema (Fig. 47–10) with peripapillary hemorrhages related to cryptococcal meningitis.[73, 74] Some cases of cryptococcal involvement of the choroid have been described in patients with disseminated cryptococcosis. The ocular manifestations of cryptococcosis respond to appropriate systemic therapy with intravenous amphotericin B or an imidazole. However, optic nerve involvement can sometimes lead to optic atrophy, even if the meningitis is well controlled by anticryptococcal therapy.

Other Opportunistic Infections

Histoplasma capsulatum retinitis has been described in highly immunodepressed patients with systemic disseminated infection.[75] *Mycobacterium avium-intracellulare* has been found in autopsy studies of patients with disseminated infection, in association with *P. carinii* infection.[76, 77] A case of *Sporothrix schenckii* endophthalmitis has been reported in an HIV-positive individual with disseminated cutaneous sporotrichosis.[78]

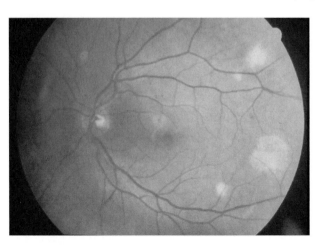

FIGURE 47–8. Pneumocystosis. (See color insert.)

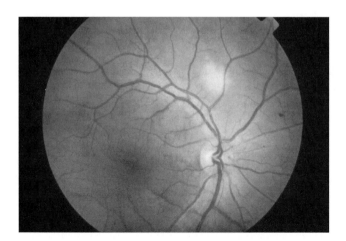

FIGURE 47–9. Ocular tuberculosis. (See color insert.)

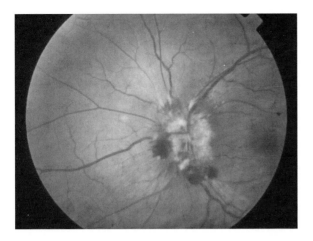

FIGURE 47–10. Papilledema in cryptococcal meningitis.

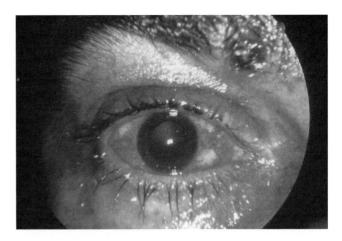

FIGURE 47–11. Herpes zoster ophthalmicus.

Other Chorioretinal Infections

Syphilis

Syphilis occurs at any degree of immunodeficiency but often when CD4+ T-cell counts are above 200/μl. This is not an opportunistic infection but is often seen in AIDS patients with multiple sexual partners. The course of syphilis in HIV-infected patients is accelerated, and neurosyphilis is more severe than in HIV-seronegative patients. Ocular syphilis manifests as retinitis with vasculitis, involvement of the optic nerve, vitritis, and inflammation of the anterior chamber, with sometimes a hypopyon.[79–82] The diagnosis is based on positive Venereal Disease Research Laboratory (VDRL), *Treponema pallidum* hemagglutination assay (TPHA), and fluorescent treponemal antibody (FTA)-absorbed tests. Therapy consists of intravenous penicillin for 15 days.

Candidiasis

Although oroesophageal candidiasis is frequent in AIDS, ocular candidiasis is rare and is not considered an opportunistic infection. It mainly occurs in intravenous drug users after use of contaminated injection equipment. CD4+ T-cell counts are variable and may often be quite high, as the patients are still active intravenous drug users. The clinical manifestations and management of such patients is the same as that of HIV-seronegative patients.

Lymphoma

Retinal lymphoma is a very rare complication of AIDS and is often misdiagnosed. It manifests as retinitis and vitritis resistant to various antibiotics. The diagnosis is based on ocular ultrasonography, oculo-orbital and cerebral magnetic resonance imaging, the presence of malignant cells, and elevated interleukin-10 levels in cerebrospinal fluid or the vitreous, and possibly on retinal biopsy.[83, 84] The prognosis is poor despite radiotherapy and chemotherapy, because of the frequent cerebral involvement.

HERPES ZOSTER OPHTHALMICUS

Herpes zoster ophthalmicus is frequent in HIV-infected patients. It occurs at an early stage of the disease, when CD4+ T-cell counts are above 200/μl. In HIV-infected patients, herpes zoster ophthalmicus is extensive (Fig. 47–11) and relapsing, and it requires intravenous acyclovir therapy. Although keratitis is the most common form of ocular involvement, anterior uveitis is frequent[85, 86] and must be aggressively treated with topical steroids and cycloplegic and monitored for the development of secondary complications. HIV-infected patients with a history of herpes zoster may be at risk of VZV retinitis.

DRUG-RELATED UVEITIS

In the context of HIV infection, rifabutin was the first medication reported to induce drug-related uveitis.[87, 88] Rifabutin is given as curative or preventive treatment for disseminated *M. avium-intracellulare*–complex infection, usually for patients with severe immunodeficiency. Rifabutin-related uveitis is total, including severe inflammation of the vitreous and anterior chamber, and occasionally a hypopyon.[89, 90] No retinal lesions are noted. In severe cases, it can manifest as endophthalmitis (Fig. 47–12). With topical steroid therapy and discontinuation of rifabutin, the uveitis disappears within a few days. The pathogenesis of rifabutin-related uveitis is unclear, but a local immunoallergic reaction to rifabutin, and *M. avium-intracellulare* antigen-antibody conflicts have been postu-

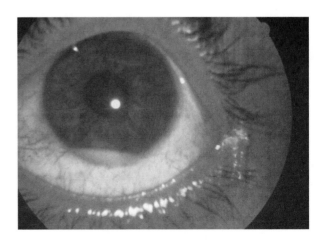

FIGURE 47–12. Rifabutin-related uveitis.

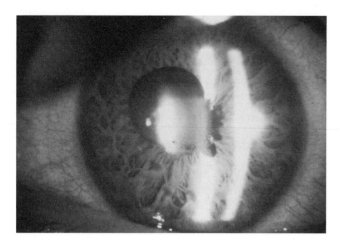

FIGURE 47–13. Cidofovir-related uveitis.

lated. The occurrence of rifabutin-related uveitis is promoted by concomitant use of fluconazole or clarithromycin, which both increase the serum concentration of rifabutin by inhibiting the cytochrome P450 system.

Cidofovir, an anti-CMV nucleoside analogue, can induce anterior uveitis, whether administered intravitreally or intravenously. The frequencies have been reported to be 26% to 32% after intravitreal administration[91, 92] and 26% to 44% after intravenous administration.[93] The uveitis is accompanied by low intraocular pressure, and sometimes by posterior synechiae (Fig. 47–13) or vitritis. These manifestations may be related to a direct toxic effect of cidofovir on the ciliary body.[93] Uveitis generally responds favorably to local steroid therapy but can relapse if cidofovir is continued.

Studies of large series are needed to determine the respective roles of PIs, microbial pathogens, immunity and coadministered drugs in the onset of drug-induced uveitis in HIV-infected patients.

SUMMARY

The profile of HIV disease has recently changed with the advent of HAART, which induces a significant restoration of the immunity. Opportunistic infections such as CMV retinitis are less frequent. Ocular inflammatory reactions can develop, especially in CMV-infected eyes. The future of HIV infection depends on the importance of resistance to HAART, and to the availability of new effective anti-HIV compounds.

References

1. Palella FJ, Delaney KM, Moorman AC, et al: Declining morbidity and mortality among patients with advanced human immunodeficiency virus infection. N Engl J Med 1998;338:853–860.
2. Autran B, Carcelain G, Li TS, et al: Positive effects of combined antiretroviral therapy on CD4 T-cell homeostasis and function in advanced HIV disease. Science 1997;277:112–116.
3. World Health Organization: AIDS—Global data: The current global situation of the HIV/AIDS pandemic. Wkly Epidemiol Rec 1993;68:9–11.
4. Holland GN, Pepose JS, Pettit TH, et al: Acquired immune deficiency syndrome: Ocular manifestations. Ophthalmology 1983;90:859–873.
5. Jabs DA, Green WR, Fox R, et al: Ocular manifestations of acquired immune deficiency syndrome. Ophthalmology 1989;96:1092–1099.
6. Jabs DA: Ocular manifestations of HIV infection. Trans Am Ophthalmol Soc 1995;93:623–683.
7. Jabs DA, Bartlett JG: AIDS in ophthalmology: A period of transition. Am J Ophthalmol 1997;124:227–233.
8. Nussenblatt RB, Lane HC: Human immunodeficiency virus disease: Changing patterns of intraocular inflammation. Am J Ophthalmol 1998;125:374–382.
9. Holland GN: Pieces of a puzzle: Toward a better understanding of intraocular inflammation associated with human immunodeficiency virus disease. Am J Ophthalmol 1998;125:383–385.
10. Freeman WR, Chen A, Henderly DE, et al: Prevalence and significance of acquired immunodeficiency syndrome-related retinal microvasculopathy. Am J Ophthalmol 1989;107:229–235.
11. Kuppermann BD, Petty JG, Richman DD, et al: Correlation between CD4+ counts and prevalence of cytomegalovirus retinitis and human immunodeficiency virus-related noninfectious retinal vasculopathy in patients with acquired immunodeficiency syndrome. Am J Ophthalmol 1993;115:575–582.
12. Kestelyn P, Van de Perre P, Rouvroy D, et al: A prospective study of the ophthalmologic findings in the acquired immune deficiency syndrome in Africa. Am J Ophthalmol 1985;100:230–238.
13. Kestelyn P, Lepage P, Perre PVD: Perivasculitis of the retinal vessels as an important sign in children with AIDS-related complex. Am J Ophthalmol 1985;100:614–615.
14. Rosberger DF, Heinemann MH, Friedberg DN, et al: Uveitis associated with human immunodeficiency virus infection. Am J Ophthalmol 1998;125:301–305.
15. Levinson RD, Vann R, Davis JL, et al: Chronic multifocal retinal infiltrates in patients infected with human immunodeficiency virus. Am J Ophthalmol 1998;125:312–324.
16. Centers for Disease Control: 1993 revised classification system for HIV infection and expanded surveillance case definition for AIDS among adolescents and adults. MMWR Morb Mortal Wkly Rep 1992;41:1–19.
17. Doan S, Cochereau I, Guvenisik N, et al: Cytomegalovirus retinitis in HIV-infected patients with and without highly active antiretroviral therapy. Am J Ophthalmol 1999;128:250–251.
18. Pertel P, Hirschtick R, Phair J, et al: Risk of developing cytomegalovirus retinitis in persons infected with the human immunodeficiency virus. J Acquir Immune Defic Syndr 1992;5:1069–1074.
19. Holland GN, Shuler JD: Progression rates of cytomegalovirus retinopathy in ganciclovir-treated and untreated patients. Arch Ophthalmol 1992;110:1435–1442.
20. Martin DF, Parks DJ, Mellow JD, et al: Treatment of cytomegalovirus retinitis with an intraocular sustained-release ganciclovir implant. Arch Ophthalmol 1994;112:1531–1539.
21. Martin DF, Kuppermenn BD, Wolitz RA, et al: Oral ganciclovir with cytomegalovirus retinitis treated with a ganciclovir implant. Roche Ganciclovir Study Group. N Engl J Med 1999;340:1063–1070.
22. Palestine AG, Polis MA, De Smet MD, et al: A randomized, controlled trial of foscarnet in the treatment of cytomegalovirus retinitis in patients with AIDS. Ann Intern Med 1991;115:665–673.
23. Holland GN, Sidikaro Y, Kreiger AE, et al: Treatment of cytomegalovirus retinopathy with ganciclovir. Ophthalmology 1987;94:815–823.
24. Jabs DA, Newman C, de Bustros S, et al: Treatment of cytomegalovirus retinitis with ganciclovir. Ophthalmology 1987;94:824–830.
25. Jacobson MA, O'Donnell JJ, Brodie HR, et al: Randomized prospective trial of CMV maintenance therapy for cytomegalovirus retinitis. J Med Virol 1988;25:339–349.
26. Jacobson MA, O'Donnell JJ, Mills J: Foscarnet treatment of cytomegalovirus retinitis in patients with the acquired immunodeficiency syndrome. Antimicrob Agents Chemother 1989;33:736–741.
27. Studies of Ocular Complications of AIDS Research Group: Mortality in patients with the acquired immunodeficiency syndrome treated with either foscarnet or ganciclovir for cytomegalovirus retinitis. N Engl J Med 1992;326:213–220.
28. The Oral Ganciclovir European and Australian Cooperative Study Group: Intravenous versus oral ganciclovir: European/Australian comparative study of efficacy and safety in the prevention of cytomegalovirus retinitis recurrence in patients with AIDS. AIDS 1995;9:471–477.
29. Squires KE: Oral ganciclovir for cytomegalovirus retinitis in patients with AIDS: Results of two randomized studies. AIDS 1996;10(Suppl 4):S13–S18.
30. Poplin M, Pollard R, Tierney M, et al: Combination therapy of cytomegalovirus (CMV) retinitis with a human monoclonal anti-CMV antibody (SDZ MSL-109) and either ganciclovir (DHPG) or

foscarnet (PFA). Ninth International Conference on AIDS. Berlin, 1993, p 54, Abstract No WS-B11-2.

31. Lalezari JP, Stagg RJ, Kuppermann BD, et al: Intravenous cidofovir for peripheral cytomegalovirus retinitis in patients with AIDS. Ann Intern Med 1997;126:264–274.

32. Brian Reed J, Schwab IR, Gordon J, et al: Regression of cytomegalovirus retinitis associated with protease-inhibitor treatment in patients with AIDS. Am J Ophthalmol 1997;124:199–205.

33. Van den Horn GJ, Meenken C, et al: Effects of protease inhibitors on the course of CMV retinitis in relation to CD4+ lymphocyte responses in HIV+ patients. Br J Ophthalmol 1998;82:988–990.

34. Jabs DA, Bolton SG, Dunn JP, et al: Discontinuing anticytomegalovirus therapy in patients with immune reconstitution after combination antiretroviral therapy. Am J Ophthalmol 1998;126:817–822.

35. Vrabec TR, Baldassano VF, Whitcup SM: Discontinuation of maintenance therapy in patients with quiescent cytomegalovirus retinitis and elevated CD4+ counts. Ophthalmology 1998;105:1259–1264.

36. Tural C, Romeu J, Sirera G, et al: Long-lasting remission of cytomegalovirus retinitis without maintenance therapy in human immunodeficiency virus-infected patients. J Infect Dis 1998;177:1080–1083.

37. Spector SA, McKinley G, Lalezari JP, et al: Oral ganciclovir for the prevention of cytomegalovirus disease in persons with AIDS. Roche Cooperative Oral Ganciclovir Study Group. N Engl J Med 1996;334:1491–1497.

38. Cantrill HL, Henry K, Melroe NH, et al: Treatment of cytomegalovirus retinitis with intravitreal ganciclovir. Long term results. Ophthalmology 1989;96:367–374.

39. Heinemann MH. Long-term intravitreal ganciclovir therapy for cytomegalovirus retinopathy. Arch Ophthalmol 1989;107:1767–1772.

40. Cochereau-Massin I, LeHoang P, Lautier-Frau M, et al: Efficacy and tolerance of intravitreal ganciclovir in cytomegalovirus retinitis in acquired immune deficiency syndrome. Ophthalmology 1991; 98:1348–1355.

41. Hodge WC, Lalonde RG, Sampalis J, et al: Once-weekly intraocular injections of ganciclovir for maintenance therapy of cytomegalovirus retinitis: Clinical and ocular outcome. J Infect Dis 1996;174:393–396.

42. Young S, Morlet N, Besen G, et al: High-dose (2000 µg) intravitreous ganciclovir in the treatment of cytomegalovirus retinitis. Ophthalmology 1998;105:1404–1410.

43. Diaz-Llopis M, Espana E, Munoz G, et al: High dose intravitreal foscarnet in the treatment of cytomegalovirus retinitis in AIDS. Br J Ophthalmol 1994;78:120–124.

44. Hatton MP, Duker JS, Reichel E, et al: Treatment of relapsed cytomegalovirus retinitis with the sustained-release ganciclovir implant. Retina 1998;18:50–55.

45. Kamal A: Sustained release intravitreal ganciclovir implant as salvage treatment in AIDS related cytomegalovirus retinitis. Br J Ophthalmol 1998;82:333.

46. Martin DF, Dunn JP, Davis JL, et al: Use of ganciclovir implant for the treatment of cytomegalovirus retinitis in the era of potent antiretroviral therapy: Recommendations of the International AIDS Society—USA panel. Am J Ophthalmol 1999;127:329–339.

47. Kirsch LS, Arevalo F, Chavez de la Paz E, et al: Intravitreal cidofovir (HPMPC) treatment of cytomegalovirus retinitis in patients with acquired immune deficiency syndrome. Ophthalmology 1995; 102:533–543.

48. Taskintuna I, Rahhal FM, Arevalo JF, et al: Low-dose intravitreal cidofovir (HPMPC) therapy of cytomegalovirus retinitis in patients with acquired immune deficiency syndrome. Ophthalmology 1997;104:1049–1057.

49. Perry CM, Balfour JA: Fomivirsen. Drugs 1999;57:375–380.

50. Freeman WR, Quiceno JI, Crapotta JA, et al: Surgical repair of rhegmatogenous retinal detachment in immunosuppressed patients with cytomegalovirus retinitis. Ophthalmology 1992;9:466–474.

51. Garcia RF, Flores-Aguilar M, Quiceno JI, et al: Results of rhegmatogenous retinal detachment repair in cytomegalovirus retinitis with and without scleral buckling. Ophthalmology 1995;102:236–245.

52. Davis JL, Serfass MS, Mei-Ying L, et al: Silicone oil in repair of retinal detachments caused by necrotizing retinitis in HIV infection. Arch Ophthalmol 1995;113:1401–1409.

53. Karavellas MP, Lowder CY, Macdonald JC, et al: Immune recovery vitritis associated with inactive cytomegalovirus retinitis: A new syndrome. Arch Ophthalmol 1998;116:169–175.

54. Karavellas MP, Plummer DJ, Macdonald JC, et al: Incidence of immune recovery vitritis in cytomegalovirus retinitis patients following institution of successful highly antiretroviral therapy. J Infect Dis 1999;179:697–700.

55. Zegans ME, Walton RC, Holland GN, et al: Transient vitreous inflammatory reactions associated with combination antiretroviral therapy in patients with AIDS and cytomegalovirus retinitis. Am J Ophthalmol 1998;125:292–300.

56. Walter KA, Coulter VL, Palay DA, et al: Corneal endothelial deposits in patients with cytomegalovirus retinitis. Am J Ophthalmol 1996;121:391–396.

57. Newsome R, Casswell T, O'Moore E, et al: Cystoid macular edema in patients with AIDS and cytomegalovirus retinitis on highly antiretroviral therapy. Br J Ophthalmol 1998;82:456–457.

58. Silverstein BE, Smith JH, Sykes SO, et al: Cystoid macular edema associated with cytomegalovirus retinitis in patients with the acquired immunodeficiency syndrome. Am J Ophthalmol 1998; 125:411–415.

59. Cassoux N, Lumbroso L, Bodaghi B, et al: Cystoid macular edema and cytomegalovirus retinitis in patients with HIV disease treated with highly active antiretroviral therapy. Br J Ophthalmol 1999;83:47–49.

60. Holland GN, Engstrom RE, Glasgow BJ, et al: Ocular toxoplasmosis in patients with the acquired immunodeficiency syndrome. Am J Ophthalmol 1988;106:653–667.

61. Cochereau-Massin I, LeHoang P, Lautier-Frau M, et al: Ocular toxoplasmosis in human immunodeficiency virus-infected patients. Am J Ophthalmol 1992;114:130–135.

62. Parke DW, Font RL: Diffuse toxoplasmic retinochoroiditis in a patient with AIDS. Arch Ophthalmol 1986;104:571–575.

63. Forster DJ, Dugel PU, Frangieh GT, et al: Rapidly progressive outer retinal necrosis in the acquired immunodeficiency syndrome. Am J Ophthalmol 1990;110:341–348.

64. Margolis TP, Lowder CY, Holland GN, et al: Varicella-zoster virus retinitis in patients with the acquired immunodeficiency syndrome. Am J Ophthalmol 1991;112:119–131.

65. Kuppermann BD, Quiceno JI, Wiley C, et al: Clinical and histopathological study of varicella zona virus retinitis in patients with the acquired immunodeficiency syndrome. Am J Ophthalmol 1994;118:589–600.

66. Engstrom RE, Holland GN, Margolis TP, et al: The progressive outer retinal necrosis syndrome. Ophthalmology 1995;101:1488–1502.

67. Rao AN, Zimmerman PL, Boyer D, et al: A clinical, histopathologic, and electron microscopic study of *Pneumocystis carinii* choroiditis. Am J Ophthalmol 1989;107:218–228.

68. Shami MJ, Freeman W, Friedberg D, et al: A multicenter study of *Pneumocystis* choroidopathy. Am J Ophthalmol 1991;112:15–22.

69. Dugel PU, Rao NA, Forster DJ, et al.: *Pneumocystis carinii* choroiditis after long-term aerosolized pentamidine therapy. Am J Ophthalmol 1990;110:113–117.

70. Muccioli C, Belfort R: Presumed ocular and central nervous system tuberculosis in a patient with the acquired immunodeficiency syndrome. Am J Ophthalmol 1996;212:217–219.

71. Recillas-Gispert C, Ortega-Larrocea G, Arellanes-Garcia L, et al: Chorioretinitis secondary to *Mycobacterium tuberculosis* in acquired immune deficiency syndrome. Retina 1997;17:437–439.

72. Campinchi-Tardy F, Darwiche A, Bergmann JF, et al: Tubercules de Bouchut et SIDA. A propos de 3 cas. J Fr Ophtalmol 1994;17:548–554.

73. Kestelyn P, Taelman H, Bogaerts J, et al: Ophthalmic manifestations of infections with *Cryptococcus neoformans* in patients with the acquired immunodeficiency syndrome. Am J Ophthalmol 1993; 116:721–727.

74. Cohen DB, Glasgow BJ: Bilateral optic nerve cryptococcosis in sudden blindness in patients with acquired immune deficiency syndrome. Ophthalmology 1993;100:1689–1694.

75. Specht CS, Mitchell KT, Bauman AE, et al: Ocular histoplasmosis with retinitis in a patient with acquired immune deficiency syndrome. Ophthalmology 1991;98:1356–1359.

76. Whitcup SM, Fenton RM, Pluda JM, et al: *Pneumocystis carinii* and *Mycobacterium avium-intracellulare* infection of the choroid. Retina 1992;12:331–335.

77. Morinelli EN, Dugel PU, Riffenburgh R, et al: Infectious multifocal choroiditis in patients with acquired immune deficiency syndrome. Ophthalmology 1993;100:1014–1021.

78. Kurosawa A, Pollock S, Collins M, et al: *Sporothrix schenckii* endophthalmitis in a patient with human immunodeficiency virus infection. Arch Ophthalmol 1988;106:376–380.

79. Bouisse V, Cochereau-Massin I, Jobin D, et al: Syphilitic uveitis and human immunodeficiency virus infection. J Fr Ophtalmol 1991;14:605–609.

80. McLeish WM, Pulido JS, Holland S, et al: The ocular manifestations of syphilis in the human immunodeficiency virus type 1-infected host. Ophthalmology 1990;97:196–203.

81. Shalaby IA, Dunn JP, Semba RD, et al: Syphilitic uveitis in human immunodeficiency virus-infected patients. Arch Ophthalmol 1997;115:469–473.

82. Kuo IC, Kapusta MA, Rao NA: Vitritis as the primary manifestation of ocular syphilis in patients with HIV infection. Am J Ophthalmol 1998;125:306–311.

83. Stanton CA, Sloan DB, Slusher MM, et al: Acquired immunodeficiency syndrome-related primary intraocular lymphoma. Arch Ophthalmol 1992;110:1614–1617.

84. Rivero ME, Kuppermann BD, Wiley CA, et al: Acquired immunodeficiency syndrome-related intraocular B-cell lymphoma. Arch Ophthalmol 1999;117:616–622.

85. Sandor EV, Millman A, Croxson TS, et al: *Herpes zoster* ophthalmicus in patients at risk for the acquired immune deficiency syndrome (AIDS). Am J Ophthalmol 1986;101:153–155.

86. Margolis TP, Milner MK, Shama A, et al: Herpes zoster ophthalmicus in patients with human immunodeficiency virus infection. Am J Ophthalmol 1998;125:285–291.

87. Shafran SD, Singer J, Zarowny DP, et al: A comparison of two regimens for the treatment of *Mycobacterium avium* complex bacteriema in AIDS: Rifabutin, ethambutol, and clarithromycin versus rifampin, ethambutol, clofazimine, and ciprofloxacin: Canadian HIV Trials Network Protocol 010 Study Group. N Engl J Med 1996;335:377–383.

88. Shafran SD, Singer J, Zarowny DP, et al: Determinants of rifabutin-associated uveitis in patients treated with rifabutin, clarithromycin, and ethambutol for *Mycobacterium avium* complex bacteriema: A multivariate analysis. Canadian HIV Trials Network Protocol 010 Study Group. J Infect Dis 1998;177:252–255.

89. Saran BR, Maguire AM, Nichols C, et al: Hypopyon uveitis in patients with acquired immunodeficiency syndrome treated for systemic *Mycobacterium avium* complex infection with rifabutin. Arch Ophthalmol 1994;112:1159–1165.

90. Jacobs DS, Piliero PJ, Kuperwaser MG, et al: Acute uveitis associated with rifabutin use in patients with human immunodeficiency virus infection. Am J Ophthalmol 1994;118:716–722.

91. Chavez de la Paz E, Arevalo JF, Kirsch LS, et al: Anterior nongranulomatous uveitis after intravitreal HPMPC (cidofovir) for the treatment of cytomegalovirus retinitis. Analysis and prevention. Ophthalmology 1997;104:539–544.

92. Akler ME, Johnson DW, Burman WJ, et al: Anterior uveitis and hypotony after intravenous cidofovir for the treatment of cytomegalovirus retinitis. Ophthalmology 1998;105:651–657.

93. Davis JL, Taskintuna I, Freeman WR, et al: Iritis and hypotony after treatment with intravenous cidofovir for cytomegalovirus retinitis. Arch Ophthalmol 1997;115:733–737.

48 ┤ MASQUERADE SYNDROMES: MALIGNANCIES

Nadia Khalida Waheed and C. Stephen Foster

INTRAOCULAR–CENTRAL NERVOUS SYSTEM LYMPHOMA

Definition

Intraocular–central nervous system (CNS) lymphoma is a rare and lethal malignancy, most commonly a diffuse, large cell lymphoma of B cells, although, rarely, it may also be of T-cell origin.[1] Several types of lymphomas can involve the eyes. These include systemic non-Hodgkin's lymphoma or systemic Hodgkin's disease, both of which can metastasize to the eye. However, intraocular Hodgkin's disease is exceptionally rare, with only a handful of reported cases, and histologic documentation in less than five eyes.[2–6] The most important of the lymphomas is non-Hodgkin's lymphoma of the eye and the CNS (or intraocular-CNS) lymphoma, also called primary CNS lymphoma, with more than 150 cases reported.

History

Intraocular-CNS lymphoma, previously termed reticulum cell sarcoma or microgliomatosis, was first described by Givner in 1955.[7] In the earlier series, definitive diagnosis of intraocular-CNS lymphoma was based on histopathologic examination of enucleated eyes, or brain biopsy and studies at autopsy.[8] In 1975, Klingele and Hogan published the first report of the use of a vitreous biopsy specimen for the diagnosis of intraocular-CNS lymphoma.[9] This has since become a widely performed procedure for the diagnosis of this condition.[7, 8, 10, 11]

Epidemiology

Although it is a rare malignancy, the incidence of intraocular-CNS lymphoma has trebled over the last decade, an increase not correlated with a correspondingly large increase in known predisposing factors.[12]

This malignancy most commonly occurs in middle to late adulthood, with a median age of 50 to 60 years[12, 13]; however, cases have been reported in children,[14, 15] and the youngest reported patient was 15 years old.[16]

The sex distribution is not clear. Although an earlier study reported no sexual predilection, some recent studies report a higher incidence in women,[11, 17–19] and one reports a higher incidence in men.[12]

Immune suppression seems to be a risk factor in the development of intraocular-CNS lymphoma. This condition has been associated with acquired immunodeficiency syndrome (AIDS)[20] and immune suppression following transplant surgery,[21] and with congenital immunodeficiencies (e.g., Wiskott-Aldrich syndrome and severe combined immunodeficiency).

Clinical Characteristics

Intraocular-CNS lymphoma arises from the eye or the brain, the spinal cord, or the leptomeninges, and then spreads throughout the CNS.[13, 22, 23] Systemic spread outside the CNS and eye is rare, occurring in only about 10% of autopsied cases.[24, 25] Ocular manifestations antedate clinically evident CNS involvement in 50% to 80% of the cases reported in the ophthalmic literature,[17, 26] although this may represent an overestimation because of a selection bias for patients with ocular involvement. Overall, around 20% of patients with primary CNS lymphoma exhibit ocular involvement at the time of diagnosis.[23]

Most of the symptoms of intraocular-CNS lymphoma are related to the posterior segment—blurred vision and/or floaters are the commonest.[24, 27] In the early stages of the disease, floaters may actually be the only symptom, without even a decrease in visual acuity. Anterior segment symptoms such as redness and pain are very rare. The initial presentation may be unilateral, although ultimate bilateral involvement is the rule.[23, 28, 29]

Examination reveals no or very mild external signs of inflammation. On slit-lamp examination, there is often mild anterior segment inflammation, with aqueous cells and flare and keratoprecipitates on the corneal endothelium.[13, 16, 21, 22, 30] The vitreous typically contains large clumps or sheets of cells, and a fundus examination shows multifocal, large, yellow, sub-retinal pigment epithelium (RPE) infiltrates with overlying solid pigment epithelium detachment[8, 17, 24, 25, 31] visualized through a hazy vitreous (Fig. 48–1A to D). Ocular findings may be in excess of those expected from clinical vision testing. Reported atypical presentations include hemorrhagic retinal vasculitis resembling a viral retinitis,[28, 32] and a normal-appearing fundus with subretinal lesions noted only by fluorescein angiography. Vitreous opacification may make the retina difficult to visualize.

Because intraocular-CNS lymphoma is more likely to involve the deep brain structures than the cerebral cortex, seizures and motor symptoms, although they do occur, are less common than in patients with other kinds of brain tumors. It has been reported that since the frontal

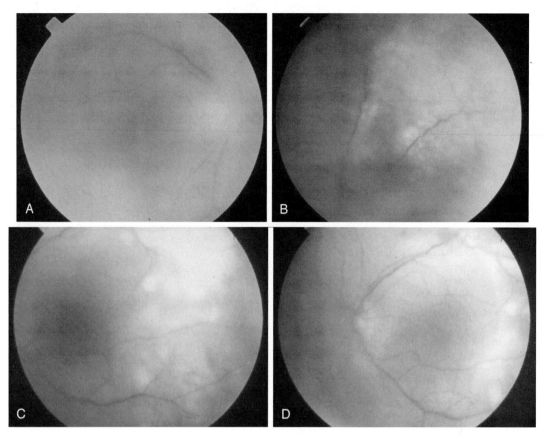

FIGURE 48–1. *A* to *D*, Intraocular-CNS lymphoma. Note the dense vitritis *(A)*, and the presence of retinal infiltrates that should raise the suspicion of intraocular-CNS lymphoma. (See color insert.)

lobe is the most commonly involved region of the brain, changes in personality and the level of alertness are common at the time of presentation.[27] CNS findings such as headaches, confusion, sensory deficits, focal weakness, diplopia, right-left confusion, poor memory, imbalance, motor weakness, and difficulty with gait have been reported.[19, 33] A history of seizures in a patient with no prior history of seizure disorder is also a strong indication of CNS involvement. Thus, careful CNS history taking and a thorough neurologic examination are vitally important, as they may indicate CNS involvement.

Systemic non-Hodgkin lymphoma presents with obvious systemic symptoms (fever, weight loss, lymphadenopathy) before ocular involvement. When ocular involvement does occur, hypopyon in an uninflamed eye,[29] hyphema, and choroidal infiltrates have been reported.[34] This is in contrast to intraocular-CNS lymphoma, which usually presents as subretinal infiltrates and thus may be confused with melanoma of the choroid. Similarly, Hodgkin's disease almost invariably presents with systemic symptoms before the eye is involved. Bilateral anterior and posterior uveitis with no retinal change[11]; uveitis with peripheral white, flat retinal deposits resembling miliary tuberculosis[9]; and anterior uveitis alone[10] have been reported in patients with ocular involvement in Hodgkin's disease.

Lymphoid hyperplasia of the uvea is another disorder that must be distinguished from intraocular-CNS lymphoma. This disorder is characterized by a well-differentiated, small lymphocytic infiltration of the uveal tract. It presents usually unilaterally as anterior uveitis, iris heterochromia, vitritis, and choroidal infiltrates,[35, 36] and it is often considered a low-grade lymphoid neoplasm; it usually responds to treatment with corticosteroids, although sometimes moderate doses of radiotherapy are needed; it has a favorable long-term prognosis.[36, 37]

Hoang-Xuan and associates have recently described a "new" masquerade syndrome in a patient presenting with histology-proven anterior and posterior scleritis and choroidal white dots, unresponsive to systemic high-dose steroids and cyclophosphamide therapy. This patient was found to have mucosal-associated lymphoid tissue lymphoma on a repeat conjunctival biopsy.[38]

Pathology, Immunology, and Pathogenesis

Most intraocular-CNS lymphomas are diffuse, large cell lymphomas of B-cell origin,[39] with a few reported cases of T-cell origin.[1] Gross specimens show large gray patches of subretinal and retinal infiltration above a thickened choroid. Collections of lymphoma cells are found between Bruch's membrane and the RPE, with reactive (mainly T) lymphocytes in the retina and choroid, surrounding the B cells.

Cytopathology specimens obtained from the vitreous of patients with intraocular lymphoma show mainly reactive T cells, histiocytes, necrotic debris, and fibrinous material, and few frankly neoplastic (B) cells. The malignant lymphoma cells are anaplastic (i.e., they have a high nuclear-to-cytoplasmic ratio), and they have lobulated nuclei with multiple small nucleoli, coarse chromatin, and mitotic figures (see Fig. 48–1). Immunohistochemistry marks them positive for B-cell markers (CD10, CD19, CD20, CD21, CD22) and for monoclonal κ and λ chains. In contrast, histiocytes have large vesicular or watery nuclei with small nucleoli and minimal clumping of the nuclear chromatin. Macrophages have much more opaque cytoplasm and somewhat eccentric nuclei, and they may contain ingested debris, including melanin granules.[19]

Cytokines play an important role in conditions involving immunologic cells, and intraocular-CNS lymphoma is no exception. Interleukin-4 (IL-4) and IL-10 are potent growth and differentiation factors for B lymphocytes, and IL-10 induces B cells to secrete large quantities of immunoglobulin G (IgG), IgA, and IgM.[40] IL-10 is also a negative regulator for IL-12–induced inflammation and has been seen primarily as a cytokine-synthesis inhibitor.[41] IL-6, a multifunctional cytokine, plays a central role in inflammatory defense mechanisms and has been found in the aqueous and vitreous of patients with non-neoplastic uveitis. The same is true of IL-12 levels, which correlate to the degree of inflammation.[42] IL-10 has been reported to be associated with the presence of malignant lymphoid neoplasms.[43, 44] The role of IL-10 levels in the diagnosis of intraocular-CNS lymphoma is discussed in the section on diagnosis.

At the genetic level, translocation of the *BCL2* gene, a proto-oncogene located on chromosome 18, is believed to be the fundamental event in many hematologic malignancies, including non-Hodgkin lymphoma,[45] where a t(14;18) translocation brings the *BCL2* gene into juxtaposition with the Ig heavy-chain promoter located on chromosome 14,[46] resulting in overexpression of the *BCL2* gene. Several investigators have also detected this immunoglobulin heavy-chain rearrangement by polymerase chain reaction (PCR) in ocular specimens of patients with intraocular-CNS lymphoma.[44, 47, 48]

Diagnosis

The three cornerstones of diagnosis in intraocular-CNS lymphoma are a thorough CNS evaluation (including a history and neurologic examination as well as magnetic resonance imaging [MRI]), CNS cytology, and a diagnostic vitrectomy. The differential diagnoses of sarcoid and, less commonly, tuberculosis, which may present in a similar way, must be excluded with appropriate investigations.

A high index of suspicion for intraocular-CNS lymphoma is necessary to avoid missing or delaying the diagnosis, especially in middle-aged or older patients presenting with chronic vitritis.[39] Findings of intense ocular inflammation (in the absence of significant pain, photophobia, or conjunctival hyperemia), and sub-RPE infiltrates, sheets and clumps of vitreous cells, and steroid resistance (after a possible initial period of steroid responsiveness), should raise suspicion for intraocular-CNS lymphoma. The reported average interval of 21 months between the onset of ocular symptoms and definitive diagnosis[11] has been shown to be reduced considerably, with most patients diagnosed between 20 and 52 weeks, if one maintains a high index of suspicion based on clinical findings.[19]

Any recent-onset CNS symptoms or findings on a neurologic examination raise the suspicion of CNS spread. An MRI is warranted, however, in all patients suspected of having CNS lymphoma, even if the history and examination are negative. On a computed tomography (CT) scan or with MRI, the appearance of an intraocular-CNS lymphoma is characteristic, with the tumor being supratentorial and multicentric in 50% of cases.[49] Unlike brain metastasis and malignant gliomas, which show ring enhancement on administration of contrast, these lesions characteristically have dense and diffuse enhancement with distinct borders.

A lumbar puncture must be performed on all patients suspected of having intraocular-CNS lymphoma, regardless of the results of the neurologic evaluation. Ten milliliters of cerebrospinal fluid (CSF) is appropriate for cytology. A repeat lumbar puncture may be required for diagnosis. Lymphoma cells are extremely fragile, and to optimize results, specimens should be transported to the laboratory immediately. Lumbar puncture can be negative in a patient with intraocular-CNS lymphoma, since CNS disease may lag ocular disease by months to years.[17] Even in the presence of CNS involvement, lumbar puncture can give false-negative results as a result of mishandling of the specimens or steroid therapy; steroids may be cytolytic in intraocular-CNS lymphoma and may even cause intraocular-CNS lymphoma lesions to decrease in size.

Vitreous biopsy of an eye with more severe vitritis or reduced vision is used to assess ocular involvement and is carried out even if the lumbar puncture results are negative. This is the gold standard for assessing ocular involvement in the disease. A standard three-port pars plana vitrectomy (PPV) is performed; before instituting the infusion, 1 ml of undiluted vitreous is obtained by a syringe and delivered immediately to the cytology laboratory.[21, 26] The specimens are fixed by mixing one part of 10% neutral-buffered formalin with one part of specimen for approximately 12 hours. A 5-ml fixed specimen is then spun at 1000 rpm for 5 minutes in a cytospin chamber to concentrate the cells onto glass slides. These are then dried and stained with a modified Papanicolaou's staining technique for cytopathologic analysis. Histochemical staining using monoclonal antibodies against the B- and T-cell markers and against κ and λ light chains is also done, and the slides are interpreted by a cytopathologist.

Total vitrectomy is then performed with infusion. Tissue culture medium enriched with 10% fetal calf serum can be added to the collection chamber of the vitrectomy machine to improve cell viability. This diluted specimen is then submitted for modified Papanicolaou's staining, histochemical staining, flow cytometry, and IL analysis. Problems encountered are similar to those of lumbar puncture specimens: the fragility of the lymphoma cells (which may be damaged by improper handling), steroid therapy (which most of these individuals were on for vitritis prior to the vitrectomy), and the high ratio of reactive cells to malignant cells. The diagnosis can easily be missed by pathologists who have had little experience with this condition. False negatives can be minimized by immediate delivery of the specimens and by the availability of an experienced cytopathologist. Even so, multiple vitreous samples may be needed to make a definitive diagnosis.[26, 50]

Ancillary diagnostic modalities include the measurement of IL levels. High IL-10 levels and an elevated ratio of IL-10 to IL-6 in vitreous specimens have been associated with intraocular-CNS lymphoma, according to some reports.[51, 52] However, a study at our center shows that IL-10 can be detected even in vitreous specimens of patients with non-neoplastic uveitis and that, conversely, IL-10 levels are not always elevated in patients with intraocular-CNS lymphoma.[53] Thus IL-10 levels are suggestive but not diagnostic of lymphoma, with vitreous biopsy cytopathology still being the only definitive means of diagnosing ocular involvement in intraocular-CNS lymphoma.

Several investigators have identified the t(14;18) locus by PCR in ocular specimens of patients with intraocular-CNS lymphoma,[47, 48] and successful amplification in both frozen and formaldehyde-fixed and paraffin-embedded samples have been reported using this method.[54, 55] Thus this promising new method may provide an additional diagnostic clue when traditional methods fail to provide an unequivocal answer.

Treatment

The optimal treatment of intraocular-CNS lymphoma is still controversial. In the case of documented CNS involvement, combined radio- and chemotherapy is recommended. Whole brain radiation with 50 gray (Gy) and an additional 10-Gy boost to the tumor side is recommended.[18, 28] However, despite high radiosensitivity, whole brain radiation alone leads to a high relapse rate, with most patients dying within 1 to 5 years of diagnosis.[28] A marked improvement in survival of patients is reported when cranial radiation is combined with intrathecal methotrexate (MTX) as systemic chemotherapy.[56] Intrathecal MTX is needed because the CNS levels of intravenous (IV) chemotherapy may be short-lived[57] and variable, despite the fact that high-dose cytosine arabinoside can lead to therapeutic levels in CSF.[32] MTX may also be delivered by an Omaya reservoir,[27] and intravitreal MTX has been employed in some patients with intraocular-CNS lymphoma with promising results.[58]

Radiation therapy has proved to be effective for ocular findings in patients with detectable involvement only in the eye and no detectable CNS involvement. A dose of 30 Gy is given, typically to both eyes, since bilateral involvement is the rule.[18, 26, 28] In these patients, there is controversy about whether to limit treatment to the eye or to prophylactically irradiate the CNS as well. Although one group of investigators has reported long-term (24 and 109 months) disease-free survival with ocular radiation only,[26] many researchers recommend prophylactic CNS radiation in addition to orbital radiation in patients with isolated ocular involvement, since these patients often have subclinical CNS involvement by the time ocular manifestations arise.[26, 59] Rouwen and colleagues[59] advise a combination of chemotherapy for CNS disease and radiotherapy for ocular disease even if CNS involvement cannot be documented by MRI and lumbar puncture, since penetration of the blood-brain barrier by chemotherapeutic agents is doubtful.

Prognosis

Prognosis of this condition is poor, despite a generally good initial response. The 5-year survival is less than 5% and median survival varies in different series from 13 to 26 months.[12, 17, 26] Char and colleagues, however, suggest that the median survival in these patients improves if a combination of intrathecal chemotherapy and radiotherapy of the CNS and orbit is employed.[26]

Complications

Cranial radiotherapy produces significant CNS toxicity in long-term survivors, which is exacerbated by chemotherapy,[13, 60] especially MTX. However, administration of chemotherapy before radiotherapy may reduce the risk of leukoencephalopathy and late toxicity.[60, 61] Some investigators recommend using systemic and intrathecal chemotherapy for intraocular-CNS lymphoma,[62] with radiotherapy used only for recurrent disease. This tends to minimize the toxicity associated with combination chemotherapy and radiotherapy usage. Survival rates may improve with a combination of intrathecal chemotherapy and radiotherapy to the orbits and whole brain.[26]

Conclusion

Intraocular-CNS lymphoma is an insidious and aggressive malignancy that presents masquerading as intraocular inflammation. A high index of suspicion, a thorough CNS evaluation, and cytologic examination of vitreous samples are the cornerstones of diagnosis. Management is controversial, but earlier diagnosis and new treatment modalities provide some hope for patients with this condition.

LEUKEMIAS

Definition

Leukemias are malignant neoplasms of the hematopoietic stem cells, characterized by diffuse replacement of the bone marrow by neoplastic cells.[63] Traditionally, leukemias are classified on the basis of the cell type involved and on the maturity of the leukemic cells into acute lymphocytic (ALL), acute myelocytic (AML), chronic lymphocytic (CLL), and chronic myelocytic (myelogenous) (CML) leukemias. The acute leukemias are characterized by the presence of very immature cells called blasts and a rapidly fatal course in untreated patients; chronic leukemias are associated, at least initially, with well-differentiated leukocytes, and with a relatively indolent course. The acute leukemias typically exhibit the characteristics of an abrupt, "stormy" onset, with symptoms related to depression of normal bone marrow function, organ infiltration, and CNS manifestations. The alteration in normal marrow function and the ability to infiltrate tissues, especially common in ALL, is responsible for many of the ocular manifestations. The chronic leukemias, although a more diverse group of disorders, do, to some extent, share the same properties.

Leukemic ophthalmopathy was apparently first established as a clinical entity in the late 19th century by Liebreich in his paper on leukemic retinopathy and central retinal artery embolism.[64] In the early 1900s, leukemic invasion of the optic nerve was considered a preterminal curiosity; however, with advances in the systemic treatments of leukemia, there was a resurgence of interest in the eye as a site where leukemic cells may escape the effects of systemic treatment and later proliferate to cause relapse.

Epidemiology

Estimates of ocular involvement in leukemia vary: Pathologic studies show a higher incidence than clinical ones and many findings are transient, waxing and waning with time and treatment. Ridgeway and associates,[65] for example, report abnormalities on ocular examination in 9% of children suffering from acute leukemias, whereas Duke-Elder[66] estimates that up to 90% of patients with leukemia demonstrate some ocular abnormality at some point in the disease course. However, it is generally accepted that the eye is involved far more often in acute than in chronic leukemias. For example, Kincaid and Green,[67] in a review of pathology specimens, report ocular involvement in 82% of cases of acute and in 75% of chronic leukemic eyes, and this difference is noted in most other studies as well.

Clinical Presentation and Diagnosis

As effective chemotherapy programs have led to longer survival times for leukemic patients, sites of extramedullary leukemic infiltration have been examined more closely because they may act as reservoirs for proliferation of leukemic cells and eventual systemic relapse. These sites have been considered "pharmacologic sanctuaries," relatively unaffected by systemic chemotherapy and requiring separate radiotherapy.[68–71] Although the CNS is one of the most frequent sites of relapse after initial induction of remission,[72] it is now generally accepted that the eye, like the CNS, is a pharmacologic sanctuary, requiring radiation for elimination of tumor cells.[65, 73]

Ocular involvement in leukemia occurs either because of infiltration of leukemic cells or because of various hemorrhagic phenomena, and practically any part of the eye can be involved. The ocular abnormalities are described next, according to the part of the eye involved. Recognizing leukemic involvement of the eye is important because it may present the first manifest signs of extramedullary relapse, and prompt identification and

initiation of treatment can be life saving, especially in acute leukemias.

Retina

Leukemic retinopathy is observed in both the acute and chronic forms of leukemia, but it is common in the acute form. It is characterized by tortuous, dilated retinal veins, which may have an irregular "boxcar" or "sausage" appearance.[74] Perivascular sheathing is often present and is thought to represent infiltration of leukemic cells.[75] Hard exudates and cotton-wool spots are also a prominent feature; the cotton-wool spots have been suggested to be either nerve fiber layer infarcts or localized collections of leukemic cells.[76]

The most striking feature of leukemic involvement of the retina, however, is the presence of retinal hemorrhages, most commonly located in the posterior pole (Fig. 48–2A, B). These hemorrhages may be at any level of the retina, including extension into the subretinal or vitreous spaces.[75] Most commonly they are intraretinal, either round or flame shaped. These intraretinal hemorrhages may appear as the classic white-centered Roth's spots, with the white centers representing cellular debris, capillary emboli, or accumulations of leukemic cells.[76, 77] Hemorrhages in the subhyaloid space are boat shaped and may break into the vitreous, thus obscuring visualization of the posterior pole. Subretinal hemorrhages are rare.

Kuwabara and Aiello[78] first described nodular retinal infiltrates, looking much like miliary nodules, associated with local necrosis and hemorrhage in a patient with chronic myelogenous leukemia, and Schachat and colleagues[79] described similar leukemic infiltrates in up to 3% of newly diagnosed ALL and AML cases. These infiltrates have been found to occur in association with elevated leukocyte counts with a high proportion of blast cells[80] and have been associated with fulminant disease and early demise.

Peripheral retinal microaneurysms are a feature of chronic leukemias, especially chronic myelogenous leukemia.[81] Prolonged leukocytosis seems to be necessary for the development of peripheral retinal microaneurysms, and this may be caused by increased lateral pressure on

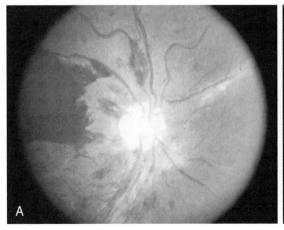
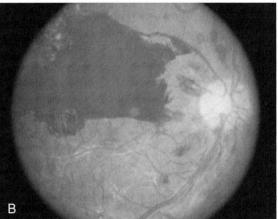

FIGURE 48–2. *A* and *B,* Fundus photographs in a patient with leukemia. Flame-shaped nerve fiber layer hemorrhages and large subhyaloid hemorrhages can be seen. (See color insert.)

the walls of vessels as a consequence of increased viscosity. Retinal neovascularization, similar to the sea-fan configuration seen in sickle cell anemia, is a rare complication that has also been found in patients with chronic myelogenous leukemia; it is associated with peripheral vascular occlusion and capillary dropout. This has been related to higher white blood cell counts and, in one case, with increased number of circulating platelets.[82–84]

Uveal Tract

CHOROID
The choroid is commonly infiltrated with leukemic cells, although this may go undetected clinically. In fact, histopathologically, the choroid may be the most commonly affected part of the eye,[67, 75] with the most striking changes observed in acute leukemias, especially ALL.[75] When visible clinically, these leukemic choroidal infiltrates may manifest as bilateral serous detachment of the retina,[67] or as single large choroidal masses and overlying serous retinal detachment in adults with chronic myelogenous leukemia.[85] This choroidal involvement can also induce secondary changes in the RPE including atrophy, hypertrophy, and hyperplasia, and occasionally giving rise to a leopard spot pattern.[67] This may occur because of either primary invasion or compressive involvement of the choriocapillaries by neoplastic cells.[86] Fluorescein angiographic changes in patients with choroidal infiltration and overlying serous retinal detachment of the retina show a multitude of RPE leakage points in the early phase of the angiogram, described as a milky-way pattern.[85] With time, these leakage points become more diffuse, and dye leaks into the subretinal space.

IRIS AND ANTERIOR SEGMENT
Anterior segment involvement in leukemias is unusual but has received increasing attention as a site of extramedullary relapse. Most cases of anterior segment involvement have had acute lymphoblastic leukemia, although cases with CLL and AML have also been reported.[87–89] Patients characteristically present with unilateral or bilateral symptoms of acute iridocyclitis with conjunctival injection, iritis, hypopyon, pseudohypopyon, or spontaneous hyphema.[65, 88, 90–93] The pseudohypopyon has, in some case reports, been defined as "shaggy, irregular, free-floating material" that fails to settle inferiorly and has a characteristic creamy-white color.[94] It consists of leukemic cells that have infiltrated into the anterior chamber and may initially respond to topical or periocular steroids, although the infiltrate recurs. Diffuse or nodular iris involvement may occur. Diffuse involvement presents as discoloration with a whitish gray film and heterochromia iridis. Nodular involvement is seen as ill-defined densities extending usually to the pupillary margin.[95] Glaucoma may occur with these findings as a result of leukemic infiltration of the trabecular meshwork, or as angle-closure glaucoma following choroidal infiltration and hemorrhage.[94, 96–98] Diagnosis is established by anterior chamber paracentesis with cytologic examination of the aqueous humor.[94] Low-dose, local anterior segment irradiation is the treatment of choice.[94, 95]

Although most patients have had meningeal or hema-tologic relapse at the time of iris infiltration, cases have been reported in which involvement of the iris may be the first, or even the only site of relapse; again, the anterior segment has been postulated as a "pharmacologic sanctuary" for leukemic cells. Bremner and Wright,[99] for example, report a case with the typical symptoms of iridocyclitis and a hypopyon, with typical "glutinous" leukemic cells in the crypt of the iris as the only site of leukemic relapse, in which symptoms resolved with local corticosteroid therapy, only to recur. Gruenewald and associates[100] and Ninane and colleagues[101] also report cases with the anterior segment as the first site of relapse. Tabbara and Beckstead[94] report the case of a 3-month-old infant with bilateral eye redness and anterior chamber pseudohypopyon as the first detected sign of acute promonocytic leukemia.

VITREOUS
Leukemic involvement of vitreous may present with a vitreous hemorrhage in the presence of retinal changes. Infiltration of the vitreous with leukemic cells without hemorrhage is uncommon, most likely reflecting the barrier function of the intact internal limiting membrane.[78] However, such cases have been reported, both in pathologic studies[67] and in case reports. Reese and Guy mention vitreous opacities in one of their cases,[102] and Swartz and Schumann[103] report the case of a patient with ALL, treated with several cycles of chemotherapy, who then presented with unilateral, progressive, painless loss of vision found to be caused by dense cellular infiltration of the vitreous, with clumping of cells and vitreous fibrils into opaque sheets as the only sign of leukemic involvement of the CNS. This patient did not receive CNS prophylactic radiation, but relapse in the eye can occur even after such radiation has been given, as seen in the case described by Bremner and Wright.[99] Diagnosis is made by a PPV with cytologic examination of the vitreous. Infections are a distinct possibility in patients with leukemia because of the leukemic state itself and the treatment received, and so endophthalmitis may have to be excluded by a Gram stain and culture of the vitrectomy specimen for bacteria and fungi. In addition, opportunistic infections commonly seen in patients with AIDS, such as cytomegalovirus retinitis, other acute necrotizing herpetic infections, and toxoplasmosis, may appear in patients with leukemia who are immunosuppressed.

Optic Nerve
Leukemic optic nerve infiltration occurs primarily in children with acute leukemias and especially ALL.[73] This is a particularly worrisome finding; like vitreous involvement, it implies CNS disease. Involvement of the optic nerve can be prelaminar, with primarily invasion of the optic nerve head, or retrolaminar. Prelaminar invasion is associated with a fluffy, edematous appearance to the nerve head with moderate edema and hemorrhage. The visual acuity may be altered only minimally, or it may be significantly impaired if edema and hemorrhage extend into the macular area.[73] Retrolaminar invasion, on the other hand, is associated with a profound decrease in vision and moderate to pronounced disc elevation and some edema and hemorrhage. This must be distinguished from

papilledema due to increased intracranial pressure, and this is done by a lumbar puncture. Differentiation is important because infiltration of either type of leukemic optic neuropathy responds dramatically to radiation therapy, whereas papilledema does not. In fact, with retrolaminar infiltration, urgent institution of radiation therapy is necessary to restore vision and to prevent permanent visual loss.

Since the recognition of the CNS as a pharmacologic sanctuary, and the eye as an extension of this pharmacologically privileged site,[68, 70, 104] it is now widely accepted that the posterior pole of the eye should be included in radiation therapy for the prophylaxis of CNS leukemic involvement.[65] Thus the frequency of optic nerve head involvement in leukemias is decreasing with the use of prophylactic posterior pole radiation and more aggressive systemic and intrathecal chemotherapy.[73]

Orbital and Lid Involvement

Approximately 11% of children with unilateral proptosis have some form of acute leukemia,[105] and leukemia accounts for 2% to 6% of orbital tumors of childhood.[106] Orbital involvement of the eyes occurs as a result of either tissue infiltration by leukemic cells or hemorrhage. Thus, patients may have infiltration of the lid, orbit, or lacrimal gland, proptosis, diplopia, motility disturbances, ecchymosis, lid hemorrhage, or retrobulbar hemorrhage, which may extend forward into the subconjunctival space. In an undiagnosed patient, biopsy may be required for diagnosis of leukemia, and in the immunocompromised leukemic patient with proptosis (especially one on chemotherapy), infection must be excluded.[107] Orbital leukemia may also present with infiltration of any other orbital structure including the lacrimal gland, the rectus muscles, the dermis, and the lacrimal draining system.[68, 108]

Granulocytic sarcoma, or chloroma, a variant of myelogenous leukemia, classically presents with tumor masses in the orbit. These may be unilateral or bilateral, and they have a greenish appearance on gross pathologic examination because of the presence of the enzyme myeloperoxidase.[109] A chloroma may manifest at any time in the course of myelogenous leukemia, sometimes preceding hematologic signs. In myeloproliferative disorders, it may be a harbinger of a blast crisis and transformation into AML.[110] Thus, in the presence of granulocytic sarcoma, the ophthalmologist must be alerted to the imminent appearance of AML. These tumors have a poor prognosis, with a survival of between 1 and 30 months after onset of ocular signs and symptoms.[111, 112]

Other Unusual Manifestations

Leukemia can present with infiltration and hemorrhage into practically any part of the eye, and thus a number of uncommon manifestations have been reported in the literature, including corneal ring ulcer in AML,[113] Sjögren's syndrome with lacrimal gland enlargement in CLL,[114] and anterior segment ischemia[115] in CML.

Pathogenesis

Various studies have attempted to relate the pathologic findings in the eyes of leukemic patients with the overall systemic changes. Although most authors have been un-

able to relate the retinal findings of leukemia to hematologic status,[80, 116] Culler[117] reports a correlation between low red cell and platelet counts and retinal hemorrhages, and the relationship between low platelet counts and hemorrhages is confirmed by two more recent prospective studies.[118, 119] Kincaid and Green[67] have suggested that the relationship between retinal findings and the blood count may be inconclusive because the blood profile in these patients varies during the disease course, and the appearance of the retinal findings may be delayed, correlating better with the blood cell counts of approximately a month earlier.

Treatment and Prognosis

The treatment and prognosis for signs and symptoms in leukemia were described in preceding sections. As long-term survival and even cure of leukemia become a possibility, increasing attention is being paid to the ocular manifestations, both as a sign of extramedullary disease relapse, and in terms of vision preservation to enhance quality of life. Although, even with irradiation and intrathecal MTX, visual outcome is not always good, new studies evaluating the ocular morbidity of acute leukemias have shown surprisingly good results in both AML and ALL patients,[120, 121] as prophylactic and treatment approaches for extramedullary leukemia continue to be refined, based on the type of leukemia, previous treatments, marrow relapse, and CSF profile.[122–124] Development of the concept of certain extramedullary sites, including the CNS and the eye, as pharmacologic sanctuaries has been a significant step in decreasing ocular as well as systemic morbidity.[65, 80, 125, 126] The most striking example of this is ALL, which now has a 90% remission rate and a 50% cure rate.[125, 126]

MALIGNANT MELANOMA

Definition

Malignant melanoma of the eye is a malignant melanocytic stromal proliferation of the choroid, the ciliary body, or the iris. Malignant melanoma of the choroid and ciliary body is the most common primary intraocular malignancy.

History

Melanoma was considered to be the most common malignancy of the eye up to the 1960s, when it was thought to have an incidence around 20 times greater than that of metastatic tumors.[127] However, with increased survival of cancer patients and with the proliferation of medical literature, it came to be recognized that malignant melanomas, although the most common primary eye malignancy, are in fact, much less common than metastatic tumors of the eye.

Epidemiology

Melanomas are the most prevalent primary eye malignancies, with posterior melanomas occurring at a higher frequency than iris melanomas. Iris lesions account for only 3.3% to 12.5% of all surgically excised melanomas[128–132]; they occur at an average age of between 40 and 50 years[128, 132–136] and with equal incidence in men and women.[128–130, 132, 135, 136] They occur more in whites and in patients with light irides than in Asians and blacks.[128, 134, 137] Most iridic melanomas (and also nevi) arise from the inferior portion of the iris, more often peripherally and temporally.[128, 134, 136]

Choroidal melanomas occur at an average age that is about 10 years above that for iris melanomas. They are eight times more common in whites than blacks[138, 139] and six times more common in whites than in some Asian populations.[140, 141]

Clinical Characteristics

In a high proportion of patients, iris melanomas arise from pre-existing lesions that suddenly undergo active growth.[129, 130, 132, 142] They present in three patterns—ring, tapioca, and diffuse melanomas. Diffuse melanomas present with unilateral acquired heterochromia and secondary glaucoma. Although they have the highest likelihood of metastasizing, they also have an excellent prognosis.[132, 142–144] Ring melanomas involve more than two thirds of the angle circumferentially, and they are associated with secondary glaucoma. Many are diagnosed incorrectly because of failure to recognize an infiltrating pigmented lesion as a cause of refractory glaucoma. Tapioca melanomas[145] are lightly pigmented or nonpigmented multifocal nodules that project into the anterior chamber. These lesions are sometimes associated with glaucoma. They were initially thought of as benign, but now it is recognized that some can be categorized histologically as melanomas,[142] and metastatic disease has been reported.[146]

Clinical differentiation between malignant and benign lesions is based on clinical features. A lesion is considered malignant if it is 3 mm or greater in diameter and 1 mm or greater in thickness and has three of the following five features[147, 148]: secondary glaucoma, secondary cataract, photographic documentation of growth, ectropion irides, and prominent vascularity. Notable tumor growth and intense vascularity have been cited as being the most reliable signs for the diagnosis of melanoma of the iris.[149]

However, these traditionally accepted concepts are now being challenged, and a recent study by Jakobiec and Silbert shows no correlation between the type of lesion and the presence of ectropion uvea, splinting or distortion of the pupil, vascularity, involvement of the chamber angle, glaucoma, or touching of the cornea.[142] This study concludes that progressive growth or involvement of the ciliary body in a ring configuration with progressive glaucoma is more commonly associated with benign tumors; nevertheless, a lesion with these features must still be scrutinized very closely.[142] Tumors with ciliary body involvement (Fig. 48–3A–D) are also associated with a higher incidence of malignancy (although neither episcleral dilatation nor sector cataract reflected malignancy or ciliary body involvement).[142]

Some studies also show that medial location and presence of pigment dispersion onto the iris or angle structures are the only features associated with tumor growth.[150] According to other studies, however, iris melanomas are more likely to be inferiorly and temporally located;[128, 134, 136] some authors believe that a superiorly located lesion is unlikely to be a melanoma[151] but may be metastatic or a ciliary body tumor. Because of clinical findings such as pigment dispersion in the anterior cham-

ber and pigment on the anterior surface of the lens, this condition can masquerade as uveitis.

Choroidal melanomas present with symptoms of visual loss, photopsias, and visual field defects, although they may be asymptomatic. Unusual presentations, including severe pain, suggest a diagnosis other than that of choroidal melanoma; but pain may occur in melanomas associated with inflammation, massive extraocular extension, or neovascular glaucoma. An ocular history of an old nevus, or systemic nonocular malignancies may be helpful in establishing a diagnosis, but one must also remember that 6% to 10% of melanoma patients have another primary neoplasm.[152, 153]

Examination is of vital importance in the diagnosis, as it has been reported that indirect ophthalmoscopy leads to a correct diagnosis of melanoma in greater than 95% of cases.[154] Visual fields are not helpful in ruling out benign lesions,[147, 155] as melanomas have no characteristic visual field changes. Scleral transillumination is blocked by melanomas but not by choroidal effusions. Melanomas appear classically as pigmented, dome- or collar button–shaped tumors with associated exudative retinal detachment that may involve the macula and thus decrease vision (see Fig. 48–3E). Although only a minority of choroidal melanomas have the collar-button configuration, breaks in Bruch's membrane are rarely seen with any other type of lesion.

Other signs include a deposition of lipofuscin at the level of the RPE, seen as an orange pigment; a tumor with an elevated, globular shape; exudative retinal detachment with a large tumor; and tumor pigmentation (although nearly one fourth of tumors are nonpigmented). Some large melanomas, especially those involving the ciliary body, may have prominent scleral vessels called sentinel vessels (see Fig. 48–3C).

Uncommon presentations include diffuse melanoma (less than 5 mm thick, covering more than 25% of the uveal tract),[156] which has a higher rate of extraocular spread. Melanomas may also present with significant anterior uveitis, especially with iridial melanomas, or posterior inflammation with choroidal and ciliary melanomas; these cases may be very similar to the presentation of sarcoid, tuberculous uveitis, or posterior scleritis, and the choroidal mass may be misdiagnosed as a granuloma.[145] Fraser and Font,[157] for example, in a series of 450 eyes with melanomas of the choroid and ciliary body, report that 22 (4.9%) had ocular inflammation: episcleritis (7 patients), anterior or posterior uveitis (14 patients), and panophthalmitis or endophthalmitis. Haddab and associates[158] report the case of a 22-year-old man with a decreased visual acuity and signs of cells and flare in the anterior chamber; keratoprecipitates, posterior synechiae, and round yellowish nodules on the iris; and elevated intraocular pressure and cataract, who was initially treated for anterior uveitis for at least 2 months before a diagnosis of ciliary body melanoma was made. Similarly, Furdova and associates[159] report the case of a 23-year-old woman with an ultimate diagnosis of malignant melanoma penetrating the optic nerve, diagnosed as intermediate uveitis and treated for a prolonged period as an outpatient, and later with a PPV, until malignant cells were found in her anterior chamber 4 months after the PPV. Thus, melanomas must be kept in mind in the case of such

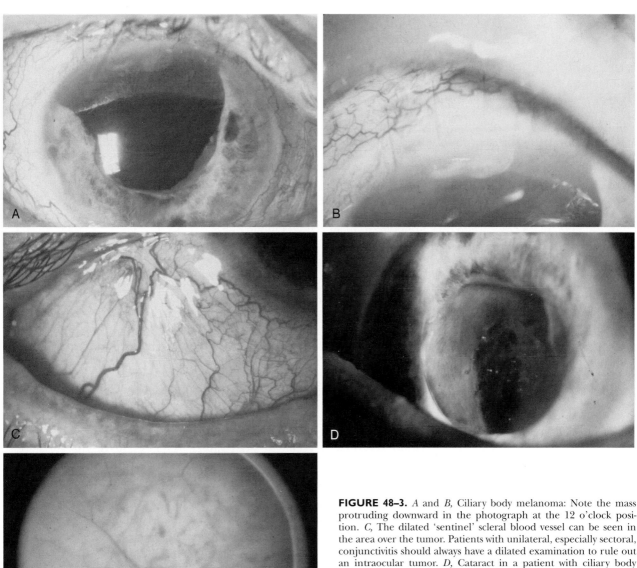

FIGURE 48–3. *A* and *B,* Ciliary body melanoma: Note the mass protruding downward in the photograph at the 12 o'clock position. *C,* The dilated 'sentinel' scleral blood vessel can be seen in the area over the tumor. Patients with unilateral, especially sectoral, conjunctivitis should always have a dilated examination to rule out an intraocular tumor. *D,* Cataract in a patient with ciliary body melanoma. *E,* Malignant melanoma. The large, elevated dome shape of the tumor seen in this picture is characteristic. Tumors may also show breaks in Bruch's membrane, giving a collar-button appearance. Although most tumors are pigmented, nearly 25% can be nonpigmented. (See color insert.)

presentations, especially if the patient does not respond to treatment.

Certain atypical findings may lead to a diagnosis other than melanoma: The presence of significant hemorrhage is seen in choroidal melanomas only when the tumor has broken through Bruch's membrane, or with large tumors; a mass lesion less than 4 mm with hemorrhage should bring to mind other possibilities (e.g., ruptured macro aneurysms, disciform lesions, and localized choroidal detachment). Multiple choroidal tumors are suggestive of metastasis or lymphoid lesions; black pigmentation is suggestive of RPE hypertrophy, hyperplasia, or melanocytoma; a pink-orange color is typical of choroidal hemangioma, hemorrhage, or osteoma; absence of pigmentation, although present in one fourth of melanomas, must

prompt one to rule out choroidal hemangiomas and metastasis.

Pigmented choroidal lesions between 1.5 and 3 mm in thickness have been termed intermediate elevated pigmented choroidal tumors and may have signs of chronicity. These lesions, however, must be carefully observed for signs of growth by sequential examinations, photography, and ultrasonography, and for the presence of growth, exudative retinal detachment, and lipofuscin, which increase the likelihood of malignancy.

Pathophysiology, Immunology, and Pathology

Sunlight exposure is thought to be important in the pathogenesis of iridial melanomas,[160] thus its predilection for light irides and Caucasians. These lesions are also thought to develop from preexisting benign nevi.[142, 161]

The histopathologic classification of iris and choroidal melanomas was originally described by Callender.[162] Uveal melanomas are assigned into the following groups based on their histopathologic features: spindle A, spindle B, fascicular, mixed, epithelioid and necrotic. Now melanomas with a spindle A histology are regarded as benign spindle cell nevi.[162, 163] This classification system has been shown to have prognostic value for ciliochoroidal melanomas, as mortality increases linearly from the spindle A cytology to the aggressive epithelioid cytology.[130, 164–166]

However, since iridic lesions have been found to behave in a much more benign fashion than melanomas of the choroid and ciliary body, iridic melanomas have been classified into a nine-part histopathologic classification by Jakobiec and Silbert[142]; these investigators argue that, based on the clinical behavior of iris melanomas, a majority of these lesions are inherently benign. However, other investigators dispute this, saying that although melanocytic iris tumors have an excellent prognosis, this is primarily because of their conspicuous location and their smaller size at diagnosis,[167] and therefore they should not be considered distinct from posterior melanomas.

Diagnosis

Iris Melanomas

Excluding primary ciliary body melanomas with iris extension is vital because of the completely different management and prognosis of these two conditions. This is done by indirect ophthalmoscopy with scleral depression, scleral transillumination, and gonioscopy. Ultrasonography is done if primary ciliary body melanoma cannot be excluded. Benign lesions simulating malignant melanoma of the iris must also be excluded. One study, for example, found that only 24% of lesions referred as presumed iris melanoma had been correctly diagnosed,[148] and the major misdiagnosed lesions in that series were primary cysts (38%) and nevi (31%).

Photographic documentation of any stromal melanocytic tumor of the iris is required; photographic evidence of progressive growth or a diffuse ring configuration point toward malignant melanoma. Similarly, glaucoma points toward a malignant lesion, as does the tendency of the lesion to spread beyond the pupillary neuroectodermal margin of the iris and, for example, to deposit on the lens or cause retrocorneal nodules. Fluorescein angiographic patterns may also help differentiate between a benign and a malignant lesion.[168–170] Benign nevi have a filigree vascular network pattern (early filling, late leaking), or they may be angiographically silent, while malignant tumors have irregular and indistinct vascular channels that fill later (i.e., in more than 30 seconds). Although these features are useful, they probably should not be used as a definitive or decision-making investigation in determining malignancy.[171] Several other tests have been suggested but not found to be useful.[147, 149]

Choroidal Melanomas

Choroidal melanoma is diagnosed on the basis of indirect ophthalmoscopy, scleral transillumination, and ultrasonography. For lesions more than 3 mm thick, combined A and B scan ultrasonography has a more than 95% accuracy in the diagnosis of choroidal melanomas.[154] The three characteristic features on B scan are an acoustically silent zone within the melanoma, choroidal excavation, and shadowing in the orbit. A scan features include medium to low vitreal echoes, with smooth attenuation and vascular pulsations within the tumor. Ultrasonography of a nevus, in contrast, shows a flat lesion with choroidal discontinuity on the B scan and medium to high internal reflectivity on the A scan. Intermediate elevated pigmented choroidal lesions (between 1.5 and 3 mm in height), although difficult to diagnose on ultrasonography, nevertheless may exhibit enlargement on sequential ultrasound exams.

Ancillary investigations include fluorescein angiography, CT, MRI, indocyanine green angiography, and radioactive phosphorus uptake. Fluorescein angiography is of limited value.[154] Larger melanomas may show an intrinsic tumor "double circulation" with extensive leakage, late staining, and multiple pin-point leaks or "hot spots" at the level of the RPE,[155, 172] but these signs are by no means very sensitive or specific. Fluorescein angiography, however, can be useful in differentiating hemorrhagic lesions (e.g., ruptured macroaneurysms, disciform lesions, and localized choroidal detachment).

High-resolution CT[173, 174] is actually less accurate than ultrasonography; MRI, nuclear MRI (NMRI), and Doppler studies still have an uncertain role. Indocyanine green angiography may be useful in the diagnosis of choroidal melanomas, hemangiomas, and uveal metastasis.[175] A radioactive phosphorus uptake test has a low sensitivity and specificity,[160–165, 176–181] and fine-needle aspiration biopsy (FNAB) is neither generally required nor a good diagnostic measure for determining cell type or differentiating melanoma from nevi or other spindle cell tumors, and it carries with it the additional possible risk of seeding of the needle tract.

Treatment

Because iris melanomas have a generally good prognosis, observation with photos every 3, 6, or 12 months, depending on clinical features, may be all that is warranted.[142, 147, 149] Surgical intervention is indicated, with complete excision usually by sector iridectomy, if the tumor growth is pronounced and/or refractory secondary glaucoma occurs, or the tumor grows over the pupillary margin and affects vision.[147, 150] Some investigators advise iridocyclectomy for peripheral lesions that either involve the chamber angle or are associated with glaucoma,[147, 149] with the potential visual consequences and even mortality with delayed tumor removal dictating this course. However, since up to 50% of patients undergoing iridocyclectomy retain no useful vision, some investigators have recommended ultrasound-guided needle biopsy for cytologic diagnosis before iridocyclectomy.[142, 150] Because it has been recognized that the prognosis of iris melanomas is good, however, there is a trend toward conservative management of iris lesions with local excision (iridocyclectomy), with follow-up every few months for spindle B histology, and enucleation is advised only if epithelioid cells are discovered on biopsy, except in the monocular patient.[152] Another surgical modality for which smaller melanomas of the ciliary body or anterior choroids may be amenable is partial lamellar sclerouvectomy.

The management of choroidal tumors is based on their size. A major advance in the treatment of choroidal tumors is that of external beam radiation. Pioneering work on this modality done by Gragoudas and associates of the Massachusetts Eye and Ear Infirmary, among others, has shown encouraging results in some laboratory and animal studies.[182, 183] Advantages of this technique are that a maximum density of ionization can be focused onto a localized volume, and thus large-sized tumors and tumors adjacent to critical structures can be treated. This modality is being used in certain centers in the United States and other countries; the major disadvantages are limited availability and cost. Concerns about its use in humans have also been raised, with a study showing the use of radiation prior to enucleation actually adversely affecting survival,[184] hypothesized to be the result of pre-existing metastases. At present, therefore, the most common modality for treating medium-sized choroidal melanomas is radiotherapy, employing either radioactive iodine (I^{125}) or ruthenium (Ru^{106}) plaques to the sclera over the base of the tumor. Transpupillary thermotherapy is an emerging modality for the treatment of small- to medium-sized tumors, pioneered by Shields and associates.[176, 177] Large tumors require enucleation except in the elderly, unfit, or monocular patients. For medium-sized tumors, distinguishing between benign and malignant lesions becomes important. General health, age, and vision in the opposite eye also have to be considered; a course of observation for growth may be justifiable in smaller tumors in older patients. In small tumors, differentiating nevus from melanoma is important, and the ratio of height to base diameter is critical; pigmentation and secondary retinal detachments also play a role. Drusenoid appearance indicates chronicity and thus may point toward a benign, slow-growing tumor. In most patients, a period of observation is adequate. Medical evaluation in patients undergoing enucleation is important not only for assessing the general health of the patient but also in looking for second malignancies and to rule out metastases.

Complications

Complications of partial resection of iris melanomas are metastatic spread, usually through the surgical wound from glaucoma filtration procedures,[185–190] and after surgical and accidental trauma. The complications associated with enucleation include infection, bleeding, and extrusion or migration of the implant, as well as the psychological consequences of loss of one eye. This is especially severe for the asymptomatic patient. Similarly, the complications of radiation have been discussed elsewhere in this chapter. Interestingly, because of the observation that few patients have metastases from uveal melanoma noted at the time of initial presentation and before enucleation, some investigators have hypothesized that enucleation may potentiate the spread of metastases.[191–194] Most surgeons have emphasized the use of techniques to minimize the possible spread due to enucleation, such as the "no touch" technique[191] and maintaining normal intraocular pressure during surgery.[192, 193]

Prognosis

Most melanocytic iris tumors behave in a benign fashion (unlike choroid and ciliary body melanomas[166, 195]) and do not metastasize. Although the controversy as to whether iris lesions are inherently benign or not continues, most iris melanomas have a good prognosis unless metastatic spread[134, 185] or extraocular extension has occurred.[188]

In malignant melanoma of the iris and ciliary body, overall mortality has been reported at 35% in 5 years and 50% in 10 years,[196] with the prognosis depending on size (largest tumor diameter in contact with sclera), pigmentation, cell type, scleral extension, mitotic activity, location of anterior margin of the tumor and optic nerve extension,[152] age at enucleation, height of tumor, and the integrity of Bruch's membrane.[153] The same studies identify a cutoff size of 10 mm as the most important marker, a size of 10 mm or less having a better prognosis than a size of more than 10 mm. The five leading predictors of survival in these studies were largest diameter of the tumor, epithelioid cells per high-power field, invasion to line of transection, location of anterior margin of the tumor, and degree of pigmentation.

Conclusions

Iris melanomas and choroidal ciliary melanomas represent two very different malignancies of the melanocytic stromal cells, which can masquerade as intraocular inflammation. Iris melanomas have a typically indolent course, whereas choroidal ciliary melanomas must be distinguished from other similar conditions, as the management and prognosis depend to a very large extent on accurate diagnosis.

RETINOBLASTOMA

Definition

A retinoblastoma is a malignancy arising from the photoreceptor precursor cells of the retina.[197, 198] It is the commonest ocular tumor of childhood.

History

The first report of retinoblastoma in medical or ophthalmic literature comes from the mid 18th century, when the case of a 3-year-old girl with bilateral ocular tumors was described. William Hey, in 1805, introduced the term fungus haematodes to describe retinoblastomas and other highly vascular, fungating tumors, but it was Wardrop, who, in his *Observations on Fungus Haematodes or Soft Cancer*, first brought together the scattered reports and descriptions of this tumor, identified its retinal origin, and distinguished it from "soft cancers" in general, on the basis of its occurring primarily in children.[199]

Virchow[200] coined the term retinal glioma, which persisted in the literature until it was recognized that the tumor arose from the neuroepithelial cells of the retina, when Verhoff, of the Massachusetts Eye and Ear Infirmary, named the tumor retinoblastoma. Retinoblastomas have been studied extensively as a part of molecular genetics, and they have been vital to our understanding of how genes cause cancer.

Epidemiology

The incidence of retinoblastoma is 1 in 20,000 infants and children. The vast majority of retinoblastomas present in children under 3 years of age—the tumor rarely presents in children over 5 years.[201] Around 40% of retinoblastomas are familial—that is, the mutation in the retinoblastoma gene is a germ-line mutation that is transmitted from the parents, and 60% are sporadic; however, not all familial cases have a positive family history. Seventy percent of these tumors are unilateral and 30% bilateral, with familial cases typically presenting bilaterally.

The familial cases are generally diagnosed earlier, many by screening examinations in infancy; bilateral cases are diagnosed at an average age of 15 months and unilateral cases at 24 months.[202]

Clinical Characteristics

The two most common modes of presentation are leukokoria and strabismus,[203, 204] highlighting the need for a dilated fundus examination in all patients with strabismus. A less common presentation is as intraocular inflammation[205]; other uncommon presentations include secondary glaucoma, proptosis, and a pinealoblastoma. Because distant metastases tend to occur late, most patients present with local signs before distant metastasis.

Intraocular inflammation may be true inflammation (i.e., an inflammatory response to necrosis of the tumor) or only simulated inflammation as tumor cells enter the anterior chamber and simulate anterior uveitis. Retinoblastoma can easily be confused with granulomatous uveitis of almost any cause, including tuberculous and syphilitic.[206, 207] Weizenblatt[207] reports a case of an 8-year-old boy, initially presenting with unilateral decreased vision, ciliary injection, balled and strand-like vitreous opacities, and a gray focus in the fundus, but with no retinal mass. The patient was initially diagnosed and managed as having uveitis, but on recurrence of symptoms, he was considered to have endophthalmitis and was evaluated for possible tuberculous, syphilitic, brucellar, tularemic, and toxoplasmic etiologies. The diagnosis of retinoblastoma was made only after the patient's death more than a year later.

Ellsworth[205] reports a case of left esotropia at birth and a typical picture of granulomatous uveitis with vitreous haze that made examination of the fundus impossible, which later proved to be a retinoblastoma with massive involvement of the choroid. And Stafford and colleagues report a case series in which nearly 40% of patients with retinoblastoma had been initially misdiagnosed with uveitis.[208] Because delay in the diagnosis of this tumor is associated with spread and a high mortality, it is essential to consider and exclude retinoblastoma in any major disease in the eye of a child that precludes a view of the fundus.

Among the uncommon presentations, secondary angle-closure glaucoma occurs as a result of mass effect closing the anterior angle. Proptosis, caused by growth of the tumor into the orbit, is a rare presentation in developed countries, but it is extremely common, and may

indeed be the most common, in developing countries.[209] Patients may also present with pinealoblastoma,[210, 211] a retinoblastoma in the pineal body, although these generally occur at a stage when patients have already been diagnosed with retinoblastoma.

Pathophysiology, Pathology, and Immunology

The genetics of retinoblastoma have been of great interest to molecular biologists studying cancer. Human cells are known to carry two copies of the retinoblastoma gene (*Rb*), a cancer suppressor or proto-oncogene, located on chromosome 13q14. According to Knudson's two-hit hypothesis, which has since been substantiated by considerable experimental evidence, both normal alleles of the *Rb* locus must be inactivated for retinoblastoma to develop. In familial cases, children are born with one normal and one defective copy of the *Rb* gene. The second copy is lost through some form of somatic mutation (point mutation, interstitial deletion of 13q14, or even complete loss of chromosome 13). Loss of both copies gives rise to retinoblastoma. Since the first mutation is a germ-line mutation inherited from an affected parent, it is present in all cells of the body, whereas the second mutation (the second hit) occurs in a retinal precursor cell whose progeny then give rise to the retinoblastoma; this mutation is thus present only in cells of the tumor itself. In sporadic cases, both normal *Rb* genes are lost by somatic mutation in one of the retinoblasts. Thus the mutations are present only in the progeny of this retinoblast, which then form the tumor.

Patients with familial retinoblastoma, who have a mutant copy of the gene in all cells of the body, are also at a greatly increased risk of developing osteosarcoma and some other soft tissue sarcomas. Interestingly, inactivation of the *Rb* locus has been observed in several other tumors, including adenocarcinoma of the breast, small cell carcinoma of the lung, and bladder cancer. Because of the familial nature of retinoblastoma, risk assessment becomes important for family members. This will be discussed later.

Spread of the retinoblastoma may be direct (into the orbital tissues from the globe), via the optic nerve into the CSF, and hematogenously to the bone marrow. Distant metastases occur late in the course of the disease (Fig. 48–4).

Diagnosis

Because a retinoblastoma is the most common intraocular malignancy of childhood, any patient with the presenting signs of leukokoria, strabismus, or uveitis must have this condition ruled out. The differential diagnosis of leukokoria includes persistent hyperplastic primary vitreous, posterior cataract, retrolental fibroplasia, retinoblastoma, coloboma of choroid or optic disc, and uveitis.[212] As mentioned, around 40% of misdiagnosed cases of retinoblastoma may initially be diagnosed as uveitis.[208] Other rare intraocular tumors of childhood (e.g., medulloepithelioma, and possibly optic gliomas) may also be diagnosed as retinoblastoma. These can generally be excluded by a thorough clinical history and examination,

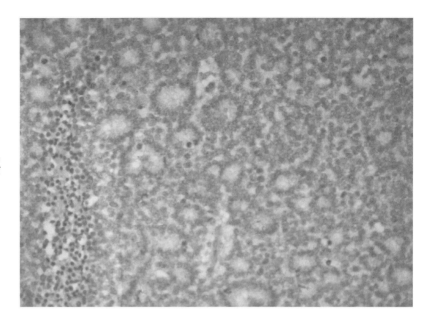

FIGURE 48–4. Flexner-Wintersteiner rosettes, which are characteristic of retinoblastoma. (Courtesy of Thadeus P. Dryja, MD.) (See color insert.)

although some patients may present a difficult diagnostic problem.

In pediatric patients suspected of this malignancy or presenting with uveitis, a family history is vital, followed by a complete eye examination, including a visual acuity and dilated fundus examination. The fundus examination is usually carried out under general anesthesia, with careful documentation of the size and location of the tumor on a large fundus drawing, which is essential for follow-up and planning radiation. Bone marrow aspiration and biopsy, and a lumbar puncture for cytocentrifuge examination, may also be performed under the same anesthesia, although the usefulness of such methods has recently been questioned.[213]

Ancillary measures include CT of the orbit and head[214] which may lead to a diagnosis of pinealoblastoma[215] but is of limited value in evaluating optic nerve involvement, because spread to the optic nerve is infiltrative and does not generally enlarge the nerve. It may, however, distinguish between an invading tumor and one merely impinging on the nerve. Occasionally, retinoblastoma calcifications may be visible on the CT scan and may help distinguish retinoblastoma from non-neoplastic conditions.[216, 217] A bone scan may identify a bone metastasis, although it is not used regularly in asymptomatic patients.[218] Reports show that MRI may help estimate differentiation in retinoblastomas.[219] Lactate dehydrogenase (LDH) levels in the aqueous humor may also be very helpful in a difficult differential diagnosis.[220] Elevated total LDH levels in the aqueous humor are very sensitive and fairly specific for retinoblastoma, although they must be interpreted with caution in patients with glaucoma or large numbers of histiocytes and neutrophils in the eye, and they may also be elevated in conditions such as Coats' disease. LDH isoenzyme patterns in the aqueous humor, and the ratio of aqueous humor to serum LDH are of doubtful value and probably not useful in establishing the diagnosis of retinoblastoma.[221–234]

Blood specimens must be obtained from the patient, parents, and siblings for DNA analysis for risk assessment. Blood samples from affected individuals are used to identify the germ-line mutation in the *Rb* gene. Searching for this mutation in the parents and siblings of the patient helps assess the risk of retinoblastoma in the siblings and future siblings of the patient. In nonfamilial cases, the germ-line mutations are not present. However, even in familial cases it is sometimes not possible to identify the germ-line mutation by direct methods, and restriction fragment length polymorphisms (RFLP) or other DNA polymorphism analysis of two or more family members affected by the disease may be necessary. If the patient is the only individual affected by the disease, these RFLPs cannot be used, but risk is predicted by a study of whether the disease was unifocal or multifocal (which includes bilateral retinoblastoma, multifocal retinoblastoma, unifocal retinoblastoma with a related primary in the CNS, and unifocal retinoblastoma with a subsequent osteosarcoma) and a genetic analysis of cells obtained from the tumor. The risk of developing retinoblastoma in offspring and siblings of the patient is then calculated and forms the basis on which these at-risk individuals are followed, if necessary, with examination under anesthesia.

Treatment

Ellsworth, in 1969, observed that in the treatment of retinoblastoma, "life is gambled for sight,"[205] and this holds true even today with the targets for treatment being the complete control of malignancy *and* the preservation of useful vision.

The most commonly used treatment in patients with good prognostic factors (Reese-Ellsworth criteria Ia, Ib, IIa, and IIb; Table 48–1)[205] is external beam radiation. Because of the numerous side effects of radiation on the normal tissue of the eye, a balance must be achieved between providing sufficiently high and extensive radiation for a realistic chance of eradicating the cancer, and minimizing the radiation exposure of normal tissue. External beam radiation therapy (EBRT), either through a Weiss[226] approach of a two-field plan (a classic split-field, an ipsilateral temporal field, and a more lightly weighted

TABLE 48-1. THE REESE-ELLSWORTH CRITERIA

Ia	Solitary tumor less than 4 dd or behind the equator
b	Multiple tumors, none larger than 4 dd, all at or behind the equator
IIa	Solitary tumor 4–10 dd, at or behind the equator
b	Multiple tumors, 4–10 dd, at or behind the equator
IIIa	Any lesion anterior to the equator
b	Solitary tumor larger than 10 dd behind the equator
IVa	Multiple tumors, some larger than 10 dd
b	Any lesion extending anteriorly to the ora serrata
Va	Massive tumor involving over half the retina
b	Vitreous seeding

dd, disc diameter.
From Ellsworth RM: The practical management of retinoblastoma. Trans Am Ophthalmol Soc 1969;67:463–534, with permission.

anterior field), or through Schipper's[227, 228] or Harnett's[229] contact lens treatment (with a temporal split-field photon approach), provides more extensive radiation; cobalt plaque approaches lead to more limited radiation exposure but are unsuitable for patients with significant vitreous seeding, two or more tumors, large (>10 mm) tumors, or tumors near or on the macula, since the potential for new tumor development or incomplete radiation of existing tumor exists.

Follow-up of patients undergoing radiotherapy is important to observe and document regression of disease. This includes examination of the patient toward the end of radiotherapy, and a repeat examination under anesthesia at 6 weeks after radiotherapy, with documentation on large retinal drawings at each visit. Successful local control following radiotherapy is defined as a failure of the tumor to enlarge. However, there are a number of different patterns of response that the tumor can show:

Type 1: Conversion of tumor to a lumpy, calcified mass—the "cottage cheese" appearance
Type 2: Change from solid, pink, or opaque and vascular, to translucent, gray, and less vascular, the "fish-flesh" appearance
Type 3: A combination of types 1 and 2
Type 4: Total loss of tumor, retina, and choroid, leaving bare sclera[230]

Larger tumors show types 1 or 3 and smaller ones types 2 or 3 patterns. Very small tumors may show a type 4 pattern. Larger tumors, however, tend not to change, or to shrink only slowly over time. As mentioned, failure to increase in size represents local success of radiotherapy.

The second modality of treatment is enucleation. Enucleation should be considered in all eyes where there is no chance of preserving useful vision.[205] Indications include unfavorable Reese-Ellsworth (see Table 48–1)[205] criteria, including tumors anterior to the ora serrata, especially with anterior segment invasion, total retinal detachment, and a posterior segment full of tumor. Relative indications include invasion of optic nerve by tumor[231] (it may be helpful to obtain a CT scan to decide whether the tumor is invading or merely impinging on the nerve), viable-looking vitreous seeds that are poorly responsive to radiation (as it is difficult to assess the viability of vitreous seeds by examination alone, attempts

to treat the eye with radiation may be made if the outcome of treatment with radiotherapy seems otherwise favorable in terms of visual rehabilitation).

Following enucleation, pathologic examination of the obtained specimen is conducted to identify spread into the orbit or globe, which may require combined radiation and chemotherapy, or very rarely an exenteration.[232] Tumor cells are obtained and used for DNA analysis to help identify the mutations causing the tumor. At the time of enucleation, a long segment of the optic nerve should be obtained in an effort to ensure removal of any optic nerve invaded by tumor, and the nerve should be examined for evidence of tumor invasion.

Photocoagulation and cryotherapy are other modalities of treatment. These are used primarily when the tumors are small, few in number, and remote from the disc and macula.[230, 233, 234] They are used as second-line treatment for recurrences after EBRT, with photocoagulation used for more posterior and cryotherapy for more anteriorly located tumors. However, these techniques are not very successful when viable tumor masses have broken from the main tumor mass during EBRT, settled along the vitreous base, and continued to grow.

Control in both these modalities (in contrast to control in radiotherapy) is defined as complete disappearance of the tumor, with formation of a flat scar.[235] This might take a few weeks to evolve, and both cryopexy and photocoagulation can be repeated if a response does not occur with the initial treatment. Photocoagulation involves using a laser to put a double row of burns around each tumor. Cryotherapy, performed trans-sclerally, involves three to four freeze-thaw cycles.

Photoactive dyes have been used in conjunction with laser or electromagnetic energy in treatment, although clinical experience with this is still limited. The technique involves absorption of photoactive dyes by the tumor mass and therefore increased vulnerability to treatment with laser,[236] ultraviolet light, or visible light.[237]

Long-term follow-up of patients is planned after the initial therapy. Examination under anesthesia is carried out every 3 months for 4 years, every 6 months for another 2 years, and then annually for an additional 2 years, when most children are old enough to tolerate annual peripheral retinal examinations without anesthesia. Regular ophthalmic screening appropriate for age is also conducted. These children must also be screened for secondary nonocular tumors associated with retinoblastoma.

Siblings in whom the risk of the hereditary retinoblastoma gene cannot be excluded must also be followed up regularly. This usually takes the form of examinations under anesthesia every 3 months up to 4 years of age, and less frequently thereafter. The frequency of examinations can be altered in those with low risk (1% to 5%), and eye examinations without anesthesia may be used in those with extremely low risk (<0.1%).

Prognosis

Overall, in countries where adequate medical care facilities for early detection and treatment of this disease are available, the prognosis of retinoblastoma is good.[238–242] More than 85% of children in developed countries have long-term survival following retinoblastoma.[202, 243] In developing countries where such facilities are not readily available, the survival rate is poor.[209]

Several prognostic indicators for retinoblastoma have been studied. The Reese-Ellsworth criteria (see Table 48–1), the present criteria of suitability for radiation using tumor control and vision preservation as end points, divide the tumor into different prognostic categories. Studies also show that local spread into the orbital tissues and the optic nerve[202, 232, 244] decreases survival, although local spread is usually still quite controllable; survival of patients with optic nerve spread depends also on the extent of posterior involvement of the nerve. Massive choroidal involvement may also have some prognostic significance.[245] Although retrobulbar spread and spread outside the orbit was traditionally considered fatal, the use of combined chemotherapy has resulted in long-term survival and apparent cure in some patients with bone marrow spread.[239–242] Pinealoblastomas, on the other hand, have a very poor prognosis, being uniformly fatal.[210, 211]

However, even if the retinoblastoma is survived, individuals with the 13q14 locus abnormalities in the germ-cell line (i.e., in hereditary retinoblastoma) have an increased risk of other malignancies, the commonest being osteosarcoma, followed by malignant melanoma. Other malignancies with a higher risk in these patients include soft tissue sarcomas, skin cancers, leukemias, lymphomas, and brain tumors—2% to 5% of these children develop tumors of the pineal region.[246–252] Because about 67% of these tumors are in the radiation field,[246] they have traditionally been considered radiation induced. However, these tumors also occur in patients who have not received radiation therapy,[246] and it has been shown that although the irradiated group initiate second tumor development approximately 5 years earlier than the nonirradiated group, the frequency of second tumor development is approximately equal with or without radiation, and furthermore that the ultimate total risk of tumors in patients with hereditary retinoblastoma is extremely high regardless of radiation therapy.[242] The extent of mortality from the second tumors is controversial, with various series reporting ranges from 59% of bilateral retinoblastoma patients dead by 35 years after diagnosis, to others with only 4% after 30 years.[248–251] This disparity may be the result of selection biases in the patient population.

Complications

Radiotherapy can potentially be associated with a large variety of complications. These include cataract formation, retinal vasculitis, changes in irradiated tissue, and possibly, second malignancies.

Cataract formation is important because, in a child, this almost always leads to amblyopia.[253] Temporal fields seem to protect against cataract formation,[201] but the newer lateral field approaches, where there is an intersection of the lens and the anterior field edge, lead to increased cataract production.[254] However, the technique developed by Weiss and colleagues,[226] mentioned previously, minimizes the risk when properly conducted.

Retinal vasculitis is another, dose-dependent, and potentially visually devastating consequence of radiation. It is the commonest initial cause of vision loss in children treated with two or more full courses of EBRT to the entire retina.[201] Plaque approaches can also cause vascular damage, hemorrhage, and subsequent vitreous opacity.[216, 217]

Effects of radiation on growing tissues include hypoplasia of temporal bone, above a threshold level of 2000 to 3500 cGy. These changes, however, if symmetrical, are not cosmetically disfiguring. This complication is markedly decreased in plaque therapy. Similarly, failure of eruption of molar teeth has been reported.

Second tumor formation, as discussed previously, has classically been attributed to radiotherapy, but there is evidence that the risk of second tumors in patients with hereditary retinoblastoma is extremely high regardless of radiation use. These tumors are believed to occur when changes at both the 13q14 loci eliminate production of the tumor suppressor gene; these tumors also follow a two-hit pattern, with the first hit in extraocular tissues being the germ-line mutation, and the second hit being caused by some other mutagen, which could be radiation. Both alleles being inactivated in a nonocular tissue gives rise to a tumor of that tissue. The role of radiation in this complication may possibly be addressed in the future by more effective neoadjuvant chemotherapy followed by more local approaches including radiation.[238, 242] However, the only hope for the elimination of such tumors lies in gene therapy that can reverse effects of the germ-line mutation.

Conclusion

Retinoblastoma is a childhood malignancy that can masquerade as uveitis. Diagnosis is important because the tumor is curable if treated early and must be ruled out in all children with uveitis. Not only is it important to treat the index case but also to determine the familial nature of the disease and to counsel and follow-up relatives.

METASTASIS

Definition

Metastatic disease is the commonest malignancy affecting the eye,[255] and its incidence is growing as patients with systemic malignancies survive longer. Metastases to the eye were first reported by Horner in 1864,[256] and they were initially believed to be uncommon.[257, 258] But in the late 1900s, it came to be recognized that metastatic malignancies were more common than previously thought, with incidences among various groups of cancer patients ranging from 4.7% to 27%.[257–259]

Epidemiology

Although ocular metastasis is rare for most cancers, its incidence is increasing as the survival time for cancers increases and as metastatic manifestations become more common and surveillance for them becomes more vigilant. Choroidal metastasis in patients dying of systemic malignancies range from 5% to 27%; this broad reported range probably reflects the variety of patients seen in any particular setting. In breast cancer patients with no ocular symptoms, for example, the incidence is 9.2%, whereas it is 27% in those with symptoms,[260] and autopsy studies report even higher incidences (37% in patients dying of breast cancer,[255] 9.3% in patients dying of all types of cancers[261]), probably reflecting the addition of cases with subclinical ocular metastasis.

The most common primary cancers for ocular metastasis are the breast,[262–266] the lungs,[127, 263, 264, 267] and "unknown," in that order. However, breast cancer metastasizes to the eye late in its course, so that it is usually clinically evident elsewhere, either in the breast itself, or as lung or disseminated metastases[260] before ocular symptoms arise. The malignancies with the highest incidence of ocular presentation preceding extraocular detection are lung and renal cell carcinoma. The incidence of lung cancer metastatic to the eye is increasing as the incidence of this cancer increases, and lung metastases are now the commonest malignancies of the iris.[268, 269] Metastases from cancers of the kidney and prostate and cutaneous melanoma are not uncommon.[127, 262, 263, 267, 270] Metastases from adenocystic cancer, Merkel's male breast cancer, and choriocarcinoma have also been reported.[271–277]

Clinical series on the incidence of ocular metastases from different primary malignancies tend to select for the less aggressive malignancies (e.g., breast), when the metastases have had time to grow and manifest as ocular symptoms, whereas autopsy studies have comparatively higher frequencies of the more aggressive malignancies, when death occurs before the ocular disease becomes clinically manifest. Interestingly, some malignancies are also associated with a higher incidence of *primary* choroidal cancers: The relationship between breast cancer and primary choroidal melanoma has been well documented.[278] This, then, indicates the need to differentiate primary choroidal cancers from metastases in a patient with a systemic malignancy.

The most frequent sites for ocular metastasis are the posterior choroid,[263, 264] the orbit, the iris, and the ciliary body,[255, 264, 279] in that order. Metastases to the retina are rare and occur in less than 1% of cases.[263, 267]

Clinical Characteristics

The patient may be asymptomatic. When symptoms are present, posterior segment symptoms such as decreased visual acuity, floaters, and field defects are the ones most often reported.[263] Metamorphopsia, diplopia, red eye, ptosis, anisocoria, and exophthalmos are other presenting signs.[263] Pain may also occur, and this along with unexplained retinal detachment, glaucoma, neovascularization, and uveitis should alert the clinician to the possibility of metastatic cancer.[267]

On examination, visual acuity is frequently decreased, but it may improve through refraction.[260] Slit-lamp examination and dilated funduscopic examination may disclose serous retinal detachment[263, 264] with a flat elevation of the retina and choroid. Choroidal metastases typically have an irregular outline, are yellow-gray to pink-white in color with edematous and detached overlying retina, are generally several disc diameters in size, and may have overlying clumps of pigment. They are frequently multiple and bilateral[260] (Fig. 48–5). Disc edema may also be present. Other possible findings include vitreous hemor-

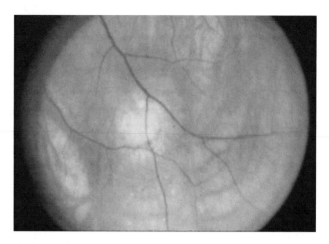

FIGURE 48–5. Metastases to the choroid. Note the multiple lesions and irregular outline. Choroidal metastases are typically multiple, have an irregular outline, are yellow-gray to pink-white in color with edematous and detached overlying retina, are generally several disc diameters in size, and may have overlying clumps of pigment. (See color insert.)

rhage, increased intraocular pressure, and anterior and posterior uveitis.

Posterior uveitis in metastatic malignant masquerade has been reported to present as clumps of pigmented or nonpigmented cells on vitreous strands, which may partially obscure the view of the retina and which are discovered to be refractory to steroid treatment.

An anterior segment presentation is less common, but patients may have symptoms of blurred vision, red eye, photophobia, pain, and (occasionally) spontaneous hyphema. Patients are reported to have iritis or anterior uveitis (in nearly half), secondary glaucoma[280] (in around two thirds), and a mass lesion of the iris (60%),[279] which is most commonly an inferiorly situated gray-white or pink nodule, although infiltrative lesions may also be present. Typical presentations include mild nongranulomatous anterior uveitis with associated increase in intraocular pressure, refractory to steroid treatment, or recurrent after the treatment is stopped.[281] Anterior segment presentations are typically associated with tumor location in the anterior segment of the eye,[262] and gonioscopy is an obviously important diagnostic step in such cases. Despite careful examination, however, no visible lesion may be detected in the eye. Denslow and Kielar, for example, reported a case in which no obvious lesions were identified in the eye, nor could a primary malignancy be found, although bone metastasis occurred later in the course of the disease.[281]

Pathophysiology, Pathology, and Immunology

Spread of tumors to the eye is via the hematogenous route, most commonly through the pulmonary circulation and then via the carotids into the ciliary arteries, and thence to the choroid. This explains the high incidence of lung metastasis (up to 85%) in people with metastatic ocular malignancy.[127] The origin of the left common carotid artery directly from the aorta has been suggested as an explanation for the preponderance of lesions in left eyes reported by some[255, 259, 262, 264, 265, 267, 282–285] but not others, and the distribution of ciliary arteries is sometimes used to explain why these lesions are more frequent at the posterior pole and temporally, where there is a greater density of these blood vessels.

Some tumor cells may, however, bypass the lungs and reach the eye via Batson's vertebral plexus of veins, or they may simply be too small to be filtered out by the pulmonary blood vessels. This has been suggested as an explanation for the absence of lung metastasis of the primary cancer in about 15% of cases.

Diagnosis

The major differential diagnosis in these patients is that of primary uveal melanoma. The distinction is important as the two conditions are managed differently and carry very different prognoses. Other major differential diagnoses of choroidal metastases are rhegmatogenous retinal detachment and choroidal granulomas. Differentiation of metastatic ocular malignancy from primary uveal melanoma is based on the characteristic clinical findings of flat, infiltrative choroidal lesions with large overlying retinal detachments in metastatic disease, which may be multifocal and bilateral.[260] There is a history of malignancy in many cases, and this is clearly very helpful in the clinical differentiation process. Diffuse choroidal infiltration and vitreous seeding with no obvious choroidal mass has also been described in malignant skin melanoma metastatic to the eye.[286, 287] Primary uveal melanomas, by contrast, are characteristically described as bulky growths with a collar-button appearance, as they rupture through the Bruch's membrane and are associated with small retinal detachments, although this is not always the case. They are generally unilateral, single lesions and have only a weak association with other malignancies (e.g., breast cancer). Serial funduscopic examinations usually show a more rapid growth in the case of metastasis. Amelanotic uveal melanomas may present a difficult differential diagnostic challenge and, while additional studies may provide clues, the clinical examination including indirect ophthalmoscopy usually provides the most reliable means of distinguishing these tumors from choroidal metastases.[154] The iris, in metastatic disease, may show prominent vascularity.

Choroidal metastases exhibit early blockage of the choroidal blood flow on fluorescein angiography, with late staining of and leakage from these vessels. Fluorescein angiography of iris metastases shows extensive leakage of the iris vessels.[288] Ultrasonography shows prominent acoustic brightness with moderate to high internal reflectivity, compared to the characteristic findings of choroidal melanomas on ultrasonography, described previously in this chapter. In the case of effusions and detachments, the metastatic lesions can be difficult to see, and therefore ultrasonography can be extremely valuable in helping to establish the diagnosis.[280]

MRI can also be useful in differentiating metastases from uveal melanomas.[289–291] Uveal melanomas have been described as having a characteristic MRI appearance with a high signal intensity resulting from short T1 relaxation times, (although this is not always the case and clinical correlation of the MRI findings is always essential to avoid misdiagnosis), whereas metastatic tumors can give a wide variety of signals.[292–294] MRI is also clearly helpful for the evaluation of the brain for metastatic lesions.[293]

For iris lesions, anterior chamber tap and cytology have been suggested for diagnosis in difficult cases.[286, 295] Cytologic features of the cells obtained by this method may help distinguish between metastatic and melanotic nodules and also provide clues about the origin of the primary tumor in the case of iris metastases with an occult primary. Direct ciliary body lesion biopsy has also been reported and found to be diagnostic in a case of carcinoid tumor metastatic to the iris.[296]

At the same time, if metastases are suspected in the absence of a known primary, the patient is also evaluated for the primary tumor. Elevated carcinoembryonic antigen (CEA) levels also suggest metastases when a primary tumor has not been identified,[281, 297] but CEA is a nonspecific marker of malignancy. CEA and gamma-glutamyl-transpeptidase levels may be used adjunctively to distinguish metastasis from amelanotic melanomas.[298]

Treatment

By far the most common treatment in patients with ocular metastatic disease is radiotherapy. The patients have metastatic (and therefore often end-stage) disease, so radiation is used for palliation and to improve vision and quality of life; most studies report around a 90% success rate with radiation in achieving stabilization of vision and improved quality of life.[260, 299–305] Radiation is also used when the lesions are causing retinal detachment, or when they are rapidly enlarging despite the fact that the patient is on systemic chemotherapy.[260]

Enucleation is indicated when metastases are suspected but primary uveal melanoma cannot be excluded (although this is rare and eye-saving measures such as needle biopsy of choroidal lesions has been reported[306]); in the case of low-grade malignancies and solitary metastasis to the eye, when excision of the primary malignancy and the solitary metastasis may effect a cure[264, 307, 308] (this may occur with carcinoid tumors or, occasionally, with renal cell carcinomas[309]); and for a blind and intractably painful eye when enucleation may improve the quality of life.

Rarely, in anterior uveal disease, local excision is useful as an eye-preserving measure. When vision is not being threatened, systemic therapy and observation are usually sufficient.[277, 310]

Complications

Complications of radiotherapy include madarosis, radiation-induced cataract, keratoconjunctivitis, and radiation retinopathy. These were discussed in some detail in the earlier section on retinoblastoma. However, many patients do not survive long enough to experience the full force of these side effects.

Prognosis

The prognosis for patients with metastatic ocular disease is poor (overall survival of 6 to 12 months[262]), as metastasis represents disseminated cancer but differs for various primary tumors and with location within the eye. Long-term survival of patients with solitary carcinoid tumor metastatic to the eye has been reported.[307, 308, 311] Breast cancer tends to metastasize late in its course, whereas lung cancer metastasizes early. Cutaneous melanomas also tend to metastasize to the eye later, and in association with widespread metastasis,[286, 287, 311–313] and therefore they have one of the worst prognoses.

Conclusion

Metastatic malignancy to the eye can masquerade as uveitis, and the uveitic masquerade may be the first presenting sign of an occult malignancy. Thus metastases must be considered, especially in the older patient presenting with uveitis refractory to or recurring after steroid therapy. Although the prognosis is poor, as metastatic disease is generally associated with advanced, pre-terminal primary cancers, the importance of making this diagnosis lies in the fact that, with early recognition, a considerable amount can be done to improve the quality of life in these patients.

PARANEOPLASTIC SYNDROMES

Definition

In patients with cancer, symptom complexes that cannot be readily explained, either by local or distant spread of the tumor or by elaboration of hormones indigenous to the tissue from which the malignancy arose, are called paraneoplastic syndromes. A number of different malignancies produce paraneoplastic syndromes with involvement of neuronal tissue—the cerebellum, the anterior horn cells, and the sensory root ganglia to name just a few—and in many of these, the pathogenic factor is the presence of antibodies to CNS antigens. Similarly, paraneoplastic neuronal degeneration of the retinal photoreceptor cells causing both rod and cone dysfunction, and associated with antibodies to certain retinal elements, has been described as cancer-associated retinopathy (CAR). Melanoma-associated retinopathy (MAR) syndrome is another visual paraneoplastic condition. MAR is very similar to CAR, but it is associated with metastases from cutaneous melanomas and with certain distinguishing clinical features. Bilateral diffuse uveal melanocytic proliferation is a recently described paraneoplastic entity characterized by a bilateral, diffuse proliferation of melanocytic cells throughout the uvea in association with a systemic malignant neoplasm.

History

CAR was first described by Sawyer and associates in 1976[314] in a case series of three patients with small cell carcinoma of the lung. These three older patients had vision loss with symptoms before the diagnosis of cancer, early visual field defects of ringlike scotomas, and retinal arteriolar narrowing. Histopathologic examination in these cases revealed widespread, severe degeneration of the outer retinal layers and mild melanophagic activity. In 1982, Kornguth and associates[315] published the first report demonstrating antiretinal ganglion cell antibodies in patients with small cell carcinoma of the lung. In 1987, Thirkill and associates[316] reported the isolation of the 23-kD CAR retinal antigen, and in 1992 they identified it as the photoreceptor component recoverin.[317] Since then, it has been recognized that malignancies other than pulmonary small cell carcinoma, and retinal proteins other than recoverin can be associated with the CAR syndrome.

Epidemiology

CAR seems to be equally common in men and women; in a summary of 28 patients with CAR,[318] 16 were men and 12 were women. The patients are generally older adults, the same summary reporting an age range between 37 and 76 years, with 22 of 28 patients being 60 years or older. Many patients with CAR are smokers, and this is consistent with the preponderance of patients having pulmonary small cell cancer. Thirkill and colleagues,[319] for example, in a series of 10 patients, identify all as heavy smokers.

The most common malignancy associated with CAR is small cell cancer of the lung, seen in about 60% of the cases; however, non–small cell pulmonary cancer, endometrial carcinoma, breast adenocarcinoma, cervical small cell carcinoma, embryonal rhabdomyosarcoma, and melanoma[318] have also been reported to be associated with CAR.

Clinical Characteristics

Characteristically, patients present with fairly rapid, unexplained vision loss occurring over several weeks to months and often associated with photopsias, night blindness, positive transient visual phenomena, and visual field disturbances. The vision loss frequently precedes the diagnosis of a systemic malignancy, thus making diagnosis of CAR less apparent. The time reported between onset of visual symptoms and the diagnosis of cancer varies from a few weeks to several months.[316, 318, 320] Gehrs and Tiedman, for example, report an interval of 18 months in one of their patients.[320]

Vision loss is often asymmetric; the presenting visual acuity may range from 20/20 to light perception.[319] Some people report frank nyctalopia, whereas others report glare and photosensitivity, possibly reflecting differences in the relative involvement of rods or cones. Color vision loss may be present at the time of presentation or may develop over the course of the disease. Transient, painless visual obscurations, including dimming of central vision and loss of peripheral vision, may last from seconds to minutes. Bizarre visual phenomena, such as halos, "floating tissue paper"[314] in the eye, "swarms of bees" over the central vision,[314] and "shimmering curtains" have been reported.

Visual field changes characteristically show initial midperipheral scotomas that eventually lead to classic ring scotomas[321] with central sparing,[319] although there are many variations on this pattern, and central defects may also occur. Arcuate defects, because they result from damage to the outer retina, do not respect the horizontal meridian.[318] These changes may be asymmetrical between the two eyes,[319] and diagnosis of the condition can easily be missed if visual-field testing is not done.

The slit-lamp examination is usually normal.[321] However, there are several reports of patients having vitritis in association with this condition. Thirkill and associates, for example, report vitreous cells in seven of a series of eight patients.[319] Although the vitreous reaction is very often mild, this case series included patients with heavy debris, 2+ cells, and peripheral vitreous clumps of cells. Ohkawa and associates[322] report a case with mild bilateral iridocyclitis and vitritis with retinopathy characterized by a mottled RPE pattern, narrowed arterioles, and several spots of hyperpigmentation.

In the CAR syndrome, the fundus can appear remarkably normal in the early stages of the disease, although subtle arteriolar narrowing is characteristic[321] and disc pallor may or may not be present.[321] Although mottling of the RPE has been described, the appearance of the fundus may be completely normal,[319] thus making diagnosis of the disease even more difficult.

Pathology

Histopathologic study of the eyes in these cases reveals widespread, severe degeneration of the outer retinal layers, and mild melanophagocytic activity. There is "severe disintegration of the photoreceptors, marked loss of nuclei from the outer nuclear layer, and macrophages containing phagocytosed granules from the RPE," with almost complete preservation of the other layers of the retina.[314] There may be variation on this basic pattern, with sparing of cones being reported on the histopathologic examination of the eyes of patients with primarily rod dysfunction clinically and on electroretinography (ERG). Clearly, then, it seems that specific cells in the retina are being targeted in this condition.

The most well-accepted mechanism for the pathogenesis of the CAR syndrome involves autoimmunity to components of the retinal photoreceptors. The most well-recognized antigen to which an autoimmune reaction is produced in CAR, especially in association with small cell carcinoma of the lung, is the 23-kD antigen recoverin, which is a component of the photoreceptor cells. Experimental evidence suggests that there is aberrant expression of recoverin in pulmonary small cell carcinoma, which results in sensitization to this photoreceptor component.[323] Retinal proteins other than the 23-kD antigen have also been implicated in CAR, including 40-kD, 45-kD, and 60-kD proteins, none of which have been cloned to provide the exact protein sequence of the retinal antigen involved.[324]

Diagnosis

The diagnosis can be difficult, especially when the ocular presentation occurs before the systemic neoplastic process has been discovered. Jacobson and associates[321] have described a characteristic triad of photosensitivity, ring scotomas, and attenuation of retinal arteriolar caliber. These, together with the other features described, especially when they occur in the older patient and when abnormalities on the examination of the eye are inconsistent with the degree of symptomatic disability of the patient, should raise the suspicion of CAR.

The ERG pattern can be extremely sensitive in making the diagnosis of CAR, showing reduced amplitudes or being totally flat in these patients; progression of the disease may be associated with progressive reductions in ERG amplitudes.[319] On the other hand, visual acuity may be normal in the presence of a flat ERG, indicating severe retinal dysfunction with relative macular sparing. The relative rod and cone dysfunction in CAR varies from patient to patient: Patients with clinical problems associated with rod dysfunction (e.g., nyctalopia, prolonged dark adaptation, and peripheral or ring scotomas) show

an abnormal scotopic ERG, whereas those with clinical features suggestive of cone dysfunction (e.g., glare and photosensitivity, decreased acuity, and dyschromatopsia) show a typically abnormal cone ERG.[319]

Immunohistochemical testing is also required in these patients, to identify the presence of the antiretinal antibodies. In any patients suspected of having CAR, and with no known malignancy, a search for the systemic malignancy must also be undertaken. Before making the diagnosis of CAR, metastatic involvement of the eye, optic nerve compression, and chemotherapy-induced toxicity need to be excluded.

MAR differs from CAR in that it usually occurs in individuals who have an established diagnosis of cutaneous melanoma, and it is usually found to be associated with metastases. Although cases have been reported in which MAR occurred in the absence of any obvious metastasis after extensive evaluation,[325] caution is advised in declaring such patients metastases free, since an occult metastasis may well become apparent later.

MAR patients are typically men, presenting with shimmering, flickering, or pulsating photopsias, with progressive visual loss over months. Progression of symptoms, although reported, appears to be uncommon. The primary manifestation in MAR is a central visual field defect, with relative sparing of the peripheral visual fields, and ERGs show a characteristic pattern (similar to congenital stationary night blindness) with a markedly reduced b-wave in the presence of a normal dark-adapted a-wave.[326] Such a pattern localizes the pathology to the inner retinal plexes rather than the photoreceptors. Indeed, MAR is not associated with recoverin hypersensitivity, and since it commonly develops long after the primary cancer is discovered, it is thought to involve a different mechanism. Studies have shown the presence of immunoglobulins that react selectively with the bipolar cells of the retina.[327] Identification of MAR is important, as it could be the first sign of metastases in a patient with a seemingly stable or cured condition.

Bilateral diffuse uveal melanocytic proliferation is another condition that frequently presents with visual symptoms prior to the diagnosis of the systemic malignancy. Dilated episcleral vessels, early maturation of cataracts, and moderate vitritis have been described as typical ocular features, with proliferation of choroidal nevus-like lesions, and the presence of round, yellow-orange lesions at the level of the RPE, associated with serous macular detachment. Fluorescein angiography shows numerous window defects of the RPE at the posterior pole. Histopathologic examination shows choroidal thickening with proliferation of benign-looking, spindle-shaped melanocytes. This condition should be suspected in patients with multiple, bilateral uveal nevi, with serous retinal detachment, vitritis, and cataracts. Diagnosis is important as it could lead to the early detection and therefore improved prognosis of a malignancy.

Treatment

Several treatment modalities have been tried with inconsistent results. Treatment is based on the premise that CAR is an autoimmune condition, and therefore immunosuppressive therapies are the mainstay of treatment.

Prednisone, plasmapheresis, and intravenous immunoglobulin have been used, with the antiretinal antibody titers used to monitor treatment.[327] It has been suggested that if antibody titers do not fall to baseline with a particular immunosuppressive agent, changing to other immunosuppressive measures may be necessary.

The treatment for patients with the MAR syndrome is similar to that of CAR.

Prognosis

The visual prognosis of paraneoplastic retinopathies, both CAR and MAR, is generally poor, with different treatment modalities showing inconsistent results. Patients may show no response even on plasmapheresis, presumably because once retinal structures have been irreversibly damaged, immunosuppressive therapy will not reverse the change. However, there have been reports of both CAR and MAR patients who have improved with treatment,[327] and of CAR patients who failed a trial of prednisone and plasmapheresis but responded dramatically to intravenous immunoglobulin.[328]

References

1. Goldey SH, Stern GA, Oblon DJ, et al: Immunophenotypic characterization to an unusual T-cell lymphoma presenting as anterior uveitis. A clinicopathologic case report. Arch Ophthalmol 1989;107:1349–1353.
2. Bishop JE, Salmonsen PC: Presumed intraocular Hodgkin's disease. Ophthalmology 1985;17:589–592.
3. Barr CC, Joondeph HC: Retinal periphlebitis as the initial clinical finding in a patient with Hodgkin's disease. Retina 1983;3:253–257.
4. Kamellin S: Uveitis associated with retinal disease: Report of a case. Arch Ophthalmol 1944;31:517–519.
5. Primbs BB, Monsees EW, Irvine AR: Intraocular Hodgkin's disease. Arch Ophthalmol 1961;66:477–482.
6. Sachs B: Eye conditions in leukemia: Report of four cases. Arch Ophthalmol 1928;57:474–479.
7. Givner I: Malignant lymphoma with ocular involvement: A clinicopathological report. Am J Ophthalmol 1955;39:29–32.
8. Barr CC, Green WR, Payne JW, et al: Intraocular reticulum cell sarcoma: Clinicopathologic study of four cases and review of the literature. Surv Ophthalmol 1975;19:224–239.
9. Klingele TG, Hogan MJ: Ocular reticulum cell sarcoma. Am J Ophthalmol 1975;79:39–47.
10. Lijung B, Char D, Miller D, Deschenes J: Intraocular lymphoma: Cytologic diagnosis and role of immunologic markers. Acta Cytologica 1988;32:840–847.
11. Whitcup SM, deSmet MD, Rubin BI, et al: Intraocular lymphoma. Clinical and histopathological diagnosis. Ophthalmology 1993;100:1399–1406.
12. Hochberg FH, Miller DC: Primary central nervous system lymphoma. J Neurosurg 1988;68:835–853.
13. DeAngelis LM, Yahalom J, Thaler H, et al: Combined modality therapy for primary CNS lymphoma. J Clin Oncol 1992;10:635–643.
14. Helle TL, Britt RH, Colby TV: Primary lymphoma of the central nervous system: Clinicopathological study of experience at Stanford. J Neurosurg 1984;60:94–103.
15. Cohen IJ, Vogel R, Matz S, et al: Successful non-neurotoxic therapy (without radiation) of a multifocal primary brain lymphoma with methotrexate, vincristine, and BCNY protocol (DEMOB). Cancer 1986;57:6–11.
16. Qualman SJ, Mendelsohn G, Mann RB, et al: Intraocular lymphomas: Natural history based on a clinicopathologic study of eight cases and review of the literature. Cancer 1983;52:878–886.
17. Freeman L, Scachat A, Knox D, et al: Clinical features, laboratory investigations and survival in reticulum cell sarcoma. Ophthalmology 1987;94:1631–1639.
18. Siegel MJ, Dalton J, Friedman AJ, et al: Ten-year experience with primary ocular reticulum cell sarcoma (large cell non-Hodgkin lymphoma). Br J Ophthalmol 1989;73:342–346.
19. Akpek EK, Ahmed I, Jakobiec FA, et al: Intraocular—central nervous system lymphoma: Clinical features, diagnosis and outcomes. Ophthalmology 1999;106:1805–1810.
20. Schanzer CM, Font RL, O'Malley RE: Primary ocular malignant lymphoma associated with the acquired immune deficiency syndrome. Ophthalmology 1991;98:88–91.
21. Johnson BL: Intraocular and central nervous system lymphoma in a cardiac transplant recipient. Ophthalmology 1992;99:987–992.
22. Appen RE: Posterior uveitis and primary cerebral reticulum cell sarcoma. Arch Ophthalmol 1975;93:123–124.
23. Rockwood EJ, Zakov ZN, Bay JW: Combined malignant lymphoma of the eye and CNS (reticulum-cell sarcoma). J Neurosurg 1984;61:369–374.
24. Henry JM, Heffner RR Jr, Dillard SH, et al: Primary malignant lymphomas of the central nervous system. Cancer 1974;34:1293–1302.
25. Murray K, Kun L, Cox JW: Primary malignant lymphoma of the central nervous system: Results of treatment of 11 cases and review of the literature. J Neurosurg 1986;65:600–607.
26. Char DJ, Ljung BM, Miller T, Phillips T: Intraocular-CNS lymphoma (ocular reticulum cell sarcoma): Diagnosis and management. Ophthalmology 1988;95:625–630.
27. Baumann MA, Ritch PS, Hande KR, et al: Treatment of intraocular lymphoma with high dose Ara-C. Cancer 1986;57:1273–1275.
28. de Smet ME, Nussenblatt RB, Davis JL, et al: Large cell lymphoma masquerading as a viral retinitis. Int Ophthalmol 1990;14:413–417.
29. Guzak SV: Lymphoma as a cause of hyphema. Arch Ophthalmol 1970;84:229–231.
30. Margolis L, Fraser R, Lichter A, Char D: The role of radiation therapy in the management of ocular reticulum cell sarcoma. Cancer 1980;45:688–692.
31. Corriveau C, Easterbrook M, Payne D: Lymphoma simulating uveitis (masquerade syndrome). Can J Ophthalmol 1986;21:144–149.
32. Gass JD, Sever RJ, Grizzard WS, et al: Multifocal pigment epithelium detachment by reticulum cell sarcoma. A characteristic funduscopic picture. Retina 1984;4:135–143.
33. Nussenblatt RB, Whitcup SM, Palestine AG: Masquerade syndromes. In: Nussenblatt RB, Whitcup SM, Palestine AG, eds: Uveitis: Fundamentals and Clinical Practice, 2nd ed. St. Louis, Mosby Year–Book, 1996, pp 385–395.
34. Fredrick DR, Char DH, Ljung BM, et al: Solitary intraocular lymphoma as an initial presentation of widespread disease. Arch Ophthalmol 1989;107:395–397.
35. Ryan SJ, Zimmerman LE, King FM: Reactive lymphoid hyperplasia: An unusual form of intraocular pseudotumor. Trans Am Acad Ophthalmol Otolaryngol 1972;76:652–671.
36. Jakobiec FA, Sacks E, Kronish JW, et al: Multifocal static creamy choroidal infiltrates: An early sign of lymphoid neoplasia. Ophthalmology 1987;94:397–406.
37. Desroches G, Abrams GW, Gass JDM: Reactive lymphoid hyperplasia of the uvea: A case with ultrasonographic and computed tomographic studies. Arch Ophthalmol 1983;101:725–728.
38. Hoang-Xuan T, Bodaghi B, Toublanc M, et al: Scleritis and mucosal-associated lymphoid tissue lymphoma: A new masquerade syndrome. Ophthalmology 1996;103:631–635
39. Brown SM, Jampol LM, Cantrill HL: Intraocular-CNS lymphoma presenting as retinal vasculitis. Surv Ophthalmol 1994;39:133–140.
40. Rousset F, Garcia E, Defrance T, et al: Interleukin 10 is a potent growth and differentiation factor for activated human B lymphocytes. Proc Natl Acad Sci U S A 1992;89:1890–1893.
41. Borish L, Rosenwasser LJ: Update on cytokines. J Allergy Clin Immunol 1996;97:719–733.
42. El-Shabrawi Y, Livir-Rallatos C, Christen W, et al: High levels of interleukin-12 in the aqueous humor and vitreous of patients with uveitis. Ophthalmology 1998;105:1659–1663.
43. Benjamin D, Kuobloch TJ, Dayton MA: Human interleukin 10: B cell lines derived from patients with AIDS and Burkitt's lymphoma constitutively secrete large quantities of interleukin 10. Blood 1992;80:1289–1298.
44. Stewart JP, Behm FG, Arrand JR, Rooney CM: Differential expression of viral and human interleukin-10 by primary B cell tumor and B cell lines. Virology 1994;200:724–732.
45. Hockenbery DM, Zutter M, Hickey W, et al: BCL2 protein is topographically restricted in tissues characterized by apoptotic cell death. Proc Natl Acad Sci U S A 1991;88:6961–6965.

46. Weiss LM, Warnke RA, Sklar J, Cleary ML: Molecular analysis of the t(14;18) chromosomal translocation in malignant lymphomas. N Engl J Med 1987;317:1185–1189.

47. Katai N, Kuroiwa S, Fujimori K, Yoshimura N: Diagnosis of intra-ocular-CNS lymphoma by polymerase chain reaction. Graefes Arch Clin Exp Ophthalmol 1997;235:431–436.

48. Shen DF, Zhuang Z, LeHoang P, et al: Utility of microdissection and polymerase chain reaction for the detection of immunoglobulin gene rearrangement and translocation in intraocular-CNS lymphoma. Ophthalmology 1998;105:1664–1669.

49. Freilich RJ, DeAngelis LM: Primary central nervous system lymphoma. Neurol Clin 1995;13:901–914.

50. Char DH, Margolis L, Newman AB: Ocular reticulum cell sarcoma. Am J Ophthalmol 1981;91:480–483.

51. Chan CC, Whitcup SC, Solomon D, Nussenblatt RB: Interleukin-10 in the vitreous of patients with primary intraocular lymphoma. Am J Ophthalmol 1995;120:671–673.

52. Whitcup SM, Stark-Vancs V, Wittes RE, et al: Association of interleukin 10 in the vitreous and cerebrospinal fluid and primary central nervous system lymphoma. Arch Ophthalmol 1997; 115:1157–1160.

53. Akpek EK, Maca S, Christen WG, Foster CS: Elevated vitreal interleukin-10 level is not diagnostic of intraocular-CNS lymphoma. Ophthalmology 1999;106:2291–2295.

54. Chen Y-T, Whitney KD, Chen Y: Clonality analysis of B-cell lymphoma in fresh-frozen and paraffin embedded tissues: The effects of variable polymerase chain reaction parameters. Mod Pathol 1994;7:429–434.

55. Abdel-Rheheim FA, Edwards E, Arber DA: Utility of a rapid polymerase chain reaction panel for the detection of molecular changes in B-cell lymphoma. Arch Pathol Lab Med 1996;120:357–363.

56. DeAngelis LM, Yahalom J, Heinemann MH, et al: Primary CNS lymphoma: Combined treatment with chemotherapy and radiotherapy. Neurology 1990;40:80–86.

57. Shapiro WR, Young DF, Tehta B: Methotrexate: Distribution in cerebrospinal fluid after intravenous, intraventricular and lumbar injections. N Engl J Med 1975;293:161–166.

58. Fishburn BC, Wilson DJ, Rosenbaum JT, Neuwelt EA: Intravitreal methotrexate as an adjunctive treatment of intraocular lymphoma. Arch Ophthalmol 1997;115:1152–1156.

59. Rouwen AJP, Wijermans PW, Boen-Tan TN, et al: Intraocular non-Hodgkin's lymphoma treated with systemic and intrathecal chemotherapy and radiotherapy: A case report and review of the literature. Graefes Arch Clin Exp Ophthalmol 1989;227:355–359.

60. Bleyer WA: Neurologic sequelae of methotrexate and ionizing radiation: A new classification. Cancer Treat Rep 1981;65(suppl 1):89–98.

61. Geyer JR, Taylor EM, Histein JM: Radiation, methotrexate, and white matter necrosis: Laboratory evidence for neural radioprotection with pre-irradiation methotrexate. Int J Radiat Oncol Biol Phys 1988;15:373–375.

62. Peterson K, Gordon KB, Heinemann M-H, et al: The clinical spectrum of ocular lymphoma. Cancer 1993;72:843–849.

63. Cotran RS, Kumar V, Robbins SL, eds: Robbins Pathologic Basis Of Disease. Philadelphia, W.B. Saunders, 1994, pp 649–663.

64. Liebreich R: Uber Retinitis Leucaemica and uber Embolie der Arteria Centralis Retinae. Dtsch Klin 1861;13:495–497.

65. Ridgeway EW, Jaffe N, Walton DS: Leukemic ophthalmopathy in children. Cancer 1976;38:1744–1749.

66. Duke-Elder S: System of Ophthalmology, vol 10. St. Louis, CV Mosby, 1967, pp 387–390.

67. Kincaid MC, Green WR: Ocular and orbital involvement in leukemia. Surv Ophthalmol 1983;27:211–232.

68. Aur RJA, Simone J, Hustu HO, et al: Central nervous system therapy and combination chemotherapy of childhood lymphocytic leukemia. Blood 1971;37:272–281.

69. Haghbin M, Tan C, Clarkson B, et al: Intensive chemotherapy in children with acute lymphoblastic leukemia (L2 protocol). Cancer 1973;33:1491–1498.

70. Hustu HO, Aur RJA, Verzosa MD, et al: Prevention of central nervous system leukemia by irradiation. Cancer 1973;32:585–597.

71. Nies B, Bodey G, Thomas LB, et al: The persistence of extramedullary leukemic infiltrates during bone marrow remission of acute leukemia. Blood 1965;26:133–141.

72. Evans AE, Gilbert ES, Zandstra R: The increasing incidence of central nervous system leukemia in children. Cancer 1970;26:404–409.

73. Rosenthal AR: Ocular manifestations of leukemia. Ophthalmology 1983;90:899–905.

74. Ballyntyne AJ, Michaelson IC: Disorders of the blood and blood forming organs. In: Ballentyne AJ, Michaelson IC, eds: Textbook of the Fundus of the Eye. Baltimore, Williams & Wilkins, 1970, pp 287–299.

75. Allen RA, Straatsma BR: Ocular involvement in leukemia-allied disorders. Arch Ophthalmol 1961;66:490–508.

76. Holt JM, Gordon-Smith EC: Retinal abnormalities in diseases of the blood. Br J Ophthalmol 1969;53:145–160.

77. Gass JDM: Differential Diagnosis of Intraocular Tumors: A Stereoscopic Presentation. St. Louis, CV Mosby, 1974, pp 159–176.

78. Kuwabara T, Aiello LM: Leukemic miliary nodules in the retina. Arch Ophthalmol 1964;72:494–497.

79. Schachat AP, Markowitz JA, Guyer DR, et al: Ophthalmic manifestations of leukemia. Arch Ophthalmol 1989;107:697–700.

80. Robb RM, Ervin LD, Sallan SE: A pathologic study of eye involvement in acute leukemia of childhood. Trans Am Ophthalmol Soc 1978;76:90–101.

81. Jampol LM, Goldberg MF, Busse B: Peripheral retinal microaneurysms in chronic leukemia. Am J Ophthalmol 1975;80:242–248.

82. Morse PH, McCready JL: Peripheral retinal neovascularization in chronic myelocytic leukemia. Am J Ophthalmol 1971;72:975–978.

83. Frank RN, Ryan SJ Jr: Peripheral retinal neovascularization with chronic myelogenous leukemia. Arch Ophthalmol 1972;87:585–589.

84. Leveille AS, Morse PH: Platelet-induced retinal neovascularization in leukemia. Am J Ophthalmol 1981;91:640–643.

85. Kincaid MC, Green WR, Kelley JS: Acute ocular leukemia. Am J Ophthalmol 1979;87:698–702.

86. Hine JE, Kingbam JD: Myclogenous leukemia and bilateral exudative retinal detachment. Ann Ophthalmol 1979;11:1867–1872.

87. Newman NM, Smith ME, Gay AJ: An unusual case of leukemia involving the eye: A clinicopathological study. Surv Ophthalmol 1972;16:316–321.

88. Perry HD, Matien FJ: Iris involvement in granulocytic sarcoma. Am J Ophthalmol 1979;87:530–532.

89. Martin B: Infiltration of the iris in chronic lymphatic leukemia. Br J Ophthalmol 1968;52:781–785.

90. Rowan PJ, Sloan JB: Iris and anterior chamber involvement in leukemia. Ann Ophthalmol 1976;8:1081–1085.

91. Holbrook CT, Elsas FJ, Crist WM, Castleberry RP: Acute leukemia and hypopyon. J Pediatr 1978;93:626–628.

92. Zakka K, Yee RD, Shorr N, et al: Leukemic iris infiltration. Am J Ophthalmol 1980;89:204–209.

93. Hinzpeter EN, Knobel H, Freund J: Spontaneous haemophthalmus in leukemia. Ophthalmologica 1978;177:224–228.

94. Tabbara KF, Beckstead JH: Acute promonocytic leukemia with ocular involvement. Arch Ophthalmol 1980;98:1055–1058.

95. Johnston SS, Ware CF: Iris involvement in leukemia. Br J Ophthalmol 1973;57:320–324.

96. Glaser B, Smith JL: Leukemic glaucoma. Br J Ophthalmol 1966;50:92–94.

97. Wolintz AH, Goldstein JU, Seligman BR, et al: Secondary glaucoma in leukemia. Ann Ophthalmol 1971;3:1211–1213.

98. Kozlowski IM, Hirose T, Jalkh AE: Massive subretinal hemorrhage with acute angle-closure glaucoma in chronic myelocytic leukemia. Am J Ophthalmol 1987;103:837–838.

99. Bremner MH, Wright J: Ocular leukemia in acute lymphoblastic leukemia of childhood. Aust J Ophthalmol 1982;10:255–252.

100. Gruenewald RL, Perry MC, Henry PH: Leukemic iritis with hypopyon. Cancer 1979;44:1511–1513.

101. Ninane J, Taylor D, Day S: The eye as a sanctuary in acute lymphoblastic leukemia. Lancet 1980;1:452–453.

102. Reese AB, Guy L: Exophthalmos in leukemia. Am J Ophthalmol 1933;16:718–720.

103. Swartz M, Schumann GB: Acute leukemic infiltration of the vitreous diagnosed by pars plana aspiration. Am J Ophthalmol 1980;90:326–330.

104. Ellis W, Little UL: Leukemic infiltration of the optic nerve head. Am J Ophthalmol 1973;75:867–871.

105. Oakhill A, Willshaw H, Mann JR: Unilateral proptosis. Arch Dis Child 1981;56:549–551.

106. Porterfield JF: Orbital tumors in children: A report on 214 cases. Int Ophthalmol Clin 1962;2:319–335.
107. Rubinfeld RS, Gootenberg JE, Chavis RM, Zimmerman LE: Early onset acute orbital involvement in childhood acute lymphoblastic leukemia. Ophthalmology 1988;95:116–120.
108. Benger RS, Frueh BR: Lacrimal drainage obstruction from lacrimal sac infiltration by lymphocytic neoplasia. Am J Ophthalmol 1986;101:242–245.
109. Davis JL, Parke DW II, Font RL: Granulocytic sarcoma of the orbit. Ophthalmology 1985;92:1758–1762.
110. Neiman RS, Barcos M, Berard C, et al: Granulocytic sarcoma: A clinicopathologic study of 61 biopsied cases. Cancer 1981;48:1426–1437.
111. Zimmerman LE, Font RL: Ophthalmologic manifestations of granulocytic sarcoma. Am J Ophthalmol 1975;80:975–990.
112. Liu P, Ishimaru T, McGregor D, et al: Autopsy study of granulocytic sarcoma in patients with myelogenous leukemia, Hiroshima-Nagasaki, 1949–1969. Cancer 1973;31:948–955.
113. Bhadresa GN: Changes in the anterior segment as a presenting feature in leukemia. Br J Ophthalmol 1971;55:133–135.
114. Gumpel JM: Chronic lymphocytic leukemia presenting as Sjögren's syndrome. Proc R Soc Med 1972;65:877–878.
115. Cullis CM, Hines DR, Bullock JD: Anterior segment ischemia: Classification and description in chronic myelogenous leukemia. Ann Ophthalmol 1979;11:1739–1744.
116. Mahneke A, Vidabaek A: On changes in the optic fundus in leukemia. Acta Ophthalmol 1964;42:201–210.
117. Culler AM: Fundus changes in leukemia. Trans Am Ophthalmol Soc 1951;49:445–473.
118. Guyer DR, Schachat A, Vitale S, et al: Leukemic retinopathy relationship between fundus lesions and hematologic parameters at diagnosis. Ophthalmology 1989;96:860–864.
119. Karesh JW, Goldman EJ, Reck K, et al: A prospective ophthalmic evaluation of patients with acute myeloid leukemia: Correlation of ocular and hematologic findings. J Clin Oncol 1989;7:1528–1532.
120. Hoover DL, Smith LEH, Turner SJ, et al: Ophthalmic evaluation of survivors of acute lymphoblastic leukemia. Ophthalmology 1988;95:151–155.
121. Weaver RG Jr, Chauvenet AR, Smith TJ, Schwartz AC: Ophthalmic evaluation of long-term survivors of childhood acute lymphoblastic leukemia. Cancer 1986;58:963–968.
122. Bunin NJ, Pui C, Hustu HO, Rivera GK: Unusual extramedullary relapses in children with acute lymphoblastic leukemia. J Pediatr 1986;109:665–668.
123. Schwartz CL, Miller NR, Wharam MD, Leventhal BG: The optic nerve as the site of initial relapse in childhood acute lymphoblastic leukemia. Cancer 1989;63:1616–1620.
124. Bleyer WA, Poplack DG: Prophylaxis and treatment of leukemia in the central nervous system and other sanctuaries. Semin Oncol 1985;12:131–148.
125. Champlin R, Gale RP: Acute lymphoblastic leukemia: Recent advances in biology and therapy. Blood 1989;73:2051–2066.
126. Niemeyer CM, Hitchcock-Bryan S, Sallan SE: Comparative analysis of treatment programs for childhood acute lymphoblastic leukemia. Semin Oncol 1985;12:122–130.
127. Ferry AP: Metastatic carcinoma of the eye and ocular adnexa. Int Ophthalmol Clin 1967;7:615.
128. Rones B, Zimmerman LE: The prognosis of primary tumors of the iris treated by iridectomy. Arch Ophthalmol 1958;60:193.
129. Raivio I: Uveal melanoma in Finland: An epidemiological, clinical, histological, and prognostic study. Acta Ophthalmol (Copenh) 1977;55(suppl):133.
130. Jensen OA: Malignant melanomas of the human uvea. Recent follow-up of cases in Denmark, 1943–1952. Acta Ophthalmol (Copenh) 1970;48:1113.
131. Holland G: Clinical features and pathology of pigment tumours of the iris. Klin Monatsbl Augenheilkd 1967;150:359.
132. Ashton N: Primary tumours of the iris. Br J Ophthalmol 1964;48:650.
133. Ashton N, Wybar K: Primary tumours of the iris. Ophthalmologica 1966;151:97.
134. Arentsen JJ, Green WR: Melanoma of the iris: Report of 72 cases treated surgically. Ophthalmol Surg 1975;6:23.
135. Duke JR, Dunn SN: Primary tumors of the iris. Arch Ophthalmol 1958;59:204.
136. Cleasby GW: Malignant melanoma of the iris. Arch Ophthalmol 1958;60:403.
137. Rootman J, Gallagher MA: Color as a risk factor in iris melanoma. Am J Ophthalmol 1984;98:558.
138. Margo CE, McLean IW: Malignant melanoma of the choroid and ciliary body in black patients. Arch Ophthalmol 1984;102:77–79.
139. Graham BJ, Duane TD: Meetings, conferences, symposia: Report of ocular melanoma task force. Am J Ophthalmol 1981;90:728–733.
140. Scotto J, Fraumeni JF, Lee JAH: Melanomas of the eye and other noncutaneous sites. J Natl Cancer Inst 1976;56:489–491.
141. Haukin T, Teppo L, Saxen F: Cancer of the eye: A review of trends and differentials. World Health Stat Q 1978;31:143–158.
142. Jakobiec FA, Silbert G: Are most iris "melanomas" really nevi? A clinicopathologic study of 189 lesions. Arch Ophthalmol 1981;99:2117.
143. Rones B, Zimmerman LE: The production of heterochromia and glaucoma by diffuse malignant melanoma of the iris. Trans Am Acad Ophthalmol Otolaryngol 1957;61:447.
144. Litricin O: Diffuse malignant ring melanoma of the iris and ciliary body. Ophthalmologica 1979;178:235.
145. Reese AB, Mund ML, Iwamoto T: Tapioca melanoma of the iris. Part 1. Clinical and light microscopy studies. Am J Ophthalmol 1972;74:840.
146. Zakka KA, Foos R, Sulit H: Metastatic tapioca melanoma. Br J Ophthalmol 1979;63:744.
147. Shields JA. Melanocytic tumors of the iris. In: Shields JA, ed: Diagnosis and Management of Intraocular Tumors. St. Louis, CV Mosby, 1983, pp 83–121.
148. Shields JA, Sanborn GE, Augsburger JJ: The differential diagnosis of malignant melanoma of the iris. Ophthalmology 1983;90:716.
149. Char DH: Anterior uveal tumors. In: Char DH, ed: Clinical Ocular Oncology. New York, Churchill-Livingstone, 1989, pp 91–149.
150. Territo C, Shields CL, Shields JA, et al: Natural course of melanocytic tumors of the iris. Ophthalmology 1988;95:1251.
151. Shields JA, Kline MW, Augsburger JJ: Primary iris cysts: A review of the literature and report of 62 cases. Br J Ophthalmol 1984;68:152.
152. Jensen OA: Malignant melanomas of the uvea in Denmark, 1943–1952: A clinical, histopathological and prognostic study. Acta Ophthalmol Suppl 1963;75:1–220.
153. Lischko AM, Seddon JM, Gragoudas ES, et al: Evaluation of prior primary malignancy as a determinant of uveal melanoma. Ophthalmology 1989;96:1716–1721.
154. Char DH, Stone RD, Irvine AR, et al: Diagnostic modalities in choroidal melanoma. Am J Ophthalmol 1980;89:223–230.
155. Gass JDM: Problems in the differential diagnosis of choroidal nevi and malignant melanomas. The 33rd Edward Jackson Memorial Lecture. Am J Ophthalmol 1977;83:299–323.
156. Font RL, Spaulding A, Zimmerman L: Diffuse malignant melanoma of the uveal tract: A clinicopathologic report of 54 cases. Trans Am Acad Ophthalmol Otolaryngol 1968;72:877–895.
157. Fraser DJ, Font RL: Ocular inflammation and hemorrhage as initial manifestation of uveal malignant melanoma. Arch Ophthalmol 1979;97:1311–1314.
158. Haddab SA, Hidayat A, Tabbara KF: Ciliary body melanoma with optic nerve invasion. Br J Ophthalmol 1990;74:123–124.
159. Furdova A, Strmen P, Olah Z: Intraocular malignant melanoma in intermediate uveitis treated conservatively and surgically for a prolonged period. Cesk Oftal 1994;50:286–291.
160. Johnson MW, Skuta GL, Kincaid MC, et al: Malignant melanoma of the iris in xeroderma pigmentosum. Arch Ophthalmol 1989;107:402.
161. Cialdini AP, Sahel JA, Jalkh AE, et al: Malignant transformation of an iris melanocytoma. Graefes Arch Clin Exp Ophthalmol 1989;227:348.
162. Callender GR: Malignant melanocytic tumors of the eye. A study of histologic types in 111 cases. Trans Am Acad Ophthalmol Otolaryngol 1931;36:131.
163. McLean IW, Zimmerman LE, Evans RM: Reappraisal of Callender's spindle: A type of malignant melanoma of choroid and ciliary body. Am J Ophthalmol 1978;86:557.
164. Wilder HC, Paul EV: Malignant melanoma of the choroid and ciliary body. A study of 2535 cases. Milit Surgeon 1962;109:370.
165. McLean IW, Foster WD, Zimmerman LE: Prognostic factors in small malignant melanomas of choroid and ciliary body. Arch Ophthalmol 1977;95:48.

166. Callender GR, Wilder HC, Ash JE: Five hundred melanomas of the choroid and ciliary body followed five years or longer. Am J Ophthalmol 1942;25:962.
167. Kersten RC, Tse DT, Anderson R: Iris melanoma—Nevus or malignancy? Surv Ophthalmol 1985;29:423.
168. Jakobiec FA, Depot MJ, Henkind P, Spencer WH: Fluorescein angiographic patterns of iris melanocytic tumors. Arch Ophthalmol 1982;100:1288.
169. Brovkina AF, Chichua AG: Value of fluorescein iridography in diagnosis of tumours of the iridociliary zone. Br J Ophthalmol 1979;63:157.
170. Demeler U: Fluorescence angiographical studies in the diagnosis and follow-up of tumors of the iris and ciliary body. Adv Ophthalmol 1981;42:1.
171. Geisse LJ, Robertson DM: Iris melanomas. Am J Ophthalmol 1985;99:638.
172. Gass JDM: Observations of suspected choroidal and ciliary body melanomas for evidence of growth prior to enucleation. Ophthalmology 1980;87:523–528.
173. Mafee MF, Peyman GA, McKusick MA: Malignant uveal melanoma and similar lesions studied by computed tomography. Radiology 1985;156:403–408.
174. Peyster RG, Augsburger JJ, Shields JA, et al: Choroidal melanoma: Comparison of CT, funduscopy, and ultrasound. Radiology 1985;156:675–680.
175. Bischoff PM, Flower RW: Ten years' experience with choroidal angiography using indocyanine green dye: A new routine examination or an epilogue? Doc Ophthalmol 1985;60:235–291.
176. Shields JA: Current approaches to the diagnosis and management of choroidal melanomas. Surv Ophthalmol 1977;21:443–463.
177. Shields JA, McDonald PR, Leonard BC, Canny CLB: The diagnosis of uveal malignant melanoma in eyes with opaque media. Am J Ophthalmol 1977;83:95–105.
178. Wollensak J, Heinrich M: In vivo and in vitro measurements of P uptake in the ocular tissue in cases of malignant melanoma. Graefes Arch Clin Exp Ophthalmol 1981;217:35–44.
179. McLean IW, Shields JA: Prognostic value of P uptake in posterior uveal melanoma. Ophthalmology 1980;87:543–548.
180. Boniuk M, Ruiz RS: Viewpoints. The P test in the diagnosis of ocular melanoma. Surv Ophthalmol 1980;24:671–678.
181. Goldberg B, Kara GB, Previtte LR: The use of radioactive phosphorus (P) in the diagnosis of ocular tumors. Am J Ophthalmol 1980;90:817–828.
182. Gragoudas ES, Char DH: Charged particle irradiation of uveal melanomas. In: Albert PM, Jakobiec FA, eds: Principles and Practice of Ophthalmology, vol 5. Philadelphia, W.B. Saunders, 1994, pp 3233–3244.
183. Gragoudas ES, Goitein M, Verhey L, et al: Proton beam irradiation of uveal melanomas: Preliminary results. Arch Ophthalmol 1978;96:1583–1591.
184. Char DH, Phillips TL, Andrejeski Y, et al: Failure of preenucleation radiation to decrease the uveal melanoma mortality. Am J Ophthalmol 1988;106:21–26.
185. Sunba MSN, Rahi AHS, Morgan G: Tumors of the anterior uvea. 1. Metastasizing malignant melanoma of the iris. Arch Ophthalmol 1980;98:82.
186. Char DH, Crawford JB, Gonzales J, Miller T: Iris melanoma with increased intraocular pressure. Differentiation of focal solitary tumors from diffuse or multiple tumors. Arch Ophthalmol 1989;107:548.
187. Grossniklaus HE, Brown RH, Stuiting RD, Blasberg RD: Iris melanoma seeding through a trabeculectomy site. Arch Ophthalmol 1990;108:1287.
188. Omulecki W, Prusczynski M, Borowski J: Ring melanoma of the iris and ciliary body. Br J Ophthalmol 1985;69:514.
189. Planten JT: An unnecessary mistake. Ophthalmologica 1970;160:369.
190. Margo CE, Groden LR: Iris melanoma with extensive corneal invasion and metastases. Am J Ophthalmol 1987;104:543.
191. Fraunfelder FT, Boozman FW III, Wilson RS, et al: No-touch technique for intraocular malignant melanomas. Arch Ophthalmol 1977;95:1616–1620.
192. Kramer KK, LaPiana FG, Whitmore PV: Enucleation with stabilization of intraocular pressure in the treatment of uveal melanomas. Ophthalmic Surg 1977;11:39–43.
193. Moses KC, LaPiana FG: Controlled enucleation. Ophthalmic Surg 1987;18:379–382.
194. Niederkorn JY: Enucleation induced metastases of intraocular melanomas in mice. Ophthalmology 1984;91:692–700.
195. Zimmerman LE: Histopathological considerations in the management of tumors of the iris and ciliary body. Ann Inst Barraquer 1971;10:27.
196. Chang M, Zimmerman LE, McLean IW: The persisting pseudomelanoma problem. Arch Ophthalmol 1984;102:726–727.
197. Zimmerman LE: Retinoblastoma and retinocytoma. In: Spencer WH, ed: Ophthalmic Pathology. Philadelphia, W.B. Saunders, 1985, p 1292.
198. Tso MOM, Zimmerman LE, Fine BS: The nature of retinoblastoma. 1. Photoreceptor differentiation: A clinical and histologic study. Am J Ophthalmol 1970;69:339–350.
199. Albert DM, Robinson N: James Wardrop: A brief review of his life and contributions. Wardrop Lecture, 1974. Trans Ophthalmol Soc UK 1974;94:892–908.
200. Duke-Elder S, Dobree JH: System of Ophthalmology, vol 10. Diseases of the Retina. St. Louis, CV Mosby, 1967, p 672.
201. Cassady JR, Sagerman RH, Tretter P, et al: Radiation therapy in retinoblastoma. Radiology 1969;93:405–409.
202. Abramson DH, Ellsworth RM, Grumbach N, et al: Retinoblastoma: Survival, age at detection, and comparison 1914–1958, 1958–1983. J Pediatr Ophthalmol Strabismus 1985;22:246–250.
203. Schappert-Kimmijser J, Hemmes GD, Nijland R: The heredity of retinoblastoma. Ophthalmologica 1966;152:197–213.
204. Shields JA, Augsburger JJ: Current approaches to the diagnosis and management of retinoblastoma. Surv Ophthalmol 1981;25:347–372.
205. Ellsworth RM: The practical management of retinoblastoma. Trans Am Ophthalmol Soc 1969;67:463–534.
206. Kuchle HJ, Remky H, Sattler R: Diagnosis of gliomatous pseudouveitis, report of a case. Am J Ophthalmol 1959;47:185.
207. Weizenblatt S: Differential difficulties in atypical retinoblastoma, report of a case. AMA Arch Ophthalmol 1957;58:699.
208. Stafford WR, Yannoff M, Parnell BL: Retinoblastoma initially misdiagnosed as primary ocular inflammation. Arch Ophthalmol 1969;82:771–773.
209. Kodilinge HC: Retinoblastoma in Nigeria: Problems in treatment. Am J Ophthalmol 1967;63:469–481.
210. Bader JL, Meadows AT, Zimmerman LE, et al: Bilateral retinoblastoma with ectopic intracranial retinoblastoma: Trilateral retinoblastoma. Cancer Genet Cytogenet 1982;5:203–213.
211. Kingston JE, Plowman PN, Hungerford JL: Ectopic intracranial retinoblastoma in childhood. Br J Ophthalmol 1985;69:742–748.
212. Howard GM, Ellsworth RM: Differential diagnosis of retinoblastoma. A statistical survey of 500 children. I: Relative frequency of the lesions which simulate retinoblastoma. II: Factors relating to the diagnosis of retinoblastoma. Am J Ophthalmol 1965;60:610–621.
213. Pratt CB, Meyer D, Chenaille P, et al: The use of bone marrow aspirates and lumbar puncture at the time of diagnosis of retinoblastoma. J Clin Oncol 1989;7:140–143.
214. Ellsworth RM: The management of retinoblastoma. Jpn J Ophthalmol 1978;22:389–395.
215. Donoso LA, Shields JA, Felberg NT, et al: Intracranial malignancy in patients with bilateral retinoblastoma. Retina 1981;1:67–74.
216. Shields JA, Michelson JB, Leonard BC, et al: B-scan ultrasonography in the diagnosis of atypical retinoblastomas. Can J Ophthalmol 1976;11:42–51.
217. Hermsen VM: Echographic diagnosis. In: Blodi FC, ed: Retinoblastoma. New York, Churchill-Livingstone, 1985, pp 111–127.
218. Pratt CB, Crom DB, Magill L, et al: Skeletal scintigraphy in patients with bilateral retinoblastoma. Cancer 1990;65:26–28.
219. Benhamou E, Borges J, Tso MOM: Magnetic resonance imaging in retinoblastoma and retinocytoma: A case report. J Pediatr Ophthalmol Strabismus 1989;26:276–280.
220. Piro P, Abramson DH, Ellsworth RM, et al: Aqueous humor lactate dehydrogenase in retinoblastoma patients. Arch Ophthalmol 1978;96:1823–1825.
221. Das A, Roy IS, Maitra TK: Lactate dehydrogenase level and protein pattern in the aqueous humour of patients with retinoblastoma. Can J Ophthalmol 1983;18:337–339.
222. Abramson DH, Piro PA, Ellsworth RM, et al: Lactate dehydrogen-

ase levels and isozyme patterns. Measurements in the aqueous humor and serum of retinoblastoma patients. Arch Ophthalmol 1979;97:870–871.

223. Jakobiec FA, Abramson D, Scher R: Increased aqueous lactate dehydrogenase in Coats' disease. Am J Ophthalmol 1978;85:686–689.

224. Dayal Y, Goyal JL, Jaffery NF, Agarwal HC: Lactate dehydrogenase levels in aqueous humor and serum in retinoblastoma. Jpn J Ophthalmol 1985;29:417–422.

225. Armstrong DI: The use of 4–6 meV electrons for the conservative treatment of retinoblastoma. Br J Radiol 1974;47:326–331.

226. Weiss DR, Cassady JR, Peterson R: Retinoblastoma: A modification in the radiation therapy technique. Radiology 1975;114:705–708.

227. Schipper J: An accurate and simple method for megavoltage radiation therapy of retinoblastoma. Radiother Oncol 1983;1:31–41.

228. Schipper J, Tan KEWP, van Peperzeel HA: Treatment of retinoblastoma by precision megavoltage radiation radiotherapy. Radiother Oncol 1985;3:117–132.

229. Harnett AN, Hungerford JL, Lambert GD, et al: Improved external beam radiotherapy for the treatment of retinoblastoma. Br J Radiol 1987;60:753–760.

230. Abramson DH: The focal treatment of retinoblastoma with emphasis on xenon arc photocoagulation. Acta Ophthalmol 1989;67(suppl 194):7–63.

231. Bedford MA, Bedotto C, McFaul PA: Retinoblastoma: A study of 139 cases. Br J Ophthalmol 1971;55:19–27.

232. Ellsworth RM: Orbital retinoblastoma. Trans Am Ophthalmol Soc 1974;72:79–88.

233. Shields JA, Augsburger JJ, Donoso LA: Recent developments related to retinoblastoma. J Pediatr Ophthalmol Strabismus 1986;23:148–152.

234. Abramson DH, Ellsworth RM, Rozakis GW: Cryosurgery for retinoblastoma. Arch Ophthalmol 1982;100:1253–1256.

235. Peterson RA: Retinoblastoma: Diagnosis and nonradiation therapies. In: Albert DM, Jakobiec FA, eds: Principles and Practice of Ophthalmology, vol 5. Philadelphia, W.B. Saunders, 1994, pp 3279–3285.

235a. Cassady JR: Radiation therapy for retinoblastoma. In: Albert DM, Jakobiec FA, eds: Principles and Practice of Ophthalmology, vol 5. Philadelphia, W.B. Saunders, 1994, pp 3285–3297.

236. Ohnishi Y, Yamana Y, Minei M: Photoradiation therapy using argon laser and a hematoporphorin derivative for retinoblastoma: A preliminary report. Jpn J Ophthalmol 1986;30:409–419.

237. Benedict WF, Lingua RW, Doiron DR, et al: Tumor regression of human retinoblastoma in the nude mouse following photoradiation therapy: A preliminary report. Med Pediatr Oncol 1980;8:397–401.

238. Grier HE, Weinstein HJ, Revesz T, et al: Cytogenetic evidence for involvement of erythroid progenitors in a child with therapy-linked myelodysplasia. Br J Hematology 1986;64:513–519.

239. Petersen RA, Friend S, Albert D: Prolonged survival of a child with metastatic retinoblastoma. J Pediatr Ophthalmol Strabismus 1987;24:247–248.

240. Keith CG: Chemotherapy in retinoblastoma management. Ophthalmic Paediatr Genet 1989;10:93–98.

241. Saleh RA, Gross S, Cassano W, et al: Metastatic retinoblastoma successfully treated with immunomagnetic-purged autologous bone marrow transplantation. Cancer 1988;62:2301–2303.

242. Grabowski EF, Abramson DH: Intraocular and extraocular retinoblastoma. Hematol Oncol Clin North Am 1987;1:721–735.

243. Sanders BM, Draper GJ, Kingston JE: Retinoblastoma in Great Britain 1969–80: Incidence, treatment and survival. Br J Ophthalmol 1988;72:576–583.

244. Goble RR, McKenzie J, Kingston JE, et al: Orbital recurrence of retinoblastoma successfully treated by combined therapy. Br J Ophthalmol 1990;74:97–98.

245. Redier LD, Ellsworth RM: Prognostic importance of choroidal invasion in retinoblastoma. Arch Ophthalmol 1973;90:294–296.

246. Abramson DH, Ellsworth RM, Kitchin D, et al: Second monocular tumors in retinoblastoma survivors: Are they radiation induced? Ophthalmology 1984;91:1351–1355.

247. Kitchen FD, Ellsworth RE: Pleitropic effects of the gene for retinoblastoma. J Med Genet 1974;11:244–246.

248. Roarty JD, McLean IW, Zimmerman LE: Incidence of second neoplasms in patients with bilateral retinoblastoma. Ophthalmology 1988;95:1583–1587.

249. Der Kinderen DJ, Koten JW, Wolterbeck R, et al: Nonocular cancer in hereditary retinoblastoma survivors and relatives. Ophthalmic Pediatr Genet 1987;8:23–25.

250. Draper GJ, Sanders BM, Kingston JE: Second primary neoplasms in patients with retinoblastoma. Br J Ophthalmol 1986;53:661–671.

251. Lueder GT, Judisch GF, O'Gorman TW: Second monocular tumors in survivors of hereditary retinoblastoma. Arch Ophthalmol 1986;104:372–373.

252. Schifter S, Vendelgo L, Jensen OM, Kaae S: Ewing's tumor following bilateral retinoblastoma. Cancer 1983;51:1746–1749.

253. Traboulski EI, Zimmerman L, Manz HJ: Cutaneous malignant melanoma in survivors of hereditable retinoblastoma. Arch Ophthalmol 1988;106:1059–1061.

254. Pesin SR, Shields JA: Seven cases of trilateral retinoblastoma. Am J Ophthalmol 1989;107:121–126.

255. Bloch RS, Gartner S: The incidence of ocular metastatic carcinoma. Arch Ophthalmol 1971;85:673.

256. Horner F: Carcinoma der Dura Mater Exophthaimus. Klin Monatsbl Augenheilkd 1864;2:186.

257. Duke-Elder S, ed: System of Ophthalmology, vol 9. Disease of the Uveal Tract. St Louis, CV Mosby, 1966, p 917.

258. Godtfredsen E: On the frequency of secondary carcinoma of the choroid. Acta Ophthalmol 1944;22:394.

259. Albert DM, Rubenstein RA, Scheie HG: Tumor metastases to the eye. Part 1. Incidence in 213 patients with generalized malignancy. Am J Ophthalmol 1967;63:723.

260. Mewis L, Young SE: Breast carcinoma metastatic to the choroid: Analysis of 67 patients. Ophthalmology 1982;89:147.

261. Nelson CC, Hertzberg BS, Klintworth GK: A histopathologic study of 716 eyes in patients with cancer at the time of death. Am J Ophthalmol 1983;95:788.

262. Ferry AP, Font RL: Carcinoma metastatic to the eye and orbit. 1. A clinicopathologic study of 227 cases. Arch Ophthalmol 1974;92:276.

263. Freedman ML, Folk JC: Metastatic tumors to the eye and orbit: Patient survival and clinical characteristics. Arch Ophthalmol 1987;105:121.

264. Stephens RF, Shields JA: Diagnosis and management of cancer metastatic to the uvea: A study of 70 cases. Ophthalmology 1979;86:1336.

265. Hart WM: Metastatic carcinoma to the eye and orbit. Int Ophthalmol Clin 1962;2:465.

266. Reese AG: Tumors of the Eye, 2nd ed. New York, Hoeber, 1963.

267. Castro PA, Albert DM, Wang WJ, Ni C: Tumors metastatic to the eye and adnexa. Int Ophthalmol Clin 1982;22:189.

268. Sanders TE: Metastatic carcinoma of the iris. Am J Ophthalmol 1938;21:646.

269. Green WR: The uveal tract. In: Spencer WH, ed: Ophthalmic Pathology: An Atlas and Textbook, 3rd ed, vol 3. Philadelphia, W.B. Saunders, 1985, pp 1352–2140.

270. Boldt HC, Nerrad JA: Orbital metastases from prostate carcinoma. Arch Ophthalmol 1988;106:1403.

271. Guttmann SM, Weiss JS, Albert DM: Choroidal metastases of adenocytic carcinoma of the salivary gland. Br J Ophthalmol 1986;70:100.

272. Small KW, Rosenwasser GO, Alexander EA III, et al: Presumed choroidal metastasis of Merkel cell carcinoma. Ann Ophthalmol 1990;22:187.

273. Mooy CM, de Jong PTVM, Verbeek AM: Choroidal metastasis of oesophageal squamous cell carcinoma. Int Ophthalmol 1990;14:63.

274. Scilletta B, Racalbuto A, Russello D, et al: Carcinoma of the male breast and ocular metastases. Ital J Surg Sci 1989;19:93.

275. Schlaen ND, Naves AE: Orbital and choroidal metastases from carcinoma of the male breast. Arch Ophthalmol 1986;104:1344.

276. Kurosawa A, Sawaguchi S: Iris metastasis from squamous cell carcinoma of the uterine cervix. Arch Ophthalmol 1987;105:618.

277. Barondes MJ, Hamilton AM, Ifungerford J, et al: Treatment of choroidal metastasis from choriocarcinoma. Arch Ophthalmol 1989;107:796.

278. Henkind P, Roth MS: Breast carcinoma and concurrent uveal melanoma. Am J Ophthalmol 1971;71:198.

279. Ferry AP, Font RL: Carcinoma metastatic to the eye and orbit. II. A clinicopathological study of 26 patients with carcinoma metastatic to the anterior segment of the eye. Arch Ophthalmol 1975;93:472.

280. Sneed SR, Byrne SF, Mieler WF, et al: Choroidal detachment associated with malignant choroidal tumors. Ophthalmology 1991;98:963.

281. Denslow GT, Kielar RA: Metastatic adenocarcinoma to the anterior uvea and increased carcinoembryonic antigen levels. Am J Ophthalmol 1978;85:363.

282. Jensen OA: Metastatic tumors to the eye and orbit. A histopathological analysis of a Danish series. Acta Pathol Microbiol Scand 1970;212:201.

283. Albert DM, Rubenstein RA, Scheie HG: Tumor metastasis to the eye. Part II. Clinical study in infants and children. Am J Ophthalmol 1967;63:727.

284. Goldberg RA, Rootman J, Cline RA: Tumors metastatic to the orbit: A changing picture. Surv Ophthalmol 1990;35:1.

285. Hutchison DS, Smith TR: Ocular and orbital metastatic carcinoma. Ann Ophthalmol 1979;11:869.

286. Char DH, Schwartz A, Miller TR, et al: Ocular metastases from systemic melanoma. Am J Ophthalmol 1980;90:702.

287. Fishman ML, Tomaszewski MM, Kuwabara T: Malignant melanoma of the skin metastatic to the eye. Arch Ophthalmol 1976;94:1309.

288. Freeman TR, Friedman AH: Metastatic carcinoma of the iris. Am J Ophthalmol 1975;80:947.

289. Peyman GA, Matee MF: Uveal melanoma and similar lesions: The role of magnetic resonance imaging and computed tomography. Radiat Clin North Am 1987;25:471.

290. Peyster RG, Shapiro MD, Haik BG: Orbital metastases: Role of magnetic resonance imaging and computed tomography. Radiat Clin North Am 1987;25:647.

291. Raymond WR IV, Char DH, Norman D: Magnetic resonance imaging evaluation of uveal tumors. Am J Ophthalmol 1991;111:633.

292. Mafee MF, Peyman GA, Peace JH, et al: Magnetic resonance imaging in the evaluation and differentiation of uveal melanoma. Ophthalmology 1987;94:341.

293. Haik BG, Saint Louis L, Smith ME, et al: Magnetic resonance imaging in choroidal tumors. Ann Ophthalmol 1987;19:218.

294. Liu KR, Peyman GA, Mafee MF, et al: False positive magnetic resonance imaging of a choroidal nevus simulating a choroidal melanoma. Int Ophthalmol 1989;13:265.

295. Scholz R, Green WR, Baranano EC, et al: Metastatic carcinoma of the iris. Diagnosis by aqueous paracentesis and response to irradiation and chemotherapy. Ophthalmology 1983;90:1524.

296. Bardenstein DS, Char DH, Jones C, et al: Metastatic ciliary body carcinoid tumor. Arch Ophthalmol 1990;108:1590.

297. Denslow GT, Kielar RA: Metastatic adenocarcinoma to the anterior uvea and elevated CEA levels. Cancer 1978;42:1504.

298. Michelson JB, Felberg NT, Shields JA: Evaluation of metastatic cancer to the eye. Carcinoembryonic antigen and gamma glutamyl transpeptidase. Arch Ophthalmol 1977;95:692.

299. Bradly LW, Shields JA, Augsberger JJ, et al: Malignant tumors of the eye. In: Mansfield CM, ed: Therapeutic Radiology, 2nd ed. New York, Elsevier, 1989.

300. Maor M, Chan RC, Young SE: Radiotherapy of choroidal metastases. Breast cancer as primary site. Cancer 1977;40:2081.

301. Dobrowsky W: Treatment of choroidal metastases. Br J Radiat 1988;61:140.

302. Minatel E, Forber L, Trovo MG, et al: The efficacy of radiotherapy in the treatment of intraocular metastases. Rays (Roma) 1988;13:95.

303. Orenstein M, Anderson D, Stein J: Choroidal metastases. Cancer 1972;29:1101.

304. Reddy S, Saxena VS, Hendrickson F, et al: Malignant metastatic disease of the eye: Management of an uncommon complication. Cancer 1981;47:810.

305. Brady LW, Shields JA, Augsburger JJ, et al: Malignant intraocular tumors. Cancer 1982;49:578.

306. Augsburger JJ: Fine needle aspiration of suspected metastatic cancers to the posterior uvea. Trans Am Ophthalmol Soc 1988;86:499.

307. Bell RM, Bullock JD, Albert DM: Solitary choroidal metastasis from bronchial carcinoid. Br J Ophthalmol 1975;59:155.

308. Rodrigues MM, Shields JA: Iris metastasis from a bronchial carcinoid tumor. Arch Ophthalmol 1978;96:77.

309. Kindermann WR, Shields JA, Eiferman RA, et al: Metastatic renal cell carcinoma to the eye and adnexa. A report of three cases and review of the literature. Ophthalmology 1981;88:1347.

310. Sierocki JS, Norman CC, Schafrank M, et al: Carcinoma metastatic to the anterior ocular segment: Response to chemotherapy. Cancer 1980;45:2521.

311. Font RL, Kaufer G, Winstanley RA: Metastases of bronchial carcinoid to the eye. Am J Ophthalmol 1966;62:723.

312. Shields JA, Shields CL, Shakin EP, et al: Metastasis of choroidal melanoma to the contralateral choroid, orbit and eyelid. Br J Ophthalmol 1988;72:456.

313. Orcutt JC, Char DH: Melanoma metastatic to the orbit. Ophthalmology 1988;95:1033.

314. Sawyer RA, Selhorst JB, Zimmerman LE, et al: Blindness caused by photoreceptor degeneration as a remote effect of cancer. Am J Ophthalmol 1976;81:606–613.

315. Kornguth SE, Klein R, Appen R, Choate J: Occurrence of anti-retinal ganglion cell antibodies in patients with small cell carcinoma of the lung. Cancer 1982;50;1289–1293.

316. Thirkill CE, Roth AM, Keltner JL: Cancer associated retinopathy. Arch Ophthalmol 1987;105:372–375.

317. Thirkill CE, Tait RC, Tyler NK, et al: The cancer-associated retinopathy antigen is a recoverin-like protein. Invest Ophthalmol Vis Sci 1992;33;2768–2772.

318. Rizzo JF, Volpe NJ: Cancer associated retinopathy. In: Pepose JS, Holland GN, Wilhelmus KR, eds. Ocular Infection and Immunity. St Louis, Mosby, 1996, pp 585–599.

319. Thirkill CE, Keltner JL, Tyler NK, Roth AM: Antibody reactions with retina and cancer-associated antigens in 10 patients with cancer associated retinopathy. Arch Ophthalmol 1993;111:931–937.

320. Gehrs K, Tiedman J: Hemeralopia in an older adult. Surv Ophthalmol 1992;37:185–189.

321. Jacobson DM, Thirkill CE, Tipping SJ: A clinical triad to diagnose paraneoplastic retinopathy. Ann Neurol 1990;28:162–167.

322. Ohkawa T, Kawashima H, Makino S, et al: Cancer associated retinopathy in a patient with endometrial cancer. Am J Ophthalmol 1996;122:740–742.

323. Klenchin VA, Kalvert PD, Mounds MD: Inhibition of rhodopsin kinase by recoverin. A further evidence for a negative feedback system in phototransduction. J Biol Chem 1995;270:16147–16152.

324. Murphy MA, Thirkill CE, Hart WM: Paraneoplastic retinopathy: A novel autoantibody reaction associated with small cell lung carcinoma. J Neuroophthalmol 1996;17:77–83.

325. Thirkill CE, Keltner JL: Commonality and diversity in melanoma-associated retinopathy (MAR). ARVO abstracts. Invest Ophthalmol Vis Sci 1998;39(suppl 4):S363.

326. Keltner JL, Thirkill CE: Cancer-associated retinopathy vs recoverin-associated retinopathy. Arch Ophthalmol 1993;111:931–937.

327. Weinstein JM, Kelman SE, Bresnick GH, Kornguth SE: Paraneoplastic retinopathy associated with antiretinal bipolar cell antibodies in cutaneous malignant melanoma. Ophthalmology 1994;101:1236–1243.

328. Guy J, Aptsiauri N: IVIg protocol: Reversal of carcinoma-associated retinopathy (CAR) induced blindness with IVIg. Neurology 1997;48(suppl):A329–A330.

MASQUERADE SYNDROMES: ENDOPHTHALMITIS

C. Michael Samson and C. Stephen Foster

Intraocular inflammations due to infections are among the most challenging entities capable of masquerading as autoimmune uveitis. Clues implicating infectious microbes can be subtle or absent. And unlike the other masquerade syndromes, initiating treatment with corticosteroids or immunomodulators in this class of disorders can result in devastating consequences.

Two forms of endophthalmitis can masquerade as non-infectious inflammation: chronic postoperative endophthalmitis and endogenous endophthalmitis. The other forms, acute postoperative endophthalmitis and traumatic endophthalmitis, are more easily recognized and rarely pose the diagnostic dilemma often associated with the aforementioned forms. This chapter addresses the characteristics of chronic postoperative and endogenous endophthalmitis, and the approach to their management.

CHRONIC POSTOPERATIVE ENDOPHTHALMITIS

Definition

Chronic postoperative endophthalmitis is a clinical syndrome characterized by recurrent episodes of low-grade inflammation secondary to microbes introduced into the eye during intraocular surgery. Some authors distinguish this syndrome from acute postoperative endophthalmitis by assigning a specific time of onset: inflammation beginning more than 1 month after surgery is defined as the chronic form, whereas inflammation beginning less than 1 month after surgery is considered acute.[1, 2] However, this is a potential source of confusion, since no single cutoff time can reliably differentiate between the two forms, which are strikingly different clinical entities.

More potential confusion can result from the term delayed-onset endophthalmitis being used synonymously with chronic postoperative endophthalmitis.[1] Although it is technically accurate, other authors have used delayed onset to describe cases of postoperative endophthalmitis that occur 8 days to 2 weeks after surgery that clinically resemble the more explosive acute form.[3] To the authors' knowledge, there is no consensus on the appropriate use of these terms. Table 49–1 displays our proposed use of these three terms based more on clinical presentation and less on arbitrarily assigned times of onset. For the purpose of this book, the definition of chronic postoperative endophthalmitis is as displayed in this table.

History

The term chronic postoperative endophthalmitis was first used by Roussel and colleagues in a report describing two cases of endophthalmitis due to *Propionibacterium acnes*.[4] The first report implicating microbes as a cause of chronic postoperative intraocular inflammation was the first case report of chronic *P. acnes* endophthalmitis, pub-

lished the previous year.[5] Since then, other case reports have identified other organisms capable of producing a clinical picture similar to that caused by *P. acnes*. These reports allowed clinicians to recognize that postoperative intraocular infection could present very differently from the well-recognized acute form.

Epidemiology

The incidence of postoperative endophthalmitis following cataract surgery has been reported as being between 0.07% and 0.33%. There are no clear estimates of the incidence of chronic postoperative endophthalmitis, because cases are rare and others go undiagnosed. No specific risk factors have been found in these patients: Most reports indicate that these subjects do not share those risk factors known to be associated with acute postoperative endophthalmitis (e.g., wound abnormality).

P. acnes was the first organism described as a cause of this disorder. It is an anaerobic gram-positive pleomorphic bacillus normally found on the skin, external ear canal, mouth, and upper respiratory tract. It has been known to cause infection of the skin, nasal passages, heart, and eye. It is a normal inhabitant of the lids and conjunctiva, and has been associated with ocular infections such as blepharitis, keratitis, canaliculitis, and orbital cellulitis.

Since the first *P. acnes* case reports, other microbes have been shown to present with a similar clinical picture. Notably, these organisms resemble *P. acnes* in that they lack the virulence factors commonly found in those microbes associated with acute postoperative endophthalmitis. The organisms associated with the chronic form include coagulase-negative *Staphylococcus*, *Corynebacterium* sp., *Actinomyces*, *Nocardia*, and *Candida* sp.

Clinical Presentation

Chronic postoperative endophthalmitis occurs following cataract extraction with intraocular lens implantation in the vast majority of cases. It may also occur following cataract surgery in which an intraocular lens is not implanted. Inflammatory episodes begin well after the im-

TABLE 49–1. DEFINITIONS OF DIFFERENT CATEGORIES OF ENDOPHTHALMITIS

Acute postoperative endophthalmitis—intraocular inflammation secondary to an infectious cause characterized by an explosive onset and occurring in the immediate postoperative period following ocular surgery (typically within 7 days of the operation)

Delayed-onset endophthalmitis—intraocular inflammation secondary to an infectious cause characterized by an explosive onset, but occurring up to four weeks after an ocular surgery

Chronic postoperative endophthalmitis—intraocular inflammation secondary to an infectious cause characterized by indolent inflammation occurring any time following an ocular surgery

mediate postoperative recovery period, first occurring from months to years after the operation.[6] It is when the delay is prolonged that clinicians may not immediately link the new-onset uveitis with potential postoperative infection. The episodes tend to run an indolent, seemingly benign course, responding well to topical or periocular steroid therapy, and uniformly recur as steroid therapy is tapered. Subsequent attacks can remain low grade or may increase in severity.[7]

The first cases of chronic postoperative endophthalmitis were presented by Meisler and colleagues in the *American Journal of Ophthalmology* in 1986, and were found be due to *P. acnes*.[5] Subsequent reports of *P. acnes* endophthalmitis shared many clinical characteristics, and it was considered by some to represent its own unique syndrome.

Ocular inflammation due to *P. acnes* is usually noted around 3 to 4 months following an uncomplicated cataract surgery.[8, 9] It resembles a granulomatous uveitis.[8] Initially, inflammation responds well to topical steroids, only to relapse when the steroids are tapered. Recurrences become progressively worse. Cases initially presenting as nongranulomatous inflammation may become granulomatous, considered by some as an ominous sign.[7, 10]

One of the signs considered to be a hallmark of the syndrome is the presence of a white plaque, usually situated between the intraocular lens and the lens capsule.[4, 9, 11, 12] The plaque can also be present on the corneal endothelium.[13, 14] It should be noted that such plaques are not unique to *P. acnes*, and have been seen in chronic postoperative endophthalmitis due to other organisms, which include *Candida, Torulopsis magnoliae, Corynebacterium* sp., and *Mycobacterium chelonae*.[15]

Other clinical signs seen in *P. acnes* endophthalmitis include hypopyon,[7, 9–12] iris nodules,[11] vitritis,[4, 9, 10, 16] and vascular occlusion with retinal hemorrhages.[9, 16] Intraocular pressure is often elevated,[10, 13, 16, 17] which is consistent with the known association of uveitic glaucoma and infectious etiologies (e.g., herpes zoster virus [HZV] keratouveitis). *P. acnes* has been known to masquerade as an intermediate uveitis.[18]

It has subsequently become clear that the classic clinical presentation first described due to *P. acnes* can occur in the setting of other bacterial species.[15, 19, 20] Notably, these organisms tend to be slow-growing gram-positive bacteria. Undoubtedly, there are more yet unidentified common pathogenic factors shared by the organisms that allow them to present in such a similar manner.

Postoperative endophthalmitis due to fungal organisms are much rarer than their bacterial counterparts. However, clinical suspicion of fungal infection should be considered in all cases of chronic postoperative inflammation, because delayed diagnosis of intraocular fungal infection is almost always associated with a poor visual outcome and, in many cases, loss of the eye.

Chronic postoperative endophthalmitis due to fungal organisms can present similarly to the picture described for *P. acnes*. Inflammation does not occur episodically but rather is constantly present. A hypopyon usually becomes apparent. Certain other clinical signs suggest a fungal etiology. An iris or ciliary body mass should make one suspicious of a fungal etiology. Also, intraocular fungal organisms have been known to produce a keratitis from within the eye. So-called fluff balls classically described to be present in the vitreous, can also be seen in the anterior chamber.[21] Fungus can also cause necrotizing scleritis. Finally, aggressive topical, periocular, or intraocular steroid therapy may exacerbate the infection and worsen the course.[21] This is an ominous sign, and would prompt the treating physician to obtain an intraocular specimen in search of fungal organisms.

Pathophysiology and Etiology

Postoperative endophthalmitis is a result of the introduction of microbes into the eye at the time of surgery. Studies examining anterior chamber specimens during cataract surgery have demonstrated a contamination rate of 26%.[22] One can show that in the majority of cases, these organisms can be isolated from conjunctival swab cultures of the same eye.[22] Despite this high rate of anterior chamber contamination, postoperative endophthalmitis, acute or chronic, remains relatively rare, and thus other factors must be involved in the development of these clinical entities.

One factor that must contribute to the unique characteristics of this syndrome is the kind of microbes known to cause it. Multiple organisms have been cited, and include *P. acnes*, coagulase-negative staphylococcus, *Corynebacterium* sp., *Actinomyces*, and *Nocardia*.[1, 9, 19, 23, 24] These organisms are thought to be less virulent than organisms that cause acute postoperative endophthalmitis. However, the seemingly less-virulent coagulase-negative micrococcus is also the most common organism found in acute postoperative endophthalmitis. Other species that are believed to be indolent, like *P. acnes*, are also capable of producing acute postoperative endophthalmitis. Although low virulence obviously plays an important part in the chronic form, other factors, like the amount of organisms inoculated and patient risk factors, may explain why some cases of endophthalmitis due to these organisms can present in the fulminant form.

Another characteristic of these organisms is their ability to cause chronic infection. Histologic studies reveal that *P. acnes* is able to persist within the capsule. Histology of the plaque demonstrates numerous intracellular and extracellular organisms adjacent to a normal lens capsule.[25] Reaction against organisms harbored in the capsule is unlikely, because no inflammatory cells are seen on microscopic examination of the capsule.[8, 25] Recurrent inflammatory episodes are most likely due to the periodic release of sequestered organisms into the anterior chamber. This is further supported by immunohistochemistry studies of vitreous samples from patients with *P. acnes*, which reveal a neutrophilic predominance and lack of lymphocytes, characteristic of an acute immune response.

Fungal organisms capable of presenting a *P. acnes*–like syndrome include *Candida parapsilosis, Candida famata (Torulopsis candida)*, and *Acermonium kiliense*.[21] Although some fungal sources can be traced to the patient's flora (e.g., *Candida*), environmental factors in the operating room can contribute to infections due to fungal organisms not normally found as commensals of the skin. One study traced the source of four cases of endophthalmitis due to *A. kiliense* to the ventilation system, after noting that all four cases were performed very early on the first operating day of the week. It was believed that the organisms were introduced into the operating room environment when the ventilation system was switched on. Phenotypically identical organisms were cultured from humidifier water in the vent above the operating room.[21]

Wound abnormalities, a well-known risk factor for acute postoperative endophthalmitis, can lead to introduction of fungus from the outside environment and the development of the chronic form. One case report describes endophthalmitis due to *Histoplasma* in a patient living in an area endemic for *Histoplasma*. The patient had a wound abnormality (vitreous wick), and testing revealed negative serology and absence of systemic infection.

Diagnosis

Diagnosis relies on isolation of the causative organisms. This is done by either demonstrating the organisms on Gram's stain or by culture of an aqueous or vitreous sample. Ideally, both procedures are performed. because neither method alone is completely reliable. Many times, the ophthalmologist is unwilling to have the patient undergo a vitreous biopsy owing to good visual acuity and control of the inflammatory episodes by topical steroids. In these cases, an anterior chamber (AC) tap alone may be initiated. Owens and colleagues reported successful culture of *P. acnes* when the AC tap needle was directed into the capsular plaque or bag.[26] One must remember that successful yield of a positive Gram's stain or culture from the aqueous is less likely than that of a vitreous specimen. Additionally, with modern instruments and good surgical technique, a vitreous biopsy does not pose an unreasonable risk to the patient in the absence of other existing ocular conditions.

Case reports of endophthalmitis by *P. acnes* have shown that multiple vitreous biopsies can yield negative results. This can be due to several reasons. First, *P. acnes* is a slow-growing organism. Reports indicate that it can take longer than 2 weeks for the specimen to grow in culture[12]; most institutions do not carry out cultures for more than 5 days. Second, as an anaerobe, it has fastidious physiologic requirements.[27] Experiments show that a delay of more than 8 hours from delivery from the operating room to the appropriate culture environment results in a significant drop in yield of organisms. Last, the bulk of the organisms reside within the confines of the capsule (at the capsular plaque, if present).[25] Many authors recommend that attempts to retrieve capsular specimens for pathologic and microbiologic examination should be made in order to maximize the chance of isolating the causative organism.[10, 28]

On the other hand, false-positive results can also be a problem. *P. acnes* is a known contaminant among blood cultures. Chern and colleagues demonstrated that it is possible to obtain false-positive *P. acnes* cultures from uninfected eyes.[29] Potential contamination sources are many, because *P. acnes* is ubiquitous. Contamination can occur at the level of the patient, the surgeon, operating room nurse and staff, or at the microbiology laboratory. Needless to say, it is important to emphasize that equal care must be taken in delivering and processing the specimen as the care needed to obtain it.

When fungal organisms are in the differential, the same techniques and approaches used for bacterial organisms will aid in finding the causative organisms. Gram's stain is not as sensitive in demonstrating fungal microbes; Giemsa's or Gomori's methenamine staining should be performed if fungal infection is suggested.[21]

Differential Diagnosis

Although this chapter has dealt primarily with infectious etiologies thus far, there are many noninfectious causes of chronic postoperative inflammation that can masquerade as chronic autoimmune uveitis (Table 49–2). Among these causes is inflammation associated with the intraocular lens implant. Lens malposition causing constant iris trauma (e.g., iris chafing) can result in chronic inflammation.[2] An intraocular lens positioned in the posterior sulcus can also cause iris chafing, either from the contact with the pupillary margin by the optic or trauma to the ciliary body by the haptics. Intraocular lens material has also been implicated as the cause of chronic cells in the anterior chamber after cataract surgery although this is becoming less common with newer and safer lenses.[2] In the past, the uveitis-glaucoma-hyphema (UGH) syndrome was associated with the trauma induced by anterior chamber lenses, although with newer manufacturing techniques and intraocular lens design, this syndrome is seen less often.

Retained cortical material associated inflammation, classically resembling acute postoperative endophthalmitis, can also result in persistent chronic low-grade inflammation.[2] Retained cortex may be present in the capsular bag (e.g., incomplete cleanup), or may be a result of cortical pieces lost into the vitreous after capsular rupture. The amount of inflammation usually parallels the amount of cortical material left in the eye, although individual factors also play a role, because some patients seem to tolerate cortex floating in the vitreous cavity for years without experiencing inflammatory episodes. Retained cataract constituents were thought to account for most chronic postoperative inflammation before the multitude of reports citing microbes as potential etiologies, so one should not become complacent and should avoid the erroneous notion that all postoperative cells are due to retained cortex.

TABLE 49–2. CAUSATIVE ORGANISMS IN ENDOGENOUS ENDOPHTHALMITIS

BACTERIA	FUNGI
Streptococcus sp.	*Candida albicans*
Staphylococcus sp.	*Aspergillus* sp.
Clostridia septicum	*Histoplasma*
Bacillus cereus	*Coccidioides*
Coagulase-negative *Staphylococcus*	*Blastomyces*
Escherischia coli	*Cryptococcus*
Klebsiella pneumoniae	*Sporothrix*
Serratia marcescens	*Pseudallescheria boydii*
Pseudomonas aeruginosa	*Bipolar hawaiiensis*
Neisseria meningitides	
Listeria monocytogenes	

Finally, the new onset of intraocular inflammation following surgery may not be related to the surgery at all. Patients may be experiencing their first episodes of uveitis from other causes. In the elderly, one should be careful to consider central nervous system/intraocular lymphoma as a possibility, because there is at least one case report in the literature of lymphoma masquerading as a chronic postoperative endophthalmitis from microbial causes.

Treatment

Winward and coauthors reviewed the management and outcomes of 22 cases of *P. acnes* endophthalmitis.[30] They found treatment with intraocular antibiotics alone resulted in a failure rate of 88%. Other investigators have shared similar poor outcomes with intravitreal antibiotics alone.[1] Winward also found that patients with *P. acnes* endophthalmitis who underwent partial removal of the capsule had a better success rate. Success in this subgroup seemed dependent on the identification and removal of a intracapsular plaque: Those in whom a plaque was not visualized often required additional surgical procedures. Winward and colleagues found that the group of patients who did best were those who underwent total capsulectomy during their initial surgery: Every patient in this group was successfully cured. The authors also found that simultaneous secondary intraocular lens implantation in this group did not seem to affect the outcome adversely.[30]

These finding suggest that organisms harbored in the capsule are somewhat protected from treatment with antibiotic injection. Histology confirms that the majority of organisms are sequestered within the capsule. This helps explain both the stuttering course of the disease, as well as the high success rate in patients who underwent total capsulectomy.

However, theories and conjecture concerning pathogenic mechanisms must ultimately stand the test of clinical experiences. Despite Winward's findings suggesting that treatment of this disorder is ultimately surgical removal of the capsule, other authors have reported successful treatment of *P. acnes* with intraocular antibiotic injection alone, intravenous antibiotics,[31] and oral antibiotics alone.[17] *P. acnes* responds best to vancomycin and is also sensitive to penicillins, cephalosporin, clindamycin, and chloramphenicol. The organism is relatively resistant to aminoglycosides.[32]

There is no consensus on the best approach to treat these cases. Some authors advocate treating with topical steroids if visual acuity is better than 20/40 and the inflammatory episodes are nonprogressive.[31] Others advocate that the disease is similar to an abscess, in which microbes are confined in a region with poor access of antibiotics, and hence, surgical treatment is required. Most authors lean toward surgical treatment with supplemental antibiotics.[6, 26] We agree with this approach.

Treatment of fungal endophthalmitis from all causes is difficult. Patients often require prolonged therapy, and in many cases, fungal organisms cannot be eradicated from the eye despite aggressive therapy. Weissgold and colleagues reported on the onset of fungal infection of the cornea in two patients who previously were thought to have had successfully treated postoperative fungal endophthalmitis.[21] It is not unusual for fungal endophthalmitis to recur despite repeat vitrectomies and intraocular amphotericin. At times, adjunctive intravenous therapy is indicated, putting the patient at significant risk of drug toxicity.

Because of the difficulty of treating such cases, it is a reminder to all surgeons that although the risk of postoperative endophthalmitis cannot be completely eliminated (at this time), careful attention to sterile technique, good operating room management of surgery supplies and media, meticulous attention to creation of the surgical wound, and education of the patient with regard to good hygiene in the immediate postoperative period, may reduce the chance of introduction of infectious organisms in the first place.

Complications

The complications are similar to those seen in other chronic uveitis entities. These complications usually occur because of the failure of diagnosis. Glaucoma, from inflammation and chronic steroid use, can be difficult to control. Severe or prolonged inflammation leads to proliferative vitreoretinopathy, at which point salvage of the eye is unlikely. Although death from subsequent sepsis has not been associated with cases of chronic postoperative endophthalmitis, it has been seen in acute postoperative endophthalmitis; the absence of reports may be due to the fact that presumably if the infectious agent had been discovered, the patient would have been cured.

Prognosis

In many cases, chronic postoperative endophthalmitis due to bacterial causes has a good outcome and is thought to have a better outcome than acute endophthalmitis due to the less virulent organisms. It is highly likely that there exist many undiagnosed patients that are being managed with chronic topical steroids who are doing well.

ENDOGENOUS ENDOPHTHALMITIS

Definition

Endogenous endophthalmitis is intraocular infection due to bacterial or fungal microbes seeded to the eye from the vascular circulation. Clinically, it presents as acute uveitis without history or evidence of penetration of the globe, and occurs in patients who have a focus of infection distant from the eye. Occasionally, signs of a systemic infection are subtle or absent, and in these cases, the condition masquerades as an autoimmune uveitis.

Epidemiology

Endogenous endophthalmitis is a uncommon entity. Study reports estimate that it accounts for between 2% and 8% of cases of all forms of endophthalmitis.[33] The overall incidence in predisposed patient populations is not known. The incidence of fungal endophthalmitis in patients with candidemia has ranged between 1% and 40%. This wide range may be due in part to some authors broadening the definition of *Candida* to include patients with fundus lesions that do not extend into the vitreous;

this does not necessarily meet the more literal terminology of endophthalmitis.[34]

Endogenous endophthalmitis often occurs in the setting of an immunocompromised patient. Predisposing medical conditions include diabetes mellitus,[33, 35–38] malignancy,[33, 38–41] sickle cell anemia,[42] systemic lupus erythematosus,[42, 43] and human immunodeficiency virus (HIV).[44–47] Iatrogenic immunosuppression in the form of chemotherapy for treating malignancy and immunosuppressives and systemic corticosteroids for organ transplant patients[33, 38, 43, 47–49] also appear to predispose the patient to endogenous bacterial endophthalmitis. Although endophthalmitis may occur as the only obvious site of infection in the immunocompromised patient, the presence of a focus of infection is the rule. Okada and colleagues found prior medical conditions in 90% of their patients with endogenous bacterial endophthalmitis.[33] Urinary tract infection, liver or gastrointestinal abscess, meningitis, cellulitis, cholecystitis, and pneumonia encompass the most commonly cited sources of infection.[33, 35]

Several other conditions that can lead to hematogenous dissemination of microbes in immunocompetent individuals have been associated with endogenous endophthalmitis. Patients who develop subacute bacterial endocarditis have been shown to be at increased risk for spread to the eye.[33, 49, 50] One series found endocarditis accounted for the source of infection in 46% of cases.[33] Periodontal infection,[51] indwelling intravenous catheters,[45, 50, 52, 53] contaminated intravenous solutions,[54] and intravenous drug abuse[33, 55–58] have also been shown as risk factors in patients with a good immune status. Endogenous *Candida* endophthalmitis has been reported following induced abortion in healthy women.[59]

Endogenous endophthalmitis can present in the neonate.[52, 60–63] The immune system is not fully matured during the first 6 months after birth and perhaps for up to 1 year. The fact that physicians overlook this fact is apparent in case reports of children undergoing enucleation for retinoblastoma, only to discover that the diagnosis was endophthalmitis. Given that in many of these cases a systemic infection was not apparent, it underscores the importance of remembering that immune function cannot be considered completely competent in an otherwise healthy-appearing neonate.

Clinical Characteristics

The onset of ocular inflammation in a patient with a systemic infection helps greatly in raising the suspicion that the microbe is also responsible for the eye disease. In most cases, patients will already be under the care of a physician for a systemic illness. The risk factors predisposing to infection are readily apparent by the medical history and the current illness. Some patients may have multiple risk factors for infection. For example, certain systemic diseases require prolonged intravenous therapy, which may predispose the patient to intravenous line–related infection. In malignancy or autoimmune disease, the specific chemotherapeutic treatment may further compromise the patient's immune status.

It is when a systemic infection is not present or obvious that ophthalmologists may overlook the possibility of an infectious etiology. Some infections are either difficult to diagnose (e.g., osteomyelitis) or are dismissed as a less serious infection (e.g., sinusitis or pneumonia misinterpreted as a common cold). In the latter case, the patient may present to the ophthalmologist focused only on the ocular symptoms, creating further potential to misdiagnosed intraocular inflammation as an autoimmune process. Unfortunately, even obvious cases can be overlooked by the ophthalmologist who does not keep infection in his differential, as illustrated by the following case:

CASE PRESENTATION

A 56-year-old dentist with a history of type II diabetes mellitus was scheduled to go on a trip to China when he began to have fever, chills, and a nonproductive cough. He took over-the-counter medications for symptomatic relief. When he arrived in China, he noted blurring vision of his left eye. Over the next 4 days, his left eye became increasingly red and painful, prompting him to seek medical attention. He was seen at the local eye clinic, where he was diagnosed with acute anterior uveitis and started on topical steroid drops and cycloplegics, and told to follow up at the hospital-based ophthalmology service. He was seen there 2 days later, with worsening of his condition: 3 plus anterior chamber cells, corneal edema, granulomatous keratic precipitates, and a hypopyon. He was also noted to be confused, for which he was transferred to the emergency room. Testing revealed a glucose level of higher than 400, and the patient was admitted for glucose control. Incidental chest radiograph revealed a pulmonary infiltrate; the patient was placed on intravenous antibiotics.

During hospitalization, the ophthalmology service started the patient on a daily regimen of periocular steroid injections, supplemented by topical atropine and steroids drops. The hypopyon resolved, but a fibrin membrane developed, covering the pupil. He was discharged on topical prednisolone, tropicamide, and timolol, with vision of light perception.

He returned to the United States and was seen at the Massachusetts Eye and Ear Infirmary and was eventually referred to the Ocular Immunology & Uveitis Service. On examination, vision of the left eye was bare light perception, with lid edema, 4 + conjunctival injection, 3 + conjunctival chemosis, corneal edema, hypopyon, and the dense fibrin membrane obscuring the pupil. We recommended urgent anterior chamber tap and vitreous biopsy to rule out infection, which was performed. Gram's stain of the anterior chamber specimen was negative, but the vitreous specimen revealed gram-negative rods. Intraocular antibiotics were injected, and the patient was placed on oral antibiotics. Twenty-four hours later, *Klebsiella pneumoniae* had grown out of culture from the vitreous specimen. By this time, the vision was no light perception, with early signs of limitation of extraocular movements. Because of the patient's unimproved ocular status and the possibility of early orbital cellulitis, the patient underwent evisceration.

As mentioned several times in this text, a detailed review of systems is an essential step in the evaluation of all patients with uveitis. Because of the previously mentioned circumstances that can lead to overlooking an infectious cause, the review of systems may provide the only clue to the ophthalmologist that an infection should be suspected.

The possibility of endophthalmitis cannot be excluded even when the review of systems is unrevealing. Use of intravenous drugs is an obvious potential source of microbes for endogenous endophthalmitis, and most patients will not readily volunteer this information during the initial encounter with the physician. Physical examination for tell-tale signs of drug use on the patient's skin may provide the only clue of this etiology.[57] This fact underscores that the ophthalmologist keen on saving the vision of a patient with uveitis of unknown etiology cannot limit the physical examination to the globe.

Finally, there are cases in which no systemic disease or predisposing risk factors can be found.[63, 64] Diagnosis in these patients relies heavily on the clinician's level of suspicion. If symptoms progress slowly in these patients, delay in diagnosis is often the rule, with one study revealing a mean duration from symptoms to diagnosis of 61 days in patients eventually found to have *Candida* endophthalmitis.[65]

The presenting symptoms and signs are similar to those of uveitis of autoimmune causes. Classically, endogenous endophthalmitis from bacteria presents more explosively than does fungal infection. Symptoms include blurred vision, pain, and photophobia. Pain however is not a constant feature.[66] Floaters are rarely a complaint in rapidly progressive cases but may be noted in cases with a more insidious onset (i.e., fungal endogenous endophthalmitis).

Examination reveals severely reduced visual acuity in the affected eye, often in the count-fingers to light perception range. Periorbital edema can vary from severe to absent. If periocular swelling is associated with proptosis, an associated orbital cellulitis may be present.[49] This may be an ominous sign in immunocompromised patients.

Usually, both anterior and posterior segments are involved. Anterior signs include cells, flare, and inferior keratic precipitates. A hypopyon is cited in most reported cases,[41] but this may be due to a selection bias, because all of these reports are retrospective cohort studies. A so-called dark hypopyon may be suggestive of *Listeria*.[40] Anterior chamber fibrin or an inflammatory membrane can also be seen. Another noted feature is corneal edema,[36, 39, 42, 67] although this feature can also be seen in severe noninfectious uveitis. Intraocular pressures may be extremely elevated,[40] which is consistent with what is found clinically in uveitis entities from other infectious organisms not normally associated with concomitant sepsis (e.g., herpesvirus, toxoplasmosis, and syphilis). Iris nodules can be seen in fungal endophthalmitis.[41, 67] Rubeosis iridis and angle-closure glaucoma can be seen in severe inflammation or in a prolonged course.

Some posterior signs can also be suggestive of an infectious process. Although vitreal cells are nonspecific, vitreal condensations of inflammatory cells, or so-called fluff balls and pearls on a string are usually associated with fungal infection.[68] This picture is even more suggestive of fungal infection when the fluff balls are localized in the posterior vitreous near the posterior pole[57] (as opposed to the anterior vitreous or inferior vitreous base). White or creamy discrete deep choroidal lesions are also seen in fungal infection, representing separate foci of disseminated organisms. Alternatively, a white chorioretinal infiltrate with indistinct borders can also be seen.[41, 67] Roth spots can be seen in both bacterial and fungal infections.[69] An inflammatory exudate may occur in either the subhyaloid or subretinal space (e.g., subretinal abscess), capable of forming a pseudohypopyon.[58, 67, 70] Disc edema,[46] subretinal abscess,[71] vasculitis,[69, 72] retinal cyst,[37] retinal necrosis,[35] and choroidal mass[73] are uncommon signs. It should be noted that although they are suggestive, none of these signs are specific: Fluff balls at the vitreous base are seen in intermediate uveitis, and pseudohypopyon has been described in syphilis and Adamantiades-Behçet disease.

Pathogenesis

The type of microbe that infects the eye is related to the patient's specific risk factors. *Streptococcus* sp. causes endophthalmitis in endocarditis patients, whereas *Klebsiella* sp. can be isolated in patients with liver abscesses and *Candida* endophthalmitis is associated with indwelling intravenous catheters and intravenous drug abuse. Gram-positive bacteria (*S. aureus* and streptococcal species) account for the majority of bacterial causes,[33] whereas *Candida* species is the most common cause of fungal endogenous endophthalmitis. A list of reported organisms can be found in Table 49–3.

The majority of infections are presumably the result of hematogenous dissemination of the organisms. Rabbit models demonstrate that disseminated microbes initially colonize the choroid, and then spread inward to the retina. Endogenous endophthalmitis has been reported in patients with meningitis, which raises the possibility that spread of organisms from the cerebral spinal fluid may represent an alternative way of infection seeding to the eye.

Diagnosis

Diagnosis relies on isolation of the causative microbes. This requires obtaining intraocular fluid, usually in the form of a vitreous biopsy. An anterior chamber tap can also isolate causative microbes but is usually performed as a supplemental procedure to the vitreous biopsy. Retinal biopsy may be necessary in selected cases.[70]

Identification of organisms from systemic infected sites is potentially useful.[73] When a patient develops endophthalmitis in the presence of a systemic infection, one

TABLE 49–3. NONINFECTIOUS CAUSES OF CHRONIC POSTOPERATIVE INTRAOCULAR INFLAMMATION

Lens-induced uveitis (phacoantigenic uveitis)
    Retained cortical material
    Retained intravitreal lens fragments
Intraocular lens–related uveitis
    Iris chafing intraocular lens implant malposition
    Uveitis-glaucoma-hyphema (UGH) syndrome
    Intraocular lens implant material related
Other causes
    Masquerade (intraocular lymphoma)
    Sympathetic ophthalmia
    Uveitis of other causes unrelated to surgery

often presumes that the causative organism of each infection is the same. However, this is not always the case. Often, the patient population at risk for endogenous endophthalmitis is predisposed to infection from multiple sources. For example, a cancer patient admitted for bacterial pneumonia may develop fungal endophthalmitis from infection of the line used for his antibiotics and other intravenous medications. Furthermore, certain organisms may be difficult to isolate from systemic sites, because one series of culture-proven endogenous fungal endophthalmitis found positive blood cultures in only two of 16 patients.[65]

Treatment

The mainstay of treatment consists of intraocular antibiotics. If Gram's and fungal staining is performed at the initial harvesting of undiluted vitreous material, therapy can be targeted against a narrower spectrum of microbes immediately. This approach, which can categorize the infection into gram-positive bacteria, gram-negative, or fungal infection at the time of biopsy, can potentially save the eye, because delay in the institution of the appropriate antimicrobial therapy of 24 hours can sometimes mean the difference between salvage of the eye and evisceration. Some authors advocate that intraocular antibiotics are not needed in all cases of endogenous endophthalmitis, citing the potential macular toxicity of these medications when given intraocularly, as well as the reports of endogenous fungal endophthalmitis successfully treated with vitrectomy and systemic fluconazole.[65] Often, when the clinical picture is suggestive, empiric intraocular antibiotics with or without steroids is given at the time of initial biopsy (see Table 49–4). Intravitreal steroid has not been associated with exacerbation of a fungal endophthalmitis when injected with intravitreal amphotericin B.[74, 75]

The use of systemic antimicrobial therapy in endogenous endophthalmitis is usually not controversial. In many cases, patients are already receiving antibiotics for the source infection. However, when a focus of infection outside the eye is not identified, the usefulness of systemic treatment for localized eye disease is not as clear. Antibiotics against bacteria in general carry little risk, and thus their use in this circumstance is rarely problematic. The benefit of systemic antifungals in isolated fungal endophthalmitis is less certain. Although they demonstrate good vitreous penetration, use of oral antifungal agents should be seriously considered given the high incidence of *Candida*.[76, 77] Intravenous amphotericin carries significant risk of renal toxicity. Futhermore, it is known that intravenous amphotericin does not penetrate the eye well. There is evidence in the literature supporting both its usefulness and its uselessness. Case reports describe patients who were successfully treated with vitrectomy and intraocular antifungals without systemic antifungals,[34, 78] as well as patients who were successfully treated with systemic antifungals without vitrectomy.[47, 48] When employed, the dosage of systemic amphotericin given is commonly around 0.5 to 1.0 mg/kg/day.

Similarly, the role of vitrectomy in the management of endogenous endophthalmitis is not clear. Reports of successful treatment both with and without surgery have been cited.[58, 66, 78–80] Although one usually assumes that vitrectomy can enhance visual recovery by both "debulking" the amount of intraocular organisms, as well as removing debris that will impair optimum visual recovery, there also exist reports of clearance of the vitreous with excellent visual acuity with systemic treatment alone.[66] Today, most experts lean toward the use of pars plana vitrectomy with intravitreal antibiotics in most cases, whereas systemic treatment alone may be considered in those with mild vitritis.

A prospective controlled clinical trial comparing the various combinations of treatment modalities is not feasible, because cases of endogenous endophthalmitis are rare and the patient population in which they occur is extremely heterogeneous. With the current available therapies, success relies heavily on prompt diagnosis, as well as the clinical judgment and experience of the treating ophthalmologist.

Complications

The most serious complication among patients with endogenous endophthalmitis is death.[52] This pertains to the subgroup of patients who have either sepsis or a systemic illness rendering them immunocompromised. Often, they are extremely ill, and sometimes terminally so. Under these circumstances, the ocular process is overshadowed by the primary systemic illness. Diagnostic surgical procedures in the operating room need to be deferred if they pose a significant risk to the patient's survival. Sometimes, the ophthalmologist may need to perform a vitreous biopsy and intravitreal injection of antibiotics at the bedside, if salvaging vision has a chance of preserving the patient's quality of life, or if eventual recovery from the systemic illness is likely.

Ocular complications from endophthalmitis are as varied as those found in other uveitic entities. Cataract formation represents a relatively mild complication, whereas neovascular glaucoma, optic neuropathy, and retinal detachment[65] represent the more severe end of the spectrum. Recurrence of infection can become a frustrating sequela, with fungal infections historically described as being able to persist in the eye even after multiple attempts at cleanup.[65] Development of orbital cellulitis by direct spread of intraocular microbes has been cited anecdotally as a reason to pursue evisceration in hopeless cases. This contention is supported by histopathologic identification of fungal organisms present within scleral emissarial canals and reports of spontaneous scleral perforation from *Klebsiella* endophthalmitis.[35]

Last, complications can occur secondary to antibiotic treatment. Intravitreal antibiotics, particularly gentamicin and vancomycin, are known to have potential macular toxicity. Systemic antimicrobial therapy may present a risk of specific organ toxicity (e.g., amphotericin and the kidneys) as well as the risk carried by the presence of an intravenous line, a significant danger in this patient population.

Prognosis

Successful treatment of endogenous endophthalmitis requires prompt diagnosis and therapy. Like acute postoperative endophthalmitis, the endogenous form can present in an explosive manner, with progression to loss of useful vision in a matter of days. Unlike postoperative or post-traumatic infection, a clear history suggesting an infectious etiology is not always present. Assumption that the process is autoimmune and ought to respond to high-dose steroids can be disastrous. Even when appropriately diagnosed, virulence of the offending microbe and poor health status of the patient may delay resolution and limit visual recovery. It is one of the masquerade syndromes that absolutely should not be overlooked in any patient presenting with intraocular inflammation of unknown etiology.

References

1. Fox GM, Joondeph BC, Flynn HW, et al: Delayed-onset pseudophakic endophthalmitis. Am J Ophthalmol 1991;111:163–173.
2. Mandelbaum S, Meisler D: Postoperative chronic microbial endophthalmitis. Int Ophthalmol Clin, 1993;3:71–79.
3. Jiraskova N, Rozsival P: Delayed-onset *Pseudomonas stutzeri* endophthalmitis after uncomplicated cataract surgery. J Cataract Refract Surg 1998;24:866–867.
4. Roussel T, Culbertson W, Jaffe N: Chronic postoperative endophthalmitis associated with *Propionibacterium acnes*. Arch Ophthalmol 1987;105:1199–1201.
5. Meisler D, Palestine AG, Vastine DW, et al: Chronic *Propionibacterium* endophthalmitis after extracapsular cataract extraction and intraocular lens implantation. Am J Ophthalmol 1986;102:733–739.
6. Posenauer B, Funk J: Chronic postoperative endophthalmitis caused by *Propionibacterium acnes*. Eur J Ophthalmol 1992;2:94–97.
7. Jaffe GJ, Whitcher JP, Biswell R, et al: *Propionibacterium acnes* endophthalmitis seven months after extracapsular cataract, extraction and intraocular lens implantation. Ophthalmic Surg 1986;17:791–793.
8. Meisler D, Mandelbaum S: *Propionibacterium*-associated endophthalmitis after extracapsular cataract extraction. Review of reported cases. Ophthalmology 1989;96:54–61.
9. Zambrano W, Flynn HW, Pfulgfelder SC, et al: Management options for *Propionibacterium acnes* endophthalmitis. Ophthalmology 1989;96:1100–1105.
10. Piest K, Apple DJ, Kincaid MC, et al: Localized endophthalmitis: A newly described cause of the so-called toxic lens syndrome. J Cataract Refract Surg 1987;13:498–510.
11. Stokes D, O'Day D: Iris nodule and intralenticular abscess associated with *Propionibacteruim acnes* endophthalmitis. Arch Ophthalmol 1992;110:921–922.
12. Omerod D, Edelstein MA, Schmidt GJ, et al: The intraocular environment and experimental anaerobic bacterial endophthalmitis. Arch Ophthalmol 1987;104:1571–1575.
13. Abrahams IW: *Propionibacterium acnes* endophthalmitis: An unusual manner of presentation. J Cataract Refract Surg 1989;15:698–701.
14. Chien AM, Raber IM, Fischer DH, et al: *Propionibacterium acnes* endophthalmitis after intracapsular cataract extraction. Ophthalmology 1992;99:487–490.
15. El-Asrar AM, Tabbara K: Chronic endophthalmitis after extracapsular cataract extraction caused by *Mycobacterium chelonae* subspecies *abcessus* [Letter]. Eye 1995;9:798–801.
16. Keyser B, Maguire J, Halperin L: *Propionibacterium acnes* endophthalmitis after *Staphylococcus epidermidis* endophthalmitis. Am J Ophthalmol 1993;116:505–506.
17. Pivetti-Pezzi P, Accorinti M: *Propionibacterium* endophthalmitis [Letter]. Ophthalmology 1992;99:1753–1754.
18. Omerod D, Puklin J, Giles C: Chronic *Propionibacterium acnes* endophthalmitis as a cause of intermediate uveitis. Ocul Immunol Inflamm 1997;4:67–68.
19. Zimmerman P, Mamalis N, Alder JB, et al: Chronic *Nocardia asteroides* endophthalmtiis after extracapsular cataract extraction. Arch Ophthalmol 1993;111:837–840.
20. Von Below H, Wilk CM, Schall KP, et al: *Rhodococcus luteus* and *Rhodococcus erythropolis* chronic endophthalmtiis after lens implantation [Letter]. Am J Ophthalmol 1991;112:596–597.
21. Weissgold DJ, Orlin SE, Sulewski ME: Delayed-onset fungal keratitis after endophthalmitis. Ophthalmology 1998;105:258–262.
22. Egger S, Huber Spitzy V, Scholda C: Bacterial contamination during extracapsular cataract extraction. Ophthalmologica 1994;208:77–81.
23. Manners RM, Canning CR: Posterior lens capsule abscess due to *Propionibacterium acnes* and *Staphylococcus epidermidis* following extracapsular cataract extraction. Br J Ophthalmol 1991;75:710–712.
24. Roussel T, Olson ER, Rice T: Chronic postoperative endophthalmitis associated with *Actinomyces* species. Arch Ophthalmol 1991;109:60–62.
25. Meisler DM, Zakov ZN, Bruner WE, et al: Endophthalmitis associated with sequestered intraocular *Propionibacterium acnes*. Am J Ophthalmol 1987;104:428–429.
26. Owens S, Lam S, Tessler HH, et al: Preliminary study of a new intraocular method in the diagnosis and treatment of *Propionibacterium acnes* endophthalmitis following cataract extraction. Ophthal Surg 1993;24:268–272.
27. Hall G, Pratt Rippin K, Meisler DM, et al: Growth curve for *Propionibacterium acnes*. Curr Eye Res 1994;13:465–466.
28. Sawusch MR, Michels RG, Stark WJ, et al: Endophthalmitis due to *Propionibacterium acnes* sequestered between IOL optic and posterior capsule. Ophthalmic Surg 1989;20:90–92.
29. Chern K, Meisler DM, Hall GS, et al: Bacterial contamination of anaerobic vitreous cultures: Using techniques employed for endophthalmitis. Curt Eye Res 1996;15:697–699.
30. Winward KE, Plugfelder SC, Flynn HW, et al: Postoperative *Propionibacterium* endophthalmitis. Ophthalmology 1993;100:447–451.
31. Brady SE, Cohen EJ, Fischer DH: Diagnosis and treatment of chronic postoperative bacterial endophthalmitis. Ophthalmic Surg 1988;19:580–584.
32. Beatty RF, Robin JB, Trousdale MD, et al: Anaerobic endophthalmitis caused by *Propionibacterium acnes*. Am J Opthalmol 1986;101:114–116.
33. Okada AA, Johnson RP, Liles WC, et al: Endogenous bacterial endophthalmitis. Report of a ten-year retrospective study. Ophthalmology 1994;101:832–838.
34. Donahue SP, Greven CM, Zuravleff JJ, et al: Intraocular candidiasis in patients with candidemia. Clinical implications derived from a prospective multicenter study. Ophthalmology 1994;101:1302–1309.
35. Liao HR, Lee HW, Leu HS, et al: Endogenous *Klebsiella pneumoniae* endophthalmitis in diabetic patients. Can J Ophthalmol 1992;27:143–147.
36. Margo CE, Mames RN, Guy JR: Endogenous *Klebsiella* endophthalmitis. Ophthalmology 1994;101:1298–1301.
37. Sipperley JO, Shore JW: Septic retinal cyst in endogenous *Klebsiella* endophthalmitis. Am J Ophthalmol 1992;94:124–125.
38. Ambler JS, Meisler DM, Zakov ZN, et al: Endogenous *Mycobacterium chelonae* endophthalmitis. Am J Ophthalmol 1989;108:338–339.
39. Davitt B, Gehrs K, Bowers T: Endogenous *Nocardia* endophthalmitis. Retina 1998;18:71–73.
40. Eliott D, O'Brien TP, Green WR, et al: Elevated intraocular pressure, pigment dispersion and dark hypopyon in endogenous endophthalmitis from *Listeria monocytogenes*. Surv Ophthalmol 1992;37:117–124.
41. Blumenkranz MS, Stevens DA: Therapy of endogenous fungal endophthalmitis. Arch Ophthalmol 1980;98:1216–1220.
42. Werner MS, Feist RM, Green JL: Hemoglobin SC disease with endogenous endophthalmitis. Am J Ophthalmol 1992;113:208–209.
43. Ishibashi Y, Watanabe R, Hommura S, et al: Endogenous *Nocardia asteroides* endophthalmitis in a patient with systemic lupus erythematosus. Br J Ophthalmol 1990;74:433–436.
44. Scherer WJ, Lee K: Implications of early systemic therapy on the incidence of endogenous fungal endophthalmitis. Ophthalmology 1997;104:1593–1598.
45. Tufail A, Weisz JM, Holland GN: Endogenous bacterial endophthalmitis as a complication of intravenous therapy for cytomegalovirus retinopathy [Letter]. Arch Ophthalmol 1996;114:879–880.
46. Glasgow BJ, Engstrom RE, Holland GN, et al: Bilateral endogenous *Fusarium* endophthalmitis associated with acquired immunodeficiency syndrome. Arch Ophthalmol 1996;114:873–877.
47. Pavan PR, Margo CE: Endogenous endophthalmitis caused by *Bipolaris hawaiiensis* in a patient with acquired immunodeficiency syndrome. Am J Ophthalmol 1993;116:644–645.
48. Graham DA, Kinyoun JL, George DP: Endogenous *Aspergillus* endophthalmitis after lung transplantation. Am J Ophthalmol 1995;119:107–109.
49. Patel AS, Hemady RK, Rodrigues M, et al: Endogenous *Fusarium* endophthalmitis in a patient with acute lymphocytic leukemia. Am J Ophthalmol 1994;117:363–368.

50. Ishak MA, Zablit KV, Dumas J: Endogenous endophthalmitis caused by *Actinobacillus actinomycetemcomitans.* Can J Ophthalmol 1986; 21:284–286.

51. Hornblass A, To K, Coden DJ, et al: Endogenous orbital cellulitis and endogenous endophthalmitis in subacute bacterial endocarditis. Am J Ophthalmol 1989;108:196–197.

52. Parke DW, Jones DB, Gentry LO: Endogenous endophthalmitis among patients with candidemia. Ophthalmology 1982;89:789–796.

53. Wolfensberger TJ, Gonvers M: Bilateral endogenous *Candida* endophthalmitis. Retina 1998;18:280–281.

54. Daily MJ, Dickey JB, Packo KH: Endogenous *Candida* endophthalmitis after intravenous anesthesia with propofol. Arch Ophthalmol 1991;109:1081–1084.

55. Lance SE, Friberg TR, Kowalski RP: *Aspergillus flavus* endophthalmitis and retinitis in an intravenous drug abuser. Ophthalmology 1988;95:947–949.

56. Gabriele P, Hutchins RK: *Fusarium* endophthalmitis in an intravenous drag abuser. Am J Ophthalmol 1996; 122:119–121.

57. Doft BH, Clarkson JG, Rebell G, et al: Endogenous *Aspergillus* endophthalmitis in drug abusers. Arch Ophthalmol 1980;98:859–862.

58. Weishaar PD, Flynn HW, Murray TG, et al: Endogenous *Aspergillus* endophthalmitis. Ophthalmology 1998;105:57–65.

59. Chen SJ, Chung YM, Liu JH: Endogenous *Candida* endophthalmitis after induced abortion. Am J Ophthalmol 1998;125:873–876.

60. Shields JA, Shields CL, Eagle RC, et al: Endogenous endophthalmitis simulating retinoblastoma. Retina 1995;15:213–219.

61. Palmer EA: Endogenous *Candida* endophthalmitis in infants. Am J Ophthalmol 1980;89:388–395.

62. Clinch TE, Duker JS, Eagle RC, et al: Infantile endogenous *Candida* endophthalmitis presenting as a cataract. Surv Ophthalmol 1989;34:107–112.

63. Friedlander SM, Raphaelian PV, Granet DB: Bilateral endogenous *Escherichia coli* endophthalmitis in a neonate with meningitis. Retina 1996;16:341–343.

64. Pfeifer JD, Grand MG, Thomas MA, et al: Endogenous *Pseudallescheria boydii* endophthalmitis. Arch Ophthalmol 1991;109:1714–1717.

65. Essman TF, Flynn HW, Smiddy WE, et al: Treatment outcomes in a 10-year study of endogenous fungal endophthalmitis. Opthalmic Surg Lasers 1997;28:185–194.

66. Luttrull JK, Wan WL, Kubak BM, et al: Treatment of ocular fungal infections with oral fluconazole. Am J Ophthalmol 1995;119:477–481.

67. Heidemann DG, Murphy SF, Lewis M: Endogenous *Listeria monocytogenes* endophthalmitis presenting as keratouveitis. Cornea 1990; 9:179–180.

68. Kostick DA, Foster RE, Lowder CY, et al: Endogenous endophthalmitis caused by *Candida albicans* in a healthy woman. Am J Ophthalmol 1992;113:593–595.

69. Gross JG: Endogenous *Aspergillus*-induced endophthalmitis. Retina 1992;12:341–345.

70. Sheu SJ, Chen YC, Kuo NW, et al: Endogenous cryptococcal endophthalmitis. Ophthalmology 1998;104:377–381.

71. Yang SS, Hsieh CL, Chen TL: Vitrectomy for endogenous *Klebsiella pneumoniae* endophthalmitis with massive subretinal abscess. Ophthalmic Surg Lasers 1997;28:147–150.

72. Jones DB, Green MT, Osato MS, et al: Endogenous *Candida albicans* endophthalmitis in the rabbit. Arch Ophthalmol 1981;99:2182–2187.

73. Berman AJ, Del Priore LV, Fischer CK: Endogenous *Ochrobactrum anthropi* endophthalmitis. Am J Ophthalmol 1997;123:560–562.

74. Gottlieb JL, McAllister IL, Guttman FA, et al: Choroidal blastomycosis. A report of two cases. Retina 1995;15:248–252.

75. Coats ML, Peyman GA: Intravitreal corticosteroids in the treatment of exogenous fungal endophthalmitis. Retina 1992;12:46–51.

76. O'Day DM: Ocular uptake of fluconazole following oral administration. Arch Ophthalmol 1999;108:1006–1008.

77. Savanyi DV, Perfect JR, Cobo LM, et al: Penetration of new azole compounds into the eye and efficacy in experimental *Candida* endophthalmitis. Antimicrob Agents Chemother 1987;31:6–10.

78. Brod RD, Flynn HW, Clarkson JG, et al: Endogenous *Candida* endophthalmitis: Management without intravenous amphotericin B. Ophthalmology 1990;97:666–674.

79. Laatikainen L, Tuominen M, von Dickhoff K: Treatment of endogenous fungal endophthalmitis with systemic fluconazole with or without vitrectomy. Am J Ophthalmol 1992;113:205–207.

80. Christmas NJ, Smiddy WE: Vitrectomy and systemic fluconazole for treatment of endogenous fungal endophthalmitis. Ophthalmic Surg Lasers 1996;27:1012–1018.

NONMALIGNANT, NONINFECTIOUS MASQUERADE SYNDROMES

Lijing Yao and C. Stephen Foster

Masquerade syndromes are defined as a group of disorders characterized by the presence of intraocular cells secondary to noninflammatory diseases, and are often misdiagnosed as chronic idiopathic uveitis.

In 1957, Cooper and Riker[1] reported the first relationship between systemic lymphoma and "uveitis." Although several subsequent reports documented cases of intracranial lymphomas associated with intraocular inflammation[2] and retinal detachments (RDs) associated with scleritis,[3] ocular masquerade syndromes were not yet given a formal ophthalmic definition. Until 1967, the term masquerade syndrome was first cited in the ophthalmic literature by Theodore to describe a case of conjunctival carcinoma that manifested as chronic conjunctivitis.[4] Today, the term masquerade syndrome is most widely accepted to describe some disorders that simulate chronic idiopathic uveitis.

Reports of masquerade syndromes are rare. Only one case of masquerade syndrome in 426 cases of uveitis was reported in a large prospective study of general uveitis.[5] Review of the literature between 1967 and most current published series discloses that the most common conditions that can masquerade as idiopathic uveitis are malignancies and infectious endophthalmitis. Other nonmalignant and noninfectious diseases, including peripheral RD, retinitis pigmentosa, intraocular foreign body, pigmentary dispersion syndrome, ocular ischemic syndrome, juvenile xanthogranuloma, and others have also been mentioned. Malignancy and endophthalmitis are discussed in the preceding chapters. In this chapter, we discuss only nonmalignant and noninfectious masquerade disorders, which can be misdiagnosed as uveitis. We stress the common and different clinical manifestations of each masquerade disorder, its diagnosis, and its differential diagnosis in more detail.

RHEGMATOGENOUS RETINAL DETACHMENT

Definition

RD is defined as a separation of the sensory retina from the retinal pigment epithelium (RPE) with an accumulation of fluid in the potential space between them. It is often classified into three distinct types: (1) rhegmatogenous, (2) traction, and (3) exudative. A primary, or spontaneous, RD is a rhegmatogenous detachment that is caused by retinal breaks—tears, holes, and dialyses in the retina, in which fluid from the vitreous cavity seeps through the retinal breaks, accumulates in the potential subretinal space, and separates the retina from the RPE. Rhegmatogenous RD is the most common form of RD. RDs secondary to other disease processes, not primarily caused by retinal holes, are termed nonrhegmatogenous detachments, which include traction and exudative RD.

A traction RD is often caused by vitreoretinal fibroproliferative membranes that mechanically pull the retina off from the underlying retinal pigment. An exudative RD results from retinal or choroidal conditions that disturb the RPE or blood-retinal barrier, accumulating fluid in the subretinal space from either the retinal or the choroidal circulation.

When a retinal tear forms idiopathically and a detached retina ensues, the fluid accumulated in the subretinal space can stimulate an inflammatory response, leading to increased vascular permeability and leakage of cells and protein into the anterior chamber and vitreous. Therefore, these inflammatory features can mask the primary RD itself.

History

The development of RD concepts can be divided into two major periods—early and modern. The early stage (1851–1918) started with the invention of the direct ophthalmoscope by von Helmholtz in 1851.[6] Shortly after that invention, Coccius first observed a retinal break in 1853.[7] Since then, numerous works and debated theories were made in an attempt to find the etiology of RD.[8–17]

Among those early studies, the theory of vitreous and retinal breaks as the possible etiology of RD suggested by de Wecker and de Jaeger in 1870,[12] Leber in 1882,[13] and de Wecker in 1888[14] was the representative landmark work. But the theory and its full importance went unrecognized until 1919, when Gonin[18] conclusively confirmed that retinal breaks cause RDs; he demonstrated that sealing retinal tears cures the detachment. Gonin's procedure received widespread acceptance in 1929.

Gonin's pioneer work between 1919 and 1935 brings the pathogenesis study and treatment of rhegmatogenous detachment into the modern era. During the modern period (1936–present), major landmark works include the method of intraocular air tamponade to displace the retina toward the eyeball wall and to provide temporary internal tamponade of retinal breaks by Rosengren in 1938[19]; the development of complete retinal examination through binocular indirect ophthalmoscopy by Schepens in 1947[20] and 1951[21]; the introduction of scleral indentation ("buckling") by Custodis in 1953[22]; the method of photocoagulation by Meyer-Schwickerath in 1954[23]; the "re-discovery" of modern buckling for treatment of RD by Schepens and colleagues in 1957[24]; the introduction of silicone oils to retinal surgery by Cibis et al in 1962[25]; the technique of modern vitrectomy by Machemer and colleagues in 1971[26]; athermal buckling by Zauberman and Garcia Rosell in 1975[27]; the first use of perfluorocarbon liquids in vitreoretinal surgery by Chang in 1987[28]; and the methods of Nd:YAG laser vitreolysis by Berglin and associates in 1987.[29]

In addition to typical features of retinal breaks and

vitreous traction, inflammatory response associated with rhegmatogenous RD was also mentioned in many of these early papers. Usually, the inflammation is mild and does not affect making the correct diagnosis. Recently, some unusual cases of rhegmatogenous RD-associated uveitis were reported, and the importance of inflammation as an accompanying clinical sign of RD and its possible diagnostic confusion with other clinical entities was gradually stressed and gained attention.[30–34]

Epidemiology

The observed incidence of rhegmatogenous RD varies because of the difference in inclusion criteria and methods of data collection. An annual incidence of 12.4 to 17.9 per 100,000 population was reported in the United States.[25–37] In Europe, the earliest report of the incidence was 3.8 per 100,000.[38] Recent reports, however, suggested that it is higher, with an annual incidence of 6.9 to 14 per 100,000 population.[39–41] The incidence of RD presents an increasing tendency in the United States and Europe; it has been suggested that increasing cataract surgery might be a significant factor for increasing the long-term cumulative probability of RD.[37, 40]

An incidence of 8.9 to 10.8 per 100,000 population was reported in Israel.[42] Two early reports from Africa revealed a low incidence rate, from 0.5 to 1.0 per 100,000 population.[43, 44] In Asia, an annual incidence of 10.4 and 10.5 per 100,000 population was reported from Japan[45] and Singapore,[46] respectively.

Although there are no reliable studies on racial differences in the incidence of rhegmatogenous RD, it has been suggested that the incidence is lower in blacks than in whites,[43, 44, 47, 48] which may be related to the relative infrequency of myopia in blacks. In Asia, the incidence was the highest in Chinese because of a higher prevalence of myopia, followed by Malays, and lowest for Indians.[46] No apparent gender preference was reported in some studies,[35, 36, 39, 49] although sex predilection at some age groups was found in others.[37, 40, 41, 45, 46, 50] Men were more prone to retinal detachment than women, which is explained by the greater liability to trauma in men.[51–60] However, a higher risk in women confined to the nontraumatic rhegmatogenous RD group was also reported.[40]

The incidence of RD increases after the age of 20 and progresses until its zenith in the 50- to 60-year-old age group for both sexes.[35–37, 51–55, 61–63] Relatively few cases were seen after the age of 70 years. The mean age of the overall rhegmatogenous RD population was reported to be about 54 to 60 years in the United States[35, 36] and Europe.[39, 40] In Israel, the average age at detachment was reported to be 48 years.[40] In Asia, the mean age was 70.2 years old for aphakic RD, and the highest risk for nontraumatic phakic RD was in the 60- to 69-year-old age group for both sexes.[45] Chinese showed the highest annual incidence of RD operations in the 40- to 50-year-old category.[46]

Clinical Features

The main symptoms of rhegmatogenous RD include floaters, flashes (photopsia), shadows or blind areas, and clouded vision. Lightning flashes last an instant or a few seconds and probably represent mechanical retinal stimulation resulting from vitreoretinal traction or tearing of the retina.[64–68, 70] The floaters often indicate vitreous hemorrhage that occurs when papillary or retinal vessels are torn by vitreous traction or when retinal vessels crossing retinal tears are avulsed. Many individuals with myopia also report vitreous floaters without RD or retinal breaks; those patients, however, note them chronically. Some patients may never experience floaters or flashes, presenting instead with the symptoms of a shadow or curtain with visual field loss or decreased visual acuity.[66, 67] Decreasing visual acuity can be secondary either to macular detachment or to ocular media clouding by pigment floaters, vitreous hemorrhage, or inflammatory debris.

A peripheral retinal break with a relatively immobile corrugated fold is a typical and primary sign of rhegmatogenous RD on fundus examination. The retinal break can commonly present as a full-thickness flap tear or a horseshoe tear caused by vitreous traction or by an atrophic round or oval hole. Almost all patients with rhegmatogenous RD have posterior vitreous detachment (PVD),[66, 67] and approximately 15% of all patients with acute PVD may develop a retinal tear.[69–74] Vitreous hemorrhage can also be seen and is found in 13% to 19% of rhegmatogenous RD patients with acute PVD,[69–72] and relative hypotony is common in patients with rhegmatogenous RD.[30, 31, 34, 75–79]

Other clinical features that may masquerade as uveitis include pigment cells ("tobacco dust")[80, 81] and inflammatory cells in the anterior chamber and vitreous. Some patients with asymptomatic or not recently symptomatic rhegmatogenous RD may show a substantial number of cells in the vitreous.[73, 82] Some degree of intraocular inflammation is always associated with rhegmatogenous RD, which may present as iridocyclitis or anterior uveitis,[64, 65, 81] posterior uveitis, and panuveitis.[31, 80] In severe cases, patients may develop aqueous flare, concentric iris folds, deepened anterior chamber, iridodonesis, posterior synechiae, hazy vitreous or vitreous cells, and detachment of the ciliary body and choroid with hypotony.[30, 31, 34]

It is not surprising, therefore, that misdiagnoses are often made when dealing with this clinical entity. Pigmented cells in the aqueous humor may lead to improper grading of anterior chamber inflammation. In some cases, the obvious features of inflammation associated with rhegmatogenous RD can lead to misdiagnosis as uveitis, and the detachment may be completely overlooked. It is important to stress here that all cases of persistent ocular inflammation with relative hypotony and a substantial number of vitreous cells should be viewed with a high index of suspicion for a possible underlying rhegmatogenous RD.

Longstanding RD with peripheral retinal tears can also present as an anterior cellular reaction with accompanying elevation of ocular pressure (Schwartz' syndrome).[77, 83–86] If the detachment is not detected, the patient may also be mistakenly treated for uveitis or glaucoma.

Pathogenesis and Etiology

The most causative conditions that may increase the risk of retinal breaks and subsequent RDs include PVD, lattice degeneration of the retina, myopia, especially axial myopia, cystic retinal tufts, degenerative retinoschisis, idiopathic retinal dialyses, a history of previous cataract surgery and trauma to the globe.

PVD usually results from age-related vitreous liquefaction (syneresis).[74, 87–92] Liquefaction of the posterior part of the vitreous and its detachment from above results in increased mobility of the posterior part of the vitreous and forms the posterior vitreous detachment. When PVD occurs with the traction forces shortly thereafter, the traction forces are transmitted to physiologic and pathologic areas of firm vitreoretinal adhesion. These areas include the vitreous base, margins of lattice retinal degeneration, cystic retinal tufts and retinoschisis, retinal dialyses, and paravascular retina. Retinal tears often occur when the traction forces are exerted on these pathologic areas. Fluid coming from the liquefied vitreous then seeps through the retinal tears and accumulates in the subretinal space and elevates the retina. The incidence of PVD is higher with increasing age[74] and in individuals with myopic eyes,[86, 93, 94] cataract surgery, and YAG capsulotomy.[35, 60, 69, 95–106] Intraocular inflammation, diabetes, trauma, and certain hereditary conditions also increase the incidence of PVD.

Lattice degeneration typically consists of equatorially oriented patches of crisscrossing white lines. The peripheral degeneration area is thinned and associated with liquefaction of the overlying vitreous gel and strong vitreoretinal adhesions along the margin of the lesions. Atrophic round holes are often present within the areas of lattice degeneration.[107] It is more common in myopic eyes,[108–111] especially in highly myopic eyes with increasing axial length.[69, 110, 112–117] Lattice degeneration causes 21% to 30% of rhegmatogenous RD.[118, 119]

Myopia increases the incidence of both lattice degeneration[69, 113] and PVD,[69, 120] and causes 34% to 40%[60, 94, 121] of rhegmatogenous RD. Some asymptomatic retinal breaks that cause clinical RD are mainly seen in young myopic patients,[12] older patients,[117, 122] and most aphakic eyes. Other factors such as choroidal ischemia,[123] thinning of the myopic retina,[121] genetic factors, or unknown variables may also be related to development of retinal breaks and detachment in myopic eyes.

Cystic retinal tufts are congenital small discrete white lesions. Histologically, they are composed of degenerated retinal cells and some glial proliferation. Cystic retinal tufts are commonly associated with retinal breaks[124–127] and may be responsible for approximately 10% of clinical rhegmatogenous detachments.[128]

Age-related degenerative retinoschisis occurs when the cysts of peripheral cystoid degeneration coalesce,[129–132] with resultant lamellar splitting of the retina, and most frequently precedes hole formation. Degenerative retinoschisis is associated with RD in 2% to 6% of rhegmatogenous RD cases.[133, 134]

Aphakic and pseudophakic eyes increase the risk of RD because of an increased rate of vitreous liquefaction, posterior vitreous detachment, vitreous loss and a destabilization effect on the vitreous. Approximately 23% to 40% of rhegmatogenous detachments occur after cataract extraction,[35, 97–100] and the risk is especially high if the eye is also myopic. Nd:YAG laser capsulotomy after extracapsular cataract extraction also increases the rate of RD,[100–105]

suggesting a direct destabilization effect on the hyaluronic acid infrastructure of the vitreous gel and the rapid loss of hyaluronic acid content.

Blunt trauma often produces a traction force at the vitreous base or other pathologic areas, which predisposes to rhegmatogenous RD in 7% to 16% of cases.[135] The incidence is especially high in an eye with high myopia or lattice degeneration.

When a retinal tear forms as a result of the vitreous traction on pathogenic areas of retina, an RD ensues. Retinal pigment granules disperse in the vitreous or anterior chamber from the RPE through the retinal tear and mimic a feature of intraocular inflammation. RD itself in some way also triggers an inflammatory response. It has been suggested that vitreous in contact with the pigment epithelium stimulates an inflammatory reaction in the choroid and subretinal fluid, causing uveitis.[136] Other studies indicate that some histamine or histamine-like substances in the subretinal fluid might be elaborated from the mast cells in the uvea and incite the inflammatory response.[30, 137] Ocular inflammation adversely increases capillary permeability, causing leakage of fluid and protein into the extravascular space, hyperemia of the choroid and ciliary body, eventual ciliary body and choroidal detachment, and subsequent hypotony.[138] Therefore, some degree of inflammatory response is always associated with rhegmatogenous RD.

Diagnosis

Diagnosis of RD depends on a detailed ophthalmic history and a thorough ophthalmic examination. Ophthalmic history should include the following:

1. Present illness—its specific symptom and duration. Light flashes or a sudden onset of floaters, or both, followed by progressive visual field loss of one eye are typical and important symptoms that strongly suggest rhegmatogenous RD.
2. Pre-existent eye diseases. Many pre-existent factors predispose to the development of rhegmatogenous RD; these include PVD, aphakia, high myopia, lattice degeneration and retinoschisis, retinal cystic degeneration, a family history of RD, prior RD in the patient's other eye, and others.
3. Current and past head or eye trauma. History of trauma should be suspected in all cases of unilateral aphakia, particularly when the contralateral eye is completely normal.
4. Family history. There is a significantly increased incidence of rhegmatogenous RD in some pedigrees with myopia and lattice degeneration. Because cataract surgery, YAG laser capsulotomy, and trauma itself can cause intraocular inflammatory reaction, when taking an ocular history, clinicians must have a clear mind that these features can also mask an underlying ocular disease.

A detailed ophthalmic examination should include visual acuity and visual field tests, slit-lamp examination, indirect ophthalmoscopy, and special tests.

The visual acuity may decrease if vitreous hemorrhage, iridocyclitis, vitritis, or detachment of the macula occur. The defects in visual field correspond to the area of detached retina and may also result from a dense vitreous hemorrhage associated with a retinal tear.

Slit-lamp biomicroscopy evaluations will stress anterior segment, anterior and posterior vitreous gel, and measurement of the intraocular pressure (IOP) by applanation tonometry. Pigment debris within the anterior chamber and anterior vitreous is regularly seen in patients with rhegmatogenous detachment.[80, 82] Other cells in the vitreous are also commonly present. The cells may be red cells from torn retinal blood vessels or inflammatory cells (white blood cells and macrophages) from coincident iridocyclitis. Liquefaction of the central vitreous gel followed by collapse and forward displacement of the posterior cortical vitreous can be visible with the slit lamp in most cases of rhegmatogenous RD.[139, 140] The ocular pressure is expected to be somewhat lower in the eye with detachment.[70, 78, 141–145] Sometimes the involved eye is hypotonous, in which case choroidal detachment may be present. The IOP may also be elevated in eyes with RD, and an association between open-angle glaucoma and detachment has been demonstrated.[76, 146–151]

Examination of both eyes with dilated indirect ophthalmoscopy is important in the evaluation of patients with uveitis. The "uveitis" may be secondary to a peripheral retinal break and RD. The presence of a detached retina and a retinal break is the typical sign of a rhegmatogenous RD. However, 5% to 10% of cases of true rhegmatogenous detachments have no definite retinal break discovered on clinically evaluation. The detached retina is slightly opaque and often has a corrugated appearance. The subretinal fluid is usually clear and nonshifting.

In certain cases, it may be difficult to diagnose and localize retinal breaks and detached retina because of opaque media such as vitreous hemorrhage. Ultrasonography and electroretinography are most valuable for these cases.

Because some degree of intraocular inflammation[30, 31, 34, 80] is often present in rhegmatogenous RD cases and occasionally may be severe,[30, 31, 34] the primary disorder can masquerade as uveitis. The diagnosis and subsequent treatment may be missed or delayed because the masquerade features resulted from the RD itself. Today, it is not surprising for us to see that, in many routine eye exams, clinicians so easily and simply classify some intraocular inflammation with no special or obvious finding of systemic disease as idiopathic uveitis, neglecting to look further for other possible underlying ocular diseases. This incorrect diagnosis may then adversely play a misleading role for other ophthalmologists when a patient who has an initial misdiagnosis seeks further consultation from other ocular services.

Accurate diagnostic strategies are very important for any disorder that may present some degree of intraocular inflammation and may masquerade as uveitis. The correct diagnostic strategies will stress a detailed ophthalmic history including predisposing conditions and clinical appearance of the disease at presentation, careful ophthalmic examination, and ultrasonography. The original diagnosis should be reviewed and the effects of any treatment must be re-evaluated periodically. If a treatment is ineffective, re-evaluation of the previous diagnosis should be considered immediately.

Differential Diagnosis

Because of the inflammatory characteristics associated with rhegmatogenous RD, the differential diagnosis should be considered between rhegmatogenous RD and an inflammatory disorder. Findings on the ophthalmic examination, including pigment and inflammatory cells in the anterior chamber and vitreous, are consistent with either a rhegmatogenous RD or an inflammatory disorder. In the absence of previous intraocular surgery or a choroidal malignant melanoma, pigmented cells or "tobacco dust" in the anterior chamber and vitreous and the presence of PVD are almost pathognomonic of RD or retinal tear[77, 83, 84] In addition, the presence of deepened anterior chamber, PVD, iridodonesis, detachment of the ciliary body and choroid with relative hypotony, and a typical break in the retina (Fig. 50–1) all favor the diagnosis of a rhegmatogenous RD.

Other diagnoses, including an inflammatory or exudative RD, traction detachment, and choroidal effusion syndromes, should also be considered. Exudative RD is caused by exudation of fluid from the choroid or retina in the absence of retinal breaks. Neoplasms such as melanoma[30, 152] and metastatic carcinoma, and inflammatory diseases such as Harada's disease[153] and scleritis[3] are the leading causes of exudative detachments.

The choroidal neoplasm can usually be found by indirect ophthalmoscopy and confirmed by fluorescein angiography and ultrasonography. In addition to the mass, other features common to exudative RD, such as shifting fluid, a biomicroscopically clear vitreous, and the absence of retinal break, are likely to be distinguished from rhegmatogenous RD.

Vogt-Koyanagi-Harada syndrome (VKH) is a bilateral uveitis associated with headache, malaise, tinnitus, nausea, and meningeal inflammation. Exudative RD is also an essential feature of VKH. Most cases of VKH respond well to high doses of systemic corticosteroids.

Posterior scleral inflammation can cause exudative RD.[154, 155] It can be differentiated by showing a thickened sclera on ultrasonography,[154] with accompanying pain.

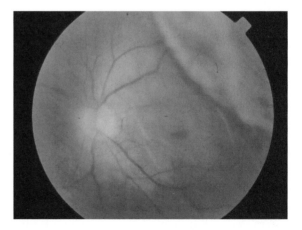

FIGURE 50–1. Peripheral retinal detachment. The detachment has progressed to the point at which it is now quite obvious. However, it has existed for approximately 6 weeks and has slowly progressed to this point. Once the detachment was repaired and the peripheral retinal break was successfully closed, the "chronic uveitis" vanished without further (medical) treatment. (See color insert.)

The inflammation usually responds well to corticosteroids or nonsteroidal anti-inflammatory drugs.[154]

The uveal effusion syndrome is an inflammatory condition characterized by peripheral choroidal separation and secondary RD.[156–159] The detached retina shows the characteristic smooth contours and shifting fluid. In rhegmatogenous RD, the retina shows a tear and a relatively immobile corrugated surface, and the vitreous usually presents inflammation. Vitreous membranes caused by proliferative retinopathies or penetrating injuries can pull the sensory retina away from the pigment epithelium, causing a traction RD. In most cases, the causative vitreous membrane can be seen ophthalmoscopically or with the three-mirror lens. The detachment may resolve after the traction ligaments are relieved by vitrectomy.

Treatment

The goal of rhegmatogenous retinal reattachment surgery is to bring the retina into contact with the choroid and sclera, to establish a chorioretinal adhesion around all retinal breaks, and to offset all important vitreoretinal traction. Operative procedures include the alteration of scleral contour, the establishment of chorioretinal adhesions, and the drainage of subretinal fluid.

The scleral contour may be altered by scleral buckling techniques, and retina can be pushed outward to contact choroid and sclera by the application of a variety of foreign materials such as intravitreal gas, silicone oil, and hyaluronic acid. Cryotherapy, diathermy, and photocoagulation may achieve chorioretinal adhesion reaction. Subretinal fluid can be drained from one or more sites internally or externally, and vitreous traction can be released by vitrectomy.

Intraocular inflammation associated with rhegmatogenous RD often clears postoperatively if the retina is successfully reattached. In eyes with marked inflammation, preoperative steroid treatment is suggested. Surgery must be postponed in some cases with severe inflammation, hypotony, and choroidal detachment until these are reversed with corticosteroid treatment. Suprachoroidal fluid is drained intraoperatively and a balanced salt solution is injected into the vitreous cavity in an eye with sizable choroidal detachments.[160]

Complications

Complications usually include intraocular inflammation, glaucoma, hemorrhage, and later development of proliferative vitreoretinopathy. Visual acuity may be damaged if the detachment involves the macula. In some complicated cases, the rhegmatogenous RD may initiate a series of exaggerated pathophysiologic changes in the eye, with the severe inflammation leading to choroidal detachment and hypotony.

Prognosis

By arriving at the correct diagnosis and using the appropriate application of surgical methods, retinal reattachment can be achieved in more than 90% of cases of rhegmatogenous RD.[160, 161] Ten to twenty percent of eyes require more than one operation to reattach the retina.[162–165] Visual recovery depends on the extent of macular damage caused by the detachment and any surgical complications. About 37% to 50% [100, 163, 166–168] of patients with successful reattachment now can achieve final visual acuity of 20/56 or better. The prognosis of surgery and visual improvement is very poor in rhegmatogenous RD complicated by severe ocular inflammation, choroidal detachment, and hypotony.[30, 34]

Conclusions

Rhegmatogenous RD is usually caused by retinal breaks, in which fluid from the vitreous cavity seeps through the breaks, accumulates in the potential subretinal space, and separates the retina from the RPE.

Peripheral breaks with a relatively immobile corrugated fold in retina are a typical feature of rhegmatogenous RD. Other clinical manifestations include posterior vitreous detachment, vitreous hemorrhage, and mild intraocular inflammation. Intraocular inflammation may be severe in some cases.

Slight proteinaceous flare and occasional cells in the anterior chamber and vitreous are common in eyes with rhegmatogenous RD. Eyes with more severe inflammation may show intense flare in the anterior chamber and debris in the vitreous. Therefore, the features of intraocular inflammation with rhegmatogenous RD can masquerade as uveitis. Misdiagnosis can be avoided by a detailed ophthalmic history and thorough ocular examination. Knowledge of the clinical features of each disease, the possible masquerade syndromes, and the diagnosis and differential diagnosis between an ocular inflammatory disorder and other ocular or systemic diseases is important for making a correct diagnosis.

RETINITIS PIGMENTOSA

Definition

Retinitis pigmentosa (RP) is a group of hereditary retinal degenerative diseases characterized by progressive degeneration of retinal photoreceptors with associated pigmented epithelial changes, which often manifest as bilateral night blindness, progressive visual field loss, and abnormal or nonrecordable findings on electroretinogram (ERG).

Classification of RP is important and complicated. At present, there is no generally agreed-upon classification for RP disorders.[169–179] In general, RP can be divided into two large groups: primary and secondary RP.[180] Primary RP is a disease confined to the eye with no other systemic manifestation, which can include rod degeneration, cone degeneration, and congenital onset disorders such as Leber's congenital amaurosis. Secondary RP is a pigmented retinal degeneration associated with single or multiple organ system diseases. The most common secondary forms of associated RP include Usher's syndrome, Bardet-Biedl syndrome, Senior-Loken syndrome and abetalipoproteinemia.[180]

Either primary or secondary RP can be inherited as an autosomal recessive, autosomal dominant, or X-linked trait, based on the features of genetic inheritance.[180] There is also another group named simplex RP or nonhereditary RP, which presents as an isolated case. Sometimes, the term multiplex is also used to describe this group of RP when more than one person is affected (e.g., in a sibling of a family).[181] Simplex RP is frequently seen in the diseases of pigmented paravenous retinochoroidopathy, nonspecific RP, unknown RP type, pericentral RP, some rod-cone degeneration, and rod degeneration forms.

RP can also be subdivided into two broad categories: typical and atypical,[182] based on clinical mode of inheritance, age of onset, rate of progression, severity, and ERG findings. Typical RP refers to those patients with an obvious hereditary pattern characterized by the onset of night blindness in childhood or young adulthood, progressive contraction of the peripheral visual field, the characteristic pigmented retinopathy, and abnormal or extinguished ERG. Atypical forms of RP often present clinical symptoms and signs that are closely related to typical RP but are often incomplete forms of the disease such as sector RP, retinitis pigmentosa sine pigmenti, and retinitis punctata albescens.[182] The hereditary pattern can be complete or uncertain in atypical RP.

Not only is the classification of RP complicated but the clinical features of RP are also various. Except for the typical symptoms and pigmentary retinopathy, patients with RP can also frequently exhibit some features consistent with underlying inflammatory disease such as pigmented vitreous cells, posterior subcapsular cataract, and cystic macular edema.[183-185] Clinically, vitreal cells and macular edema may occur in all age groups and in patients with typical pigmentary changes, but with a higher incidence in younger patients and in the cases with minimal retinopathy.[182] These features can masquerade as ocular inflammatory disease, especially in some patients with no defined hereditary history. For this reason, today, with the increase of some isolated or atypical cases, RP has been considered as one of the masquerade syndromes of ocular inflammatory disease.

History

The development of RP concepts is consistent with a number of clinical observations, fundus examinations, and the hereditary nature of the disease over the years. The early observations of familial complicated night blindness were first made by Ovelgün in 1744.[186] Since then, other clinical features, including poor vision and pigmented lesions in the retina, were also reported.[187, 188] Shortly after the invention of the ophthalmoscope by von Helmholtz in 1851, some cases that most assuredly represented the characteristics of RP were further confirmed.[189, 190] But no defined term was offered until 1855 and 1857, when Donders first used the term retinitis pigmentosa to describe the disease.[191, 192] Other terms, such as tapetoretinal degeneration,[193] pigmentary retinopathy, primary pigmentary retinal degeneration, and rod-cone dystrophy, have also been used to describe the disorder, but the term retinitis pigmentosa is still widely accepted as describing the entire class of inherited pigmentary degenerations of the retina.

The hereditary and consanguineous nature of RP was subsequently noted[169, 194-197] soon after the recognition of the clinical features of RP. Over the years, the clear hereditary pedigree of typical RP, including autosomal recessive, autosomal dominant, and X-linked transmission, has been further reported and confirmed in more

studies of large populations in various parts of the world.[172, 174, 198-221] Abnormal to extinguished ERG associated with RP was also observed by Karpe in 1945.[221] Since then, numerous ERG documentation studies[220-238] and other spectral sensitivity studies, including the early receptor potential of ERG,[239] electro-oculogram (EOG),[240-245] dark adaptation,[246-250] perimetry,[251-254] psychophysical flicker testing,[255, 256] and color vision,[257-260] have been done, with a peak period for these types of studies from the 1950s to the 1980s.

From the early 1970s to the present, ultrastructural and genetic studies of RP explored the pathogenesis of the disease. During this period, one of the most striking concepts for RP pathogenesis was dysfunction of the integration between retinal photoreceptors and pigment epithelia. It has been suggested that micrometabolic disorders of the outer segment portions of the photoreceptors and dysfunction of RPE in the maintenance of photoreceptor cell homeostasis may cause degeneration, either primarily or secondarily, of rods, cones, or a combination of both.[261-276]

Gene defects and point mutations in the rhodopsin gene on chromosomes 3, 6, 7 and 8 in patients with autosomal dominant retinitis pigmentosa (ADRP) have been reported in many studies.[277-282] At present, at least 80 or more genes causing retinal degenerative diseases have been identified.[271-318] In addition, advanced studies in immunology also further improve the recognition of immunologic or autoimmunologic processes associated with RP. Some antiretinal antibodies in RP patients have been reported.[319-321] It has been suggested that ocular inflammation associated with RP may be due to a secondary immunologic reaction against retinal antigens released into the vitreous as the retina degenerates; and these antibodies might also be related to cystoid macular edema in RP patients.[319-325] For this reason, recently, the possible immune mechanism and associated inflammation with RP, especially seen in atypical cases, has been stressed as a possible uveitis masquerade syndrome.

Epidemiology

The incidence of RP is estimated to be as high as 1 in 3500 to 4000 worldwide.[326-337] In Switzerland,[326] a low prevalence of RP was found (1 in 7000), whereas in American Navajo Indians, 1 in 1878 has the disease.[338]

In various surveys of the genetic types of RP, the estimates of percentage of autosomal recessive cases of RP have been reported to be from 13% to 69% (average: 41% in the United States, 15% in England, and 33% in China).[329-332, 336, 337, 339, 340] Autosomal dominant RP is believed to account for 10% to 24% of cases (16% in the United States, 24% in England, and 11% in China).[329-332, 336, 337, 339, 340] X-linked RP represents from 5% to 21% of cases (9% in the United States, 18% in England, and 8% in China).[179, 329-332, 337, 339, 340]

Although most RP cases are believed to be genetic, the frequency of simplex or multiplex cases with no family history of affected relatives has also been reported to range from 15% to 63% (the average across studies is 35% in the United States, 42% in England, and 48% in China).[179, 329-332, 337, 339, 340] Some atypical disorders are also often seen in routine eye clinics. The high rate of simplex cases and the rising rate of atypical RP cases has increased the diagnostic challenges for clinicians.

Clinical Features

Night blindness is one of the most common early symptoms in patients with RP. Usually, patients with typical RP have poor vision and constricted visual fields in the dark beginning in childhood or adolescence (autosomal recessive and X-linked recessive) or young adulthood (autosomal dominant). As the disease progresses, patients gradually lose their far-peripheral field of vision, typically leaving a small central field of vision until eventually even central vision is affected.[340–343] Central visual acuity can be seriously affected early in the course of the disease by cystoid macular edema, macular atrophy, or the development of a posterior subcapsular cataract.[169, 174, 184, 185, 343–349] Ten percent to 15% of patients may not be aware of symptoms until central vision is affected.[182, 343] In addition, some RP patients may have severe myopia and astigmatism, especially seen in X-linked RP and the congenital form.[340–344, 350, 351] Other complaints such as headache (53%) and light flashes (35%) can be associated with RP in the early course of the disease.[352]

At early stages of RP, fundus examination usually reveals granularity or tiny focal depigmented spots in the midperiphery and far periphery. Retinal vessels may be relatively normal or mildly attenuated. As the disease progresses, widespread hypopigmentation, peripheral pigment migration and clumping, and the characteristic bone-spicule pattern of retinal pigment are consistently found in a midperipheral annular zone of both eyes (Fig. 50–2). The retinal vessels, particularly the arteries, continue to become more narrow, and the optic disc appears waxy and pale. The entire midperipheral and far peripheral fundus is replaced by dense bone-spicule pigmentary formations, which present a reticular or lobular structural appearance in advanced RP. The retinal vessels become quite constricted and appear threadlike. The optic nerve head becomes pale. In some cases with severe RPE loss, the overall fundus may appear yellow or white, with greater visibility of underlying choroidal vessels.[340–344]

The anterior segment, vitreous, and macula also frequently show abnormalities in patients with RP. Posterior subcapsular opacity is common in most types of RP. The vitreous changes include dustlike reflective particles, cells, posterior vitreous separation, cottonball-like opacities, interwoven filaments in the retrocortical space, and spindle-shaped vitreous condensations.[340–344, 352, 353] Asteroid hyalosis can also be seen. Macular changes may include early broadening or loss of foveal reflexes; as the disease progresses, cystoid macular edema,[185, 313, 354–362] diffuse retinal vascular leakage,[363] wrinkling of the internal limiting membrane,[184] and macular preretinal fibrosis can also sequentially occur.[185, 189, 362, 364, 365]

In some patients with RP, the vitreous changes may be the earliest finding, and bilateral macular edema can also occur in the early stage of the disease. Most patients with macular edema have 1+ or 2+ vitreous cells.[182] Because of these features of anterior chamber cells and macular edema, consistent with ocular inflammatory features, it is not surprising that the inflammation associated with RP can masquerade as idiopathic uveitis. In some conditions, especially when RP occurs as an isolated case with a negative family history or in atypical cases in which the symptoms and characteristic retinopathy are minimal in the early course of the disease, patients may initially be seen with only visual loss secondary to ocular inflammation and macular edema; the underlying diagnosis of RP may be missed. Therefore, in routine eye clinic examinations, correct recognition of the features of the disease is very important. Because the classification of RP is complicated and the clinical features associated with RP are various at different stages, any inflammation involving both eyes with subtle retinal pigmented changes or macular edema should be highly suspect as a masquerade syndrome that may be confounding the diagnosis.

Pathogenesis and Etiology

RP may result from a primary defect in the rod and cone photoreceptors and dysfunction of retinal pigmented epithelium cells.[366] Numerous histopathologic studies of patients' eyes with RP have corroborated this idea.[265, 268, 269, 275, 276, 367] In the degenerative area of RP, there is loss of outer segments and a decrease in photoreceptor numbers. Other histopathologic changes include degeneration of the retinal receptor elements; depigmentation of the RPE; migration of RPE cells into the overlying retina, particularly in the perivascular areas; hyalinization and thickening of the retinal vessel walls; diffuse atrophy of the whole retina; and gliosis. These changes are usually most prominent in the midperipheral fundus.[265, 268, 269, 273, 275, 366, 367]

At present, the concept of the photoreceptors as the primary degeneration site in RP has been further supported by advanced molecular biologic techniques. At least 50 or more different mutations in rhodopsin in families with ADRP have been identified.[278–320] It has been suggested that alteration and dysfunction of various genes coding for proteins that are specific for the function or structure of the photoreceptor or pigment epithelium

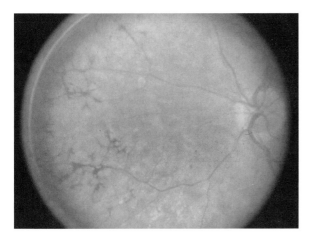

FIGURE 50–2. Retinitis pigmentosa. Note in particular the bone-spicule, mid and far peripheral retinal pigmentary changes, and retinal arteriolar narrowing. This patient had had chronic vitritis for 2 years before the appearance of the characteristic, diagnostic retinal pigmentary changes. (See color insert.)

can lead to the degenerative changes of these cells and the final common pathologic picture of RP.

Ultrastructural studies of the vitreous of patients with RP show the presence of RPE cells; uveal melanocytes; retinal astrocytes; lymphocytes, which are mostly T cells; and macrophage-like cells.[266, 368–370] The presence of these inflammatory cells indicates possible immunologic or autoimmunologic processes involved in the pathogenesis of photoreceptor degeneration in RP. Retinal outer segments and pigment epithelia are known to be antigenic,[371–375] and an immune response to these antigens may cause an inflammatory reaction and retinal edema in patients with genetically determined retinal degeneration.[323] Antibodies directed against photoreceptors,[320–322] elevation of serum IgM,[324, 375] the presence of circulating immune complexes, and reduction in the total number of T cells in RP patients have been reported.[376–382] It has been suggested that ocular inflammation associated with RP may be due to the increase of vascular permeability to immune complexes or to a secondary immune reaction against retinal antigens released into the vitreous as the retina degenerates; and this mechanism has also been considered as a factor in cystoid macular edema associated with RP. Although the exact role of immune or autoimmune responses in the pathogenesis of RP has not been confirmed,[171, 291, 292, 345, 346] the features of a variable amount of cellular infiltration in vitreous and the detectable antiretina antibodies associated with RP reported in recent studies have increased the complexity of the disease concepts, and this clearly needs to be carefully evaluated by clinicians dealing with RP patients, because it can mimic an ocular inflammatory disease.

Diagnosis

The diagnosis of RP is based on a complete ocular, systemic, and family history, a thorough ocular examination, and laboratory evaluation. The detailed history should include information regarding the nature of the symptoms, age of onset, progression, systemic associations, and family pedigree.[340, 343, 352] Bilateral involvement, night blindness, and progressive loss of peripheral vision starting in childhood or adolescence, with a feature of family and consanguinity occurrence, are the typical symptoms and history for considering the diagnosis.[343]

When the symptoms of blindness or very low vision with nystagmus, sluggish pupillary reaction, and high hyperopia occur at birth, the diagnosis of a congenital form of RP such as Leber's amaurosis is considered.[182, 228, 343, 352] Systemic symptoms, including sensorineural hearing loss, cerebellar dysfunction, various nutritional deficiencies, valvular heart disease or vascular insufficiency, exposure to drugs or toxins,[347] and possible immunologic or autoimmunologic processes are most helpful in diagnosing typical or atypical RP associated with systemic disorders (such as Usher's syndrome) and in excluding other diagnoses (infectious disease such as syphilis or viral infection). Medical or neurologic examination and consultation are recommended in patients with RP associated with these systemic symptoms, in order to avoid misdiagnosis and delayed therapy.[181, 343]

Abnormal signs of typical RP on ocular examination usually include narrowed retinal vessels, depigmentation of RPE, intraretinal bone spicule pigmentation, waxy pallor of the optic discs, and the presence of posterior subcapsular cataract. Vitreous abnormalities, and cystoid macular edema in some cases, are consistent with the diagnosis of RP.[340–344]

ERG is invaluable in assessing retinal function and progression, and in providing prognostic information for patients with RP. It is clearly useful for all patients in whom the diagnosis of RP is in question. In patients with typical RP, the ERG shows a diminished amplitude of the a-wave and b-wave in individuals with early disease, or extinguished a-wave and b-wave responses in patients with advanced RP, particularly in the dark adapted state, with a delay in b-wave implicit time.[175, 221, 228–230, 239, 383–390] Quantitative diminishment of the ERG over time, with comparison of serial visual field testing, especially provides valuable information regarding the course of progression.[337]

Progressive visual field loss is one of the cardinal features of typical RP. In the early stage of RP, visual field loss usually begins as a group of isolated ring scotomas in the midperiphery. As the disease progresses, multiple scotomas gradually coalesce to form partial to full-ring scotomata. In advanced disease, the superior and nasal field can be completely lost, leaving a small oval of intact central island of field.[239, 384, 391, 392] The periodic evaluation of visual field function in RP is most useful for RP diagnosis and differential diagnosis.

Other electrophysiologic methods as aids for diagnosis of RP include the dark-adaptation test, the electro-oculogram (EOG), the visually evoked response (VER), and contrast sensitivity testing. The observed abnormalities of these tests in patients with RP can include low ratio of light peak to dark in the EOG test,[241, 242, 244, 256] prolonged dark adaptation thresholds,[246–250] and poor contrast sensitivity.[251, 253] These tests are not specific and are not recommended when the diagnosis of RP is otherwise clear.

Fluorescein angiography can also be valuable in documenting early deterioration of the RPE in patients with RP, and especially in female carriers of X-linked RP.[337, 343] It also has a role in the evaluation of patients with possible cystoid macular edema and some atypical pigmentary patterns.[353]

Although complete ocular, systemic, and family history and other various laboratory methods described earlier help in the diagnosis of RP, the challenge for clinicians to make a correct diagnosis is greatly increased with the increasing clinical reports of atypical and isolated RP cases. Many cases present as an atypical form or show nonhereditary family history. These atypical symptoms and signs and negative family history can manifest or mimic the features of other diseases. In general, the possible masquerade features of RP include simplex case presence with a poor hereditary family history, the absence of pigment migration in an initial stage of the disease, shorter duration of symptoms, less severe night blindness, and less impairment of the ERG. Other features include the presence of vitreous cells, posterior subcapsular cataract (PSC), and cystoid macular edema. Because the visual decrease or loss secondary to vitreous opacity, PSC, or cystoid macular edema may be an initial reason for RP patients to have a routine eye examination, when the pigment migration is minimal, these RP patients may be misdiagnosed as having uveitis. Therefore, in routine eye examinations, clinicians must have a high index of suspicion for the possible underlying RP in any patient with persistent visual loss with bilateral ocular inflammation.

Differential Diagnosis

There are a number of disorders that may produce a pigmentary retinopathy and mimic RP. Clinically, these disorders are called pseudoretinitis pigmentosa. The main pseudoretinitis pigmentosa cases include retinal infectious or inflammatory diseases; drug toxicities such as chloroquine, thioridazine, and chlorpromazine[393–406]; some hereditary vitreoretinopathy diseases such as pigmented paravenous retinochoroidal atrophy; and uniocular retinitis pigmentosa.[181, 342]

Rubella retinopathy, the most common ocular manifestation of congenital rubella, can be mistaken for a panretinal degeneration such as RP.[340, 407] Rubella retinopathy commonly produces scattered pigmentary deposits, or on occasion, the pigmentation may be bone spicule–like; more often one sees subretinal clumps or salt-and-pepper pigmentation, and the retinal vessel caliber tends to be normal.[181, 340, 408] The correct diagnosis can usually be established by a combination of clinical features and the ERG, which is either normal or only mildly depressed in rubella retinopathy, but which is almost invariably severely to profoundly abnormal in RP. Some rubella patients can also present with full or partial deafness, which can masquerade as Usher's syndrome, but the lack of progression of the visual field does not favor this diagnosis.

Both congenital syphilis with pigmentary retinopathy and attenuated visual field and acquired syphilis–associated chorioretinitis can mimic the features of RP.[181, 340, 409] However, congenital syphilis usually also includes interstitial keratitis, and pigmentary changes in the fundus appear more patchy and postinflammatory in nature.[340] Most patients with luetic retinopathy have no relevant family history, and the change of visual field is often asymmetric. Moreover, symptoms and signs of underlying systemic disease are usually present. These features, together with positive serology for syphilis, serve to distinguish the disease from RP.

Other infectious or inflammatory entities that occasionally result in pigmentary retinopathy are also considered in the differential diagnosis, including measles retinopathy, cytomegalovirus infection, toxoplasmosis, herpes infection, birdshot retinochoroidopathy, advanced cases of Harada's disease, disseminated choroiditis, chorioretinitis, and serpiginous or geographic atrophy.[181, 340] However, most of these conditions present with asymmetric ocular involvement, and the absence of a genetic component in the nature of the diseases also distinguishes these disorders from RP.[181]

Ocular abnormalities resulting from drug toxicities may present with blurring of central vision, poor night vision, a brownish discoloration to the vision, and retinopathy,[403–406] which can mimic RP. However, most patients with drug toxicity retinopathy have a long history of therapy for underlying chronic diseases such as collagen vascular disorders and arthritis. Most drug toxicity retinopathy appears to regress when the drug is stopped, although continuous progressive cases such as thioridazine and chloroquine toxicity have also been reported.[181, 404]

Pigmented paravenous retinochoroidal atrophy is a pigmentary retinopathy without a definite inheritance pattern.[181, 410–415] The cause and pathophysiologic mechanisms of this condition are presently poorly understood, but may represent an acquired response pattern to an infectious or inflammatory disease.[412–419] Almost all of the cases are sporadic.[341] The characteristic fundus appearance is that of pigmentary changes closely associated with retinal veins.[341] The ERG in this disease is usually only mildly to moderately abnormal, if at all,[340, 414, 415, 419–421] but the EOG is usually abnormal[420] and can be severely so.[421] The features of isolated presence and paravenous retinopathy are the criteria for correct diagnosis.

Unilateral pigmentary retinopathy exhibits regional or generalized loss of the RPE with migration into the retinal layers. The most common cause of unilateral pigmentary retinopathy is traumatic injury.[181, 340, 422] The positive traumatic history and uniocular involvement can differentiate this condition from RP.

Treatment

Because a definitive or effective therapeutic strategy has not been established for RP, the main efforts in management of RP include improvement of visual function, periodic routine ocular examination and evaluation, and psychological and genetic consultation.[328, 340, 342, 343, 423]

Most patients can benefit from the treatment of complications such as refractive errors and cataracts and from use of a variety of optical aids for peripheral visual loss and preserved central vision.[328, 342, 343, 414] In RP patients with cystoid macular edema (CME), peribulbar or oral steroids and carbonic anhydrase inhibitors (acetazolamide and methazolamide) can be considered to reduce the edema and improve visual acuity.[340, 424–426] Periodic visual field and ERG evaluation with compassionate explanation of visual field defects can help patients appreciate the rate of progression and hence plan for future disability.[340] Psychological consultation, genetic counseling, and support groups are often of great benefit for patients to gain more knowledge about the disorder and learn various skills for handling low vision.[181, 340]

Combined deficiency of vitamins A and E may cause nyctalopic and progressive retinal degeneration in humans.[427, 428] Vitamin A administered orally or by injection has been used for many years as therapy for RP.[429] However, the effect of vitamin A treatment for RP is still controversial,[328, 430–431] and at present, there is no proven effective treatment to slow the loss of visual function in patients with retinitis pigmentosa.[432–434] It is conceivable that vitamin A therapy is helpful in retinal degeneration from abetalipoproteinemia.[435–437] Large doses of vitamin A have been reported to return dark-adaptation thresholds and ERG responses to normal in the early stages of this disorder.[438] Vitamin E has also been advocated to prevent the progression of this retinal degeneration.[439]

Complications/Prognosis

Cataract and CME can occur with RP. Recurrent serous detachment of the pigment epithelium and retina can also occur as a complication in patients with RP.[181, 340] RP's chronic course extends over many years.[181, 340] Eventually, patients with RP may experience profound visual loss and blindness in middle or later life.

Conclusions

Retinitis pigmentosa is a group of hereditary retinal degenerative diseases characterized by progressive degeneration of retinal photoreceptors with associated pigmented epithelial changes, which often first manifest as bilateral night blindness, progressive visual field loss, and an abnormal or nonrecordable ERG.

RP can occur as a primary disorder inherited in an autosomal dominant, autosomal recessive, or X-linked recessive manner, or it may occur in systemic diseases that usually present as an autosomal recessive pattern. However, clinical observation has revealed that more than 50% of cases of RP occur as simplex cases with no family history of the disorder.

In addition to the characteristic fundus changes (narrowed retinal vessels, depigmentation of RPE, intraretinal bone spicule pigmentation, waxy pallor of the optic discs), patients with RP also have other signs, including posterior subcapsular cataract, vitreous cells, and cystoid macular edema. The vitreous changes and macular edema can occur in the early stage of RP, and patients with RP may initially be seen with only visual loss secondary to the media opacity and edema. Clinically, because these initial symptoms and signs associated with RP are consistent with features of uveitis, the disease can be misdiagnosed as uveitis. Especially with the increase in the number of nonhereditary cases and atypical cases that have less severe symptoms of night blindness and minimal retinopathy, the masquerade features of these atypical presentations have greatly challenged the ability of clinicians to establish a correct diagnosis. It is important to stress here that clinicians must be suspicious that any persistent visual loss with bilateral ocular inflammation and minimal pigment changes might represent RP. Further evaluation and examination, as well as retinal function evaluation, are crucial in clarifying the suspicious initial diagnosis and in excluding other entities.

INTRAOCULAR FOREIGN BODY

Definition

A foreign body within the eye after a penetrating ocular injury is called intraocular foreign body (IOFB). The site of an IOFB varies with its point of entry and velocity. IOFBs may lodge in both the anterior segment (cornea, anterior or posterior chamber, anterior chamber angle, iris and ciliary body, lens, and anterior vitreous) and the posterior segment (choroid, vitreous, retina, and optic nerve). Most IOFBs are magnetic (iron, steel, nickel)[440] or nonmagnetic (aluminum, copper, magnesium, lead, silicon and zinc, gold, and silver) metals and are associated with activities involving striking metal against metal[441-443] or the use of motorized machines.[444] Other

materials, such as vegetable material (thorn, wood, soil) and non-magnetic substances (glass, plastic, stone, coal, sand) may also be found.[441, 443, 445-449] The size of retained IOFBs varies, but as a general rule, they are usually small and sharp, thereby leaving a relatively small entry site that may be self-sealing.[442, 448]

Retained IOFBs can cause various degrees of inflammation. Persistent anterior or posterior uveitis is one of the most common complications associated with IOFBs. It has been reported that the inflammatory feature secondary to an IOFB may masquerade as uveitis.[450, 451] Therefore, intraocular foreign bodies should always be considered in the differential diagnosis of uveitis.

History and Epidemiology

Retained intraocular foreign bodies have been reported since the early 1800s.[448] As social and industrial economies developed, ocular injuries have become so common that their social and economic burdens involving a huge cost in human unhappiness, economic inefficiency, and monetary loss have received a great deal of attention by ophthalmologists over the past 3 decades.[441, 448, 452]

Epidemiologic data concerning intraocular foreign bodies are incomplete and not well organized in the ophthalmic literature, but studies of general injuries have been investigated. It has been reported that in the United States, approximately 2.4 million general ocular injuries occur each year.[453, 454] The annual incidence of general ocular injuries was estimated to be 7.7 to 13.2 per 100,000 population.[455-459] A report from other countries indicated an annual incidence of 8.1 per 100,000 individuals in Scotland,[460] 6.1 per 100,000 in Sweden,[461] and 15.2 per 100,000 in Australia.[462] In Singapore, an annual incidence rate of open globe injury was 3.7 per 100,000 population, and nearly 15% of open globe injuries were associated with an IOFB.[463] A study on IOFB has shown that 15% of IOFBs after a penetrating injury may lodge in the anterior chamber, 8% in the lens, and 70% in the posterior segment.[448] There are high rates of ocular injury in young adults,[464-467] with a peak age-incidence from about 18 to 25 years of age and an additional peak rate after age 70.[456, 458] Males have a higher incidence than females.[455-459, 468-470]

Clinical Features

The clinical features following the entrance of a foreign body into the eye vary with the size, composition, and location of the particle concerned. Most foreign bodies are relatively small and sharp, and the globe is not disorganized. Patients can have a transient stinging sensation with a history of a high-risk activity such as hammering metal on metal. Little pain may be experienced at the time of impact.[448] If a particle is large, vision may be immediately blurred owing to the collapse of the anterior chamber, or lost owing to an intraocular hemorrhage either into the anterior chamber or the vitreous. If the particle is small, no further symptoms may arise, and the patient's vision may remain normal for weeks or years.

Unless the entry wound is extensive, it usually heals rapidly. Patients with an IOFB may or may not have a clinically detectable corneal or scleral perforation site or a readily detectable intraocular foreign body. A corneal wound, however, always leaves a permanent track, and although it may eventually become inconspicuous, it can be seen by slit-lamp biomicroscopy. Seidel's test can be used to evaluate a corneal wound.[443] A conjunctiva-scleral wound tends to become invisible unless it has been of considerable size, when its presence may be betrayed by the migration of uveal pigment to the surface.[448] Other possible associated signs of IOFBs, including iris hole, localized iris hemorrhage, iris distortion or transillumination defect, an irregular pupil, rupture in the lens capsule, cataract, vitreous hemorrhage, and decreased IOP, may also be detected by slit-lamp biomicroscopy.

When a foreign body in the anterior or the posterior segment is irritative, an anterior or posterior uveitis can be excited. A particle in the vitreous may cause the gel to degenerate and become turbid. Small vitreous hemorrhages can eventually become organized into a fibrous band. The contraction of the band may eventually lead to a detachment of the retina, which ultimately causes general distortion, disorganization, and atrophy of the globe. When a foreign body strikes the retina and the choroid, a retinal tear can occur; the vitreous usually becomes adherent to the wound and fills the gap by a plug of newly formed fibrous tissue. The foreign body becomes partially or completely encapsulated. Occasionally, the foreign body may lodge in the optic disc and cause an inflammatory reaction involving the optic nerve. The inflammatory reaction can also produce an exudative proliferation of fibrous tissue around the optic disc and cause further damage to the optic nerve.

Metallic foreign bodies such as iron and copper are electrolytically dissociated or react with the tissue-fluids to form decomposition products, usually by oxidation, and tend to cause specific toxic reactions such as siderosis and chalcosis. Siderosis affects virtually all ocular structures, but the most characteristic changes involve the iris, lens, and retina, causing rusty brown deposits and discoloration in corneal stroma, iris, and lens, and degenerative pigmentary changes of the retina.[442, 448, 471] Other signs include mydriasis, uveitis, optic disk hyperemia, and pallor,[443] and narrowed arterioles can also occur. Chronic open-angle glaucoma can be a complication of siderosis due to iron-containing phagocytes and cell debris blocking the trabecular meshwork. The clinical feature of chalcosis includes a greenish blue ring in the peripheral cornea (Kayser-Fleischer ring), a sunflower anterior subcapsular cataract, metallic refractile particles in the aqueous humor, a greenish coloration of the iris and sometimes the vitreous, and a brilliant and highly refractile deposit on the surface of the retina, usually in the macula.[442, 448, 472]

Most foreign bodies, especially nonorganized particles, can be chemically inert for an indefinite time,[441, 462, 464-475] sometimes becoming encapsulated in the eye, with tolerance of eye tissues toward the presence of the foreign body. The tolerance of the separate tissues of eyes varies considerably. The uveal tissues, especially the ciliary body, usually show the greatest reaction to injury of any kind, even though the foreign body is inert. This reaction may slowly and cumulatively develop into a chronic and persistent uveitis, which can eventually lead to atrophy and shrinkage of the globe with complete loss of func-

tion.[448] The clinical picture of uveitis secondary to an IOFB can present with ocular pain, redness, photophobia, fine keratic precipitates, fibrin dusting of the endothelium, anterior chamber, cells and flare,[450] and localized imprints with pigmentary degeneration associated with vitreous opacities,[447] as well as local inflammatory reactions mimicking granulomatous uveitis.[476] In many situations, the insidious and recalcitrant uveitis may be the only major complaint. Significant other clinical signs in patients with an IOFB, especially when the foreign particle is inert and tolerated, may be minimal, and an ophthalmologist may make a misdiagnosis of idiopathic uveitis, particularly when patients have no recall of recent ocular trauma.[450, 451] It is particularly important to stress here that any unexplained and persistent uveitis, especially when the uveitis is refractory, should raise suspicion for the possibility of an IOFB.

Pathogenesis and Pathophysiology

Mechanical and chemical or toxic, as well as inflammatory, injuries are the major pathophysiologic mechanisms of the eye to IOFBs. This pathophysiologic reaction of eye tissues varies within wide limits with the composition of the particles.[448] Most nonorganic and nonmagnetic substances (e.g., stone, rock, sand, coal, glass, plaster, rubber, porcelain, carbon, clay, gold, silver, lead, platinum, and tantalum) cause nonspecific inflammation by mechanical irritation to the involved tissues. The mechanical effect is essentially exudative and fibroblastic in type, in order to isolate and encapsulate the foreign body.[448] Usually, these mechanical effects on the involved eye tissues are chronic and primarily depend on the locations of particles. The exudative reaction in the ocular anterior segment often causes a chronic and persistent iridocyclitis. The mechanical effect on the posterior segment may produce persistent posterior uveitis, opacification, liquefaction and shrinkage of the vitreous gel, and exudative and proliferative changes in the retina and optic nerve, which eventually may cause RD.

Chemical injuries to eye tissues resulting from an IOFB primarily come from various irritative metal materials such as iron, copper, lead, and zinc. The mechanism of chemical damage is thought to be electrolytic dissociation of the metal or reaction with tissue fluids, usually by oxidation, causing diffusion and spread of the toxic products to various ocular structures.[442, 446, 448] Toxic metal ions can deposit on the cornea, iris and lens epithelia, and retina, and cause degeneration of those tissues and damage retinal photoreceptors and pigment epithelium, which finally leads to siderosis (iron) and chalcosis (copper).

Most organic materials such as vegetable particles can produce a considerable tissue-reaction of the foreign body granulomatous type. The pathologic reaction of ocular tissues to vegetable substances often presents with a low-grade chronic inflammatory response of a fibroblastic and proliferative nature, characterized by the presence of giant cells, which tend to wall off the foreign material and attempt to phagocytize it.[448, 477, 478]

In general, the pathophysiologic reactions of eyes to an IOFB primarily produce chronic inflammatory responses. The more vascular the tissue and the higher its metabolic activity, the lower the tolerance.[448] The uveal tissues, especially the ciliary body, usually show the greatest reaction to injury of any kind and the lowest tolerance even though the foreign body is inert.

Diagnosis

An accurate and detailed history is vital for making the correct diagnosis and providing effective management for IOFBs. Current and past ocular history regarding the exact activities and the amount of time of the patient involvement in high-risk work such as hammering metal on metal should be carefully recorded. Complete ocular examinations, including the visual-acuity assessment and careful evaluation for a possible wound of entry, are always required. Slit-lamp biomicroscopy is an especially important examination step for IOFBs, including checking the lens for disruption, cataract, or embedded foreign body (Fig. 50–3). Most anterior segment IOFBs can be seen directly with a slit lamp.[442] If an IOFB is suspected to be lodged in the anterior chamber angle, gonioscopy should be performed (Fig. 50–4). Dilated retinal examination using indirect ophthalmoscopy is essential for evaluating an IOFB in the retina and optic disc. Careful biomicroscopic evaluation of the nonpenetrated eye should also be part of the ocular examination.

Special tests, including plain film radiography, computed tomography (CT) scanning, ultrasonography, ERG, and EOG testing, can all be useful for identification and localization of suspected IOFBs.[452, 479–485] Plain radiography is particularly helpful in the detection of intraocular metallic materials. It has been reported that the rate of detection of metallic IOFB by plain radiography ranges between 40% and 90%.[486, 487]

Because CT scanning can enhance resolution, it has been suggested that it has largely supplanted plain radiography.[488] Thin-section CT scanning can provide precise localization of metallic IOFBs as small as 0.7 mm in diameter.[489–496] Nonmetallic IOFBs such as plastic materials, glass, wood, insect fragments, and objects located adjacent to the scleral wall may be visualized with less reliability by CT.[491, 497–499]

Magnetic resonance imaging (MRI), however, with the

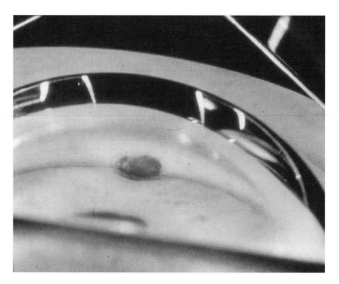

FIGURE 50–4. A tiny pebble of sand resting in the inferior angle. Its presence was not inert but rather created continuing iris trauma with stimulation of chronic anterior chamber cells. (See color insert.)

feature of offering superb soft tissue definition, can be more useful for detection of vegetable, glass, or plastic IOFBs, especially when CT scanning fails to reveal a suspected IOFB.[500, 501] But MRI is generally contraindicated for metallic IOFBs because of the risk of intraocular movement of metallic materials.[502–505]

Modern A-scan and B-scan ultrasonography can give a general idea of the presence and relative position of an IOFB and will be especially useful in eyes with small particles, opaque media, poor patient cooperation, or hidden location (Fig. 50–5).[442, 506, 507]

ERG and EOG testing have been used to study the degree of ocular injury from metallosis, especially for

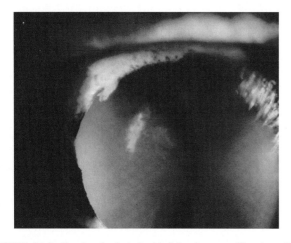

FIGURE 50–3. Foreign body imbedded in the crystalline lens. Note also the small tear of the iris sphincter. This intraocular foreign body had caused chronic intraocular inflammation. (See color insert.)

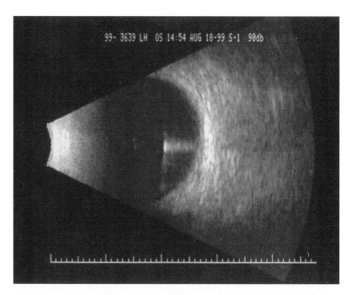

FIGURE 50–5. B-scan ultrasonogram showing the presence of an intraocular foreign body in the vitreous cavity in this patient who had not been adequately examined with a depressed, dilated funduscopic examination, and therefore the presence of the intraocular foreign body had been missed.

evaluating retinal function and for monitoring ocular recovery after metallic foreign body removal.[508–514] The ERG abnormalities in siderosis are characterized by a decrease in b-wave amplitude or complete flattening of the ERG curves in untreated eyes. Up to 50% b-wave reduction appears to be reversible.[508]

Differential Diagnosis

Some patients with IOFB may present without any history of trauma. Therefore, IOFB should always be considered in the differential diagnosis of chronic uveitis. Usually, chronic inflammation associated with IOFBs does not respond to standard medical treatment. A detailed history and thorough ocular examination, with some additional tests including ultrasound, radiography, and CT can distinguish this entity from uveitis.

Treatment

Management of IOFBs depends on several factors, including the type and location of the IOFB. In general, most metallic and magnetic IOFBs are considered toxic (such as copper) and relatively toxic (such as iron, steel, lead, zinc, nickel, and aluminum), and should be removed promptly.[444, 515–528] Vegetable matter such as wood has a high risk of microbial endophthalmitis (bacterial and fungal)[442, 449, 528, 529] and should also be removed without delay. Bacterial contamination by metallic intraocular foreign bodies has been reported,[530–532] and surgical removal is always considered for these contaminated materials.

Most nonorganic and nonmetallic IOFBs such as glass and plastic materials are usually inert and well tolerated in the eye[445] and need a less emergent approach. However, a large foreign body in the visual axis, even if inert, should be removed promptly.[533] Well-encapsulated IOFBs, including most nonmetallic matter (glass, stone, and plastic) and even metallic particles (copper, iron, aluminum), can often be inert or protected against metal dissociation and toxicity and retained within the eyes for months to years without any signs and symptoms of toxicity (metallosis bulbi) or other problem.[445, 534, 535] A conservative approach has been suggested for those inert and chronic IOFBs,[449] but any foreign body associated with severe recurrent inflammation should be surgically removed.[533] Periodic follow-up for many years is required for the inert and encapsulated IOFBs, and special attention needs to be directed toward a possible delayed inflammatory reaction.[533] Because modern microsurgical techniques and instrumentation have lessened the operative risks and increased the efficacy of IOFB removal, it has been recommended in recent years that most IOFBs undergo surgical removal.[442]

Current surgical methods for removing IOFBs include external magnets and vitrectomy. Electromagnets have been used to remove magnetic IOFBs for more than 100 years.[535] The magnet techniques, including small, hand-held, practical electromagnets, magnetic forceps, and tips with more or less magnetic force, have been improved over the years.[443, 536–548] Magnetic extraction can also be used with iron-containing foreign bodies, especially with magnetic forceps and tips that can grasp the foreign body. Vitrectomy is used to deal with most cases of nonmagnetic, large, or subretinal IOFBs, eyes with opaque media,

or whenever IOFBs cannot be removed by a magnet.[442] Vitrectomy offers the advantage of clearing the media and operating under the microscope with good visualization and full control over the extraction process.[442]

IOFBs are usually removed through the limbus, pars plana, or posterior sclera.[520, 521, 549–555] The proper surgical procedure of extraction mainly depends on the location, composition, and associated ocular injuries of the IOFBs. When an IOFB is lodged in the anterior chamber, limbal extraction is generally used. Pars plana extraction is mostly used for IOFBs suspended in the vitreous, or lying on the pars plana, ciliary body, retina, and optic nerve. When a magnetic IOFB is lodged in the retina, choroid, or sclera, extraction through the sclera posterior to the pars plana has been suggested.[521, 530]

Complications

An intraocular hemorrhage can occur associated with an immediate mechanical effect by a foreign body on the injured eye. Sometimes, the hemorrhage is so small as to escape clinical notice. If the hemorrhage has been profuse, local or massive bands of fibrous tissue may be formed. Vitreous organization, fibrous proliferation, subretinal neovascularization, and epimacular fibrosis[445] may lead to RD or eventually to gross cicatricial distortion of the globe.

Most vegetable IOFBs are contaminated and can carry pathogens such as *Bacillus cereus* and fungi.[445, 556, 557] Bacillus or fungus endophthalmitis is commonly associated with vegetable or soil intraocular foreign bodies, and has a rapid onset and poor visual prognosis. Endophthalmitis caused by *Staphylococcus epidermidis* and mixed species *(S. aureus* and *S. epidermidis)* has also been reported.[557] An IOFB of pure copper can induce an acutely destructive, violent inflammation.[445, 558] Endophthalmitis caused by graphite pencil lead has also been reported in a recent article.[559]

Although the incidence of sympathetic ophthalmia following the retention of an IOFB is exceedingly low,[477] it still may occur following the retention of every type of foreign body.[448] Sympathetic uveitis can develop many years after an IOFB has been retained.

Prognosis

Penetrating eye injuries with retained intraocular foreign bodies result in better final visual acuity in general than occurs with other injuries with ocular perforation.[451] Many factors, including the size, the material, and the location of IOFBs, influence the final visual recovery after removal of IOFBs. Small IOFBs with clear media and an IOFB location in the vitreous or overlying the retina or pars plana usually indicate favorable outcome.[442, 560] Sixty percent of eyes with an IOFB have been reported to have final visual acuity greater than or equal to 24/40 after magnetic extraction of the IOFB, and three fourths have a final acuity of 20/200 or better.[441, 444, 448, 516, 523, 561–564] With modern vitreous surgery, approximately one third of injured eyes with IOFBs can have recovery of visual acuity of 20/40 or better. Two thirds recover to 20/200 or better, and three fourths have ambulatory vision (5/200 or better).[549, 563–566] The advent of vitreous surgery with computed tomography and the use of the intraocular magnet have decreased the postoperative complication rate and provided a more favorable prognosis.[442, 557, 567]

A favorable prognosis of IOFBs also depends on the correct diagnosis and early surgical intervention.[567] Any delay or misdiagnosis increases the risk of ocular complications such as infectious endophthalmitis and proliferative vitreoretinopathy and brings a less favorable prognosis. Persistent and chronic uveitis is a particular masquerade syndrome associated with IOFBs, and misdiagnosis may occur.

Conclusion

Retained IOFBs can cause various degrees of inflammation. Persistent anterior or posterior uveitis is the most common complication associated with IOFBs. The uveal tissues, especially the ciliary body, show the greatest reaction to injury of any kind, even though the foreign body is inert. This reaction may slowly and cumulatively develop into a chronic and persistent uveitis, which can be misdiagnosed as idiopathic uveitis.

Ophthalmologists must remember that any unexplained and persistent uveitis, especially when the uveitis is refractory to treatment, raises a high level of suspicion for the possibility of an IOFB masquerading as idiopathic uveitis. A favorable prognosis of IOFBs depends on the correct diagnosis and early surgical intervention.

PIGMENT DISPERSION

Definition

Pigment dispersion syndrome (PDS) is characterized by release of pigment from the pigmented epithelium of the iris or ciliary body, or both, particularly in the midperipheral region in both eyes, with an attendant deposition of pigment on intraocular structures such as the back of the cornea, the trabecular meshwork, the iris, and the lens.[568] PDS can occur with or without elevation of IOP.

The dispersion of particles into the anterior chamber can mimic the presence of cells, and some cases of PDS have been mistaken for uveitis.[569] Therefore, in recent years, the disease has been considered as one of the uveitis masquerade syndromes.

History

The presence of pigment in the aqueous outflow system was first observed by von Hippel in early 1901.[570] The possible mechanism that suggested pigment release to different parts of the eye from the pigmented epithelium of the iris was then suggested by Levinsohn in 1909.[571] Although some studies supported and debated the concept,[572–576] the defined concept and its clinical significance for this entity were not established until 1940, when Sugar described one patient with glaucoma who had degeneration of the pigment epithelium of the iris and ciliary body and marked deposition of pigment on the anterior segment surfaces. Based on the observation of the case, Sugar first hypothesized the possible relationship between the accumulation of the pigment and glaucoma.[577] Subsequently, in 1949, Sugar and Barbour further reported the details of this entity and applied the term pigmentary glaucoma (PG) to this clinical condition.[578] When the typical findings of pigment depositions on anterior segment surfaces without associated glaucoma are observed, the term PDS has been advocated.[579]

Epidemiology and Risk Factors

The true prevalence of PDS is not known. Most cases of mild PDS probably are never detected.[580] The important risk factors for the development and progression of PDS include young age, male gender (male-to-female ratio of approximately 2:1), myopia (62% to 78%), and white race.[578, 579, 581–585] The spectrum of pigmentary disorders generally affects young adults, ages 20 to 45 years.[578, 579, 582] The mean age at the time of diagnosis of patients with pigmentary dispersion syndrome for men is about 35 to 45 years and for women is 40 to 50 years old.[583, 586] Although it has been suggested that PDS also may be seen in older individuals,[582] there is a tendency for it to decrease in severity or disappear later in life.[582, 587]

The ratio of males to females with PDS with normal IOP may be equal or may show a greater proportion of women.[583] But PDS with glaucoma tends to be more common in men than in women.[583, 584] Most PDS patients have deep anterior chambers,[586, 587] and usually, but not always, are myopic and white.[578, 579, 581, 586, 588–591] The disease is rare in blacks and Asians. A hereditary basis of this disease,[579, 581, 586, 588–591] with probable autosomal dominant inheritance[592, 593] and autosomal recessive inheritance,[594] has been suggested, but this factor has not been clearly established.

Accumulation of pigment may result in transient elevation of IOP or irreparable damage to the meshwork accompanied by uncontrolled glaucoma. Patients with PDS may go for years (12 to 20 years) before developing PG,[568, 579, 595, 596] or may never have a rise in IOP. The majority of patients with PDS do not develop glaucoma.[568, 579, 595, 596] It has been reported that the transition from PDS to PG was found in 20% to 35% of PDS patients.[595, 597] When glaucoma does occur, it tends to develop bilaterally, more often in men (2.4:1) and at a younger age than in women (average 37 years versus 51 years).[598] The main risk factors for the transition from PDS to PG were ocular hypertension and myopia. PG is thought to constitute 1% to 1.5% of the glaucoma cases in the Western world.[583, 599]

Clinical Features

The most important clinical feature of PDS is the deposition of pigment throughout the ocular anterior segment, including on the lens, zonules, iris surface (Fig. 50–6), corneal endothelium, and trabecular meshwork. The deposition of pigment on the corneal endothelium is generally accumulated in a central, vertical spindle-shaped pattern due to aqueous convection currents,[579] producing the Krukenberg spindle.[600, 601] The spindle can vary from 1 to 6 mm in length and can be approximately 3 mm in width. Pigment deposition on the cornea occasionally occurs as more diffusely distributed punctate deposits,[601] but there is no significant difference in central endothelial cell density and corneal thickness in patients with PDS.[602, 603]

Pigment dispersion is produced by a loss of pigment from the pigmented epithelium of the iris, particularly in the midperipheral region, which results in radial transillumination defects in the iris and dispersion of melanin

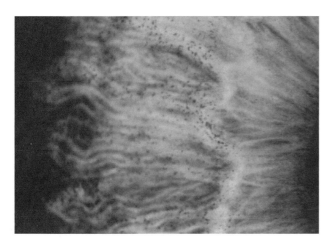

FIGURE 50–6. A patient with pigmentary dispersion syndrome. Note the pigmentary granules deposited on the iris surface. This patient had been treated for multiple episodes of recurrent uveitis. In fact, the cells in the anterior chamber were pigment granules. (See color insert.)

pigment into the aqueous humor.[604, 605] The defect can be dotlike or splinter-like, and occasionally two adjacent defects can form a V, with its apex oriented either centrally or peripherally.[606] As the disease progresses, the number of defects can increase, sometimes to the point where there is a full ring of discrete defects of iris.[606] Some patients with PDS or PG may not present with transillumination defects because of having especially dark and thick iris stroma.

The anterior chamber in patients with PDS is characteristically deep, and the peripheral iris is slightly concave. Gonioscopic examination usually shows an open angle. The most striking gonioscopic finding is a heavy, dark brown to almost black band of hyperpigmentation in the full circumference of the trabecular meshwork (Fig. 50–7). The dispersed pigment may also accumulate along Schwalbe's line, especially inferiorly, creating a thin dark band (Sampaolesi line).[600] IOP can be entirely normal or elevated.

Another constant characteristic in PDS is the deposi-

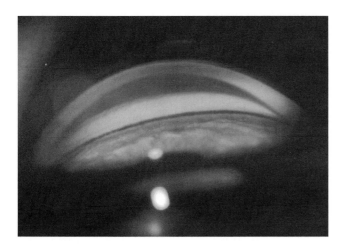

FIGURE 50–7. Another patient with pigmentary dispersion syndrome. Note the diagnostic presence of extreme amounts of pigment deposited in the angle. (See color insert.)

tion of a ring of pigmentation (complete or incomplete) on the posterior peripheral surface of the lens.[605, 607] The pigment line on the lens is usually located at the insertion of the zonular fibers on the posterior capsule, which usually is not seen on routine slit-lamp examination even if the pupil is dilated but is easily seen gonioscopically, especially with pupillary dilation.

Iris heterochromia and anisocoria can also be seen in eyes with PDS. The iris heterochromia results from pigment granules on the stroma of the iris, which may give the iris a progressively darker appearance and create heterochromia in asymmetric cases.[582] In addition, other findings, including RD (6.4% in one study),[583] lattice degeneration (20%),[608] and full-thickness retinal breaks (11.7%),[609] have also been reported in patients with PDS.

Pigment granules can mimic the appearance of inflammatory cells in the anterior chamber, that is, uveitis. Pigment particles in patients with PDS are often seen floating in the anterior chamber, especially following pupillary dilation, and they may be mistaken for inflammatory cells. In some cases, a rapid rise in IOP associated with PDS as a result of exercise[598] can cause corneal edema and halo vision. This feature may further confuse the unsuspecting ophthalmologist who is evaluating the PDS patient with this problem. In addition, iris atrophy can also be seen with herpes zoster and with herpes simplex uveitis, giving additional potential for a misdiagnosis.[606] PDS should always be suspected when the pigment deposition is in multiple locations in both eyes, with iris atrophy and heterochromia, normal or elevated IOP, keratic precipitates in a central, vertical, spindle-shaped pattern, and a heavily pigmented trabecular meshwork.

Pathogenesis and Pathophysiology

Change and loss of pigment epithelium, including focal atrophy, degeneration of the iris neuroepithelium, and hyperplasia of the dilator muscles, have been suggested as the mechanism of pigment dispersion.[610–613] Pigment granules may be dislodged mechanically from the pigmented epithelium of the iris by a back-and-forth rubbing due to a backward bowing of the posterior peripheral iris surface against zonules that insert anteriorly on the lens surface.[600, 614] The radial folds of iris pigment epithelium rubbing against the lens capsule itself may also be an additional mechanism of pigment release.[581, 601] Electron microscopy studies have confirmed that the iris defects in PDS consistently coincide with the location of the zonular fibers.[615] Biometric and ultrasound biomicroscopic studies of the anterior segment[587, 616–622] have revealed a deeper anterior chamber with corresponding concavity of the iris posteriorly and flatter lenses in eyes with PDS, further supporting the mechanical theory of the iris rubbing.

Released pigment is usually carried to the trabecular meshwork, where a small amount of pigment can quickly be phagocytized by the endothelial cells that line the trabecular beams,[613, 614, 623–627] and it may not obstruct outflow sufficiently to elevate the IOP. However, if the particulate load is heavy, pigment cells migrate further along the outflow pathway and downstream into the juxtacanalicular region, either obstructing the intertrabecular spaces or migrating into Schlemm's canal.[606, 623] Trapped pigment in the meshwork can cause enough obstruction of the outflow facility to elevate the IOP, resulting in PG.

The release of pigment from the posterior surface of the iris causes the pigment particles floating in the anterior chamber, which can mimic the cells seen in uveitis. However, although macrophages may be called forth into the stroma of the iris, the floating of pigment in the aqueous lumen does not invoke an inflammatory response in eyes with PDS.[606] The inflammatory signs such as ciliary injection or synechias are always absent in the eye with PDS. This noninflammatory pathologic feature in eyes with PDS can be important in distinguishing PDS from an inflammation event.

Diagnosis

The diagnosis of PDS is essentially a clinical one, based on a thorough ophthalmic history and ocular examination. Affected patients tend to be young white men with myopia. Ocular characteristics associated with PDS usually include peripheral slitlike iris transillumination defects, increased trabecular meshwork pigmentation, Krukenberg's spindle on the posterior surface of the cornea, a posterior concave iris, and normal or elevated IOP. The presence of pigment particles in the anterior chamber with increased pigmentation of both eyes, and the absence of synechiae and ciliary injection serve to solidify the diagnosis. One should also be able to discriminate between inflammatory cells and pigment cells and granules.

A typical transillumination defect presenting as a radial and slitlike or wedgelike pattern in the midperipheral iris has been suggested to be an essential feature in the diagnosis of PDS.[606] Examination for transillumination defects should be considered as a routine part of the ophthalmic examination in patients with uveitis. The defects are best seen with low magnification and narrow slit-lamp beam, which is positioned coaxial to the observer in the patient's pupil. A shielded fiberoptic transilluminator and Koeppe gonioscope lens are also good for testing the loss of pigment from the posterior layer of the iris.[606] In some patients, however, with a dark and thick iris stroma that may prevent transillumination of the defects, the absence of this finding does not rule out the diagnosis of PDS. A digitizing infrared videographic technique usually allows visualization of discrete iris transillumination defects that were not visible by slit-lamp examination.[628]

Gonioscopy is an important and essential step in making a diagnosis of PDS and grading the extent of pigment dispersion. The most essential gonioscopic finding is a dense, dark or almost black pigment band, which covers at least the posterior three fifths of the trabecular meshwork in the full circumference.[606] The dispersed pigment may also accumulate along Schwalbe's line, especially inferiorly, creating a thin, dark band. Other findings in gonioscopy include a deep anterior chamber with a concave posterior iris. The angle of the anterior chamber in the eye with PDS or PG is wide and open all around. A detailed examination of an increase or decrease in the degree of pigmentation within the trabecular meshwork

can be observed consistently by a pigment scale gonioscopy lens.[606, 629]

High-frequency, high-resolution anterior segment ultrasound biomicroscopy can also provide a cross-sectional view of the peripheral iris configuration and define the relationships of the iris to the anterior chamber and lens surface in patients with PDS or PG.[621, 622, 630–635] The examination by ultrasound biomicroscopy in the living eye has confirmed the original postmortem histologic studies that showed iridozonular contact,[621] which will be helpful in making a diagnosis and considering further treatment for PDS or PG.[606]

Tomography for facility of outflow determination can document the facility at the time of presentation; decreased facility correlates with disease progression, and this worsens with episodes of active dispersion of pigment. This method has been suggested as an additional test for longitudinal monitoring.[606, 636]

Fundus examination is most helpful in evaluating optic nerve damage in PDS patients with elevation of IOP and in excluding other conditions associated with increased anterior segment pigmentation, including some forms of uveitis, trauma, ocular melanosis, and melanoma. The optic nerve is usually normal in most patients with PDS but can be damaged if elevation of IOP occurs. The peripheral retina can be normal or abnormal in patients with PDS. RDs, lattice degeneration, and full-thickness retinal breaks are common abnormal findings on fundus examination in eyes with PDS.[583, 608, 609]

The increase of pigmentation in multiple parts of the anterior segment of both eyes, with no inflammatory features throughout the ophthalmic examination, is particularly helpful in considering a correct diagnosis of PDS and differentiating this disease from uveitis.

Differential Diagnosis

In addition to PDS, other abnormal conditions in which pigment is disseminated into the anterior chamber include some forms of uveitis, cysts of the iris and ciliary body, dispersion of melanoma cells, postoperative conditions, trauma, and aging changes.[600] These conditions constitute the differential diagnosis for PDS.

Pigment granules associated with PDS are often seen floating in the anterior chamber and depositing on the surface of the lens and cornea; this may mimic uveitis. Inflammatory diseases involving the posterior surface of the iris occasionally can disperse a moderate amount of pigment, often settling into the inferior angles; and local patches of pigment loss can also be seen in patients with severe uveitis. The inflammatory signs and symptoms, such as pain, photophobia, ciliary injection, or synechiae, are typically absent in eyes with PDS.

Patients with peripheral iris or ciliary body cysts occasionally may produce a moderate amount of pigment in the anterior chamber and trabecular meshwork,[637, 638] similar to the feature of PDS. However, the presence of the characteristic peripheral iris irregularities, the absence of typical Krukenberg's spindle, and the feature of less dense pigment in the trabecular meshwork can distinguish this entity from PDS.

Iris, ciliary body, or even posterior segment melanoma (if the anterior hyaloid face is disrupted) can be associated with dispersed pigment. The pigmented tumor cells, or pigment-laden macrophages, may cause considerable darkening of the anterior and posterior segments.[606, 639] Melanoma usually has an apparent intraocular mass with only monocular involvement, and the typical signs of PDS, such as Krukenberg's spindle and transillumination defects, are absent.

Pigment dispersion associated with postoperative conditions or trauma usually presents irregular patches of iris loss. In addition, most cases occur unilaterally and have characteristic features of surgical or traumatic history, which can be easily distinguished from PDS.

With the increase of age, cells on the posterior surface of the iris occasionally release small amounts of pigment, which can deposit in the trabecular meshwork and gradually darken the structure. However, the degree of pigmentation within the trabecular meshwork generally is less dense than that seen in PDS, with an uneven distribution throughout the circumference of the trabecular meshwork.[600]

PDS with elevation of IOP (PG) must be distinguished from the pseudoexfoliation syndrome, the glaucoma disorder most similar to PG. Like PG, exfoliation syndrome with glaucoma is characterized by a loss of pigment from the iris neuroepithelium and has the same clinical symptoms, including iris transillumination defects, Krukenberg's spindle, clumping of pigment in the angles, and elevation of IOP. However, pseudoexfoliation syndrome is usually seen in the older patient, without preference to sex, race, and refractive error. Pigmentation of the trabecular meshwork in exfoliation is less intense than in PG, and the iris transillumination defects are located more at the pupillary border rather than in the midperiphery of the iris. Most patients (50%) with exfoliation syndrome have only one eye involved, compared with patients with pigmentary dispersion, which is usually bilateral.[600] In addition, pseudoexfoliation syndrome, as its name implies, is characterized by the presence of white flakes of exfoliation material at the pupillary border and on the anterior lens surface, the hallmark of the exfoliation in the pseudoexfoliation syndrome.

Treatment

Regular examination and follow-up are the most important management strategies for patients with PDS. Patients with early pigment dispersion should be followed with a careful evaluation of the number of iris transillumination defects, the configuration of the iris, and the degree of pigmentation in the various areas of the eye, especially in the trabecular meshwork by gonioscopy. IOP, facility of outflow changes, optic nerve, and visual fields should be measured regularly. Therapeutic interventions should be considered and performed appropriately if PG develops. A general treatment approach to PG has been suggested: medical treatment first, laser therapy second, and incisional surgical intervention third. Medical therapy for PD includes adrenergic antagonists and agonists, and mitotic agents, which typically suffice for mild cases. Laser surgery, including laser trabeculoplasty[583, 640] and peripheral iridotomy,[598, 641] has proved to be effective in eyes with PD or PG. If adequate control cannot be ob-

tained by medication or laser surgery, then filtration surgery should be undertaken.[606]

Complications/Prognosis

The transition from PDS to PG has been found to be 20% to 35%.[595, 597] Patients with PDS may go for years (12 to 20 years) before developing PG,[568, 579, 595, 596] or may never have a rise in IOP. A majority of patients with PDS may not develop glaucoma.[568, 579, 595, 596]

Slow regression over the years, as the amount of pigment released from the posterior surface of the iris decreases, has been reported in PDS and PG.[606] In some patients, it has been reported that pigmentation and damage to the trabecular meshwork may be partially or almost totally reversible.[584, 618] Remission of PG has also been reported after glaucoma surgery[583] and lens subluxation.[642] PDS patients who have a normal tonographic facility of outflow on initial presentation have a good prognosis.[568] If intraocular pressure cannot be controlled and the trabecular function does not improve, irreversible damage to the optic nerve and visual field loss eventually develop. It has been reported that visual field loss in pigment dispersion with glaucoma is high.[642]

Conclusions

PDS is characterized by release of pigment from the pigmented epithelium of the iris or ciliary body, or both, particularly in the midperipheral region in both eyes, with an attendant deposition of pigment on intraocular structures such as the back of the cornea, the trabecular meshwork, the iris, and the lens. Affected patients tend to be young white men with myopia. Ocular characteristics associated with PDS usually include peripheral slit-like iris transillumination defects, increased trabecular meshwork pigmentation, Krukenberg's spindle, a posterior concave iris, and normal or elevated IOP. Pigment granules associated with PDS are often seen floating in the anterior chamber, and these granules may mimic the features of inflammatory diseases and masquerade as uveitis.

OCULAR ISCHEMIC SYNDROME

Definition

Ocular ischemic syndrome (OIS) is a rare condition of chronic vascular insufficiency in which abnormalities may occur in both the anterior and posterior segments of eyes as a result of reduced orbital blood flow secondary to severe carotid artery occlusive disease.[643, 644]

Usually, the gradual diminution in the blood supply to eyes secondary to severe carotid artery obstruction predominantly affects the posterior segment, causing peripheral retinal hemorrhages, peripheral microaneurysms, narrowed retinal arteries, and dilated retinal vessels. However, this disorder may progress to cause anterior segment ischemia.[644-647] Red eye, pain, anterior chamber cells, and flare are the common manifestations of the advanced form of this disorder. These features may mimic anterior uveitis. Hence, OIS should be considered as one of the masquerade syndromes in dealing with any ocular inflammatory disorder.[644, 648, 649]

History and Epidemiology

OIS secondary to severe carotid artery obstruction was first reported by Kearns and Hollenhorst in 1963.[643, 650]

The disorder was initially described as venous stasis retinopathy by an observation of hemorrhage retinopathy from retinal hypoperfusion at an abnormally low arterial pressure in approximately 5% of patients with severe carotid artery insufficiency or thrombosis.[643, 650] Since then, a number of additional alternative terms have been proposed, including ischemic ocular inflammation,[644] ischemic oculopathy,[651] and ocular ischemic syndrome.[652, 653] Because histopathologic examination of eyes with the entity generally does not reveal inflammation,[654, 656] currently, the term ocular ischemic syndrome has been documented to appropriately describe the features of ocular ischemic disorders secondary to carotid artery occlusive diseases.[655]

OIS is a rare disorder. The prevalence of this disease has not been extensively studied, but an annual incidence of 7.5 OIS cases per million population has been reported.[645] It has been estimated that a number of misdiagnosed cases in clinics may exist that probably contribute to the low estimated incidence.[650] The mean age of patients with OIS is about 65 years old, with a range generally from age 50 to 80 years old.[645, 646, 650–653, 656] No racial predilection has been identified, and men are affected more than women by a ratio of about 2:1.[650, 653, 656] Either unilateral (80%) or bilateral disease can occur, and approximately 20% of patients have bilateral ocular involvement.[650]

Clinical Characteristics

Visual loss and ocular pain are the most frequent presenting ocular complaints. More than 90% of patients with OIS have a history of visual loss in the affected eye or eyes.[653] The episodes of visual loss may be fleeting, including amaurosis fugax (15%), gradual (28%), or sudden (41%),[657] but generally occur over weeks to months.[653] The degree of visual loss is variable, with visual acuity ranging from 20/20 to 20/50 or 20/200, or from counting fingers to no light perception in the later stage of the disease secondary to neovascular glaucoma.[658, 659] Ocular pain is characteristically described as a dull ache in the periocular or orbital region in about 40% of cases,[653] which is thought to be due either to the ischemia itself or to the secondary neovascular glaucoma.[653, 659]

Anterior segment signs with OIS by slit-lamp biomicroscopy examination usually show episcleral vascular congestion; corneal edema and striae; keratic precipitate; mid-dilated, sluggish, or unreactive pupil; anterior chamber cells and flare (18% of eyes); and rubeosis iridis (67% of eyes) with secondary neovascular glaucoma (35%).[647, 651, 653, 657, 659] About two thirds of eyes with OIS have rubeosis iridis at the time of initial examination.[651, 653, 657]

Posterior segment changes with OIS, characterized by hypoperfusion retinopathy and choroidal perfusion defects, primarily result in narrowed retinal arteries, dilated but nontortuous retinal veins, dot and blot retinal hemorrhages and microaneurysms, and optic disc and retinal neovascularization (35% and 8% of eyes, respectively).[651] Retinal hemorrhages are seen in about 80% of affected eyes with OIS, and are most commonly present in the midperiphery, but can also extend into the posterior pole.[651, 653] Other signs, including cherry-red spot (12%)

of eyes), cotton-wool spots (6% of eyes), spontaneous pulsation of the central retinal artery in 4%, a change in the ophthalmic-artery pressure in 4%, vitreous hemorrhage in 4%, cholesterol emboli within the retinal arteries in 2%, and anterior ischemic optic neuropathy in 2%, can also be seen by fundus examination.[644, 647, 651, 653, 657–660]

Usually, most ocular ischemic syndrome manifestations begin in the posterior segment.[643, 661] If it is left unchecked, this clinical entity may progress to the anterior segment and cause panocular ischemia, which can eventually cause iris neovascularization, neovascular glaucoma, and ultimately blindness.[644, 647, 662]

In addition to ocular abnormalities, systemic diseases, primarily including atherosclerosis and systemic arterial hypertension as well as diabetes mellitus, can be seen in patients who have OIS.[651, 657] Nearly 38% to 50% of patients may also have evidence of ischemic heart disease, whereas about 25% to 31% of patients have been reported to have a history of a previous stroke or transient ischemic attack.[651, 657, 663]

The inflammatory features with which OIS patients primarily present are those of anterior uveitis. Iritis has been reported in approximately 20% of eyes with OIS, although it is usually fairly mild.[651, 653] Iritis is characterized by the presence of anterior chamber cells and flare, and rubeosis iridis is routinely associated with flare in the anterior chamber. The cellular response is typically mild, never exceeding grade 2 as per the Schlaegel classification.[653, 664] Iritis, with other clinical symptoms of OIS, such as red eye and pain, iris atrophy with an irregularly dilated and poorly responsive pupil, hypotony, rapidly progressive cataracts, corneal edema, keratic precipitates, and Descemet's folds, may mimic a primary ocular inflammatory disease.[476, 644, 649, 665] In addition, clinically, the syndrome of ocular inflammation secondary to chronic ischemia is uncommon, and neither ophthalmologists nor other specialists dealing with patients with carotid artery disease have much experience of this disorder, which further increases the difficulty of diagnosis.[646] Without a correct cognition of this disorder, the clinical features, especially the inflammation, result in OIS masquerading as uveitis. Ophthalmologists must pay particular attention to any patient over the age of 50 years with a new-onset iritis, especially with the observation of rubeosis iridis in an individual without diabetic history and without any evidence of venous obstructive disease or other obvious predisposing cause, with a high index of suspicion of OIS.

Pathogenesis and Etiology

Carotid artery stenosis or obstruction is one of the major causes of OIS. In general, a 90% or greater stenosis of the ipsilateral carotid arterial system is present in patients with OIS.[651, 653] The obstruction can occur within the common carotid or internal carotid artery. It has been shown that 90% carotid stenosis will slowly reduce the ipsilateral central retinal artery perfusion pressure by about 50%.[651, 666–668] The subsequent chronic reduction in blood flow in the ophthalmic artery leads to increasing ocular ischemia, tissue hypoxia and varying degrees of focal ischemic necrosis, and neovascularization.[647, 652, 667] Moreover, the decreased flow in the ophthalmic artery can increase blood viscosity and red blood cell aggregation and decrease red blood cell deformation.[669] The subsequent tissue hypoxia may further damage the endothelial cells of vessels and cause loss of endothelial cells and pericytes that may lead to the increased permeability.[654, 655] All of these factors could cause chronic intermittent ischemic symptoms and ocular inflammatory reactions, eventually leading to rubeosis iridis and subsequent neovascular glaucoma.[647, 652]

Partial or complete thrombosis of the internal carotid artery secondary to atherosclerosis is one of the major causes for most OIS cases.[670] Atheromatous plaques of the aorta and carotid arteries are the most common sources of emboli to the internal carotid. Other systemic disorders, such as dissecting aneurysm of the carotid artery,[671] giant cell arteritis,[672, 673] fibromuscular dysplasia,[674] Adamantiades-Behçet's disease,[675] trauma,[676] and inflammatory entities that cause carotid artery obstruction,[651] also have been reported as causes of carotid artery stenosis. Diabetes mellitus and systemic arterial hypertension, as well as the manifestations of cardiac ischemia such as myocardial infarction, angina, heart failure, peripheral vascular disease requiring bypass surgery, and cerebrovascular accident, have been proposed as possible risk factors for the development of atherosclerotic vascular disease.[656]

Diagnosis

Diagnosis of chronic ocular ischemia can usually be made clinically, based on a detailed medical and ocular history, complete ophthalmic examination, and carotid artery evaluation. New-onset unilateral visual loss and the presence of the characteristic ischemic symptoms in the eye of an elderly person are all important clues to suggest the diagnosis. The past medical history of atherosclerotic vascular disease and other risk factors for the development of atherosclerotic vascular disorders such as diabetes mellitus and systemic arterial hypertension are highly suggestive for considering a possible diagnosis of OIS.

Laboratory and ancillary testing, including fluorescein angiography, electroretinography, ultrasonography, carotid Doppler, and angiography studies (arteriography or intravenous digital subtraction angiography), are usually necessary to establish the diagnosis of OIS.

Fluorescein angiography is most helpful in visualizing a number of signs that are highly suggestive of ocular ischemic syndrome. The most prominent findings on fluorescein angiography in patients with OIS include prolonged arm-to-choroid time and delayed or patchy choroidal filling in 60% of patients,[651, 653, 677] increased retinal arteriovenous transit time (in 95% of patients),[651, 653] late staining of the retinal vessels, particularly the arteries (in 85% of patients),[653] macular edema,[678, 679] microaneurysms, and retinal capillary nonperfusion.[654, 655] Insufficiency of ocular blood flow and tissue hypoxia and endothelial damage within small retinal and choroidal vessels may account for the abnormalities presented on fluorescein angiography.

ERG usually, but not always, reveals a diminution or absence of the amplitude of both a- and b-waves in the eyes with OIS.[652, 653] A delayed recovery time of b wave in the affected eye after exposure to bright light has also

been reported.[679] It has been suggested that the abnormality of recovery time of the b wave in the ERG may be a valuable test for the detection of minor degrees of ischemic damage to retina caused by insufficiency of the retinal and choroidal circulation.[680] Visual evoked potentials have also been used to study eyes with severe carotid artery stenosis.[653] The recovery time of the amplitude of the major positive peak after photostress has been shown to improve in patients with severe stenosis after endarterectomy.[681]

Noninvasive assessment of carotid artery circulation, such as by duplex ultrasonography, should be obtained to verify the clinical suspicion.[649] Continuous-wave Doppler sonography is helpful in establishing whether or not a significant stenosis is present at the carotid bifurcation.[646, 682] Real-time ultrasound can reveal the presence of atheromatous plaques even if they do not have a significant hemodynamic effect.[646, 683] Oculoplethysmography and ophthalmodynamometry assess carotid artery patency by detection of the ophthalmic artery pulse pressure. The test usually reveals a decreased ocular perfusion pressure in the eye with OIS.[646, 683, 684] Noninvasive tests have been reported to have an accuracy of approximately 95% to 97% in detecting carotid stenosis of 75% or greater.[685–689]

If clinical symptoms and signs strongly suggest OIS, or the suspicion of significant stenotic carotid vascular disease has been detected by noninvasive carotid studies, the possibility of chronic ophthalmic artery obstruction should be confirmed by conventional carotid arteriography or intravenous digital subtraction angiography.[665, 690] Arteriography is the most reliable method of revealing carotid artery lesions. It has been reported that carotid angiography typically discloses a 90% or greater obstruction of the ipsilateral internal or common carotid artery in patients with OIS,[691] but this test has a complication rate of approximately 3.7%.[692] Intravenous digital subtraction angiography is safer and has been reported in as many as 96% of selected cases to show a lesion at the carotid bifurcation.[692]

Differential Diagnosis

OIS may be confused with diabetic retinopathy and central retinal vein obstruction. Differentiation from diabetic retinopathy can be difficult in some instances, because many patients with OIS may also have diabetes mellitus, and the retinal manifestations of both disorders may be superimposed.[691, 693] However, the retinopathy in OIS is usually unilateral (80% unilateral eye) in the older age group from 50 to 80 years old, whereas diabetic retinopathy is usually bilateral with a population of variable ages. The midperipheral location of retinopathy is the typical feature with OIS, whereas diabetic retinopathy is more often seen first in the posterior pole and macular area. In addition, delayed fluorescein choroidal filling and retinal arterial fluorescein staining, as well as decreased ophthalmodynamometry reading, are generally absent in eyes with diabetic retinopathy, whereas they are the characteristic manifestations in OIS.

Both OIS and central retinal vein obstruction can be unilateral and occur in the older age population. However, in OIS, the retinal veins are typically dilated but not tortuous, whereas venous tortuosity is commonly seen in central retinal vein occlusion.[65] Furthermore, in contrast to OIS, the retinal arterial perfusion pressure is normal in eyes with central retinal vein obstruction. In addition, both entities usually have a prolonged retinal arteriovenous transit time; however, choroidal filling defects and prominent retinal arterial staining are usually absent on fluorescein angiography in eyes with central retinal vein obstruction.[666]

The obstruction caused by an embolus within the central retinal artery can also present the same fundus appearance as OIS. However, in contrast to OIS, fluorescein angiography of eyes with central retinal artery obstruction rarely shows late vascular staining. In addition, the ERG usually reveals that the b wave is diminished and the a wave is unaffected in the eye with central artery obstruction. However, in the eye with OIS, choroidal compromise and outer retinal ischemia are also presented, and both a and b wave can be affected.[666]

Treatment

The major therapeutic goal for patients with OIS is to preserve visual function and reduce carotid artery stenosis. Full-scatter panretinal laser photocoagulation has been advocated to decrease the ocular oxygen requirements and reduce the ischemic drive for neovascularization.[650, 694–697] This approach does not improve circulation to the needy eye, but it does reduce the metabolic demand.[649] Approximately 36% of eyes with OIS have been reported to demonstrate regression of iris neovascularization after full-scatter treatment.[694] However, this method is not indicated if the anterior chamber angle is completely closed by fibrovascular tissue. Cyclocryotherapy, cyclodiathermy, or filtering procedures can be considered as further therapy for the elevation of IOP with a closed angle.[650]

Carotid endarterectomy is generally used to reverse the carotid stenosis in order to maintain or improve the vision in eyes with OIS.[657, 698, 699] The treatment is recommended only if there is partial occlusion of the internal carotid artery, and it would not be useful for a patient who has 100% carotid artery obstruction, because in this situation, a thrombus usually propagates distally, thus generally precluding a successful endarterectomy.[650, 651, 691] A paradoxical worsening may occur after carotid endarterectomy. The increased perfusion of the carotid obstruction may improve ciliary body perfusion and increase aqueous formation, causing a marked elevation in IOP and an increase in the size and the number of retinal hemorrhages. Although it has been reported that stabilization or amelioration of vision occurs in about 25% of eyes following endarterectomy,[658] clinical data and their value concerning the benefit of this treatment for this entity are still controversial and varied.[647, 700–702]

Complications and Prognosis

The progression of OIS varies considerably by individual. The early retinopathy may resolve spontaneously or a stable course may persist for years, with the development of collateral circulation despite hypoperfusion.[649, 661] Significant loss of vision due to OIS is irreversible when tissue infarction occurs.[645, 703] Rubeosis may be present in two thirds of patients with OIS. Of those patients with rubeosis, approximately one half will develop neovascular glaucoma.[659] The visual prognosis in ocular ischemic syndrome is generally poor, particularly in the presence of rubeosis.[656, 658]

OIS-associated cardiovascular disease (63%) is the major cause of mortality or significant morbidity in these patients, whereas stroke is second. Other associated diseases include systemic arterial hypertension, diabetes mellitus, and peripheral vascular diseases.[658] The 5-year mortality rate secondary to associated systemic disease has been reported to be approximately 40% in OIS patients.[656]

Conclusion

OIS is a rare condition of chronic vascular insufficiency in which abnormalities may occur in both the anterior and posterior segments of the eyes as a result of reduced blood flow secondary to severe carotid artery occlusive disease.[643, 644]

Iritis with red eye and pain is one of the clinical symptoms associated with OIS, and this may mimic uveitis. Because OIS is an uncommon disorder, diagnosis may be delayed or missed. A detailed systemic and ophthalmic history, as well as ancillary tests, with the discovery of extensive peripheral anterior synechiae associated with rubeosis in one eye of a patient older than 50 years of age with a new-onset iritis should make one suspicious. Although the prognosis for the eyes affected by chronic ischemia is generally poor, early and correct diagnosis with treatment has been reported to improve the prognosis. Furthermore, discovery of the underlying carotid pathology provides an opportunity for therapy that may improve the outlook for the patient's overall well-being and longevity.

JUVENILE XANTHOGRANULOMA

Definition

Juvenile xanthogranuloma (JXG) is a benign inflammatory disorder occurring in infants and young children, mainly affecting skin, characterized by multiple cutaneous papules. It occasionally involves the eye. Although ocular involvement in this disorder is not frequent, JXG has been reported to affect the iris and ciliary body,[671, 704–706] eyelid,[707] epibulbar area,[708] cornea, conjunctiva, sclera,[709] optic nerve, disc, retina, and choroid,[710] as well as the orbit.[704, 707–712] The iris is the structure most commonly involved clinically in JXG, characterized by the presence of an asymptomatic fleshy iris nodule, spontaneous hyphema, unilateral glaucoma, heterochromia iridis, and red eye with signs of uveitis.[705] Without a complete recognition of this disorder, the clinical features involving the iris in JXG may produce confusion with anterior uveitis in childhood, and misdiagnosis may consequently occur.

History and Epidemiology

Juvenile xanthogranuloma was first reported as causing cutaneous lesions in infants and young children by Adamson in 1905,[713] who called the condition congenital multiplex xanthoma. The disorder was further described as a separate clinical entity under the name of nevoxanthoendothelioma by McDonaugh in 1909.[714] Since then, numerous studies about this disease involving skin have been documented.[706, 715–717] Ocular involvement of this disorder was first recognized and described by Blank et al in 1949.[718] The term of juvenile xanthogranuloma was then proposed by Helwig and Hackney in 1954.[719] However, it was not until 1965 that Maumenee first reported this disease in the ophthalmic literature.[720] Since then many single case reports and series have reported the location, diagnosis, and management of this disease involving the eye.[705, 721–728]

JXG is a rare disease that primarily affects skin. There are no obvious racial or gender predilections for this disorder.[729] It has been reported that approximately 75% of the patients with JXG have skin lesions only. Extracutaneous lesions most frequently involve the eye but may also involve the lungs, testes, spleen, gastrointestinal tract, pericardium, and bone.[719, 730–732] Most patients with JXG are younger than 2 years of age at presentation.[733] It has been reported that 85% of patients with intraocular involvement present during the first year of life, and patients with skin lesions tend to be older at the time of diagnosis.[705, 721] JXG is rarely seen in adults.[26, 734–738] Ocular lesions with JXG are usually unilateral.[739] Most lesions regress within months to a few years.

Clinical Features

The clinical features of intraocular involvement with JXG vary with the tissue affected.[740] Iris infiltration, which represents the most frequent ophthalmic manifestation, is characterized by either an asymptomatic localized tumorous nodule or a diffuse thickening of iris stroma.[705, 725] The iris lesions may be highly vascular, which can cause spontaneous hemorrhage into the anterior chamber (hyphema) and secondary glaucoma due to either tumor infiltration in the anterior chamber angle or to obstruction of aqueous outflow by blood in the anterior chamber.[705, 740] Hyphema is the initial clinical sign of JXG in many cases. Diffuse iris infiltration by the disease process or blood can cause heterochromia iridis.[705, 740]

Other ocular manifestations of JXG may include a salmon pink or yellow lymphomatous infiltration in conjunctiva, sclera, and cornea; nodules in the lids; and proptosis due to orbital granuloma.[705] Massive infiltration of the optic nerve can lead to obliteration of the central retinal vein and artery with hemorrhagic necrosis of the retina and serosanguineous detachment of retina.[709] Chorioretinal infiltration in JXG may present as multiple subretinal lesions in the posterior pole with associated exudative detachment.[741] However, involvement of those sites, especially the optic disc, choroid, retina, and orbit, is exceedingly rare.

Ocular manifestations may occur concomitantly with, or more rarely without, the skin lesions.[705, 721] Skin lesions may or may not be associated with the ocular manifestations at first presentation, and sometimes do not appear until weeks to months and sometimes years after ocular involvement. The skin lesions usually consist of single or multiple, discrete, yellowish or pink nodules up to 1 cm in diameter, most commonly located on the scalp, head, and neck.[705, 735] Cutaneous lesions usually regress spontaneously and very rarely are associated with systemic involvement.

JXG can also present with a red eye, anterior chamber flare, and cells, as well as local inflammatory reactions mimicking iridocyclitis.[705] Without a correct recognition of this disorder, the feature of inflammation, with other clinical manifestations associated with JXG such as heterochromia iridis, hyphema, and secondary glaucoma, may masquerade as uveitis in childhood.[741] It is of paramount importance to suspect JXG in any infant or very young child with unilateral spontaneous hyphema and glaucoma, heterochromia iridis, and an inflamed eye with signs of uveitis.

Histopathology

Microscopic examination reveals that the ocular lesion in JXG is characterized by iris infiltration with normal-appearing histiocytes, along with occasional inflammatory cells, including lymphocytes, eosinophils, and multinucleated giant cells, typically of the Touton type (giant cells with a lipid cytoplasm ringed by nuclei).[671, 705, 740] Nuclear morphology shows no abnormal mitoses.[742] Many large, thin-walled capillaries throughout the lesion can also be seen, and spontaneous hemorrhages are caused by rupture of these thin-walled vessels.[743] Skin lesions have the same histopathologic features as those in the eye, but Touton giant cells are often greater in number in the skin than in typical iris lesions.[705, 740]

Diagnosis

Diagnosis of ocular involvement with JXG should be considered in any child who has the typical skin lesions and a diffuse or nodular iris or ciliary lesion with hyphema or secondary glaucoma. Clinical diagnosis can often be confirmed by skin biopsy. However, in some cases, the ocular involvement may occur without the presence of cutaneous lesions.[705, 740] Also, the diagnosis may be more difficult, and detailed ophthalmic examination and histopathologic examinations are required for establishing the diagnosis in this situation. Aqueous paracentesis with or without iris biopsy, with careful histopathologic examination, reveals foamy histiocytes and Touton giant cells, confirming the diagnosis of ocular involvement with JXG.[735, 740, 744, 745] In some cases with advanced buphthalmos, diagnosis has been established following enucleation of the blind eye.[705, 740]

Because JXG is a rare disorder, and many ophthalmologists may be insufficiently familiar with the clinical features, misdiagnosis or delay in providing optimal therapy can occur. Red eye with inflammatory reaction in the anterior chamber and recurrent hyphema and unilateral secondary glaucoma are the common symptoms and signs in JXG masquerade.[721, 741] Complete ophthalmic and systemic examination, as well as correct recognition of the clinical features, will always be helpful in making a correct diagnosis.

Differential Diagnosis

An asymptomatic iris mass in JXG should be differentiated from an amelanotic melanoma, iris leiomyoma, hemangioma, or lymphangioma.[742] The orbital involvement in JXG should also be differentiated from rhabdomyosarcoma, fibrosarcoma, idiopathic orbital inflammation, teratoma, or other rare congenital orbital tumors.[704] The diagnosis for these disorders is generally based on histopathologic features of a biopsy.

Treatment

If patients with JXG present only skin lesions, no active intervention is indicated, but careful ophthalmologic follow-up is strongly recommended.[746] The management of patients with ocular involvement with JXG depends on the condition of the involved eye. Ocular involvement limited to the eyelid or the epibulbar tissue also does not require specific treatment. But when there is uveal infiltration, prompt treatment is necessary.[747] Early treatment of iris involvement is important because without it, uncontrolled glaucoma, corneal blood staining, or amblyopia may occur.[742] The major principles of treatment are to limit or stop the inflammatory reaction in the anterior chamber and to reduce elevated IOP. Several methods of therapy, including steroids, local excision, irradiation, and combined irradiation and corticosteroids, have been advocated in ocular involvement with JXG.

Topical or subconjunctival steroids are generally recommended as the initial treatment for a JXG uveal lesion without glaucoma.[740, 742, 747, 748] Antiglaucoma therapy with acetazolamide can be added, if necessary.[749, 750] In some cases with mild ocular involvement, spontaneous regression might occur with simple observation or a short course of steroids. Systemic steroids,[724, 735] low dose irradiation (300 to 400 cGy),[750–753] or a combination of irradiation and steroids[739] should be considered further if the initial treatment cannot prevent recurrent hyphema and secondary glaucoma. An excisional biopsy of the lesion, if it is smaller than one quadrant in size, has also been advocated.[724, 754, 755] Surgical excision of the lesion can provide a pathologic specimen when diagnosis is in doubt, but surgery may increase the risk of hyphema and lens trauma, especially if IOP is significantly elevated with ocular inflammation.[705, 720, 725, 746] It has been suggested by Cadera that in most instances, the risks of surgery outweigh any advantage, especially because the lesions are extremely sensitive to both steroids and radiation.[746] We agree that it is probably unwise to operate on an eye for recurrent spontaneous hyphema unless all other treatments have failed.[748]

Complications and Prognosis

The prognosis for life in patients with JXG is excellent. JXG is a benign inflammatory process that is generally self-limited.[740] However, the visual prognosis is variable and depends on the condition of ocular involvement. In cases with mild ocular involvement, the condition might completely resolve with simple observation or with a short course of steroids. The visual outcome can be very poor in severe cases with iris and ciliary body involvement and complicated secondary glaucoma, corneal blood staining, and amblyopia.[740]

Conclusion

Juvenile xanthogranuloma is a rare disorder of unknown etiology in infants and very young children. The lesions primarily involve the skin and, occasionally, the eye, especially the iris and ciliary body. The clinical manifestations of ocular involvement in JXG mainly include an asymptomatic iris mass with unilateral spontaneous hyphema or secondary glaucoma, heterochromia iridis, and signs of uveitis. The diagnosis of JXG is challenging for ophthalmologists, especially when a skin lesion is absent, because the clinical features of JXG can mimic those of a primary uveitis. The correct diagnosis can be established from a correct recognition of this disorder and inclusion of it in the differential diagnosis of uveitis in infants and very young children, and from the histologic appearance by skin or iris biopsy.

References

1. Cooper EL, Riker JL: Malignant lymphoma of the uveal tract. Am J Ophthalmol 1951;34:1152.
2. Givner I: Malignant lymphoma with ocular involvement: A clinicopathologic report. Am J Ophthalmol 1955;39:29.
3. Sears ML: Choroidal and retinal detachments associated with scleritis. Am J Ophthalmol 1964;58:764–766.
4. Theodore FH: Conjunctival carcinoma masquerading as chronic conjunctivitis. Eye Ear Nose Throat Monthly 1967;46:1419–1420.
5. McCannel CA, Holland GN, Helm CJ, et al: Causes of uveitis in the general practice of ophthalmology. Am J Ophthalmol 1996;121:35–46.
6. Von Helmholtz H: Beschreibung eines Augenspiegels zur Untersuchung der Netzhaut im lebenden auge. (Description of an eye-mirror for the investigation of the retina in the living eye.) Berlin, A Forstner, 1851.
7. Coccius A: Über die Anwendung des Augenspiegels nebst angabe eines neuen Instruments. Leipzig, Immanuel Muller, 1853, pp 130–131, 150–156.
8. Von Graefe A: Notiz über die Ablösungen der Netzhaut von der Chorioidea. Graefes Arch Clin Exp Ophthalmol 1854;1:362–371.
9. Arlt F: Die Krankheiten des Auges, für praktischer Arzt, Vol 2. Prag, Czechoslovakia, Credner & Kleinbub, 1854, pp 158–184.
10. Müller H: Anatomische Beitrage zur Ophthalmologie. 7. Beschreibung einiger von Prof. V. Graefe exstirpirter Augapfel. Graefes Arch Clin Exp Ophthalmol 1858;4:363–388.
11. Iwanoff: Beiträge zur normalen und pathologischen Anatomie des Auges. 1. Beiträge zur Abloösung des Glaskörpers. Graefes Arch Clin Exp Ophthalmol 1869;15:1–69.
12. de Wecker L, de Jaeger E: Traité des maladies du fond de l'oeil et atlas d'ophthalmoscopie. Paris, Adrien Delahaye, 1870, pp 151–158.
13. Leber T: Über die Entstehung der Netzhautablösung. Ber Dtsch Ophthalmol Ges 1882;14:18–45.
14. de Wecker L: Quel but doit poursuivre le traitement du décollement de la rétine? Reprinted by Arruga H: Un document historique relatif au décollement de la rétine. Ophthalmologica 1888;98:1–6.
15. Leber T: Über die Entstehung der Netzhautablösung. Ber Dtsch Ophthalmol Ges 1908;35:120–134.
16. Dufour M, Gonin J: Maladies de la rétine. XXI. Décollement rétinien. In: Lagrange F, Valude E, eds: Encyclopédie Francaise d'Ophthalmologie, Vol 6. Paris, Octave Doin, 1906, pp 975–1025.
17. Gonin J: Pathogénie et anatomie pathologique des décollements rétiniens (à l'exclusion des décollements traumatiques, néoplastiques et parasitaires). Bull Mem Soc Fr Ophthalmol 1920;33:1–120.
18. Gonin J: Le traitement de décollement rétinien. Ann d'Ocul 1921;158:175.
19. Rosengren B: Results of treatment of detachment of the retina with diathermy and injection of air into the vitreous. Acta Ophthalmol 1938;16:573–579.
20. Schepens CL: A new ophthalmoscope demonstration. Trans Am Acad Ophthalmol Otolaryngol 1947;51:298–301.
21. Schepens CL: Examination of the ora serrata region: Its clinical significance. Acta XVI Concilium Ophthalmologicum (Britannia, 1950) 1951;2:1384–1393.
22. Custodis E: Bedeutet die plombenaufnahung auf die Sklera einen

Fortschritt im der operation Behandlung der Netzhautablosung? Ber Dtsch Ophthalmol Ges 1953;58:102.

23. Meyer-Schwickerath G: Light-coagulation: A new method for the treatment and prevention of retinal detachment. XVII Concilium Ophthalmol 1954;1:404.

24. Schepens CL, Okamura ID, Brockhurst RJ: The scleral buckling procedures. I. Surgical techniques and management. Arch Ophthalmol 1957;58:797–811.

25. Cibis PA, Becker B, Okun E, et al: The use of detachment surgery. Arch Ophthalmol 1962;68:590–599.

26. Machemer R, Buettner H, Norton EWD, et al: Vitrectomy: A pars plana approach. Trans Am Acad Ophthalmol Otolaryngol 1971;15:813–820.

27. Zauberman H, Garcia Rosell F: Treatment of retinal detachment without inducing chorioretinal lesions. Trans Am Acad Ophthalmol Otolaryngol 1975;79:835–844.

28. Chang S: Low viscosity liquid fluorochemicals in vitreous surgery. Am J Ophthalmol 1987;103:38–43.

29. Berglin L, Stenkula S, Crafoord S, et al: A new technique of treating rhegmatogenous retinal detachment using the Q-switched Nd:YAG laser. Ophthalmic Surg 1987;18:890–892.

30. Graham PA: Unusual evolution of retinal detachments. Trans Ophthalmol Soc UK 1958;78:359–371.

31. Böke W, Hübner H: Acute retinal detachment with severe uveitis and hypotony of the eyeball. Mod Probl Ophthalmol 1972;10:245–9.

32. Gottlieb F: Combined choroidal and retinal detachment. Arch Ophthalmol 1972;88:481–486.

33. Seelenfreund MH, Kraushar MS, Schepens CL, et al: Choroidal detachment associated with primary retinal detachment. Arch Ophthalmol 1974;91:254–258.

34. Jarrett WH: Rhegmatogenous retinal detachment complicated by severe intraocular inflammation, hypotony, and choroidal detachment. Trans Am Ophthalmol Soc 1981;79:664–683.

35. Haimann MH, Burton TC, Brown CK: Epidemiology of retinal detachment. Arch Ophthalmol 1982;100:289–292.

36. Wilkes SR, Beard CM, Kurland LT, et al: The incidence of retinal detachment in Rochester, Minnesota, 1970–1978. Am J Ophthalmol 1982;94:670–673.

37. Rowe JA, Erie JC, Baratz KH, et al: Retinal detachment in Olmsted County, Minnesota, 1976 through 1995. Ophthalmology 1999;106:154–159.

38. Böhringer HR: Statistisches zu Häufigkeit und Risiko der Netzhautablösung. Ophthalmologica 1956;131:331.

39. Laatikainen L, Tolppanen EM, Harju H: Epidemiology of rhegmatogenous retinal detachment in a Finnish population. Acta Ophthalmol (Copenh) 1985a;63:59–64.

40. Tornquist R, Stenkula S, Tornquist P: Retinal detachment: A study of a population-based patient material in Sweden, 1971–1981. Acta Ophthalmol 1987;65:213–222.

41. Algvere PV, Jahnberg P, Textorius O: The Swedish retinal detachment register. I. A database for epidemiological and clinical studies. Graefe's Arch Clin Exp Ophthalmol 1999;273:137–144.

42. Michaelson IC, Stein R, Barkai S, et al: A study in the prevention of retinal detachment. Ann Ophthalmol 1969;1:49–55.

43. Brown PR, Thomas RP: The low incidence of primary retinal detachment in the Negro. Am J Ophthalmol 1965;60:109–110.

44. Av-Shalom A, Berson D, Gombos GM, et al: Some comments on the incidence of idiopathic retinal detachment among Africans. Am J Ophthalmol 1967;64:384–391.

45. Sasaki k, Ideta H, Yonemoto J, et al: Epidemiologic characteristics of rhegmatogenous retinal detachment in Kumamoto, Japan. Graefes Arch Clin Exp Ophthalmol 1995;233:772–776.

46. Wong TY, Tielsch JM, Schein OD: Racial difference in the incidence of retinal detachment in Singapore. Arch Ophthalmol 1999;117:379–383.

47. Douglas WHG: Retinal detachment in the Negro of southern Africa. S Afr Arch Ophthalmol 1973;1:79.

48. Weiss H, Tasman WS: Rhegmatogenous retinal detachment in blacks. Ann Ophthalmol 1978;10:799.

49. The Eye Disease Case-control Study Group: Risk factors for idiopathic rhegmatogenous retinal detachment. Am J Epidemiol 1993;137:749–757.

50. Schepens CL, Marden D: Data on the natural history of retinal detachment: I. Age and sex relationships. Arch Ophthalmol 1961;66:631–642.

51. Bagley CH: Retinal detachment. Am J Ophthalmol 1948;31:285.

52. Robertson RW: Statistical study of retinal detachment. Trans Canad Ophthalmol Soc 1952;5:122.

53. Shapland CD: Retinal detachment techniques. Trans Ophthalmol Soc UK 1960;80:677.

54. Amsler M, Schiff-Wertheimer S: Le décollement de la rétine. In: P Bailliart, ed: Traité d'Ophthalmologie, Vol 5. Paris, Masson & Cie, 1939, pp 559–576.

55. Arruga H: Etiologia y patogenia del desprendimiento de la retina, Acta XIV Concil Ophthalmol Hispania 1933;2:1–191.

56. Stallard HB: Some observations on the causes and treatment of simple detachment of the retina. Br J Ophthalmol 1930;14:1.

57. Bartels AJH: Statistik der Fälle von Netzhautablösung. Klin Monatsbl Augenheilk 1936;96:687.

58. Dunnington JH, Macnie JP: Detachment of the retina. Arch Ophthalmol 1937;18:532.

59. Shapland CD: Retinal detachment and its treatment by surgical methods. Br J Ophthalmol 1934;18:1.

60. Ashrafzadeh MT, Schepens CL, Elzeneiny IT, et al: Aphakic and phakic retinal detachment. Arch Ophthalmol 1973;89:476.

61. Dollfus MA, Raeymaecheckers G: La galvano-cautérisation à pointe fine dans le traitement du décollement de la rétine. Ann Oculist 1960;193:385.

62. Jeandelize P, Baudot R, Gault A: Résultat du traitement du décollement rétinien par la diathermo-coagulation. Bull Soc Franc Ophthalmol 1936;49:269.

63. De Roeth A: Bilateral detachment of the retina. Arch Ophthalmol 1939;22:809.

64. Schutz JS: Retinal Detachment Surgery, Strategy and Tactics. New York, Raven Press, 1984, pp 1–12.

65. Benson WE: Primary retinal detachment. In: Benson WE, eds: Retinal Detachment. Diagnosis and Management. Philadelphia, JB Lippincott, 1998, pp 1–15.

66. Tasman WS: Posterior vitreous detachment and peripheral retinal breaks. Trans Am Acad Ophthalmol Otolaryngol 1968;72:217.

67. Lindner B: Acute posterior vitreous detachment and its retinal complications. Acta Ophthalmol 1966;87(Suppl):1.

68. Morse PH, Scheie HG, Aminlari A: Light flashes as a clue to retinal disease. Arch Ophthalmol 1974;91:179.

69. Delaney WV Jr, Oates RP: Retinal detachment in the second eye. Arch Ophthalmol 1978;96:629–34

70. Jaffe NS: Vitreous detachments. In: Jaffe NS, ed: The Vitreous in Clinical Ophthalmology. St. Louis, CV Mosby, 1969, pp 83–98.

71. Lindner B: Acute posterior vitreous detachment. Am J Ophthalmol 1975;80:44.

72. Tabotabo MD, Karp LA, Benson WE: Posterior vitreous detachment. Ann Ophthalmol 1980;12:59.

73. Boldrey EE: Risk of retinal tears in patients with vitreous floaters. Am J Ophthalmol 1983;96:783.

74. Foos RY, Wheeler NC: Vitreoretinal juncture: Synchysis senilis and posterior vitreous detachment. Ophthalmology 1982;89:1502.

75. Linner E: Intraocular pressure in retinal detachment. Arch Ophthalmol (Suppl) 1966;84:101.

76. Langham ME, Regan CDJ: Circulatory changes associated with onset of primary retinal detachment. Arch Ophthalmol 1969;81:820.

77. Schwartz A: Chronic open-angle glaucoma secondary to rhegmatogenous retinal detachment. Am J Ophthalmol 1973;75:205.

78. Burton TC, Arafat NI, Phelps CD: Intraocular pressure in retinal detachment. Int Ophthalmol 1979;1:147.

79. Phelps CD: Glaucoma associated with retinal disorders. In: Ritch R, Shields MB, eds: The Secondary Glaucoma. St. Louis, CV Mosby, 1982, p 150.

80. Stratford TP, Shafer DM: General discussion. In: Schepens CL, Regan CDJ, eds: Controversial Aspects of the Management of Retinal Detachment. Boston, Little, Brown and Company, 1965, p 51.

81. Hamilton AM, Taylor W: Significance of pigment granules in the vitreous. Br J Ophthalmol 1972;56:700.

82. Boldrey EE: Vitreous cells as an indicator of retinal tears in asymptomatic or not recently symptomatic eyes. Am J Ophthalmol 1997;123:263–264.

83. Takabatake M, Matsuo N, Okabe S, et al: Two cases of retinal detachment with ocular hypertension and many outer segments of visual cells in the anterior chamber. Acta Soc Ophthalmol Jpn 1980;84:282.

84. Matsuo N, Takabatake M, Ueno H: Application of electron microscopy to diagnosing eye disease. Electron microscopy of the floating cells in the anterior chamber in Schwartz syndrome. J Clin Electron Microscopy 1981;14:519.

85. Ueno H, Matsuo N, Koyama T, et al: A case of Schwartz syndrome. Jpn Rev Clin Ophthalmol 1981;75:1456.

86. Matsuo N, Takabatake M, Ueno H, et al: Photoreceptor outer segments in the aqueous humor in rhegmatogenous retinal detachment. Am J Ophthalmol 1986;101:673–679.

87. Sebag J: Aging of the vitreous. Eye 1987;1:254.

88. Balazs EA, Denlinger JL: Aging changes in the vitreous. In: Sekuller R, Kline D, Dismukes K, eds: Aging and Human Visual Function. New York, Alan R. Liss, 1982.

89. Eisner G: Gross anatomy of the vitreous body. Graefes Arch Klin Exp Ophthalmol 1975;193:33–56.

90. O'Malley P: The pattern of vitreous synersis. A study of 800 autopsy eyes. In: Irvine AR, O'Malley C, eds: Advances in Vitreous Surgery. Springfield, IL, Charles C Thomas, 1976.

91. Larsson L, Osterlin S: Posterior vitreous detachment. A combined clinical and physicochemical study. Graefes Arch Clin Exp Ophthalmol 1985;223:92.

92. Flood MT, Balazs EA: Hyaluronic acid content in the developing and aging human liquid and gel vitreous. Invest Ophthalmol Vis Sci Suppl 1977;16:67.

93. Goldmann H: Zur Biomikroskopie des Glaskorpers. Ophthalmologica 1954;127:334.

94. Gurtin BJ: The Myopias. New York, Harper & Row, 1985.

95. Osterlin S: Vitreous changes after cataract extraction. In: Freeman HM, Hirose T, Schepens CL, eds: Vitreous Surgery and Advances in Fundus Diagnosis and Treatment. Boston, Appleton-Century-Crofts, 1975, p 15.

96. Hauer Y, Barkay S: Vitreous detachment in aphakic eyes. Br J Ophthalmol 1964;48:341.

97. Heller MD, Straatsma BR, Foos RY: Detachment of the posterior vitreous in phakic and aphakic eyes. Mod Probl Ophthalmol 1972;10:23.

98. Hagler WS: Pseudophakic retinal detachment. Trans Am Ophthalmol Soc 1982;80:45–63.

99. Schepens CL: Retinal detachment and aphakia. Arch Opthalmol 1951;45:1.

100. Norton EWD: Retinal detachment in aphakia. Am J ophthalmol 1964;58:111.

101. McPherson AR, O'Malley RE, Bravo J: Retinal detachment following late posterior capsulotomy. Am J Ophthalmol 1983;95:593.

102. Wilkinson CP, Anderson LS, Little JH: Retinal detachment following phacoemulsification. Ophthalmology 1978;85:151.

103. Winslow RL, Taylor BC: Retinal complications following YAG laser capsulotomy. Ophthalmology 1985;92:785.

104. Ober RR, Wilkinson CP, Fiore JV, et al: Rhegmatogenous retinal detachment after neodymium-YAG laser capsulotomy in phakic and pseudophakic eyes. Am J Ophthalmol 1986;101:81.

105. Coonan P, Fung WE, Webster RG: The incidence of retinal detachment following extracapsular cataract extraction. A ten-year study. Ophthalmology 1985;92:1096.

106. Hurite FG, Byer N: Changes and prognosis of lattice degeneration of the retina. Trans Am Acad Ophthalmol Otolaryngol 1974;78:114.

107. Byer N: Changes and prognosis of lattice degeneration of the retina. Trans Am Acad Ophthalmol Otolaryngol 1974;78:114.

108. Schepens CL, Bahn GC: Examination of the ora serrata: its importance in retinal detachment. Arch Ophthalmol 1950;44:677.

109. Deleted.

110. Karlin DB, Curtin BJ: Axial length measurements and peripheral fundus changes in the myopia eye. In: Pruett RC, Regan CDJ, eds: Retina Congress. New York, Appleton-Century-Crofts, 1972, p 629.

111. Bohringer HR: Statistisches zu Haufigheit und Risiko der Netzhautablosung. Ophthalmologica 1956;131:331.

112. Karlin DB, Curtin BJ: Peripheral chorioretinal lesions and axial length of the myopic eye. Am J Ophthalmol 1976;81:625.

113. Byer N: Clinical study of lattice degeneration of the retina. Trans Am Acad Ophthalmol Otolaryngol 1965;69:1064.

114. Byer NE: Lattice degeneration of the retina. Surv Ophthalmol 1979;23:213.

115. Straatsma BR, Zeegen PD, Foos RY, et al: Lattice degeneration of the retina. Trans Am Acad Ophthalmol Otolaryngol 1974;78:87.

116. Morse PH: Lattice degeneration of the retina and retinal detachment. Am J Ophthalmol 1974;78:930.

117. Tolentino F, Schepens CL, Freeman HM: Vitreoretinal Disorders, Diagnosis and Management. Philadelphia, WB Saunders, 1976.

118. Benson WE, Morse PH: The prognosis of retinal detachment due to lattice degeneration. Ann Ophthalmol 1978;10:1197.

119. Straatsma BR, Allen RA: Lattice degeneration of the retina. Trans Am Acad Ophthalmol Otolaryngol 1962;66:600.

120. Hyams SW, Neumann E, Friedman Z: Myopia-aphakia. II. Vitreous and peripheral retina. Br J Ophthalmol 1975;59:483.

121. Schepens CL, Marden D: Data on the natural history of retinal detachment. Further characterization of certain unilateral nontraumatic cases. Am J Ophthalmol 1966;61:213.

122. Byer NE: Clinical study of retinal breaks. Trans Am Acad Ophthalmol Otolaryngol 1967;71:461.

123. Tolentino FI, Lapus JV, Novalis G, et al: Fluorescein angiography of degenerative lesions of the peripheral fundus and rhegmatogenous retinal detachment. Int Ophthalmol Clin 1976;16:13.

124. Foos RY: Vitreous base, retinal tufts, and retinal tears: pathogenetic relationships. In: Duane TD, ed: Clinical Ophthalmology, Vol 3. New York, Harper & Row, 1986.

125. Byer NE: Cystic retinal tufts and their relationship to retinal detachment. Arch Ophthalmol 1981;99;1788.

126. Murakami-Nagasako F, Ohba N: Phakic retinal detachment associated with cystic retinal tuft. Graefes Arch Clin Exp Ophthalmol 1982;219:188.

127. Foos RY: Zonular traction tufts of the peripheral retina in cadaver eyes. Arch Ophthalmol 1969;82:620.

128. Byer ME: Relationship of cystic retinal tufts to retinal detachment. Dev Ophthalmol 1981;2:36–42.

129. Straatsma BR, Foos RY, Feman SS: Degenerative diseases of the peripheral retina. In: Duane TD, ed: Clinical Ophthalmology, Vol 3. Philadelphia, Harper & Row, 1986, p 1.

130. Rutnin U, Schepens CL: Fundus appearance in normal eyes. Part III: Peripheral degenerations. Am J Ophthalmol 1967;64:1040.

131. O'Malley PF, Allen RA: Peripheral cystoid degeneration of the retina: Incidence and distribution in 1000 autopsy eyes. Arch Ophthalmol 1967;77:769.

132. Foos RY, Feman SS: Reticular cystoid degeneration of the peripheral retina. Am J Ophthalmol 1970;69:392.

133. Dobbie JG: Cryotherapy in the management of senile retinoschisis. Trans Am Acad Ophthalmol Otolaryngol 1969;73:1047–1060.

134. McPherson A, O'Malley R, Beltangady SS: Management of the fellow eyes of patients with rhegmatogenous retinal detachment. Ophthalmology 1981;88:922.

135. Malbran E, Dodds R, Hulsbus R: Traumatic retinal detachment. Mod Probl Ophthalmol 1972;10:479.

136. Kaufman PL, Podos SM: Subretinal fluid butyrylcholinesterase. Am J Ophthalmol 1973;75:627–636.

137. Dobbie JG: Prognosis based on the preoperative examination: General discussion. In: Schepens CL, Regan CDJ, eds: Controversial Aspects of the Management of Retinal Detachment. Boston, Little, Brown and Company, 1965, pp 73–74.

138. Alajmo A, Cilento A: Ulteriori osservazioni sul contenuto in istamina del liquido sottoretinico e sul suo significato clinico nel distacco di retina idiopatico. Gior Ital Oftal 1956;9:302–311.

139. Reichling W: Über die Herkunft und Entstehungsweise der subretinalen Flüssigkeit. Ber Dtsch Ophthal Ges 1955;59:92–97.

140. Pischel DK: Detachment of the vitreous as seen by slit lamp examination: With notes on the technique of slit lamp microscopy of the vitreous cavity. Am J Ophthalmol 1953;36:1497.

141. Pischel DK: Slit-lamp examination of the fundus. Arch Ophthalmol 1958;60:811.

142. Dobbie JG: A study of the intraocular fluid dynamics in retinal detachment. Acta Ophthalmol 1963;69:159.

143. Syrdalen P: Intraocular pressure and ocular rigidity in patients with retinal detachment. I. Preoperative study. Acta Ophthalmol 1970;48:1024.

144. Ehlers N, Osterby E: On the prognostic value of intraocular pressure in treatment of retinal detachment. Acta Ophthalmol 1970;48:181.

145. Ehlers N, Osterby E: Prognostic value of intraocular pressure in treatment of retinal detachment. Ophthalmol Digest 1971;33:13.

146. Ringvold A: Evidence that hypotony in retinal detachment is due to subretinal juxtapapillary fluid drainage. Arch Ophthalmol 1980;58:652.

147. Smith JL: Retinal detachment and glaucoma. Trans Am Acad Ophthalmol Otolaryngol 1963;67:731.

148. Phelps CD, Burton TC: Glaucoma and retinal detachment. Arch Ophthalmol 1977;95:418.

149. Schepens CL: Retinal Detachment and Allied Diseases, Vol 2. Philadelphia, WB Saunders, 1983, pp 963–965.

150. Schwartz A: Surgical management of glaucoma: Glaucoma and retinal detachment. Int Ophthalmol Clin 1963;3:185.

151. Sebestyen JG, Schepens CL, Rosenthal ML: Retinal detachment and glaucoma. I. Tonometric and gonioscopic study of 160 cases. Arch Ophthalmol 1962;67:736.

152. Klien BA: Concerning conditions simulating an intraocular tumor. Am J Ophthalmol 1937;20:812–819.

153. Duke-Elder S, Perkins ES: Diseases of the uveal tract: Viral uveitis, In: Duke-Elder S: System of Ophthalmology, Vol 9. St. Louis, CV Mosby, 1966, pp 373–383.

154. Benson WE, Shields JA, Tasman W, et al: Posterior scleritis. Arch Ophthalmol 1979;97:1482.

155. Feldon SE, Sigelman J, Albert DM, et al: Clinical manifestations of brawny scleritis. Am J Ophthalmol 1978;85:781–787.

156. Gass JDM, Jallow S: Idiopathic serous detachment of the choroid, ciliary body, and retina (uveal effusion syndrome). Ophthalmology 1982;89:1018.

157. Schepens CL, Brockhurst RJ: Uveal effusion. I. Clinical picture. Arch Ophthalmol 1963;70:189.

158. McDonald PR, de la Paz V, Sarin LK: Non-rhegmatogenous retinal separation associated with choroidal detachment. Trans Am Ophthalmol Soc 1964;62:226–247.

159. Rosen E, Lyne A: Uveal effusions. Am J Ophthalmol 1968;65:509–518.

160. Michels RG, Wilkinson CP, Rice TA: Results of retinal reattachment surgery. In: Michels RG, Wilkinson CP, Rice TA, eds: Retinal Detachment. St. Louis, CV Mosby, 1990, pp 917–957.

161. Kreiger AE, Hodgkinson BJ, Frederick AR, et al: The results of retinal detachment surgery: Analysis of 268 operations with a broad scleral buckle. Arch Ophthalmol 1971;86:385.

162. Rachal WF, Burton TC: Changing concepts of failure after retinal detachment surgery. Arch Ophthalmol 1979;97:480.

163. Wilkinson CP, Bradford RH, Jr: Complications of draining subretinal fluid. Retina 1984;4:1.

164. Chignell AH, Fison LG, David EWG, et al: Failure in retinal detachment surgery. Br J Ophthalmol 1973;57:525.

165. Lincoff H: Should retinal breaks be closed at the time of surgery? In: Brockhurst RJ, Boruchof SA, Hutchinson BT, Lessell S, eds: Controversy in Ophthalmology. Philadelphia, WB Saunders, 1977, pp 582–568.

166. Hilton GF, Mclean EB, Norton EWD: Retinal Detachment. Rochester, American Academy of Ophthalmology, 1979.

167. Tani P, Robertson DM, Langworthy A: Prognosis for central vision and anatomic reattachment in rhegmatogenous retinal detachment with macula detached. Am J Ophthalmol 1981;92:611.

168. Johnston GP, Arribas NP, Okun E, et al: Visual prognosis following successful retinal detachment surgery. In: Pruett RC, Regan CDJ, eds: Retina Congress. New York, Appleton-Century-Crofts, 1972, p 617.

169. Bell J: Retinitis pigmentosa and allied diseases of the eye. In: Pearson K, ed: Treasury of Human Inheritance. London, Cambridge University, Cambridge, 1922.

170. Kobayashi VA: Genetic study on retinitis pigmentosa. Jpn J Ophthalmol 1960;7:82–88.

171. Francois J: Heredity in Ophthalmology. St. Louis, CV Mosby, 1961.

172. Sorsby A: Choroid and retina. Mod Ophthalmol 1964;3:287–293.

173. Sunga RN, Sloan LL: Pigmentary degeneration of the retina: Early diagnosis and natural history. Invest Ophthalmol 1967;6:309–325.

174. Duke-Elder S, Dobree JH: Disease of the retina: The peripheral dystrophies. In Duke-Elder S, ed: System of Ophthalmology, Vol 10. St. Louis, CV Mosby, 1967, pp 577–628.

175. Kurimoto S, Suyama T, Kimura Y, et al: A classification of retinitis pigmentosa. Acta Soc Ophthalmol Jpn 1967;71:1439–1457.

176. Berson EL, Gouras P, Gunkel RD: Progressive cone degeneration. Arch Ophthalmol 1968;80:68–76.

177. Berson EL, Gouras P, Gunkel RD: Progressive cone degeneration, dominantly inherited. Arch Ophthalmol 1968;80:77–83.

178. Carr RE, Siegel IM: The vitreo-tapeto-retinal degenerations. Arch Ophthalmol 1970;84:436–445.

179. Deutman AF: The Craig Lecture: Genetically determined retinal and choroidal disease. Trans Ophthalmol Soc UK 1974;94:1014–1032.

180. Heckenlively JR: Retinitis pigmentosa. In: Heckenlively JR, ed: Retinitis Pigmentosa. Philadelphia, JB Lippincott, 1988, p 1.

181. Heckenlively JR: Simplex retinitis pigmentosa (nonhereditary pigmentary retinopathies). In: Heckenlively JR, ed: Retinitis Pigmentosa. Philadelphia, JB Lippincott, 1988, p 188.

182. Gass JDM: Heredodystrophic disorders affecting the pigment epithelium and retina: Retinitis pigmentosa. In: Gass JDM, ed: Stereoscopic Atlas of Macular Diseases: Diagnosis and Treatment. St. Louis, Mosby, 1987, p 235.

183. Heckenlively JR: The frequency of posterior subcapsular cataract in the hereditary retinal degeneration. Am J Ophthalmol 1982;93:733–738.

184. Fetkenhour CL, Choromokos E, Weinstein J, et al: Cystoid macular edema in retinitis pigmentosa. Trans Am Acad Ophthalmol Otolaryngol 1977;83:515–521.

185. Fishman GA, Maggiero JM, Fishman M: Foveal lesions seen in retinitis pigmentosa. Arch Ophthalmol 1977;95:1993–1996.

186. Ovelgün R: Nyctalopia haerediotria. Acta Physics Med (Nuremberg) 1744;7:76–77.

187. Schon M: Handbuch der pathologischen anatomie des menschlichen auges. Hamburg, 1828 (Vinken).

188. Von Ammon FA: Klinische Darstellungen der Krankheiten und Bildungsfehler des menschlichen Auges, der Augenlider und der Thränen werkzeuge; nach eigenen Beoboch tungen und Untersuchungen. Berlin, G Reimer, 1883 (Vinken).

189. Van Trig AC: De Oogspiegel, Nederlandisch Lancet, 3d series, 2d JB 417–509. Netherlands, The Hague, 1852–1853.

190. Ruete CGT: Bildliche Darstellung der krankheiten des menschlichen auges. Teubner, Leipzig, 1854.

191. Donders FC: Torpeur de la rétine congénital et héréditaire. Ann Ocul (Paris) 1855;34:270–273.

192. Donders FC: Beiträge zur pathologischen anatomie des auges. Graefes Arch Clin Exp Ophthalmol 1855;3:139–165.

193. Laber T: Die pigment degeneration der netzhaut und die mit ihr verwandten erkrankungen. Graefe-Saemich Handbuch Ges Augenheilkd 1916;2:1025–1076.

194. Von Grafe A: Exceptionnelles verhalten des gesichtsfeldes bei pigmententartung der netzhaut. Graefes Arch Clin Exp Ophthalmol 1858;4:250–253.

195. Liebreich R: Abkunft aus ehen unter blutsverwandstenals grund von retinitis pigmentosa. Dtsch Klin 1861;1:53–55.

196. Nettleship E: On retinitis pigmentosa and allied diseases. R Lond Ophthal Hosp Rep 1907/1908;17(I):1–56; (II):151–166; (III):333–427.

197. Usher CH: On the inheritance of retinitis pigmentosa with notes of cases. R Lond Ophthal Hosp Rep 1914;19:1930–2036.

198. Gonin J: Nouvelles observations de scotome annulaire dans la dégénérescence pigmentaire de la rétine. Ann Oculist (Paris) 1902;128:90–107.

199. Diem M: Retinitis punctata albescens et pigmentosa. Klin Moatsbl Augenheilkd 1914;53:371–379.

200. Wibaut F: Studien über retinitis pigmentosa. Klin Monatsbl Augenheilkd 1931;87:298–307.

201. Francois J: Dégénérescence pigmentaire de la rétine à hérédité dominante. Bull Soc Belge Ophthalmol 1935;70:79–86.

202. McQuarrie MD: Two pedigrees of hereditary blindness in man. J Genet 1935;30:147–53.

203. Biro I: Ueber den Zusammenhang von Degeneratio pigmentosa retinae und Storungen des Gehörs. Ophthalmologica 1944;107:149–57.

204. Falls HF, Cotterman C: Choroidal degeneration: a sex-linked form in which heterozygous women exhibit a tapetal-like retinal reflex. Arch Ophthalmol 1948;40:683–703.

205. Mackenzie DS: The inheritance of retinitis pigmentosa in one family. Trans Ophthalmol Soc NZ 1951;5:79–82.

206. Ammann F, Klein D, Böhringer HR: Résultats préliminaires sur la fréquence et la distribution géographique des dégénerescences tapéto-rétiniennes en Suisse (étude de cinq cantons). J Genet Hum 1961;10:99–127.

207. Francois L: Chorioretinal heretodegeneration. Proc R Soc Med 1961;54:1109–18.

208. Francois L: Chorioretinal degeneration or retinitis pigmentosa of

intermediate sex-linked heredity. Doc Ophthalmol 1962;16:111–27.

209. Ammann F, Klein D, Franceschgetti A: Genetic and epidemiological investigations on pigmentary degeneration of the retina and allied disorders in Switzerland. J Neurol Sci 1965;2:183–196.

210. Motohashi A: The prevalence of pigment degeneration of the retina. Jpn J Clin Ophthalmol 1968;22:27–35.

211. Panteleeva OA: On the hereditary tapeto-retinal degenerations. Vestn Oftalmol 1969;1:53–56.

212. Sorsby A: Ophthalmic Genetics. London, Butterworths, 1970.

213. Botermans CHG: Primary pigmentary retinal degeneration and its association with neurological diseases. In: Vinken PJ, Bruyn GW, eds: Handbook of Clinical Neurology: Neuroretinal Degenerations, Vol 13. New York, American Elsevier, 1972, pp 148–378.

214. Krill AE: Retinitis pigmentosa: A review. Sight Sav Rev 1972;42:20–28.

215. Tanabe U: Genetic study of retinal pigmentary dystrophy (retinitis pigmentosa) in Japan. Jinrui Idengaku Zasshi 1972;16:119–154.

216. Imaizumi K: Retinitis pigmentosa: genetic carriers and early cases. S Afr Arch Ophthalmol 1974;2:257–269.

217. Bird A: X-linked retinitis pigmentosa. Br J Ophthalmol 1972;59:177–199.

218. Jay B: Recent advances in ophthalmic genetics: Genetic counseling. Br J Ophthalmol 1974;58:427–437.

219. Jay B: Retinitis pigmentosa in childhood—diagnosis, counseling and prevention. Metab Ophthalmol 1978;2:221.

220. Fishman GA: Retinitis pigmentosa. Genetic percentages. Arch Ophthalmol 1978;96:822–826.

221. Karpe G: The basis of clinical electroretinography. Acta Ophthalmol (Kbh) 1945;24(Suppl):1–118.

222. Björk A, Karpe G: The clinical electroretinogram. V. The electroretinogram in retinitis pigmentosa. Acta Ophthalmol 1951;29:361–371.

223. Armington JC, Schwab GJ: Electroretinogram in nyctalopia. Arch Ophthalmol 1954;52:725–733.

224. Franceschetti A, Dieterle P: Die differential diagnostische bedeutung des elektroretinogrammes bei tapeto-retinalen degenerationen. Bibl Ophthalmol 1957;48:161–182.

225. Henkes HE, Van der Twel LH, Denier van der Gon JJ: Selective amplification of the electroretinogram. Ophthalmologica (Basel) 1956;132:140.

226. Armington JC, Gouras P, Tepas DI, et al: Detection of the electroretinogram in retinitis pigmentosa. Exp Eye Res 1961;1:74–80.

227. Gouras P, Carr RE: Electrophysiological studies in early retinitis pigmentosa. Arch Ophthalmol 1964;72:104–110.

228. Berson EL, Gouras P, Hoff M: The temporal aspects of the electroretinogram. Arch Ophthalmol 1969;81:207–214.

229. Berson EL, Gouras P, Gunkel RD, et al: Dominant retinitis pigmentosa with reduced penetrance. Arch Ophthalmol 1968;81:226–234.

230. Berson EL, Gouras P, Gunkel RD, et al: Rod and cone responses in sex-linked retinitis pigmentosa. Arch Ophthalmol 1969;81:215–225.

231. Gouras P: Electroretinography: some basic principals. Invest Ophthalmol 1970;9:557–569.

232. Krill AE: Rod-cone dystrophies. In: Krill AE, Archer DB, eds: Krill's Hereditary Retinal and Choroidal Disease. Hagerstown, MD, Harper & Row, 1977.

233. Berson EL: Hereditary retinal diseases: Classification with the full-field electroretinogram. Doc Ophthalmol 1977;13:149–171.

234. Berson EL, Simonoff EA: Dominant retinitis pigmentosa with reduced penetrance: Further studies of the electroretinogram. Arch Ophthalmol 1979;97:1286–1297.

235. Berson EL, Rosen JB, Simonoff EA: Electroretinographic testing as an aid in detection of carriers of X-chromosome-linked retinitis pigmentosa. Am J Ophthalmol 1979;87:460–468.

236. Arden GB, Carter RM, Hogg CR, et al: A modified ERG technique and the results obtained in X-linked retinitis pigmentosa. Br J Ophthalmol 1983;67:419–430.

237. Berson EL, Sandberg MA, Bosner B, et al: Course of retinitis pigmentosa over a three-year interval. Am J Ophthalmol 1985;99:240–251.

238. Marmor MF: The electroretinogram in retinitis pigmentosa. Arch Ophthalmol 1999;97:1300–1304.

239. Berson EL, Goldstein EB: The early receptor potential in sex-linked retinitis pigmentosa. Invest Ophthalmol 1970;9:58–63.

240. Riggs LA: Electroretinography in cases of night blindness. Am J Ophthalmol 1954;38:70–78.

241. Arden GB, Fojas MR: Electrophysiological abnormalities in pigmentary degenerations of the retina. Arch Ophthalmol 1962;68:369–389.

242. Arden GB, Barrada A, Kelsey JH: New clinical test of retinal function based upon the standing potential of the eye. Br J Ophthalmol 1962;46:449–467.

243. Steinberg RH: Interactions between the retinal pigment epithelium and neural retina. Doc Ophthalmol 1985;60:327–346.

244. Weleber RG, Eisner A: Retinal function and physiological studies. In: Newsome DA, ed: Retinal Dystrophies and Degeneration. New York, Raven Press, 1988, p 21.

245. Weleber RG: Fast and slow oscillations of the EOG in retinal dystrophies. Arch Ophthalmol 1989;107:530–537.

246. Alexander KR, Fishman GA: Prolonged rod dark adaptation in retinitis pigmentosa. Br J Ophthalmol 1984;68:561–569.

247. Krill AE, Smith VC, Blough R, et al: An absolute threshold defect in the inferior retina. Invest Ophthalmol Vis Sci 1968;7:701–707.

248. Weinstein GW, Maumenee AE, Hyvarinen L: On the pathogenesis of retinitis pigmentosa. Ophthalmologica 1971;62:82–97.

249. Weinstein GW, Lowell GG, Hobson RR: A comparison of electroretinographic and dark adaptation studies in retinitis pigmentosa. Doc Ophthalmol 1976;10:291–302.

250. Seiff SR, Heckenlively JR, Pearlman JT: Assessing the risk of retinitis pigmentosa with age-of-onset data. Am J Ophthalmol 1982;94:38–43.

251. Zeavin BH, Wald G: Rod and cone vision in retinitis pigmentosa. Am J Ophthalmol 1956;42:253–269.

252. Massof RW, Finkelstein D: Subclassifications of retinitis pigmentosa from two-color scotopic static perimetry. Doc Ophthalmol 1981;26:219–225.

253. Massof RW, Finkelstein D: Two forms of autosomal dominant primary retinitis pigmentosa. Doc Ophthalmol 1981;51:289–346.

254. Ernst W, Faulkner DJ, Hogg CR, et al: An automated static perimeter/adaptometer using light emitting diodes. Br J Ophthalmol 1983;67:431–442.

255. Tyler CW, Ernst W, Lyness AL: Photopic flicker sensitivity losses in simplex and multiplex retinitis pigmentosa. Invest Ophthalmol 1984;25:1035–1042.

256. Ernst W, Tyler CW, Clover GC, et al: X-linked retinitis pigmentosa: Reduced rod flicker sensitivity in heterozygous females. Invest Ophthalmol 1981;20:812–816.

257. Benson WE: An introduction to color vision. In: Duane TD, Jaeger EA, eds: Clinical Ophthalmology. Philadelphia, Harper & Row, 1985.

258. Verriest G: Les déficiences acquisés de la discrimination chromatiques. Mem Acad R Med Belg 1964;2:35–327.

259. Fishman GA, Young RSL, Vasquez V, et al: Color vision defects in retinitis pigmentosa. Ann Ophthalmol 1981;13:609–618.

260. Heckenlively JR, Martin DA, Rosales TO: Telangiectasia and optic atrophy in cone-rod degenerations. Arch Ophthalmol 1981;99:1981–1991.

261. Feeney L: Lipofuscin and melanin of human retinal pigment epithelium: Fluorescence, enzyme cytochemical and ultrastructural studies. Invest Ophthalmol Vis Sci 1978;17:583–600.

262. Wing GL, Blanchard GC, Weiter JJ: The topography and age relationship of lipofuscin concentration in the retinal pigment epithelium. Invest Ophthalmol Vis Sci 1978;17:601–607.

263. Wolter JR: Retinitis pigmentosa. Arch Ophthalmol 1971;57:539–553.

264. Kolb H, Gouras P: Electron microscopic observations of human retinitis pigmentosa, dominantly inherited. Invest Ophthalmol 1974;13:489–498.

265. Szamier RB, Berson EL: Retinal ultrastructure in advanced retinitis pigmentosa. Invest Ophthalmol Vis Sci 1977;16:947–962.

266. Sarks SH: Aging and degeneration in the macular region: A clinicopathological study. Br J Ophthalmol 1976;60:324–341.

267. Szamier RB, Berson EL, Klein R, et al: Sex-linked retinitis pigmentosa: Ultrastructure of photoreceptors and pigment epithelium. Invest Ophthalmol Vis Sci 1979;18:145–160.

268. Rayborn ME, Moorhead LC, Hollyfield JG: A dominantly inherited chorioretinal degeneration resembling retinitis pigmentosa. Ophthalmology 1982;89:1441–1453.

269. Runge P, Calver D, Marshall J, et al: The histopathology of two

distinct pigmentary retinopathies: one associated with the Kearns-Sayre syndrome, the other with Laurence-Moon-Biedl syndrome. Br J Ophthalmol 1986;70:782–796.

270. Bunt-Milam AH, Kalina RE, Pagon RA: Clinical-ultrastructural study of a retinal dystrophy. Invest Ophthalmol Vis Sci 1983; 24:458–469.

271. Cogan DG: Symposium: primary choroiretinal aberrations with night blindness. Trans Am Acad Ophthalmol Otolaryngol 1950;54:629–661.

272. Eichholtz W: Histologie der retinopathia pigmentosa cum et sine pigmento. Klin Monatsbl Augenheilkd 1974;164:467–475.

273. Lucas DR: Retinitis pigmentosa: pathological findings in two cases. Br J Ophthalmol 1956;40:14–23.

274. Mizuno K, Nashida S: Electron microscopic studies of human retinitis pigmentosa. Am J Ophthalmol 1967;63:791–803.

275. Szamier RB, Berson EL: Retinal histopathology of a carrier of X-chromosome-linked retinitis pigmentosa. Ophthalmology 1985; 92:271–278.

276. Levin PS, Green WR, Victor DI, et al: Histopathology of the eye in Cockayne's syndrome. Arch Ophthalmol 1983;101:1093–1097.

277. Bhattacharya SS, Wright AF, Clayton JF, et al: Close genetic linkage between X-linked retinitis pigmentosa and a restriction fragment length polymorphism identified by recombinant DNA probe L1.28. Nature 1984;309:253.

278. McWilliam P, Farrar GJ, Kenna P, et al: Autosomal dominant retinitis pigmentosa (ADRP): Localization of an ADRP gene to the long arm of chromosome 3. Genomics 1989;5:619.

279. Farrar GJ, McWilliam P, Bradley DG: Autosomal dominant retinitis pigmentosa: Linkage to rhodopsin and evidence for genetic heterogeneity. Genomics 1990a;8:35.

280. Inglehearn CF, Jay M, Lester DH, et al: The evidence for linkage between late onset autosomal dominant retinitis pigmentosa and chromosome 3 locus D2547 (C17): Evidence for genetic heterogeneity. Genomics 1990;6:168.

281. Blanton SH, Heckenlively JR, Cottingham AW, et al: Linkage mapping of autosomal dominant retinitis pigmentosa (RP1) to the pericentric region of human chromosome 8. Genomics 1991;11:857.

282. Kajiwara K, Hahn L, Mukai S, et al: Mutations in the human retinal degeneration slow gene in autosomal dominant retinitis pigmentosa. Nature 1991;354:480.

283. Nathans J, Piantanida TP, Eddy RL, et al: Molecular genetics of inherited variation in human color vision. Science 1986;232:203.

284. Sparkes RS, Klisak I, Kaufman D, et al: Assignment of the rhodopsin gene to human chromosome three, region 3q21-3q24 by in situ hybridization studies. Curr Eye Res 1986;5:797.

285. Musarella MA, Burghes A, Anson-Cartwright L, et al: Localization of the gene for X-linked recessive type of retinitis pigmentosa (XLRP) to Xp21 by linkage analysis. Am J Hum Genet 1988;43:484.

286. Chen JD, Halliday F, Keith G, et al: Linkage heterogeneity between X-linked retinitis pigmentosa and a map of 10 RFLP loci. Am J Hum Genet 1989;45:401.

287. Berson EL: Ocular findings in a form of retinitis pigmentosa with a rhodopsin gene defect. Trans Am Ophthalmol Soc 1990;88:355.

288. Dryja TD, McGee TL, Reichel E: A point mutation in the rhodopsin gene in one form of retinitis pigmentosa. Nature 1990;343:364.

289. Cremers FP, van de Pol DJ, van Kerkhoff LP, et al: Cloning of a gene that is rearranged in patients with choroideremia. Nature 1990;347:674.

290. Berson EL, Rosner B, Sandberg MA, et al: Ocular findings in patients with autosomal dominant retinitis pigmentosa and rhodopsin gene defect (Pro23His). Arch Ophthalmol 1991;109:92.

291. Berson EL, Rosner B, Sandberg MA, et al: Ocular findings in patients with autosomal dominant retinitis pigmentosa and rhodopsin, proline-347-leucine. Am J Ophthalmol 1991;111:614.

292. Berson EL, Sandberg MA, Dryja TP: Autosomal dominant retinitis pigmentosa with rhodopsin, valine-345-methionine. Trans Am J Ophthalmol Ophthalmol Soc 1991;89:117.

293. Bhattacharya S, Lester D, Keen TJ, et al: Retinitis pigmentosa and mutations in rhodopsin. Lancet 1991;337:185.

294. Bhattacharya SS, Inglehearn CF, Keen J, et al: Identification of novel rhodopsin mutations in patients with autosomal dominant retinitis pigmentosa. Invest Ophthalmol Vis Sci (suppl) 1991; 32:890.

295. Dryja TP, McGee TL, Hahn LB, et al: Mutations within the rhodop-

296. Dryja TP, Huhn LB, Cowley GS, et al: Mutation spectrum of the rhodopsin gene among patients with autosomal dominant retinitis pigmentosa. Proc Natl Acad Sci USA 1991;88:9370.

297. Farrar GJ, Kenna P, Jordan S, et al: A three-base-pair deletion in the peripherin-RDS gene in one form of retinitis pigmentosa. Nature 1991;354:478.

298. Farrar GJ, Kenna P, Redmond R, et al: Autosomal dominant retinitis pigmentosa: A mutation in codon 178 of the rhodopsin gene in two families of Celtic origin. Genomics 1991;11:1170.

299. Fishman GA, Stone EM, Gilbert LD, et al: Ocular findings associated with a rhodopsin gene codon 58 transversion mutation in autosomal dominant retinitis pigmentosa. Arch Ophthalmol 1991;109:1387.

300. Fujiki K, Hotta Y, Shiono T, et al: Codon 347 mutation of the rhodopsin gene in a Japanese family with autosomal dominant retinitis pigmentosa. Am J Hum Genet 1991;49(Suppl):187.

301. Gal A, Artlich A, Ludwig M, et al: Pro347Arg mutation of the rhodopsin gene in autosomal dominant retinitis pigmentosa. Genomics 1991;11:468.

302. Heckenlively JR, Rodriguez JA, Daiger SP: Autosomal dominant sectoral retinitis pigmentosa: Two families with transversion mutation in codon 23 of rhodopsin. Arch Ophthalmol 1991;109:84.

303. Inglehearn CF, Bashir R, Lester DH, et al: A 3-bp deletion in the rhodopsin gene in a family with autosomal dominant retinitis pigmentosa. Am J Hum Genet 1991;48:26.

304. Jacobson SG, Kemp CM, Sung CH, et al: Retinal function and rhodopsin levels in autosomal dominant retinitis pigmentosa with rhodopsin mutations. Am J Ophthalmol 1991;112:256.

305. Keen TJ, Inglehearn CF, Lester DH, et al: Autosomal dominant retinitis pigmentosa: Four new mutations in rhodopsin, one of them in the retinal attachment site. Genomics 1991;11:199–205.

306. Richards JE, Kuo CY, Boehnke M, et al: Rhodopsin Thr58Arg mutation in a family with autosomal dominant retinitis pigmentosa. Ophthalmology 119;98:1797.

307. Sheffield VC, Fishman GA, Beck JS, et al: Identification of novel rhodopsin mutations associated with retinitis pigmentosa by GC-clamped denaturing gradient gel electrophoresis. Am J Hum Genet 1991;49:699.

308. Sorscher EJ, Huang Z: Diagnosis of genetic disease by primer-specified restriction map modification, with application to cystic fibrosis and retinitis pigmentosa. Lancet 1991;337:1115.

309. Stone EM, Kimura AE, Nichols BE, et al: Regional distribution of retinal degeneration in patients with the proline to histidine mutation in codon 23 of the rhodopsin gene. Ophthalmology 1991;98:1806.

310. Sung CH, Davenport CM, Hennessey JC, et al: Rhodopsin mutations in autosomal dominant retinitis pigmentosa. Proc Natl Acad Sci USA 1991;88:6481.

311. Sung CH, Schneider BG, Agarwal N, et al: Functional heterogeneity of mutation rhodopsins responsible for autosomal dominant retinitis pigmentosa. Proc Natl Acad Sci USA 1991;88:8840.

312. Artlich A, Horn M, Lorenz B, et al: Recurrent 3bp deletion at codon 255/256 of the rhodopsin gene in a German pedigree with autosomal dominant retinitis pigmentosa. Am J Hum Genet 1992;50:867.

313. Bahir R, Inglehearn CF, Keen TJ, Lindsey J, et al: Exclusion of chromosomes 6 and 8 in nonrhodopsin linked adRP families: Further locus heterogeneity in adRP. Genomics 1992;14:191.

314. Bhattacharya SS: Exclusion of chromosomes 6 and 8 in non-rhodopsin linked adRP families: Further locus heterogeneity in adRP. Genomics 1992;14:191.

315. Bell C, Converse CA, Clooins MF, et al: Autosomal dominant retinitis pigmentosa (adRP)—a rhodopsin mutation in a Scottish family. J Med Genet 1992;29:667.

316. Fishman GA, Stone EM, Sheffield VC, et al: Ocular findings associated with rhodopsin gene codon 17 and codon 182 transition mutations in dominant retinitis pigmentosa. Arch Ophthalmol 1992;110:54.

317. Hargrave PA, O'Brien PJ: Speculations on the molecular basis of retinal degeneration in retinitis pigmentosa. In: Anderson RE, Hollyfield JG, La Vail MM, eds: Retinal Degenerations. Boca Raton, CRC Press, 1991.

318. Rosenfeld PH, Cowley GS, McGee TL, et al: Null mutations within

the rhodopsin gene as a cause of rod photoreceptor dysfunction and autosomal recessive retinitis pigmentosa. Nat Genet 1992;1:209.

319. Heckenlively JR, Solish AM, Chant SM, et al: Autoimmunity in hereditary retinal degeneration. II. Clinical studies: antiretinal antibodies and fluorescein angiogram findings. Br J Ophthalmol 1985;69:758–764.

320. Heckenlively JR, Aptsiauri N, Nusinowitz S, et al: Investigations of antiretinal antibodies in pigmentary retinopahty and other retinal degenerations. Trans Am Ophthalmol Soc XCIV 1996;179–206.

321. Heckenlively JR, Jordan RL, Aptsiauri N: Association of antiretinal antibodies and cystoid macular edema in patients with retinitis pigmentosa. Am J Ophthalmol 1999;127:565–573.

322. Char DH, Bergsma DR, Rabson AS, et al: Cell mediated immunity to retinal antigens in patients with pigmentary retinal degeneration. Invest Ophthalmol Vis Sci 1974;13:198–203.

323. Spalton DJ, Rahi AHS, Bird AC: Immunologic studies in retinitis pigmentosa associated with retinal vascular leakage. Br J Ophthalmol 1978;62:183–187.

324. Brinkman CJJ, Pinckers AJLG, Broekhuyse RM: Immune reactivity to different retinal antigens in patients suffering from retinitis pigmentosa. Invest Ophthalmol Vis Sci 1980;19:743–750.

325. Chant SM, Heckenlively JR, Meyers-Eliott RH: Autoimmunity in hereditary retinal degeneration. I. Basic studies. Br J Ophthalmol 1985;69:19–24.

326. Ammann F: Klein D, Franceschetti A: Genetic and epidemiological investigations on pigmentary degeneration of the retina and allied disorders in Switzerland. J Neurol Sci 1965;2:183–196.

327. Bell J: a determination of the consanguinity rate in the general hospital population of England and Wales. Ann Eugen 1940;10:370–391.

328. Merin S, Auerbach E: Retinitis pigmentosa. Survey Ophthalmology. 1976;20:303–346.

329. Boughman JA, Conneally PM, Nance WE: Population genetic studies of retinitis pigmentosa. Am J Hum Genet 1980;32:223–235.

330. Boughman J: Genetic analysis of heterogeneity and variation in retinitis pigmentosa. Birth Defects 1982;18:151–160.

331. Hu DN: Genetic aspects of retinitis pigmentosa in China. Am J Med Genet 1982;12:51–56.

332. Jay M: On the heredity of retinitis pigmentosa. Br J Ophthalmol 1982;66:405–416.

333. Bundy S, Crews SJ: Wishes of patients with retinitis pigmentosa concerning genetic counseling. J Med Genet 1982;19:317.

334. Newsome DA, Milton RC, Frederique G: High prevalence of eye disease in a Haitian locale. J Trop Med Hyg 1983;86:37–46.

335. Boughman JA, Fishman GA: A genetic analysis of retinitis pigmentosa. Br J Ophthalmol 1983;67:449–454.

336. Bunker CH, Berson EL, Bromley WC, et al: Prevalence of retinitis pigmentosa in Maine. Am J Ophthalmol 1984;97:347–365.

337. Heckenlively JR: The diagnosis and classification of retinitis pigmentosa. In: Heckenlively JR, ed: Retinitis Pigmentosa. Philadelphia, JB Lippincott, 1988, p 6.

338. Heckenlively J, Friederich R, Friederich R, et al: Retinitis pigmentosa in the Navajo. Metab Pediatr Ophthalmol 1981;5:201–206.

339. Pearlman JT: Mathematical models of retinitis pigmentosa: A study of the rate of progress in the different genetic forms. Trans Am Ophthalmol Soc 1979;77:643–656.

340. Weleber RG: Retinitis pigmentosa and allied disorders. In: Ryan SJ, ed: Retina. St. Louis, CV Mosby, 1994, p 335.

341. Heckenlively JR: Clinical findings in retinitis pigmentosa. In: Heckenlively JR, ed: Retinitis Pigmentosa. Philadelphia, JB Lippincott, 1988, p 68.

342. Berson EL: Retinitis pigmentosa and allied diseases. In: Albert DM, Jakobiec FA, eds: Principles and Practice of Ophthalmology. Philadelphia, WB Saunders, 2000, p 2262.

343. Pagon RA: Retinitis pigmentosa. Surv Ophthalmol 1988;33:137–177.

344. Newsome DA: Retinitis pigmentosa, Usher's syndrome, and other pigmetnary retinopathies. In: Newsome DA, ed: Retinal Dystrophies and Degenerations. New York, Raven Press, 1988, pp 161–194.

345. Franceschetti A, Francois J, Babel J: Les Héredodégenerescences Choriorétiniennes. Paris, Masson, 1963.

346. Deutman AF: Rod cone dystrophy: Primary hereditary, pigmentary

retinopathy, retinitis pigmentosa. In: Krill AE, Archer DB, eds: Krill's Hereditary Retinal and Choroidal Disease, Vol 2, Clinical Characteristics. New York, Harper & Row, 1977.

347. Marmor MF, Aguirre G, Arden G, et al: Retinitis pigmentosa: A symposium on terminology and methods of examination. Ophthalmology 1983;90:126.

348. Pruett RC: Retinitis pigmentosa: Clinical observations and correlations. Trans Am Ophthalmol Soc 1983;81:693.

349. Heckenlively JR: The frequency of posterior subcapsular cataract in the hereditary retinal degenerations. Am J Ophthalmol 1982;93:733.

350. Sieving PA, Fishman GA: Refractive errors of retinitis pigmentosa patients. Br J Ophthalmol 1978;52:625.

351. Berson EL, Rosner B, Simonoff EA: Risk factors for genetic typing and detection in retinitis pigmentosa. Am J Ophthalmol 1980;89:763.

352. Heckenlively JR, Yoser SL, Friedman LJ, et al: Clinical findings and common symptoms in retinitis pigmentosa. Am J Ophthalmol 1198;105:504–511.

353. Newsome DA, Hewitt AT, Swartz M: Cellular and molecular changes in RP vitreous. Invest Ophthalmol Vis Sci 1984; 25(Suppl):198.

354. Merin S: Macular cysts as an early sign of tapeto-retinal degeneration. J Pediatr Ophthalmol 1970;7:225–228.

355. Gass JDM: Stereoscopic Atlas of Macular Diseases: A Funduscopic and Angiographic Presentation. St. Louis, CV Mosby, 1970.

356. Ffytche TJ: Cystoid maculopathy in retinitis pigmentosa. Trans Ophthalmol Soc UK 1972;92:265–283.

357. Francois J, De Laey JJ, Verbraeken H: L'oedeme kystoide de la macula. Bull Soc Belge Ophthalmol 1972;161:708–721.

358. Bonnet M, Pingault MC: Cystoid macular edema and retinitis pigmentosa. Bull Soc Ophthalmol Fr 1973;73:715–718.

359. Fishman GA, Lam BL, Anderson RJ: Racial differences in the prevalence of atrophic-appearing macular lesions between black and white patients with retinitis pigmentosa. Am J Ophthalmol 1994;118:33–38.

360. Fishman GA, Fishman M, Maggiano J: Macular lesions associated with retinitis pigmentosa. Arch Ophthalmol 1977;95:798–803.

361. Spalton DJ, Bird AC, Cleary PE: Retinitis pigmentosa and retinal edema. Br J Ophthalmol 1978;62:174–182.

362. Shahidi M, Fishman G, Ogura Y, et al: Foveal thickening in retinitis pigmentosa patients with cystoid macular edema. Retina 1994;14:243–247.

363. Geltzer AI, Berson EL: Fluorescein angiography of hereditary retinal degenerations. Arch Ophthalmol 1969;81:776–782.

364. Hansen RI, Friedman AH, Gartner S, et al: The association of retinitis pigmentosa with preretinal macular gliosis. Br J Ophthalmol 1977;61:597–600.

365. Gartner S, Henkind P: Pathology of retinitis pigmentosa. Ophthalmology 1982;89:1425–1432.

366. Marshall J, Heckenlively JR: Pathologic findings and putative mechanisms in retinitis pigmentosa. In: Heckenlively JR, ed: Retinitis Pigmentosa. Philadelphia, JB Lippincott, 1988.

367. Santos-Anderson RM, Tso MOM, Fishman GA: A histopathologic study of retinitis pigmentosa. Ophthalmol Pediatr Genet I: 1982;151–168.

368. Albert DM, Pruett RC, Craft JL: Transmission electron microscopic observations of vitreous abnormalities in retinitis pigmentosa. Am J Ophthalmol 1986;101:665–672.

369. Gouras P: Transmission electron microscopic observations of vitreous abnormalities in retinitis pigmentosa. Am J Ophthalmol 1987;103:345.

370. Newsome DA, Michels RG: Detection of lymphocytes in the vitreous gel of patients with retinitis pigmentosa. Am J Ophthalmol 1988;105:596–602.

371. Meyers RL: Experimental allergic uveitis: Induction by retinal rod outer segments and pigment epithelium. Proceedings of the 1st symposium on immunology and immunopathology of the eye. Modern Problems in Ophthalmology 1974;16:41–50.

372. Reich D'Almeira F, Rahi AHS: Antigenic specificity of retinal pigment epithelium and non-immunological involvement in retinal dystrophy. Nature 1974;252:307–308.

373. Wacker WB, Kalsow CM: The role of uveal and retinal antigens in experimental ocular pathology. Proceedings of the 1st symposium on immunology and immunopathology of the eye. Modern Problems in Ophthalmology 1974;16:12–20.

374. Rahi AH, Lucas DR, Waghe M: Experimental immune retinitis: Induction by isolated photoreceptors. Mod Probl Ophthalmol 1976;16:30–40.

375. Rahi AHS: Autoimmunity and the retina: II. Raised serum IgM levels in retinitis pigmentosa. Br J Ophthalmol 1973;57:904–909.

376. Fessel WJ: Serum protein disturbance in retinitis pigmentosa. Am J Ophthalmol 1962;53:640.

377. Heredia CD, Vich JM, Huguet J, et al: Altered cellular immunity and suppressor cell activity in patients with primary retinitis pigmentosa. Br J Ophthalmol 1981;65:850.

378. Heredia CD, Huguet J, Cols N, et al: Immune complexes in retinitis pigmentosa. Br J Ophthalmol 1984;68:811–814.

379. Galbraith GMP, Fudenberg HH: One subset of patients with retinitis pigmentosa has immunologic defects. Clin Immunol Immunopathol 1984;31:254.

380. Hooks JJ, Detrick-Hooks B, Geis S, et al: Retinitis pigmentosa associated with a defect in the production of interferon-gamma. Am J Ophthalmol 1983;96:755–758.

381. Newsome DA, Nussenblatt RB: Retinal S antigen reactivity in patients with retinitis pigmentosa and Usher's syndrome. Retina 1984;4:195–199.

382. Hendricks RL, Fishman GA: Lymphocyte subpopulations and S-antigen reactivity in retinitis pigmentosa. Arch Ophthalmol 1985;103:61–65.

383. Goodman G, Gunkel RD: Familial electroretinographic and adaptometric studies in retinitis pigmentosa. Am J Ophthalmol 1958;46:142.

384. Berson EL, Gouras P, Gunkel RD: Rod responses in retinitis pigmentosa, dominantly inherited. Arch Ophthalmol 1968;80:58.

385. Berson EL: Retinitis pigmentosa and allied diseases: Electrophysiologic findings. Trans Am Acad Ophthalmol Otolaryngol 1976;81:659.

386. Berson EL: Electroretinographic findings in retinitis pigmentosa. Jpn J Ophthalmol 1987;31:327.

387. Berson EL: Light pigmentosa and allied diseases. Applications of electroretinographic testing. Int Ophthalmol 1981;4:7–22.

388. Berson EL, Sandberg MA, Rosner B, et al: Natural course of retinitis pigmentosa over a three-year interval. Am J Ophthalmol 1985;99:240–251.

389. Fishman GA: Electrophysiology and inherited retinal disorders. Doc Ophthalmologica 1985;60:107–119.

390. Fishman GA, Farber MD, Derlacki DJ: X-linked retinitis pigmentosa. Profile of clinical findings. Arch Ophthalmol 1988;106:369–375.

391. Ross DF, Fishman GA, Gilbert LD, et al: Variability of visual field measurements in normal subjects and patients with retinitis pigmentosa. Arch Ophthalmol 1984;102:1004–1010.

392. Krauss HR, Heckenlively JR: Visual field changes in cone-rod degenerations. Arch Ophthalmol 1982;100:1784–1790.

393. Siddal JR: The ocular toxic findings with prolonged and high dosage chlorpromazine intake. Arch Ophthalmol 1965;74:460–464.

394. Nylander ULF: Ocular damage in chloroquine therapy. Acta Ophthalmol 1965;44:335–348.

395. Mathalone MBR: Eye and skin changes in psychiatric patients treated with chlorpromazine. Br J Ophthalmol 1967;51:86–93.

396. Burns CA: Indomethacin, reduced retinal sensitivity and corneal deposits. Am J Ophthalmol 1968;66:825–835.

397. Carr RE, Henkind P, Rothfield N, et al: Ocular toxicity of antimalarial drugs. Am J Ophthalmol 1968;66:738–744.

398. Henkes HE, Va Lith GHM, Canta LR: Indomethacin retinopathy. Am J Ophthalmol 1972;73:846–856.

399. Cameron ME, Lawrence JM, Olrich JG: Thioridazine (Mellaril) retinopathy. Br J Ophthalmol 1972;56:131–134.

400. Francois J, De Rouck A, Cambie E: Retinal and optic evaluation in quinine poisoning. Ann Ophthalmol 1972;4:177–185.

401. Carr RE, Siegel IM: Retinal function in patients treated with indomethacin. Am J Ophthalmol 1973;75:302–306.

402. Davidorf FH: Thioridazine pigmentary retinopathy. Arch Ophthalmol 1973;251–255.

403. Meredith TA, Aaberg TM, Willerson WD: Progressive chorioretinopathy after receiving thioridazine. Arch Ophthalmol 1978;96:1172–1176.

404. Brinkley JR, Dubois EL, Ryan RJ: Long-tern course of chloroquine retinopathy after cessation of medication. Am J Ophthalmol 1979;88:1–11.

405. Marks JS: Chloroquine retinopathy: Is there a safe daily dose? Ann Rheum Dis 1982;41:52–58.

406. Infante R, Martin DA, Heckenlively JR: Hydroxychloroquine and retinal toxicity. Doc Ophthalmol Pro Ser 1983;37:121–126.

407. Cooper IZ, Krugman S: Clinical manifestations of postnatal and congenital rubella. Arch Ophthalmol 1967;77:434–439.

408. Metz HS, Harkey ME: Pigmentary retinopathy following maternal measles (Morbilli) infection. Am J Ophthalmol 1968;66:1107–1110.

409. Heckenlively JR: Secondary retinitis pigmentosa (syphilis). Doc Ophthalmol 1976;13:245–255.

410. Heckenlively JR, Kokame GT: Pigmented paravenous retinochoroidal atrophy; clinical and electrophysiological findings. Doc Ophthalmol 1985;40:235–241.

411. Foxman SG, Heckenlively JR, Sinclair SH: Rubeola retinopathy and pigmented paravenous retinochoroidalatrophy. Am J Ophthalmol 1985;99:605–606.

412. Brown TH: Retino-choroiditis radiata. Br J Ophthalmol 1937;21:645–648.

413. Franceschetti A: A curious affection of the fundusocul: lation to pigmentary paravenous chorioretinaldegeneration. Doc Ophthalmol 1962;16:81–110.

414. Krill AE: Incomplete rod-cone degeneration. In: Krill AE, Archer DB, eds: Krill's Hereditary Retinal and Choroidal Diseases, Vol 2, Clinical Characteristics. Hagerstown, MD, Harper & Row, 1977, pp 577–643.

415. Noble KG, Carr RE: Pigmented paravenous chorioretinal atrophy. Am J Ophthalmol 1978;86:65–75.

416. Hsin-Hsiang C: Retinochoroiditis radiata. Am J Ophthalmol 1948;31:1485–1487.

417. Takei Y, Harda M, Mizuno K: Pigmented paravenous retinochoroidal atrophy. Jpn J Ophthalmol 1977;21:311–317.

418. Breageat P, Amalric P: Postmeningoencephalitis bilateral paravenous chorioretinal degeneration. In: Henkind P, Shimizu K, Blodi FC, et al (eds): XXIV International Congress of Ophthalmology, Vol 1. Philadelphia, JB Lippincott, 1983, pp 454–457.

419. Miller SA, Stevens TS, Myers F, et al: Pigmented paravenous retinochoroidal atrophy. Ann Ophthalmol 1978;10:1478–1488.

420. Hirose T, Miyake Y: Pigmentary paravenous chorioretinal degeneration. Ann Ophthalmol 1979;11:709–718.

421. Lessel MR, Thaler A, Heilig P: ERG and EOG in progressive paravenous retinochoroidal atrophy. Doc Ophthalmol 1986;62:25–29.

422. Bastek JV, Foos RY, Heckenlively JR: Traumatic pigmentary retinopathy. Am J Ophthalmol 1981;92:621–624.

423. Heckenlively JR, Silver J: Management and treatment of retinitis pigmentosa. In: Heckenlively JR, ed: Retinitis Pigmentosa. Philadelphia, JB Lippincott, 1988, p 90.

424. Chen JC, Fitzke FW, Bird AC: Long-term effect of acetazolamide in a patient with retinitis pigmentosa. Invest Ophthalmol Vis Sci 1990;31:1914–1918.

425. Cox SN, Hay E, Bird AC: Treatment of chronic macular edema with acetazolamide. Arch Ophthalmol 1988;106:1190–1195.

426. Fishman CA, Gilbert LD, Fiscella RG, et al: Acetazolamide for treatment of chronic macular edema in retinitis pigmentosa. Arch Ophthalmol 1989;107:1445–1452.

427. Cogan DG, Rodrigues M, Chu FC, et al: Ocular abnormalities in abetalipoproteinemia: A clinicopathologic correlation. Ophthalmology 1984;91:991–998.

428. Berger AS, Tychsen L, Rosenblum JL: Retinopathy in human vitamin E deficiency. Am J Ophthalmol 1991;111:774–775.

429. Campbell DA, Harrison R, Tonks EL: Retinitis pigmentosa vitamin A serum levels in relation to clinical findings. Exp Eye Res 1964;3:412–426.

430. Chatzinoff A, Millmann N, Oroshnik W, et al: 11-*cis* vitamin A in the prevention of retinal rod degeneration: An animal study. Am J Ophthalmol 1958;46:205–210.

431. Chatzinoff A, Nelson E, Stahl N, et al: 11-*cis* vitamin A in the treatment of retinitis pigmentosa: A negative study. Arch Ophthalmol 1968;80:417–419.

432. Berson EL, Rosner B, Sandberg MA, et al: A randomized trial of vitamin A and vitamin E supplementation for retinitis pigmentosa. Arch Ophthalmol 1993;111:761–772.

433. Marmor MF: A randomized trial of vitamin A and vitamin E supplementation for retinitis pigmentosa. Arch Ophthalmol 1993;111:1460–1461.

434. Massof RW, Finkelstein D: Supplemental vitamin A retards loss of ERG amplitude in retinitis pigmentosa. Arch Ophthalmol 1993;111:751–754.

435. Wolff OH, Lloyd JK, Tonks EL: A-β-lipoproteinemia with special reference to the visual defect. Exp Eye Res 1964;3:439–442.

436. Carr RE: Vitamin A therapy may reverse degenerative retinal syndrome. Clin Trends 1970;8:8.

437. Sperling MA, Hiles DA, Kennerdell JS: Electroretinographic responses following vitamin A therapy in α-β-lipoproteinemia. Am J Ophthalmol 1972;73:342–351.

438. Gouras P, Carr RE, Gunkel RD: Retinitis pigmentosa in abetalipoproteinemia: Effects of vitamin A. Invest Ophthalmol Vis Sci 1971;10:784.

439. Bishara S, Merin S, Cooper M, et al: Combined vitamin A and E therapy prevents retinal electrophysiological deterioration in abetalipoproteinemia. Br J Ophthalmol 1982;66:767.

440. Smith VH: The incidence of intraocular foreign bodies. Int Ophthalmol Clin 1968;8:137–146.

441. Percival SPB: A decade of intraocular foreign bodies. Br J Ophthalmol 1972;56:454–461.

442. Smiddy WE, Stark WJ: Anterior segment intraocular foreign bodies. In: Shingleton BJ, Hersh PS, Kenyon KR, eds: Eye Trauma. St. Louis, Mosby–Year Book, 1991.

443. Hersh PS, Zagelbaum BM, Shingleton BJ, Kenyon KR: Anterior segment trauma. In: Albert DM, Jakobiec FA, eds: Principles and Practice of Ophthalmology. Philadelphia, WB Saunders, 2000, p 5201.

444. Coleman DJ, Kucas BC, Rondeau MN, et al: Management of intraocular foreign bodies. Ophthalmology 1987;94:1647–1673.

445. Wirotsko WJ, Mieler WF, McCabe CM, Dieckert JP: Intraocular foreign bodies. In: Albert DM, Jakobiec FA, eds: Principles and Practice of Ophthalmology. Philadelphia, WB Saunders Company, 2000, p 5241.

446. Barry DR: Effects of retained intraocular foreign bodies. Int Ophthalmol Clin 1968;8:153–170.

447. Neubauer H: Management of nonmagnetic intraocular foreign bodies. In: Freeman HM, ed: Ocular Trauma. New York, Appleton-Century-Crofts, 1979.

448. Duke-Elder S, Macfaul PA: Intra-ocular foreign bodies. In: Duke-Elder S, Macfaul PA, eds: System of Ophthalmology, Vol. XIV, part 1: Mechanical injuries. St. Louis, CV Mosby, 1972.

449. Spoor TC, Nesi FA: Management of Ocular, Orbital, and Adnexal Trauma. New York, Raven Press, 1988.

450. Kamath MG, Nayak IV, Satish KR: Case report: intraocular foreign body in the angle masquerading as uveitis. Ind J Ophthalmol 1991;39:138–139.

451. Alexandrakis G, Balachander R, Chaudhry NA, et al: An intraocular foreign body masquerading as idiopathic chronic iridocyclitis 1998;29:336–337.

452. Dieckert JP: Posterior segment trauma. In: Albert DM, Jakobiec FA, eds: Principles and Practice of Ophthalmology. Philadelphia, WB Saunders, 2000, p 5221.

453. Negrel AD, Massembo-Yako B, Botaka E, et al: Prévalence et causes de la cécité au Congo. Bull WHO 1990;68:237.

454. Dana MR, Tielsch JM, Enger C, et al: Visual impairment in a rural Appalachian community. JAMA 1990;264:2400.

455. Morris RE, Witherspoon CD, Helms HA Jr, et al: Eye injury registry of Alabama (preliminary report): Demographics and prognosis of severe eye injury. South Med J 1987;80:810.

456. Tielsch JM, Parver L, Shankar B: Time trends in the incidence of hospitalized ocular trauma. Arch Ophthalmol 1989;107:519.

457. Klopfer J, Tielsch JM, Vitale S, et al: Ocular trauma in the United States: Eye injuries resulting in hospitalization, 1984 through 1987. Arch Ophthalmol 1992;110:838.

458. Karlson TA, Klein BEK: The incidence of acute hospital-treated eye injuries. Arch Ophthalmol 1989;104:1473.

459. Katz J, Tielsch JM: Lifetime prevalence of ocular injuries from the Baltimore Eye Survey. Arch Ophthalmol 1993;111:1564.

460. Bdesai P, MacEwen CJ, Baines P, et al: Incidence of cases of ocular trauma admitted to hospital and incidence of blinding outcome. Br J Ophthalmol 1996;80:592.

461. Blomdahl S, Norell S: Perforating eye injury in the Stockholm population: An epidemiological study. Acta Ophthalmol 1984; 62:378.

462. Fong LP: Eye injuries in Victoria, Australia. Med J Aust 1995;162:64.

463. Wong TY, Tielsch JM: A population-based study on the incidence of severe ocular trauma in Singapore. Am J Ophthalmol 1999;128:345–351.

464. Dannenberg AL, Parver LM, Brechner RJ, et al: Penetrating eye injuries in the workplace. Arch Ophthalmol 1992;110:843.

465. Liggett PE, Pince KJ, Barlow W, et al: Ocular trauma in an urban population. Ophthalmology 1990;97:581.

466. Schein OD, Hibberd PL, Shingleton BJ, et al: The spectrum and burden of ocular injury. Ophthalmology 1988;95:300.

467. MacEwen CJ: Eye injuries: A prospective survey of 5671 cases. Br J Ophthalmol 1989;73:888.

468. Glunn RJ, Seddon JM, Berlin BM: The incidence of eye injuries in New England adults. Arch Ophthalmol 1988;106:785.

469. Koval R, Teller J, Belkin M, et al: The Israeli ocular injuries study, a nationwide collaborative study. Arch Ophthalmol 1988;106:776.

470. Canavan YM, O'Flaherty MJ, Archer DB, et al: A 10-year survey of eye injuries in Northern Ireland, 1967–76. Br J Ophthalmol 1980;64:618.

471. Sneed SR: Ocular siderosis. Arch Ophthalmol 1988;106:997.

472. Delaney WV Jr: Presumed ocular chalcosis: A reversible maculopathy. Ann Ophthalmol Vis Sci 1986;27:226–236.

473. Reeh MJ: Use of the Goniolens for diagnosis of retained foreign body in the anterior chamber. Am J Ophthalmol 1948;31:336.

474. Trantas. Bull Soc Hellen Ophthal 1938;7:166, 207.

475. Archer DB, Davies MS, Kanski JJ: Non-metallic foreign bodies in the anterior chamber. Br J Ophthalmol 1969;53:453–6.

476. Smith RE, Nozik RA: Masquerade syndromes. In: Smith RE, Nozik RA, eds: Uveitis: A Clinical Approach to Diagnosis and Management. Baltimore, Williams & Wilkins, 1989, pp 194–196.

477. Wilder HC: Intraocular foreign bodies in soldiers. Am J Ophthalmol 1948;31:57–64.

478. Duszynski LR: The contamination of operative wounds with cotton fibrils and talc. Trans Am Acad Ophthalmol Otolaryngol 1951;55:110.

479. Irvine AR: Old and new techniques combined in the management of intraocular foreign bodies. Ann Ophthalmol 1981;13:41.

480. Coleman DJ, Jack RL, Franzen LA: Ultrasonography in ocular trauma. Am J Ophthalmol 1973;75:279.

481. Fisher YL: Contact B-scan ultrasonography: A practical approach. Int Ophthalmol Clin 1979;19:103.

482. Awschalom L, Meyers SM: Ultrasonography of vitreal foreign bodies in eyes obtained at autopsy. Arch Ophthalmol 1982;100:979.

483. Wilhelm JL, Zakov ZN, Weinstein MA, et al: Localization of suspected intraocular foreign bodies with a modified Delta 2020 scanner. Ophthalmic Surg 1981;12:633.

484. Ossoinig KC: Standardized echography: Basic principles, clinical applications, and results. Int Ophthalmol Clin 1979;19:127.

485. Bertenyi A: Localization of intraocular and intraorbital foreign bodies by means of A-scan ultrasonography. Ultrasonics 1976;14:183.

486. Benson WE: Intraocular foreign bodies. In: Tasman W, Jaeger EA, eds: Duane's Clinical Ophthalmology, Vol 5. Philadelphia, JB Lippincott, 1991, pp 1–15.

487. Bryden FM, Pyott AA, Bailey M, et al: Real time ultrasound in the assessment of intraocular foreign bodies. Eye 1991;5:751–754.

488. Kollarits CR, Di Chiro G, Christiansen J, et al: Detection of orbital and intraocular foreign bodies by computerized tomography. Ophthalmic Surg 1977;8:45–53.

489. Barr CC, Vine AK, Martonyi CL: Unexplained heterochromia. Intraocular foreign body demonstrated by computed tomography. Surv Ophthalmol 1984;28:409.

490. Gaster RN, Duda EE: Localization of intraocular foreign bodies by computed tomography. Ophthalmic Surg 1980;11:25.

491. Etherington RJ, Hourihan MD: Localization of intraocular and intraorbital foreign bodies using computed tomography. Clin Radiol 1989;40:610.

492. Zinreich SJ, Miller NR, Aguayo JB, et al: Computed tomographic three-dimensional localization and compositional evaluation of intraocular and orbital foreign bodies. Arch Ophthalmol 1986; 104:1477.

493. Bhimani S, Virapongse C, Sarwar M, et al: Computed tomography in penetrating injury to the eye. Am J Ophthalmol 1984;97:583.

494. Trinkmann R, Runde H: Demonstration and localization of intraocular metallic foreign bodies by computerized tomography. Klin Monatsbl Augenheilkd 1984;184:18.

495. Lobes LA, Grand MG, Reece J, et al: Computerized axial tomography in the detection of intraocular foreign bodies. Ophthalmology 1981;88:26.

496. Totsuka K, Takao M: CT scanner and the reliable limit of detection on intraocular foreign bodies. Acta Soc Ophthalmol Jpn 1978;82:388.

497. Duker JS, Fischer DH: Occult plastic intraocular foreign body. Ophthalmic Surg 1989;20:169.

498. Topilow HW, Ackerman AL, Zimmerman RD: Limitations of computerized tomography in the localization of intraocular foreign bodies. Ophthalmology 1984;91:1086.

499. Preisova J, Riebel O, Vlkov AE, et al: Moth fragments as intraocular foreign bodies. Klin Monatsbl Augenheilkd 1988;192:30.

500. LoBue TD, Deutsch TA, Lobick J, et al: Detection and localization of nonmetallic intraocular foreign bodies by magnetic resonance imaging. Arch Ophthalmol 1988;106:260–261.

501. Salminen L: Intraocular foreign body from a Healon syringe. Am J Ophthalmol 1987;104:427.

502. Williamson TH, Smith FW, Forrester JV: Magnetic resonance imaging of intraocular foreign bodies. Br J Ophthalmol 1989;73:555.

503. Kelly WM, Paglen PG, Pearson JA, et al: Ferromagnetism of intraocular foreign body causes unilateral blindness after MR study. AJNR 1986;7:243.

504. Zheutlin JD, Thompson JT, Shofner RS: The safety of magnetic resonance imaging with intraorbital metallic objects after retinal reattachment or trauma. Am J Ophthalmol 1987;103:831.

505. Williams S, Char DH, Dillon WP, et al: Ferrous intraocular foreign bodies and magnetic resonance imaging. Am J Ophthalmol 1988;105:398.

506. Coleman DJ, Rondeau MJ: Diagnostic imaging of ocular and orbital trauma. In Shingleton BJ, Hersh PS, Kenyon KR (eds): Eye Trauma. St. Louis, Mosby-Year Book, 1991.

507. Deramo VA, Shah GK, Baumal CR, et al: Ultrasound biomicroscopy as a tool for detecting and localizing occult foreign bodies after ocular trauma. Ophthalmology 1999;106:301–305.

508. Knave B: Electroretinography in eyes with retained intraocular metallic foreign bodies: A clinical study. Acta Ophthalmol 1959;100(Suppl):1–63.

509. Knave B: The ERG and ophthalmological changes in experimental metallosis in the rabbit. II. Effects of steel, copper and aluminum particles. Acta Ophthalmol 1970;48:159–173.

510. Good P, Gross K: Electrophysiology and metallosis: Support for an oxidative (free radical) mechanism in the human eye. Ophthalmologica 1988;196:204.

511. Schmidt JGH, Nies C, Mansfeld-Nies R: On the recovery of the electroretinogram after removal of intravitreal zinc particles. Doc Ophthalmol 1987;65:471.

512. Schmidt JGH: Intravitreal cupriferous foreign bodies: Electroretinograms and inflammatory responses. Doc Ophthalmol 1988;67:253.

513. Schmidt JGH, Mansfeld-Nies R, Nies C: On the recovery of the electroretinogram after removal of intravitreal copper particles. Doc Ophthalmol 1987;65:135.

514. Brunette JR, Wagdi S, Lafond G: Electroretinographic alterations in retinal metallosis. Can J Ophthalmol 1980;15:176.

515. Tolentino FI, Liu HS, Freeman HM, et al: Vitrectomy in penetrating ocular trauma: An experience study using rabbits. Ann Ophthalmol 1979;11:1763.

516. Heimann K, Paulmann H: Vitrectomy after perforating injuries. Mod Probl Ophthalmol 1977;18:242.

517. Neubauer H: Ocular metallosis. Trans Ophthalmol Soc UK 1979;99:502.

518. Khan MD, Kundi N, Mohammed Z, et al: A 6½-year survey of intraocular and intraorbital foreign bodies in the northwest frontier province, Pakistan. Br J Ophthalmol 1987;71:716.

519. Treister G, Keren G: Operative difficulties in removal of retained intraocular foreign body by vitreous surgery. Ophthalmologica 1981;183:136.

520. Hutton WL, Snyder WB, Vaiser A: Surgical removal of non-magnetic foreign bodies. Am J Ophthalmol 1975;80:838.

521. Michels RG: Surgical management of nonmagnetic intraocular foreign bodies. Arch Ophthalmol 1975;93:1003.

522. Boldrey EE, Haidt SJ: Early vitrectomy for retained intraocular foreign body. Ann Ophthalmol 1978;10:1441.

523. Ross WH, Tasman WS: The management of magnetic intraocular foreign bodies. Can J Ophthalmol 1975;10:168.

524. Zagorski Z, Palacz O, Grabowsko J, et al: Comparative studies in chronic ocular chalcosis. Klin Oczna 1989;91:73.

525. Rosenthal AR, Appleton B, Zimmerman R, et al: Intraocular copper foreign bodies. Use of dexamethasone to suppress inflammation. Arch Ophthalmol 1976;94:1571.

526. Rosenthal AR, Marmor MF, Leuenberger P, et al: Chalcosis: A study of natural history. Ophthalmology 1979;86:1956.

527. Schmidt JGH, Maz M: Surface area sizes of intravitreal iron wires: Their effects on the electroretinograms of rats. Ophthalmologica 1988;67:263.

528. Schmidt JGH, Ehring EWG: On the recovery of the electroretinogram of rats after removal of intravitreal lead particles. Ophthalmologica 1986;62:181.

529. Fortuin ME, Blanksma LJ: An unusual complication of perforating wounds of the eye. Ophthalmologica 1986;61:197–203.

530. Mieler WF, Ellis MK, Williams DF, et al: Retained intraocular foreign bodies and endophthalmitis. Ophthalmology 1990;97:1532–1538.

531. Reich ME, Hanselmayer H: Bacterial contamination of intraocular metallic foreign bodies. Klin Monatsbl Augenheilkd 1980;176:119.

532. Behrens-Baumann W, Praetorius G: Intraocular foreign bodies: 297 consecutive cases. Ophthalmologica 1989;198:84.

533. Cullom RD Jr, Chang B: Intraocular foreign body. In: Cullom RD Jr, Chang B, eds: The Wills Eye Manual. Philadelphia, JB Lippincott Company, 1994.

534. Rao NA, Tso MOM, Rosenthal R: Chalcosis in the human eye: A clinicopathologic study. Arch Ophthalmol 1976;94:1379–1384.

535. Hirschberg J: Der Electromagnet in der Augenheilkunde. Leipzig, Veit, 1885, pp 88–91.

536. McCaslin MF: An improved hand electromagnet for eye surgery. Trans Ophthalmol Soc 1958;56:571–605.

537. Robinson A: Powerful new magnet material found. Science 1984;223:920–922.

538. Bronson NR II: Practical characteristics of ophthalmic magnets. Arch Ophthalmol 1968;79:22–27.

539. Wilson DL: A new intraocular foreign body retriever. Ophthalmic Surg 1974;6:64.

540. Lancaster WB: Stronger eye magnets. Trans Ophthalmol Soc 1975;14:168–183.

541. Neubauer H: Intraocular foreign bodies. Trans Ophthalmol Soc UK 1975;95:496–501.

542. Hutton WL: Vitreous foreign body forceps. Am J Ophthalmol 1977;84:430.

543. Hickingbotham D, Parel JM, Machemer R: Diamond-coated all-purpose foreign-body forceps. Am J Ophthalmol 1981;91:267–268.

544. Coleman DJ: A magnet tip for controlled removal of magnetic foreign bodies. Am J Ophthalmol 1978;85:256–258.

545. Crock GW, Janakiraman P, Reddy P: Intraocular magnet of parel. Br J Ophthalmol 1986;70:879.

546. Nishi O: Magnetic device for removal of intraocular foreign bodies. Ophthalmic Surg 1987;18:232.

547. May DR, Noll F, Munoz R: A 20-gauge intraocular electromagnetic tip for simplified intraocular foreign-body extraction. Arch Ophthalmol 1989;107:281–282.

548. McCuen BW, Hickingbotham D: A new retractable micromagnet for intraocular foreign body removal. Arch Ophthalmol 1989;100:1819.

549. Machemer R, Norton EWD: A new concept for vitreous surgery. 3. Indications and results. Am J Ophthalmol 1972;74:1034–56.

550. Peyman GA, Raichand M, Goldberg MF, et al: Vitrectomy in the management of intraocular foreign bodies and their complications. Br J Ophthalmol 1980;64:476.

551. Kingham JD: A microsurgical approach to the management of intraocular foreign bodies with massive tissue damage. Ann Ophthalmol 1981;13:1083.

552. Castier P, Fallas P, Lenski C, et al: The effect of mass in the prognosis of intraocular foreign bodies. Bull Mem Soc Fr Ophthalmol 1983;95:144–8.

553. Machemer R: A new concept for vitreous surgery: Two instrument techniques in pars plana vitrectomy. Arch Ophthalmol 1974;92:407.

554. Percival SPB: Late complications from posterior segment intraocular foreign bodies: With particular reference to retinal detachment. Br J Ophthalmol 1980;90:317.

555. Hanscom TA, Landers MB: Limbal extraction of posterior segment foreign bodies. Am J Ophthalmol 1979;88:777.

556. Thompson JT, Parver LM, Enger CL, et al: Infectious endophthalmitis after penetrating injuries with retained intraocular foreign bodies. Ophthalmology 1993;100:1468–1474.

557. Souza De, Howcroft MJ: Management of posterior segment intraocular foreign bodies: 14 years' experience. Can J Ophthalmol 1999;34:23–29.

558. Micovic V, Milenkovic S, Opric M: Acute aseptic panophthalmitis caused by a copper foreign body. Fortschr Ophthalmol (Germany) 1990;87:362–363.

559. Hamanaka N, Ikeda T, Inokuchi N, et al: A case of an intraocular foreign body due to graphite pencil lead complicated by endophthalmitis. Ophthalmic Surg Lasers 1999;30:229–231.

560. Brinton GS, Aaberg TM, Reeser FH, et al: Surgical results in ocular trauma involving the posterior segment. Am J Ophthalmol 1982;93:271–278.

561. Roper HJ: Review of 555 cases of intraocular foreign body with special reference to prognosis. Br J Ophthalmol 1954;38:65–99.

562. Bronson NR II: Management of intraocular foreign bodies. Am J Ophthalmol 1968;66:279–284.

563. Shock JP, Adams D: Long-term visual acuity results after penetrating and perforating ocular injuries. Am J Ophthalmol 1985;100:714–718.

564. Williams DF, Mieler WF, Abrams GW, et al: Results and prognostic factors in penetrating ocular injuries with retained intraocular foreign bodies. Ophthalmology 1988;95:911.

565. Slusher MM, Sarin LK, Federman JL: Management of intraretinal foreign bodies. Ophthalmology 1982;89:369–373.

566. Conway BP, Michels RG: Vitrectomy techniques in the management of selected penetrating ocular injuries. Trans Am Acad Ophthalmol Otolaryngol 1978;85:560–583.

567. Diblik KP: Management of posterior segment foreign bodies and long-term result. Eur J Ophthalmol 1995;5:113–118.

568. Epstein DL: Pigment dispersion and pigmentary glaucoma. In: Epstein DL, Allingham RR, Schuman JS, eds: Chandler and Grant: Glaucoma. Philadelphia, Williams & Wilkins, 1986, p 201.

569. Nussenblatt RB, Whitcup SM, Palestine AG: Masquerade syndromes. In: Nussenblatt RB, Whitcup SM, Palestine AG, eds: Uveitis: Fundamentals and Clinical Practice. St. Louis, Mosby, 1996, pp 385–395.

570. Von Hippel E: Zur pathologischen anatomie des glaucoma. Arch Ophthalmol 1901;52:498.

571. Levinsohn G: Beitrag zur pathologische anatomie und pathologie des glaukomas. Arch Augenheilkd 1909;62:131.

572. Koeppe L: Die Rolle des irispigment beim glaukom. Ber Dtsch Ophthalmol Ges 1916;40:478.

573. Jess A: Zur Frage des pigmentglaukoma. Klin Monatsbl Augenheilkd 1923;71:175.

574. Vogt A: Atlas der spaltlampenmikroskopie. Klin Monatsbl Augenheilkd 1928;81:711.

575. Birch-Hirschfeld A: Menschlichen auges durch röntgenstrahlen. Z Augenheilkd 1921;45:199.

576. Evans WH, Odom RE, Wenass EJ: Krukenberg's spindle: A study of 202 collected cases. Arch Ophthalmol 1941;26:1023.

577. Sugar HS: Concerning the chamber angle. I: Gonioscopy. Am J Ophthalmol 1940;23:853.

578. Sugar HS, Barbour FA: Pigmentary glaucoma: A rare clinical entity. Am J Ophthalmol 1949;32:90.

579. Sugar HS: Pigmentary glaucoma. A 25-year review. Am J Ophthalmol 1966;62:499.

580. Hoskins HD, Kass MA: Secondary open-angle glaucoma. In: Hoskins HD, Kass MA: Becker-Shaffer's Diagnosis and Therapy of the Glaucoma. St. Louis, CV Mosby, 1989.

581. Sugar S: Pigmentary glaucoma and the glaucoma associated with the exfoliation-pseudoexfoliation syndrome: Update. Ophthalmology 1984;91:307.

582. Lichter PR: Pigmentary glaucoma—current concepts. Trans Am Acad Ophthalmol Otol 1974;79:309.

583. Scheie HC, Gameron JD: Pigment dispersion syndrome: A clinical study. Br J Ophthalmol 1981;65:264.

584. Speakman JS: Pigmentary dispersion. Br J Ophthalmol 1981; 65:249.

585. Ritch R: Nonprogressive low-tension glaucoma with pigmentary dispersion. Am J Ophthalmol 1982;94:190.

586. Kaiser-Kupfer MI, Kupfer C, McCain L: Asymmetric pigment dispersion syndrome. Trans Am Ophthalmol Soc 1983;81:310.

587. Davidson JA, Brubaker RF, Ilstrup DM: Dimensions of the anterior chamber in pigment dispersion syndrome. Arch Ophthalmol 1983;101:81.

588. Seissinger J: Weitere Beiträge zur kenntnis der axenfeld Krukenberg'schen pigmentspindel. Klin Monatsbl Augenheilkd 1926; 77:37.

589. Strebel J, Steiger O: Korrelation der vererbung von augenleiden (Ectopia lentis cong, Ectopia pupillae, Myopie) und song nicht angeborenen herzfehlern. Arch Augenheilkd 1915;78:208.

590. Vogt A: Weitere ergebnisse der spaltlampenmikroskopie des vorderen bulbaschnittes (Cornea, vorderer glaskörper, Conjunctiva, Lidrander). I: abschnitt, Hornhaut. Arch Ophthalmol 1921;106:63.

591. Mauksch H: Zerfall des retinalen pigmentblattes der iris bei zwei brüdern. Z Augenheilkd 1925;57:262.

592. Mandelkorn RM, Hoffman ME, Olander KW, et al: Inheritance and the pigmentary dispersion syndrome. Ann Ophthalmol 1983;15:577–82.

593. McDermott JA, Ritch R, Berger A, et al: Inheritance of pigmentary dispersion syndrome. Invest Ophthalmol Vis Sci Suppl 1987; 28;153.

594. Stankovic J: Den beitrag zur kenntnis der vererbung des pigmentglaukom. Klin Monatsbl Augenheilkd 1961;139:165.

595. Migliazzo CV, Shaffer RN, Nykin R, et al: Long-term analysis of pigmentary dispersion syndrome and pigmentary glaucoma. Ophthalmology 1986;93:1528.

596. Sugar HS: Symposium: glaucoma—discussion of the three preceding papers. Trans Am Acad Ophthalmol Otolaryngol 1974;78:328.

597. Richter CU, Richardson TM, Grant WM: Pigmentary dispersion syndrome and pigmentary glaucoma: A prospective study of the natural history. Arch Ophthalmol 1986;104:211.

598. Kolker AE, Hetherington J Jr: Pigmentary glaucoma and pigment dispersion syndrome. In: Kolker AE, Hetherington J Jr, eds: Becker-Shaffer's Diagnosis and Therapy of the Glaucoma. St. Louis, CV Mosby, 1983, p 263.

599. Mapstone R: Pigment release. Br J Ophthalmol 1981;65:258.

600. Richardson TM, Ausprunk DH: Pigmentary dispersion syndrome and glaucoma. In: Albert DM, Jakobiec FA, eds: Principles and Practice of Ophthalmology. Philadelphia, WB Saunders, 2000, p 2731.

601. Shields MB: Glaucoma associated with disorders of the iris. In: Shields MB, ed: Textbook of Glaucoma. Baltimore, Williams & Wilkins, 1987, p 235.

602. Lehto I, Ruusuvaara P, Setala K: Corneal endothelium in pigmentary glaucoma and pigment dispersion syndrome. Acta Ophthalmol 1990;68:703.

603. Shihab Z, Murrell WJ, Lamberts DW, et al: The corneal endothelium and central corneal thickness in pigmentary dispersion syndrome. Arch Ophthalmol 1986;104:845.

604. Scheie HG, Fleischauer HW: Idiopathic atrophy of the epithelial layers of the iris and ciliary body. Arch Ophthalmol 1958;59:216.

605. Donaldson DD: Transillumination of the iris. Trans Am Ophthalmol Soc 1974;72:88–106.

606. Campbell DG, Schertzer RM: Pigmentary glaucoma. In: Ritch R, Shields MB, Krupin T, eds: The Glaucoma Clinical Science. St. Louis, CV Mosby, 1989, p 981.

607. Zentmayer W: Association of an annular band of pigment on the posterior capsule of the lens with a Krukenberg spindle. Arch Ophthalmol 1938;20:52.

608. Weseley P, Liebmann J, Walsh JB, et al: Lattice degeneration of the retina and the pigment dispersion syndrome. Am J Ophthalmol 1992;114:539.

609. Piccolino FC, Calabria G, Polizzi A, et al: Pigmentary retinal dystrophy associated with pigmentary glaucoma. Graefes Arch Clin Exp Ophthalmol 1989;227:335.

610. Brini A, Porte A, Roth A: Atrophie des couches épithéliales de l'iris: Étude d'un cas de glaucome pigmentaire au microscope optique et au microscope électronique. Doc Ophthalmol 1969;26:403.

611. Fine BS, Yanoff M, Scheie HG: Pigmentary "glaucoma." A histologic study. Trans Am Acad Ophthalmol Otolaryngol 1974;78:314.

612. Kupfer C, Kuwabrar T, Kaiser-Kupfer M: The histopathology of pigmentary dispersion syndrome with glaucoma. Am J Ophthalmol 1975;80:857.

613. Rodrigues MM, Spaeth GL, Weinreb S, et al: Spectrum of trabecular pigmentation in open-angle glaucoma: A clinicopathologic study. Trans Am Acad Ophthalmol Otolaryngol 1976;81:258.

614. Campbell DG: Pigmentary dispersion and glaucoma: A new theory. Arch Ophthalmol 1979;97:1667.
615. Kampik A, Green WR, Quigley HA, et al: Scanning and transmission electron microscopic studies of two types of pigment dispersion syndrome. Am J Ophthalmol 1981;91:573.
616. Strasser G, Hauff W: Pigmentary dispersion syndrome: A biometric study. Acta Ophthalmol 1985;63:721.
617. Richardson TM: Pigmentary glaucoma. In: Rich R, Shields MB, eds: The Secondary Glaucoma. St. Louis, CV Mosby, 1982, p 84.
618. Ritch R, Manusow D, Podos SM: Remission of pigmentary glaucoma in a patient with subluxed lenses. Am J Ophthalmol 1982;94:812.
619. Karickhoff, JR: Pigmentary dispersion syndrome and pigmentary glaucoma: A new mechanism concept, a new treatment, and a new technique. Ophthalmic Surg 1992;23:269.
620. Pavlin CJ, Macken P, Trope G, et al: Ultrasound biomicroscopic features of pigmentary glaucoma. Can J Ophthalmol 1994;29:187.
621. Potash SD, Tello C, Liebmann J, et al: Ultrasound biomicroscopy in pigment dispersion syndrome. Ophthalmology 1994;101:332.
622. Pavlin CJ, Harasiewicz K, Foster FS: Posterior iris bowing in pigmentary dispersion syndrome caused by accommodation. Am J Ophthalmol 1994;118:114–16.
623. Rohen JW, Van der Zypen EP: The phagocytic activity of the trabecular meshwork endothelium: An electron microscopic study of the vervet (Cercopithecus aethiops). Graefes Arch Clin Exp Ophthalmol 1968;175:143.
624. Bill A: Blood circulation and fluid dynamics in the eye. Pharmacol Physiol Rev 1975;55:383.
625. Richardson TM, Hutchinson BT, Grant WM: The outflow tract in pigmentary glaucoma: A light and electron microscopic study. Arch Ophthalmol 1977;95:1015.
626. Sherwood M, Richardson TM: Evidence for in vivo phagocytosis by trabecular endothelial cells. Invest Ophthalmol Vis Sci 1980;21(Suppl):66.
627. Campbell DG: Iridotomy and pigmentary glaucoma. Humphrey Lecture. Richmond, University of Virginia Press, 1991.
628. Alward WLM, Munden PM, Verdick RE, et al: Use of infrared videography to detect and record iris transillumination defects. Arch Ophthalmol 1990;108:748.
629. Boys-Smith J, Woods WD, Alken DG, et al: A new gonioscopy lens for the gradation of trabecular meshwork pigmentation. Invest Ophthalmol Vis Sci 1984;25(Suppl):173.
630. Pavlin CJ, Sherar MD, Foster FS: Subsurface ultrasound microscopic imaging of the intact eye. Ophthalmology 1990;97:244.
631. Pavlin CJ, Harasiewicz K, Sherar MD, et al: Clinical use of ultrasound biomicroscopy. Ophthalmology 1991;98:287–295.
632. Pavlin CJ, Ritch R, Foster FS: Ultrasound biomicroscopy in plateau iris syndrome. Am J Ophthalmol 113:390, 1992.
633. Pavlin CJ, Harasiewicz K, Foster FS: Ultrasound biomicroscopy of anterior segment structures in normal and glaucomatous eyes. Am J Ophthalmol 1992;113:381.
634. Tello C, Chi T, Shepps G, et al: Ultrasound biomicroscopy in pseudophakic malignant glaucoma. Ophthalmology 1993;100:1330–1334.
635. Tello C, Liebmann J, Potash SD, et al: Measurement of ultrasound biomicroscopy images: Intraobserver and interobserver reliability. Invest Ophthalmol Vis Sci 1994;35:3549–3552.
636. Epstein DL, Boger WP II, Grant WM: Phenylephrine provocative testing in the pigmentary dispersion syndrome. Am J Ophthalmol 1978;85:43.
637. Chandler PA, Braconier HE: Spontaneous intra-epithelial cysts of iris and ciliary body with glaucoma. Am J Ophthalmol 1958;45:64.
638. Chandler PA, Grant WM: Lectures on Glaucoma. Philadelphia, Lea and Febiger, 1965.
639. Van Buskirk EM, Leure-duPree AE: Pathophysiology and electron microscopy of melanomalytic glaucoma. Am J Ophthalmol 1978;85:160.
640. Lichter PR, Shaffer RN: Iris processes and glaucoma. Am J Ophthalmol 1970;70:905.
641. Breingan PJ, Esaki K, Ishikawa H, et al: Iridolenticular contact decreases following laser iridotomy for pigment dispersion syndrome. Arch Ophthalmol 1999;65:249.
642. Spaeth GL: Early primary open-angle glaucoma: Diagnosis and treatment. Int Ophthalmol Clin 1979;19:168.
643. Kearns TP, Hollenhorst RW: Venous-stasis retinopathy of occlusive disease of the carotid artery. Mayo Clin Proc 1963;38:304–312.
644. Knox DL: Ischemic ocular inflammation. Am J Ophthalmol 1965;60:995–1002.
645. Sturrock GD, Mueller HR: Chronic ocular ischemia. Br J Ophthalmol 1984;68:716–723.
646. Jacobs NA, Ridgway AE: Syndrome of ischemic ocular inflammation: Six cases and a review. Br J Ophthalmol 1985;69:681–687.
647. Ros MA, Magargal LE, Hedges TR, et al: Ocular ischemic syndrome: Long-term ocular complications. Ann Ophthalmol 1987;19:270.
648. Nicholas PJ: Anterior uveitis syndromes. In: Nicholas PJ, ed: Uveitis. Boston, Butterworth-Heinemann, 1998.
649. Rizzo JF III: Neuroophthalmologic disease of the retina. In: Albert DM, Jakobiec FA, eds: Principles and Practice of Ophthalmology. Philadelphia, WB Saunders, 2000, p 4083.
650. Brown GC: Ocular ischemic syndrome. In: Guyer DR, Yannuzzi LA, Chang S, et al, eds: Retina-Vitreous-Macula. Philadelphia, WB Saunders, 1999, p 372.
651. Young LHY, Appen RE: Ischemic oculopathy, a manifestation of carotid artery disease. Arch Neurol 1981;38:358–361.
652. Brown GC, Magargal LE, Simeone FA, et al: Arterial obstruction and ocular neovascularization. Ophthalmology 1982;89:139–146.
653. Brown GC, Magargal LE: The ocular ischemic syndrome. Clinical fluorescein angiographic and carotid angiographic features. Int Ophthalmol Clin 1988;11:239–251.
654. Michelson PE, Knox DL, Green WR: Ischemic ocular inflammation: A clinicopathologic case report. Arch Ophthalmol 1971;86:274–280.
655. Kahn M, Green WR, Knox DL, et al: Ocular features of carotid occlusive disease. Retina 1986;6:239–252.
656. Sivalingam A, Brown GC, Magargal LE, et al: The ocular ischemic syndrome. II. Mortality and systemic morbidity. Int Ophthalmol Clin 1989;13:187–191.
657. Mizener JB, Podhajsky P, Hayreh SS: Ocular ischemic syndrome. Ophthalmology 1997;104:859–864.
658. Sivalingam A, Brown GC, Magargal LE: The ocular ischemic syndrome. III. Visual prognosis and the effect of treatment. Int Ophthalmol Clin 1991;15:15–20.
659. Destro M, Gragoudas ES: Arterial occlusions. In: Albert DM, Jakobiec FA, eds: Principle and Practice of Ophthalmology. Philadelphia, WB Saunders, 1994.
660. Waybright EA, Selhorts JB, Combs J: Anterior ischemic optic neuropathy with internal carotid artery occlusion. Am J Ophthalmol 1982;93:42–47.
661. Hedges TR Jr: Ophthalmolscopic findings in internal carotid artery occlusion. Am J Ophthalmol 1963;55:1007–1012.
662. Hoefnagels KLJ: Rubeosis of the iris associated with occlusion of the carotid artery. Ophthalmologica 1964;148:196–200.
663. Brown GC: Anterior ischemic optic neuropathy occurring in association with carotid artery obstruction. J Clin Neuroophthalmol 1986;6:39–42.
664. Schlaegel T: Symptoms and signs of uveitis. In: Duane TD, eds: Clinical Ophthalmology, Vol 4. Hagerstown, MD, Harper & Row, 1983, pp 1–7.
665. Bullock JD, Falter RT, Downing JE, et al: Ischemic ophthalmia secondary to an ophthalmic artery occlusion. Am J Ophthalmol 1972;74:486–493.
666. Kearns TP: Ophthalmology and the carotid artery. Am J Ophthalmol 1979;88:714–722.
667. Kobayashi S, Hollenhorst RW, Sundt TM Jr: Retinal arterial pressure before and after surgery for carotid artery stenosis. Stroke 1971;2:569–575.
668. Smith VH: Pressure changes in the ophthalmic artery after carotid occlusion (an experimental study in the rabbit). Br J Ophthalmol 1961;45:1–26.
669. Ross RT, Morrow IM: Ocular and cerebral mechanisms in disease of the internal carotid artery. Can J Neurol Sci 1984;11:262–268.
670. Green WR: The uveal tract. In: Spencer WH, ed: Ophthalmic Pathology. Philadelphia, WB Saunders, 1985, p 1352.
671. Duker JS, Belmont JB: Ocular ischemic syndrome secondary to carotid artery dissection. Am J Ophthalmol 1988;106:750–752.
672. Hamed LM, Guy JR, Moster ML, et al: Giant cell arteritis in the ocular ischemic syndrome. Am J Ophthalmol 1992;113:702–705.
673. Hwang JM, Girkin CA, Perry JD, et al: Bilateral ocular ischemic syndrome secondary to giant cell arteritis progressing despite corticosteroid treatment. Am J Ophthalmol 1999;127:102–104.

674. Effeney DJ, Krupski WC, Stoney RJ, et al: Fibromuscular dysplasia of the carotid artery. Aust N Z J Surg 1983;53:527–531.

675. Dhobb M, Ammar F, Bensaid Y, et al: Arterial manifestations in Behçet's disease: Four new cases. Ann Vasc Surg 1986;1:249–252.

676. Sadun AA, Sebag J, Bienfang DC: Complete bilateral internal carotid artery occlusion in a young man. J Clin Neuroophthalmol 1983;3:63–66.

677. Ridley M, Walker P, Keller A, et al: Ocular perfusion in carotid artery disease. Poster presentation. New Orleans, American Academy of Ophthalmology, 1986.

678. Brown GC: Macular edema in association with severe carotid artery obstruction. Am J Ophthalmol 1986;102:442–448.

679. Campo RV, Reeser FH: Retinal telangiectasia secondary to bilateral carotid artery occlusion. Arch Ophthalmol 1983;101:1211–1213.

680. Russell RW, Ikeda H: Clinical and electrophysiological observations in patients with low pressure retinopathy. Br J Ophthalmol 1986;70:651–656.

681. Banchini E, Franchi A, Magni R, et al: Carotid occlusive disease. An electrophysiological investigation. J Cardiovasc Surg 1987; 28:524–527.

682. Jones AM, Biller J, Cowley AR, et al: Extracranial carotid artery arteriosclerosis. Diagnosis with continuous wave doppler and real time ultrasound studies. Arch Neurol 1982;39:393–394.

683. Weibers DO, Folger GS, Younge BR, et al: Ophthalmodynamometry and ocular pneumoplethysmography for detection of carotid occlusive disease. Arch Neurol 1982;39:690–691.

684. Kearns TP: Differential diagnosis of central retinal vein obstruction. Ophthalmology 1983;90:475–480.

685. Bosley TM: The role of carotid noninvasive test in stroke prevention. Semin Neurol 1986;6:194–203.

686. Castaldo JE, Nicholas GG, Gee W, et al: Duplex ultrasound and ocular pneumoplethysmography concordance in detecting severe carotid stenosis. Arch Neurol 1989;46:518–522.

687. Müller HR: Doppler sonography of the carotid vascular system. Internist (Berl) 1976;17:570–579.

688. Reutern GM, Büdingen HJ, Hennerici M, et al: The diagnosis of stenoses and occlusions of the carotid arteries by means of directional Dopplersonography. Arch Psychiatr Nervenkr 1976; 222:2–3, 191–207.

689. Diener HC, Dichgans J: Atraumatic diagnosis of extracranial vascular stenoses and occlusions. Internist 1979;20:531–538.

690. Madsen PH: Venous-stasis retinopathy insufficiency of the ophthalmic artery. Acta Ophthalmol 1966;44:940–947.

691. Brown GC: Ocular ischemic syndrome. In: Ryan SJ, eds: Retina. St. Louis, CV Mosby, 1994, p 1515.

692. Campo RV, Aaberg TM: Digital subtraction angiography in the diagnosis of retinal vascular disease. Am J Ophthalmol 1983;96:632–640.

693. Ino-ue M, Azumi A, Kajiura-Tsukahara T, et al: Ocular ischemic syndrome in diabetic patients. Jpn J Ophthalmol 1999;43:31–35.

694. Johnston ME, Gonder JR, Canny CL: Successful treatment of the ocular ischemic syndrome with panretinal photocoagulation and cerebrovascular surgery. Can J Ophthalmol 1988;23:114–119.

695. Eggleston TF, Bohling CA, Eggleston HC, et al: Photocoagulation for ocular ischemia associated with carotid artery occlusion. Ann Ophthalmol 1980;12:84–87.

696. Carter JE: Panretinal photocoagulation for progressive ocular neovascularization secondary to occlusion of the common carotid artery. Ann Ophthalmol 1984;16:572–576.

697. Duker J, Brown GC, Bosley TM, et al: Asymmetric proliferative diabetic retinopathy and carotid artery disease. Ophthalmology 1990;97:869–874.

698. Kearns TP, Sicken RG, Sundt TM Jr: The ocular aspects of bypass surgery of the carotid artery. Mayo Clin Proc 1979;54:3–11.

699. Kearns TP, Younge BR, Peipgras DG: Resolution of venous stasis retinopathy after carotid artery bypass surgery. Mayo Clin Proc 1980;55:342–346.

700. European Carotid Surgery Trialists' Collaborative Group: MRC European carotid surgery trial: interim results for symptomatic patients with severe (70–99%) or with mild (0–29%) carotid stenosis. Lancet 1991;337:1235–1243.

701. Mayberg MR, Wilson SE, Yatsu F, et al: Carotid endarterectomy and prevention of cerebral ischemia in symptomatic carotid stenosis. JAMA 1991;266:3289–3294.

702. North American Symptomatic Carotid Endarterectomy Trial Collaborators: Beneficial effect of carotid endarterectomy in symptomatic patients with high-grade carotid stenosis. N Engl J Med 1991;325:445–453.

703. Brown GC, Magargal LE, Shields JA, et al: Retinal arterial obstruction in children and young adults. Ophthalmology 1981;88:18–25.

704. Shields CL, Shields JA, Buchanon H: Solitary orbital juvenile xanthogranuloma. Ophthalmology 1990;108:1587–1589.

705. Zimmerman LE: Ocular lesions of juvenile xanthogranuloma. Nevoxanthoendothelioma. Trans Am Acad Ophthalmol Otolaryngol 1965;69:412–439.

706. Cleasby GW: Nevoxanthoendothelioma (juvenile xanthogranuloma) of the iris: Diagnosis by biopsy and treatment with x-ray. Arch Ophthalmol 1961;66:26–28.

707. Fleischmajer R, Hyman AB: Juvenile giant cell granuloma (Nevoxanthoendothelioma). In: Fleischmajer R, ed: The Dyslipidoses. Springfield IL, Thomas, 1960, pp 329–372.

708. Lewis JR, Drummond GT, Mielke BW, et al: Juvenile xanthogranuloma of the corneoscleral limbus. Can J Ophthalmol 1990;25:351–354.

709. Wertz FD, Zimmerman LE, McKeown CA, et al: Juvenile xanthogranuloma of the optic nerve, disc, retina, and choroid. Ophthalmology 1982;89:1331–1335.

710. Staple TW, McAlister WH, Sanders TE, et al: Juvenile xanthogranuloma of the orbit: report of a case with bone destruction. AJR Am J Roentgen 1964;91:629–632.

711. Gaynes PM, Cohen GS: Juvenile xanthogranuloma of the orbit. Am J Ophthalmol 1967;63:755–757.

712. Sanders TE, Miller JE: Infantile xanthogranuloma of the orbit. Trans Am Acad Ophthalmol Otolaryngol 1965;69:458–464.

713. Adamson HG: Society intelligence: the Dermatologic Society of London. Br J Dermatol 1905;17:222.

714. McDonaugh JER: Spontaneous disappearance of endotheliomata (nevo-xanthoma). Br J Derm 1909;21:254.

715. Adamson HG: A note on multiple eruptive xanthoma in infants: naevo-xanthoendothelioma (McDonagh). Br J Derm 1936;48:366.

716. Senear FE, Caro MR: Nevoxantho-endothelioma or juvenile xanthoma. Arch Dermatol 1936;34:195.

717. Nomland R: Nevoxantho-endothelioma of benign xanthomatous disease of infants and children. J Invest Dermatol 1954;22:207.

718. Blank H, Eglick PG, Beerman H: Nevoxanthoendothelioma with ocular involvement. Pediatrics 1949;4:349–54.

719. Helwig EB, Hackney VC: Juvenile xanthogranuloma (nevoxanthoendothelioma) Am J Ophthalmol J Path 1954;30:625.

720. Maumenee AE: Ocular lesions of nevoxanthoendothelioma (infantile xanthoma disseminatum). Trans Am Acad Ophthalmol Otolaryngol 1956;60:401–405.

721. Sanders TE: Intraocular juvenile xantho-granuloma (nevoxanthoendothelioma): A survey of 20 cases. Am J Ophthalmol 1962; 53:455–462.

722. Sanders TE: Infantile xanthogranuloma of the orbit: A report of three cases. Am J Ophthalmol 1966;61:1299–1306.

723. Maumenee AE, Longfellow DW: Treatment of intraocular nevoxanthoendothelioma (juvenile xanthogranuloma). Am J Ophthalmol 1960;49:1–7.

724. Gass JDM: Management of juvenile xanthogranuloma of the iris. Arch Ophthalmol 1964;71:344–347.

725. Moore JG, Harry J: Juvenile xanthogranuloma. Report of a case. Br J Ophthalmol 1965;49:71–75.

726. Smith ME, Sanders TE, Bresnick GH: Juvenile xanthogranuloma of the ciliary body in an adult. Arch Ophthalmol 1969;81:812–814.

727. Hedges CC: Nevoxanthoendothelioma of eye treated with superficial x-ray therapy. Am J Ophthalmol 1959;47:683–684.

728. Howard GM: Spontaneous hyphema in infancy and childhood. Arch Ophthalmol 1962;68:615–620.

729. De Villez RL, Limmer BL: Juvenile xanthogranuloma and urticaria pigmentosa. Arch Dermatol 1975;111:365–366.

730. Grice K: Juvenile xanthogranuloma (nevoxanthoendothelioma). Clin Exp Dermatol 1978;3:327–329.

731. Lamb JH, Lain ES: Nevo-xanthogranuloma-endothelioma: Its relationship to juvenile xanthoma. South Med J 193;30:585–594.

732. Webster SB, Reister HC, Harman LE Jr: Juvenile xanthogranuloma with extracutaneous lesions: a case report and review of the literature. Arch Dermatol 1966;93:71–76.

733. Tahan SR, Pastel-Levy C, Bhan AK, et al: Juvenile xanthogranuloma: Clinical and pathologic characterization. Arch Pathol Lab Med 1989;113:1057–1061.

734. Fishman SJ, Brodie S, Popkin G: Juvenile xanthogranuloma. Gate 1973;11:499–501.

735. Harley RD, Romayananda N, Chan GH: Juvenile xanthogranuloma. J Pediatr Ophthalmol Strabismus 1982;19:33–39.

736. Bruner WE, Stark WJ, Green WR: Presumed juvenile xanthogranuloma of the iris and ciliary body in an adult. Arch Ophthalmol 1982;100:457–456.

737. Brenkman RF, Oosterhuis JA, Manschot WAL: Recurrent hemorrhage in the anterior chamber caused by a (juvenile) santhogranuloma of the iris in an adult. Doc Ophthalmol 1977;42:329–333.

738. Hamburg A: Juveniles xanthogranuloma uveae beieinem erwachsenen. Ophthalmologica 1976;72:273–281.

739. Hadden OB: Bilateral juvenile xanthogranuloma of the iris. Br J Ophthalmol 1975;59:699–702.

740. Shields JA, Shields CL: Fibrous and histiocytic tumors. In: Shields JA, Shields CL, eds: Intraocular Tumors. Philadelphia, WB Saunders, 1992, p 295.

741. DeBarge LR, Chan CC, Greenberg SC, et al: Chorioretinal, iris, and ciliary body infiltration by juvenile xanthogranuloma masquerading as uveitis. Survey of Ophthalmology 1994;39:65–71.

742. Cassteels I, Olver J, Malone M, et al: Early treatment of juvenile xanthogranuloma of the iris with subconjunctival steroids. Br J Ophthalmol 1993;77:57–60.

743. Duke-Elder S: Disease of the uvea: Juvenile xanthogranuloma. In: Duke-Elder S, ed: System of Ophthalmology. St. Louis, CV Mosby, 1966, pp 656–662.

744. Shields MB: Glaucomas associated with elevated episcleral venous pressure. In: Shields MB, ed: Textbook of Glaucoma. Baltimore, Williams & Wilkins, 1987, p 278.

745. Schwartz LW, Rodrigues MM, Hallett JW: Juvenile xanthogranuloma diagnosed by paracentesis. Am J Ophthalmol 1974;77:243–246.

746. Cadera W, Silver MM, Burt L: Juvenile xanthogranuloma. Can J Ophthalmol 1983;18:169–174.

747. Clements DB: Juvenile xanthogranuloma treated with local steroids. Br J Ophthalmol 1966;50:663–665.

748. Smith JLS, Ingram RM: Juvenile oculodermal xanthogranuloma. Br J Ophthalmol 1968;52:696–703.

749. Stern SD, Arenberg IK: Infantile nevoxanthoendothelioma of the iris treated with topical steroids and antiglaucoma therapy. J Pediatr Ophthalmol Strabismus 1970;7:100–102.

750. Thieme R, Lukassek B, Keinert K: Problems in juvenile xanthogranuloma of the anterior uvea. Klin Monatsbl Augenheilkd 1980;176:893–898.

751. Hertzberg R: Nevoxantho-endothelioma (juvenile xanthogranuloma) of the eye cured with x-ray therapy. Med J Aust 1964;2:24–28.

752. MacLeod PM: Case report: Juvenile xanthogranuloma of the iris managed with superficial radiotherapy. Clin Radiol 1986;37:295–296.

753. Müller RP, Busse H: Radiotherapy in juvenile xanthogranuloma of the iris. Klin Monatsbl Augenheilkd 1986;189:15–18.

754. Newell FW: Nevoxanthoendothelioma with ocular involvement. Arch Ophthalmol 1957;58:321–327.

755. Shusterman M: Nevoxanthoendothelioma with ocular involvement: Report of a case. Trans Canad Ophthalmol Soc 1959;22:206–215.

Part V

51 — TRAUMATIC UVEITIS

Quan Dong Nguyen

Intraocular inflammation can occur after any ocular trauma, directly or indirectly. The common causes of traumatic uveitis include sports injuries,[1-3] combat injuries,[4] household accidents, and various recreational activity injuries, including those from water balloon slingshots.[5] In a study of 125 patients with ocular injuries secondary to engaging in sports, 48 suffered traumatic uveitis.[3] The great majority of patients were injured while participating in unsupervised sporting activities without wearing protective eyewear.[3] A 2-year study from New Zealand disclosed that about 30% of all sports injuries to the eye evaluated at a major hospital were caused by indoor cricket; traumatic iridocyclitis was one of the most common presentations.[1] During Operations Desert Shield and Desert Storm led by the United States in 1991, ocular injury and disease accounted for 14% (108/767) of the visits by the soldiers to the emergency department at a combat support hospital, Fitzsimmons Army Medical Center in Aurora, Colorado. Eight of the 108 patients incurred traumatic uveitis.[4] In some cases, the evaluation and management of the traumatic uveitis may unmask occult uveitic conditions or the presence of underlying diseases, infections, malignancy (melanoma),[6] or intraocular foreign body[7, 8] which may be associated with the uveitis.

Ocular inflammation also can occur after any ocular surgical procedure. During the postoperative period, it is important to differentiate infectious causes of uveitis from other causes of intraocular inflammation, as infectious etiologies such as bacterial and fungal endophthalmitis require prompt treatment with antimicrobial therapy. Patients with preexisting uveitis typically have exacerbation of their intraocular inflammation after ocular trauma or surgery, even though the uveitis has been brought to remission prior to the event.

POSTSURGICAL UVEITIS

A surgical procedure can markedly exacerbate intraocular inflammation in an eye that previously had uveitis.[9] The flare-up of the uveitis usually occurs 3 to 7 days after the surgery, and it may occur earlier in patients who do not receive proper perioperative immunosuppressants. The uveitis can be substantial, with severe pain and hypopyon, and it can be misdiagnosed as infectious endophthalmitis. Noninfectious uveitis associated with intraocular surgery is often low grade and self-limited.[10] The uveitis may be of three different forms: the acute and early uveitis that resolves quickly, the late-occurring uve-

itis, and the chronic, recurring uveitis.[11] Prolonged mild traumatic iritis, secondary to surgery, has been shown to cause abnormal corneal endothelial configuration.[12] The possible etiologies of postsurgical uveitis are listed in Table 51-1.

Cystoid Macular Edema

The cystoid macular edema that occurs after ocular surgery such as cataract extraction has a higher incidence in more severely traumatized eyes.[13] It is characterized by increased perifoveal capillary permeability that may be related either to prior vasoconstriction or to vasodilation, and it may be accompanied by a cellular inflammatory response either in the ciliary body, the vitreous, or the retina, or in combination.[13] Most of the physiologic, metabolic, and morphologic responses to trauma may be secondary to the liberation of endogenous mediators such as prostaglandins. Adequate prophylaxis may be provided by cyclo-oxygenase inhibitors or corticosteroids. However, "atraumatic" surgery with minimal disruption of the blood-ocular barrier is probably the best prophylaxis for this mostly iatrogenic disease.

Infectious Endophthalmitis

Infectious endophthalmitis may occur following any type of intraocular surgery; it is one of the true ophthalmic

TABLE 51-1. ETIOLOGIES OF POSTSURGICAL INTRAOCULAR INFLAMMATION

Postoperative day 1 to day 30
  Bacterial endophthalmitis
  Sterile endophthalmitis
  Recurrence or increased activity of previous uveitis
  Phacogenic (lens-related) uveitis
  Reaction to intraocular lens
  Responses to laser procedure
  New onset of idiopathic or previously unrecognized uveitis
Postoperative day 15 to years
  Fungal endophthalmitis
  Propionibacterium acnes or other anaerobic endophthalmitis
  Low virulence aerobic bacterial endophthalmitis
  Phacogenic (lens-related) uveitis
  Sympathetic ophthalmia
  Reaction to intraocular lens
  Iris–ciliary body irritation related to physical contact with
    intraocular lens
  New onset of idiopathic or previously unrecognized uveitis

Modified from Nussenblatt RB, Whitcup SM, Palestine AG: Postsurgical uveitis. In: Nussenblatt RB, Whitcup SM, Palestine AG, eds: Uveitis: Fundamentals and Clinical Practice, 2nd ed. St. Louis, Mosby-Yearbook, 1996, pp 256–261.

emergencies. The three common types of postsurgical endophthalmitis include acute bacterial endophthalmitis, chronic bacterial endophthalmitis, and fungal endophthalmitis. Infectious endophthalmitis is described in detail in Chapter 49.

POST-TRAUMATIC UVEITIS

Penetrating Ocular Trauma

Trauma to the eye can lead to numerous ocular complications. When the injury is penetrating, the consequences are often more severe. Early complications include hyphema, ocular hypertension, iridocyclitis, lens dislocation or rupture, corneal and scleral lacerations, endophthalmitis, choroidal rupture, retinal detachments—every ocular damage is possible, depending on the nature of injury. Late sequelae may include narrow-angle glaucoma, sympathetic ophthalmia, and retinal and choroidal neovascularization. Traumatic uveitis can coexist with any of these conditions. When ocular trauma has occurred, the patient will need annual ophthalmologic follow-up throughout life even if there are no complications, and more frequent visits if there are complications, as the number of potential future ocular problems is high.

Choroidal neovascularization is a potentially sight-threatening complication of penetrating ocular trauma.[14] The growth of new choroidal vessels beneath the retinal pigment epithelium may be stimulated, in part, by inflammatory mediators and the loss of integrity of the Bruch's membrane–retinal pigment epithelium (RPE) photoreceptor complex arising in the context of trauma. Wilson and colleagues described histopathologically the focal choroidal granulomatous inflammation as a result of penetrating ocular trauma;[15] this finding is thought to represent a reaction to a foreign body. Another devastating complication after trauma in the human eye is the development of proliferative vitreoretinopathy (PVR). In a study of 1654 injured eyes, 71 (4%) developed PVR, which is often the primary cause of retinal detachment and visual loss.[16] Severe traumatic uveitis with persistent intraocular inflammation, long and posteriorly located wounds, and vitreous hemorrhage were the strongest independent predictive factors for the development of PVR.

When there is traumatic angle recession or traumatic uveitis, fluorescein gonioangiography may be helpful in detecting newly formed vessels in the anterior chamber angle;[17] these vessels often originate from the ciliary body, and they extend predominantly onto the surface of the angle wall via the ciliary body band. Occasionally, funduscopic fluorescein angiography may be helpful to examine changes in the retina and vascular coating in traumatic and post-traumatic conditions.[18]

In some cases, the penetrating ocular injury is so small that the entrance and presence of a foreign body may be missed; an occult intraocular foreign body is an important and frequently overlooked differential diagnostic consideration in the work-up of unilateral uveitis. Meyer and Ritchey reported a case of persistent post-traumatic inflammation with the development of a vitreous mass.[19] Histologic examination of the enucleated eye showed that the lens had been replaced by a wooden foreign body

that filled the pupillary space and was surrounded by lens capsule.

Cases of penetrating ocular trauma that lead to persistent, chronic, occasionally fulminant, intraocular inflammation require additional investigations (e.g., anterior chamber paracentesis, scleral biopsy, and diagnostic vitrectomy) to find the cause of the traumatic uveitis. Cases of post-traumatic iridocyclitis secondary to *Mycobacterium lepra*,[20] *Enterobacter agglomerans*,[21] *Exophiala jeanselmei*,[22] *Sporothrix schenckii*,[23] *Pseudomonas aeruginosa*,[24] *Klebsiella oxytoca*,[24] *Aeromonas caviae*,[24] and *Flavobacterium odoratum*,[24] among others, have been reported. The common organisms that cause traumatic endophthalmitis are *Bacillus* species (post-traumatic)[25, 26] and *Staphylococcus epidermidis* (postoperative).[27] Among children with post-traumatic endophthalmitis, the most common isolates are streptococcal and staphylococcal species.[28] In addition, ocular trauma is known to cause reactivation of herpes (simplex or zoster) keratitis and keratouveitis.

Endophthalmitis associated with penetrating injury often represents a distinct kind of intraocular infection. The preceding trauma, infective agents, and inflammatory changes determine the functional outcome. In a recent retrospective study,[29] the risk factors for penetrating traumatic endophthalmitis that were found to be significant were a purely corneal wound, surgical primary repair more than 24 hours after injury, and initiation of intravenous antibiotic therapy later than 24 hours after trauma. A twofold increase in relative risk was related to the presence of an intraocular foreign body, lens injury, or a wound length less than 5 mm.

Punnonen examined 48 eyes enucleated after a perforating eye injury.[30] The time between injury and enucleation varied from 0 to 1145 days. The inflammatory signs were most marked in eyes with a corneoscleral or double perforation. Proliferation of the RPE cells or fibrous proliferation from the wound or ciliary body was found 9 to 10 days after trauma, and epiretinal membranes from the optic nerve head or from the surface of the retina were found after 1 month. Massive fibrous proliferation was seen in 94% of eyes enucleated 1 month or later after injury.

Sympathetic Ophthalmia

Sympathetic ophthalmia is an uncommon but well-known complication of ocular trauma. It is probably the intraocular inflammatory condition best known to practitioners outside ophthalmology. Although the number of patients afflicted with this condition per year is small, the concern of losing not only the involved eye but the contralateral, untouched eye as well, in a potentially sight-threatening process, is understandably great.

The bilateral granulomatous uveitis in sympathetic ophthalmia can begin as early as several days after the penetrating insult and up to decades later, with the clinical diagnosis becoming apparent in 80% of cases approximately 3 months after injury to the exciting eye.[31] Sympathetic ophthalmia seems to occur more often after nonsurgical trauma. Liddy and Stuart reported that the disorder occurred in 0.2% of nonsurgical wounds,[32] whereas Holland found the condition in 0.5% of eyes with trauma.[33] In one study, the incidence of this disease is estimated to be less than 10 cases per 100,000 surgical penetrating wounds.[31] Gass gathered data from a survey of 26 eye pathology laboratories during a 5-year period from 1975 to 1980; sympathetic ophthalmia was diagnosed in 53 eyes (2 of every 1000 eyes examined); 29 eyes (55%) were post-traumatic.[34]

Recent studies have shown that serum beta-2-microglobulin[35] and sialic acid[36] may parallel the disease severity of sympathetic ophthalmia. Interestingly, there was no significant elevation of either marker in patients with traumatic uveitis. However, the levels were increased significantly in patients with sympathetic ophthalmia and decreased during the remission stage. When the sympathetic ophthalmia relapsed, the serum beta-2-microglobulin and sialic acid levels again were elevated. The authors suggested that beta-2-microglobulin and sialic acid levels may be used as a diagnostic aid when the diagnosis of sympathetic ophthalmia remains equivocal on clinical grounds. In addition, they also suggested that a rise in serum levels of beta-2-microglobulin and sialic acid in patients with traumatic uveitis may point to the onset of sympathetic ophthalmia.[35, 36]

Indocyanine green angiography (ICGA) has been used to follow patients with posterior uveitis, including sympathetic ophthalmia. Bernasconi and colleagues reported various patterns of ICGA in patients with sympathetic ophthalmia, which were confirmed by histopathologic examination of the eyes that were eventually enucleated.[37] The ICGA showed numerous hypofluorescent dark dots visible at the intermediate phase; some became isofluorescent during the late phase and resolved after long-term corticosteroid therapy, and others remained hypofluorescent until the late phase. The pattern of hypofluorescence that persisted throughout the angiography was interpreted as resulting from cicatricial, inactive lesions, whereas the hypofluorescence that faded in the late phase was thought to represent active lesions.[37] The characteristics, diagnosis, and management of sympathetic ophthalmia are discussed in Chapter 66.

Nonpenetrating Ocular Trauma

Penetrating ocular trauma is a well-recognized cause of uveitis.[38] In some cases, severe uveitis can develop even after minor, nonpenetrating ocular trauma. The nonpenetrating traumatic iridocyclitis may present in association with hyphema, miosis, ocular hypotony, ciliary flush, or hemorrhage with excessive fibrin in the anterior chamber.[39] In such cases, evaluation for underlying causes of the uveitis should be initiated. Cases of significant anterior uveitis following minor corneal trauma have been described.[40] Investigation revealed ankylosing spondylitis in the patients who previously had not experienced any uveitis. Thus, the possibility of occult disease should be considered in cases of a disproportionately large amount of intraocular inflammation following minor ocular trauma. Sorr and Goldberg reported a case of traumatic iritis in an 8-year-old black boy who suffered blunt, nonpenetrating trauma to his brow and globe.[41] Secondary glaucoma and perimacular edema as well as central retinal artery occlusion also were present. Evaluation revealed that the child had sickle cell trait.

Rosenbaum and colleagues reported that nearly 5% of patients attending a uveitis referral clinic attributed their inflammation to nonpenetrating trauma.[42] Patients with nonpenetrating trauma were more often male, were more likely to have unilateral disease, and were younger than the majority of patients in the uveitis clinic. Many of the patients had an identifiable cause of uveitis, such as ankylosing spondylitis, Reiter's syndrome, sarcoidosis, or acute retinal necrosis, but most patients had no known predisposition. The authors suggested that nonpenetrating trauma may precipitate intraocular inflammation. In some cases, the inflammation may have preceded the trauma and the trauma merely brought to attention a disease process that had begun insidiously and therefore had been undetected. In other cases, the trauma may have had a more causal role. In the same study, there were cases of bilateral inflammation after unilateral nonpenetrating trauma. These cases suggest coincidence rather than causality. The early onset and brief duration of the inflammation make sympathetic ophthalmia seem unlikely.

Other benign nonpenetrating eye trauma such as eye rubbing also exerts an inflammatory effect. Greiner and associates reported their studies on rats.[43] Immediately after eye rubbing, the conjunctival epithelium was histologically disrupted and 50% of the mast cells showed evidence of degranulation. At 4 hours after trauma, the increase in the number of neutrophils was more than 2300%. Neutrophils were in the margins in the conjunctival vessels, had migrated into the substantia propria, and were aligned subjacent to the epithelial basement membrane.

LENS-INDUCED UVEITIS

Lenticular trauma, especially when the lens is luxated posteriorly and severely traumatized, can lead to lens-induced uveitis with granulomatous inflammatory reaction. Such reaction has been observed in humans[44] as well as animals (e.g., owl).[45, 46] In a mouse model of lens-induced uveitis, intraperitoneal injection of dimethyl sulfoxide resulted in a reduction of retinal vasculitis, hemorrhage, and necrosis.[47] Morphometric analysis of choroidal inflammation also revealed significant reduction of choroidal thickness in the treated animals. These findings suggest that hydroxyl radicals may play a role in producing ocular tissue damage in the acute Arthus-type of ocular inflammation. In some cases, the inflammation from the phacoanaphylaxis is so severe that it can lead to phthisis and enucleation.[48] Histopathology revealed lymphogranulomatous inflammation with epithelioid cells and polynuclear giant cells near the lens capsule, confirming the clinical diagnosis of a lens-induced endophthalmitis.[48]

Lens-induced uveitis is a potentially curable ocular inflammation. Early lens removal in cases of traumatic cataract with lenticular capsular rupture would lead to resolution of inflammation and better visual results.[44] Readers are encouraged to review Chapter 76 for more information.

LASER-INDUCED UVEITIS

Yttrium-aluminum-garnet (YAG) laser capsulotomy, a common procedure in patients who have had cataract extraction and intraocular lens implantation, has been associated with initiating low-grade inflammation or worsening of pre-existent uveitis.[49] The shock wave created by the laser is capable of causing a physical alteration in the blood-ocular barrier. There have been several cases of patients with a history of ongoing intraocular inflammation in which the YAG laser capsulotomy caused a significant increase in inflammation.[10] Therefore, increased topical, periocular, or even systemic corticosteroids may be required at the time of the laser procedures in some patients. In addition, YAG laser iridectomy has been reported to induce endophthalmitis.[10]

PATHOGENESIS AND PATHOLOGY

Ocular tissues, like those of other organs, exhibit limited morphologic reactions to trauma (e.g., hyperemia, abrupt vasodilation, increased blood flow, increased permeability of blood vessels, edema, increased tissue pressure [disrupted blood-ocular barrier], and, later, a cellular inflammatory response).[13] Serum fibrin degradation products are elevated in patients with acute idiopathic anterior uveitis but not in those with traumatic anterior uveitis.[50] Intraocular inflammation after ocular surgeries and trauma are mediated by leukotrienes, prostaglandins, cytokines, and growth factors, and it can be inhibited by prostaglandin inhibitors.[51] Using radioimmunoassay technique, Latanza and colleagues showed elevations in leukotrienes B_4 and C_4 in the aqueous humor of eyes of rabbits subjected to blunt ocular trauma.[52] Such increases in leukotriene levels preceded the infiltration of neutrophils into the aqueous humor.

Miyano and Chiou induced ocular inflammation using lens protein to mimic the traumatic injury of the eyes.[53] They noted that pretreatment of the eyes with indomethacin resulted in marked reduction of the ocular inflammation in the early phase. Pretreatment of the eyes with phenidone and nordihydroguaiaretic acid, on the other hand, reduced ocular inflammation during both early and late phases. These results indicate that prostaglandins are involved in the early phase of the inflammation, and that this can be reduced with cyclo-oxygenase inhibitors such as indomethacin. Further, leukotrienes are responsible primarily in the later phase; they are suppressed by lipo-oxygenase inhibitors such as phenidone and nordihydroguaiaretic acid.[53]

Other serologic markers that have been found to be elevated in post-traumatic uveitis include circulating immune complexes formed by the retinal S antigen and S antibodies,[54] and red blood cell surface immune complex rosette.[55] There is a higher CD4+/CD8+ cell ratio in the aqueous and blood samples of patients who suffered from traumatic iridocyclitis than in the samples of patients with cataract.[56] Interestingly, there is no difference in ratio between the aqueous and blood samples of the traumatized patients. It is possible that one of the most important factors in maintaining a lower CD4+/CD8+ cell ratio in normal aqueous compared to peripheral blood is an intact blood-aqueous barrier.

Prostaglandins E_2 (PGE_2) and $PGF_{2\alpha}$ are released from iris and other tissues.[57] These prostaglandins are leukotactic and induce vasodilation, increased capillary permeability, and an increase in protein content of the aqueous.

The influx of leukocytes also leads to increased concentration of PGE_1. Thus, the cascade of molecular and cellular events seen in ocular inflammation of various origins seem to result in a reaction largely mediated by prostaglandins.[57] Prostaglandins in small doses administered topically or intraocularly produce some of the responses of injury and inflammation, such as hyperemia, miosis, breakdown of the blood-aqueous barrier, and rise in intraocular pressure.[58] E-type prostaglandins administered topically with histamine (but not the individual components) cause cellular infiltration and produce edema in conjunctival tissues. Nonsteroidal aspirin-like drugs at concentrations that inhibit prostaglandin biosynthesis markedly block injury responses but have only a moderate inhibitory effect on acute inflammatory reactions of the eye. Studies have suggested that prostaglandins as well as the intermediates of arachidonic acid metabolism, especially hydroxy fatty acids, may play a role in inflammatory responses.[58] Prostaglandins also have been shown to mediate, at least in part, x-ray–induced inflammation.[59]

Interestingly, topical administration of PGE_1 and $PGF_{2\alpha}$ prior to ocular trauma has been shown to reduce the ocular inflammatory response in rabbits.[60] The model of ocular trauma consisted of puncture of the cornea without aspiration of aqueous. Pretreatment with PGE_1 and $PGF_{2\alpha}$ led to a lower rise in the aqueous PGE_2 concentration and a reduced inflammatory response after corneal puncture; the increase in the aqueous protein concentration was smaller and the aqueous ascorbate level was higher. The smaller increase in the aqueous PGE_2 concentration after pretreatment with prostaglandins correlated with reduced changes in intraocular pressure. The authors suggested that PGE_1 and $PGF_{2\alpha}$ reduced the trauma-induced inflammatory response by decreasing the formation of endogenous prostaglandins, as reflected by their concentration in aqueous.[60]

Inflammation may involve a feedback loop that ordinarily does not terminate without treatment intervention. In a predisposed eye, trauma may initiate this positive feedback loop. Several conditions—the HLA-B27 spectrum of disease, sarcoidosis, and acute retinal necrosis—seem particularly predisposed to being triggered by trauma. Trauma has been observed to initiate iritis associated with HLA-B27 and ankylosing spondylitis[40] as well as HLA-B27-associated joint disease.[61] The relative contribution of trauma in initiating inflammation outside the eye is also difficult to ascertain. For example, in rheumatoid arthritis, the role of trauma is not well determined.[62] In one study, about 5% of the patients with rheumatoid arthritis had previous trauma.[63]

Rahi and colleagues reported the histopathologic and immunologic findings in 10 cases of post-traumatic granulomatous and six cases of nongranulomatous uveitis.[64] Most cases of granulomatous uveitis showed evidence of cell-mediated immunity to uveoretinal antigens. Three patients with post-traumatic nongranulomatous uveitis showed a positive immunologic response to ocular antigens, and two of these later developed clinical evidence of sympathetic (granulomatous) ophthalmitis, which suggests that post-traumatic nongranulomatous uveitis in such cases may represent a presympathetic or modified stage of the disease. Grishina and colleagues also showed the presence of cellular reaction in eyes with traumatic uveitis, indicating that there is an autoimmune process developed in response to release of the antigenic tissue substances of the eye into the blood flow, and reactive flow of immunocompetent cells toward ocular tissues because of injury to the blood-eye barrier.[65]

TREATMENT

Treatment of traumatic uveitis follows the guidelines and principles used for treating other types of uveitis. A stepladder algorithm of different intensities of therapy is applied. In general, traumatic uveitis responds well to corticosteroids. In many cases, topical prednisolone may be sufficient to suppress the inflammation. In others, periocular steroid injection or oral prednisone may be required. A topical cycloplegic agent such as atropine sulfate 1% or scopolamine hydrobromide 0.25% is often used in conjunction with corticosteroids; cycloplegia helps to relieve ocular discomfort secondary to the inflammation and to prevent the formation of pupillary synechiae. Evaluation for herpes virus reactivation caused by the ocular trauma should be performed if the patient is treated with steroids. If there is reactivation of dendritic keratitis or keratouveitis, antherpetic therapy, topically and/or systemically, is indicated. In some cases, antiglaucoma medications may be employed to control ocular hypertension, which is secondary to the uveitis, the structural changes of the angle and/or trabecular meshwork caused by the trauma, or the use of steroids. It is rare that a steroid-sparing agent is required in managing traumatic uveitis. If the traumatic uveitis persists despite steroid therapy, evaluations for possible underlying diseases should be performed thoroughly. If such is found, control of the primary condition is required to suppress the secondary uveitis.

Any patient with a history of uveitis requires close observation and immunosuppressive therapy in the perioperative period. Depending on the status of the uveitis and the duration between the most recent flare-up of the uveitis and the surgery, the patients may require intensive topical or oral corticosteroids prior to surgery. Prednisolone acetate (1% solution) may be initiated hourly 3 days prior to surgery. Prednisone (1 mg/kg) can be instituted 2 days prior to surgery. Intraoperatively, patients with uveitis often receive intravenous steroids, typically 60 mg to 80 mg of solumedrol, and subconjunctival injection of dexamethasone at the end of the procedure. The steroid therapy is tapered in the postoperative period; the tapering rate is based on the degree of inflammation.

In cases of persistent posterior post-traumatic uveitis, vitrectomy may be indicated in an effort to elucidate the possible underlying etiology or to achieve regression of the uveitis.[66] If vitrectomy is performed, proper evaluations of the vitreous, including microbiologic, serologic, immunologic, and cytologic studies, should be performed. In one review study of diagnostic pars plana vitrectomies,[67] bacteria were identified from the vitreous in six (18%) of 34 cases of post-traumatic ocular inflammation.

Whenever there is a strong suspicion that the uveitis may be secondary to an infection or that infectious etiology also contributes to the ocular inflammation, aggressive therapy with antimicrobial therapy is indicated to prevent the development of infectious, often bacterial, endophthalmitis. In recent studies, the combination of intraocular vancomycin and amikacin, and systemic ciprofloxacin appears to be an adequate regimen for the treatment of suspected bacterial endophthalmitis resulting from ocular trauma.[68, 69] With respect to the use of intraocular steroids in a setting of ocular trauma, no categorical recommendation can be made, as it depends on the clinical context. For example, it is often difficult to exclude the possibility that a traumatic wound might be contaminated by fungus, particularly if the injury was caused by an organic substance. In such settings, the use of corticosteroids clearly should be avoided. In other settings, when the history is reliable and the presence of organic intraocular material can be excluded, the use of intraocular steroids may be quite beneficial.

Traumatic endophthalmitis in association with retinal breaks or detachments is known to have uniformly poor visual and anatomic outcomes. However, attention to the possibility of infection, selective use of broad-spectrum antibiotics, and prompt surgical intervention may help to improve the visual outcome.[70]

In cases of severe traumatic uveitis, enucleation is often debated as a potential approach to prevent the development of sympathetic ophthalmia. In a study from Russia, Valeeva and colleagues analyzed 37 cases with significant traumatic uveitis with poor prognosis.[71] In 10 patients, signs of sensitization to ocular tissues were detected at various times after the injury, using the leukocyte migration inhibition test. The authors regarded the results as indicating a response to release of tissue antigens in the blood because of impairment of the blood-eye barrier caused by the trauma. Thus, they suggested that the results of the leukocyte migration inhibition test in traumatic uveitis may be regarded, together with the clinical symptoms, as an additional indication for enucleation.

CONCLUSIONS

Traumatic uveitis categorizes any ocular inflammation resulting from direct or indirect penetrating or nonpenetrating trauma to the eye. Ocular trauma encompasses ocular surgical procedures, laser applications, and violence to the eyes. Primary traumatic uveitis is ocular inflammation directly secondary to the trauma; there is no associated underlying disease. Secondary traumatic uveitis refers to ocular inflammation that is associated with or secondary to a systemic disease or an infection, which is unmasked or worsened by the trauma. Often, trauma to the eye, especially if there is penetration, can lead to bacterial or fungal endophthalmitis, which may present initially with marked ocular inflammation. Sympathetic ophthalmia is a rare but devastating complication of ocular trauma.

Prostaglandins and leukotrienes are among the important factors that play a role in mediating the inflammation in traumatic uveitis. Inhibitors of cyclo-oxygenases and lipo-oxygenases seem to be able to halt or improve the ocular inflammation.

It is important to identify any actual etiology of the traumatic uveitis, as such knowledge will dictate proper therapy. Primary traumatic uveitis often responds well to steroid therapy—topical, oral, or by periocular injection. On the other hand, secondary traumatic uveitis necessitates therapy for the underlying diseases. Infectious endophthalmitis requires prompt and aggressive antimicrobial treatment. Any patient with a history of uveitis needs to be evaluated carefully for immunosuppressive therapy in the perioperative period, as the uveitis often worsens or reactivates after surgery.

References

1. Aburn N: Eye injuries in indoor cricket at Wellington Hospital: A survey January 1987 to June 1989. N Z Med J 1990;103:454–456.
2. MacEwen CJ: Sport associated eye injury: A casualty department survey. Br J Ophthalmol 1987;71:701–705.
3. Orlando RG, Doty JH: Ocular sports trauma: A private practice study. J Am Optom Assoc 1996;67:77–80.
4. Heier JS, Enzenauer RW, Wintermeyer SF, et al: Ocular injuries and diseases at a combat support hospital in support of Operations Desert Shield and Desert Storm. Arch Ophthalmol 1993;111:795–798.
5. Bullock JD, Ballal DR, Johnson DA, Bullock RJ: Ocular and orbital trauma from water balloon slingshots. A clinical, epidemiologic, and experimental study. Ophthalmology 1997;104:878–887.
6. Kline LB, Bright M, Brownstein S: Uveal melanoma presenting as post-traumatic choroidal hemorrhage and panophthalmitis. Can J Ophthalmol 1977;12:226–229.
7. Alexandrakis G, Balachander R, Chaudhry NA, Filatov V: An intra-ocular foreign body masquerading as idiopathic chronic iridocyclitis. Ophthalmic Surg Lasers 1998;29:336–337.
8. Felder KS, Gottlieb F: Reversible chalcosis. Ann Ophthalmol 1984;16:638–641.
9. Foster CS, Fong CP, Singh G: Cataract surgery and intraocular lens implantation in patients with uveitis. Ophthalmology 1989;96:281.
10. Nussenblatt RB, Whitcup SM, Palestine AG: Postsurgical uveitis. In: Nussenblatt R, Whitcup S, Palestine A, eds: Uveitis: Fundamentals and Clinical Practice, 2nd ed. St. Louis, Mosby-Yearbook, 1996, pp 256–261.
11. Saracco JB, Paulo F, Sarles C, et al: Postoperative uveitis following extra-capsular extraction and posterior chamber implantation. Bull Soc Ophtalmol Fr 1989;89:433–436.
12. Landshman N, Ben-Hanan I, Ban-Chaim O, et al: A model of corneal re-endothelialization after surgical trauma. Curr Eye Res 1985;4:555–561.
13. Sears ML: Aphakic cystoid macular edema. The pharmacology of ocular trauma. Surv Ophthalmol 1984;28:525–534.
14. Dolan BJ: Choroidal neovascularization not associated with age-related macular degeneration. Optom Clin 1996;5:55–76.
15. Wilson MW, Grossniklaus HE, Heathcote JG: Focal posttraumatic choroidal granulomatous inflammation. Am J Ophthalmol 1996;121:397–404.
16. Cardillo JA, Stout JT, LaBree L, et al: Post-traumatic proliferative vitreoretinopathy. The epidemiologic profile, onset, risk factors, and visual outcome. Ophthalmology 1997;104:1166–1173.
17. Kimura R: Fluorescein gonioangiography of newly formed vessels in the anterior chamber angle. Tohoku J Exp Med 1983;140:193–196.
18. Kashnikov VV, Forofonova TI, Balishanskaia TI: Fluorescein angiography in the diagnosis of injuries of internal ocular membranes. Vestn Oftalmol 1990;106:28–34.
19. Meyer RF, Ritchey CL: Migration of a wooden foreign body into the lens: Report of a case. Can J Ophthalmol 1975;10:408–411.
20. Michelson JB, Roth AM, Waring GO: Lepromatous iridocyclitis diagnosed by anterior chamber paracentesis. Am J Ophthalmol 1979;88:674–679.
21. Mason GI, Bottone EJ, Podos SM: Traumatic endophthalmitis caused by an *Erwinia* species. Am J Ophthalmol 1976;82:709–713.
22. Hammer ME, Harding S, Wynn P: Post-traumatic fungal endophthalmitis caused by *Exophiala jeanselmei*. Ann Ophthalmol 1983;9:853–855.
23. Witherspoon CD, Kuhn F, Owens SD, et al: Endophthalmitis due to *Sporothrix schenckii* after penetrating ocular injury. Ann Ophthalmol 1990;22:385–388.
24. Janknecht P, Lindeman S, Pelz K: Post-traumatic endophthalmitis with multiple water pathogens. Klin Monatsbl Augenheilkd 1997;210:388–391.
25. Affeldt JC, Flynn HW, Forster RK, et al: Microbial endophthalmitis resulting from ocular trauma. Ophthalmology 1987;94:407–413.
26. Verbraeken H, Rysselaere M: Post-traumatic endophthalmitis. Eur J Ophthalmol 1994;4:1–5.
27. Nobe JR, Gomez DS, Liggett P, et al: Post-traumatic and postoperative endophthalmitis: A comparison of visual outcomes. Br J Ophthalmol 1987;71: 614–617.
28. Alfaro DV, Roth DB, Laughlin RM, et al: Paediatric post-traumatic endophthalmitis. Br J Ophthalmol 1995;79:888–891.
29. Schmidseder E, Mino de Kaspar H, Klauss V, Kampik A: Post-traumatic endophthalmitis after penetrating eye injuries. Risk factors, microbiological diagnosis and functional outcome. Ophthalmologe 1998;95:153–157.
30. Punnonen E: Pathological findings in eyes enucleated because of perforating injury. Acta Ophthalmol (Copenh). 1990;68:265–269.
31. Marak GE: Recent advances in sympathetic ophthalmia. Surv Ophthalmol 1979;24:141–156.
32. Liddy N, Stuart J: Sympathetic ophthalmia in Canada. Can J Ophthalmol 1972;7:157–159.
33. Holland G: About the indication and time for surgical removal of an injured eye. Klin Monatsbl Augenheilkd 1964;145:732–740.
34. Gass JDM: Sympathetic ophthalmia following vitrectomy. Am J Ophthalmol 1982;93:552–558.
35. Sen DK, Sarin GS, Mathur MD: Serum beta-2 microglobulin level in sympathetic ophthalmitis. Acta Ophthalmol (Copenh) 1990;68:200–204.
36. Lamba PA, Pandey PK, Sarin GS, Mathur MD: Serum sialic acid levels in patients with sympathetic ophthalmitis. Acta Ophthalmol (Copenh) 1993;71:833–835.
37. Bernasconi O, Auer C, Zografos L, Herbort CP: Indocyanine green angiographic findings in sympathetic ophthalmia. Graefes Arch Clin Exp Ophthalmol 1998;236:635–638.
38. Lubin JR, Albert DM, Weinstein M: Sixty-five years of sympathetic ophthalmia. Ophthalmology 1980;87:109.
39. Gelatt KN: Traumatic hyphema and iridocyclitis in the horse. Mod Vet Pract 1975;56:475–479.
40. Seymour R, Ramsey MS: Unusually severe traumatic uveitis associated with occult ankylosing spondylitis. Can J Ophthalmol 1991;26:156–158.
41. Sorr EM, Goldberg RE: Traumatic central retinal artery occlusion with sickle cell trait. Am J Ophthalmol 1975;80:648–652.
42. Rosenbaum JT, Tammaro J, Robertson JE: Uveitis precipitated by nonpenetrating ocular trauma. Am J Ophthalmol 1991;112:392–395.
43. Greiner JV, Peace DG, Baird RS, Allansmith MR: Effects of eye rubbing on the conjunctiva as a model of ocular inflammation. Am J Ophthalmol 1985;100:45–50.
44. Perlman EM, Albert DM: Clinically unsuspected phacoanaphylaxis after ocular trauma. Arch Ophthalmol 1977;95:244–246.
45. Miller WW, Boosinger TR, Maslin WR: Granulomatous uveitis in an owl. J Am Vet Med Assoc 1988;193:365–366.
46. Pfleghaar S, Schaffer EH: Lens-induced uveitis (endophthalmitis phakoanaphylactica) in domestic animals. Tierarztl Prax 1992;20:7–18.
47. Rao NA, Bowe Be, Sevanian A, et al: Modulation of lens-induced uveitis by dimethyl sulfoxide. Ophthalmic Res. 1986;18:193–198.
48. Necker HP, Weidle EG, Steuhl KP: Endophthalmitis phakoanaphylactica with anterior uveitis of the partner eye. Klin Monatsbl Augenheilkd 1989;195:248–253.
49. Flohr MJ, Robin AL, Kelley JS: Early complications following Q-switched neodymium YAG laser posterior capsulotomy. Ophthalmology 1985;92:360–363.
50. Sen DK, Sarin GS, Mathur MD: Serum fibrin degradation products in acute idiopathic anterior uveitis. Acta Ophthalmol (Copenh) 1986;64:632–636.
51. Huang K, Paeyman GA, McGetrick J, et al: Indomethacin inhibition of prostaglandin mediated inflammation following intraocular surgery. Invest Ophthalmol Vis Sci 1977;16:1760–1762.
52. Latanza L, Alfaro DV, Bockman R, et al: Leukotriene levels in the aqueous humor following experimental ocular trauma. Retina 1988;8:199–204.
53. Miyano K, Chiou GC: Pharmacological prevention of ocular inflammation induced by lens proteins. Ophthalmic Res 1984;16:256–263.

54. Slepova OS, Kodzov MB, Bykovskaia GN: Specific immune complexes formed by retinal S antigen and S antibodies in infectious-allergic and post-traumatic uveitis. Vestn Oftalmol 1991;107:28–31.
55. Hou M: A study on RBC immunofunction in experimental traumatic uveitis. Chung Hua Yen Ko Tsa Chih 1993;29:233–235.
56. Avunduk AM, Avunduk MC, Tekelioglu Y, Kapicioglu Z: CD4+ T cell/CD8+ T cell ratio in the anterior chamber of the eye after penetrating injury and its comparison with normal aqueous samples. Jpn J Ophthalmol 1998;42:204–207.
57. Nelson EL: Prostaglandins and inflammation in the eye. Mod Probl Ophthalmol 1976;16:125–130.
58. Bhattacherjee P: Prostaglandins and inflammatory reactions in the eye. Methods Find Exp Clin Pharmacol 1980;2:17–31.
59. Bito LZ, Klein EM: The role of the arachidonic acid cascade in the species-specific x-ray-induced inflammation of the rabbit eye. Invest Ophthalmol Vis Sci 1982;22:579–587.
60. Hoyng PF, Verbey N, Thorig L, van Haeringen NJ: Topical prostaglandins inhibit trauma-induced inflammation in the rabbit eye. Invest Ophthalmol Vis Sci 1986;27:1217–1225.
61. Olivieri I, Gemignani G, Christou C, Giampiero P: Trauma and seronegative spondyloarthropathy. Report of two more cases of peripheral arthritis precipitated by physical injury. Ann Rheum Dis 1989;48:520.
62. Wallace DJ: The role of stress and trauma in rheumatoid arthritis and systemic lupus erythematosus. Semin Arthritis Rheum 1987;16:153.
63. Short CL, Bauer W, Reynolds WE: Rheumatoid Arthritis. Cambridge, MA, Harvard University Press, 1957.
64. Rahi A, Morgan G, Levy I, Dinning W: Immunological investigations in post-traumatic granulomatous and non-granulomatous uveitis. Br J Ophthalmol 1978;62:722–728.
65. Grishina VS, Valeeva T, Iluridze SL, Isaeva RT: Immunological reactions in pathogenesis of posttraumatic uveitis and eyeball subatrophy. Vestn Oftalmol 1997;113:30–34.
66. Freyler H, Velikay M: Vitrectomy in uveitis. Klin Monatsbl Augenheilkd 1984;185:263–267.
67. Palexas GN, Green WR, Goldberg MF, Ding Y: Diagnostic pars plana vitrectomy report of a 21-year retrospective study. Trans Am Ophthalmol Soc 1995;93:308–314.
68. Alfaro DV, Davis J, Kim S, et al: Experimental *Bacillus cereus* post-traumatic endophthalmitis and treatment with ciprofloxacin. Br J Ophthalmol 1996;80:755–758.
69. Okhravi N, Towler HM, Hykin P, et al: Assessment of a standard treatment protocol on visual outcome following presumed bacterial endophthalmitis. Br J Ophthalmol 1997;81:719–725.
70. Mieler WF, Glazer LC, Bennett SR, Han DP: Favourable outcome of traumatic endophthalmitis with associated retinal breaks or detachment. Can J Ophthalmol 1992;27:348–352.
71. Valeeva RG, Grishina VS, Iluridze SL: Clinical aspects of traumatic uveitis and causes of enucleation. Vestn Oftalmol 1997;113:38–41.

Part VI

THE UVEITIS SYNDROMES:
Autoimmune

52 — SERONEGATIVE SPONDYLOARTHROPATHIES

Maite Sainz de la Maza

Anterior uveitis is the most prevalent form of intraocular inflammatory disease. It accounts for approximately three fourths of cases, with an annual incidence rate of 8.1 new cases per population of 100,000. The differential diagnosis of anterior uveitis includes many disorders (Table 52–1). Some conditions that can cause panuveitis, such as sarcoidosis, Behçet's disease, toxoplasmosis, and bacterial endophthalmitis, may begin as anterior uveitis. The challenge to the ophthalmologist caring for a patient with anterior uveitis is to elucidate treatable causes so as to limit long-term sequelae of intraocular inflammation. In cases that are associated with systemic disease, the physician must arrange appropriate management with other specialists to minimize permanent disability or life-threatening sequelae. A careful history, complete review of systems, ophthalmologic and general medical examination, and ancillary laboratory testing are clearly all important steps in the management of patients with anterior uveitis.

There is a definitive correlation between the prevalence of certain systemic diseases (seronegative spondyloarthropathies) associated with anterior uveitis and the

TABLE 52–1. DIFFERENTIAL DIAGNOSIS IN ANTERIOR UVEITIS

Seronegative spondyloarthropathies
  Ankylosing spondylitis
  Reiter's syndrome
  Psoriatic arthritis
  Enteropathic arthritis
    Idiopathic inflammatory bowel disease
    Whipple's disease
  Juvenile rheumatoid arthritis
HLA-B27–associated anterior uveitis (ocular only)
Fuchs' heterochromic iridocyclitis
Herpetic uveitis
Glaucomatocyclitic crisis
Lens-related iridocyclitis
Intraocular lens–related iridocyclitis
Traumatic iridocyclitis
Syphilis
Tuberculosis
Renal disease–associated anterior uveitis
Kawasaki disease
Schwartz' disease
Anterior segment ischemia
Malignancy
Idiopathic

HLA-B27 haplotype. However, there is also a correlation between the prevalence of anterior uveitis and HLA-B27 even without an associated systemic condition. In one study, 47% of anterior uveitis patients had HLA-B27–associated anterior uveitis; only a quarter of these had an associated systemic condition such as one of the seronegative spondyloarthropathies. HLA-B27–associated anterior uveitis (ocular involvement only) appears to be a distinct clinical disorder that differs from idiopathic anterior uveitis. Patients with HLA-B27–associated uveitis are more often male and they tend to develop uveitis at a younger age than do patients who are HLA-B27 negative. However, some studies indicate that the long-term visual prognosis is similar for both groups.

The spondyloarthropathies are a group of disorders that share many clinical, pathologic, and immunogenetic features.[1] These features include (1) radiographic sacroiliitis with or without accompanying spondylitis, (2) inflammatory asymmetric peripheral arthritis with lack of rheumatoid nodules, (3) absence of rheumatoid factor or antinuclear antibodies, (4) strong association with HLA-B27, (5) tendency for ocular inflammation (mainly anterior uveitis), (6) variable mucocutaneous lesions, and (7) occasional cardiac abnormalities. These disorders include ankylosing spondylitis, Reiter's syndrome (RS), psoriatic arthritis (PA), enteropathic arthritis (idiopathic inflammatory bowel disease [IBD] and Whipple's disease), and a form of juvenile chronic arthritis (juvenile-onset spondyloarthropathy). The term seronegative contrasts these diseases from rheumatoid arthritis, as most patients with rheumatoid arthritis have a positive serum test for rheumatoid factor.

ANKYLOSING SPONDYLITIS

Ankylosing spondylitis (AS) (Bechterew's disease, Marie-Strümpell disease, rheumatoid spondylitis) is a chronic systemic disease of unknown cause, characterized primarily by inflammation of both sacroiliac joints and the spine, and also by a variety of extra-articular manifestations. Anterior uveitis, the most common extra-articular manifestation of AS, occurs in approximately 25% of patients either before the onset of the AS or at some point thereafter.[2, 3] Conversely, AS is the most common systemic condition known to be associated with anterior uveitis in men: 17% to 31% of men with anterior uveitis have AS.[4] Once considered a rare disease, affecting primarily men and progressing to total spinal fusion, AS is now recognized as relatively common, affecting about 1% of the general population; it has a more equal sex distribution, although it is frequently more severe in males.

History

AS has been described in Egyptian mummies and even more ancient skeletons,[5–8] although many of those may in fact have been cases of diffuse idiopathic skeletal hyperostosis or other spondyloarthropathies such as psoriatic spondylitis or RD.[9] The first documented case was the classic skeleton unearthed by the Irish medical student Bernard Connor in Paris in 1691.[10] Detailed case reports were described separately by Bechterew, Strümpell, and Marie in the second half of the 19th century.[11]

Epidemiology

AS has a prevalence of about 1% in the general population. It is seen mainly in whites and is exceptionally rare in Japanese and black Africans.[12] Onset is more frequent in the second or third decade of life. Clinical evidence of AS is three to four times more frequent in men than in women. However, the prevalence of AS in women may approach that of men. The fact that AS is diagnosed less frequently in women is partly explained by the fact that the disease is less severe and progressive in women, presenting with more peripheral joint involvement and less dramatic spinal changes.[13] There is a definitive correlation between the prevalence of the disease and the presence of HLA-B27.[14] Approximately 96% of white patients with AS and 52% of their first-degree relatives have the HLA-B27 haplotype, compared with 6% of a control population.[14, 15] Nevertheless, only 1.3% of all HLA-B27–positive individuals and 20% to 30% of the HLA-B27–positive first-degree relatives of AS patients will have the disease.[16]

Clinical Features

Systemic Manifestations

AS begins with an insidious onset of low back pain and stiffness. About half of the patients are initially relatively asymptomatic and often deny or minimize the nature and extent of their complaints. The pain is dull in character, felt deep in the gluteal region or the lumbosacral area, and it is unilateral or intermittent at first, although persistent and bilateral within a few months. Low back pain duration is usually greater than 3 months before medical attention is sought. Both the pain and the stiffness, usually worse in the morning after resting, improve with a hot shower, mild activity, or exercise. Direct pressure over the sacroiliac joints frequently, but not always, elicits pain. Findings in advanced disease include ankylosing of the sacroiliac joints and spine (Fig. 52–1), with loss of lumbar lordosis, marked dorsocervical kyphosis, and decreased chest expansion; however, few patients progress to the end stage of "bamboo spine" now, because of the earlier recognition and better treatment of AS today compared with 30 years ago.

Peripheral arthritis may be the initial manifestation of AS in 20% of patients. Although any joint may be involved, the hips, shoulders, and knees are most frequently

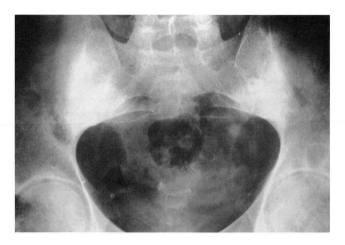

FIGURE 52–1. Pelvic x-ray studies showing the closure or sclerosis of sacroiliac joints in a patient with ankylosing spondylitis.

affected. In one study, 10% of patients had temporomandibular involvement.[17] Peripheral arthritis occurs in 35% of AS patients at some point of the disease and may start many years after spinal inflammation.[18] Enthesopathy, such as Achilles tendonitis, plantar fasciitis, intercostal muscle tendonitis, and dactylitis, is common and may be painful and recurrent.[19]

Although extra-articular systemic manifestations are uncommon in AS patients, aortic regurgitation,[20] upper lobe pulmonary fibrosis,[21] chronic prostatitis,[22] cauda equina syndrome,[23–26] and amyloid deposition[27, 28] may appear, especially after years of active disease. A few patients may have constitutional symptoms such as low-grade fever, anorexia, fatigue, and weight loss.[29]

Ocular Manifestations

Anterior uveitis, the most common ocular manifestation in AS, is typically unilateral but is recurrent and can be bilateral or alternating. The main symptoms are sudden onset of ocular pain, photophobia, and blurred vision, although it may be mild or even asymptomatic. The main signs are limbal hyperemia, fine whitish gray keratic precipitates, and prominent cellular reaction with fibrinous exudation in the anterior chamber that contributes to the formation of posterior synechiae.[30] The cellular response can be severe enough to cause hypopyon (Fig. 52–2). In fact, AS and other HLA-B27–associated arthropathy disorders are much more commonly associated with hypopyon uveitis than is Adamantiades-Behçet's disease, at least in western Europe and America. Secondary glaucoma and cataract may appear. The posterior segment is usually spared, but severe vitreous inflammation, papillitis, and retinal vasculopathy may occasionally occur.[31, 32] Cystoid macular edema may be associated with prolonged or severe cases of anterior uveitis.

The presence of anterior uveitis does not correlate with the severity of the spondylitis. AS is frequently undiagnosed before the onset of the ocular disease, especially in women, who appear to have more atypical spondyloarthropathies.[33]

Although anterior uveitis is the most common manifestation in AS, conjunctivitis and scleritis may occasionally

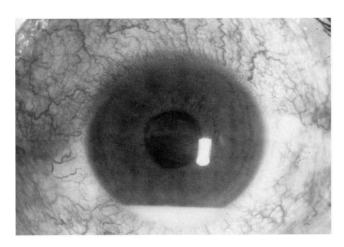

FIGURE 52–2. Hypopyon, in a patient with HLA-B27–associated uveitis in the context of ankylosing spondylitis. (See color insert.)

occur. The reported incidence of AS in patients with scleritis ranges from 0.34% to 0.93%.[34–36] Scleritis in AS generally takes the form of mild to moderate diffuse anterior scleritis without corneal lesions or decrease in visual acuity.[34, 37, 38] Although scleritis may be the initial manifestation of AS, it usually occurs after years of active AS disease, especially in patients with marked articular and extra-articular manifestations. Anterior uveitis may appear following the onset of scleritis, in which case it is impossible to know whether the uveitis is a consequence of the associated scleritis or it represents an independent effect of the disease, or both.

Pathology and Pathogenesis

The primary pathologic site for AS is at the insertion of ligaments and capsules into bone (enthesopathy). Those lesions lead to a process of ossification in the apophyseal and sacroiliac joints as well as in the intervertebral discs.[39]

The reason for the association between HLA-B27 and AS remains unknown. The fact that infections with gram-negative bacteria such as *Klebsiella pneumoniae* or *Shigella flexneri* are associated with the development of the arthritis in AS has led to several hypotheses. The cross-tolerance or molecular mimicry hypothesis suggests that an antigenic similarity exists between bacterial and HLA-B27 structures, and an immune response to *Klebsiella* therefore could cause autoimmune disease.[40] The receptor hypothesis suggests that HLA-B27 is a receptor for the infectious agent or for factors released by bacteria.[41] The chemotaxis hypothesis suggests that enhanced neutrophil chemotaxis found in HLA-B27 individuals with and without AS and reactive arthritis may contribute to susceptibility to spondyloarthropathy.[42–44] Another hypothesis suggests that proteoglycans could act as autoantigens.[45, 46] These ideas help one to think about the pathogenesis of the arthritis in AS, but the reasons for the associated anterior uveitis remain obscure.

Diagnosis

The presence of a recurrent, alternating, nongranulomatous, acute anterior uveitis in a 30- to 40-year-old man with lower back pain is suggestive of anterior uveitis associated with AS.

Although the diagnosis of longstanding AS with typical articular deformities is straightforward, early disease may be overlooked. Currently, the widely used criteria (modified New York criteria, 1984)[47] for diagnosis include the following: (1) a history of inflammatory back pain of at least 3 months' duration, improved by exercise and not relieved by rest, (2) limitation of motion of the lumbar spine in both the sagittal and frontal planes, (3) limited chest expansion, and (4) definite radiologic evidence of sacroiliitis. Definite diagnosis of AS is established by the presence of definite radiographic sacroiliitis and any one of the other three clinical criteria (Table 52–2).

The diagnosis of AS depends, therefore, on history, clinical evaluation, and radiologic confirmation. Bone scanning or magnetic resonance imaging (MRI) may be helpful if plain films are normal. HLA-B27 typing in AS with or without anterior uveitis is useful only as an adjunct to diagnosis, as the majority of HLA-B27 individuals in the general population remain unaffected, and AS may occasionally occur in HLA-B27–negative individuals. Furthermore, no significant differences in ocular complications and visual outcomes are found between HLA-B27–positive and HLA-B27–negative acute anterior uveitis patients.[48] HLA-B27 documentation is most helpful in patients with clinical criteria of AS who have not yet developed radiologic sacroiliitis.

Differential Diagnosis

The anterior uveitis associated with AS usually has a presentation similar to the anterior uveitis associated with other systemic diseases that are also characterized by sacroiliitis and spondylitis, such as RS or PA. It occurs as a unilateral, alternating, recurrent, acute iritis with symptoms such as pain, photophobia, and blurred vision, and signs such as redness, intense anterior chamber reaction, and frequent posterior synechiae. Differentiation between those systemic diseases depends on the presence or absence of the clinical and radiologic characteristics.

Treatment

Acute episodes of anterior uveitis associated with AS usually respond to short courses of frequent topical cortico-

---

TABLE 52–2. MODIFIED NEW YORK CRITERIA, 1984 FOR ANKYLOSING SPONDYLITIS

1. Clinical criteria
   1.1. Low back pain and stiffness for more than 3 months improved by exercise and not relieved by rest
   1.2. Limitation of motion of the lumbar spine in sagittal and frontal planes
   1.3. Chest expansion decreased relative to normal values for age and sex
2. Radiologic criteria*
   2.1. Sacroiliitis grade 2 to 4 bilaterally or grade 3 to 4 unilaterally

Definitive Diagnosis: Radiologic criteria associated with any one of the three clinical criteria.

Probable Diagnosis: Three clinical criteria without the radiologic sacroiliitis or radiologic sacroiliitis without any of the clinical criteria.

---

*Radiologic grading of sacroiliitis:
0, normal; 1, suspicious; 2, minimal abnormality—small localized areas or erosion or sclerosis without alteration in the joint width; 3, unequivocal abnormality—erosions, sclerosis, change in joint width or partial ankylosis; and 4, severe abnormality—total ankylosis.

steroids (one drop every hour) and cycloplegic/mydriatic agents started at the onset. If treatment is delayed or insufficient, it can become difficult to achieve control with topical treatment only. Particularly in severe cases, or in those that have associated cystoid macular edema, periocular injections of triamcinolone (40 mg/1 ml) or short-term systemic corticosteroid therapy may be required. Although data from large controlled trials are lacking, frequent recurrent disease may be treated with a maintenance course of oral nonsteroidal anti-inflammatory drugs (NSAIDs) to slow the frequency of the attacks.[49] Refractory cases may be controlled with weekly, low-dose methotrexate (e.g., 7.5–15 mg/week) or daily azathioprine (1–2 mg/kg/day); careful monitoring for side effects and complications of immunosuppressive therapy is required.

It is very important to detect the AS in patients with anterior uveitis, because if the disease is treated early, spinal deformity can be prevented. Patient education should start with the diagnosis. Physical therapy, including posturing exercises, local heat, and job modification, is designed to maintain muscle strength and flexibility even if ossification and ankylosing progress. Oral NSAIDs are helpful in decreasing acute inflammation and relieving pain.[50]

Natural History, Prognosis, and Complications

The typical course of anterior uveitis associated with AS is characterized by recurrent bouts of acute inflammation, usually affecting only one eye at a time, with a disease-free interval ranging from weeks to years. The prognosis is generally good if the episodes are treated with early and aggressive therapy. Severe or refractory cases may have associated cataract, glaucoma, or cystoid macular edema.

Although progressive impairment of spinal mobility occurs in at least half the cases of AS, functional outcome with physical and anti-inflammatory therapies is often satisfactory.[51] The disease-related mortality is related to the presence of cervical spinal subluxation, aortic regurgitation, respiratory failure, and amyloidosis.

REITER'S SYNDROME

RS is classically defined as a clinical triad consisting of arthritis, urethritis, and conjunctivitis (in 98%, 74%, and 58% of patients, respectively, in one large study).[52] However, the arthritis is frequently accompanied by only one of the other characteristic manifestations. Other common findings include mucocutaneous lesions such as keratoderma blennorrhagica, balanitis circinata, and other genital or oral mucosal lesions. Although ocular involvement most commonly consists of conjunctivitis, anterior uveitis may occur in 3% to 12% of the patients.

History

Hans Reiter, in 1916, described the classic triad of arthritis, nongonococcal urethritis, and conjunctivitis following a dysenteric episode (in a lieutenant in the Prussian army who developed first urethritis and conjunctivitis, and later arthritis, after abdominal pain and diarrhea).[53] However, a search of the literature discloses that even before, in 1776, Stoll demonstrated that those three characteristics may follow dysentery,[54] and in 1818 Sir Benjamin Brodie found the same to be true following a venereal infection.[55] In 1947, Harkness reaffirmed that RS may follow both dysenteric and venereal infections.[56] Two major epidemics of RS, one described by Paronen[57] in 1948 and the other by Noer[58] in 1966, have conclusively linked epidemic dysentery with the onset of the disease.

Epidemiology

Accurate epidemiologic studies in RS are difficult to perform because there are no definitive diagnostic tests, it frequently occurs in young patients who tend to be mobile and difficult to follow, venereal or dysenteric episodes may be mild or silent or may have been forgotten, cervicitis in women may be asymptomatic, or ocular or mucocutaneous lesions may be clinically inapparent or silent. Furthermore, some cases have been misdiagnosed as seronegative rheumatoid arthritis, whereas others were diagnosed as AS because of overlapping features. Finally, as RS is a multisystem disorder, care is often fragmented and the patient may be followed independently by an ophthalmologist, rheumatologist, urologist, or other subspecialty physician.

Nevertheless, a few studies have shown that RS is a relatively common rheumatic disease: RS develops in 1% to 3% of men following a nonspecific urethritis caused by *Chlamydia trachomatis*,[59] in 1% to 4% of individuals following enteric infections caused by *Shigella, Salmonella,* and *Campylobacter*,[60] and in a higher proportion of patients following enteric infection caused by *Yersinia*.[61-65]

The onset of symptoms is most frequently between the ages of 18 and 40 years. It has been reported, however, in children and in octogenarians.[66, 67] The sex distribution shows a definitive male predilection, but the extent of this is unclear because the diagnosis in females is more difficult to establish.[66] Postvenereal RS is more common in men, whereas postdysenteric RS affects men and women equally.[60, 66, 68] The histocompatibility antigen HLA-B27 is present in about 75% to 90% of patients with RS and in only 6% of normal control western white populations.[66] RS is rarely reported in black populations, probably reflecting the lower incidence of HLA-B27; in fact, when RS occurs in black patients, they usually are HLA-B27 negative.[69]

Clinical Features

Systemic Manifestations

ARTICULAR INVOLVEMENT

The symptoms of reactive arthritis typically develop within a month of the inciting episode of urethritis or diarrhea. However, despite careful questioning, many patients fail to recall prodromal urethral or enteric symptomatology. Arthritis is usually of acute onset, chronic or recurrent, migratory, asymmetric, and oligoarticular.[66] Lower extremity joints (i.e., knees, ankles, and toes) are the joints most commonly affected. Articular involvement may later progress in an additive fashion to affect the joints of the upper extremities, particularly the fingers or wrists, and the sacroiliac and spine joints leading to sacroiliitis or

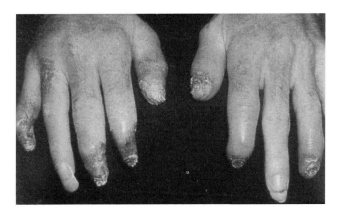

FIGURE 52–3. Dactylitis, with so-called sausage digit formation in a patients with Reiter's syndrome. (See color insert.)

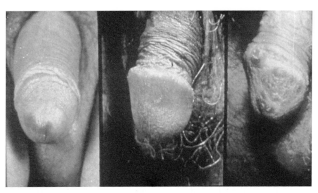

FIGURE 52–5. Circinate balanitis in three patients with Reiter's syndrome. (See color insert.)

spondylitis. Sacroiliitis and spondylitis are most common in the most severely affected individuals with chronic disease; sacroiliitis develops in 20% to 30% of patients overall and is related to the presence of HLA-B27.[1] RS should always be suspected in a young man who presents with subacute arthritis of the knees, chronic hindfoot pain, metatarsalgia, and tenderness in the low back over the sacroiliac joints.

Other rheumatologic manifestations involve ligaments, tendons, and fascias (enthesopathy); they include dactylitis ("sausage" digits) (Fig. 52–3), Achilles tendonitis, plantar fasciitis or calcaneal periostitis (painful heel syndrome) (Fig. 52–4), and chest wall pain.

EXTRA-ARTICULAR INVOLVEMENT

Constitutional symptoms include malaise, fatigue, and weight loss; fever, if present, is low grade and without accompanying chills.

Genitourinary involvement occurs in RS regardless of whether the disease follows a venereal or enteric infection. The most common problem, occurring in 90% of patients, is urethritis; prostatitis, seminal vesiculitis, epididymitis, cystitis, orchitis, and urethral strictures may also occur. Women may have cervicitis, vaginitis, or urethritis, all of which are usually asymptomatic.[66]

Mucocutaneous lesions occur in over 50% of RS patients. The most frequent skin lesion, described in 23% of patients, is circinate balanitis, which presents as vesicles that rupture to form large, shallow ulcerations or plaques on the glans or shaft of the penis with a serpiginous border (circinate) (Fig. 52–5). Keratoderma blennorrhagicum, while less frequent (12% to 14% of patients), is a characteristic hyperkeratotic skin lesion that affects primarily soles (Fig. 52–6), palms, and glans penis, and less often limbs, trunk, scrotum, and scalp. It begins as small macules that evolve into papules, vesicles, or pustules that coalesce to form hyperkeratotic scaly nodules, which usually heal without scarring after days, weeks, or months but can recur. Oral mucosal lesions are seen in about 10% of the patients; they begin as vesicles and progress to painless, small, shallow, sometimes confluent ulcers that heal within a few days or weeks. Nail changes are common and often appear as onycholysis (Fig. 52–7), yellowish discoloration, or subungual hyperkeratosis.[66]

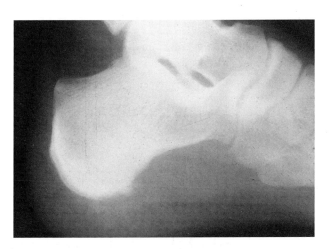

FIGURE 52–4. Periostitis of the calcaneus, with spur formation in a patient with Reiter's syndrome.

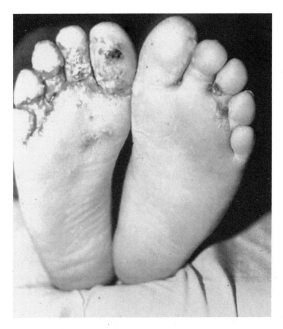

FIGURE 52–6. Keratoderma blennorrhagica in a patient with Reiter's syndrome. (See color insert.)

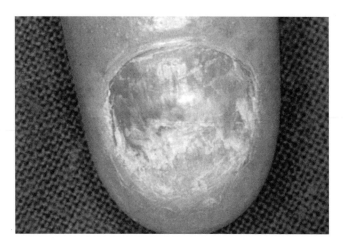

FIGURE 52–7. Onycholysis in a patient with Reiter's syndrome. (See color insert.)

Other, less common extra-articular systemic manifestations include cardiac involvement (cardiac conduction abnormalities, pericarditis, aortitis), amyloidosis, thrombophlebitis, pleuritis, nonspecific diarrhea, neuropathy, and meningoencephalitis. As in AS, vasculitis in RS is predominantly a large-vessel arteritis.

Ocular Manifestations

Anterior uveitis occurs in 3% to 12% of patients with RS.[52] The initial attack is always acute and unilateral, but recurrent episodes often affect the other eye. It is usually nongranulomatous, with fine to medium-size white keratic precipitates, a mild cellular reaction, and flare. Posterior synechiae and some cells in the vitreous are occasionally seen. Hypopyon may occur in severe cases. Secondary glaucoma can develop from posterior synechiae (pupillary block), peripheral anterior synechiae, or trabeculitis.[52, 53] Anterior uveitis is more frequent in patients who are HLA-B27 positive and/or who have sacroiliitis.[70] Conjunctivitis is the most common ocular problem in RS, occurring in 58% of patients.[52] It usually appears within a few weeks of the onset of arthritis or urethritis but occasionally may be the first manifestation of the disease.[70] The conjunctivitis is mild and bilateral, and it occurs with a mucopurulent discharge and a papillary or follicular reaction. It lasts 7 to 10 days without treatment, and cultures are negative. Rarely, a small, nontender, enlarged preauricular lymph node and mild symblepharon formation may occur.

Although conjunctivitis and anterior uveitis are the most common ocular manifestations in RS, scleritis and episcleritis may occasionally occur.[36] Diffuse anterior scleritis, although rare, is the most frequent type of scleritis in patients with RS.[71] It usually occurs in the later stages of the disease, and after conjunctivitis and/or anterior uveitis have developed. Diffuse anterior scleritis may be recurrent but it never progresses to necrotizing scleritis. Episcleritis is also rare in RS.[36, 52, 70, 72] It may take the form of simple or nodular episcleritis and, like scleritis, it usually appears after years of active RS. Keratitis in RS may be isolated but more frequently occurs associated with conjunctivitis and, less often, with anterior uveitis. It

consists of punctate epithelial lesions that may coalesce to form an ulcer. Occasionally, subjacent anterior stroma infiltrates and disciform keratitis occur.[73, 74] Disc edema, recurrent retinal edema, and retinal vasculitis have been reported rarely in RS.[75, 76]

Pathology and Pathogenesis

As in AS, the primary site of articular inflammation in RS is at the insertion of ligaments and capsules into bone (enthesopathy). This explains the frequently found Achilles tendonitis, plantar fasciitis, and arthralgias.[66]

Although the disease mechanism remains unknown, a specific genetic background and several different infective agents are now recognized. The reason for the association between HLA-B27 and RS remains unknown. The fact that enteric (caused by *Shigella*, *Salmonella*, *Yersinia*, and *Campylobacter* species) and urogenital infections (caused by *Chlamydia* or *Ureaplasma* species) are associated with the development of the arthritis in RS has led to several hypotheses. The cross tolerance or molecular mimicry hypothesis,[77–79] the receptor hypothesis,[80] the peptide-presenting hypothesis (HLA-B27, as a class I major histocompatibility antigen, could present antigenic peptides to cytotoxic T lymphocytes and induce arthritis),[81] and the chemotaxis hypothesis[82] are some of them. These data help to understand the pathogenesis of the arthritis in RS, but the reasons for the associated anterior uveitis remain obscure.

Diagnosis

The diagnosis of RS is essentially clinical. One classification system includes as major manifestations arthritis, conjunctivitis or anterior uveitis, urethritis or cervicitis, and mucocutaneous lesions (Table 52–3). The presence of arthritis and at least two of the other manifestations establishes the definite diagnosis of RS.

The diagnosis of RS depends, therefore, on history, clinical evaluation, and radiologic confirmation. Bone scanning or MRI may be helpful if plain films are normal. As in AS, the finding of HLA-B27 positivity increases the probability that the presumptive diagnosis is correct but does not establish the diagnosis.

TABLE 52–3. DIAGNOSTIC CRITERIA FOR REITER'S SYNDROME*

MAJOR CRITERIA	MINOR CRITERIA
Polyarthritis	Plantar fasciitis, Achilles tendonitis,
Conjunctivitis or anterior uveitis	lower back pain, sacroiliitis,
Urethritis/cervicitis	spondylitis
Balanitis circinata or	Keratitis
keratoderma blennorrhagicum	Cystitis, prostatitis
	Psoriasiform eruptions, oral ulcers,
	nail changes
	Diarrhea, leukocytosis, increased
	serum globulins, inflammation
	in the synovial fluid

*Reiter's syndrome (RS) diagnosis (modified from Ref. 52): definite RS: arthritis (seronegative asymmetric) and two or more other criteria; probable RS: two major and two minor (found in different systems) criteria; possible RS: two major and one minor criteria.

Differential Diagnosis

The anterior uveitis associated with RS usually has a presentation similar to anterior uveitis associated with AS or PA. It occurs as a unilateral, alternating, recurrent, acute iritis characterized by pain, photophobia, blurred vision, redness, intense anterior chamber reaction sometimes leading to hypopyon, and frequent posterior synechiae. Differentiation between those diseases depends on the specific clinical and radiologic characteristics. Hypopyon, anterior uveitis, arthritis, and oral ulcers can occur in Behçet's disease; however, in Behçet's disease the retina and choroid are frequently involved, oral ulcers are painful, and genital lesions are ulcerative.

Treatment

Anterior uveitis can be treated with short courses of frequent topical corticosteroids and cycloplegic/mydriatic agents. Hypopyon, cystoid macular edema, or the rare instances of disc or retinal involvement may also be treated with periocular injections of triamcinolone (40 mg/1 ml) and/or short-term systemic corticosteroid therapy. Although data from large controlled trials are lacking, frequent recurrent disease may be treated with a maintenance course of oral NSAIDs to slow the frequency of the attacks.[49] Corticosteroid-refractory and -intolerant patients and those with severe chronic disease may benefit from weekly, low-dose methotrexate (a total of 7.5 to 15 mg/week) or daily azathioprine (1 to 2 mg/kg/day); careful monitoring for side effects and complications is required.

Oral NSAIDs are helpful in suppressing the systemic signs and symptoms; indomethacin, sulindac, naproxen, diclofenac, phenylbutazone, and enteric-coated salicylates may be beneficial. Control of "triggering" infections may be necessary for those patients with sexually acquired reactive arthritis. A large percentage of these patients have *Chlamydia*-induced arthritis that responds to doxycycline, tetracycline, or lymecycline therapy.[83–85] Whether there are benefits of antibiotic therapy in patients with postdysenteric or idiopathic RS is unknown, but it is unlikely.

Natural History, Prognosis, and Complications

Anterior uveitis associated with RS is characterized by recurrent episodes of unilateral, often alternating, acute inflammation with intervals between exacerbations ranging from weeks to years. Prognosis is generally good if the episodes are treated with early and aggressive therapy. Severe or refractory cases may have associated cataract, glaucoma, or cystoid macular edema.

The natural history of the systemic disease is highly variable and related to the particular infective organism.[1, 66] Most patients have an initial episode of arthritis with or without extra-articular disease of 2 to 3 months' duration; whereas some patients experience recurrent attacks with prolonged disease-free intervals, 20% to 50% have a chronic course of peripheral arthritis with the potential for progressive spondylitic changes resembling those seen in AS.[1] Severe disability occurs in less than 15% of patients and is frequently secondary to unrelenting lower extremity disease, aggressive axial involvement, or progressive visual impairment.[86] The disease-related mortality is related to the presence of cardiac complications or amyloidosis.[1, 66]

PSORIATIC ARTHRITIS

Psoriatic arthritis is defined as the triad of psoriasis (skin and/or nail); a chronic, recurrent, erosive polyarthritis (peripheral and/or spinal); and a negative test for rheumatoid factor.[87]

History

The French must be credited with initiating the concept of PA. While Alibert in 1818 was the first to draw attention to the association between psoriasis and arthritis,[88] Pierre Bazin in 1860 was the first to use the term psoriatic arthritis ("psoriasis arthritique").[89] Charles Bourdillon in 1888 provided a detailed description of psoriasis-associated arthritis.[90] It was not until the association of rheumatoid factor and rheumatoid arthritis was described in 1948 that the seronegative PA was accepted as a true, independent entity.[91] Large, well-conducted surveys performed by Wright[92] and by Baker and colleagues[93] helped to establish the definite characteristics of PA.

Epidemiology

Psoriasis occurs in 1% to 2% of the white population and affects individuals in the second or third decade of life. PA occurring in about 5% to 7% of patients with psoriasis[94] has an estimated prevalence in the population of 0.1%.[95] The onset is most frequent between 30 and 40 years of age, and women are slightly more frequently represented (1.04:1). Psoriasis also may occur in children between 9 and 12 years of age, more commonly in girls.[96] A positive family history may be obtained in one third of patients, implying a role for genetic and/or environmental factors. Psoriasis and PA are reportedly associated with *HLA-A2, B17*,[97] *B38, B39*,[98, 99] *Cw6*,[100] and *DR7a*[101] genes. The association of HLA-B27 is with psoriatic sacroiliitis and spondylitis (50%) but not with psoriatic peripheral arthritis or psoriasis.[102]

There is a well-recognized association between trauma to a joint and a flare of PA in that same joint[103]; the frequent involvement of the distal interphalangeal joints suggests that excessive microtrauma may predispose to the development of PA.

Clinical Features

Systemic Manifestations

PA is characterized by skin and articular involvement. Other systemic findings such as amyloidosis, apical pulmonary fibrosis, and aortic insufficiency are seen only rarely.[1] Constitutional signs and symptoms, such as fever and fatigue, may occur. Pustular skin lesions, caused by small vessel vasculitis, may occasionally appear.

In most cases, the skin disease precedes the articular involvement by many years, but in about 15% to 20% of patients the psoriasis develops after the arthritis.[104, 105]

Skin lesions in patients with PA do not follow a particular pattern. They may vary from small hidden patches in the axilla, under the breast, umbilicus, or genitalia to a generalized exfoliation involving elbows, legs, scalp,

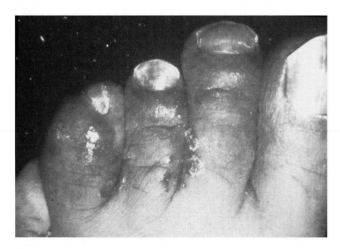

FIGURE 52–8. Psoriatic arthritic nail changes with so-called sausage digits and onycholysis. (See color insert.)

abdomen, and back.[106, 107] Nail changes are more frequent in patients with PA (80%) than in patients with psoriasis without arthritis (15% to 30%).[107] They are characterized by onycholysis, pitting, ridging, and nail discoloration or fragmentation. A synchronous flare of the joints and nails occurs more commonly than a flare of the joints and skin. Patients with more severe arthritis tend to have greater nail involvement.[108]

There are at least five patterns of joint involvement in PA: (1) Asymmetric monoarticular arthritis (5% to 10%) involves the distal interphalangeal joints of the fingers and toes and is often associated with diffuse swelling of the digits (sausage digits) and with nail lesions (Fig. 52–8); (2) chronic asymmetric oligoarticular arthritis (50% to 70%) affects two or three joints at a time; (3) chronic symmetric polyarthritis (15% to 25%) resembles rheumatoid arthritis but the test for rheumatoid factor is negative; (4) spondyloarthritis (20% to 30%) is characterized by sacroiliitis with or without spondylitis, is more common in men than in women, and has a strong association with HLA-B27; (5) arthritis mutilans (5%) shows a progression to osteolysis with resulting severe deformities and ankylosing of joints. Apart from this deforming group, the arthritis of PA is not severe; the pain and disability are much less than those produced by rheumatoid arthritis.[109]

Ocular Manifestations

Anterior uveitis occurs in 7% to 20% of patients with PA.[110, 111] It is usually acute and nongranulomatous, occurring with fine endothelial keratic precipitates and a mild cellular reaction, similar to the anterior uveitis associated with AS or RS. Hypopyon,[112] posterior synechiae, mild vitritis, and secondary cystoid macular edema are occasionally seen. Anterior uveitis is more frequent in patients who are HLA-B27 positive or who have sacroiliitis or spondylitis, mainly in the male subset of patients with deforming arthritis.

Other eye lesions in PA may occur, including conjunctivitis in 20%, episcleritis in 2%, and scleritis in 1% to 2%.[71, 73, 110] Episcleritis and scleritis usually appear after many years of active disease. Although diffuse anterior scleritis is often seen,[113] it may take almost any form of scleritis, including the anterior necrotizing and the posterior types.[71] Mild retinal vasculitis has been reported rarely in PA.

Pathology and Pathogenesis

The primary pathologic lesion in the arthritis of PA is a synovitis that is generally indistinguishable from that of rheumatoid arthritis.[114] There are also microvascular abnormalities in both normal and involved skin, including excessive capillary tortuosity and coiling.[115] Nail-fold capillary microscopy shows a decrease in the number of vessels with engorged capillary tufts.[116]

Although the disease mechanism remains unknown, a specific genetic background (50% of patients with psoriatic spondylitis have HLA-B27) and some infective agents (*Streptococcus* and *Staphylococcus* species in psoriatic plaques and nails)[117–119] appear to play a role. The finding of increased HLA-DR expression on keratinocytes from psoriatic plaques has led to the hypothesis that keratinocytes might process bacterial antigens and activate T cells directly.[120] These data help to understand the pathogenesis of the arthritis in PA but the reasons for the associated anterior uveitis remain obscure.

Diagnosis

The diagnosis of PA is essentially clinical. It is characterized by the presence of psoriasis or psoriatic nail disease and a seronegative inflammatory peripheral arthritis, with or without sacroiliitis or spondylitis. Radiologic changes compatible with PA are (1) erosions, with widening of the joint space and expansion of the base of the terminal phalanx in distal interphalangeal joints; (2) terminal phalangeal osteolysis; (3) dissolution of bones, especially the metatarsal (arthritis mutilans) resulting in a "pencil-in-cup" appearance or "fish tail" deformity; and (4) sacroiliitis and spondylitis. Elevated circulating immune complexes have been found in 50% of patients with PA.[121] As in AS or Reiter's disease, the finding of HLA-B27 positivity increases the probability that the presumptive diagnosis is correct but does not establish the diagnosis.

Differential Diagnosis

The anterior uveitis associated with PA usually has a presentation similar to the anterior uveitis associated with AS or RS. Differentiation between those diseases depends on the specific clinical and radiologic characteristics. The differentiation of PA from RS is particularly difficult, because both diseases are associated with HLA-B27 and involve the sacroiliac joint and the spine, and because keratoderma blennorrhagicum is indistinguishable both clinically and histologically from pustular psoriasis. A helpful clinical distinction is the greater likelihood of upper extremity involvement in PA.

Treatment

Anterior uveitis can be treated with topical corticosteroids and cycloplegic/mydriatic agents. Cystoid macular edema may be also treated with periocular injections of triamcinolone (40 mg/1 ml) and/or short-term systemic corticosteroid therapy.[111] Although data from large controlled trials are lacking, frequent recurrent disease may be treated with a maintenance course of oral NSAIDs to slow the frequency of the attacks. Corticosteroid-refractory and -intolerant patients and those with chronic or recurrent disease may benefit from weekly, low-dose methotrexate (a total of 7.5 to 15 mg/week)[122] or daily cyclosporin (2.5–5 mg/kg/day)[123, 124]; careful monitoring for side effects and complications is required.

Oral NSAIDs are helpful in suppressing the systemic signs and symptoms. When NSAID-resistant or progressive erosive deforming peripheral arthritis develops, methotrexate, cyclosporine, leflunomide, etanercept, and photochemotherapy (methoxypsoralen and long-wave ultraviolet-A light [PUVA]) may assist in managing both the joint and the skin disease.

Natural History, Prognosis, and Complications

The ocular prognosis is generally good. Severe or refractory cases may have associated cataract, glaucoma, or cystoid macular edema.

The systemic prognosis is generally benign. Apart from the deforming group of arthritis mutilans (5% of patients), the arthritis of PA is not severe; most patients have relatively asymptomatic periods with episodic flares of synovitis. The mortality in PA is usually caused by unrelated disease, but fatal complications from treatment with cytotoxic drugs may occur.[125]

ENTEROPATHIC ARTHRITIS

Enteropathic arthritis can be defined as arthritis induced by or occurring with intestinal disease. Some forms, mainly the idiopathic IBDs and Whipple's disease, are included in the concept of spondyloarthropathies because they are characterized by the absence of rheumatoid factor, by both sacroiliitis (with or without spondylitis) and inflammatory peripheral arthritis (usually pauciarticular and asymmetric), by ligament and tendon involvement (enthesopathy), by strong association with HLA-B27, by mucocutaneous lesions, and by tendency for ocular manifestations, including anterior uveitis.

Idiopathic Inflammatory Bowel Disease–Associated Arthritis

Crohn's disease (CD) and ulcerative colitis (UC) are IBDs that may have articular manifestations such as peripheral arthritis or spondyloarthropathy.[126] Both diseases may have ocular manifestations, including anterior uveitis.

History and Epidemiology

Although described in 1895,[127] joint manifestations in UC were not appreciated until much later.[128, 129] Similar observations were made in CD.[130–132]

Peripheral arthritis appears in 20% of patients with CD[132, 133] and in 10% of patients with UC,[134] usually those with other extraintestinal manifestations. It most commonly begins between the ages of 25 and 45 years, and women and men are equally involved.[135] Sacroiliitis with or without spondylitis appears in 10% of patients with CD or UC and affects men more commonly than women. This form of arthritis is strongly associated with HLA-B27, which is present in 50% to 70% of patients.[136, 137]

Clinical Features

SYSTEMIC MANIFESTATIONS

Gastrointestinal and articular manifestations are the hallmarks of IBD-associated arthritis. Other systemic manifestations include skin lesions (erythema nodosum or pyoderma gangrenosum), oral ulcerations, hepatobiliary disorders, urogenital involvement (ureteral obstruction, nephrolithiasis, or prostatitis), and thrombophlebitis. Some of these manifestations, particularly the skin lesions, are caused by small-size-vessel vasculitis.

Gastrointestinal symptoms in CD include relapsing right-lower-quadrant colicky pain associated with diarrhea, constipation, nausea, vomiting, fever, anorexia, and weight loss. Patients with UC present with left-lower-quadrant cramping pain, relapsing bloody mucoid diarrhea leading to dehydration and electrolyte imbalance, fever, anorexia, and weight loss.

Peripheral arthritis usually occurs 6 months to several years after the onset of intestinal manifestations, although occasionally it may appear at the same time as, or preceding, the colitis.[138] Clinically, the arthritis is usually of acute onset, mono- or pauciarticular, and primarily affecting the knees and the ankles, and it resolves within a few weeks without residual joint damage. Other joints that may be involved are the metacarpophalangeal and metatarsophalangeal joints, hips, shoulders, elbows, and wrists. The arthritis waxes and wanes with the intestinal activity and is more common in patients with severe bowel disease or when associated systemic complications are present, such as skin lesions, mouth ulcerations, and uveitis.[135] Joint involvement in UC is more frequent in patients with colon disease than in patients with isolated rectal involvement. In CD, arthritis is more common in patients with colon disease than in patients with small bowel involvement.[139] Surgical removal of an inflamed colon has a therapeutic effect in many patients with UC but in only a small number of patients with CD.[126, 137] Enthesopathy (Achilles tendinitis or plantar fasciitis), clubbing of fingers (up to 30%), and periostitis may appear.[140, 141]

Sacroiliitis with or without spondylitis, indistinguishable from AS, frequently precedes overt evidence of bowel involvement and progresses independently of the intestinal disease or proctocolectomy.[126]

OCULAR MANIFESTATIONS

Ocular manifestations, occurring in 1.9% to 11.8% of the patients with IBD, include most commonly anterior uveitis, episcleritis, scleritis, and keratitis.[142–145] Eye lesions are more frequent in IBD patients with colitis or ileocolitis than in those with isolated small bowel or rectal involvement. They are also more common in IBD patients with arthritis or other extraintestinal manifestations such as anemia, skin lesions, oral ulcerations, and hepatobiliary disease.[142, 143, 146] The degree of ocular inflammation tends to parallel the activity of the intestinal or articular disease.[142–147] In some patients with UC, proctocolectomy has resulted in resolution of the ocular disease; however, removal of the diseased bowel does not necessarily prevent recurrences of the ocular inflammation.[142]

Anterior uveitis, occurring in about 2% to 11% of IBD patients, is usually insidious in onset, bilateral, recurrent or chronic, nongranulomatous, with fine white keratic precipitates, moderate cells, and flare.[142, 143] Cystoid macular edema may be associated in severe cases. Episcleritis, scleritis, and glaucoma may accompany the uveitis. Anterior uveitis may occur before, during, or after the initial bowel attack, and it is associated with the presence of arthritis, particularly spondylitis. Posterior uveitis, much less frequent, may also occur, and it is characterized by granulomatous panuveitis with choroidal infiltrates.[148] Retinal vasculitis can develop and may be secondary to immune complex vasculitis or thromboembolic disease.[149, 150] Other posterior segment manifestations include serous retinal detachment, retrobulbar neuritis, and papillitis.[146]

Episcleritis is common in patients with IBD, particularly in those with CD.[144, 146, 151, 152] Knox and coworkers[144] reported that the presence of episcleritis in UC is a good indicator to consider changing the diagnosis to CD, because, in their experience, episcleritis is associated only with CD. The reported incidence of IBD in patients with episcleritis (all of them with CD) is 3.19%.[36] Although episcleritis may precede bowel disease,[151] it usually occurs some years after the onset of gut symptoms, particularly during active episodes.[146] Episcleritis is more commonly associated with the presence of arthritis and other extraintestinal manifestations (anemia, skin lesions, oral ulcerations, or hepatobiliary disease).[142, 144, 146]

The reported incidence of IBD in patients with scleritis ranges from 2.06% to 9.67%.[35, 36, 71, 153] Although scleritis may appear prior to the onset of the intestinal involvement, it usually occurs after some years of bowel disease, especially during periods of disease exacerbation.[145, 146, 151] Scleritis is more commonly associated with the presence of arthritis and other extraintestinal manifestations.[144, 146] It may be diffuse anterior, nodular anterior, necrotizing anterior, scleromalacia perforans anterior, or posterior, and it is usually recurrent.[38, 113, 146, 154, 155] Systemic or surgical treatment of the bowel manifestations may or may not control the scleritis.

Keratitis in IBD may take the form of peripheral, small, round, subepithelial, white-to-gray infiltrates, probably the result of acute inflammation,[156] which may lead to limbal thinning.[157] It also may take the form of peripheral nebulous subepithelial infiltrates, probably the result of scarring.[156]

Other, less common ocular manifestations are conjunctivitis, orbital pseudotumor, extraocular muscle paresis, orbital cellulitis, and orbital myositis.[146, 151, 158]

Pathology and Pathogenesis

CD is a chronic focal granulomatous disease characterized by transmural inflammation of the gastrointestinal tract, predominantly the ileum and cecum. UC is a chronic inflammatory disease that affects the colonic mucosa and submucosa, predominantly the rectosigmoid area.[126]

The etiology of IBD is unknown and the relationship between gut and joint inflammation is not fully understood. There is evidence of genetic predisposition in IBD-associated sacroiliitis and spondylitis, because 50% to 70% of those patients possess HLA-B27. The pathogenesis of IBD-associated peripheral arthritis could be related to increased gut permeability permitting exogenous factors to enter the body, and to a defective local immunoregulatory mechanism; the latter could act by inducing a switch of the protective local IgA response to a more systemic IgG and IgE response, and by enhancing T-cell–dependent immune reactions.[159] Peptides shared by colon, joint, and eye may provide further understanding of the association of anterior uveitis and IBD-associated arthritis.[160]

Diagnosis

The diagnosis of IBD is made on the basis of tissue biopsy from colonoscopy. Clinical signs and symptoms combined with radiologic studies including barium enema and upper gastrointestinal series support the diagnosis.[161] In CD, radiologic studies show deep ulcerations (collar button), long strictured segments (string sign) and skip areas, and biopsy shows granuloma formation with transmural inflammation. In UC, radiologic studies show lack of haustral markings, fine serrations, large ulcerations, and pseudopolyps, and biopsy shows microabscesses of the crypts of Lieberkühn and macroscopic ulcerations with inflammation limited to the mucosa. Radiographs of involved joints in IBD-associated arthritis show minimal destructive signs such as cystic changes, narrowing of the joint space, and erosions. As in AS, RS, and PA, HLA-B27 positivity increases the probability that the presumptive diagnosis is correct but does not establish the diagnosis.

Differential Diagnosis

Anterior uveitis in IBD-associated arthritis patients is usually nongranulomatous, with fine white keratic precipitates, moderate cells, and flare; these characteristics may be similar to the ones of anterior uveitis associated with other spondyloarthropathies including AS, RS, or PA. Anterior uveitis in IBD-associated arthritis patients may also be insidious in onset, bilateral, and chronic in duration; these characteristics are in contrast to the ones of anterior uveitis associated with the other spondyloarthropathies, which is usually acute in onset, unilateral, and limited in duration. Differential diagnosis of posterior involvement in IBD includes various causes of intermediate uveitis, pars planitis, idiopathic retinal vasculitis, Behçet's disease, and sarcoidosis. Episcleritis, scleritis, and glaucoma more commonly accompany the anterior uveitis in IBD-associated arthritis than the anterior uveitis in the other spondyloarthropathies.[162] Differentiation between those systemic diseases depends on the presence or absence of the clinical and radiologic characteristics.

Anterior uveitis and bowel manifestations can also be noted in Whipple's disease, giardiasis, and amebiasis. Whipple's disease is associated with more constitutional symptoms, normal radiologic studies, and a characteristic small intestine biopsy. Stools for ova and parasite can help differentiate parasitic diseases.

Treatment

Anterior uveitis can be treated with topical corticosteroids and cycloplegic/mydriatic agents. Cystoid macular edema and posterior segment involvement may also be treated with periocular injections of triamcinolone (40 mg/1 ml) and/or short-term systemic corticosteroid therapy.[163] Frequent recurrent disease may be treated with a maintenance course of oral NSAIDs to slow the frequency of the attacks. Corticosteroid-refractory and -intolerant cases and those with severe chronic disease may benefit from weekly, low-dose methotrexate (a total of 7.5 to 15 mg/week); careful monitoring for side effects and complications is required.

Oral NSAIDs are helpful in suppressing the systemic signs and symptoms, although they may occasionally cause exacerbation of diarrhea and colitis. Sulfasalazine may assist in controlling bowel inflammation and sometimes also benefits the arthritis,[164] but it has no effect on the uveitis. Corticosteroids can be successfully used intra-articularly or orally; they might have an effect on the peripheral arthritis but not on the axial joint involvement. They should be used only as necessary to control the bowel disease. Surgical excision of the inflamed bowel might assist in managing the extraintestinal symptoms, including peripheral arthritis and ocular manifestations.[142] When resistant cases develop, methotrexate, azathioprine, and/or anti–TNF-α agents may assist in managing both the bowel and the joint disease.[165] As in AS, physiotherapy is mandatory to prevent deforming ankylosing in patients with spinal disease and in some patients with peripheral joint disease.

Natural History, Prognosis, and Complications

The ocular prognosis is generally good. Severe or refractory cases may have associated cataract, glaucoma, or cystoid macular edema.

Whipple's Disease

Whipple's disease is a rare systemic infectious disorder characterized by malabsorption causing chronic diarrhea. Identification of the organism, *Tropheryma whippelii*, has led to earlier diagnosis and a better understanding of the pathogenesis of the disease. Seronegative sacroiliitis and spondylitis may be present. Based on this and the increased prevalence of HLA-B27, Whipple's disease is classified as a spondyloarthropathy.

History

In 1907, Whipple described a case of a 36-year-old male physician with diarrhea and malabsorption, wasting, joint inflammation, mesenteric lymphadenopathy, and widespread intestinal fat infiltration as "intestinal lipodystrophy."[166] Whipple hypothesized the cause was infectious, as rod-shaped organisms were detected in silver-stained sections. In 1948, Black-Schaffer first reported the histologic criteria for diagnosing Whipple's disease and described positive periodic acid–Schiff (PAS) staining of macrophages throughout the lamina propria of the intestines.[167] He proposed changing the name suggested by Whipple (intestinal lipodystrophy) to Whipple's disease. In 1960, the organism was visualized under electron microscopy as bacillary, gram-positive bacteria, located intracellularly and extracellularly.[168] The mechanism responsible for malabsorption was bacterial invasion of the intestinal epithelium. Molecular biology techniques have allowed identification and classification of the gram-positive actinomycete *Tropheryma whippelii*.[169]

Epidemiology

Whipple's disease is a rare disorder occurring mainly in middle-aged (average age, 49 years) white (99%) men (9:1 male-to-female ratio). Familial cases have been observed and the incidence of *HLA-B27* is 30%.[170] Many of the patients (66%) have an occupation with soil or animal contact.

Clinical Features

Gastrointestinal manifestations, mainly diarrhea with malabsorption (steatorrhea) and ill-defined abdominal pain, are the most prominent symptoms. Other common systemic findings include weight loss, hypotension, lymphadenopathy (including mesenteric and retroperitoneal), fever, peripheral edema, endocarditis, pneumonia, pleurisy, hyperpigmentation of the skin, and migratory polyarthritis.[171] Central nervous system manifestations including dementia, ophthalmoplegia, and myoclonus have also been reported.[172]

Seronegative peripheral oligoarthritis or polyarthritis is present in 90% of the patients. It may precede other disease manifestations by decades, is often migratory, and involves large joints. Arthritis activity fluctuates independently of intestinal symptoms. Sacroiliitis is present in 7% and spondylitis in 4% of the cases.[173]

Ocular manifestations were first reported in 1949.[174] They are usually neuro-ophthalmic findings such as ophthalmoplegia (external, internal, supranuclear), gaze palsies, pupillary abnormalities, nystagmus, and papilledema.[175] Other eye findings are anterior uveitis, choroiditis, retinitis, vitritis, retinal vasculitis, conjunctivitis, and keratitis.[176–179]

Pathology and Pathogenesis

Granules of PAS-positive material and rod-shaped bacteria can be seen within macrophages of the intestinal villi on jejunal biopsy and in other involved tissues.[168] Opacities in the vitreous consist of macrophages that have migrated from the inner layers of the retina into the vitreous body.

Whipple's disease is caused by an unculturable microbe, a gram-positive actinomycete that is not closely related to any other microbe. The mechanism responsible for malabsorption seems to be bacterial invasion of the intestinal epithelium and not blockage of the lymphatics.

Diagnosis

Patients with anterior and/or posterior uveitis or retinal vasculitis associated with abdominal pain, diarrhea, weight loss, and migratory arthralgias should be suspected of having Whipple's disease. Jejunal biopsy demonstrates an abundance of macrophages filled with PAS-positive granules and bacilliform gram-positive microorganisms in the lamina propria of the small intestine.[171] Vitrectomy may be diagnostic.[179] Polymerase chain reaction (PCR) has been used to identify *Tropheryma whippelii* from intestinal tissue[168] as well as from vitreous fluid.[180] PCR is available to investigators, but it is not routinely performed in commercial laboratories to diagnose Whipple's disease.

Differential Diagnosis

The differential diagnosis must include idiopathic IBD, because both disorders may have gastrointestinal manifestations, and uveitis. Systemic lupus erythematosus, polyarteritis nodosa, Behçet's disease, and sarcoidosis can have multisystemic involvement, retinal vasculitis, and uveitis. Jejunal biopsy may be crucial to the differentiation.

Treatment

Ten to 14 days of intravenous penicillin and streptomycin followed by a year of trimethoprim/sulfamethoxazole is the treatment of choice.[170, 171] Clinical experience with ceftriaxone is limited although promising. Other alternative agents are tetracycline or doxycycline. Intraocular inflammation can be controlled with topical, regional, or oral corticosteroids.

Natural History, Prognosis, and Complications

A correct diagnosis is essential, because the condition responds well to appropriate antibiotic therapy, and, untreated, Whipple's disease can be fatal.[171] Relapse after short courses of antibiotics (less than 1 year) are frequent. Death occurs in about 26% of cases, either because of lack of treatment, relapse, or predisposing factor for other illness.

JUVENILE ARTHRITIS

Uveitis may occur in association with juvenile arthritis. Chronic inflammatory arthritis in childhood is a heterogeneous group of disorders for which there is no universally agreed upon classification. The American College of Rheumatology (ACR) differentiates juvenile spondyloarthropathies, juvenile rheumatoid arthritis (JRA), and other arthritides in childhood (sarcoidosis and neonatal onset multisystem inflammatory disease).[181] In practice, however, early recognition and differentiation of juvenile spondyloarthropathies from JRA is difficult. Sacroiliac inflammation and spondylitis are late manifestations of these diseases.[182] Initial presentation with inflammation in a lower limb peripheral joint may be consistent with subsequent development of juvenile spondyloarthropathy.[182, 183] Because of that, I will focus not only on juvenile spondyloarthropathies, which are the subject of this chapter, but also on JRA. The ACR classification will be used.

Juvenile-Onset Spondyloarthropathies

Juvenile-onset spondyloarthropathy, occurring in children under the age of 16 years, includes juvenile AS, cervical spondylitis in girls, RS, PA, and IBD-associated arthritis. As for the adult spondyloarthropathies, the characteristics of these diseases include (1) radiographic sacroiliitis with or without accompanying spondylitis, (2) inflammatory asymmetric peripheral arthritis with lack of rheumatoid nodules, (3) absence of rheumatoid factor or antinuclear antibodies, (4) strong association with *HLA-B27*, (5) a tendency for ocular inflammation (mainly anterior uveitis), and (6) variable mucocutaneous lesions.[183]

Epidemiology

Spondylitis is uncommon in children. Difficulties in diagnosis make the actual incidence of juvenile spondyloarthropathies hard to determine. Children with inflammation of the lumbosacral spine and sacroiliac joints

have a high frequency of the histocompatibility antigen HLA-B27. American surveys show that about 20% of both boys and girls who are HLA-B27 positive will develop AS.[184, 185] These rates are higher than for European populations.[183] In children with AS, HLA-B27 is associated with unilateral anterior uveitis of sudden onset.

Clinical Features

JUVENILE ANKYLOSING SPONDYLITIS

Juvenile AS is a chronic arthropathy that most frequently affects boys (2:1 male-to-female ratio) after the age of 10 years. All patients ultimately develop back pain with radiographic involvement of the lumbosacral spine and sacroiliac joints; however, peripheral arthritis, which usually affects hips, knees, ankles, or heels, together with enthesitis (especially around the knees and feet) may precede spondyloarthropathy by years.[183] Because HLA-B27 is positive in about 91% of these patients, the presence of peripheral arthritis in an HLA-B27–positive boy without radiographic evidence of sacroiliac involvement could be compatible with a future development of AS. By the definition of spondyloarthropathy, tests for rheumatoid factor and antinuclear antibodies are negative. Recurrent attacks of acute anterior uveitis, in contrast to the chronic progressive iridocyclitis of JRA, occur in 5% to 15% of these children.[186, 187] The attacks are usually unilateral, although either eye may be involved at different times. Topical corticosteroids and, if necessary transseptal injections of corticosteroids are effective. The long-term visual prognosis is good.

CERVICAL SPONDYLITIS IN GIRLS

Cervical apophyseal joint fusion and symmetric destructive polyarthritis involving small joints of the hands and wrists with deformities of the fingers and fusion of the wrists are seen in HLA-B27–positive girls.[188] Cervical apophyseal joint fusion is clinically indistinguishable from cervical joint disease in JRA. Most of the patients (65%) are seronegative for rheumatoid factor and for antinuclear antibodies. HLA-B27–positive and antinuclear antibody–negative patients are more likely to develop recurrent attacks of acute anterior uveitis, in contrast to the chronic progressive iridocyclitis of JRA. On the other hand, HLA-B27–positive and antinuclear antibody–positive patients are more likely to develop chronic progressive iridocyclitis similar to the one seen in JRA.

JUVENILE REITER'S SYNDROME

RS is extremely infrequent in children.[189] However, when present, it exhibits the same pathogenetic and clinical characteristics seen in RS in adults. By the definition of spondyloarthropathy, tests for rheumatoid factor and antinuclear antibodies are negative, and HLA-B27 is positive for close to 90% of children. About 2% of patients develop acute anterior uveitis.[190] The attacks are usually unilateral, although either eye may be involved at different times. Topical corticosteroids and, if necessary, transseptal injections of corticosteroids are effective. The long-term visual prognosis is good.

PSORIATIC ARTHRITIS

Juvenile PA can be defined as arthritis occurring with psoriasis or with three of the following criteria: dactylitis, nail pitting, family history of psoriasis, or a rash that is not entirely typical of psoriasis. It is more frequent in girls (3:2 female-to-male ratio), with a mean age of onset of psoriasis of about 9 years and a mean age of onset of arthritis of about 11 years. Arthritis is typically mono-articular at presentation, most frequently involving the knees, although over time, asymmetric polyarthritis may develop. Rheumatoid factor is negative. Antinuclear antibodies may be positive. There is no particular HLA association, except in those children with sacroiliitis who are likely to be HLA-B27 positive. Between 8% and 15% of children with PA develop a chronic iridocyclitis similar to the one seen in JRA. These patients are usually antinuclear antibody positive (80%), with oligoarticular disease presenting at earlier age (about 3 years) and dermatologic disease presenting at older age (about 13 years). In these cases, an initial diagnosis of oligoarticular JRA is usual before dermatologic disease appears.

JUVENILE IBD-ASSOCIATED ARTHRITIS

IBD-associated arthritis is uncommon in children.[193] It is usually mild and pauciarticular and affects primarily large joints. A less frequent articular manifestation is spondylitis and sacroiliitis, which is chronic and associated with HLA-B27. Anterior uveitis may be acute or chronic; while acute anterior uveitis is more common in HLA-B27–positive children, chronic anterior uveitis is more frequent in children with peripheral joint disease. In children with CD, anterior uveitis is more common in those with arthritis and in those with colon disease (rather than small bowel involvement).

Juvenile Rheumatoid Arthritis

JRA is defined as a chronic seronegative peripheral arthritis in a child under the age of 16, and it can be classified by type of onset into oligoarticular, polyarticular, and systemic JRA.[194]

History

An early adolescent skeleton with changes compatible with JRA was entombed in the Andes of Peru between AD 900 and 1050.[195] Although children with polyarthritis were first described by Cornil in 1864[196] and by Diament-

berger in 1890,[197] it was not until 1897, that George Frederick Still provided the basis to establish the disease as JRA.[198] Ocular inflammation in JRA has been recognized since Ohm's first description in 1910.[199]

Epidemiology

JRA has an estimated prevalence of about 113.4 per 100,000 children in the United States.[200] No race or climate is excluded from its attack. It is much more common in girls (70% to 75%) than in boys. The oligoarticular (pauciarticular) onset type is the most common (about 50%), followed by the polyarticular (40%), and the systemic (10%) onset; each of those categories has its own clinical characteristics (Table 52–4).[194] Genetic factors play a role in the association between arthritis and uveitis. HLA-DR5 is associated with uveitis in children with oligoarticular JRA.[201] Conversely, HLA-DR1 and HLA-DR4 are negatively associated with uveitis.

Clinical Features

ARTICULAR MANIFESTATIONS

Oligoarticular (Pauciarticular) Onset JRA. Oligoarticular (pauciarticular) onset JRA accounts for at least 50% of children with JRA. It is common in girls (5:1) with a peak age of onset at 2 years. Oligoarticular onset JRA involves four or fewer joints during the first 6 months of the disease; the knees and, less frequently, the ankles and wrists may exhibit painless swelling. The arthritis may be evanescent, rarely destructive, and radiologically insignificant. About 75% of these patients test positive for antinuclear antibody. This mode of onset is rarely associated with systemic signs.

Polyarticular Onset JRA. Polyarticular onset JRA accounts for at least 40% of children with JRA. It is common in girls (3:1) with a peak age of onset at 3 years. Polyarticular onset JRA involves five or more joints during the first 6 months of the disease; small joints of the hand are characteristically inflamed but larger joints of the knee, ankle, or wrist may also become involved. The asymmetric polyarthritis may be acute or chronic and may be destructive in 15% of the patients. IgM rheumatoid factor is present in 10% of children with this subgroup of JRA and is associated with the presence of subcutaneous nodules, erosions, and a poor prognosis. About 40% of these patients test positive for antinuclear antibody. Systemic

TABLE 52–4. CHARACTERISTICS OF JUVENILE RHEUMATOID ARTHRITIS BY TYPE OF ONSET

	OLIGOARTICULAR	POLYARTICULAR	SYSTEMIC
Frequency of cases	50%	40%	10%
Number of joints involved	Less than five	More than four	Variable
Age at onset	Early childhood	Throughout childhood	Throughout childhood
	Peak: 2 yr	Peak: 3 yr	No peak
Sex ratio (F:M)	5:1	3:1	1:1
Systemic involvement	None	Moderate	Prominent
Chronic anterior uveitis	20%	5%	Rare
Rheumatoid factor present	Rare	10%	Rare
Antinuclear antibody present	75% to 85%	40% to 50%	10%
Prognosis	Good to excellent*	Fair to good	Poor to good

*Visual prognosis may be guarded
Modified from Cassidy JT, Petty RE: Textbook of Pediatric Rheumatology, 3rd ed. Philadelphia, W.B. Saunders, 1994.

symptoms, including anorexia, anemia, and growth retardation, are moderate.

Systemic Onset JRA. Systemic onset JRA accounts for at least 10% of children with JRA. It occurs with equal frequency in boys and girls and can appear at any age. In addition to symmetric polyarthritis, children have fever (39°C or 40°C during the evening and normal during the morning), macular rash, leukocytosis, lymphadenopathy, and hepatomegaly; pericarditis, pleuritis, splenomegaly, and abdominal pain are less frequently observed.[202] Articular disease is symmetric and may be destructive in 25% of patients; hands, wrists, feet, ankles, elbows, knees, hips, shoulders, cervical spine, and jaw may be involved. Antinuclear antibody is positive in only 10% of the patients.

OCULAR MANIFESTATIONS

About 20% of children with the oligoarticular JRA and 5% of children with the polyarticular JRA develop anterior uveitis.[182] Because oligoarticular JRA is more commonly associated with anterior uveitis, known risk factors for the presence of anterior uveitis are young age, female sex, antinuclear antibody positivity, rheumatoid factor seronegativity, and oligoarticular onset.[203] Joint inflammation usually precedes anterior uveitis by several years, but occasionally eye inflammation may precede the development of arthritis by months to years.

JRA-associated uveitis is usually a chronic, nongranulomatous, bilateral (75%) iridocyclitis, and it is often asymptomatic until damage to intraocular structures becomes substantial.[204] The keratic precipitates are usually nongranulomatous, small to medium in size, and localized in the inferior half of the corneal endothelium. Many hundreds of minute keratic precipitates (endothelial dusting) may appear during exacerbations of ocular inflammation. Mutton fat and Koeppe nodules may (rarely) be present. Anterior chamber reaction, usually graded from 1 to 2+ cells, and associated chronic flare are characteristic. Anterior chamber cells and not flare should be used as an indicator of inflammatory activity or need for treatment. Because the severity of uveitis is unrelated to the exacerbation of joint inflammation, articular disease should not be used as a proxy indicator of ocular inflammation. Both eyes are usually involved either simultaneously or within a few months of each other.[182] The onset of uveitis is usually asymptomatic (over 50%) and its presence is often initially detected by routine slit-lamp biomicroscopic examination or school vision screening detection of impaired vision. Frequently, the first sign of uveitis is an irregular pupil as a result of posterior synechiae. Although the eye is usually noninjected, even during exacerbations (Fig. 52–9), it is important to emphasize to parents that a red eye should not be dismissed as conjunctivitis. Sometimes, the initial presentation of uveitis includes visual loss, cataract, band keratopathy, and glaucoma. Therefore, girls with oligoarticular arthritis, who are antinuclear antibody positive and rheumatoid factor negative, should be screened every 3 to 4 months for the development of chronic iridocyclitis.[205]

Ocular complications may be sight threatening and include glaucoma, cataract, cyclitic membrane and hypotony, and band keratopathy.[206–210] Glaucoma may be

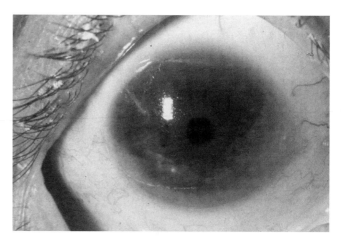

FIGURE 52–9. The typical quiet eye of a patient with active juvenile rheumatoid arthritis–associated iridocyclitis with an undilatable pupil secondary to dense posterior synechial formation. (See color insert.)

present in up to 20% of patients and may be caused by pupillary block or from chronic inflammation with presumed damage to the trabecular meshwork. Cataract formation may occur in 42% to 92% of patients and in children may lead to amblyopia. Cyclitic membrane formation and ocular hypotony can develop in longstanding inflammation in the presence of posterior synechiae and a small pupil (Fig. 52–10), or after eye surgery. Band keratopathy is present in about 41% of these children and can cause significant visual loss (Fig. 52–11). Although uveitis in JRA is usually anterior, vitritis, cystoid macular edema, and optic nerve edema may be seen.

Pathology and Pathogenesis

Pathologic findings show that the synovium becomes hyperplastic, with subsynovial lymphocytic infiltration, vascular endothelial hyperplasia, and edema.[211] Similar histologic pictures are seen in the eyes of these patients. Lymphocytes, plasma cells, and scattered giant cells infiltrate the iris and ciliary body.[212, 213]

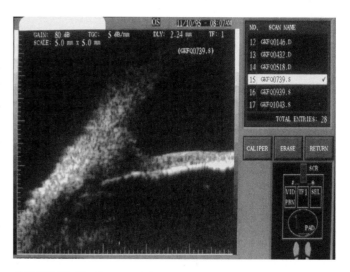

FIGURE 52–10. Ultrasound biomicroscopy of a patient with juvenile rheumatoid arthritis–associated iridocyclitis. Note the membrane on the ciliary body.

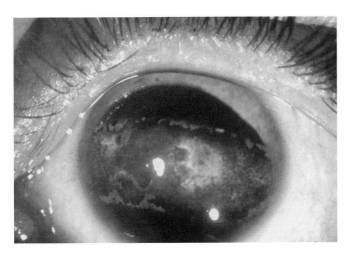

FIGURE 52–11. Band keratopathy in a patient with juvenile rheumatoid arthritis–associated iridocyclitis.

The cause of uveitis and arthritis in JRA is unknown. Immunity to ocular antigens (S antigen or iris antigen)[214–216] has been studied, but whether the immune reactions play a role in the pathogenesis or whether they are simply responses to damage by other mechanisms is unknown.

Diagnosis

Oligoarticular, polyarticular, and systemic onset JRA have their own clinical and serologic characteristics (see Table 52–4). Routine ocular examinations by an ophthalmologist are mandatory every 3 or 4 months to early detect and treat chronic iridocyclitis. Antinuclear antibody positivity is present in almost all children with oligoarticular onset JRA and uveitis, but is present in up to 80% of those without uveitis. Therefore, the antinuclear antibody negativity may be of some help in predicting that a child will not develop uveitis, but its positivity does not assist in the prediction of the development of uveitis.

Differential Diagnosis

Ocular sarcoidosis in children is the disease that most closely mimics uveitis in JRA, because both entities may develop skin, joint, and eye manifestations without radiographic evidence of pulmonary disease.[217] Antinuclear antibody positivity, characteristic distribution of involved joints, and chronic nongranulomatous iridocyclitis and band keratopathy can help diagnose JRA. Skin biopsy showing noncaseating granulomas may prove sarcoidosis.

Anterior uveitis associated with the spondyloarthropathies is characterized, unlike the chronic iridocyclitis, by acute, symptomatic onset of anterior uveitis, limited course, unilateral involvement, and good visual prognosis without vision-threatening complications.

Other diseases to consider in the differential diagnosis of juvenile arthritis and uveitis are Lyme disease, trauma, keratouveitis caused by herpes simplex or herpes zoster, and Kawasaki disease.

Treatment

Patients with uveitis associated with JRA need to be seen by an ophthalmologist regularly, every 3 or 4 months. The mainstay of therapy for the ocular inflammation in these patients consists of topical corticosteroids and mydriatics. Topical corticosteroids should be used frequently (up every to 1 to 2 hours) during exacerbations, and tapered as the inflammation resolves. It is important to find the lowest dose required to keep the iridocyclitis under control and minimize complications such as cataract formation or glaucoma. Eyes that have flare but no cells in the anterior chamber do not require corticosteroids, because these agents would increase the chances of secondary cataract or glaucoma. A short-acting mydriatic such as tropicamide is preferred to the longer-acting agents, to keep the pupil mobile and help prevent the formation of posterior synechiae. In patients who cannot be controlled with topical therapy alone, regional corticosteroids (triamcinolone 40 mg/1 ml) can be useful; however, this may be difficult to deliver in this age group and frequently requires general anesthesia. Oral NSAIDs have been shown to help control both articular and ocular inflammation and can help decrease the amount of topical corticosteroid needed to control the uveitis.[218, 219] Tolmetin or naproxen are the NSAIDs more commonly used in children. Short courses of oral corticosteroids (1 mg/kg/day) can be used in severe cases and tapered according to the clinical response. However, they should not be used chronically because of their multiple and severe side effects in children. Refractory cases may be controlled with weekly, low-dose methotrexate; careful monitoring for side effects and complications of immunosuppressive therapy is required.

Since 1950, the prevalence of blindness in children with JRA-associated uveitis has dropped from approximately 50% to its current 12% level as a result of two important sea-changes in medicine and ophthalmology: the advent of corticosteroid therapy and the widening recognition of the importance of regular slit-lamp examinations of children with JRA. It is my impression that the next revolutionary change in this matter is already underway. Increasing numbers of ophthalmologists and pediatric rheumatologists are recognizing the long-term benefits of early intervention with low-dose, once weekly methotrexate therapy, and the extraordinary safety record of this treatment approach, compared with chronic steroid or NSAID therapy.[220, 221] I have the very distinct impression, as I travel to diverse regions to lecture and to see patients, that in those areas that are well served with modern-trained pediatric rheumatologists there are many fewer children with JRA-associated uveitis that has produced or is producing ocular damage, compared with the numbers of such children seen in areas devoid of such specialists. I attribute this to the more proactive therapeutic intervention, especially with low-dose systemic methotrexate, by the collaborative liaisons between ophthalmologists and pediatric rheumatologists in some communities.

This is incredibly gratifying, given the extraordinarily cruel toll JRA-associated uveitis has "silently" extracted from its victims over the past half century: "silently" because of its nearly imperceptibly slow vision-robbing damage. Indeed, far too few ophthalmologists seem to be aware of eloquent documentation of researchers from many different countries on this silent epidemic.

Medical management of glaucoma is difficult. Topical

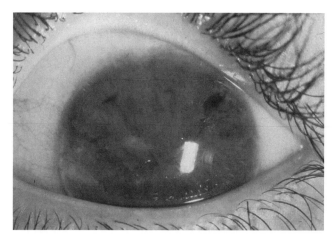

FIGURE 52–12. Left eye of a young woman with juvenile rheumatoid arthritis–associated iridocyclitis, status post cataract extraction with implantation of a posterior chamber lens implant. Note not only the pupillary seclusion but also the obvious inflammatory membrane cocoon around the lens implant. Contraction of this membrane is displacing the lens implant anteriorly and is detaching the ciliary body, producing progressive hypotony. (See color insert.)

β-blockers and sympathomimetic agents may be sufficient, but many patients require carbonic anhydrase inhibitors. Laser iridotomy is indicated in glaucoma caused by pupillary block with iris bombé.

Surgery is often needed in uveitis associated with JRA. Cataract removal should be performed only in eyes that have been without inflammation for at least 3 months. Phacoemulsification combined with pars plana vitrectomy or pars plana lensectomy/vitrectomy can be used.[209, 222] Intraocular lenses are contraindicated in these patients (Fig. 52–12). Aggressive anti-inflammatory therapy before and after surgery is recommended.[209] Traditional glaucoma surgery with trabeculectomy has shown poor results because of both the low scleral rigidity and the fibrous proliferation seen at the filtration site in young patients.[202] The use of aqueous drainage devices such as Molteno implants may improve success rates.[223] Chemical chelation with topical application of ethylenediaminetetraacetic acid (EDTA) solution after debridement of the epithelium with 70% alcohol and scraping is helpful in removing band keratopathy. The excimer laser may have some role.

Prognosis

The severity of intraocular inflammation that is observed on the initial examination correlates with the degree of final vision loss and with the extent of ocular complications. However, earlier detection and earlier and aggressive treatment improve visual outcome and decrease ocular complications.

Factors that correlate with poor visual prognosis are onset of uveitis before onset of arthritis, oligoarticular arthritis, young age at onset, female sex, antinuclear antibody positivity, and rheumatoid factor negativity. In children with uveitis associated with JRA, 10% develop mild uveitis, 15% moderate uveitis, 50% moderate to severe uveitis, and 25% are unresponsive to therapy. Overall, 75% of children with moderate to severe uveitis experience visual loss resulting from ocular complications.[222]

A team approach including pediatricians, rheumatologists, orthopedists, and ophthalmologists offers the greatest potential for limitation of both ocular and articular complications in JRA.

References

1. Arnett FC: Seronegative spondyloarthropathies. Bull Rheum Dis 1987;37:1.
2. Khan MA: Ankylosing spondylitis. In: Calin A, ed: Spondyloarthropathies. Orlando, FL, Grune & Stratton, 1984, p 69.
3. Bluestone R: Ankylosing spondylitis. In: McCarthy DJ, ed: Arthritis and Allied Conditions, 10th ed. Philadelphia, Lea & Febiger, 1985, p 819.
4. Brewerton DA, Caffrey M, Hart FD, et al: Ankylosing spondylitis and HLA-B27. Lancet 1973;1:904.
5. Raymond P: Les maladies de nos ancêtres à l'age de la piètre [The diseases of our ancestors in the stone age]. Aeschlape 1912;2:121.
6. Ruffer MA, Rietti A: On osseous lesions in ancient Egyptians. J Pathol Bacteriol 1912;16:439.
7. Bourke JB: A review of the palaeopathology of arthritic diseases in antiquity. In: Drothwell D, Sardison AT, eds. Springfield, IL, Charles C Thomas, 1967, p 352.
8. Short CL: The antiquity of rheumatoid arthritis. Arthritis Rheum 1974;17:193.
9. Rogers J, Watt I, Deppe P: Paleopathology of spinal osteophytosis, vertebral ankylosis spondylitis, and vertebral hyperostosis. Ann Rheum Dis 1985;44:113–120.
10. Connor B: Sur la Continuité de Plusieurs Os, à l'Occasion d'un Tronc de Squelette Humain, où les Côtes, l'Os Sacrum, et les Os de Siles, qui Naturellement sont Distincts et Separés, ne Font qu'un Seul Os Continu et Inséparable. Rheims 1691.
11. Bywaters EGL: Historical introduction. In: Moll JMH, ed: Ankylosing Spondylitis. Edinburgh, Churchill Livingstone, 1980, p 1.
12. Calin A: Ankylosing spondylitis. In: Kelley WN, Harris ED, Ruddy S, Sledge CB, eds: Textbook of Rheumatology, 2nd ed, vol II. Philadelphia, W.B. Saunders, 1985, p 993.
13. Calin A, Fries JF: The striking prevalence of ankylosing spondylitis in "healthy" W27 positive males and females. A controlled study. N Engl J Med 1975;293:835.
14. Woodrow JC: Genetic aspects of spondyloarthropathies. Clin Rheum Dis 1985;11:1.
15. Brewerton DA, Caffrey M, Hart FD, et al: Ankylosing spondylitis and *HLA-B27*. Lancet 1973;1:904.
16. Van der Linden S, Valkenburg HA, Cats A: Evaluation of diagnostic criteria for ankylosing spondylitis: A proposal for modification of the New York criteria. Arthritis Rheum 1984;27:361.
17. Davidson C, Wojtulewski JA, Bacon PA, et al: Temporomandibular joint disease in ankylosing spondylitis. Ann Rheum Dis 1975;34:87.
18. Cohen MD, Ginsburg WW: Late-onset peripheral joint disease in ankylosing spondylitis. Ann Rheum Dis 1982;41:574.
19. Mau W, Zeidler H, Mau R, et al: Clinical features and prognosis of patients with possible ankylosing spondylitis. Result of a 10-year follow-up. J Rheumatol 1988;15:1109.
20. Bulkley BH, Roberts WC: Ankylosing spondylitis and aortic regurgitation. Description of the characteristic cardiovascular lesions from a study of eight necropsy patients. Circulation 1973;18:1014.
21. Hamilton KA: Pulmonary disease manifestations of ankylosing spondilarthritis. Ann Intern Med 1949;31:216.
22. Mason RM, Murray RS, Oates JK, et al: Prostatitis and ankylosing spondylitis. Br Med J 1958;1:748.
23. Bowie EA, Glasgow GL: Cauda equina lesions associated with ankylosing spondylitis: Report of three cases. Br Med J 1961;2:24.
24. Hauge T: Chronic rheumatoid spondylitis and spondyloarthritis associated with neurological symptoms and signs occasionally simulating an intraspinal expansive process. Acta Chir Scand 1961;120:395.
25. Tullous MW, Skerhult HEI, Story JL, et al: Cauda equina syndrome of long-standing ankylosing spondylitis. Case report and review of the literature. J Neurosurg 1990;73:441.
26. Mitchell MJ, Sartoris DJ, Moody D, et al: Cauda equina syndrome complicating ankylosing spondylitis. Radiology 1990;175:521.
27. Jayson MIV, Salmon PR, Harrison W: Amyloidosis in ankylosing spondylitis. Rheum Phys Med 1971;1:78.
28. Lance NJ, Curran JJ: Amyloidosis in a case of ankylosing spondylitis with a review of the literature. J Rheumatol 1991;18:100.

29. Hart FD: The stiff aching back. The differential diagnosis of ankylosing spondylitis. Lancet 1968;1:740.

30. Rosenbaum JT: Characterization of uveitis associated with spondyloarthritis. J Rheumatol 1989;16:792.

31. Rodriguez A, Akova YA, Pedroza Seres M, et al: Posterior segment ocular manifestations in patient with *HLA-B27*–associated uveitis. Ophthalmology 1994;101:1267.

32. Castillo A, Sayagues O, Grande C, et al: *HLA-B27*–associated uveitis presenting with diffuse vitritis. Ophthalmic Surg Lasers 1996;27:321.

33. Tay Kearney ML, Schwam BL, Lowder C, et al: Clinical features and associated systemic disease of *HLA-B27* uveitis. Am J Ophthalmol 1996;121:47.

34. Watson PG, Hayreh SS: Scleritis and episcleritis. Br J Ophthalmol 1976;60:163.

35. Tuft SJ, Watson PG: Progression of scleral disease. Ophthalmology 1991;98:467.

36. Sainz de la Maza M, Jabbur NS, Foster CS: Severity of scleritis and episcleritis. Ophthalmology 1994;101:389.

37. Hakin KN, Watson PG: Systemic associations of scleritis. Int Ophthalmol Clin 1991;31:111.

38. Foster CS, Sainz de la Maza M: The Sclera. New York, Springer-Verlag, 1994.

39. Resnick D, Niwayama G: Ankylosing spondylitis. In: Resnick D, Niwayama G, eds: Diagnosis of Bone and Joint Disorders. Philadelphia, W.B. Saunders, 1988, p 1103.

40. Ebringer A, Cox NL, Abuljadayel I: *Klebsiella* antibodies in ankylosing spondylitis and *Proteus* antibodies in rheumatoid arthritis. Br J Rheumatol 1988;27:72.

41. Geczy AF, Alexander K, Bashir HV: A factor(s) in *Klebsiella* filtrates specifically modifies an *HLA-B27* associated cell-surface component. Nature 1980;283:782.

42. Leirisalo M, Repo H, Tiilikainen A, et al: Chemotaxis in *Yersinia* arthritis: *HLA-B27*–positive neutrophils show high stimulated motility in vitro. Arthritis Rheum 1980;23:1036.

43. Pease CT, Fordham JN, Currey HLF: Polymorphonuclear cell motility, ankylosing spondylitis, and *HLA-B27*. Ann Rheum Dis 1984;43:279.

44. Pease CT, Fennell M, Brewerton DA, et al: Polymorphonuclear leukocyte motility in men with ankylosing spondylitis. Ann Rheum Dis 1989;48:35.

45. Golds EE, Stephen IBM, Esdaile JM, et al: Lymphocyte transformation to connective tissue antigens in adult and juvenile rheumatoid arthritis, osteoarthritis, ankylosing spondylitis, systemic lupus erythematosus, and a nonarthritic control population. Cell Immunol 1983;82:196.

46. Dayer E, Mathai L, Glan TT, et al: Cartilage proteoglycan-induced arthritis in BALB/c mice. Arthritis Rheum 1990;33:1394.

47. The HSG, Steven MM, van der Linden SM, et al: Evaluation of diagnostic criteria for ankylosing spondylitis: A comparison of the Rome, New York, and modified New York criteria in patients with a positive clinical history screening test for ankylosing spondylitis. Br J Rheumatol 1985;24:242.

48. Linssen A, Meenken C: Outcomes of *HLA-B27*–positive and *HLA-B27*–negative acute anterior uveitis. Am J Ophthalmol 1995;120:351.

49. Rosenbaum JT: Characterization of uveitis associated with spondyloarthritis. J Rheumatol 1989;16:792.

50. Khan MA: Medical and surgical treatment of seronegative spondyloarthropathy. Curr Opin Rheumatol 1990;2:592.

51. Carette S, Graham D, Little H, et al: The natural course of ankylosing spondylitis. Arthritis Rheum 1983;26:186.

52. Lee DA, Barker SM, Su WPD, et al: The clinical diagnosis of Reiter's syndrome. Ophthalmology 1986;93:350.

53. Reiter H: Ueber eine bisher unerkannte Spirochaeteninfektion (Spirochaetosis arthritica). Dtsch Med Wochenschr 1916;42:1435.

54. Stoll M (1776): Cited by Huette, in De l'arthrite dysenterique. Arch Gen Med 1869;14:29.

55. Brodie BC: Pathologic and Surgical Observations on Disease and Joints. London, Longman, 1818.

56. Harkness AH: Reiter's disease. Br Med J 1947;1:72.

57. Paronen I: Reiter's disease: A study of 344 cases observed in Finland. Acta Med Scand 1948;131:1.

58. Noer HR: An ''experimental'' epidemic of Reiter's syndrome: JAMA 1966;198:693.

59. Keat A, Maini RN, Nkwazi GC, et al: Role of *Chlamydia trachomatis* and *HLA-B27* in sexually acquired reactive arthritis. Br Med J 1978;1:605.

60. Lahesmaaa-Rantala R, Toivanen A: Clinical spectrum of reactive arthritis. In: Toivanen A, Toivanen P, eds: Reactive Arthritis. Boca Raton, FL, CRC Press, 1988, p 1.

61. Arvaston B, Damgaard K, Winblad S: Clinical symptoms of infection with *Yersinia enterocolitica*. Scand J Infect Dis 1971;3:37.

62. Leino R, Kalliomaki JL: Yersiniosis as an internal disease. Ann Intern Med 1974;81:458.

63. Tertti R, Granfors K, Lehtonen OP, et al: An outbreak of *Yersinia pseudotuberculosis* infection. J Infect Dis 1984;149:245.

64. Sievers K, Ahvonen P, Aho K: Epidemiological aspects of *Yersinia* arthritis. Int J Epidemiol 1972;1:45.

65. Aho K, Leirisalo-Repo M, Repo H: Reactive arthritis. Clin Rheum Dis 1985;11:25.

66. Keat A: Reiter's syndrome and reactive arthritis in perspective. N Engl J Med 1983;309:1606.

67. Khan MA, van der Linden SM: A wider spectrum of spondyloarthropathies. Semin Arthritis Rheum 1990;20:107.

68. Phillips PE: The role of infectious agents in the spondyloarthropathies. Scand J Rheumatol 1988;17:435.

69. Stein M, Davis P, Emmanuel J, et al: The spondyloarthropathies in Zimbabwe: A clinical and immunogenetic profile. J Rheumatol 1990;17:1337.

70. Ostler HB, Dawson CR, Schachter J, et al: Reiter's syndrome. Am J Ophthalmol 1971;71:986.

71. Sainz de la Maza M, Foster CS, Jabbur NS: Scleritis associated with systemic vasculitic diseases. Ophthalmology 1995;102:687.

72. Weinberger HW, Ropes MW, Kulka JP, et al: Reiter's syndrome, clinical and pathological observations: A long-term study of 16 cases. Medicine 1962;41:35.

73. Luxenberg MN: Reiter's keratoconjunctivitis. Arch Ophthalmol 1990;108:280.

74. Mark DB, McCulley JB: Reiter's keratitis. Arch Ophthalmol 1982;100:781.

75. Mattson R: Recurrent retinitis in Reiter's disease. Acta Ophthalmol 1955;33:403.

76. Conway RM, Graham SL, Lassere M: Incomplete Reiter's syndrome with focal involvement of the posterior segment. Aust N Z J Ophthalmol 1995;23:63.

77. Schwimmbeck PL, Yu DTY, Oldstone MBA: Autoantibodies to *HLA-B27* patients with ankylosing spondylitis and Reiter's syndrome: Molecular mimicry with *Klebsiella pneumoniae* nitrogenase reductase as potential mechanisms of autoimmune disease. J Exp Med 1987;166:173.

78. Stieglitz H, Fosmire S, Lipsky PE: Identification of a 2-Md plasmid from *Shigella flexneri* associated with reactive arthritis. Arthritis Rheum 1989;32:937.

79. Lahesmaa R, Skurnik M, Vaara M, et al: Molecular mimicry between *HLA-B27* and *Yersinia, Salmonella, Shigella* and *Klebsiella* with the same region of HLA alpha1 helix. Clin Exp Immunol 1991;86:399.

80. Seager K, Bashir HV, Geczy AF, et al: Evidence for a specific B27-associated cell surface marker on lymphocytes of patients with ankylosing spondylitis. Nature 1979;227:68.

81. Kievitis F, Ivanyi P, Krimpenfort P, et al: HLA restricted recognition of viral antigens in HLA trangenic mice. Nature 1987;329:447.

82. Leirisalo-Repo M, Lauhio A, Repo H: Chemotaxis and chemiluminescence responses of synovial fluid polymorphonuclear leucocytes during acute reactive arthritis. Ann Rheum Dis 1990;49:615.

83. Pott HG, Wittenborg A, Junge-Hulsing G: Long-term antibiotic treatment in reactive arthritis. Lancet 1988;1:245.

84. Bardin T, Enel C, Lathrop MG: Treatment by tetracycline or erythromycin of urethritides allows significant prevention of post-venereal arthritic flares in Reiter's syndrome patients. Arthritis Rheum 1990;33:S26.

85. Lauhio A, Leirisalo-Repo M, Lahdevirta J, et al: Double-blind, placebo-controlled study of three-month treatment with lymecycline in reactive arthritis, with special reference to *Chlamydia* arthritis. Arthritis Rheum 1991;34:6.

86. Kaarela K, Lehtinen K, Luukkainen R: Work capacity of patients with inflammatory joint disease: An eight year follow-up study. Scand J Rheumatol 1987;16:403.

87. Gerber HL, Espinoza LR: Psoriatic Arthritis. Orlando, FL, Grune & Stratton, 1985.

88. Alibert JL: Precis Theorique et Pratique sur les Maladies de la Peau. Paris, Caille et Ravier, 1818.

89. Bazin P: Leçons Theoriques et Cliniques sur les Affections Cutanees de Nature Arthritique et Arthreux. Paris, Delahaye, 1860, p 154.

90. Bourdillon C: These de Paris. No 298. 1888.

91. Baker H: Epidemiologic aspects of psoriasis and arthritis. Br J Dermatol 1966;78:249.

92. Wright V: Psoriasis and arthritis. Ann Rheum Dis 1956;15:348.

93. Baker H, Golding DN, Thompson M: Psoriasis and arthritis. Ann Intern Med 1963;58:909.

94. Leczinsky CG: The incidence of arthropathy in a ten-year series of psoriasis cases. Acta Derm Venereol (Stockh) 1948;28:483.

95. Wright V: Psoriatic arthritis. In: Kelley WN, Harris ED, Ruddy S, Sledge CB, eds: Textbook of Rheumatology, 2nd ed, vol II. Philadelphia, W.B. Saunders, 1985, p 1060.

96. Southwood TR, Petty RE, Malleson PN, et al: Psoriatic arthritis in children. Arthritis Rheum 1989;32:1007.

97. Hamilton ML, Gladman DD, Shore A, et al: Juvenile psoriatic arthritis and HLA antigens. Ann Rheum Dis 1990;49:694.

98. Beauleiu AD, Roy R, Mathon G, et al: Psoriatic arthritis: Risk factors for patients with psoriasis—A study based on histocompatibility antigens frequencies. J Rheumatol 1983;10:633.

99. Gladman D, Anhorn K, Schachter R, et al: HLA antigens in psoriatic arthritis. J Rheumatol 1986;13:586.

100. Murray C, Mann DL, Gerber LN, et al: Histocompatibility allontigens in psoriasis and psoriatic arthritis. Evidence for the influence of multiple genes in the major histocompatibility complex. J Clin Invest 1980;66:670.

101. Sakkas LI, Loqueman N, Bird H, et al: HLA class II and T cell receptor gene polymorphisms in psoriatic arthritis and psoriasis. J Rheumatol 1990;17:1487.

102. Suarez-Almazor ME, Russell AS: Sacroiliitis in psoriasis: Relationship to peripheral arthritis and HLA-B27. J Rheumatol 1990;17:804.

103. Langevitz P, Buskila D, Gladman DD: Psoriatic arthritis precipitated by physical trauma. J Rheumatol 1990;17:695.

104. Gladman DD, Shuckett R, Rusell ML, et al: Psoriatic arthritis (PSA)—An analysis of 220 patients. Q J Med 1987;62:127.

105. Biondi Oriente C, Scarpa R, Pucino A, et al: Psoriasis and psoriatic arthritis. Dermatological and rheumatological co-operative clinical report. Acta Derm Venereol (Stockh) 1989;146:69.

106. Moll JM, Wright V: Psoriatic arthritis. Semin Arthritis Rheum 1973;3:55.

107. Scarpa R, Oriente P, Pucino A, et al: Psoriatic arthritis in psoriatic patients. Br J Rheumatol 1984;23:246.

108. Baker H, Golding DN, Thompson M: The nails in psoriatic arthritis. Br J Derm 1964;76:549.

109. Roberts MET, Wright V, Hill AGS, et al: Psoriatic arthritis: A follow-up study. Ann Rheum Dis 1976;35:206.

110. Lambert JR, Wright V: Eye inflammation in psoriatic arthritis. Ann Rheum Dis 1976;35:354.

111. Knox DL: Psoriasis and intraocular inflammation. Trans Am Ophthalmol Soc 1979;127:210.

112. Iijima S, Iwata M, Otuska F: Psoriatic arthritis and hypopyon-iridocyclitis. Possible mechanism of the association of psoriasis and anterior uveitis. Dermatology 1996;193:295.

113. Watson PG, Hazleman BL: The Sclera and Systemic Disorders. Philadelphia, W.B. Saunders, 1976, p 206.

114. Espinoza LR, Vasey FB, Espinoza CG, et al: Vascular changes in psoriatic synovium: A light and electron microscopic study. Arthritis Rheum 1982;25:677.

115. Ryan TJ: Microcirculation in psoriasis: Blood vessels, lymphatics, and tissue fluid. Pharmacol Ther 1980;10:27.

116. Zaric D, Worm AM, Stahl D, et al: Capillary microscopy of the nailford in psoriatic and rheumatoid arthritis. Scand J Rheumatol 1981;10:249.

117. Vasey FB, Deitz C, Fenske NA, et al: Possible involvement of Group A streptococci in the pathogenesis of psoriatic arthritis. J Rheumatol 1982;9:719.

118. Mustakallio KK, Lassus A: Staphylococcal alpha-antitoxin in psoriasis arthropathy. Br J Dermatol 1964;76:544.

119. Rahman MU, Ahmen S, Schumacher HR, et al: High levels of antipeptidoglycan antibodies in psoriatic and other seronegative arthritides. J Rheumatol 1990;17:621.

120. Gottlieb AB, Fu SM, Carter DM, et al: Marked increase in the frequency of psoriatic arthritis in psoriasis patients with HLA-DR + keratinocytes. Arthritis Rheum 1987;30:901.

121. Hall RP, Gerber LH, Lawley TJ: IgA-containing immune complexes in patients with psoriatic arthritis. Clin Exp Rheumatol 1984;2:221.

122. Black RL, O'Brien WM, Van Scott EJ, et al: Methotrexate therapy in psoriatic arthritis. JAMA 1964;189:743.

123. Ellis CH, Gorsulowsky DC, Hamilton TA, et al: Cyclosporine improves psoriasis in a double-blind study. JAMA 1986;256:3110.

124. Faulds D, Goa KL, Benfield P: Cyclosporin. A review of its pharmacodynamic and pharmacokinetic properties, and therapeutic use in immunoregulatory disorders. Drugs 1993;45:953.

125. Roberts MET, Wright V, Hill AGS, et al: Psoriatic arthritis: Follow-up study. Ann Rheum Dis 1976;35:206.

126. Palumbo PJ, Ward LE, Sauer WG: Musculoskeletal manifestations of IBD: Ulcerative and granulomatous colitis and ulcerative proctitis. Mayo Clin Proc 1973;48:411.

127. White MH: Colitis. Lancet 1895;1:583.

128. Bywaters EGL, Ansell BM: Arthritis associated with ulcerative colitis. Ann Rheum Dis 1958;17:169.

129. Wright V, Watkinson G: Articular complication of ulcerative colitis. Am J Proctol 1966;17:107.

130. Van Patter WN, Barger JA, Dockerty MB, et al: Regional enteritis. Gastroenterology 1954;26:347.

131. Acheson ED: An association between ulcerative colitis, regional enteritis, and ankylosing spondylitis. Q J Med 1960;29:489.

132. Ansell BM, Wigley RAD: Arthritis manifestations in regional enteritis. Ann Rheum Dis 1964;23:64.

133. Münch H, Purman J, Reis HE, et al: Clinical features of inflammatory joint and spine manifestations in Crohn's disease. Hepatogastroenterology 1986;33:123.

134. Greenstein AJ, Janowitz HD, Sachar DB: The extraintestinal complications of Crohn's disease and ulcerative colitis: A study of 700 patients. Medicine 1976;55:401.

135. Gravallese EM, Kantrowitz FG: Arthritic manifestations of inflammatory bowel disease. Am J Gastroenterol 1988;83:703.

136. Mallas EC, McIntosh P, Asquith P, et al: Histocompatibility antigens in inflammatory bowel disease: Their clinical significance and their association with arthropathy with special reference to HLA-B27. Gut 1976;17:906.

137. Van Den Berg-Loonen, Dekker-Saeys BJ, Meuwissen SGD, et al: Histocompatibility antigens and other genetic markers in ankylosing spondylitis and inflammatory bowel disease. J Immunogenet 1977;4:167.

138. Haslock I, Wright V: The musculoskeletal complications of Crohn's disease. Medicine 1973;52:217.

139. Isdale A, Wright V: Seronegative arthritis and the bowel. Baillières Clin Rheumatol 1989;3:285.

140. Anderson DO, Mullinger MA, Bagoch A: Regional enteritis involving the duodenum with clubbing of the fingers and steatorrhea. Gastroenterology 1957;32:917.

141. Kitis G, Thompson H, Allan RN: Finger clubbing in inflammatory bowel disease: Its prevalence and pathogenesis. Br Med J 1979;2:825.

142. Hopkins DJ, Horan E, Burton IL, et al: Ocular disorders in a series of 332 patients with Crohn's disease. Br J Ophthalmol 1974;58:732.

143. Wright R, Lumsden K, Luntz MH, et al: Abnormalities of the sacroiliac joints and uveitis in ulcerative colitis. Q J Med 1965;34:229.

144. Knox DL, Schachat AP, Mustonen E: Primary, secondary, and coincidental ocular complications of Crohn's disease. Ophthalmology 1984;91:163.

145. Billson FA, de Dombal FT, Watkinson G, et al: Ocular complications of ulcerative colitis. Gut 1967;8:102.

146. Salmon JF, Wright JP, Murray ADN: Ocular inflammation in Crohn's disease. Ophthalmology 1991;98:480.

147. Ellis PO, Gentry JH: Ocular complications of ulcerative colitis. Am J Ophthalmol 1964;58:779.

148. Salmon JF, Wright JP, Bowen RM, et al: Granulomatous uveitis in Crohn's disease. Arch Ophthalmol 1989;107:718.

149. Ruby AJ, Jampol LM: Crohn's disease and retinal vascular disease. Am J Ophthalmol 1990;110:349.

150. Duker JS, Brown GC, Brooks L: Retinal vasculitis in Crohn's disease. Am J Ophthalmol 1987;103:664.

151. Petrelli EA, McKinley M, Troncale FJ: Ocular manifestations of inflammatory bowel disease. Ann Ophthalmol 1982;14:356.

152. Macoul KL: Ocular changes in granulomatous ileocolitis. Arch Ophthalmol 1970;84:95.

153. Lyne AJ, Pitkeatheley DA: Episcleritis and scleritis. Arch Ophthalmol 1968;80:171.

154. Jameson Evans P, Eustace P: Scleromalacia perforans associated with Crohn's disease. Br J Ophthalmol 1973;57:330.

155. Sainz de la Maza M, Foster CS: Necrotizing scleritis after ocular surgery. A clinicopathologic study. Ophthalmology 1991;98:1720.

156. Knox DL, Snip RC, Stark WJ: The keratopathy of Crohn's disease. Am J Ophthalmol 1980;90:862.

157. Geerards AJ, Beekhuis WH, Remeyer L, et al: Crohn's colitis and the cornea. Cornea 1997;16:227.

158. Durno CA, Ehrlich R, Taylor R: Keeping an eye on Crohn's disease: Orbital myositis as the presenting symptom. Can J Gastroenterol 1997;11:497.

159. Kirsner JB, Shorter RG: Shorter developments in "nonspecific" inflammatory bowel disease. N Engl J Med 1982;306:775.

160. Bhagat S, Das KM: A shared and unique peptide in the human colon, eye, and joint detected by a monoclonal antibody. Gastroenterology 1994;107:103.

161. Clark RL, Muhletaler CA, Margulies SI: Colitic arthritis: Clinical and radiographic manifestations. Radiology 1971;101:585.

162. Lyons JL, Rosenbaum JT: Uveitis associated with inflammatory bowel disease compared with uveitis associated with spondyloarthropathy. Arch Ophthalmol 1997;115:61.

163. Soukiasian SH, Foster CS, Raizman MB: Treatment strategies for scleritis and uveitis associated with inflammatory bowel disease. Am J Ophthalmol 1994;118:601.

164. Mielants H, Veys EM: HLA-B27 related arthritis and bowel inflammation. Part I: Sulphasalazine (Salazopyrin) in HLA-B27 related reactive arthritis. J Rheumatol 1985;12:287.

165. Wilke WS: Methotrexate use in miscellaneous inflammatory diseases. Rheum Dis Clin North Am 1997;23:855.

166. Whipple GH: A hitherto undescribed disease characterized anatomically by deposits of fat and fatty acids in the intestinal and mesenteric lymphatic tissues. Johns Hopkins Hosp Bull 1907;18:382.

167. Black-Schaffer B: Tinctoral demonstration of glycoprotein in Whipple's disease. Proc Soc Exp Biol Med 1949;72:225.

168. Cohen AS, Schimmel EM, Holt PR, et al: Ultrastructural abnormalities in Whipple's disease. Proc Soc Exp Biol Med 1960;105:411.

169. Relman DA, Schmidt TM, MacDermott RP, et al: Identification of the uncultured bacillus of Whipple's disease. N Engl J Med 1992;327:293.

170. McKinley R, Grace CS: Whipple's disease in an HLA-B27 positive female. Aust N Z J Med 1985;15:758.

171. Maizel H, Ruffin JM, Dobbins WO III: Whipple's disease: A review of 19 patients from one hospital and a review of the literature since 1950. Medicine 1970;49:175.

172. Dobbins WO III: Whipple's disease. In: Mandell GL, Douglas RG Jr, Bennett JE, eds: Principles and Practice of Infectious Diseases, 3rd ed. New York, Churchill Livingstone, 1990.

173. Canoso JJ, Saini M, Hermos JA: Whipple's disease and ankylosing spondylitis. Simultaneous occurrence in HLA-B27 male. J Rheumatol 1978;5:79.

174. Jones FA, Paulley JW: Intestinal lipodystrophy (Whipple's disease). Lancet 1949;1:214.

175. Badenoch J, Richards WCD, Oppenheimer DR: Encephalopathy in a case of Whipple's disease. J Neurol Neurosurg Psychiatry 1963;26:203.

176. Leland TM, Chambers JK: Ocular findings in Whipple's disease. South Med 1978;71:335.

177. Disdier P, Harle JR, Vidal-Morris D, et al: Chemosis associated with Whipple's disease. N Engl J Med 1991;112:217.

178. Avila MP, Jalkh AE, Feldman E, et al: Manifestations of Whipple's disease in the posterior segment of the eye. Arch Ophthalmol 1984;102:384.

179. Durant WJ, Flood T, Goldberg MF, et al: Vitrectomy and Whipple's disease. Arch Ophthalmol 1984;102:848.

180. Rickman L, Freeman WR, Green WR, et al: Brief report: Uveitis caused by *Tropheryma whippelii* (Whipple's bacillus). N Engl J Med 1995;332:363.

181. Kanski JJ, Petty RE: Chronic childhood arthritis and uveitis. In: Pepose JS, Holland GN, Wilhelmus KR, eds: Ocular Infection and Immunity. St. Louis, Mosby, 1996, p 485.

182. Kanski JJ: Juvenile arthritis and uveitis. Surv Ophthalmol 1990;31:253.

183. Calabro JJ: Clinical aspects of juvenile and adult ankylosing spondylitis. Br J Rheum 1983;22:104.

184. Calin A, Fries JF, Schurman D, et al: The close correlation between symptoms and disease expression in HLA-B27 positive individuals. J Rheumatol 1977;4:277.

185. Cohen LM, Mital KK, Schmid FR, et al: Increased risk for spondylitis stigmata in apparently healthy HLA-W27 men. Ann Intern Med 1976;84:1.

186. Hafner R: Die juvenile Spondarthritis. retrospektive Untersuchung an 71 patients. Manatsschr Kinderheilkd 1987;135:41.

187. Schaller J: Ankylosing spondylitis of childhood onset. Arthritis Rheum 1977;20:398.

188. Arnett FC, Bias WB, Stevens MB: Juvenile onset chronic arthritis: Clinical and roentgenographic features of a unique HLA-B27 subset. Am J Med 1980;69:369.

189. Rosenberg AM, Petty RE: Reiter's disease in children. Am J Dis Child 1979;133:394.

190. Iveson JMI, Nanda BS, Hancock JAH, et al: Reiter's disease in three boys. Ann Rheum Dis 1975;34:364.

191. Shore A, Ansell BM: Juvenile psoriatic arthritis: An analysis of 60 cases. J Pediatr 1982;100:529.

192. Southwood TR, Petty RE, Malleson PN: Juvenile psoriatic arthritis—An analysis of 60 cases. Arthritis Rheum 1989;32:1007.

193. Lindsley CB, Schaller JG: Arthritis associated with inflammatory bowel disease in children. J Pediatr 1974;84:16.

194. Cassidy JT, Petty RE: Textbook of Pediatric Rheumatology, 3rd ed. Philadelphia, W.B. Saunders, 1994.

195. Buikstra JE, Poznanski A, Cerna ML, et al: A case of juvenile rheumatoid arthritis from pre-Columbian Peru. In: Buikstra JE, ed: A Life in Science: Papers in Honor of J Lawrence Angel. Kampsville IL, Center for American Archeology, 1990, p 99.

196. Cornil MV: Mémoire sur des coincidences pathologiques du rhumatisme articulaire chronique. C R Mém Soc Biol (Paris) 1864;4:3.

197. Diamantberger S: Du rhumatisme noueux (polyarthrite déformante) chez les infants. Paris, Lecrosnier et Babe, 1890.

198. Still GF: On a form of chronic joint disease in children. Med Chir Trans 1897;80:47. (Reprinted in Arch Dis Child 1941;16:156.)

199. Ohm J: Bandformiae Hornhauttrubung bei einem nainjahrigen madchen und ihre Behandlung mit subkonjunktivalen jodkaliumeinsptritzungen. Klin Monatsbl Augenheilkd 1910;48:243.

200. Towner SR, Michet CJ Jr, O'Fallon WM, et al: The epidemiology of juvenile rheumatoid arthritis in Rochester, Minnesota. Arthritis Rheum 1983;26:1208.

201. Malagon C, Van Kerckhove C, Giannini EH, et al: The iridocyclitis of early onset pauciarticular juvenile rheumatoid arthritis: Outcome in immunogenetically characterised patients. J Rheumatol 1992;19:160.

202. O'Brien JM, Albert DM: Therapeutic approaches for ophthalmic problems in juvenile rheumatoid arthritis. Rheum Dis Clin North Am 1989;15:413.

203. Dana MR, Merayo Lloves J, Schaumberg DA, et al: Visual outcomes prognosticators in juvenile rheumatoid arthritis associated uveitis. Ophthalmology 1997;104:236.

204. Petty RE: Current knowledge of the etiology and pathogenesis of chronic uveitis accompanying juvenile rheumatoid arthritis. Rheum Dis Clin North Am 1987;13:19.

205. Boone MI, Moore TL, Cruz OA: Screening for uveitis in juvenile rheumatoid arthritis. J Pediatr Ophthalmol Strabismus 1998;35:41.

206. Key SW III, Kimura SJ: Iridocyclitis associated with juvenile rheumatoid arthritis. Am J Ophthalmol 1975;80:425.

207. Wolf MD, Lichter PR, Ragsdale CG: Prognostic factors in the uveitis of juvenile rheumatoid arthritis. Ophthalmology 1987;94:1242.

208. Rosenberg AM: Uveitis associated with juvenile rheumatoid arthritis. Semin Arthritis Rheum 1987;16:158.

209. Tugal Tutkun I, Havrlikova K, Power WJ, et al: Changing patterns in uveitis of childhood. Ophthalmology 1996;103:375.

210. Foster CS, Barrett F: Cataract development and cataract surgery in patients with juvenile rheumatoid arthritis associated iridocyclitis. Ophthalmology 1993;100:809.

211. Bywaters EGL: Pathologic aspects of juvenile chronic polyarthritis. Arthritis Rheum 1977;20:271.

212. Merrian JC, Chylack LT, Albert DM: Early onset pauciarticular

juvenile rheumatoid arthritis: A histopathologic study. Arch Ophthalmol 1983;101:1085.

213. Sabates R, Smith T, Apple D: Ocular histopathology in juvenile rheumatoid arthritis. Ann Ophthalmol 1979;733:737.

214. Petty RE, Hunt DWC, Rollins DF, et al: Immunity to soluble retinal antigen in patients with uveitis accompanying juvenile rheumatoid arthritis. Arthritis Rheum 1987;30:287.

215. Gupta D, Singh VK, Rajasingh J, et al: Cellular immune responses of patients with juvenile chronic arthritis to retinal antigens and their synthetic peptides. Immunol Res 1996;15:74.

216. Hunt DW, Petty RE, Millar F: Iris protein antibodies in serum of patients with juvenile rheumatoid arthritis and uveitis. Int Arch Allergy Immunol 1993;100:314.

217. Sakurai Y, Nakajima M, Kamisue S, et al: Preschool sarcoidosis mimicking juvenile rheumatoid arthritis: The significance of gallium scintigraphy and skin biopsy in the differential diagnosis. Acta Pediatr Jpn 1997;39:74.

218. Olson NY, Lindsley CB, Godfrey WA: Nonsteroidal anti-inflammatory drug therapy in chronic childhood iridocyclitis. Am J Dis Child 1988;142:1289.

219. Lovell DJ, Giannini EW, Brewer EJ Jr: Time course of response to nonsteroidal antiinflammatory drugs in juvenile rheumatoid arthritis. Arthritis Rheum 1984;27:1433.

220. Foster CS: Ocular manifestations of childhood arthritis. Womens Health Primary Care 1998;1:823–833.

221. Nguyen QD, Foster CS: Saving the vision of children with juvenile rheumatoid arthritis–associated uveitis. JAMA 1998;280:1133–1134.

222. Diamond JG, Kaplan HG: Lensectomy and vitrectomy for complicated cataract secondary to uveitis. Arch Ophthalmol 1978; 96:1798.

223. Valimaki J, Airaksinen PJ, Tuulonen A: Molteno implantation for secondary glaucoma in juvenile rheumatoid arthritis. Arch Ophthalmol 1997;115:1253.

53 | SYSTEMIC LUPUS ERYTHEMATOSUS

Harvey Siy Uy and Pik Sha Chan

DEFINITION

Systemic lupus erythematosus (SLE) is an autoimmune disease characterized by the production of numerous autoantibodies. Many of the clinical manifestations of SLE, such as lupus nephritis and arthritis, result from tissue damage attributed, at least in part, to the deposition of pathogenic immune complexes. Other manifestations, such as hemolytic anemia, thrombocytopenia, and the antiphospholipid syndrome, arise from the direct effects of autoantibodies on cell surface molecules or serum components. SLE is not organ specific and can affect multiple (if not all) organ systems. The wide distribution of systemic involvement is a result of the fact that the majority of the autoantibodies are targeted against components of the cell nuclei. Arthritis, glomerulonephritis, and dermatitis are the primary clinical manifestations; however, hematologic and neurologic disturbances are also common.

The ocular manifestations of SLE include lid dermatitis, keratitis, scleritis, secondary Sjögren's syndrome, retinal and choroidal vascular lesions, and neuro-ophthalmic lesions. Eye involvement may precede systemic symptoms. Early recognition of ocular lupus erythematosus by the ophthalmologist may prevent not only the blinding complications of SLE but also can lead to timely institution of systemic therapy that may prolong the patient's life and improve its quality.

HISTORY

Lupus dermatitis was first described in 1845 by a dermatologist, Hebra, who regarded it as a benign, local skin condition.[1] Kaposi, in 1872, conducted the first autopsy on a patient with SLE, and he reported that this condition was in fact a systemic illness with potentially life-threatening consequences.[1] The first report of ocular lesions in a patient with SLE was in 1929, with Bergmeister's description of the classic retinal findings of cotton-wool exudates, irregular white patches along the retinal veins, and disc hyperemia.[2] Semon and Wolff conducted histologic examinations of the eyes of patients with SLE in 1933 and found mild choroiditis and subretinal exudation.[3] Baehr and colleagues reported, in 1935, that 50% of patients with SLE developed retinal lesions.[4, 5] Maumenee also conducted histologic studies, which revealed retinal cytoid bodies, superficial retinal hemorrhages, and mild choroiditis in the eyes of patients with SLE retinopathy.[6]

In 1971, the American Rheumatic Association published a report, "The Preliminary Criteria for the Classification of Systemic Lupus Erythematosus," which provided the first published criteria for the diagnosis of SLE. This was followed in 1982 by "The 1982 Revised Criteria for the Classification of Systemic Lupus Erythematosus," which incorporated serologic abnormalities, such as antibodies to DNA, antinuclear antibodies, serum complement, and other serologic and immunopathologic assays

(Table 53–1). These criteria are widely accepted and currently provide the basis for standardized diagnosis of SLE in clinical and research work.[7]

EPIDEMIOLOGY

The prevalence of SLE varies worldwide. The prevalence in North America and Northern Europe is 40 per 100,000 population. The female-to-male ratio is about 9:1. Black Americans and Hispanics appear to have higher incidence rates. Over 80% of cases involve women in their childbearing years. SLE may affect up to 1 in 1000 young women (1 in 250 black women). The prevalence in children and older adults is approximately 1 per 100,000.[8]

CLINICAL CHARACTERISTICS

Systemic Manifestations

The systemic manifestations of SLE are diverse.[8, 9] To aid in establishing a diagnosis, the American Rheumatism Association has established 11 diagnostic criteria for SLE (see Table 53–1). A diagnosis of SLE can be made when four of these criteria are met. It should be emphasized that these criteria were primarily intended for the use of clinical investigators. For patient management, a clinical diagnosis may be made even when less than four criteria are met.

Cutaneous disease affects approximately 85% of patients. The characteristic butterfly rash across the nose and cheeks, known as the malar flush, is the most common finding, appearing as flat or slightly raised, fixed erythema over the malar eminences, usually sparing the nasolabial folds (Fig. 53–1). Discoid lupus erythematosus consists of erythematous raised areas with adherent keratotic scaling and follicular plugging (Fig. 53–2). Cutaneous ulcers, splinter hemorrhages, purpuric skin lesions, and alopecia are other dermatologic manifestations that occur frequently as well. Less common skin lesions include maculopapular eruptions, lupus profundus, hypertrophic discoid lesions (Fig. 53–3), bullae, and urticarial

TABLE 53–1. THE 1982 REVISED CRITERIA FOR THE CLASSIFICATION OF SYSTEMIC LUPUS ERYTHEMATOSUS

1. Malar rash
2. Discoid rash
3. Photosensitivity
4. Oral ulcers
5. Arthritis (nonerosive, two or more peripheral joints)
6. Serositis (pleuritis, pericarditis)
7. Renal disorder (proteinuria, nephritis)
8. Neurologic disorder (seizures, psychosis)
9. Hematologic disorder (hemolytic anemia, leukopenia, lymphopenia, thrombocytopenia)
10. Immunologic disorder (positive LE cell prep, anti-native DNA, anti-Sm, false-positive test for syphilis)
11. Antinuclear antibody (in the absence of drugs associated with "drug-induced" lupus)

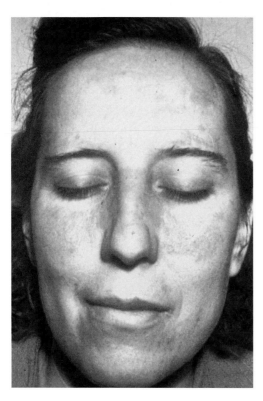

FIGURE 53–1. Lupus mask or butterfly rash. Note the erythematous dermatitis over the malar eminences of the cheeks and the bridge of the nose. (See color insert.)

skin lesions. Painless oral ulcers may be found in 30% to 40% of patients. Initiation or exacerbation with sun exposure is characteristic of lupus erythematosus skin lesions. Raynaud's phenomenon occurs in about 20% of patients.

Arthritis is a very common initial symptom; it may afflict up to 85% of SLE patients. Lupus arthritis presents as painful or tender peripheral joint involvement or nondeforming, migratory polyarthritis. Other, less frequent musculoskeletal manifestations include cutaneous nodules, myalgias, and myositis.

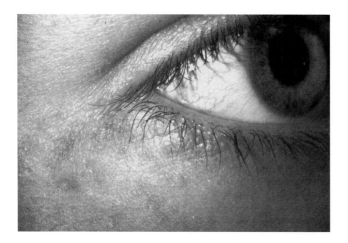

FIGURE 53–2. Discoid lupus in a patient with chronic blepharitis. Note the subtle erythematous lesions of the skin of the lower eyelid. (See color insert.)

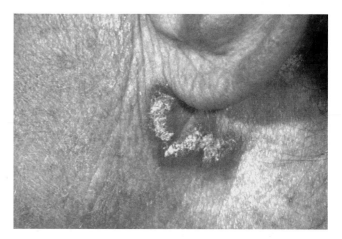

FIGURE 53–3. Hypertrophic discoid lupus. Note the hypertrophic lesion under the patient's left ear, with silvery keratinization on the surface. (See color insert.)

Nonspecific systemic symptoms such as fatigue, fever, and weight loss affect most patients with SLE.

Renal involvement occurs in approximately half of the patients and may take the form of either nephrotic syndrome with proteinuria or glomerulonephritis producing "active" urinary sediment. Mesangial disease, focal proliferative nephritis, diffuse proliferative nephritis, and membranous glomerulonephritis may manifest in lupus patients. Lupus nephritis is the major cause of morbidity and mortality in patients with SLE.

Cardiac involvement may occur, with pericarditis (seen in approximately 20% of lupus patients), myocarditis, and Libman-Sacks endocarditis. Libman-Sacks endocarditis is associated with the presence of phospholipid antibody. Potential pulmonary lesions include pleuritis and pneumonitis. Hepatosplenomegaly and adenopathy, while not part of the diagnostic criteria, can be seen in many patients with SLE.

Neuropsychiatric manifestations occur in about a third of patients with SLE. Seizures, organic brain syndrome, and psychosis may occur. Transverse myelitis is a rare manifestation, occurring in only 4% of patients with SLE, but it is often seen in association with optic neuritis. Peripheral neuropathy and cranial nerve palsies are less commonly seen.

Hematologic abnormalities are frequently detected in patients with SLE. Chronic anemia or autoimmune hemolytic anemia, leukopenia, lymphopenia, and thrombocytopenia are commonly observed. In addition, lupus patients are prone to thrombotic episodes.

Ocular Manifestations

SLE can involve the eye and adnexae. SLE should be considered in the differential diagnosis of mucocutaneous disease, episcleritis, scleritis, keratoconjunctivitis sicca, keratopathy, uveitis, retinal and choroidal microangiopathy, papillitis, and neuro-ophthalmic disease.[10]

The eyelids may manifest the inflammatory and scaly lesions of discoid lupus erythematosus. The patients complain of recurrent eyelid irritation and redness, more prominent over the lateral third of the lower eyelids. Discoid lupus erythematosus of the eyelids may be pres-

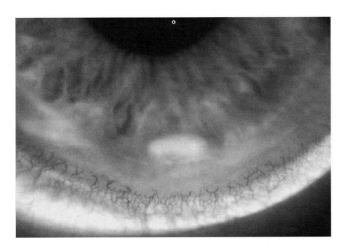

FIGURE 53–4. Peripheral keratitis in a patient with systemic lupus erythematosus. Note the perilimbal, circumferential mid to deep stromal infiltrate in the corneal stroma. (See color insert.)

ent for years, until a skin biopsy is performed. Histopathologic features include hyperkeratosis, basal cell vacuolation, perivasculitis, and dermal inflammation.[11] We have described a distinct hypertrophic variant of discoid lupus erythematosus involving the conjunctiva.[12]

Secondary Sjögren's syndrome, or keratoconjunctivitis sicca, occurs in approximately 20% of patients with SLE and is indistinguishable from the sicca complex seen in other connective tissue diseases.[13–15] Abnormal Schirmer and rose bengal staining tests may show reduced tear flow and staining of the corneal and conjunctival epithelia. Filamentary conjunctivitis may also develop as part of the sicca syndrome.[10, 16] In addition to keratoconjunctivitis sicca, Halmay and Ludwig in 1965 described a grayish white, band-shaped infiltration in the central corneal stroma (Fig. 53–4).[17] Reeves described a similar diffuse white haze, which progressed to a granular lesion despite topical steroid treatment.[18]

Scleritis is frequently associated with systemic vascular diseases such as SLE. In a review of 172 patients with scleritis, Sainz de la Maza and coauthors found systemic vasculitic disease present in 82 patients (48%) including seven with systemic lupus erythematosus (4%).[19] Of these seven patients, four manifested with diffuse anterior, two with nodular, and one with posterior scleritis. Scleritis in a patient with systemic lupus generally has a good ocular prognosis, because necrotizing scleritis rarely develops in patients with SLE.

Episcleritis may also be associated with SLE. In a review of 100 patients with episcleritis, Akpek and coauthors noted SLE as an underlying disease in 4 of 36 (11%) patients with an identifiable systemic illness. Although episcleritis is generally considered a benign, self-limited disease, a careful review of systems and an ocular examination should still be conducted in patients with episcleritis, so as not to miss an associated ocular or underlying systemic condition.[20]

Angle-closure glaucoma secondary to uveal effusion may be an initial manifestation of SLE. Recently, Wisotsky and colleagues reported a case of bilateral pleural and uveal effusions with secondary angle-closure and elevated

intraocular pressures. Intraocular pressures were refractory to antiglaucoma medications and laser therapy. Drainage of the choroidal effusion via sclerotomies resulted in resolution of the angle-closure glaucoma.[21]

Perhaps the most well recognized ocular manifestation of SLE is lupus retinopathy.[22–27] This potentially blinding condition is considered an important marker of disease activity by rheumatologists. Visual loss from lupus retinopathy is viewed as an important index of disease severity.[28] Since the initial report by Bergmeister in 1929, numerous authors have described lupus retinopathy.[2, 3, 6, 10, 29] In the presteroid era, retinopathy was present in up to half of SLE patients.[4] However, with the advent of steroid and immunosuppressive therapy, the incidence of retinopathy has declined considerably. The prevalence of lupus retinopathy ranges from 3% in an outpatient population with mild to absent disease,[11] to 29% among patients with active disease.[30] However, in patients on maintenance therapy with chloroquine, Klinkhoff and associates detected retinopathy in 7 of 43 (16%) patients. Systemic lupus activity was present in five of these seven patients (71%). The onset of retinopathy may be associated with exacerbation of systemic SLE.[29]

The lesions of lupus retinopathy are varied in appearance but most are believed to arise from retinal vasculitis. The different manifestations of lupus retinopathy and their complications are listed in Table 53–2. These funduscopic findings may be classified into the five following, closely related categories.[10, 22–25, 31–33]

Vasculitis

Inflammation of the retinal vasculature may lead to focal leakage from the retinal capillaries and arterioles. Funduscopic signs of vasculitis include retinal arterial sheathing (Fig. 53–5). Fluorescein angiography reveals dye leakage from the retinal blood vessels (Fig. 53–6). Vasculitis of the optic nerve vessels may lead to optic nerve head swelling and subsequent ischemic optic neuropathy.

Vaso-occlusion

MICROVASCULAR OCCLUSION

Cotton-wool spots are the classic lesions of lupus retinopathy (Fig. 53–7, and Tables 53–2 and 53–3). These represent focal areas of ischemia where there is interruption

TABLE 53–2. SIGNS OF LUPUS RETINOPATHY

1. Cotton-wool spots
2. Retinal hemorrhage: dot, blot, flame-shaped
3. Preretinal hemorrhage
4. Microaneurysms
5. Focal narrowing of retinal vasculature
6. Arterial occlusion with focal deposits
7. Central/branch retinal arterial occlusion with cherry red spot
8. Central/branch venous occlusion
9. Retinal neovascularization
10. Anterior segment ischemia
11. Vitreous hemorrhage
12. Traction retinal detachment
13. Neovascular or hemorrhagic glaucoma
14. Hypertensive changes (arteriolar narrowing, hard exudates, flame hemorrhages, papilledema)
15. Optic disc vasculitis

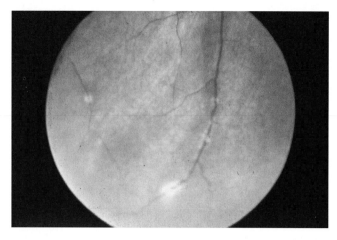

FIGURE 53–5. Retinal arteritis in a patient with systemic lupus erythematosus. Note the periarteriolar inflammatory cell infiltrate. (See color insert.)

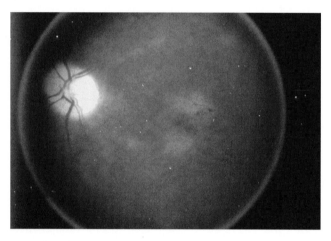

FIGURE 53–6. Fluorescein angiogram, late phase, in a patient with arteriolitis secondary to systemic lupus erythematosus. In addition to late vascular staining, note also the fluorescein dye leakage into the macula (cystoid macular edema).

TABLE 53–3. INTRAOCULAR FINDINGS IN PATIENTS WITH SYSTEMIC LUPUS ERYTHEMATOSUS

Cotton-wool spots	168/1473 (11.4)
Retinal hemorrhages	111/1473 (7.5)
Arterial narrowing	86/1473 (5.8)
Papilledema	13/1473 (0.9)
Retinal edema	9/1473 (0.6)
Uveitis	6/1473 (0.4)

From Gold DH, Morris DA, Henkind P: Ocular findings in systemic lupus erythematosus. Br J Ophthalmol 1972; 56:800.

of axoplasmic flow within the nerve fibers of the retina, resulting in accumulation of axoplasmic material and swelling of the nerve fiber. Cotton-wool spots in SLE are believed to result from occlusion of the small retinal arterioles, or endarterioles, by infiltrating inflammatory cells. They may occur singly and be asymptomatic or they may be extensive in number and cause visual loss when the macula is involved. On fluorescein angiography, cotton-wool spots correspond to areas of focal nonperfusion (Fig. 53–8). In contrast to retinal nonperfusion from hypertension and diabetes, the ischemia produced in lupus retinopathy is often not as extensive and is not associated with widespread arterial narrowing.[26, 31]

ARTERIAL OCCLUSION

Arterial occlusion is a rare form of lupus retinopathy characterized by occlusion of the central retinal artery causing widespread retinal ischemia and severe, permanent visual loss.[30] The clinical characteristics of central retinal artery occlusion include rapid-onset, painless blurring of vision, a Marcus-Gunn afferent pupil defect, retinal arterial attenuation, and macular edema and whitening that result in a cherry-red spot appearance of the fovea. The prognosis for this type of lesion is as poor as it is for central retinal artery occlusion.[27, 31] Sudden visual loss with central retinal artery occlusion in a young patient should prompt the clinician to include SLE and other collagen diseases in the list of differential diagnosis. Multifocal branch arterial occlusion or the larger retinal

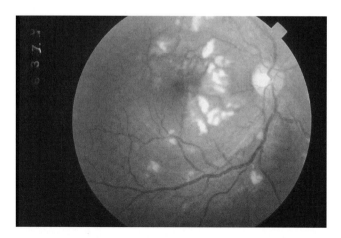

FIGURE 53–7. Extensive lupus retinopathy, with arteriolitis, arteriolar occlusion, and retinal infarcts, with extensive cotton-wool lesions in the nerve fiber layer of the retina. (See color insert.)

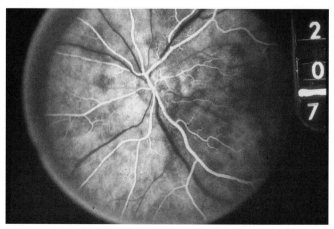

FIGURE 53–8. Fluorescein angiogram, arterial phase, in a patient with systemic lupus erythematosus. Note the patchy pattern of choroidal filling, indicative of choroidal involvement in the vasculitis process.

arteries may also occur, leading to larger areas of retinal ischemia and edema.[24, 34]

VENOUS OCCLUSION

Although lupus retinopathy is not principally a venous disease, central retinal vein occlusion has been reported to occur in association with SLE. It may be that an initial arterial occlusion causes secondary venous stasis and engorgement leading to central or branch vein occlusion. Subsequent reperfusion of the arteries, coupled with inflammatory damage to the venous endothelium, may lead to retinal and papillary hemorrhage. Venous occlusion is a rare manifestation of lupus retinopathy but can be a cause of permanent visual loss.[26, 35, 36]

Vasodisruption

Intraretinal hemorrhages are frequent findings in lupus retinopathy. Other vascular abnormalities that develop uncommonly in lupus retinopathy include microaneurysm formation, vascular leakage with retinal edema, and preretinal hemorrhages.[23, 25] The pathogenesis of these changes is unknown. Stafford-Brady and coauthors believe that the presence of retinal hemorrhages is a significant finding because it is associated with a greater risk of mortality.[33]

ISCHEMIC SEQUELAE

Severe retinal ischemia from either arterial or venous occlusive disease may result in retinal neovascularization.[25, 32] The complications of severe ischemia, such as vitreous hemorrhage, traction retinal detachment, and secondary neovascular or hemorrhagic glaucoma, are sight threatening.

HYPERTENSIVE SEQUELAE

Renal involvement by SLE will generally lead to secondary hypertension. When prolonged, the retina may develop hypertensive retinopathy characterized by bilateral retinal arterial narrowing, arteriovenous crossing changes, intraretinal hemorrhages, hard exudate formation, and hypertensive papilledema. Rarely, multiple areas of choroidal infarction (Elschnig's spots) may appear as localized brown-red areas ophthalmoscopically. These foci show underlying choriocapillaris nonperfusion on fluorescein angiography and may be associated with transudation of subretinal fluid and neurosensory retinal detachment.[14, 34, 37]

A review of 1473 SLE patients from several published series[10] revealed the frequencies of ocular findings shown in Table 53–3. In a large prospective study of 550 patients designed to examine the relationship of lupus retinopathy to systemic disease, Stafford-Brady and co-workers found that 41 patients (7.5%) exhibited lupus retinopathy. Of these patients, 34 had microangiopathy (cotton-wool spots in 20 patients; hemorrhages in 7; both cotton-wool spots and hemorrhages in 7), and 3 exhibited transient papilledema.[33]

Fluorescein angiography is useful for visualizing the retinal vasculature and often demonstrates abrupt termination of retinal arteries and arterioles, producing areas of poor capillary-bed perfusion. The areas of retinal nonperfusion are often located around the disc or within the macula, suggesting precapillary arteriole occlusion. Other findings include focal areas of capillary dropout corresponding to cotton-wool spots, irregular retinal artery caliber, and arterial and venous dye leakage (Fig. 53–9). The veins may exhibit marked stasis with segmentation of the blood column and sometimes late dye extravasation. Neovascular tufts may also be seen as points of early dye leakage on fluorescein angiography.[22, 24, 38]

As seen in diabetic retinopathy, an early lesion in lupus retinopathy may be retinal capillary microaneurysms. A fluorescein angiographic study of ambulatory, moderately active and inactive SLE patients revealed microaneurysms and/or retinal capillary dilation that leaked fluorescein in 13 of 50 consecutive patients (24%). Only drusen were seen ophthalmoscopically in three of these patients. It is unclear whether these microaneurysms represent the earliest lesions or residual lesions from previous inflammatory episodes.[24, 39]

Another large series of fluorescein angiograms performed on 50, mostly in-patients at the Hammersmith Hospital[30] compared angiographic findings of asymptomatic patients, patients with intermediately active disease (arthralgias, mild skin rash, pleuritis, alopecia, and malaise), and patients with severely active disease (arthritis, nephritis, cerebral disease, extensive cutaneous vasculitis). Ten of the 26 patients (38%) with highly active disease had cotton-wool spots, papillitis, or vascular leakage. In the intermediate group, 2 of 13 patients (15%) had angiographic changes (vascular leakage). Only 1 of 11 asymptomatic patients (9%) manifested angiographic changes (disc vasculitis). One of the 50 patients exhibited severe arterial occlusive disease with retinal neovascularization, and another had extensive venous disease. This study concluded that angiographic changes in SLE are more frequently found in patients with active disease. However, the authors were careful to point out previous reports that emphasized that severe retinal vasculitis may occur without systemic illness.[40] This study failed to find an association between retinopathy and cerebral disease.[30]

Choroidopathy is an even more rare manifestation of SLE, with only about a dozen cases reported in the English literature. Lupus choroidopathy presents as single or

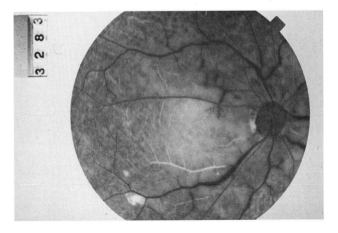

FIGURE 53–9. Fluorescein angiogram in a patient with systemic lupus erythematosus demonstrating arteriolitis and irregular arteriolar and venular caliber with capillary dropout around areas of retinal infarction.

TABLE 53–4. SYMPTOMS AND SITES OF NEURO-OPHTHALMIC INVOLVEMENT IN PATIENTS WITH SYSTEMIC LUPUS ERYTHEMATOSUS

Neuro-ophthalmic symptoms
    Transient amaurosis
    Cortical blindness
    Visual field defects
    Papilledema
    Optic atrophy
    Strabismus
    Pseudotumor cerebri
    Visual hallucinations
Sites of neuro-ophthalmic involvement in SLE
    Extraocular muscle involvement
    Optic neuritis
    Retrobulbar neuritis
    Ischemic optic neuropathy
    Retrochiasmal tract involvement
    Occipital lobe infarct
    Cerebrum

multiple areas of serous elevation of the retinal pigment epithelium and sensory retina with associated retinal pigment epithelial mottling.[41] Fluorescein angiography reveals focal areas of fluorescein leakage through the retinal pigment epithelium, with dye pooling under the sensory retina. Lupus choroidopathy is highly associated with systemic involvement. In the 12 patients reported, six manifested with hypertension and nephritis, three with systemic vasculitis, one with CNS lupus, and one with disseminated intravascular coagulopathy and thrombotic thrombocytopenic purpura. The ocular prognosis for lupus choroidopathy is relatively good when systemic immunosuppressive treatment is given. Eleven of the 12 described patients subsequently experienced resolution or improvement of the choroidopathy.[24, 29, 41–44]

Whereas central nervous system (CNS) disease in SLE is well known, neuro-ophthalmic involvement is probably underrecognized (Table 53–4). Extraocular muscle problems may result from either cranial nerve or muscle involvement. Optic nerve involvement may take several forms. Papilledema is observed frequently but is rarely associated with visual loss.[45, 46] Optic neuritis,[47] ischemic optic neuropathy,[48] and inflammation of the optic chiasm, retrochiasmal tracts, and occipital lobes may cause visual disturbances and blindness.[49] In optic disc vasculitis, the visual field loss is either complete or an altitudinal hemianopia, and the visual prognosis is poor, whereas in optic neuritis, visual field defects are either central or patchy, and visual recovery is generally considerable.[30]

Cerebral involvement may take the form of visual hallucinations and field loss.[49] Histopathologic studies reveal at least two types of nervous tissue involvement: The first type consists of microangiopathy resulting in focal demyelination, axonal damage, and optic nerve infarcts.[45, 50–52] The second type is inflammation of the nervous tissues. Transverse myelitis is present in more than half of patients with lupus optic neuropathy.[47] Other rare manifestations include pseudotumor cerebri[53] and neuromyelitis optica, a form of multiple sclerosis characterized by spinal cord demyelination and optic atrophy.[50]

PATHOPHYSIOLOGY

SLE is generally believed to result from a complex interplay of genetic, infectious, and immunologic factors. Familial aggregation of autoimmune diseases and the association with the HLA types HLA-DR2 and HLA-DR3 suggest a genetic predisposition. A greater concordance rate of 30% to 50% in monozygotic twins has been reported. Histocompatibility antigens may play a role in the pathogenesis of SLE and discoid lupus erythematosus. HLA-B8 is associated with SLE in females, whereas HLA-B7 and HLA-B8.42 are associated with discoid lupus erythematosus.[8, 54]

An animal model of lupus exists in the MRL-*lpr* mouse, in which a gene for lymphoproliferation has been bred. In this model, accumulation of CD3+CD4-CD8- T lymphocytes and autoreactive CD4+ T cells leads to massive lymphadenopathy and development of autoimmunity. It is believed that these autoreactive T cells stimulate the growth and differentiation of autoreactive B cells, which in turn produce autoantibodies that cause arthritis and nephritis in these mice. When neonatal MRL-*lpr* mice are thymectomized, autoimmunity does not develop, further strengthening the theory that T cells are important in the development of autoimmunity. The *lpr* gene, also identified as the *fas* gene, is involved in the process of apoptosis (cell death), which has been implicated in the clonal deletion of self-reactive lymphocytes.[54, 55] Inheritance of a defective second component of complement (C2) can also produce a lupus-like syndrome.[56]

A viral etiology is suspected in the development of human and experimental SLE. Type C virus expression has been identified in NZB mice as well as in the lymphocytes and kidneys of some SLE patients.[46] NZB mice are deficient in CD8 cytotoxic/suppressor T cells. This defect may lead to decreased immune surveillance and allow infection by oncogenic viruses. These viruses may then incorporate their genomes into the host cell genome. These genetic changes may then incite development of antibodies against the now altered host DNA. Viral antigens on infected cell surfaces may provoke development of autoantibodies in an exaggerated humoral response against these infected cells, which are now considered by the immune system as nonself.[54] Aside from an infectious agent, drugs and environmental triggers such as radiation may damage normal body constituents, resulting in the formation of immunogens. Because these immunogens resemble normal human constituents, an immunologic response may be induced against these normal structures in a process called molecular mimicry.[8]

SLE is characterized by suppressor T-cell dysfunction, B-cell hyperreactivity, polyclonal B-cell activation, hypergammaglobulinemia, loss of immune tolerance, and autoantibody production. These autoantibodies include antinuclear antibodies, antibodies to DNA, both single-stranded DNA (anti-ssDNA) and double-stranded or native DNA (anti-dsDNA or anti-nDNA), and antibodies to cytoplasmic components. These autoantibodies enter the circulation and are deposited in various target organs throughout the body, where they form pathogenic immune complexes that incite inflammatory responses and activate the complement system. The resulting inflammation then causes organ damage and clinical disease such as vasculitis, nephritis, and arthritis. A variety of autoantibodies are produced by patients with SLE, and different autoantibody "profiles" (antinuclear antibodies, anti-

Smith, anti-ribonucleoprotein, anti-histone) appear to be somewhat predictive of the clinical pattern of the patient's disease.[56] Recent studies suggest that a wider than previously appreciated array of autoantibodies are produced in patients with SLE,[57] including autoantibodies against annexias,[58] the CD45 cell surface glycoprotein,[59] calreticulin,[60] and nucleosomes.[61] Indeed, it may be that the loss of tolerance for nucleosomes is a primary event, with aberrant apoptosis resulting in their systemic release, and nucleosomes then driving the autoimmune response, with nucleosome-specific CD4 T cells inducing anti-dsDNA and anti-histone antibody production. It appears that nucleosomal antigens (histone and DNA) complexed to anti-dsDNA are very efficient at binding to renal glomerular basement membrane and inducing nephritis. Monocyte-macrophage function is depressed in early SLE, and because these cells participate in the processing of antigen and in lymphokine activity, this defect could result in depressed cellular immunity.[62]

Vasculitis is believed to be the starting point in the pathogenesis of tissue and organ damage in SLE. As early as 1932, Goldstein and Wexler demonstrated extensive fibrinoid necrosis of the vessel walls.[40] Perivascular inflammatory infiltrates have been demonstrated in eyes with SLE vasculitis. Immunoglobulin and complement deposits have been demonstrated in the retinal and cerebral blood vessel walls,[63] ciliary body, choroid, and conjunctival basement membrane of SLE patients.[64]

An animal model of uveal and retinal vasculitis exists. When antigen is injected into the vitreous of hyperimmune rabbits, intense vasculitis develops. Immunohistochemical studies reveal immune complex deposition within the vessel walls. These immune complexes can activate the complement system and trigger rapid neutrophilic infiltration, which in turn causes vascular occlusion and ischemia. This mechanism may occur in lupus retinopathy, leading to vaso-occlusion.[65]

Vascular lesions in the eye may mirror vascular alterations in other parts of the body. Intimal and medial thickening of the retinal vessel walls, as well as deposition of fibrinoid material causing vaso-occlusion in the superficial and deep nerve fiber layers, has been observed by Maumenee[7] and by Clifton and Greer.[39] In severe vascular involvement, widespread necrosis of the retina with lymphocytic and plasma cell infiltration may be observed. The similarities between pathologic lesions of the retinal and CNS vasculature are well described and may account for the association between retinal and CNS involvement.[6, 40, 66]

DIAGNOSIS
The diagnosis of SLE is based on a combination of clinical and laboratory findings (see Table 53–1). The detection of antinuclear antibodies is a good screening test for SLE, as it occurs in 95% of patients. However, antinuclear antibodies are present in most other rheumatic diseases, as well as in autoimmune liver and thyroid disease, and thus should be considered a nonspecific test. More specific antibodies for the diagnosis of SLE include antibodies to dsDNA and to Smith antigen.[8]

Occasionally, ocular manifestations may precede systemic findings. The ophthalmologist should be suspicious of any young patient with cotton-wool spots or hemorrhages. An appropriate referral to a rheumatologist or internist should then be made. Funduscopy and indirect ophthalmoscopy are the most important means of detecting lupus retinopathy. Fluorescein angiography is of limited value in the initial definitive diagnosis of SLE. Angiographic findings in lupus retinopathy are nonspecific and may be mirrored by other retinal vasculitides or vaso-occlusive diseases such as Adamantiades-Behçet's disease, diabetic and hypertensive retinopathy, and other collagen vascular diseases. Angiographic findings are not predictive of cerebral disease but may indicate systemic activity. No relationship has been found between retinal and cutaneous vasculitis.[31] There has been no prospective study that has investigated the prognostic value of fluorescein angiography. Angiography, however, may be used to evaluate retinal perfusion and detect retinal neovascularization or edema that may be amenable to laser treatment or cryotherapy. Angiography is also useful in confirming the diagnosis of lupus choroidopathy.

The Farnsworth 100 hue test may detect abnormalities in hue discrimination among patients with SLE retinopathy and should be performed in cases of suspected lupus retinopathy. This test, however, is nonspecific and its interpretation should be made cautiously, especially when antimalarial treatment is being given, as these medicines may also affect hue discrimination.[29]

The differential diagnosis for multifocal retinal vascular occlusive disease includes Adamantiades-Behçet's disease, polyarteritis nodosa, Takayasu's disease, Wegener's granulomatosis, and syphilis. Cotton-wool spots may be seen in diabetes, hypertension, and radiation retinopathy.

Antiphospholipid antibodies are present in approximately 17% of SLE patients, and these are associated with thrombotic disorders, such as deep vein thrombophlebitis and strokes. Lupus anticoagulant is related to other antiphospholipid antibodies, including the anticardiolipin antibody and the biologic false-positive test for syphilis. Lupus anticoagulant is an immunoglobulin that reacts in vitro with negatively charged phospholipids (platelet factor 3), thereby inhibiting the generation of prothrombin activator complex. Lupus anticoagulant together with other related antiphospholipid antibodies, such as the anticardiolipin antibodies, are associated with thrombotic events. Circulating lupus anticoagulant may be found in some patients with SLE. While the role of antiphospholipid antibodies is unclear, it is hypothesized that they may cause thrombotic phenomena by means of induction of platelet aggregation or by inhibition of prostacyclin production by the vascular endothelium.[67–69]

TREATMENT
Immunosuppressive therapy is the mainstay of treatment for both systemic and ocular lupus. The choice of treatment is dependent on the organ involved and on the severity of the lesions. When only arthritis or serositis is present, nonsteroidal anti-inflammatory agents may be sufficient to control the disease. Antimalarials are primarily used in the treatment of skin disease. Chloroquine retinopathy may result from chloroquine treatment. This may take the form of macular pigmentary changes, blurred vision, and paracentral visual field depression.

Steroids are usually reserved for hematologic, renal, and CNS involvement. Long-term steroid-sparing maintenance therapy may necessitate the use of systemic immunosuppressive agents such as cyclophosphamide or azathioprine.[8, 9, 70] It should be noted that ocular relapse or activity may occur independently of systemic signs,[26, 28] and that the onset of scleritis or retinal vasculitis in a patient with otherwise apparently well controlled SLE is a very ominous sign, portending a lupus flare unless the vigor of therapy is increased considerably.

Laser photocoagulation in cases of severe vaso-occlusive disease may be successful in ameliorating the ischemic complications of lupus retinopathy. Care should be taken during panretinal photocoagulation, as anterior segment ischemia can develop after laser treatment. Full control systemically of the SLE may be advisable prior to laser treatment. Vitreoretinal surgery may be indicated for patients with vitreous hemorrhage or traction retinal detachment.[26]

PROGNOSIS

With current methods of treatment, the 10-year survival rate of SLE patients approaches 90%. The risk factors for poorer prognosis include nephritis, hypertension, onset at younger age, male sex, and the presence of antibodies to native DNA.[9]

While retinal lesions may occur frequently in SLE, they are rare causes of visual impairment. Poor visual outcome is associated with severe vaso-occlusive disease, retinal vasculitis, central retinal artery occlusion, central retinal venous occlusion, and traction retinal detachment. Jabs and colleagues[26] and Gold and coworkers[25] have demonstrated that severe retinal vascular disease correlated with CNS disease and not with hematologic and renal involvement. Both groups believe that severe retinal involvement should be considered a marker for CNS disease. In contrast, Klinkoff and colleagues[30] and Lanham and coworkers[31] could not find an association between less severe lupus retinopathy and CNS disease in their series.

In a large prospective series of 550 patients conducted by Stafford-Brady and coworkers, 88% of patients with lupus retinopathy had active lupus at the time retinopathy was diagnosed. Active CNS lupus was present in 73% of patients with retinopathy. The CNS manifestations included organic brain syndrome, focal neurologic deficit, psychoneurosis, intractable headaches, psychosis, and seizures. Renal disease was present in 63.5% of patients. The study also found that 34% of patients who developed lupus retinopathy died, whereas only 10.8% of patients without retinopathy expired. Patients who developed retinal hemorrhages had the highest risk for mortality (50%). The visual prognosis among these SLE patients was excellent—only 5 of 550 (0.9%) developed blindness. Microangiopathy or transient papilledema was not associated with permanent visual loss. Loss of vision resulted from ischemic optic neuropathy, central retinal vein occlusion, central retinal artery occlusion, or serous retinal detachment. The frequency of lupus anticoagulant among all SLE patients was found to be 17%. An increased frequency of lupus anticoagulant (38%) was detected among patients with lupus retinopathy.[34] The study concluded that lupus retinopathy carries a good prognosis for vision but a poor prognosis for survival.[27] Other authors have suggested that the incidence of retinal thrombosis may occur independently of systemic disease activity.[34, 68, 70]

CONCLUSIONS

SLE is an autoimmune, multisystem disorder with a propensity for involving ocular tissues. Although ocular involvement is generally benign, potentially blinding complications may occur. When lupus retinopathy or neuro-ophthalmic involvement is detected in a patient, the prudent ophthalmologist should also conduct a thorough search for systemic involvement and refer the patient to the appropriate clinical services. Early recognition of SLE and timely institution of systemic therapy may minimize morbidity and mortality from this disease.

References

1. Hebra F, Kaposi M: On Disease of the Skin Including the Exanthemata. Translated and Edited by W. Tay. London, The New Sydenham Society, 1875.
2. Bergmeister R: Uber primare and miliare Tuberkulose der Retina. Wien Med Schnschr 1929;79:1116.
3. Semon HC, Wolff E: Acute lupus erythematosus with fundus lesions. Proc R Soc Med 1933;27:153.
4. Baehr G, Klemperer P, Schifrin A: A diffuse disease of the peripheral circulation (usually associated with lupus erythematosus and endocarditis). Trans Assoc Am Physicians 1935;50:139.
5. Klemperer P, Baehr G, Schifrin A: Pathology of lupus erythematosus. Arch Path 1941;32:569.
6. Maumenee AE: Retinal lesions in lupus erythematosus. Am J Ophthalmol 1940;23:971.
7. Tan EM, Cohen AS, Fries JF, et al: The 1982 revised criteria for the classification of systemic lupus erythematosus. Arthritis Rheum 1982;25:1271.
8. Mills JA: Systemic lupus erythematosus. N Engl J Med 1994;330:1871.
9. Steinberg AD: Management of systemic lupus erythematosus. In: Kelly WN, Harris ED, Ruddy S, et al, eds: Textbook of Rheumatology, 2nd ed. Philadelphia, W.B. Saunders, 1985, p 1130.
10. Gold DH, Morris DA, Henkind P: Ocular findings in systemic lupus erythematosus. Br J Ophthalmol 1972;56:800.
11. Huey C, Jakobiec FA, Iwamoto T, et al: Discoid lupus erythematosus of the eyelids. Ophthalmology 1983;90:1389.
12. Uy HS, Pineda R 2nd, Shore JW, et al: Hypertrophic discoid lupus erythematosus of the conjunctiva. Am J Ophthalmol 1999;127:604.
13. Alarcon-Segovia D, Ibanez G, Hernandez-Ortiz I, et al: Sjögren's syndrome in progressive systemic scleroderma. Am J Med 1974;57:78.
14. Steinberg AD, Talal N: The coexistence of Sjögren's syndrome and systemic lupus erythematosus. Ann Intern Med 1971;74:55.
15. Whaley K, Webb J, McAvoy BA, et al: Sjögren's syndrome. 2. Clinical associations and immunological phenomena. Q J Med 1974;42:513.
16. Grennan DM, Forrester J: Involvement of the eye in SLE and scleroderma. Ann Rheum Dis 1977;36:152.
17. Halmay O, Ludwig K: Bilateral band-shaped deep keratitis and iridocyclitis in systemic lupus erythematosus. Br J Ophthalmol 1964;48:558.
18. Reeves J: Keratopathy associated with systemic lupus erythematosus. Arch Ophthalmol 1965;74:159.
19. Sainz de la Maza M, Foster CS, Jabbur NS: Scleritis associated with systemic vasculitic diseases. Ophthalmology 1995;102:687.
20. Akpek EK, Uy HS, Christen W, et al: Severity of episcleritis and systemic disease association. Ophthalmology 1999;106:729.
21. Wisotsky BJ, Magat-Gordon CB, Puklin JE: Angle-closure glaucoma as an initial presentation of systemic lupus erythematosus. Ophthalmology 1998;105:1170.
22. Bishko F: Retinopathy in systemic lupus erythematosus. Arthritis Rheum 1972;15:57.
23. Coppeto J, Lessell S: Retinopathy in systemic lupus erythematosus. Arch Ophthalmol 1977;95:794.

24. Gold D, Feiner L, Henkind P: Retinal arterial occlusive disease in systemic lupus erythematosus. Arch Ophthalmol 1977;95:1580.

25. Jabs DA, Fine SL, Hochberg MC, et al: Severe retinal vaso-occlusive disease in systemic lupus erythematosus. Arch Ophthalmol 1986;104:558.

26. Silverman M, Lubeck MJ, Briney WG: Central retinal vein occlusion complicating systemic lupus erythematosus. Arthritis Rheum 1978;21:839.

27. Wong K, Ai E, Jones JV, Young D: Visual loss as the initial symptom of systemic lupus erythematosus. Am J Ophthalmol 1981;92:238.

28. Committee on Prognosis Studies in SLE: Prognosis studies in SLE: An activity index (abstract). Arthritis Rheum 1986;29(suppl 4):S93.

29. Klinkhoff AV, Beattie CW, Chalmers A: Retinopathy in systemic lupus erythematosus: Relationship to disease activity. Arthritis Rheum 1986;29:1152.

30. Lanham JG, Barrie T, Kohner EM, Hughs RV: SLE retinopathy: Evaluation by fluorescein angiography. Ann Rheum Dis 1982;41:473.

31. Dougal MA, Evans LS, McClellan KR, Robinson J: Central retinal arterial occlusion in systemic lupus erythematosus. Ann Ophthalmol 1983;15:38.

32. Kayazawa F, Honda A: Severe retinal vascular lesions in systemic lupus erythematosus. Ann Ophthalmol 1981;13:1291.

33. Stafford-Brady FJ, Urowitz MB, Gladman DD, Easterbrook M: Lupus retinopathy: Patterns, associations, and prognosis. Arthritis Rheum 1988;31:1105.

34. Hammami H, Streiff E: Changes of retinal vessels in a case of lupus erythematosus disseminatus: Development following treatment with immunosuppressive agents. Ophthalmologica 1973;166:16.

35. Ellis CJ, Hamer DB, Hunt TW, et al: Medical investigation of retinal vascular occlusion. Br Med J 1964;2:1093.

36. Harvey AM, Shulman LE, Tumulty PA, et al: Systemic lupus erythematosus: Review of the literature and clinical analysis of 138 cases. Medicine 1954;33:291.

37. Carpenter MT, O'Doyle JE, Enzenauer RV, et al: Choroiditis in systemic lupus erythematosus. Am J Ophthalmol 1994;117:535–536.

38. Clifton F, Greer CH: Ocular changes in acute systemic lupus erythematosus. Br J Ophthalmol 1955;39:1.

39. Santos R, Barojas E, Alarcon-Segovia D, Ibanez G: Retinal microangiopathy in systemic lupus erythematosus. Am J Ophthalmol 1975;80:249.

40. Goldstein I, Wexler D: Retinal vascular disease in a case of acute lupus erythematosus disseminatus. Arch Ophthalmol 1932;8:852.

41. Jabs DA, Hanneken AM, Schachat AP, Fine SL: Choroidopathy in systemic lupus erythematosus. Arch Ophthalmol 1988;106:230.

42. Diddie KR, Aronson AJ, Ernest JT: Chorioretinopathy in a case of systemic lupus erythematosus. Trans Am J Ophthalmol Soc 1977;75:122.

43. Gass JDM: A fluorescein angiographic study of macular dysfunction secondary to retinal vascular disease: VI. X-ray irradiation, carotid artery occlusion, collagen vascular disease, and vitritis. Arch Ophthalmol 1968;80:606.

44. Kinyoun JL, Kalina RE: Visual loss from choroidal ischemia. Am J Ophthalmol 1986;101:650.

45. Hackett ER, Martinez RD, Larson PF, Paddison RM: Optic neuritis in systemic lupus erythematosus. Arch Neurol 1974;31:9.

46. O'Conner JF, Musher DM: Central nervous system involvement in systemic lupus erythematosus. Study of 150 cases. Arch Neurol 1966;14:157.

47. Jabs DA, Miller NR, Newman SA, et al: Optic neuropathy in systemic lupus erythematosus. Arch Ophthalmol 1986;104:564.

48. Hayreh SS: Posterior ischemic optic neuropathy. Ophthalmologica 1981;182:29.

49. Lessell S: The neuro-ophthalmology of systemic lupus erythematosus. Doc Ophthalmol 1979;47:13.

50. April RS, Vansonnenberg E: A case of neuromyelitis optica (Devic's syndrome) in systemic lupus erythematosus. Neurology 1976;26;1066.

51. Kinney EL, Berdoff RL, Rao NS, Fox LM: Devic's syndrome and systemic lupus erythematosus: A case report with necropsy. Arch Neurol 1979;36:643.

52. Shepherd DI, Downie AW, Best PV: Systemic lupus erythematosus and multiple sclerosis. Arch Neurol 1074;30:423.

53. Carlow TJ, Glaser JS: Pseudotumor cerebri syndrome in systemic lupus erythematosus. JAMA 1974;228:197.

54. Abbas AK, Lichtman AH, Pober JS: Self tolerance and autoimmunity. In: Abbas AK, Lichtman AH, Pober JS, eds: Cellular and Molecular Immunology, 2nd ed. Philadelphia, W.B. Saunders, 1994, p 384.

55. Theofilopoulous AN, Kofler R, Singer PA, Dixon FJ: Molecular genetics of murine lupus models. Adv Immunol 1989;46:61.

56. Douglass MC, Lamberg SI, Lorincz AI, et al: Lupus erythematosus-like syndrome with a familial deficiency of C2. Arch Dermatol 1976;112:671.

57. Jayaram N, Sharma BK, Sehgal S: Autoantibody profile in systemic lupus erythematosus. Indian J Pathol Microbiol 1990;33:57–63.

58. Bastian BC: Annexias in cancer and autoimmune diseases. Cell Mol Life Sci 1997;53:554–556.

59. Mamoune A, Saroux A, Delaunoy JL, et al: Autoantibodies to CD45 in systemic lupus erythematosus. J Autoimmune 1998;11:485–488.

60. Boehm J, Orth T, Van Nguyen P, Solig HD: Systemic lupus erythematosus is associated with increased autoantibody titers against calreticulin and grp94, but calreticulin is not the Ro/SS-A antigen. Eur J Clin Invest 1994;24:248–257.

61. van Bruggen MC, Kramers C, Berden JH: Autoimmunity against nucleosomes and lupus nephritis. Ann Med Interne (Paris) 1996;147:485–489.

62. Landry M: Phagocyte function and cell-mediated immunity in systemic lupus erythematosus. Arch Dermatol 1977;113:147.

63. Karpik AG, Schwartz MM, Dickey LE, et al: Ocular immune reactants in patients dying with systemic lupus erythematosus. Clin Immunol Immunopathol 1985;35:295.

64. Aronson AJ, Ordonez NG, Diddie KR, Ernest JT: Immune complex deposition in the eye in systemic lupus erythematosus. Arch Intern Med 1979;139:1312.

65. Levine RA, Ward PA: Experimental acute immunologic ocular vasculitis. Am J Ophthalmol 1972;69:1023.

66. Graham EM, Spalton DJ, Barnard RO, et al: Cerebral and retinal vascular changes in systemic lupus erythematosus. Ophthalmology 1985;92:444–448.

67. Boey MI, Colaco CB, Gharavi AE, et al: Thrombosis in systemic lupus erythematosus: Striking association with the presence of circulating lupus anticoagulant. Br Med J 1983;287:1021.

68. Harris EN, Gharavi AE, Boey ML, et al: Anticardiolipin antibodies: Detection by radioimmunoassay and association with thrombosis in systemic lupus erythematosus. Lancet 1983;2:1211.

69. Petri M, Rheinshmidt M, Whiting-O'Keefe Q, et al: The frequency of lupus anticoagulant in systemic lupus erythematosus. Ann Intern Med 1987;106:524.

70. Felson DT, Anderson J: Evidence for the superiority of immunosuppressive drugs and prednisone over prednisone alone in lupus nephritis. N Engl J Med 1984;311:1528.

SCLERODERMA

Anthony S. Ekong, Stefanos Baltatzis,
and C. Stephen Foster

DEFINITION

Scleroderma is a multisystem connective tissue disease characterized by severe alterations in the microvasculature,[1] prominent inflammatory and immunologic alterations, and excessive deposition of collagen and other intracellular matrices in the skin and internal organs, including the lungs, kidneys, and gastrointestinal tract.[2] Scleroderma exists in two forms: a benign form localized to the skin, characterized clinically by thickening and fibrosis (scleroderma), and a systemic form (systemic sclerosis [SSc]) when there is visceral involvement.

Localized scleroderma (morphea and linear scleroderma) primarily affects children and young adults, mostly females.[2] Morphea is characterized by one or more isolated areas of sclerotic plaques that, after several months to years, spontaneously soften with a residual area of hyperpigmentation or hypopigmentation.[3] The lesions may become multiple or confluent, with a benign clinical course, in which case the term generalized morphea is used. In linear scleroderma, the sclerotic lesions appear as linear streaks or bands, primarily on the extremities. When the face or scalp is involved, usually unilaterally, the term en coup de sabre is used. The term evolved because the lesion may resemble a scar from a wound caused by a sabre. This can cause facial asymmetry, with hemifacial atrophy that is indistinguishable from Parry-Romberg syndrome. The relationship between progressive hemifacial atrophy (Parry-Romberg syndrome) and en coup de sabre is unclear. There is considerable overlap between morphea and linear scleroderma; both types coexist in many patients. Progression of localized scleroderma to the systemic form of the disease is rare but has been reported.[4-6]

SSc has been divided into two subgroups of limited or diffuse disease. This division is based solely on the degree and extent of skin thickening. The subgroup characterized by diffuse cutaneous involvement usually presents with rapid widespread thickening of the skin affecting the distal and proximal extremities, and patients with the diffuse involvement are at increased risk of early development of visceral involvement. In contrast, patients with limited cutaneous involvement have skin thickening limited to the distal extremities, with an interval of one or more decades before visceral involvement.[2] Facial skin thickening occurs in both systemic forms and is not a distinguishing feature.

There is clinical relevance in classifying patients into the limited or diffuse forms of the disease. Patients with the limited form tend to have a better prognosis, although severe pulmonary hypertension is more common in the late stage.[7] Pulmonary fibrosis may occur in both limited and diffuse disease but is more common in the late diffuse type. The risk of developing severe end organ complications, especially retinal involvement end death, is higher in patients with the diffuse disease.[8]

HISTORY

The initial description of scleroderma is found in a monograph written by Carlo Curzio and published in Naples in 1753.[9, 10] Rodnan[11] described Curzio's account of a young woman who presented with complaint of excessive tension and hardness of the skin. In 1847, Gintrac,[12] after a review of the earlier cases, introduced the term scleroderma (skleros—hard, derma—skin), emphasizing that the skin was the most obvious organ involved. Raynaud documented the association of abnormal vasoconstriction with scleroderma in 1862,[13] and Weber first recorded the coexistence of cutaneous calcinosis and scleroderma in 1878.[14] Subsequently, other associations were observed, such as esophageal dysmotility, sclerodactyly, and telangiectasia. Despite the fact that many patients with scleroderma were known to die from systemic complications after the development of cutaneous complaints, the visceral involvement was generally believed to be unrelated to the hardening of the skin.

The existence of visceral involvement was first clearly documented in 1924 by Matsui,[15] who described sclerosis of the lungs, gastrointestinal tract, and kidney of five patients. Goetz presented a detailed review of the systemic manifestations in 1945 and proposed that the term scleroderma be replaced by progressive SSc (generalized scleroderma).[16]

Subsequently, SSc was classified into progressive systemic sclerosis (PSS) and the CREST syndrome, the latter consisting of sclerosis, Raynaud's phenomenon, esophageal dysmotility, sclerodactyly, and telangiectasia. The current classification of SSc into diffuse and limited diseases was introduced to replace the above-mentioned classification, which was found unsatisfactory for many reasons.[17] First, skin involvement in the diffuse variant (the PSS form) is not progressive; rather, it tends to worsen over a 3- to 5-year period, then frequently stabilizes and may even regress. Also the internal organ manifestation is progressive only in a small portion of diffuse disease patients. Second, although the stigmata of the acronym CREST do develop in patients with the limited disease irrespective of the duration, they can also occur in patients with the late stage of diffuse disease. Disregarding the association of renal disease with diffuse scleroderma and pulmonary hypertension with limited scleroderma, there is little difference between these subgroups in very late disease.

EPIDEMIOLOGY

Scleroderma is a rare disease. Criteria for the classification and diagnosis of the disease were not formulated until 1980 by the American Rheumatism Association, now the American College of Rheumatology, and therefore, available epidemiologic data using current criteria are sparse (Table 54–1). Data based on the two largest studies reported after the publication of these criteria and cov-

TABLE 54–1. PRELIMINARY CRITERIA FOR SCLERODERMA*

MAJOR CRITERION

Sclerodermatous skin changes (tightness, thickening, and nonpitting induration, excluding localized forms of scleroderma) proximal to the metacarpophalangeal or metatarsophalangeal joints

MINOR CRITERIA

(In the absence of proximal scleroderma)

Sclerodactyly; sclerodermatous skin changes of fingers or toes

Digital pitting scars of fingertips or loss of substance of the distal finger pad

Bibasilar pulmonary fibrosis not attributable to primary lung disease

---

*One major or two minor criteria have a sensitivity of 97% and a specificity of 98% when compared with patients with systemic lupus erythematosus, polymyositis/dermatomyositis, or Raynaud's phenomenon.

From the Subcommittee for Scleroderma Criteria of the American Rheumatism Association Diagnostic and Therapeutic Criteria Committee: Preliminary criteria for the classification of systemic sclerosis (scleroderma). Arthritis Rheum 1980;23:581.

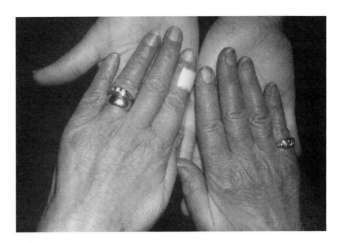

FIGURE 54–1. Raynaud's phenomenon in a patient with progressive systemic sclerosis. Note the "cyanotic" appearance of all of the digits on the right hand, and the distal portions of the digits on the left hand.

ering only a period of two decades place the incidence at approximately 19 cases per million,[18, 19] with a prevalence of 240 cases per million.[19]

SSc affects more women than men, with a ratio ranging between 3:1 and 8:1, depending on the age of the patient; the ratio is higher during the childbearing years and considerably lower in later adult life.[20] Disease onset is highest between ages 30 and 50 years, with a peak onset at about 50 years.[21]

A higher proportion of black patients may have the diffuse rather than the limited form of the disease, and it may occur at an earlier age than in whites.[21, 22] Most cases occur sporadically irrespective of season, occupation, or socioeconomic status. There is an association of scleroderma with exposure to environmental toxins. The disease has a worldwide distribution although it is less frequent in Asia.[23] Familial cases have rarely been reported, and a weak correlation with the human leukocyte antigens HLA-DQ1, HLA-DRB1, and HLA-DPB1 exists.

CLINICAL CHARACTERISTICS

Systemic

The initial symptom in most patients with scleroderma is Raynaud's phenomenon, occurring in 90% of cases. Raynaud's phenomenon is characterized by the sequential development of pallor, cyanosis, and rubor of the digits on cold exposure or emotional stress, or both (Fig. 54–1). These symptoms may be present for years before the occurrence of other systemic manifestations, in patients with limited SSc. Both vasospasm and structural abnormalities of the arteriolar and arterial tree have been implicated.[24] An early manifestation of SSc, especially in individuals with the diffuse disease, is bilateral symmetric painless swelling or thickening of the fingers and hands and sometimes the ankle and the feet.[2] This edematous phase, which may result from multiple factors including microvascular disruption, local inflammatory reactions, and deposition of hydrophilic glycosaminoglycan in the dermis, may last for a few weeks to several months. The longer the duration of the edematous changes, the more favorable the long-term prognosis. Subsequently, as the induration phase develops, sclerodactyly (Fig. 54–2), and

the classic pursed-mouth, pinched nose, tight face appearance of patients with SSc (Fig. 54–3) are produced. This is followed by the atrophic phase in which the skin may actually soften. With prolonged disease duration, telangiectasias and subcutaneous calcinosis may develop; this occurs more frequently in patients with limited cutaneous scleroderma. Polyarthralgias of small and large joints and occasional polyarthritis are commonly present early in diffuse scleroderma, often leading to the erroneous diagnosis of rheumatoid arthritis.

Involvement of the gastrointestinal tract ranks only behind Raynaud's phenomenon and scleroderma skin changes as common manifestations of SSc. Esophageal dysfunction is extremely common, occurring in approximately 50% of patients.[25, 26] Heartburn, dysphagia with solid food, and reflux that can lead to peptic esophagitis, Barrett's metaphasia, and esophageal strictures may occur (Fig. 54–4). Both the diffuse and limited disease subtypes are similarly affected. Histopathologically, there is fibrosis and smooth muscle atrophy of both the lower two thirds of the esophagus and the lower esophageal sphincter.

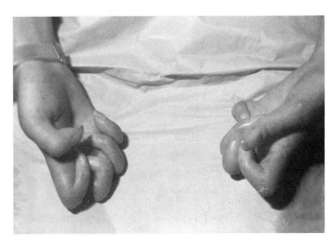

FIGURE 54–2. Sclerodactyly in a patient with progressive systemic sclerosis. Note not only the contractures and deformity of the digits but also the dermatologic abnormalities and the shiny character to some of the areas of the skin.

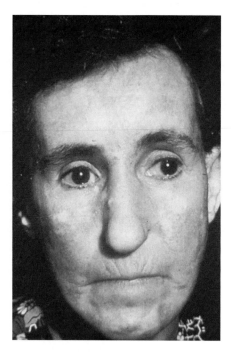

FIGURE 54-3. Full-face photograph of a patient with progressive systemic sclerosis who has blepharophimosis and, most obvious, the pursed-lip features of a patient with scleroderma; the patient is unable to open her mouth to any appreciable degree.

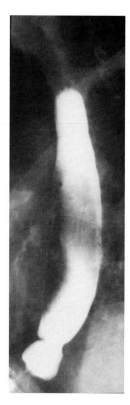

FIGURE 54-4. Esophageal stricture in the distal portion of the esophagus, as demonstrated by barium swallow radiography, in a patient with progressive systemic sclerosis. The area of stricture is quite apparent.

Delayed gastric emptying is often associated with esophageal dysfunction. In addition, the patient may complain of nausea, vomiting, or diffuse epigastric discomfort. Small bowel hypomotility can complicate long-standing limited SSc, leading to fecal stagnation with bacterial overgrowth and secondary malabsorption.[25, 26] Symptoms include intermittent abdominal bloating, distention, pain, diarrhea, and weight loss. The colon may also undergo fibrotic changes, with constipation being the leading symptom. Rectal prolapse and fecal incontinence reflect SSc involvement of the anal sphincter.

The two major pulmonary manifestations of SSc are pulmonary hypertension (PHTN) and interstitial fibrosis (Fig. 54-5).[27] Isolated pulmonary hypertension is more common in patients with limited cutaneous sclerosis.[7] These patients may present with rapidly progressive dyspnea, although approximately one third may be asymptomatic.[28] Some patients with PHTN may present with symptoms of right-sided heart failure, including pedal edema and congestive hepatomegaly with abdominal discomfort. The most common abnormality on pulmonary function testing is reduced diffusing capacity for carbon monoxide.[29] PHTN may occur in patients with diffuse disease, usually in association with advanced interstitial fibrosis.

Interstitial fibrosis is responsible for significant rates of morbidity and mortality among scleroderma patients. Exertional dyspnea and nonproductive cough are the usual complaints, with bibasilar crackles on auscultation. Pulmonary function tests reveal a restrictive pattern, with a decreased forced vital capacity (FVC). Patients with either limited or diffuse disease can be affected, although the disease tends to be more severe in the diffuse subset. Bronchoalveolar lavage reveals increased proportions of

neutrophils, lymphocytes, and occasionally, eosinophils in most patients.[30]

Cardiac involvement in SSc is common but rarely clinically signficant.[31] It can be manifested as pericarditis, conduction problems, arrhythmias, myocardial disease, and congestive heart failure[32] (from renal and pulmonary involvement).

Scleroderma renal crisis (SRC) was the leading cause of death among patients with diffuse disease before the introduction of angiotensin-converting enzyme (ACE) inhibitors.[33] Patients in SRC, without warning, develop a renin-mediated malignant arterial hypertension and oli-

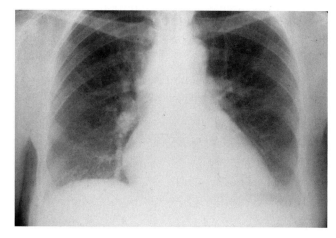

FIGURE 54-5. Pulmonary interstitial fibrosis, with the increased interstitial markings on plain chest x-ray study in a patient with scleroderma.

guric acute renal failure.[34] SRC is a medical emergency. Azotemia, proteinuria, and hypertension independent of renal crisis are seen in many patients with scleroderma.[35]

The nervous system can be (uncommonly) involved in patients with scleroderma. Carpal tunnel syndrome, peripheral neuropathy, autonomic dysfunction and trigeminal neuralgia have been described.[36] Thyroid gland fibrosis with hypothyroidism has also been reported.[37] Impotence occurs in a high proportion of men with scleroderma and may represent penile vascular ischemia.[38]

Ocular

Scleroderma frequently affects the eyelids and the periorbital tissue. The most commonly reported lid findings relate to fibrotic changes, with stiffness or tightness, resulting in an indurated quality of the lids, sometimes leading to difficulty with lid eversion and blepharophimosis.[39–41] Lid telangiectasia and madarosis can also occur.[39, 41] Morphea of the eyelids has been described.[42] Periorbital edema in association with PSS, as well as linear scleroderma and localized disease, may be early clinical signs. As with the extremities, this edema, which may persist for months, is followed by an atrophic phase.[43–45]

Reduced tear secretion, measured by Schirmer test and rose bengal staining, with associated keratoconjunctivitis sicca (KCS) is common in patients with SSc.[40] In one series, clinical signs of dry eye were found in 75% of patients with scleroderma.[46]

The majority of corneal changes result from KCS. Corneal opacification has been induced by cold in patients with Raynaud's disease associated with SSc.[47] Conjunctival fornix foreshortening in the absence of clinically evident conjunctival inflammation has been reported (Fig. 54–6).[39] This is not surprising, given the fact that SSc is characterized by generalized dermal and subepithelial fibrosis. Telangiectasia and sludging of the conjunctival vessels have been observed[41]; this, too, is not surprising given the underlying vascular abnormalities observed in arteries, arterioles, and capillaries.[1]

Orbital involvement is limited to the extraocular muscles in both PSS and localized scleroderma, and it has been associated with ocular myopathy, most notably in-

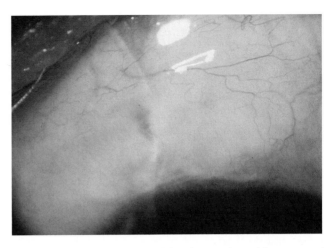

FIGURE 54–7. An area of scleral loss in a patient with en coup de sabre or linear scleroderma involving the face, including eyelids. The area of scleral involvement is in a direct line with the dermatome involved.

volving the superior rectus muscle.[48] Ocular involvement may also occur along the meridian of an en coup de sabre, involving deep and superficial structures, implicating abnormal embryonal neural crest migration and proliferation in lesion development.[49] We reported the unusual case of a 43-year-old woman with progressive facial hemiatrophy associated with a linear en coup de sabre who presented with spontaneous sclera perforation in the ipsilateral eye (Fig. 54–7). The location of the scleral loss was exactly on the line of the en coup de sabre atrophy. She did not have detectable antinuclear antibody titers, and histopathologic examination of the affected sclera revealed no inflammatory cells.[50]

Systemic microvascular abnormalities are the hallmark of SSc, and so it is not surprising that the choroidal vasculature is affected in a large proportion of patients. Greenan and Forster[51] found that 5 of 10 patients with scleroderma had patchy areas of nonperfusion of the choroidal vasculature on fluorescein angiography; one patient showed abnormalities of the retina vasculature with microaneurysmal dilatation of the terminal venules in one quadrant.

Serup and colleagues[52] performed ophthalmoscopy and fluorescein angiography on 21 patients with generalized (limited) scleroderma. None of these patients had any history of concomitant vascular diseases, including hypertension, diabetes or renal disease, and ophthalmoscopy revealed no abnormalities. However, seven (33%) of the 21 angiograms were assessed as definitely abnormal. The abnormalities consisted of variable hyperfluorescence of the pigment epithelium layer in the late phase, which may represent damage to the choriocapillaris with atrophy of the overlying retinal pigment epithelium (Fig. 54–8).[52–54] Interestingly, the retina vasculature was not affected. The authors speculated that the absence of neural supply and internal elastic membrane in the retinal arterioles might render them less sensitive to damage.

Farkas and associates[55] performed a postmortem ocular study of one patient with SSc. They showed by electronmicroscopy and histochemistry that the choroidal

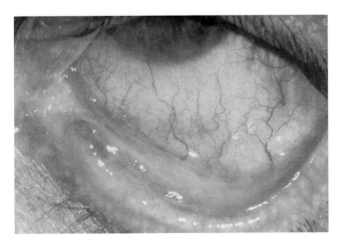

FIGURE 54–6. Foreshortening of the inferior fornix, with obvious subepithelial fibrosis, in a patient with scleroderma.

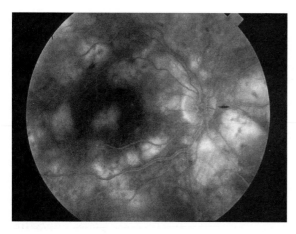

FIGURE 54–8. Late phase of a fluorescein angiogram performed on a patient with choroidal involvement in scleroderma. Note the choroidopathy, as evidenced by late staining in a patchy pattern of the areas of choroidal inflammation.

vasculature was grossly affected, with diffuse endothelial cell swelling and necrosis obstructing the lumen of capillaries. Also, basement membrane thickening and deposition of mucopolysaccharide material in and around the endothelium were found. In contrast, only minor abnormalities of retinal arterioles were noted. These changes are typical of the vascular endothelial abnormalities found elsewhere in patients with SSc. Retinopathy, including cotton wool spots, intraretinal edema, venous thrombosis, hemorrhage, exudate and parafoveal telangiectasia in association with CREST syndrome has been described.[55–58] These findings appear in advanced disease and may not be primarily due to SSc itself but rather may be secondary consequences of systemic hypertension frequently found in these patients. In general most patients with SSc have minimal funduscopic findings.

PATHOPHYSIOLOGY, IMMUNOLOGY, PATHOLOGY, AND PATHOGENESIS

The susceptible host–external agent–immune response model has been suggested for SSc.[59] In this model, a genetically susceptible individual is exposed to some environmental stimulus, which serves as a trigger to incite the immune system to produce vascular injury by a heretofore unclear mechanism. Cytokines are released that may cause further endothelial activation or injury and stimulate fibroblast proliferation and production of collagen.

The evidence for genetic influence in SSc is not very strong. Certain class II HLA genes are overrepresented in the patient population with SSc, with HLA-DR1, (DRB1*1302) DR3, and DR5 (HLA-DQB1*0501) being the most commonly reported haplotypes.[60] HLA-DQw7, (HLA-DQB1*0301) and DQW5 genes may also be important in predisposing an individual to the development of SSc, especially with anticentromere autoantibody production.[61]

Clinical variants of SSc have been described in patients after exposure to certain environmental stimuli. Silica dust, polyvinyl chloride, silicone breast implant, ingestion of toxic rapeseed oil, various drugs such as bleomycin,

carbidopa, L-tryptophan, cocaine, and appetite suppressants have been implicated.[31, 62]

Both humoral and cellular immune dysfunction with increased production of certain cytokines and autoantibodies have been found in patients with scleroderma. As in most other connective tissue diseases, antinuclear antibodies (ANAs) are present in sera of most patients with SSc.[63] The antibody titers can be very high but do not correlate with disease activity. Unlike the other connective tissue diseases, the intracellular antigen targets of the ANAs in SSc are different. These SSc-specific ANAs are directed against DNA topoisomerase 1 (topo-1); chromosomal centromere; RNA polymerase (RNAP) I, II, and III; and some nucleolar components. Anticentromere antibodies (specific for limited scleroderma and found in 57% of patients with CREST syndrome), and Scl-70 or antitopoisomerase-1 (specific for diffuse scleroderma and present in 40%) are the two most common SSc marker antibodies. Approximately 40% of SSc patients are likely to have neither antibody present.[64]

The presence of a dense mononuclear cell infiltrate in the dermis and along blood vessels in the early stage of SSc[65] implicates lymphocytes and monocytes as major mediators in the evolution of this disease. Activation of the lymphocytes is evidenced by increased serum levels of factors and receptors associated with T cells. Increased serum levels of interleukins (IL) 2, 4, 6, and 8 and transforming growth factor beta (TGF-β)[66–69] have been reported, and these appear to play an important role in fibroblast proliferation as well as collagen synthesis. In addition, elevated levels of IL-2 and soluble IL-2 receptor (CD25 molecule) in the serum of patients with SSc correlate with disease activity and extent of internal organ involvement.[70]

Blood vessel abnormalities are central to the pathema seen in SSc patients. In every affected organ, there is remarkable thickening of the intima of arterioles and smaller arteries, with narrowing of the vascular lumen and, in many instances, obliteration of the small arterioles. Endothelial cell injury with reduplication of basement membrane material is routinely observed on histopathologic and ultrastructural studies. Endothelin, the most potent vasoconstrictor yet identified, is present in higher than normal amounts in the blood of patients with SSc,[71] and implicates endothelial cell injury. This cytokine is synthesized by vascular endothelial cells; however, the primary signals responsible for inducing upregulation and perpetuation of endothelin synthesis are not well understood. The ability of lymphocytes to adhere to endothelial cells is strongly mediated by cellular adhesion molecules (CAMs).[72] In SSc, elevated levels of different CAMs such as intracellular adhesion molecule 1 (ICAM-1),[73] endothelial leukocyte adhesion molecule 1 (ECAM-1),[74] and vascular cell adhesion molecule 1 (VCAM-1), P-selectin, and E-selectin, have been detected and correlated with both their in situ expression and clinical disease activity in patients with SSc.[75]

Mast cells have been considered as potential pathogenic participants in scleroderma, too. Increased numbers of mast cells are found in a variety of fibrotic conditions, including graft-versus-host disease (characterized by collagen proliferation and fibrosis), interstitial fibrosis, and also in the conjunctiva of patients with scleroderma.[46] Increased eosinophil granule proteins are present in the skin of some patients with SSc.[76]

A reasonable working hypothesis for the pathogenesis of SSc probably should also involve abnormalities of the vascular endothelium, and of both the immune and connective tissue systems.[77] Perhaps there is lymphocyte sensitization to antigens, such as type IV collagen or skin along with subsequent proliferation of dermal fibroblasts, an overproduction of immature collagen, and vascular overgrowth. Many factors are implicated in the pathogenesis of SSc; their relative roles or contributions are speculative, making targeted, specific therapy difficult.

Histopathologic features of SSc are influenced by the stage of the disease. In the early phase, there is mild lymphocytic and monocytic cell infiltrate, mainly around small blood vessels and in the dermis. Subsequently, a marked increase in collagen and other extracellular matrix components, such as fibronectin and glycosaminoglycans, are observed in the dermis and extend into the subcutaneous fat. In the atrophic phase of the disease, there is a paucity of cellular infiltrate, thinning of the epidermis with loss of rete pegs, and increased collagen contraction corresponding to the clinically observed fibrosis.

DIAGNOSIS

There is no single diagnostic test for SSc. Diagnosis is made on clinical grounds, based on criteria established by the American Rheumatism Association (Table 54–1) that are about 97% sensitive and 98% specific.[78]

The major criterion is sclerodermatous skin changes in any location proximal to the metacarpophalangeal joints. Minor criteria include sclerodactyly (sclerosis affecting only the fingers or toes), digital pitting scars of fingertips or loss of substance of the distal pad, and bibasilar pulmonary fibrosis not attributable to primary lung disease.

A disease can be classified as scleroderma if the major criterion or if two of the three minor criteria are present.

TREATMENT

Organ-specific therapy and disease-modifying agents are the main modalities in use at present. Raynaud's phenomenon (RP) has been treated with both nonpharmacologic and pharmacologic methods. Avoiding cold exposure, keeping the entire body warm, and total abstinence from smoking are usually effective in mild to moderate cases. Calcium channel blockers are the first-line drug therapy in complicated cases. Short-acting nifedipine has been shown to be highly effective in improving digital blood flow and inducing healing of digital ulcers.[79] Other vasodilating agents, including nitrates and sympatholytics, have been employed in patients with SSc and RP. ACE inhibitors have been used with increased success in improving survival and reversing renin-mediated SRC.[33] Borderline or frank hypertension has also been successfully treated with ACE inhibitors.

The use of proton pump inhibitors (e.g., omeprazole) and prokinetic agents (e.g., cisapride) has ameliorated many esophageal dysmotility and delayed gastric emptying symptoms in cases not amenable to life style modifi-

cations.[80] Antacids are useful in relieving symptoms associated with the esophageal reflux. Patients with esophageal strictures benefit from periodic dilatation.

No therapy has proved effective in decreasing the mortality or progression of pulmonary hypertension in patients with SSc. Vasodilators, specifically calcium channel blockers, have been used with varying success.[81] Similarly, interstitial lung disease (ILD) has been difficult to treat except in those cases in which bronchoalveolar lavage shows inflammatory alveolitis. Silver and colleagues[82] reported improved FVC in patients with moderately severe ILD with active alveolitis who were treated with oral daily cyclophosphamide (approximately 100 mg per day) and low-dose prednisone.

Ocular involvement, especially dry eyes, can be treated with artificial tears, lubricating ointments, punctal occlusion, and topical cyclosporin A. Topical corticosteroid cream may provide some relief to skin involvement around the eye. Systemic steroids can be used to treat inflammatory ocular myopathy. In general, the retinal pigment epithelium (RPE) epitheliopathy resulting from choroidal vasculature abnormalities does not affect visual function in the cases reported so far. However, because loss of visual function can result when there is extensive RPE atrophy with degeneration of the retinal layers, we believe periodic fluorescein angiography should be obtained in patients with SSc.

Disease-modifying agents have focused on halting the fibrotic and inflammatory responses characteristic of SSc with limited success. Relatively minimal effort has been directed at the mediators of vascular dysfunction in SSc. D-penicillamine (DPA), has been used since the 1960s for the treatment of diffuse SSc based on anecdotal reports of effectiveness and on its interference with cross-linking of collagen. In a double-masked, randomized controlled clinical trial involving 134 patients, all of whom had diffuse disease of less than 18 months, high-dose DPA (750 to 1000 mg per day) was compared with low-dose DPA (125 mg every other day).[83] During a mean follow-up of 4 years, skin thickness score, incidence of scleroderma renal disease, and mortality were not different between the two groups. There was a greater improvement in skin scores in the low-dose group than in the high-dose group (not statistically significant). Furthermore, of the 20 adverse events necessitating drug withdrawal, 80% occurred in the high-dose group. It appears from this study that there might not be much advantage in using this therapy.

Interferon alfa (IFN-α) and interferon gamma (IFN-γ) both have antifibrotic potential and have been evaluated in patients with SSc. So far, only IFN-α has been subjected to a randomized double-masked study comparing its efficacy versus placebo in patients with early diffuse SSc.[84] There were more treatment withdrawals because of drug toxicity, and a greater deterioration was noted in the treatment group in skin score, FVC, diffusing capacity for carbon monoxide (DLCO) and renal function, raising concerns about the benefit of this drug in the treatment of SSc. Another antifibrotic agent under study is recombinant human relaxin, given its ability to inhibit collagen production through increased collagenase activity.[85]

The real promise for major advance in the care of patients with SSc may lie in the areas of immunomodulatory therapy. This is not surprising, given the prominent abnormalities of cellular and humoral immune function present at early stages of the disease. So far, methotrexate (MTX) has shown promising results. In a double-masked trial, 29 limited and diffuse SSc patients were randomized to receive 15 mg of MTX per week or placebo.[86] After 24 weeks, 8 of 17 patients in the MTX group versus 1 of 12 patients in the placebo group were judged to have improvement in skin scores, creatinine clearance, and general well-being (outcomes were not statistically significant). Similarly, a double-masked, placebo-controlled trial examining the safety and efficacy of low-dose tissue plasminogen activator (t-PA) in the treatment of SSc concluded that low-dose recombinant human t-PA is safe and is accompanied by modest improvement in symptoms in a subset of scleroderma patients.[87] Other immunomodulatory therapies that have been used in patients with SSc have included intravenous dexamethasone pulses,[88] oral cyclophosphamide,[82, 89] and plasmapheresis and oral daily 2.5mg/kg cyclophosphamide therapy.[90] Several other immunomodulatory agents including thalidomide, an inhibitor of tumor necrosis factor alpha (TNF-α) and oral type 1 collagen[8] are under study.

PROGNOSIS

The presence and extent of internal organ involvement are the main determinants of morbidity and mortality in patients with scleroderma. Those with the diffuse disease are known to have a high incidence of internal organ manifestations and have a slightly worse prognosis. Scleroderma renal crisis was once regarded as one of the features associated with the worst prognosis. Because of its association with hyperreninemia, ACE inhibitors have been very successful in reversing SRc and improving survival.[33] Pulmonary complications associated with pulmonary hypertension and interstitial fibrosis have emerged as the most difficult to treat end-organ involvement and are the principal cause of morbidity and mortality in late SSc. Pulmonary hypertension has a particularly poor prognosis,[7] with most patients dying within 2 years. The disease is usually detected during the moderate to severe, irreversible stage. None of the current noninvasive studies (chest radiography, pulmonary function test, echocardiography) are sensitive in detecting early, potentially reversible, mild degree of PHTN.[29]

CONCLUSION

SSc is a multisystem disorder of connective tissue disease characterized clinically by fibrosis of the skin and internal organs, including the heart, lungs, kidneys, and gastrointestinal tract. Its etiology and pathogenesis are unknown, rendering effective treatment of the systemic complications difficult.

Most of the ocular manifestations do not lead to significant visual impairment, unlike many other connective tissue diseases, and they can usually be managed symptomatically. It is conceivable that scleroderma choroidopathy, if extensive, can have a deleterious effect on the outer retinal function. We have recommended periodic fluorescein angiography to monitor patients for scleroderma choroidopathy. One may question the relevance of this test given that no treatment is available if evidence of progressive scleroderma choroidopathy is observed on the angiogram. The real benefits of obtaining periodic angiograms may have to do with learning more about the natural history of this choroidopathy.

References

1. Heron GS, Romero LI: Vascular abnormalities in scleroderma. Semin Cutan Med Surg 1998;17:12.
2. Leroy EC, Silver RM: Systemic sclerosis and related syndromes. In: Schumacher HR, ed: Primer on Rheumatic Diseases, 10th ed. Atlanta, Georgia, Arthritis Foundation, 1993, p 118.
3. Peterson LS, Nelson AM, Su WP: Classification of morphea. Mayo Clin Proc 1995;70:1068.
4. Christiansen HB, Dorsey CS, O'Leary PA, et al. Localized scleroderma: A clinical study of two hundred and thirty-five cases. Arch Dermatol 1956;74:629.
5. Curtis AC, Jansen TG: The prognosis of localized scleroderma. Arch Dermatol 1958;78:749.
6. Birdi N, Laxer RM, Thorner P, et al: Localized scleroderma, progressing to systemic disease: A case report and review of the literature. Arthritis Rheum 1993;36:410.
7. Stupi AM, Steen VD, Owens GR, et al: Pulmonary hypertension in the CREST syndrome variant of multiple sclerosis. Arthritis Rheum 1986;29:515.
8. Leroy EC, Black C, Fleischmajer R, et al: Scleroderma (systemic sclerosis): classifications, onsets and pathogenesis. J Rheumatol 1988;15:202.
9. Curzio C: a) Discussioni anatomico-pratiche di un raro, e stravagante morbo cutaneo in une giovane donna felicemente curato in questo grande Ospedale degl'Incurabili, Giovanni di Simone, Napoli, 1753
10. Dissertation anatomique et pratique sur une malade de la peau, d'une epsece fort rare et fort singuliare, translated by Vandermonde, Vincent, Paris, 1755.
11. Rodnan GP, Benedek TG: An historical account of the study of progressive systemic sclerosis (diffuse scleroderma). Ann Intern Med 1962;57:305.
12. Gintrac E: Note sur la sclérodermie. Rev Med Chir 1847:2:263.
13. Raynaud M: De l'asphyxie locale et de la gangrene symétrique des extrémités. Paris, Rignoux, 1862.
14. Weber H: Case presentation. Correspondentzlbart Schweiz. Aertze 1878;8:623.
15. Matsui S: Über die Pathologie und Pathogenese von Sklerodermia universalis. Mitt Med Fakult Kaiserl Univ Tokyo 1924;31:55.
16. Goetz RH: Pathology of progressive systemic sclerosis (generalized scleroderma) with special reference to changes in the viscera. Clin Proc 1945;4:337.
17. Mayes MD: Classification and epidemiology of scleroderma. Semin Cutan Med Surg 1998;17:22.
18. Steen VD, Conte C, Santoro D, et al: Twenty year incidence survey of systemic sclerosis. (Abstract.) Arthritis Rheum 1988;31 (Suppl):S57.
19. Mayes MD, Laing TJ, Gillespie BW, et al: Prevalence, incidence and survival rates of systemic sclerosis in Detroit metropolitan area. (Abstract.) Arthritis Rheum 1996;39(suppl):S150.
20. Silman AJ: Scleroderma—demographics and survival. J Rheumatol 1997;24(Suppl 48):58.
21. Laing TJ, Gillespie BW, Toth MB, et al: Racial differences in scleroderma among women in Michigan. Arthritis Rheum 1997;40:734.
22. Steen VD, Oddis CV, Conte CG, et al: Incidence of systemic sclerosis in Allegheny County, Pennsylvania. A twenty year study of hospital diagnosed cases, 1963–1982. Arthritis Rheum 1997;40:441.
23. Tamaki T, Mori S, Takahara K, et al: Epidemiological study of patients with systemic sclerosis in Tokyo. (Abstract.) Arch Dermatol Res 1991;283:366.
24. Wigley FM, Flavahan NA: Raynaud's phenomenon. Rheum Dis Clin North Am 1996;22:765.
25. Sjögren RW: Gastrointestinal features of scleroderma. Curr Opin Rheumatol 1996;8:569.
26. Lock G, Holstege A, Lang B, et al: Gastrointestinal manifestations of progressive systemic sclerosis. Am J Gastroenterol 1997;92:763.

27. Silver RM: Scleroderma: Clinical problems; the lungs. Rheum Dis Clin North Am 1996;22:825.
28. Sullivan WD, Hurst DJ, Harmon CE, et al: A prospective evaluation emphasizing pulmonary involvement in patients with mixed connective tissue disease. Medicine 1984;63:92.
29. Ungerer RG, Tashkin DP, Furst D, et al: Prevalence and clinical correlates of pulmonary arterial hypertension on progressive systemic sclerosis. Am J Med 1983;75:65.
30. Silver RM, Miller KS, Kinsella MB, et al: Evaluation and management of scleroderma lung disease using bronchoalveolar lavage. Am J Med 1990;88:470.
31. Perez MI, Kohn SR: Systemic sclerosis. Am Acad Dermatol 1993;28:525.
32. Deswal A, Follansbee WP: Cardiac involvement in scleroderma. Rheum Dis Clin North Am 1996;22:841.
33. Steen VD, Constantino JP, Shapiro AP, et al: Outcome of renal crisis in systemic sclerosis: Relation to availability of angiotensin converting enzyme (ACE) inhibitors. Ann Intern Med 1990;113:352.
34. Steen VD: Scleroderma renal crisis. Rheum Dis Clin North Am 1996;22:861.
35. Tuffanelli DL, Winkelman RK: Systemic scleroderma: A clinical study of 727 cases. Arch Dermatol 1961;84:359.
36. Cerinic MM, Generini S, Pignone A, et al: The nervous system in systemic sclerosis (scleroderma). Rheum Dis Clin North Am 1996;22:879.
37. Gordon MB, Klein L, Dekker A, et al: Thyroid disease in progressive systemic sclerosis: Increased frequency of glandular fibrosis and hypothyroidism. Ann Intern Med 1981;95:431.
38. Nowlin NS, Brick JE, Weaver DJ, et al: Impotence in scleroderma. Ann Intern Med 1986;104:794.
39. Horan EC: Ophthalmic manifestations of progressive systemic sclerosis. Br J Ophthalmol 1969;53:388.
40. Kirkham TH: Scleroderma and Sjögren's syndrome. Br J Ophthalmol 1969;53:131.
41. West RH, Barnett AJ: Ocular involvement in scleroderma. Br J Ophthalmol 1979;63:845.
42. El-Baba F, Frangieh GT, Iliff WJ, et al: Morphea of the eyelids. Ophthalmology 1982;89:1285.
43. Long PR, Miller OF 3rd, et al: Linear scleroderma: report of a case presenting as persistent unilateral lid edema. J Am Acad Dermatol 1982;7:541.
44. Stone RA, Scheie HG: Periorbital scleroderma associated with heterochromia iridis. Am J Ophthalmol 1980;90:858.
45. Dorwart BB: Periorbital edema in progressive systemic sclerosis. Ann Intern Med 1974;80:273.
46. Mancel E, Janin A, Gosset D, et al: Conjunctival biopsy in scleroderma and primary Sjögren's syndrome. Am J Ophthalmol 1993;115:792.
47. McWhae JA, Andrews AM: Transient corneal opacification induced by cold in Raynaud's disease. Ophthalmology 1991;98:666.
48. Arnett FC, Michels RG: Inflammatory ocular myopathy in systemic sclerosis (scleroderma). Arch Intern Med 1973;132:740.
49. Serup J, Serup L, Sjo O, et al: Localized scleroderma "coup de sabre" with external eye muscle involvement at the same line. Clin Exp Dermatol 1984;9:196.
50. Hoang-Xuan T, Foster CS, Jakobiec FA, et al: Romberg's progressive hemifacial atrophy: An association with scleral melting. Cornea 1991;10:361.
51. Grennan AM, Forrester J: Involvement of the eye in SLE and scleroderma. A study using fluorescein angiograph in addition to clinical ophthalmic assessment. Ann Rheum Dis 1977;36:152.
52. Serup L, Serup J, Hagdrup H, et al: Fundus fluorescein angiography in generalized scleroderma. Ophthalmic Res 1987;19:303.
53. Hesse RJ, Slagle DF: Scleroderma choroidopathy: Report of an unusual case. Ann Ophthalmol 1982;14:524.
54. Kraus A, Guerra-Bautista G, Espinoza G, et al: Defects of the retinal pigment epithelium in scleroderma. Br J Rheumatol 1991;30:112.
55. Farkas TG, Sylvester V, Archer D, et al: The choroidopathy of progressive systemic sclerosis (scleroderma). Am J Ophthalmol 1972;74:875.
56. Pollack IP, Becker B: Cystoid bodies of the retina in a patient with scleroderma. Am J Ophthalmol 1962;54:655.
57. Agatston HJ: Scleroderma with retinopathy. Am J Ophthalmol 1953;36:120.

58. Proctor B, Chang T, Hay D, et al: Parafoveal telangiectasia in association with CREST syndrome. Arch Ophthalmol 1998;116:814.
59. Furst DE, Clements PJ: Hypothesis for the pathogenesis of systemic sclerosis. J Rheumatol 1977;24:53.
60. Arnett FC, Reveille JD, Goldstein R, et al: Auto antibodies to fibrillarin in systemic sclerosis (scleroderma). An immunogenetic, serologic, and clinical analysis. Arthritis Rheum 1996;39:1151.
61. Arnett FC: HLA and autoimmunity in scleroderma. Int Rev Ophthalmol 1995;12:107.
62. Haustein UF, Haupt B: Drug-induced scleroderma and scerlodermiform conditions. Clin Dermatol 1998;16:353.
63. Okano Y: Antinuclear antibodies in systemic sclerosis. Rheum Dis Clin North Am 1996;22:709.
64. Spencer-Green G, Alter D, Welch HG, et al: Test performance in systemic sclerosis: Anti-centromere and anti-Scl-70 antibodies. Am J Med 1997;103:242.
65. Prescott RJ, Freemon AJ, Jones CJ, et al: Sequential dermal microvascular and perivascular changes in the development of scleroderma. J Pathol 1992;166:255.
66. Salmon-Her V, Serpier H: Expression of interleukin-4 in scleroderma skin specimens and scleroderma fibroblasts cultures. Potential role in fibrosis. Arch Dermatol 1996;132:802.
67. Gurram M, Pahwa S, Frieri M, et al: Augmented interleukin-6 secretion in collagen stimulated peripheral blood mononuclear cells from patients with systemic sclerosis. Ann Allergy 1994;73:493.
68. Higley H, Perischitte K, Chu S, et al: Immunocytochemical localization and in situ detection of transforming growth factor beta 1. Association with type 1 procollagen and inflammatory cell markers in diffuse and limited systemic sclerosis, morphea and Raynaud's phenomenon. Arthritis Rheum 1994;37:278.
69. Southcott AM, Jones KP, Li D, et al: Interleukin-8 differential expression in lung fibrosing alveolitis and systemic sclerosis. Am J Respir Crit Care Med 1995;151:604.
70. Patrick MR, Kurkham BW, Graham M, et al: Circulating interleukin-1 beta and soluble interleukin-2 receptor: Evaluation as markers of disease activity in scleroderma. J Rheumatol 1995;22:654.
71. Belongia EA, Hedberg CW, Gleich GH, et al: An investigation of the cause of the eosinophilia-myalgia syndrome associated with tryptophan use. N Engl J Med 1990;323:357.
72. Cronstein B, Weissman G: The adhesion molecules of inflammation. Arthritis Rheum 1993;36:147.
73. Sfikakis PP, Tesar J, Baraf H, et al: Circulating intercellular adhesion molecule 1 in patients with systemic sclerosis. Clin Immunol Immunopathol 1993;68:88.
74. Carson WE, Beall LD, Hunder GG, et al: Serum ELAM-1 is increased in vasculitis scleroderma. J Rheumatol 1993;20:809.
75. Grushwitz MS, Hornstein OP, von Den Driesch P, et al: Correlation of soluble adhesion molecules in the peripheral blood of scleroderma patients in their in situ expression and with disease activity. Arthritis Rheum 1995;38:184.
76. Cox D, Earle L, Jiminez SA, et al: Elevation levels of eosinophil major protein in the sera of patients with systemic sclerosis. Arthritis Rheum 1995;38:939.
77. Foster CS: Systemic lupus erythematosus, discoid lupus erythematosus, and progressive systemic sclerosis. Int Ophthalmol Clin 1997;37:93.
78. Subcommittee for Scleroderma Criteria of the American Rheumatism Association, Diagnostic and Therapeutic Criteria Committee: Preliminary criteria for the classification of systemic sclerosis (scleroderma). Arthritis Rheum 1980;23:581.
79. Finch MB, Dawson J, Johnston GD, et al: The peripheral vascular effects of nifedipine in Raynaud's syndrome associated with scleroderma. A double-blind crossover study. Clin Rheumatol 1986;5:493.
80. Stone JH, Wigley FM: Management of systemic sclerosis: The art and science. Semin Cutan Med Surg 1998;17:55.
81. Sfikakis PP, Kyriakidis MK, Vergos CG, et al: Cardiopulmonary hemodynamics in systemic sclerosis and response to nifedipine and captopril Am J Med 1991;90:541.
82. Siver RM, Warrick JH, Kinsella MB, et al: Cyclophosphamide and low-dose prednisone therapy in patients with systemic sclerosis (scleroderma) with interstitial lung disease. J Rheumatol 1993;20:838.
83. Clements PJ, Furst DE, Wong WK, et al: High-dose versus low-dose

D-penicillamine in early diffuse systemic sclerosis. Analysis of a two-year double-blind, randomized, controlled clinical trial. Arthritis Rheum 1999;42:1194.

84. Silman A, Herrick A, Denton C, et al: Alpha interferon does not improve patient outcome in early diffuse scleroderma. Arthritis Rheum 1997;40:S123.

85. Siebold JR, Korn J, Simms R, et al: Controlled trial of recombinant human relaxin in diffuse scleroderma. Arthritis Rheum 1997;40:S123.

86. van den Hoogen FH, Boerbooms AM, Swaak AJ, et al: Comparison of methotrexate in the treatment of systemic sclerosis: a 24 week randomized double-blind trial, followed by a 24 week observational trial. Br J Rheumatol 1996;35:364.

87. Wilson D, Edworthy SM, Hart DA, et al: The safety and efficacy of low-dose tissue plasminogen activator in the treatment of sclerosis. J Dermatol 1995;22:637.

88. Pai BS, Srivas CR, Sabitha L, et al: Efficacy of dexamethasone pulse therapy and progressive systemic sclerosis. Int J Dermatol 1995;34:726.

89. Akesson A, Scheja A, Lundin A, et al: Improve pulmonary function in systemic sclerosis after treatment with cyclophosphamide. Arthritis Rheum 1994;37:729.

90. Dau PC, Callahan JP: Immune modulation during the treatment of systemic sclerosis with plasmapheresis and immunosuppressive drugs. Clin Immunol Immunopathol 1994;70:159.

91. McKown KM, Carbone LD, Bustillo JM, et al: Open trial of oral type 1 collagen in patients with systemic sclerosis (SSC). Arthritis Rheum 1997;40:S100.

55 GIANT CELL ARTERITIS

Jean Yang and C. Stephen Foster

DEFINITION

Giant cell arteritis (GCA), also known as temporal arteritis, is a systemic granulomatous vasculitis that involves medium- and large-sized arteries. The disease has certain characteristic manifestations, including headache, temporal tenderness or reduced pulsation, jaw claudication, and scalp tenderness. Involvement of the ophthalmic and posterior ciliary arteries can lead to permanent partial or complete vision loss. Blindness can be potentially prevented by prompt treatment with corticosteroids.

HISTORY

Ali-ibn-Isa of Baghdad first described GCA in the 10th century and made the association between this disease and vision loss.[1] In the English literature, Hutchinson in 1890 described the disease in a man in his 80s who "had red streaks on his head which were painful and prevented him wearing his hat. The red streaks proved, on examination, to be his temporal arteries."[2] Horton and colleagues, in 1932, first described the pathologic features of the arteritis.[3] In 1938, Jennings reported loss of vision as a result of the disease.[4]

GCA is also known as temporal arteritis,[3] cranial arteritis,[5] and granulomatous arteritis.[6] In Europe, the disease is sometimes called Horton's giant cell arteritis. Giant cell arteritis is the preferred name for the disease because of its systemic nature.

EPIDEMIOLOGY

GCA usually occurs in individuals aged 50 or older, and the incidence of the disease increases with age. Women are two to three times more frequently involved than men.[7-9] Most epidemiologic studies have shown the disease to be prevalent predominantly in whites of European origin. The reported incidence is variable, ranging from 0.49 to 33.6 per 100,000 aged 50 and older.[7-26] Comparison of results between studies is difficult because of differences in diagnostic and inclusion criteria. The incidence of biopsy-proven GCA ranges from 0.49[12] to 25.4[22] per 100,000 aged 50 and older. The incidence is highest in Scandinavia (23.3 to 33.6 per 100,000 over age 50[15, 18, 22]) and Minnesota (19.1 to 24.1 per 100,000 over age 50).[8, 13] A much lower incidence is reported in Israel (0.49 to 0.86 per 100,000 over age 50[12]) and Tennessee (1.58 per 100,000 over age 50).[14] Several studies showed an age-specific incidence rate increasing from 2.1 to 6.6 per 100,000 in the sixth decade, to 48.9 to 70.7 per 100,000 in the ninth decade.[7, 23]

Significant increases in the annual incidence rate of GCA have been reported in several series from different countries and regions.[8-10, 21, 23, 26] The reason for this increase is unclear. In some of these studies, the increase in incidence is observed only in women and therefore cannot be explained by increased clinical awareness of physicians and improved diagnostic tests alone.[8, 9] Salvarani and colleagues[23] and Elling and coworkers[24] showed fluctuations of incidence rate in a cyclic pattern with "epidemics" occurring every 6 to 7 years, and they speculated an infectious cause for this disease. Elling and colleagues correlated peak incidences of GCA with two epidemics of *Mycoplasma pneumoniae* infection,[24] and Gabriel and associates note that the cycles of GCA epidemic-like peaks mimics that of parvovirus B19 epidemic cycles.[27]

Autopsy histopathologic studies found arteritis lesions in the temporal artery or aorta in 1.5 to 1.7 % of autopsies performed.[28, 29] This suggests that subclinical GCA may be more prevalent than the epidemiologic data indicate.

CLINICAL MANIFESTATIONS

Systemic Features

The disease often begins insidiously, with constitutional symptoms such as malaise, anorexia, weight loss, night sweats, myalgia, and fever. The prodromal period may last from several weeks to months. The most common symptom is headache,[10, 11, 30] which is usually temporal or occipital, and can be either unilateral or bilateral. The headache can gradually increase in severity and is usually worse in the evening and with exposure to cold temperatures.[31] Other cranial symptoms include scalp and temporal tenderness, jaw claudication, facial pain, earache, toothache, tongue and palate pain, and odynophagia.[30-34]

Given the potentially devastating visual consequences of GCA, and the fact that this disease is one of the treatable causes of blindness, it is important to be reminded of what Paulley and Hughes once stated, "When elderly people begin to fail mentally and physically, this should be one of the first disorders to be considered, and not one of the last."[32] It is especially incumbent on clinicians to be vigilant of the "silent" presentation, or the occult form of the disease. In occult GCA, the classic symptoms may be minimal or absent, or they may appear long after the ocular phase of the disease.[35] In 8%[7] to 34%[35] of cases, patients present with only vague constitutional symptoms, which makes the diagnosis difficult. In one study, atypical, silent presentation of the disease in a group of patients resulted in a mean delay in diagnosis of 21.5 days, in contrast to a delay of 8.5 days in the group with typical presentations.[36] A recent study showed 21% of 85 patients had ocular involvement without any systemic symptoms and signs of GCA.[37]

Many neurologic diseases are associated with GCA. Caselli and colleagues reported neurologic problems occurring in 31% of 166 patients with GCA.[38] Cerebrovascular disease is thought by some to be the most common cause of death in patients with GCA.[40, 41] It is difficult to assess the frequency of cerebrovascular disease, which has been reported to be 1% to 25% in a number of series.[31, 38-40] Other associated neurologic diseases include peripheral neuropathies, neuro-otologic syndromes, neuropsychiatric syndromes, seizures, and myopathy.[32, 34, 38, 41-45] Neuro-ophthalmic manifestations will be discussed later.

Large vessels such as the aorta and its major branches can be involved. The cardiovascular involvement of GCA may not be readily recognized because the involvement can be asymptomatic, and atherosclerosis often coexists with GCA. Severe involvement can lead to aortic incompetence, aortic aneurysm, aortic arch syndrome, aortic rupture, and myocardial infarction.[32, 45–50] Involvement of other large vessels can result in claudication of an extremity, paresthesias, and Raynaud's phenomenon. In a study of 248 patients with GCA, 34 had evidence of aortic or other large vessel disease.[46]

Other less common systemic manifestations include pulmonary abnormalities such as cough,[51, 52] pleural effusion,[53] pulmonary thrombosis, and infarction[54, 55]; gastroenterologic complications such as intestinal fistula formation and perforation[56, 57]; renal vasculitis and renal failure[58, 59]; and dermatologic diseases such as scalp necrosis,[34, 60] gangrene, and erythema nodosum–like lesions on the lower extremities.[61, 62]

Relationship to Polymyalgia Rheumatica

The relationship between GCA and polymyalgia rheumatica (PMR) is unclear. PMR is a syndrome characterized by morning stiffness, pain and stiffness in pelvic and shoulder girdles, elevated erythrocyte sedimentation rate (ESR), and a rapid response to small doses of corticosteroids. Like GCA, it is a disease of the elderly, involving predominantly whites, and is more common in women by a ratio of 2 or 3 to 1. GCA and PMR are often present in the same patient. Furthermore, arteritis was found in clinically asymptomatic temporal arteries in patients with PMR.[63] It is believed by some that the two diseases are different manifestations of the same underlying pathology.[64]

The incidence of PMR is reported to be 53.7 per 100,000 aged 50 and older in Olmstead County, Minnesota,[13] and 28.6 per 100,000 aged 50 and older in Goteborg, Sweden.[65] In the Minnesota study, GCA was found in 15 of 96 patients (16%) with PMR. In other series, positive temporal artery biopsy in patients with PMR ranges from 0% in New York[66] to 41% in some Scandinavian countries.[45, 67] The low rate of positive biopsy in New York is thought to be a result of the Jewish descent of many of the patients studied, because it corresponds to the low incidence of GCA reported in Israel.[68] In a large prospective study in Norway, random biopsies of 68 patients with PMR revealed inflammatory changes in only three patients (4.4%).[69] A recent study identified the best predictors of arteritis in patients with PMR as a new-onset headache, clinically abnormal temporal arteries, jaw claudication, elevated liver enzymes, and age greater than 70 years at disease onset.[70] Among the patients with GCA, approximately half develop PMR.[10]

GCA and PMR have different clinical courses that suggest that they are indeed two separate diseases. Unlike GCA, PMR responds to small doses of corticosteroids. Also PMR can be chronic and recurrent, while late recurrence of GCA is very uncommon.

Ophthalmic Features

Anterior Ischemic Optic Neuropathy

The reported rate of ocular involvement in GCA varies greatly, from 14% to 70%.[8, 10, 11, 22, 31, 37, 38, 40, 71, 72] Likely explanations for the differences in reported incidences are differences in diagnostic criteria, and probable selection bias in favor of cases with ophthalmic involvement in some of the earlier series. More important, the decreasing incidence of ophthalmic involvement in later studies probably should be credited to increased clinical awareness and prompt treatment.

The most common and devastating ocular symptom of GCA is vision loss, either partial or complete. The rate of vision loss is difficult to ascertain, with reported incidence wildly ranging from 8% to 65%.[8, 10, 11, 30, 31, 37, 38, 40, 71] The use of corticosteroids and, again, increased clinical awareness may account for the lower rate of vision loss in the later series. The most common etiology of vision loss is anterior ischemic optic neuropathy (AION). Other causes include central or branch retinal artery occlusion, cilioretinal artery occlusion, posterior ischemic optic neuropathy (PION), choroidal infarction, and, rarely, anterior segment ischemia and cortical blindness. The vision loss in GCA may be either unilateral or bilateral, and it is usually sudden, painless, and permanent. Often the loss of vision is found on waking up in the morning. Amaurosis fugax is an ominous sign of impending AION, which occurs in 10%[11, 38] to 18%[73] of cases. When the second eye is involved, the time interval between vision loss of two eyes is 7[11] to 23[73] days. Fleeting visual blurring with heat or exercise, or Uhthoff's phenomenon, has been described in GCA.[74]

AION results from ischemia of the optic nerve head, which is mainly supplied by the posterior ciliary arteries. AION is divided into the arteritic type, caused by GCA, and the nonarteritic type, which has other causes such as hypertension, diabetes mellitus, atherosclerosis, carotid artery disease, and collagen vascular disease.[75] Nonarteritic AION also includes those cases with no apparent cause. The majority of AION is nonarteritic, accounting for 87.5% to 91% of cases.[75–77] AION presents with sudden painless loss of vision, although visual acuity can range from 20/20 to no light perception.[78] Relative afferent pupillary defect can be found. Fundus examination shows optic disc edema, which may be accompanied by splinter hemorrhages at the disc margin (Fig. 55–1). A chalky white edematous optic disc is highly suggestive of arteritic AION, and it is very rare in the nonarteritic type (Fig. 55–2).[79] Similarly, the presence of cilioretinal artery occlusion is also almost diagnostic of arteritic AION (Fig. 55–3).[79] In nonarteritic AION, a small "crowded" optic disc cup is often found in the fellow eye, which is not characteristic of arteritic AION.[80] Visual field perimetry typically shows inferior altitudinal defect, inferior nasal sectoral defect or central scotoma, and a variety of other defects.[73, 78] Fluorescein angiogram reveals filling defects of the optic disc, peripapillary choroid, and choroidal watershed zones. Extensive choroidal nonfilling is very characteristic of arteritic AION (Fig. 55–4).[79] With time, the optic disc edema usually resolves, in about 2 months, and it is followed by sectoral general optic atrophy. Bilateral involvement is more common in arteritic AION, by a factor of 1.9 according to one study.[77]

It is important to distinguish arteritic from nonarteritic AION. Hayreh described a set of criteria to differentiate the two types.[75] Arteritic AION can be differentiated from

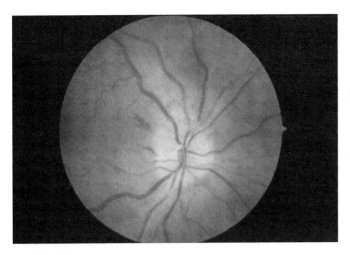

FIGURE 55–1. Giant cell arteritis, with abrupt loss of vision, left eye, with disc edema and splinter hemorrhages adjacent to the disc. (Courtesy of Simmons Lessell, MD.)

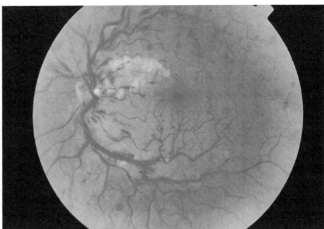

FIGURE 55–3. Giant cell arteritis with occlusion of a cilioretinal artery, and associated intraretinal hemorrhages. (Courtesy of John I. Loewenstein, MD.) (See color insert.)

nonarteritic AION by the previously described classic systemic symptoms, visual symptoms (especially amaurosis fugax and diplopia), elevated ESR and C-reactive protein (CRP), early massive visual loss; the presence of chalky white optic disc edema, cilioretinal artery occlusion, massive choroidal nonfilling of the choroid on fluorescein angiogram, and positive temporal artery biopsy findings.[75]

Posterior Ischemic Optic Neuropathy

PION, also referred to as retrobulbar ischemic optic neuritis, is caused by ischemia of the posterior part of the optic nerve. PION is a less common complication of GCA and is usually a diagnosis of exclusion. The disease is manifested as visual loss with an afferent pupillary defect but with no apparent fundus abnormality.[81, 82] The optic nerve head shows atrophic changes 5 to 6 weeks later. A recent color Doppler ultrasonography study showed decreased blood flow in a patient with arteritic PION.[83]

Central Retinal Artery Occlusion

Central retinal artery occlusion (CRAO) is another potential complication of GCA. The incidence of CRAO in

GCA in the literature ranges from 4% to 21%.[11, 39, 73, 84] It was shown that central retinal artery and one or more of the posterior ciliary arteries often arise from a common branch from the ophthalmic artery.[85] Therefore, it is not surprising that in cases of CRAO in GCA, there is involvement of the posterior ciliary arteries. Hayreh demonstrated, by fluorescein angiogram, that the majority of the CRAO cases in GCA were accompanied by a combined occlusion of the posterior ciliary artery.[78] This is also supported by color Doppler ultrasonography findings of decreased flow in the posterior ciliary arteries in a patient with CRAO caused by GCA.[83] Another color Doppler study showed significantly reduced flow velocities in central retinal and short posterior ciliary arteries in all the patients with GCA studied.[86] Cilioretinal artery is also a branch of the posterior ciliary artery. Occlusion of the cilioretinal artery is usually associated with AION, and its occlusion is a differential feature of arteritic AION from the nonarteritic type.[75]

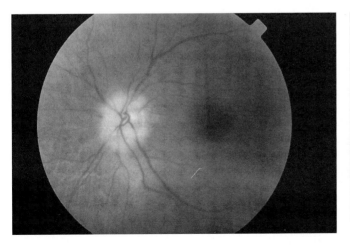

FIGURE 55–2. Giant cell arteritis, in a patient who demonstrates the chalky white form of disc edema. (Courtesy of Joseph F. Rizzo III, MD.) (See color insert.)

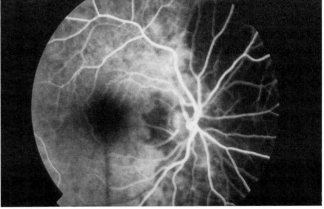

FIGURE 55–4. Giant cell arteritis, fluorescein angiogram, demonstrating extensive delayed filling of multiple areas of the choroid, which is indicative of choroidal involvement in this systemic arteritic disease. (Courtesy of Joseph F. Rizzo III, MD.)

Branch Retinal Artery Occlusion

Branch retinal artery occlusion has also been reported in GCA.[87] However, Hayreh argued that many cases of branch retinal artery occlusion in GCA are probably misdiagnosed cilioretinal artery occlusions, as GCA is not a disease that involves arterioles.[88] Recently, another case of GCA presenting with branch retinal artery occlusion as the initial sign was reported.[89] The authors speculated that the inflammation or thrombosis of the ophthalmic artery or central retinal artery reduces blood flow in retinal arterioles and predisposes the development of branch retinal artery occlusion. This speculation is supported by the observation of cotton-wool spots in GCA, which is a sign of focal retinal ischemia caused by retinal arteriolar obstruction.[90]

Choroidal Ischemia

Choroidal ischemia is another manifestation of occlusion of the posterior ciliary artery, because the choroid is supplied by the posterior ciliary arteries. Choroidal ischemia is often found only on fluorescein angiogram, and it remains asymptomatic.[79] However, it may lead to decreased vision: It was the cause of vision loss in 6% of cases in one study.[73] Choroidal ischemia may not have any obvious retinal findings. When the macula is involved, choroidal ischemia may have the appearance of a whitish lesion involving the peripapillary region, which probably represents degenerated pigment epithelium.[79] Choroidal ischemia may also appear as scattered yellow-white lesions at the level of the retinal pigment epithelium.[91] Areas of choroidal infarcts resulting from choroidal ischemia later appear as peripheral chorioretinal degenerative lesions. These areas are often found in the midperipheral region, and they tend to be triangular in shape, with the base toward the equator and the apex toward the posterior pole.[79, 92]

Neuro-ophthalmic

Diplopia is a frequently reported finding in GCA, with an incidence of 2% to 17%.[10, 31, 34, 38, 40, 71, 93] Diplopia may occur during and after the headache, and it can precede visual loss.[71, 93] It has been noted that diplopia may be present without any evident extraocular muscle abnormalities.[31, 71, 94] Hollenhorst reported that only 12 of 22 patients with diplopia had demonstrable extraocular muscle abnormalities.[31] Hollenhorst also noted that the vertically acting extraocular muscles are more frequently affected. The oculomotor nerve appears to be the most commonly involved, usually sparing the pupil.[93, 95] Other cranial nerves frequently involved are the abducens (CN VI) and the trochlear (CN IV).[11, 39, 95, 96] The cause of diplopia is generally thought to be neurogenic in nature. However, some have suggested that the ophthalmoplegia is due to muscle ischemia. Barricks and colleagues showed autopsy findings of muscle ischemia in a patient with GCA and ophthalmoplegia.[97] Sibony and Lessell reported transient oculomotor synkinesis in GCA, and argued that this was evidence that the ophthalmoplegia was neurogenic rather than myogenic in nature.[98] In contrast to the visual loss in this disease, which often is permanent, diplopia usually resolves with time, sometimes even without steroid treatment.[11, 71, 93]

Other neuro-ophthalmologic abnormalities associated with GCA include ptosis,[99] nystagmus,[31] and internuclear ophthalmoplegia.[100] Pupillary abnormalities associated with GCA include, most commonly, a relative afferent pupillary defect, tonic pupil,[101, 102] and Horner's syndrome.[103]

Uveitis

Anterior segment ischemia[104, 105] and uveitis[106, 107] are less common in GCA. Ocular hypotony,[108] corneal edema,[109] marginal corneal ulceration,[110] episcleritis and scleritis,[111] neovascular glaucoma,[112] and orbital pseudotumor[113] have all been reported.

Cerebral ischemia may rarely produce visual loss.[39, 114] Characteristic visual field defects such as homonymous hemianopia probably results from ischemic postchiasmal lesions.[31] Cortical blindness caused by infarction of the occipital lobes and associated with vertebral arteritis has been described.[115, 116]

PATHOLOGY

The most commonly involved vessels in GCA are the superficial temporal, occipital, vertebral, ophthalmic, and posterior ciliary arteries.[116] The reason for the frequency of involvement of the cranial vessels is not clear. Other arteries, especially the aorta and coronary arteries, can be involved.[46] It has been noted that intracranial arterial involvement is less frequent, and the vertebral arteries that are severely affected show no evidence of the disease shortly after entering the dura.[116] It has been postulated that the inflammation in GCA is correlated with the amount of the elastic tissue in the arteries, which would explain why intracranial arteries are less involved, because they contain less elastic fibers.[117]

All three layers of the arterial wall may be involved by granulomatous inflammation, although the inflammation can be located mainly in the media and intima.[33, 118] The involved area is infiltrated with epithelioid macrophages, lymphocytes, and multinucleated giant cells. The intima is thickened with edema and fibrosis, and the lumen may be markedly narrowed as a result. Fragmentation and destruction of the internal elastic lamina are frequently seen. Multinucleated giant cells are often seen adjacent to the internal elastic lamina. Although giant cells are characteristic of this disease, their presence is not a prerequisite to make the histopathologic diagnosis. Although focal areas of intimal and medial necrosis can be observed, extensive necrosis is unusual and should suggest other diagnoses.[119] Healed arteritis is characterized by irregular intimal and medial fibrosis, scattered chronic inflammatory cells, and small blood vessel formation in the vessel walls.[120]

Skip areas, or segments of normal artery, can be present between the arteritic lesions.[121] Therefore, a negative biopsy cannot sufficiently exclude the diagnosis.

IMMUNOLOGY AND PATHOGENESIS

Despite the great interest and extensive immunologic studies on GCA, the etiology of this disease remains unclear. Studies have suggested the role of a humoral immunologic mechanism in the pathogenesis of GCA, but increasing evidence points to its being a cell-mediated disease.

An early report speculated that the immune reaction of the disease was directed toward elastin.[118] This was derived from the observation of the degradation of the internal elastic lamina and associated granulomatous inflammation, especially the concentration of giant cell reaction in the region of the internal elastic lamina. Occasionally, giant cells also appeared to have phagocytosed elastin,[118] although this was not generally confirmed by electron microscopy.[122, 123] The speculation of elastin being the target of the inflammatory activity is supported by the fact that intracranial arteries, which contain fewer elastic fibers, are less frequently affected.[116] Furthermore, the basal and stimulated elastolytic activity of monocytes was shown to be increased in GCA.[124] Deposition of leukocyte elastase was found along the fragmented internal lamina.[125] Elevated serum levels of neutrophil elastase in GCA patients was reported.[126] However, anti-elastin antibodies have not been demonstrated in the serum of GCA patients.[127] A recent study investigated the reaction of peripheral blood mononuclear cells from patients with GCA and controls, to elastase-derived elastin peptides. A proliferative response was found in 12 of 13 patients with GCA, and only in 3 of 34 of controls.[128] Another study found actinic elastotic degeneration in the posterior ciliary arteries of 68% of subjects aged 70 to 90 years. Particularly, one of these eyes showed giant cells on degenerate lamina, which was thought to be preclinical GCA.[129]

Another postulated pathogenic mechanism is an immune reaction to degenerated smooth muscle cells, with a secondary degradation of the elasticum and the formation of giant cells.[130] This hypothesis is supported by the finding, by electron microscopy, of macrophages and giant cells closely attached to the smooth muscle cells.[131] In addition, adhesion molecules, such as intercellular adhesion molecule-1 (ICAM-1), have been found to be expressed on the smooth muscle cells of the media.[132]

There may be a genetic predisposition to GCA, given the observation that the disease predominantly involves the white population. Increased prevalence of human leukocyte antigens HLA-DR3, HLA-DR4, HLA-B8, HLA-DRB1, and HLA-Cw3 (which is linked to HLA-DR4) have been found in patients with GCA.[133–137] There were also reports indicating that HLA-DR4 is increased only in those GCA patients who also have PMR, but not in patients with GCA alone.[138, 139] Of note is that the molecule encoded by HLA-DRB1 is intimately involved in antigen presentation to T cells.[140]

Earlier reports suggested that humoral autoimmunity may play a role in the pathogenesis of this disease. Elevated serum immunoglobulins and complement were reported.[141] Some reported circulating immune complexes,[142] as well as certain correlation between this finding and clinical disease activity,[143, 144] However, others did not corroborate the prevalence of circulating immune complexes in patients with GCA compared to controls.[145] Deposition of immunoglobulins and complement in the arterial wall were demonstrated by some,[146–148] although others found the deposition in many fewer biopsy samples.[149–151] Antibodies against intermediate filaments

were also demonstrated, which was thought to be a supportive finding for an autoimmune process.[152]

Cellular immunity is suggested by the infiltrating cell types, consisting of lymphocytes, monocytes, interdigitating reticulum cells, histiocytes, and giant cells. The majority of the lymphocytes in the arteritic lesions of GCA are T lymphocytes, with an absence of or very few B lymphocytes.[149, 152–154] A study of five patients who developed GCA after the onset of chronic lymphocytic leukemia found no leukemic B cells, known for their ability to diffusely seed organs, in the arteritic lesions.[155] This finding suggests that B cells are actively excluded in the inflammatory process. Monoclonal antibody studies in most of the reports indicated a predominance of CD4 + helper/inducer subsets over CD8 + cytotoxic/suppressor subset,[150, 153, 154] except for one report, in which equal numbers of each were observed.[147] Interdigitating reticulum cells were observed in 41% of the patients in one study and were associated with a shorter duration of disease activity.[154]

Some of the infiltrating macrophages and T lymphocytes were shown to express class II major histocompatibility antigen HLA-DR and transferrin receptors, which suggests that these lymphocytes are immunologically activated.[153, 154, 156] A higher percentage of T lymphocytes in the arterial wall expressed HLA-DR than those of the peripheral blood, indicating a high degree of local T-cell activation.[156] Infiltrating T lymphocytes also expressed interleukin-2 (IL-2) receptors.[153, 154, 156] In one of the studies, the IL-2 receptor expression decreased from 87.5% to 14% after the treatment with corticosteroids.[154] Most of T lymphocytes expressed the integrin receptors, such as lymphocyte function-associated antigens-1 (LFA-1) and very late activation molecules (VLA-1).[157] Strong expressions of ICAM-1 and LFA-3 were found on macrophages, epithelioid cells, and giant cells in the granulomatous lesion.[132]

There is evidence indicating that T cells involved in the disease are of selected clonotypes. T cells of identical T-cell receptor (TCR) V beta chains were isolated from distinct inflammatory foci of the same patient.[158, 159] When inflamed arteries are implanted into severe combined immunodeficiency (SCID) mice, T cells with identical TCRs were expanded in different mice with the same tissue grafts from the same patient.[160] This selective proliferation suggests that there is a locally expressed antigen that is recognized by a small fraction of CD4 T cells.

In situ production of cytokines, including IL-1 beta, IL-6, transforming growth factor-beta (TGF-β), interferon-gamma (IFN-γ), and IL-2, were detected in the vasculitic lesions of GCA.[161] IL-2 was also found in the biopsy specimens from patients with PMR, but TGF-β was not.[161] In the GCA artery-implanted SCID mice, it was shown that T-cell depletion led to decreased production of IL-1 beta and IL-6, and adoptive transfer of tissue-derived T cells enhanced the production of IL-2 and IFN-γ.[160] Further studies showed different patterns of cytokine production correlated with different patterns of clinical manifestations. For example, ischemic symptoms, such as jaw claudication and visual symptoms, were associated with higher concentrations of IFN-γ and IL-1.[162] An elevated serum IL-6 level has been reported in GCA, and higher levels were found to correlate with disease activity.[163, 164] Tumor necrosis factor was demonstrated in the artery walls, and it was localized to giant cells and macrophages.[165] Platelet-derived growth factor-A (PDGF-A) and PDGF-B were produced by macrophages, smooth muscle cells, and giant cells at the media-intima border. PDGF expression was associated with concentric intimal hyperplasia.[166] Serum levels of soluble IL-2 receptors and CD23 were found to be elevated during the active phase of the disease.[167, 168] The effect of corticosteroids on the cytokine production was studied in artery-SCID mice chimeras, which revealed that the treatment reduced tissue concentrations of IL-2, IL-1-beta, and IL-6 mRNA. Synthesis of IFN-γ mRNA was only slightly decreased, and that of TGF-β1 was unaffected.[169] The persistent TGF-β1 transcription may explain the chronicity of the disease.

Macrophages in arterial walls were found to contain proteolytic enzymes, including gelatinases such as matrix metalloproteinases (MMPs), which are type IV collagenases. Specimens from GCA patients showed enhanced immunostaining for MMP-9 and MMP-2 in the media and near internal elastic lamina.[170, 171] Serum MMP-9 titers were also significantly increased in patients with GCA.[172] The detection of MMP-9 suggests that degradation of intercellular matrix, especially elastic fibers, may take place in GCA.

A recent study demonstrated that the strongest inflammatory infiltration was in the adventitia, and a higher concentration of macrophages, HLA-DR, ICAM-1, and IL-2 were seen in the outer than in the inner half of the intima. This distribution was thought to indicate that the majority of the inflammatory cells enter the arterial wall from adventitial microvessels, migrate through the media, and aggregate at the peripheral intima and internal elastic membrane.[173] In another study, different subsets of macrophages were found at different areas of the arterial wall. The TGF-β1-expressing subset exhibited a strong preference for the adventitia, whereas the inducible nitric oxide synthase–expressing subset was almost exclusively found in the intimal layer, and the collagenase-expressing subset preferred the intima-media junction.[174] This finding suggests that the TGF-β1-expressing subset may function as a pro-inflammatory mediator, whereas the inducible nitric oxide synthase– and the collagenase-expressing macrophages are involved in tissue destruction in the center of pathology.

CD8+ lymphocytes in the peripheral blood of patients with GCA and PMR have been noted to be decreased in both absolute numbers and relative percentages.[175-177] Some studies indicate that the decrease of CD8+ lymphocytes is related to disease activity.[175, 177] Low percentages of CD8+ T cells in the peripheral blood of healthy relatives of patients with GCA suggest that this might be a hereditary characteristic.[178] The peripheral blood CD8+ T cells in patients with GCA were found to have a restricted repertoire with a distinct J beta gene segment usage, indicating that selectively expanded CD8+ cells may be of functional importance in the pathogenesis.[179]

A recent study detected parvovirus B19 DNA, by polymerase chain reaction, in the temporal artery biopsy tissue from patients with GCA. Parvovirus B19 DNA was detected in 7 of 13 specimens with histologic diagnosis of GCA, but it was not found in 33 of the 37 negative biopsy specimens, therefore suggesting a possible role of parvovirus B19 in the pathogenesis of this disease.[27]

DIAGNOSIS

The diagnosis of GCA is largely based on clinical impression. The American College of Rheumatology 1990 criteria for the classification of GCA are listed in Table 55–1.[180] The fulfillment of three of the five criteria is associated with a sensitivity of 93.5% and a specificity of 91.2%. Laboratory tests, particularly an elevated ESR, elevated serum fibrinogen, and soluble IL-2 receptor, can strongly support the diagnosis. Histopathologic evidence of GCA is still regarded as definitive.

Hematologic Tests

ESR is the most widely used, and remains the most valuable, laboratory test in the diagnosis of GCA. The Westergren technique is commonly used, as it is more sensitive than the Wintrobe technique, especially to increases in asymmetric macromolecules.[181] It is, for example, directly correlated with serum fibrinogen levels. In most series, ESR is elevated in 90% to 100% of cases.[10, 31, 32] The mean ESR value in the acute phase of GCA ranges from 83 to 107 mm/hour.[10, 11, 45, 73] However, normal values of ESR in biopsy-proven GCA are well documented,[40, 182] and ESR values less than 30 or 50 mm/hour have been found in 22.5% to 26% of cases in some series.[73, 183] Therefore, a normal ESR value does not exclude the diagnosis of GCA. The ESR level usually correlates well with disease activity

TABLE 55–1. 1990 AMERICAN COLLEGE OF RHEUMATOLOGY CRITERIA FOR THE CLASSIFICATION OF GIANT CELL ARTERITIS (TRADITIONAL FORMAT)

CRITERION	DEFINITION
1. Age at disease onset, ≥50 years	Development of symptoms or findings beginning at age 50 or older
2. New headache	New onset of or new type of localized pain in the head
3. Temporal artery abnormality	Temporal artery tenderness to palpation or decreased pulsation, unrelated to arteriosclerosis of cervical arteries
4. Elevated erythrocyte sedimentation rate	Erythrocyte sedimentation rate ≥50 mm/hr by the Westergren method
5. Abnormal artery biopsy	Biopsy specimen with artery showing vasculitis characterized by a predominance of mononuclear cell infiltration or granulomatous inflammation, usually with multinucleated giant cells

Clinical diagnosis of GCA is made if at least three of these five criteria are present. The presence of any three or more criteria yields a sensitivity of 93.5% and a specificity of 91.2%.

From Hunder GG, Bloch DA, Michel BA, et al: The American College of Rheumatology 1990 criteria for the classification of giant cell arteritis. Arthritis Rheum 1990;33:1122–1128.

and therefore is useful in monitoring treatment.[184, 185] ESR may be affected by anemia. An inverse relationship between ESR and hematocrit has been reported.[186]

CRP is a protein produced by hepatocytes, and it can be elevated in acute inflammatory disorders. Unlike ESR, CRP is not affected by anemia or the concentrations of other plasma proteins.[94, 187] CRP has been reported to be elevated in acute GCA, and its level correlates well with clinical disease activity.[184, 185, 187, 188] Compared with ESR and other hematologic tests, CRP tends to normalize more rapidly following corticosteroid treatment.[184, 187, 189] Opinions differ as to which is a better diagnostic test in GCA. Whereas ESR is regarded by some as a better indicator of clinical disease activity,[184, 185, 190] others consider CRP as more sensitive in the diagnosis of GCA[191] and in assessing the adequacy of corticosteroid treatment.[187]

Other hematologic tests including plasma viscosity, blood count, and various acute-phase reactants may also be helpful in the diagnosis of GCA. Plasma viscosity often is raised in GCA and is found to correlate well with ESR.[189, 192] Plasma viscosity combined with ESR may improve the diagnostic accuracy.[192] Normochromic normocytic anemia is commonly seen in GCA,[13, 193–195] and thrombocytosis is also documented.[195] Serum fibrinogen is typically elevated in GCA, which decreases rapidly following corticosteroid treatment.[184, 189] Von Willebrand factor can also be raised in GCA, and it may persist after corticosteroid treatment.[196] One study showed raised von Willebrand factor persisted during the first 2 years of treatment but normalized in patients in long-term remission.[197] Other proteins that may be raised in GCA include haptoglobin,[184, 190] orosomucoid,[190] α-1-antichymotrypsin,[188] and α-1-antitrypsin.[190] Anticardiolipin antibodies have been found to be prevalent in GCA patients.[198–201] The findings of some studies suggested that patients with PMR and/or GCA with elevated levels of anticardiolipin antibodies had increased risk of developing GCA or other major vascular complications.[199, 200]

Liver Function Tests

Liver function is frequently abnormal in GCA.[10, 13, 195] A common abnormality is an elevated alkaline phosphatase level, although transaminases may also be elevated.[13, 195, 202] Alkaline phosphatase is usually modestly elevated and tends to normalize with treatment.[203] The etiology of liver dysfunction is unclear. Although hepatic arteritis,[204] hepatic granuloma,[205] hepatocyte necrosis,[206] and intrahepatic cholestasis, suggesting immune complex deposition,[207] have all been reported in association with GCA, many liver biopsies appeared normal or showed nonspecific changes.[203] Radionuclide liver scans showed abnormal uptake in 7 of 29 patients with PMR or GCA, and this persisted even when liver function returned to normal after treatment.[203] Patients with abnormal liver scans were more likely to have raised alkaline phosphatase.

Other Diagnostic Studies

Fluorescein Angiogram

Fluorescein angiography shows a delay in arm-to-retina circulation time, and massive choroidal nonfilling.[79] This pattern of choroidal nonfilling is considered almost diagnostic of arteritic AION.[88] The medial posterior ciliary artery is involved more frequently than the lateral posterior ciliary artery.[79]

Color Doppler Ultrasonography

Color Doppler ultrasonography has been found to be a useful noninvasive tool in the diagnosis of GCA. Using this technique, studies of temporal arteries showed decreased blood flow velocity, thickening of the vessel wall, and stenosis or occlusions of the temporal arteries.[208, 209] One of the studies revealed a dark halo around the lumen of the temporal arteries in patients with GCA, which was thought to be caused by edema of the artery wall. The dark halo was a specific sign, and it disappeared after corticosteroid treatment.[208] Color Doppler studies of the orbit showed undetectable blood flow, reduced flow velocities in central retinal and short posterior ciliary arteries, high velocity and turbulent flow at presumed focal stenotic lesions, reversal of flow within the ophthalmic artery, and reduced and truncated time-velocity waveforms.[210, 211] Some of these observed changes are unique for, or more frequent in, GCA compared to nonarteritic AION.

Temporal Artery Biopsy

A positive temporal artery biopsy provides the definitive diagnosis of GCA. Because the diagnosis of GCA commits the patient to long-term corticosteroid treatment, which is associated with significant morbidity, a biopsy of the temporal artery is strongly advised to definitively secure the diagnosis.

The rate of positive biopsies varies among different series, ranging from 60% to 95% of clinical cases of GCA,[31, 44, 212–217] with rates greater than 90% in several series.[31, 45, 212–217] Negative biopsies cannot exclude the diagnosis of GCA, because skip areas, areas in between segments of arteritic lesions that show little or no sign of inflammation, may have been obtained at biopsy.[121] False-negative biopsies can be decreased by obtaining longer biopsy specimens (2 to 3 cm), and by careful serial sectioning.[88, 94, 121] If the biopsy is negative but there is a strong clinical suspicion, biopsy of the contralateral temporal artery should be performed.[88] Immunofluorescence microscopy studies were compared to light microscopy, and the former was not found to be more sensitive.[218]

The treatment with corticosteroids should not be delayed pending the results of temporal artery biopsy, although the biopsy should be performed within 1 week after the beginning of the treatment. Histopathologic changes may persist for months after the initiation of steroids.[45, 219] Although some data suggested the positivity rates of biopsy were similar in corticosteroid-treated and untreated patients,[212] one study showed the rate of a positive biopsy result falls from 82% in the untreated patients to 60% in patients who were treated for less than 1 week.[213]

Various signs and symptoms of GCA have been studied to determine which would best predict the diagnosis. The combination of a recent-onset headache, jaw claudication, and abnormalities of the temporal arteries on physical examination was associated with a specificity of 94.8% with respect to the histologic diagnosis, and 100% with respect to final diagnosis.[217] Another study also indicated that a history of jaw claudication and a palpably abnormal temporal artery were more common in cases with positive biopsies.[215] A more recent study identified jaw claudication, CRP above 2.45 mg/dl, neck pain, and an ESR of 47 or above as the clinical criteria most strongly suggestive of GCA.[191]

TREATMENT

Corticosteroids should be started immediately when there is a high suspicion of GCA. The use of corticosteroids was shown by Birkhead and colleagues in 1957 to be effective in the treatment of GCA, especially in reducing the rate of blindness.[219] In this study, 16 eyes of 55 patients presented with blindness, and two additional eyes became blind following corticosteroids treatment. This outcome was compared to 53 patients who were treated prior to the introduction of steroids, of which 16 eyes were blind at presentation, and eight more eyes became blind during follow-up. Corticosteroids also significantly relieved many other systemic symptoms. The prompt symptomatic relief is so characteristic that it is used by some as a diagnostic criterion.[8, 220]

There are no controlled prospective trials addressing the dosage and duration of treatment. Usually, a high initial dosage of corticosteroids, 80 to 120 mg/day of prednisone, is given. It has been noted that ophthalmologists tend to use higher dosages than rheumatologists, which probably is a result of different disease characteristics encountered by different subspecialties.[94] A lower dose of steroids, 40 mg/day of prednisolone, was used by some rheumatologists to achieve adequate control in most patients with GCA.[221] A retrospective evaluation studied patients treated with three different dose regimens: 30 to 40 mg/day, 40 to 60 mg/day, and over 60 mg/day, and similar efficacies were found. However, the group treated with over 60 mg/day had fewer flare-ups during the first year.[222] In cases of acute visual loss, high-dose intravenous corticosteroids are used by some to prevent the further visual loss or involvement of the fellow eye.[88] Although some data suggest high-dose intravenous corticosteroids may diminish the likelihood of fellow-eye involvement,[73] cases of severe visual loss in the fellow eye despite this treatment regimen were also reported.[223] It is unclear if visual improvement can be achieved with high-dose intravenous corticosteroids. Reports of visual improvement following high-dose intravenous corticosteroids have been anecdotal[11, 224, 225] and are viewed with skepticism by some.[88] Alternate-day oral corticosteroid therapy has been tried but found to be less effective.[226]

There are no generalized rules regarding the rate of steroid reduction once the disease is stabilized. Usually the steroid dose is adjusted based on the clinical response and the decrease in ESR. Other tests such as CRP and color Doppler ultrasonography may also aid in assessing the disease activity. The lowest dose of steroids that achieves disease quiescence and the lowest possible ESR is used as the maintenance dose. The steroid taper should be gradual to prevent exacerbation. Relapses can occur while the patients are on steroids,[40] especially when the steroid reduction is too rapid.[10, 45] Relapses usually occur

within the first year or within 3 months after withdrawal of treatment, but they can occur as late as 10 years after.[227] In a majority of cases, the dose of steroid can be decreased to below 7.5 mg/day of prednisone after 1 year of therapy.[227, 228] The duration of therapy should be individualized. A review of literature indicates that in many studies, the treatment is needed for at least 2 years,[11, 45, 229, 230] with 30% to 40% of patients in some European studies requiring longer or even indefinite treatment.[39, 227] The duration of treatment is somewhat shorter in the American studies.[10, 13] There are some reports indicating that the percentage of peripheral CD8+ lymphocytes remained decreased after 6 months or 1 year of corticosteroid treatment, even when the disease was under control symptomatically, and ESR and CRP were significantly decreased.[175, 231] One study showed that those patients who had a lower percentage of CD8+ at 6 months of treatment required a significantly longer course of corticosteroid treatment and more relapses, suggesting CD8+ percentage may be a useful monitoring parameter.[231]

Azathioprine has been used in an attempt to reduce the maintenance dose of steroids in patients with PMR and GCA, and in one study it was found to have a modest effect.[232] However, another study found methotrexate to be superior than azathioprine.[233] There are several reports indicating a steroid-sparing effect of methotrexate.[234, 235] However, one controlled study of PMR and GCA, with only six GCA patients included, failed to demonstrate this.[236] There have been some anecdotal reports of cyclosporine being an effective adjuvant therapy,[237] and of cases of steroid-resistant GCA that were responsive to cyclophosphamide treatment.[238]

If parvovirus B19 is confirmed to be a pathogenic factor, then the treatment with intravenous immunoglobulin (IVIg) may become plausible, as IVIg is effective in controlling chronic parvovirus B19 infection in immunocompromised individuals, and in patients with systemic necrotizing vasculitis possibly related to parvovirus B19 infection.[239]

PROGNOSIS

General Prognosis

GCA is a systemic vasculitis that can result in serious, life-threatening complications, such as cerebral vascular accidents, aortic rupture, and myocardial infarction. Prior to the introduction of corticosteroids, in one report, three of the seven patients with GCA died.[240] With the use of corticosteroids, several large series with long-term follow-up indicate that life expectancy in patients with GCA is the same as that of the general population,[10, 11, 240, 241] with one study showing an even lowered mortality rate.[227] On the other hand, a study from Sweden showed an increased mortality rate from vascular diseases during the first year, while the overall mortality rate after the first year, and over a 10-year period, was not higher than that in the general population. The increased first-year mortality rate was attributed to inadequate corticosteroid treatment.[242] Another report also considered inadequate treatment as an important contributory factor to the cause of deaths.[243] On the contrary, high maintenance steroid dose and visual loss were associated with a short-ened life span in another study.[39] The authors suggested that the steroid treatment itself contributed to the increased mortality, because the clinical features in this group of patients were not more severe. A Danish study reported a significantly higher mortality rate in GCA patients.[244]

Although the maintenance corticosteroid doses used in treating this disease are relatively low, the reported side effects are nonetheless numerous. Common side effects include cushingoid appearance, weight gain, osteoporosis, compression fractures, hypertension, diabetes, peptic ulcer disease, immunosuppression and infections, ischemic necrosis of the femoral head, proximal muscle weakness, elevated intraocular pressure, and cataracts.[10, 11, 227, 245] One study showed that serious corticosteroid-related complications are significantly more frequent in the group of patients on an average daily maintenance prednisone dose of 26.3 mg, compared with those on a daily dose of 13 mg.[245]

Visual Prognosis

In the earlier reports, the rate of visual loss was as high as 60%,[11, 31, 40, 71, 219] with the rate of bilateral visual loss being 20%.[11, 71, 219] With corticosteroid treatment and increased clinical awareness of the disease, the rate of visual loss in more recent studies ranges from 6% to 22%.[8, 30, 38, 73, 84] It has been reported that 6% to 13% of patients with visual loss lose vision while on corticosteroids treatment.[73, 84] The visual loss in GCA is usually permanent, although there are reports of improved vision, including with high-dose intravenous corticosteroid treatment.[11, 224, 225]

CONCLUSION

GCA is a systemic disease of the elderly that may result in profound, irreversible loss of vision. GCA is also a disease for which the treatment with corticosteroids is effective, and therefore loss of vision can be prevented by prompt diagnosis and initiation of treatment. The disease requires long-term corticosteroid treatment, which is associated with significant corticosteroid-related side effects. Alternative treatment with corticosteroid-sparing agents remains to be further explored. Although there have been significant new advances in the understanding of the immunopathology of GCA, the exact etiology of the disease remains unclear. Further understanding of the immunopathogenesis of the disease in the future may result in treatment with more disease-specific immunomodulators.

References

1. Wood CA: A memorandum book of a tenth century oculist, a translation of Tadkivate Ali Ibn Isa. Chicago, Northwestern University Press, 1936, 225–226.
2. Hutchinson J: Disease of the arteries. 1: On a peculiar form of thrombotic arteritis of the aged which is sometimes productive of gangrene. Arch Surg (London) 1890;1:323–329.
3. Horton BT, Magath TB, Brown GE: An undescribed form of arteritis of the temporal vessels. Lancet 1932;7:700–701.
4. Jennings GH: Arteritis of the temporal vessels. Lancet 1938;1:424–428.
5. Kilbourne ED, Wolff HG: Cranial arteritis: A critical evaluation of the syndrome of "temporal arteritis" with report of a case. Ann Intern Med 1946;24:1–10.
6. Cohen DN: Granulomatous arteritis. Compr Ther 1975;1:60–63.
7. Bengtsson BA, Malmvall BE: The epidemiology of giant cell arteritis including temporal arteritis and polymyalgia rheumatica. Incidences of different clinical presentations and eye complications. Arthritis Rheum 1981;24:899–904.
8. Machado EB, Michet CJ, Ballard DJ, et al: Trends in incidence and clinical presentation of temporal arteritis in Olmsted County, Minnesota, 1950–1985. Arthritis Rheum 1988;31:745–749.
9. Nordborg E, Bengtsson BA: Epidemiology of biopsy-proven giant cell arteritis (GCA). J Intern Med 1990;227:233–236.
10. Huston KA, Hunder GG, Lie JT, et al: Temporal arteritis: A 25-year epidemiologic, clinical, and pathologic study. Ann Intern Med 1978;88:162–167.
11. Jonasson F, Cullen JF, Elton RA: Temporal arteritis. A 14-year epidemiological, clinical and prognostic study. Scott Med J 1979;24:111–117.
12. Friedman G, Friedman B, Benbassat J: Epidemiology of temporal arteritis in Israel. Isr J Med Sci 1982;18:241–244.
13. Chuang TY, Hunder GG, Ilstrup DM, et al: Polymyalgia rheumatica: A 10-year epidemiologic and clinical study. Ann Intern Med 1982;97:672–680.
14. Smith CA, Fidler WJ, Pinals RS: The epidemiology of giant cell arteritis. Report of a ten-year study in Shelby County, Tennessee. Arthritis Rheum 1983;26:1214–1219.
15. Boesen DR, Sorensen SF: Giant cell arteritis, temporal arteritis, and polymyalgia rheumatica in a Danish county. A prospective investigation, 1982–1985. Arthritis Rheum 1987;30:294–299.
16. Gonzalez EB, Varner WT, Lisse JR, et al: Giant cell arteritis in the southern United States. An 11-year retrospective study from the Texas Gulf Coast. Arch Intern Med 1989;149:1561–1565.
17. Salvarani C, Macchioni P, Zizzi F, et al: Epidemiologic and immunogenetic aspects of polymyalgia rheumatica and giant cell arteritis in northern Italy. Arthritis Rheum 1991;34:351–356.
18. Noltorp S, Svensson B: High incidence of polymyalgia rheumatica and giant cell arteritis in a Swedish community. Clin Exp Rheumatol 1991;9:351–355.
19. Berlit P: Clinical and laboratory findings with giant cell arteritis. J Neurol Sci 1992;111:1–12.
20. Franzen P, Sutinen S, von Knorring J: Giant cell arteritis and polymyalgia rheumatica in a region of Finland: An epidemiologic, clinical and pathologic study, 1984–1988. J Rheumatol 1992;19:273–276.
21. Sonnenblick M, Nesher G, Friedlander Y, et al: Giant cell arteritis in Jerusalem: A 12-year epidemiological study. Br J Rheumatol 1994;33:938–941.
22. Baldursson O, Steinsson K, Bjornsson J, et al: Giant cell arteritis in Iceland. An epidemiologic and histopathologic analysis. Arthritis Rheum 1994;37:1007–1012.
23. Salvarani C, Gabriel SE, O'Fallon WM, et al: The incidence of giant cell arteritis in Olmsted County, Minnesota: Apparent fluctuations in a cyclic pattern. Ann Intern Med 1995;123:192–194.
24. Elling P, Olsson AT, Elling H: Synchronous variations of the incidence of temporal arteritis and polymyalgia rheumatica in different regions of Denmark: Association with epidemics of mycoplasma pneumoniae infection. J Rheumatol 1996;23:112–119.
25. Gran JT, Myklebust G: The incidence of polymyalgia rheumatica and temporal arteritis in the county of Aust Agder, south Norway: A prospective study 1987–94. J Rheumatol 1997;24:1739–1743.
26. Gonzalez-Gay MA, Blanco R, Sanchez-Andrade A, et al: Giant cell arteritis in Lugo, Spain: A more frequent disease with fewer classic features. J Rheumatol 1997;24:2166–2170.
27. Gabriel SE, Espy M, Erdman DD, et al: The role of parvovirus B19 in the pathogenesis of giant cell arteritis. Arthritis Rheum 1999;42:1255–1258.
28. Ostberg G: Temporal arteritis in a large necropsy series. Ann Rheum Dis 1971;30:224–225.
29. Ostberg G: On arteritis with special reference to polymyalgia arterica. Acta Pathol Microbiol Scand 1993;sect A273(suppl):1–59.
30. Font C, Cid MC, Coll-Vinent B, et al: Clinical features in patients with permanent visual loss due to biopsy-proven giant cell arteritis. Br J Rheumatol 1997;36:251–254.
31. Hollenhorst RW, Brown JR, Wagener HP, et al: Neurologic aspects of temporal arteritis. Neurology 1960;10:490–498.
32. Paulley JW, Hughes JP: Giant-cell arteritis, or arteritis of the aged. Br Med J 1960;2:1562–1567.

33. Hamilton CR, Shelley WM, Tumulty PA: Giant cell arteritis: Including temporal arteritis and polymyalgia rheumatica. Medicine 1971;50:1–27.

34. Russel RWR: Giant-cell arteritis: A review of 35 cases. Q J Med 1959;28:471–489.

35. Simons RJ, Cogan DG: Occult temporal arteritis. Arch Ophthalmol 1962;68:38–48.

36. Desmet GD, Knockaert DC, Bobbaers HJ: Temporal arteritis: The silent presentation and delay in diagnosis. J Intern Med 1990;227:237–240.

37. Hayreh SS, Podhajsky PA, Zimmerman B: Occult giant cell arteritis: Ocular manifestations. Am J Ophthalmol 1998;125:521–526.

38. Caselli R, Hunder GG, Whisnant JP: Neurologic disease in biopsy-proven giant cell (temporal) arteritis. Neurology 1988;38:352–359.

39. Graham E, Holland A, Avery A, et al: Prognosis in giant cell arteritis. Br Med J 1981;282:269–271.

40. Whitfield AG, Bateman M, Cooke WT: Temporal arteritis. Br J Ophthalmol 1963;47:555–566.

41. Reich KA, Giansiracusa DF, Strongwater SL: Neurologic manifestations of giant cell arteritis. Am J Med 1990;89:67–72.

42. Warrel DA, Godfrey S, Olsen EGJ: Giant-cell arteritis with peripheral neuropathy. Lancet 1968;1:1010–1013.

43. Pascuzzi RM, Roos KL, Davis TE: Mental status abnormalities in temporal arteritis: A treatable cause of dementia in the elderly. Arthritis Rheum 1989;32:1308–1311.

44. Andrews JM: Giant-cell arteritis: A disease with variable clinical manifestations. Neurology 1966;16:963–971.

45. Fauchald P, Rygvold O, Oystese B, et al: Temporal arteritis and polymyalgia rheumatica: Clinical and biopsy findings. Ann Intern Med 1972;77:845–852.

46. Klein RG, Hunder GG, Stanson AW, et al: Large artery involvement in giant cell (temporal) arteritis. Ann Intern Med 1975;83:806–812.

47. Sorensen PS, Lorenzen I: Giant cell arteritis, temporal arteritis and polymyalgia rheumatica: A retrospective study of 63 patients. Acta Med Scand 1977;201:207–213.

48. Lie JT: Aortic and extracranial large vessel giant cell arteritis: A review of 72 cases with histopathologic documentation. Semin Arthritis Rheum 1995;24:422–431.

49. Liu G, Shupak R, Chiu BK: Aortic dissection in giant-cell arteritis. Semin Arthritis Rheum 1995;25:160–171.

50. Evans JM, O'Fallon WM, Hunder GG: Increased incidence of aortic aneurysm and dissection in giant cell (temporal) arteritis. A population-based study. Ann Intern Med 1995;122:502–507.

51. Larson TS, Hall S, Hepper NG, et al: Respiratory tract symptoms as a clue to giant cell arteritis. Ann Intern Med 1984;101:594–597.

52. Olopade CO, Sekosan M, Schraufnagel DE: Giant cell arteritis manifesting as chronic cough and fever of unknown origin. Mayo Clin Proc 1997;72:1048–1050.

53. Gur H, Ehrenfeld M, Izsak E: Pleural effusion as a presenting manifestations of giant cell arteritis. Clin Rheumatol 1996;15:200–203.

54. Lardrin I, Chassagne P, Bouaniche M, et al: Pulmonary artery thrombosis in giant cell arteritis. A new case and review of literature. Ann Med Interne 1997;148:315–316.

55. de Heide LJ, Pieterman H, Hennemann G: Pulmonary infarction caused by giant cell arteritis of the pulmonary artery. Neth J Med 1995;46:36–40.

56. Lagrand WK, Hoogendoorn M, Bakker K, et al: Aortoduodenal fistula as an unusual and fatal manifestations of giant-cell arteritis. Eur J Vasc Endovasc Surg 1996;11:502–503.

57. Tsuyuoka R, Takahashi T, Shinoda E, et al: Intestinal perforation in temporal arteritis, associated with paroxysmal nocturnal hemoglobinuria. Intern Med 1996;35:159–161.

58. Lenz T, Schmidt R, Scherberich JE, et al: Renal failure in giant cell arteritis. Am J Kidney Dis 1998;31:1044–1047.

59. Govil YK, Sabanathan K, Scott D: Giant cell arteritis presenting as renal vasculitis. Postgrad Med J 1998;74:170–171.

60. Currey J: Scalp necrosis in giant cell arteritis and review of the literature. Br J Rheumatol 1997;36:814–816.

61. Goldberg JW, Lee ML, Sajjad SM: Giant cell arteritis of the skin simulating erythema nodosum. Ann Rheum Disease 1987;46:706–708.

62. Lie JT, Tokugawa DA: Bilateral lower limb gangrene and stroke as initial manifestations of systemic giant cell arteritis in an African-American. J Rheumatol 1995;22:363–366.

63. Alestig K, Barr J: Giant cell arteritis. Lancet 1963;1:1228–1230.

64. Bengtsson BA: Epidemiology of giant cell arteritis. Baillieres Clin Rheumatol 1991;5:379–385.

65. Bengtsson BA, Malmvall BE: Giant cell arteritis. Acta Med Scand 1982;658(suppl):18–28.

66. Spiera H, Davison S: Treatment of polymyalgia rheumatica. Arthritis Rheum 1982;25:120.

67. Hamrin B: Polymyalgia rheumatica. Acta Med Scand 1972;533(suppl):1–164.

68. Healey LA: Relation of giant cell arteritis to polymyalgia rheumatica. Baillieres Clin Rheumatol 1991;5:371–378.

69. Myklebust G, Gran JT: A prospective study of 287 patients with polymyalgia rheumatica and temporal arteritis: Clinical and laboratory manifestations at onset of disease and at the time of diagnosis. Br J Rheumatol 1996;35:1161–1168.

70. Rodriguez-Valverde V, Sarabia JM, Gonzalez-Gay MA, et al: Risk factors and predictive models of giant cell arteritis in polymyalgia rheumatica. Am J Med 1997;102:331–336.

71. Wagener HP, Hollenhorst RW: The ocular lesions of temporal arteritis. Am J Ophthalmol 1958;45:617–630.

72. Healey LA, Wilske KR: Manifestations of giant cell arteritis. Med Clin North Am 1977;61:261–270.

73. Liu GT, Glaser JS, Schatz NJ, et al: Visual morbidity in giant cell arteritis, clinical characteristics and prognosis for vision. Ophthalmology 1994;101:1779–1785.

74. Raymond LA, Sacks JG, Choromokos E, et al: Short posterior ciliary artery insufficiency with hyperthermia (Uhthoff's symptom). Am J Ophthalmol 1980;90:619–623.

75. Hayreh SS: Anterior ischaemic optic neuropathy, differentiation of arteritic from non-arteritic type and its management. Eye 1990;4:25–41.

76. Guer DR, Miller NR, Auer CL, et al: The risk of cerebrovascular and cardiovascular disease in patients with anterior ischemic optic neuropathy. Arch Ophthalmol 1985;103:1136–1142.

77. Beri M, Klugman MR, Kohler JA, et al: Anterior ischemic optic neuropathy. VII. Incidence of bilaterality and various influencing factors. Ophthalmology 1987;94:1020–1028.

78. Hayreh SS, Podhajsky P: Visual field defects in anterior ischemic optic neuropathy. Doc Ophthalmol Proc Ser 1979;19:53–71.

79. Hayreh SS: Anterior ischemic optic neuropathy II. Fundus on ophthalmoscopy and fluorescein angiography. Br J Ophthalmol 1974;58:964–980.

80. Beck RW, Servais GE, Hayreh SS: Anterior ischemic optic neuropathy. IX. Cup-to-disc ratio and its role in pathogenesis. Ophthalmology 1989;94:1503–1508.

81. Hayreh SS: Posterior ischemic optic neuropathy. Ophthalmologica 1981;182:29–41.

82. Gladstone GJ: The afferent pupillary defect as an early manifestation of occult temporal arteritis. Ann Ophthalmol 1982;14:1088–1091.

83. Ghanchi FD, Williamson TH, Lim CS, et al: Colour Doppler imaging in GCA: Serial examination and comparison with nonarteritic anterior ischemic optic neuropathy. Eye 1996;10:459–464.

84. Aiello PD, Trautmann JC, McPhee TJ, et al: Visual prognosis in giant cell arteritis. Ophthalmology 1993;100:550–555.

85. Singh S, Dass R: The central artery of the retina I. Origin and course. Br J Ophthalmol 1960;44:193–212.

86. Ho AC, Sergott RC, Regillo CD, et al: Color Doppler hemodynamics of giant cell arteritis. Arch Ophthalmol 1994;112:938–945.

87. Cullen JF: Occult temporal arteritis. Br J Ophthalmol 1967;51:513–525.

88. Hayreh SS: Ophthalmic features of giant cell arteritis. Baillieres Clin Rheumatol 1991;5:431–459.

89. Fineman MS, Savino PJ, Federman JL, et al: Branch retinal artery occlusion as the initial sign of giant cell arteritis. Am J Ophthalmol 1996;122:428–430.

90. Melberg NS, Grand MG, Dieckert JP, et al: Cotton wool spots and the early diagnosis of giant cell arteritis. Ophthalmology 1995;102:1611–1614.

91. Quillen DA, Cantore WA, Schwartz, et al: Choroidal nonperfusion in giant cell arteritis. Am J Ophthalmol 1993;116:171–175.

92. Amalric P: Acute choroidal ischemia. Trans Ophthalmol Soc U K 1972;91:305–322.

93. Meadows SP: Temporal or giant cell arteritis. Proc R Soc Med 1966;59:329–333.

94. Ghanchi FD, Dutton GN: Current concepts in giant cell arteritis. Surv Ophthalmol 1997;42:99–123.
95. Russell RWR: Giant-cell arteritis: A review of 35 cases. Q J Med 1959;28:471–489.
96. Simmons RJ, Cogan DG: Occult temporal arteritis. Arch Ophthalmol 1962;68:8–18.
97. Barricks ME, Traviesa DB, Glaser JS, et al: Ophthalmoplegia in cranial arteritis. Brain 1977;100:209–221.
98. Sibony PA, Lessell S: Transient oculomotor synkinesis in temporal arteritis. Arch Neurol 1984;41:87–88.
99. Dimant J, Grob D, Brunner NG: Ophthalmoplegia, ptosis, and miosis in temporal arteritis. Neurology 1980;30:1054–1058.
100. Crompton JL, Burrow DJ, Iyer PV: Bilateral internuclear ophthalmoplegia—An unusual initial presenting sign of giant cell arteritis. Aust N Z J Ophthalmol 1989;17:71–74.
101. Coppeto JR, Greco T: Mydriasis in giant-cell arteritis. J Clin Neuroophthalmol 1989;9:267–269.
102. Currie J, Lessell S: Tonic pupil with giant cell arteritis. Br J Ophthalmol 1984;68:135–138.
103. Bell TAG, Gibson RA, Tullo AB: A case of giant-cell arteritis and Horner's syndrome. Scott Med J 1980;25:302.
104. Birt CM, Slomovic A, Motolko M, et al: Anterior segment ischemia in giant cell arteritis. Can J Ophthalmol 1994;29:93–94.
105. Zion VM, Goodside V: Anterior segment ischemia with ischemic optic neuropathy. Surv Ophthalmol 1974;19:19–30.
106. Dasgupta B, Pitzalis C, Panayi GS: Inflammation of the uveal tract as a presenting feature of temporal arteritis. Ann Rheum Dis 1989;48:964–965.
107. Coppeto JR, Monteiro ML, Sciarra R: Giant-cell arteritis with bilateral uveitic glaucoma. Ann Ophthalmol 1985;17:299–302.
108. Radda TM, Bardach H, Riss B: Acute ocular hypotony. A rare complication of temporal arteritis. Ophthalmologica 1981;182:148–152.
109. Nielsen NV, Eriksen JS, Olsen T: Corneal edema as a result of ischemic endothelial damage: A case report. Ann Ophthalmol 1982;14:276–278.
110. Gerstle CC, Friedman AH: Marginal corneal ulceration (limbal guttering) as a presenting sign of temporal arteritis. Ophthalmology 1980;87:1173–1176.
111. Long RG, Friedmann AI, James DG: Scleritis and temporal arteritis. Postgrad Med J 1976;52:689–692.
112. Wolter JR, Phillips RL: Secondary glaucoma in cranial arteritis. Am J Ophthalmol 1965;59:625–634.
113. Nassani S, Cocito L, Arcuri T, et al: Orbital pseudotumor as a presenting sign of temporal arteritis. Clin Exp Rheumatol 1995;13:367–369.
114. Heptinstall RH, Porter KA, Barkley H: Giant cell (temporal) arteritis. J Pathol Bacteriol 1954;67:507–519.
115. Symonds C, Mackenzie I: Bilateral loss of vision from cerebral infarction. Brain 1957;80:415–455.
116. Wilkinson IM, Russell RW: Arteries of the head and neck in giant cell arteritis. A pathological study to show the pattern of arterial involvement. Arch Neurol 1972;27:378–391.
117. Healey LA: The spectrum of polymyalgia rheumatica. Clin Geriatr Med 1988;4:323–331.
118. Kimmelstiel P, Gilmour MT, Hodges HH: Degeneration of elastic fibers in granulomatous giant cell arteritis (temporal arteritis). Arch Pathol 1952;54:157–168.
119. Ashton-Key M, Gallagher PJ: Surgical pathology of cranial arteritis and polymyalgia rheumatica. Baillieres Clin Rheumatol 1991;5:387–404.
120. Lie JT, Brown AL, Carter ET: Spectrum of aging changes in temporal arteritis. Arch Pathol 1970;90:278–285.
121. Albert DM, Ruchman MC, Keltner JL: Skip areas in temporal arteritis. Arch Ophthalmol 1976;94:2072–2077.
122. Parker F, Healy LA, Wilske KR, et al: Light and electron microscopic studies on human temporal arteries with special reference to alterations related to senescence, atherosclerosis and giant cell arteritis. Am J Pathol 1975;79:57–80.
123. Chemnitz J, Christensen BC, Christoffersen P: Giant-cell arteritis. Histological, immunohistochemical and electronmicroscopic studies. Acta Pathol Microbiol Immunol Scand 1987;95:251–262.
124. Jensen HS, Mogensen HH, Mikkelsen AG: Basal and stimulated elastolytic activity of blood monocytes is increased in glucocorticoid-treated giant cell arteritis. Scand J Rheumatol 1990;19:251–256.
125. Velvart M, Felder M, Fehr K, et al: Temporal arteritis in polymyalgia rheumatica: Immune complex deposits and the role of the leukocyte elastase in the pathogenesis. Z Rheumatol 1983;42:320–327.
126. Genereau T, Peyri N, Berard M, et al: Human neutrophil elastase in temporal (giant cell) arteritis: Plasma and immunohistochemical studies. J Rheumatol 1998;25:710–713.
127. Hunder GG: More on polymyalgia rheumatica and giant cell arteritis. West J Med 1984;141:68–70.
128. Gillot JM, Masy E, Davril M: Elastase derived elastin peptides: Putative autoimmune targets in giant cell arteritis. J Rheumatol 1997;24:677–682.
129. O'Brien JP, Regan W: Actinically degenerate elastic tissue: The prime antigen in the giant cell (temporal) arteritis syndrome? Clin Exp Rheumatol 1998;16:39–48.
130. Reinecke RD, Kuwabara T: Temporal arteritis. I. Smooth muscle cell involvement. Arch Ophthalmol 1969;82:446–453.
131. Shiiki H, Shimokama T, Watanabe T: Temporal arteritis: Cell composition and the possible pathogenetic role of cell-mediated immunity. Hum Pathol 1989;20:1057–1064.
132. Wawryk SO, Ayberk H, Boyd AW, et al: Analysis of adhesion molecules in the immunopathogenesis of giant cell arteritis. J Clin Pathol 1991;44:497–501.
133. Armstrong RD, Behn A, Myles A, et al: Histocompatibility antigens in polymyalgia rheumatica and giant cell arteritis. J Rheumatol 1983;10:659–661.
134. Lowenstien MB, Bridgefore PH, Vasey FB, et al: Increased frequency of HLA-DR3 and DR4 in polymyalgia rheumatica-giant cell arteritis. Arthritis Rheum 1983;26:925–927.
135. Hazleman B, Goldstone A, Voak D: Associated of polymyalgia rheumatica and giant cell arteritis with HLA-B8. Br Med J 1977;2:989–991.
136. Hansen JA, Healey LA, Wilske KR: Association between giant cell (temporal) arteritis and HLA-Cw3. Hum Immunol 1985;13:193–198.
137. Combe B, Sany J, Le Quellec A, et al: Distribution of HLA-DRB1 alleles of patients with polymyalgia rheumatica and giant cell arteritis in a Mediterranean population. J Rheumatol 1998;25:94–98.
138. Cid MC, Ercilla G, Vilaseca J, et al: Polymyalgia rheumatica: A syndrome associated with HLA-DR4 antigen. Arthritis Rheum 1988;31:678–682.
139. Richardson JE, Gladman DD, Fam A, et al: HLA-DR4 in giant cell arteritis: Association with polymyalgia rheumatica syndrome. Arthritis Rheum 1987;30:1293–1297.
140. Weyand CM, Hicok KC, Hunder GG, et al: The HLA-DRB1 locus as a genetic component in giant cell arteritis: Mapping of a disease-linked sequence motif to the antigen-binding site of the HLA-DR molecule. J Clin Invest 1992;90:2355–2361.
141. Malmvall B, Bengtsson B, Kaijser B, et al: Serum levels of immunoglobulin and complement in giant-cell arteritis. JAMA 1976;236:1876.
142. Espinoza LR, Bridgeford P, Lowenstein M, et al: Polymyalgia rheumatica and giant cell arteritis: Circulating immune complexes. J Rheumatol 1982;9:556–560.
143. Papaioannou CC, Gupta RC, Hunder GG, et al: Circulating immune complexes in giant cell arteritis and polymyalgia rheumatica. Arthritis Rheum 1980;23:1021–1025.
144. Park JR, Jones JG, Harkiss GD: Circulating immune complexes in polymyalgia rheumatica and giant cell arteritis. Ann Rheum Dis 1981;40:360–365.
145. Malmvall BE, Bengtsson BA, Nilsson LA, et al: Immune complexes, rheumatoid factors, and cellular immunological parameters in patients with giant cell arteritis. Ann Rheum Dis 1981;40:276–280.
146. Waaler E, Tonder O, Milde EJ: Immunological and histological studies of temporal arteries from patients with temporal arteritis and/or polymyalgia rheumatica. Acta Pathol Microbiol Scand 1976;84:55–63.
147. Wells KK, Folberg R, Goeken JA, et al: Temporal artery biopsies. Correlation of light microscopy and immunofluorescence microscopy. Ophthalmology 1989;96:1058–1064.
148. Park JR, Hazleman BL: Immunological and histological study of temporal arteries. Ann Rheum Dis 1978;37:238–243.
149. Chess J, Albert DM, Bhan AK: Serologic and immunopathologic findings in temporal arteritis. Am J Ophthalmol 1983;96:283–289.
150. Banks PM, Cohen MD, Ginsburg WW, et al: Immunohistologic

and cytochemical studies of temporal arteritis. Arthritis Rheum 1983;26:1201–1207.

151. Gallagher P, Jones K: immunohistochemical findings in cranial arteritis. Arthritis Rheum 1982;25:75–79.

152. Dasgupta B, Duke O, Kyle V: Antibodies to intermediate filaments in polymyalgia rheumatica and giant cell arteritis: A sequential study. Ann Rheum Dis 1987;46:746–749.

153. Andersson R, Jonsson R, Tarkowski A, et al: T cell subsets and expression of immunological activation markers in the arterial walls of patients with giant cell arteritis. Ann Rheum Dis 1987;46:915–923.

154. Cid MC, Campo E, Ercilla G, et al: Immunohistochemical analysis of lymphoid and macrophage cell subsets and their immunologic activation markers in temporal arteritis. Influence of corticosteroids treatment. Arthritis Rheum 1989;32:884–893.

155. Martinez-Tabodada V, Brack A, Hunder GG, et al: The inflammatory infiltrate in giant cell arteritis selects against B lymphocytes. J Rheumatol 1996;23:1011–1014.

156. Andersson R, Hansson GK, Soderstrom T, et al: HLA-DR expression in the vascular lesion and circulating T lymphocytes of patients with giant cell arteritis. Clin Exp Immunol 1988;73:82–87.

157. Schaufelberger C, Stemme S, Andersson R, et al: T lymphocytes in giant cell arteritic lesions are polyclonal cells expressing alpha beta type antigen receptors and VLA-1 integrin receptors. Clin Exp Immunol 1993;91:421–428.

158. Weyand CM, Schonberger J, Oppitz U, et al: Distinct vascular lesions in giant cell arteritis share identical T cell clonotypes. J Exp Med 1994;179:951–960.

159. Martinez-Taboada VM, Hunder NN, Hunder GG, et al: Recognition of tissue residing antigen by T cells in vasculitic lesions of giant cell arteritis. J Mol Med 1996;74:695–703.

160. Brack A, Geisler A, Martinez-Taboada VM, et al: Giant cell arteritis is a T cell-dependent disease. Mol Med 1997;3:530–543.

161. Weyand CM, Hicok KC, Hunder GG, et al: Tissue cytokine patterns in patients with polymyalgia rheumatica and giant cell arteritis. Ann Intern Med 1994;121:484–491.

162. Weyand CM, Tetzlaff N, Bjornsson J, et al: Disease patterns and tissue cytokine profiles in giant cell arteritis. Arthritis Rheum 1997;40:19–26.

163. Dasgupta B, Panayi GS: Interleukin-6 in serum of patients with polymyalgia rheumatica and giant cell arteritis. Br J Rheumatol 1990;29:456–458.

164. Roche NE, Fulbright JW, Wagner AD, et al: Correlation of interleukin-6 production and disease activity in polymyalgia rheumatica and giant cell arteritis. Arthritis Rheum 1993;36:1286–1294.

165. Field M, Cook A, Gallagher G: Immuno-localisation of tumour necrosis factor and its receptors in temporal arteritis. Rheumatol Int 1997;17:113–118.

166. Kaiser M, Weyand CM, Bjornsson J, et al: Platelet-derived growth factor, intimal hyperplasia, and ischemic complications in giant cell arteritis. Arthritis Rheum 1998;41:623–633.

167. Salvarani C, Boiardi L, Macchioni P, et al: Role of peripheral CD8+ lymphocytes and soluble IL-2 receptors in predicting the duration of corticosteroids treatment in polymyalgia rheumatica and giant cell arteritis. Ann Rheum Dis 1995;54:640–644.

168. Roblot P, Morel F, Lelievre E, et al: Serum soluble CD23 levels in giant cell arteritis. Immunol Lett 1996;53:41–44.

169. Brack A, Rittner HL, Younge BR, et al: Glucocorticoids-mediated repression of cytokine gene transcription in human arteritis-SCID chimeras. J Clin Invest 1997;99:2842–2850.

170. Nikkari ST, Hoyhtya M, Isola J, et al: Macrophages contain 92-kd gelatinase (MMP-9) at the site of degenerated internal elastic lamina in temporal arteritis. Am J Pathol 1996;159:1537–1533.

171. Tomita T, Imakawa K: Matrix metalloproteinases and tissue inhibitors of metalloproteinases in giant cell arteritis: An immunocytochemical study. Pathology 1998;30:40–50.

172. Sorbi D, French DL, Nuovo GJ, et al: Elevated levels of 92-kd type IV collagenase (matrix metalloproteinase 9) in giant cell arteritis. Arthritis Rheum 1996;39:1747–1753.

173. Nordborg E, Nordborg C: The inflammatory reaction in giant cell arteritis: An immunohistochemical investigation. Clin Exp Rheumatol 1998;16:165–168.

174. Weyand CM, Wagner AD, Bjornsson J, et al: Correlation of the topographical arrangement and the functional pattern of tissue-infiltrating macrophages in giant cell arteritis. J Clin Invest 1996;98:1642–1649.

175. Dasgupta B, Duke O, Timms AM, et al: Selective depletion and activation of CD8+ lymphocytes from peripheral blood of patients with polymyalgia rheumatica and giant cell arteritis. Ann Rheum Dis 1989;48:307–311.

176. Benlahrache C, Segond P, Auquier L, et al: Decrease of the OKT8 positive T cell subset in polymyalgia rheumatica. Lack of correlation with disease activity. Arthritis Rheum 1983;26:1472–1480.

177. Elling H, Elling P: Decreased level of suppressor/cytotoxic T cells (OKT8+) in polymyalgia rheumatica and temporal arteritis: relation to disease activity. J Rheumatol 1985;12:306–309.

178. Johansen M, Elling P, Elling H: A genetic approach to the aetiology of giant cell arteritis: Depletion of the CD8+ T-lymphocyte subset in relatives of patients with polymyalgia rheumatica and arteritis temporalis. Clin Exp Rheumatol 1995;13:745–748.

179. Martinez-Taboada VM, Goronzy JJ, Weyand CM: Clonally expanded CD8+ T cells in patients with polymyalgia rheumatica and giant cell arteritis. Clin Immunol Immunopathol 1996;79:263–270.

180. Hunder GG, Bloch DA, Michel BA, et al: The American College of Rheumatology 1990 criteria for the classification of giant cell arteritis. Arthritis Rheum 1990;33:1122–1128.

181. Goodman BW: Temporal arteritis. Am J Med 1979;67:839–852.

182. Wong RL, Korn JH: Temporal arteritis without an elevated erythrocyte sedimentation rate. Am J Med 1986;80:959–964.

183. Ellis ME, Ralston S: ESR in the diagnosis and management of polymyalgia rheumatica/giant cell arteritis syndrome. Ann Rheum Dis 1983;42:169–170.

184. Andersson R, Malmvall BE, Bengtsson BA: Acute phase reactants in the initial phase of giant cell arteritis. Acta Med Scand 1986;220:365–367.

185. Kyle V, Cawston TE, Hazleman BL: Erythrocyte sedimentation rate and C reactive protein in the assessment of polymyalgia rheumatica/giant cell arteritis on presentation and during follow up. Ann Rheum Dis 1989;48:667–671.

186. Jacobson DM, Slamovits TL: Erythrocyte sedimentation rate and its relationship to hematocrit in giant cell arteritis. Arch Ophthalmol 1987;105:965–967.

187. Eshaghian J, Goeken JA: C-reactive protein in giant cell (cranial, temporal) arteritis. Ophthalmology 1980;87:1160–1166.

188. Pountain GD, Calvin J, Hazleman BL: Alpha 1-antichymotrypsin, C-reactive protein and erythrocyte sedimentation rate in polymyalgia rheumatica and giant cell arteritis. Br J Rheumatol 1994;33:550–554.

189. Gudmundsson M, Nordborg E, Bengtsson BA, et al: Plasma viscosity in giant cell arteritis as a predictor of disease activity. Ann Rheum Dis 1993;52:104–109.

190. Park JR, Jones JG, Hazleman BL: Relationship of the erythrocyte sedimentation rate to acute phase proteins in polymyalgia rheumatica and giant cell arteritis. Ann Rheum Dis 1981;40:493–495.

191. Hayreh SS, Podhajsky PA, Raman R, et al: Giant cell arteritis: Validity and reliability of various diagnostic criteria. Am J Ophthalmol 1997;123:285–296.

192. Brittain GPH, McIlwaine GG, Bell JA, et al: Plasma viscosity or erythrocyte sedimentation rate in the diagnosis of giant cell arteritis? Br J Ophthalmol 1991;75:656–659.

193. Weiss LM, Gonzales E, Miller SB, et al: Severe anemia as the presenting manifestation of giant cell arteritis. Arthritis Rheum 1995;38:434–436.

194. Healy LA, Wilske KR: Presentation of occult giant cell arteritis. Arthritis Rheum 1980;23:641–643.

195. Malmvall BE, Bengtsson BA: Giant cell arteritis. Clinical features and involvement of different organs. Scand J Rheumatol 1978;7:154–158.

196. Federici AB, Fox RI, Espinoza LR, et al: Elevation of von Willebrand factor is independent of erythrocyte sedimentation rate and persists after glucocorticoid treatment in giant cell arteritis. Arthritis Rheum 1984;27:1046–1049.

197. Cid MC, Monteagudo J, Oristrell J, et al: Von Willebrand factor in the outcome of temporal arteritis. Ann Rheum Dis 1996;55:927–930.

198. Espinoza LR, Jara LJ, Silveira LH: Anticardiolipin antibodies in polymyalgia rheumatica-giant cell arteritis: Associated with severe vascular complications. Am J Med 1991;90:474–478.

199. McLean RM, Greco TP: Anticardiolipin antibodies in the polymyalgia rheumatica-giant cell arteritis syndromes. Clin Rheumatol 1995;14:191–196.

200. Chakravarty K, Pountain G, Merry P, et al: A longitudinal study of anticardiolipin antibodies in polymyalgia rheumatica and giant cell arteritis. J Rheumatol 1995;22:1694–1697.
201. Duhart P, Berruyer M, Pinede L, et al: Anticardiolipin antibodies and giant cell arteritis: A prospective, multicenter case-control study. Arthritis Rheum 1998;41:701–709.
202. Kyle V, Wraight EP, Hazleman BL: Liver scan abnormalities in polymyalgia/giant cell arteritis. Clin Rheumatol 1991;10:294–297.
203. Kyle V: Laboratory investigations including liver in polymyalgia rheumatica/giant cell arteritis. Baillieres Clin Rheumatol 1991;5:475–484.
204. Ogilvie AL, James PD, Toghill PJ: Hepatic involvement in polymyalgia arteritica. J Clin Pathol 1981;34:769–772.
205. Litwack KD, Bohan A, Silverman L: Granulomatous liver disease and giant cell arteritis. Case report and literature review. J Rheumatol 1977;4:307–312.
206. Leong AS-Y, Alp MH: Hepatocellular disease in giant cell arteritis/polymyalgia rheumatica syndrome. Ann Rheum Dis 1981;40:92–95.
207. MaCormack LR, Astarita RW, Foroozan P: Liver involvement in giant cell arteritis. Digest Dis 1978;23:728–745.
208. Schmidt WA, Draft HE, Vorpahl K, et al: Color duplex ultrasonography in the diagnosis of temporal arteritis. N Engl J Med 1997;337:1336–1342.
209. Lauwerys BR, Puttemans T, Houssiau FA, et al: Color Doppler sonography of the temporal arteries in giant cell arteritis and polymyalgia rheumatica. J Rheumatol 1997;24:1570–1574.
210. Ghanchi FD, Williamson TH, Lim CS, et al: Colour Doppler imaging in giant cell (temporal) arteritis: Serial examination and comparison with non-arteritic anterior ischaemic optic neuropathy. Eye 1996;10:459–464.
211. Ho AC, Sergott RC, Regillo CD, et al: Color Doppler hemodynamics of giant cell arteritis. Arch Ophthalmol 1994;112:938–945.
212. Achkar AA, Lie JT, Hunder GG, et al: How does previous corticosteroids treatment affect the biopsy findings in giant cell arteritis? Ann Intern Med 1994;120:987–992.
213. Allison MC, Gallagher PJ: Temporal artery biopsy and corticosteroids treatment. Ann Rheum Dis 1984;43:416–417.
214. Allsop CJ, Gallagher PJ: Temporal artery biopsy in giant cell arteritis. A reappraisal. Am J Surg Pathol 1981;5:317–313.
215. Hall S, Persellin S, Lie JT, et al: The therapeutic impact of temporal artery biopsy. Lancet 1983;2:1217–1220.
216. Hedges TR, Gieger GL, Albert DM: The clinical value of negative temporal artery biopsy specimens. Arch Ophthalmol 1983;101:1251–1254.
217. Vilaseca J, Gonzalez A, Cid MC, et al: Clinical usefulness of temporal artery biopsy. Ann Rheum Dis 1987;46:282–285.
218. Cohen DN: Temporal arteritis: Improvement in visual prognosis and management with repeat biopsies. Trans Am Acad Ophthalmol Otolaryngol 1973;77:74–85.
219. Birkhead NC, Wagener HP: Treatment of temporal arteritis with adrenal corticosteroids: Results in fifty-five cases in which lesion was proved at biopsy. JAMA 1957;163:821–827.
220. Jones JG, Hazleman BL: Prognosis and management of polymyalgia rheumatica. Ann Rheum Dis 1981;40:1–5.
221. Kyle V, Hazleman BL: Treatment of polymyalgia rheumatica and giant cell arteritis. I. Steroid regimens in the first two months. Ann Rheum Dis 1989;48:548–551.
222. Nesher G, Rubinow A, Sonnenblick M: Efficacy and adverse effects of different corticosteroid dose regimens in temporal arteritis: A retrospective study. Clin Exp Rheumatol 1997;15:303–306.
223. Cornblath WT, Eggenberger ER: Progressive visual loss from giant cell arteritis despite high-dose intravenous methylprednisolone. Ophthalmology 1997;104:854–858.
224. Rosenfeld SI, Kosmorsky GS, Klingele TG: Treatment of temporal arteritis with ocular involvement. Am J Med 1986;80:143–145.
225. Diamon JP: Treatable blindness in temporal arteritis. Br J Ophthalmol 1991;75:432.
226. Hunder GG, Sheps SG, Allen GL, et al: Daily and alternate-day corticosteroid regimens in treatment of giant cell arteritis: Comparison in a prospective study. Ann Intern Med 1975;82:613–618.
227. Bengtsson BA, Malmvall BE: Prognosis of giant cell arteritis including temporal arteritis and polymyalgia rheumatica. Acta Med Scand 1981;209:337–345.
228. Kyle V, Hazleman BL: The clinical and laboratory course of polymyalgia rheumatica/giant cell arteritis. Br J Rheumatol 1988;27(suppl):7.
229. Bahlas S, Ramos-Remus C, Davis P: Clinical outcome of 149 patients with polymyalgia rheumatica and giant cell arteritis. J Rheumatol 1998;25:99–104.
230. Fernandez-Herlihy L: Duration of corticosteroid therapy in giant cell arteritis. J Rheumatol 1980;7:361–364.
231. Salvarani C, Boiardi L, Macchioni P, et al: Role of peripheral CD8+ lymphocytes and soluble IL-2 receptor in predicting the duration of corticosteroid treatment in polymyalgia rheumatica and giant cell arteritis. Ann Rheum Dis 1995;54:640–644.
232. De Silva M, Hazleman BL: Azathioprine in giant cell arteritis/polymyalgia rheumatica: A double-blind study. Ann Rheum Dis 1986;45:136–138.
233. Settas L, Dimitriadis G, Sfetsios T, et al: Methotrexate versus azathioprine in polymyalgia rheumatica-giant cell arteritis: A double blind, cross over trial. Arthritis Rheum 1991;34(suppl):S72.
234. Hernandez C, Fernandez B, Ramos P, et al: Giant cell arteritis therapy: MTX as steroid-sparing agent. Arthritis Rheum 1991;34(suppl):S73.
235. Krall PL, Mazanec DJ, Wilke WS: Methotrexate for corticosteroid-resistant polymyalgia rheumatica and giant cell arteritis. Cleve Clin J Med 1989;56:253–257.
236. van der Veen MJ, Dinant HJ, van Booma-Frankfort C, et al: Can methotrexate be used as a steroid sparing agent in the treatment of polymyalgia rheumatica and giant cell arteritis? Ann Rheum Dis 1996;55:218–223.
237. Wendling D, Hory B, Blanc D: Cyclosporine: A new adjuvant therapy for giant cell arteritis? Ann Rheum Dis 1985;28:1078–1079.
238. Utsinger PD: Treatment of steroid non-responsive giant cell arteritis (GCA) with cytoxan. Arthitis Rheum 1982;25(suppl):S31.
239. Cooke WT, Cloake PCP, Govan ADT, et al: Temporal arteritis: A generalized vascular disease. Q J Med 1946;15:47.
240. Matteson EL, Gold KN, Bloch DA, et al: Long-term survival of patients with giant cell arteritis in the American College of Rheumatology giant cell arteritis classification criteria cohort. Am J Med 1996;100:193–196.
241. Gonzalez-Gay MA, Blanco R, Abraira V: Giant cell arteritis in Lugo, Spain, is associated with low longterm mortality. J Rheumatol 1997;24:2171–2176.
242. Nordborg E, Bengtsson BA: Death rates and causes of death in 284 consecutive patients with giant cell arteritis confirmed by biopsy. Br Med J 1989;299:549–550.
243. Soderbergh J, Malmvall BE, Andersson R, et al: Giant cell arteritis as a cause of death. Report of nine cases. JAMA 1986;255:493–496.
244. Bisgard C, Sloth H, Keiding N, et al: Excess mortality in giant cell arteritis. J Intern Med 1991;230:119–123.
245. Rubinow A, Brandt KD, Cohen AS, et al: Iatrogenic morbidity accompanying suppression temporal arteritis by adrenal corticosteroids. Ann Ophthalmol 1984;16:258–265.
246. Schneider HA, Weber AA, Ballen PH: The visual prognosis in temporal arteritis. Ann Ophthalmol 1971;3:1215–1228.

ADAMANTIADES-BEHÇET DISEASE

Panayotis Zafirakis and C. Stephen Foster

DEFINITION

Adamantiades-Behçet disease (ABD) is a chronic, relapsing inflammatory disorder of unknown etiology, historically characterized by the triad of recurrent oral and genital aphthous ulcers, ocular inflammation, and skin lesions such as erythema nodosum and acneiform eruptions. ABD frequently involves the joints, the central nervous system (CNS), and the gastrointestinal tract as well. Furthermore, ABD may be the best example of a disease characterized mainly by retinal vasculitis associated with devastating effects on the patient's visual outcome. There is not a universally accepted diagnostic test for this disorder. Thus, the diagnosis of ABD relies on the identification of several sets, or combinations, of its more typical clinical features.

HISTORY

The first description of the symptoms of the disease was probably reported by Hippocrates, 5th century BC, in his third book of epidemiology[1]:

There were other forms of fever. . . . Many developed aphthae, ulcerations. Many ulcerations about the genital parts . . . watery ophthalmies of a chronic character, with pains; fungus excretions of the eyelids externally, internally which destroyed the sight of many persons. . . . There were fungous growth on ulcers, and on those localized on the genital organs. Many anthraxes through the summer . . . other great affections; many large herpetes.

Since that time, isolated symptoms of the ABD were described during the 19th century, and concomitant symptoms were reported in 1895 and 1906.[2] Isolated symptoms were recognized by Blüthe,[3] Planner,[4] and Shigeta.[5]

In 1930, Benedictos Adamantiades,[6] a Greek ophthalmologist, presented at the Medical Society of Athens the case of a 20-year-old man who suffered from recurrent iritis with hypopyon resulting in blindness, associated with phlebitis, mouth ulcers, genital ulcers, and knee arthritis. Synovial fluid from the knee was tested and found to be sterile and transparent. Based on these observations, Adamantiades concluded that "recurrent iritis with hypopyon constitutes a discrete clinical entity."[6] One year later, in 1931, he published this case in the Annales d'Oculistique.[7] In 1932, Dascalopoulos, another Greek ophthalmologist, reported a new case with the same symptoms in the Annales d'Oculistique journal.[8] Six years later in 1937, H. Behçet, a Turkish professor in dermatology, described three patients with this constellation of findings of oral and genital ulcers and recurrent iritis; the disease is known by his name primarily because of the wider distribution of his paper in the medical literature.[9–11] Godde-Jolly,[12] Bietti-Bruna,[13] and others long ago suggested that the disease should probably more appropriately be called Adamantiades-Behçet disease, to better reflect the important contributions both these physicians

made, and this chapter adopts that attitude and philosophy.

Despite the fact that Adamantiades's first patient did suffer from phlebitis with leg ulcer, it was only in 1946 that he described what he named the fourth symptom, "thrombophlebitis" of retinal vessels, the limbs, or both.[14] Later, additional signs were described worldwide regarding other body organs.

EPIDEMIOLOGY

Geographic and Ethnic Distribution

ABD has a worldwide distribution but is most common in the countries of the Eastern Mediterranean and in the Eastern rim of Asia. The disease is predominately reported between the 30° and 45° north latitudes in Asian and European populations, which corresponds to the old Silk Route used by traders from the East to Europe.[15] The exact incidence, prevalence, and family occurrence of the disease are unknown, but the prevalence of ABD appears to have increased during the last 40 years, the highest prevalence being 80 to 300 cases per 100,000 population in Turkey.[16, 17] The prevalence of ABD[14] was 8 to 10 cases per 100,000 population in Japan in the late 1970s.[18] It is postulated that there are approximately 15,000 patients in Japan with ABD, 11,000 of them being treated currently.[15] ABD was diagnosed in more than 20% of the patients with uveitis examined in the uveitis clinic of the University of Tokyo's Department of Ophthalmology between 1965 and 1977.[18] The annual incidence of ABD in Iran is approximately 345 patients in a population of 60 million,[19] and the prevalence is 16 to 100 cases in 100,000.[20] The prevalence of ABD in Greece is 6 cases per 100,000 population.[21] The prevalence of the disease in Germany (West Berlin) was 1.6 cases in 100,000 in 1989, and this has risen to 2.26 cases in 100,000 in 1994.[22] In the United States, the prevalence is 4 patients per 1 million population,[23] with ABD representing 0.2 to 0.4 percent of uveitis cases in this country.[24] The increased prevalence may be related to a better awareness of the illness, and in some countries to migration (Table 56–1).

Sex

Many reports, mainly from the Mediterranean basin and the Far East, have shown a preponderance of males to females.[24–27] More recent evidence, however, suggests a more even distribution of the disease between the sexes. In the series of Colvard and colleagues,[28] only 13 of the 32 patients were male. In 1971, in a series of 10 patients from North America, only 3 were male.[29] Sakamoto and colleagues[30] reported a 2:1 male-to-female ratio in Japan. Other data have shown that men predominate in Lebanon (11:1), Greece (7.9:1), Egypt (5.3:1), Israel (3.8:1), Turkey (3.4:1) and Iran (1.2:1), whereas women predominate in Germany (1:0.9), Brazil (1:0.7), and the United States (1:0.2). Although discrepancies in the reported

TABLE 56–1. PREVALENCE OF ADAMANTIADES-BEHÇET DISEASE PER 100,000 INHABITANTS

COUNTRY	PREVALENCE
Turkey	80–300
Japan	8–10
Iran	16–100
Germany	2.26
USA	0.4

male-to-female ratios may reflect a change in the nature of the disease, it is more likely that in previous years, women in many countries were embarrassed to visit a physician with complains related to the cluster of signs and symptoms that make up ABD. The complete type of ABD (see the later section on clinical features) is more frequent in males; the incomplete type has equal frequency in both sexes. Although the disease is believed to have a worse overall prognosis in males than in females[31] in the Mediterranean basin and in the Middle and Far East, no such difference has been noted in Western European and American studies.

Age
The age of onset of the first symptom varies in many studies. Most authors consider the onset of the disease to be the age at which the patient fulfilled the diagnostic criteria of the disease. The mean age of onset is 25 to 35 years worldwide, with a range of 2 months to 72 years. In Germany the mean age of onset is estimated to be approximately 25 for men and 24.5 for women.[32]

Heredity and Sexual Transmission
ABD sometimes affects more than one member in the same family. Although several familial cases[33–35] and a pair of monozygotic brothers[36] concordant for the disease have been reported, no consistent inheritance pattern has been confirmed.[37, 38] Furthermore, no transmission of the disease from husband to wife or vice versa has been reported.

CLINICAL FEATURES

Diagnostic Criteria and Clinical Types of the Disease
The diagnosis of ABD is based on the presence of a set of clinical findings, and diagnostic criteria were first suggested in 1969.[39] There followed suggested criteria, published by the Research Committee of Japan and by O'Duffy,[41] Zhang,[42] Dilsen and colleagues,[43] James,[44] and lately the International Study Group.[45]

One diagnostic system has been suggested by the Behçet's Research Committee of Japan (Table 56–2).[40] In this diagnostic system there are four major and five minor criteria. The major criteria include recurrent aphthous ulcers of oral mucosal, skin lesions (similar to those of erythema nodosum or acne, and a pathergy test), genital ulcers, and ocular inflammatory disease. The minor criteria include arthritis, intestinal ulcer, epididymitis, vascular disease, and neuropsychiatric symptoms. Combinations of these criteria lead to four types of ABD: (1) the complete type (four major symptoms simultaneously or at different

TABLE 56–2. DIAGNOSTIC SYSTEM OF ADAMANTIADES-BEHÇET DISEASE SUGGESTED BY BEHÇET'S RESEARCH COMMITTEE OF JAPAN

Major criteria
  Recurrent oral aphthae
  Skin lesion
  Recurrent genital ulcers
  Inflammation of the eye
Minor criteria
  Arthritis
  Ulceration of the bowel
  Epididymitis
  Vasculitis/vasculopathy
  Neuropsychiatric symptoms
Types of ABD
  Complete (4 major)
  Incomplete (3 major, or ocular involvement with 1 other major)
  Suspect (2 major, no eye involvement)
  Possible (1 major)

Modified from Newman NM, Hoyt WF, Spencer WH: Macula-sparing monocular blackouts: Clinical and pathologic investigation of intermittent choroidal vascular insufficiency in a case of periarteritis nodosa. Arch Ophthalmol 1974;91:367–370.

times); (2) the incomplete type (three major symptoms simultaneously or at different times, or typical recurrent ocular disease with one other major criterion); (3) the suspect type (two major symptoms excluding ocular); and (4) the possible type (one main symptom).

The committee also identified several special clinical types of ABD, depending on the predominant manifestation; namely, neuro-Behçet, oculo-Behçet, intestinal-Behçet or vasculo-Behçet.

Three laboratory tests have also been included in this system: a pathergy (skin-prick) test, human leukocyte antigen (HLA) testing for HLA-B51, and a screening of nonspecific factors indicative of immune system activation (elevated erythrocyte sedimentation rate, positive C-reactive protein, and an increase in peripheral blood leukocytes). The same diagnostic system has been advocated by Nussenblatt and colleagues[46]

The diagnostic system that has been suggested by the International Study Group for Behçet's Disease[45] requires the presence of oral ulceration in all patients plus any two of the following: genital ulceration, typically defined eye lesion, typically defined skin lesion, or a positive pathergy test (Table 56–3). Thus, the International Study Group for Behçet's Disease stresses the importance of oral aphthae in the diagnosis of ABD, whereas the Behçet's Research Committee classification stresses the importance of ocular symptomatology.

TABLE 56–3. DIAGNOSTIC SYSTEM OF ADAMANTIADES-BEHÇET DISEASE SUGGESTED BY THE INTERNATIONAL STUDY GROUP FOR BEHÇET'S DISEASE

Recurrent oral aphthae (at least 3 times per year), plus 2 of the following:

Recurrent genital ulcers	Skin involvement
Ocular inflammation	Positive pathergy test

Modified from Gold DH: Ocular manifestations of connective tissue (collagen) diseases. In: Tasman W, Jaeger AE, eds: Duane's Clinical Ophthalmology, vol 5. Philadelphia, J.B. Lippincott, 1989, pp 17–19.

The International Study Group for Behçet's Disease suggested that there are several clinical findings that may be important and may aid in the diagnosis of ABD, but as their frequency is low, they are not included in their criteria. The reason was to simplify the list, thus reducing the chance of subjective error. Undoubtedly, all the diagnostic systems have some degree of uncertainty, as any of the criteria may be manifested at different times during the clinical course of the disease.

Nonocular Manifestations

Oral Aphthae

Oral aphtha is the most frequent finding in ABD (Fig. 56–1). These ulcers produce a significant amount of discomfort and are recurrent. Although the number of individuals with oral aphthae in the general population is quite high, the lesions in ABD may occur in clusters and may be located anywhere in the oral cavity: the lips, gums, palate, tongue, uvula, and posterior pharynx. They can be small and very painful. The characteristic oral lesions are discrete, round or oval, white ulcerations 3 to 15 mm in diameter with a red rim. They may recur every 5 to 10 days, or every month, or even years apart without following any rule. They usually last for approximately 7 to 10 days and may heal without scarring, although they may produce scarring when they are numerous and large.

The aphthae of ABD should be differentiated from those seen in Stevens-Johnson and Reiter's syndromes,[47] in which they are painless, with irregular rims or heaped-up edges and they usually occur on the palate, pharynx, and tonsils, structures rarely involved in ABD. Oral aphthae can also be found in some individuals after eating certain type of foods, or they may be provoked by trauma to the oral mucosa.

Skin Lesions

Cutaneous involvement is frequent in ABD. Painful, recurrent lesions of erythema nodosum may appear in groups not only over the tibia, which is the most frequent location, but also on the face, neck, buttocks, and elsewhere (Fig. 56–2). The lesion usually disappears, without

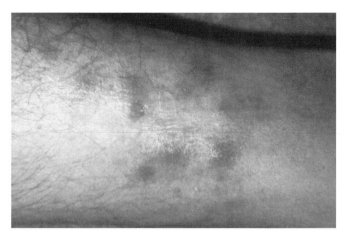

FIGURE 56–2. Erythema nodosum–like lesions on anterior tibial surface. (See color insert.)

any scarring, after several weeks, but they may indeed leave scars. It is not uncommon to find hyperpigmented or hypopigmented scars in the wake of erythema nodosum in ABD. This may be a helpful physical sign.

Superficial thrombophlebitis can occur in the upper or lower extremities. It can be migratory or it may occur after an injection or the drawing of a blood sample. This phenomenon should be evaluated carefully, because it may denote a more systemic vascular disorder.

Skin eruptions resembling acne vulgaris or folliculitis frequently appear on the upper thorax and face. Approximately 40% of patients with ABD exhibit a cutaneous phenomenon termed pathergy, in which sterile pustules develop at sites of spontaneous or induced trauma (venipuncture, injection of sterile saline).[48] This phenomenon is not pathognomonic of ABD, although some investigators believe that it is an important criterion that can be used for the diagnosis.[45] Dermatographia, another dermatologic phenomenon of cutaneous hypersensitivity, can also be found in one third to one half of the patients.

Genital Ulcers

The gross appearance of the genital ulcers is similar to that of the oral aphthous ulcers. In male patients they can occur on the scrotum (Fig. 56–3) or penis (Fig. 56–4). In female patients they can appear on the vulva and vaginal mucosa.[49] Such ulcers can also be found on the perianal areas. They may be painless in women. Sometimes, however, they are very painful, leading initially to misdiagnose them as herpetic in origin. Vulvar lesions frequently occur premenstrually.[46]

Genital lesions can be deep, scarring as they heal. Therefore, examination of the genital area in a patient suspected as having ABD can be helpful, since signs of healed lesions may be present.

Vascular Disorders, Cardiac Involvement

Although vasculitis as the presenting symptom of ABD is rare, vessels of any size can be affected. Müftüoglou and colleagues[50] observed vascular involvement in 24% of the 531 patients with ABD in whom the deep and the superficial thrombophlebites of the leg were the most frequent vascular alterations. In other series of patients, thrombo-

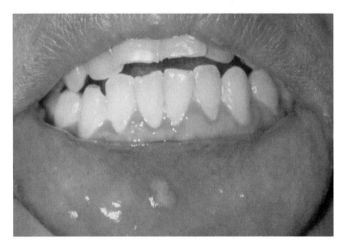

FIGURE 56–1. Aphthous oral ulcer on the inner surface of the inferior lip. (See color insert.)

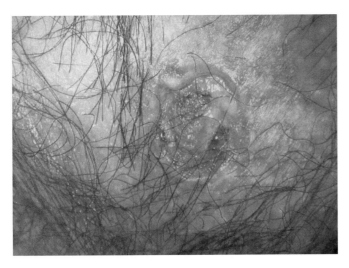

FIGURE 56–3. ABD lesion on the scrotum.

phlebitis occurred in 10%.[43] During the disease course, the frequency ranges from 8%[51] to 38%.[43]

Four types of vascular lesions are recognized: arterial occlusion, aneurysms, venous occlusion, and varices. Vasculitis occurring simultaneously in multiple vessels has been reported.[52, 53] Not only have both deep and superficial venous thrombosis been reported but also varicose veins, arterial obstruction, aneurysms, and Budd-Chiari syndrome.[54] The frequency of deep arteriovenous thrombosis was found to be 10% in a study from India.[55] Obstructive vasculitis of veins and arteries have also been documented.[56–59] Aneurysms are not uncommon, and they have a worse prognosis than that of occlusive lesions, with a death rate estimated to reach 60%,[60] because aneurysmal rupture leads to severe hemorrhage.[59] Although 14% of ABD patients were documented to have venous manifestations, only 2% had arterial manifestations in one large series.[61] Both arterial and venous involvement have been found in nearly all body vessels.[61]

Cardiac involvement includes granulomatous endocarditis,[62] recurrent ventricular arrhythmias,[63] myocarditis,[64] endomyocardial fibrosis,[65, 66] myocardial infarction,[67] silent myocardial ischemia,[68] valvular regurgitation, coronary arteritis, and pericarditis.[69] The incidence of heart lesions usually ranges from 5% to 10% of ABD cases.[66] However, in the Japanese autopsy registry, the frequency of heart manifestations was found to be 17%.[65]

Neurologic Involvement, Psychiatric Disturbances

Nervous system involvement (often termed neuro-ABD) is one of the most serious manifestations of ABD. Although any part of the neuraxis can be involved and CNS involvement is quite well recognized, there is no clear evidence that the associated peripheral nervous system symptoms or signs are a direct result of the ABD process. Therefore, they should be cautiously incorporated into ABD. The nervous system involvement either is caused by primary neural parenchymal lesions (neuro-ABD) or is secondary to major vascular involvement (vasculo-ABD).

The reported frequency of CNS involvement in cases of ABD ranges from 3% to 10%,[27] and computed tomography (CT) findings have been correlated with clinical variables.[70] The onset of the neurologic picture generally appears 4 to 6 years after the onset of ABD. However, some patients develop neuro-ABD simultaneously with or prior to the full-blown picture of ABD, and this may cause confusion in the diagnosis. Approximately 10% of patients with neuro-ABD show ocular involvement, whereas up to 30% of patients with ocular-ABD have neuro-ABD. However, in a recent study from Japan,[71] only 6.6% of 317 patients with ocular-ABD developed CNS symptoms. In the same study, the incidence of neuro-ABD in patients who did not take cyclosporine-A (Cs-A) was only 3.3% (9 of 270), but 12 (25.5%) of the 47 patients who were on Cs-A developed neurologic manifestation. The authors concluded that Cs-A may exhibit neurotoxicity in patients with ABD or may accelerate the development of neuro-ABD.

The following neuro-ophthalmic changes have been noted in ABD[72]: (1) palsies (usually transient) of cranial nerves VI and VII; (2) central scotomas caused by papillitis and visual field defects[73]; and (3) papilledema[74] resulting from pseudotumor cerebri caused by thrombosis of the intradural venous sinuses.[75]

Neuro-ABD is mainly a disease of the motor compartment of the CNS, frequently accompanied by mental changes. CNS involvement may be acute, with clinical signs suggestive of meningoencephalitis, which may resolve spontaneously.[76] Headaches usually are related to widespread vasculitis, which induces brain lesions.[77] The main signs of CNS involvement are pyramidal brain stem lesions and seizure. The clinical course of CNS involvement is relapsing, with recurrences to be the rule, in 40% of cases, whereas 30% have a secondary progressive course and 16% a primary progressive course.[78] Although the prognosis in older series was poor,[79] with death occurring in 10% of cases,[78] today the outcome generally is good because of early diagnosis and aggressive treatment with immunosuppressive or immunomodulating drugs.[80]

Men are affected more often than women.[78] Sphincter disturbances, pseudobulbar syndrome, intracranial hypertension, and deep sensory abnormalities may be seen, and a few cases of aseptic meningitis have been reported.[78] Psychiatric manifestations include confusion,

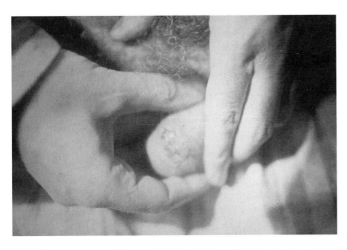

FIGURE 56–4. ABD lesion on the penis. (See color insert.)

hallucinations, and agitation. Audiovestibular involvement may be seen in patients with ABD and may induce sudden deafness.[81]

CT, magnetic resonance imaging (MRI), single-photon emission computed tomography, brain angiography, and analysis of cerebrospinal fluid (CSF) offer assistance in the diagnosis of CNS involvement in ABD. However, MRI is more sensitive than CT in detecting abnormalities in neuro-ABD.[77] The lesions shown by MRI or CT usually show contrast enhancement in the acute period, which usually resolves in the passage of time.[70, 77] CSF usually has a high protein content and/or pleocytosis with lymphocyte predominance.[78, 82]

Genitourinary Involvement

The reported incidence of epididymitis in patients with ABD ranges from 4%[83] to 11%.[19] Recurrent episodes of pain and swelling of the area are the cardinal signs of epididymal involvement.

Kidney involvement includes acute glomerulonephritis,[69] IgA nephropathy,[84] and amyloidosis.[85] Acute glomerulonephritis has been found in 11% of ABD cases,[19] and amyloidosis has been described in 2% of patients with ABD.[85] Renal vein thrombosis, diffuse crescentic, or focal and segmental necrotizing glomerulonephritis have also been reported.[84]

Gastrointestinal Involvement

Gastrointestinal lesions include single or multiple ulcers of the esophagus, stomach, or intestine. The reported frequency varies in different countries, with a low frequency in Turkey[86] and a high frequency in Japan (50%–60% of ABD cases).[51] These patients usually complain of diarrhea and hemorrhages.[51] Intestinal perforation can also be seen.[51] In a large series of ABD patients, digestive lesions were found in 16%, whereas ulcerative colitis was noted in 1%.[87] No difference in frequency of *Helicobacter pylori* was found between ABD patients and controls.[88]

Pulmonary Involvement

The main pathologic feature of respiratory involvement is pulmonary arteritis, which may present as a tuberculosis-like shadow.[89] However, the lungs can also be affected secondary to superior vena caval and/or other mediastinal vascular lesions. The consequences are pulmonary embolisms, infarctions, or aneurysmal bronchial fistula.[90, 91] Pulmonary hypertension, pleural effusion due to biopsy proven vasculitis, and cor pulmonale can also be seen in patients with pulmonary involvement.[90, 91] Recurrent hemoptysis, dyspnea, cough, chest pain, and fever are the cardinal symptoms.[92] When the hemoptysis is massive, it may require emergency surgery.[93] CT or MRI may reveal asymptomatic aneurysmal dilatations. The prognosis of patients with aneurysms is poor. The frequency of pulmonary involvement in some studies is estimated to be up to 18%.[85]

Joint Involvement

At least half of the patients with ABD manifest arthritis at some time during the clinical course of the disease, with the knee being the most common joint affected (50%).[46] Arthritis as a first symptom in ABD patients has been reported in 13% in the series of Kaklamani and colleagues,[94] in 9% in the series of Gharibdoost and colleagues,[95] and in 14% in the series from Germany.[32] Peripheral arthritis may be monoarticular, oligoarticular, or polyarticular. It mainly affects the joints of the lower extremities, it recurs occasionally, and it rarely is chronic. The arthritis is usually nonmigrating and nondestructive and may be symmetrical (86%)[55] or asymmetrical.[96] However, in rare cases, loss of cartilage and pannus formation with erosive damage have been found.[39, 51, 97]

Ankylosing spondylitis has been reported in 10%[98] and sacroiliitis in 34%[99] of ABD cases. Other investigators have found a lower frequency of sacroiliitis.[39] This discrepancy may be attributed to more frequent use of CT today. Joint lesions can be found more often with CT scans than with plain radiographs.[99] Based on these observations, it had been suggested that ABD should be added in the seronegative arthritis group.[100]

Ocular Manifestations

The onset of ocular involvement, frequently termed ocular-ABD, has extremely serious implications. Recurrences are common and the recurrent attacks of ocular inflammation lead to severe, permanent ocular damage unless effective treatment is instituted. Each attack damages the eye. The involvement of the eye occurs in 43%[55] to 72%,[83] and loss of sight occurs in 25% of ABD patients.[101] The reported frequency of ocular involvement in cases of ABD is 83% to 95% in men and 67% to 73% in women.[102] The disease is more severe in men,[22] and bilateral disease occurs in 80% of patients. Eye involvement as the first presenting manifestation of ABD is uncommon, ranging from 10%[85] to 13%.[95] The time from the onset of buccal and genital lesions to ocular involvement is estimated to be between 3 and 4 years.[103] The initial ocular manifestations may be unilateral, but progression to bilateral involvement is the rule, occurring in at least two thirds of the cases.[104]

Nongranulomatous inflammation with necrotizing obliterative vasculitis may be found either in the anterior or the posterior segment, or, more commonly, in both.

Anterior Segment

Anterior uveitis may be the only ocular manifestation of ABD. The classic finding of iridocyclitis with hypopyon (Fig. 56–5) is present in only 19% to 31% of ABD cases.[18, 104] Mamo and Baghdassarian[26] reported that hypopyon has become an uncommon finding in ABD. They attributed this apparent decline to the advent of steroid management, which has resulted in dampening inflammatory responses.

The inflammatory response in the anterior chamber in ABD is nongranulomatous in nature. The patients often complain of redness, periorbital pain, photophobia, and blurred vision. Tearing may occur, but ocular discharge is rare. Slit-lamp biomicroscopic examination reveals conjunctival injection, ciliary flush in the perilimbal area, cells and flare in the anterior chamber, and fine keratic precipitates. The cells can be seen to move freely in the anterior chamber, following the currents of aqueous movement caused by the temperature differential

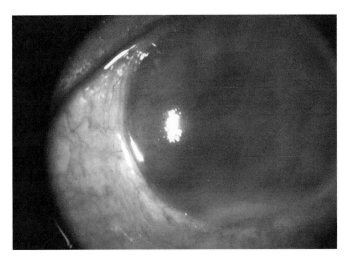

FIGURE 56–5. Hypopyon in a patient with ABD. (See color insert.)

between the front and the back portions of the chamber. A typical finding with the hypopyon of ABD is that it may shift with gravity as the patient changes head positions. In eyes with severe iridocyclitis, in which hypopyon is not seen by direct examination with slit-lamp biomicroscopy, a small layering of leukocytes can be observed in the angle by gonioscopy. This is termed angle hypopyon. A more common presentation is iridocyclitis without hypopyon, which is found in two thirds of cases.[18]

The anterior uveitis may resolve spontaneously over 2 to 3 weeks even if therapy is not instituted. Chronic inflammation is not characteristic of this disorder. It is explosive in nature, appearing very rapidly. Some patients with ABD may change from feeling perfect one moment to having very severe inflammation 2 hours later. However, this anterior segment inflammation may not be accompanied by posterior segment involvement. Structural changes of the anterior portion of the eye, including posterior synechiae, iris atrophy, and peripheral anterior synechiae, may develop during the course of repeated ocular inflammatory attacks. The presence of peripheral anterior synechiae or iris bombé from pupillary seclusion may lead to secondary glaucoma. Neovascularization of the iris can occur as a result of posterior segment involvement (see later). It is also an ominous sign, a prognosticator of poor outcome.

Other, less frequent anterior segment findings are cataract, episcleritis, scleritis, subconjunctival hemorrhage, filamentary keratitis, conjunctival ulcers,[18] and corneal immune ring opacity.[105]

Posterior Segment

White cell infiltration of the vitreous body, ranging from a moderate number of cells suspended on the vitreous fibrils to a dense plasmoid reaction with sheets of inflammatory cells, is always present during the acute phase. An isolated vitreous inflammatory reaction is not characteristic of ABD. However, Horiuchi and colleagues[106] reported that the most frequent sign of the involvement of the posterior segment was irreversible changes of the vitreous, and that the most important of these changes was posterior vitreous detachment. They

found that posterior vitreous detachment occurred at an early stage of ocular involvement, in 92% of the affected eyes.

The essential retinal finding is an obliterative, necrotizing vasculitis that affects both the arteries and veins in the posterior pole.[104, 107] Fundus examination reveals venous and capillary dilation with engorgement. Involvement of the retinal vessels in the form of acute periphlebitis or thromboangiitis obliterans may lead to massive retinal and vitreous hemorrhage.[104] Patchy perivascular sheathing with inflammatory whitish yellow exudates surrounding retinal hemorrhages may be seen (Fig. 56–6). They usually accumulate in the deeper retinal layers during acute episodes, while the overlying retina shows turbidity and edema. Retinal edema is present in 10% to 20% of cases, especially in the macula.[104] Retinal atrophy frequently is present after the retinal exudates and hemorrhage resolve, offering stark testimony to the prior ischemia. Sheathing of the veins often precedes sheathing of the arteries. Choroidal vascular involvement occurs as well, and choroidal infarcts are probably more common than is generally appreciated.

Severe vasculitis may lead to ischemic retinal changes because of vascular occlusion. This vascular occlusion causes tissue hypoxia, which stimulates the growth of new vessels at the optic nerve (neovascularization of disc [NVD]) or elsewhere (NVE). Both NVD and NVE can rupture and bleed, causing the vitreous cavity to fill with blood. Bleeding into the vitreous cavity can lead to organization with membrane formation. These membranes may contract and pull the retina, causing retinal tears with subsequent retinal detachment.

Neovascular glaucoma occurs in as many as 6% of patients with ABD. This often results in phthisis bulbi, which may occur in the presence or absence of central retinal vein or artery occlusion. Central or branch retinal vein (Fig. 56–7) or artery occlusions may be present.[108, 109]

The optic nerve is affected in at least one fourth of ABD patients.[104] Hyperemia of the optic disc with blurring of the margins (papillitis) is the most frequently observed

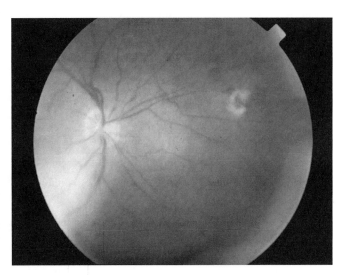

FIGURE 56–6. Fundus photograph of a retinal lesion with accompanying intraretinal hemorrhages and vasculitis. (See color insert.)

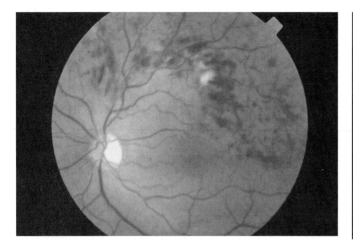

FIGURE 56–7. Fundus photograph with a branch retinal vein occlusion in a patient with ABD.

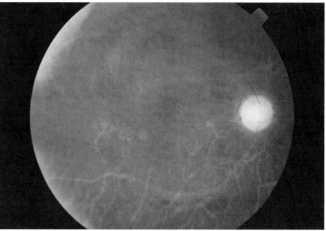

FIGURE 56–9. End stage of repeated ABD attacks of posterior pole. Note the retinal atrophy associated with vessel attenuation and an optic disc atrophy. (See color insert.)

lesion of the optic disc. Papilledema is not frequent, but it may occur (Fig. 56–8A,B).[110] Progressive optic atrophy may occur as a result of microvasculitis of the arterioles supplying the optic nerve.

Repeated inflammatory bouts are of major concern, with the most vision-robbing pathology located in the posterior pole, with fibrotic, attenuated retinal arterioles, narrowed and occluded "silver-wired" vessels (Fig. 56–9), a variable degree of chorioretinal scars (Fig. 56–10), retinal pigment epithelial alternations, and optic nerve atrophy being the consequences of repeated inflammatory assaults (see Fig. 56–9).

ADAMANTIADES-BEHÇET DISEASE IN CHILDREN
Several reports describing ABD in children have been published.[111–116] ABD in neonates whose mothers had oral and genital ulcers during pregnancy have also been described.[117] Recently, a case of transient neonatal ABD with life-threatening complications was reported.[118] The incidence of ABD in childhood in Japan is approximately 1.5% of all reported cases of ABD, and there are some differences in these cases compared to adult cases. Dur-

ing the course of the disease, uveitis and arthritis are seen more frequently in children, whereas genital and oral ulcers are less frequent. The first disease manifestation in children with ABD is oral aphthae in 55%, and uveitis in 31% of cases.[115] However, periphlebitis has not been described in childhood ABD yet. In another study from Turkey, children showed lower vascular, neurologic, and ocular manifestations than did adults.[113]

ADAMANTIADES-BEHÇET DISEASE IN PREGNANCY
Fetal and pregnancy outcomes were generally considered good in a recent study by Marsal and colleagues, in which 59 pregnancies in 54 women with ABD were analyzed.[119] No changes regarding disease activity during pregnancy were noted in 47%, exacerbation of the disease was observed in 34%, and symptomatic improvement was reported in 26%. After delivery, stable disease was noted in 43%, improvement was observed in 31%, and disease deterioration was found in 19%. Ten miscarriages occurred.[119] However, in another study, in which 27 women were enrolled, exacerbation of ABD during pregnancy

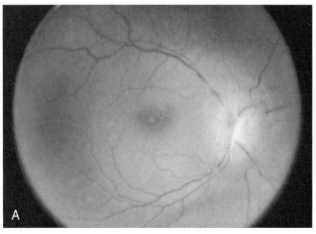

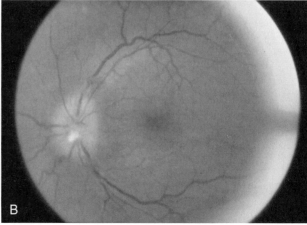

FIGURE 56–8. *A* and *B*, Bilateral optic disc edema in a patient with ABD. (See color insert.)

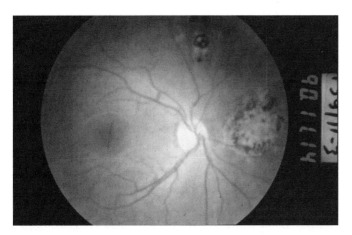

FIGURE 56–10. Fundus photograph from a patient with repeated attacks of ABD showing a scar in the nasal area of the posterior pole. (See color insert.)

was noted in 18 pregnant women (67%).[120] In a recent study, fetal and pregnancy outcomes were generally considered good. In addition, disease manifestations were not worsened, and the frequencies of spontaneous abortions, congenital malformation, and perinatal death in babies born to ABD patients were not significantly different from those of healthy women with recurrent oral ulcerations.[121] Finally, the first case of Budd-Chiari syndrome during puerperium was described.[122]

PATHOGENESIS AND IMMUNOLOGY OF ABD

The cause of ABD remains unknown. Environmental factors, infectious agents, immune mechanisms, and genetic factors have been studied intensively. Many environmental factors have been implicated but not proved.[123]

Infectious Agents

Epidemiologic data[124] as well as familial incidence incriminate an infectious cause for ABD. However, no microorganism has been reproducibly isolated from lesions of patients with ABD.

In a limited number of patients, herpes simplex virus type 1 was found in the peripheral blood by using polymerase chain reaction (PCR). A positive reaction for herpes simplex was detected in biopsy samples from genital[125] and intestinal ulcers,[126] but a large number of patients is needed to confirm such results. Not only herpes simplex virus but also hepatitis C virus has been incriminated as a causative factor for ABD.[127] Although parvovirus B19 has been reported to be associated with vasculitis, recent findings do not support a role for parvovirus B19 in the pathogenesis of ABD.[128]

Elevated serum antibody titers for antistreptococcal antibodies against certain serotypes of *Streptococcus sanguis* have been found in patients with ABD,[129] and ABD patients showed a greater frequency of *S. sanguis* in their oral flora compared with controls.[130] This observation could explain the decision of some investigators who treat oral ulcers with penicillin.

Immunoglobulin A isotype of antibodies specific for *Mycobacterium tuberculosis* heat shock protein-65, which can cross-react with certain serotypes of *S. sanguis*, have been

isolated from patients with ABD.[131] However, the pathogenic role of this protein has not been accepted.

Immune Mechanisms

Although there are disagreements as to whether ABD should be considered an autoimmune disease, autoimmune mechanisms are incriminated in the pathogenesis of ABD.[132] However, there are many ways in which ABD differs from a classic autoimmune disease. The most important differences lie in the male preponderance, the lack of association with other autoimmune diseases, the absence of autoantibodies, the lack of association with HLA-alleles usually seen in autoimmune diseases, the hyperactivity of B cells, and the lack of definite T-cell hypofunction in ABD. Since the most popular research interest in ABD is directed toward immunologic mechanisms, Emmi and colleagues[133] recently described the immunologic aspects of ABD.

The main microscopic finding at most sites of active ABD is an occlusive vasculitis (see later).[134] At the cellular level, few reports have correlated T-cell changes with ABD disturbances,[135] but current observations suggest that during the active stage of ABD, T cells are activated (overexpression of CD25), HLA class II (HLA-DR) expression on T cells is down-regulated, whereas both helper (CD4) and suppressor-cytotoxic (CD8) T cells have cytophilic IgA bound to their surfaces. In addition, an increased percentage of T-cell receptor (TCR) γδ has been found in the circulation of patients with ABD.[136, 137] The significance of this increase in γδ T cells in circulation and their effect in inflammation in ABD is unclear. Nonetheless, recently it has been shown that the ABD-specific heat shock protein peptides predominately stimulate the γδ T-cell populations.[136]

Natural killer cells and neutrophils are also increased in number and activity. Sera from patients with ABD enhanced the adherence of neutrophils to vascular endothelial cell monolayer in vitro.[138] This finding could explain the mechanism responsible for neutrophil accumulation at injury sites.

Evidence is emerging that immune response caused by Th1/Th2 (Th0) cells is critical in the development of the pathologic/inflammatory response.[139] However, the role of Th0 cell cytokines in human autoimmune diseases has rarely been studied. In ABD, various proinflammatory interleukins (ILs), such as IL-1a, IL-6, IL-8, tumor necrosis factor-α (TNF-α), and soluble IL-2 receptors have been reported to be elevated in the sera of patients with ABD.[140–143] IL-8 has a potent effect on neutrophils,[141] and increased chemotactic activity of neutrophils has been observed in ABD disease.[144, 145] It is unclear how anti-inflammatory cytokines IL-4, LI-10, and IL-13 (the Th2 response) regulate secretion of proinflammatory cytokines IL-1a, IL-6, IL-8, and TNF-α in ABD.[140–143] Recently, it has been shown that the immune system in ABD may be characterized by a divergent cytokine production profile of mixed Th1/Th2 (Th0) cell type, and interferon-γ (INF-γ) is critical in modulating the IL-4, IL-10, and IL-12 cytokine network pathway in this disease.[146]

Initial concepts of immune alternations in patients with ABD concerned immune complexes. Circulating immune complexes (CIC) have been associated with uveitis[147] and found in ocular specimens.[148] Thus, the finding of CIC in ABD patients supports such an association for its ocular complications.[149] Serum levels of immunoglobulins A, E, and M are increased in ABD patients. These antibodies found in patients with ABD have been used in an attempt to define the disease itself.[150–152] Immune complex formation has been detected in the tissues, particularly in active stages of ABD. Furthermore, Kasp and colleagues[153] have reported that patients with elevated levels of CIC had a better visual prognosis than did patients without CIC. They have theorized that CIC may have a protective value, as opposed to a destructive role, inasmuch as they may help to eliminate potentially harmful initiators of the immune reaction. These findings are in agreement with those reported by Charteris and colleagues,[154] who suggested that cell-mediated immunity, rather than immune complex deposition was responsible for the perpetuation of the ocular inflammation in ABD and that CD4 T cells played a central role in this.

Sera of patients with ABD were examined for the presence of antiphospholipid antibodies.[155, 156] There was a statistically significant association between these antibodies and the retinal vascular disease in ABD patients. Antibodies against the endothelium have also been detected in the sera of patients with ABD and active thrombophlebitis or retinal vasculitis. Antithrombin III, protein C, and protein S are major natural inhibitors of coagulation, and it is well known that deficiency of those proteins causes thrombotic disorders. However, antithrombin III, protein C, and protein S deficiencies are not a probable cause of thrombotic manifestations in ABD.[157, 158] Endothelial damage may be induced by increased levels of von Willebrand factor, which was increased in ABD patients, particularly those with vasculitis.[159]

Genetic Factors

The fact that certain racial groups appear to be at increased risk for ABD suggests a genetic predisposition to the disease. Indeed, HLA-B5 phenotype and its subtype HLA-Bw51[160] have been found in a significantly higher proportion of patients suffering from ABD than in the general population. This strong association has been confirmed in many different ethnic groups from the Middle East to the Far East, such as Japan,[18, 161] Turkey,[162] Germany,[22] and Greece,[163] but not in whites living in the United States and England.[164, 165] The HLA-B51 gene has recently been identified to comprise seven alleles, B*5101 to B*5107.[166, 167] However, ABD was found to be strongly associated with the HLA-B*5101 alleles in Japan[168] and in Greece.[169]

On the other hand, HLA-DR1 and HLA-DQw1 have been shown to be significantly decreased in patients with ABD. This may indicate that an individual who carries these antigens is resistant to develop the disease. These results suggest that not only disease susceptibility but also resistant genes play an important role in the immunogenetic mechanisms of ABD.[170]

Specific associations between HLA type and clinical manifestations of ABD have also been found. Thus, HLA-B12 is associated with mucocutaneous lesions, HLA-B27 with arthritis, and HLA-B5 with ocular lesions.[171] Such associations, however, were not found in a study from Turkey.[172] Furthermore, in a Asian report, patients with ABD and refractory ocular lesions were strongly associated with HLA-DQw3, and the onset of the disease was earlier than in the HLA-DQw3–negative patients.[173]

The reason for the association between HLA-B51 and ABD is not clear. It is possible that the HLA specificity is a marker for the different immune response gene found in ABD patients, as the genomic region that encodes the HLA antigens is the same as the one that controls the immune response. Another hypothesis suggests that HLA antigens may function as targets themselves, either for exogenous agents or for endogenous autoimmune reactions.

Taking into account these findings, a model explaining the etiopathogenesis of ABD was proposed by Emmi and associates.[133] An exogenous factor (e.g., a microbe) is internalized by antigen-presenting cells (APC) (e.g., macrophages, dendritic cells), where it undergoes processing in an acidic vesicular compartment. Processing ensures that portions of a protein (the immunodominant peptides) will bind to class II major histocompatibility complex (MHC) molecules, forming an immunogenic complex that is then expressed on the surface of the APC, where it is recognized by CD4+ T cells. Activated Th1 cells produce ILs (IL-2, INF-γ, and TNF-β) and induce B cell proliferation. INF-γ activates macrophages and they release TNF-α, IL-1, and IL-8. These cytokines are responsible for the expression of adhesion molecules on the endothelial cells. IL-8 also induces chemotaxis and activates neutrophils. Both factors are necessary for the increased vascular permeability and the passage of neutrophils and activated T cells through the endothelium to the inflammatory area. Genetic factors may also be responsible for the expression and perpetuation of the illness.[174] Thus, inflammation and B-cell proliferation in a genetically susceptible individual can lead to ABD.

PATHOLOGY

Even though ABD can cause blindness, few reports on the ocular immunohistopathology of ABD have been published.[152, 154, 175, 176] In contrast, many histopathologic studies have been performed on other tissues involved with ABD. It is primarily an inflammatory disorder involving small blood vessels, particularly venules. The early lesions resemble a delayed type hypersensitivity reaction, whereas the late lesions resemble an immune complex type reaction. The role of immune complexes in causing venulitis is, however, questionable, as immunoglobulins are not routinely found in vessel walls.

Histopathology

The common underlying histopathologic lesion in all affected organs is both leukocytoclastic and monocytic occlusive vasculitis that is responsible for organ failure. However, the level of occlusion may reflect the age of the lesion and the type of cells that participate in such a lesion.[177] The principal pathologic features are perivascular infiltrates of lymphocytes and mononuclear cells, swelling and proliferation of small vessels, and fibrinoid degeneration. In postmortem examination of the brain, demyelination is the most common finding, followed by encephalomalacia at multiple sites, accompanied by perivascular cell infiltration in the brain stem, spinal cord, cerebrum, and cerebellum.[65] The histologic characteristics of erythema nodosum are areas that are infiltrated by lymphocytes and a few histiocytes.[178] Histopathology of the mucocutaneous lesions in ABD are characterized by the presence of neutrophils, fibrinoid necrosis, and a mixed perivascular infiltrate.[179] Increased numbers of mast cells have also been reported in the cellular infiltrates of the recurrent mucocutaneous ulcers.[180]

Ocular histopathologic changes are similar to those found in other organs, as was described previously. During the acute inflammation, the iris, ciliary body, and choroid show diffuse infiltration with neutrophils, and later with lymphocytes, monocytes, and mast cells. In the more chronic stage, with many recurrences, increased collagen is present, which can lead to iris atrophy and posterior synechiae, cyclitic membrane formation, and thickening of the choroid and sometimes hypotony and phthisis bulbi. In the retina, vasculitis with marked infiltration of leukocytes, and plasma cells in and around blood vessels and into retinal tissue is the most prominent finding. Veins are more affected than arteries. During the inflammatory process, the retinal vascular endothelial cells become swollen, neutrophils migrate, and thrombus formation begins. Rods and cones in areas of involvement are destroyed, and fibrosis of the inner nuclear layer is present. Retinal pigment epithelium destruction is minimal. In more advanced cases, there is fibrosis of the blood vessels and sometimes complete vascular obliteration. The optic nerve vessels can also be affected by the vasculitic process, which can lead to optic neuritis, ischemia, and, in more severe chronic cases, optic atrophy.

Immunopathology

Immunopathology of the affected organs has shown that the T cell is the predominant inflammatory cell type, suggesting that cell-mediated immunity plays a central role in ABD.[135, 154, 181] Immunohistologic study of the pathergy test site shows infiltration similar to that observed in a delayed-type hypersensitivity reaction.[182] Furthermore, immunopathology of the conjunctival biopsy of patients with inactive ABD has revealed that both neutrophils and T cells are involved in response to surgical trauma, along with overexpression of E-selectin and intracellular adhesion molecule-1, suggesting a hyperreaction in areas that are not primarily involved during the disease process.[176]

DIAGNOSIS

Diagnosis of ABD is based on clinical observations only. Therefore, the criteria defined either by the International Study Group of Behçet's disease or the Japanese Research Committee of Behçet's disease should be applied. Although there are no laboratory tests that are specific for the diagnosis of ABD, some are helpful for evaluation.

Fluorescein Angiography and Indocyanine Green Angiography

Fluorescein angiography (FA) demonstrates marked dilation and occlusion of the retinal capillaries in patients with ABD. In a recent study from Turkey, FA disclosed incipient fundus changes in 6.3% of patients with ABD who had no abnormal finding on fundus examination as well as no visual complains.[183] Fundus FA is *mandatory* in the study and longitudinal care of patients with ocular ABD. It should be used to monitor the extent of damage to the vasculature of the retina and the optic nerve[184] so that therapy can be adjusted on the basis of these subclinical signs rather than solely on vision loss, clearly an irreversible clinical finding.

During acute inflammation, there is diffuse fluorescein leakage from the retinal capillaries (Fig. 56–11), the larger engorged vessels, and the optic disc. Persistent, diffuse dye leakage is seen even with resolution of inflammatory episodes. In addition, FA may show late staining of the vasculature, evidence of large zones of capillary nonperfusion, collateral vascular formation, secondary retinal telangiectasia, and retinal neovascularization. Macular alterations (macular ischemia, cystoid macular edema [Fig. 56–12], macular hole, and epiretinal membrane), which may be responsible for poor vision, can be seen by FA.[185] Evidence of retinal pigment epithelial involvement is rarely seen in this disorder. However, Matsuo and colleagues[186] reported that patients with ABD have choroidal abnormalities that were revealed only with indocyanine green angiography (ICG), and not with funduscopy or FA. Thus, simultaneous ICG and FA would be useful for examining choroidal lesions in ABD. FA and/ or ICG, together with slit-lamp fundus biomicroscopy should be used to evaluate the response to medical treatment.

Electrophysiology

Flash electroretinography together with pattern visually evoked potentials may be good indicators for monitoring posterior segment changes as well as for predicting visual prognosis.[187]

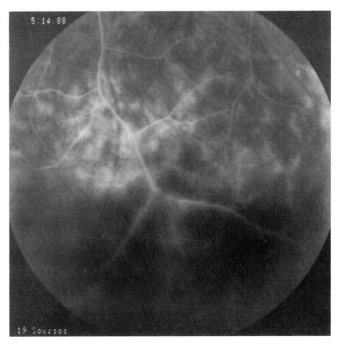

FIGURE 56–11. Fluorescein angiography (same patient of Figure 56–10) revealing substantial leakage of dye from peripheral retinal vessels due to peripheral retinal vasculitis.

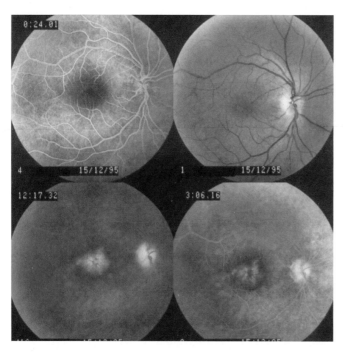

FIGURE 56–12. Fluorescein angiography with the characteristic angiographic pattern of prominent cystoid macular edema. Note the accumulation of fluorescein in the cystoid spaces of Henle's layer.

Serologic Studies

The erythrocyte sedimentation rate, C-reactive protein, and other acute-phase reactants, such as properdin factor b and α_1-acid glycoprotein, may be elevated during the acute phase of ABD.[188] Additionally, longitudinal monitoring of soluble CD25 molecules in the serum (soluble IL-2 receptor [sIL-2r]) along with these acute-phase reactants, to be quite useful, since a rise in these markers often precedes the development of a clinically obvious recurrence, thereby providing the clinician the opportunity for a preemptive therapeutic strike. The levels of ILs and adhesion molecules, and the role of the imaging techniques have already been discussed in the relevant sections.

Hence, diagnosis and assessment of disease activity are based on clinical findings on examination. Decreased fluorescein leakage indicates a favorable response to therapy. The longitudinal assessment strategy and the treatment philosophy described here are extremely important, because ABD is categorically a blinding disease, and usually bilateral.[18, 189, 190] The second eye is generally affected within 1 year of disease onset in the first eye, although this may not occur for as long as 7 years.

DIFFERENTIAL DIAGNOSIS

It is important to consider other types of uveitis in the differential diagnosis of ABD, particularly when the presentation is incomplete or atypical, since other illness may have ocular manifestations similar to those found in ABD.

Severe recurrent iridocyclitis with hypopyon can be found in HLA-B27-associated anterior uveitis. In contrast to ABD, this uveitis is usually unilateral and the hypopyon is less mobile.

Reiter's syndrome can resemble the incomplete form of ABD. However, Reiter's syndrome is generally not associated with vasculitis, and the oral ulcers are usually painless.

Although sarcoidosis may have posterior segment lesions similar to those found in ABD, the uveitis in ABD has an explosive nature. Even though vasculitis can be found in sarcoidosis, it is usually not occlusive, and it more frequently affects veins in a sectional manner, in contrast to ABD, which affects both arteries and veins in a diffuse manner.

Other forms of vasculitis such as systemic lupus erythematosus (SLE), polyarteritis nodosa (PAN), and Wegener's granulomatosis (WG) should also be included in the differential diagnosis of ABD. In the evaluation of a patient with multisystem illness and possible vasculitis, it is useful to take an organized system approach to the history and examination. The specific pattern of tissue involvement can be used to focus on potential diagnoses and subsequent diagnostic tests. For example, the presence of oral ulcers in the setting of a systemic process may suggest ABD but also WG, Crohn's disease, Reiter's syndrome, or SLE. Specific eye findings may help to focus the diagnostic evaluation.

SLE, like ABD, produces multisystem involvement, and definitive criteria are available with the detection of extractable antinuclear antibodies, and in particular anti-DNA antibodies. The retinal features of SLE are caused by arterial occlusion, and the characteristic findings are cotton-wool spots, larger retinal infarcts, and optic disc infarction. Thus, unlike ABD, in which arteries and veins can both be involved, veins are not involved in SLE, and there are no inflammatory changes in the anterior chamber or vitreous.

PAN is a necrotizing vasculitis that involves medium-sized macular arteries and smaller arterioles. Retinal vasculitis of PAN resembles the vasculitis found in ABD, but vitritis is not so prominent. In addition, nephropathy is commonly found in PAN but is very rare in ABD.

Retinal vasculitis can also be found in WG. However, the presence of upper and lower respiratory involvement, the concomitant glomerulonephritis, and a positive antineutrophil cytoplasmic antibody test are highly specific for WG. In contrast to the occlusive vasculitis found in ABD, the vasculitis of WG is a necrotizing granulomatous vasculitis.

Finally, the retinitis of ABD can be suggestive of a viral retinitis. Acute retinal necrosis mimics the rapid progression and severity of ABD. However, the lesions of ABD rarely begin as uniformly in the periphery and are often associated with systemic symptoms and signs.

TREATMENT

The goal of therapy is to treat the acute disease, but, perhaps even more important, to prevent or at least to decrease the number of repetitive ocular inflammatory episodes of the posterior pole (Figs. 56–13 and 56–14). The choice of medication is based on the severity of the disease. In general, treatment should be more aggressive whenever the following are present: complete ABD, involvement of the CNS, vascular involvement, retinal

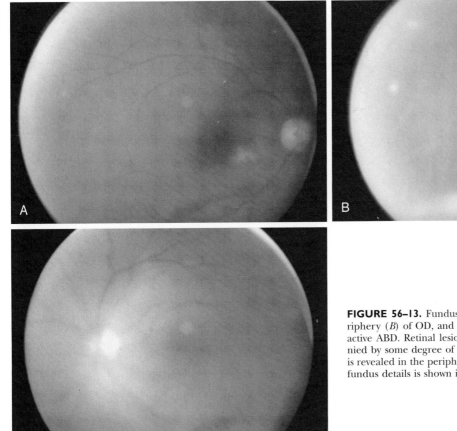

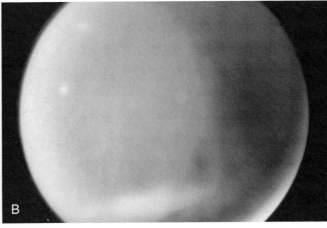

FIGURE 56–13. Fundus photographs of posterior pole (*A*) and periphery (*B*) of OD, and posterior pole of OS (*C*) from a patient with active ABD. Retinal lesion located in the inferior quadrant accompanied by some degree of vitritis is noted in OD (*A*). Snow bank lesion is revealed in the periphery of OD (*B*). Extensive vitritis that obscures fundus details is shown in OS (*C*). (See color insert.)

and bilateral involvement, male sex,[18] and a geographic origin in the Mediterranean basin or Far East.[18]

Many treatment modalities have been tried in ocular ABD with varying claims of success. Evaluation of all these treatment modalities is very difficult because of the unpredictable and intermittent course of the symptoms. The frequency of exacerbations can be influenced by drugs for various periods of time, but systematic study of the influence of these treatment modalities on the final outcome and the final visual acuity has been very limited.

The most commonly used agents today are corticosteroids, cytotoxic drugs, colchicine, Cs-A, and tacrolimus (FK-506).

Corticosteroids

Although many forms of uveitis are initially treated with corticosteroids, ABD usually becomes "resistant" to corticosteroid therapy.[191] Systemic or topical corticosteroids have a beneficial effect on the acute ocular inflammation. Despite the fact that corticosteroids alone have failed to prevent vision loss in patients with ABD,[18, 24, 26, 104, 191, 192] systemic corticosteroids (1 to 1.5 mg/kg of prednisone per day) are especially useful in quickly controlling acute inflammation, but they appear to have little effect, if any, on the late sequelae. The addition of corticosteroid to a therapeutic regimen for treatment of the ocular manifestations of ABD is not well accepted in Japan. However, it is appropriate to use systemic corticosteroids for patients being treated with immunosuppressive drugs for acute

posterior segment inflammation, because their immediate anti-inflammatory action is of benefit while waiting for the full effect of the cytotoxic drugs. Then the corticosteroids are gradually tapered. Intravenous administration of a high dose of corticosteroids may be beneficial in selected case of acute severe inflammation.[193] In select cases, low-dose corticosteroids (15 to 30 mg/day) may be required chronically in combination with immunosuppressive agents for controlling the uveitis. This combination is beneficial for reducing the adverse effects of either drug.[194] More will be said later about the art of the polypharmacologic approach to treating ABD. In anterior segment inflammation, topical corticosteroids, with or without periocular corticosteroids, are required.

Cytotoxic Agents

Immunosuppressive treatment is required for severe uveitis with retinal involvement. Several reports from the Mediterranean area have underlined the efficacy of cytotoxic agents in controlling ABD ocular inflammation.[195–197] Immunosuppressive drugs that are currently used in the treatment of ocular ABD include azathioprine, chlorambucil, cyclophosphamide, methotrexate, cyclosporine, tacrolimus, and mycophenolate mofetil.

Azathioprine

Azathioprine is an immunosuppressive drug that interferes with purine incorporation into DNA, and hence it affects rapidly proliferating cells such as activated lymphocytes.

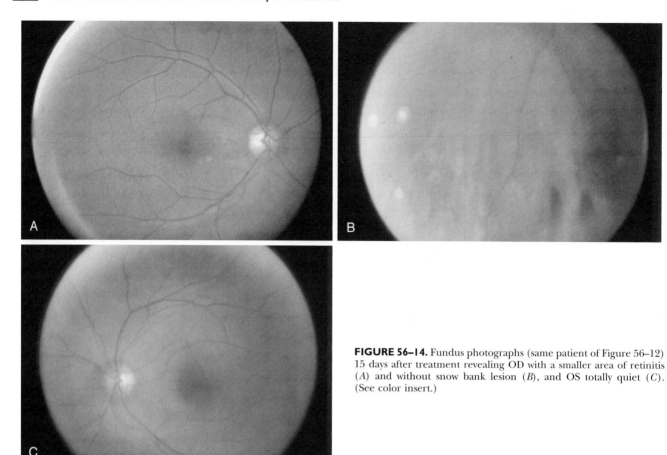

FIGURE 56–14. Fundus photographs (same patient of Figure 56–12) 15 days after treatment revealing OD with a smaller area of retinitis (*A*) and without snow bank lesion (*B*), and OS totally quiet (*C*). (See color insert.)

Although earlier reports of treatment with azathioprine (2.5 mg/kg/day) gave inconclusive results,[104, 198] a double-blind study from Turkey showed that azathioprine was useless in restoring compromised vision, but it was superior to placebo in preserving visual acuity in those with established eye disease.[189] Azathioprine was also effective in treating oral and genital ulcers, and arthritis.[189] My results with azathioprine alone are less impressive. Indeed, as will be emphasized later, I rarely, if ever, rely on any single agent for patients with ABD posterior segment manifestations at the Massachusetts Eye and Ear Infirmary.

Chlorambucil

Chlorambucil, a slow-acting alkylating agent, was the first immunosuppressive drug to be used in patients with ocular ABD. It was employed in 1970 by Mamo and Azzam because corticosteroids failed to prevent visual deterioration in their patients with ABD in Lebanon.[199] Although its side effects are essentially the same as those of cyclophosphamide, the rationale behind its use was that it was slower acting than cyclophosphamide and could be administered more safely on an outpatient basis. Godfrey and colleagues[200] as well as Pivetti-Pezzi and colleagues[201] also reported on the effectiveness of chlorambucil in the treatment of ABD, and Tessler and Jennings[202] reported that high-dose, short-term chlorambucil treatment for ABD also produced favorable results.

However, Tabbara[203] reported long-term results with chlorambucil that were disappointing, with 75% of eyes in patients treated with chlorambucil as monotherapy having visual acuity of 20/200 or less. These results could be explained by the fact that chlorambucil, a slow-acting agent, suppresses the immune system slowly, which would be a disadvantage, as rapid immunosuppression is usually desirable for patients with ABD. To understand Tabbara's results, it would be helpful to have comparative data on the vigor of therapy and the level of immunosuppression of the patients.

The usual starting dose of chlorambucil is 0.1 mg/kg/day. One to 3 months of therapy is usually required before its immunosuppressive action is apparent. The drug dose is adjusted to maintain clinical remission for approximately 1 year. Proper hematologic monitoring can be complex and must be done by a chemotherapist experienced in chlorambucil therapy. Azoospermia in men cannot be avoided, and therefore sperm banking, when available, should be offered. Amenorrhea in women can often be avoided by induction of menopause during the course of treatment through the use of leuprolide acetate (Lupron).

Cyclophosphamide

Cyclophosphamide, a fast-acting alkylating agent, has been utilized widely in Japan with favorable results in controlling uveitis, preventing ocular attacks, and maintaining good visual acuity for long periods in patients with ABD.[197] It has been shown that cyclophosphamide is superior to steroids in suppressing ocular inflammation in patients with ABD.[204] Similarly, oral cyclophosphamide produced ocular and systemic improvement in patients with ABD who had been previously unresponsive to systemic corticosteroids.[205] Although chlorambucil may be the single most efficacious agent in management of ABD, capable of inducing long-term disease remission, intravenous cyclophosphamide may be a highly attractive alternative. Intravenous cyclophosphamide (750 to 1000 mg/sq m every 4 weeks) has been used by Baer and colleagues[104] in cases refractory to chlorambucil and in severe vasculitis with favorable results. Foster and colleagues[206] as well as Fain and colleagues[207] have shown both cyclophosphamide and chlorambucil to be superior to Cs-A in management of the posterior segment manifestations of ABD. However, in a study from Turkey in which intravenous cyclophosphamide was compared with oral Cs-A, cyclophosphamide was found to be less effective, especially during the first 6 months of the treatment.[208]

Cyclosporine-A

The mechanisms by which Cs-A acts are not completely understood, attesting to the enormous complexity underlying T-cell activation. It is believed that Cs-A disrupts the transmission of signals from the T-cell receptor to genes that encode for multiple lymphokines and enzymes necessary for activation of resting T cells and cytoaggression while leaving the T-cell priming reaction unaffected.[209]

Nussenblatt and colleagues of the National Eye Institute were first to report the efficacy of Cs-A at doses of 10 mg/kg/day in patients with intractable uveitis of various etiologies, including ABD refractory to corticosteroid and cytotoxic agents.[210–214] This observation was subsequently corroborated by other investigators in treatment of ABD.[215] However, a dose of 10 mg/kg/day that was initially used is now known to be associated with a 100% incidence of renal toxicity, and it has been suggested that the more prudent dose should be 5 mg/kg/day.[216] Later studies have shown that combination of a low dose of Cs-A with corticosteroids was more effective in improving visual acuity than the higher dose of Cs-A alone.[217–220] A very slow tapering of the medication is usually advisable since a rebound phenomenon has been observed in some cases when discontinuation of Cs-A was abrupt.[220] Nevertheless, Foster and colleagues[206] as well as Chavis and colleagues[221] have shown that less toxic doses of Cs-A are distinctly inferior to cytotoxic agents (azathioprine, cyclophosphamide, and chlorambucil) in management of the posterior segment manifestations and inflammatory recurrences in patients with ABD. I have successfully employed Cs-A at low doses in combination with azathioprine as a steroid-sparing strategy in the treatment of ABD. However, it is extremely difficult to wean patients off Cs-A without recurrent disease, even when they have been on this medication for over 2 years. The definitive efficacy and long-term outcome of combined Cs-A regimens with prednisone and other immunosuppressive agents (e.g., azathioprine) in ABD await critical evaluation in prospective, randomized trials.

Tacrolimus

Tacrolimus (FK-506) is a newly developed immunosuppressive drug. Its action is very similar to that of Cs-A: It selectively suppresses CD4+ T lymphocytes. The Japanese FK-506 Study Group on Refractory Uveitis reported favorable results in 75% of 53 patients with refractory uveitis, including 41 patients with ABD.[79] The therapy was switched to FK-506 (0.10 to 0.15 mg/kg/day) because of therapeutic failures and adverse side effects with systemic corticosteroids, colchicine, cyclophosphamide, and Cs-A. However, FK-506 is associated with not infrequent occurrence of disconcerting side effects such as renal, gastrointestinal, and neurologic problems.[222] On the other hand, hirsutism, gingival hypertrophy, and coarsening of facial features have not been reported in patients treated with FK-506.

Colchicine

Colchicine exhibits both anti-inflammatory and antimitotic properties, mediated mainly through its inhibition of microtubular formation.[223] Because enhanced neutrophil migration is a characteristic feature of ABD, colchicine (0.6 mg/day) is most useful in prophylaxis of recurrent inflammatory episodes (rather than in treatment of active disease) or in the rare patients with mild, unilateral involvement in whom the clinician wishes to defer immunosuppressive therapy.[224] Colchicine can also be used in combination with other drugs in treating all forms of ocular and systemic manifestations of ABD.[144, 197, 225] It is not effective as monotherapy in treating ocular symptoms, but it may form part of a polypharmacologic "recipe" for patients with ABD.

Mycophenolate Mofetil

Mycophenolate mofetil is a novel immunosuppressive agent that blocks DNA synthesis by the inhibition of the enzyme inosine monophosphate dehydrogenase.[226] Mycophenolate mofetil, unlike Cs-A and FK-506, does not inhibit the early production of interleukin-2 or the production of cytokines of T-helper-cell clones belonging to the Th0 and Th2 subsets.[227] Because mycophenolate mofetil works at a later stage in the T-cell cycle, it acts synergistically with other immunosuppressives.[228] More recently, Larkin and Lightman[229] successfully treated two ABD patients by adding mycophenolate mofetil to their therapeutic regiments. These patients responded inadequately to steroids used concomitantly with Cs-A.

Other Treatment Modalities

Other treatment modalities that have been tried in ocular ABD with some benefit include interferons,[230–233] plasmapheresis,[161, 234] pentoxyphilline,[235] penicillin,[236] thalidomide,[237] and interferon-α2b.

ABD is a complex disorder for which no best therapeutic agent has yet been described. Although one patient may respond well to combination low-dose prednisone and cyclosporin, another, with seemingly identical ABD manifestations, may not. Azathioprine may be just the right additional ingredient in the nonresponding patient's therapeutic recipe to result in stability and freedom from relapses, or it may not. The patient may need to be advanced to alkylating therapy with chlorambucil or cyclophosphamide to induce disease remission. The following case description, contributed by Dr. C. Stephen Foster of Boston, is an example of the complexities and difficult decisions that the physician and patient may need to make throughout the course of ABD.

CASE REPORT

A 22-year-old white man presented to the Ocular Immunology and Uveitis Service of the Massachusetts Eye and Ear Infirmary in November, 1997, referred from his local ophthalmologist with a 6-week history of bilateral uveitis, treated with topical and systemic steroids. The presenting visual acuity was 20/80 in each eye (OU). Review of systems disclosed a history of recurrent aphthous mouth ulcers, seasonal allergies, and acneiform skin lesions.

The ophthalmic examination disclosed panuveitis, with posterior segment involvement much greater than anterior segment manifestations, with papillitis string-of-pearls vitreal exudates, and substantial narrowing of the arterioles. FA disclosed late disc and arteriolar staining; areas of nonperfusion with infarction were present.

Serologic studies disclosed a white count of 14,000 with a hemoglobin of 15, lymphopenia, with atypical lymphocytes, and both IgM and IgA serologic titers for positive for antibodies directed against *Toxocara*. The patient had significant dog and puppy contact.

Because of treatment resistance and the unusual appearance, as well as progression to hand-movement acuity in the left eye (OS), a diagnostic pars plana vitrectomy was performed. Results of an HLA-B51 test, received after the vitrectomy, were positive. Because the cytology of the harvested vitreal cells were not indicative of a malignant process, and because PCR analysis did not indicate an infectious etiology, therapy was begun with combination prednisone, cyclosporin, and azathioprine. Visual acuity of the right eye improved to 20/25, and that of the left eye improved to 20/100. With prednisone tapering, however, the patient's Adamantiades-Behçet's disease, with primarily retinal manifestations, recurred abruptly over a period of 36 hours, diminishing the acuity of the right eye to 20/100 and diminishing hand-movement acuity in the left. The cyclosporin and azathioprine therapy was stopped. Regional steroid injection, intravenous pulse steroid therapy (250 mg of methylprednisolone intravenously 5 times a day), and pulse cyclophosphamide therapy were instituted. This combination was associated with a complete abrogation of the active inflammation and recovery of vision to 20/25 OD and 20/200 OS. Noncompliance for appointments for repeated cyclophosphamide infusions resulted in an additional hypopyon uveitis with retinal vaso-occlusive vasculitis and loss of acuities to hand movements OD and counting fingers OS.

Hospitalization once more, with emergency intravenous cyclophosphamide and steroid therapy, along with intraocular dexamethasone 400 μg and plasmapheresis, was associated with recovery of visual acuities of 20/40 OD and 20/70 OS. The patient was then maintained (with relative stable visual acuity and freedom from such explosive episodes) over the next 8 months with intermittent cyclophosphamide infusions, approximately every 3 to 6 weeks. Two more episodes of recurrence were managed in the same way, with plasmapheresis employed urgently. An additional recurrence in June of 1999 appeared to have slightly different characteristics from previous ones, with unusual areas of peripheral retinitis. Urgent diagnostic pars plana vitrectomy with PCR and culture analysis of the harvested material disclosed herpes simplex virus; the intraoperative appearance of the right eye was that of peripheral acute retinal necrosis. Intravitreal and high-dose intravenous acyclovir therapy was employed.

Because of this new turn of events, we did not feel comfortable with the idea of continued control of the ABD with intravenous pulse cyclophosphamide therapy. Therefore, we began subcutaneous interferon-α2b, 3 million units subcutaneously 3 times weekly. For 4 months, the patient was maintained on this therapeutic technique without evidence of relapse. The visual acuities as of the date of this report, February, 2001, were 20/80 OD and 20/60 OS.

This case report illustrates some of the challenges faced by the physician caring for a patient with ABD. There is no best treatment. There is as much art as science involved in discovering a recipe that induces long-lasting remission in each individual patient. Those physicians most experienced with such patients may be best prepared, by virtue of that experience, to deal with the intricacies of ocular ABD cases, adapting to the changing characteristics of the case as it evolves, adjusting the therapeutic recipe based on the characteristics of the patient and knowledge of new and evolving technology and medications. Finding such physicians in regions where ABD is uncommon is especially difficult.

MANAGEMENT OF OCULAR COMPLICATIONS

Ophthalmic complications such as cataract, cystoid macular edema, glaucoma, neovascularization, and vitreous hemorrhage are not rare in patients with ABD, and they produce vision loss if not treated correctly.

Cataract formation is especially common, both because of the recurrent inflammation and as a consequence of the steroid treatment. Cataract removal should be performed in the quieted eye for two reasons. The first is for visual acuity improvement. The second is so that the physician can observe the posterior segment of the eye to monitor disease activity and treatment effect, and the cataract may obscure that view. Successful cataract surgery with minimal postoperative inflammation will be most likely if the uveitis has been inactive for 3 months, prophylactic perioperative treatment with corticosteroids is employed, immunosuppressive drugs are continued, complete removal of cortical material is performed, and a posterior chamber intraocular lens is placed into the capsular bag if an intraocular lens is implanted.[238–240] Systemic and topical corticosteroids should be administered 1 week prior to any surgical intervention and should continue postoperatively.[238] It is important to remember that even if one understands and abides by the principles of operating only on quiet eyes, the visual prognosis may be extremely guarded, regardless of surgical skills and elegance, if posterior segment complications of ABD have already occurred prior to surgery.[241, 242]

Yoshikawa and colleagues[243] reported that uveitic cystoid macular edema resolved with periocular injections of corticosteroids in approximately 50% of the cases. However, management of pseudophakic cystoid macular edema associated with ABD is more difficult than management of uveitic cystoid macular edema in general.

Secondary and neovascular glaucoma may be responsible for profound loss of vision in patients with ABD. Initial medical therapy with topical and systemic antiglaucoma medications may not suffice. Treatment decisions require consideration of the status of the optic nerve and the visual field. Evaluation of the visual fields can be difficult. The coexistence of neuro-ABD or other ocular complications such as cataract and posterior segment disease can cause visual field defects that are difficult to distinguish from those seen because of glaucoma. If medical treatment is inadequate to control the intraocular pressure and stabilize the visual field, surgical intervention must be considered. Trabeculectomy with localized antimitotic therapy or use of a drainage tube such as the Ahmed or Molteno valve tube shunt are the most reasonable options.

Vitreous hemorrhages are very frequent in ABD cases with severe retinal disease. Hemorrhages may resolve spontaneously, but in some cases vitrectomy is required. Visual outcome after vitrectomy may be disappointing because of coexisting macular damage. In patients with multiple episodes of retinal disease, areas of atrophic retina are present. Retinal detachments are therefore common in the later stages of the disease. Phthisis bulbi with or without iris neovascularization usually follows retinal detachment.

Development of retinal and/or optic disc neovascularization is a major complication of the repeated attacks on the retinal vasculature. This neovascularization is attributed to the ABD vasculopathy leading to retinal hypoxia. Thus, meticulous evaluation of the retina is very important for the early diagnosis of neovascularization and treatment with laser photocoagulation.[244] However, concerns about the efficacy of such treatment exist: Some investigators believe that laser photocoagulation may release antigens from the retina, which can be responsible for systemic sensitization and exacerbation of the ABD. Therefore, patients with signs of recurrence should be aggressively treated.

Cataract surgery and other operations such as vitrectomy and scleral buckling procedure are well tolerated in patients with inactive ABD.[18, 104, 239, 240, 245]

PROGNOSIS FOR VISION

Visual prognosis in ABD is a subject of much controversy. Some authors have reported loss of vision in many of their patients and others have reported little loss of vision.[191, 246] The use of immunosuppressive drugs as well as genetic predisposition for severe ABD may explain such discrepancies. Today, no definitive prognostic factors for visual outcome have been identified, although Sakamoto and colleagues[30] did try to determine such prognostic factors. They concluded that skin lesions, arthritis, and posterior uveitis attacks were linked to loss of vision, whereas female sex, disease free interval, and anterior attacks were related to retention of vision. Accurate prognostic factors for visual outcome could be valuable for deciding the most appropriate type of treatment. Thus,

if the patient with ABD is at high risk for visual loss, very aggressive treatment should be instituted. On the other hand, if the patient is at low risk, a mild treatment with few potential side effects should be recommended. In addition, Demiroglu and colleagues[247] reported that age of 30 years or less, male sex, vascular thrombosis, and CNS involvement were risk factors for ocular disease. It is clear that the key to preserving good vision is prompt and aggressive treatment with very close surveillance and monitoring, as ABD is a chronic disease with exacerbations after long periods of remissions.

CONCLUSION

ABD is a chronic, recurrent, multisystem inflammatory disorder, mainly characterized by the classic triad of recurrent ocular inflammation, skin lesions, and recurrent oral and genital ulcers. It frequently involves the joints, the CNS, and the gastrointestinal tract. It is most common in Turkey and the Far East, and in countries along the old Silk Route connecting the Far East with the Mediterranean basin. Children are rarely affected. Infectious agents, immune mechanisms, and genetic factors are implicated in the etiopathogenesis of the disease, which remains to be elucidated. The pathology of the lesions consists of widespread vasculitis. There is not a universally accepted diagnostic test for this disorder. Thus, the diagnosis of ABD relies on the identification of several combinations of its more typical clinical features. The prognosis of the disease has improved, even when vital organs are involved, because of early diagnosis and treatment. However, untreated, the natural history of ocular ABD for useful vision appears to be very poor.

Therapy with cytotoxic medications such as cyclophosphamide and chlorambucil has been shown to be efficacious in treating ABD. In fact, chlorambucil is the only medication that has resulted in complete remission and "cure" of ABD. On the other hand, Cs-A showed promising results in preserving good vision in patients with ABD, but the initial work was performed with doses that are now known to be associated with 100% incidence of nephrotoxicity, and subsequent results with smaller doses have been disappointing. Treatment is a complicated issue and needs to be individualized to the patient, balancing the risks of therapy with the putative efficacy of a given approach.

References

1. Kaktos, ed: Hippocrates: Third Book on Epidemiology. Case 7. 1993;13:209.
2. Dilsen N: History and development of Behçet's disease. VII International Conference on Behçet's Disease. Rev Rhum Engl Ed 1996;63:512–519.
3. Blüthe L: Zur Kenntnis des recidivereden hypopyon. Inaugural Thesis, Heidelberg, 1908.
4. Planner R: Behçet's disease. In: Manacelli M, Nazaro P, eds. Behçet's Disease. Basel, Karger, 1966.
5. Shigeta T: Recurrent iritis with hypopyon and its pathological findings. Acta Soc Ophthalmol Jpn 1924;28:516.
6. Adamantiades B: A case of recurrent hypopyon iritis. Medical Society of Athens, 1930:586–593.
7. Adamantiades B: Sur un cas d'iritis à hypopyon récidivante. Ann Ocul (Paris) 1931;168:271–274.
8. Dascalopoulos N: Sur deux cas de uveite récidivante. Ann Ocul (Paris) 1932;169:387–389.
9. Behçet H: Über rezidivierende aphthose, durch ein Virus verur-

648

CHAPTER 56: ADAMANTIADES-BEHÇET DISEASE

sachte Geschwure am Mud, am Auge und an den Genitalien. Derm Wochenschr 1937;36:1152–1157.

10. Behçet H: Considerations sur les lesions aphteuses de la bouche et des parties genitales, ainsi que sur les manifestations oculaires d'origine probablement virutique et observations concernant leur foyer d'infection. Bull Soc Fr Dermatol Syph 1940;45:420–433.

11. Behçet H: Some observations on the clinical pictures of the so-called triple symptom complex. Dermatologica 1940;81:73–78.

12. Godde-Jolly D: Sur le syndrome Adamantiades-Behçet's. Bull Soc Fr Ophthalmol 1961;4(suppl):125.

13. Bietti-Bruna F: An ophthalmic report on Behçet's disease. In: Manacelli M, Nazaro P, eds. Behçet's Disease. Basel, Karger, 1966, pp 79–110.

14. Adamantiades B: La thrombophlébite comme quatriéme symptome de l'iritis rècidivante à hypopyon. Ann Ocul (Paris) 1946;179:143–148.

15. Ohno S: Behçet's disease in the world. In: Lehner T, Barnes CG, eds: Recent Advances in Behçet's Disease. London, Royal Society of Medicine Service, 1986.

16. Yazici H: Behçet's syndrome. In: Klippel JH, Dieppe PA, eds: Rheumatology 6.20.1–6.20.6. London, Mosby, 1994.

17. Yurdakul S, Gunaydin I, Tuzun Y, et al: The prevalence of Behçet's syndrome in a rural area in Northern Turkey. J Rheumatol 1988;15:820.

18. Mishima S, Masuda K, Izawa Y, et al: Behçet's disease in Japan: Ophthalmologic aspects. Trans Am Ophthalmol Soc 1979;76:225–279.

19. Shahram F, Davatchi F, Akbarian M, et al: The 1996 survey of Behçet's disease in Iran, study of 3153 cases. In: VIIth International Conference on Behçet's Disease [Abstract CO4]. Rev Rhum Engl Ed 1996;63:538.

20. Davatchi F, Shahram F, Akbarian M, et al: The prevalence of Behçet's disease in Iran. In: Nasution AR, Darmawan J, Isbagio H, eds. Proceedings of the 7th APLAR Congress of Rheumatology. Japan KK: Churchill Livingstone, 1992, pp 95–98.

21. Palimeris G, Papakonstantinou P, Mantas M: The Adamantiades-Behçet's syndrome in Greece. In: Saari KM, ed. Uveitis Update. Amsterdam, Excerpta Medica, 1984, p 321.

22. Zouboulis CC, Kotter I, Djawari D, et al: Epidemiological features of Adamantiades-Behçet's disease in Germany and in Europe. Yonsei Med J 1997;38:411–422.

23. O'Duffy JD: Behçet's disease. In: Kelly WN, Harris ED, Ruddy S, Sledge CB, eds. Textbook of Rheumatology. Philadelphia, W.B. Saunders, 1985, pp 1174–1178.

24. Chajek T, Fainaru M: Behçet's disease: Report of 41 cases and a review of the literature. Medicine 1975;54:179–196.

25. Hamdi M, Abdalla MI: Ocular manifestations of Behçet's disease. Bull Ophthalmol Soc Egypt 1974;67:73–83.

26. Mamo JG, Baghdassarian A: Behçet's disease: A report of 28 cases. Arch Ophthalmol 1964;71:4–14.

27. Shimizu T: Clinical and immunological studies on Behçet's syndrome. Folia Ophthalmol Jpn 1971;22:801–810.

28. Colvard MD, Robertson DM, O'Duffy JD: The ocular manifestations of Behçet's disease. Arch Ophtalmol 1977;95:1813–1817.

29. O'Duffy JD, Carney JA, Deodhar S: Behçet's disease: Report of ten cases, three with new manifestations. Ann Intern Med 1971;75:561–570.

30. Sakamoto M, Akazawa K, Nishioka Y, et al: Prognostic factors of vision in patients with Behçet's disease. Ophthalmology 1995;102:317–321.

31. Stratigos AJ, Laskaris G, Stratigos JD: Behçet's disease. Semin Neurol 1992;12:346–357.

32. Zouboulis CC, Djawari D, Kirch W: Adamantiades-Behçet's disease in Germany. In: Godeau P, Wechsler B, eds. Behçet's Disease. New York, Elsevier Science, 1993, pp 193–196.

33. Dundar SV, Gencalp U, Simsek H: Familial cases of Behçet's disease. Br J Dermatol 1985;113:319–321.

34. Villanueva JL, Gonzalez-Dominguez J, Gonzalez-Fernanders R, et al: HLA antigen familial study in complete Behçet's syndrome affecting three sisters. Ann Rheum Dis 1993;52:155–157.

35. Vaiopoulos G, Sfikakis PP, Hatzinikolaou P, et al: Adamantiades-Behçet's disease in sisters. Clin Rheumatol 1996;15:382–384.

36. Hamuryudan V, Yurdakul S, Ozbakir F, et al: Monozygotic twins concordant for Behçet's syndrome. Arthritis Rheum 1991;34:1071–1072.

37. Mizuki N, Ohno S, Tanaka H, et al: Association of HLA B-51 and lack of association of class II alleles with Behçet's disease. Tissue Antigens 1992;40:22–30.

38. Stewart B: Genetic analysis of families of patients with Behçet's syndrome: Data incompatible with autosomal recessive inheritance. Ann Rheum Dis 1986;45:265–268.

39. Mason RM, Barnes CG: Behçet's syndrome with arthritis. Ann Rheum Dis 1969;28:95–103.

40. Behçet's Disease Research Committee of Japan: Behçet's disease: Guide to diagnosis of Behçet's disease. Jpn J Ophthalmol 1974;18:291–294.

41. O'Duffy JD: Suggested criteria for diagnosis of Behçet's disease. J Rheumatol 1974;1(suppl):18.

42. Zhang XQ: Criteria for Behçet's disease. Chin J Intern Med 1980;19:1–20.

43. Dilsen N, Konice M, Aral O: Our diagnostic criteria for Behçet's disease. In: Hamza M, ed. Behçet's Disease. Proceedings of the Third Mediterranean Congress of Rheumatology, May 1986, pp 11–15.

44. James DG: Behçet's disease. In: Fitzpatrick TB, Eizen AZ, Wolff K, et al, eds. Dermatology in General Medicine. New York, McGraw-Hill, 1986, p 1242.

45. International Study Group for Behçet's Disease: Criteria for diagnosis of Behçet's disease. Lancet 1990;335:1078–1080.

46. Nussenblatt RB, Whitcup SM, Palestine AG: Behçet's disease. In: Craven L, Buckwalter, eds. Uveitis: Fundamentals and Clinical Practice, 2nd ed. St. Louis, Mosby, 1996, pp 334–353.

47. Michaelson JB, Chisari FV: Behçet's disease. Surv Ophthalmol 1982;26:190–203.

48. Curth HO: Behçet's syndrome, abortive form(?): Recurrent aphthous oral lesions and recurrent genital ulcerations. Arch Derm Syph 1946;54:179–196.

49. Kobayashi T, Matsumaya E, Sugimoto T: Gynecological aspect of muco-cutaneous-ocular syndromes. World Obstet Gynecol 1959;11:995–999.

50. Müftüoglou Ü, Yurdakul S, Yazici H, et al: Vascular involvement in Behçet's disease—a review of 129 cases. In: Lehner T, Barnes CG, eds. Recent Advances in Behçet's Disease. London, Royal Society of Medicine Service, 1986.

51. Shimizu T, Ehrlich GE, Inaba G, Hayashi K: Behçet's disease (Behçet's syndrome). Semin Arthritis Rheum 1979;8:223–260.

52. O'Duffy JD: Vasculitis in Behçet's disease. Rheumat Dis Clin North Am 1990;16:423–431.

53. Sechas MN, Liapis CD, Gougoulakis AG: Vascular manifestations of Behçet's disease. Int Angiol 1989;8:145–150.

54. Hatzinicolaou P, Vayopoulos G, Mauropoulos S, et al: Vascular manifestations of Behçet's disease. Br J Rheumatol 1992;31:284–285.

55. Pande I, Uppal S, Kailash S, et al: Behçet's disease in India: A clinical, immunological, immunogenetic and outcome study. Br J Rheumatol 1995;34:825–830.

56. Cooper AM, Naughton MN, Williams BD: Chronic arterial occlusion associated with Behçet's disease. Br J Rheumatol 1994;33:170–172.

57. Bastounis E, Maltezos C, Giabouras S, et al: Arterial aneurysms in Behçet's disease. Int Angiol 1994;13:196–201.

58. Little AG, Zarin CK: Abdominal aortic aneurysm and Behçet's disease. Surgery 1982;91:359–362.

59. Thi Huong DL, Wechsler B, Papo Th, et al: Arterial lesions in Behçet's disease: A study of 25 patients. J Rheumatol 1995;22:2103–2113.

60. Urajama A, Sakuragi S, Sakai F, et al: Angio Behçet's syndrome. In: Inaba GI, ed. Proceedings of the International Conference of Behçet's Disease. Tokyo, University of Tokyo Press, 1980, pp 171–176.

61. Kuzu MA, Ozaslan C, Koksoy C, et al: Vascular involvement in Behçet's disease: 8-years audit. World J Surg 1994;18:948–954.

62. Huycke E, Robinowitz M, Cohen IS, et al: Granulomatous endocarditis with systemic embolism in Behçet's disease. Ann Intern Med 1985;102:791–793.

63. Schiff S, Moffatt R, Mandel WJ, Rubin SA: Acute myocardial infarction and recurrent ventricular arrhythmias in Behçet's syndrome. Am Heart J 1982;103:438–440.

64. Lie JT: Cardiac and pulmonary manifestations of Behçet's syndrome. Pathol Res Pract 1988;183:347–352.

65. Lakhanpal SH, Tani K, Lie JT, et al: Pathologic features of Behçet's syndrome: A review of Japanese autopsy registry data. Hum Pathol 1985;16:790–795.
66. Bletry O, Mohattane A, Wechsler B, et al: Atteinte cardiaque de la maladie de Behçet: Douze observations. Presse Med 1988;17:2388–2391.
67. Ioakimidis D, Georganas C, Panagoulis C, et al: A case of Adamantiades-Behçet's syndrome presenting as myocardial infarction. Clin Exp Rheumatol 1993;11:183–186.
68. Gullu I, Benekli M, Muderrisoglu H, et al: Silent myocardial ischemia in Behçet's disease. J Rheumatol 1996;23:323–327.
69. Hamuryudan V, Yardakul S, Kural AR, et al: Diffuse proliferative glomerulonephritis in Behçet's syndrome. Br J Rheumatol 1991;30:63–64.
70. Herskowitz S, Lipton R, Landos G: Neuro-Behçet's disease: CT and clinical correlates. Neurology 1988;38:1714–1720.
71. Kotake S, Higashi K, Yoshikawa K, et al: Central nervous system symptoms in patients with Behçet's disease receiving cyclosporine therapy. Ophthalmology 1999;106:586–589.
72. Anaba G: Clinical features of neuro-Behçet's syndrome. In: Lehner T, Barnes CG, eds. Recent Advances in Behçet's Disease. London, Royal Society of Medicine Service, 1986, pp 235–246.
73. James DG, Spiteri MA: Behçet's disease. Ophthalmology 1982;89:1279–1284.
74. Pamir MN, Kansu T, Erbengi A, Zileli T: Papilledema in Behçet's syndrome. Arch Neurol 1981;38:643–645.
75. Wechsler B, Bousser MG, Du LTH, et al: Central venous sinus thrombosis in Behçet's disease (Letter). Mayo Clin Proc 1985;60:891.
76. Hirohata SH, Kamoshita H, Taketani T: Spontaneous remission in meningoencephalitis in Behçet's disease. J Rheumatol 1989;16:1283–1284.
77. Akman-Demir G, Kurt BB, Serdaloglu P, et al: Seven-year follow-up of neurologic involvement in Behçet's syndrome. Arch Neurol 1996;53:691–694.
78. Akman-Demir G, Serdaroglou P, Tasci B, et al: Neurological involvement in Behçet's disease. In: VIIth International Conference on Behçet's Disease [Abstract GO2]. Rev Rhum Engl Ed 1996;63:549.
79. Wolf SM, Schotland DL, Phillips LL: Involvement of nervous system in Behçet's syndrome. Arch Neurol 1965;12:315–325.
80. O'Duffy JD, Goldstein NP: Neurological involvement in seven patients with Behçet's disease. Am J Med 1976;61:170–178.
81. Shahram F, Sabeti F, Davatchi F, et al: Audiovestibular involvement in Behçet's disease (in patients with disease duration more than 5 years). In: VIIth International Conference on Behçet's Disease [Abstract GO3]. Rev Rhum Engl Ed 1996;63:550.
82. El Rahami K, Bohlega S, Al Kawi MZ, et al: Cerebrospinal fluid analysis (CSF) in Behçet's disease. In: VIIth International Conference on Behçet's Disease [Abstract GO2]. Rev Rhum Engl Ed 1996;63:552.
83. Benamour S, Zeroual B, Bennis R, et al: Maladie de Behçet 316 cas. La Presse Med 1990;19:1485–1489.
84. Hemmen T, Perez-Canto A, Distler A, et al: IgA nephropathy in a patient with Behçet's syndrome: Case report and review literature. Br J Rheumatol 1997;36:696–699.
85. Dilsen N, Konice K, Aral O, et al: Risk factors for vital organ involvement in Behçet's disease. In: Godeau P, Wechsler B, eds. Behçet's Disease. New York, Elsevier Science, 1993;165–169.
86. Yurdakul S, Tuzuner N, Yurdakul I, et al: Gastrointestinal involvement in Behçet's syndrome: A controlled study. Ann Rheum Dis 1996;55:208–210.
87. Benamour S, Zeroual B, Bettal S, et al: Digestive manifestations of Behçet's disease based on a series of 74 cases. In: Godeau P, Wechsler B, eds. Behçet's Disease. New York, Elsevier Science, 1993;255–260.
88. Ormeci N, Gurler A, Cakir M, et al: Prevalence of *H. pylori* in Behçet's disease. In: VIIth International Conference on Behçet's Disease [Abstract J14]. Rev Rhum Engl Ed 1996;63:558.
89. Erkan F, Çavdar T: Pulmonary vasculitis in Behçet's disease. Am Rev Respir Dis 1992;146:232–239.
90. Raz I, Okon E, Chajek-Shaul T: Pulmonary manifestations in Behçet's syndrome. Chest 1989;95:585–589.
91. Tunaci A, Berkmen YM, Gokmen E: Thoracic involvement in Behçet's disease: Pathologic, clinical, and imaging features. AJR Am J Roentgenol 1995;164:51–56.

92. O'Duffy JD: Behçet's syndrome. N Engl J Med 1990;322:326–327.
93. Bradbury AW, Milne AA, Murie JA: Surgical aspects of Behçet's disease. Br J Surg 1994;81:1712–1721.
94. Kaklamani VG, Vaiopoulos G, Kaklamanis PG: Behçet's disease. Semin Arthritis Rheum 1998;27:197–217.
95. Gharibdoost F, Davatchi F, Shahram F, et al: Clinical manifestations of Behçet's disease in Iran: Analysis of 2176 cases. In: Godeau P, Wechsler B, eds. Behçet's Disease. New York, Elsevier Science, 1993, 153–158.
96. Calguneri M, Kiraz S, Ertenli I, et al: The effect of prophylactic penicillin treatment on the course of arthritis episodes in patients with Behçet's disease: A randomized clinical trial. Arthritis Rheum 1996;39:2062–2065.
97. Yurdakul S, Yazici H, Tuzun Y, et al: The arthritis of Behçet's disease: A prospective study. Ann Rheum Dis 1983;42:505–515.
98. Tosun M, Uslu T, Ibraim-Imanoglou H, et al: Coexisting ankylosing spondylitis and Behçet's disease. Clin Rheumatol 1996;15:619–620.
99. Oliviery I, Gemignani G, Camerini E, et al: Computed tomography of the sacroiliac joints in four patients with Behçet's syndrome: Confirmation of sacroiliitis. Br J Rheumatol 1990;29:264–7.
100. Dilsen N, Konice M, Aral O: Why Behçet's disease should be accepted as a seronegative arthritis. In: Lehner T, Barnes CG, eds. Recent Advances in Behçet's Disease. London, Royal Society of Medicine Services (International Congress and Symposium Series no. 103), 1986, pp 281–284.
101. Hazleman BL: Rheumatic disorders of the eye and the various structures involved. Br J Rheumatol 1996;35:258–68.
102. Masuda K, Inaba G, Mizushima H, et al: A nation-wide survey of Behçet's disease in Japan. Jpn J Ophthalmol 1975;19:278–285.
103. Imai Y: Studies on prognosis and symptoms of Behçet's disease in long-term observation. Jpn J Clin Ophthalmol 1971;25:665–694.
104. Baer JC, Raizman MB, Foster CS: Ocular Behçet's disease in the United States: Clinical presentation and visual outcome in 29 patients. In: Masahiko U, Shigeaki O, Koki A, eds. Proceedings of the 5th International Symposium on the Immunology and Immunopathology of the Eye, Tokyo, 13–15 March. New York, Elsevier Science, 1990, p 383.
105. Cohen S, Kremer I, Tiqva P: Bilateral corneal immune ring opacity in Behçet's syndrome. Arch Ophthalmol 1991;109:324–325.
106. Horiuchi T, Yoneya S, Numaga T: Vitreous involvement may be crucial in the prognosis of Behçet's disease. In: Blodi F, Brancato R, Cristini G, et al, eds. Acta XXV Concilium Ophthalmologicum. Rome, Kugler and Ghedini, 1986, pp 2624–2631.
107. Ehrlich GE: Vasculitis in Behçet's disease. Int Rev Immunol 1997;14:81–88.
108. Richards RD: Simultaneous occlusion of the central retinal artery and vein in Behçet's disease. Trans Am Ophthalmol Soc 1979;77:191–209.
109. Bonamour G, Grange JD, Bonnet M: Retinal vein involvement in Behçet's disease. In: Dilsen N, Konice M, Ovul C, eds. Behçet's Disease. Proceedings of an International Symposium on Behçet's Disease, Istanbul, September 29–30, 1977. Amsterdam, Excerpta Medica, 1979, pp 142–144.
110. Kalbian VV, Challis MT: Behçet's disease. Report of twelve cases with three manifesting as papilledema. Am J Med 1970;49:823–829.
111. Uziel Y, Brike R, Padeh S, et al: Juvenile Behçet's disease in Israel. The Pediatric Rheumatology Study Group of Israel. Clin Exp Rheumatol 1998;16:502–505.
112. Bahabri SA, al-Mazyed A, al-Balaa S, et al: Juvenile Behçet's disease in Arab children. Clin Exp Rheumatol 1996;14:331–335.
113. Sarica R, Azizlerli G, Kose A, et al: Juvenile Behçet's disease among 1784 Turkish Behçet's patients. Int J Dermatol 1996;35:109–111.
114. Hamza M: Juvenile Behçet's disease. In: Godeau P, Wechsler B, eds. Behçet's Disease. New York, Elsevier Science, 1993, pp 377–380.
115. Shafaie N, Shahram F, Davatchi F, et al: Behçet's disease in children. In: Godeau P, Wechsler B, eds. Behçet's Disease. New York, Elsevier Science, 1993, pp 381–383.
116. Vaiopoulos G, Kaklamanis VG, Markomichelakis NN, et al: Clinical features of juvenile Adamantiadis-Behçet's disease in Greece. Clin Exp Rheumatol 1990;17:146–149.
117. Fain O, Mathieu E, Lachassinne E, et al: Neonatal Behçet's disease. Am J Med 1995;98:310–311.
118. Stark AC, Bhakta B, Chamberlain MA, et al: Life-threatening transient neonatal Behçet's disease. Br J Rheumatol 1997;36:700–702.
119. Marsal S, Falga C, Simeon CP, et al: Behçet's disease and pregnancy relationship study. Br J Rheumatol 1997;36:234–238.

120. Nadji A, Shahram F, Davatchi F, et al: Behçet's disease and pregnancy. In: VIIth International Conference on Behçet's Disease [Abstract B10]. Rev Rhum Engl Ed 1996;63:536.

121. Bang D, Chun YS, Haam IB, et al: The influence of pregnancy on Behçet's disease. Yonsei Med J 1997;38:437–443.

122. Sciuto M, Porciello G, Occhipinti G, et al: Multiple and reversible osteolytic lesions: An unusual manifestation of Behçet's disease. J Rheumatol 1996;23:564–566.

123. O'Duffy JD, Lehner T, Barnes CG: Summary of the Third International Conference on Behçet's Disease, Tokyo, Japan, October 23–24, 1981. J Rheumatol 1983;10:154–158.

124. Hamza M: Foreword. In: VIIth International Conference on Behçet's Disease. Rev Rhum Engl Ed 1996;63:508.

125. Bang D, Cho YH, Choi H-J, et al: Detection of herpes simplex virus DNA by polymerase chain reaction in genital ulcer of patients with Behçet's disease. In: VIIth International Conference on Behçet's Disease [Abstract B19]. Rev Rhum Engl Ed 1996;63:532.

126. Lee ES, Lee S, Bang D, Sohn S: Herpes simplex virus detection by polymerase chain reaction in intestinal ulcer of patients with Behçet's disease. In: VIIth International Conference on Behçet's Disease [Abstract B18]. Rev Rhum Engl Ed 1996;63:531.

127. Cantini F, Emmi L, Niccoli L, et al: Lack of association between chronic hepatitis C virus infection and Behçet's disease. Clin Exp Rheumatol 1997;15:338–339.

128. Kiraz S, Ertenli I, Benekli M, Calguneri M: Parvovirus B19 infection in Behçet's disease. Clin Exp Rheumatol. 1996;14:71–73.

129. Mizushima Y: Behçet's disease. Curr Opin Rheumatol 1991;3:32–35.

130. Isogai E, Ohno S, Kotake S, et al: Chemiluminescence of neutrophils from patients with Behçet's disease and its correlation with an increased proportion of uncommon serotypes of *Streptococcus sanguis* in the oral flora. Arch Oral Biol 1990;35:43–48.

131. Pervin K, Childerstone A, Shinnick T, et al: T cell epitope expression of mycobacterial and homologous human 65-kilodalton heat shock protein peptides in short term cell lines from patients with Behçet's disease. J Immunol 1993;151:2273–2282.

132. Yazici H: The place of Behçet's syndrome among the autoimmune diseases. Int Rev Immunol 1997;14:1–10.

133. Emmi L, Brugnolo F, Salvati G, Marchione T: Immunopathological aspects of Behçet's disease. Clin Exp Rheumatol 1995;13:687–691.

134. Valente RM, Hall S, O'Duffy JD, Conn DL: Vasculitis and related disorders: Behçet's disease. In: Kelley WN, Harris ED, Rudy S, Sledge CB, eds. Textbook of Rheumatology, 5th ed. Philadelphia, W.B. Saunders, 1997, pp 1114–1122.

135. Valesini G, Pivetti-Pezzi P, Mastrandrea F, et al: Evaluation of T cell subsets in Behçet's syndrome using anti-T cell monoclonal antibodies. Clin Exp Immunol 1985;60:55–60.

136. Hasan A, Fortune F, Wilson A, et al: Role of γδ T cells in pathogenesis and diagnosis of Behçet's disease. Lancet 1996;347:789–794.

137. Suzuki Y, Hoshi K, Tatsada T, Mizushima Y: Increased peripheral blood γδ+ T cells and natural killer cells in Behçet's disease. J Rheumatol 1992;19:588–592.

138. Sahin S, Akoglu T, Direskeneli H, et al: Neutrophil adhesion to endothelial cells and factors affecting adhesion in patients with Behçet's disease. Ann Rheum Dis 1996;55:128–133.

139. Mosmann TR, Sad S: The expanding universe of T cell subset: Th1, Th2 and more. Immunol Today 1996;17:138–146.

140. Sayinalp N, Ozcebo O, Ozdemir O, et al: Cytokines in Behçet's disease. J Rheumatol 1996;23:321–322.

141. Al-Dalaan A, Al-Sedairy S, Al-Balla S, et al: Enhanced interleukin 8 secretion in circulation of patients with Behçet's disease. J Rheumatol 1995;22:904–907.

142. Sanake T, Suzuki N, Ueda Y: Analysis of interleukin-2 activity in patients with Behçet's disease. Arthritis Rheum 1986;29:371–378.

143. Hamzaoui K, Hamza M, Ayed K: Production of TNF-γ and IL-1 in active Behçet's disease. J Rheumatol 1990;17:1428–1429.

144. Matsumura N, Mizushima Y: Leukocyte movement and colchicine treatment in Behçet's disease. Lancet 1975;2:813.

145. Sobel JD, Haim S, Obedeanu N, et al: Polymorphonuclear leukocyte function in Behçet's disease. J Clin Pathol 1977;30:250–253.

146. Raziuddin S, Al-Dalaan A, Bahabri S, et al: Divergent cytokine production profile in Behçet's disease. Altered Th1/Th2 cell cytokine pattern. J Rheumatol 1998;25:329–333.

147. Char DH, Stein P, Masi R, et al: Immune complexes in uveitis. Am J Ophthalmol 1979;87:678–681.

148. Dernouchamps JP, Vaerman JP, Michels J, et al: Immune complexes in the aqueous humor and serum. Am J Ophthalmol 1977;84:24–31.

149. Levinsky RJ, Lehner T: Circulating soluble immune complexes in recurrent oral ulceration and Behçet's syndrome. Clin Exp Immunol 1978;32:193–198.

150. Klok AM, de Vries J, Rothova A, et al: Antibodies against ocular and oral antigens in Behçet's disease associated with uveitis. Curr Eye Res 1989;8:957–962.

151. Michaelson JB, Chisari FV, Kansu T: Antibodies to oral mucosa in patients with ocular Behçet's disease. Ophthalmology 1985;92:1277–1281.

152. Mullaney J, Collum LM: Ocular vasculitis in Behçet's disease: A pathologic and immunohistochemical study. Int Ophthalmol 1985;7:183–191.

153. Kasp E, Graham EM, Stanford MR, et al: Retinal autoimmunity and circulating immune complexes in ocular Behçet's disease. In: Lehner T, Barnes CG, eds. Recent Advances in Behçet's Disease. London, Royal Society of Medicine Services, 1986, 67–72.

154. Charteris DG, Barton K, McCartney AC, Lightman SL: CD4+ lymphocyte involvement in ocular Behçet's disease. Autoimmunity 1992;12:201–206.

155. Hull RG, Harris EN, Gharavi AE, et al: Anticardiolipin antibodies: Occurrence in Behçet's syndrome. Ann Rheum Dis 1984;43:746–748.

156. Zouboulis CC, Buttner P, Tebbe B, Orfanos CE: Anticardiolipin antibodies in Adamantiades-Behçet's disease. Br J Dermatol 1993;128:281–284.

157. Lenk N, Ozet G, Alli N, et al: Protein C and protein S activities in Behçet's disease as risk factors of thrombosis. Int J Dermatol 1998;37:124–125.

158. Nalcaci M, Pekcelen Y: Antithrombin III, protein C and protein S plasma levels in patients with Behçet's disease. J Int Med Res 1998;26:206–208.

159. Yazici H, Hekim N, Ozbakir F, et al: Von Willebrand factor in Behçet's syndrome. J Rheumatol 1987;14:305–306.

160. Ohno S, Ohguchi M, Hirose S, et al: Close association of HLA-Bw51 with Behçet's disease. Arch Ophthalmol 1982;100:1455–1458.

161. Raizman MB, Foster CS: Plasma exchange in the therapy of Behçet's disease. Graefes Arch Clin Exp Ophthalmol 1989;227:360–363.

162. Yazici H, Chamberlain MA, Schieuder I, et al: HLA antigens in Behçet's disease: A reappraisal by a comparative study of Turkish and British patients. Ann Rheum Dis 1980;39:344–348.

163. Zervas J, Vayopoulos G, Sakellaropoulos N, et al: HLA antigens and Adamantiades-Behçet's disease (A-BD) in Greeks. Clin Exp Rheumatol 1988;6:277–280.

164. Ohno S, Char DH, Kimura SJ, et al: Studies on HLA antigens in American patients with Behçet's disease. Jpn J Ophthalmol 1978;22:58–61.

165. O'Duffy JD, Taswell HF, Elveback LR: HL-A antigens in Behçet's disease. J Rheumatol 1976;3:1–3.

166. Arnett KL, Parham P: HLA class I nucleotide sequences. Tissue Antigens 1995;46:217–257.

167. Curran MD, Williams F, Rima BK, et al: A new HLA-B51 allele, B*5107 in RCE55 detected and characterized by PCR-SSOP, cloning and nucleotide sequence determination. Tissue Antigens 1996;48:228–230.

168. Mizuki N, Inokoko H, Ando H, et al: Behçet's disease associated with one of the HLA-B51 subantigens, HLA-B*5101. Am J Ophthalmol 1993;116:406–409.

169. Koumantaki Y, Stavropoulos K, Spyropoulou M, et al: HLA-B*5101 in Greek patients with Behçet's disease. Hum Immunol 1998;59:250–255.

170. Numaga J, Matsuki M, Mochizuki M, et al: An HLA-D region restriction fragment associated with refractory Behçet's disease. Am J Ophthalmol 1988;105:528–533.

171. Lehner T, Barnes CG: Criteria for diagnosis and classification of Behçet's syndrome. In: Lehner T, Barnes CG, eds. Behçet's Syndrome: Clinical and Immunological Features. Proceedings of a Conference Sponsored by Royal Society of Medicine, February 1979. London, Academic Press, 1979, pp 1–9.

172. Möftöoglou AU, Yazici H, Yurdakul S, et al: Behçet's disease: Lack of correlation of clinical manifestations with HLA antigens. Tissue Antigens 1981;17:226–230.

173. Matsuki K, Tuji T, Tokunago K, et al: HLA antigens in Behçet's disease with refractory ocular attacks. Tissue Antigens 1987;29:208–213.

174. Mizuki N, Ohno S: Immunogenetic studies of Behçet's disease. In: VIIth International Conference on Behçet's Disease. Rev Rhum Engl Ed 1996;63:520–527.

175. Charteris DG, Champ C, Rosenthal AR, et al: Behçet's disease: Activated T lymphocytes in retinal perivasculitis. Br J Ophthalmol 1992;76:499–501.

176. Tugal-Tutkun I, Urgancioglu M, Foster CS: Immunopathologic study of the conjunctiva in patients with Behçet's disease. Ophthalmology 1995;102:1660–1668.

177. Inoue C, Itoh R, Kawa Y, et al: Pathogenesis of mucocutaneous lesions in Behçet's disease. J Dermatol 1994;21:474–480.

178. Su WPD, Chun S, Lee S, Rogers RS III: Histopathological spectrum of erythema nodosum lesions in Behçet's disease. In: O'Duffy JD, Kokmen E, eds. Behçet's Disease. New York, Marcel Dekker, 1991, pp 229–240.

179. Kienbaum S, Zouboulis CC, Waibel M, Orfanos CE: Chemotactic neutrophilic vasculitis: A new histopathological pattern of vasculitis found in mucocutaneous lesions of patients with Adamantiades-Behçet's disease. In: Godeau O, Wechsler B, eds. Behçet's Disease. New York, Elsevier Science, 1993, pp 337–341.

180. Shikano S: Ocular pathology of Behçet's syndrome. In: Moracelli M, Nazzaro P, eds. International Symposium on Behçet's Disease. Karger, Basel, 1966, pp 111–136.

181. Yamana S, Jones SL, Aoi K, et al: Lymphocytic subset in erythema nodosum-like lesions from patients with Behçet's disease. In: Lecher T, Barnes CG, eds. Recent Advances in Behçet's Disease. London, Royal Society of Medicine, 1986, pp 117–121.

182. Gul A, Esin S, Dilsen N, et al: Immunopathology of skin pathergy reaction in Behçet's disease. Br J Dermatol 1995;132:901–907.

183. Atmaca LS: Fundus changes associated with Behçet's disease. Graefes Arch Clin Exp Ophthalmol 1989;227:340–344.

184. Matsuo N, Ojima M, Kumashiro O, et al: Fluorescein angiographic disorders of the retina and the optic disc in Behçet's disease. In: Inaba G, ed. Behçet's Disease: Pathogenic Mechanism and Clinical Future. Proceedings of the International Conference on Behçet's Disease. Tokyo, October 23–24, 1981. Tokyo, University of Tokyo Press, 1982;161–170.

185. Bentley CR, Stanfort MR, Shilling JS, et al: Macular ischemia in posterior uveitis. Eye 1993;7:411–414.

186. Matsuo T, Sato Y, Shiraga F, et al: Choroidal abnormalities in Behçet's disease observed by simultaneous indocyanine green and fluorescein angiography with scanning laser ophthalmoscopy. Ophthalmology 1999;106:295–300.

187. Cruz CD, Adachi-Usami E, Kakisu Y: Flash electroretinograms and pattern visually evoked cortical potentials in Behçet's disease. Jpn J Ophthalmol 1990;34:142–148.

188. Ozoran K, Duzgun N, Tutkak H, et al: Fibronectin and circulating immune complexes in Behçet's disease. Rheumatol Int 1996;15:221–224.

189. Yazici H, Pazarli H, Barnes C, et al: A controlled trial of azathioprine in Behçet's syndrome. N Engl J Med 1990;322:281–285.

190. Michelson JB, Dhisari FV: Behçet's disease. Surv Ophthalmol 1982;26:190–203.

191. BenEzra D, Cohen E: Treatment and visual prognosis in Behçet's disease. Br J Ophthalmol 1986;70:589–592.

192. Pazarli H, Ozyazgan Y, Actunc T: Clinical observations on hypoyon attacks of Behçet's disease in Turkey. In: VIIth International Conference on Behçet's Disease. [Abstracts], Rochester MN, September 14–15, 1979.

193. Reed BJ, Morse LS, Schwab IR: High-dose intravenous pulse methylprednisolone hemisuccinated in acute Behçet's retinitis. Am J Ophthalmol 1998;125:410–411.

194. Santamaria J: Steroidal agents: The systemic and ocular complications. Ocul Inflamm Ther 1988;1:19–25.

195. Mamo JD: Treatment of Behçet's disease with chlorambucil. A follow-up report. Arch Ophthalmol 1976;94:580–583.

196. Trichoulis D: Treatment of Behçet's disease with chlorambucil. Br Ophthalmol 1976;60:55–57.

197. Hijikata K, Masuda K: Visual prognosis in Behçet's disease: Effects of cyclophosphamide and colchicine. Jpn J Ophthalmol 1978;22:506–519.

198. Nussenblatt RB, Palestine AG: Cyclosporine: Immunology, pharmacology and therapeutic uses. Surv Ophthalmol 1986;31:159–169.

199. Mamo JG, Azzam SA: Treatment of Behçet's disease with chlorambucil. Arch Ophthalmol 1970;84:446–450.

200. Godfrey WA, Epstein WV, O'Connor GR, et al: The use of chlorambucil in intractable idiopathic uveitis. Am J Ophthalmol 1974;78:415–428.

201. Pivetti-Pezzi P, Gasparri V, De Liso P, et al: Prognosis in Behçet's disease. Ann Ophthalmol 1985;17:20–25.

202. Tessler HH, Jennings T: High-dose short term chlorambucil for intractable sympathetic ophthalmia and Behçet's disease. Br J Ophthalmol 1990;74:353–357.

203. Tabbara KF: Chlorambucil in Behçet's disease. A reappraisal. Ophthalmology 1983;90:906–908.

204. Oniki S, Kurakazu K, Kawata K: Immunosuppressive treatment of Behçet's disease with cyclophosphamide. Jpn J Ophthalmol 1976;20:32–40.

205. Gills JP, Buckley CE: Cyclophosphamide therapy of Behçet's disease. Ann Ophthalmol 1970;2:399–405.

206. Foster CS, Baer JC, Raizman MB: Therapeutic responses to systemic immunosuppressive chemotherapy agents in patients with Behçet's syndrome affecting the eyes. In: O'Duffy JD, Kokmen E, eds. Behçet's disease: Basic and clinical aspects. New York, Marcel Dekker, 1991, pp 581–588.

207. Fain O, Du LTH, Wechsler B: Pulse cyclophosphamide in Behçet's disease. In: O'Duffy JD, Kokmen E, eds. Behçet's disease: Basic and clinical aspects. New York, Marcel Dekker, 1991, pp 569–573.

208. Ozyazgan Y, Yurdakul S, Yazici H, et al: Low dose cyclosporin A versus pulsed cyclophosphamide in Behçet's syndrome: A single masked trial. Br J Ophthalmol 1992;76:241–243.

209. Sigal NH, Dumont FJ: Cyclosporine A, FK-506, and rapamycin: Pharmacologic probes of lymphocyte signal transduction. Ann Rev Immunol 1992;10:519–560.

210. Nussenblatt RB, Palestine AG, Chan CC, et al: Effectiveness of cyclosporin therapy for Behçet's disease. Arthritis Rheum 1985;28:671–679.

211. Nussenblatt RB, Palestine AG, Rook AH, et al: Treatment of intraocular inflammation with cyclosporine A. Lancet 1983;1:235–238.

212. Nussenblatt RB, Palestine AG, Chan CC: Cyclosporin A in the treatment of intraocular inflammatory disease resistant to systemic corticosteroids and cytotoxic agents. Am J Ophthalmol 1983;96:275–282.

213. Nussenblatt RB, Palestine AG, Chan CC, et al: Improvement of uveitis and optic nerve disease by cyclosporin in a patient with multiple sclerosis. Am J Ophthalmol 1984;97:790–791.

214. Nussenblatt RB, Palestine AG, Chan CC: Cyclosporin therapy for uveitis: Long-term follow up. J Ocul Pharmacol 1985;1:369–382.

215. Binder AI, Graham EM, Sanders MD, et al: Cyclosporine A in the treatment of severe Behçet's uveitis. Br J Rheumatol 1987;76:285–291.

216. BenEzra D, Nussenblatt RB, Timonen P: Optimal use of Sandimmune in endogenous uveitis. Berlin, Springer-Verlag, 1988.

217. Whitcup SM, Salvo EC, Nussenblatt RB: Combined cyclosporine and corticosteroid therapy for sight-threatening uveitis in Behçet's disease. Am J Ophthalmol 1994;118:39–45.

218. Sajjadi H, Soheilian M, Ahmadieh H, et al: Low dose cyclosporin-A therapy in Behçet's disease. J Ocul Pharmacol 1994;10:553–560.

219. Atmaca LS, Batioglu F: The efficacy of cyclosporin-A in the treatment of Behçet's disease. Ophthalmic Surg 1994;25:321–327.

220. Hayasaka S, Kawamoto K, Noda S, et al: Visual prognosis in patients with Behçet's disease receiving colchicine, systemic corticosteroid or cyclosporin. Ophthalmologica 1994;208:210–213.

221. Chavis PS, Antonios SR, Tabbara KF: Cyclosporine effect on optic nerve and retinal vasculitis in Behçet's disease. Doc Ophthalmol 1992;80:133–142.

222. Martin DF, DeBarge LR, Nussenblatt RB, et al: Synergistic effect of rapamycin and cyclosporine A on the inhibition of experimental autoimmune uveoretinitis. Invest Ophthalmol Vis Sci 1993;34:S1476.

223. Insel PA: Analgesic-antipyretics and antiinflammatory agents: Drugs employed in the treatment of rheumatoid arthritis and gout. In: Gilman AG, Rall TW, Nies AS, Taylor P, eds. Goodman and Gilman's The Pharmacological Basis of Therapeutics. New York, Pergamon Press, 1990, pp 674–676.

224. Nussenblatt RB, Plestin AG: Uveitis, Fundamentals and Clinical Practice. Chicago, Year Book Medical, 1989, pp 116–144.

225. Raynor A, Akari AD: Behçet's disease and treatment with colchicine. J Am Acad Dermatol 1980;2:396–400.

226. Allison AC, Eugui EM: Mycophenolate mofetil (RS-61443): Mode of action and effects on graft rejection. In: Thompson AW, Starzl TE, eds. Immunosuppressive Drugs: Developments in Anti-rejection Therapy. Boston, E Arnold, 1994, 141–159.

227. Allison AC, Eugui EM: Immunosuppressive and other effects of mycophenolic acid and an ester prodrug mycophenolate mofetil. Immunol Rev 1993;136:5–28.

228. Siconolfi L: Mycophenolate mofetil (CellCept): Immunosuppression on the cutting edge. AACN Clin Issues 1996;7:390–402.

229. Larkin G, Lightman S: Mycophenolate mofetil: A useful immunosuppressive in inflammatory eye diseases. Ophthalmology 1999;106:370–374.

230. Alpsoy E, Yilmaz E, Basaran E, et al: Interferon therapy for Behçet's disease. J Am Acad Dermatol 1994;31:617–619.

231. O'Duffy JD, Calamia K, Cohen S, et al: Interferon-γ treatment of Behçet's disease. J Rheumatol 1998;25:1938–1944.

232. Zouboulis CC, Orfanos CE: Treatment of Adamantiades-Behçet's disease with systemic interferon-γ. Arch Dermatol 1998;134:1010–1016.

233. Kotter I, Eckstein AK, Stubiger N, Zierhut M: Treatment of ocular symptoms of Behçet's disease with interferon alpha 2a: A pilot study. Br J Ophthalmol 1998;82:488–494.

234. Wizemann AJ, Wizemann V: Therapeutic effects of short-term plasma exchange in endogenous uveitis. Am J Ophthalmol 1984;97:565–572.

235. Yasui K, Ohta K, Kobayashi M, et al: Successful treatment of Behçet's disease with pentoxifylline. Ann Intern Med 1996; 124:891–893.

236. Calguneri M, Kiraz S, Ertenli I, et al: The effect of prophylactic penicillin treatment on the course of arthritis episodes in patients with Behçet's disease. A randomized clinical trial. Arthritis Rheum 1996;39:2062–2065.

237. Gardner-Medwin JM, Smith NJ, Powell RJ: Clinical experience with thalidomide in the management of severe oral and genital ulceration in conditions such as Behçet's disease: Use of neurophysiological studies to detect thalidomide neuropathy. Ann Rheum Dis 1994;53:828–832.

238. Rojas B, Zafirakis P, Foster CS: Cataract surgery in patients with uveitis. Curr Opin Ophthalmol 1997;8:6–12.

239. Foster CS, Fong LP, Singh G: Cataract surgery and intraocular lens implantation in patients with uveitis. Ophthalmology 1988;96:281–288.

240. Tabbara KF, Chavis PS: Cataract extraction in Behçet's disease. Ocul Immunol Inflamm 1997;5:27–32.

241. Ciftci OU, Ozdemir O: Cataract extraction in Behçet's disease. Acta Ophthalmol Scand 1996;74:74–76.

242. Yazici H, Tuzun YU, Pazarli H: Influence of age of onset and patient's sex on the prevalence and severity of manifestations of Behçet's syndrome. Ann Rheum Dis 1984;43:783–789.

243. Yoshikawa K, Ichiishi A, Kotake S, et al: Posterior sub-Tenon's space injection of repository corticosteroids in uveitis patients with cystoid macular edema. Nippon Ganka Gakkai Zasshi 1993; 97:1070–1074.

244. Atmaca LS: Experience with photocoagulation in Behçet's disease. Ophthalmic Surg 1990;21:571–576.

245. Minura Y: Surgical results of complicated cataract in Behçet's disease. In: Reports of the Behçet's Disease Research Committee. Japan, Ministry of Health and Welfare, 1976, pp 152–159.

246. Mamo JG: The rate of visual loss in Behçet's disease. Arch Ophthalmol 1970;84:451–452.

247. Demiroglu H, Barista I, Dündar S: Risk factor assessment and prognosis of eye involvement in Behçet's disease in Turkey. Ophthalmology 1997;104:701–705.

POLYARTERITIS NODOSA

Masoud Soheilian

DEFINITION

Polyarteritis nodosa (PAN) (also called periarteritis and polyangiitis) is a group of rare multisystemic diseases with necrotizing vasculitis but without granulomatous features (as in Wegener's granulomatosis). They are characterized by patchy but widespread involvement of small to medium-sized muscular arteries and sometimes even small vessels such as arterioles, capillaries, and venules. Involvement leads to focal signs that result from local circulatory disturbances and ischemia, caused by thrombosis, embolism, or rupture of the vessel wall. There are two forms of systemic PAN: macroscopic PAN (MaPAN) and microscopic PAN (MiPAN).

HISTORY AND CLASSIFICATION

The term nodosa in PAN reflects the characteristic nodular appearance of the diseased vessels. It was first described by Kussmaul and Maier in 1866.[1] They described a 27-year-old tailor's apprentice with nephritis, mononeuritis multiplex, and abdominal pain, and they named this condition periarteritis nodosa, noting extensive inflammation, thrombosis, and fibrosis of small and medium-sized arteries resulting in aneurysmal thickening of arteries, resembling a string of knots. Periarteritis nodosa was renamed polyarteritis nodosa in 1903 by Ferrari, who emphasized the transmural and multifocal nature of the inflammation.[2]

A number of different clinical and pathologic types of vasculitis were described over the next 50 years. In 1948, Zeek and colleagues[3] were the first to propose a classification scheme for vasculitis. They categorized five types of necrotizing vasculitis based on clinical and pathologic features and size and type of vessel involvement.

The American College of Rheumatology Subcommittee on Classification of Vasculitis developed a standard vasculitis classification and selected seven forms of vasculitis.[4] Subsequently the Chapel Hill Consensus Conference on the Nomenclature of Systemic Vasculitis set out to correct the problem of a lack of standardized diagnostic terms and definitions.[5] According to the Chapel Hill classification, PAN is a disease affecting all arteries and therefore all systems. However, because involvement of small vessels such as arterioles and venules has been described in PAN, the 19th century classification of PAN needed to be revised and reclassified. The classification system proposed by this group limits the definition to exclude involvement of small vessels and glomerulonephritis. These cases are designated as microscopic polyangiitis or polyarteritis (MiPAN). However, some authorities argue that this distinction is unwarranted because there is no clear biologic evidence to support the existence of two different disease entities.

EPIDEMIOLOGY

PAN is an uncommon disease that affects mostly 40- to 60-year-old adults; men are twice as likely to be affected as women.[6] Exact appreciation of the incidence of systemic PAN is difficult to achieve. Estimates of the annual incidence of PAN-type systemic vasculitis in a general population range from 4.6 per million in England,[7] to 9.0 per million in Minnesota,[8] to 77 per million in a hepatitis B hyperendemic Alaskan Eskimo population.[9] Another published study has shown a prevalence rate of 7 per million.[10] The estimated annual mortality rate for PAN in New York City in 1950 was 1.2 to 1.5 per million.[11] It should be emphasized that most studies of PAN in the past were likely to include both microscopic and macroscopic forms.

CLINICAL CHARACTERISTICS

Systemic Manifestations

Polyarteritis nodosa is a systemic illness that can affect almost any organ. The onset is variable depending on the organ system affected. The general signs and symptoms of serum sickness may occur, including fever, malaise, weight loss, myalgias, and arthralgias. Certain main clinical presentations have been distinguished:[12]

1. A nonspecific subacute or chronic pyrexial wasting illness
2. An atypical abdominal illness
3. A primary renal disorder
4. A combination of polyneuritic and polymyositic features

The order and progress of system involvement are variable. Sometimes, only one organ or system may be involved for a long period. More commonly, multisystem involvement occurs early.

Renal Involvement

Renal manifestations[13, 14] are eventually present in three of every four patients with PAN. Vascular lesions such as microaneurysms with vessel stenosis and thrombosis may lead to cortical infarction. These pathologic findings may preclude renal biopsy because of the risk of vessel rupture.[15] Kidney involvement with or without hypertension is a primary cause of death in patients with systemic PAN.

Cardiovascular Involvement

Cardiovascular manifestations are as frequent as renal involvement and are the second leading cause of death in patients with PAN.[12] Hypertension, a consequence of renal involvement, is an almost constant accompanying feature. Coronary thrombosis, pericarditis, intrapericardial hemorrhage, and acute aortitis can occur. Myocardial involvement may lead to dysrhythmias, heart failure, and infarction.

Cutaneous Involvement

Approximately one fifth to one half of patients with systemic PAN have cutaneous manifestations.[12] The most significant clinical sign is the presence of cutaneous or subcutaneous nodules, which occur in groups along the course of superficial arteries. They are found around the knee, anterior lower leg, and dorsum of the foot (Fig. 57–1).[16] They are the result of local necrosis of the arterial wall at points of bifurcation. Pulsatile aneurysms result from healing by fibrosis. Local rupture may give rise to a local intracutaneous hematoma or ecchymosis. Peripheral embolization of thrombi causes infarction of the tissues, and the fingers and toes in particular may be affected by small infarcts, splinter hemorrhage, Osler's nodes, and gangrene.[12] Infarcts in the skin may present as tender nodules, purpuric plaques, or hemorrhagic bullae. A cutaneous localized form of PAN characterized by cutaneous nodules and livedo reticularis exists; however, patients with systemic disease usually do not manifest this type of lesion.[17]

Gastrointestinal Involvement

Abdominal pain is caused by polyarteritic lesions in the submucous and muscular layers of the intestine, or by mesenteric thrombosis (Fig. 57–2) or infarcts in the liver and spleen, giving rise to perihepatitis and perisplenitis. Gangrene of the bowel, peritonitis, perforation, and intra-abdominal hemorrhage are other features. Steatorrhea may occur as a result of the scarred bowel.[18] Acute pancreatitis and pancreatic fibrosis may occur.

Musculoskeletal Involvement

Nondeforming and nonerosive arthritis and arthralgia, resembling that in rheumatic fever, may occur without gross physical signs. Bony changes in the form of periosteal thickening of the tibia and fibula may also occur.

A true myopathy may occur in PAN. In some cases, the disorder may be confined to the skin and muscle, presenting with pain in the legs.[19]

Neurologic Involvement

Neurologic manifestations are usually the result of involvement of the arteries of the vasa nervorum and are usually limited to the peripheral nervous system. Both motor and sensory changes occur. Mononeuritis multi-

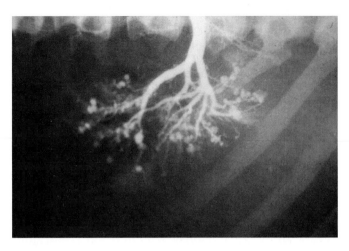

FIGURE 57–2. Abdominal aortic angiogram in a patient with recurrent scleritis and episodic abdominal pain. Note the sacular aneurysms of the mesenteric artery, nearly a pathognomonic feature of polyarteritis nodosa. (Courtesy of C. Stephen Foster, M.D.)

plex is a symptom complex of pain, paresthesia, or paresis of a single peripheral nerve occurring secondary to interruption of the blood supply to that nerve. Other manifestations of neurologic involvement vary widely, from a Guillain-Barré–like syndrome to hemiplegia, convulsion, or multiple sclerosis–like features.[15]

Genitourinary Involvement

Epididymal pain is an extremely suggestive clinical feature and is virtually pathognomonic of polyarteritis nodosa in the appropriate clinical context. Biopsy of the involved epididymis unequivocally establishes the diagnosis in cases where other tissue is unavailable for sampling or the diagnosis is uncertain.

Ocular Manifestations

PAN can involve almost every tissue of the eye, depending on which vessels are affected by the vasculitic process. Ocular manifestations appear in 10% to 20% of PAN patients, and it can be the first manifestation of the disease.[20–22] The ophthalmologist may play an important role in the diagnosis and management of a patient with this potentially lethal vasculitic disease.

Anterior Segment Manifestations

The conjunctiva may be hyperemic and edematous, with occasional subconjunctival hemorrhages. Sjögren's syndrome with keratoconjunctivitis sicca has been described in association with PAN. Conjunctival infarction may produce pale yellow, raised, and friable conjunctival lesions with subconjunctival hemorrhages.[23]

Vascular inflammation of episcleral, scleral, and limbal vessels may lead to episcleritis, scleritis, and sclerokeratitis.[24–27] The incidence of PAN in patients with scleritis ranges from 0.68 to 6.45.[28–30] Necrotizing anterior scleritis, often associated with peripheral ulcerative keratitis (PUK), is the most frequent type of scleritis in patients with PAN.[21, 26, 27] The scleritis becomes extremely painful and is highly destructive unless the correct diagnosis is made and control of the underlying systemic disease is

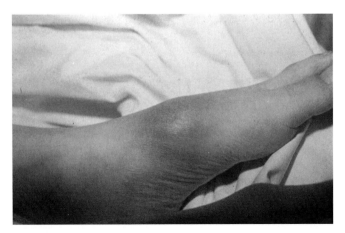

FIGURE 57–1. Subcutaneous nodule, dorsal aspect of the foot of a patient who subsequently was biopsied (see Figure 57–7), with histopathologically proven polyarteritis nodosa. (Courtesy of C. Stephen Foster, M.D.) (See color insert.)

achieved (Fig. 57–3). The PUK corneal ulceration is progressive, both circumferentially and centrally, with undermining of the central edge of the ulcer that results in an overhanging lip of the cornea. However, scleral involvement helps to distinguish classic Mooren's ulcer from the sclerokeratitis-associated vasculitic diseases such as PAN. On occasion, episcleritis may be seen in patients with PAN, but it is less common or ominous than scleritis.[24, 29, 31] In most cases, sclerokeratitis presents after PAN has been diagnosed, but it occasionally may be the presenting manifestation of the disease.[20–22]

Cogan's syndrome (nonluetic interstitial keratitis with audiovestibular disease) has been described in association with PAN.[32]

Uveoretinal Manifestations

Involvement of iris vasculature may produce acute, nongranulomatous iritis with leakage of protein into the anterior chamber.[23, 25] A vitritis may also be noted.[33] Diffuse bilateral nongranulomatous panuveitis associated with retinal vasculitis has also been described in PAN.[34] The most common ocular findings in PAN are choroidal and retinal vasculitis[24] (Figs. 57–4 and 57–5). Choroidal vasculitis is the most frequent histologic abnormality,[35–37] but the presence of yellow subretinal patches is less often appreciated clinically. Involvement of the posterior ciliary arteries and choroidal vessels may manifest as choroidal infarcts and exudative retinal detachments.[38] The retinopathy of PAN is sometimes secondary to coexistent hypertension, but it may occur as a result of retinal vasculitis.

Subhyaloid hemorrhage, retinal hemorrhages, edema, lipid exudate, cotton-wool spots, marked irregularity of the caliber of retinal vessels, and exudative retinal detachment have all been described. Vascular occlusion, particularly central retinal artery occlusion, is not uncommon.[25, 39]

Fluorescein angiography has shown a normal retinal circulation with delayed choroidal filling,[40] and an arteritis with staining of involved arterial segments, dilated and tortuous capillaries both in the peripapillary region and

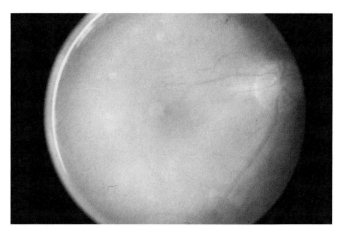

FIGURE 57–4. Retinal vasculitis, right eye, in a patient with polyarteritis nodosa. Note the slightly hazy view of the fundus, because of the presence of vitreal cells. Frank arteritis is clinically obvious, and fluorescein angiogram confirmed this (see Figure 57–6). (Courtesy of C. Stephen Foster, M.D.)

in the vicinity of the diseased arteries, and thrombosis of the retinal vein, usually without evidence of a retinal periphlebitis[41] (Fig. 57–6). However, Morgan and colleagues reported a case of biopsy-proven PAN in which the patient presented with bilateral iritis, vitritis, and retinal vasculitis involving both the retinal arteries and veins, demonstrated clinically and by fluorescein angiography.[38] Leakage through diseased vessel walls may also be noted.[41]

Neurophthalmic Manifestations

Optic nerve involvement takes several different forms. Papilledema or papillitis due to optic nerve vasculitis may occur. In one study, papilledema was present in 10% of patients.[39]

Orbital involvement may produce exophthalmos or a pseudotumor condition as a result of inflammation of orbital vessels[39, 42–45] and sometimes assumes the picture of an orbital neoplasm.[44]

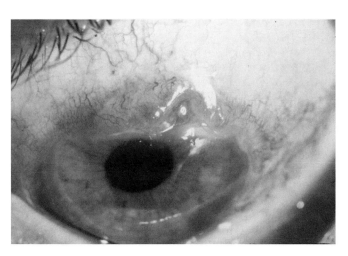

FIGURE 57–3. Left eye of patient described in Figure 57–2, with resolving scleritis but now with the onset of peripheral ulcerative keratitis prior to the institution of adequate doses of cyclophosphamide therapy. (Courtesy of C. Stephen Foster, M.D.) (See color insert.)

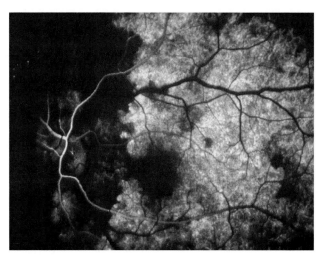

FIGURE 57–5. Fluorescein angiogram of the same patient as shown in Figure 57–4, illustrating the focal areas of delayed choroidal filling, which are indicative of choroidal involvement from the arteritic process. (Courtesy of C. Stephen Foster, M.D.)

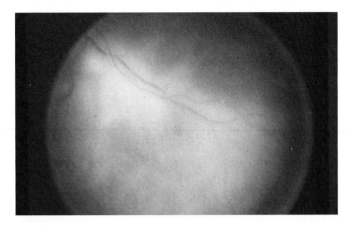

FIGURE 57–6. Fluorescein angiogram of the same patient as shown in Figure 57–4, late phase, demonstrating the extensive leakage from the inflamed retinal arterioles. (Courtesy of C. Stephen Foster, M.D.)

Arteritis of the posterior ciliary vessels with intermittent choroidal vascular insufficiency may be responsible for recurrent episodes of monocular constriction of the visual field with sparing of central vision.[40]

Vasculitic involvement of central and peripheral nervous system may produce third, fifth, sixth, and seventh nerve palsies, hemianopia, nystagmus, amaurosis fugax, diplopia,[45] and Horner's syndrome.[39]

PATHOGENESIS AND ETIOLOGY

The etiology of polyarteritis nodosa and the cause of the arteritis are unknown. Some evidence supports a role for immune complex–mediated vessel damage, because circulating immune complexes are found frequently[46] and (less commonly) serum complement is also diminished.[47] However, immune deposits of immunoglobulins and complement are seldom found in involved tissue in PAN.[48] It is likely that various antigens may trigger a circulating immune complex–mediated vasculitis. Viruses may contribute to the pathogenesis of arteritis, with the most commonly associated virus being hepatitis B. Between 30% and 70% of patients with PAN have antihepatitis B antibodies.[49] Recently other viruses such as human immunodeficiency virus (HIV),[50] cytomegalovirus,[51] hepatitis A and C,[52] human T-cell leukemia-lymphoma virus,[53] and parvovirus[54] have been associated with PAN.

Viruses can infect endothelial cells and alter their functions, including induction of receptors for the Fc portion of IgG, induction of receptors for C3B, and promotion of leukocyte adherence.[55] Infected endothelial cells express class 2 antigens and are capable of producing interleukin-1 (IL-1).[56] Finally, as a result of viral infection, the biology of endothelial cells is altered, permitting the endothelial cells to participate in a chronic inflammatory process.

Other known factors associated with PAN include drug abuse,[57] hyposensitization treatment,[58] B-cell neoplasm,[59] and acute otitis media.[60]

Antiendothelial cell antibodies may have a pathogenic role in PAN in the presence of factors such as tumor necrosis factor (TNF), IL-1, and interferon-gamma (IFN-γ).[61]

It is possible that PAN could be a result of several etiologic agents' having a final common pathway of inducing necrotizing vasculitis.

Inflammation of the arterial wall, induced by immune complexes, direct organism invasion, or antibodies toward endothelial cells, injures and perturbs the endothelial cells, resulting in an elevation of Von Willebrand factor and factor VIII in the blood of patients, just as in other systemic vasculitis diseases. The injured endothelial cells may release platelet-activating factor, which may influence the chemotaxis of neutrophils and eosinophils plus the release of other cytokines.[62] IL-1 and TNF that may be released from endothelial cells can convert a normally anticoagulant endothelial cell surface to a procoagulant surface. Finally, adherence of endothelial cells by neutrophils, monocytes, and lymphocytes increases. Consequently, the injured endothelial cells, by release of a variety of cytokines, become the promoter and the focus of an immune response, clot formation, and cellular proliferation.

Injury to the endothelium of blood vessels also diminishes its modulating effect on underlying smooth muscle tone that is usually mediated by the production of a dilator substance—endothelially derived relaxing factor (which may be nitric oxide)[63, 64]—and ultimately alters blood vessel contractility. Consequently, although in the healthy state, the endothelium produces factors that relax the underlying smooth muscle in response to numerous mediators and physiologic conditions; in the diseased endothelium, vasoconstrictive events may dominate.

Coagulation abnormalities such as hyperfibrinogenemia, thrombocytosis, and diminished fibrinolytic activity may occur in systemic vasculitic disorders, such as PAN, which result in arterial occlusive changes.[61]

In summary, the effect of inflammation on the blood vessels, and specifically on the endothelium, is a net increase in vasoconstriction, platelet aggregation, clot formation, and release of growth factors that may result in luminal occlusion. The proliferation of endothelial and smooth muscle cells triggered by inflammation may be as important as the inflammation itself in determining the outcome of the pathologic changes in the artery.

PATHOLOGY

MaPAN is a necrotizing segmental vasculitis involving small and medium-sized arteries, principally at branching and bifurcation points. The involvement may be so focal that only a solitary microscopic lesion is found in a large tissue section. The segmental necrotizing vasculitis is characterized by fibrinoid changes of the media with destruction of the internal elastic lamina, accompanied by infiltration of the media and adventitia, initially by neutrophils and later by mononuclear cells, the latter imparting a frankly granulomatous morphology to some of more chronic vascular lesions (Fig. 57–7). Fibroblastic proliferation ensues, with secondary thrombosis and resultant organ infarction. A subsequent reparative medial response occurs, characterized by replacement of the medial wall by granulation tissue and intimal fibrosis. A disruption of normal architecture of the entire vessel wall results in the typical aneurysmal dilations that give the disease its name. It must be appreciated that in PAN, diagnostic histopathology will not be obtained from su-

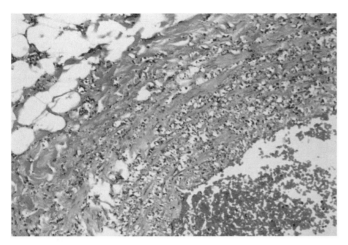

FIGURE 57–7. Histopathology, H & E section, 800 ×, from the biopsy of the subcutaneous nodule of the patient shown in Figure 57–1. Note the neutrophil invasion of the media of this artery, with fibrinoid necrosis of the vessel wall. (Courtesy of C. Stephen Foster, M.D.) (See color insert.)

perficial biopsies of the cutaneous lesions. Diagnostic changes in muscular arteries are usually seen in tissue from muscle, kidney, or even testes or occasionally from deep incisional skin biopsies.[17, 65]

DIAGNOSIS

The diagnosis of systemic PAN is generally based on clinical and histopathologic grounds. General laboratory evaluation is nonspecific and only supportive of clinical diagnosis. Any patient with PUK, scleritis, or occlusive retinal vasculitis should be reviewed for systemic evidence of PAN. A tissue diagnosis is usually necessary for confirmation. Muscle, renal, skin, peripheral nerve, testicular, or epididymal tissue is often required.[66, 67] Biopsy of involved tissue may demonstrate a hemorrhagic vasculitis and fibrinoid necrosis, which establishes the diagnosis.[68] Testicular and skin biopsy can confirm the diagnosis in 50% to 80% of patients.[69, 70] Autopsy studies have shown vascular inflammation in the testes in 86% of patients when the entire testis is sectioned and examined thoroughly.[70] Blind biopsy of asymptomatic organs rarely establishes the diagnosis.[31, 71]

Laboratory Findings

Most laboratory tests are nonspecific and reflect only the systemic nature of the disease. The erythrocyte sedimentation rate (ESR), neutrophil count, and serum globulin levels are usually elevated. Eosinophilia may be present. When the urinary sediment reveals red cells, red cell casts, or proteinuria, renal disease must be suspected. Hypocomplementemia may reflect a more active disease. Approximately one third of patients with PAN have hepatitis-B antigenemia.[72] Cryoglobulins may be present, and circulating immune complexes may be detected. Rheumatoid factor and antinuclear antibody are usually negative, but antineutrophil cytoplasmic antibody (ANCA) may be positive. In a review of published studies, the average diagnostic sensitivity of c-ANCA for MaPAN was 5%, and of p-ANCA it was 15%.[73]

The angiographic finding of small, aneurysmal dila-

tion in renal, hepatic, and gastrointestinal vessels may be helpful in establishing the diagnosis, although they may be found in systemic lupus erythematosus[74] and fibromuscular dysplasia.[75]

DIFFERENTIAL DIAGNOSIS

Important entities to exclude in the differential diagnosis of polyarteritis nodosa include obvious systemic diseases associated with retinal vasculitis, such as Adamantiades-Behçet's disease, systemic lupus erythematosus, mixed connective tissue disease, dermatomyositis, and progressive systemic sclerosis. Dermatomyositis and progressive systemic sclerosis can usually be differentiated on the basis of systemic features. The clinical picture and serologic abnormalities are distinct for systemic lupus erythematosus and for mixed connective tissue diseases. While both entities may manifest buccal mucosal ulcerations, the aphthous lesions of Adamantiades-Behçet's disease are distinct, they may also appear on the external genitalia, and these patients frequently have associated arthralgias and erythema nodosum.

TREATMENT

This group of disorders is potentially fatal[34, 68] and yet there is no completely satisfactory treatment for either the systemic or the ocular components. As in other vasculitic diseases, the ocular manifestations of PAN are reliable signs of systemic vasculitis and represent a clear indication for immunosuppressive therapy. These patients must be treated with systemic cyclophosphamide and corticosteroids, and it is important to treat the patient rather than the laboratory abnormalities, although the ESR is a useful indication of activity. The combination of prednisolone (60 to 120 mg) with cyclophosphamide (1 to 2 mg/kg/day) results in an 80% to 96% 5-year survival rate.[76, 77] If the patient is intolerant to cyclophosphamide, other immunosuppressants should be used in an effort to save not only the patient's eye but the patient's life as well. Such alternatives include azathioprine, methotrexate, cyclosporine A, and, recently, tacrolimus.[78] Sulfapyridine therapy has also been shown to induce remissions in patients with predominantly cutaneous disease.[79]

The use of antiplatelet drugs concomitantly with the initiation of corticosteroid treatment might modify the potential vasospastic and platelet-aggregation effects of the disease. Comorbid diseases, such as hypertension, diabetes mellitus, and hyperlipidemia, must be vigorously treated. Agents inhibiting cytokines, growth factors, and cellular proliferation may play a therapeutic role in the future. Intravenous gamma globulins and monoclonal antibody therapy have been helpful in some patients. IFN-α has been effective in patients with PAN associated with hepatitis B.[80]

PROGNOSIS

Prior to the advent of new immunosuppressive chemotherapies, systemic PAN was usually fatal and was associated with a progressive course, leading to death from renal or cardiac complications. Without therapy, classic PAN carries an 80% to 90% 5-year mortality rate. Corticosteroids have reduced this rate to 50%, and the addition of cyclophosphamide has profoundly improved survival.[76]

Poor prognostic factors at the time of diagnosis include gastrointestinal vasculitis and older age (over 50 years) at diagnosis.[7, 31, 81] Other identified factors indicative of a poor prognosis include renal, cardiac, and neuropathic involvement.[7, 81, 82]

Microscopic Polyarteritis Nodosa

MiPAN, also called polyangiitis, is now distinguishable from MaPAN by the criteria established at the Chapel Hill Conference on Nomenclature (Table 57–1).[5] Based on this recent classification of vasculitis syndromes, MiPAN histologically refers to a necrotizing vasculitis involving capillaries, venules, and arterioles along with a focal segmental necrotizing glomerulonephritis and sometimes crescent formation. Pulmonary involvement can occur as a result of capillaritis and is characterized clinically by hemoptysis and histologically by a neutrophilic capillaritis. This combination of renal and pulmonary disease often suggests the diagnosis of Goodpasture's syndrome.[83] Nasopharyngeal involvement is frequent, with oral ulcers, sinusitis, and epistaxis among the more common manifestations. Skin involvement is also frequent. Involvement of small and medium-sized arteries does not exclude the diagnosis of MiPAN. The p-ANCA (antibody to myeloperoxidase) autoantibody pattern, a marker for MiPAN, is found in 50% to 80% of affected patients; about 40% have the c-ANCA (antibody to proteinase 3) autoantibody pattern,[84] with few or no immune deposits in involved vessels. Positive ANCA and negative serologic tests for hepatitis B help differential MiPAN from MaPAN. MiPAN differs histopathologically from Wegener's granulomatosis by the absence of extravascular inflammation.

Ocular manifestations in MiPAN are uncommon but may include conjunctival injection, nodular lesions of the conjunctiva, peripheral corneal thinning or ulceration, scleritis, PUK, sicca syndrome, eyelid edema, and nodular lesions of the skin of the eyelid margin with an ulcerative surface.[85] Review of the literature after the Chapel Hill classification on Nomenclature of Systemic Vasculitis disclosed only one case of uveitis with retinal vasculitis and vitreous hemorrhage reported in pure MiPAN.[78]

The 5-year survival of MiPAN is approximately 60%. Death is caused by uncontrolled active disease or superimposed infection. Factors contributing to early demise are older age and renal failure. The usual treatment for patients with MiPAN and renal involvement or significant lung involvement is prednisone (60 mg/day) and cyclophosphamide (1 to 2 mg/kg/day). Intravenous gamma globulin has been successfully used in the treatment of cyclophosphamide-resistant MiPAN.[68]

CONCLUSIONS

The classification system of patients suspected of having PAN has changed recently. MaPAN is diagnosed when necrotizing inflammation of medium-sized or small arteries is observed without glomerulonephritis or vasculitis in arterioles, capillaries, or venules. Whenever necrotizing vasculitis, affecting small vessels (i.e., capillaries, venules, or arterioles) with few or no immune deposits, is found, MiPAN is diagnosed, even if concurrent small and medium-sized artery involvement exists. Ocular involvement is seen in 10% to 20% of patients with PAN but is less commonly observed in MiPAN. Both c-ANCA and p-ANCA patterns are serologically demonstrable in nearly half of the patients with MiPAN, whereas they have low diagnostic sensitivities and specificities for MaPAN.

Several inflammatory conditions can be mistaken for either MaPAN and MiPAN: Wegener's granulomatosis, Adamantiades-Behçet's disease, systemic lupus erythematosus (including some forms of rheumatoid arthritis with widespread arterial changes), and other forms of systemic vasculitis. The clinical features and tissue biopsy can help differentiate PAN from other entities.

The current therapy for PAN involves a combination of oral cyclophosphamide and corticosteroids. Systemic corticosteroids alone are not effective in controlling ocular inflammation in PAN. Ophthalmologists should be familiar with the clinical features of this rare disease, as this potentially fatal disorder may present initially with ocular involvement. A close collaboration with a team of other treating physicians (such as a rheumatologist, dermatologist, nephrologist, hematologist, or pulmonary physician), especially in the comanagement of immunosuppressive therapy, ensures the best possible care for these patients.

TABLE 57–1. CLINICAL FORMS OF SYSTEMIC POLYARTERITIS NODOSA (PAN) ADOPTED BY THE CHAPEL HILL CONSENSUS CONFERENCE ON THE NOMENCLATURE OF SYSTEMIC VASCULITIS

Macroscopic polyarteritis nodosa (MaPAN)	Necrotizing inflammation of medium-sized or small arteries without glomerulonephritis or vasculitis in arterioles, capillaries, or venules.
Microscopic polyarteritis nodosa (MiPAN)	Necrotizing vasculitis with few or no immune deposits affecting small vessels (capillaries, venules, or arterioles). Necrotizing arteritis involving small and medium-sized arteries may be present. Necrotizing glomerulonephritis is very common. Pulmonary capillaritis often occurs.

References

1. Kussmaul A, Maier R: Ueber eine bisher nicht beshriebene eigenthumliche Arterienerkrankung (Periarteritis Nodosda), die mit Morbus Brightii und rapid Fortschreitender allgemeiner Muskellahmung einhergeht. Dtsch Arch Klin Med 1866;1:484–518.
2. Ferrari E: Ueber Poly-arteritis Acuta Nodosa (Sogennannte Arteritis Nodosa) und ihre Beziehungen zur Polymyositis und Polyneuritis acuta. Beitr Pathol Anat 1903;34:350–386.
3. Zeek PM, Smith CC, Wector JC: Studies on periarteritis nodosa: III. The differentiation between the vascular lesions of periarteritis nodosa and of hypersensitivity. Am J Pathol 1948;24:889–917.
4. Hunder GG, Arend WP, Bloch DA, et al: The American College of Rheumatology 1990 criteria for the classification of vasculitis: Introduction. Arthritis Rheum 1990;33:1065–1067.
5. Jennette JC, Falk RJ, Andrassy K, et al: Nomenclature of systemic vasculitides. Arthritis Rheum 1994;37:187–192.
6. Foster CS, Forstot SL, Wilson LA: Mortality rate in rheumatoid arthritis patients developing necrotizing scleritis of peripheral ulcerative keratitis. Ophthalmology 1984;91:1253.
7. Scott DGI, Bacon PA, Elliot PJ, et al: Systemic vasculitis in a district general hospital 1972–1980: Clinical and laboratory features, classification and prognosis of 80 cases. Q J Med 1982;203:292.
8. Kurland LT, Chuang TY, Hunder GH: Epidemiology of the rheumatic diseases. New York, Gower, 1984.

9. McMahon BJ, Heyward WL, Templin DW, et al: Hepatitis B-associated polyarteritis nodosa in Alaskan Eskimos: Clinical and epidemiologic features and long-term follow-up. Hepatology 1989;9:97.

10. Kurland LT, Hauser WA, Ferguson RH, et al: Epidemiologic features of diffuse connective tissue disorders in Rochester, Minn., 1951 through 1967 with special reference to systemic lupus erythematosus. Mayo Clin Proc 1969;44:649–663.

11. Masi AT: Population studies in rheumatic disease. Annu Rev Med 1967;18:185.

12. Ryan TJ: Cutaneous vasculitis. In: Rook A, Wilkinson DS, Ebling FJG, et al, eds: Textbook of Dermatology, vol. 3. London, Blackwell, 1992, p 1947.

13. Davson J, Ball J, Platt R: The kidney in periarteritis nodosa. Q J Med 1948;17:175–202.

14. Platt R, Davson J: A clinical and pathological study of renal disease. Q J Med 1950;19:33–55.

15. Verztman L: Polyarteritis nodosa. Clin Rheum Dis 1980;6:297–317.

16. Fisher I, Orkin M: Cutaneous form of periarteritis nodosa—An entity? Arch Dermatol 1964;89:180–189.

17. Jorizzo JL: Polyarteritis nodosa. In: Demis DJ, ed: Clinical dermatology, vol 1. Philadelphia, J.B. Lippincott, 1991, unit 5–6.

18. Carron DB, Douglas AP: Steatorrhoea in vascular insufficiency of the small intestine. Q J Med 1965;34:331–40.

19. Golding DN: Polyarteritis presenting with leg pains. Br Med J 1970;1:277–278.

20. Foster CS: Immunosuppressive therapy for external ocular inflammatory disease. Ophthalmology 1980;87:140.

21. Wise GN: Ocular periarteritis nodosa. AMA Arch Ophthalmol 1952;48:1.

22. Moore JG, Sevel D: Corneoscleral ulceration in periarteritis nodosa. Br J Ophthalmol 1966;50:651.

23. Purcell JJ Jr, Birkenkamp R, Tsai CC: Conjunctival lesions in periarteritis nodosa: A clinical and immunopathologic study. Arch Ophthalmol 1984;102:736.

24. Goar EL, Smith LS: Polyarteritis nodosa of the eye. Am J Ophthalmol 1952;35:1619.

25. Sheehean B, Harriman DG, Bradshaw JP: Polyarteritis nodosa with ophthalmic and neurological complications. AMA Arch Ophthalmol 1958;60:537.

26. Herbert F, McPherson SD: Scleral necrosis in periarteritis nodosa. Am J Ophthalmol 1947;30:727.

27. Cogan DG: Corneoscleral lesions in periarteritis nodosa and Wegener's granulomatosis. Trans Am Acad Ophthalmol 1955;53:321.

28. Lyne AJ, Pitkeathley DA: Episcleritis and scleritis. Arch Ophthalmol 1968;80:171.

29. Watson PG, Hayreh SS: Scleritis and episcleritis. Br J Ophthalmol 1976;60:163.

30. Tuft SJ, Watson PG: Progression of scleral disease. Ophthalmology 1991;98:467.

31. Cohen RD, Conn DL, Ilstrup DM: Clinical features, prognosis, and response to treatment in polyarteritis. Mayo Clin Proc 1980;55:146–155.

32. Gilbert WS, Talbot FJ: Cogan's syndrome. Signs of polyarteritis nodosa and cerebral venous sinus thrombosis. Arch Ophthalmol 1969;82:633.

33. Opremcak EM: Uveitis: A clinical manual for ocular inflammation. New York, Springer-Verlag, 1995.

34. Akova YA, Jabbur NS, Foster CS: Ocular presentation of polyarteritis nodosa. Clinical course and management with steroid and cytotoxic therapy. Ophthalmology 1993;100:1775.

35. Hakin KN, Watson PG: Systemic association of scleritis. Int Ophthalmol Clin 1991;31:111.

36. Goldstein I, Wexler D: The ocular pathology of periarteritis nodosa. Arch Ophthalmol 1929;2:288.

37. King RT: Ocular involvement in a case of periarteritis nodosa. Trans Ophthalmol Soc UK 1935;55:246.

38. Morgan CM, Foster CS, D'Amico JD, et al: Retinal vasculitis in polyarteritis nodosa. Retina 1986;6:205–209.

39. Ford RG, Siekert RG: Central nervous system manifestations of periarteritis nodosa. Neurology 1965;15:114.

40. Newman NM, Hoyt WF, Spencer WH: Macula-sparing monocular blackouts: Clinical and pathologic investigation of intermittent choroidal vascular insufficiency in a case of periarteritis nodosa. Arch Ophthalmol 1974;91:367–370.

41. Rosen ES: The retinopathy in polyarteritis nodosa. Br J Ophthalmol 1968;52:903.

42. Friedenwald JS, Rones B: Ocular lesions in septicemia. Arch Ophthalmol 1931;5:175.

43. Gaynon IE, Asbury MK: Ocular findings in a case of peripheral nodosa. Am J Ophthalmol 1943;23:1072.

44. Van Wien S, Merz EH: Exophthalmos secondary to periarteritis nodosa. Am J Ophthalmol 1963;56:204.

45. Gold DH: Ocular manifestations of connective tissue (collagen) diseases. In: Tasman W, Jaeger AE, eds: Duane's Clinical Ophthalmology, vol. 5. Philadelphia, J.B. Lippincott, 1989, pp 17–19.

46. Leib ES, Hibrawi H, Chia D, et al: Correlation of disease activity in systemic necrotizing vasculitis with immune complexes. J Rheumatol 1981;8:258.

47. Conn DL, McDuffie FC, Holley KE, et al: Immunologic mechanisms in systemic vasculitis. Mayo Clin Proc 1976;51:511.

48. Ronco P, Verroust P, Mignon F, et al: Immunopathological studies of polyarteritis nodosa and Wegener's granulomatosis: A report of 43 patients with 51 renal biopsies. Q J Med 1983;52:212.

49. Gocke DJ, Hsu K, Morgan C, et al: Association between polyarteritis nodosa and Australia antigen. Lancet 1970;2:1149.

50. Calabrese LH, Estes M, Yen-Leieberman B, et al: Systemic vasculitis in association with human immunodeficiency virus infection. Arthritis Rheum 1989;32:569.

51. Curtis JL, Egbert BM: Cutaneous cytomegalovirus vasculitis: An unusual clinical presentation of a common opportunistic pathogen. Hum Pathol 1982;13:1138.

52. Inman RD, Hodge M, Johnson MEA, et al: Arthritis, vasculitis, and cryoglobulinemia associated with relapsing hepatitis A virus infection. Ann Intern Med 1986;105:700.

53. Haynes BF, Miller SE, Palker TJ, et al: Identification of human T-cell leukemia virus in a Japanese patient with adult T-cell leukemia and cutaneous lymphomatous vasculitis. Proc Natl Acad Sci USA 1983;80:2054.

54. Li Loong TC, Coyle PV, Anderson MJ, et al: Human serum parvovirus associated vasculitis. Postgrad Med J 1986;62:493.

55. Friedman HM: Infection of endothelial cells by common human viruses. Rev Infect Dis 1989;2(suppl 4):700.

56. Bielke MA: Vascular endothelium in immunology and infectious disease. Rev Infect Dis 1989;2:273.

57. Citron BP, Halpern M, McCarron M, et al: Necrotizing angiitis associated with drug abuse. N Engl J Med 1970;283:1003–1011.

58. Phanuphak P, Kohler PF, Stanford RE, et al: Onset of polyarteritis nodosa during allergic hyposensitization treatment. Am J Med 1980;68:479–485.

59. Elkon KB, Hughs GRV, Catovsky CJP, et al: Hairy cell leukemia with polyarteritis nodosa. Lancet 1979;2:280–282.

60. Sargent JS, Christian CL: Necrotizing vasculitis after acute serous otitis media. Ann Intern Med 1974;81:195–199.

61. Conn DL: Polyarteritis. In: Rheumatic Disease Clinics of North America, vol 16. Philadelphia, W.B. Saunders, 1990, pp 341–362.

62. Braquet P, Hosford D, Braquet M, et al: Role of cytokines and platelet-activating factor in microvascular immune injury. Int Arch Allergy Appl Immunol 1989;88:88.

63. Palmer RMJ, Ashton DS, Moncada S: Vascular endothelial cells synthesize nitric oxide from L-arginine. Nature 1988;333:664.

64. Vanhoutte PM: The endothelium-modulator of vascular smooth-muscle tone (editorial). N Engl J Med 1988;319:512.

65. Patalano VJ, Sommers SC: Biopsy diagnosis of polyarteritis nodosa. Arch Pathol 1961;72:1–7.

66. Diaz-Perez JL, Winkelmann RK: Cutaneous periarteritis nodosa. Arch Dermatol 1974;110:407.

67. Dyck PJ, Conn DL, Okazaki H: Necrotizing angiopathic neuropathy: Three-dimensional morphology of fiber degeneration related to sites of occluded vessels. Mayo Clin Proc 1972;47:461.

68. Valente RM, Hall S, O'Duffy JD, Conn DL: Vasculitic syndromes. In: Kelly WN, Harris ED Jr, Ruddy S, Sledge CB, eds: Textbook of Rheumatology, 5th ed, vol. 2, Philadelphia, W.B. Saunders, 1997, pp 1079–1122.

69. Maxeiner SR Jr, McDonald JR, Kirklin JW: Muscle biopsy in the diagnosis of periarteritis nodosa: An evaluation. Surg Clin North Am 1952;10:1225.

70. Dahl EV, Baggenstoss AH, DeWeerd JH: Testicular lesions of periarteritis nodosa, with special reference to diagnosis. Am J Med 1960;28:222.

71. Sizeland PC, Bailey RR, Lynn KI, Robson RA: Wegener's granulomatosis with renal involvement: A 14-year experience. N Z Med J 1990;103:366–367.

72. Duffy J, Lidsky MD, Sharp JT, et al: Polyarthritis, polyarteritis, and hepatitis B. Medicine 1976;55:19–37.

73. Kallenberg CG, Brouwer E, Weening JJ, Cohen Tervaert JW: Antineutrophil cytoplasmic antibodies: Current diagnostic and pathophysiological potential. Kidney Int 1994;46:1–15.

74. Longstreth PL, Lorobkin M, Palubinskas AJ: Renal microaneurysms in a patient with systemic lupus erythematosus. Radiology 1974;113:65.

75. McKusick VA: Buerger's disease: A distinct clinical and pathologic entity. JAMA 1962;181:93.

76. Fauci AS, Doppman JL, Wolff SM: Cyclophosphamide-induced remission in advanced polyarteritis nodosa. Am J Med 1978;64:890.

77. McCauley RL, Johnston MR, Fauci AS: Surgical aspects of necrotizing vasculitis. Surgery 1985;97:104–110.

78. Sloper CM, Powell RJ, Dua HS: Tacrolimus (FK506) in the treatment of posterior uveitis refractory to cyclosporine. Ophthalmology 1999;106:723–728.

79. Diaz-Perez JL, Winkelmann RK: Cutaneous periarteritis nodosa: A study of 33 cases. In: Wolff K, Winkelmann RK, eds: Major Problems in Dermatology. Philadelphia: WB Saunders Co., 1980, pp 273–284.

80. Guillevin L, Lhote F, Leon A, et al: Treatment of polyarteritis nodosa related to hepatitis B virus with short-term steroid therapy associated with antiviral agents and plasma exchanges: A prospective trial in 33 patients. J Rheumatol 1993;20:289–298.

81. Guillevin L, Du LTH, Godeau P, et al: Clinical findings and prognosis of polyarteritis nodosa, and Churg-Strauss angiitis: A study in 165 patients. Br J Rheumatol 1988;27:258.

82. Sack M, Cassidy JT, Bole GG: Prognostic factors in polyarteritis. J Rheumatol 1975;2:411.

83. Harman LE, Margo CE: Wegener's granulomatosis. Surv Ophthalmol 1998;42:458–480.

84. Geffriaud-Ricouard C, Noel LH, Chauveau D, et al: Clinical spectrum associated with ANCA of defined antigen specificities in 98 selected patients. Clin Nephrol 1993;39:125–136.

85. Caster JC, Shetlar DJ, Pappolla MA, Yee RW: Microscopic polyangiitis with ocular involvement. Arch Ophthalmol 1996;114:346–348.

58 — WEGENER'S GRANULOMATOSIS

Sarkis H. Soukiasian

DEFINITION

Wegener's granulomatosis is a distinct systemic clinicopathologic entity characterized by granulomatous vasculitis of the upper and lower respiratory tract with frequent involvement of the kidneys, the latter being a major determinant of poor outcome.[1-4] Ocular involvement is seen in about 50% of cases.[5-8]

Wegener's granulomatosis is usually classified within the spectrum of systemic necrotizing vasculitis (of the small arteries and veins), a group of disorders that may exhibit nonspecific features in the early stages but may evolve over time to more clinically recognizable patterns.[9-11] A number of classification systems for systemic vasculitis have been proposed and modified, each with limitations, as an understanding of the pathogenicity of most of the clinically recognized entities has been lacking, and tissue sampling errors, chronicity of disease, and partial therapy can greatly impact the pathologic features.[12-17] Nonetheless, a useful classification has been formulated by Lie,[18] which is partly based on the size of the involved blood vessels (Table 58–1).

The classic diagnostic criteria for Wegener's granulomatosis was based on the initial detailed clinical[19] and pathologic[20] findings presented by Godman and Churg in 1954, which included the triad of necrotizing granulomas of the upper and lower respiratory system, systemic vasculitis, and necrotizing glomerulonephritis. These classic criteria correlate with a complete and fulminant form of the disease, which historically had been nearly always fatal. However, it is apparent that Wegener's granulomatosis is a continuum of disease, where various combinations of the three major anatomic sites (the upper and lower respiratory tract and the kidney) can produce a spectrum of disease,[21] and that in many patients some features of the disease may be absent. In the incomplete or limited form of Wegener's granulomatosis,[22] the kidneys are usually spared (Table 58–2).[23-26] Although any organ system may be involved in limited Wegener's granulomatosis, the upper or lower respiratory system is the most common. A very limited form of the disease, with clinical involvement of a single organ such as the eye, has also been described.[27] Ophthalmic involvement can manifest as orbitopathy, conjunctivitis, episcleritis, scleritis, keratitis, uveitis, and vasculitis.

HISTORY

Klinger was the first to describe this disease as a form of polyarteritis nodosa.[28] However, Frederich Wegener, a German pathologist, recognized the unique nature of the condition and established Wegener's granulomatosis as a distinct clinicopathologic entity with his description of three patients with necrotizing granulomatous arteritis of the upper and lower respiratory tract, including the sinuses, middle ear, and nasopharynx.[29, 30] The classic diagnostic criteria for Wegener's granulomatosis were based on the detailed clinicopathologic description of Godman and Churg in their 1954 publication and included the triad of (1) necrotizing granulomatous vasculitis of the upper and lower respiratory tract, (2) focal necrotizing glomerulonephritis, and (3) systemic necrotizing vasculitis involving both arteries and veins.[20]

This classic form of the disease was almost always fatal prior to introduction of cytotoxic immunosuppressive therapy.[19, 31] The use of systemic cytotoxic immunosuppressive agents heralded a new era in the treatment of Wegener's granulomatosis. The effectiveness of combined cyclophosphamide and corticosteroid therapy in producing partial and complete remissions was demonstrated prospectively at the National Institutes of Health (NIH)

TABLE 58–1. CLASSIFICATION OF VASCULITIS

Primary vasculitides
  Affecting large-, medium-, and small-sized vessels
    Takayasu's arteritis
    Giant cell arteritis
    Isolated angiitis of the central nervous system
  Affecting predominantly medium- and small-sized blood vessels
    Polyarteritis nodosa
    Churg-Strauss syndrome
    Wegener's granulomatosis
  Affecting predominantly small-sized blood vessels
    Microscopic angiitis
    Schönlein-Henoch syndrome
    Cutaneous leukocytoclastic angiitis
  Miscellaneous conditions
    Behçet's syndrome
    Beurger's disease
    Cogan's syndrome
    Kawasaki disease
Secondary vasculitides
  Infection-related vasculitis
  Vasculitis secondary to connective tissue disease
  Drug hypersensitivity–related vasculitis
  Vasculitis secondary to essential mixed cryoglobulinemia
  Malignancy-related vasculitis
  Hypocomplementemic urticarial vasculitis
  Post–organ transplant vasculitis
  Pseudovasculitic syndromes (antiphospholipid syndrome, atrial myxoma, endocarditis, Sneddon's syndrome)

Modified from Lie JT: Illustrated histopathologic classification criteria for selected vasculitis syndromes: American College of Rheumatology Subcommittee on Classification of Vasculitis. Arthritis Rheum 1990;33:1074–1087, with permission.

TABLE 58–2. WEGENER'S GRANULOMATOSIS— DIAGNOSTIC CRITERIA

Classic triad or complete form
  Necrotizing granuloma of the upper and lower respiratory tract
  Systemic vasculitis
  Focal necrotizing glomerulonephritis
Incomplete or limited form
  Common
    Localized, cavitary necrotic pneumonitis with sparing of the kidneys, with or without other organ involvement
  Less Common
    Isolated organ involvement sparing both the lungs and kidneys

in 1973,[32] and it has profoundly changed the outlook for this previously universally fatal disease.

More recently, the demonstration of antibodies directed against neutrophil and monocyte cytoplasmic target antigens (antineutrophil cytoplasmic antibodies [ANCAs]) (see Diagnosis section, later) has resulted in a highly specific and sensitive laboratory test for active Wegener's granulomatosis, which has facilitated its earlier diagnosis, especially in anatomically limited cases, thus favorably impacting morbidity.

EPIDEMIOLOGY

Wegener's granulomatosis is a rare inflammatory disease and the exact incidence is unclear. A preliminary estimate from Rochester, Minnesota, was 0.4 cases per 100,000.[33] Although it has been suggested that the incidence of Wegener's granulomatosis is increasing, this may simply represent the availability of ANCA testing, enabling more frequent diagnosis.[34] The peak incidence is typically in the fourth and fifth decades of life,[7, 19, 31, 35] although the disease has been observed across the whole spectrum of life, with patients as young as 3 months[22] and as old as their eighties.[36] A slight male predominance has been reported in some series,[31, 37] but a recent large study of 158 patients found an equal number of men and women.[35] Wegener's granulomatosis can be seen in any racial group, although the disease is most frequently reported in white patients.[35, 37] Although a seasonal association has been reported (the most frequent onset beginning in the winter months),[38] a more recent study found no seasonal differences.[39]

CLINICAL CHARACTERISTICS

Systemic

The clinicopathologic criteria for the classic or complete form of Wegener's granulomatosis was detailed by Godman and Churg in 1954[20] and included the triad of necrotizing granuloma of upper and lower respiratory system, systemic vasculitis, and necrotizing glomerulonephritis. However, the limited form of Wegener's granulomatosis is more common,[25] can be more indolent, may at times have a protracted clinical course,[40] and may also have a better prognosis than the complete form.[22] The disease can begin with limited organ involvement and then evolve with variable speed to a more generalized form with nose, lung, and kidney involvement.[41] Because increased awareness of the disease has made earlier diagnosis possible, the limited form may be even more common than first suspected. Although no specific criteria are established for the limited form, and any organ can be involved, the most common clinically recognized presentation is that of upper or lower respiratory system involvement, with sparing of the kidneys, with or without systemic vasculitis (see Table 58–2).

The clinical presentation of patients with Wegener's granulomatosis often includes nonspecific signs and symptoms of a systemic illness, such as fever, malaise, weight loss, arthralgias, and myalgias.[37] The earliest complaints and the most common reason for seeking medical care are usually referable to the upper respiratory tract and may include symptoms such as sinus pain, purulent nasal discharge, epistaxis resulting from chronic sinusitis and rhinitis, nasal ulceration, and serous otitis media. These can result in suppurative otitis, mastoiditis, a saddle-nose defect, and hearing loss[1, 3, 21, 35, 37] (Fig. 58–1). If a physician discovers that a patient has ulceration of the nasal mucosa, palatal ulcers, or destructive sinusitis, Wegener's granulomatosis should be strongly considered.[26] Ultimately, over 90% of patients have upper respiratory involvement.[35] Secondary bacterial infections often develop in the sinuses and are usually caused by *Staphylococcus aureus*. It has been proposed that relapse is more common in patients who are chronic nasal carriers of *S. aureus*.[42] Some laboratory evidence suggests that chronic stimulation of phagocytes by infectious agents may result in the generation of a humoral response against phagocyte cytoplasmic components.[43]

A significant proportion of patients present with pulmonary findings.[37, 44] Symptoms include cough, hemoptysis, dyspnea, and, less commonly, pleuritic chest pain and tracheal obstruction. Unilateral or bilateral pulmonary infiltrates, nodules, or both, which are the most characteristic features, are present in nearly 50% of patients initially,[35, 45] with lung disease eventually developing in 85% of patients[35] (Fig. 58–2). Pleural effusion may be found in 12% of cases.[45] However, about one third of patients will have radiographs showing infiltrates and nodules but no clinical symptoms.[35] One of the most frequent causes of diffuse pulmonary hemorrhage is Wegener's granulomatosis, and this is associated with significant morbidity.[13]

Although renal involvement is clinically evident in only 11% to 20% of cases at presentation, glomerulonephritis eventually develops in 77% to 85% of patients, usually within the first 2 years of disease onset.[35, 37] Thus, it is important for the physician not to have a false sense of security that the patient has a limited form of disease,

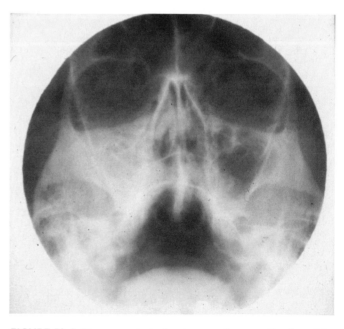

FIGURE 58–1. Sinus x-ray study showing complete opacification of the maxillary sinus on the right, and partial opacification with some bony destruction in the maxillary sinus on the left in this patient with Wegener's granulomatosis.

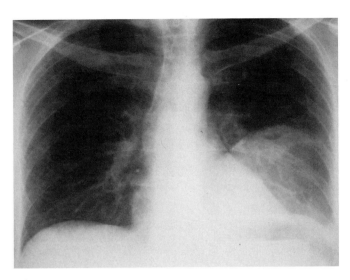

FIGURE 58–2. Chest x-ray study demonstrating pulmonary infiltrates, which is a characteristic presenting feature in a significant percentage of patients with Wegener's granulomatosis.

but rather to monitor the patient closely for more ominous renal signs. Findings ultimately include proteinuria, hematuria, red blood cell casts, and renal insufficiency. Hypertension is relatively uncommon.

Dermatologic involvement is seen in about half of the patients, although at presentation only about 13% have such findings.[35] The most common finding is purpura involving the lower extremities, with trunk and upper extremities involved infrequently. Less commonly, ulcers, vesicles, papules, subcutaneous nodules, and lesions resembling those of pyoderma may be seen. The lesions may or may not be pruritic.[46]

Arthralgias and myalgias, which occur early in the course of the disease, are common and may be seen in as many as 70% of patients.[35] They resolve without residual effects. Joint swelling and nondeforming arthritis are less commonly seen. An incorrect diagnosis of rheumatoid arthritis may be made in the presence of a false-positive rheumatoid factor (seen in 60% of patients).[35]

Nervous system involvement is seen in about one third of patients. Peripheral neuropathies, such as mononeuritis multiplex, are the most common.[47] Cranial neuropathies (most commonly of cranial nerves II, VI, and VII), external ophthalmoplegia, seizures, cerebritis, and stroke syndromes are important findings. Diabetes insipidus may occur when granulomas extend from the sinuses into the pituitary gland.[47]

Cardiac involvement is rare, with pericarditis being the most frequent (6%). Myocarditis or arteritis is relatively rare. Other infrequently involved organs are the parotid gland, breast, urethra, cervix, vagina, and gut.[35]

Pediatric patients have clinical features similar to those of adult-onset disease but with subglottic stenosis and nasal deformities being more frequent.[48–50]

Ophthalmic

Straatsma's review of the literature was the first large series of autopsy-confirmed cases of Wegener's granulomatosis published, in which ocular involvement was noted

in 43% (19 of 44) of these cases.[5] Subsequent studies report similar findings, with ophthalmic involvement ultimately present in about half of the patients (29% to 79%) (Table 58–3),[6, 7, 35, 51] although ocular abnormalities may have been noted in only 13% to 15% at presentation.[7, 35] Ocular disease can be a presenting or even the only clinically apparent manifestation of Wegener's granulomatosis.[52–61] A very limited form of the disease, with clinically apparent involvement of a single organ such as the eye, has been reported.[27] Eye and systemic disease can follow a parallel course.

The ocular manifestations of Wegener's granulomatosis are diverse and essentially any ocular tissue may be involved (see Table 58–3). Straatsma classified the ocular findings as contiguous if there was direct extension from the adjacent involved sinuses, or primary (noncontiguous) when there was lack of continuity.[5] Contiguous orbital disease may result in severe orbital pseudotumor, abscess, or cellulitis. Noncontiguous or focal disease results from a focal vasculitis, which may involve both the anterior and posterior segments of the eye and occasionally the orbit. Multiple ocular structures may simultaneously be involved. Severe ocular morbidity with vision loss or total blindness may be seen in 8% to 37% of patients, especially if the disease has been longstanding or inadequately treated, or when there has been a delay in diagnosis.[36, 51] The ocular symptoms or findings may be the presenting feature or even the only clinically apparent findings, especially in limited Wegener's granulomatosis.[7, 27, 53, 54, 56–61]

Orbital involvement is one of the most frequently reported ocular finding of Wegener's granulomatosis[5–7, 35, 51] and is usually secondary to contiguous sinus or nasal disease (Fig. 58–3). Damage may result from mass compression, vascular occlusion, or spread of an orbital cellulitis.[6] Proptosis, which is frequently painful, is a common ocular manifestation in up to one third of cases involving the eye or orbit.[35] Pseudotumor of the orbit or an orbital mass are common findings, with cranial nerve involvement and entrapment of extraocular muscle resulting in diplopia.[62] Orbital involvement can frequently result in vision loss or blindness, usually from a compressive ischemic optic neuropathy.[5, 6, 19, 20, 35] In the most recent published experience from the NIH, in a group of 158 patients with Wegener's granulomatosis, about one half of the patients with retro-orbital pseudotumors lost vision (8% of the total).[35] Nasolacrimal duct obstruction, which is seen less frequently, is a late finding and is usually associated with nasal involvement.[7, 58] Although most findings may be relatively nonspecific, proptosis in the setting of upper or lower airway disease or glomerulonephritis is strongly suggestive of Wegener's granulomatosis.[35]

Although recurrent conjunctivitis and episcleritis are frequent ocular findings in patients with Wegener's granulomatosis, they are relatively benign. In contrast, scleritis and peripheral ulcerative keratitis can lead to significant ocular morbidity, with vision loss and even blindness, if treatment is inadequate. The globe can perforate and may require enucleation. Scleritis may be nodular, diffuse, or necrotizing (Fig. 58–4). Keratitis, which is sometimes associated with scleritis, can begin as peripheral

TABLE 58-3. OPHTHALMIC INVOLVEMENT IN WEGENER'S GRANULOMATOSIS

STUDY	TOTAL (N)	OCULAR INVOLVEMENT	CONJUNCTIVA[a]	EPISCLERITIS/ SCLERITIS	KERATITIS/ PUK	UVEITIS	OPTIC NERVE	RETINAL ARTERY/VEIN OCCLUSION ± VASCULITIS OR RETINITIS	ORBITAL	NLD OBSTRUCTION
Straatsma[5]	44	19 (43)[b]	6 (32)	3 (16)	2 (11)	3 (16)	NA	1 (5)	6 (32)	NA
Haynes et al.[6]	29	14 (48)	5 (38)	4 (29)	NA	NA	4 (29)	1 (5)	7 (50)	2 (14)
Haynes et al.[6] (review of lit)	342	131 (38)	—	46 (35)[c]	—	6 (5)	—	23 (18)[d]	52 (40)	9 (7)
Spalton et al.[53]	8	—	3 (38)	3 (38)	4 (50)	3 (38)[e]	1 (13)	1 (13)	3 (38)	
Bullen et al.[7]	140	40 (28.6)	6 (15)	15 (38)	NA	4 (10)	9 (22)	7 (18)	18 (45)	10 (25)
Pinching et al.[8]	18[f]	14 (78)	7 (39)	8[g] (44)	NA	2 (11)	2 (11)[h]	Retinal vasculitis (clinical) 10 (71)[i]	—	

[a]Conjunctivitis and conjunctival hemorrhages.
[b]The number of eyes is followed by the percent of eyes in parentheses.
[c]Combined conjunctivitis, episcleritis, scleritis, and corneoscleral ulcer.
[d]Presented as retinal and optic nerve vasculitis.
[e]2 of 3 patients had associated marginal keratitis or scleritis.
[f]Study reviewed patients with severe retinal disease.
[g]Noted only episcleritis.
[h]Papilledema was the type of optic nerve involvement.
[i]Clinically diagnosed as vasculitis. Patients had hemorrhages and exudates, and fluorescein angiography showed leaking vessels. Some of the patients were hypertensive and probably had hypertensive retinopathy.
PUK, peripheral ulcerative keratitis; NLD, nasolacrimal duct.

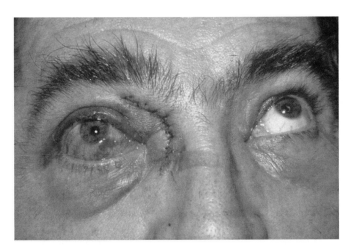

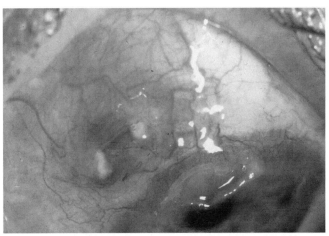

FIGURE 58–3. Orbital involvement in a patient with Wegener's granulomatosis with proptosis and limitation of extraocular movement.

FIGURE 58–4. Necrotizing scleritis with associated peripheral keratitis in a patient with Wegener's granulomatosis. (See color insert.)

intrastromal infiltrates, ultimately ulcerating, and progressing circumferentially and centrally. Scleritis, with or without peripheral ulcerative keratitis, can be a presenting, or at times the only apparent, clinical feature of Wegener's granulomatosis.[5, 27, 51–53, 58–61, 63] It has been proposed that necrotizing scleritis with peripheral ulcerative keratitis may characterize systemic vasculitis.[64, 65] Interestingly, a recent study has reported that the sera of 46% of Wegener's granulomatosis patients had autoantibodies to one of two corneal antigens.[66] Wegener's granulomatosis–associated necrotizing scleritis appears to correlate best with systemic involvement,[63] and the onset of scleritis may portend the development of systemic disease.[37]

Lid edema and granuloma, as well as sicca syndrome with positive SS-A/SS-B antibodies, have also been reported.[51, 67, 68]

The uveitis associated with Wegener's granulomatosis is nonspecific, is unilateral or bilateral, and can be anterior, intermediate, or posterior, with or without vitritis[5, 7, 24, 51, 69–71] (Fig. 58–5). Although about 10% of

patients with Wegener's granulomatosis and ocular involvement have been reported to have uveitis (the majority having a nonspecific anterior uveitis), many have undoubtedly been associated with scleritis or keratitis.[6, 51, 59, 60, 71, 72] Foster and Sainz de la Maza reported that 42% of their 14 patients with Wegener's granulomatosis–associated scleritis had anterior uveitis.[60] However, the incidence was no different than in 158 scleritis patients without Wegener's granulomatosis, thus leading them to conclude that there was no association, per se, between Wegener's granulomatosis and anterior uveitis.[60] In contrast to scleritis, uveitis has usually not been the presenting manifestation of Wegener's granulomatosis, as most patients had established disease or had previously presented with other symptoms and signs attributable to Wegener's granulomatosis.

Intermediate uveitis with "peripheral snowballs" has been reported, although one of two cases also had diffuse scleritis.[7] Choroidal folds with uveal thickening[73] and chorioretinal ischemia with infarction presenting clini-

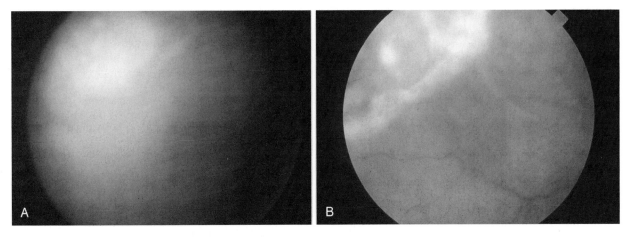

FIGURE 58–5. *A*, Posterior uveitis, with retinal vasculitis and frank retinal infarct in a patient with Wegener's granulomatosis. Note in particular the hazy view as a consequence of cells in the vitreous. *B*, Same patient as in Figure 58–5*A*, with partial resolution after institution of cyclophosphamide therapy. Note the clearing of the vitreous and a clearer view of the area of retina, which has now been destroyed through infarction. (See color insert.)

cally as single or multiple, white or creamy lesions at the level of the retinal pigment epithelium have also been reported.[74]

Retinal involvement is a relatively uncommon ophthalmic manifestation of Wegener's granulomatosis (5% to 12%), with retinal hemorrhages in the posterior or peripheral retina being the most common finding.[5–8, 24, 51] Vitreous hemorrhage may result.[24] Both central retinal artery and vein occlusions have been reported[6–8, 51]; however, the exact etiology, whether vasculitic, embolic, thrombotic, or a retro-orbital process, has not always been clearly defined. Retinal vasculitis, in the form of arteritis or periphlebitis, is an uncommon but often-reported finding[7, 24, 51] and may, at times, be seen with associated scleritis.[24, 73] Bullen and colleagues identified four patients with retinal vasculitis manifesting as retinal hemorrhages and edema, cotton-wool exudates, and choroidal thickening.[7] One of the four had hypertensive renal failure. Of the 10 patients reported by Pinching and colleagues to have clinical retinal vasculitis, all had severe renal disease and some were hypertensive, with six of six fluorescein angiograms revealing only "vascular leakage."[8] Thus, some reported cases may be the result of hypertensive retinopathy. Other reported findings have included pigment epithelial atrophy with disc edema,[51] unilateral or bilateral choroidal detachments,[51] and a case of combined detachment of the choroid and retina in conjunction with scleritis and vitritis.[71]

Retinitis with retinal vasculitis, exudates, and retinal necrosis have been reported in an occasional patient being treated with cytotoxic agents and prednisone for systemic Wegener's granulomatosis.[70, 75] Both patients in these two reports had concomitant systemic cytomegalovirus (CMV) infection. One was treated with ganciclovir with resolution of the retinitis.[75] Later, a retinal biopsy was obtained (to differentiate CMV from Wegener's granulomatosis vasculitis) at the time of repair of a complete rhegmatogenous retinal detachment.[75] The biopsy disclosed perivascular immune complex deposition without cellular infiltration and with no cytomegalic cells or viral inclusions.[75] These two cases most likely represented CMV retinitis, although vasculitis secondary to Wegener's granulomatosis cannot be excluded. These cases also highlight the importance of considering an infectious cause for the uveitis. Secondary iris neovascularization from severe uveitis or retinal vascular occlusions may result in neovascular glaucoma.[24, 51]

PATHOGENESIS/IMMUNOPATHOLOGY

The cause of Wegener's granulomatosis is unknown. A hypersensitivity phenomenon has been proposed by some because the pathologic reaction manifested by granulomatous vasculitis and glomerulonephritis is characteristic of hypersensitivity states described in animals and man.[5, 19, 31, 76] Because respiratory tract disease usually precedes renal and systemic involvement, it has been postulated that the upper and lower airways are the initial sites of stimulation in an individual susceptible to certain airborne substances. Various allergies, including allergic skin reactions, allergic rhinitis, asthma, and drug allergies, are reported to be more common in patients with Wegener's granulomatosis.[77] It is possible that infectious

agents, such as parvovirus B19[78, 79] and *Staphylococcus aureus*, may play a role by providing an antigenic primer, especially because some relapses are associated with a preceding or concurrent infection.[8, 43, 80] The role of superantigens in the pathogenesis of vasculitis has been considered, because superantigen-producing microorganisms have regularly been found in patients with Wegener's granulomatosis.[81] However, the evidence for an infectious contribution to the pathogenesis of Wegener's granulomatosis is speculative and some studies have not found an association.[32] To date, no offending antigen, microbe, chemical, or noxious agent has been isolated.

Circulating immune complexes and glomerular subepithelial immune deposits have infrequently been reported, thus being termed pauci-immune, and cryoglobulin levels are seldom elevated.[82–84] The presence of granulomas suggests a delayed-type hypersensitivity reaction and involvement of T cells. Activated T cells, predominantly CD4, are found in biopsy specimens,[85] and soluble interleukin-2 (IL-2)–receptor levels are elevated during active Wegener's granulomatosis, even when other markers of disease activity such as C-reactive protein (CRP) are normal.[86, 87] Circulating T cells obtained from patients with Wegener's granulomatosis seem to have a predominantly Th1-type profile[88, 89] with conserved T-cell-receptor-beta motifs.[90] A recent study has shown that CD4+ T cells from active Wegener's granulomatosis patients overproduce interferon-gamma and tissue necrosis factor-alpha, thus resulting in an unbalanced TH1-type profile, probably as a result of dysregulated IL-12 secretion.[91] The dose-dependent inhibition of interferon-gamma by exogenous IL-10 may have therapeutic implications for this disease.[91]

Wegener's granulomatosis has been observed in siblings.[92] A higher frequency of certain human leukocyte antigen markers (B2, B8, DR1, DR2, and DqW7) than in control subjects has been reported, without a consistent relationship to disease.[93, 94]

Role of ANCA in Wegener's Granulomatosis

It is unclear whether ANCAs play a pathologic role in Wegener's granulomatosis. The majority of the target antigens for ANCA have proteolytic activities. Studies of the interactions between ANCA and its target antigens have produced mixed results (i.e. agonistic, antagonistic, or nil [reviewed in Hoffman and Specks[95]]). Because all patients with Wegener's granulomatosis are not ANCA positive, it is unlikely that ANCAs are essential for disease pathogenesis. However, evidence suggests that they may still play an important role by enhanced neutrophil oxidative bursts and degranulation, enhanced neutrophil adhesion to endothelial cells, and synthesis and release of IL-1β from neutrophils and IL-8 from monocytes, thus enhancing the recruitment of more inflammatory cells to the site of active inflammation (reviewed in Hoffman and Specks[95]). The increased surface expression of proteinase-3 (PR3) on neutrophils, which was reported to correlate with disease activity, suggests that the interaction of ANCA with expressed PR3 may have a role in the disease.[96]

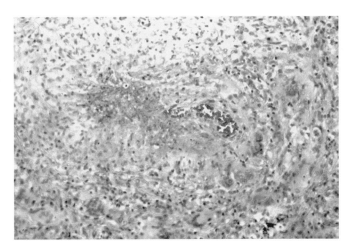

FIGURE 58–6. Lung biopsy demonstrating granulomatous inflammation in a patient with Wegener's granulomatosis. (See color insert.)

PATHOLOGY

General

Wegener, in his original report,[30] emphasized that Wegener's granulomatosis is not only a vasculitis but also a necrotizing granulomatosis. The earliest lesion of the condition in the lung has been shown to be a focus of injury and necrosis evolving into a necrotizing, palisading granuloma without the involvement of vessels.[97] Arteries, veins, and capillaries can all be affected.[98] Arteritis is typically characterized by chronic inflammation, although acute inflammation with fibrinoid necrosis may be seen in 11%. Venulitis is seen in 76% and tissue eosinophilia is seen in 63% of cases.[98] In open lung biopsies, about 90% of specimens have been found to have combination of granulomas and vasculitis, or vasculitis, necrosis, and granulomatous inflammation[98] (Fig. 58–6). In contrast, in only 7% of transbronchial biopsies is vasculitis identified.[98] Vasculitis, although present in most cases, is not necessary for the diagnosis of Wegener's granulomatosis and may not be central to the disease pathogenesis.[41, 99, 100]

The pathology of head and neck tissue differs from that of the lung, possibly because of sampling errors resulting from the small amount of tissue available from biopsies. The combination of vasculitis, necrosis, and granulomatous inflammation is found in only 16%.[101] The presence of all three features establishes the diagnosis of Wegener's granulomatosis. However, when less than the three features are present, clinical correlation is required.[102]

The most common renal lesion in Wegener's granulomatosis is focal necrotizing glomerulonephritis, with the spectrum extending from diffuse proliferative glomerulonephritis and interstitial nephritis to hyalinization of glomeruli.[35, 103, 104] Granulomatous inflammation around glomeruli and necrotizing vasculitis of small renal arteries are not common, being seen in only about 5% of cases,[11, 35–37] thus emphasizing the lack of diagnostic usefulness of a percutaneous renal biopsy.

It is imperative to exclude infectious etiologies such as *Mycobacterium*, *Nocardia*, and fungi, which may have similar histopathologic features, by using special stains and appropriate cultures. The clinical features are important for differentiating other diseases with similar histopathologic changes, such as Churg-Strauss granulomas, rheumatoid nodules, and tuberculous granulomas.

Eye Pathology

Orbital tissue demonstrates evidence of acute and chromic inflammation, with or without granulomatous vasculitis.[37, 54]

Limited ocular tissue, especially of the retina and choroid (which usually becomes available after enucleation or postmortem), may be available for systematic histopathologic evaluation. The majority of tissue is from the sclera and conjunctiva, with the latter being less specific. Necrotizing granuloma with or without inflammatory microangiopathy is very suggestive of Wegener's granulomatosis,[60] even if the classic necrotizing, granulomatous vasculitis is rarely seen[105] (Fig. 58–7). Although a recent study was able to differentiate between necrotizing scleritis that was associated with systemic autoimmune disease from those that were not by identifying the presence of zonal necrotizing granulomatous inflammation, the investigators could not differentiate between rheumatoid arthritis (the most common disease) and other systemic conditions including Wegener's granulomatosis.[106] This study was limited by the fact that, for Wegener's granulomatosis and other systemic autoimmune diseases, only a single case of each was included. Hence, the possibility remains that other differentiating features might have been detected if additional specimens had been studied.

The histopathologic findings in uveitis cases show evidence of nonspecific vasculitis and granulomatosis.[5, 52] Chronic necrotizing granulomatous reaction of the uvea and peripheral retina; perivascular leukocytoclastic infiltration of the episclera, sclera, and retinal vessels; and chronic choroiditis have been reported.[51, 59, 107] In severe cases, necrosis of the ciliary body and the iris root may be seen.[59]

DIAGNOSIS

Establishing the diagnosis of Wegener's granulomatosis is essential, because therapy with cyclophosphamide is

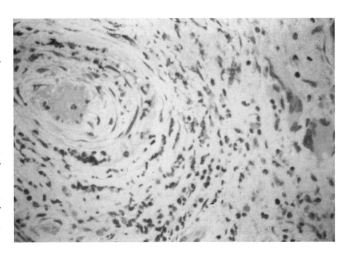

FIGURE 58–7. Photomicrograph of scleral tissue from a patient with limited Wegener's granulomatosis demonstrating granulomatous foci with collagen necrosis. (See color insert.)

required for this entity, whereas some other forms of vasculitis may be treated with corticosteroids alone. The diagnosis of Wegener's granulomatosis has historically been made using the clinicopathologic criteria of granulomatous involvement of the upper and lower respiratory tract, glomerulonephritis, and varying degrees of systemic vasculitis.[20] Various diagnostic criteria have been proposed and continue to evolve.[37, 13, 21, 108] Given the wide range of clinical presentations, including those patients with mild and indolent disease, diagnosis may be delayed. In the NIH cases, the median and mean times from the onset of symptoms to the diagnosis of Wegener's granulomatosis were 4.5 and 15 months, respectively, with 8% of the patients being diagnosed 5 to 16 years later.[35]

After reviewing their data, Fauci and colleagues at the NIH recommended that to establish a definitive diagnosis of Wegener's granulomatosis, a patient should have clinical evidence of disease in at least two of three areas (upper airways, lung, and kidney), and biopsy results that show disease in at least one and preferably two of these organ systems.[37] The American College of Rheumatology has established the following criteria for the diagnosis of the Wegener's granulomatosis and to distinguish it from other vasculitides: (1) a urinary sediment containing red blood cell casts or more than five red blood cells per high-power field, (2) abnormal findings on the chest radiograph (e.g., nodules, cavities, or fixed infiltrates), (3) oral ulcers or nasal discharge, and (4) granulomatous inflammation on biopsy.[13] The presence of two or more of these four criteria was associated with an 88% sensitivity and a 92% specificity. These criteria were based on cases that had demonstrated vasculitis. However, the earliest lesion of the condition has been shown to be a focus of injury and necrosis evolving into a necrotizing, palisading granuloma without the participation of vessels.[97] Thus, cases in the granulomatous phase without vasculitis could be misclassified.

The ELK classification system proposed by DeRemee and colleagues (E = ears, nose, and throat, or upper respiratory tract; L = lung; and K = kidney) utilizes ANCA results.[21, 116] Under this system, any typical manifestation in the E, L, or K supported by typical histopathology or a positive c-ANCA test (see next section) qualifies for the diagnosis of Wegener's granulomatosis.[108]

Most laboratory findings are generally nonspecific and indicate a systemic inflammatory illness (such as normochromic, normocytic anemia; moderate leukocytosis without eosinophilia; thrombocytosis; hypergammaglobulinemia; elevated erythrocyte sedimentation rate [ESR]; and elevated CRP).[35, 37] ESR correlates better with disease activity than does CRP.[35] Levels of all immunoglobulins may be elevated, especially IgE.[109] Rheumatoid factor has been reported to be elevated in more than 50% of patients, being present most often in patients with extensive disease.[8, 35] However, antinuclear antibodies and cryoglobulins are usually absent, with complement C3 levels usually being normal. Abnormal urinary sediment, proteinuria, and creatinine clearance may denote glomerular involvement.

Antineutrophil Cytoplasmic Antibody Testing

Until the mid 1980s, there was no specific laboratory test for Wegener's granulomatosis. After the first reports of ANCAs in the early 1980s in patients with necrotizing glomerulonephritis[110] and systemic vasculitis with pulmonary symptoms,[111] ANCAs have been recognized to be both sensitive and specific for Wegener's granulomatosis.[112–115]

ANCAs are antibodies directed against cytoplasmic azurophil granules of neutrophils and monocytes. The original and still most widely used method of detection is by indirect immunofluorescence (IIF), which demonstrates two fluorescence patterns of staining on ethanol-fixed neutrophils: a granular, centrally accentuated, cytoplasmic pattern termed c-ANCA, and a perinuclear staining pattern termed p-ANCA (Fig. 58–8). The specific target antigens for ANCA responsible for each pattern of staining have been identified (Table 58–4). Enzyme-linked immunosorbent assay (ELISA) is currently used

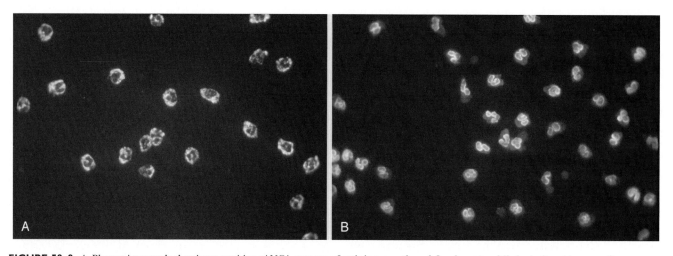

FIGURE 58–8. *A,* Photomicrograph showing a positive cANCA pattern of staining on ethanol fixed neutrophils by indirect immunofluorescence. This centrally accentuated cytoplasmic pattern of staining is characteristic for patients with Wegener's granulomatosis and is almost always due to antibodies directed against proteinase 3 (PR3). *B,* This photomicrograph demonstrates a pANCA (paranuclear) pattern of staining by indirect immunofluorescence. A variety of target antigens can produce this pattern of staining including those that are nonspecific. Myeloperoxidase (MPO) is the target antigen (as demonstrated by ELISA) with the most utility, because it is frequently associated with Wegener's granulomatosis, microscopic polyangiitis, and pauci-immune glomerulonephritis. (See color insert.)

TABLE 58–4. TARGET ANTIGENS FOR ANCA AND DISEASE ASSOCIATION

IMMUNOFLUORESCENCE PATTERN	DISEASE ASSOCIATION	TARGET ANTIGEN
c-ANCA	WG (very rarely CSS)	PR3
p-ANCA	WG, microscopic polyarteritis[195, 196] (very rarely CSS)	MPO
	Systemic vasculitis—unspecified	Azurocidin, BPI
	Rheumatic autoimmune disease (RA [16%–35%], SLE, SS, polymyositis and dermatomyositis, RP, APAS, juvenile chronic arthritis, etc.)	Lactoferrin, elastase, lysozyme, cathepsin G, MPO (rare), elastase, unidentified antigens
	IBD	
	Ulcerative colitis (40%–83%)	Cathepsin G, LF, elastase, lysozyme, and BPI
	Crohn's disease (10%–40%)	Not identified
	Other autoimmune disease	
	Primary sclerosing cholangitis (64%–87%)	
	Autoimmune hepatitis (type I)	
	Drugs	
	Hydralazine-induced lupus	MPO, elastase
	Hydralazine-induced vasculitis	MPO, lactoferrin
	Minocycline-induced arthritis, fever, livedo reticularis	MPO
	Propylthiouracil- vasculitis	PR3, MPO, elastase
	Infection[a]	
	HIV (or atypical cANCA)	Undefined
	Bacterial infection in CF	BPI
	Chromomycosis[a]	Undefined
	Malaria[b]	PR3

[a]Some with atypical c-ANCA pattern.
[b]Included here for categorization reasons.
ANCA, antineutrophil cytoplasmic antibodies; PR3, proteinase 3; c-ANCA, classic cytoplasmic ANCA; p-ANCA, perinuclear ANCA; MPO, myeloperoxidase; BPI, bactericidal/permeability-increasing protein; CSS, Churg-Strauss syndrome; RA, rheumatoid arthritis; SLE, systemic lupus erythematosus; RP, relapsing polychondritis; APAS, antiphospholipid antibody syndrome; SS, Sjögren's syndrome; IBD, inflammatory bowel disease; CF, cystic fibrosis; WG, Wegener's granulomatosis.
Modified from Hoffman GS, Specks U: Antineutrophil cytoplasmic antibodies. Arthritis Rheum 1998;41:1521–1537, with permission.

for antigen-specific ANCA determination. The c-ANCA pattern is almost always produced by antibodies against PR3[116–118] and very rarely by antibodies to other antigens (see review by Hoffman and Specks[95]), and this makes it both sensitive and specific for Wegener's granulomatosis. However, antibodies against a variety of target antigens can produce the p-ANCA fluorescence pattern, including antibodies directed against myeloperoxidase (MPO), elastase, cathepsin G, azurocidin, lactoferrin, lysozyme, and bactericidal/permeability-increasing protein, with the target antigen being elusive in many cases.[95] MPO is the target antigen with the greatest clinical utility because of its frequent association with Wegener's granulomatosis, microscopic polyangiitis, and pauci-immune glomerulonephritis.[119, 120] A p-ANCA staining result needs to be further evaluated by ELISA to assess whether the target antigen is MPO or another nonspecific antigen.

Because testing methodology and titer readings differ from laboratory to laboratory, with no international standards, values from one laboratory cannot always be compared to those from another, and thus serial titer determinations for any given patient should be performed at a single laboratory. Ideally, the IIF results should be corroborated with antigen-specific testing for PR3 and MPO (although c-ANCA by IIF is nearly always due to anti-PR3). The identification of other target antigens is of unclear clinical significance at this time.

Between 80% and 95% of all ANCA found in Wegener's granulomatosis is c-ANCA; the remainder is p-ANCA directed against MPO.[120–123] ANCA specificity is about 98%, but the sensitivity depends on disease activity and extent.[124] For patients with active generalized disease, it is about 95% sensitive, but this decreases to 41% when

the disease is in remission. The sensitivity for active limited disease is about 65%, but it is only 35% when the disease is in remission.[124]

Numerous studies have reported a relationship between ANCA titers and disease activity,[112, 114, 116, 124, 125] with the disappearance of ANCA being associated with clinical remission.[114, 126] However, this association has not been universal and cannot be relied on solely.[127–129] Despite clinical remission, elevated ANCA titers may persist in up to 40% of patients, and ANCA titer changes with disease activity in only 64% of patients.[35, 124, 126–130] Because of the time differential of months and possibly years between serologic and clinical relapse in some patients, the direct cause-and-effect relationship of ANCA titer to disease activity becomes less certain.[128, 131, 132] The lack of reversion of ANCA titers in clinical remission may be a prognosticator for early relapse as reported by Power and associates in cases of Wegener's granulomatosis–associated scleritis.[129] Thus, an ANCA titer is more predictive of activity in the serial follow-up of an individual patient than in the general comparison of groups of patients.

ANCA in Ocular Inflammation

There have been numerous studies published on the use of ANCA in patients with ocular inflammation, with either type of ANCA being present.[58, 61, 72, 73, 129, 133–135] A positive ANCA appears to be very sensitive and specific for Wegener's granulomatosis–associated scleritis.[61] Of my study of 24 patients with scleritis in whom ANCA titers were obtained, all seven with a positive ANCA had clinical and pathologic evidence of Wegener's granulomatosis. However, in none of the patients who were ANCA negative could the diagnosis of Wegener's granulomatosis eventually be established. Nölle and colleagues also found c-ANCA testing to be very specific in 72 patients with Wegener's granulomatosis and various forms of ocular inflammation.[135] The sensitivity or specificity in patients with uveitis alone is unclear. Young found a positive ANCA by IIF in 11 of 98 cases with uveitis.[133] Of the three patients who had a positive c-ANCA, two had retinal vasculitis but neither of these had Wegener's granulomatosis (one had Behçet's disease, the other had "mild colitis").[133] The remaining eight were p-ANCA positive, but the specific target antigen was not determined, and the specific clinical diagnosis was not specified. These results, from nearly a decade ago, employing IIF testing rather than ELISA, are of uncertain significance. ANCA testing in patients with contiguous orbital involvement may have a sensitivity and specificity profile similar to that reported for limited Wegener's granulomatosis.

Thus, ANCA testing is a useful adjunct for establishing the clinical diagnosis and in the management of Wegener's granulomatosis, but there are certain limitations. Therefore, neither a positive nor a negative ANCA result can be solely relied on. Patients presenting with scleritis or proptosis with associated respiratory or renal symptoms and a positive ANCA with antibodies to PR3 or MPO must be considered to have Wegener's granulomatosis, most likely, even in the absence of tissue diagnosis. The specificity of a positive ANCA is less clear in patients with isolated uveitis or retinal vasculitis, so other clinical findings and a supportive biopsy are required for the diagnosis to be established.

Evaluation of Patients

The evaluation of patients suspected to have Wegener's granulomatosis should include a complete, meticulous review of systems, laboratory testing (ANCA, ESR, CRP, complete blood count, blood urea nitrogen, creatinine, and urine analysis), a chest radiograph, and a radiograph or computed tomography scan of the sinus. Referral to a medical subspecialist and otolaryngology consultant may be required based on the ophthalmologic evaluation. Histopathologic tissue should be sought whenever possible.

TREATMENT

Historically, a variety of treatment modalities, including antibiotics,[31] chelating agents,[136] and local irradiation,[31, 137] were tried without success. The prognosis for most patients with generalized Wegener's granulomatosis, untreated or ineffectively treated with corticosteroids alone, was dismal, particularly after the recognition of functional renal impairment.[8, 31, 138] The average life expectancy for a patient with Wegener's granulomatosis without treatment was only 5 months,[31] with a 1-year survival rate of less than 20%.[10, 11, 35, 37] Steroids alone only slightly more than doubled the life expectancy to about 12 months,[138] with a 1-year survival of 34%.[11] Alternative therapies using nitrogen mustard, chlorambucil, and other cytotoxic agents suggested a better outcome.[19, 138–143]

The introduction of combination treatment with low-dose cyclophosphamide and corticosteroids dramatically altered the prognosis for this fatal disease.[10, 11, 32, 35, 37, 144] The landmark prospective study and long-term follow-up

of Wegener's granulomatosis patients at the NIH has demonstrated long-term remission rates of 93%, lasting from 7 months to 13.2 years (mean, 48 months), with a median time to remission of 12 months.[32, 35, 37] However, nearly half the patients who have achieved remission later experience at least one relapse,[35] reinforcing the importance of careful long-term follow-up.

The classic regimen from the NIH,[35, 37] which is not unlike that currently used, consists of daily oral therapy with cyclophosphamide, 2 mg/kg body weight, and prednisone, 1 mg/kg body weight. Higher doses may be used in patients with fulminant and rapidly progressive disease. The daily prednisone dose is continued for 4 weeks and changed to an alternate day regimen. The prednisone dosage is gradually tapered according to individual response to therapy. Cyclophosphamide is continued for at least 1 year after the patient has achieved complete remission. Cyclophosphamide is then tapered by 25-mg decrements every 2 to 3 months until discontinuation, or until disease recurrence requires a dose increase. The cyclophosphamide dosage may need to be adjusted to maintain acceptable blood counts (particularly a leukocyte count above 3000/mm^3).

Both oral and intravenous cyclophosphamide have been used successfully,[126, 145–149] with equal effectiveness, in combination with corticosteroids.[126] Although intermittent pulse cyclophosphamide is less toxic than daily oral cyclophosphamide and the overall monthly dose may be less, relapse may occur more frequently with the intravenous route.[11, 35, 126] The intravenous pulse cyclophosphamide dose is 15 mg/kg given in a single intravenous pulse every 4 to 6 weeks.

Because of the rarity of Wegener's granulomatosis and the sufficiently compelling results of cyclophosphamide therapy compared with the predictable natural history of the disease, no controlled randomized comparative drug trials have been conducted. However, the significant morbidity associated with cyclophosphamide therapy (see later) has prompted the use of alternative therapies, although they are still considered second-line.

Azathioprine has shown some success, but it is less effective than cyclophosphamide and should not be used as first-line therapy. It should only be considered in patients experiencing adverse side effects or when fertility concerns arise.[38, 150–154] Disease relapse has occurred when therapy has been converted from cyclophosphamide to azathioprine.

Methotrexate has also been used for the treatment of Wegener's granulomatosis without significant side effects.[155–160] Low-dose weekly methotrexate, with or without concomitant corticosteroids, has been used successfully for the maintenance of cyclophosphamide-induced remission (about 90% of the cases were successfully maintained in remission).[158] Low-dose weekly methotrexate has also been used successfully for non–life-threatening Wegener's granulomatosis, as either primary therapy or when cyclophosphamide therapy was not effective or had caused significant toxicity, with remission rates of 59% to 74%.[35, 155, 158–160] However, Stone and colleagues found a high rate of disease relapse with methotrexate, and a need to maintain patients on long-term chronic therapy.[160]

Other therapies that show promise include cyclosporine, monoclonal antibody, intravenous immunoglobulin, and protein A immunoadsorption.[161–166]

Trimethoprim-sulfamethoxazole (T/S) has been reported to be of benefit[167–172] in patients with the limited form of Wegener's granulomatosis where there is no renal involvement. The mechanism of action is unclear, and both an antimicrobial effect (which would prevent infections that would trigger relapses) and an anti-inflammatory/immunosuppressive effect are theorized. A case of very limited Wegener's granulomatosis, with a positive conjunctival biopsy, MPO-positive p-ANCA, and presenting with scleritis as the only clinically apparent manifestation, was successfully treated with oral T/S with clinical improvement and normalization of serial p-ANCA titers.[172] The anecdotal nature of such reports, the questionable diagnosis, the failure to rule out infections, and the use of concurrent immunosuppressive therapy do not provide convincing evidence of the efficacy of T/S in Wegener's, so the use of this therapy should be approached with caution.[35, 173]

Patients should be treated and appropriately monitored for myelosuppression and the potential complications of corticosteroid and cyclophosphamide or other cytotoxic agent therapy by individuals with training and experience in the use of chemotherapeutic agents.

Therapy of patients with limited disease and ophthalmic involvement should be approached with the same philosophy as patients with the complete form of the disease. Because the onset of ocular inflammation may herald systemic disease, careful review of systems and appropriate referral to a medical subspecialist to carefully assess systemic involvement is critical.

Conjunctivitis and episcleritis, which are usually not vision threatening, may be treated with local corticosteroid therapy with careful monitoring for the development of more severe ophthalmic disease. T/S may be considered, with the reservations noted.

However, the frequent failure of localized, severe, vision-threatening ophthalmic disease (orbital disease, scleritis [especially necrotizing], peripheral ulcerative keratitis, uveitis, and retinal and optic nerve vasculitis) to respond to local therapy alone[58, 59, 73, 174] and the not infrequent progression to other organ involvement with its associated morbidity require the use of systemic cytotoxic immunosuppressive therapy, as for any patient with Wegener's granulomatosis.[144] Systemic prednisone alone is not effective.[63] Thus, a systemic regimen of cyclophosphamide with the adjunctive use of systemic and local or regional corticosteroids, using the guidelines noted, should be used.

Surgical intervention may be required in patients with orbital disease (e.g., decompression and drainage), and appropriate consultation should be obtained. Tectonic scleral grafting may be required in patients with impending globe perforation from necrotizing scleritis.

Although some investigators feel that a rise in an ANCA titer in a patient with stable disease portends a clinical exacerbation[132] and justifies immunosuppressive therapy, this is not universally accepted.[35] Patients in clinical remission whose ANCA titers do not revert to normal may also be at increased risk of recurrence.[129] Power and colleagues reported on eight patients with scleritis;

disease relapse occurred in four of the five patients in whom ANCA titers had not normalized. None of the three patients whose ANCA titers normalized had a relapse.[129] Thus, close monitoring of clinically inactive patients with persistently high or rising ANCA titers is imperative.

Complications of Disease and Systemic Cytotoxic Therapy

Disease-related morbidity was seen in 86% of patients at the NIH. These complications included chronic renal insufficiency (42%), hearing loss (usually partial unilateral or bilateral) (35%), cosmetic and functional nasal deformities usually associated with chronic sinus disease (28%), tracheal stenosis (13%), and vision loss (8%).[35] Disease- and therapy-related morbidity included chronic sinus dysfunction (47%) and pulmonary insufficiency (17%).[35]

Cyclophosphamide is associated with the potential for side effects and complications. Opportunistic infections (particularly herpes zoster) may occur, as can sterility (57%), cyclophosphamide-induced cystitis (43%), bladder cancer (2.8%), and myelodysplasia (2%). Glucocorticosteroid-induced cataracts (21%), fractures (11%), aseptic necrosis of the femoral head (3%), infection, hair loss, diabetes mellitus, hypertension, Cushing's syndrome, and peptic ulcer disease may arise as a consequence of corticosteroid therapy.

There is a 2.4-fold overall increase in malignancies in patients with Wegener's granulomatosis. A 33-fold increase in bladder cancer is noted, with a latency of 7 months to 10 years after discontinuing cyclophosphamide. Thus, serial urinalyses should be obtained even after discontinuation of cyclophosphamide therapy, and the presence of hematuria warrants cystoscopy. An 11-fold increase of lymphomas is also noted. Neoplasms such as lymphocytic leukemias have been observed in patients with Wegener's granulomatosis who were treated for long periods with cytotoxic agents.[175–178]

PROGNOSIS

The outcome of Wegener's granulomatosis had dramatically improved with the introduction of daily cyclophosphamide combined with glucocorticosteroids. The prognosis for limited Wegener's granulomatosis is better than for the complete form.[22] Patients with severe renal disease, even with cytotoxic immunosuppressive therapy, have a guarded prognosis with a higher mortality.[8, 179] In the study by Pinching and colleagues of 18 patients with severe renal disease, 11 (61%) had died at 5 years, highlighting the importance for early diagnosis.[8] In the NIH series of 158 patients who had been followed from 6 months to 24 years, 91% experienced a marked improvement, and 75% achieved a complete remission.[35] Although 50% of patients in remission may have one or more relapses, 44% of patients do have remissions of greater than 5 years.[35] However, there is significant associated morbidity from the disease (86%) or side effects from the therapy (42%).[35] The socioeconomic and quality-of-life impacts of Wegener's granulomatosis are also significant.[180]

The visual prognosis depends on the severity and chronicity of the eye disease and, in general, is good when treated appropriately with systemic cytotoxic therapy. Vision loss or total blindness may be seen in 8% to 37% of patients, especially if the disease has been longstanding or inadequately treated, or when there has been a delay in diagnosis.[35, 51] Frequently, the causes are compressive optic neuropathy, retinal and optic nerve vasculitis, and globe perforation from necrotizing scleritis and peripheral ulcerative keratitis. Complications of chronic uveitis, such as cystoid macular edema, can also permanently affect vision. These findings emphasize the importance of rapid diagnosis and the institution of appropriate therapy.

CONCLUSION

Wegener's granulomatosis is no longer a universally fatal disease; rather, it is eminently treatable, with a very high chance of remission and long-term survival. Despite this dramatic improvement in prognosis, there can still be significant morbidity and even death from delays in diagnosis and from the systemic cytotoxic therapy. The importance of rapid diagnosis prior to the onset of renal disease and the initiation of appropriate therapy by a trained expert cannot be overstated. Better understanding of the immunopathogenesis of Wegener's granulomatosis, such as the role of T cells and dysregulated IL-12 secretion, may lead to more novel and selective treatment strategies, including the use of monoclonal antibodies and cytokines.

The utility of ANCA as a very sensitive diagnostic laboratory test, especially in patients with very limited disease, has greatly facilitated earlier diagnosis and may help in the clinical management of Wegener's granulomatosis, including the ocular inflammation.

The ophthalmologist must be exceedingly familiar with Wegener's granulomatosis, not only because of the diversity of ocular inflammatory manifestations present in about 50% of affected patients, but also because ocular involvement can be the only or the predominant presenting feature of the disease. The presence of corneoscleral disease may be an indicator of systemic vasculitis, so a careful systemic evaluation and timely therapy may reduce not only ocular morbidity but also systemic morbidity. Although uveitis and retinal vasculitis are less frequently encountered than scleritis or orbital disease, and they are often found in association with scleral inflammation, they can cause significant vision loss. The treatment of ocular inflammation should be similar to the approach used in other clinical variants of limited or generalized Wegener's granulomatosis. Local therapy is not effective for vision-threatening disease, nor is the use of systemic corticosteroids alone. Cytotoxic immunosuppressive agents, such as cyclophosphamide, are mandatory. The visual prognosis with appropriate therapy remains good.

References

1. Wolf SM, Fauci AS, Horn RG, Dale DC: Wegener's granulomatosis. Ann Intern Med 1974;81:513–525.
2. Falk RJ, Jennette JC: ANCA small-vessel vasculitis. J Am Soc Nephrol 1997;8:314–322.
3. Serra A, Cameron HS, Turner DR, et al: Vasculitis affecting the kidney: Presentation, histopathology and long-term outcome. Q J Med 1984;53:181–207.
4. Hogan S II, Nachman PH, Wilkman AS, et al: Prognostic markers in patients with antineutrophil cytoplasmic autoantibody-associated microscopic polyangiitis and glomerulonephritis. J Am Soc Nephrol 1996;7:23–32.
5. Straatsma BR: Ocular manifestations of WG. Am J Ophthalmol 1957;44:789.
6. Haynes BF, Fishman ML, Fauci AS, Wolff SM: The ocular manifestations of Wegener's granulomatosis. Fifteen years experience and review of the literature. Am J Med 1977;63:131–141.
7. Bullen CL, Liesegang TJ, McDonald TJ, DeRemee RA: Ocular complications of WG. Ophthalmology 1983;90:279–290.
8. Pinching AJ, Lockwood CM, Pussell BA, et al: Wegener's granulomatosis: Observations on 18 patients with severe renal disease. Q J Med 1983;208:435–460.
9. Zeek PM: Periarteritis nodosa and other forms of necrotizing angiitis. N Engl J Med 1953;248:764.
10. Fauci AS, Haynes BF, Katz P: The spectrum of vasculitis: Clinical, pathologic, immunologic, and therapeutic considerations. Ann Intern Med 1978;89:660.
11. Cupps TR, Fauci T: The Vasculitides. Philadelphia, W.B. Saunders, 1981.
12. Hunder GG, Arend WP, Bloch DA, et al: The American College of Rheumatology 1990 criteria for the classification of vasculitis: Introduction. Arthritis Rheum 1990;33:1065–1067.
13. Leavitt RY, Fauci AS, Bloch DA, et al: The American College of Rheumatology 1990 criteria for the classification of Wegener's granulomatosis: Introduction. Arthritis Rheum 1990;33:1101–1107.
14. Jennette JC, Falk RJ, Andrassy K, et al: Nomenclature of systemic vasculitides: Proposal of an international consensus conference (review). Arthritis Rheum 1994;37:187–192.
15. deShazo RD, Levinson AI, Lawless OJ, et al: Systemic vasculitis with coexistent large and small vessel involvement: A classification dilemma. JAMA 1977;238:1940–1942.
16. Lie JT: Illustrated histopathologic classification criteria for selected vasculitis syndromes: American College of Rheumatology Subcommittee on Classification of Vasculitis. Arthritis Rheum 1990;33:1074–1087.
17. Rao JK, Allen NB, Pincus T: Limitations of the 1990 American College of Rheumatology classification criteria in the diagnosis of vasculitis. Ann Intern Med 1998;129:345–352.
18. Lie JT: Nomenclature and classification of vasculitis: Plus ça change, plus c'est la meme chose (editorial). Arthritis Rheum 1994;37:181–186.
19. Fahey J, Leonard E, Churg H, Godman G: Wegener's granulomatosis. Am J Med 1954;17:168.
20. Godman CC, Churg J: Wegener's granulomatosis: Pathology and review of the literature. Arthritis Pathol 1954;58:533.
21. DeRemee RA, McDonald TJ, Harrison EG Jr, Coles DT: Wegener's granulomatosis: Anatomic correlates, a proposed classification. Mayo Clin Proc 1976;51:777–781.
22. McDonald TJ, DeRemee RA, Kern EB, Harrison EG Jr: Nasal manifestations of WG. Laryngoscope 1974;84:2101–2112.
23. Carrington CB, Leibow AA: Limited forms of angiitis and granulomatosis of Wegener's type. Am J Med 1966;41:497–527.
24. Cassan SM, Coles DT, Harrison E: The concept of limited forms of Wegener's granulomatosis. Am J Med 1970;49:366.
25. Coutu RE, Klein M, Lessell S, et al: Limited form of WG: Eye involvement as a major sign. JAMA 1975;233:868–871.
26. Liebow AA: Pulmonary angiitis and granulomatosis (Burns Amberson lecture). Am Rev Respir Dis 1973;108:1–18.
27. Niffenegger JH, Jakobiec FA, Foster CS, et al: Pathologic diagnosis of very limited (ocular or orbital) Wegener's granulomatosis. (In press)
28. Klinger H: Grenzformen der periarteritis Nodosa. Z Pathol 1931;42:455.
29. Wegener F: Über eine eigenartige rhinogene Granulomatose mit besonderer Beteilgung des Arteriensystems und der Nieren. Beitr Pathol Anat 1939;102:36.
30. Wegener F: Über generalisierte, septische Gefässerkrankungen. Verh Dtsch Ges Pathol 1936;29:202–210.
31. Walton EW: Giant-cell granuloma of the respiratory tract (Wegener's granulomatosis). Br Med J 1958;2:265.
32. Fauci AS, Wolff SM: WG: Studies in 18 patients and a review of the literature. Medicine (Baltimore) 1973;52:535.

33. Scott DG, Watts RA: Classification and epidemiology of systemic vasculitis. Br J Rheumatol 1994;33:897–900.

34. Andrews M, Edmunds M, Campbell A, et al: Systemic vasculitis in the 80s: Is there an increasing incidence of Wegener's granulomatosis and microscopic polyarteritis. J R Coll Phys 1990;24:284.

35. Hoffman GS, Kerr GS, Leavitt RY, et al: Wegener's granulomatosis: An analysis of 158 patients. Ann Intern Med 1992;116:448.

36. Valente RM, Hall S, O'Duffy JD, Conn DL: Vasculitis and related disorders. In: Kelley WN, Harris ED, Ruddy S, Sledge CB, eds: Textbook of Rheumatology, 5th ed. Philadelphia, W.B. Saunders, 1977, pp 1079–1122.

37. Fauci AS, Haynes BF, Katz P, Wolff SM: Wegener's granulomatosis: Prospective clinical and therapeutic experience with 85 patients for 21 years. Ann Intern Med 1983;98:76.

38. Raynauld JT, Bloch DA, Fries JF: Seasonal variation in the onset of Wegener's granulomatosis, polyarteritis nodosa, and giant cell arteritis. J Rheumatol 1992;20:1524.

39. Dana GF, Cotch MF, Galperin C, et al: Wegener's granulomatosis: Role of environmental exposures. Clin Exp Rheumatol 1998;16:669–674.

40. Fienberg R: The protracted superficial phenomenon in pathergic (Wegener's) granulomatosis. Hum Pathol 1981;12:458–467.

41. Specks U, DeRemee RA: Granulomatous vasculitis: Wegener's granulomatosis and Churg-Strauss syndrome. Rheum Dis Clin North Am 1990;16:377.

42. Stageman CA, Cohen Tervaert JW, Sluiter WJ, et al: Association of chronic nasal carriage of *Staphylococcus aureus* and higher relapse rates in Wegener's granulomatosis. Ann Intern Med 1994;120:12.

43. Forde AM, Feighery C, Jackson J: Anti-phagocyte antibodies and infection. Autoimmunity 1998;28:5–14.

44. Leavitt RY, Fauci AS: Pulmonary vasculitis. Am Rev Respir Dis 1986;134:149–166.

45. Cordier JF, Valeyre D, Guillevin L, et al: Pulmonary Wegener's granulomatosis: A clinical and imaging study of 77 cases. Chest 1990;97:906.

46. Frances C, Du LTH, Piette JC, et al: Wegener's granulomatosis: Dermatological manifestations in 75 cases with clinicopathologic correlation. Arch Dermatol 1994;130:861.

47. Nishino H, Rubino PA, DeRemee RA, et al: Neurological involvement in Wegener's granulomatosis: An analysis of 324 consecutive patients at the Mayo Clinic. Ann Neurol 1993;33:4.

48. Moorthy AV, Chesney RW, Segar WE, Groshong T: Wegener's granulomatosis in childhood: Prolonged survival following cytotoxic therapy. J Pediatr 1977;91:616.

49. Orlowski JP, Clough JD, Dyment PG: Wegener's granulomatosis in the pediatric age group. Pediatrics 1978;61:83.

50. Rottem M, Fauci AS, Hallahan CW, et al: Wegener's granulomatosis in children and adolescents: Clinical presentation and outcome. J Pediatr 1993;122:26.

51. Spalton DJ, Graham EM, Page NGR, Sanders MD: Ocular changes in limited forms of Wegener's granulomatosis. Br J Ophthalmol 1981;65:553–563.

52. Cogan D: Corneoscleral lesions in periarteritis nodosa and WG. Trans Am Ophthalmol Soc 1955;53:321–344.

53. Ferry AP, Leopold IH: Marginal (ring) corneal ulcer as presenting manifestation of Wegener's granuloma. A clinicopathologic study. Trans Am Acad Ophthalmol Otolaryngol 1970;74:1276.

54. Blodi FC, Gass JDM: Inflammatory pseudotumor of the orbit. Br J Ophthalmol 1968;52:79–93.

55. Weiter J, Farkas TG: Pseudotumor of the orbit as a presenting sign in WG. Surv Ophthalmol 1972;17:106–119.

56. Allen JC, France TD: Pseudotumor as the presenting sign of Wegener's granulomatosis in a child. J Pediatr Ophthalmol Strabismus 1977;14:158–159.

57. Parelhoff ES, Chavis RM, Friendly DS: WG presenting as orbital pseudotumor in children. J Pediatr Ophthalmol Strabismus 1985;22:100–104.

58. Kalina PH, Garrity JA, Herman D, et al: Role of testing anticytoplasmic autoantibodies in the differential diagnosis of scleritis and orbital pseudotumor. Mayo Clin Proc 1990;65:1110–1117.

59. Brubaker R, Font RL, Shepherd EM: Granulomatous sclerouveitis: Regression of ocular lesions with cyclophosphamide and prednisone. Arch Ophthalmol 1971;86:517–524.

60. Foster CS, Sainz de la Maza M: The Sclera. New York, Springer-Verlag, 1994.

61. Soukiasian SH, Foster CS, Niles JL, et al: Diagnostic value of antineutrophil cytoplasmic antibodies in scleritis associated with Wegener's granulomatosis. Ophthalmology 1992;99:123–132.

62. Cassan SM, Divertie MB, Hollenhorst TW, Harrison E: Pseudotumor of the orbit in limited Wegener's granulomatosis. Ann Intern Med 1970;72:687.

63. Charles SJ, Meyer PA, Watson PG: Diagnosis and management of systemic Wegener's granulomatosis presenting with anterior inflammatory disease. Br J Ophthalmol 1991;75:201–207.

64. Watson PG, Mason S: Fluorescein angiography in the differential diagnosis of sclerokeratitis. Br J Ophthalmol 1987;71:145–151.

65. Watson PG: Vascular changes in peripheral corneal destructive disease. Eye 1990;4:65–73.

66. Reynolds I, John SL, Tullo AB, et al: Characterization of two corneal epithelium-derived antigens associated with vasculitis. Invest Ophthalmol Vis Sci 1998;39:2594–2601.

67. Schmidt R, Koderisch J, Krastel H, et al: Sicca syndrome in patients with Wegener's granulomatosis. Lancet 1989;1:904–914.

68. Andrassy K, Darai G, Koderisch J, Ritz E: Immunologic abnormalities in Wegener's granulomatosis. Ann Intern Med 1983;99:127–128.

69. Samuelson TW, Margo CE: Protracted uveitis as the initial manifestation of Wegener's granulomatosis. Arch Ophthalmol 1990;108:478–479.

70. Tanihara H, Nakayama Y, Honda Y: Wegener's granulomatosis with rapidly progressive retinitis and anterior uveitis. Acta Ophthalmol 1993;71:853–855.

71. Marcus DM, Frederick AR, Raizman MB, Shore JW: Choroidal and retinal detachment in antineutrophil cytoplasmic antibody-positive scleritis. Am J Ophthalmol 1995;119:517–519.

72. de Keizer RJW, van der Woude FJ: cANCA test and the detection of Wegener's disease in sclerokeratitis and uveitis. Curr Eye Res 1990;9:59–61.

73. Pulido JS, Goeken JA, Nerad JA, et al: Ocular manifestations with circulating antineutrophil cytoplasmic antibodies. Arch Ophthalmol 1990;108:845–850.

74. Kinyoun JL, Kalina RE, Klein ML: Choroidal involvement in systemic necrotizing vasculitis. Arch Ophthalmol 1987;105:939.

75. Freeman WR, Stern WH, Gross JG, et al: Pathologic observations made by retinal biopsy. Retina 1990;10:195–204.

76. Blatt IM, Holbrooke SS, Rubin P, et al: Fatal granulomatosis of the respiratory tract (lethal midline granuloma-WG). AMA Arch Otolaryngol 1959;70:707.

77. Cuadrado MJ, D'Cruz F, Lloyd N, et al: Allergic disorders in systemic vasculitis: A case-controlled study. Br J Rheumatol 1994;33:749–753.

78. Finkel TH, Torok TJ, Ferguson PJ, et al: Chronic parvovirus B19 infection and systemic necrotizing vasculitis: Opportunistic infection or aetiological agent? Lancet 1994;343:1255–1258.

79. Niccari S, Mertsola H, Korvenrantra H, et al: Wegener's granulomatosis and parvovirus B19 infection. Arthritis Rheumatol 1994;37:1717.

80. Pinching AJ, Rees AJ, Pussel BA, et al: Relapses in Wegener's granulomatosis: Role of infection. Br Med J 1980;281:836–838.

81. Cohen Tervaert JW, Popa ER, Bos NA: The role of superantigens in vasculitis. Curr Opin Rheumatol 1999;11:23–33.

82. Ronco P, Verroust P, Mignon F, et al: Immunopathological studies of polyarteritis nodosa and WG: A report of 43 patients with 51 renal biopsies. Q J Med 1983;52:212–223.

83. Horn G, Fauci AS, Rosenthal AS, et al: Renal biopsy pathology in WG. Am J Pathol 1974;74:423.

84. Howell SB, Epstein WV: Circulating immunoglobulin complexes in WG. Am J Med 1976;60:259.

85. Brouwer E, Cohen Tervaert JW, Horst G, et al: Predominance of IgG1 and IgG4 subclasses of antineutrophil cytoplasmic autoantibodies (ANCA) in patients with WG and clinically related disorders. Clin Exp Immunol 1991;83:379–386.

86. Stegman CA, Cohen Tervaert JW, Huitema MG, et al: Serum markers of T cell activation in relapses of WG. Clin Exp Immunol 1993;91:415.

87. Schmitt WH, Heesen C, Csernok E, et al: Elevated serum levels of soluble interleukin-2 receptor in patients with WG. Arthritis Rheum 1992;35:1088.

88. Gross WL, Trabandt A, Csernok E: Pathogenesis of Wegener's granulomatosis. Ann Med Interne (Paris) 1998;149:280–286.

89. Moosig F, Csernok E, Wang G, Groos WL: Costimulatory molecules in Wegener's granulomatosis (WG): Lack of expression CD28 and preferential up-regulation of its ligands B7-1 (CD80) and B7-2 (CD86) on T cells. Clin Exp Immunol 1998;114:113–118.

90. Grunewald J, Halapi E, Wahlstrom J, et al: T-cell expansions with conserved T-cell receptor beta chain motifs in the peripheral blood of HLA-DRB1*0401 positive patients with necrotizing vasculitis. Blood 1889;92:3737.

91. Ludviksonn BR, Sneller MC, Chua KS, et al: Active Wegener's granulomatosis is associated with HLA-DR+ CD4+ T cells exhibiting an unbalanced TH1-type T cell cytokine pattern: Reversal with IL-10. J Immunol 1998;160:3602–3609.

92. Hay EM, Beaman M, Ralston AH, et al: WG occurring in siblings. Br J Rheumatol 1991;30:144.

93. Papiha SS, Murty GE, Ad'Hia A, et al: Association of WG with HLA antigens and other genetic markers. Ann Rheum Dis 1992;41:246–248.

94. Elkon KB, Sutherland DC, Rees AJ, et al: HLA-A antigens of patients with WG. Tissue Antigens 1978;11:129.

95. Hoffman GS, Specks U: Antineutrophil cytoplasmic antibodies. Arthritis Rheum 1998;41:1521–1537.

96. Muller Kobold AC, Kallenberg CG, Tervaert JW: Leukocyte membrane expression of proteinase 3 correlates with disease activity in patients with Wegener's granulomatosis. Br J Rheumatol 1998;37:901–907.

97. Feinberg R: A morphologic and immunohistologic study of the evolution of the necrotizing palisading granuloma of pathergic (Wegener's) granulomatosis. Semin Respir Med 1989;10:126–132.

98. Travis WH, Hoffman GS, Leavitt RY, et al: Surgical pathology of the lung in WG. Review of 87 open lung biopsies from 67 patients. Am J Surg Pathol 1991;15:315–333.

99. Mark EJ, Matsabara O, Tan-Liu Ns, Feinberg R: The pulmonary biopsy in the early diagnosis of Wegener's (pathergic) granulomatosis: A study based on 35 open lung biopsies. Hum Pathol 1988;19:1065–1071.

100. Wegener F: WG: Thoughts and observations of a pathologist. Eur Arch Otorhinolaryngol 1990;247:133–142.

101. Devaney KO, Travis WD, Hoffman G, et al: Interpretation of head and neck biopsies in WG. A pathologic study of 126 biopsies in 70 patients. Am J Surg Pathol 1990;14:555–564.

102. Colby TV, Tazelaar HD, Specks U, et al: Nasal biopsy in Wegener's granulomatosis (editorial). Hum Pathol 1992;22:101.

103. Antonovych TT, Sabnis SG, Tuur SM, et al: Morphological differences between polyarteritis and WG using light, electron and immunohistochemical techniques. Mod Pathol 1989;2:349–359.

104. Weiss MA, Crissman JD: Renal biopsy findings in WG: Segmental necrotizing glomerulonephritis with glomerular thrombosis. Hum Pathol 1985;15:943–956.

105. Fong LP, Sainz de la Maza M, Rice BA, et al: Immunopathology of the sclera. Ophthalmology 1991;98:472.

106. Rioano WP, Hidayat AH, Rao NA: Scleritis: A clinicopathologic study of 55 cases. Ophthalmology 199;106:1328–1333.

107. Lee AF, Wu JS, Huang DF, et al: Choroidal involvement in Wegener's granulomatosis: A case report. Chung Hua I Hsueh Tsa Chih (Taipei) 1998;61:496–499.

108. DeRemee RA: The nosology of Wegener's granulomatosis utilizing the ELK format augmented by c-ANCA. Adv Exp Med Biol 1993;336:209–215.

109. Conn DL, Gleich GJ, DeRemee RA, et al: Raised serum immunoglobulin E in Wegener's granulomatosis. Ann Rheum Dis 1976;35:377.

110. Davies DJ, Moran JE, Niall JF, Ryan GB: Segmental necrotizing glomerulonephritis with antineutrophil antibody: Possible arbovirus aetiology? Br Med J 1982;282:606.

111. Hall JB, Wadham BM, Wood CJ, et al: Vasculitis and glomerulonephritis: A subgroup with an antineutrophil cytoplasmic antibody. Aust N Z Med 1984;12:277–278.

112. Van der Woude FJ, Rasmussen N, Lobatto S: Autoantibodies against neutrophils and monocytes: Tool for diagnosis and marker of disease activity in Wegener's granulomatosis. Lancet 1985;1:425–429.

113. Savage COS, Winearls CG, Jones S, et al: Prospective study of radioimmunoassay for the diagnosis of systemic vasculitis. Lancet 1987;1:1389–1393.

114. Specks U, Wheatly CL, McDonald TJ, et al: Anticytoplasmic autoantibodies in the diagnosis and follow-up of Wegener's granulomatosis. Mayo Clin Proc 1989;64:28–36.

115. Lillington GA: Serodiagnosis of Wegener's granulomatosis: Pathobiologic and clinical implications. Mayo Clin Proc 1989;64:119–122.

116. Lüdemann J, Csernok E, Ulmer M, et al: Anti-neutrophil cytoplasmic antibodies in Wegener's granulomatosis: Immunodiagnostic value, monoclonal antibodies and characterization of target antigen. Neth J Med 1990;36:157–162.

117. Jennette JC, Hoidal HR, Falk RJ: Specificity of anti-neutrophil cytoplasmic antibodies for proteinase 3. Blood 1990;75:226–304.

118. Niles J, Ahmad MR, McCluskey RT: Specificity of anti-neutrophil cytoplasmic antibodies for proteinase 3 (letter). Blood 1990;75:22–64.

119. Falk RJ, Jennette JC: Anti-neutrophil cytoplasmic autoantibodies with specificity for myeloperoxidase in patients with systemic vasculitis and idiopathic necrotizing glomerulonephritis. N Engl J Med 1988;25:1652–1657.

120. Cohen Tervaert JW, Goldschmeding R, Elema HD, et al: Association of autoantibodies to myeloperoxidase with different forms of vasculitis. Arthritis Rheum 1990;33:1264–1272.

121. Hauschild S, Schmitt WH, Cserniok E, et al: ANCA in systemic vasculitides, collagen vascular diseases, rheumatic disorders and inflammatory bowel diseases. Adv Exp Med Biol 1993;336:245–251.

122. Venning MC, Quinn A, Broomhead V, Bird AG: Antibodies directed against neutrophils (c-ANCA and p-ANCA) are of distinct diagnostic value in systemic vasculitis. Q J Med 1990;77:1287–1296.

123. Savige JA, Gallicchio M, Georgiou T, Davies D: Diverse target antigens recognized by circulating antibodies in antineutrophil cytoplasmic antibody-associated renal vasculitides. Clin Exp Immunol 1990;82:238–243.

124. Nölle B, Specks U, Lüdemann J, et al: Anticytoplasmic antibodies: Their immunodiagnostic value in WG. Ann Intern Med 1989;111:28–40.

125. Cohen Tervaert JW, van der Woude FJ, Fauci AS, et al: Association between active Wegener's granulomatosis and anticytoplasmic antibodies. Arch Intern Med 1989;149:2461.

126. Falk RJ, Hogan S, Carey TS, et al: Clinical course of anti-neutrophil cytoplasmic autoantibody-associated glomerulonephritis in systemic vasculitis. Ann Intern Med 1990;113:656.

127. Geffriaud-Ricouard C, Noel LH, Chauveau D, et al: Clinical spectrum associated with ANCA of defined antigen specificities in 98 selected patients. Clin Nephrol 1993;39:125.

128. Kerr GS, Fleisher TA, Hallahan CW, et al: Limited prognostic value of changes in antineutrophil cytoplasmic antibody titer in patients with Wegener's granulomatosis. Arthritis Rheum 1993;36:365.

129. Power WJ, Rodriguez A, Neves RA, et al: Disease relapse in patients with ocular manifestations of Wegener's granulomatosis. Ophthalmology 1995;102:154–160.

130. Cohen Tervaert JW, Stegman CA, Kallenberg CGM: Serial ANCA testing is useful in monitoring disease activity of patients with ANCA-associated vasculitides. Sarcoidosis Vasc Diffuse Lung Dis 1996;13:241–245.

131. Pettersson E, Heigl Z: Antineutrophil cytoplasmic antibody titers in relation to disease activity in patients with necrotizing vasculitis: A longitudinal study. Clin Nephrol 1992;37:219.

132. Cohen Tervaert JW, Huitema MG, Hene RJ, Sluiter WJ: Prevention of relapses in Wegener's granulomatosis by treatment based on antineutrophil cytoplasmic antibody titer. Lancet 1990;336:709–711.

133. Young DW: The antineutrophil antibody in uveitis. Br J Ophthalmol 1991;75:208–211.

134. Cheung NT, Young DW: The ANCA test in ocular inflammation (letter). Acta Ophthalmol 1994;72:651–652.

135. Nölle B, Coners H, Dunker G: ANCA in ocular inflammatory disorders. Adv Exp Med Biol 1993;336:305–307.

136. Hansotia P, Peters H, Bennett M, Brown R: Chelation therapy in WG. Treatment with EDTA. Ann Otol Rhinol Laryngol 1969;78:388.

137. Merrill MD: Roentgen therapy in WG. Am J Roentgenol 1961;85:96.

138. Hollander D, Manning RT: The use of alkylating agents in the treatment of WG. Ann Intern Med 1967;67:393–398.

139. Aungst CW, Lessman EM: WG treated with nitrogen mustard. N Y J Med 1962;62:3302.

140. McIlvanie SK: WG: Successful treatment with chlorambucil. JAMA 1966;197:90–94.

141. Novack SN, Pearson CM: Cyclophosphamide therapy in Wegener's granulomatosis. N Engl J Med 1971;284:938–942.

142. Raitt JW: Wegener's granulomatosis: Treatment with cytotoxic agents and adrenocorticoids. Ann Intern Med 1971;74:344–356.

143. Isreal HL, Patchefsky AS: Wegener's granulomatosis of the lung: Diagnosis and treatment experience with 12 cases. Ann Intern Med 1971;74:881–891.

144. Reza MJ, Dornfeld L, Goldberg LS, et al: Wegener's granulomatosis. Long-term follow-up of patients treated with cyclophosphamide. Arthritis Rheum 1975;18:501–506.

145. Grotz W, Wanner C, Keller E, et al: Crescentic glomerulonephritis in Wegener's granulomatosis: Morphology, therapy, outcome. Clin Nephrol 1991;35:243–251.

146. Gross WL, Rasmussen N: Treatment of WG: The view from two non-nephrologists. Nephrol Dial Transplant 1994;9:1219–1225.

147. Hoffman GS, Leavitt RY, Fleisher TA, et al: Treatment of WG with intermittent high dose intravenous cyclophosphamide. Am J Med 1990;89:405–410.

148. Cupps TR: Cyclophosphamide: To pulse or not to pulse? Am J Med 1990;89:399–402.

149. Haubitz M, Schellong S, Gobel U, et al: Intravenous pulse administration of cyclophosphamide versus daily oral treatment in patients with antineutrophil cytoplasmic antibody-associated vasculitis and renal involvement: A prospective, randomized study. Arthritis Rheum 1998;41:1835–1844.

150. Bonroncle BA, Smith EJ, Cuppage FE: Treatment of Wegener's granulomatosis with Imuran. Am J Med 1967;42:314–318.

151. Steinman TI, Jaffe BF, Monaco AP, Wolff SM: Recurrence of Wegener's granulomatosis after kidney transplantation: Successful re-induction of remission with cyclophosphamide. Am J Med 1980;68:458–460.

152. Fairley KF, Barrie UJ, Johnson W: Sterility and testicular atrophy related to cyclophosphamide therapy. Lancet 1972;4:568–569.

153. Miller JJ, Williams GF, Leissring JC: Multiple lasting complications of cyclophosphamide, including ovarian destruction. Am J Med 1971;50:530–535.

154. Israel HL, Patchefsky AS, Saldana MJ: Wegener's granulomatosis, lymphomatoid granulomatosis, and benign lymphocytic angiitis and granulomatosis of the lung. Recognition and treatment. Ann Intern Med 1977;87:691.

155. Capizzi RL, Bertino JR: Methotrexate therapy of Wegener's granulomatosis. Ann Intern Med 1971;74:74–79.

156. Hoffman GS, Leavitt RY, Kerr GS, Fauci AS: The treatment of Wegener's granulomatosis with glucocorticoids and methotrexate. Arthritis Rheum 1992;35:1322–1329.

157. Bottlieb BS, Miller LC, Howite NT: Methotrexate treatment of Wegener granulomatosis in children. J Pediatr 1996;129:604–607.

158. de Groot K, Reinhold-Keller E, Tatsis E, et al: Therapy for the maintenance of remission in sixty-five patients with generalized Wegener's granulomatosis. Methotrexate versus trimethoprim/sulfamethoxazole. Arthritis Rheum 1996;39:2052–2061.

159. de Groot K, Muhler M, Reinhold-Keller E, et al: Induction of remission in Wegener's granulomatosis with low dose methotrexate. J Rheumatol 1998;25:492–495.

160. Stone JH, Tun W, Hellman DB: Treatment of non-life threatening Wegener's granulomatosis with methotrexate and daily prednisone as the initial therapy choice. J Rheumatol 1999;26:1134–1139.

161. Haubitz M, Koch KM, Brunkhorst R: Cyclosporin for the preven-

tion of disease reactivation in relapsing ANCA-associated vasculitis. Nephrol Dial Transplant 1998;13:2074–2076.

162. Jayne DRW, Davies MJ, Fox CJV, et al: Treatment of systemic vasculitis with pooled intravenous immunoglobulin. Lancet 1991;337:1137–1139.

163. Tuso P, Moudgil A, Hay J, et al: Treatment of antineutrophil cytoplasmic autoantibody positive systemic vasculitis and glomerulonephritis with pooled intravenous gammaglobulin. Am J Kidney Dis 1992;20:504.

164. Rossi F, Jayne DRW, Lockwood CM, Kazatchkine MD: Antiidiotypes against anti-neutrophil cytoplasmic antigen autoantibodies in normal human polyspecific IgG for therapeutic use and in the remission sera of patients with systemic vasculitis. Clin Exp Immunol 1991;83:298–303.

165. Lockwood CM, Thiru S, Isaacs HO, et al: Long-term remission of intractable systemic vasculitis with monoclonal antibody therapy. Lancet 1993;341:1620–1622.

166. Lockwood CM: Refractory Wegener's granulomatosis: A model for shorter immunotherapy of autoimmune disease. J R Coll Physicians Lond 1998;32:473–478.

167. De Remee RA, McDonald TJ, Weiland LH: WG: Observations on treatment with antimicrobial agents. Mayo Clin Proc 1985;60:27–32.

168. West BC, Todd HR, King JW: WG and trimethoprim-sulfamethoxazole. Ann Intern Med 1987;106:840–842.

169. Yuasa K, Tokitsu M, Goto H, et al: WG: Diagnosis by transbronchial lung biopsy, evaluation by gallium scintigraphy and treatment with sulfamethoxazole/trimethoprim. Am J Med 1988;84:371–372.

170. De Remee RA: The treatment of WG with trimethoprim/sulfamethoxazole: Illusion or vision? Arthritis Rheum 1988;31:1068–1072.

171. Israel HL: Sulfamethoxazole-trimethoprim therapy for WG. Arch Intern Med 1988;148:2293–2295.

172. Soukiasian SH, Jakobiec FA, Niles JL, Pavan-Langston D: Trimethoprim-sulfamethoxazole for scleritis associated with limited Wegener's granulomatosis: Use of histopathology and anti-neutrophil cytoplasmic antibody (ANCA) test. Cornea 1993;12:174–180.

173. Leavitt TY, Hoffman GS, Fauci AS: Response: The role of trimethoprim/sulfamethoxazole in the treatment of WG. Arthritis Rheum 1988;31:1073–1074.

174. Brady HR, Israel MR, Lewin WH: WG and corneo-scleral ulcer. JAMA 1965;193:248.

175. Wheeler GE: Cytoxan-associated leukemia in WG. Ann Intern Med 1991;94:361.

176. Westberg NS, Swolin B: Acute myelogenous leukemia appearing in two patients after prolonged continuous chlorambucil therapy for WG. Acta Med Scand 1976;199:373.

177. Chang H, Geary CB: Therapy-linked leukemia (letter). Lancet 1997;1:97.

178. Sant GR, Ucci AA, Meared EM: Renal immunoblastic sarcoma complicating immunosuppressive therapy for WG. Urology 1983;21:632–634.

179. Brandwein S, Esdaile J, Danoff D, et al: Wegener's granulomatosis. Clinical features and outcome in 13 patients. Arch Intern Med 1983;143:476.

180. Hoffman GS, Drucker Y, Cotch MF, et al: Wegener's granulomatosis: Patient-reported effects of disease on health, function, and income. Arthritis Rheum 1998;41:2257–2262.

59 — EYE DISEASE AND SYSTEMIC CORRELATES IN RELAPSING POLYCHONDRITIS

Richard Paul Wetzig

DEFINITION

Relapsing polychondritis (RP) is a rare autoimmune disease with protean manifestations. It frequently affects the eye, typically with episcleritis, scleritis, uveitis, vasculitis, or some related pathology. Although certain laboratory parameters may be abnormal, none are diagnostic of the disease. The diagnosis is therefore based on clinical grounds. The most distinguishing features include inflammatory episodes of auricular, nasal, or laryngotracheal cartilage and an inflammatory arthritis. Isolated findings are not sufficient to make the diagnosis of RP and can often be associated with other distinct syndromes. Rather, a particular array of signs and symptoms defines the disease, often presenting in a staggered relapsing and remitting pattern over time. It can run a relatively benign course, or it can be fatal.

The criterion of McAdam and colleagues[1] for RP, as revised by Damiani and Levine[2] and later by Isaak and colleagues,[3] is the presentation of three or more of the following six signs: recurrent chondritis of both auricles, chondritis of nasal cartilage, nonerosive inflammatory polyarthritis, inflammation of ocular structures, chondritis of the respiratory tract, or cochlear or vestibular damage. Any of these signs and a positive biopsy is also considered diagnostic. Finally, the diagnosis can be made based on chondritis in two or more separate anatomic locations, with response to corticosteroids or dapsone.

HISTORY

RP was first described by Jaksch-Wartenhorst in 1923. He called it polychondropathia.[4] In subsequent years, the disease was called polychondritis, perichondritis, chondritis, and eventually relapsing polychondritis for the first time by Pearson and coworkers in 1960.[5]

The first reported ocular histologic findings were described by Verity and colleagues in an episcleritis specimen. They included a decrease in basophilia and fragmentation of elastic tissue with an accumulation of mast cells, plasma cells, and lymphocytes around episcleral vessels.[6]

It has been noted that phylogenetically the sclera has associations with cartilage, as cartilaginous plates have been found in the sclera of lower vertebrates but not of humans. Because cartilage appears to be a primary target of the destructive immune response in RP, it has been postulated that scleral components sharing antigenicity with cartilage are the targets in ocular disease.[7] Sequestration of these ocular antigens could play a part in the pathology of RP as proposed by Magargal and coworkers.[8] Various experimental models for the immunologic privilege of the eye have been studied.[9–12]

Because of the wide variety of its clinical manifestations, an understanding of RP requires a multidisciplinary approach. Over 550 cases of RP have been reported in a broad spectrum of specialties throughout the worldwide literature.[13]

EPIDEMIOLOGY

Most series reporting findings in RP indicate an equal male-to-female ratio, a predilection for white persons, an average age of onset in the fourth decade, and multisystem involvement at the time of presentation.[3, 14, 15] In one series, the mean delay between the onset of symptoms and diagnosis was 2.9 years.[16]

CLINICAL CHARACTERISTICS

In a retrospective study of 112 patients with RP attending the Mayo Clinic, 21 had ocular symptoms at onset and 57 developed ocular symptoms during the course of the disease.[3] The authors describe ocular findings of episcleritis, scleritis, iridocyclitis, corneal infiltrates and thinning, proptosis, lid edema, retinopathy, and optic neuritis. Consistent with other investigators, they reported characteristic features of otorhinolaryngeal, respiratory, arthritic, renal, cardiovascular, dermatologic, and neurologic findings. In a study of 62 patients with RP, Zeuner and coworkers reported that 85.1% showed intermittent inflammatory episodes, and 12.9% had symptoms that persisted during follow-up.[17]

Auricular chondritis presents initially in roughly half the patients with RP and eventually develops in 80% to 90%, whereas saddle-nose deformity presents in about 20% to 25% and subsequently evolves in 30% to 60% (Fig. 59–1).[3, 17] Patients with these symptoms are seen initially by the otolaryngologist.[18] Auricular and nasal chondritis are painful, with inflammation of cartilage in ear and nose; some patients may develop epistaxis.[16]

Approximately 30% of patients with RP develop laryngotracheal involvement. Beginning with hoarseness or aphonia and local tenderness, this is the result of inflammation of cartilage, with inflammatory edema and narrowing or collapse of the airway (Fig. 59–2).[3, 16, 17] Iatrogenic airway obstruction has been reported with attempted bronchoscope, intubation, and tracheostomy.[19] Hughes and coworkers reported that, overall, 50% of deaths resulting from complications of RP were related to airway lesions.[15] Impairment of lower airway mucociliary function and a poor cough reflex may also occur as a result of inflammation of bronchial cartilage, leading to bronchitis or pneumonia.[16, 20]

General constitutional symptoms and signs, including fever, weight loss, fatigue, night sweats, and enlarged inguinal lymph nodes occur in 20% to 35% of patients with RP at disease onset; eventually, 45% to 60% are affected.[3, 17] Nondeforming, nonerosive rheumatoid factor–negative oligoarthritis or polyarthritis can occur periodically over the course of RP.[21] Virtually any joint can be involved. Anterior flail chest has resulted from joint dissolution caused by costochondritis.[16]

Both sensorineural and conductive hearing loss occur in roughly 20% to 30% of RP patients.[3, 17]

Cardiovascular disease is the second leading cause of death in patients with RP, although a causative link is not always found. Regurgitation resulting from involvement of the aortic ring, mitral regurgitation, aortic aneurysms, conduction defects, myocarditis, pericarditis, and myocardial infarction are reported.[16, 17, 22]

Skin lesions can be associated with RP, at times in the form of a nonspecific dermatitis and at other times in the form of a more characteristic leukocytoclastic vasculitis.[3, 17, 23]

Renal complications can be lethal in RP, with deaths due to glomerulonephritis reported.[3]

Associations with inflammatory bowel disease,[24] autoimmune hemolytic anemia,[25] myeloproliferative syndrome,[26] autoimmune thyroiditis,[27, 28] and insulin-dependent diabetes mellitus[27, 28] have rarely been reported.

Of particular note is the occasional association between RP and collagen vascular diseases such as rheumatoid arthritis, confusing the differential diagnosis at times, yet adding valuable insights into the pathology.[17]

CLINICAL MANIFESTATIONS OF OCULAR INVOLVEMENT

Numerous case reports of ocular inflammation in patients with RP have appeared in the literature.[29–31] Ocular mani

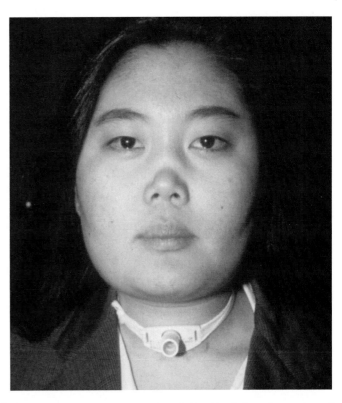

FIGURE 59–2. Relapsing polychondritis with obvious destruction of nasal cartilage, with collapse and saddle nose deformity. Note also that the patient has developed tracheal involvement as a consequence of undertreatment, with resultant need for permanent tracheostomy. (Courtesy of C. Stephen Foster, MD.) (See color insert.)

festations in 11 patients with RP and scleritis treated on the Immunology Service at the Massachusetts Eye and Ear Infirmary included necrotizing scleritis, nodular scleritis, diffuse inflammation, peripheral ulcerative keratitis, descemetocele, iritis, vitritis, retinopathy, papilledema, muscle palsy, ptosis, peripheral corneal infiltrates, and episcleritis.[32] In one large series, nonspecific ocular involvement was the first manifestation of RP in 19% of cases, whereas most patients with inflammatory eye disease tended to develop multiple systemic manifestations.[3] The data obtained by Isaak and colleagues[3] and by Zeuner and coworkers[17] are in approximate agreement, with 20% to 30% of patients with RP reported to have ocular symptoms at the time of RP onset, and around 50% ultimately developing ocular symptoms during the course of the disease. The most common eye presentations are conjunctivitis, episcleritis, and scleritis, each appearing in more than 10% of involved eyes. In addition, 5% to 10% had iritis, retinopathy, muscle paresis, or peripheral corneal thinning. Less common were lid edema, orbital inflammation, peripheral corneal infiltrates, keratitis sicca, and papilledema.[3] Overlap syndromes and ocular manifestations are too nonspecific to be used alone to make the diagnosis of RP.

Scleritis can be a sight-threatening manifestation of RP. It is either diffuse, nodular, or necrotizing.[8, 32] Scleral thinning or scleromalacia can occur, but posterior scleritis is infrequent.[33, 34] Sainz de la Maza reported, in a series of 113 eyes with scleritis, that 47.7% of the patients had

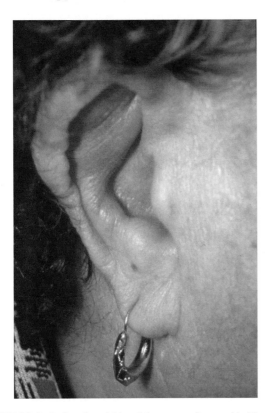

FIGURE 59–1. Active chondritis of the external ear, with 'floppiness' of that same ear as a consequence of prior episodes of chondritis with loss of cartilage. (Courtesy of C. Stephen Foster, MD.) (See color insert.)

associated systemic vasculitic disease, including 32 with rheumatoid arthritis, 14 with Wegener's granulomatosis, 11 with RP, 7 with arthritis and inflammatory bowel disease, and 7 with systemic lupus erythematosus (SLE).[35] It was observed that diffuse scleritis tended to occur without systemic vasculitis and that necrotizing scleritis tended to accompany systemic vasculitis. The occurrence of nodular scleritis did not correlate with the presence or absence of systemic vasculitis. Some investigators have noticed a parallel between scleritis or episcleritis and disease activity in RP elsewhere, most commonly the nose and joints.[3]

Iridocyclitis may be recurrent and may occur in up to 30% of RP patients, often in association with inflammation of the cornea or sclera.[1, 3, 31] Isaak and coworkers found 10 patients with iritis, 1 with choroiditis, and 9 with "retinopathy" in a cohort of 112 patients with relapsing polychodritis,[3] and Matoba and colleagues reported on another 10 patients with uveitis, 5 of whom did not have scleritis.[30] Three of the patients in the latter study developed uveitis *prior to* the development of any other symptoms of RP, and in nearly all of the patients the diagnosis of RP had not been established prior to the onset of uveitis, emphasizing the importance of the ophthalmologist in establishing the diagnosis.

Conjunctival inflammation in the form of nonspecific bilateral redness, irritation, and itching occurred in 3 of 112 patients with RP in the Mayo Clinic series, and 2 of 112 had nonspecific conjunctival hemorrhage. The same series reported mild keratoconjunctivitis sicca in several patients, with severe dry eyes in two patients with Sjögren's syndrome.[3]

Corneal thinning and ulceration have been associated with relapsing polychondritis.[3, 36–38] In addition, focal peripheral epithelial or stromal corneal infiltrates associated with ulceration, pannus, peripheral corneal thinning, perforation, or corneal edema can occur.[3, 29, 30, 36, 39] Neurosensory or exudative retinal detachments as well as retinal infiltrates and chorioretinitis with uveitis are reported in patients with RP.[1, 3, 8, 33] Isolated reports of retinal artery occlusion have appeared.[40, 41] Rarely, retinal pigment epithelial defects or retinal vein occlusion is seen.[3, 8] Cataracts, most frequently posterior subcapsular, often occur in patients with RP.[1, 3, 16] They may be caused either by the disease itself or by the corticosteroids used in its treatment.

Various neuro-ophthalmologic presentations infrequently appear with relapsing polychondritis. Extraocular muscle paresis, perhaps caused by an underlying vasculitis, are the most common and can cause ophthalmoplegia and diplopia.[13, 16, 33, 42] RP has been seen with ptosis[43] and Horner's syndrome.[15, 44]

Optic neuritis and ischemic optic neuropathy sometimes occur.[13, 33, 45, 46] Optic atrophy has been reported.[47] Also, visual field defects, perhaps caused by cerebral vasculitis, may occur.[3] Other neurologic symptoms that may present include headaches, encephalopathy, ataxia, hemiplegia, seizures, and a temporal arteritis vasculitis.[17] Papilledema may be observed.[3, 48]

Proptosis and chemosis, possibly caused by posterior orbital inflammation of cartilage, are the most common ocular adnexal findings in RP and can mimic pseudotumor.[3, 16, 33, 49–51] Other adnexal findings include lid edema that can mimic cellulitis, as well as tarsitis and dacryocystitis.[3] Secondary glaucoma sometimes occurs in the setting of keratitis or iridocyclitis.[30, 52]

End-stage eye disease in RP can unfortunately result in panophthalmitis and blindness.[36, 53]

PATHOPHYSIOLOGY/IMMUNOLOGY/ PATHOLOGY/PATHOGENESIS

No histopathologic pattern is pathognomonic for RP, and unless perichondral tissue at marginal sites of involvement is sampled, only nonspecific granulation tissue is found.[16] Any cartilage, including the elastic cartilage of the ears and nose, the hyaline cartilage of peripheral joints, the fibrocartilage at axial sites, and the cartilage of the tracheobronchial tree together with other proteoglycan-rich structures in the eye, heart, blood vessels, and inner ear may be inflamed.[16] Histologically, there is loss of basophilic staining of the cartilage matrix, perichondral inflammation at the cartilage–soft tissue interface, fibrocytic and capillary endothelial cell proliferation, perivascular mononuclear and neutrophil infiltrates, and vacuolated necrotic chondrocytes with replacement by fibrous tissue.[15, 54, 55] Biopsy of cartilage may produce structural damage and cosmetic deformity; a posterior auricular approach is the least destructive.[16]

Conjunctival biopsy in a patient with RP and scleritis showed mast cells and chronic inflammatory cells such as plasma cells and lymphocytes in the substantia propria. Additionally, there was a vasculitis defined by conjunctival vessel wall invasion with neutrophils and deposition of IgG, IgM, and complement component C3 in the vessel walls on immunofluorescent study.[32] In an eye obtained at autopsy from a patient with RP and iridocyclitis, chronic inflammatory cells and fibroblasts were found in the anterior segment, forming a cyclitic membrane.[56] In a blind eye enucleated following hypopyon uveitis, marginal keratitis and perforation, and inflammatory cellular infiltration of the corneal stroma and iris were found.[36] Additional regional findings have been perivascular lymphocytic cuffing in a biopsy of inflamed conjunctiva from one patient with episcleritis, and granulomatous inflammation of the sclera and choroid with vasculitis of the conjunctiva in another.[57] In another globe obtained at autopsy, mononuclear inflammatory cells and plasma cells were scattered about episcleral vessels.[55] Vasculitis affects a wide range of organ systems and vessels of all sizes in patients with relapsing polychondritis, from aortitis with aortic rupture to microscopic angiitis of dermatologic, renal, neural, audiovestibular, and episcleral tissue.[58]

Several lines of evidence indicate that RP might be an autoimmune disease.[59] Autoantibodies to native collagens type II[60–63] and types IX and XI[64] have been reported. Immunofluorescence microassays show granular immunoglobulin G (IgG), IgA, IgM, and complement at the junction of fibrous and cartilaginous tissue, suggesting the presence of immune complexes.[3, 65–67] Additionally, cell-mediated immune response to collagen has been reported.[68, 69] Five of 11 patients with scleritis and RP had circulating immune complexes, 5 of 11 had antinuclear antibodies, and 3 of 11 had abnormal serum complement levels in one series.[32] Patients have been reported with low titers of cytoplasmic antibody or perinuclear cytoplasmic antibody that are sometimes correlated with coexisting vasculitis.[70] In one study, cellular infiltrates were predominantly human lymphocyte antigen (HLA)-DR–positive antigen-presenting cells, with a significant number of CD4 + T lymphocytes.[71] One study of RP patients reported 8 of 21 patients with elevated anticardiolipin antibodies, 1 of 21 with elevated antiphosphatidylserine antibodies, and none with elevated anti-beta-2-glycoprotein I antibodies; the investigators suggested that, when high levels of antiphospholipid do exist, they are more likely to reflect SLE because RP patients showed no clinical signs or symptoms of antiphospholipid syndrome.[72] Circulating antibodies to corneal epithelium have been detected by immunofluorescence before and after treatment in a RP patient.[73] It has been suggested by some that immune complex deposition in the eye could explain aspects of inflammatory eye disease in patients with RP.[8]

A highly significant association between RP and the major histocompatibility locus HLA-DR4 has been found, with no statistically significant link to any of its DRB1*04 subtype alleles.[17, 18, 74] No significant association between HLA-DR4 and any specific manifestations of RP was found, and HLA-DR1 was not statistically linked to patients even when they were HLA-DR4 negative.[17] Furthermore, the extent of organ involvement was negatively correlated with HLA-DR6 in this series. The frequency of HLA-DR4 is also quite high in rheumatoid arthritis patients, although Gregerson and coworkers implicate a different role for this than for RP.[17, 75] To date, no association between RP and either the HLA-A or HLA-B loci has been detected.[74, 76] In animal models, rats or mice immunized with native type II collagen developed auricular chondritis with arthritis and positive findings on immunofluorescence, similar to those seen in humans with RP.[77, 78] The response occurs in some strains of rats or mice but not in others, suggesting immunogenetic restriction.[79, 80]

Altogether, strong evidence supports the hypothesis that RP is an autoimmune disease with vasculitis as the cause of ocular, cardiovascular, dermatologic, neurologic, and audiovestibular inflammation.[3, 17]

DIAGNOSIS

Trentham and Le enumerated various aspects of the differential diagnosis in RP.[16] The initial presentation of a painful, tender, and swollen ear in isolation is usually misdiagnosed as infectious perichondritis and needs to be distinguished from trauma, insect bite, or exposure to excessive heat or cold.[16] The ears can become floppy and soft with internal calcific deposits detectable on radiographs after repeated episodes of RP.[16] Nasal pain, hoarseness, throat pain, and difficulty talking are common presenting symptoms, as are joint pain with or without swelling caused by a seronegative nondeforming arthritis of virtually any synovial joint.[1, 2, 16] Conductive hearing loss can occur when chondritis causes closure of the external auditory canal from collapse or edema, whereas sensorineural hearing loss can result from vasculitis occurring in the vestibular or cochlear branch of the internal auditory artery.[1, 2, 16] As presenting signs in RP, the abrupt onset of hearing loss, dizziness, ataxia, nausea, and vomiting can mimic a posterior circulation stroke.[16]

Acute vestibular symptoms usually improve, but hearing loss is often permanent.[16] Recurring episcleritis or scleritis may occur early in RP but are not diagnostic in isolation and may even mistakenly suggest a reactive arthritis or spondyloarthropathy when coincident with joint symptoms.[16] Included in the differential diagnosis for RP are rheumatoid arthritis, Sjögren's syndrome, Reiter's syndrome, sarcoidosis, polyarteritis nodosa, Adamantiades-Behçet disease (ABD), Still's disease, solitary scleritis, Cogan's syndrome with interstitial keratitis plus audiovestibular symptoms, and Wegener's granulomatosis, which is distinguishable through its early involvement of noncartilaginous tissue and granulomas on biopsy.[1–3, 16]

Although biopsy and laboratory tests are nondiagnostic, nearly all patients with RP have increased nonspecific inflammatory activity as manifested by elevated erythrocyte sedimentation rate (ESR), C-reactive protein, and serum protein electrophoresis.[3, 16, 17] When rheumatoid factor or antinuclear antibodies are positive, there is usually a collagen vascular disease such as rheumatoid arthritis or SLE associated with RP.[16, 17] Out of 61 patients with RP, including two with glomerulonephritis in Zeuner's series, all had a creatinine level below 1.5 mg/dl.[17] The diagnosis of RP continues to rest on clinical findings.

Magnetic resonance imaging, computed tomography, and roentgenograms can be useful in following the course of RP, particularly with respect to laryngotracheal function.[3, 81–83] Imaging studies have also been useful in detecting abnormalities in lobar and segmental bronchi[84] and cerebral arteritis[85] in the setting of RP. Pulmonary function tests may be useful in following lower airway involvement.[20]

Roughly 25% of patients in recent large series of RP have associated collagen vascular disease such as SLE, rheumatoid arthritis, ABD, Sjögren's syndrome, or mixed connective tissue disease, whereas some are hypothyroid or have myelodysplastic syndromes.[16, 17]

TREATMENT

Topical steroids do little to alleviate ocular symptoms in RP; systemic steroids are necessary at the very least, and immunosuppressives are used in refractory cases.[16]

Dapsone is felt to be efficacious in treating extraocular manifestations of moderately severe RP.[86, 87] Azathioprine and penicillamine also have been used.[88, 89] RP has been treated with plasma exchange[90] and anti-CD4 monoclonal antibody.[91, 92] Investigators using methotrexate in RP found a steroid-sparing effect, improvement in symptoms, and increased longevity.[16, 93] One patient who developed toxicity to methotrexate improved on oral minocycline, which is sometimes used in rheumatoid arthritis.[94] RP with ocular involvement has responded to cyclosporin A.[95, 96] Cyclophosphamide has been a mainstay in the treatment of severe refractory RP.[1, 97] With respect to ocular manifestations of RP, Hoang-Xuan reported that diffuse scleritis was controlled by either indomethacin, dapsone, or cyclophosphamide, nodular scleritis was controlled by either steroids or azathioprine, and necrotizing scleritis responded only to cyclophosphamide.[32] Mortality is low with systemic chemotherapy.[98]

Lamellar keratectomy and keratoepithelioplasty are surgical approaches reported to be effective in preventing recurrence of a corneal marginal ulcers in patients with RP.[38, 99]

PROGNOSIS

It has been reported that the average duration of RP is 8 years.[16] Its course may be relatively indolent and benign, or rapidly fatal. Recent series seem to indicate a trend toward more favorable outcomes than earlier studies, perhaps because of a combination of less referral bias and improved modern treatment modalities.[14, 27] A recent series reported a survival rate of 94% over an average disease duration of 8 years,[16] whereas an earlier series reported a 5-year survival of 74%, with the most common cause of death being infection, usually in the form of pneumonia.[3] At final follow-up, Michet and colleagues[27] did not find that most patients still had symptoms requiring steroids, in contrast to Hughes and coworkers.[15] The former group noted that anemia at diagnosis was overall a bad prognostic sign for all, while saddle-nose deformity and systemic vasculitis were the worst prognostic signs for patients under 51 years of age.[27] The prognosis in RP worsens with delay in diagnosis.[3, 27]

Sainz de la Maza and colleagues reported that, in their series of patients with scleritis, the outcome of scleritis with systemic vascular disease was worse than the outcome of scleritis without systemic vasculitis.[35] It was found that scleritis associated with Wegener's granulomatosis was the most severe, scleritis with SLE or spondyloarthropathies was usually benign and self limiting, and scleritis with rheumatoid arthritis or RP was of intermediate severity.

Mortality from vascular-related events is higher when necrotizing scleritis occurs in the setting of rheumatoid arthritis.[100, 101] It might be inferred that outcomes in RP with severe ocular disease would be improved with aggressive immunosuppressive therapy.

CONCLUSIONS

Chronic debilitating diseases such as RP can extract a devastating emotional and physical toll on patients. Goldsmith notes that this is particularly true in patients with immunologic and collagen vascular diseases or cancer, motivating them to spend more time than most treating physicians will ever have to investigate their particular illness on the internet.[102] One website for uveitis in RP reads: fever, inflammatory episodes of cartilage (ear, nose, trachea, costochondritis) with arthritis (McAdam's criteria), and cardiac, renal, and skin vasculitis (http://www.uicedu/com/eye/department/guptabook/emuveitis6.htm). Patients have access to information beyond the scientific database as well. The result is a concerted distillation of information through the internet with respect to a disease process, leading to "virtual communities" of patients.[101] Instead of being steered by managed care, patients are flooded with information regarding where they should go for treatment. Physicians need not see increased patient activism as an adversarial trend. A future symbiosis between patient advocacy and provider leadership might influence free market forces in America to evolve into a kinder and gentler health care system. Perhaps it would not even be too much to hope for better education, stronger research and development, and an approach toward universal coverage as a result.

Acknowledgments

The author gratefully appreciates the help of the staff at the Webb medical library at Penrose Hospital in Colorado Springs and the staff at the Dennison medical library at the University of Colorado Health Sciences Center in Denver for valuable assistance in performing the literature search for this chapter. I also thank my wife Melissa for help with the word processing in preparation of the manuscript.

References

1. McAdam LP, O'Hanlan MA, Bluestone R, et al: Relapsing polychondritis: Prospective study of 23 patients and a review of the literature. Medicine 1976;55:193–215.
2. Damiani JM, Levine HL: Relapsing polychondritis—Report of ten cases. Laryngoscope 1979;89:929–946.
3. Isaak BL, Liesgang TJ, Michet CJ Jr: Ocular and systemic findings in relapsing polychondritis. Ophthalmology 1986;93:681–689.
4. Jaksch-Wartenhorst R: Polychondropathia. Wien Arch Intern Med 1923;6:93–100.
5. Pearson CM, Kline HM, Newcomer VD: Relapsing polychondritis. New Engl J Med 1960;263:51–58.
6. Verity MA, Larson WM, Madden SC: Relapsing polychondritis. Report of two necropsied cases with histochemical investigation of the cartilage lesion. Am J Pathol 1963;42:251–269.
7. Anderson B: XXIII Edward Jackson Memorial Lecture. Ocular lesions in relapsing polychondritis and other rheumatoid syndromes. Trans Am Acad Ophthalmol Otol 1967;71:227–242.
8. Magargal LE, Donoso LA, Goldberg RE, et al: Ocular manifestations of relapsing polychondritis. Retina 1981;1:96–97.
9. Wacker WB, Donoso LA, Kalsow CM, et al: Experimental allergic uveitis, isolation, characterization and localization of a soluble uveito-pathogenic antigen from bovine retina. J Immunol 1978;19:1949–1958.
10. Wetzig RP, Foster CS, Greene MI: Ocular immune responses. Priming of A/J mice in the anterior chamber with azobenzene arsonate-derivatized cells induces second-order-like suppressor T-cells. J Immunol 1982;128:1753.
11. Foster CS, Monroe JG, Campbell R, et al: Ocular immune responses. II. Priming of A/J mice in the vitreous induces either enhancement or suppression of subsequent hapten-specific DTH responses. J Immunol 1986;36:2787.
12. Holland EJ, Chan CC, Wetzig RP, et al: Clinical and immunohistologic studies of corneal graft rejection in the rat keratoplasty model. Cornea 1991;7:809.
13. Myasaka LS, de Andrade A, Bueno CE, et al: Relapsing polychondritis. Rev Paul Med 1998;116:1637–1642.
14. Dolan DL, Lemmon GB, Teitelbaum SL: Relapsing Polychondritis; analytical literature review and studies of pathogenesis. Am J Med 1966;41:285–299.
15. Hughes RA, Berry CL, Seifert M, et al: Relapsing polychondritis; Three cases with a clinico-pathological study and literature review. Q J Med 1972;41:363–380.
16. Trentham DE, Le CH: Relapsing polychondritis: Clinical review. Ann Intern Med 1998;129:114–122.
17. Zeuner M, Straub RH, Rauh G, et al: Relapsing polychondritis: Clinical and immunogenetic analyses of 62 patients. J Rheumatol 1997;24:96–101.
18. McCaffrey TV, McDonald TJ, McCaffrey LA: Head and neck manifestations of relapsing polychondritis: Review of 29 cases. Otolaryngology 1978;86:473–478.
19. Purcelli FM, Nahum A, Monell C: Relapsing polychondritis with tracheal collapse. Ann Otol Rhinol Laryngol 1962;71:1120–1129.
20. Mohsenifar Z, Taskin DP, Carson SA, et al: Pulmonary function in patients with relapsing polychondritis. Chest 1982;81:711–717.
21. O'Hanlan M, McAdam L, Bluestone R, et al: The arthropathy of relapsing polychondritis. Arthritis Rheum 1976;19:191–194.
22. Cipriano PR, Alonso DR, Baltaxe HA, et al: Multiple aortic aneurysms in relapsing polychondritis. Am J Cardiol 1976;37:1097–1102.
23. Maestres CA, Igual A, Botey A, et al: Relapsing polychondritis with glomerulonephritis and severe aortic insufficiency surgically treated with success. Thorac Cardiovasc Surg 1983;31:307–309.

24. Asuncion AM, Federman DG, Kirshner RS: Swelling of the ear in a patient with ulcerative colitis. Arthritis Rheum 1994;37:432–434.

25. Itabashi H, Hishinuma A, Yoshida K, et al: A case of relapsing polychondritis associated with hemolytic anemia. Jpn J Med Sci Biol 1990;29:91–93.

26. Diebold J, Rauh G, Jaeger K, et al: Bone marrow pathology in relapsing polychondritis: High frequency of myelodysplastic syndromes. Br J Haemotol 1995;89:820–830.

27. Michet CJ, McKenna CH, Harvinder S, et al: Relapsing polychondritis. Survival role of early disease manifestations. Ann Intern Med 1986;104:74–78.

28. Takamatsu K, Nishiyama T, Nkauchi Y, et al: A case of insulin dependant diabetes mellitus associated with relapsing polychondritis, Hashimoto's thyroiditis, and pituitary adrenocortical insufficiency in succession. Jpn J Med Sci Biol 1989;28:232–236.

29. Bergaust B, Abrahamsen A: Relapsing polychondritis. Report of a case presenting multiple ocular complications. ACTA Ophthalmol 1969;47:174–181.

30. Matoba A, Plager S, Barber J, et al: Keratitis in relapsing polychondritis. Ann Ophthalmol 1984;16:367–370.

31. Zierhut M, Foster CS: Uveitis and relapsing polychondritis. In: Dernouchamps JP, Verougstraete C, Caspers-Velu L, Tassighin MJ, eds: Recent Advances in Uveitis. Amsterdam, Kugler, 1993, pp 487–489.

32. Hoang-Xuan T, Foster C, Rice B: Scleritis in relapsing polychondritis. Response to therapy. Ophthalmology 1990;97:892–898.

33. McCay DA, Watson PG, Lyne AJ: Relapsing polychondritis and eye disease. Br J Ophthalmol 1974;58:600–605.

34. Turut P, Malthieu D, Leroux JL: Scleromalacia in a case of chronic atrophic polychondritis. Bull Soc Ophthalmol Fr 1981;81:589–592.

35. Sainz de la Maza M, Foster CS, Jabbur NS: Scleritis associated with systemic vasculitic diseases. Ophthalmol 1995;102:687–692.

36. Barth WF, Berson EL: Relapsing chondritis, rheumatoid arthritis and blindness. Am J Ophthalmol 1968;66:890–896.

37. Zion VM, Brakup AH, Weingeist S: Relapsing polychondritis, erythema nodosum and sclerouveitis. A case report with anterior segment angiography. Surv Ophthalmol 1974;19:107–114.

38. Martin NF, Stark WJ, Maumenee AE: Treatment of Mooren's and Mooren-like ulcer by lamellar keratectomy: Report of six eyes and literature review. Ophthalmic Surg 1987;18:564–569.

39. Michelson JB: Melting corneas with collapsing nose. Surv Ophthalmol 1984;29:148–154.

40. Hemry DA, Moss AJ, Jacox RF: Relapsing polychondritis, a "floppy" valve and migratory polytendinitis. Ann Intern Med 1972;77:576–580.

41. Ridgway HB, Hansotia PL, Schorr WP: Relapsing polychondritis. Arch Dermatol 1979;115:43–45.

42. Rucker CW, Ferguson RH: Ocular manifestations of relapsing polychondritis. Arch Ophthalmol 1965;73:46–48.

43. Dupond JL, Humbert P, Mallet H: Chronic atrophic polychondritis and exophthalmos. Ann Med Interne (Paris) 1989;140:64–65.

44. Lang H: Recurrent iridocyclitis purulenta with secondary glaucoma and recurring chondritis of the external ear, nasal cartilage and larynx. Ber Zusammenkunft Dtsch Ophthalmol Ges 1974;72:521–525.

45. Killian PJ, Susae J, Lawless OJ: Optic neuropathy in relapsing polychondritis. JAMA 1978;239:49–50.

46. Sundoram MB, Rajput AH: Nervous system complications of relapsing polychondritis. Neurology 1983;33:513–515.

47. Eckardt CE: Seltene form der Augenbeteiligung bei rezidivierender Polychondritis. Klin Monatsbl Augenheilkd 1981;178:368–372.

48. Stiles MC, Khan JA: Relapsing polychondritis. Arch Ophthalmol 1989;107:277.

49. Crovato F, Nigro A, De Marchi R, et al: Exophthalmos in relapsing polychondritis. Arch Ophthalmol 1965;73:46–48.

50. Rucker CW, Ferguson RH: Ocular manifestations of relapsing polychondritis. Arch Ophthalmol 1965;73:46–48.

51. Rosen SW, MacKenzie MR, Cohen PJ, et al: A syndrome resembling polychondritis in a patient with ulcerative colitis. Gastroenterology 1969;56:323–330.

52. Neild GH, Cameron JS, Lessof MH: Relapsing polychondritis with crescentic glomerulonephritis. Br J Med 1978;1:743–745.

53. Czarnowski J: Systemic cartilage disease. Otolaryngol Pol 1986;40:59–64.

54. Herman JH: Polychondritis. In: Kelly WN, Harrid ED, Ruddy S, et al, eds: Textbook of Rheumatology, 3rd ed. Philadelphia, W.B. Saunders, 1993, pp 134–138.

55. Trentham DE: Relapsing polychondritis. In: McCarty DJ, Koopman WJ, eds: Arthritis and allied conditions: A Textbook of Rheumatology, 12th ed. Philadelphia, Lea & Febiger, 1993, pp 1369–1375.

56. Matas BR: Iridocyclitis associated with relapsing polychondritis. Arch Ophthalmol 1970;84:474–476.

57. Anderson B: Ocular lesions in relapsing polychondritis and other rheumatoid syndromes. Am J Ophthalmol 1967;64:35–50.

58. Michet CJ: Vasculitis and relapsing polychondritis. Rheum Dis Clin North Am 1990;16:441–444.

59. Giroux L, Paquin F, Guerard-Desjardins MJ, et al: Relapsing polychondritis: An autoimmune disease. Semin Arthritis Rheum 1983;13:182–187.

60. Foidart JM, Abe S, Martin GR, et al: Antibodies to type II collagen in relapsing polychondritis. N Engl J Med 1978;299:1203–1207.

61. Meyer O, Cyna J, Dryll A, et al: Relapsing polychondritis– Pathogenic role of anti-native collagen type II antibodies: A case report with immunological and pathological studies. J Rheumatol 1981;8:820–824.

62. Terako K, Shimozuru Y, Katayama K, et al: Specificities to antibodies to type II collagen in rheumatoid arthritis. Arthritis Rheum 1990;33:1493–1500.

63. Yang CL, Brinkman J, Rui HF, et al: Autoantibodies to collagens in relapsing polychondritis. Arch Dermatol Res 1993;285:245–249.

64. Alsalemeh S, Mollenhauer J, Scheuplein F, et al: Preferential cellular and humoral immune reactivities to native and denatured collagen types IX and XI in a patient with fatal relapsing polychondritis. J Rheumatol 1993;20:1419–1424.

65. Dolan DL, Lemmon GB, Teitelbaum SL: Relapsing polychondritis. Analytical literature review and studies on pathogenesis. Am J Med 1966;41:285–298.

66. Kindblom LJ, Dalen P, Edmar G, et al: Relapsing polychondritis: A clinical pathologic-anatomic and histochemical study of 2 cases. Acta Pathol Microbiol Immunol Scand 1974;85:656–664.

67. Valenzuela R, Cooperrider PA, Gogate P: Relapsing polychondritis: Immunomicroscopic findings in cartilage ear biopsy specimens. Hum Pathol 1980;11:19–22.

68. Herman JH, Dennis MV: Immunopathologic studies in relapsing polychondritis. J Clin Invest 1973;52:549–558.

69. Rajapake DA, Bywaters EG: Cell-mediated immunity to cartilage proteoglycan in relapsing polychondritis. Clin Exp Immunol 1974;16:497–502.

70. Papo T, Piette JC, Le Thi Huong Du, et al: Antineutrophil cytoplasmic antibodies in polychondritis [letter]. Ann Rheum Dis 1993;52:384–385.

71. Svenson KG, Holmdahl R, Klareskog L, et al: Cyclosporin A treatment in a case of relapsing polychondritis. Scand J Rheumatol 1984;13:329–333.

72. Zeuner M, Straub RH, Schlosser U: Anti-phospholipid antibodies in patients with relapsing polychondritis. Lupus 1998;7:12–14.

73. Albers FW, Majoor MH, Vander Gaag R: Corneal autoimmunity in a patient with relapsing polychondritis. Eur Arch Otorhinolaryngol 1992;249:296–299.

74. Lang B, Rothenfusser A, Lauchbury JS, et al: Susceptibility to relapsing polychondritis is associated with HLA-DR4. Arthritis Rheum 1993;36:660–664.

75. Gregerson PK, Silver J, Winchester RJ: The shared epitope hypothesis. An approach to understanding the molecular genetics of susceptibility to rheumatoid arthritis. Arthritis Rheum 1988;30:1205–1213.

76. Luthra HS, McKenna CH, Terasaki PI: Lack of association of HLA-A and B locus antigens with relapsing polychondritis. Tissue Antigens 1981;17:442–443.

77. Cremer MA, Pitcock JA, Stuart JM, et al: Auricular chondritis in rats: An experimental model of relapsing polychondritis induced with type II collagen. J Exp Med 1981;154:535–540.

78. McCune WJ, Schiller AL, Dynesius-Trentham RA, et al: Type II collagen-induced auricular chondritis. Arthritis Rheum 1982;25:266–273.

79. Wooley PH, Dillon AM, Luthra HS, et al: Genetic control of type II collagen-induced arthritis in mice: Factors influencing disease susceptibility and evidence for multiple MHC-associated gene control. Transplant Proc 1983;15:180–185.

80. Griffiths MM: Immunogenetics of collagen-induced arthritis in rats. Int Rev Immunol 1988;4:1–15.

81. Eng J, Sabanathan S: Airway complications in relapsing polychondritis. Ann Thorac Surg 1991;51:686–692.

82. Fornadley JA, Seibert DJ, Ostrov BE, et al: The role of MRI when relapsing polychondritis is suspected but not proven. Int J Pediatr Otorhinolaryngol 1995;31:101–107.

83. Cossu ML, Rovasios S, Iannucelli A, et al: A case of relapsing polychondritis presenting as mediastinal syndrome, diagnosed by CT scans of the trachea and head. Panminerva Med 1997;39:233–236.

84. Davis SD, Berkmen YM, King T: Peripheral bronchial involvement in relapsing polychondritis: Demonstration by thin-section CT. Am J Radiol 1989;153:953–954.

85. Massry GG, Chung SM, Selhorst JB: Optic neuropathy, headache, and diplopia with MRI suggestive of cerebral arteritis in relapsing polychondritis. J Neuroophthalmol 1995;15:171–175.

86. Ridgway HB, Hansotia PL, Schorr WF: Relapsing polychondritis: Unusual neurological findings and therapeutic efficacy of dapsone. Arch Dermatol 1979;115:43–45.

87. Barranco VP, Minor DB, Soloman H: Treatment of relapsing polychondritis with dapsone. Arch Dermatol 1976;112:1286–1288.

88. Mohnesifar Z, Taskin DP, Carson SA, et al: Pulmonary function in patients with relapsing polychondritis. Chest 1982;81:711–717.

89. Crockford MP, Kerr IH: Relapsing polychondritis. Clin Radiol 1988;39:386–390.

90. Neilly JB, Winter JH, Stevensen RD: Progressive tracheobronchial polychondritis: Need for early diagnoses. Thorax 1985;40:78–79.

91. Choy EH, Chikanza IC, Kingsley GH, et al: Chimeric anti-CD4 monoclonal antibody for relapsing polychondritis [Letter]. Lancet 1991;338:450.

92. Van der Lubbe PA, Mittenburg AM, Breedveld FC: Anti-CD4 monoclonal antibody for relapsing polychondritis [Letter]. Lancet 1991;337:349.

93. Park J, Gowin KM, Schumacher HR: Steroid sparing effect of methotrexate in relapsing polychondritis. J Rheumatol 1996;23:937–938.

94. Trentham DE, Dynesius-Trentham RA: Antibiotic therapy for rheumatoid arthritis. Scientific and anecdotal appraisals. Rheum Dis Clin North Am 1995;21:817–834.

95. Priori R, Pardi MP, Luan FL, et al: Cyclosporin A in the treatment of relapsing polychondritis with severe recurrent eye involvement. Br J Rheumatol 1992;32:352.

96. Kung AW, Lau CS, Wu PC: Grave's ophthalmopathy and relapsing polychondritis. Clin Exp Rheumatol 1995;13:501–503.

97. Ruhlen JL, Huston KA, Wood WG: Relapsing polychondritis with glomerulonephritis. Improvement with prednisone and cyclophosphamide. JAMA 1981;245:847–848.

98. Foster CS, Forstot SL, Wilson LA: Mortality rate in rheumatoid arthritis patients developing necrotizing scleritis or peripheral ulcerative keratitis: Effects of systemic immunosuppression. Ophthalmology 1984;91:1253–1263.

99. Kato T, Yamaguchi T, Hamanaka T, et al: Corneal marginal ulcer in relapsing polychondritis: Treatment with keratoepithelioplasty. Ophthalmic Surg Lasers 1998;29:767–769.

100. Foster CS: Immunosuppressive therapy for external ocular inflammatory disease. Ophthalmology 1980;87:140–150.

101. Tuft SJ, Watson PG: Progression of scleral disease. Ophthalmology 1991;98:467–471.

102. Goldsmith J: The future of medicine. Colorado Medical Society Interim Conference, Denver, CO, Feburary 26–27, 1996.

Elisabetta Miserocchi and C. Stephen Foster

DEFINITION

Antiphospholipid syndrome (APS) is a hypercoagulable disorder with highly variable symptoms that include ocular manifestations. It is characterized by recurrent venous and arterial thrombosis, fetal losses, and thrombocytopenia associated with raised levels of antiphospholipid antibodies (aPL), which are the serologic markers of this clinical entity. Clinically, the most important aPL are anticardiolipin antibodies (aCL) and lupus anticoagulant (LAC). The presence of this heterogeneous group of antibodies was first reported in patients affected by systemic lupus erythematosus (SLE), but aPL were subsequently detected in patients without any clinical or laboratory evidence of SLE. This led investigators to define primary antiphospholipid syndrome (PAPS) as occurring in subjects without any associated medical disorder,[1-4] as opposed to secondary APS, which is associated with SLE and other collagen diseases,[5] or with certain therapeutic drugs[6,7] and infections.[6]

HISTORY

Current concepts about aPL date to the first part of this century with the development of the nontreponemal serologic tests for syphilis. Syphilis and other infections caused by *Treponema pallidum* induce antibodies that give a highly positive serologic test for syphilis.[8] But it later became clear that two types of biologic false-positive serologic tests for syphilis could occur: acute, most frequently associated with viral or other infections, and chronic, often associated with the presence of collagen vascular disease.[6,9] In the early 1940s, Mary Pangborn[9a] identified the antigenic component of the tissue used in these tests as an anionic phospholipid, which she named cardiolipin.[10] Subsequent studies characterized cardiolipin structure and found that the antibodies present in patients with syphilis have a cross reactivity with synthetic cardiolipin analogues and anionic phospholipids.[11]

In 1952, Conley and Hartmann[12] reported the occurrence of a circulating anticoagulant (synonym: inhibitor) in the setting of SLE. They also concluded that the anticoagulant was associated with clinical bleeding. Subsequently, a number of reports appeared describing no association of this inhibitor with bleeding complications, but rather a paradoxical association with thrombosis.[13] The term lupus anticoagulant was given to this inhibitor by Feinstein and Rapaport in 1972.[14]

It was then determined that patients with LAC may also have a false-positive result on a serologic tests for syphilis, with the association between SLE and the biologic false-positive serologic test for syphilis being so strong that this latter test was included in the diagnostic criteria for SLE.[15] This phenomenon was explained with the development of a radioimmunoassay that detected antibodies against the cardiolipin substrate of the syphilis test.

Finally, in 1993, G. R. Hughes[16] demonstrated a corre-lation between elevated anticardiolipin antibody levels and the presence of LAC in patients with venous and arterial thromboses, recurrent pregnancy loss, and thrombocytopenia. The association of these signs and symptoms was called antiphospholipid antibody syndrome or Hughes' syndrome.[1]

EPIDEMIOLOGY

The epidemiology of APS is still unclear because of the relatively low incidence of the disease and the poor standardization of diagnostic tests to identify the antibodies. The aPL are not specific for APS. The prevalence of aCL in the general population ranges from 0% to 14%,[17-19] with a prevalence of less than 5%.[20] The prevalence of aCL increases with age, which may reflect a normal phenomenon of aging rather than an increased risk of disease. In SLE patients, Love and Santoro found the frequency of LAC and aCL to be 34% and 44%, respectively.[21]

Occasionally, aPL may be present, although in low titers, in various autoimmune disorders other than SLE, such as Sjögren's syndrome, Adamantiades-Behçet disease (ABD), and rheumatoid arthritis. Positive levels of IgG or IgM aCL[6] in patients with rheumatoid arthritis ranged from 8% to 33%, and 13 of 70 patients with ABD were positive for aCL in a study by Sammaritano and colleagues.[6]

Other conditions that can be associated with the presence of aPL include common viral infections, such as adenovirus, rubella, chicken pox, mumps, and mycoplasma, and nonviral infections, such as syphilis, Lyme disease, Q fever, angina or adenoid vegetation treated with penicillin, and typhoid fever.[6,22,23]

Infection with the human immunodeficiency virus has been associated with aPL; the incidence of aPL in this population ranges from 20% to 42%.[6] In addition, some authors found a correlation between chronic hepatitis C and APS.[24] The presence of aPL has also been reported in cases of lymphoma and dysglobulinemia.[22] The prevalence of PAPS is still unknown.[1]

The frequent correlation between vascular complications such as stroke and myocardial infarction and the presence of aPL gave rise to many studies in patients with arteriosclerotic cardiovascular disease. The prevalence of aPL is higher in patients with stroke and myocardial infarction than in normal controls, ranging from 10% to 20%[6]; this suggest a causal role of aPL in arteriosclerotic cardiovascular disease. In addition patients with aPL have a higher frequency of recurrent stroke.

In a 1989 study of 70 patients with APS, the ratio of women to men was about 2:1 for the primary form and 9:1 for cases associated with SLE.[25] However, when patients with recurrent fetal loss were excluded, distribution between women and men was fairly equal.[6,26] APS occurs most often in relatively young patients; the median age in most series is between 35 and 45 years.[6,27] Familial occurrence of elevated levels of aPL as well as an association with human lymphocyte antigen (HLA) DR4, DR7, DQw7, and DQw53 types have been reported.[28]

CLINICAL CHARACTERISTICS

Systemic Features

The primary clinical features of APS are thrombosis, fetal loss, and thrombocytopenia, although this disease is a multisystemic disorder involving any organ system (Table 60–1). The presentation varies from the subacute (recurrent migraine, visual disturbance, and occasional dysarthria with a possible history of chorea, deep vein thrombosis, or recurrent early miscarriage) to the acute (accelerated cardiac valve failure, thrombocytopenia, major stroke, and widespread thrombosis).[16]

Thrombotic

The main associated feature is thrombosis, both venous and arterial, the latter distinguishing it from many other hypercoagulable disorders, and with the majority of symptoms being related to the location of the thrombosis. Vessels of any size can be involved: the aortic arch, the carotid artery, pulmonary vessels, and smaller skin vessels. The most common site of venous thrombosis in APS is deep venous thrombosis of the lower extremities. Other sites of venous thrombosis include retinal vein, renal vein, and hepatic veins. Lechemer and Pabinger-Fashing[29] found that venous thrombosis accounted for 71% of thrombosis in APS. In a study of 100 patients with verified venous thrombosis, 24% had aCL and 4% had LAC.[30]

Arterial thrombosis is less prevalent than venous thrombosis in patients with APS,[26] with one notable exception: The central nervous system has a special predilection for arterial thrombosis in patients with APS. Strokes and transient ischemic attacks are the most common thrombotic central nervous system (CNS) manifesta-

tions. Lechemer and Pabinger-Fashing reported the prevalence of cerebral thrombosis to be 25% and that of peripheral arterial thrombosis to be 16%.[29] Some cerebral arterial events in APS, however, are probably embolic, with mitral valve vegetation being the leading cause.[31] Rarer arterial lesions that have been described include digital and extremity gangrene and cardiac, intestinal, hepatic, and adrenal thrombosis.[6, 26]

Cardiac

Angina and myocardial infarction due to thrombosis have been reported in APS patients with aPL. The frequency of myocardial infarction is unknown, although one study found that a fifth of all young patients with myocardial infarction had aPL.[32]

Verrucous endocarditis (similar to that found in Libman-Sacks endocarditis), particularly involving the mitral valve, has been detected in patients with APS and sometimes requires valvular replacement. Khamashta and colleagues found that 38% of patients with aPL had valve abnormalities.[33] Pulmonary hypertension and pulmonary emboli are also a feature of APS.[16] In addition, intracardiac thrombi that can mimic atrial myxoma, and diffuse cardiomyopathy have been reported in these patients.[31] A screening echocardiography should be performed in all APS patients with arterial thrombosis, especially those with lesions in the cerebral or ocular distribution, because these patients seem more likely to have valvular abnormalities than do patients with venous thrombosis.[6, 26] Also, a potential role for aPL in atherosclerosis was suggested by a study that showed cross reaction between aPL and oxidized low-density lipoprotein antibodies.[34]

Neurologic

Although the most common neurologic findings of APS are ischemic strokes and transient ischemic attacks due to vascular thrombosis, or secondary to embolic events, some other neurologic conditions have been described not necessarily related to the thrombosis.

Chorea is a classic neurologic manifestation of APS.[35, 36] In addition, transverse myelopathy is associated with APS; it is the result of cord infarcts that are detectable by magnetic resonance imaging.[26, 37]

Migraine headache is a common finding in patients with APS and often precedes the diagnosis of APS by many years. Other manifestations include epilepsy, psychiatric features, and cognitive function deficit. In some untreated patients, recurrent cerebral ischemia leads to multi-infarct dementia.[16]

An association between multiple sclerosis and aPL has also been reported. In one study,[38] 22% of patients with definite or probable multiple sclerosis had a positive anticardiolipin antibody test.

Renal

Different mechanisms of renal involvement in patients with APS can lead to a variety of clinical patterns ranging from isolated hypertension to malignant hypertension, severe proteinuria, and renal failure, including cortical necrosis. Renal vein and arterial thromboses are most common features in patients with APS associated with SLE.[16] Gluek and colleagues found a higher prevalence

TABLE 60–1. SYSTEMIC MANIFESTATIONS OF THE ANTIPHOSPHOLIPID SYNDROME

Rheumatology	SLE, discoid lupus, Sjögren's syndrome, RA, vasculitis, Adamantiades-Behçet disease
Neurology	Cerebral ischemia, stroke, migraine, epilepsy, chorea, transverse myelopathy, multiple sclerosis, dementia, epilepsy, psychiatric features
Cardiology	Angina, myocardial infarction, intracardiac thrombi, verrucous endocarditis, pulmonary hypertension, atherosclerosis
Nephrology	Renal vein-arterial thrombosis, glomerular thrombosis, thrombotic microangiopathy, renal vasculitis, malignant hypertension
Dermatology	Livedo reticularis, leg ulcers, Sneddon's syndrome, skin nodules
Endocrinology	Addison's disease from adrenal thrombosis
Gastroenterology	Gut ischemia, hematemesis, liver vein thrombosis, Budd-Chiari syndrome
Hematology	Thrombocytopenia, hemolytic anemia Coombs' positive, idiopathic thrombocytopenic purpura
Obstetrics	Recurrent fetal losses
Intensive care	ARDS, acute collapse, jaundice, death

SLE, systemic lupus erythematosus; RA, rheumatoid arthritis; ARDS, acute respiratory distress syndrome.

of glomerular thrombosis in patients with aPL than in those without these antibodies.[39] Amigo and coworkers found renal disease in 25% of patients with primary APS, and the biopsy findings were consistent with thrombotic microangiopathy characterized by different degrees of severity. Thrombosis and ischemia, rather than inflammatory vasculitis, seem to have been the pathogenic mechanisms.[40]

Dermatologic

About 25% to 40% of patients with APS have cutaneous lesions. A common (if not the hallmark) cutaneous sign is livedo reticularis, occurring in 20% to 30% of patients.[27] This purple lacelike rash, most prominent on the extremities, is probably secondary to thrombosis in superficial capillaries and venulae. Other common cutaneous signs include superficial thrombophlebitis, skin nodules, and chronic leg ulcers.[16, 26] Early recognition of these relatively benign signs is important because they can be the precursor of later major thrombotic events in patients.

Patients with Sneddon-Wilkinson syndrome, which comprises the triad of livedo reticularis, cerebrovascular disease, and labile hypertension, may represent a subset of the APS.[6]

Endocrine

There has been an increasing number of reports of Addison's disease in association with aPL in recent years. The mechanism is uncertain but may involve suprarenal hemorrhage or thrombosis.[41]

Hematologic

Thrombocytopenia is a common manifestation, found in about 15% to 20% of APS patients. However, the deficit in platelet counts is often transient, and paradoxically these patients are at risk of thrombosis.[6]

Hemolytic anemia and leukopenia with a positive Coombs test have been described in patients with APS.[6, 16, 26]

Gastroenterologic

Thrombosis of the hepatic circulation can occur in patients with APS and can lead to Budd-Chiari syndrome. Recent studies report that APS is the second most common cause of this hepatic disease.[16, 42]

Obstetric

Fetal loss can occur at any stage of pregnancy, although in late stages it is more specific for APS. Diagnosis of APS as a cause of first trimester loss requires a high index of suspicion, as first trimester losses from other causes are common, occurring in about 10% of clinically recognized pregnancies.[26, 43]

Musculoskeletal

A small number of patients with primary APS develop avascular necrosis of bone. This was primarily observed in patients following orthopedic surgery.[44]

Intensive Care

Occasionally, APS occurs dramatically as "catastrophic" APS of unknown etiology.[16] There is multiple organ involvement with acute collapse, thrombocytopenia, adult respiratory distress syndrome, jaundice, and death.

TABLE 60–2. OCULAR MANIFESTATIONS OF ANTIPHOSPHOLIPID SYNDROME

Ocular symptoms	Transient blurry vision, decreased vision, transient diplopia, amaurosis fugax, transient visual field loss, headache, asymptomatic photopsia
Conjunctiva	Telangiectasias, aneurysm, episcleritis
Cornea	Keratoprecipitates, limbal keratitis
Anterior chamber	Mild flare, few cells in anterior chamber
Vitreous	Vitritis, vitreous hemorrhages
Retina	Arterial and venous thrombosis (BRVO, BRAO, CRVO, CRAO), venous tortuosity, aneurysms, cotton-wool spots, vasculitis, vascular sheathing, macular serous detachment, acute retinal necrosis, peripheral drusen, retinal ischemia, retinal neovascularization
Optic nerve	Optic disc edema, anterior ischemic optic neuropathy

BRVO, branch retinal vein occlusion; BRAO, branch retinal artery occlusion; CRVO, central retinal vein occlusion; CRAO, central retinal artery occlusion.

Ocular Features

In recent years, numerous research groups have devoted much interest to ocular APS findings. Only a few cases have been reported in the ophthalmologic literature, because the pathogenetic mechanism of aPL is still unclear and it is difficult to make an exact correlation between ocular features and the presence of aPL antibodies.

Ocular manifestations occurring during the course of primary and secondary APS include a broad clinical picture. Vaso-occlusive retinopathy and neuro-ophthalmologic symptoms are considered the hallmarks (Table 60–2).[2]

Anterior segment involvement is usually mild and relatively uncommon. It includes conjunctival telangiectasia or conjunctival microaneurysms, simple episcleritis, limbal keratitis, and keratoprecipitates with mild anterior chamber inflammation[45] (Fig. 60–1).

In addition, some authors have described a correlation

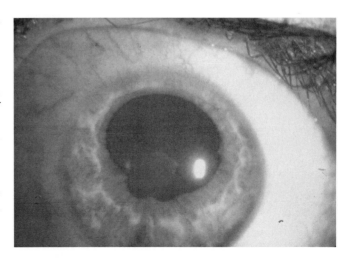

FIGURE 60–1. Anterior uveitis with pupillary membrane and posterior synechia in a patient with antiphospholipid syndrome.

between the presence of aCL and several uveitis entities. These include SLE with retinal vasculitis, acute retinal necrosis, idiopathic retinal vasculitis, and syphilis with posterior uveitis.[46]

Some patients may be symptomatic, but most patients with ocular involvement in APS present with visual symptoms such as transient blurring of vision, decreased vision, transient diplopia, amaurosis fugax, and transient field loss associated with headache and photopsia.[22, 45] In a study of 17 patients with high titers of IgG aCL antibodies, 59% presented visual symptoms.[45] In the same study, posterior segment abnormalities were found in 88% of the patients, and these included vitreous hemorrhage, vitreous cells, and swelling of the optic disc. Retinal abnormalities included venous tortuosity, vascular inflammation, pigment abnormalities, flame-shaped hemorrhages, cotton-wool spots (Fig. 60–2), microaneurysms, serous macular detachment, intraretinal microvascular abnormalities, and peripheral drusen.[45]

Vaso-occlusive Retinopathy

Many authors have reported the development of retinal vascular thrombosis in patients affected by APS. Retinal artery occlusion, venous occlusion, and capillary nonperfusion, in particular, have been described in patients suffering from primary or secondary APS.[2, 3, 22]

Retinal vaso-occlusive entities reported in the literature include central retinal vein occlusion,[47, 48] branch retinal vein occlusion,[49] central retinal artery occlusion,[50] branch retinal artery occlusion,[51] and cilioretinal artery occlusion.[23]

Retinal fluorescein angiography demonstrates a variety of patterns of vaso-occlusive retinopathy, including window defects and blocked fluorescence in the choroidal phase, areas of capillary nonperfusion, vascular obstruction, leakage, retinal neovascularization, and vascular caliber alterations such as microaneurysms, capillary ectasia, and tortuosity. Optic disc leakage may also be evident on the fluorescein angiography.[49]

The prevalence of vasculopathic eye disease involving

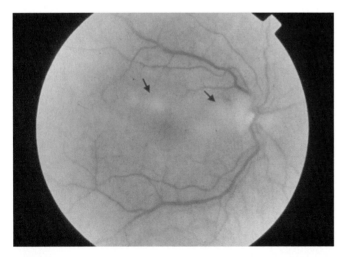

FIGURE 60–2. Posterior segment involvement in a patient with antiphospholipid syndrome. The arrows show presence of retinal cotton-wool spots. (See color insert.)

retinal and choroidal vessels in patients with PAPS is high, around 17%,[45] whereas patients with secondary APS associated with SLE are more likely to have retinal thrombotic complications.[45]

In contrast to these results, Glacet-Bernard and colleagues, in a prospective study of 75 patients, concluded that aPL antibodies are present in only 5% of patients with retinal vein occlusion, without significant difference from the control group. But, when present, especially in young patients with features of APS or SLE, aPL may constitute a contributory factor for the occlusive phenomenon.[22]

Others studies reported that vaso-occlusive retinopathy in the course of APS occurs rarely, with an incidence ranging from 0.5% to 8%.[52] Although this retinal vascular abnormality cannot be included among the classic clinical manifestations of the syndrome, its presence in association with significant serum levels of aPL, and in the absence of well-recognized risk factors, may be considered diagnostic for APS.[53]

It is also possible that a classic clinical manifestation of APS does not occur in patients with vaso-occlusive retinopathy and aPL. Nevertheless, these patients should be considered to be affected by APS, since retinal thrombosis could be the first clinical manifestation of the syndrome.[2] It is also possible that these patients will develop other thrombotic events later, such as pulmonary emboli or cerebral stroke, if correct therapy has not been implemented. Interestingly, some studies have documented an association between occlusive retinal vascular disease and cerebrovascular disease in SLE patients with raised levels of aCL.[52]

Neuro-ophthalmologic Manifestations

Central nervous system involvement in the course of the APS is not uncommon. Both visual sensory symptoms (such as monocular or bilateral transient visual loss or transient visual field loss) and visual sensory lesions (such as ischemic optic neuropathy or progressive optic atrophy) may be observed.[2, 45]

APS should be included in the differential diagnosis of optic atrophy. Support for the diagnosis of primary APS includes the insidious onset of pallor and visual loss, which would not be expected in optic neuropathy associated with temporal arteritis, ischemic optic neuropathy, or collagen vascular disease, and the lack of any other positive tests supporting alternative diagnoses.[54]

The presence of IgG aCL antibodies in patients suffering from arteritic anterior ischemic optic neuropathy, and their absence in patients with nonarteritic forms of the disease, raised questions as to their possible involvement in the pathogenesis of giant cell arteritis. It may be that antibodies deposited on the walls of arteries affected by giant cell arteritis initiate a microvascular thrombosis in the posterior ciliary arteries and peripapillary choroidal vasculature.[54, 55]

In addition, aPL might interact with nervous system phospholipids, causing spinal cord disease, such as transverse myelitis (TM).[2] Interestingly, TM is the most frequently found neurologic disease in SLE patients affected by optic neuropathy. Devic's syndrome is the name used to describe TM with optic neuritis in SLE patients. Jabs and colleagues reported that TM is the most common disorder occurring in SLE patients with optic neuropathy, reported in 54% of cases.[56]

IMMUNOLOGY

The aPL antibodies are a family of immunoglobulins (IgG, IgM, and IgA, or a mixture thereof) with varying affinities for phospholipid-protein complexes. Included in this family are LAC, aCL, and antibodies causing a biologic false-positive serologic test for syphilis.[57] LAC antibodies are recognized by their ability to interfere with phospholipid-dependent coagulation reactions, whereas aCL antibodies are known for their ability to interact with negatively charged phospholipid such as cardiolipin and phosphatidylinositol in solid-phase immunoassays.[58] In addition, different autoantibodies have been described in patients with APS.[10] These include antinuclear, anti-ssDNA, antimitochondrial, antiplatelet, antierythrocyte, antiprothrombin, anti–protein C, anti–protein S, antiendothelial cell,[59] and anti–β2-glycoprotein I (GPI) antibodies. This has led some investigators to suggest that APS is a complex autoimmune disorder in which several autoantibodies coexist with aPL.

LAC

LACs are immunoglobulins (IgG, IgM, IgA, or a mixture) that interfere with one or more of the in vitro phospholipid-dependent coagulation tests (e.g., activated partial thromboplastin time [APTT], dilute prothrombin time [dPT], kaolin clotting time [KCT], Textarin time), causing a prolongation of coagulation.[14] Several protein targets for LAC have been identified, including β2-GPI, human prothrombin, annexin V, high- and low-molecular-weight kininogens, and other vitamin K–dependent proteins, including protein C and protein S.[14]

Although the presence of an anticoagulant suggests a bleeding diathesis, only a small minority of patients with LAC experience hemorrhagic difficulties.[12] In these patients, the bleeding complications are associated with thrombocytopenia or an acquired deficiency of prothrombin.[14] The paradoxical association between the presence of antibodies prolonging phospholipid-dependent clotting tests in vitro (LAC) and the occurrence of thrombotic complications in vivo has not been elucidated. One hypothesis[60] that may explain this LAC in vitro phenomenon is an antibody-mediated agglutination of phospholipid in suspension, which would limit the surface available for coagulation reactions. When a more physiologic surface such as endothelial cells is used for the assembly of the prothrombinase complex, the agglutination of phospholipid cannot take place. In addition, the antibodies that inhibit the prothrombinase activity exert their action via binding to phospholipid-bound prothrombin. This limits the amount of prothrombin available for the prothrombinase and leads to thrombotic events.[60]

LAC has been found in patients with a variety of benign conditions, as well in healthy persons with no known systemic disease. It has also been found in patients with autoimmune diseases or infections, and after the use of certain drugs (Table 60–3).[14] In most cases, drug-induced LAC is not associated with thromboembolic complica-

TABLE 60–3. PRINCIPAL DRUGS CAUSING LUPUS ANTICOAGULANT ACTIVITY

Antibiotics	Penicillin
	Streptomycin
Antiarrhythmics	Procainamide
	Quinidine
Antihypertensives	Acebutolol
	Hydralazine
	Propranolol
Antipsychotics	Chlorpromazine
	Haloperidol
	Fluphenazine

tions. There are, however, some exceptions, including chlorpromazine, phenytoin (Dilantin), quinidine, and alpha-interferon.[14]

In the pediatric population, the presence of LAC is most often a result of intercurrent infections.[61] In the young adult and middle-aged population, LAC antibodies are most frequently identified in women, reflecting the greater incidence of autoimmune disease in this population,[14] whereas in the geriatric population many cases of LAC are drug related.[14]

The aCL Antibodies

Although aCL antibodies are so named because they bind to immobilized cardiolipin in an enzyme-linked immunosorbent assay (ELISA), they cross-react with a variety of negatively charged phospholipids besides cardiolipin, including phosphatidylserine, phosphatidylinositol, and phosphatic acid.[62] The association of aCL with the thrombotic predisposition in APS has been considered causal because of the effect of these antibodies on different components within the circulation. Thus aCL antibodies have been shown to activate cultured endothelial cells,[63] promote platelet aggregation and activation, induce tissue factor expression, and affect various coagulation pathways.[62]

The conceivable targets of aCL were thought to be negatively charged phospholipids. However, several authors recently reported that the binding of autoimmune aCL to phospholipid depended on the presence of a plasma cofactor, β2-GPI.[64]

Nonautoimmune aCL antibodies also exist, binding to negatively charged phospholipid and not depending on β2-GPI for binding. These nonautoimmune antibodies explain the aCL detected in patients with infections, and they, unlike those with APS, carry little risk of thrombosis.[26]

The β2-GPI Cofactor

In 1990, several authors found that the antigen for the antibodies detected by the ELISA test was not cardiolipin but rather a plasma protein, β2-GPI (also termed apolipoprotein H), captured on cardiolipin.[64] This finding was based on the observation that following purification of aPL autoantibodies, these antibodies do not bind to phospholipid unless incubated with human plasma or human serum.[10, 65, 66]

β2-GPI is a 50-kD glycoprotein that is present in normal plasma at a concentration of 100 to 300 μg/ml. The amino acid sequence of β2-GPI was determined by Lozier and colleagues,[62] and its complementary DNA was cloned. Its physiologic function is not known. Structurally, β2-GPI is a member of the complement control protein family, with five of the consensus repeats ("sushi" domains) that characterize this group of molecules.[65, 67] A fraction of β2-GPI circulates in association with lipoproteins, which is why it has also been termed apolipoprotein H. β2-GPI binds to anionic phospholipids, and lysine-rich segments in the fifth domain have been implicated as a phospholipid-binding region. There is evidence that β2-GPI undergoes a conformational change upon binding to anionic phospholipid, and the resulting presentation of neoepitopes has been thought to be responsible for the aCL binding.[65]

In vitro, β-GPI inhibits prothrombinase activity, contact pathway activation, ADP-induced platelet aggregation, and factor Xa generation by platelets.[67, 68] Although these data suggest that β2-GPI functions as a natural anticoagulant, deficiency of this protein is not clearly associated with an increased risk of thrombosis.[69] Recent data indicate that β2-GPI binding to membranes containing physiologic concentrations of anionic phospholipid is relatively weak; thus, normal plasma levels of β2-GPI probably have little effect on hemostatic reactions in vivo.[70] Most aPL antibodies associated with APS are directed against epitopes expressed on β2-GPI, not on cardiolipin, and the anti–β2-GPI antibodies have been reported by several authors to be a more specific serologic marker for thrombotic events than aCL in patients with APS.[71]

IMMUNOPATHOGENESIS

Despite the remarkable interest in this syndrome in the last few years, there is no sufficient explanation for the immune response that leads to the development of aPL. The most credible hypothesis is that T lymphocytes play an important role in autoantibody production and disease pathogenesis.[10] Also, aPL antibodies are directed against antigens involved in the maintenance of normal hemostasis.[26] Many of these antigens circulate in the plasma or are associated in enzyme-cofactor complexes assembled on phospholipid membranes (e.g., protein C and protein S), and therefore they can be attached by the antibodies.[1, 26] Such complexes can be in vivo immunogens and lead to the autoimmune response in APS. The mechanisms by which such complexes become immunogenic are not known.[1, 10]

Thrombosis

The pathophysiology of thrombosis in APS is also unclear. Research supports the hypothesis that the implicated autoantibodies not only are an important marker of the disease[72] but also play a direct role in the development of thrombosis, fetal losses, and thrombocytopenia.[10] Observations that support this hypothesis[73] include the facts that many of the antigens targeted by aPL are involved in thrombosis and hemostasis, that the autoantibodies and antigens are accessible to one another in circulating plasma or on cell surfaces exposed to circulating plasma (blood cells, vascular endothelium, placental trophoblast), and that antibody levels correlate with clinical risk.[10] Among the many thrombogenic mechanisms involved in APS, some of the most remarkable involve inhibition of the protein C pathway, an important anticoagulant protein. Also, autoantibodies to β2-GPI, protein S, and thrombomodulin have all been implicated in the inhibition of this pathway.[1, 26, 72]

Increased platelet aggregation is another potential mechanism for thromboembolism in APS.[26] The aPL antibodies have a direct stimulatory effect on platelets, and they promote the synthesis of the inducible form of cyclooxygenase in endothelial cells.[74] In addition, these antibodies can induce the expression of adhesion molecules on endothelial surfaces and enhance monocyte adhesion to endothelial cells.[75]

Fetal Losses

The most credible hypothesis for spontaneous abortion in APS is placental thrombosis. The immediate cause of fetal death is hypoxia due to insufficient uteroplacental blood. Histologic studies reveal that a vasculopathy of the maternal spiral artery is the most important cause of placental infarction.[26] Autoantibodies reactive with trophoblast cells have also been implicated.[76]

Thrombocytopenia

The pathogenesis of thrombocytopenia in APS is not understood; aPL may interact directly with surface proteins like β2-GPI and CD36, a membrane glycoprotein expressed on platelets and endothelial cells. This interaction may lead to increased platelet uptake and aggregation.[10]

DIAGNOSIS

Laboratory Investigations

The LAC and anticardiolipin tests are generally accepted confirmatory tests for APS.[77] The aPL, aCL, and LAC antibodies can be detected by a variety of tests, and their identification is one of the most controversial points in the management of APS because of the lack of standardization in the laboratory test and because of the numerous assays used for diagnosis.

Detection of aCL is done by ELISA; most kits use cardiolipin as the target antigen.[78, 79] This test presents a number of advantages: First, it is relatively easy to perform and also identifies the titer and isotype of the antibodies.[80] Assay results are usually reported as anticardiolipin antibody units. Values are reported in standardized units: GPL for IgG aCL and MPL for IgM aCL; aCL values are classified as low (10 to 20 units), medium (>20 to 80 units), or high (>80 units). Values below 10 units are considered negative.[81]

The anticardiolipin test is positive in more than 80% to 90% of patients with APS when performed appropriately. However, it is not specific: It may be positive in a number of disorders other than APS.[81] Therefore, new, more specific tests have been developed. Several authors have reported that the anti–β2-GPI test is more specific for detection of APS.[77] Its sensitivity varies from 40% to 90%.[77] Other investigators have found that an ELISA kit utilizing a mixture of phospholipids as antigen (APhL ELISA Kit, QUANTA LITE™ ELISA, Specialty Laboratories, Inc., Santa Monica, CA) has enabled more specific detection of patients with APS.[82] The specificity of this test is 99% (versus 96% of the standard ELISA), and its sensitivity is 90%.[81]

The LAC is less frequently positive for APS and it is regarded as the more specific test.[82] The most sensitive assays for LAC detection seems to be the KCT and the Russell viper venom time. The APTT, probably the most commonly used test in clinical studies, is less sensitive than either of the former.[14, 78]

Diagnostic Criteria

Preliminary classification criteria for the APS were established during an international workshop in October 1998 in Sapporo, Japan.[83, 84] Definite aPL antibody syndrome is considered if at least one of the clinical criteria is present, and one of the laboratory criteria in the following steps.

Clinical Criteria

1. Vascular thrombosis: One or more clinical episodes of arterial, venous, or small-vessel thrombosis in any tissue or organ. Thrombosis must be confirmed by imaging or Doppler studies or histopathology, with the exception of superficial venous thrombosis. For histopathologic confirmation, thrombosis should be present without significant evidence of vessels wall inflammation.
2. Pregnancy morbidity:
   a. One or more unexplained deaths of a morphologically normal fetus at or beyond the 10th week of gestation, with normal fetal morphology documented by ultrasound or by direct examination of the fetus, or
   b. One or more premature births of a morphologically normal neonate at or before the 34th week of gestation because of severe preeclampsia or eclampsia, or severe placental insufficiency, or
   c. Three or more unexplained consecutive spontaneous abortions before the 10th week of gestation, with maternal anatomic or hormonal abnormalities and paternal and maternal chromosomal causes excluded.

Laboratory Criteria

1. Anticardiolipin antibody of IgG and/or IgM isotype in blood, present in medium or high titer, on two or more occasions, at least 6 weeks apart, measured by a standardized ELISA for β2-GPI–dependent aCL.
2. LAC present in plasma on two or more occasions at least 6 weeks apart, detected according to the guidelines of the International Society on Thrombosis and Hemostasis, in the following steps:
   a. Prolonged phospholipid-dependent coagulation demonstrated on a screening test (e.g., APTT, KCT, DVVT [dilute viper venom time], dPT, Textarin time).
   b. Failure to correct the prolonged coagulation time on the screening test by mixing with normal, platelet-poor plasma.
   c. Shortening or correction of the prolonged coagulation time on the screening test by the addition of excess phospholipid.

   d. Exclusion of other coagulopathies (e.g. factor VIII inhibitor or heparin, as appropriate).

TREATMENT

Many aspects of treatment of APS remain controversial. Current management varies significantly and is based on disease manifestations. The most commonly used drugs in the different trials are anticoagulants, antiplatelet agents, and immunosuppressants.

Primary Prophylaxis

Patients who are positive for the presence of aPL but who do not have a history of thrombosis or other manifestations of APS should not be treated. But it is important for these asymptomatic patients to reduce other risk factors for thrombosis, such as lowering elevated cholesterol levels, maintaining ideal weight and well-controlled blood pressure levels, avoiding oral contraception and discontinuing smoking.[26, 85]

Hydroxychloroquin has been used as a prophylactic agent against deep venous thrombosis in hip surgery[26, 86] and also in symptomatic SLE patients with high titers of aPL antibodies, in the latter case with successful results in controlling both risk of thrombosis and cutaneous and musculoskeletal manifestations of SLE.[26] Different opinions have been expressed about the prophylactic treatment with daily low-dose (80 mg) aspirin and nonsteroidal anti-inflammatory agents, but the majority of studies did not show benefits from the use of these drugs.[87]

Secondary Prophylaxis—Treatment of Thrombotic Event

The most recent and largest retrospective study for the treatment of APS patients after a venous or arterial thrombotic event is that of Khamashta and colleagues.[87] In this series, treatment with intensive warfarin to maintain an international normalization ratio (INR) greater than 3, with or without low-dose aspirin, was more effective than low-intensity warfarin (INR, 2 to 3) in the prevention of recurrent thrombosis.[87]

Aspirin is often used in secondary prophylaxis of APS patients, but there is inadequate evidence to support its use.[1] The optimal degree and duration of anticoagulation is controversial. Both the Rosove and Brewer[88] and the Khamashta and colleagues series[87] recommended lifelong warfarin therapy, and concluded that the high risk of recurrent thrombosis outweighed the risk of major, even life-threatening bleeding incurred with high-dose warfarin treatment. The use of heparin in APS patients is limited to acute anticoagulation after the thrombotic event, but long-term anticoagulation with heparin should be avoided because of the high risk of osteoporosis.[1, 26]

Treatment of Thrombocytopenia

Paradoxically, thrombocytopenic patients with APS remain at risk for thrombosis. Patients whose platelet count falls below 50,000 (or especially below 35,000) are also at increased risk for bleeding. The current opinion[87] is to treat patients who have profound thrombocytopenia with corticosteroids and, if necessary, intravenous immunoglobulins to achieve a platelet count of greater than 50,000.

Treatment in Pregnancy

A pregnant patient in whom aCL or LAC is found, and who does not have a history of miscarriages, does not require treatment; these women can have a successful pregnancy even in the presence of aPL.[89] Warfarin is contraindicated in pregnancy because of its teratogenic potential. High doses of prednisone should be avoided given the risk of high incidence maternal complications such as preeclampsia, diabetes, infections, and osteoporosis. The most common protocol for APS pregnant patients suggests the use of a combination of subcutaneous heparin and aspirin[90] to help prevent thrombosis and decidual vasculopathy.

Treatment of Ocular Complications

Given the severity of the thrombotic complications in many patients with aPL, the ophthalmologist must be alert to their presence and start prompt therapeutic intervention. Once the vaso-occlusive event has occurred, anticoagulant therapy must begin as soon as possible, consisting of intravenous heparin followed by oral warfarin, and in most cases given for a prolonged period of time.[91] The duration of the anticoagulant therapy with or without the combination of low-dose aspirin are still controversial. In some patients, the retinopathy appeared to worsen when the anticoagulant therapy was decreased, whereas it stabilized when full anticoagulation was reinstituted.[91] Therefore, it is probably prudent to continue the anticoagulant therapy for many years after the occurrence of the vaso-occlusive retinopathy, perhaps for patient's lifetime. The role of corticosteroids is unclear. Conley and Hartmann[12] observed that steroids can suppress the LAC activity. However, retinal thrombosis has occurred or recurred in LAC patients on steroid therapy. If the diagnosis of retinal artery or vein thrombosis excludes a vasculitis cause, medical therapy should not include corticosteroids. Conversely, corticosteroids and immunosuppressants, such as cyclophosphamide or azathioprine, should be given to any patient who might continue to have active retinal thrombosis despite adequate anticoagulation and antiplatelet therapy.[91, 92] Besides the medical therapy, modalities employed in the treatment of complications arising from vaso-occlusive retinopathy are similar to the approach used in the treatment of other ischemic ocular disorders, including panretinal photocoagulation and vitreous surgery. Mild degrees of nonprogressive peripheral preretinal neovascularization without marked vitreous hemorrhage or traction do not require laser therapy and can be managed by periodic assessement.[93] In eyes with extensive peripheral neovascularization and vitreous hemorrhage, peripheral scatter photocoagulation is usually effective in causing regression of the new vessels.[93]

With regard to the treatment of optic neuropathy, Giorgi and colleagues[2] believe that visual improvement after intravenous administration of cyclophosphamide could be caused by a vasculitic component in its pathogenesis. Conversely, if the optic neuropathy is caused by severe thrombotic occlusion of the ciliary vessels in relation to aPL, the ischemia may be so acute that it leads to irreversible axonal necrosis, despite the administration of immunosuppressant agents: In these patients, an anticoagulant therapy is required to achieve visual improvement.

The treatment for optic neuritis in patients with secondary APS associated with SLE is oral corticosteroids. Most patients respond to this treatment, but in some patients, the response is partial, transitory, or unsuccessful, with progression to permanent blindness; in these patients, immunosuppressive therapy with intravenous cyclophosphamide has been effective.[94]

PROGNOSIS

The natural history of APS is related to the severity of its major clinical manifestation, in particular the risk and the rate of recurrences of thrombotic events.

In a prospective study of 360 patients, Finazzi and colleagues[85] found a total incidence of thrombotic complications of 9.4%. Thromboses were spontaneous, triggered by infections, pregnancy or immobilization; 73% of these thromboses were recurrences, 68% of which occurred in the same vascular district. In accordance with others authors, Finazzi and colleagues[85] found a correlation between the levels and isotypes of aPL and the severity of clinical manifestations.[6, 26, 85, 95] Generally, patients with moderate to high levels of IgG aCL are more susceptible to thrombotic complications than are those with IgM or IgA isotypes. In addition, a history of previous thrombosis associated with high levels of aPL carries an increased risk for thrombosis; therefore these patients require long-term therapy. Conversely, asymptomatic subjects with aPL have a low incidence of thrombosis.[26, 85]

The incidence of major bleeding ranges from 1.7% to 1.8% and included menometrorrhagia, macrohematuria, muscle hematoma, gastrointestinal and retroperitoneal hematoma, and fatal cerebral bleeding.[85] The causes of bleeding were both thrombocytopenia and anticoagulant therapy.[85]

Although cancer is not usually considered a characteristic feature of APS patients, neoplastic disorders, in particular hematologic neoplasias such as leukemias and non-Hodgkin's lymphoma, have been found as important causes of morbidity and mortality.[85]

With respect to pregnancy losses, the risk factors identified as significant predictors are elevated levels of IgG aCL, a history of miscarriages, and underlying SLE or lupus-like syndrome.[16, 85] Today, fetal survival for APS women is approximately 80%, although the prematurity rate of successful pregnancies and the rate of intrauterine growth retardation are still high.[76]

In addition, the risk of arterial or venous thrombosis and fetal losses is higher in patients that present three isotypes of aCL and LAC antibodies together.[95]

CONCLUSIONS

The APS is a rare disorder characterized by the presence of arterial and venous thrombosis, fetal losses, and thrombocytopenia. LAC and aCL are the serologic markers of the syndrome. The exact pathogenesis of thrombosis is not completely understood, but it may involve β2-GPI (a natural anticoagulant), platelet aggregation, the protein C pathway, or endothelial cell function.

The multisystemic presentation of APS mostly depends on the site of thrombosis and may also include striking ocular features. Vaso-occlusive retinopathy and neuro-ophthalmologic disorders are the most important ocular manifestations. Therefore, in the presence of a venous or arterial thrombosis, it is important for the ophthalmologist to include APS in the differential diagnosis of the hypercoagulable disorders, and to rule out other conditions that display the same clinical manifestations or laboratory finding.

The diagnosis of APS is based on clinical characteristics and on the laboratory evidence of the aPL. The difficulty in laboratory technique standardization is probably one of the important causes of misdiagnosis of APS patients. The early recognition of patients with APS allows appropriate therapy to be instituted, reducing the risk of future thrombosis.

The treatment following a thrombotic event includes intravenous heparin for the acute phase, followed by long-term high-dose warfarin with or without aspirin, maintaining an INR greater than 3. The duration of the anticoagulation treatment is still controversial. Corticosteroids and intravenous immunoglobulins can be used for thrombocytopenia. Pregnant women with APS can be treated with subcutaneous heparin and aspirin.

The prognosis of patients with APS is mostly related to the site of thrombosis, the rate of recurrences of thrombotic events, and the potential side effects of anticoagulant therapy.

References

1. Goel N: Antiphospholipid antibody syndrome: Current concepts. Hosp Pract 1998;15:129–149.
2. Giorgi D, Balacco Gabrieli C, Bonomo L: The clinico-ophthalmological spectrum of antiphospholipid syndrome. Ocul Immunol Inflamm 1998;6:269–273.
3. Acheson JF, Gregson RMC, Merry P, et al: Vaso-occlusive retinopathy in the primary antiphospholipid syndrome. Eye 1991;5:48–55.
4. Alarcon-Segovia D, Sanchez-Guerrero J: Primary antiphospholipid syndrome. J Rheumatol 1989;16:482–488.
5. Harris EN, Gharavi AE, Loizou S, et al: Crossreactivity of antiphospholipid antibodies. J Clin Lab Immunol 1985;16:1–6.
6. Sammaritano LR, Gharavi AE, Lockshin MD: Antiphospholipid antibody syndrome: Immunologic and clinical aspects. Semin Arthritis Rheum 1990;20:81–96.
7. Zarrabi MJ, Zuker S, Derman RM, et al: Immunologic and coagulation disorders in chlorpromazine treated patients. Ann Intern Med 1979;91:194–199.
8. Moore JE, Lutz WB: The natural history of systemic lupus erythematosus: An approach to its study through chronic biology false positive reactors. J Chronic Dis 1955;1:297–316.
9. Harvey AM, Shulman LE: Connective tissue disease and the chronic biologic false-positive test for syphilis (BFP reaction). Med Clin North Am 1966;50:1271–1279.
9a. Pangborn MC: Isolation and purification of a serologically active phospholipid beef heart. J Biol Chem 1942;143:247–256.
10. Roubey RAS: Immunology of the antiphospholipid antibody syndrome. Arthritis Rheum 1996;39:1444–1454.
11. Inoue G, Nojima S: Immunochemical studies of phospholipids. IV. The reactives of antisera against natural cardiolipin and synthetic cardiolipin analogues-containing antigens. Chem Phys Lipids 1969;3:70–77.
12. Conley CL, Hartmann RC: A hemorrhagic disorder caused by circulating anticoagulant in patients with disseminated SLE. J Clin Invest 1952;31:621–622.
13. Bowie EJW, Thompson JH, Pascuzzi CA, et al: Thrombosis in SLE despite circulating anticoagulants. J Lab Clin Med 1963;62:416–430.
14. Feinstein DI, Rapaport SL: Acquired inhibitors of blood coagulation. Prog Hemost Thromb 1972;1:75–95.
15. Tan EM, Choen AS, Fries JF, et al: The 1982 revised criteria for the classification of systemic lupus erythematosus. Arthritis Rheum 1982;25:1271–1277.
16. Hughes GR: The antiphospholipid syndrome: Ten years on. Lancet 1993;342:341–344.
17. Lockwood CL, Romero R, Feinberg RF, et al: The prevalence and biologic significance of lupus anticoagulant and anticardiolipin antibodies in a general obstetric population. Am J Obstet Gynecol 1989;161:369–373.
18. Kalunian KC, Peter JB, Middlekauff HR, et al: Clinical significance of a single test for anticardiolipin antibodies. Am J Med 1988;85:602–608.
19. Fort JG, Cowchock S, Abruzzo JL, et al: Anticardiolipin antibodies in patients with rheumatic diseases. Arthritis Rheum 1987;30:752–760.
20. Vila P, Hernandez MC, Lopez-Fernandez MF, et al: Prevalence, follow up and clinical significance of the anticardiolipin antibodies in normal subjects. Thromb Haemost 1994;72:209–213.
21. Love PE, Santoro SA: Antiphospholipid antibodies: Anticardiolipin and the lupus anticoagulant in systemic lupus erythematosus (SLE) and in non SLE disorders: Prevalence and clinical significance. Ann Intern Med 1990;112:682.
22. Glacet-Bernard A, Bayani N, Chretien P, et al: Antiphospholipid antibodies in retinal vascular occlusion. Arch Ophthalmol 1994;112:790–795.
23. Dori D, Gelfand YA, Brenner B, et al: Cilioretinal artery occlusion: An ocular complication of primary antiphospholipid syndrome. Retina 1997;17:555–557.
24. Alric L, Oskman F, Sanmarco M, et al: Association of antiphospholipid syndrome and chronic hepatitis C. Br J Rheumatol 1998;37:589–590.
25. Asherson RA, Khamashta MA, Ordi-Ros J, et al: The primary antiphospholipid syndrome: Major clinical and serological features. Medicine (Baltimore) 1989;68:366–372.
26. Petri M: Pathogenesis and treatment of the antiphospholipid antibody syndrome. Med Clin North Am 1997;81:151–176.
27. Lockshin MD. Antiphospholipid antibody syndrome. Rheum Dis Clin North Am 1994;20:45–59.
28. Panzer S, Pabinger I, Gschwandtner ME, et al: Lupus anticoagulants: Strong association with the major histocompatibility complex class II and platelet antibodies. Br J Hematol 1997;98:342–345.
29. Lechener K, Pabinger-Fashing I: Lupus anticoagulant and thrombosis: A study of 25 cases and review of literature. Haemostasis 1985;15:254–262.
30. Bick RL, Jakway J, Baker WF: Deep vein thrombosis: Prevalence of etiologic factors and results of management in 100 consecutive patients. Semin Thromb Hemost 1992;18:276–274.
31. Anderson D, Bell D, Lodge R, et al: Recurrent cerebral ischemia and mitral valve vegetation in a patient with antiphospholipid antibodies. J Rheumatol 1987;14:839–841.
32. Hamsten A, Norberg R, Bjorkholm M, et al: Antibodies to cardiolipin in young survivors of myocardial infarction: An association with recurrent cardiovascular events. Lancet 1986;331:113–116.
33. Khamashta MA, Cervera R, Asherson RA, et al: Association of antibodies against phospholipid with heart valve disease in systemic lupus erythematosus. Lancet 1990;335:1541–1544.
34. Lecerf V, Alhenc-Gelas M, Laurian C, et al: Antiphospholipid antibodies and atherosclerosis. Am J Med 1992;92:575–576.
35. Asherson RA, Derksen RH, Harris EN, et al: Chorea in systemic lupus and lupus like disease: Association with antiphospholipid antibodies. Semin Arthritis Rheum 1987;16:253–259.
36. Levine SR, Welch KMA: Cerebrovascular ischemia associated with lupus anticoagulants. Stroke 1987;18:257–263.
37. Lavalle C, Pizarro S, Drenkard C, et al: Transverse myelitis: A manifestation of systemic lupus erythematosus strongly associated with antiphospholipid antibodies. J Rheumatol 1990;17:34–37.
38. Lolli F, Mata S, Baruffi MC, et al: Cerebrospinal fluid anticardiolipin antibodies in antibodies in neurological disease. Clin Immunol Immunopathol 1991;59:314.
39. Glueck HI, Kant KS, Weiss MA, et al: Thrombosis in systemic lupus erythematosus: Relation to the presence of circulating anticoagulant. Arch Intern Med 1985;145:1389–1395.
40. Amigo MC, Garcia-Torres R, Robles M, et al: Renal involvement in primary antiphospholipid syndrome. J Rheumatol 1992;19:1181–1185.
41. Gonzalez G, Gutierrez M, Ortiz M, et al: Association of APS with primary adrenal insufficiency. J Rheumatol 1996;23:1286–1287.
42. Pelletier S, Landi B, Piette JC, et al: The antiphospholipid syndrome as the second cause of non malignant Budd-Chiari syndrome. Arthritis Rheum 1992;35(suppl):S238.
43. Branch DW: Thoughts on the mechanism of pregnancy loss associated with the antiphospholipid syndrome. Lupus 1994;3:275–280.
44. Asherson RA, Liote F, Page B, et al: Aseptic necrosis of bone

and antiphospholipid antibodies in systemic lupus erythematosus. J Rheumatol 1993;20:284–288.

45. Castañon C, Amigo MC, Bañales JL, et al: Ocular vaso-occlusive disease in primary antiphospholipid syndrome. Ophthalmology 1995;102:256–262.

46. Klok AM, Geertzen R, Rothova A, et al: Anticardiolipin antibodies in uveitis. Curr Eye Res 1992;11:209–213.

47. Boey ML, Colaco CB, Gharavi AE, et al: Thrombosis in systemic lupus erythematosus: Striking association with the presence of circulating lupus anticoagulant. Br Med J 1983;287:1021–1023.

48. Pulido JS, Ward LM, Fishman GA, et al: Antiphospholipid antibodies associated with retinal vascular disease. Retina 1987;7:215–218.

49. Wiechens B, Schroder JO, Potzsch B: Primary antiphospholipid antibody syndrome and retinal occlusive vasculopathy. Am J Ophthalmol 1997;123:848–850.

50. Jonas J, Kolbe K, Volker HE, et al: Central retinal artery occlusion in Sneddon's disease associated with antiphospholipid antibodies. Am J Ophthalmol 1986;102:37–40.

51. Levine SR, Crofts JW, Lesser GW, et al: Visual symptoms associated with the presence of a lupus anticoagulant. Ophthalmology 1988;95:686–692.

52. Asherson RA, Merry P, Acheson JF, et al: Antiphospholipid antibodies: A risk factor for occlusive ocular vascular disease in systemic lupus erythematosus and the primary antiphospholipid syndrome. Ann Rheum Dis 1989;48:358–361.

53. Giorgi D, Vaccaro F: Vaso-occlusive retinopathy: Is it a classical clinical manifestation of the antiphospholipid syndrome? Lupus 1997;6:617.

54. Gerber SL, Cantor LB: Progressive optic atrophy and the primary antiphospholipid syndrome. Am J Ophthalmol 1990;110:443–444.

55. Watts T, Greaves M, Rennie IG, et al: Antiphospholipid antibodies in the aetiology of ischemic optic neuropathy. Eye 1991;5:75–79.

56. Jabs DA, Miller NR, Newman SA, et al: Optic neuropathy in SLE. Arch Ophthalmol 1986;104:564–568.

57. Guglielmone HA, Fernandez E: Distribution of lupus anticoagulant and anticardiolipin antibody isotypes in a population with antiphospholipid syndrome. J Rheumatol 1999;26:86–90.

58. McNeil HP, Chesterman CN, Krilis SA: Immunology and clinical importance of antiphospholipid antibodies. Adv Immunol 1991;49:193–280.

59. Navarro M, Cervera R, Teixido M, et al: Antibodies to endothelial cells and to β2-GPI in the antiphospholipid syndrome: Prevalence and isotype distribution. Br J Rheumatol 1996;35:523–528.

60. Oostig JD, Derksen RHWM, Bobbink IWG, et al: Antiphospholipid antibodies directed against a combination of phospholipids with prothrombin, protein C, or protein S: An explanation for their pathogenetic mechanism. Blood 1993;81:2618–2625.

61. Manco-Johnson MJ, Nuss P: Lupus anticoagulant in children with thrombosis. Am J Hematol 1995;48:240–243.

62. Lozier J, Takahashi N, Putnam FW: Complete amino acid sequence of human plasma beta 2-glycoprotein I. Proc Natl Acad Sci U S A 1984;81:3640–3704.

63. Simantov RJ, La Sala SK, Gharavi AE, et al: Activation of cultured endothelial cells by antiphospholipid antibodies. J Clin Invest 1995;96:2211.

64. Galli M, Comfurius P, Maassen C, et al: Anticardiolipin antibodies directed not to cardiolipin but to a plasma protein cofactor. Lancet 1990;335:1544.

65. Arnout J, Vermylen J: Mechanism of action of β2-GPI dependent lupus anticoagulants. Lupus 1998;(suppl 2):S23–S28.

66. McIntyre JA, Wagenknecht DR, Sugi T, et al: Phospholipid binding plasma proteins required for antiphospholipid antibody detection—An overview. Am J Reprod Immunol 1997;37:101–110.

67. Hunt JE, McNeil HP, Morgan GJ, et al: A phospholipid β2-GPI complex is an antigen for anticardiolipin antibodies occurring in autoimmune disease but not with infection. Lupus 1992;1:75–81.

68. Shi W, Chong BH, Hogg PJ, et al: Anticardiolipin antibodies block the inhibition by β2-GPI of the factor Xa generating activity of platelets. Thromb Haemost 1993;70:342–345.

69. Bancsi LFJMM, Van der Liden JK, Bertina RM: β2-GPI deficiency and the risk of thrombosis. Thromb Haemost 1992;67:649–653.

70. Roubey RAS, Harper MF, Lentz BR: The interaction of β2-GPI with phospholipid membranes. Arthritis Rheum 1995;38(suppl 9):S211.

71. Inanc M, Donohoe S, Ravirajan CT, et al: Anti β2-GPI, anti-pro-thrombin and anticardiolipin antibodies in a longitudinal study of patients with systemic lupus erythematosus and the antiphospholipid syndrome. Br J Rheumatol 1998;37:1089–1094.

72. Guerin J, Feighery C, Sim RB, et al: Antibodies to β2 glycoprotein I: A specific marker for the antiphospholipid syndrome. Clin Exp Immunol 1997;109:304–309.

73. Roubey RAS: Mechanism of autoantibody-mediated thrombosis. Lupus 1998;7(suppl.2):S114–119.

74. Lellouche F, Martinuzzo M, Said P, et al: Imbalance of thromboxane/prostacyclin biosynthesis in patients with lupus anticoagulant. Blood 1991;78:2894–2899.

75. Carreras LO, Maclouf J: Antiphospholipid antibodies and eicosanoids. Lupus 1994;3:271–274.

76. Lockshin MD: Pregnancy loss and antiphospholipid antibodies. Lupus 1998;7(suppl 2):S86–S89.

77. Harris EN, Pierangeli SS, Gharavi AE: Diagnosis of the antiphospholipid syndrome: A proposal for use of laboratory tests. Lupus 1998;7(suppl 2):S144–S148.

78. Loizou S, McCrea JD, Rudge AC, et al: Measurement of anticardiolipin antibodies by an enzyme linked immunosorbent assay (ELISA): Standardization and quantificaton of result. Clin Exp Immunol 1985;62:738–745.

79. Piette JC: Towards improved criteria for the antiphospholipid syndrome. Lupus 1998;7(suppl 2):S149–S157.

80. Tincani A, Spatola L, Cinquini M, et al: Anti β2-GPI antibodies: Clinical significance. Lupus 1998;7(suppl 2):S107–S108.

81. Merkel PA, Yuchiao C, Pierangeli S: Comparison between two standard anticardiolipin antibody test and a new phospholipid test in patients with connective tissue diseases. J Rheumatol 1999;26:591–596.

82. Harris EN, Pierangeli SS: A more specific ELISA assay for the detection antiphospholipid antibodies. Clin Immunol News 1995;15:26–28.

83. Brandt JT, Triplett DA, Alving B, et al: Criteria for the diagnosis of the lupus anticoagulants: An update. Thromb Haemost 1995;74:1185–1190.

84. Wilson WA, Gharavi AE, Koike T, et al: International consensus statement on preliminary classification criteria for definite antiphospholipid syndrome. Report of an international workshop. Arthritis Rheum 1999;7:1309–1311.

85. Finazzi G, Brancaccio V, Moia M, et al: Natural history and risk factors in 360 patients with antiphospholipid antibodies: A four-year prospective study from the Italian registry. Am J Med 1996;100:530–536.

86. Loudon JR: Hydroxychloroquin and postoperative thromboembolism after total hip replacement. Am J Med 1988;85:57–61.

87. Khamashta MA, Cuardado MJ, Mujic F, et al: The management of thrombosis in the antiphospholipid syndrome. N Engl J Med 1995;332:993–997.

88. Rosove MH, Brewer PMC: Antiphospholipid thrombosis: Clinical course after the first thrombotic event in 70 patients. Ann Intern Med 1992;117:303–308.

89. Out HJ, Bruinse HW, Christiaens GC, et al: A prospective, controlled multicenter study on the obstetric risks of pregnant women with antiphospholipid antibodies. Am J Obstet Gynecol 1992;167:26–32.

90. Cowchock FS, Reece EA, Balaban D, et al: Repeated fetal losses associated with antiphospholipid antibodies: A collaborative randomized trial comparing prednisone with low-dose heparin treatment. Am J Obstet Gynecol 1992;166:1318–1323.

91. Kleine RC, Najarian LV, Schatten S, et al: Vaso-occlusive retinopathy associated with antiphospholipid antibodies (lupus anticoagulant retinopathy). Ophthalmology 1989;96:896–904.

92. Ingram SB, Goodnight SH, Bennet RM: An unusual syndrome of a devastating non-inflammatory vasculopathy associated with anticardiolipin antibodies. Arthritis Rheum. 1987;30:1167–1172.

93. Vine AK: Severe periphlebitis, peripheral retinal ischemia, and preretinal neovascularization in patients with multiple sclerosis. Am J Ophthalmol 1992;113:28–32.

94. Galindo-Rodriguez G, Avina-Zubieta A, Pizarro S, et al: Cyclophosphamide pulse therapy in optic neuritis due to systemic lupus erythematosus: An open trial. Am J Med 1999;106:65–69.

95. Guglielmone H, Fernandez EJ: Distribution of lupus anticoagulant and anticardiolipin antibody isotypes in a population with antiphospholipid syndrome. J Rheumatol 1999;26:86–90.

FUCHS' HETEROCHROMIC IRIDOCYCLITIS

Charalampos Livir-Rallatos

DEFINITION

Fuchs' heterochromic iridocyclitis (FHI) is a low-grade, chronic, nongranulomatous uveitis of unknown origin. This mostly unilateral disease is characterized by a relative absence of redness of the external eye, small stellate keratic precipitates scattered on the entire corneal endothelium, iris atrophy with or without heterochromia, abnormal angle vessels, and a lack of posterior synechiae. Cataract and glaucoma are considered to be the major complications. This limited, classic description of FHI has been challenged recently. More recent reviews have suggested that the clinical spectrum of FHI is wider than what has been previously defined, and that the clinical course is more variable. Some authors use the term Fuchs' uveitis syndrome, as the term heterochromic does not apply to all patients with the disease and the disease may affect other parts of the eye as well.

HISTORY

A review of the medical literature suggests that Lawrence[1] was the first to describe some components of this entity, reporting on four patients with cataract and heterochromia in 1843. Other components of this condition were published later by Weill[2] in 1904. It was Ernst Fuchs,[3] professor of ophthalmology at the University of Vienna, however, who expanded on the work of Weill to describe both the clinical and pathologic features of the disease with an accuracy remarkable for 1906, a time prior to the availability of the slit-lamp biomicroscope. His group of 38 patients was very large, considering the paucity of eyes in the previous reports. The constellation of signs, which was originally named complicated heterochromia by Fuchs, now bears his name and has provoked the interest of many ophthalmologists in the succeeding years. Kimura and colleagues,[4] in their description of 23 patients with FHI, were one of the first groups to recognize other features of the disease and the fact that multiple portions of the eye can be affected by this inflammatory process. Franceschetti[5] expanded the criteria of FHI and described them in more detail, based on a series of 62 patients. Loewenfeld and Thompson,[6, 7] in 1973, reviewed FHI, referring to over 700 publications. From 1973 to 2000, additional series of patients have been reported, expanding the clinical spectrum of the disease.

EPIDEMIOLOGY

The prevalence of FHI in uveitis populations varies from 1.2% to 4.5% in several reported series.[8–11] The true prevalence is probably higher, given the fact that heterochromia can be absent or very subtle and therefore difficult to detect, especially in patients with brown irides. The disease has no racial or sexual predilection and can affect patients at all ages.[12–14] Although the condition is mostly unilateral, bilateral cases are seen in approximately 10% of patients.[13, 14]

On several occasions, more than one member of a family have been noted to have FHI,[15, 16] and the disease has been described in a pair of monozygotic twins.[17] But familial reports of FHI account for only a tiny minority of the large number of patients now reported, and recently discordance has been described in proven monozygotic twins.[18]

Although several types of uveitis have been associated with human lymphocyte antigens (HLA), none have been associated with FHI. An association with HLA-B18 has been reported in one series,[19] but this has not been substantiated by others.[20, 21] A decreased frequency of both HLA-Cw3 and HLA-DRw53 has been found in some studies,[20, 21] but a larger number of patients is required to confirm such association. Recently, the HLA-A2 antigen was found to have a statistically significant negative association with FHI.[22]

CLINICAL MANIFESTATIONS AND COMPLICATIONS

Most patients with FHI present in early adulthood, although the disease may commence in childhood. The condition is customarily unilateral but bilateral involvement can be seen. Many patients are unaware of their disease, which is discovered during the course of a routine eye examination. The most common symptoms reported are floaters caused by vitreous opacities, and visual deterioration caused by cataract. Pain and perilimbal injection are rare. Awareness of heterochromia prior to diagnosis is seen in the minority of patients. Some patients may complain of symptoms associated with recurrent hyphema (blurred vision, floaters) or symptoms consistent with elevated intraocular pressure (mild pain, blurred vision, colored haloes around lights).

Classical teaching seems to stress the paramount importance of heterochromia in FHI. This emphasis is imprudent and can lead to underdiagnosis of the disease. Heterochromia can be subtle or absent in darkly pigmented irides (in blacks,[23] whites,[24] or Asians[25]) and when there is bilateral involvement. Typically, heterochromia is caused by atrophy of the anterior border layer of the iris[13, 26] (Figs. 61–1 and 61–2). This progressive atrophy will make the brown iris appear less brown, whereas in the light blue iris it will cause an apparent deepening of the blue color because of the revealing of the underlying iris pigmented epithelium.[13] Sometimes stromal atrophy may become so severe that the iris pigmented epithelium can be observed directly. The result is a paradoxical or "reverse heterochromia" with the involved eye becoming the darker eye.

FHI causes atrophy and depigmentation of all iris layers: anterior border layer, stroma proper, and pigmented epithelium. However, the vast majority of patients have a significant loss of anterior border layer, usually seen early

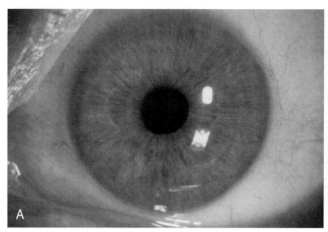 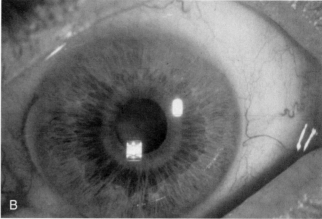

FIGURE 61–1. Right and left eye of a patient with Fuchs' heterochromic iridocyclitis (right eye, *A*; left eye, *B*). Note the difference in apparent color of the irides. The left eye is the eye with the iridocyclitis. (Courtesy of C. Stephen Foster, MD.) (See color insert.)

in the course of the disease. Stromal atrophy results in a somewhat moth-eaten appearance resulting from blunting of the surface rugae. Advanced atrophy may lead to the exposure of deeper structures such as the iris vasculature, the sphincter pupillae, and the underlying pigmented epithelium. Atrophy of the latter can be demonstrated only when it has advanced far enough to result in transillumination defects which are usually noted in the area adjacent to the pupil. However, sector atrophy, such as that seen in herpes infection, does not occur in FHI.[26, 27] The pupillary ruff is particularly vulnerable, having gaps in the majority of patients. Atrophy of the sphincter and dilator pupillae may cause anisocoria, with the affected pupil being larger or smaller than the unaffected side. In general, FHI causes atrophy of the iris, which highlights rather than hides its architecture. This is appreciated when comparison with the fellow eye is performed at the slit-lamp biomicroscope.[26]

Iris nodules in FHI can be either pupillary (Koeppe) or stromal (Busacca). Iris nodules are quite common in FHI in some series,[14, 23] whereas in others they are not.[12, 28] These nodules are small and transparent and therefore may be overlooked, or when noted they may lead to a misdiagnosis of other types of chronic granulomatous iridocyclitis, especially in black patients.[29] Other minute, crystalline, highly refractile deposits on the surface of the iris (termed Russell bodies) are a rare biomicroscopic finding in eyes with FHI.[30, 31] These crystals probably represent plasma cells filled with immunoglobulin.

Posterior synechiae do not generally form in patients with FHI. However, posterior synechiae can occur after anterior segment surgery.[12, 13, 32] Moreover, transient synechiae may occur in association with Koeppe nodules, but they are evanescent and leave radial residual pigment on the anterior lens capsule.[28]

The incidence of iris and anterior chamber angle neovascularization in FHI has been a subject of debate. This is because it is difficult to interpret normal variations of iris vasculature and because iris atrophy may increase the visibility of pre-existing, although possibly altered, iris vessels. Such vessels may become straighter, narrower, and infarcted, as demonstrated with fluorescein angiography.[6, 7, 33–35] Although uncommon, frank rubeosis over the anterior chamber angle and iris surface has been reported by several authors.[12, 13, 23, 24, 33, 36] The fragile blood vessels in the iridocorneal angle (Fig. 61–3) and iris may be responsible for the occurrence of hyphema after anterior chamber paracentesis[37] (Amsler's sign). Hyphema in FHI, which has been termed filiform hemorrhage, may also occur spontaneously, or after trivial nonpenetrating eye injury. It has been described after the use of Honan balloon[38] prior to cataract surgery, after applanation tonometry,[13] after gonioscopy, and perioperatively in patients undergoing cataract surgery.[39–45]

Not all patients with FHI have signs of active inflammation. Anterior chamber inflammation when present is mild and is characterized by the presence of a moderate number of cells and little flare. The keratic precipitates in FHI are virtually pathognomonic of this condition. They are small and stellate, with fibrillary extensions and tiny interspersed fibrils (Figs. 61–4 and 61–5). They are translucent, nonpigmented, and scattered over the entire

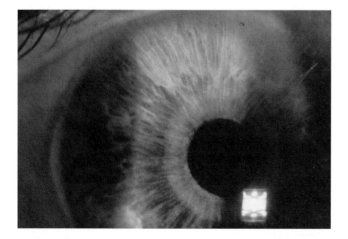

FIGURE 61–2. Higher magnification of the left eye shown in Figure 61–1*B*. Note the loss of iris substance in the anterior layers of the iris, allowing the pigment epithelium to be more apparent. (Courtesy of C. Stephen Foster, MD.) (See color insert.)

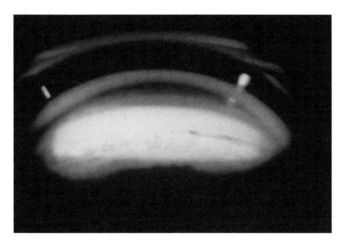

FIGURE 61–3. Gonioscopic photograph of a patient with Fuchs' heterochromic iridocyclitis. Note the very subtle vascular anomalies in the angle. (Courtesy of C. Stephen Foster, MD.) (See color insert.)

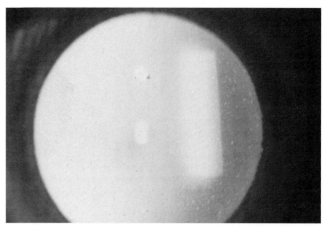

FIGURE 61–5. Same eye as shown in Figure 61–4; retroillumination photo, which allows one to see slightly more clearly the small fibrils that connect adjacent KPs. (Courtesy of C. Stephen Foster, MD.) (See color insert.)

corneal endothelium. The distribution of keratic precipitates in the upper part of the cornea is also pathognomonic of FHI. However, they can have a triangular distribution in the inferior cornea in some patients. The cellular activity in the anterior chamber varies over time. Some authors have noted that intraocular inflammation may disappear after cataract surgery.[5, 13] It is not known whether this is because the disease may go into remission after lens removal or because it represents a quiet period between episodes of active inflammation.

Cataract formation is a common complication of FHI. It usually commences as posterior subcapsular cataract that progresses to maturity with variable speed.[13]

Secondary glaucoma is undoubtedly the most damaging complication of FHI. The prevalence of glaucoma in FHI is reported to be as high as 59%, and it is the most common cause of permanent visual loss in these patients.[4–6, 10, 12, 23] The glaucoma is typically the chronic open-angle type.[28] However, peripheral anterior synechiae, neovascularization of the chamber angle,[36, 46] phaco-

lytic glaucoma,[47, 48] trabeculitis,[36, 49] and corticosteroid-induced glaucoma[50] have been described as possible causes of secondary glaucoma in FHI.

Vitreous opacification is seen in the majority of patients with FHI.[13, 14] In general, profound cellular activity in the vitreous is not a feature of the disease, but there are exceptions, and severe inflammation with snowball formation can be seen.[13, 14] In contrast to intermediate uveitis, macular edema is never seen in FHI.[4, 12, 13, 23, 24]

Peripheral inflammatory chorioretinal scars resembling those caused in *Toxoplasma* retinochoroiditis are seen in a few patients with FHI. The prevalence of such scars varies from 7.2% to 65% according to various reports.[13, 51, 52] These lesions are usually small (one-half disc diameter) atrophic scars with hyperpigmented borders, often located in the periphery. They can be seen in the affected eye, in the unaffected contralateral eye, or in both eyes. Chorioretinal scars consistent with ocular histoplasmosis have also been noted in patients with FHI. However, a causal relationship with infectious agents is still unproved.

PATHOLOGY

Fuchs first described the histopathologic findings in specimens obtained from six patients. He reported anterior stromal depigmentation of the iris, hyalinization and endothelial cell proliferation of the blood vessel walls, and cellular infiltration with lymphocytes, plasma cells and Russell bodies.[3] These findings have been confirmed by others.[6, 53]

Electron microscopy studies demonstrate endoplasmic reticulum damage, a decreased number of melanocytes with no dendritic processes and with melanosomes that are smaller and irregular in size and shape, and degeneration of adrenergic nerve fibers.[26, 54, 55] It is not known whether the structural changes in nerve endings and melanocytes are caused by chronic inflammation or by a primary defect of adrenergic innervation leading to defective production of melanin granules.

There is a paucity of light- and electron-microscopic studies on the trabecular meshwork of Fuchs' patients with secondary glaucoma, and these are controversial. An

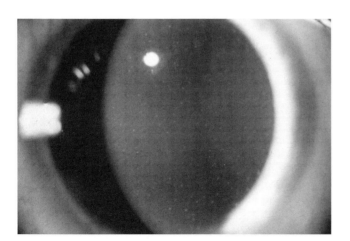

FIGURE 61–4. Typical keratic precipitate (KP) distribution and configuration in a patient with Fuchs' heterochromic iridocyclitis. Note that the KPs are distributed throughout the entire extent of the corneal endothelium and that many have a fibrillar or stellate character to them. (Courtesy of C. Stephen Foster, MD.) (See color insert.)

increased outflow resistance with sclerosis of the trabecular meshwork was reported by Huber,[56] whereas Benedict and colleagues[57] noted a collapse of the canal of Schlemm with atrophy of its wall.

The overall histopathologic appearance of FHI is that of chronic mononuclear inflammation, which does not differentiate it from other types of chronic iridocyclitis.

ETIOLOGY AND PATHOGENESIS

The etiology of the disease remains elusive. Ernst Fuchs assumed that the syndrome was caused by a noxious factor of unknown origin, which was present from fetal or early postnatal life.[3] Since then, many theories concerning the cause of FHI have been proposed, including genetic, sympathetic, infectious, and immunologic-inflammatory theories. Nevertheless, at present there is no adequate evidence to formulate a pathophysiologic mechanism that can explain all features of the disease.

Genetic theories emerged from the fact that other types of heterochromia, namely "simple" uncomplicated heterochromia and heterochromia in Waardenburg's syndrome, are dominantly inherited. Loewenfeld and Thompson, in their review of 1500 cases with FHI, found only five families with two cases of FHI.[7] In another review of 550 cases, Dernouchamps found six familial cases with FHI.[10] Although the disease has been reported to occur in monozygotic twins,[17] there is no strong familial association to provide adequate proof for the hereditary theory in FHI. Furthermore, studies on HLA typing have not shown any strong association of FHI with human leukocyte antigens. At present, neither familial concurrence nor HLA association supports the hypothesis of a genetic basis of the disease, although the concept of genetic predisposition remains open.

The association of peripheral chorioretinal scars with FHI has raised the hypothesis of an infectious agent causing FHI. Such scars were described both by Fuchs[3] and Kimura and coworkers[4] but were noticeably absent in a large number of patients reported by Loewenfeld and Thompson.[6, 7] Liesegang, in his review of 54 patients with FHI, found only two patients with chorioretinal scars.[12] In 1982, de Abreu and coworkers[58] reported a high incidence (56.5%) of chorioretinal scars consistent with ocular toxoplasmosis and confirmed serologic evidence for *Toxoplasma gondii* infection. He suggested that *T. gondii* could be a possible cause of FHI. Other investigators have also reported an association of toxoplasmosis-like scars and seropositivity for *T. gondii* infection with FHI.[23, 59–62] There are various possible reasons for the variation in the reported prevalence of toxoplasmosis-like scars in FHI: methods of examinations, diagnostic criteria both for FHI and toxoplasmosis-like scars, and prevalence of toxoplasmosis in different populations. Therefore, it was of paramount importance that a control group of the same population be studied simultaneously under the same methods. When that was done, a significantly higher prevalence of chorioretinal scarring was observed in FHI patients than in control groups.[51, 52, 62, 63] In a recent study, La Hey and associates[51] analyzed the association between FHI and toxoplasmosis by studying humoral and cell-mediated immunity against *T. gondii* in blood and aqueous humor of patients with FHI, other types of uveitis,

and controls. They concluded that there is no association between FHI and toxoplasmosis, although there is an association between FHI and toxoplasmosis-like chorioretinal scars. However, the authors acknowledged that there were no active chorioretinal lesions in patients with FHI at the time of blood sampling or at the time when the aqueous humor was obtained. Until now, few sporadic cases of FHI with an active *Toxoplasma* lesion or with a well-documented history of congenital toxoplasmosis have been reported.[52, 58, 59, 63–65] These case reports support the hypothesis that infection with *T. gondii* may lead to FHI, but this may concern only a small number of patients with FHI. It is also possible that ocular toxoplasmosis can create a chronic condition that resembles FHI, as suggested by Schwab.[52]

Theories that relate FHI to the sympathetic nervous system arise from the fact that damage to the adrenergic innervation of the iris may lead to iris hypochromia. Bistis was the first to propose that some "trophic" defect in the sympathetic nervous system could inhibit the process of iris pigmentation.[65] Thus, congenital Horner's syndrome was initially thought to be the cause of FHI.[66] In 1973, Loewenfeld and Thompson[7] reviewed 1746 cases with FHI and found only 25 cases (1.4%) with Horner's syndrome. This figure was considered to be too low to implicate a causal relation between FHI and Horner's syndrome. However, since 1973, additional cases of FHI and ipsilateral Horner's syndrome have been published.[67] Furthermore, FHI and Horner's syndrome developed in the same eye after stellate ganglionectomy.[68] Two other conditions, the Parry-Romberg syndrome of progressive hemifacial atrophy and the "status dysraphicus," the unilateral syndrome of dysmorphism and asymmetry, have been associated with FHI and sympathetic defect.[13, 69–71] Finally, electron microscopic studies have suggested that defective production of melanin granules resulting from inadequate function of adrenergic nerves may cause iris hypochromia.[55] Furthermore, defective adrenergic innervation of blood vessels in FHI may increase vascular permeability (as has been demonstrated with iris fluorescein angiography) with subsequent leakage of proteins and inflammatory mediators into the anterior chamber.

Various immunologic abnormalities have been noted in patients with FHI. Cellular and humoral immune responses to a corneal antigen (54 kD) have been found with high frequency in patients with FHI.[72, 73] This finding, in combination with the fact that corneal endothelial cells have immunomodulating capacities (ability to express major histocompatibility complex class II antigens and immune adhesion molecules)[74, 75] may explain the diffuse distribution of keratic precipitates and the endothelial abnormalities demonstrated on specular microscopy in some patients.[76]

Arffa and Schlaegel have described patients with toxoplasmosis-like scars and negative titers for toxoplasmosis in undiluted serum.[62] They proposed that chorioretinal lesions could result from autoimmunity against retinal or choroidal antigens.[62] In accordance with this hypothesis, La Hey and colleagues found that a significantly higher percentage of patients with FHI had a positive cellular autoimmune response to S-retinal antigen than healthy controls and other patients with anterior uveitis.[77] However, they also found patients with no chorioretinal scars but with positive immune response to S-retinal antigen.[77] It is unknown whether the immune sensitization against corneal and retinal antigens observed in FHI is the cause of the disease or represents a secondary autoimmune epiphenomenon. No autoantibodies to iris components were found in the sera of patients with FHI.[77]

In a recent study, the cellular phenotypes and the cytokine profile in the aqueous humor in patients with FHI and idiopathic anterior uveitis (IAU) were compared.[78] CD8+ T cells were higher in FHI, whereas CD4+ T cells were higher in IAU. INF-γ and interleukin (IL)-10 levels were higher and IL-12 levels were lower in FHI than in IAU. The authors suggest that the predominance of CD8+ T cells and the lower levels of IL-12 in FHI may account for the low-grade inflammation and the better outcome of this disease in comparison with IAU. In another study, an increased level of soluble IL-2 receptor, a marker of T-cell activation was found in peripheral blood of FHI patients.[79]

Intraocular production of immunoglobulin G (IgG), mainly the IgG_1 subclass, has been found in approximately 60% of patients with FHI.[80–82] However, an antigenic stimulus for this oligoclonal B-cell response has not yet been identified. This increased B-lymphocyte activity may be caused by the local production of IL-6 in the aqueous humor, as it has been demonstrated in 63% of patients with FHI.[82] Although deposits of immunoglobulins and complement have been found in the vascular wall of iris biopsy specimens obtained from patients with FHI, there is still no adequate evidence to support the concept of immune complex vasculitis as the cause of the disease.[83]

The many pathogenetic mechanisms that have been proposed, in addition to the fact that the disease has been reported in combination with toxoplasmosis, Horner's syndrome, Parry-Romberg syndrome, a retinitis pigmentosa-like picture,[84, 85] ocular trauma,[59, 86] subclavian steal syndrome,[87] and Möbius' syndrome,[88] make it difficult to believe that FHI has a single etiology. It is therefore possible that various stimuli (e.g., infectious, immunologic, and neurogenic) trigger the eye to a particular pathway, the clinical end result of which is FHI.

DIAGNOSIS

The diagnosis of FHI is important to make for the following reasons: (1) Patients with FHI are at a significant risk for developing glaucoma and need to be followed regularly for early glaucoma detection. (2) Although corticosteroids can reduce the clinical signs of inflammation, they do not produce any change in the clinical course and on a long-term basis can hasten the formation of cataract and induce glaucoma in steroid responders. (3) As a relatively mild form of chronic uveitis, FHI has a fairly good prognosis for the patient.

There are no laboratory tests to confirm the diagnosis of FHI. The diagnosis is essentially a clinical one, based on a thorough ophthalmic examination. Although there are no universally established diagnostic criteria for FHI, I suggest that the following are sufficient to make the diagnosis (Table 61–1): (1) the absence of acute symptoms of severe pain, redness, photophobia, (2) the pres-

TABLE 61–1. DIAGNOSTIC CRITERIA FOR FUCHS' HETEROCHROMIC IRIDOCYCLITIS

Absence of acute symptoms of severe pain, redness, photophobia
Presence of small, white, stellate keratic precipitates distributed across the endothelium
Low-grade anterior chamber inflammation
Diffuse iris stromal atrophy with or without heterochromia
Absence of posterior synechiae prior to cataract surgery
Presence of cells and opacities in the anterior vitreous

ence of characteristic small, white, stellate, keratic precipitates distributed widely across the endothelium, (3) low-grade anterior chamber inflammation, (4) diffuse iris stromal atrophy with or without heterochromia, (5) the absence of posterior synechiae prior to cataract surgery, and (6) the presence of cells and opacities in the anterior vitreous. Cataract and glaucoma can be present but are not essential criteria for the diagnosis of FHI.

In a typical case of FHI, the diagnosis of the disease is usually straightforward. However, in atypical cases the differential diagnosis includes disorders that produce iris heterochromia. Hypopigmentary causes of heterochromia such as "simple" uncomplicated heterochromia, heterochromia in association with Horner's syndrome, Duane's syndrome, and Waardenberg's syndrome do not generally produce a problem because they are not accompanied by inflammation.[89, 90] Iris heterochromia can be seen in chronic anterior uveitis caused by herpes zoster infection, but the pattern of iris atrophy, the patient's history, and the laboratory work-up will help to make the correct diagnosis. Hyperchromic causes of heterochromia, such as ocular melanosis, iris nevus syndrome, iris melanoma, siderosis bulbi, and xanthochromia, have typical features that can exclude them from the differential diagnosis.

Posner-Schlossmann syndrome and neovascular glaucoma can cause ocular disease that resembles FHI complicated by secondary glaucoma. In addition, glaucomatocyclitic crisis can also cause iris heterochromia.[91] However, the intraocular pressure rise in Posner-Schlossmann syndrome dramatically responds to topical steroids, something that is not seen in FHI.

Intermediate uveitis frequently presents with symptoms of floaters and blurred vision, often unilaterally in an age group similar to that for FHI. Furthermore, nongranulomatous anterior chamber inflammation and inflammatory aggregates in the anterior vitreous and peripheral retina are the hallmark of the disease. However, neither the pars plana exudates nor macular edema has been noted in FHI, whereas in intermediate uveitis these features are quite common.

TREATMENT AND PROGNOSIS

In the vast majority of patients with FHI, the inflammatory activity in the anterior chamber is mild and can fluctuate over time. Assuming that minimal inflammatory activity in FHI is not harmful for the intraocular structures, and taking into account the side effects of the long-term use of topical steroids, therapy is usually not indicated. However, FHI can be associated with pain and floaters and an increase in anterior segment inflammation that may contribute to the development of glaucoma.[92] These cases may warrant treatment with topical steroid for a short period. We know of no studies to support the use of oral anti-inflammatory medication in FHI.

Cataract formation is a virtually constant feature of the disease. Several studies have addressed the problems encountered during and after cataract surgery in FHI patients. Some have suggested that cataract surgery is typically uneventful, whereas others have found a higher incidence of operative and postoperative complications. The early encouraging results of Franceschetti[5] and Kimura and colleagues[4] during the era of intracapsular cataract surgery were disputed by Ward and Hart,[39] who reported patients having extensive complications with intracapsular surgery, including vitreous loss, hyphema, vitreous hemorrhage, uveitis, and progressive glaucoma. Corneal decompensation with peripheral and central bullous keratopathy with intracapsular surgery has also been described.[12] Although many eyes with FHI have tolerated iris-fixated or anterior chamber intraocular lenses for many years, there were patients in whom enucleation was performed for intractable glaucoma. Most experts today would agree that iris touch with an intraocular lens is undesirable in patients with a history of uveitis.

Cataract surgery in eyes with FHI has evolved concurrently with cataract surgery in general. Several papers have been published on extracapsular cataract extraction with posterior chamber intraocular lens implantation in FHI patients.[40, 93–98] Although the incidence of postoperative complications may differ in these studies, the visual outcome is excellent for a high proportion of patients in most of them. According to these reports, the most common complications in eyes undergoing modern extracapsular cataract extraction with intraocular lens implantation are hyphema, glaucoma, pigment deposits on the lens surface, vitreous opacities, and posterior capsule opacification. Intraocular hemorrhage is rarely significant enough to interfere with surgery. Although glaucoma is part of the natural history of the disease, cataract surgery may provoke its onset or worsen its course. Vitreous opacities are an integral part of the syndrome and, in some instances, these may be so profound as to necessitate vitrectomy.[99] Advanced cataract at presentation can obscure the detection of vitreous opacities, so the high frequency of vitreous opacification after cataract surgery is probably not related to the surgery itself. Posterior capsule opacification in FHI is felt to be higher than in the normal cataract population, and glaucoma precipitated by both surgical and yttrium-aluminum-garnet capsulotomy has occurred.[99] Severe iris atrophy with substantial transillumination defects, abnormalities of iris vasculature, and glaucoma are considered preoperative markers of guarded prognosis according to Jones.[43] These markers are indicators of severe disease and are associated with increased postoperative inflammation.

In conclusion, cataract surgery in patients with FHI is usually uneventful, although occasionally it may have a compromised outcome. Preoperative and postoperative control of inflammation with topical steroids is of paramount importance for a successful surgical outcome. A posterior chamber intraocular lens placed in the capsular bag is probably most appropriate.[97] The long-term efficacy and safety of foldable intraocular lenses in the era of phacoemulsification in patients with FHI have yet to be addressed. Secondary glaucoma remains the major complication of cataract surgery in FHI because of its high frequency and uncertain prognosis. Preoperative markers should alert the surgeon for increased vigilance in detecting and treating both secondary glaucoma and recurrent uveitis.

Treatment of glaucoma is the most difficult aspect in the management of FHI. When the intraocular pressure rise is intermittent and associated with increased intraocular inflammation, as may happen in the early stages of the disease, topical steroids are beneficial. However, antiglaucoma medications are required later in the course of the disease. The reported success rate of maximal medical treatment of glaucoma in FHI varies among authors. Jones[93] reported that 63% of glaucomatous patients with FHI responded to topical medication alone over a follow-up period of 10.2 years, a figure that does not significantly differ from that encountered in primary open-angle glaucoma. However, La Hey and colleagues[101] noted that maximal medical treatment was unsuccessful in 73% of glaucomatous patients with FHI.

Glaucoma filtration surgery is unavoidable in patients unresponsive to topical medication. Such surgery carries all the attendant risks associated with glaucoma surgery in uveitis patients, including bleb failure. However the use of fibrosis-inhibiting drugs (5-fluorouracil, mitomycin C) seems to have improved the success rate of filtration surgery in FHI patients and is currently recommended as an adjunct to the first surgical procedure.[92, 100] Patients who do not respond to filtration surgery may require shunt implantation. Rarely, patients have undergone enucleation for absolute or rubeotic glaucoma.[46, 93]

The prognosis of FHI is variable and depends on the clinical spectrum of the disease. With prolonged follow up, 40% of patients maintain a visual acuity of 20/40 or better.[12] Cataract formation is the most common cause of decreased vision in FHI, and of course this is potentially restorable. Glaucoma development is the most common cause of permanent visual loss in a significant number of patients, with prognosis less favorable than that of primary open-angle glaucoma.

CONCLUSIONS

FHI is a chronic low-grade uveitis, the diagnosis of which is entirely clinical. It is underdiagnosed because of its variable clinical spectrum. Although it can mimic various forms of uveitis, it is important to make the correct diagnosis because both management and prognosis differ from those of other uveitides. While its etiology remains unknown, it is possible that the disease has multiple causes that lead through different pathogenetic mechanisms to the same clinical entity. Although many patients do not require treatment, it is not a benign condition as often perceived. The high incidence of glaucoma makes it mandatory that all patients should be screened at regular intervals, even if they are not being actively treated and are relative asymptomatic.

References

1. Lawrence W: Changes in color in the iris. In: Hays I, ed: A Treatise on Diseases of the Eye. Philadelphia, Lea & Blanchard, 1843, pp 411–416.
2. Weill G: Über heterophthalmus. Z Augenheilkd 1904;11:165–176
3. Fuchs E: Über Komplicationen der Heterochromie. Z Augenheilkd 1906;15:191–212.
4. Kimura SJ, Hogan MJ, Thygeson P: Fuchs' syndrome of heterochromic cyclitis. Arch Ophthalmol 1955;54:179–186.
5. Franceschetti A: Heterochromic cyclitis (Fuchs' syndrome). Am J Ophthalmol 1955;39:50–58.
6. Loewenfeld IE, Thompson S: Fuchs' heterochromic cyclitis. A critical review of the literature I. Clinical characteristics of the syndrome. Surv Ophthalmol 1973;17:394–457
7. Loewenfeld IE, Thompson S: Fuchs' heterochromic cyclitis. A critical review of the literature II. Etiology and mechanisms. Surv Ophthalmol 1973;18:2–61.
8. Bloch-Michel E: Physiopathology of Fuchs heterochromic cyclitis. Trans Ophthalmol Soc U K 1981;101:384–386.
9. Chung YM, Yeh TS, Liu JH: Endogenous uveitis in Chinese—An analysis of 240 cases in a uveitis clinic. Jpn J Ophthalmol 1988;32:64–69.
10. Dernouchamps JP: Fuchs heterochromic cyclitis: An IUSG study on 550 cases. In: Saari KM, ed: Uveitis Update. Amsterdam, Excerpta Medica, 1984, pp 129–135.
11. Weiner A, BenEzra D: Clinical patterns and associated conditions in chronic uveitis. Am J Ophthalmol 1991;112:151–158.
12. Liesegang TJ: Clinical features and prognosis in Fuchs uveitis syndrome. Arch Ophthalmol 1982;100:1622–1626.
13. Jones NP: Fuchs' heterochromic uveitis: A reappraisal of the clinical spectrum. Eye 1991;5:649–661.
14. Fearnley IR, Rosenthal AR: Fuchs' heterochromic iridocyclitis revisited. Acta Ophthalmol Scand 1995;73:166–170.
15. Becker J: Heterochromiglaukom bei Mutter and Tochter. Klin Monatsbl Augenheilkd 1927;78:707.
16. Strieff EB: Sur l'hérédité de l'hétérochromie. Arch Klaus-Stiftung Vererb-Forsch 1947;22:256–260.
17. Makley TA: Heterochromic cyclitis in identical twins. Am J Ophthalmol 1956;41:768–772.
18. Jones NP, Read AP: Is there a genetic basis for Fuchs heterochromic uveitis? Discordance in monozygotic twins. Br J Ophthalmol 1992;76:22–24.
19. Pivetti Pezzi P, Catarinelli G, Paroli MP, et al: Fuchs' heterochromic iridocyclitis: II. Immunogenetic aspects. Clin Oculist Patol Oculare 1990;11:123–127.
20. De Bruyere M, Dernouchamps J-P, Sokal G: HLA antigens in Fuchs' heterochromic iridocyclitis. Am J Ophthalmol 1986;102:392–393.
21. Saari M, Vuorre I, Tiilikainen A, et al: Genetic background in Fuchs' heterochromic cyclitis. Can J Ophthalmol 1978;13:240–246.
22. Munoz G, Lopez-Corell MP, Taboada JF, et al: Fuchs' heterochromic cyclitis and HLA histocompatibility antigens. Int Ophthalmol 1994;18:127–130.
23. Tabbut BR, Tessler HH, Williams D: Fuchs' heterochromic iridocyclitis in blacks. Arch Ophthalmol 1988;106:1688–1690.
24. Jain IS, Gupta A, Gangwar DN, et al: Fuchs' heterochromic cyclitis: Some observations on clinical picture and on cataract surgery. Ann Ophthalmol 1983;15:640–642.
25. Kimura SJ: Fuchs' syndrome of heterochromic cyclitis in brown-eyed patients. Trans Am Ophthalmol Soc 1978;76:76–89.
26. McCartney AC, Bull TB, Spalton DJ: Fuchs' heterochromic cyclitis: An electron microscopy study. Trans Ophthalmol Soc U K 1986;105:324–329.
27. Jones NP: Fuchs' heterochromic uveitis: An update. Surv Ophthalmol 1993;37:253–272.
28. O'Connor GR: Heterochromic iridocyclitis. Trans Ophthalmol Soc U K 1985;104:219–231.
29. Rothova A, La Hey E, Baarsma S, et al: Iris nodules in Fuchs heterochromic uveitis. Am J Ophthalmol 1994;118:338–342.
30. Lam S, Tessler H, Winchester K, et al: Iris crystals in chronic iridocyclitis. Br J Ophthalmol 1993;77:181–182.
31. Zamir E, Margalit E, Chowers I, et al: Iris crystals in Fuchs' heterochromic iridocyclitis. Arch Ophthalmol 1998;116:1394.
32. Soheilian M, Karimian F, Javadi MA, et al: Surgical management of cataract and posterior chamber intraocular lens implanta-

tion in Fuchs' heterochromic iridocyclitis. Int Ophthalmol 1997;21:137–141.
33. Berger BB, Tessler HH, Kottow MH: Anterior segment ischemia in Fuchs' heterochromic cyclitis. Arch Ophthalmol 1980;98:499–501.
34. Bernsmeier H, Kluxen G, Friedberg D: Fluorescence angiographical findings in complicated heterochromia of Fuchs. Ber Zusammenkunft Dtsch Ophthalmol Ges 1981;78:49–52.
35. Verma LV, Arora R: Clinico-pathologic correlates in Fuchs' heterochromic iridocyclitis—An iris angiographic study. Indian J Ophthalmol 1990;38:159–161.
36. Perry HD, Yanoff M, Scheie HG: Rubeosis in Fuchs' heterochromic iridocyclitis. Arch Ophthalmol 1975;93:337–339.
37. Amsler M: New clinical aspects on the vegetative eye. Trans Ophthalmol Soc U K 1948;68:45–74.
38. Feldman ST, Deutsch TA: Hyphema following Honan balloon use in Fuchs' heterochromic iridocyclitis. Arch Ophthalmol 1986;104:967.
39. Ward DM, Hart CT: Complicated cataract extraction in Fuchs' heterochromic uveitis. Br J Ophthalmol 1967;51:530–538.
40. Baarsma GS, De Vries J, Hammudoglou CD: Extracapsular cataract extraction with posterior chamber lens implantation in Fuchs' heterochromic cyclitis. Br J Ophthalmol 1991;75:306–308.
41. Gee SS, Tabbara KF: Extracapsular cataract extraction with posterior chamber lens implantation in Fuchs' heterochromic iridocyclitis. Am J Ophthalmol 1989;108:310–314.
42. Hooper PL, Rao NA, Smith RE: Cataract extraction in uveitis patients: Surv Ophthalmol 1990;35:120–144.
43. Jones NP: Extracapsular cataract surgery with and without intraocular lens implantation in Fuchs' heterochromic uveitis. Eye 1990;4:145–150.
44. Jakeman CM, Jordan K, Keast-Butler J, et al: Cataract surgery with intraocular lens implantation in Fuchs' heterochromic cyclitis. Eye 1990;4:543–547.
45. Mills KB, Rosen ES: Intraocular lens implantation following cataract extraction in Fuchs' heterochromic uveitis. Ophthalmic Surg 1982;13:467–469.
46. Lerman S, Levy C: Heterochromic cyclitis and neovascular glaucoma. Am J Ophthalmol 1964;57:479.
47. Uemura A, Sameshima M, Nakao K: Complications of hypermature cataract. Spontaneous absorption of lens material and phacolytic glaucoma associated retinal perivasculitis. Jpn J Ophthalmol 1988;32:35.
48. Muller H: Phacolytic glaucoma and phacogenic ophthalmia. Trans Ophthalmol Soc U K 1963;83:691.
49. Roussel TJ, Coster DJ: Fuchs' heterochromic cyclitis and posterior capsulotomy. Br J Ophthalmol 1985;69:449.
50. David DS, Berkowitz JS: Ocular effects of topical and systemic corticosteroids. Lancet 1969;2:149.
51. La Hey E, Rothova A, Baarsma S, et al: Fuchs' heterochromic iridocyclitis is not associated with ocular toxoplasmosis. Arch Ophthalmol 1992;110:806–811.
52. Schwab IR: The epidemiologic association of Fuchs' heterochromic iridocyclitis and ocular toxoplasmosis. Am J Ophthalmol 1991;111:356–362.
53. Goldberg MF, Erozan YS, Duke JR, et al: Cytopathologic and histopathologic aspects of Fuchs' heterochromic iridocyclitis. Arch Ophthalmol 1965;74:604–609.
54. Wobmann P: Fuchs' heterochromic cyclitis: Electron microscopic study of nine iris biopsies. Albrecht von Graefes Arch Ophthalmol 1976;199:167–178.
55. Melamed S, Lahav M, Sandbank U, et al: Fuchs' heterochromic iridocyclitis: An electron microscopic study of the iris. Invest Ophthalmol Vis Sci 1978;17:1193–1198.
56. Huber A: Das Glaukom bei komplizierter Heterochromie Fuchs. Ophthalmlologica 1961;142:66.
57. Benedict O, Roll P, Zirm M: Das Glaucom bei der heterochromiezyklitis Fuchs. Gonioscopische befunde und ultrastrukturelle untersuchungen des Trabekelwerkes. Klin Monatsbl Augenheilkd 1978;173:523.
58. De Abreu MT, Belfort R, Hirata PS: Fuchs heterochromic cyclitis and ocular toxoplasmosis. Am J Ophthalmol 1982;93:739–744.
59. Saraux H, Laroche L, Le Hoang P: Secondary Fuchs heterochromic cyclitis: A new approach to an old disease. Ophthalmologica 1985;190:193–198.
60. Silva HS, Orefice F, Pinheiro SRA: Study of 132 cases of heterochromic cyclitis of Fuchs. Arq Bras Oftalmol 1988;51:160–162.

61. Schwab IR: Fuchs' heterochromic iridocyclitis. Int Ophthalmol Clin 1990;30:252–256.
62. Arffa RC, Schlaegel TF: Chorioretinal scars in Fuchs' heterochromic iridocyclitis. Arch Ophthalmol 1984;102:1153–1155.
63. Pezzi PP, Niutta A, Abdulariz M, et al: Fuchs' heterochromic iridocyclitis and toxoplasmic retinochoroiditis. Int J Ophthalmol 1987;1/2:97–101.
64. La Hey E, Rothova A: Fuchs' heterochromic cyclitis in congenital ocular toxoplasmosis. Br J Ophthalmol 1991;6:372–373.
65. La Hey E, Baarsma S: Contralateral active ocular toxoplasmosis in Fuchs' heterochromic cyclitis. Br J Ophthalmol 1993;77:455–456.
66. Bistis J: La paralyse du sympathique dans l'étiologie de l'héterochromie. Arch Ophthalmol 1912;32:578–583.
67. Regenbogen LS, Naveh-Floman N: Glaucoma in Fuchs' heterochromic cyclitis associated with congenital Horner's syndrome. Br J Ophthalmol 1987;71:844–849.
68. Makley TA, Abbot K: Neurogenic heterochromia: Report of an interesting case. Am J Ophthalmol 1965;59:927–928.
69. Passow A: Hornersyndrom, Heterochromie und status Dysrapficus, ein Symptomenkomplex. Arch Augenheilkd 1933;197:1–151.
70. Fulmek R: Hemiatrophia progressiva faciei (Romberg Syndrom) mit gleichseitiger Heterochromia complicata (Fuchs' Syndrom). Klin Monatsbl Augenheilkd 1974;164:615–628.
71. La Hey E, Baarsma S: Fuchs' heterochromic cyclitis and retinal vascular abnormalities in progressive hemifacial atrophy. Eye 1993;7:426–428.
72. La Hey E, Baarsma S, Rothova A, et al: High incidence of corneal epithelium antibodies in Fuchs' heterochromic cyclitis. Br J Ophthalmol 1988;72:921–925.
73. Van der Gaag R, Broersma L, Rothova A, et al: Immunity to a corneal antigen in Fuchs' heterochromic cyclitis patients. Invest Ophthalmol Vis Sci 1989;30:443–448.
74. Foets BJJ, van den Oord JJ, Billiau A, et al: Heterogeneous induction of MHC class II antigens on corneal endothelium by INF-γ. Invest Ophthalmol Vis Sci 1991;32:341–345.
75. Foets BJJ, van den Oord JJ, Volpes R, et al: In situ immunohistochemical analysis of cell adhesion molecule on human corneal endothelial cells. Br J Ophthalmol 1992;76:205–209.
76. Alanko HI, Vuorre I, Saari KM: Characteristics of corneal endothelial cells in Fuchs' heterochromic cyclitis. Acta Ophthalmol 1986;64:623–631.
77. La Hey E, Broersma L, van der Gaag R, et al: Does autoimmunity to S-antigen play a role in Fuchs' heterochromic cyclitis? Br J Ophthalmol 1993;77:436–439.
78. Muhaya M, Calder V, Towler HMA, et al: Characterization of T cells and cytokines in the aqueous humour in patients with Fuchs' heterochromic cyclitis and idiopathic anterior uveitis. Clin Exp Immunol 1998;111:123–128.
79. Arocker-Mettinger E, Asenbauer T, Ulbrich S, et al: Serum interleukin-2 receptor levels in uveitis. Curr Eye Res 1990;9(suppl):25–29.
80. Bloch-Michel E, Lampin P, Debbia M, et al: Local production of IgG and IgG subclasses in the aqueous humour of patients with Fuchs' heterochromic cyclitis, herpetic uveitis and toxoplasmic chorioretinitis. Int Ophthalmol 1997;21:187–194.
81. Murray PI, Hoekzema R, Luyendijk L, et al: Analysis of aqueous humour immunoglobulin G in uveitis by enzyme-linked immunosorbent assay, isoelectric focusing, and immunoblotting. Invest Ophthalmol Vis Sci 1990;31:2129–2135.
82. Murray PI, Hoekzema R, van Haren MA, et al: Aqueous humour analysis in Fuchs' heterochromic cyclitis. Curr Eye Res 1990;9(suppl):53–57.
83. La Hey E, Mooy CM, Baarsma GS, et al: Immune deposits in iris biopsy specimens from patients with Fuchs' heterochromic iridocyclitis. Am J Ophthalmol 1992;113:75–80.
84. Vourre I, Saari M, Tilikainen I, et al: Fuchs' heterochromic cyclitis associated with retinitis pigmentosa: A family study. Can J Ophthalmol 1979;14:10–16.
85. van der Born LI, van Schooneveld JM, de Jong TVM, et al: Fuchs' heterochromic uveitis associated with retinitis pigmentosa in a father and son. Br J Ophthalmol 1994;78:504–505.
86. Vadot E: Cyclite heterochromique de Fuchs post-traumatique. Bull Soc Ophthalmol Fr 1981;81:665–667.
87. Donoso LA, Eiferman RA, Magargal LE: Fuchs' heterochromic cyclitis associated with subclavian steal syndrome. Ann Ophthalmol 1981;13:1153–1155.
88. Huber A, Kraus-Mackiw E: Heterochromiezyklitis Fuchs bei Möbius Syndrom. Klin Monatsbl Augenheilkd 1981;178:182–185.
89. Pietruschka G, Priesz G: Clinical problems of different forms of heterochromia. Klin Monatsbl Augenheilkd 1975;166:494–498.
90. Raab EL: Clinical features of Duane's syndrome. J Pediatr Ophthalmol Strabismus 1986;23:64–68.
91. Posner A, Schlossmann A: Syndrome of unilateral recurrent attacks of glaucoma with cyclitis symptoms. Arch Ophthalmol 1948;39:517.
92. Jones NP: Glaucoma in Fuchs heterochromic uveitis: Aetiology, management, outcome. Eye 1991;5:662–667.
93. Razzak A, Al-Samarrai A: Intraocular lens implantation following cataract extraction in Fuchs' heterochromic uveitis. Ophthalmic Res 1990;22:134–136.
94. Chung YM, Yeh TS: Intraocular lens implantation following cataract extraction in uveitis. Ophthalmic Res 1990;21:272–276.
95. Jakeman CM, Jordan K, Keast-Butler J, et al: Cataract surgery with intraocular lens implantation in Fuchs' heterochromic cyclitis. Eye 1990;4:543–547.
96. Swewood DR, Rosenthal AR: Cataract surgery in Fuchs' heterochromic iridocyclitis. Br J Ophthalmol 1992;76:238–240.
97. Jones NP: Cataract surgery using heparin surface-modified intraocular lenses in Fuchs' heterochromic uveitis. Ophthalmic Surg 1995;26:49–52.
98. Foster RE, Lowder CY, Meisler DM, et al: Extracapsular cataract extraction and posterior chamber intraocular lens implantation in uveitis patients. Ophthalmology 1992;99:1234–1241.
99. Jones NP: Cataract surgery in Fuchs' heterochromic uveitis: Past, present and future. J Cataract Refract Surg 1996;22:261–268.
100. La Hey E, de Vries J, Langerhorst CT, et al: Treatment and prognosis of secondary glaucoma in Fuchs' heterochromic iridocyclitis. Am J Ophthalmol 1993;116:327–340.

Nikos N. Markomichelakis

DEFINITION

Multiple sclerosis (MS) is a chronic, inflammatory, demyelinating disease of the central nervous system (CNS) mostly affecting young adults. The hallmark of the disease is dissemination in time and space (i.e., multiple episodes of dysfunction and multiple areas of involvement within the CNS), although the homogeneity of MS as a disease entity has been a long-debated issue.[1] The disease is divided into benign, relapsing-remitting, and chronic progressive (primary and secondary) forms.[2, 3] The clinical picture is determined by the location of foci of demyelination within the CNS. Classic features include fatigue, cognitive dysfunction, dysarthria, decreased perception of vibration and position sense, ataxia and intention tremor, weakness or paralysis of one or more limbs, spasticity, bladder problems, sexual dysfunction, and pain. The eyes are frequently affected, with optic neuritis, extraocular muscle disturbances, uveitis, and retinal periphlebitis among the ophthalmic signs of the disease. Although the etiology of MS remains unknown, two types of disease processes have been postulated: direct infection of the CNS with a neurotropic agent, and autoimmunity.

HISTORY

Although the word sclerosis is derived from the Greek word scleros (hard), Greek or Roman physicians did not describe MS. Sir Augustus d'Esti, grandson of King George III of England, clearly described MS in 1822 in his diary.[4] In the mid 1800s, Carswell in London and Cruveilhier and Charcot in Paris published detailed illustrations of MS plaques and sclerosis (in the French literature the disease was called sclerose en plaques). These observers documented the intermittent and seemingly random neurologic symptoms and the variable evolution of the disease.[5]

In 1835, Charcot reported a woman with MS and "feebleness of vision," illustrating a link between optic neuritis and MS. Later, in 1866, Vulpian and Charcot emphasized the importance of ocular signs in MS, and in 1885, Uhthoff and Parinaud associated optic neuritis with MS. Sequin published the first American reports of "disseminated cerebrospinal sclerosis," including cases of optic neuritis with subacute transverse myelitis.[5] Adie, Denny-Brown, and McAlpine[6] all stated that unilateral retrobulbar neuritis was a symptom of MS. Retinal venous sheathing in patients with MS was first described clinically by Rucker[7] in 1944. In 1965, Archambau and colleagues[8] mentioned patients with MS who had associated uveitis. Breger and Leopold[9] reported that ocular inflammation in patients with MS has the form of intermediate uveitis.

EPIDEMIOLOGY

The first episode of MS usually occurs between ages 20 and 40 years. Onset of the disease before age 14 or beyond age 60 is uncommon. Women outnumber men by about 1.8 to 1.[10] There is a striking geographic variation in the prevalence of MS. The disease is rare in equatorial regions and becomes increasingly more common in higher latitudes in either hemisphere. The prevalence in northern Europe, Canada, New Zealand, and southern Australia is more than 30 cases in 100,000 population.[11] In the Mediterranean basin and southern South America, the prevalence is moderate (5 to 29 in 100,000).[11] In Asia, India, Africa, the Caribbean, Central America, Mexico, and northern South America, MS is rare (less than five new cases each year per 100,000 persons).[11] It is estimated that over 100,000 persons in the United States are afflicted with MS.[12] However, northern states have a prevalence of over 100 in 100,000, in contrast to southern states, where it is only 20 in 100,000.[10] Several investigators have shown that the number of cases in some locales may be increasing.[13–15]

Optic neuritis is a common manifestation of MS; it may be the initial expression or it may occur later in the course of the disease. Approximately 15% to 25% of cases of definite MS present with optic neuritis, and an additional 40% to 73% will suffer an attack of optic neuritis at some point.[16–18] Conversely, 30% of patients with optic neuritis will develop clinically definite MS, as reported by the Optic Neuritis Study Group.[19] The longer patients with optic neuritis are followed, the greater the prevalence of subsequent demyelinative signs and symptoms. In a population-based study in Olmsted County, Minnesota, the life-table analysis showed that of 95 patients with isolated optic neuritis in the prevalence cohort, 39% had progressed to clinically definite MS by 10 years of follow-up, 49% had done so by 20 years, 54% by 30 years, and 60% by 40 years.[20] The same study reported equal risks of developing MS in men and women, in contrast to a study in New England,[21] in which the risk rate was 3.4 times greater for women.

The reported frequency of uveitis among patients with MS varies widely, from 0.4% to 26.9%.[8, 9, 21–24] These extreme differences may reflect the variations in patient populations, diagnostic criteria, and examination techniques. As uveitis may develop as late as 17 years after the onset of MS,[25] it is apparent that the longer the follow-up, the higher the prevalence. The prevalence of MS in the total uveitic population has been reported to be 1% to 2%,[23, 24, 26, 27] with a higher prevalence among patients with intermediate uveitis, ranging from 7.8% to 14.8%.[25, 28–30] The prevalence of MS in patients with uveitis at the Massachusetts Eye and Ear Infirmary is 1.3%, and 8% in the subgroup of patients with intermediate uveitis.[31]

CLINICAL FEATURES

Systemic Manifestations

MS lesions in the brain and spinal cord can potentially damage every function of the CNS.

Fatigue

This is the most common symptom in MS and is seen in all stages of the condition.[32] Fatigue is sometimes unprovoked (lassitude), or it can develop rapidly after only minimal activity. It is usually worse in high temperature or high humidity or in the afternoon; the body temperature is slightly higher in all of these situations. This extreme sensitivity to heat is called Uhthoff's phenomenon.

Sensory Disturbance

Sensory symptoms are common and are characteristically difficult for the patient to describe. Tingling, numbness, a tight band, pins and needles, a dead feeling, ice inside the leg, standing on broken glass, and something "not right" are common descriptions patients employ in their attempts to describe the sensory symptoms. Paresthesias typically begin in a hand or foot, progress over several days to involve the entire limb, and then resolve over several weeks. One third of MS patients experience Lhermitte's sign, described as the feeling of an electric shock or vibration running from the neck down the spine, especially if the examiner exerts pressure on the patient's inion at the back of the skull or with flexion of the neck.[33]

Pain

Pain is only recently recognized as a frequent symptom in patients with MS. Up to two thirds of patients with MS complain of pain at some time during the course of their disease. Pain may be acute or chronic. The spectrum of pain is broad and includes trigeminal neuralgia, headaches, radicular pain, musculoskeletal pain, dysesthesias, tonic seizures, spasms, and clonus.

Poor Mobility

Weakness often affects the legs and sometimes the arms. Patients complain of weakness, stiffness, a foot-drop, or tripping. On examination, the hip flexors are often weak. Hyperreflexia, spasticity, and the Babinski sign are common.

Bladder/Bowel/Sexual Dysfunction

Bladder dysfunction, including hesitancy, urgency, frequency, and incontinence, is common; it is the initial symptom in 5% and develops later in 90% of patients.[34] Equally common is bowel dysfunction, particularly constipation.[35] Women are more likely to complain of loss of genital sensation and occasionally develop anorgasmia.[36]

Cognitive Dysfunction

This is well established as a common problem in MS patients. A recent study has demonstrated that the impairment of memory is a factor for poor prognosis.[37]

Speech or Swallowing Disturbance

The cerebellum or its pathways are damaged in 50% of patients with MS. Intention tremor of the limbs, head or trunk titubation, and dysarthria can be totally disabling.

Psychiatric Disturbance

The incidence of depression is increased in MS patients and their families.[38] Euphoria, when it occurs, indicates widespread cerebral disease and is often associated with dementia.

Ocular Manifestations

Diplopia or Nystagmus

Diplopia may occur because the third or sixth cranial nerve pathways are damaged along their course within the CNS. Medial rectus weakness is usually part of an internuclear ophthalmoplegia (INO) that is caused by medial longitudinal fasciculus lesions. INO is paresis or weakness of adduction ipsilateral to the medial longitudinal fasciculus lesion and dissociated nystagmus of the abducting eye. Bilateral INO in a young patient is nearly pathognomonic of MS.[39] Nystagmus is common but usually inconsequential.[40] Horner's syndrome is also occasionally present.

Optic Neuritis

The optic nerves are frequently involved, especially in younger patients.[41] Optic neuritis is considered a forme fruste of MS and a harbinger of underlying neurologic disease. Optic neuritis typically begins with rapid loss of vision, partial or total, usually in one eye. Although central scotoma is more common, virtually any field defect can be seen. Color perception and contrast sensitivity disturbance is seen in virtually all patients and is often out of proportion to the reduction in visual acuity. Pain in or behind the eye accompanies optic neuritis and sometimes precedes the visual loss. The pain is present at rest, on voluntary movement, and with pressure on the globe. A unilateral afferent pupil defect is usually seen.

The fundus is normal in cases with retrobulbar neuritis. Fewer than half of optic neuritis patients show papillitis. Slitlike defects in the peripapillary nerve fiber layer have been described in patients with MS with and without a history of acute optic neuritis. Retinal nerve fiber layer defects can best be seen with red-free light. Retinal venous sheathing may accompany optic neuritis.

Visual acuity usually begins to improve 2 weeks after the onset of optic neuritis, and resolution continues over several months. Complete recovery of visual acuity is common, but other disturbances of vision may persist, such as visual blurring, drab colors, and red or blue desaturation. The reduction of apparent light intensity is often associated with an ipsilateral Marcus Gunn pupillary response. Bright lights cause a prolonged afterimage, a "flight of colors." Eye movements sometimes cause fleeting flashes of light (movement phosphenes), which may correspond to Lhermitte's sign. Depth perception is impaired and is worse with moving objects (Pulfrich phenomenon). Increased body temperature can amplify all of these symptoms and may diminish visual acuity (Uhthoff's phenomenon). After the neuritis resolves, the disc is usually pale (optic pallor), commonly in its temporal aspect.

Uveitis

Intermediate uveitis is the form of ocular inflammation most commonly encountered in patients with MS. The differences from the idiopathic form of pars planitis (PP) are minimal. Nussenblatt and colleagues[42] note that patients with MS typically develop a granulomatous anterior uveitis with formation of mutton-fat keratic precipitates, in contrast to patients with idiopathic intermediate uveitis, who have minimal anterior segment inflammation. According to Bamford and coworkers,[43] special signs in MS patients have been observed: vascular sheathing in the posterior pole (and not near the affected pars plana) and absence of macular edema (in contrast to idiopathic PP). In my experience at the Massachusetts Eye and Ear Infirmary and the General Hospital of Athens, there are similarities in clinical findings, course, and outcome of patients with PP with no evidence of an underlying systemic disease and those with MS (unpublished data). Posterior synechiae formation tends to be more common among patients with MS (29% versus 14%). Periphlebitis in MS can be found either in the posterior pole or in the retinal periphery. Although the incidence of periphlebitis in intermediate uveitis is independent of the coexistence of MS, the involvement of vessels in the posterior pole is more common in MS (41% versus 26%). I have not observed any difference in the incidence of macular edema or epiretinal membrane among PP patients with or without MS. In my experience, retinal vasculitis in MS ranges from mild venous sheathing to severe retinal involvement with vascular occlusion, neovascularization, and vitreous hemorrhage. Similar findings have been reported by Graham and colleagues.[44] Optic neuritis may either precede or follow the onset of intermediate uveitis.[27, 29]

Anterior uveitis is rare in patients with MS.[45–47] When present, it takes the form of granulomatous iridocyclitis with iris nodule formation.[48] Posterior uveitis associated with MS has been reported only sporadically,[8] although pathologic reports showed increased incidences of choroiditis (11.5%)[49] and retinitis (6.4%).[50]

Retinal venous sheathing has been described in MS patients with and without concomitant uveitis,[43, 44, 51] as well as in patients with optic neuritis.[29, 52]

COMPLICATIONS

The most common ocular complication of MS is atrophy of the optic nerve and inner retinal layers. The disc is usually pale (optic pallor), commonly in its temporal aspect. Clinical detection of retinal nerve fiber layer atrophy is possible only after a 50% loss of neural tissue in a given area. The varying degrees of atrophy are secondary to retrograde degeneration of axons in plaques of the pregeniculate pathways in MS.[49] Several authors have reported disc pallor in upwards of 50% of cases (Fig. 62–1).[53, 54]

Complications of intermediate uveitis, as shown in many large series of patients, include, in decreasing order of frequency, cataract formation, cystoid macular edema, epiretinal membrane formation, glaucoma, retinal detachment, and neovascularization with and without vitreous hemorrhage. Whether these complications occur differently in intermediate uveitis associated with MS has been, until recently, unclear. Breger and Leopold,[9] in a series of 14 patients, reported only one patient with lenticular opacities, and three patients with possible macular edema (absent foveal reflex). Chester and coworkers,[28] using fluorescein angiograms (FA), found three of seven patients with central leakage. At the Massachusetts Eye and Ear Infirmary and the General Hospital of Athens, in a series of 17 patients (34 eyes) with intermediate uveitis and definite MS, the following complications were

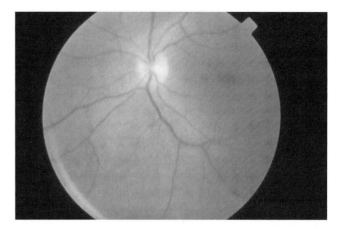

FIGURE 62–1. Optic nerve pallor following optic neuritis. (See color insert.)

found: cataract formation (44%), chronic cystoid macular edema (28%), optic pallor (23%), severe epiretinal membrane (12%), elevated intraocular pressure (12%), retinal schisis (6%), and vitreous hemorrhage (3%). With the exception of optic disc atrophy due to optic neuritis, the frequencies of complications are comparable with those in idiopathic PP and sarcoidosis.

ETIOLOGY

The cause of MS remains unknown despite decades of intense research. Hundreds of epidemiologic and genetic studies, pathologic analyses, and animal models have suggested several etiologies, but none are universally accepted. There appears to be an autoimmune attack against myelin and myelin-forming cells in the brain and spinal cord. MS, however, has been difficult to definitively classify as a true autoimmune disease.[55] T-cell and antibody reactivity have been tested against numerous brain antigens, but no target antigen has been clearly and consistently demonstrated. Cloned T cells from MS patients show excessive reactions to myelin antigens in some studies but not in others. It is possible that the immune response evolves through epitope spreading, generating responses to a number of CNS antigens. The lack of a causative antigen suggests that regulation of immune responses may be abnormal and that oligodendroglia are innocent bystanders that are damaged by unregulated inflammation.

The heterogeneity of the disease suggests that a variety of causes may be involved in the etiology. Migration, ethnic, and twin studies suggest that both genes and environment affect the development of MS.

Many viruses have been implicated as the cause of MS. The list includes rabies virus, measles virus, rubella virus, mumps virus, coronaviruses, canine distemper virus, herpesvirus (herpes simplex virus, varicella-zoster virus, Epstein-Barr virus), simian-virus-5, Marek's virus, JC virus, and tick-borne encephalitis virus.[56] The most recent candidates are human herpesvirus-6 (a member of the β-herpes virus family) and MS-associated retrovirus (a member of the endogenous retrovirus-9 family).[56] Unfortunately, none of these claims has withstood intense scrutiny and the test of time. The question remains as to whether a virus, directly or indirectly, triggers the immune reaction seen in MS, or whether this arises from autoantigenic stimulus independent of viral infection, whether it be systemic or local.

Bacteria also have been implicated in the etiology of MS.[57] Experimental allergic encephalomyelitis (EAE), the experimental analogue of MS, is induced by mixing tissue cells with adjuvant that contains *Mycobacterium tuberculosis*. Additionally, clinical studies show that there is a three-fold increase in exacerbations after bacterial infections.[58]

Environmental causes have been suggested, but none is clearly a direct cause of MS. Seasonal variations in MS frequency differ in various locales.[59] Other putative environmental etiologies include nutrition, high consumption of animal fat and low intake of fish products,[60, 61] latitude,[62] sunlight,[63] exposure to wool or sheep, and high socioeconomic status.[60]

There are multiple genetic influences on the development of MS. First-degree relatives have a 10- to 70-fold increased risk of developing MS compared to the general population.[64] Although this could be interpreted as reflecting an environmental exposure rather than a genetic predisposition, the monozygotic concordance rate is 30% and the dizygotic rate is 5%, indicating that there is a genetic component to MS.[65] Familial cases do not follow Mendelian genetics. Chataway and colleagues suggest that MS depends on independent or epistatic effects of several genes, each with small individual effects.[66] The most prevalent human leukocyte antigen (HLA) determinants found in the MS population of northern European origin are DR15 (the subtype of DR2 that expresses DRB1*1501) and DQ6.[67] Weinshenker and colleagues, in Olmsted County, Minnesota, found a positive association between MS susceptibility and the DR15-DQ6 and DR13-DQ7 haplotypes; however, they did not find any association with disease severity.[68] Barcellos and colleagues found a significant effect of a single locus on chromosome 19q13.2 in Caucasian patients with MS.[69] The consensus view is that it is polygenetic—the major histocompatibility complex being the most important but not the only genetic factor.

PATHOGENESIS AND PATHOLOGY

An MS plaque is formed after activated peripheral T cells adhere to CNS postcapillary venules. The T cells pass through the endothelial cells and migrate into the periventricular parenchyma. An equivalent number of monocytes are also present at this early stage. The inflammation is associated with destruction of the inner myelin lamellae and dysfunction of oligodendroglia.

Immune activation in the periphery may precede neurologic problems and possibly magnetic resonance imaging (MRI) abnormalities. A complex imbalance in both cytokine and the Fas-FasL system is present in MS.[70] In active MS, lymphocytes express excessive levels of activation proteins (HLA-DR, CD71, SLAM+) and costimulatory molecules (B7-1 and B7-2).[70, 71] The data from several studies indicate that different cytokine profiles may be observed in patients with acute or stable disease. High levels of interleukin (IL)-10 and transforming growth factor (TGF)-β are present in the cerebrospinal fluid (CSF) of patients in a stable phase of MS, whereas elevated levels of tissue necrosis factor (TNF)-α and granulocyte-macrophage colony-stimulating factor (GM-CSF) are observed in the active phase.[72] Expressions of TNF-α, interferon (INF)-γ, and IL-10 mRNA are higher in the CSF and white blood cells of MS patients.[73–75] Vandervyner and colleagues found that TNF-α and INF-γ mRNA levels are significantly elevated among myelin basic protein reactive T-cell clones derived from HLA-DR2–positive MS patients.[76]

The role of apoptosis in MS has been investigated with regard to the oligodendrocyte, the myelinating cell and the CNS, and the lymphocyte. The issue is still controversial in MS. However, with EAE, modulation of apoptosis in transgenic animals has been shown to influence the course of the disease.[77]

Taken together, these data suggest that, more likely than not, MS develops in the genetically susceptible individual who is exposed to some trigger (e.g., a microbe), with subsequent T-cell activation or loss of self-tolerance. Several different mechanisms may play a role in the initiation and perpetuation of the inflammation through T-cell activation. A myelin basic protein (MBP) peptide or superantigens can activate T cells. Exogenous antigens, and even self-antigens, sharing sequence similarities with MBP peptide can activate MBP-specific T cells (molecular mimicry). Superantigens, which are microbial proteins, can also activate T cells expressing a given Vβ family member. Another potential mechanism is the activation of autoreactive T cells, which can be triggered either through the T-cell antigen receptor or through an antigen-independent mechanism during the course of an inflammatory reaction.[77]

The nature of the relation between PP and MS is not clear. Many questions arise from the association: Do PP and MS have a common pathogenetic mechanism? Or does the coexistence of PP with MS represent the tendency of more than one disease of immune etiology to occur in certain individuals? Edelsten and colleagues reported an increased prevalence of HLA-B7 in patients with MS and symptomatic uveitis.[78] Malinowski and colleagues found an association with HLA-B8, B51, and DR2 in their group of PP patients.[79] Most recently, Tang and coworkers[80] and Raja and colleagues[81] demonstrated a strong association of HLA-DR15 and intermediate uveitis, and they mentioned the lack of any association between HLA-DR16 (the other "split" epitope of HLA-DR2) and expression of the PP phenotype.

Uveitis has been observed in EAE produced by immunization with CNS homogenates.[82, 83] EAE has been observed by immunizing with uveal tissue, although uveitis was not produced.[82] Thus, similar antigens may exist in the CNS and uvea or retina, and these findings could be explained by an autoimmune response to a common factor in MS. Ohguro and coworkers[84] found serum antibodies to arrestin (retinal S-antigen) in 8 of 14 patients with MS without any evidence of uveitis. The antibody titers were higher during relapses than during remissions, and the authors suggest that antibodies reactive with arrestin may be related to the clinical course of MS. These findings could also explain the development of uveitis in some patients with MS.

Lucchinetti and colleagues described at least five distinct patterns of MS pathology, based mainly on the preservation or loss of oligodendrocytes.[85] In pathologic studies of eyes from patients with MS, observation of uveal tract inflammation has been rare, in contrast to studies of vascular inflammation.[49, 50] According to Arnold and colleagues,[50] retinal phlebitis is not a secondary response to uveitis or a passive extension of a CNS infiltrate but a concurrent part of a multifocal process in neural tissue.

DIAGNOSIS

The established clinical criteria for the diagnosis of MS depend on the clinical demonstration of lesions disseminated in both time and space in separate portions of the white matter of the CNS. Patients are also expected to have clinically appropriate MS-like symptoms. Criteria that must be satisfied to establish a diagnosis of clinically definite MS include a reliable history of at least two episodes of neurologic deficit and objective clinical signs of lesions at more than one site within the CNS.[86] Demonstration of a second lesion by paraclinical and laboratory tests, in concert with one objective clinical lesion, also fulfills the criteria.[87]

An MRI, examination of the CSF, and evaluation of evoked potentials are performed to establish a diagnosis of MS. Other ancillary testing, such as FA, is useful in evaluating ocular signs or detecting subclinical ocular manifestations.

Magnetic Resonance Imaging

MRI abnormalities can clearly support the diagnosis of MS. The plaques typically appear as areas of increased signal intensity on T2-weighted and proton density images, and sometimes as areas of decreased signal intensity on T1-weighted images (Fig. 62–2). The current feeling is that for an MRI to be strongly suggestive of MS there should be three lesions, at least one periventricular, or four or more lesions. Lesions larger than 6 mm in diameter are more specific for MS than smaller lesions. Lesions that arise from the corpus callosum and infratentorial lesions or oval-shaped lesions have high specificity for the diagnosis of MS. If a lesion of a specific type or location suggestive of MS is found, in addition to the three or four lesions just indicated, the specificity for MS probably increases.[88]

Laboratory Testing

The CSF shows elevated protein; a moderate increase in white blood cells (often containing occasional blasts in active disease); increased immunoglobulin G (IgG), IgG/albumin index, and IgG synthesis rate; and oligoclonal bands. An index ratio of CSF antibodies to measles, rubella, and herpes zoster may improve sensitivity.[89]

Electrophysiology

Evoked potentials are occasionally helpful (e.g., when the MRI and CSF are normal), but they should not be used for the routine diagnosis of MS. The frequency of abnormal evoked potentials in definite MS is as follows: visual = 90%, auditory = 80%, and somatosensory = 70%. In patients with optic neuritis, visual evoked potentials are always abnormal in the affected eye, but 35% of patients return to normal within 2 years.[90]

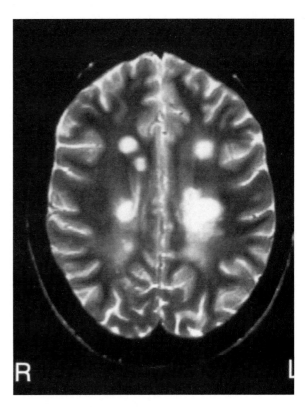

FIGURE 62–2. MRI abnormalities.

Fluorescein Angiography

FA is helpful in delineating the presence of vasculitis. Dye leakage or staining of vessel walls corresponding to areas of sheathing indicates active periphlebitis. Sheathing without fluorescein abnormality was observed in patients with venous sclerosis.[43] The most prominent finding on angiography is dye leakage from the retinal venules and capillaries late in the study, which results in cystoid macular and retinal edema.

Other Ancillary Tests

Visual field testing is helpful in detecting optic neuritis. Perimetry shows scotomata that are usually diffuse or central but sometimes are peripheral. Contrast sensitivity tests, flight of colors tests, and color vision tests are useful to detect subclinical optic tract lesions in patients with MS and normal visual acuity but no history of optic neuritis.[91] Color vision abnormalities are traditionally most pronounced with red light; acutely, blue/yellow defects may be more common.[92]

A diagnosis of MS should be questioned, judiciously, when there are (1) no eye findings, (2) no remissions, (3) localized disease, (4) no sensory or bladder symptoms, and (5) normal CSF.[93]

DIFFERENTIAL DIAGNOSIS

Other diseases that may mimic MS must be excluded (Table 61–1). Inflammatory systemic diseases that produce encephalomyelopathy, optic neuritis, ophthalmoplegia, retinal vasculitis, and uveitis include neurosyphilis, neuroborreliosis, viral infections, Adamantiades-Behçet disease (ABD), and sarcoidosis.

TABLE 62–1. DISEASES THAT MAY MIMIC MULTIPLE SCLEROSIS

Central nervous system (CNS) lymphoma
CNS vasculitis
Syphilis
Lyme disease
Sarcoidosis

Neurosyphilis, both the meningovascular type and tabes dorsalis, may mimic MS. The classic ocular finding is the Argyll Robertson pupil. Also, disc edema or optic atrophy, and oculomotor palsies are frequently found. However, uveitis and retinal vasculitis are rare.[94] Moreover, the clinical history, together with positive serology for syphilis, reactive CSF Venereal Disease Research Laboratory (VDRL) test, and MRI evidence, serve to distinguish this entity from MS.

Lyme neuroborreliosis may mimic MS clinically and on MRI. Intermediate uveitis, vasculitis, and optic neuritis have been reported in Lyme disease.[95] The presence of erythema migrans is a single pathognomonic criterion. Serum and intrathecal production of anti–*Borrelia burgdorferi* antibody occurs frequently. A positive enzyme-linked immunosorbent assay is suggestive for Lyme disease, but this should be confirmed by Western blotting.

Herpes family viruses may produce encephalitis. Uveitis (acute retinal necrosis syndrome[96, 97] or frosted branch angiitis[98]) may occur at the same time, or following infection as a result of reactivation of virus. These disorders are monophasic, in contrast with MS. Detection of virus in ocular fluids or in CSF by polymerase chain reaction could confirm the diagnosis of a viral infection.

Human T-cell leukemia/lymphoma virus (HTLV)-1 has been implicated in the etiology of MS, and this virus has been associated with intermediate uveitis.[99] Therefore, in endemic areas HTLV-1 may be included in the differential diagnosis.

ABD can cause episodic, multifocal CNS lesions that can be confused with MS clinically and on MRI. However, ABD is associated with genital and oral ulcers and meningoencephalitis. Uveitis is anterior with hypopyon, or posterior with areas of retinal infraction with hemorrhage and edematous retina. Patients experience multiple explosive inflammatory episodes. PP has been reported in ABD,[30] but this is relatively rare. Optic neuropathy may be seen, but it has the form of papillitis.[100]

Sarcoidosis may involve all components of the nervous system.[101] Rarely, multiple lesions that mimic MS, spinal cord abnormalities, and peripheral neuropathy can occur. Optic neuritis,[102] intermediate uveitis,[25] and periphlebitis[103] are common manifestations of sarcoidosis. Sarcoidosis must be excluded in the evaluation of patients with uveitis who are suspected of having MS.

NATURAL COURSE AND PROGNOSIS

The course of MS varies. The Advisory Committee on Clinical Trials of New Agents in MS of the National Multiple Sclerosis Society has specified consensus definitions of the clinical course of MS.[104] The recommended course labels are relapsing-remitting, primary progressive, secondary progressive, and progressive-relapsing MS.

These categories are not immutable; patients frequently drift from one type of MS to another, become stable, or suddenly develop active disease.

The clinical prognosis of optic neuritis in patients with MS is surprisingly good. The Optic Neuritis Study Group[105] has recently reported the visual changes and frequency of recurrent optic neuritis in the first 5 years after enrollment in the Optic Neuritis Treatment Trial. According to these results, contrast sensitivity is more often abnormal than is visual acuity, visual field, or color vision. Visual acuity is generally well preserved even if it is severely reduced at presentation.

In large populations, 20% to 40% have "benign disease," defined as having less than moderate disability after 10 years. Half will develop progressive MS within 10 years. Patients with the greatest risk of disability are those with primary progressive disease, and relapsing-remitting patients who are older at onset.[106]

The prognosis of intermediate uveitis associated with MS is not well documented. In a series of nine patients,[23] visual acuity was 6/9 or better in all 17 eyes, color vision was impaired in only 1 of 17 eyes, and optic atrophy was present in 6 of 17 eyes. Malinowski and colleagues[29] found an overall favorable visual prognosis in 54 patients with PP, among them 8 patients with definite MS. In my experience, the course and the final outcome of intermediate uveitis associated with MS are comparable with those of idiopathic intermediate uveitis. Among our 17 PP patients with MS, and with a follow-up ranging from 3 to 15 years, the average number of exacerbations per year was 0.65. More than half of our patients experienced final visual acuity better than 20/40, and one fourth had 20/20. Poor visual outcome was attributed to recurrent attacks of retrobulbar neuritis, leading to optic atrophy.

THERAPY

Many approaches to the treatment of MS have been employed, but no treatment completely halts the disease.[107] Glucocorticoids, such as oral prednisone and adrenocorticotropic hormone, temporarily ameliorate many of the symptoms of MS by reducing edema and inflammation, but they do not alter the course of the disease.[108] High-dose intravenous methylprednisolone lessens recurrences of optic neuritis and prevents the development of MS only during the first 2 years.[109] Azathioprine produces modest benefits with respect to relapse rates and disease progression after 2 or more years of treatment.[110] Cyclophosphamide, because of its modest impact on disease progression and its potentially severe side effects, is generally reserved for patients with aggressive relapsing/remitting or chronic progressive disease in whom other treatments have failed.[111] Methotrexate causes slight improvement on a composite score of neurologic function. In patients with rapidly progressive disease, it might be worth considering.[112] Cladribine, a nucleoside drug, targets both resting and dividing lymphocytes and may be able to destroy the activated T cells that induce CNS demyelination, thus producing stabilization or improvement in chronic MS.[113] In an 18-month clinical trial, MRI lesions that enhanced after gadolium administration were completely suppressed in the cladribine-treated patients by the sixth month of treatment.[114] At present, there is no evidence to support the use of intravenous immunoglobulins in secondary or primary progressive MS.[115] Sulfasalazine causes early improvement but no long-term benefit.[116] Linomide (quinoline 3-carboxamide) is a synthetic immunomodulator that can stimulate various lymphocyte subpopulations[117] and increase the activity of natural killer cells.[118] Up-regulation of naive T cells and parallel down-regulation of memory T lymphocytes may represent one main mechanism by which Linomide inhibits MS activity. Clinical trials have revealed that Linomide not only significantly reduces clinical and MRI activity in secondary progressive[117] or relapsing/remitting[119] MS, but it also prevents the appearance of new active lesions on the MRI scan in secondary progressive MS.[118] However, Linomide failed to induce remyelination in a viral model of MS.[120]

Recent studies have shown that INF-β-1b[121] delays sustained neurologic deterioration in patients with secondary progressive MS, while INF-β-1a[122] alters the course of relapsing/remitting MS. Copolymer-1 (glatiramer acetate) also reduces clinical disease activity in relapsing/remitting MS.[123] However, a 2-year longitudinal study showed that it had no effect on cognitive function in relapsing/remitting MS.[124]

It remains unclear whether the various therapeutic modalities used in the treatment of MS are effective against MS-associated uveitis. Clinical trials describing the natural course and treatment results specifically of uveitis associated with MS have not been reported to date.

Currently, MS-associated intermediate uveitis and its complications are treated in the same manner as idiopathic intermediate uveitis. I treat these cases with a stepladder approach, basing the decision to treat not only on the level of visual acuity but on the presence or absence of uveitis, even at low intensity. When visual acuity is less than 20/30 and there is active inflammation, I use transseptal injections of corticosteroids. If this fails or when aggressive inflammation is present, I administer methotrexate, azathioprine, cyclosporine-A, or INF-1β, depending on the bias of the patient's neurologist.

CONCLUSIONS

MS is an immunologically mediated disorder in which inflammation of the CNS is the prominent feature, resulting in various neurologic signs and symptoms. MS mainly affects young females from the northern part of the globe. The most frequent ocular manifestations of the disease are optic neuritis, intermediate uveitis, and periphlebitis. Prognosis of the ocular disease is surprisingly good. Although there are new treatment modalities with promising results, their influence on the ocular disease is not yet known.

References

1. Baker AB: Problems in the classification of multiple sclerosis. In: Alter M, Kurtzke JF, eds: The Epidemiology of Multiple Sclerosis. Springfield, IL: Charles C Thomas, 1968, pp 14–25.
2. Filippi M, Campi A, Martinelli V, et al: Brain and spinal cord MR in benign multiple sclerosis: A follow-up study. J Neurol Sci 1996;143:143–149.
3. Weinshenker BG, Miller D: Multiple sclerosis: One disease or many? In: Paty D, Ebers GC, eds: Multiple Sclerosis. Philadelphia: FA Davis, 1997, pp 37–46.
4. Firth D: The Case of Augustus d'Esti. Great Britain, Cambridge University Press, 1948, 1–59.
5. DeJong RN: Multiple sclerosis. History, definition and general considerations. In: Vinken PJ, Bruyn GW, eds: Handbook of Clinical Neurology. Multiple Sclerosis and Other Demyelinating Diseases. New York, Elsevier, 1970, pp 45–62.
6. Kurtzke JF: Clinical manifestations of multiple sclerosis. In: Vinken PJ, Bruyn GW, eds. Handbook of Clinical Neurology. Multiple Sclerosis and Other Demyelinating Diseases. New York, Elsevier, 1970, pp 161–216.
7. Rucker CW: Sheathing of the retina veins in multiple sclerosis. JAMA 1945;127:970–973.
8. Archambau PL, Hollenhurst RW, Rucker CW: Posterior uveitis as a manifestation of multiple sclerosis. Mayo Clin Proc 1965;40:544–551.
9. Breger BC, Leopold IH: The incidence of uveitis in multiple sclerosis. Am J Ophthalmol 1966;62:540–545.
10. Kurtzke JF, Beebe GW, Norman JE Jr: Epidemiology of multiple sclerosis in U.S. veterans: 1. Race, sex, and geographic distribution. Neurology 1979;29:1228–1235.
11. Kurtzke JF: A reassessment of the distribution of multiple sclerosis. Part one. Acta Neurol Scand 1975;51:110–136.
12. Jacobson DL, Gange SJ, Rose NR, Graham NM: Epidemiology and estimated population burden of selected autoimmune diseases in the United States. Clin Immunol Immunopathol 1997;84:223–243.
13. Kurtzke JF: Multiple sclerosis: Changing times. Neuroepidemiology 1991;10:1–8.
14. Wynn DR, Rodriguez M, O'Fallon WM, Kurland LT: A reappraisal of the epidemiology of multiple sclerosis in Olmsted County, Minnesota. Neurology 1990;40:780–786.
15. Midgard R, Riise T, Svanes C, et al: Incidence of multiple sclerosis in More and Romsdal, Norway, from 1950 to 1991. An age-period-cohort analysis. Brain 1996;119:203–211.
16. Shibasaki H, McDonald WI, Kuroiwa Y: Racial modification of clinical picture of multiple sclerosis: Comparison between British and Japanese patients. J Neurol Sci 1981;49:243.
17. Francis DA, Compston DA, Batchelor JR, et al: A reassessment of the risk of multiple sclerosis developing in patients with optic neuritis after extended follow-up. J Neurol Neurosurg Psychiatry 1987;50:6.
18. Cantore WA: Optic neuritis. Pa Med 1996;99(suppl):96–98.
19. Optic Neuritis Study Group. The 5-year risk of MS after optic neuritis. Experience of the Optic Neuritis Treatment Trial. Neurology 1997;49:1404–1418.
20. Rodriguez M, Siva A, Cross SA, et al: Optic neuritis: A population-based study in Olmsted County, Minnesota. Neurology 1995;45:244–250.
21. Porter R: Uveitis in association with multiple sclerosis. Br J Ophthalmol 1972;54:478–481.
22. Ardouin M, Urvoy M, Clement J, Oger J: Uvéite et sclérose en plaques: Mythe ou réalité? J Fr Ophthalmol 1979;2:127–130.
23. Graham EM, Francis DA, Sanders MD, Rudge P: Ocular inflammatory changes in established multiple sclerosis. J Neurol Neurosurg Psychiatry 1989;52:1360–1363.
24. Biousse V, Trichet C, Bloch-Michel E, Roullet E: Multiple sclerosis associated with uveitis in two large clinic-based series. Neurology 1999;52:179–181.
25. Zierhut M, Foster CS: Multiple sclerosis, sarcoidosis and other diseases in patients with pars planitis. Dev Ophthalmol 1992;23:41–47.
26. Rothova A, Buitenhuis HJ, Meenken C, et al: Uveitis and systemic disease. Br J Ophthalmol 1992;76:137–141.
27. McCannel CA, Holland GN, Helm CJ, et al: Causes of uveitis in the general practice of ophthalmology. UCLA Community-based uveitis study group. Am J Ophthalmol 1996;121:35–46.
28. Chester GH, Blach RK, Cleary PE: Inflammation in the region of the vitreous base: Pars planitis. Trans Ophthalmol Soc U K 1976;96:151–197.
29. Malinowski SM, Pulido JS, Folk JC: Long term visual outcome and complications associated with pars planitis. Ophthalmology 1993;100:818–825.
30. Palimeris G, Markomichelakis N, Konstantinidou V, Trakaniari AN: Intermediate uveitis. What is the natural course of the disease and its relationship with other systemic diseases? Eur J Ophthalmol 1994;3:223–227.

31. Rodriguez A, Calogne M, Pedroza-Seres M, et al: Referral patterns of uveitis in a tertiary eye care center. Arch Ophthalmol 1996;114:593–599.

32. Reder AT, Antel JP: Clinical spectrum of multiple sclerosis. Neurol Clin 1983;1:573–599.

33. Archibald CJ, McGrath PJ, Ritvo PG, et al: Pain prevalence, severity and impact in a clinic sample of multiple sclerosis patients. Pain 1994;58:89–93.

34. Andrews KL, Husmann DA: Bladder dysfunction and management in multiple sclerosis. Mayo Clin Proc 1997;72:1176–1183.

35. Stark ME: Challenging problems presenting as constipation. Am J Gastroenterol 1999;94:567–574.

36. Foley FW, Sanders A: Sexuality, multiple sclerosis and women. MS Management 1997;4:1–7.

37. Kujala P, Portin R, Ruuitiain J: The progress of cognitive decline in multiple sclerosis: A controlled 3-year follow-up. Brain 1997;120:289–297.

38. Fassbender K, Schmidt R, Mossner R, et al: Mood disorders and dysfunction of the hypothalamic-pituitary-adrenal axis in multiple sclerosis. Arch Neurol 1998;55:66–72.

39. Muri RM, Meienberg O: The clinical spectrum of internuclear ophthalmoplegia in multiple sclerosis. Arch Neurol 1985;42:851.

40. Gresty MA, Ell JJ, Findley LJ: Acquired pendular nystagmus: Its characteristics, localizing value and pathophysiology. J Neurol Neurosurg Psychiatry 1982;45:431.

41. Reder AT. Optic neuritis. In: Gilman S, ed: Neurobase, 4th ed. San Diego, Arbor, 1998.

42. Nussenblatt RB, Whitcup SM, Palestine AG: Intermediate uveitis. In: Uveitis: Fundamentals and Clinical Practice, 2nd ed. St. Louis, Mosby, 1996, 58–68.

43. Bamford CR, Gantly JP, Sibley WA, Laguna JF: Uveitis, perivenous sheathing and multiple sclerosis. Neurology 1978;28:119–124.

44. Graham EM, Stanford MR, Sander MD, et al: A point prevalence study of 150 patients with idiopathic retinal vasculitis: 1. Diagnostic value of ophthalmological features. Br J Ophthalmol 1989;73:714–721.

45. Curless RG, Bray PF: Uveitis and multiple sclerosis in an adolescent. Am J Dis Child 1972;123:149–150.

46. Meisler DM, Tomsak RL, Khoury S, et al: Anterior uveitis and multiple sclerosis. Cleve Clin J Med 1989;56:535–538.

47. Lim JI, Tessler HH, Goodwin JA: Anterior granulomatous uveitis in patients with multiple sclerosis. Ophthalmology 1991;98:142–145.

48. Bachman DM, Rosenthal AR, Beckingsale AB: Granulomatous uveitis in neurological disease. Br J Ophthalmol 1985;69:192–196.

49. Kerrison JB, Flynn T, Green WR: Retinal pathologic changes in multiple sclerosis. Retina 1994;14:445–451.

50. Arnold AC, Pepose JS, Hepler RS, Foos RY: Retinal periphlebitis and retinitis in multiple sclerosis. I. Pathologic characteristics. Ophthalmology 1984;91:255–262.

51. Engell T: Neurological disease activity in multiple sclerosis patients with periphlebitis retinae. Acta Neurol Scand 1986;73:168–172.

52. Lightman S, McDonald WI, Bird AC, et al: Retinal venous sheathing in optic neuritis: Its significance for pathogenesis of multiple sclerosis. Brain 1987;100:405.

53. Frisen L, Hoyt WF: Insidious atrophy of retinal nerve fibers in multiple sclerosis. Arch Ophthalmol 1974;92:91–97.

54. Elbol P, Work K: Retinal nerve fiber layer in multiple sclerosis. Acta Ophthalmol (Copenh) 1990;68:481–486.

55. Reder AT: Multiple sclerosis. In: Gilman S, ed: Neurobase, 4th ed. San Diego, Arbor, 1998.

56. Monteyne P, Bureau JF, Brahic M: Viruses and multiple sclerosis. Curr Opin Neurol 1998;11:287–291.

57. Janeway CH, Travers P: Immunobiology. The immune system in health and disease. London: Current Biology Ltd/Garland, 1994, chap. 11.

58. Rapp NS, Gilroy J, Lerner AM: Role of bacterial infection in exacerbation of multiple sclerosis. Am J Phys Med Rehabil 1995;4:415–418.

59. Goodkin DE, Hertsgaard D: Seasonal variation of multiple sclerosis exacerbations in North Dakota. Arch Neurol 1989;46:1015–1018.

60. Ben-Shlomo Y: Dietary fat in the epidemiology of multiple sclerosis: Has the situation been adequately assessed? Neuroepidemiology 1992;11:214–225.

61. Ghadirian P, Jain M, Ducic S, et al: Nutritional factors in the etiology of multiple sclerosis: A case-control study in Montreal, Canada. Int J Epidemiol 1998;27:845–852.

62. Esparza ML, Sasaki S, Kesteloot H: Nutrition, latitude, and multiple sclerosis mortality: An ecologic study. Am J Epidemiol 1995;142:733–737.

63. Hutter CD, Laing P: Multiple sclerosis: Sunlight, diet, immunology and etiology. Med Hypotheses 1996;46:67–74.

64. Hogancamp WE, Rodriguez M, Weinshenker BG: The epidemiology of multiple sclerosis. Mayo Clin Proc 1997;72:871–878.

65. Sadovnick AD, Armstrong H, Rice GPA, et al: A population-based study of multiple sclerosis in twins: Update. Ann Neurol 1993;33:281–285.

66. Chataway J, Feakes R, Coraddu F, et al: The genetics of multiple sclerosis: Principles, background, and updated results of the United Kingdom systematic genome screen. Brain 1998;121:1869–1887.

67. Martin RJ: Genetics of multiple sclerosis—How could disease-associated HLA-types contribute to pathogenesis? Neural Transm Suppl 1997;49:177–194.

68. Weinshenker BG, Santrach P, Bissonet AS, et al: Major histocompatibility complex class II alleles and the course and outcome of MS: A population-based study. Neurology 1998;51:742–747.

69. Barcellos LF, Thomson G, Carrington M, et al: Chromosome 19 single-locus and multilocus haplotype association with multiple sclerosis. Evidence of a new susceptibility locus in Caucasian and Chinese patients. JAMA 1997;15:1256–1261.

70. Ferrante P, Fusi ML, Saresella M, et al: Cytokine production and surface marker expression in acute and stable multiple sclerosis: Altered IL-12 production and augmented signaling lymphocytic activation molecule (SLAM)-expressing lymphocytes in acute multiple sclerosis. J Immunol 1998;160:1514–1521.

71. Genc K, Reder AT: Increased B7-1+ B cells in active multiple sclerosis, and reversal by interferon beta-1b therapy. J Clin Invest 1997;99:2664–2671.

72. Carrieri PB, Provitera V, De Rosa T, et al: Profile of cerebrospinal fluid and serum cytokines in patients with relapsing-remitting multiple sclerosis: A correlation with clinical activity. Immunopharmacol Immunotoxicol 1998;11:293–298.

73. Calabresi PA, Tranquill LR, McFarland HF, Cowan EP: Cytokine gene expression in cells derived from CSF of multiple sclerosis patients. J Neuroimmunol 1998;89:198–205.

74. Monteyne P, Sindic CJ: Data on cytokine mRNA expression in CSF and peripheral blood mononuclear cells from MS patients as detected by PCR. Mult Scler 1998;4:143–146.

75. Rieckmann P, Albrecht M, Kitze B, et al: Cytokine mRNA levels in mononuclear blood cells from patients with multiple sclerosis. Neurology 1994;44:1523–1526.

76. Vandervyner C, Motmans K, Stinissen P, et al: Cytokine mRNA profile of myelin basic protein reactive T-cell clones in patients with multiple sclerosis. Autoimmunity 1998;28:77–89.

77. Libau RS, Fontaine B: Recent advances in immunology in multiple sclerosis. Curr Opin Neurol 1998;11:293–298.

78. Edelsten C, Stanford MR, Ormerod I, Welsh KI: Prevalence of HLA B7 in MS with symptomatic uveitis. Lancet 1992;339:942.

79. Malinowski SM, Pulido JS, Goeken NE, et al: The association of HLA-B8, B51, DR2, and multiple sclerosis in pars planitis. Ophthalmology 1993;100:1199–1205.

80. Tang WM, Pulido JS, Eckels DD, et al: The association of HLA-DR15 and intermediate uveitis. Am J Ophthalmol 1997;123:70–75.

81. Raja SC, Jabs DA, Dun JP, et al: Pars planitis. Clinical features and class II HLA associations. Ophthalmology 1999;106:594–599.

82. Bullington RJ, Waksman BH: Uveitis in rabbits with experimental allergic encephalomyelitis. Arch Ophthalmol 1958;59:435–445.

83. Von Sallman L, Myers RE, Lerner EM II, Stone SH: Vasculo-occlusive retinopathy in experimental allergic encephalomyelitis. Arch Ophthalmol 1967;78:112–120.

84. Ohguro H, Chiba S, Igarashi Y, et al: β-Arrestin and arrestin are recognized by autoantibodies in sera from multiple sclerosis patients. Proc Natl Acad Sci USA 1993;90:3241–3245.

85. Lucchinetti CF, Bruck W, Rodriguez M, Lassmann H: Distinct patterns of multiple sclerosis pathology indicate heterogeneity in pathogenesis. Brain Pathol 1996;6:259–274.

86. Schumacher GA, Beebe G, Kilber RF, et al: Problems of experimental trials of therapy in multiple sclerosis: Report by the panel on the evaluation of experimental trials of therapy in multiple sclerosis. Ann N Y Acad Sci 1965;122:552–568.

87. Poser CM, Paty DW, Scheinberg I, et al: New diagnostic criteria for

multiple sclerosis: Guidelines for research protocols. Ann Neurol 1983;13:227–231.

88. Paty DW, Li DKB: Diagnosis of multiple sclerosis 1998: Do we need new diagnosis criteria? In: Paty D, Ebers GC, eds: Multiple Sclerosis. Philadelphia, FA Davis, 1997, pp 47–50.

89. Felgenhauer K, Reiber H: The diagnostic significance of antibody specificity indices in multiple sclerosis and herpes virus induced diseases of the nervous system. Clin Invest 1992;70:28–37.

90. Heinrichs IH, McLean DR: Evolution of visual evoked potentials in optic neuritis. Can J Neurol Sci 1988;15:394–396.

91. van Diemen HAM, Lanting P, Koetsier JC, et al: Evaluation of the visual system in multiple sclerosis: A comparative study of diagnostic tests. Clin Neurol Neurosurg 1992;94:191–195.

92. Katz B: The dyschromatopsia of optic neuritis: A descriptive analysis of data from the optic neuritis treatment trial. Trans Am Ophthalmol Soc 1995;93:685–708.

93. Rudick RA, Schiffer RB, Schwetz KM, Herndon RM: Multiple sclerosis. The problem of incorrect diagnosis. Arch Neurol 1986;43:578–583.

94. Nussenblatt RB, Whitcup SM, Palestine AG: Uveitis. Fundamentals and Clinical Practice, 2nd ed. St Louis, Mosby, 1996, pp 160–168.

95. Balcer LJ, Witenkorn JM, Galetta SL: Neuro-ophthalmic manifestations of Lyme disease. J Neuroophthalmol 1997;17:108–121.

96. Culbertson WW, Blumenkrantz MS, Pepose JS, et al: Varicella zoster virus is a cause of the acute retinal necrosis syndrome. Ophthalmology 1986;93:559–569.

97. Lewis MI, Culbertson WW, Pepose JS, et al: Herpes simplex virus type I: A cause of ARN syndrome. Ophthalmology 1989;96:875–878.

98. Chatzoulis DM, Theodosiadis PG, Apostolopoulos MN, et al: Retinal perivasculitis in an immunocompetent patient with systemic herpes simplex infection. Am J Ophthalmol 1997;123:699–702.

99. Mochizuki M, Watanabe T, Yamaguchi K, et al: Uveitis associated with human T-cell lymphotropic virus type I. Am J Ophthalmol 1992;114:123–129.

100. Tabara KF, Al Balla S: Ocular manifestations of Behçet's disease. Asia-Pacific Ophthalmol 1991;3:8–11.

101. Siltzbach LE, James DG, Neville E, et al: Course and prognosis of sarcoidosis around the world. Am J Med 1974;57:847–852.

102. Rush JA: Retrobulbar optic neuropathy in sarcoidosis. Ann Ophthalmol 1980;12:390–394.

103. Obenauf CD, Shaw HE, Sydnor CF, et al: Sarcoidosis and its ophthalmic manifestations. Am J Ophthalmol 1978;86:648–655.

104. Loublin F, Reingold SC: Defining the clinical course of multiple sclerosis: Results of an international survey. National Multiple Sclerosis Society (USA) Advisory Committee on Clinical Trials of New Agents in Multiple Sclerosis. Neurology 1996;46:907–911.

105. The Optic Neuritis Study Group: Visual function 5 years after optic neuritis. Experience of the Optic Neuritis Treatment Trial. Arch Ophthalmol 1997;115:1545–1552.

106. Weinshenker BG: The natural history of multiple sclerosis. Neurol Clin 1995;13:119–146.

107. Hunter SF, Weinshenker BG, Carter JL, Noseworthy JH: Rational clinical immunotherapy for multiple sclerosis. Mayo Clin Proc 1997;72:765–780.

108. Becker CC, Gidal BE, Fleming JO: Immunotherapy in multiple sclerosis, Part 1. Am J Health Syst Pharm 1995;52:1985–2000.

109. Bek RW, Trabe JD: What we have learned from the Optic Neuritis Treatment Trial. Ophthalmology 1995;102:1504–1508.

110. Milanese C, La Manitia L, Salmaggi A, Eoli M: A double blind study on azathioprine efficacy in multiple sclerosis: Final report. J Neurol 1993;240:295–298.

111. Noseworthy JH, Ebers GC, Roberts R: Cyclophosphamide and MS. Neurology 1994;44:579–581.

112. Van Oosten BW, Truyen L, Barkhof F, Polman CH: Choosing drug therapy for multiple sclerosis. Drugs 1998;56:555–563.

113. Sipe JC, Romine JS, Koziol JA, et al: Development of cladribine treatment in multiple sclerosis. Mult Scler 1996;1:295–299.

114. Romine JS, Sipe JC, Koziol JA, et al: A double-blind, placebo-controlled, randomized trial of cladribine in relapsing-remitting multiple sclerosis. Proc Assoc Am Physicians 1999;111:35–44.

115. Lisak RP: Intravenous immunoglobulins in multiple sclerosis. Neurology 1998;51:S25–29.

116. Noseworthy JH, O'Brien P, Erickson BJ, et al: The Mayo Clinic–Canadian Cooperative trial of sulfasalazine in active multiple sclerosis. Neurology 1998;51:1342–1352.

117. Abramsky O, Lehmann D, Karussis D: Immunomodulation with Linomide: Possible novel therapy for multiple sclerosis. Mult Scler 1996;2:206–210.

118. Karussis DM, Meiner Z, Lehmann D, et al: Treatment of secondary progressive multiple sclerosis with the immunomodulator Linomide: A double-blind, placebo controlled pilot study with monthly magnetic resonance imaging evaluation. Neurology 1996;47:341–346.

119. Drescher KM, Rivera-Quinones C, Lucchinetti CF, Rodriguez M: Failure of treatment with Linomide or oral myelin tolerization to ameliorate demyelination in a viral model of multiple sclerosis. J Neuroimmunol 1998;88:111–119.

120. Andersen O, Lycke J, Tollesson PO, et al: Linomide reduces the rate of active lesions in relapsing-remitting multiple sclerosis. Mult Scler 1996;1:348.

121. Placebo-controlled multicentre randomized trial of interferon beta-1b in treatment of secondary progressive multiple sclerosis. European Study group on interferon beta-1b in secondary progressive MS. Lancet 1998;352:1491–1497.

122. PRISMS (Prevention of Relapses and Disability by Interferon Beta-1a Subcutaneously in Multiple Sclerosis) Study Group. Randomised double-blind placebo-controlled study of interferon beta-1a in relapsing/remitting multiple sclerosis. Lancet 1998;352:1498–1504.

123. Johnson K, Brooks BR, Cohen JA, et al: Copolymer 1 reduces the relapse rate and improves disability in relapsing/remitting multiple sclerosis: Results of a phase III multicenter, double-blind, placebo-controlled trial. Neurology 1995;45:1268–1276.

124. Weinstein A, Schwid SI, Schiffer RB, et al: Neuropsychologic status in multiple sclerosis after treatment with glatiramer. Arch Neurol 1999;56:319–324.

63 SARCOIDOSIS

Panagiota Stavrou and C. Stephen Foster

DEFINITION AND HISTORY

Sarcoidosis is a multisystem granulomatous disease that was first described by Jonathan Hutchinson in 1878.[1] In 1899, Cesar Boeck demonstrated that noncaseating granulomatous inflammation was the pathologic hallmark of sarcoidosis.[2] He found no microorganisms and postulated that the cause of the disease was defective blood formation or autointoxication. In 1909, Heerfordt reported an association between uveitis, enlargement of the lacrimal glands, and cranial nerve palsies.[3] Schumacher in 1909 and Bering in 1910 reported iritis in association with cutaneous lesions and Schaumann in 1914 recognized the multisystem nature of the disease.[4, 5] In 1916, Boeck observed the lack of cutaneous reaction to tuberculin in patients with sarcoidosis and an absence of mycobacteria in guinea pigs inoculated with sarcoidal tissue.[6]

The clinical manifestations of sarcoidosis are variable and its course can be unpredictable. The organs affected more often are the lungs, skin, and eyes. However, the severity of organ involvement varies between individuals and among ethnic groups with differential expression of disease severity. It has been suggested that the clinical course may occasionally correlate with the type and character of disease presentation.[7] An acute onset with erythema nodosum or asymptomatic bilateral hilar lymphadenopathy usually follows a self-limiting course, whereas an insidious onset, especially with multiple extrapulmonary lesions, is often followed by relentless, progressive fibrosis of the lungs and other organs. The spectrum of ocular manifestations is wide; almost every part of the eye and other orbital structures can be affected. Ocular involvement may coexist with asymptomatic systemic disease, or it may *precede* systemic involvement by several years.

Definitive diagnosis is made by the demonstration of noncaseating granuloma by tissue biopsy. When a diagnosis of sarcoidosis is suspected but no affected tissue amenable to biopsy is identifiable, circumstantial evidence of the diagnosis may be obtained through noninvasive investigations, including measurement of serum angiotensin converting enzyme (ACE) and lysozyme, radiograph and computed tomography (CT) of the chest, gallium (Ga) scintillography, pulmonary function tests, bronchoalveolar lavage (BAL), and measurement of serum and urinary calcium.

EPIDEMIOLOGY

Sarcoidosis is characterized by a great diversity in its incidence in various parts of the world, racial predilection, and clinical course and prognosis. Differences in the global prevalence of sarcoidosis between the hemispheres, as well as between the northern and southern regions of countries such as Italy and Japan, have also been reported.[7] It has been suggested that sarcoidosis is more common in certain geographic areas such as the southeastern part of the United States, but when case-matched controls have been used, these geographic differences are less striking. In the United States, the majority of patients are blacks, with a prevalence of 40 per 100,000, compared to 5 per 100,000 among whites. In Europe, the disease affects mostly whites, but there is great variation in prevalence among different countries: The prevalence per 100,000 is 64 in Sweden, 10 in France, 3 in Poland, and an extraordinary 200 for Irish women living in London. In contrast, the disease is rare in India, Southeast Asia, New Zealand, and mainland China.

Diab and colleagues[8] reported on 20 Arab patients with sarcoidosis in Kuwait. All of them had thoracic lesions. When compared to westerners, these patients were older, and they more frequently demonstrated constitutional symptoms and presented with thoracic involvement with rare ocular and central nervous system manifestations. Pietinalho and colleagues[9] reported that in 1984, the prevalence of sarcoidosis was 28.2 per 100,000 in Finland and 3.7 per 100,000 in Hokkaido, Japan. In Hokkaido, the area with the highest incidence in Japan, patients were significantly younger at diagnosis and eye symptoms were more frequent (45% vs 7%). However, respiratory and joint symptoms and erythema nodosum were more frequent in Finland.

A change in the pattern of organ involvement has been reported in Japan, with an increase in the proportion of patients with ocular involvement (from 41.6% to 58.7% in women); an increase in the number of middle-aged and elderly patients is also noted.[10] Gupta and Gupta[11] reported on 125 cases of biopsy-proven sarcoidosis seen between 1972 and 1990 in Calcutta, India. The authors described that the presentation, clinical course, and radiologic features were considerably different from those seen in the West; elderly men over 40 years were more prevalent in this patient sample, and a previously unreported high susceptibility of medical personnel as well as doctors (8%) and their close relations (8.8%) was noted. Ocular symptoms (20%) included acute or chronic uveitis, corneal opacities, and lacrimal gland enlargement, but keratoconjunctivitis sicca secondary to lacrimal gland involvement was not as prevalent in this Indian study group as in prior reports of patient groups in western countries. There was no case of conjunctival involvement despite routine "blind" biopsy in a large number of patients. The sex ratios largely depend on the age at diagnosis, the mode of detection, and geography.[7] When the data include large numbers of early, asymptomatic cases detected by mass x-ray screening efforts, male predominance is found. When the data deal with symptomatic cases, on the other hand, a slight female predominance is observed. Swedish and Japanese studies show that the incidence in both sexes is usually highest in the second and third decades, often forming a bimodal curve with the second peak in middle age, especially in women.[7] Although most patients present between the ages of 20 and 40 years, clinically evident disease onset can occur in children and in the elderly.

Several cases of familial sarcoidosis (including in monozygotic twins) have been described, as well as husband-and-wife pairs. This, together with geographic clusters of sarcoidosis occurring among unrelated individuals living closely within a community, argues for environmental factors in the pathogenesis of the disease.[12]

As the pathophysiology of sarcoidosis probably involves antigen recognition, processing, and presentation, there has been significant interest in finding possible associations with human leukocyte antigen (HLA)-related genes. Although no consistent association has been found, the HLA-B8 has been associated with patients who present acutely with erythema nodosum and who show early resolution of sarcoidosis.[12–15] Epidemiologic studies attempting to link sarcoidosis to various environmental or occupational factors have been inconclusive. However, in 1992, tuberculosis mycobacterial DNA was demonstrated by polymerase chain reaction in BAL samples in 50% of patients with sarcoidosis, and nontuberculosis mycobacterial DNA in a further 20% of the sarcoidosis patients.[16] Another study showed tuberculosis mycobacterial rRNA in sarcoid splenic tissues by liquid-phase DNA/RNA hybridization, suggesting that mycobacteria may play a part in the cause of sarcoidosis.[17] Unlike many diseases in which lungs are involved, sarcoidosis favors nonsmokers.

CLINICAL FEATURES

Systemic Manifestations

The lung is the most frequently affected organ in patients with sarcoidosis. Histologically, the lesions are distributed primarily along the lymphatics around bronchi and blood vessels, although alveolar lesions are also seen. The relative frequency of granulomas in the bronchial submucosa accounts for the high diagnostic yield of bronchoscopic biopsies. Lymph nodes are involved in almost all cases, especially the hilar and mediastinal nodes. The majority of patients are asymptomatic, although others may complain of cough or dyspnea.

The spleen is clinically enlarged in only 18% of cases, although microscopic evidence of sarcoid granulomas in splenic tissue is present in three quarters of patients. Although the liver is affected less often than the spleen, elevated liver enzymes in a patient suspected of having sarcoidosis may prompt percutaneous liver biopsy in the search for histopathologic confirmation of the diagnosis. Renal insufficiency has been reported in patients with histologic involvement of the kidneys and has been attributed to hypercalcemia and interstitial granulomatous nephritis.[18] Radiographic abnormalities of the bones can be identified in about one fifth of patients. The radiologically visible lesions are usually seen in the phalangeal bones of the hands and feet, creating small, circumscribed areas of bone resorption within the marrow cavity (Fig. 63–1).

Skin lesions are found in 9% to 37% of patients. They may be specific, showing histologically noncaseating granulomas, or nonspecific (e.g., erythema nodosum). The specific skin lesions include lupus pernio, infiltrated plaques, maculopapular eruptions, subcutaneous nod-

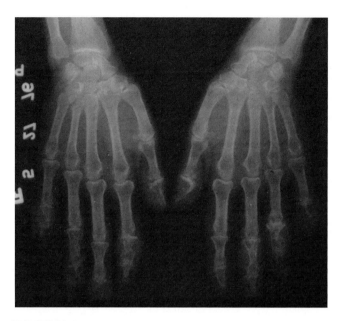

FIGURE 63–1. X-ray study of hands of a patient with sarcoidosis showing circumscribed areas of bone resorption within the marrow cavity.

ules, and infiltration of old scars (Figs. 63–2 and 63–3). Lupus pernio and plaques are associated with more severe systemic involvement and a more chronic course, whereas erythema nodosum is the hallmark of acute and benign disease.[19] Lesions may also appear on the mucous membranes of the oral cavity, larynx, and upper respiratory tract.

Although direct cardiac involvement is seen in only 5% of patients, cor pulmonale is common in patients with severe pulmonary sarcoidosis. Cardiac complications include conduction abnormalities, myocardiopathy, pericarditis, and pericardial effusion.

The clinical course of sarcoidosis may be acute or chronic. Acute disease develops over a few weeks and is characterized by constitutional symptoms such as fever, erythema nodosum, arthralgias, and parotid enlargement or uveitis in 25% to 50% of patients. Acute disease may resolve with minimal residual sequelae or may progress

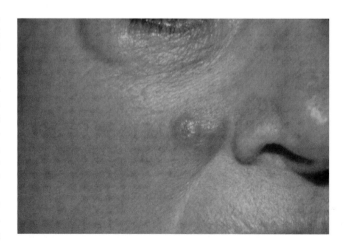

FIGURE 63–2. Umbilicated sarcoid skin lesion in a patient who presented with uveitis. (See color insert.)

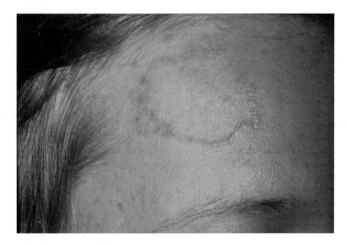

FIGURE 63–3. Sarcoid plaque–like skin lesion in a patient with sarcoidosis. (See color insert.)

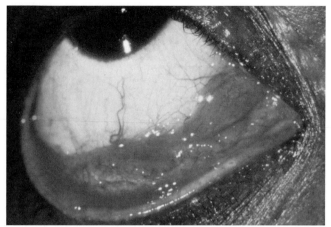

FIGURE 63–4. Conjunctival nodules in sarcoidosis. (See color insert.)

to chronic sarcoidosis. In 40% to 70% of patients, sarcoidosis develops insidiously over several months. These patients usually present with respiratory symptoms and lack constitutional complaints. A summary of the extraocular organ involvement in patients with sarcoidosis is shown in Table 63–1.

Ocular Manifestations

Anterior Segment

The frequency of ocular involvement ranges from 26% to 50%. This statistic is based on studies with varying population and geographic distributions and nonuniform criteria for diagnosis and follow-up, making comparisons between studies difficult and resulting in a wide range of reported ocular involvement. Anterior segment pathology is the most common ocular manifestation and is seen in 85% of patients with ocular sarcoidosis. Conjunctival involvement has been reported in 6.9% to 70% of patients with ocular sarcoidosis.[20–25] Sarcoid granulomas have been described as solitary, yellow, "millet-seed" nodules (Fig. 63–4).[26] These may be difficult to differentiate clinically from lymphoid follicles; however, they are often larger, tend to be evenly distributed, and they show a characteristic disposition to confluence.[25] Although most patients are asymptomatic, diplopia from a large conjunc-

tival granuloma has been reported,[22] and cicatrizing changes with symblepharon formation may occur.[21] Hunter and Foster[24] reported a higher incidence of conjunctival involvement in patients younger than 35 years of age. Conjunctival chalky deposits were reported in 5 of 69 (7.2%) patients by Crick and colleagues.[25] Only one of these five patients had uveitis, prompting the authors to suggest that the calcium deposits were secondary to hypercalcemia rather than to chronic inflammation; indeed, the deposits disappeared with a low calcium diet.

Anterior uveitis has been reported in 22% to 70% of patients with ocular involvement, and it is usually granulomatous (Fig. 63–5) and chronic.[20, 22–25] Karma and colleagues[21] classified the possible course of uveitis as being either monophasic, relapsing, or chronic. The visual prognosis was related to the course of uveitis, being better in patients exhibiting the monophasic type. Anterior uveitis is reported to be more common among black patients in the Netherlands.[22]

Iris nodules (Figs. 63–6 and 63–7) have been reported in up to 12.5% of patients with sarcoidosis-associated

TABLE 63–1. ORGAN INVOLVEMENT AT NECROPSY IN PATIENTS WITH SARCOIDOSIS

ORGAN	PERCENT OF PATIENTS
Lymph nodes	78
Lung	77
Liver	67
Spleen	50
Heart	20
Skin	16
Brain	8
Kidney	7
Eye	6

Adapted from Branson JH, Park JH: Sarcoidosis: Hepatic involvement. Ann Intern Med 1954;40:11.

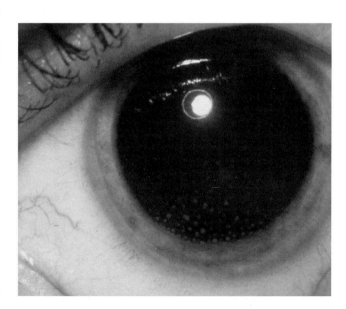

FIGURE 63–5. Mutton fat keratic precipitates. (See color insert.)

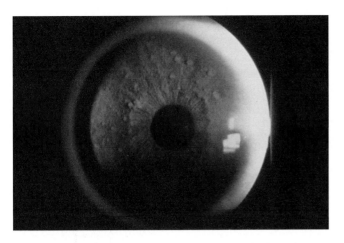

FIGURE 63–6. Busacca iris nodules. (See color insert.)

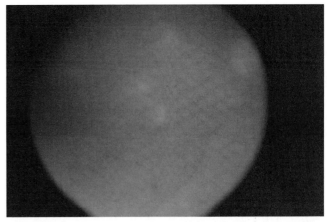

FIGURE 63–8. Vitritis, snow balls, and perivenular exudates in a patient with sarcoidosis. (See color insert.)

uveitis.[20, 21, 23] Exacerbations of granulomatous uveitis are often associated with an appearance of fresh iris or fundus nodules. A large iris sarcoid nodule touching the corneal endothelium and extending to the pupil centrally, producing posterior synechiae and sector cortical cataract, was reported by Mader and colleagues,[27] and secondary glaucoma due to occlusion of the angle by an iris nodule was observed by Crick and colleagues.[25]

Posterior synechiae have been reported in 20% to 26%,[21, 24] cataract in 4% to 35%,[20–25, 28, 29] and glaucoma in 4% to 33%[20–25, 29, 30] of patients with sarcoidosis-associated uveitis. Corneal band keratopathy develops in 4.5% to 11% of patients,[20, 21, 23, 25] and it is associated with hypercalcemia in the majority of the cases.[20, 21] Scleritis is a relatively rare manifestation. Scleral plaques have been reported in up to 2% of patients.[23, 24]

Posterior Segment

Involvement of the posterior segment is seen in 25% of patients with ocular sarcoidosis, and it can be the sole manifestation of the disease in 5% of patients. The most common manifestations of sarcoidosis involving the posterior segment are vitritis (Fig. 63–8), occurring in 3%

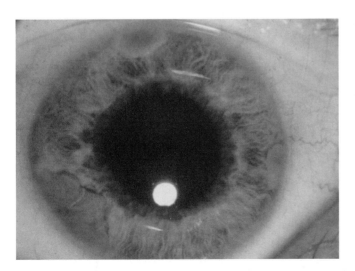

FIGURE 63–7. True iris nodule in sarcoidosis. (See color insert.)

to 62%,[20, 23, 24] intermediate uveitis in 16% to 38%,[24, 30] panuveitis in 9% to 30%,[22, 25, 30] posterior uveitis in 12%,[30] retinal vasculitis in 9% to 34%,[20, 23, 24] and optic nerve involvement in 7.4% to 34%[20, 24] of patients. Periphlebitis is a hallmark, although not pathognomonic, of sarcoidosis and may be associated with yellow perivenous exudates ("taches de bougie" or candle wax drippings). Cellular infiltration of the vitreous may occur in clumps ("snowballs") in the inferior vitreous or in chains ("string of pearls").

Other manifestations include choroidal nodules[20, 23] and exudative retinal detachment,[21, 23] which may result in phthisis.[21] Clinical and/or angiographic cystoid macular edema (CME) has been reported in 19% to 72% of patients[24, 29, 30] and was noted to be more common in patients with posterior uveitis; it was correlated with the duration of active uveitis and delay in seeking treatment.[30]

Rothova and colleagues[22] reported that sarcoidosis-associated posterior uveitis was usually chronic and was more common in white women with late onset of the disease. The same investigators noted that uveitis was an early feature of sarcoidosis, seen in 25 of 29 (86%) patients; moreover, in 9 of the 25 cases, ocular inflammation preceded any systemic signs of sarcoidosis by more than 1 year. Overall, patients with chronic posterior uveitis and panuveitis have significantly more complications than do patients with anterior uveitis.[21, 22, 30]

Vrabec and colleagues[31] reported "taches de bougie" in 22 patients with sarcoidosis. The authors described two clinical patterns, each with a different visual prognosis. The first and more frequent type, in the active phase, is associated with vitritis and segmental venous "sheathing" or perivenular exudates (Fig. 63–9). Small, discrete white spots occur in clusters around retinal venules, often limited to one or two retinal quadrants, frequently the inferior and nasal. This presentation may be indistinguishable from multifocal choroiditis and panuveitis. These lesions evolve into areas of cobblestone-like chorioretinal atrophy approximately one-third the disc area in size. Spots may develop several years after the initial presentation in some patients. The second type is characterized by yellow-orange lesions located at the level of the choroid, predominantly in the posterior and nasal fundus, simulating the

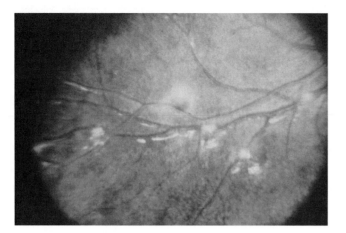

FIGURE 63–9. Perivenular exudates in sarcoidosis. (See color insert.)

lesions of birdshot chorioretinopathy. These are discrete and depigmented but not atrophic. They have no surrounding retinal pigment epithelial (RPE) clumping and they are not associated with retinal vasculitis or retinal vascular obstruction. Visual prognosis is thought to be better in patients with the latter type because of absence of retinal inflammation.

Other studies have also reported on the "punched-out" multifocal lesions (Fig. 63–10) seen in patients with uveitis secondary to sarcoidosis.[21, 29, 32] These lesions may correspond to those described in a clinicopathologic correlation by Gass and Olson.[33] The authors reported intraretinal epithelioid cell nodules which, in some areas, extended from the retinal veins through the internal limiting membrane into the vitreous or beneath the RPE. Some retinal vessels appeared obliterated by the inflammatory reaction.

Severe retinal vasculitis and ischemic retinopathy with neovascularization, requiring scatter photocoagulation, has been described in some patients.[22, 30] Duker and colleagues[34] reported seven patients (11 eyes) with proliferative sarcoid retinopathy. All of them displayed retinal neovascularization. In addition, two eyes developed optic disc neovascularization, and one developed rubeosis

iridis. In all cases, there was concomitant peripheral retinal capillary nonperfusion. Although retinal neovascularization occurs in patients who show areas of nonperfusion by fluorescein angiography, it can also occur in response to inflammation alone. In these patients, anti-inflammatory treatment may induce involution of the neovascular tissue.

Fluorescein angiography in patients with sarcoidosis may show retinal vascular staining, CME, and retinal or optic disc neovascularization. A recent study characterized the indocyanine green angiographic features in 19 patients with sarcoidosis-associated posterior uveitis into four patterns.[35] These are hypofluorescent choroidal lesions, focal hyperfluorescent pinpoints, fuzzy choroidal vessels with leakage, and diffuse late zonal choroidal hyperfluorescence. The authors reported that all 19 patients were found to have choroidal involvement by indocyanine green angiography, yet eight patients had no evidence of retinal or choroidal involvement on clinical examination or fluorescein angiography.

Other, less frequent complications of sarcoidosis-associated uveitis include peripapillary[36] and subfoveal[37] choroidal neovascularization, posterior scleritis with annular ciliochoroidal detachment causing angle-closure glaucoma,[38] branch vein occlusion,[39] and solitary choroidal mass without inflammation.[40] In one report, central retinal vein occlusion leading to a painful blind eye secondary to neovascular glaucoma was found on histopathologic examination to be caused by a large noncaseating granuloma of the ciliary body.[41] Other unusual presentations of sarcoidosis include serpiginous choroiditis[42] and birdshot-like chorioretinopathy.[43, 44]

Neurosarcoidosis

Posterior segment involvement may be accompanied by disease of the central nervous system in 25% to 30%.[20, 45] Brinkman and Rothova[43] described six patients with neurosarcoidosis and uveitis. All patients had posterior uveitis or panuveitis consisting of multifocal chorioretinal lesions, optic nerve granulomas (Fig. 63–11), periphlebitis, and papilledema. The neurologic features included Babinski reflexes, spinal cord compression, myasthenia,

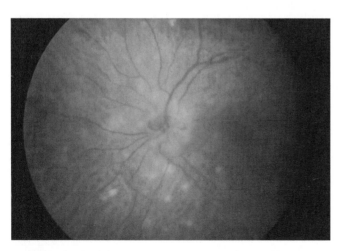

FIGURE 63–10. Vitritis, disc edema, disc neovascularization, nerve fiber layer hemorrhages, and multiple atrophic chorioretinal lesions in sarcoidosis. (See color insert.)

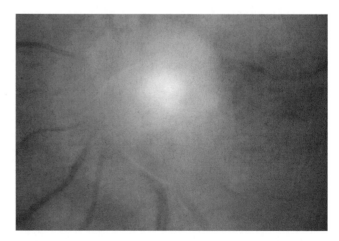

FIGURE 63–11. Optic nerve granuloma in a patient with sarcoidosis. (See color insert.)

"schizophrenia," cranial nerve paresis (V, VII, XI, XII [VII being the most common]), hypothalamic-pituitary gland dysfunction, visual field loss, and normal pressure hydrocephalus. Optic atrophy with or without uveitis [20, 46] and optic neuropathy [20, 47] have also been reported.

Orbit and Lids

Although sarcoid granulomas have been described in several areas inside the orbit, the lacrimal gland appears to be the organ most commonly affected (Fig. 63–12). The frequency of lacrimal gland involvement varies from 7% to 69%.[20–25] This range results from the diversity of criteria used in various studies, including palpable lacrimal gland enlargement, dry eye, and diagnosis by biopsy. Obenauf and colleagues[20] and Rothova and colleagues[22] reported lacrimal gland involvement in 15.8% and 38%, respectively, of patients with ocular sarcoidosis and noted that it was more frequent among black patients. Dry eye can occur with or without palpable lacrimal gland enlargement,[23] and histologic confirmation of the disease has been reported from a gland that was not palpable.[25] Obenauf and colleagues[20] reported bilateral acute dacryoadenitis in one patient, and nine patients who had bilateral lacrimal gland enlargement without any other ocular manifestations of sarcoidosis.

The nasolacrimal drainage system (NLDS) may also become involved in patients with sarcoidosis. Dacryostenosis or total obstruction due to histologically proven sarcoidosis of the NLDS has been reported.[21, 22, 48] The patients usually present with epiphora and nasal congestion that is due to coexistent paranasal and intranasal disease.[48]

Extraocular muscle involvement can occur; it presents with diplopia or painful external ophthalmoplegia.[49, 50] Evaluation of these patients by magnetic resonance imaging shows extraocular muscle enlargement; biopsy of the affected muscle is indicated to establish the diagnosis. Bilateral orbital, lid, and extraocular muscle involvement, together with thickening of the optic nerve sheath, has also been reported.[51] Painless unilateral orbital swelling caused by sarcoid granulomas of the soft tissue around the eye outside the lacrimal gland was observed in two

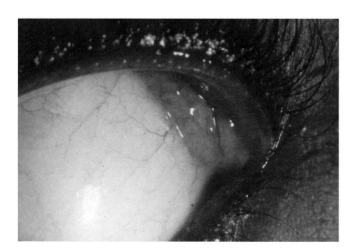

FIGURE 63–12. Lacrimal gland enlargement in a patient with sarcoidosis. (See color insert.)

TABLE 63–2. OCULAR MANIFESTATIONS IN PATIENTS WITH SARCOIDOSIS

MANIFESTATION	PERCENT OF PATIENTS	REFERENCES
Anterior segment	85	
Conjunctival involvement	6.9–70	20–25
Anterior uveitis	22–70	20, 22–25
Iris nodules	11.4–12.5	20, 21, 23
Posterior synechiae	20–26	21, 24
Cataract	4–35	20–25, 28, 29
Glaucoma	4–33	20–25, 29, 30
Band keratopathy	4.5–11	20, 21, 23, 25
Posterior segment	25	
Vitritis	3–62	20, 23, 24
Intermediate uveitis	16–38	24, 30
Panuveitis	9–30	22, 25, 30
Posterior uveitis	12	30
Retinal vasculitis	9–34	20, 23, 24
Cystoid macular edema	19–72	24, 29, 30
Optic nerve involvement	7.4–34	20, 24
Orbit	26	
Lacrimal gland involvement	7–69	20–25

patients by Peterson and colleagues.[52] This regressed with oral prednisone therapy. Hunter and Foster[24] described eyelid nodules in one of their 86 patients. A summary of the ocular manifestations in patients with sarcoidosis is shown in Table 63–2.

Sarcoidosis in Childhood

Early onset or preschool sarcoidosis seen in children younger than 5 years of age is relatively rare. The classic triad of symptoms consists of skin, eye, and joint lesions; pulmonary involvement is rare, at least initially. It can be easily misdiagnosed as juvenile rheumatoid arthritis (JRA), as the latter also presents with symptoms related to the joints and eyes.[53, 54] However, children with JRA-associated uveitis usually suffer from pauciarticular arthritis, are antinuclear antibody (ANA) positive, and rarely develop skin lesions,[55] whereas children with sarcoidosis usually develop polyarthritis, are ANA negative, have elevated serum ACE, and often exhibit skin lesions in the form of erythema nodosum. Sarcoidosis has been described in a 7-month-old child.[53]

The ocular manifestations in children are similar to those seen in adults and include iridocyclitis, posterior uveitis, periphlebitis, macular edema, branch retinal vein occlusion, interstitial keratitis, and multiple corneal limbal nodules.[39, 56–59] Bilateral lower motor neuron facial palsy and bilateral hearing loss have also been reported.[60] Histologic diagnosis has been made by biopsy of parotid gland, lung, and cutaneous lesions. Ga scanning showed the typical "panda" appearance in a child of preschool age with posterior uveitis.[57] Oral steroids have been used with good response of the ocular inflammation and other symptoms.

Characteristic Presentations

Heerfordt's syndrome (uveoparotid fever), described in 1909 by Heerfordt, consists of uveitis, parotitis, fever, and facial or other cranial nerve palsies.[3] It was not until 1936 that Bruins Slot linked the findings with sarcoidosis.[61]

Lofgren's syndrome consists of erythema nodosum, febrile arthropathy, and bilateral hilar lymphadenopathy. It was described by Lofgren in 1946 and is reported to be associated with a favorable prognosis.[62]

The combination of salivary and lacrimal gland inflammatory enlargement with xerostomia is called *Mikulicz's syndrome.* This term includes all forms of involvement of these glands including sarcoidosis, leukemia, and lymphoma.

HISTOLOGY

Non-necrotizing (noncaseating) granulomas are the hallmark of sarcoidosis. Histiocytes, epithelioid cells, and multinucleated giant cells make up the center of the granuloma, surrounded by lymphocytes, plasma cells, and fibroblasts in the periphery (Fig. 63–13). Gross necrosis is not a feature of sarcoidosis, and suggests alternative diagnoses (e.g., tuberculosis, fungal infection, vasculitis), but occasional granulomas may show central fibrinoid necrosis.[63] The epithelioid cells are transformed bone marrow monocytes and are therefore members of the mononuclear phagocyte system. In contrast to macrophages, the epithelioid cells have marked secretory activity that includes over 40 different cytokines and other mediators. Among the enzymes and other chemicals secreted by granulomas are ACE, lysozyme, glucuronidase, collagenase, and calcitriol.

Deposits of immunoglobulins and various inclusion bodies, such as asteroid, Schaumann's bodies, or Wesenberg-Hamazaki bodies, may be seen. They are found predominantly within giant cells but may be seen in the extracellular space. Asteroid bodies are seen in 2% to 9% of cases, are formed from accumulations of cytoskeletal filaments, and contain lipoprotein. Schaumann's bodies are concentric, laminated, blue calcified structures. They are seen in 48% to 88% of cases and indicate chronic granulomatous disease. Schaumann's bodies represent accumulations of oxidized lipid within lysosomes. Wesenberg-Hamazaki bodies, observed in 11% to 68% of lymph nodes with sarcoidosis, are giant lysosomes and are usually present extracellularly or within macrophages. They are yellow, ovoid, periodic acid–Schiff–positive inclusions,

probably representing large lysosomes containing iron and protein material. They are not specific to sarcoidosis.

Kveim-Siltzbach Test

In 1941, Kveim reported the use of a suspension derived from the spleen of a patient with sarcoidosis that, when injected intracutaneously into patients with biopsy-proven sarcoidosis, yielded a cutaneous papule containing noncaseating epithelioid granulomas.[64] The test was later labeled the Kveim-Siltzbach (KS) test in recognition of Siltzbach's contributions. Four to 6 weeks after subcutaneous injection of the KS reagent, the typical positive KS lesion presents as a red or brownish raised papule ranging from a few millimeters to up to 1.5 cm in diameter. Histopathologic analysis of the biopsied lesion reveals a granuloma composed of epithelioid cells, occasional Langhans' cells, and scattered lymphocytes at its center, with a surrounding cuff of mononuclear cells, primarily lymphocytes. Pierard and colleagues[65] have suggested that the KS reaction parallels the evolution of pulmonary sarcoidosis, with exuberant reaction during overt pulmonary granulomatous infiltration and a more bland response during chronic fibrotic disease. Positive KS tests are reported in almost all patients with sarcoidosis who present with erythema nodosum and hilar lymphadenopathy with clear lung fields.

The KS test has been reported to be positive in approximately 80% of patients with sarcoidosis, with less than 1% false-positive results when a properly prepared and validated KS reagent is used. A negative result does not exclude the diagnosis. Steroids suppress KS reactivity, and therefore the test should not be performed in patients receiving systemic steroids or in those who will require treatment prior to the 4- to 6-week development period of the KS lesion.

In recent years, the KS test has fallen into disuse because of the potential risks inherent in the use of human tissue (transmission of infectious agents such as hepatitis B, human immunodeficiency virus, and the virus of the Creutzfeldt-Jakob syndrome),[66] the meticulous care required for the production and validation of the KS reagent, and the evolution of other diagnostic techniques to assess patients suspected of having sarcoidosis, such as BAL, Ga scanning, chest CT scanning, and measurement of serum ACE.

Cutaneous Anergy

In 1916, Boeck first described cutaneous anergy to tuberculin in patients with sarcoidosis.[6] Later it was realized that this phenomenon was not limited to tuberculin alone, but that anergy to a variety of other skin test antigens such as *Candida,* mumps protein, streptococcal protein, and tetanus toxoid was also typical. In 1994, Kataria and Holter proposed a mechanism for the cutaneous anergy seen in sarcoidosis.[67] Compartmentalization of the immune response is well recognized in sarcoidosis. At sites of granulomatous inflammation, there is a predominance of T-helper lymphocytes, which proliferate and secrete large amounts of lymphokines, including interleukin (IL)-2, monocyte chemotactic factor (MCF), and migration inhibition factor (MIF). These lymphokines induce and amplify the immune response by en-

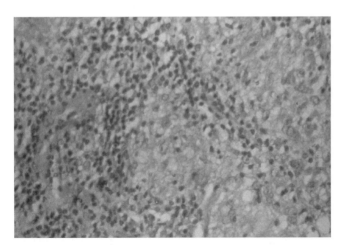

FIGURE 63–13. Non-necrotizing granuloma in sarcoidosis. Histiocytes, epithelioid cells, and multinucleated giant cells are surrounded by lymphocytes, plasma cells, and fibroblasts. (See color insert.)

hancing T-lymphocyte proliferation as well as by recruiting and retaining monocytes from the circulation. The concentration of lymphokines and monokines produced at sites of granulomatous inflammation is highest locally. Nevertheless, the protein molecules diffuse into blood, establishing a concentration gradient between the granulomatous inflammatory site and the remote site of the delayed-type hypersensitivity (DTH) skin test. As a result, the traffic of T-helper lymphocytes and monocytes is preferentially directed toward sites of granuloma formation. That leads to a preponderance of suppressor cells in the peripheral blood and competitively depletes the T-helper cells and monocytes available to sites of DTH.

Although the initial cellular influx of DTH is similar to that of the early stages of granulomatous inflammation, the availability of the deposited antigen is only transient, and the DTH response must compete for the same cellular elements at multiple granulomatous sites in the body. The granulomatous sites have the advantage of steeper cytokine gradients to attract T-helper cell and monocyte traffic. As a result, comparatively few cells migrate to the site of soluble recall antigens. Cutaneous anergy therefore is an epiphenomenon of active sarcoidosis, a nonspecific process that is seen in other granulomatous inflammations and that resolves when the underlying granulomatous disease activity wanes.

Collagen alteration has been noted at KS antigen injection sites,[68] but not in normal volunteers injected with KS antigen,[69] suggesting that these collagen changes are limited to patients with sarcoidosis who harbor cognate lymphocytes. In patients with sarcoidosis, the antigen may bind to the altered collagen, immobilizing lymphocytes at the injection site for a focused immune response. Of particular interest is the initial mononuclear cell influx with T-helper lymphocytes and monocyte-macrophages, a process pathologically analogous to the mononuclear cell alveolitis that antedates granuloma formation in the lung.

ETIOLOGY AND PATHOGENESIS

The processes involved in the pathogenesis of sarcoidosis in the lungs include accumulation of CD4+ lymphocytes at the affected site. The cytokines and factors secreted by these cells account for the influx of monocytes, alveolitis, and noncaseating granuloma formation in the lung, and for the resulting progressive fibrosis, all characteristic features of pulmonary sarcoidosis. Sarcoidosis is characterized by "compartmentalization" of the T cells, such that the relative proportion of CD4+ T cells in blood is reduced (e.g., CD4/CD8 = 0.8), while the reverse relation is observed in affected tissue (e.g., CD4/CD8 = 1.8 in lung). The CD4+ cells in the involved organs are "activated" and thus are releasing IL-2 and other mediators, while the CD4+ cells in other sites, such as blood, are quiescent. The result systemically (among other consequences) is a generalized immunologic dysregulation, as evidenced by hyperglobulinemia, autoantibody production, and impairment of T-cell–mediated DTH responses (anergy).

In 1992, Holter and colleagues[69] demonstrated a Kveim-like granulomagenic activity in nonviable autologous BAL cells (NABC) recovered soon after symptomatic onset or relapse of sarcoidosis, but not in patients with chronic stable sarcoidosis. The authors suggested that macrophages bearing the putative granulomagenic factor become tightly interdigitated into the granuloma matrix as they differentiate into epithelioid cells, rendering them unrecoverable by lavage. This is consistent with the "walling-off" function of granulomatous inflammation.

The same group of investigators demonstrated a Kveim-like granulomagenic activity of peripheral blood monocytes, the progenitors of the alveolar macrophage.[68] These findings suggest that the circulating monocyte is already primed with the granulomagenic factor before differentiation into alveolar macrophage. A monocyte source of the factor explains the multisystem distribution of granulomas in sarcoidosis. Consistent with these findings are recent reports of sarcoidosis recurring in recipients of allogeneic normal lung transplants[70] and the development of sarcoidosis in the recipient of bone marrow harvested from a patient with sarcoidosis.[71]

This evidence indicates that antigen processing and presentation triggers the T-lymphocyte activation and proliferation in the first place. Lymphocyte activation and proliferation antedate granuloma formation at the KS skin test sites and in the lung, and granulomagenic activity has been shown in autologous monocyte-macrophage preparations. These findings suggest that sarcoidosis represents a unique type of autoimmune disease, in which a monocyte-associated autoantigen is attacked by cell-mediated immune mechanisms rather than by the traditional humoral ones.[68]

Chest Radiology

Sulavik and colleagues[72] suggested the following roentgen staging of sarcoidosis: 0 = normal chest radiograph; 1 = bilateral symmetric hilar lymphadenopathy (BSHL) only; 2 = BSHL with bilateral symmetric lung infiltration (Fig. 63–14); 3 = bilateral symmetric lung infiltration only; 4a = BSHL with bilateral symmetric lung infiltration indicative of pulmonary fibrosis (BSIF); and 4b = BSIF only (Table 63–3). Roentgen findings used to

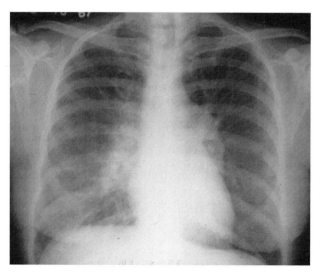

FIGURE 63–14. Chest x-ray study in a patient presenting with uveitis showing bilateral symmetric hilar lymphadenopathy and bilateral lung infiltration.

TABLE 63–3. RADIOGRAPHIC STAGING OF PULMONARY SARCOIDOSIS

STAGE	FINDINGS
0	Normal chest radiograph
1	Bilateral symmetric hilar lymphadenopathy (BSHL) only
2	BSHL with bilateral symmetric lung infiltration
3	Bilateral symmetric lung infiltration only
4a	BSHL with bilateral symmetric lung fibrosis
4b	Bilateral symmetric lung fibrosis only

Adapted from Sulavik SB, Spencer RP, Palestro CJ, et al: Specificity and sensitivity of distinctive chest radiographic and/or ^{67}Ga images in the noninvasive diagnosis of sarcoidosis. Chest 1993;103:403.

indicate pulmonary fibrosis include (1) bilateral, usually mid- and upper lung field fibrobullous change; (2) bilateral retraction of fissures or hila upward, associated with significant volume loss; and (3) bilateral "honey-combing," defined as well-demarcated ringlets approximately 3 to 12 mm in diameter. The clinical use of stage 4 has been disputed by other authors, as identification of this stage may be inconsistent between observers.

A worldwide survey reported in 1976[73] revealed the following frequencies of lung involvement in 3654 patients: stage 0 = 8%; stage 1 = 51%; stage 2 = 29%; stage 3 = 12%.

The lymphadenopathy in sarcoidosis is primarily hilar, with frequent involvement of the right paratracheal chain. Involvement of the other mediastinal lymph nodes, and particularly the anterior mediastinal ones, should lead to consideration of other diseases (e.g., lymphoma or metastatic malignancy). A recent report has evaluated the use of CT and mediastinoscopy in the diagnosis of sarcoidosis.[74] CT is superior to plain roentgenograms as the mediastinum, as well as the lung parenchyma, can be better visualized.

Gallium Scan

A gallium scan (^{67}Ga) is performed 48 to 72 hours after intravenous injection of 5 to 8 mCi ^{67}Ga citrate. Abnormal uptake is assessed in relation to liver activity. Although it has been suggested that activated lymphocytes and macrophages play a role in the localization of ^{67}Ga, the exact mechanism of ^{67}Ga uptake is not well known. A whole-body ^{67}Ga scan is recommended in the evaluation of patients with suspected sarcoidosis, as there have been reports of extrapulmonary uptake.[75] It is also valuable in localizing sites for possible biopsy and may reduce the need for more invasive diagnostic procedures. Karma and colleagues[21] reported that only 4 of 12 patients with chronic ophthalmic changes had increased ^{67}Ga uptake over the orbits, and they thus concluded that (limited) ^{67}Ga scanning was not valuable in the assessment of activity of chronic sarcoidosis.

Sulavik and colleagues[76] have called the combined abnormal bilateral symmetric ^{67}Ga uptake of the lacrimal and parotid glands (with or without submandibular gland ^{67}Ga uptake) as the "panda" image or pattern (Fig. 63–15). The presence and pattern of ^{67}Ga uptake in both (1) the parahilar and infrahilar bronchopulmonary lymph nodes and (2) the right paratracheal (azygous) mediastinal lymph nodes is called the "lambda" image after its

resemblance to the Greek letter λ. The "lambda" pattern has been reported in 72% of patients with sarcoidosis but in none of 540 patients with other diseases.[76] Sulavik and colleagues[72] also reported that a "lambda" image (usually associated with a "panda" image) or a "panda" ^{67}Ga uptake image together with BSHL or BSIF on chest radiography are highly specific in the noninvasive diagnosis of sarcoidosis.

Pulmonary uptake of ^{67}Ga is sensitive but not specific in the diagnosis of pulmonary sarcoidosis, as it can occur in a wide variety of other inflammatory and neoplastic diseases. Abnormal ^{67}Ga uptake in salivary and lacrimal glands may also occur in Sjögren's syndrome and tuberculosis, and after radiation therapy. However, the combination of raised serum ACE and positive ^{67}Ga uptake increases the specificity to 99%[77, 78] and the sensitivity to 73%.[78] Weinreb and colleagues[79] reported positive limited ^{67}Ga uptake in patients with granulomatous uveitis with and without elevated serum ACE.

Angiotensin Converting Enzyme

ACE cleaves the terminal dipeptide histine-leucine from the C-terminus of angiotensin I, converting it to angiotensin II. ACE is normally present in the vascular endothelium of many organs (lung, kidney, small intestine, uterus, prostate, thyroid, testes, adrenals) and in macrophages. It is the latter source that is thought to be responsible for elevated ACE levels in patients with sarcoidosis, reflecting granuloma "load." The induction of ACE synthesis in epithelioid cells and macrophages is caused by a soluble ACE-inducing factor (AIF). AIF activity has been detected in vivo in serum and BAL fluid of patients with active sarcoidosis, and has been generated in vitro by co-culture of monocytes with autologous T lymphocytes, where the activity was present in the cell-free media.[80] In healthy controls, serum ACE is age dependent; individuals younger than 21 years of age have higher levels than those older than 21 years.[81]

ACE is elevated in 60% to 90% of patients with active sarcoidosis. A normal serum ACE does not exclude the diagnosis, especially if the disease is in its early stages and localized to a small area (e.g., the eye), and therefore has a small epithelioid cell population. False low values are also measured in patients taking ACE inhibitors or in patients with endothelial abnormalities, such as deep vein

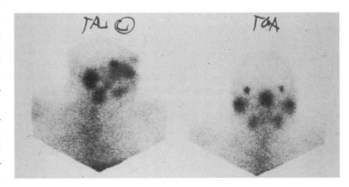

FIGURE 63–15. Panda sign in a patient with sarcoidosis. Bilateral symmetric ^{67}Ga uptake of the lacrimal, parotid, and submandibular glands.

thrombosis, and in patients who have had chemotherapy or radiation. Treatment with systemic steroids or other immunosuppressive agents can also affect ACE levels, with values normalizing when there is adequate control of intraocular inflammation.

Other disorders associated with elevated serum ACE include Gaucher's disease, leprosy, chronic pulmonary disease, rheumatoid arthritis, spondylitis, primary biliary cirrhosis, tuberculosis, histoplasmosis, histiocytic medullary fibrosis, hyperthyroidism, and diabetes mellitus (Table 63–4). However, most of these are not associated with uveitis, with the exception of tuberculosis, leprosy, and histoplasmosis. A careful history and ophthalmologic and systemic examination combined with other appropriate investigations should help to distinguish between these disorders.

Serum ACE levels probably parallel the total body mass and activity of granulomas. Its levels may vary throughout the disease course in patients with chronic uveitis, from normal to elevated, reflecting underlying disease activity.[32] ACE may not be elevated in patients with subclinical disease even in the presence of active uveitis. Karma and colleagues[21] reported that serum ACE was elevated in a significantly larger number of patients with ophthalmic sarcoidosis than with isolated pulmonary sarcoidosis or resolved disease.

Power and colleagues[78] reported a sensitivity of an initially raised serum ACE in diagnosing sarcoidosis of 73% and a specificity of 83%. The sensitivity can increase to 84% and the specificity to 95% when ACE levels of greater than 50 units/liter (i.e., the mean plus the standard deviation) are used.[81] Power and colleagues[78] found no association between ocular disease activity and initial serum ACE levels. They found elevated ACE in patients with uveitis caused by other diseases including Adamantiades-Behçet disease, HLA-B27–associated uveitis, syphilis, systemic lupus erythematosus, JRA, tuberculosis, sympathetic ophthalmia, acute retinal necrosis, intraocular lymphoma, birdshot chorioretinopathy, Lyme disease, Vogt-Koyanagi-Harada syndrome, and Wegener's granulomatosis.

TABLE 63–4. FREQUENCY OF INCREASED SERUM ANGIOTENSIN-CONVERTING ENZYME IN DISEASES OTHER THAN SARCOIDOSIS

DISEASE	PERCENT OF PATIENTS
Gaucher's disease	90
Hyperthyroidism	70
Berylliosis	44
Silicosis	42
Leprosy	34
Primary biliary cirrhosis	24
Cirrhosis	23
Diabetes mellitus	22
Histoplasmosis	16
Asbestosis	15
Allergic alveolitis	9
Tuberculosis	7
Coccidioidomycosis	6
Pulmonary fibrosis	5
Hodgkin's disease	5

ACE levels in tears have been reported to be elevated in patients with ocular sarcoidosis; however, the test is not specific for sarcoidosis.[82] Weinreb and colleagues[83] reported on the value of measuring ACE levels in aqueous humor of patients with granulomatous uveitis and suspected sarcoidosis. The authors found high aqueous ACE levels in these patients, compared with controls; they also reported one patient in whom the serum ACE was normal but the aqueous humor ACE was elevated.

Pulmonary Function Tests

Pulmonary function tests are useful in the initial diagnosis and follow-up of patients with sarcoidosis. Their sensitivity in disease with and without radiographic evidence of parenchymal involvement has been reported as 70% and 40%, respectively. The most common abnormalities seen early in the course of the disease are an increase after exercise in the alveolar-arterial oxygen gradient and diffusing capacity and a reduction in lung compliance. Moderate parenchymal involvement is associated with reduced inspiratory capacity, reduced total lung capacity, decreased diffusing capacity at rest, widened alveolar-arterial oxygen gradient, decreased partial pressure of oxygen in the blood, and increased respiratory rate. Late stages may be complicated by airways distortion, which may manifest as obstructive lung disease. Pulmonary hypertension is a late manifestation seen in a small proportion of patients.

Bronchoalveolar Lavage

The introduction of the fiberoptic bronchoscope in the early 1970s facilitated the study of the inflammatory process involved in sarcoidosis by the use of BAL. The earliest pathologic finding in patients with sarcoidosis is a mononuclear alveolitis composed of increased CD4+ lymphocytes (with an increased CD4/CD8 ratio), monocyte-macrophages, and rare B lymphocytes. Indirect evidence of heightened antigen-mediated activity is apparent from increased percentages of alveolar macrophages expressing DR antigens and increased density of human leukocyte antigen D surface antigens on sarcoid alveolar macrophages. In addition, lymphocytes rosetting about macrophages are seen in BAL specimens and in cells sloughed from in vitro–cultured intact sarcoid granulomas.

Sarcoid alveolar macrophages express increased intercellular adhesion molecules (ICAM-1) and leukocyte function-associated antigen (LFA-1) to facilitate the process. Lung macrophages spontaneously release IL-1. BAL lung T cells and in vitro–cultured intact cutaneous sarcoid granulomas spontaneously release IL-2. These finding suggest that active antigen presentation is central in the pathogenesis of sarcoidosis. The consequence of antigen presentation to specific T lymphocytes is amplification of the immune response through proliferation of T lymphocytes and their production of cytokines. Monocytes are the predominant cellular resource required for granuloma architecture. Lung T lymphocytes produce about 25 times more MCF per cell than the autologous peripheral blood T lymphocytes. Another lymphokine, MIF, prevents the migration of monocyte-macrophages accumulated at the site of the granuloma formation. In addition, the supernatants of sarcoid skin granulomas contain an inhibitor of monocyte leukotaxis with properties similar to the leukotactic inhibitor in the plasma of untreated sarcoid patients.

Recruited monocytes become activated, and sequentially differentiate into macrophages, epithelioid cells, and Langhans' giant cells. Further development of granuloma structure appears to require the induction of inter-epithelioid adhesion molecules such as LFA-1 and ICAM-1. Interferon (INF)-γ mediates the process and is known to be increased at sites of disease activity in sarcoidosis. Moller and colleagues[84] found dominant T_H1 cytokine expression in BAL patients from patients with sarcoidosis. T_H1 cells is the subgroup of CD4+ T cells that mediate cellular immune responses, characteristically during infections caused by intracellular bacteria. They produce IL-2, INF-γ, and tumor necrosis factor (TNF)-β.

Transbronchial Lung Biopsy

Tissue for biopsy from the bronchial mucosa or the adjacent lung is obtained through a fiberoptic bronchoscope. The procedure does not require general anesthesia, has a low complication rate, and is comfortable for the patient. The specimens obtained are small, but special fixation techniques permit accurate histologic diagnosis in most cases.[85] Gilman and Wang[86] recommended that four biopsies, obtained at each bronchoscopy, increased the diagnostic yield to 90%. Noncaseating granulomas have been reported in 54% to 88% of patients who underwent transbronchial lung biopsy (TBLB).[85, 87] The rate of positive findings by TBLB is higher in patients with radiologic evidence of pulmonary infiltration, and it is approximately 60% among patients with hilar lymphadenopathy whose chest radiographs show normal lung parenchyma.[85] Leonard and colleagues[87] reported that simultaneous TBLB, transbronchial needle aspiration, and BAL gave a diagnostic sensitivity of 100% in the 13 patients examined.

TBLB has been reported to show noncaseating granulomas in 37 of 60 patients (61.7%) with intraocular inflammation compatible with a diagnosis of sarcoidosis, who did not show bilateral hilar lymphadenopathy and had sparse contributory evidence for sarcoidosis.[88] The authors reported no complications apart from segmental pneumothorax in one patient.

Hypercalcemia

Hypercalcemia has been reported in 10% to 15% of patients with sarcoidosis and is related to increased serum concentrations of 1,25-dihydroxy-vitamin D_3 (calcitriol). Hypercalcemia is not specific for sarcoidosis and is seen in other granulomatous diseases such as tuberculosis, leprosy, coccidioidomycosis, histoplasmosis, and berylliosis. Calcitriol is produced at sites of active disease by alveolar macrophages and possibly T lymphocytes.[89] Elevated serum levels of calcitriol in hypercalcemic patients with sarcoidosis lead to increased absorption of calcium and phosphate from the gastrointestinal tract, which leads to hypercalcemia and hypercalciuria.

Recent studies have shown a role of calcitriol in modulating the immune response. Activated lymphocytes and cells of monocyte-macrophage lineage express receptors for calcitriol. Calcitriol promotes the differentiation of monocyte-macrophages, stimulates the proliferation of blood monocytes, and favors the formation of multinucleated giant cells. Calcitriol also enhances the cytotoxic function and mycobacterial killing of monocytes and their production of IL-1, TNF, and prostaglandin E_2.

Hypercalciuria is two to three times more common than hypercalcemia and is assessed by 24-hour urinary calcium determination. Hypercalcemia is always associated with hypercalciuria, while hypercalciuria may be present without hypercalcemia.[89] Persistent hypercalcemia is associated with risk of nephrocalcinosis[18] and is an indication for treatment. Systemic steroids are effective in normalizing serum calcium levels usually within 2 weeks, and they decrease serum calcitriol levels even faster.[89] Patients with hypercalcemia should be advised to avoid a high calcium diet, vitamin D supplements, and exposure to sunlight.

Lysozyme

Lysozyme is an enzyme normally secreted by monocytes and polymorphonuclear leukocytes. In healthy controls, serum lysozyme levels are age dependent, with an increase seen in subjects over 60 years of age.[81] Several reports have shown that the levels of serum lysozyme are raised in patients with sarcoidosis and may be related to disease activity. Raised lysozyme levels have been reported in parallel to raised serum ACE levels. It is thought that the epithelioid cell of the sarcoid granuloma is the source for both lysozyme and ACE. In contrast to ACE, the lysozyme concentration is also high in patients with erythema nodosum.[89] The values of both biochemical markers return to normal levels with successful treatment of sarcoidosis. Abnormal values of serum lysozyme have been reported in tuberculosis, silicosis, asbestosis, and berylliosis.

Baarsma and colleagues[81] reported that a lysozyme level of more than the mean plus two standard deviations has a sensitivity of 60%, a specificity of 76%, and a predictive value of only 12%. The predictive value of a positive test of 100% was reached at lysozyme levels seven standard deviations above the mean. The authors concluded that lysozyme levels have a limited value in the diagnosis of sarcoidosis.

Other biochemical markers used in the investigation of patients suspected of having sarcoidosis include $β_2$-microglobulin, IL-2 receptors, hyaluronan, fibronectin, collagenase, histamine, and platelet-activating factor. These have not been studied in relation to eye disease.

Tissue Biopsy

Conjunctival Biopsy

Conjunctival biopsy is of particular importance in everyday clinical practice because the tissue is easily accessible, the procedure is simple, and there is a low complication rate. The lower fornix is the preferred site and topical anesthesia is sufficient. The technique usually consists of retraction of the lower lid and excision of a strip of stretched conjunctiva with Westcott scissors. Topical antibiotic is instilled and pressure is applied for 5 to 10 min to avoid hemorrhage and soft-tissue edema. The optimal size of biopsy is approximately 1 cm long by 3 mm wide. No suturing is required. Although there have been no reports of infection or symblepharon, Karma and colleagues[21] noted minute scars at the site of the previous conjunctival biopsy in some patients.

The efficacy of the technique in the diagnosis of sarcoidosis remains controversial. The positive yield of conjunctival biopsy ranges from 14% to 40.4% and is based on studies performing unilateral or bilateral biopsies in patients with histologically confirmed nonocular sarcoidosis, sarcoidosis suspects, patients with and without ocular involvement, and patients who had or had not been initiated on treatment for their disease.[21, 26, 90–92]

Spaide and Ward[90] reported positive biopsies in 19 of 47 untreated patients (40.4%) and described higher yield in patients with follicles, those with ocular abnormality consistent with sarcoidosis, and those with pulmonary infiltrates. Crick and colleagues[25] also reported higher yield in patients with follicles and those with histologically confirmed nonocular sarcoidosis. Clinical interpretation of nodules may be difficult, as true sarcoid granulomas may be too small to be detected with slit-lamp examination, whereas more prominent nodules may turn out to be large follicles, an ectopic lacrimal gland, or foreign body fibrosis rather than noncaseating granulomas. These observations have led some investigators to perform blind (nondirected) biopsy, which has been reported to be positive in 55% to 71.4% of patients with biopsy-proven extraocular sarcoidosis[92, 26] and in 28.5% of patients with suspected sarcoidosis.[26] Repeat biopsy may be useful in patients in whom the initial biopsy was negative, as it can be positive, revealing a previously false-negative result.[21] Furthermore, bilateral conjunctival biopsies with examination of multiple sections of each specimen are also recommended, as granulomas may be present in limited numbers, so they may be missed if the number of sections is not adequate.[92]

Lacrimal Gland Biopsy

Lacrimal gland biopsy is considered in patients with clinically enlarged lacrimal glands and in those with positive ^{67}Ga uptake by the lacrimal glands. The biopsy can be performed either through a conjunctival or external (skin) approach. Transconjunctival biopsy of the palpebral lobe carries the risk of damage of the lacrimal gland ductules, which may lead to dry eye syndrome.

Skin Biopsy

As mentioned, skin lesions in sarcoidosis may be specific, showing histologically noncaseating granulomas such as lupus pernio, maculopapular eruptions, and subcutaneous nodules, or nonspecific (e.g., erythema nodosum). Biopsy of coexisting skin lesions is indicated in patients with ocular findings suggestive of sarcoidosis so that a histologic diagnosis can be made.

DIAGNOSIS

The definitive diagnosis of sarcoidosis requires histologic confirmation. Sometimes, sarcoidosis may manifest itself first in the eye, with uveitis, and clinically detectable extraocular manifestations may evolve slowly over several years.[22] Pursuit of such "sarcoid suspects," we believe,

should be vigorous and should be repeated annually, despite the bias of health maintenance organization "gate keepers" toward economy and parsimony, because the disease carries generally poor ocular prognosis, and one may well be faced with the decision about long-term immunomodulatory therapy. Clearly, a commitment to long-term therapy is best made in the context of a clear, definite diagnosis.

The evaluation of patients with uveitis caused by suspected sarcoidosis can be staged from noninvasive laboratory and radiologic tests to invasive ones, depending on the ease or difficulty of diagnosis. Initial assessment consists of chest radiograph, serum ACE, lysozyme, serum and urine calcium, and liver enzymes. At this stage, biopsy of clinically suspicious, easily accessible tissue (conjunctiva, skin) is advised. If these initial studies are negative, chest CT, whole-body ^{67}Ga scan, and pulmonary function tests should be performed. Chest CT and whole-body ^{67}Ga scan are advised in the presence of elevated serum ACE, lysozyme, or serum and urine calcium. If the chest radiograph, chest CT, or ^{67}Ga scan findings are characteristic of sarcoidosis, BAL and TBLB are advised. Open lung biopsy is reserved for patients with radiologic evidence of sarcoidosis in whom histologic proof is lacking despite systematic evaluation as previously outlined. An algorithm of the assessment of patients with suspected sarcoidosis is given in Figure 63–16.

DIFFERENTIAL DIAGNOSIS

The differential diagnosis of ocular sarcoidosis depends on the primary anatomic site involved. Sarcoidosis may simulate anterior, intermediate, and posterior uveitis and those uveitides associated with vitritis and multiple chorioretinal lesions such as multifocal choroiditis, birdshot retinochoroidopathy, Vogt-Koyanagi-Harada syndrome, sympathetic ophthalmia, tuberculosis, syphilis, toxoplasmosis, serpiginous chorioretinopathy, lymphoma, leukemia, and Whipple's disease (Table 63–5). A solitary choroidal mass appearing in an eye with sarcoidosis must be differentiated from metastatic tumor or a choroidal melanoma. Similarly, an optic nerve mass in a patient with sarcoidosis can be differentiated from a solitary granuloma due to tuberculosis or leprosy by a careful review of systems and skin testing with purified protein derivative. Central nervous system involvement secondary to sarcoidosis producing increased intracranial pressure and papilledema must be differentiated from other space-occupying lesions such as neoplasia or infections. Proliferative sarcoid retinopathy is distinguishable from other potential causes of retinal ischemia with neovascularization, such as Adamantiades-Behçet disease, central retinal vein occlusion, diabetes mellitus, and sickle-cell retinopathy, based on careful clinical examination and ocular and systemic history. Periphlebitis appearing in sarcoidosis needs to be differentiated from that seen in multiple sclerosis, systemic lupus erythematosus, Eales' disease, and frosted branch angiitis. Finally, vitritis, together with focal or multifocal chorioretinal involvement, are features common to both sarcoidosis and many of the posterior uveitic entities listed in Table 63–5. For example, both sarcoidosis and birdshot retinochoroidopathy manifest vitritis and vasculitis, and the appearance of the choroidal

Initial studies

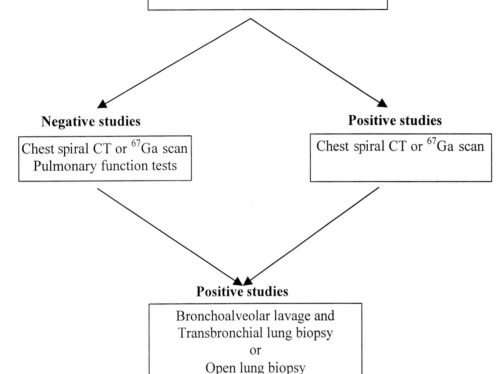

FIGURE 63–16. Algorithm for evaluation of patients with suspected sarcoidosis.

granuloma seen in ocular sarcoid may be confused with typical birdshot lesions.

TREATMENT

Ocular sarcoidosis is a potentially blinding disease that warrants aggressive treatment.[21, 22, 93] Mild anterior uveitis is treated by topical steroids and cycloplegics. Crick and colleagues[25] reported that prompt use of systemic steroids may save vision in patients with severe inflammation of the posterior segment. They noted that topical steroids were ineffective in posterior uveitis and reported one patient (who received only that treatment) who went totally blind within weeks of the onset of symptoms.

Systemic steroids are indicated in anterior uveitis that does not respond to topical steroids, and in patients with posterior uveitis, neovascularization, or orbital disease with visual symptoms or optic nerve compromise. Peribulbar steroids may also be useful. Patients who are refractory to steroids may respond to the addition of oral nonsteroidal anti-inflammatory drugs. If inflammation persists, immunosuppressive chemotherapy may be required. Successful results have been reported with aza-

thioprine, cyclosporine, and cyclophosphamide.[21, 28, 30] Dev and colleagues[94] reported that low-dose methotrexate was effective in controlling previously uncontrolled inflammation in 20 eyes from 11 patients with sarcoidosis-associated panuveitis, allowed elimination of corticosteroids in certain patients, and permitted successful cata-

TABLE 63–5. DIFFERENTIAL DIAGNOSIS OF SARCOIDOSIS

Anterior uveitis	Posterior uveitis
HLA-B27–associated iridocyclitis	Toxoplasmosis
Fuchs' heterochromic cyclitis	Toxocariasis
Herpes simplex virus	Histoplasmosis
Varicella zoster virus	Tuberculosis
Syphilis	Syphilis
Tuberculosis	Birdshot retinochoroidopathy
Juvenile rheumatoid arthritis	Serpiginous choroidopathy
Idiopathic	Vogt-Koyanagi-Harada syndrome
Intermediate uveitis	Intraocular lymphoma
Pars planitis	Sympathetic ophthalmia
Multiple sclerosis	Adamantiades-Behçet disease
Lyme borreliosis	Whipple disease

ract surgery in patients in whom it had previously been impossible.

Guidelines on the preparation of patients with sarcoidosis for cataract surgery have been described by Akova and Foster.[28] The preoperative medications employed by these investigators included periocular steroids (71%), systemic nonsteroidal anti-inflammatory drugs (71%), oral prednisone (57%), azathioprine (7%), and cyclosporine (7%). Secondary glaucoma not responding to medical treatment has been treated by trabeculectomy and cryoablative therapy.[28, 30] Laser trabeculoplasty and conventional filtering procedures are usually not effective in these patients. Drainage devices or trabeculectomy enhanced by antimetabolites may be necessary. Retinal neovascularization with evidence of ischemia on angiography responds well to panretinal photocoagulation.[22, 30, 34] Topical injection of steroids has been used successfully in the management of large sarcoid iris nodules.[27]

COMPLICATIONS

As mentioned, posterior segment involvement in sarcoidosis is associated with more severe visual loss than is anterior segment involvement.[21, 22] The major cause of poor visual outcome in these patients is macular pathology (CME, epiretinal membrane, macular hole). Optic atrophy may occur either in association with uveitis or in patients with sarcoidosis of the central nervous system. Secondary glaucoma is another important cause of visual loss in patients with sarcoidosis and may be the result of "trabeculitis," angle closure from peripheral anterior synechiae, or posterior synechiae and formation of iris bombé, or it may be steroid induced.[23, 28] Vitreous hemorrhage secondary to retinal neovascularization can also cause visual morbidity. Cataract and vitreous opacities may be managed by cataract extraction and vitrectomy. Visually significant band keratopathy may require its removal with chelating agents.

PROGNOSIS

In 1996, Rothova and colleagues[93] reported that sarcoidosis was the leading systemic disease associated with unilateral blindness, seen in 8 of 56 patients (14%). Severe visual loss (20/200 or less) has been reported in 6% to 23.8% of patients with ocular sarcoidosis and is more common in patients with chronic posterior uveitis.[21, 22] Glaucoma is another complication leading to significant visual loss in these patients.[23, 28]

Dana and colleagues[30] reported that visual acuity worse than 20/40 was related to black race, delay of more than 1 year between onset of symptoms and presentation to a uveitis subspecialist, development of glaucoma, and presence of posterior or intermediate uveitis.

Akova and Foster[28] reported that visual acuity worse than 20/40 was seen in 39% of patients with ocular sarcoidosis following cataract extraction and lens implantation. The causes of reduced visual acuity were CME, epiretinal membrane, glaucomatous optic nerve damage, central retinal vein occlusion, and peripapillary neovascularization secondary to optic disc granuloma.

CONCLUSIONS

Ocular involvement occurs in 26% to 50% of patients with confirmed diagnosis of sarcoidosis and, when pres-

ent, is generally seen early in the course of disease. The ocular manifestations are variable, as any part of the eye and the other orbital structures can be affected. All patients who present with uveitis, lid lesions, proptosis, extraocular nerve palsies, or optic nerve disease should be assessed carefully with a complete review of systems and appropriate radiologic, serologic, and other ancillary tests as outlined in the Diagnosis section so that sarcoidosis is excluded. Histologic confirmation of sarcoidosis should be sought in patients with clinical or other evidence suggestive of the disease. Periodic reevaluation is advised in patients with chronic uveitis in whom the initial investigations are negative. Persistent ocular sarcoidosis is vision robbing and may lead to blindness. Aggressiveness of treatment should be adjusted according to the type and nature of the ocular manifestations and may range from short courses of topical corticosteroids to long-term immunomodulation.

References

1. Hutchinson J: Anomalous disease of the skin of the fingers: Papillary psoriasis. In: Hutchinson J: Illustrations of Clinical Surgery. London, J & A Churchill, 1878, p 24.
2. Boeck C: Multiple benign sarkoid of the skin. J Cutan Genitour 1899;17:543.
3. Heerfordt CF: Uber eine: Febris uveo-parotidea subchronica, an der Glandula parotis und der Uvea des auges lokalisiert und haufig mit paresen cerebrospinaler nerven kompliziert. Albrecht von Graefes Arch Klin Exp Ophthalmol 1909;70:254.
4. Sharma OP: Sarcoidosis. Dis Mon 1990;36:469.
5. Elias JA, Daniele RP: Systemic sarcoidosis. In: Baum GL, Wolinsky E, eds: Textbook of Pulmonary Diseases, 4th ed. Boston, Little, Brown, 1989, p 663.
6. Boeck C: Nochmals zur Klinik und zur Stellung des "benignen Miliarlupoids." Arch Dermatol Syph (Wien) 1916;121:707.
7. Hosoda Y, Yamaguchi M, Hiraga Y: Global epidemiology of sarcoidosis. What story do prevalence and incidence tell us? Clin Chest Med 1997;18:681.
8. Diab SM, Karnik AM, Ouda BA, et al: Sarcoidosis in Arabs: The clinical profile of 20 patients and review of the literature. Sarcoidosis 1991;8:56.
9. Pietinalho A, Hiraga Y, Hosoda Y, et al: The frequency of sarcoidosis in Finland and Hokkaido, Japan. A comparative epidemiological study. Sarcoidosis 1995;12:61.
10. Yamaguchi M, Hosoda Y, Sasaki R, et al: Epidemiological study on sarcoidosis in Japan. Recent trends in incidence and prevalence rates and changes in epidemiological features. Sarcoidosis 1989;6:138.
11. Gupta SK, Gupta S: Sarcoidosis in India: A review of 125 biopsy-proven cases from eastern India. Sarcoidosis 1990;7:43.
12. Rybicki BA, Maliarik MJ, Major M, et al: Genetics of sarcoidosis. Clin Chest Med 1997;18:707.
13. Martinetti M, Tinelli C, Kolek V, et al: The sarcoidosis map: A joint survey of clinical and immunogenetic findings in two European countries. Am J Respir Crit Care Med 1995;152:557.
14. Bresnitz EA, Strom BL: Epidemiology of sarcoidosis. Epidemiol Rev 1983;5:124.
15. Smith MJ, Turton CW, Mitchell DN, et al: Association of HLA-B8 with spontaneous resolution in sarcoidosis. Thorax 1981;36:296.
16. Saboor SA, Johnson NM, McFadden J: Detection of mycobacterial DNA in sarcoidosis and tuberculosis with polymerase chain reaction. Lancet 1992;339:1012.
17. Mitchell IC, Turk JL, Mitchell DN: Detection of mycobacterial rRNA in sarcoidosis with liquid-phase hybridisation. Lancet 1992;339:1015.
18. McCurley T, Salter J, Glick A: Renal insufficiency in sarcoidosis. Arch Pathol Lab Med 1990;114:488.
19. Mañá J, Marcoval J, Graells J, et al: Cutaneous involvement in sarcoidosis. Relationship to systemic disease. Arch Dermatol 1997;133:882.
20. Obenauf CD, Shaw HE, Sydnor CF, et al: Sarcoidosis and its ocular manifestations. Am J Ophthalmol 1978;86:648.

21. Karma A, Huhti E, Poukkula A: Course and outcome of ocular sarcoidosis. Am J Ophthalmol 1988;106:467.

22. Rothova A, Alberts C, Glasius E, et al: Risk factors for ocular sarcoidosis. Doc Ophthalmol 1989;72:287.

23. Jabs DA, Johns CJ: Ocular involvement in chronic sarcoidosis. Am J Ophthalmol 1986;102:297.

24. Hunter DG, Foster CS: Ocular manifestations of sarcoidosis. In: Albert DM, Jakobiec FA, eds: Principles and Practice of Ophthalmology. Philadelphia, W.B. Saunders, 1994, pp 443–450.

25. Crick RP, Hoyle C, Smellie H: The eyes in sarcoidosis. Br J Ophthalmol 1961;45:461.

26. Karcioglu ZA, Brear R: Conjunctival biopsy in sarcoidosis. Am J Ophthalmol 1985;99:68.

27. Mader TH, Chismire KJ, Cornell FM: The treatment of an enlarged sarcoid iris nodule with injectable corticosteroids. Am J Ophthalmol 1988;106:365.

28. Akova YA, Foster CS: Cataract surgery in patients with sarcoidosis-associated uveitis. Ophthalmology 1994;101:473.

29. Lardenoye CWTA, Van der Lelij A, de Loos WS, et al: Peripheral multifocal chorioretinitis. A distinct clinical entity? Ophthalmology 1997;104:1820.

30. Dana M-R, Merayo-Lloves J, Schaumberg DA, et al: Prognosticators for visual outcome in sarcoid uveitis. Ophthalmology 1996;103:1846.

31. Vrabec TR, Augsburger JJ, Fisher DH, et al: Taches de bougie. Ophthalmology 1995;102:1712.

32. Stavrou P, Linton S, Young DW, et al: Clinical diagnosis of ocular sarcoidosis. Eye 1997;11:365.

33. Gass JDM, Olson CL: Sarcoidosis with optic nerve and retinal involvement. Arch Ophthalmol 1976;94:945.

34. Duker JS, Brown GC, McNamara JA: Proliferative sarcoid retinopathy. Ophthalmology 1988;95:1680.

35. Wolfensberger TJ, Herbort CP: Indocyanine green angiographic features in ocular sarcoidosis. Ophthalmology 1999;106:285.

36. Gragoudas ES, Regan CDJ: Bilateral subretinal neovascularization in presumed sarcoidosis. Arch Ophthalmol 1981;99:1194.

37. Inagaki M, Harada T, Kiribuchi T, et al: Subfoveal choroidal neovascularization in uveitis. Ophthalmologica 1996;210:229.

38. Dodds EM, Lowder CY, Barnhorst DA, et al: Posterior scleritis with annular ciliochoroidal detachment. Am J Ophthalmol 1995;120:677.

39. Ohara K, Okubo A, Sasaki H, et al: Branch retinal vein occlusion in a child with ocular sarcoidosis. Am J Ophthalmol 1995;119:806.

40. Tingley DP, Gonder JR: Ocular sarcoidosis presenting as a solitary choroidal mass. Can J Ophthalmol 1992;27:25.

41. DeRosa AJ, Margo CE, Orlick ME: Hemorrhagic retinopathy as the presenting manifestation of sarcoidosis. Retina 1995;15:422.

42. Edelsten C, Stanford MR, Graham EM: Serpiginous choroiditis: An unusual presentation of ocular sarcoidosis. Br J Ophthalmol 1994;78:70.

43. Brinkman CJJ, Rothova A: Fundus pathology in neurosarcoidosis. Int Ophthalmol 1993;17:23.

44. Priem HA, Oosterhuis JA: Birdshot chorioretinopathy: Clinical characteristics and evolution. Br J Ophthalmol 1988;72:646.

45. Gould H, Kaufman HE: Sarcoid of the fundus. Arch Ophthalmol 1961;65:453.

46. Wall M, Newman S, Slavin M, et al: Optic atrophy. Surv Ophthalmol 1991;36:51.

47. Galetta S, Schatz NJ, Glaser JS: Acute sarcoid optic neuropathy with spontaneous recovery. J Clin Neuroophthalmol 1989;9:27.

48. Wong RJ, Gliklich RE, Rubin PA, et al: Bilateral nasolacrimal duct obstruction managed with endoscopic techniques. Arch Otolaryngol Head Neck Surg 1998;124:703.

49. Simon EM, Zoarski GH, Rothman MI, et al: Systemic sarcoidosis with bilateral orbital involvement: MR findings. AJNR Am J Neuroradiol 1998;19:336.

50. Cornblath WT, Elner V, Rolfe M: Extraocular muscle involvement in sarcoidosis. Ophthalmology 1993;100:501.

51. Imes RK, Reifschneider JS, O'Connor LE: Systemic sarcoidosis presenting initially with bilateral orbital and upper lid masses. Ann Ophthalmol 1998;20:466.

52. Peterson EA, Hymas DC, Pratt DV, et al: Sarcoidosis with orbital tumor outside the lacrimal gland: Initial manifestation in 2 elderly white women. Arch Ophthalmol 1998;116:804.

53. Cancrini C, Angelini F, Colavita M, et al: Erythema nodosum: A presenting sign of early onset sarcoidosis. Clin Exp Rheumatol 1998;16:337.

54. Sahn EE, Hampton MT, Garen PD, et al: Preschool sarcoidosis masquerading as juvenile rheumatoid arthritis: Two case reports and a review of the literature. Pediatr Dermatol 1990;7:208.

55. O'Brien JM, Albert DM, Foster CS: Juvenile rheumatoid arthritis. In: Albert DM, Jakobiec FA, eds: Principles and Practice of Ophthalmology: Clinical Practice. Philadelphia, W.B. Saunders, 1993, p 2873.

56. Hegab SM, al-Mutawa SA, Sheriff SM: Sarcoidosis presenting as multifocal limbal corneal nodules. J Pediatr Ophthalmol Strabismus 1998;35:323.

57. Lennarson P, Barney NP: Interstitial keratitis as presenting ophthalmic sign of sarcoidosis in a child. J Pediatr Ophthalmol Strabismus 1995;32:194.

58. Sakurai Y, Nakajima M, Kamisue S, et al: Preschool sarcoidosis mimicking juvenile rheumatoid arthritis: The significance of gallium scintigraphy and skin biopsy in the differential diagnosis. Acta Paediatr Jpn 1997;39:74.

59. Ukae S, Tsutsumi H, Adachi N, et al: Preschool sarcoidosis manifesting as juvenile rheumatoid arthritis: A case report and a review of the literature of Japanese cases. Acta Paediatr Jpn 1994;36:515.

60. Vaphiades MS, Eggenberger E: Childhood sarcoidosis. J Neuroophthalmol 1998;18:99.

61. Bruins Slot WJ: Ziekte van Besnier-Boeck en febris uveoparotidea (Heerfordt). Ned Tijdschr Geneeskd 1936;80:2859.

62. Lofgren S: Erythema nodosum: Studies on etiology and pathogenesis in 185 adult cases. Acta Med Scand 1946;124(suppl):1.

63. Kobzik L, Schoen FJ: The lung. In: Cotran RS, Kumar V, Robbins SL, eds: Robbins Pathologic Basis of Disease, 5th ed. Philadelphia, W.B. Saunders, 1994, pp 673–734.

64. Kveim A: En ny og spesifikk kutan-reaksjon ved Boeck's sarcoid. Nord Med 1941;9:169.

65. Pierard GE, Damseaux M, Franchimont C, et al: The histological structure of Kveim tests parallels the evolution of pulmonary sarcoidosis. Am J Dermatopathol 1982;4:17.

66. Wigley RD: Moratorium on Kveim tests. Lancet 1993;341:1284.

67. Kataria YP, Holter JF: Cutaneous anergy in sarcoidosis. In: James DG, ed: Sarcoidosis and Other Granulomatous Disorders (vol 73, Lung Biology in Health and Disease). New York, Marcel Dekker, 1994, p 181.

68. Kataria YP, Holter JF: Immunology of sarcoidosis. Clin Chest Med 1997;18:719.

69. Holter JF, Park HK, Sjoerdsma KW, et al: Nonviable autologous bronchoalveolar lavage cell preparations induce intradermal epithelioid cell granulomas in sarcoidosis patients. Am Rev Respir Dis 1992;145:864.

70. Martinez FJ, Orens JB, Deeb M, et al: Recurrence of sarcoidosis following bilateral allogeneic lung transplantation. Chest 1994;106:1597.

71. Heyll A, Meckenstock G, Aul C, et al: Possible transmission of sarcoidosis via allogeneic bone marrow transplantation. Bone Marrow Transplant 1994;14:161.

72. Sulavik SB, Spencer RP, Palestro CJ, et al: Specificity and sensitivity of distinctive chest radiographic and/or ^{67}Ga images in the noninvasive diagnosis of sarcoidosis. Chest 1993;103:403.

73. James DJ, Neville E, Siltzbach LE, et al: A worldwide review of sarcoidosis. Proceedings of the Seventh International Conference on Sarcoidosis and Other Granulomatous Disorders. Ann N Y Acad Sci 1976;278:321.

74. Kosmorsky GS, Meisler DM, Rice TW, et al: Chest computed tomography and mediastinoscopy in the diagnosis of sarcoidosis-associated uveitis. Am J Ophthalmol 1998;126:132.

75. Sulavik SB, Palestro CJ, Spencer RP, et al: Extrapulmonary sites of radiogallium accumulation in sarcoidosis. Clin Nucl Med 1990;15:876.

76. Sulavik SB, Spencer RP, Weed DA, et al: Recognition of distinctive patterns of gallium-67 distribution in sarcoidosis. J Nucl Med 1990;31:1909.

77. Nosal A, Schleissner LA, Mishkin FS, et al: Angiotensin-1-converting enzyme and gallium scan in noninvasive evaluation of sarcoidosis. Ann Intern Med 1979;90:328.

78. Power WJ, Neves RA, Rodriguez A, et al: The value of combined serum angiotensin-converting enzyme and gallium scan in diagnosing ocular sarcoidosis. Ophthalmology 1995;102:2007.

79. Weinreb RN, Barth R, Kimura SJ: Limited gallium scans and angiotensin converting enzyme in granulomatous uveitis. Ophthalmology 1980;87:202.

80. Conrad AK, Rohrbach MS: An in vivo model for the induction of angiotensin-converting enzyme in sarcoidosis. Am Rev Respir Dis 1987;135:396.
81. Baarsma GS, La Hey E, Glasius E, et al: The predictive value of serum angiotensin converting enzyme and lysozyme levels in the diagnosis of ocular sarcoidosis. Am J Ophthalmol 1987;104:211.
82. Immonen I, Friberg K, Sorsila R, et al: Concentration of angiotensin-converting enzyme in tears of patients with sarcoidosis. Acta Ophthalmol 1987;65:27.
83. Weinreb RN, Sandman R, Ryder MI, et al: Angiotensin-converting enzyme activity in human aqueous humor. Arch Ophthalmol 1985;103:34.
84. Moller DR, Forman JD, Liu MC, et al: Enhanced expression of IL-12 associated with Th1 cytokine profiles in active pulmonary sarcoidosis. J Immunol 1996;156:4952.
85. Mitchell DM, Mitchell DN, Collins JV, et al: Transbronchial lung biopsy through fibreoptic bronchoscope in diagnosis of sarcoidosis. Br Med J 1980;280:679.
86. Gilman MJ, Wang KP: Transbronchial lung biopsy in sarcoidosis. An approach to determine the optimal number of biopsies. Am Rev Respir Dis 1980;122:721.
87. Leonard C, Tormey VJ, Okeane C, et al: Bronchoscopic diagnosis of sarcoidosis. Eur Respir J 1997;10:2722.
88. Ohara K, Okubo A, Kamata K, et al: Transbronchial lung biopsy in the diagnosis of suspected ocular sarcoidosis. Arch Ophthalmol 1993;111:642.
89. Costabel U, Teschler H: Biochemical changes in sarcoidosis. Clin Chest Med 1997;18:827.
90. Spaide FR, Ward DL: Conjunctival biopsy in the diagnosis of sarcoidosis. Br J Ophthalmol 1990;74:469.
91. Hershey JM, Pulido JS, Folberg R, et al: Non-caseating conjunctival granulomas in patients with multifocal choroiditis and panuveitis. Ophthalmology 1994;101:596.
92. Nicholls CW, Eagle RC, Yanoff M, et al: Conjunctival biopsy as an aid in the evaluation of the patients with suspected sarcoidosis. Ophthalmology 1980;87:287.
93. Rothova A, Suttorp-van Schulten MSA, Treffers WF, et al: Causes and frequency of blindness in patients with intraocular inflammatory disease. Br J Ophthalmol 1996;80:332.
94. Dev S, McCallum RM, Jaffe GJ: Methotrexate treatment for sarcoid-associated panuveitis. Ophthalmology 1999;106:111.

64 TUBULOINTERSTITIAL NEPHRITIS AND UVEITIS SYNDROME

Vakur Pinar, Nicolette Gion, and C. Stephen Foster

DEFINITION

Acute tubulointerstitial nephritis (ATIN) is an important cause of renal failures. It may be idiopathic or associated with drug hypersensitivity, infections, and immunologic diseases.[1] Idiopathic acute tubulointerstitial nephritis and uveitis (TINU) is an uncommon syndrome involving the kidney and the eye. It occurs mainly in children and young adults, and females are affected more often than males.[2–4] Patients usually present with systemic symptoms including fatigue, malaise, anorexia, abdominal pain, fever, and anemia. The nephritis usually precedes the uveitis, although simultaneous onset in both organs has been described.[2, 5, 6] The nephropathy typically resolves spontaneously or responds favorably to systemic steroid therapy,[2, 6–10] but the uveitis often becomes chronic and is treatment resistant.[2, 9–19]

HISTORY

The association of idiopathic ATIN and uveitis was first described by Dobrin and associates in 1975.[2] They reported two adolescent girls (ages 14 and 17) with severe eosinophilic interstitial nephritis and renal failure. Both patients had bilateral anterior uveitis, and bone marrow granulomas were found on bone marrow biopsy, with one patient also having lymph node granulomas. The authors proposed that these cases represented a "new syndrome" because extensive investigation for an etiologic agent was unrevealing and neither patient's condition could be classified as a known disease entity. In most of the cases reported since then, the infiltration of eosinophils in the renal interstitium was not as marked, and bone marrow or lymph node granulomas were reported only in two subsequent cases.[20, 21] Thus, the term renal-ocular syndrome, or more recently, TINU syndrome seems to be more suitable for the clinicopathologic entity. In 1988, Rosenbaum's article on five patients with bilateral uveitis associated with interstitial nephritis drew attention to this syndrome in the ophthalmic literature.[6]

EPIDEMIOLOGY

TINU syndrome is a rare and relatively new syndrome, but it may have been underrecognized. Since the initial description in 1975, about 60 cases have been reported in the ophthalmologic and nephrologic literature. In Rosenbaum's study, 5 of 244 patients with uveitis were found to suffer from TINU, which ranked as the sixth most common systemic illness associated with uveitis in his clinic.[6] BenEzra, in a letter to the editor of the *American Journal of Ophthalmology*, argued with this prevalence of 2% and estimated the prevalence to be 0.5% in most uveitis clinics.[8] The diagnosis, and hence prevalence studies, may be difficult because (1) definite diagnosis requires kidney biopsy, (2) nephropathy can resolve sponta-

neously, and (3) systemic complaints are nonspecific. TINU syndrome is an illness of childhood and adolescence but can appear at any age.[2–4, 17, 19–22] There is a marked female predominance; most of the reported young patients and all, except one,[17] of the adult patients (aged 23–74) have been females.[2–4, 19]

CLINICAL FEATURES

TINU is a systemic disease. Most patients have systemic complaints that include fatigue, malaise, anorexia, weight loss, abdominal pain, and fever and there is usually a typical time sequence for the appearance of these clinical features in TINU syndrome.[5] These first nonspecific signs and symptoms usually precede the nephropathy by up to 1 month. Nausea, vomiting, headache, and myalgia can also form a part of the initial group of symptoms. After a few weeks, the disease is fully developed, with a triad consisting of an inflammatory syndrome, nephropathy, and somewhat later, usually uveitis. The inflammatory syndrome is always present and consists of a markedly increased sedimentation rate, high plasma proteins (mainly hypergammaglobulinemia), and anemia. The nephropathy generally appears a few weeks later. Proteinuria is a constant feature. Laboratory findings of tubulointerstitial damage include normoglycemic (renal) glycosuria, leucocyturia, aminoaciduria, microhematuria, and increased urinary excretion of β_2-microglobulin. Most urine casts, when seen, are granular, hyaline, or leukocyte casts. Diuresis is maintained, and polyuria may even be prominent, sometimes causing nocturia. There is also a low glomerular filtration rate (GFR) with elevated blood urea nitrogen (BUN) and creatinine levels. Hypertension is typically absent. The nephritis usually resolves or responds to steroid or immunosuppressive therapy, but nephrotic syndrome may develop, and chronic renal failure may occur. A few patients eventually require dialysis.

Uveitis, the third component of the triad, usually occurs a few weeks to several months after the onset of the renal disease, not infrequently when renal function is recovering and initial symptoms are waning. Uveitis may precede or occur simultaneously with nephropathy. It is typically bilateral, anterior, acute, and nongranulomatous (Table 64–1). Pain, photophobia, ciliary injection, a mild to severe degree of anterior chamber cells, and flare are usually present, and posterior synechiae can occur. Hausmann and colleagues reported a 53-year-old woman with TINU syndrome who presented with bilateral granulomatous anterior uveitis,[15] and we also saw a 13-year-old girl with TINU syndrome who presented with granulomatous anterior uveitis to the Immunology and Uveitis Service of the Massachusetts Eye and Ear Infirmary. A 14-year-old boy with bilateral nongranulomatous panuveitis

Bilateral anterior uveitis
Acute onset in one or both eyes
Usually nongranulomatous
Recurrences are common
Usually responds to topical corticosteroid therapy

was also examined on our service. Panuveitis, pars planitis, and posterior uveitis in the relapsing disease have been described in some patients with TINU syndrome.[2, 6–29] A 15-year-old boy who developed unilateral posterior uveitis with papillitis, optic disc hemorrhage, and macular plicae 1 month after bilateral anterior uveitis has been described.[30] Acute posterior multifocal placoid pigment epitheliopathy (APMPPE) has been reported in association with acute nephritis in one patient, but renal biopsy was not done owing to spontaneous recovery of the nephropathy.[18]

As a summary of clinical features, a typical patient profile is an adolescent girl or adult woman with bilateral, recurrent anterior uveitis who has had systemic complaints and laboratory findings or a history of ATIN.

PATHOLOGY, IMMUNOLOGY, AND PATHOGENESIS

The histologic picture of renal biopsy specimens in ATIN is characterized by cellular infiltration and edema of the interstitium.[31–33] The majority of the inflammatory cells are T lymphocytes. The remaining cells (forming up to half of the cellular infiltrate) are monocytes and macrophages, with very few cells expressing B lymphocyte markers. Plasma cells. granulocytes, neutrophils, and eosinophils may be seen. The eosinophilic component, emphasized originally by Dobrin,[2] is variable and may be minimal or absent. The tubules show some edema with patchy epithelial degeneration, focal necrosis, and dilation or atrophy. Fibrosis is occasionally seen, but there are no glomerular or vascular changes present. Occasionally granulomas are found.[5, 13]

Immunofluorescence microscopic studies are negative for fibrinogen, immunoglobulins, and complement components. Circulating immune complexes have been detected in only a minority of cases, and in the patients studied, immune complexes were detected in the aqueous and the serum.[6, 7, 13, 16, 34] There are several reports of elevated immunoglobulin G (IgG) levels in the serum of TINU patients.[11, 13, 21, 35] Immunohistopathologic studies reveal that the majority of the infiltrating cells were CD4+ (helper or inducer) T lymphocytes, suggesting the involvement of T-cell–mediated delayed type hypersensitivity[33, 35–37] in the pathogenesis of TINU. Dominant infiltration of CD8+ (suppressor/cytotoxic) T cells in the renal interstitium was found in some studies.[21, 22] There is no clear explanation for this discrepancy at present. Chan and coworkers reported that CD4+ T-cell subtype is predominant in ocular infiltrates during the early stages of experimental autoimmune uveitis (EAU)—and sympathetic ophthalmia—whereas CD8+ T cells predominate in the later stages.[25, 26] This subset change was explained

as a reflection of the kinetics and regulation of the inflammatory response in autoimmune diseases, but the actual cause of this phenomenon is still controversial. Yoshioka and coworkers demonstrated the expression of the interleukin-2 (IL-2) receptor on infiltrating mononuclear cells, which is expressed mainly and transiently on recently activated T cells.[36] Three of the four patients with TINU syndrome, seen on the Immunology and Uveitis Service of the Massachusetts Eye and Ear Infirmary,[28] showed elevated soluble IL-2 receptor (sIL-2R) levels. Rodriguez-Perez and colleagues found a clear predominance of activated memory T lymphocytes (CD45RO+) in the interstitial infiltration.[29] Increased immunologic reactivity in the renal tissue was also demonstrated, together with a suppressed peripheral T-cell function both in vivo (anergy to skin test) and in vitro (decreased lymphokine secretion).[29] It is noteworthy that four patients reported in that study were studied during remission of the disease. In contrast, a temporary depression of the cellular immunity was observed in the acute phase, as opposed to the strongly positive tuberculin reaction before illness and during remission in Van Acker and coworkers' study.[4]

Birnbacher and associates found cytotoxic T-cell, macrophage, and granulocyte activation in blood immunologic analysis and serum analysis of a 14-year-old boy with TINU syndrome.[24] They interpreted these findings as either a significant role in its pathogenesis or as part of a microbe-triggered immune response. Antineutrophil cytoplasmic antibodies (ANCAs), both with a cytoplasmic and a perinuclear pattern, were detected in three patients, suggesting autoimmunity.[30–32] However, ANCAs were not regularly examined in previous studies, and they were not detected in 13 cases (not yet published).[30–34] The presence of ANCAs has been reported in some patients with uveitis of various etiologies, albeit with a low prevalence and questionable pathogenic significance.[33, 34] Various human leukocyte antigen (HLA) associations have been described. Tissue typing for HLA-A, -B, -C, and -DR antigens in the study conducted by Iitsuka and coworkers revealed identical HLA-CW3 in three patients and identical HLA-A24 in all four cases, whereas Gafter and colleagues found a high frequency of HLA-DR6 in three patients.[30, 37] Interestingly, BenEzra noted that three of his four patients with interstitial nephritis and bilateral anterior uveitis were HLA-B27 positive, but this might be a random association because there are no other reports of HLA-B27 positivity in TINU patients described in the literature.[8]

The etiology and pathogenesis of TINU syndrome is still unknown. Search for an infectious agent has been negative, despite extensive culture and serologic testing. Abnormalities of both humoral and cellular immunity have been reported emphasizing an immunologic disorder, accompanying or causing this syndrome. An immunologic disorder, probably T-cell–mediated, is most likely because (1) the interstitial infiltrate consists mainly of T lymphocytes; (2) granulomas are seen occasionally; (3) immunofluorescence studies are mostly negative for tubulointerstitial deposits; (4) hypergammaglobulinemia, circulating immune complexes, and ANCAs were detected in some patients; and (5) there is a favorable response to steroid treatment in most cases. A possible role of chlamydia infection has been suggested based on the course of the antichlamydial antibody titers in a 38-year-old woman with TINU.[38] In our series of six TINU patients, abnormal findings included Epstein-Barr virus IgG, highly elevated anticardiolipin-IgM and increased complement 4 (C4) in one patient, antinuclear antibody (ANA) positivity and decreased total complement levels in another patient, and elevated sIL-2R levels in three patients.[28] HLA-typing in one case showed HLA-A9, -A33, -B65, and -Cw8.

DIAGNOSIS AND DIFFERENTIAL DIAGNOSIS

The first step in the diagnosis of TINU syndrome is perhaps an awareness of the entity itself and a high index of suspicion. Anterior uveitis is the most common form of intraocular inflammation, and it is frequently associated with systemic diseases such as HLA-B27–associated seronegative spondyloarthropathies, juvenile rheumatoid arthritis, sarcoidosis, and diabetes mellitus. TINU syndrome takes its place on this list, albeit as a rare cause. All patients with bilateral anterior acute uveitis in association with systemic symptoms such as fatigue, fever, headache, anorexia, weight loss, and abdominal or flank pain should undergo careful evaluation of renal function. The interval between systemic signs and renal and ocular symptoms may range between 0 and 14 months[28]; hence, the importance of careful history taking. Laboratory findings of high sedimentation rate, normochromic normocytic anemia, elevated serum creatinine and BUN levels, abnormal urinalysis findings (renal glycosuria, proteinuria, aminoaciduria, microhematuria) support the diagnosis, and nephrology consultation should be requested. TINU syndrome is a clinicopathologic entity, and definitive diagnosis is established by kidney biopsy. Because nephropathy can recover spontaneously in some cases and kidney biopsy is not a routine procedure, the definitive diagnosis of TINU syndrome may be unfortunately missed in some cases.

The differential diagnosis (Table 64–2) must include diseases associated with uveitis and interstitial nephritis, which may be either isolated or accompanied by glomerulonephritis. The concurrence of uveitis and ATIN is uncommon. Potential causes include sarcoidosis, Sjögren's syndrome, Adamantiades-Behçet disease, IgA nephropathy (Berger's disease), Kawasaki's disease, systemic lupus erythematosus, tuberculosis, syphilis, toxoplasmosis, brucellosis, and leptospirosis. Drug hypersensitivity (e.g., nonsteroidal anti-inflammatory drugs, antibiotics, diuret-

ics) is the most common cause of ATIN in adults and can be rarely associated with anterior uveitis.[39] The possibility of drug-induced ATIN, with the incidental (or drug-induced) findings of anterior uveitis, should be considered in the presence of maculopapular rash, arthralgia, eosinophilia, and eosinophiluria. Bilateral, recurrent anterior uveitis of sudden onset, similar to that seen in TINU syndrome, has been described in association with past streptococcal infection, which is also a common cause of ATIN in children.[40–42] Most of these differential diagnoses can be excluded by a detailed history, physical examination, and serologic tests. The TINU syndrome can be regarded as distinct from these and other oculorenal syndromes on the basis of clinical features, pathology, and natural history.

TREATMENT AND PROGNOSIS

In most cases, topical steroids have been adequate in controlling the uveitis, whereas some patients require systemic steroid treatment.[6, 23] In steroid-resistant patients and in those who exhibit recurrent attacks of uveitis after discontinuation of steroids, immunomodulatory agents can achieve control of the inflammation and prevent relapses.

In general, the outcome of TINU syndrome is favorable. The interstitial nephritis usually resolves completely, either spontaneously or after systemic corticosteroid treatment.[1, 6, 13, 43] The aim of steroid therapy is to alter the course of the acute renal failure by achieving a rapid improvement of renal function and to minimize any residual damage. Full recovery occurs in children, and relapse of nephritis is not seen. The course of ATIN may be less predictable and more guarded in adults. Cases of nephrotic syndrome, relapsing nephritis, and development of chronic renal failure, despite the use of systemic steroids and other immunosuppressants (chlorambucil and cyclophosphamide), have been reported.[1, 11, 12] In a review of the literature, Cacoub and coworkers described one adult patient who developed terminal renal failure and two patients with deterioration of renal function who were not treated with corticosteroids; interstitial fibrosis and tubular atrophy were correlated with poor renal function prognosis.[10] Rodriguez-Perez and colleagues reported on five patients with a 1-year follow-up, whose renal function and uveitis responded dramatically to steroid treatment maintained for a period of 6 to 9 months.[29] Gafter and associates reported on four patients with TINU syndrome (one adolescent and three adult females) who were treated with systemic prednisone.[13] There was a favorable response of the renal disease in all cases, as indicated by the decrease of serum creatinine and disappearance of proteinuria. Treatment lasted from 5 to 12 months because a rapid taper in the prednisone dosage was associated with a rise in serum creatinine. After cessation of treatment, there was no exacerbation of nephritis during a follow-up period of 2.5 to 9.5 years. In contrast, the anterior uveitis relapsed many times in all patients. Its response to systemic steroid treatment was regarded as inconsistent, with several exacerbations occurring during steroid treatment. No controlled studies to date confirm whether use of systemic corticosteroids is truly beneficial in the treatment of ATIN in TINU syn-

TABLE 64–2. DIFFERENTIAL DIAGNOSIS OF TINU SYNDROME

Sarcoidosis	Adamantiades-Behçet disease
Sjögren's syndrome	Syphilis
Post streptococcal uveitis	Tuberculosis
Juvenile rheumatoid arthritis (JRA)	Brucellosis
IgA nephropathy (Berger's disease)	Leptospirosis
Vasculitides (e.g., systemic lupus erythematosus, Wegener's granulomatosis)	

drome. Clearly, all patients with TINU syndrome should be managed in collaboration with a nephrologist, particularly if ATIN occurs simultaneously with uveitis or follows it.

Bilateral anterior uveitis usually responds well to topical corticosteroid treatment. It should be treated aggressively initially (e.g., one drop every hour while awake), with slow tapering. In case of failure, the compliance of the patient and dosing schedule should be checked before advancing to a more aggressive treatment (e.g., periocular injection; per oral route). Cycloplegic and mydriatic agents should be used to prevent posterior synechiae and to relieve pain. Cyclopentolate is better avoided, because it has been shown to be a chemoattractant for leukocytes in one study.[44] Should there be an ocular hypertensive response to local steroids, another preparation (e.g., fluorometholone, rimexolone) or topical antiglaucomatous agents (beta blockers, carbonic anhydrase inhibitors) can be used. Complications such as posterior synechiae, cystoid macular edema, and progression of intraocular inflammation to the posterior segment (optic disc edema, pars planitis, and panuveitis) have been reported.[28]

If uveitis persists in both eyes despite topical steroid therapy or posterior segment complications develop, systemic corticosteroid treatment should be considered. Serious side effects of long-term steroid treatment, particularly in children, are well-known, and monitoring of these side effects as well as the clinical response to the therapy should be done regularly. Steroid-sparing strategies should be considered in steroid-dependent cases. This is usually achieved by use of other immunosuppressive agents such as methotrexate (7.5 mg to 20 mg/week), cyclosporine A (3 mg to 5 mg/kg/day), or azathioprine (1 mg to 2.5 mg/kg/day), either alone or in combination, in order to increase efficiency and decrease toxicity. To our knowledge, the report by Sanchez Roman and coworkers is the first to describe the use of steroid-sparing agents in a patient with posterior uveitis in the TINU syndrome.[45] The authors described several relapses of uveitis despite the use of oral steroids, which persisted after addition of azathioprine. Their patient responded favorably to cyclosporine A as monotherapy. At the Immunology and Uveitis Service of the Massachusetts Eye and Ear Infirmary, we examined six patients who were referred to us because of recurrences of uveitis despite treatment with topical, regional, and systemic steroids, and in one patient, methotrexate. Introduction or addition of immunosuppressants such as methotrexate, azathioprine, or cyclosporine A in five of six patients achieved control of the ocular inflammation and prevented relapses over a mean follow-up period of 19.66 months.[28] Methotrexate alone (in three patients) or in combination with cyclosporine A (in one patient) was successful in controlling the uveitis. One patient did not respond to the combination of methotrexate and systemic steroids, and developed steroid-induced side effects. He responded well to a combination of cyclosporine A and azathioprine. All patients tolerated the chemotherapy well, apart from one patient who complained of nausea and abdominal pain after taking methotrexate. These symptoms resolved after dividing the dose of methotrexate on two successive days.

Our case series confirms and extends the observation of Sanchez Roman and associates that the introduction of immunosuppressive agents can achieve control of the intraocular inflammation and prevent relapses in TINU patients.[45] Because no "best drug" is known for TINU syndrome, the selection of the most effective immunosuppressant must follow a "sequential stepladder approach," with low-dose once-weekly methotrexate generally being the first step, followed by cyclosporine A or azathioprine. As always, the use of such immunomodulatory therapy should be under the management of an individual (ophthalmologist, nephrologist, oncologist) who is, by virtue of training and experience, expert in such management.

CONCLUSION

TINU syndrome is a distinct clinicopathologic entity characterized by acute tubulointerstitial nephritis with nonoliguric acute renal failure accompanied or followed by bilateral anterior acute nongranulomatous uveitis, which tends to be relapsing and treatment resistant. TINU is most frequently seen in children and adult women, but it can occur at any age. The differential diagnosis includes systemic diseases and oculorenal syndromes associated with anterior uveitis. TINU syndrome is probably an immunologic disorder involving the kidney and eye, but its etiology and pathogenesis are still unknown. In general, the outcome of TINU syndrome is favorable. Nephropathy resolves either spontaneously or after systemic corticosteroid treatment and does not relapse. The uveitis usually responds to topical steroid therapy, but some patients require systemic steroid treatment or the introduction of immunosuppressive agents, or both, to achieve control of the ocular inflammation and to prevent relapses.

References

1. Smoyer WE, Kelly CJ, Kaplan BS: Tubulointerstitial nephritis. In: Holliday MA, Barrat TM, Avner ED, eds: Pediatric Nephrology, 3rd ed. Baltimore, Williams & Wilkins, 1994, p 890.
2. Dobrin RS, Vernier RL, Fish AJ: Acute eosinophilic interstitial nephritis and renal failure with bone marrow–lymph node granulomas. A new syndrome. Am J Med 1975;59:325.
3. Steinman TI, Silva P: Acute interstitial nephritis and iritis. Renalocular syndrome. Am J Med 1984;77:189.
4. Van Acker KJ, Buyssens N, Neetens A, et al: Acute tubulointerstitial nephritis with uveitis. Acta Paediatr Belg 1980;33:171.
5. Vanhaesebrouck P, Carton D, De Bel C, et al: Acute tubulointerstitial nephritis and uveitis syndrome (TINU syndrome). Nephron 1985;40:418.
6. Rosenbaum JT: Bilateral anterior uveitis and interstitial nephritis. Am J Ophthalmol 1988;105:534.
7. Rosenbaum JT: Uveitis. An internist's view. Arch Intern Med 1989;149:1173.
8. BenEzra D: Bilateral anterior uveitis and interstitial nephritis. Am J Ophthalmol 1988;106:766.
9. Burnier M, Jaeger P, Campiche M, et al: Idiopathic acute interstitial nephritis and uveitis in the adult. Am J Nephrol 1986;6:312.
10. Cacoub P, Deray G, Le Hoang P, et al: Idiopathic acute interstitial nephritis associated with anterior uveitis in adults. Clin Nephrol 1989;31:307.
11. Riminton S, O'Donnel J: Tubulo-interstitial nephritis and uveitis (TINU) syndrome in an adult. Aust NZ J Med 1993;23:57.
12. Salu P, Stempels N, Vanden Houte K, et al: Acute tubulointerstitial nephritis and uveitis syndrome in the elderly. Br J Ophthalmol 1990;74:53.
13. Gafter U, Ben-Basat M, Zevin D, et al: Anterior uveitis, a presenting symptom in acute interstitial nephritis. Nephron 1986;42:249.
14. Itami N, Akutsu Y, Yasoshima K, et al: Acute tubulointerstitial nephritis with uveitis. Arch Intern Med 1990;150:688.

15. Hausmann N, Neyer U, Hammerle W: Akut rezidivierende Uveitis und idiopathische interstitielle Nephritis—eine nosologische Einheit (TINU-Syndrom). Klin Monatsbl Augenheilk 1988;193:35.

16. Burghard R, Brandis M, Hoyer PF, et al: Acute interstitial nephritis in childhood. Eur J Paediatr 1984;142:103.

17. Waeben M, Boven K, D'Heer B, et al: Tubulo-interstitial nephritis-uveitis (TINU) syndrome with posterior uveitis. Bull Soc Belge Ophtalmol 1996;261:73.

18. Laatikainen LT, Immonen IJR: Acute posterior multifocal placoid pigment epitheliopathy in connection with acute nephritis. Retina 1988;8:122.

19. Savir H: Uveitis and interstitial nephritis. In: Regenbogen LS, Eliahou HE, eds: Diseases Affecting the Eye and the Kidney. Basel, S Karger AG, 1993, p 381.

20. Iida H, Terada Y, Nishino A, et al: Acute interstitial nephritis with bone marrow granulomas and uveitis. Nephron 1985;40:108.

21. Kobayashi Y, Honda M, Yoshikawa N, et al: Immunohistological study in sixteen children with acute tubulointerstitial nephritis. Clin Nephrol 1998;50:14.

22. Pamukcu R, Moorthy AV, Singer JR, et al: Idiopathic acute interstitial nephritis: Characterization of the infiltrating cells in the renal interstitium as T helper lymphocytes. Am J Kidney Dis 1984;4:24.

23. Hirano K, Tomino Y, Mikami H, et al: A case of acute tubulointerstitial nephritis and uveitis syndrome with a dramatic response to corticosteroid therapy. Am J Nephrol 1989;9:499.

24. Birnbacher R, Balzar E, Aufricht C, et al: Tubulointerstitial nephritis and uveitis: An immunological disorder? Pediatr Nephrol 1995;9:193.

25. Chan CC, Mochizuki M, Palestine AG, et al: Kinetics of T-lymphocyte subsets in the eyes of Lewis rats with experimental autoimmune uveitis. Cell Immunol 1985;96:430.

26. Chan CC, BenEzra D, Rodrigues MM, et al: Immunohistochemistry and electron microscopy of choroidal infiltrates and Dalen-Fuchs nodules in sympathetic ophthalmia. Ophthalmology 1985;92:580.

27. Derzko-Dzulyhsky L, Rabinovitch T: Tubulointerstitial nephritis and uveitis with bilateral multifocal choroiditis. Am J Ophthalmol 2000;129:807–809.

28. Gion N, Stavron P, Foster CS: Immunomodulatory therapy for chronic tubulointerstitial nephritis–associated uveitis. Am J Ophthalmol 2000;107:764.

29. Rodriguez-Perez JC, Cruz-Alamo M, Perez-Aciego P, et al: Clinical and immune aspects of idiopathic acute tubulointerstitial nephritis and uveitis syndrome. Am J Nephrol 1995;15:386.

30. Gafter U, Kalechman Y, Zevin D, et al: Tubulointerstitial nephritis and uveitis: Association with suppressed cellular immunity. Nephrol Dial Transplant 1993;8:821.

31. Simon AH, Alves-Filho G, Ribeiro-Alves MA: Acute tubulointerstitial nephritis and uveitis with antineutrophil cytoplasmic antibody. Am J Kidney Dis 1996;28:124.

32. Chen HC, Sheu MM, Tsai JH: Acute tubulo-interstitial nephritis and uveitis with anti-neutrophil cytoplasmic antibodies in an adult: An immune disorder? Nephron 1998;78:372.

33. Okada K, Okamato Y, Kagami S: Acute interstitial nephritis and uveitis with bone marrow granulomas and anti-neutrophil cytoplasmic antibodies. Am J Nephrol 1995;15:337.

34. Hagen EC, van de Vijver-Reenalda H, de Keizeer RJ, et al: Uveitis and anti-neutrophil cytoplasmic antibodies. Clin Exp Immunol 1994;95:56.

35. Young DW: The antineutrophil antibody in uveitis. Br J Ophthalmol 1991;75:208.

36. Yoshioka K, Takamova T, Kanasaki M, et al: Acute interstitial nephritis and uveitis syndrome: Activated immune cell infiltration in the kidney. Pediatr Nephrol 1991;5:232.

37. Iitsuka T, Yamaguchi N, Kobayashi M, et al: HLA tissue types in patients with acute tubulointerstitial nephritis accompanying uveitis. Nippon Jinzo Gakkai Shi 1993;35:723.

38. Stupp R, Mihatsch MJ, Matter L, et al: Acute tubulo-interstitial nephritis with uveitis (TINU syndrome) in a patient with serologic evidence for chlamydia infection. Klin Wochenschr 1990;68:971.

39. Tilden ME, Rosenbaum JT, Fraunfelder FT: Systemic sulfonamides as a cause of bilateral anterior uveitis. Arch Ophthalmol 1991;109:67.

40. Cokingtin CD, Han DP: Bilateral nongranulomatous uveitis and a poststreptococcal syndrome. Am J Ophthalmol 1991;112:595.

41. Leiba H, Barasch J, Pollack A: Poststreptococcal uveitis. Am J Ophthalmol 1998;126:317.

42. Holland GN: Recurrent anterior uveitis associated with streptococcal pharyngitis in a patient with a history of poststreptococcal syndrome. Am J Ophthalmol 1999;127:346.

43. Bunchman TE, Bloom JN: A syndrome of acute interstitial nephritis and anterior uveitis. Pediatr Nephrol 1993;7:520.

44. Tsai E, Till GO, Marak GE Jr: Effects of mydriatic agents on neutrophil migration. Ophthalmic Res 1988;20:14.

45. Sanchez Roman J, Gonzalez Reina I, Castillo Palma MH, Rocha Castilla JL: Posterior uveitis associated with acute tubulointerstitial nephritis with favorable response to cyclosporin. Pathogenic implications. Med Clin (Barc) 1995;104:118.

Albert T. Vitale

DEFINITION

Birdshot retinochoroidopathy (BSRC) is a clinically distinct, uncommon form of chronic intraocular inflammation characterized by vitritis and multiple, bilateral, hypopigmented, postequatorial fundus inflammatory lesions. Although its etiology remains unknown, a putative autoimmune mechanism is likely to play an important pathogenic role given the demonstration of retinal autoantigen reactivity and the very strong association with the human leukocyte antigen (HLA)-A29 phenotype unique to this disease.

HISTORY

The term birdshot retinochoroidopathy was coined in 1980 by Ryan and Maumenee[1] in their initial description of a group of 13 patients who shared certain similarities with the pars planitis syndrome. These patients were remarkable for the notable absence of a pars plana exudate and the unique presence of multiple, hypopigmented lesions at the level of the retinal pigment epithelium (RPE) reminiscent of the scatter pattern seen with birdshot fired from a shotgun onto a paper target. Undoubtedly, the striking clinical appearance of these spots must have inspired Gass[2] in 1981 to describe this same entity as vitiliginous choroiditis, given the similarity of the fundus lesions to cutaneous vitiligo. Indeed, two patients were thought to have developed vitiligo after the onset of visual symptoms in his series.[2]

In the absence of a specific etiology, other descriptive names have been used to describe this entity. Priem and Oosterhuis[3] note that the earliest report of this disease was probably by Franceschetti and Babel[4] in 1949 who named it chorioretinopathie en taches de bougies to describe the fundus of a 63-year-old woman with characteristic features of birdshot retinochoroidopathy but with systemic features of sarcoidosis. Likewise, Aaberg[5] dubbed this condition salmon patch choroidopathy, and Amalric and Cuq[6] preferred chorioretinopathie en grans de riz, seeing in it a rice grain pattern.

Although the term birdshot retinochoroidopathy is graphically descriptive and is currently the most widely accepted nomenclature, Opremcak[7] suggests that the term birdshot retinochoroiditis be advanced to more specifically reflect the essential inflammatory nature of this condition.

EPIDEMIOLOGY

BSRC is an uncommon disease. The largest series reported in the literature to date consists of 102 patients (203 eyes) collected from 14 European ophthalmology clinics between 1980 and 1986.[3] In the United States, Henderly and coworkers[8] reported only seven cases of BSRC among a population of 600 patients referred to a specialized uveitis clinic. The emergence of BSRC as a "new" uveitic entity is reflected by our experience in caring for 19 such individuals, representing 7.9% of 240 patients with posterior uveitis referred to the Immunology Service of the Massachusetts Eye and Ear Infirmary from 1982 to 1992.[9]

In contrast to most other uveitic entities in which the onset of disease is in younger age groups, BSRC typically occurs during middle age, presenting at an average age of 50, with a range of between 35 and 70 years of age.[1–3, 9–11] The reason for this age shift is unclear.

BSRC is found almost exclusively among whites, with a higher incidence in those of Northern European descent.[1–3, 11, 12] Finally, an apparent gender preference is observed in some series, with women representing up to 70% of reported cases,[1, 2, 12] whereas no significant predilection for sex is found in others.[3, 9, 13, 14]

CLINICAL FEATURES

Patients with BSRC present most commonly with varying degrees of gradual, painless visual loss, frequently complaining of floaters. The onset of visual symptoms may initially involve only one eye, but over time the fellow eye is almost always affected, albeit asymmetrically. Photophobia, some degree of nyctalopia, and disturbances in color vision are frequently reported.[2, 11] Visual complaints are not infrequently dramatically out of proportion to the measured visual acuity, with some patients complaining of debilitating visual loss in the face of 20/20 Snellen acuity.[7, 12] Such symptoms are indicative of diffuse retinal dysfunction underlying this disease, documented by electroretinography (see later).

In general, BSRC occurs in otherwise healthy patients. However, careful medical history, examination, and review of symptoms may reveal associated systemic pathology. Priem and Oosterhuis[3] noted an unusually high prevalence of vascular disease in their series of 102 patients with BSRC; 16 had systemic hypertension, 5 had coronary artery disease, 2 had suffered a cerebrovascular accident, and 3 had evidence of central retinal vein occlusion. Likewise, my group noted systemic hypertension in 3 of our 19 patients with BSRC.[15]

Although Gass initially forged the association of BSRC with vitiligo, the hypopigmented spots observed on the arms and legs of his patients with vitiliginous choroiditis appear to be more closely related to idiopathic guttate hypomelanosis than to vitiligo.[16] Only one patient in both the series of my group[15] and that of Priem and Oosterhuis[3] had evidence of cutaneous depigmentation. Moreover, evidence of BSRC was found in only one of 223 patients with vitiligo examined by Wagoner and associates.[17]

Other systemic associations include case reports of patients with autoimmune sensorineural hearing loss,[18] myelodysplasia syndrome,[19] and psoriasis[20] together with funduscopic lesions typical of BSRC. Although these may be coincidental findings, it is interesting to note that both the ocular and cutaneous problems of the patient with psoriasis resolved following treatment with aromatic retinoids.[20]

In their original description of BSRC, Ryan and Maumenee[1] cited the following diagnostic criteria: (1) a quiet (i.e., externally uninflamed), nonpainful eye, (2) minimal to no anterior uveitis, (3) vitritis without pars plana exudate (in contradistinction to pars planitis), (4) retinal vascular leakage, particularly involving the perifoveal capillaries leading to cystoid macular edema (CME) and occasionally to disc edema, (5) distinctive, discrete, cream-colored or depigmented spots scattered throughout the posterior fundus.

Examination of the anterior segment reveals a quiet eye without conjunctival injection or circumlimbal flush. While a mild nongranulomatous iritis with fine keratic precipitates on the corneal endothelium may be present in approximately 25% of cases,[7] iridocapsular synechiae, posterior subcapsular cataract, and ocular hypotony secondary to ciliary body hyposecretion are unusual. In my experience, intraocular pressures are typically normal. However, Priem and Oosterhuis noted a 19% incidence of open angle glaucoma unassociated with pigment dispersion or elevated episcleral venous pressure.[3] No other study has reported such an association.

Biomicroscopic examination consistently reveals the presence of diffuse inflammatory cells in both the anterior and posterior vitreous body. The severity and location of the vitreous cellular infiltration varies, being more pronounced during earlier stages of the disease,[21] sometimes forming "mutton fat" precipitates on the posterior vitreous face during periods of disease activity.[2] Alternative diagnoses should be considered in the absence of vitritis.[7]

Funduscopic examination highlights the multiple, bilateral, cream-colored birdshot lesions scattered throughout the postequatorial retina, characteristic of this entity. These spots tend to be round to ovoid, varying in size from 50 to 1500 μm[7, 16] (Fig. 65–1). Occasionally, they may become confluent, producing large areas of geographic depigmentation and even a blond appearance to the fundus.[1, 16] BSRC lesions are often best appreciated with indirect ophthalmoscopy, as their borders are indistinct and not sharply demarcated. The distribution pattern of these spots is variable throughout the posterior

pole and midperiphery, but they are often more easily visualized in the inferonasal quadrant.[22] BSRC lesions may be diffuse or asymmetric, they may be macular sparing or macular involving, and they frequently assume a radial orientation peripherally, being distributed along the large choroidal vessels.[3, 10] The lesions are not associated with significant hyperpigmentation within or at their margins.[16]

Biomicroscopic examination discloses that these lesions are at the level of the outer retina, RPE, and inner choroid. The overlying retina appears normal during the early stages of depigmentation, with large choroidal vessels frequently visible within the lesion. Absence of visible choroidal vessels within the BSRC spots, either during episodes of severe vitritis or early in the evolution of depigmentation, may give the appearance of an elevated choroidal inflammatory infiltrate.[16] Such lesions have been described as having "substance" and interpreted as evidence of inflammatory activity.[12] As will be discussed later, these early lesions frequently show no angiographic abnormality. Later in their evolution, BSRC spots may be associated with atrophy of both the overlying retina and the RPE as demonstrated biomicroscopically and angiographically. Hyperpigmentation may rarely be observed in some lesions in the later stages of the disease.[7, 16]

Other clinical features indicative of chronic intraocular inflammation in BSRC include vasculitis, involving predominantly the retinal venules, manifested by sheathing and associated vascular leakage on fluorescein angiography (FA).[10] Vascular incompetence as a result of retinal vasculitis and posterior segment inflammation is a consistent feature of this disease and may produce marked thickening of the retina on biomicroscopic examination. Cystoid macular edema, either diffuse or focal, and optic nerve head swelling are commonly observed. Progressive papillitis may develop into optic atrophy. Attenuation of retinal arterioles and vascular tortuosity,[1, 21, 22] nerve fiber layer hemorrhages,[21, 22] retinal and subretinal neovascularization,[3, 23, 24] and epiretinal membranes[3, 15] have also been reported.

COMPLICATIONS

The most common complication of BSRC is chronic cystoid macular edema, occurring in upward of 50% of cases, and this is the most frequent cause of reduced central visual acuity.[3, 15] Its presence is important in establishing the diagnosis[12] and is itself an indication for therapeutic intervention so that permanent structural damage to the macula (cystic macula) is averted and good visual function is preserved.[15]

Epiretinal membrane formation occurs in up to 10% of cases[3] and may be responsible for significant visual compromise.[15] Macular pucker has been observed to progress as part of a cicatricial phenomenon during resolution of intraocular inflammation.[13, 22]

Any pathologic process (including intraocular inflammation) that disrupts the integrity of the choriocapillaries–RPE–Bruch's membrane complex, creates an environment that permits the development of choroidal neovascularization (CNV). Priem and Oosterhuis reported both macular and peripapillary subretinal neovascularization in 6% of their 102 cases of BSRC.[3] Likewise,

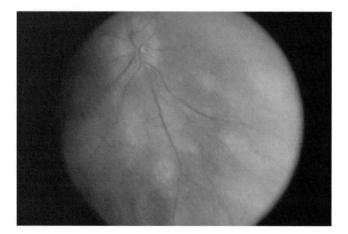

FIGURE 65–1. Typical appearance of birdshot lesions in the posterior pole consisting of scattered cream-colored spots varying in size from 50 to 1500 μm. (See color insert.)

serous neurosensory elevation associated with juxtapapillary subretinal new vessels has been described in BSRC patients by Soubrane and colleagues.[25] Choroidal neovascular membranes involving the macula may arise adjacent to classic depigmented lesions between 6 months and 5 years after the onset of disease.[24] No specific study has been performed to evaluate the efficacy of laser photocoagulation in the treatment of CNV in eyes affected by BSRC. However, based on the experience with other macular diseases complicated by CNV for which abundant data exist, laser therapy, performed under fluorescein and/or indocyanine green (ICG) guidance, is recommended to prevent loss of central vision.[3, 22, 24, 25]

Of the 203 eyes studied by Priem and Oosterhuis, retinal neovascularization located on the optic disc and in the retinal periphery occurred in 2 and 13 eyes, respectively, apparently in the absence of retinal capillary nonperfusion.[3] Retinal neovascularization has been reported in uveitic eyes without evidence of capillary nonperfusion,[26, 27] presumably caused by the release of vasogenic substances by inflammatory mediators. In contrast, peripheral retinal neovascularization associated with capillary closure and localized vitreous hemorrhage in a patient with BSRC was described by Barondes and associates.[23]

Other late complications include optic atrophy, either as a sequela to chronic inflammation or secondary to acute ischemic anterior neuropathy,[28] cataract, rubeosis iridis, glaucoma, or rhegmatogenous retinal detachment.[10, 15]

ETIOLOGY

The etiology of BSRC remains elusive. Although the disease has been reported to occur in monozygotic twins,[29] there is no strong familial association or established mode of inheritance. BSRC is unique in having the strongest association between an HLA and a disease that has ever been described. Specifically, the HLA-A29 phenotype is present in 80% to 98% of white patients with BSRC, compared to 7% of controls.[14, 30–33] The relative risk of developing BSRC in a patient bearing the HLA-A29 phenotype is between 50 and 224 times greater than that with other phenotypes.[32, 33] The sensitivity (96%) and specificity (93%) of HLA type in BSRC patients can be useful in confirming the diagnosis.[34] Feltkamp has calculated that the probability of a diagnosis of BSRC rises from 70% to 97% in HLA-A29–positive patients and drops from 70% to 8.5% in HLA-A29–negative individuals.[35] The strength of this HLA association with BSRC points to an underlying genetic predisposition for the development of the disease.

The HLA-A29 antigen can be divided into two subtypes, A29.1 and A29.2, as described by Yang.[36] The distribution of these subtypes varies with ethnicity: The A29.1 subtype is found more commonly among populations from Southeast Asia (where BSRC has not been reported),[22, 37] whereas the A29.2 subtype is observed in approximately 90% of healthy whites of Northern European extraction.[38] In their analysis of a subgroup of 33 patients with BSRC, Le Hoang and colleagues found the A29.2 subtype in all subjects (100%).[14] The significant absence of the A29.1 subtype in this population of patients has been interpreted as representing a possible "resistance motif" associated with this molecule by Tabary and coworkers.[39] They found that whereas the sequence of HLA-A29.2 was identical both in BSRC patients and in healthy control subjects, a single substitution in the extracellular domain differentiated the two HLA-A29 subtypes. As the mutation observed in HLA-A29.1 is unique to that molecule, these authors suggest that the ancestral type is HLA-A29.2, with resistance to BSRC being conferred by the more recently mutated HLA-A29.1 subtype. They further postulate that the nature of the HLA-A29.1 mutation might influence the binding of the CD8 T-cell glycoprotein, or another accessory molecule, impeding its interaction with the T-cell receptor, and so impairing T-cell activation.[12, 22, 39]

De Waal and coworkers, on the other hand, found that the distribution of HLA-A29 subtypes in their group of 20 Northern European patients with birdshot chorioretinopathy did not differ from that found among healthy controls.[38] Whereas both subtypes were found among BSRC patients, HLA-29.2 was more frequently identified because of its overwhelming prevalence (90%) in this particular study population. These authors suggest that disease susceptibility is conferred by a common determinant expressed on both variants of HLA-A29, but the possibility exists that a gene in tight linkage disequilibrium with both subtypes may be involved in the pathogenesis of the disease.[38]

PATHOGENESIS AND PATHOLOGY

It is well established that the class I major histocompatibility (MHC) molecules play an important regulatory role in the immune response, controlling the selection, degradation, and presentation of antigens within antigen presenting cells and their recognition by effector T cells.[40] Retinal autoimmunity may play an important pathogenetic role in the development and perpetuation of intraocular inflammation for HLA-A29–positive individuals, as a result of a genetic error of immune regulation. Evidence in support of this notion is found in the strong in vitro cell-mediated responses to a variety of retinal autoantigens, including S-antigen (S-Ag) and interphotoreceptor retinoid binding protein (IRBP) observed in 92% of patients with BSRC.[32, 41] Opremcak and Cowans reported a frequency of between 4 and 7 S-Ag–specific T cells/10^6 peripheral blood lymphocytes in patients with BSRC.[42] Furthermore, these autoreactive T cells were found to produce interleukin 2 (IL-2) in response to autoantigens, and such cells were not detectable during disease quiescence or during therapy with cyclosporine.

Animals immunized with S-Ag develop severe intraocular inflammation termed experimental autoimmune uveitis (EAU), a disease not dissimilar to that seen in the human patient with BSRC, replete with specific humoral and cellular immune responses to autoantigen.[43] Finally, lymphocytes specifically primed to these autoantigens will produce EAU when adoptively transferred into naive recipients.[44]

The histopathologic findings of a single, phthisical eye enucleated from a patient with BSRC, who also exhibited a positive in vitro lymphocyte proliferative response to retinal S-Ag, has been reported.[32] Examination of the iris and ciliary body revealed a mild lymphocytic infiltration, whereas the retina was involved with a diffuse, chronic granulomatous inflammation with giant cells, epithelioid cells, lymphocytes, and plasma cells in the outer retinal layers. The inflammatory response in the choroid was likewise granulomatous, but it was milder and thought to be a secondary response. Similar histopathologic findings are observed in S-Ag–induced EAU in primates.[45] These histopathologic similarities, as well as those seen clinically between S-Ag–induced EAU and that of BSRC, strongly implicate a role for S-Ag and autoimmunity in the pathogenesis of this disease.[32]

The precise mechanisms or inciting events that might lead to the development of retinal autoimmunity or to the abnormal expression of an immune determinant during the course of the inflammatory reaction are unknown. Whereas autoimmunity may represent an epiphenomenon that develops after an unrelated insult to the retina, the work of Nussenblatt[32, 45] and others[46] strongly suggests its bona fide role in the pathogenesis of this disease. Alternatively, autoimmune phenomena may act to perpetuate the inflammatory disease process rather than initiate it.[22]

Several theories have been proposed to explain the genesis of autoimmunity in a genetically predisposed individual.[12, 40, 47, 48] One such theory invokes a receptor mechanism in which the MHC antigens provide a specific cell surface marker for the binding of an inciting infectious agent. HLA-A29 patients would develop disease by providing the necessary receptor to a putative "birdshot pathogen." Alternatively, an "altered self" model proposes that the host's immune system recognizes the HLA-A29 MHC-antigen complex as foreign, having been distorted as a result of binding with an exogenous pathogen (i.e., a virus, antigen, or hapten).

The potential role of such HLA disease mechanisms in the pathogenesis of BSRC is intriguing, especially in the light of recent reports of patients with BSRC and serologic evidence of concomitant infection with a variety of microorganisms.[49, 50] Suttorp-Schulten and associates[50] found antibodies to *Borrelia burgdorferi* in 3 of 11 patients with BSRC, all of whom carried the HLA-A29 antigen. Further investigation will be necessary to determine whether these results represent false-positive reactions or if, in fact, *B. burgdorferi* plays a causative role in the pathogenesis of BSRC. Likewise, Kuhne and colleagues[49] speculate on the pathogenetic role of *Coxiella burnetii* in their two patients with retinal vasculitis and Q fever. Although one of these patients was HLA-A29 positive, a causative role for this organism in BSRC could not be demonstrated.

Finally, the role of the pineal gland in the pathogenesis of BSRC has been questioned, based on direct evidence of its involvement in EAU and on indirect evidence surrounding the function of this organ. The retina and the pineal gland share a common embryologic origin and, not surprisingly, common antigens, namely S-Ag and IRBP.[51, 52] Moreover, animals immunized with S-Ag and IRBP develop not only EAU, but also pinealitis.[53, 54] In healthy individuals, the pineal gland is responsible for the secretion of melatonin in a diurnal fashion, a hormone that is thought to control the level of dermal pigmentation.[55] Opremcak postulates that intercurrent inflammation of the pineal gland in patients with BSRC may play a role in the development of vitiliginous BSRC lesions and in the disturbances in the sleep cycles and mood often observed in these patients.[7] Indeed, patients with chronic posterior uveitis, including those with BSRC, show a decrease in the nocturnal peak plasma melatonin levels by approximately 45%.[56]

DIAGNOSIS

The diagnosis of BSRC is essentially a clinical one, based on a thorough ophthalmic and medical history, review of systems, and ocular examination revealing the characteristic funduscopic picture (Table 65–1). The absence of significant anterior inflammatory sequelae (synechiae), and the presence of vitritis and/or CME without pars plana exudation, all serve to solidify the diagnosis. Except for atypical cases, laboratory and ancillary testing are usually not necessary to establish the diagnosis of BSRC, but they are most useful in confirming the initial clinical impression and in excluding other differential diagnostic considerations.

Laboratory Investigations

A directed laboratory work-up to rule out likely infectious (syphilis, tuberculosis) and noninfectious (sarcoidosis, masquerade syndromes) causes of uveitis is essential at presentation, prior to the commencement of any systemic therapy. It includes the following: complete blood count with differential, fluorescent treponemal antibody absorption and rapid plasma reagin tests, skin testing for anergy and with purified protein derivative, tests for angiotensin-converting enzyme and serum lysozyme, and a chest radiograph.

Extended laboratory investigations, unless clinically indicated, are rarely fruitful. Despite the putative autoimmune etiology, autoantibody studies have not provided further insights into BSRC pathogenesis and are not useful diagnostically. For example, while anticardiolipin anti-

TABLE 65–1. BIRDSHOT RETINOCHOROIDOPATHY: DIAGNOSTIC FEATURES

Patient characteristics
  Whites
  Average age, 50 years
Ocular examination
  Anterior segment
    Mild nongranulomatous iridocyclitis
    Iridocapsular synechiae rare
  Posterior segment
    Vitritis
    Pars plana snowbank absent
    Multiple, postequatorial, ovoid, deep, cream-colored
      (depigmented) lesions 50 to 1500 μm
    Retinal vascular leakage, cystoid macular edema
    Subretinal, retinal neovascularization
Ancillary tests
  HLA-A29 positive
  Retinal autoantigen reactivity
  Abnormal electroretinogram, electro-oculogram, dark adaptation
    thresholds
  Enhanced visualization of choroidal lesions on indocyanine green
    angiography

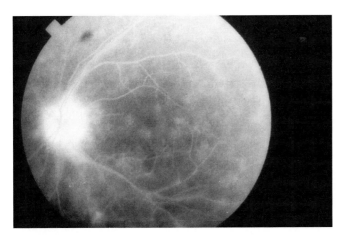

FIGURE 65–2. Late-phase fluorescein angiogram depicting diffuse leakage and cystoid macular edema.

bodies have been associated with thrombosis and retinal vasculitis, only 3 of 24 patients with retinal vasculitis and none of 10 patients with BSRC were positive for this antibody in a study by Klok and associates.[57] These authors discourage the routine use of this test for diagnostic purposes.

Fluorescein Angiography

FA is most helpful in delineating the extent of retinal vascular leakage and in following the clinical course. Indeed, the most prominent findings on angiography include hyperfluorescence of the optic disc, and dye leakage from the retinal venules and capillaries late in the study, resulting in cystoid macular and retinal edema (Fig. 65–2).[1, 3, 11, 32] Apparent large-vessel perfusion abnormalities are manifested by a delay in the retinal artery filling time, by prolongation of the arteriovenous transit time, and by varying degrees of subnormal fluorescence of the retinal vessels during the course of the study.[2, 16] Interestingly, although the arteriovenous circulation time was observed to be delayed in four patients with BSRC studied by FA, it was found to be nearly normal when viewed with ICG angiography in a report by Guex-Crosier and Herbort.[58] The authors conclude that the apparent increased retinal circulation time seen on FA is caused by gradual tissue permeation and delayed venous reabsorption of small molecules such as fluorescein (in contradistinction to larger, highly protein-bound ICG molecules) as a result of a deranged blood-retinal barrier rather than as a true reflection of the intravascular hemodynamics.

In contrast to their striking appearance when viewed by indirect ophthalmoscopy, the birdshot lesions are far less conspicuous, fewer in number, and manifest inconsistent findings on FA. The angiographic heterogeneity of these lesions seems to depend on their age and associated degree of activity, as well as on the presence of many lesions at different stages of evolution within the same eye.[22]

Not infrequently, the early, cream-colored lesions may show no angiographic abnormality, remaining silent throughout all stages of the angiogram.[16, 59] On the other hand, these early lesions, particularly those interpreted as being active, may mask fluorescence in the early phase

of the angiogram and stain in the late phase.[2, 3, 15] In the former situation, angiographic silence would be predicted by a deep location of the lesions or by those very early in their evolution, such that the overlying RPE and choriocapillaries remain unaffected.[22] An inflammatory infiltrate at the level of the outer choroid associated with large choroidal vessels might, in the latter scenario, disrupt the choriocapillaries' perfusion and cause a secondary alteration in the RPE, producing early hypofluorescence with subsequent late-phase hyperfluorescence.[3, 22, 59] Later in their evolution, the typical focally depigmented or atrophic-appearing BSRC lesions demonstrate uniform hypofluorescence in the early phase of the angiogram, with visualization of the large choroidal vessels through an attenuated RPE and nonperfused choriocapillaries. Diffuse hyperfluorescence and staining of these lesions are seen in the late phases.[2, 16, 22]

Indocyanine Green Angiography

Whereas retinal vascular abnormalities are better studied with FA, ICG angiography provides the additional dimension of choroidal analysis in BSRC. ICG reveals well-delineated hypofluorescent choroidal spots in the mid-phase of the study, which not only correspond to the location of the birdshot lesions but also are far more numerous than those seen either on FA or clinically (Fig. 65–3).[59, 60] This again underscores the diffuse nature of the disease process. A one-to-one correspondence in terms of the size of the hypofluorescent dark spots seen

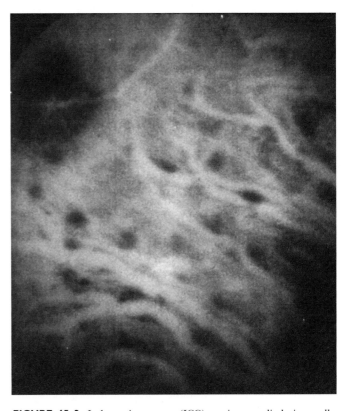

FIGURE 65–3. Indocyanine green (ICG) angiogram disclosing well-delineated hypofluorescent choroidal spots, which not only correspond to the location of the birdshot lesions but also are far more numerous than those seen either on fluorescein angiography or clinically.

on ICG and the size of the lesions seen clinically or on the red-free photographs is not observed.[61] These hypofluorescent choroidal lesions assume a vasotropic orientation, being bordered by large to medium-sized choroidal vessels, a configuration that appears to be specific to BSRC.[60, 62, 63] The choroidal vessels themselves are normal, without evidence of large-vessel choroidal inflammatory involvement.[61] The hypofluorescent nature of these lesions may represent hypoperfusion of the choriocapillaris.[22, 59] Alternatively, they may represent nonvascularized inflammatory foci, as evidenced by the observation that (occasionally) hypofluorescent areas on ICG, especially those corresponding to early lesions, may mask fluorescence from underlying choroidal vessels.[59] In other cases, hyperfluorescent spots in the late phases of the ICG study have been demonstrated in patients with active inflammation.[62]

Electrophysiology

Although the electroretinogram (ERG) is a mass response to light stimuli, the pattern of that response is distinct in BSRC, pointing to topographic retina pathology.[11, 64, 65] The a-wave of the ERG is well preserved, whereas the b-wave exhibits a reduction in amplitude and an increased latency time.[64, 65] This negative b-wave configuration is indicative of pathology affecting the inner neural retinal layer with little or no involvement of the photoreceptors, a pattern also seen in central retinal artery occlusion, congenital retinoschisis, and congenital stationary night blindness.[64] These findings are consistent with the marked retinal vasculopathy seen clinically and on FA in patients with BSRC. Depending on the severity and stage of the disease, abnormalities may range from the mere absence of oscillatory potentials to a nonrecordable ERG.[3, 64, 65] Similarly, abnormal ratios of slow oscillations (light rise versus dark trough [L/D < 1.85]) have been reported in the vast majority of patients with BSRC.[2, 3, 11, 64, 65] Although both the slow (L/D) and fast (D/L) oscillations are thought to reflect changes in the degree of polarization of the RPE, the slow oscillation appears to be affected by vasculopathy affecting the inner retina, whereas the fast oscillation is not.[65, 66]

Other commonly observed electrophysiologic abnormalities include elevation of the dark adaptation thresholds,[3, 11, 64, 65] and reduced amplitudes and delayed responses in the pattern-evoked cortical potentials.[65]

Other Ancillary Tests

Laser flare-cell photometry of four patients with BSRC demonstrated maintenance of the integrity of the blood aqueous barrier (5.7 ± 1.1 photons/msec versus 4.7 ± 0.16 photons/msec for controls).[67] This finding is consistent with the absence of flare seen clinically and the paucity of anterior segment findings seen in patients with BSRC.

Finally, visual field testing has revealed a variety of defects, including constriction of the peripheral visual field, central and paracentral scotomata, and enlargement of the blind spot.[2, 3, 10, 65] Acquired dyschromatopsias, mainly of the blue-yellow type,[65] have been reported, while some patients may exhibit both blue-yellow and red-green defects.[3]

DIFFERENTIAL DIAGNOSIS

The diagnosis of BSRC is relatively straightforward in patients manifesting vitritis and the classic funduscopic appearance. In these individuals, the differential diagnosis includes the so-called white dot syndromes as well as systemic infectious and noninfectious diseases that produce panuveitis and light-colored fundus lesions at some stage in their clinical course (Table 65–2).

As in any case of posterior uveitis, exclusion of potentially treatable infectious causes of intraocular inflammation is imperative. Both syphilis and tuberculosis can produce vitritis and choroiditis with light-colored fundus lesions.[68, 69] However, these lesions tend not to be ovoid, and they develop varying degrees of RPE hyperplasia. Moreover, signs and symptoms of underlying systemic disease are usually present. These findings, together with positive serology for syphilis, positive intradermal skin testing, and abnormal chest radiographic findings of tuberculosis, serve to distinguish these entities from BSRC.

Other presumably infectious entities producing white dots to be considered in the differential diagnosis include diffuse unilateral subacute neuroretinitis (DUSN) and the ocular histoplasmosis syndrome (OHS). While DUSN may present with scattered, deep, gray-white fundus lesions and a moderate vitritis, as the name implies, the pathology is unilateral.[70] In addition, the disease is caused by a nematode, which may leave subretinal tracks, massive RPE disruption, and optic atrophy in its wake.[71] *Histoplasma capsulatum* is the presumed etiologic agent in OHS, which is characterized by the following cardinal clinical features: peripheral histo spots, peripapillary pigmentary changes, maculopathy, and a quiet vitreous.[72] In contradistinction to the classic BSRC lesions, histo spots are punched out, well delineated, relatively small (200 µm), and may be associated with pigment clumping centrally.[73] Furthermore, the absence of vitritis clearly separates OHS from BSRC.

Sarcoidosis must be excluded in the work-up of patients suspected of having BSRC. This is particularly important in the absence of anterior segment stigmata of granulomatous inflammation (mutton-fat keratic precipi-

TABLE 65–2. BIRDSHOT RETINOCHOROIDOPATHY: DIFFERENTIAL DIAGNOSIS

White dots present
  Infectious
    Tuberculosis
    Syphilis
    Ocular histoplasmosis syndrome
    Diffuse unilateral subacute neuroretinitis
  Noninfectious
    Sarcoidosis
    Vogt-Koyanagi-Harada syndrome
    Sympathetic ophthalmia
    Multifocal choroiditis and panuveitis
    Punctate inner choroidopathy
    Multiple evanescent white dot syndrome
    Acute posterior multifocal placoid pigment epitheliopathy
White dots absent
  Retinal vasculitis
  Pars planitis
  Idiopathic (senile) vitritis
  Intraocular lymphoma

tates and Koeppe or Busacca iris nodules), as both entities manifest vitritis and vasculitis, and the appearance of the choroidal granulomata seen in ocular sarcoid may be confused with typical birdshot lesions. In 22 patients with sarcoidosis, Vrabec and colleagues observed two patterns of "taches de bougie" (candle wax spots), one of which (the large, posterior, pale yellow-orange streak) developed in six patients and was indistinguishable from the lesions of BSRC.[74] Priem and Oosterhuis examined 38 patients in their series of 102 patients with BSRC for evidence of sarcoidosis and identified one individual with biopsy-proven sarcoid.[3] Brinkman and Rothova[75] described six patients with neurosarcoidosis, all of whom had vitritis, disc edema, periphlebitis, and multifocal chorioretinal lesions similar to those seen in BSRC. Likewise, Brod[76] and Kuboshiro and Yoshioka[77] each reported patients exhibiting characteristic ocular signs of BSRC who, in fact, had systemic, biopsy-confirmed sarcoidosis.

Patients with Vogt-Koyanagi-Harada (VKH) disease may have choroidal lesions in the active phase and present with bilateral intraocular inflammation similar to BSRC.[78] Exudative retinal detachment is an essential feature of VKH, as is the predominance of choroidal versus retinal vascular inflammation appreciated clinically and angiographically. Furthermore, VKH is a systemic disease with characteristic extraocular differentiating features, including poliosis, vitiligo, hearing loss, and meningeal symptoms.

Sympathetic ophthalmia, like VKH, is another form of chronic uveitis in which multiple cream-colored choroidal inflammatory foci (Dalen-Fuchs nodules) are observed.[79] Although these lesions tend to be more discrete, it is the context of their appearance in the fellow eye after trauma or surgery and inflammation in the inciting eye that distinguishes them from those of BSRC.

Multifocal choroiditis and panuveitis syndrome (MCP), punctate inner choroidopathy (PIC), multiple evanescent white dot syndrome (MEWDS), and acute posterior multifocal placoid pigment epitheliopathy (APMPPE) are other white dot syndromes to be distinguished from BSRC. MCP, as its name implies, is characterized by multiple bilateral, postequatorial lesions of 50 to 200 μm in diameter at the level of the RPE or inner choroid, together with vitritis, and frequently anterior segment inflammation.[80] Except for the presence of inflammation, the funduscopic appearance of MCP and OHS share many similarities that clearly differentiate them from BSRC—namely, the presence of hyperpigmented scars surrounding the peripapillary region, and the smaller, discrete, punched-out peripheral lesions. Likewise, PIC, which shares the ocular characteristics of MCP except for the presence of inflammation, can be distinguished from BSRC.[81] MEWDS typically presents in young women as a sudden unilateral loss of vision and is characterized by multiple small (100 to 200 μm) white dots at the level of the outer retina or RPE, particularly in the perifoveal and peripheral macula.[82] Not only are the size, color, location, and ephemeral nature of these white dots distinct from those seen in BSRC, but vitritis is minimal and visual recovery is usually observed after 7 weeks in patients with MEWDS. APMPPE, like MEWDS, presents in otherwise healthy adults as acute transient visual loss with minimal

vitritis. But the process is bilateral, albeit asymmetric, in APMPPE.[83] In contrast to those seen in BSRC, the cream-colored lesions of APMPPE have a plaque-like morphology and are located predominantly in the posterior pole. Moreover, the FA features of these plaques (i.e., early blockage and late staining) are characteristic and distinct from those of BSRC. Finally, resolution of the acute lesions in APMPPE is usually accompanied by hyperpigmentation and visual recovery.

Difficulties in the diagnosis of BSRC may arise in the absence of classic clinical features early in the disease course, in mildly affected eyes, or before the evolution of typical hypopigmented fundus lesions. Priem and Oosterhuis noted that in 5 of their 102 patients, clear-cut evidence of BSRC spots did not develop until several years after their initial presentation with varying degrees of vitritis, papillitis, and retinal vasculitis.[3] This peculiar pattern of late-developing hypopigmented spots, as long as 8 years after the onset of vitritis, papillitis, and retinal vasculitis in patients with BSRC, was subsequently reported.[84, 85] Soubrane and colleagues[85] suggest HLA-A29 antigen assessment in cases of longstanding uveitis and vasculitis in an effort to avoid misdiagnosis of idiopathic retinal vasculitis in BSRC patients with late-evolving lesions.

Further insight into the evolution of BSRC lesions and the prognostic significance of the HLA-A29 phenotype in patients with retinal vasculitis is provided by Bloch-Michel and Frau[86] in their study of 20 patients with BSRC (95% of whom were HLA-A29 positive) and 36 patients with retinal vasculitis (62% HLA-A29 positive). Among the 22 patients with retinal vasculitis followed for an average of 8 years who carried the HLA-A29 phenotype, only one developed fundus lesions consistent with BSRC. Patients with BSRC were found to have a more severe disease course than those with idiopathic retinal vasculitis. However, among patients with idiopathic retinal vasculitis, those with the HLA-A29 phenotype tended to have bilateral disease, more posterior involvement, and a poorer visual prognosis than those without the HLA-A29 phenotype, who had more peripheral vascular involvement. Whether BSRC and HLA-A29–positive retinal vasculitis represent different stages of the same disease or two separate entities is not currently known. Bergink and colleagues[87] suggest classifying patients with the HLA-A29 phenotype and retinal vasculitis who have not yet developed depigmented fundus lesions typical of BSRC as having HLA-A29–positive idiopathic vasculitis.

Patients with the pars planitis variant of intermediate uveitis and idiopathic senile vitritis may present with bilateral vitreal inflammation. Unlike patients with BSRC, those with pars planitis are younger and present with inflammatory cells located predominantly in the anterior vitreous with characteristic changes in the peripheral retina and vitreous base known as snowballs or snowbanks.[88] Idiopathic senile vitritis occurs in older individuals, and, as is the case with pars planitis, it is not characterized by fundus lesions, further distinguishing these entities from BSRC.[89]

Finally, masquerade syndromes, particularly intraocular large-cell lymphoma, may present with bilateral multiple, yellow subretinal/sub-RPE infiltrates and a vitritis that is typically only partially responsive to systemic steroids.[90] Usually, the clinical context, together with the smaller size, larger number, and subretinal location of the lesions distinguishes this entity from BSRC. While many patients with intraocular lymphoma may present with central nervous system disease, a high index of suspicion is necessary to make the diagnosis, beginning with a thorough history and neurologic exam. A systemic work-up, including hematology testing, lumbar puncture, and magnetic resonance imaging, should be performed. Diagnostic vitrectomy is often essential in making the definitive diagnosis.

TREATMENT

A definitive therapeutic strategy for the care of patients with BSRC has yet to be formulated, given its uncertain natural history, and the relatively small number of individuals with this disease. The mainstay of treatment has been the use of periocular and systemic steroids, but their efficacy is inconsistent, with an unclear effect on the long-term visual prognosis.[1–3, 10, 32] Although some patients may experience a dramatic initial improvement in visual acuity in response to relatively high doses of systemic prednisone (1.0 mg/kg daily) or periocular triamcinolone (40 mg/ml), others may not. The benefits of periocular steroid therapy are transient, providing short-term reduction in vitreal inflammation and hastening the resolution of CME. Hence, the use of regional corticosteroids is mainly adjunctive, employed in the treatment of inflammatory exacerbations for patients on systemic therapy or in cases of asymmetric disease. Of those patients treated with systemic steroids, less than 15% achieve an adequate clinical response and are able to be maintained on low to moderate doses of prednisone.[7] This, together with steroid intolerance and concerns regarding the highly undesirable side effects associated with prolonged administration, limit the utility of systemic steroids in the treatment of BSRC. Similarly, nonsteroidal anti-inflammatory drugs[91] and various cytotoxic agents have been employed without substantiated efficacy.[1, 2, 11]

Cyclosporine A (CSA), a fungal metabolite that prevents the production of IL-2, and thus helper T-cell function, has been of value in treating retinal S-Ag–induced experimental autoimmune uveitis,[92] and posterior uveitis in humans.[93] Because retinal autoimmunity is thought to play an important role in the pathogenesis of BSRC, one might expect CSA to be efficacious in its treatment. Nussenblatt and colleagues[93, 94] reasoned in this manner and treated a small group of patients with BSRC with CSA, reporting good results. These findings were corroborated by Le Hoang and associates,[13] who treated 21 patients (42 eyes) suffering from BSRC with CSA. A marked reduction of vitritis was reported in all eyes, improved visual acuity in 23 (54.8%) eyes, and stabilization of vision in 11 (26.2%) eyes. These reports, other uncontrolled studies,[95–97] two nonrandomized[98, 99] and one randomized clinical trial,[100] each reporting the efficacy of CSA in the treatment of various forms of noninfectious uveitis, all employed doses of 10 mg/kg daily, a dose that is now known to be associated with a very high incidence of untoward nephrotoxic and hypertensive effects.

In an effort to curtail these and other secondary complications of CSA therapy, low-dose regimens (2.0 to 5.0 mg/kg daily), with vigilant monitoring for toxicity, have been advocated.[101] Studies employing low-dose CSA alone,[102, 103] in combination with low-dose prednisone,[104–107] or with other immunosuppressive agents[15, 94, 108–110] have demonstrated anti-inflammatory efficacy while reducing, but not eliminating, CSA-associated toxicity. Indeed, with careful monitoring, renal side effects were well tolerated and vision improved or stabilized in 76% of 22 uveitis patients treated with long-term (mean, 7 years), low-dose (0.75 to 2.0 mg/kg daily) CSA.[111] However, systemic hypertension occurred in 81% of 16 previously normotensive patients with idiopathic autoimmune uveitis treated with low-dose CSA (5.0 mg/kg daily) for at least 2 years. Blood pressure was controlled with a single medication in all but two patients.[112]

In our study of 19 patients with BSRC, a favorable visual outcome, inflammatory control, and a lack of demonstrable CSA-associated nephrotoxicity with few secondary side effects were achieved employing very low initial doses of CSA (2.5 mg/kg daily), alone or in combination with azathioprine as a steroid-sparing agent.[15] Vitreous inflammation was controlled in 23 eyes (88.5%) treated according to this strategy. Visual acuity improved or stabilized in 20 eyes (83.3%) receiving CSA alone or in combination with azathioprine, whereas 6 of 11 eyes (54%) receiving only periocular steroids experienced a significant deterioration in visual acuity.

Serum creatinine levels were virtually unchanged from baseline during the follow-up period (median, 36 months) and it was necessary to discontinue CSA because of hypertension in only one patient. The paucity of hypertensive side effects and renal toxicity, as reflected by the change in the serum creatinine from baseline, may have been the result of the very low initial dose of CSA (2.5 mg/kg daily) employed and subsequent escalation to the target range of 3.0 to 5.0 mg/kg daily, and to vigilant monitoring of these parameters.

Finally, a philosophy of zero tolerance for even low-grade inflammation and a limited tolerance for steroid use in patients for whom alternative anti-inflammatory medication is a reasonable option, to limit permanent ocular structural damage, underlies our approach to uveitis patients in general and those with BSRC in particular. Given the uncertain natural history and visual prognosis, the presence of intraocular inflammation rather than an arbitrary visual acuity level was the primary indication for the initiation of low-dose CSA. This parameter also determined the threshold for subsequent dosage adjustments and for the addition of azathioprine as a steroid-sparing agent. In this way, perhaps patients with BSRC may achieve long-term benefits from low-dose CSA therapy early in the course of their disease, even when the visual acuity is better than 20/40 prior to the onset of visually limiting sequelae.

NATURAL HISTORY AND PROGNOSIS

The natural history of BSRC is unknown. The disease is chronic, marked by multiple exacerbations and remissions that may extend over a period of decades. Although some investigators believe that BSRC has a tendency to stabilize over a 3- to 4-year period and go into remission,[10] others are more pessimistic about the long-term visual prognosis.[1-3, 15, 32] Some patients may have relatively good visual acuity on presentation, but as many as 20% may experience a reduction in visual acuity of three Snellen lines or more, with greater than one third of such eyes reaching a level of 20/200 or worse in at least one eye.[1-3, 10, 11, 32] Visual loss is most commonly the result of CME and optic atrophy.[21] The long-term outcome of treatment with various low-dose CSA regimens for BSRC is unknown. Given the rationale for the use of CSA in this disease entity, it is hoped that permanent ocular structural damage can be limited by its use in achieving complete control of intraocular inflammation and thus an improved visual outcome in patients suffering from BSRC.

CONCLUSIONS

BSRC is a recently recognized, distinct, uveitic entity characterized by the presence of vitritis, retinal vascular incompetence, and a striking funduscopic picture of multiple hypopigmented lesions. ICG angiography reveals many more of these lesions than are appreciated on either FA or on clinical exam, reflecting the diffuse nature of the disease process. Although its etiology is unknown, autoimmune mechanisms are likely to play an important role, given the demonstration of retinal autoantigen reactivity and the strong association with HLA-A29. Untreated, the natural history for useful vision in at least one eye appears to be poor, and therapy with corticosteroids is of inconsistent efficacy and is associated with an uncertain visual prognosis.

Given the putative autoimmune pathogenesis, a rationale exists for the use of CSA in the treatment of BSRC. Clinical experience suggests that low-dose regimens of CSA, used alone or in combination with other immunosuppressive agents, are both safe and effective, and offer a useful steroid-sparing strategy in the management of BSRC, provided vigilant monitoring for potential drug-induced toxicities is exercised.

References

1. Ryan SJ, Maumenee AE: Birdshot retinochoroidopathy. Am J Ophthalmol 1980;89:31.
2. Gass JDM: Vitiliginous chorioretinitis. Arch Ophthalmol 1981;99:1978.
3. Priem HA, Oosterhuis JA: Birdshot chorioretinopathy: Clinical characteristics and evolution. Br J Ophthalmol 1988;72:646.
4. Franceschetti A, Babel J: La chorio-rétinite en "tâches de bougie" manifestation de la maladie de Besnier-Boek. Ophthalmologica 1949;118:701.
5. Aaberg TM: Diffuse inflammatory salmon patch choroidopathy syndrome. International Fluorescein Macula Symposium. Carmel, CA, 1979.
6. Amalric P, Cuq G: Une forme très particulière de choriorétinopathie en grans de riz. Bull Soc Ophtalmol Fr 1981;81:131.
7. Opremcak EM: Birdshot retinochoroiditis. In: Albert DM, Jakobiec FA, eds: Principles and Practice of Ophthalmology, vol 1. Philadelphia, W.B. Saunders, 1994, p 475.
8. Henderly DE, Genstler AJ, Smith RE, et al: Changing patterns of uveitis. Am J Ophthalmol 1987;103:131.
9. Rodriguez A, Calonge M, Pedroza-Seres M, et al: Referral patterns of uveitis in a tertiary eye care center. Arch Ophthalmol 1996;114:593.
10. Fuerst DJ, Tessler HH, Fishman GA, et al: Birdshot retinochoroidopathy. Arch Ophthalmol 1984;102:214.
11. Kaplan HJ, Aaberg TM: Birdshot retinochoroidopathy. Am J Ophthalmol 1980;90:773.
12. Nussenblatt RB, Whitcup SM, Palestine AG: Birdshot retinochoroidopathy. In: Nussenblatt RB, Whitcup SM, Palestine AG, eds: Uveitis: Fundamentals and Clinical Practice, 2nd ed. St Louis, Mosby–Year Book, 1996, p 325.
13. Le Hoang P, Girard B, Keray G, et al: Cyclosporine in the treatment of birdshot retinochoroidopathy. Transplant Proc 1988;20(suppl 4):128.
14. Le Hoang P, Ozdemir N, Benhamou A, et al: HLA-A29.2 subtype associated with birdshot retinochoroidopathy. Am J Ophthalmol 1992;113:33.
15. Vitale AT, Rodriguez A, Foster CS: Low-dose cyclosporine therapy in the treatment of birdshot retinochoroidopathy. Ophthalmology 1994;101:822.
16. Gass JDM: Inflammatory diseases of the retina and choroid. In: Stereoscopic Atlas of Macular Diseases, Diagnosis and Treatment, 4th ed, vol II. St Louis, Mosby–Year Book, 1997, p 710.
17. Wagoner MD, Albert DM, Lerner AB, et al: New observations on vitiligo and ocular disease. Am J Ophthalmol 1983;96:16.
18. Heaton JM, Mills RP: Sensorineural hearing loss associated with birdshot retinochoroidopathy. Arch Otolaryngol Head Neck Surg 1993;119:680.
19. Noble KG, Greenberg J: Appearance of birdshot retinochoroidopathy in a patient with myelodysplasia. Am J Ophthalmol 1998;125:108.
20. Hesse S, Berhis P, Chemila JF, et al: Psoriasis and birdshot chorioretinopathy: A response to aromatic retinoids. Dermatology 1923;187:137.
21. Ryan SJ, Dugel PU, Stout TJ: Birdshot retinochoroidopathy. In: Ryan SJ, ed: Retina, 2nd ed, vol 2, Medical Retina. St. Louis, Mosby–Year Book, 1994, p 1677.
22. Le Hoang P, Ryan SJ: Birdshot retinochoroidopathy. In: Pepose JS, Holland GN, Wilhelmus KR, eds: Ocular Infection and Immunity. St Louis, Mosby–Year Book, 1996, p 570.
23. Barondes MJ, Fastenberg DM, Schwartz PL, et al: Peripheral retinal neovascularization in birdshot retinochoroidopathy. Ann Ophthalmol 1989;21:306.
24. Brucker AJ, Deglin EA, Bene C, et al: Subretinal choroidal neovascularization in birdshot retinochoroidopathy. Am J Ophthalmol 1985;99:40.
25. Soubrane G, Coscas G, Binaghi M, et al: Birdshot retinochoroidopathy and subretinal new vessels. Br J Ophthalmol 1983;67:461.
26. Felder KS, Brockhurst RJ: Neovascular fundus abnormalities in peripheral uveitis. Arch Ophthalmol 1982;100:750.
27. Shorb SB, Irvine AR, Kimura SL, et al: Optic disk neovascularization associated with chronic uveitis. Am J Ophthalmol 1967;82:175.
28. Caballero-Presencia A, Diaz-Guia E, Lopez-Lopez JM: Acute anterior ischemic optic neuropathy in birdshot retinochoroidopathy. Ophthalmologica 1988;196:87.
29. Fich M, Rosenberg T: Birdshot retinochoroidopathy in monozygotic twins. Acta Ophthalmol 1992;70:693.
30. Baarsma GS, Kijlstra A, Oosterhuis JA, et al: Association of birdshot retinochoroidopathy and HLA-A29 antigen. Doc Ophthalmol 1986;61:267.
31. Baarsma GS, Priem HA, Kijlstra A: Association of birdshot retinochoroidopathy and HLA-A29 antigen. Curr Eye Res 1990;9:63.
32. Nussenblatt RB, Mittal KK, Ryan S, et al: Birdshot retinochoroidopathy associated with HLA-A29 antigen and immune responsiveness to retinal S-antigen. Am J Ophthalmol 1982;94:147.
33. Priem HA, Kijlstra A, Noens L, et al: HLA typing in birdshot chorioretinopathy. Am J Ophthalmol 1988;105:182.
34. Feltkamp TEW: Ophthalmological significance of HLA associated uveitis. Eye 1990;4:839.
35. Feltkamp TEW: HLA and uveitis. Int Ophthalmol 1990;14:327.
36. Yang SY: Population analysis of class I HLA antigens by one-dimensional isoelectric focusing gel electrophoresis: Workshop summary report. In: Dupont B, ed: Immunobiology of HLA. New York, Springer-Verlag, 1989, p 309.
37. Tabary T, Le Hoang P, Betuel H, et al: Susceptibility to birdshot choroidopathy is restricted to the HLA-A29.2 subtype. Tissue Antigens 1990;36:177.
38. de Waal LP, Lardy NM, van der Horst AR, et al: HLA-A29 subtypes and birdshot retinochoroidopathy. Immunogenetics 1992;35:51.
39. Tabary T, Prochnicka-Chalufour A, Cornillet P, et al: HLA subtypes and "birdshot" choroido-retinopathy susceptibility: A possible "resistance motif" in the HLA-A29.1 molecule. C R Acad Sci III 1991;313:599.

40. Svejgaard A: HLA and disease. In: Rose NR, Friedman H, eds: Manual of Clinical Immunology, 2nd ed. Washington, DC, American Society of Microbiology, 1980, p 1049.

41. de Smet MD, Yamamoto JH, Mochizuki M, et al: Cellular immune responses of patients with uveitis to retinal antigens and their fragments. Am J Ophthalmol 1990;110:135.

42. Opremcak EM, Cowans AB: Limiting dilution analysis of S-antigen specific IL-2 secreting autoimmune T-lymphocytes in patients with uveitis. Invest Ophthalmol Vis Sci 1990;32(suppl):66.

43. Wacker WB, Donoso LA, Kalsow CM, et al: Experimental allergic uveitis. Isolation, characterization, and localization of a soluble uveitopathogenic antigen from bovine retina. J Immunol 1977;119:1949.

44. Mochizuki M, Kuwabara T, McAllister C, et al: Adoptive transfer of experimental autoimmune uveoretinitis in rats: Immunopathogenic mechanisms and histologic features. Invest Ophthalmol Vis Sci 1985;26:1.

45. Nussenblatt RB, Kuwabara T, de Montasterio F, et al: S-antigen uveitis in primates: A new model for human disease. Arch Ophthalmol 1981;99:1090.

46. Jobin D, Thillaye B, de Kozak Y, et al: Severe retinochoroidopathy: Variations of humoral and cellular immunity to S-antigen in a longitudinal study. Curr Eye Res 1990;9(suppl):91.

47. Bejamin R, Parham P: HLA-B27 and ankylosing spondylitis. Immunol Today 1990;11:132.

48. Tiwari JC, Terasaki PI: Guilt by Association. HLA and Disease Association. New York, Springer-Verlag, 1989, pp 25 and 264.

49. Kuhne F, Morlat P, Riss I, et al: Is A29, B12 vasculitis caused by the Q fever agent (*Coxiella burnetii*)? J Fr Ophthalmol 1992;15:315.

50. Suttorp-Schulten MS, Luyendijk L, van Dam AP, et al: Birdshot chorioretinopathy and Lyme borreliosis. Am J Ophthalmol 1993;115:149.

51. Kalsow CM, Wacker WB: Pineal gland involvement in retina-induced experimental allergic uveitis. Invest Ophthalmol Vis Sci 1978;17:774.

52. Rodrigues MM, Hackett J, Gaskins R, et al: Interphotoreceptor retinoid-binding protein in retinal rod cells and pineal gland. Invest Ophthalmol Vis Sci 1986;27:844.

53. Gery I, Wiggert B, Redmond TM, et al: Uveoretinitis and pinealitis induced by immunization with IRBP. Invest Ophthalmol Vis Sci 1986;27:1296.

54. Mochizuki M, Charley J, Kuwabara T, et al: Involvement of the pineal gland in rats with experimental autoimmune uveitis. Invest Ophthalmol Vis Sci 1983;24:1333.

55. Lewy AJ: The pineal gland. In: Wyngaarden JB, Smith LH, Bennett JC, eds: Cecil Textbook of Medicine, 19th ed, vol II. Philadelphia, W.B. Saunders, 1992, p 1246.

56. Touitou Y, Le Hoang P, Claustrat B, et al: Decreased nocturnal plasma melatonin peak in patients with a functional alteration of the retina in relation with uveitis. Neurosci Lett 1986;70:170.

57. Klok AM, Geertzen R, Rothova A, et al: Anticardiolipin antibodies in uveitis. Curr Eye Res 1992;11(suppl):709.

58. Guex-Crosier Y, Herbort CP: Prolonged retinal arterio-venous circulation time by fluorescein but not by indocyanine green angiography in birdshot retinochoroidopathy. Ocul Immunol Inflamm 1997;5:203.

59. Howe LJ, Stanford MR, Graham EM, et al: Choroidal abnormalities in birdshot retinochoroidopathy: An indocyanine green angiography study. Eye 1997;11:554.

60. Chang B, Goldstein DA, Rabb MF, et al: Indocyanine green angiographic features in birdshot retinochoroidopathy. Invest Ophthalmol Vis Sci 1995;36:S782.

61. Coscas G: Personal communication, Paris, 1999.

62. Herbort CP, Borruat F, de Couten C, et al: Angiographie au vert d'indocyanine dans les uvéites postérieures. Klin Monatsbl Augenheilkd 1996;208:321.

63. Yannuzi LA, Sorenson JA, Guyer DR, et al: Indocyanine green angiography: Current status. Eur J Ophthalmol 1994;4:69.

64. Hirose T, Katsumi O, Pruett RC, et al: Retinal function in birdshot retinochoroidopathy. Acta Ophthalmol 1991;69:327.

65. Priem HA, De Rouck A, De Laey JJ, et al: Electrophysiological studies in birdshot chorioretinopathy. Am J Ophthalmol 1998;106:430.

66. De Rouck A, Kayembe D: A clinical procedure for the simultaneous recording of fast and slow EOG oscillations. Int Ophthalmol 1981;3:179.

67. Guex-Crosier Y, Pittet N, Herbort CP: Evaluation of laser flare-cell photometry in the appraisal and management of intraocular inflammation in uveitis. Ophthalmology 1994;101:728.

68. Helm CJ, Holland GN: Ocular tuberculosis. Surv Ophthalmol 1993;38:229.

69. Tamesis RR, Foster CS: Ocular syphilis. Ophthalmology 1990;97:1281.

70. Gass JDM, Scelfo R: Diffuse unilateral subacute neuroretinitis. J R Soc Med 1978;71:95.

71. Kazacos KR, Vestre WA, Kazacos EA, et al: Diffuse unilateral subacute neuroretinitis syndrome: A probable cause. Arch Ophthalmol 1984;102:967.

72. Woods AC, Whalen HE: The probable role of benign histoplasmosis in the etiology of granulomatous uveitis. Am J Ophthalmol 1960;49:205.

73. Smith RE, Ganley JP, Knox DL: Presumed ocular histoplasmosis. II. Patterns of peripheral and peripapillary scarring in persons with nonmacular disease. Arch Ophthalmol 1972;85:251.

74. Vrabec TR, Augsburger JJ, Fischer DH, et al: Taches de bougie. Ophthalmology 1995;102:1712.

75. Brinkman CJ, Rothova A: Fundus pathology in neurosarcoidosis. Int Ophthalmol 1993;17:23.

76. Brod RD: Presumed sarcoid choroidopathy mimicking birdshot retinochoroidopathy. Am J Ophthalmol 1990;109:357.

77. Kuboshiro T, Yoshioka H: Birdshot retinochoroidopathy: A possible relationship to ocular sarcoidosis. Krume Med J 1998;35:193.

78. Moorthy RS, Inomata H, Rao NA: Vogt-Koyanagi-Harada syndrome. Surv Ophthalmol 1995;39:265.

79. Marak GE: Recent advances in sympathetic ophthalmia. Surv Ophthalmol 1979;24:141.

80. Nozik RA, Dorsch W: A new chorioretinopathy associated with anterior uveitis. Am J Ophthalmol 1973;76:758.

81. Watzke RC, Packer AJ, Folk JC, et al: Punctate inner choroidopathy. Am J Ophthalmol 1984;98:572.

82. Jampol LM, Sieving PA, Pugh D, et al: Multiple evanescent white dot syndrome. 1. Clinical findings. Arch Ophthalmol 1984;102:671.

83. Gass JDM: Acute posterior multifocal placoid pigment epitheliopathy. Arch Ophthalmol 1968;80:177.

84. Godel V, Baruch E, Lazar M: Late development of chorioretinal lesions in birdshot retinochoroidopathy. Ann Ophthalmol 1989;21:49.

85. Soubrane G, Bokobza R, Coscas G: Late developing lesions in birdshot retinochoroidopathy. Am J Ophthalmol 1970;109:204.

86. Bloch-Michel E, Frau E: Birdshot retinochoroidopathy and HLA-A29 + and HLA-A29–idiopathic retinal vasculitis: Comparative study of 56 cases. Can J Ophthalmol 1991;26:361.

87. Bergink GJ, Ooyman FM, Maas S, et al: Three HLA-A29 positive patients with uveitis. Acta Ophthalmol Scand 1996;74:81.

88. Brockhurst RJ, Schepens CL, Okamura ID: Uveitis. II. Peripheral uveitis. Clinical description, complications, and differential diagnosis. Am J Ophthalmol 1960;49:1257.

89. Brinton GS, Osher RH, Gass JD: Idiopathic vitritis. Retina 1983; 3:95.

90. Whitcup SM, de Smet MD, Rubin BI, et al: Intraocular lymphoma: Clinical and histopathologic diagnosis. Ophthalmology 1993; 100:1399.

91. Hofman HM, Feicht B: Birdshot chorioretinopathy: Systemic therapy with corticosteroids and nonsteroidal anti-inflammatory drugs. Klin Monatsbl Augenheilkd 1990;197:159.

92. Nussenblatt RA, Rodrigues MM, Wacker WB, et al: Cyclosporine A. Inhibition of experimental autoimmune uveitis in Lewis rats. J Clin Invest 1981;67:1228.

93. Nussenblatt RB, Palestine AG, Chan CC: Cyclosporine therapy in the treatment of intraocular inflammatory disease resistant to systemic corticosteroids and cytotoxic agents. Am J Ophthalmol 1983;96:275.

94. Nussenblatt RB, Palestine AG, Chan CC: Cyclosporine therapy for uveitis: Long-term followup. J Ocul Pharmacol 1985;1:369.

95. Binder AI, Graham EM, Sanders MD, et al: Cyclosporine A in the treatment of severe Behçet's uveitis. Br J Rheumatol 1987;26:285.

96. Graham EM, Sanders MD, James DG, et al: Cyclosporine A in the treatment of posterior uveitis. Trans Ophthalmol Soc U K 1985;104:146.

97. Wakefield D, McCluskey P: Cyclosporine: A therapy in inflammatory eye disease. J Ocul Pharmacol 1991;7:221.

98. de Vries J, Baarsma GS, Zaal MJW, et al: Cyclosporine in the treatment of severe chronic idiopathic uveitis. Br J Ophthalmol 1990;74:344.

99. Masuda K, Nakajima A, Urayama A, et al: Double-masked trial of cyclosporine versus colchicine and long-term open study of cyclosporine in Behçet's disease. Lancet 1989;1:1093.

100. Nussenblatt RB, Palestine AG, Chan CC, et al: Randomized, double-masked study of cyclosporine compared to prednisolone in the treatment of endogenous uveitis. Am J Ophthalmol 1991;112:138.

101. Benezra D, Nussenblatt RB, Timonen P: Optimal use of Sandimmune in endogenous uveitis. Berlin, Springer-Verlag, 1988.

102. Cohen E, Raz J, Maftzir G, et al: Low-dose cyclosporine A in uveitis: A long term follow-up. Ocul Immunol Inflamm 1993;1:195.

103. Towler HM, Cliffe AM, Whiting PH, et al: Low dose cyclosporine A therapy in chronic posterior uveitis. Eye 1989;3:282.

104. Bielory L, Holland C, Gaslon P, et al: Uveitis, cutaneous and neurosarcoid: Treatment with low-dose cyclosporine A. Transplant Proc 1998;20(suppl 4):144.

105. Diaz-Llopis M, Cervera M, Menezo JL: Cyclosporine A treatment of Behçet's disease: A long-term study. Curr Eye Res 1990;9(Suppl):17.

106. Towler HM, Lightman SL, Forrester JV: Low-dose cyclosporine therapy of ocular inflammation: Preliminary report of a long-term follow-up study. J Autoimmun 1992;5(suppl A):259.

107. Towler HM, Whiting PH, Forrester JV: Combination low dose cyclosporine A and steroid therapy in chronic intraocular inflammation. Eye 1990;4:514.

108. Hooper PL, Kaplan HJ: Triple agent immunosuppression in serpiginous choroiditis. Ophthalmology 1991;98:944.

109. Nussenblatt RB, Palestine AG, Chan CC, et al: Improvement of uveitis and optic nerve disease by cyclosporine in a patient with multiple sclerosis. Am J Ophthalmol 1984;97:790.

110. Vitale AT, Rodriguez A, Foster CS: Low-dose cyclosporine A therapy in treating chronic, noninfectious uveitis. Ophthalmology 1996;103:365.

111. Callanan DG, Cheung MK, Martin DF, et al: Outcome of uveitis patients treated with long term cyclosporine. Invest Ophthalmol Vis Sci 1994;35:2094.

112. Deray G, Benhmida M, Le Hoang P, et al: Renal function and blood pressure in patients receiving long-term, low-dose cyclosporine therapy for idiopathic autoimmune uveitis. Ann Intern Med 1992;117:578.

66

SYMPATHETIC OPHTHALMIA

William J. Power

DEFINITION

Sympathetic ophthalmia is probably the best-known intraocular inflammatory condition to practitioners outside of ophthalmology. It is a bilateral granulomatous uveitis that occurs after either surgery or penetrating trauma to one eye. The traumatized eye is called the exciting eye and the noninjured eye is called the sympathizing eye. Although not a common disease, it remains one of the most feared complications in ophthalmology today because of its potentially blinding effects in both eyes. Newer observations have helped put this disorder into perspective.

HISTORY

Sympathetic ophthalmia has stimulated enormous interest since its clinical description by William MacKenzie in the middle of the 19th century.[1] In his series of six patients, all of whom followed penetrating trauma, he found that the recurrent attacks of inflammation led to eventual blindness and that no treatment was effective for the condition. MacKenzie postulated that the inflammatory process spread from the exciting to the sympathizing eye via the optic nerve and optic chiasm.

Ernest Fuchs has been credited with the first detailed histopathologic description of the disease and established it as a separate disease entity, distinct from other ocular inflammatory disorders.[2] He described a mixed-cell inflammatory infiltration of the uveal tract particularly affecting the choroid. He and Dalen independently described the inflammatory nodular aggregates (Dalen-Fuchs nodules) that now bear their names.[3]

INCIDENCE AND EPIDEMIOLOGY

There are numerous reports in the literature regarding the incidence of sympathetic ophthalmia, but in many purported cases pathologic proof of the diagnosis is lacking. In the older literature in particular, sympathetic ophthalmia was probably often confused with other forms of uveitis.

Sympathetic ophthalmia occurs more often after non-surgical trauma. Liddy and Stuart reported the disorder as occurring in 0.2% of nonsurgical wounds,[4] and Holland found it in 0.5% of eyes with trauma.[5] Marak has estimated the incidence of this disease to be less than 10 cases per 100,000 surgical penetrating wounds.[6] Sympathetic ophthalmia has occurred after intraocular procedures such as paracentesis, iridectomy, iris inclusions, cyclodialysis, transscleral neodymium:YAG (yttrium aluminum garnet) cyclodestruction, cataract extraction, evisceration, retinal detachment repair, and pars plana vitrectomy.[7–12] Gass[12] reports that the prevalence of sympathetic ophthalmia is 0.01% following routine pars plana vitrectomy but 0.06% when pars plana vitrectomy is performed in the context of other penetrating wounds, suggesting that the clinical impression of an increased prevalence of sympathetic ophthalmia following multiple surgical pro-

cedures[13] may in fact be accurate. It has also been reported to have occurred following proton beam irradiation, and after helium ion therapy for choroidal melanoma.[14, 15]

No cases of sympathetic ophthalmia were seen as a result of trauma suffered during the Vietnam War, the Korean Conflict, or the Six Days' War.[13] This is in contrast to the older literature suggesting an incidence of about 2%. Duke-Elder and Perkins claimed an unreferenced incidence of over 16% occurring during the American Civil War.[16] It must be borne in mind that there were no specialized ophthalmologists among the physicians in the Civil War, and so this figure is almost certainly an overestimate of the true incidence. Indeed, during the last century, and in particular over the last 30 years, there has been a dramatic decrease in the incidence of sympathetic ophthalmia, resulting in large part from the advent of corticosteroids and antibiotics, together with improved surgical management of traumatic ocular injuries.[4, 17, 18]

It is thought to be more common in men, almost certainly because of their higher incidence of ocular trauma. It is also thought to be more common in lighter-skinned races, but this may be because of better reporting and recognition of the disease.

CLINICAL FEATURES

Sympathetic ophthalmia is a bilateral panuveitis. The onset of inflammation in the sympathizing eye is quite often insidious. The latent period is usually between 2 weeks and 3 months, but cases have been reported as early as 5 days and as late as 66 years after the initial incident.[19, 20] Ninety percent of cases become manifest in the first year after the injury.

The inflammatory response seen in the anterior chamber is granulomatous in the classic case, with mutton-fat keratic precipitates on the corneal endothelium and findings of an acute anterior uveitis (Fig. 66–1). There is generally a moderate to severe vitritis accompanied by posterior segment abnormalities. Of particular note are multiple white-yellow lesions seen in the periphery of the choroid, sometimes becoming confluent (Fig. 66–2). These represent the clinical appearance of the Dalen-Fuchs nodule. Papillitis can be most prominent and circumpapillary choroidal lesions may be seen as well. It should be remembered that the clinical appearance of sympathetic ophthalmia represents a spectrum, which can range from very mild to severe. Alopecia, poliosis, vitiligo, dysacousia, and cells in the cerebrospinal fluid, typically found in Vogt-Koyanagi-Harada syndrome (VKH), may rarely be associated with sympathetic ophthalmia. The sequelae of the inflammation noted in sympathetic ophthalmia are quite variable, depending on the severity of the ocular inflammation and whether therapy has been instituted. Secondary glaucoma as well as cataract can be seen. In addition, retinal and optic atrophy may occur, which may be seen in association with retinal detachment or subretinal fibrosis and underlying choroidal atrophy.

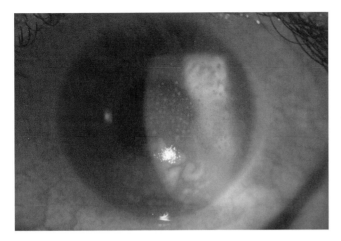

FIGURE 66–1. Granulomatous anterior uveitis in a patient with acute sympathetic ophthalmia.

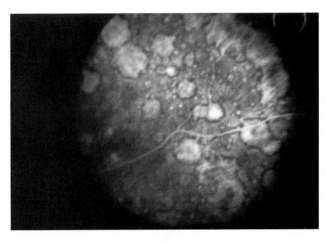

FIGURE 66–3. Multiple areas of hyperfluorescence on fluorescein angiography. The smaller areas of hyperfluorescence corresponded to the clinically observed Dalen-Fuchs nodules.

In the acute phase of sympathetic ophthalmia, the fluorescein angiogram typically demonstrates multiple hyperfluorescent sites of leakage at the level of the retinal pigment epithelium during the venous phase, and, like those seen in VKH, they persist. In severe cases, these foci may coalesce, with pooling of dye beneath areas of exudative neurosensory detachment. Less commonly, the angiogram demonstrates multiple hypofluorescent areas followed by late staining, as seen in acute posterior multifocal placoid pigment epitheliopathy. The sites of early blocked fluorescence generally correspond to the clinically observed Dalen-Fuchs nodules (Fig. 66–3). It is probably the status of the pigment epithelium overlying the Dalen-Fuchs nodules or the integrity of the choriocapillaris that determines the hyperfluorescent or hypofluorescent nature of these lesions on angiography. The optic nerve head may demonstrate leakage in the later stages of the angiogram. B-scan ultrasonography can be used to demonstrate the marked choroidal thickening seen in cases of sympathetic ophthalmia (Fig. 66–4).

PATHOLOGY AND PATHOGENESIS

The histopathology of the inflammatory changes in sympathetic ophthalmia are identical in the exciting and sympathizing eyes.[21] A diffuse granulomatous infiltration is seen throughout the uveal tract, with marked thickening in the posterior choroid (Fig. 66–5). Classically, the choriocapillaris is spared and there is a relative lack of retinal involvement. However, atypical histopathologic features in the history of sympathetic ophthalmia have been reported. Specifically, variable degrees of retinal involvement, including perivasculitis, retinitis, detachment, and gliosis, have been described.[8]

The other characteristic histopathologic finding in sympathetic ophthalmia is that of Dalen-Fuchs nodules, which are present in about one third of eyes.[22] These nodules represent collections of lymphocytes, histiocytes, and altered pigment epithelial cells that lie just internal to Bruch's membrane. Jakobiec and coworkers[22] and Chan and colleagues[23] have used monoclonal antibodies to demonstrate that Dalen-Fuchs nodules are composed of a mixture of Ia+ cells, OKM1 cells (presumably histiocytes), and depigmented retinal pigment epithelial cells that are Ia− and OKM1−. The subsets of infiltrating lymphocytes in the choroid have also been identified

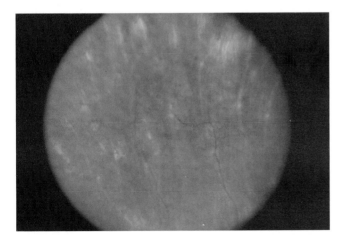

FIGURE 66–2. Multiple cream-colored lesions scattered throughout the midequatorial region of the fundus in a patient with sympathetic ophthalmia. (See color insert.)

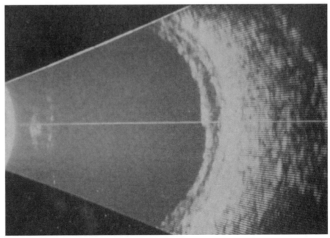

FIGURE 66–4. B-scan ultrasonography demonstrating marked choroidal thickening.

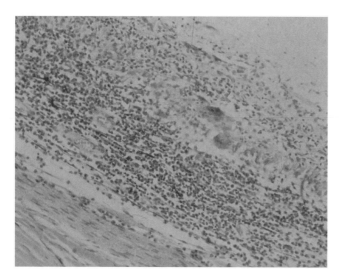

FIGURE 66–5. Histopathologic examination of an eye with sympathetic ophthalmia shows an intense mononuclear cell infiltrate in the choroid with relative sparing of the choriocapillaris. (H&E original magnification × 80.) (See color insert.)

using immunohistochemical techniques. While Jakobiec and colleagues[22] noted a predominance of CD8 cells in the choroid of patients in eyes removed well after the initial surgical trauma, Chan and colleagues[23] have noted there is a predominance of CD4 T cells in an eye enucleated only several months after initial nonsurgical trauma. They later found that the sympathizing eye of the same patient, which ultimately came to be studied, had a predominance of CD8 cells. These changes in T-cell subsets over time may reflect a dynamic situation in which there is an attempt to down-regulate the immune response with the influx of suppressor T cells.

Another highly characteristic histopathologic feature of sympathetic ophthalmia is pigment phagocytosis by the epithelioid cells in the absence of uveal necrosis.

The frequency of phacoantigenic uveitis (PAU) associated with sympathetic ophthalmia has been well documented.[25] In a review of 105 cases by Lubin and coworkers,[21] 46% demonstrated histopathologic evidence of PAU. All the eyes with PAU had sustained a break in the lens capsule. It is interesting to note that in their series of cases, spanning the years 1913 to 1978, only one case of PAU associated with sympathetic ophthalmia was detected after 1949. The authors attribute this to the introduction of corticosteroid therapy and the more complete treatment that lens injuries currently receive. It has been suggested that the strong association between the two conditions may indicate a predisposition to autoimmune disease in certain patients, or that there are some common antigens shared between the lens and uveal tissue.[26]

ETIOLOGY

The concept that an autoimmune inflammatory response is the basis of this disorder is not a new one, having been proposed by Elschnig in 1910 with uveal pigment being thought of as the putative antigenic stimulus.[26] In vitro cell culturing techniques have been used to evaluate responses of lymphocytes from patients with sympathetic

ophthalmia. The patients have demonstrated a positive proliferative response to uveal or uveoretinal preparations, underscoring the predominance of T-cell responses in this disorder.[28] In contrast, humoral immune mechanisms are not thought to be pathogenetic, as demonstrated by Chan and colleagues who found no circulating antiretinal S-antigen antibodies in a group of patients with sympathetic ophthalmia using the enzyme-linked immunosorbent assay technique.[29] Although no exact experimental model for sympathetic ophthalmia yet exists, the induction of uveitis with the ocular antigens interphotoreceptor retinoid binding protein and S-antigen produces a disease in monkeys that has many of the characteristics of sympathetic ophthalmia, including the development of Dalen-Fuchs nodules. An important factor in the development of sympathetic ophthalmia may be that penetrating trauma permits access to lymphatics and the presentation of ocular antigens to the systemic immune system in a different way from the usual, setting the stage for autoimmune inflammatory sequelae.

The Role of the Penetrating Wound

Any theory on the pathogenesis of sympathetic ophthalmia must take into account the fact that sympathetic ophthalmia develops almost exclusively after a penetrating wound. To study this more closely, Rao and colleagues used the retinal S-antigen uveitis model to compare intraocular antigen presentation with extraocular antigen presentation.[29] Intraocular antigen presentation represents a situation comparable to nonpenetrating trauma, and extraocular antigen presentation a situation comparable to a penetrating wound with uveal prolapse. None of the animals injected intraocularly developed contralateral inflammation, whereas 4 of 10 injected subconjunctivally developed chorioretinal lesions in both eyes 14 to 16 days after sensitization.

Animals receiving subconjunctival injections of antigen had evidence of cell-mediated hypersensitivity as well as precipitating antibodies to retinal S-antigen, whereas the animals receiving intraocular inoculations had no immune responses to retinal S-antigen detected by the screening tests employed. Rao and coworkers suggested that the penetrating wound participated in the development of sympathetic ophthalmia by exposing uveoretinal antigens to the conjunctival lymphatics and thereby inducing a subsequent immunopathologic response.[29]

It has long been postulated that an infectious agent may be required concurrently with the antigen to initiate an immune response resulting in sympathetic ophthalmia.[31] Active proliferation of the organism may in fact not be necessary. Products such as bacterial cell wall, which may be present in the wound, could act as immunostimulators and thereby up-regulate a local immune response. The possible adjuvant role of an infectious agent correlates well with the strong association between sympathetic ophthalmia and perforating wounds with uveal prolapse and its lack of association with nonperforating injuries.

Immune Privilege of the Eye

The immune privilege of the eye has been recognized for over a century: Early investigators discovered that tumor tissue injected into the anterior chamber of the eye survived for an unusually long time, whereas tumor tissue taken from one animal and grafted subcutaneously into another was quickly destroyed. The lack of a recognizable lymphatic drainage pathway was identified as a common anatomic feature of the anterior chamber of the eye, brain, ovary, and testis. It was concluded that antigenic material was sequestered in these immunologically privileged sites and was probably ignored by the immune system. But we now know that immune privilege in the anterior chamber of the eye is not the result of immunologic ignorance of the antigen but of an active regulation of immunity that suppresses cell-mediated immunity while promoting humoral immunity.[32] This anterior chamber–associated immune deviation (ACAID) depends on unique features of both the spleen and the eye for its initiation.[33] In particular, cells from the iris and ciliary body are able to down-regulate the earliest events of antigen presentation and lymphocyte activation, thereby initiating a selective impairment of delayed hypersensitivity.

Mizuno and coworkers have demonstrated that mice and rats develop ACAID when S-antigen is injected uniocularly.[33] In an effort to determine whether the induction of ACAID could prevent experimental autoimmune uveitis, susceptible animals were pretreated with a uniocular injection of retinal S-antigen. When these rats were subsequently injected subcutaneously with S-antigen, minimal uveitis was noted. Thus, an experimentally induced suppression of S-antigen–specific delayed hypersensitivity was able to prevent the subsequent development of S-antigen–specific retinitis.

One might wonder whether there might be, in certain genetically susceptible individuals, and under certain immunologically stimulating conditions with bacterial adjuvant stimulation, loss of immune tolerance and induction of autoimmune uveitis called sympathetic ophthalmia.

Genetic Predisposition to Sympathetic Ophthalmia

Many studies have shown associations between specific histocompatibility antigenic determinants in a variety of ocular diseases. Typically, there is a statistically significant increase in the incidence of one particular histocompatibility antigen in the patient population with a specific disease, compared with a matched control population. Reynard and colleagues have demonstrated an increased

frequency of the human leukocyte antigen (HLA) A11 in a group of 20 patients with histopathologically proven sympathetic ophthalmia.[34] The relative risk in the disease group compared to the control group was 11. This association suggests that a genetic factor may play an important role in the pathogenesis of sympathetic ophthalmia.

HLA-DR4 (and the closely linked HLA-DQw3 in Americans and HLA-DRw53 in Japanese) is over-represented in populations of patients with sympathetic ophthalmia.[36] These same alleles are overrepresented in Japanese and American patients with VKH, and in patients with a variety of nonocular autoimmune diseases, lending support to the idea that a genetic susceptibility factor is operative, at least in some patients with sympathetic ophthalmia.

It is possible to hypothesize that the perforating injury permits several events to take place. The first is that drainage of antigen from the eye can occur through the lymphatics, an event that does not occur under normal conditions. The second is that small amounts of adjuvant, such as bacterial cell wall or other immunostimulators, might now enter the eye. These products may then profoundly upgrade the local immune response, causing it to bypass certain inherent suppressor mechanisms in genetically prone individuals. This leads then to the inflammatory response that ultimately leads to the clinical entity that is recognized as sympathetic ophthalmia.

DIFFERENTIAL DIAGNOSIS

The diagnosis of sympathetic ophthalmia is a clinical one depending essentially on the history of ocular injury by surgery or trauma followed by bilateral granulomatous uveitis. The pathologic diagnosis is defined by characteristic features, as mentioned previously, including a predominant T-cell inflammatory infiltrate in the uvea, the early phagocytosis of pigment granules, and the presence of Dalen-Fuchs nodules.

Occasionally, it may be difficult to distinguish sympathetic ophthalmia from VKH (Table 66–1). But patients with VKH have no history of trauma. Typically, they have bilateral localized serous detachments of the retina, which are not seen in sympathetic ophthalmia. VKH is also more prevalent in certain racial and ethnic groups. It has been estimated to constitute approximately 8% of all cases of endogenous uveitis in Japan.[37] It appears to be extremely rare in patients of northern European extraction. In the typical case of sympathetic ophthalmia,

TABLE 66–1. COMPARISON OF SYMPATHETIC OPHTHALMIA AND VOGT-KOYANAGI-HARADA SYNDROME

	SYMPATHETIC OPHTHALMIA	VOGT-KOYANAGI-HARADA SYNDROME
Age	All ages	20–50 years
Racial predisposition	None	Asian and black
Penetrating trauma	Always present	Absent
Skin changes	Uncommon	Common (60% to 90%)
CNS findings	Uncommon	Common (85%)
Hearing dysfunction	Uncommon	Common (75%)
Retinal serous detachment	Rare	Frequently seen
Choriocapillaris involvement	Usually absent	Frequently seen
CSF findings	Usually normal	Pleocytosis (84%)

CNS, central nervous system; CSF, cerebrospinal fluid.

no laboratory studies are necessary for diagnosis. If it is necessary to differentiate the syndrome from VKH, a lumbar puncture should be performed early in the course of the disease. This reveals a pleocytosis in 84% of cases of VKH, with mostly lymphocytes and monocytes present.[38] Sarcoidosis, when it produces multiple small foci of choroiditis, may also (rarely) be confused with postoperative sympathetic ophthalmia.

PREVENTION AND MANAGEMENT

Surgical Treatment

The only known prevention for sympathetic ophthalmia is enucleation, and this must be performed *prior to* the development of the autoimmune response if it is to be effective. The classic teaching has been that enucleation within 14 days after ocular injury protects the second eye from the development of sympathetic ophthalmia. Exceptions to this rule do occur but are rare.[39]

Controversy still exists regarding the advisability of enucleating the exciting eye once sympathetic ophthalmia has commenced. The review by Lubin and coworkers would suggest that enucleation within 2 weeks of the initiation of the inflammatory response may beneficially affect the visual outcome of the remaining eye.[21] Reynard and associates, in their retrospective clinicopathologic study, also noted that enucleation within 2 weeks of the beginning of symptoms resulted in a fairly benign course—specifically, less frequent and milder relapses and a good visual outcome (visual acuity better than 20/50).[39] In contrast, another review indicates no benefit to the sympathizing eye from enucleation of the exciting eye, whether performed immediately before, concomitant with, or subsequent to the development of sympathetic ophthalmia at various elapsed intervals following injury.[8] It must be stressed that enucleation should be considered only when the visual prognosis is nil for the eye being considered for enucleation, because not uncommonly the exciting eye may ultimately be the one with better vision.

Sympathetic ophthalmia may occur after evisceration probably as a result of remaining uveal tissue in the scleral emissary channels.[9] It would seem prudent not to perform eviscerations except perhaps in cases of endophthalmitis or in patients whose general condition is very poor.

Medical Treatment

Corticosteroids

If the decision has been made to intervene with anti-inflammatory therapy, the initial approach, in most cases, should be with corticosteroids. They may be given topically, by sub-Tenon or transseptal injection, and systemically. Systemic steroids are recommended on a daily basis, beginning with a high dose of a short-acting agent (e.g., 1.0 to 1.5 mg/kg/day prednisone). Three months is a sensible time frame in which to evaluate whether the therapeutic approach has worked, the clinical criteria for improvement depending largely on the seriousness of the inflammatory response. If steroid therapy is effective, then a slow taper should be initiated. However, in some patients, the disease may not be controlled with this approach, because of either persistent disease activity or the necessity for long-term maintenance with systemic steroids with attendant intolerable side effects. In a long-term follow-up of sympathetic ophthalmia patients treated with steroids, Makley and Azar found that 65% of eyes had a stable visual acuity of 20/60 or better.[40] Others have reported similar success rates.[22, 40]

Cyclosporine

Other forms of immunosuppressive therapy have been tried with success in steroid-resistant cases of sympathetic ophthalmia. In a group of five patients, Nussenblatt and Palestine[41] used systemic cyclosporine and noted that the inflammatory response appeared to respond well to this agent. Thirty-two patients with sympathetic ophthalmia were followed at the National Eye Institute (Bethesda, MD) over a 10-year period.[43] Seven required a combination of cyclosporine and oral prednisone to control their disease. Towler and colleagues also reported good results with cyclosporine and corticosteroid combination therapy in patients with sympathetic ophthalmia.[43]

Cytotoxic Agents

Jennings and Tessler found chlorambucil to be particularly effective in those patients with severe disease in a series of 20 patients with sympathetic ophthalmia.[44] They noted that the subsidence of inflammation coincided with a decrease in white blood cell count. Despite previous reports of major complications with chlorambucil, they had no complications with this form of treatment, although evaluations of fertility were not conducted. Azathioprine, at a dose of 50 mg three times a day, has also been used effectively in combination with low-dose corticosteroids.[45] Use of these agents must be performed by individuals who by virtue of their training and experience are truly expert in the indications for and side effects of treatment with such medications. To this end, collaborative management with an internist, rheumatologist, or hematologist is advisable.

PROGNOSIS

The relapsing nature of sympathetic ophthalmia and the potential toxicity of treatment modalities warrant a careful long-term follow-up of patients with this disease. Spontaneous improvement is rare. The use of corticosteroid and other immunosuppressive agents, together with state-of-the-art microsurgical techniques for wound repair, have improved the prognosis of sympathetic ophthalmia such that good vision can be expected in the sympathizing eye. Cataract, secondary glaucoma, and chronic maculopathy are the major causes of visual loss. Fortunately, sympathetic ophthalmia is a relatively rare condition; but it remains an enigmatic disease with the potential for bilateral blindness.

References

1. MacKenzie W: A practical treatise on diseases of the eye, 3rd ed. London, Longmans, 1840, pp 523–534.
2. Fuchs E: Uber sympathisierende Entzundung (Zuerst Bermerkunen uber serose traumatische Iritis). Graefes Arch Clin Exp Ophthalmol 1905;61:365–456.
3. Dalen A: Zur Kenntnis der sogenannten Choroiditis sympathetica. Mitt Augenklin Carolin Med-Chirurg Inst Stockholm 1904;6:1.

4. Liddy N, Stuart J: Sympathetic ophthalmia in Canada. Can J Ophthalmol 1972;7:157–159.

5. Holland G: About the indications and time for surgical removal of an injured eye. Klin Monatsbl Augenheilkd 1964;145:732–740.

6. Marak GE: Recent advances in sympathetic ophthalmia. Surv Ophthalmol 1979;24:141–156.

7. Rao NA: Sympathetic ophthalmia. In: Ryan SJ, ed: Retina, vol. 2: Medical Retina. St Louis, CV Mosby, 1989, pp 715–721.

8. Winter FC: Sympathetic uveitis: A clinical and pathologic study of the visual result. Am J Ophthalmol 1955;39:340–347.

9. Green WR, Maumenee AE, Sanders TE, Smith ME: Sympathetic uveitis following evisceration. Trans Am Acad Ophthalmol Otolaryngol 1972;76:625–644.

10. Lam S, Tessler HH, Lam BL, Wilensky JT: High incidence of sympathetic ophthalmia after contact and noncontact neodymium: YAG cyclotherapy. Ophthalmology 1992;12:1818–1822.

11. Wang WJ: Clinical and histopathological report of sympathetic ophthalmia after retinal detachment surgery. Br J Ophthalmol 1983;67:150–152.

12. Gass JDM: Sympathetic ophthalmia following vitrectomy. Am J Ophthalmol 1982;93:552–558.

13. Albert DM, Diaz-Rohena R: A historical review of sympathetic ophthalmia and its epidemiology. Surv Ophthalmol 1989;34:1–14.

14. Margo CE, Pautler SE: Granulomatous uveitis after treatment of a choroidal melanoma with proton-beam irradiation. Retina 1990;10:140–143.

15. Fries PD, Char DH, Crawford JB, Waterhouse W: Sympathetic ophthalmia complicating helium ion irradiation of a choroidal melanoma. Arch Ophthalmol 1987;105:1561–1564.

16. Duke-Elder ES, Perkins EA: Diseases of the uveal tract. In: Duke-Elder WS, ed: System of Ophthalmology, vol 9. St. Louis, CV Mosby, 1966, pp 558–593.

17. Wykes WN: A ten-year survey of penetrating eye injury in Gwent, 1979–1985. Br J Ophthalmol 1988;72:607–611.

18. Green WR: The uveal tract. In: Spencer WH, ed: Ophthalmic Pathology: An Atlas and Textbook, 3rd ed, vol 3. Philadelphia, W.B. Saunders, 1986, pp 1915–1956.

19. Verhoeff F: An effective treatment for sympathetic uveitis. Arch Ophthalmol 1927;56:28.

20. Easom HA, Zimmerman LE: Sympathetic ophthalmia and bilateral phacoanaphylaxis: A clinicopathological correlation of the sympathogenic and sympathizing eyes. Arch Ophthalmol 1964;72:9–15.

21. Lubin JR, Albert DM, Weinstein M: Sixty-five years of sympathetic ophthalmia: A clinicopathological review of 105 cases (1913–1978). Ophthalmology 1980;87:109–121.

22. Jakobiec FA, Marboe CC, Knowles DM II, et al: Human sympathetic ophthalmia. An analysis of the inflammatory infiltrate by hybridoma monoclonal antibodies, immunohistochemistry, and correlative electron microscopy. Ophthalmology 1983;90:76–95.

23. Chan CC, Ben Ezra D, Rodrigues MM, et al: Immunohistochemistry and electron microscopy of choroidal infiltrates and Dalen-Fuchs nodules in sympathetic ophthalmia. Ophthalmology 1985;92:690–695.

24. de Veer JA: Bilateral endophthalmitis phacoanaphylactica. Arch Ophthalmol 1953;49:607–632.

25. Blodi FC: Sympathetic uveitis as an allergic phenomenon. Trans Am Acad Ophthalmol Otolaryngol 1959;63:642–649.

26. Elschnig A: Studien zur sympathischen ophthalmie. Die antigene Wirkung des Augenpigmentes. Arch Ophthalmol 1910;76:509.

27. Wong VG, Anderson R, O'Brien PJ: Sympathetic ophthalmia and lymphocyte transformation. Am J Ophthalmol 1971;72:960–965.

28. Chan CC, Palestine AG, Nussenblatt RB, et al: Antiretinal autoantibodies in Vogt-Koyanagi-Harada syndrome, Behçet's disease, and sympathetic ophthalmia. Ophthalmology 1985;92:1025–1028.

29. Rao NA, Robin J, Hartmann D, et al: The role of the penetrating wound in the development of sympathetic ophthalmia. Experimental observations. Arch Ophthalmol 1983;101:102–104.

30. Joy HH: Sympathetic ophthalmia: The history of its pathogenic studies. Am J Ophthalmol 1953;36:1100–1120.

31. Streilein JW, Niederkorn JY, Shadduck JA: Systemic immune unresponsiveness induced in adult mice by anterior chamber presentation of minor histocompatibility antigens. J Exp Med 1980;152:112–125.

32. Williamson JSP, Bradley D, Streilein JW: Immunoregulatory properties of bone marrow derived cells in the iris and ciliary body. Immunology 1989;67:96–102.

33. Mizuno K, Clark AF, Streilein JW: Ocular injection of retinal S antigen: Suppression of autoimmune uveitis. Invest Ophthalmol Vis Sci 1989;30:182–184.

34. Reynard M, Schulman IA, Azen SP, Minckler D: Histocompatibility antigens in sympathetic ophthalmia. Am J Ophthalmol 1983;95:216–221.

35. Sugiura S: Vogt-Koyanagi-Harada disease. Jpn J Ophthalmol 1978;22:9–35.

36. Davis JL, Mittal KK, Freidlin V, et al: HLA association and ancestry in VKH and sympathetic ophthalmia. Ophthalmology 1990;97:1137–1142.

37. Ohno S, Minakawa R, Matsuda H: Clinical studies on Vogt-Koyanagi-Harada's disease. Jpn J Ophthalmol 1988;32:334–343.

38. Gion N, Stavrou P, Foster CS: Immunomodulatory therapy for chronic tubulointerstitial nephritis associated uveitis (TINU). Am J Ophthalmol 2000;129:764–768.

39. Reynard M, Riffenburgh RS, Maes EF: Effect of corticosteroid treatment and enucleation on the visual prognosis of sympathetic ophthalmia. Am J Ophthalmol 1983;96:290–294.

40. Makley TA, Azar A: Sympathetic ophthalmia: A long term follow up. Arch Ophthalmol 1978;96:257–262.

41. Nussenblatt RB, Palestine AG: Sympathetic ophthalmia. In: Uveitis Fundamentals and Clinical Practice. Chicago, Year Book, 1989, pp 257–271.

42. Chan CC, Roberge FG, Whitecup SM, et al: Thirty-two cases of sympathetic ophthalmia: A retrospective study at the National Eye Institute, USA from 1982–1992. Arch Ophthalmol 1995;113:597–600.

43. Towler HMA, Whiting PH, Forrester JV: Combination low-dose cyclosporin A and steroid therapy in chronic intraocular inflammation. Eye 1990;4:514–520.

44. Jennings T, Tessler H: Twenty cases of sympathetic ophthalmia. Br J Ophthalmol 1989;73:140–145.

45. Hakin KN, Pearson RV, Lightman SL: Sympathetic ophthalmia: Visual results with modern immunosuppressive therapy. Eye 1992;6:453–455.

67

VOGT-KOYANAGI-HARADA SYNDROME

Nattaporn Tesavibul

DEFINITION AND HISTORY

Vogt-Koyanagi-Harada syndrome (VKH), formerly known as uveomeningitic syndrome, is a systemic disorder involving multiple organ systems, including the ocular, auditory, nervous, and integumentary systems. Severe bilateral panuveitis associated with exudative retinal detachment is the hallmark of ocular disease. It was first described by a Persian physician, Ali-ibn-Isa (940 to 1010 AD),[1] who reported whitening of the eyelashes, eyebrows, and hair (poliosis) associated with inflammation of the eyes. In 1873, this association was reported again by Schenkl,[2] followed by Hutchinson[3] in 1892 and Vogt in 1906.[4] In 1926, Einosuke Harada described a posterior uveitis associated with exudative retinal detachment and cerebrospinal fluid (CSF) pleocytosis.[5] Koyanagi in 1929 described patients with bilateral iridocyclitis associated with vitiligo, alopecia, and poliosis accompanied by tinnitus and deafness.[6] In 1932, Babel,[7] and later in 1949 Bruno and McPherson,[8] consolidated the descriptions of Vogt, Koyanagi, and Harada and suggested that these signs and symptoms are manifestations in a spectrum of the same underlying disease process, and that only the intensity and distribution varies from patient to patient. Since then, the term uveomeningo-encephalitic syndrome has been commonly replaced by VKH.

EPIDEMIOLOGY

The disease has a worldwide distribution but has a predilection for darkly pigmented races such as Asians, Hispanics, and Native Americans. In the United States, Nussenblatt and coworkers reported that 44% of the patients in their series were blacks.[9] VKH is uncommon in whites.[10] It is a common cause of endogenous uveitis in Japan, constituting at least 8% of cases.[10] This is also true for certain parts of Latin America, particularly Brazil. In the United States, it accounts for 1% to 4% of all uveitis referrals.[11, 12]

There appears to be some global variation in gender predilection of these patients, but most studies suggest that women are affected somewhat more frequently than men.[11–16]

Most patients are in the second to fifth decades of life at the onset of the disease,[10–13, 16] although Cunningham and colleagues reported a 4-year-old boy with the disease.[17]

CLINICAL MANIFESTATIONS

The clinical course has been divided into four distinct phases.[10] The *prodromal phase* mimics a systemic viral infection. Symptoms include fever, headache, nausea, vertigo, orbital pain, and neurologic involvement such as meningismus. Tinnitus is a characteristic clinical symptom. Additionally, less common neurologic symptoms include ataxia, confusion, and focal neurologic signs. Symptoms usually last for a few days and are followed by an *acute uveitic phase* that may last for several weeks. Seventy per-

cent of VKH patients present to ophthalmologic attention during this phase with bilateral uveitis.[10] In 30%, there may be a delay of 1 to 3 days before the second eye becomes involved. Thickening of the posterior choroid, manifested as an elevation of the peripapillary retinochoroidal layer, and disc hyperemia are early findings.[18] Subsequent retinal pigment epithelium (RPE) barrier breakdown causes subretinal fluid accumulation and multiple serous retinal detachments (Fig. 67–1).

As the disorder evolves, optic nerve head swelling is noted in 87% of the cases,[19] usually accompanying severe inflammation. The findings associated with posterior uveitis, serous retinal detachment, and CSF pleocytosis in the absence of extraocular manifestations are often termed Harada's form of this syndrome. Early in the course of the disease, exudative retinal detachment may appear as retinal striae secondary to choroidal folds. In addition, exudative maculopathy may vary from loculated to multifocal to frank bullous exudative retinal detachment, the pathophysiology being choroidal inflammation leading to RPE derangement and subsequent exudative retinal detachment.

Eventually the inflammation, which is usually granulomatous, extends to the anterior segment, causing muttonfat keratic precipitates and iris nodules (Fig. 67–2). Early on, the anterior chamber may be shallow[20] because of ciliary edema,[21, 22] serous detachment of the ciliary body,[23–25] and forward displacement of the lens-iris diaphragm, which resolves after the inflammation subsides. This may cause a moderate rise in intraocular pressure[20] and acute angle-closure glaucoma.[22, 26] Corneal anesthesia, tonic pupils, and accommodative impairment have been reported in one case.[27] Bilateral iridocyclitis associated with vitiligo, poliosis, and auditory problems are widely known as the Vogt-Koyanagi form of this disease.

The *convalescent phase* follows gradually, with skin and uveal depigmentation. Sugiura's sign or perilimbal vitiligo is the earliest depigmentation to occur, often within 1

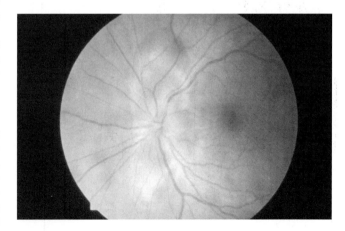

FIGURE 67–1. Optic disc edema and exudative retinal detachment in early VKH syndrome. (See color insert.)

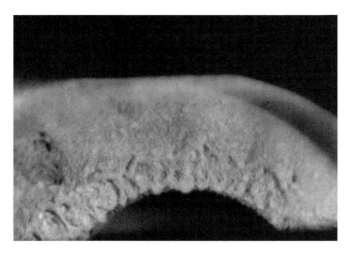

FIGURE 67–2. Multiple iris Koeppe nodules in a patient with VKH syndrome. (Courtesy C. S. Foster, M.D.)

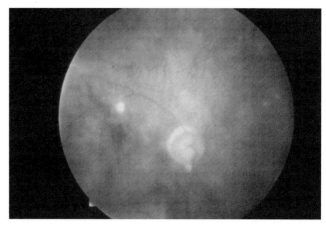

FIGURE 67–4. "Blond" appearance of fundus in Asian patient after the active inflammatory stage of VKH syndrome. (See color insert.)

month of disease onset.[28] This form of depigmentation is reported to occur in 85% of Japanese patients and is virtually unheard of in white patients (Fig. 67–3).[19] Depigmentation of the choroid causing sunset-glow appearance of the fundus occurs 2 or 3 months after the uveitic phase and is more common in Asian patients (Fig. 67–4).[18] Foci of hyperpigmentation from RPE alterations can be found, especially in Hispanic patients.[29] Yellow-white, well-circumscribed lesions similar to Dalen-Fuchs nodules in sympathetic ophthalmia are common, usually in the mid periphery (Fig. 67–5). The convalescent phase may last for several months.

This stage may be interrupted by the *chronic recurrent phase,* which manifests as a recurrent, mainly anterior uveitis. Recurrent posterior uveitis is uncommon. These episodes of granulomatous uveitis are often resistant to steroid therapy. Another characteristic finding in recurrent disease is the development of iris nodules. Focal pigment atrophy of the iris may also occur. Complications of chronic inflammation such as glaucoma, cataract, neovascularization of the retina and disc, arteriovenous anas-

tomosis,[30] and subretinal neovascular membrane (SRNVM) formation usually develop during this stage.

EXTRAOCULAR MANIFESTATIONS

Because VKH is a systemic disease with no confirmatory laboratory tests, the presence of extraocular manifestations is very important in securing the diagnosis. Some authors assert that even with ocular findings typical of this disease, VKH cannot be definitively diagnosed without concurrent extraocular findings.[9] However, the incidence of extraocular manifestations varies markedly in different reported series, which may reflect racial differences in the expression of these findings.

Integumentary System

Integumentary system involvement is seen at various stages of the disease. Seventy-two percent of patients report sensitivity to touch of the hair and skin in the prodromal stage.[10, 19] Alopecia has been reported in 73% of VKH patients in one study[31] but in only 13% of patients reported by Beniz and coworkers.[13] Poliosis and vitiligo usually occur during the convalescent stage. The occurrence of vitiligo varies from 10% to 63% between races

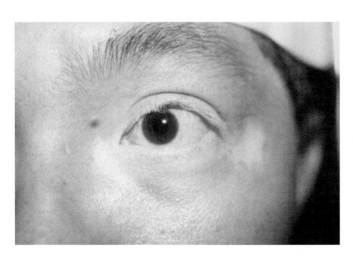

FIGURE 67–3. Periocular vitiligo in an Asian patient with VKH syndrome. Note also the poliosis of cilia nasally, upper lid. (See color insert.)

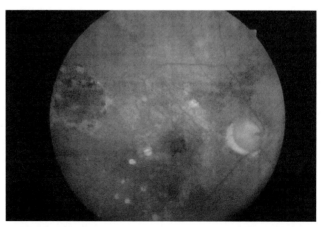

FIGURE 67–5. Fundus photo from the same patient demonstrating advanced glaucomatous optic disc cupping, severe chorioretinal scar with severe RPE alteration, and old Dalen-Fuchs nodules. (See color insert.)

(see Fig. 67–3 and Fig. 67–6).[13, 31] Hispanic people have a lower incidence of dermatologic involvement,[13] whereas Asians are more commonly affected. Axillary involvement of vitiligo is frequently overlooked by patients and physicians alike (see Fig. 67–4).

Neurologic Manifestations

Headache, confusion, orbital pain, and stiff neck are common in the prodromal stage. Headache was by far the most common neurologic complaint in a study reported by Beniz and coworkers.[13] CSF pleocytosis with a predominance of lymphocytes and monocytes and normal glucose have been found in more than 80% of patients with VKH and may persist for up to 8 weeks.[10, 11] Focal neurologic signs such as cranial neuropathies, hemiparesis, aphasia, transverse myelitis, and ganglionitis, although rare, have been reported.[32, 33]

Auditory Manifestations

Auditory problems occur in 75% of the patients, often concomitant with active ocular disease.[31, 34] Hearing loss usually involves the high frequencies but may affect all frequencies in the early stage.[35] Improvement is often noted in 2 to 3 months, although persistent alterations may occur.[10] Vestibular dysfunction is uncommon.[18]

ETIOLOGY AND PATHOGENESIS

Although the exact etiology of VKH is unknown, the disease is thought to be a primarily inflammatory condition directed against melanin-containing cells or a common antigen expressed therein and shared by the skin, eye, meninges, and ear. Alternatively, some investigators have invoked a primary infectious etiology, and others postulate a microbe as initiating or triggering the autoimmune process.

Several studies have suggested that the inflammation in VKH may represent a cellular immune process directed against melanocytes.[10, 36–39] Close contact between lymphocytes and uveal melanocytes as seen on electron microscopy with locally associated choroidal basement membrane destruction has been demonstrated.[36] Lymphocytes from peripheral blood and CSF of patients with the disease have been shown to be cytotoxic to the B-36 mela-

noma cell line.[37, 40] McClellan and coworkers also found interleukin (IL)-2–dependent T cells with specificity toward normal melanocytes, as well as melanoma cells.[41] These studies suggest that autoimmunity to melanocytes in the uveal tract and integumentary system may be pathogenetic in the development of inflammation in the eyes, other parts of the nervous system, and skin in VKH patients.

Attempts to identify antigens causing ocular inflammation in VKH have yielded contradictory results. DeSmet and colleagues[42] found no lymphocyte proliferation in the presence of retinal antigens in patients with chronic VKH, whereas a study by Naidu and colleagues showed a positive response to retinal S-antigen and interphotoreceptor retinoid binding protein in untreated patients with active disease.[43] Autoantibodies against photoreceptor outer segments and Müller cells have been detected in the sera of VKH patients.[44] However, these antibodies could be a secondary response that follows retinal damage in patients with this disease.

HISTOPATHOLOGY

The major histopathologic feature of VKH is a diffuse granulomatous inflammation of the uveal tract with a preponderance of lymphocytes and epithelioid cells. Some investigators reported a nongranulomatous inflammation.[38, 45–48] Dalen-Fuchs nodules, consisting of epithelioid cells, macrophages, lymphocytes, and altered RPE cells, are often present in the chronic stage.[47] In longstanding cases, the retina may be gliotic, with areas of RPE alteration. The choriocapillaris is usually but not always involved, followed by the disappearance of choroidal melanocytes, chorioretinal scarring,[47, 49, 50] and, occasionally, choroidal neovascularization.[51] Although much has been said about the differences histologically between VKH and sympathetic ophthalmia, with choriocapillaris sparing in the former, it is clear that standard histologic study cannot definitively differentiate one from the other. Recent studies of sympathetic ophthalmia and VKH suggest that anti-inflammatory products secreted by the RPE, including transforming growth factor-beta (TGF-β) and RPE protective protein, may allow preservation of the retina and choriocapillaris by the suppression of oxidant release in the inflamed choroid. This may save the uvea from necrotic damage and extensive inflammatory cell infiltration.[52]

Immunocytology

Immunohistochemical studies in active VKH revealed an increased ratio of T-helper to T-suppressor cells, and activated T lymphocytes with CD25 and CD26 markers within choroidal inflammatory foci.[38, 45, 53] The same results were also reported on skin biopsy specimens from vitiligo patches of these patients.[54] In contrast, patients in the convalescent stage of VKH, evaluated by Inomata and Sakamoto[46] and Sakamoto and coworkers,[55] demonstrated a ratio of 2:3 for CD4+ cells to CD8+ cells. This has also been demonstrated in studies by Ariga and coworkers[56] and Nonaka and coworkers.[57] The disappearance of choroidal melanocytes has also been reported.[46, 55] Choroidal melanocytes do not normally express more than minimal amounts of class II major histocompatibility

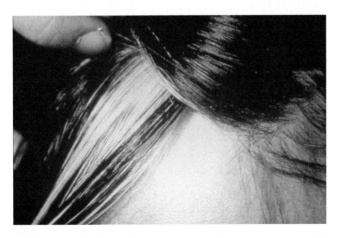

FIGURE 67–6. Vitiligo of hair (white forelock) in a patient with VKH. (Courtesy C. S. Foster, M.D.) (See color insert.)

(MHC) proteins. However, these proteins have been found in large quantity in the choroidal melanocytes and the endothelium of the choriocapillaris of VKH patients.[38] This suggests that T-cell–mediated delayed-type hypersensitivity against choroidal melanocytes that aberrantly express class II MHC antigens may contribute to the autoimmune inflammatory process.

CD4+ cells are reported to be more numerous than CD8+ cells in the aqueous humor of patients with acute disease. This proportion is reversed in convalescent disease.[58] The majority of CD4+ lymphocytes in aqueous humor and CSF from patients with active VKH disease expressed memory marker and Fas antigen.[59, 60] Okubo and coworkers reported a decrease in the total number of T cells (OKT3+), helper T cells (OKT4+), and suppressor T cells (OKT11+) in the peripheral blood of patients with active disease.[61] Liu and Sun noted that the CD4/CD8 ratio was increased in patients with active recurrent disease.[62] Okubo and coworkers also reported an increased number of cells with DR expression in patients whose disease recurred.[61]

High levels of IL-2 and interferon-gamma (IFN-γ) in patients' serum,[63] and increased levels of IL-6 in aqueous humor[58] during active disease have also been reported. T-cell clones from aqueous humor of VKH patients were found to produce significantly larger amounts of IL-8, IL-6, and IFN-γ than T-cell clones from healthy donors. These results suggest that cytokines produced by T cells infiltrating in the eye may play a role in the pathogenesis of VKH.[64]

GENETIC FACTORS
Among Chinese, Japanese, and Hispanic persons, there is a strong association between HLA-DR4 and -Dw53 with VKH.[65–69] HLA-DR4 has also been reported to be related to VKH disease in Italian and Brazilian patients.[70, 71] Martinez and colleagues reported HLA-DRw52 in VKH patients of Cherokee ancestry.[72] The role of genetics in VKH is strengthened by reports of familial cases (siblings and monozygotic twins).[73–75]

DIAGNOSIS
Patients with VKH who manifest all the ocular and extraocular manifestations pose little diagnostic uncertainty, but unfortunately they are rare. Given the wide variation in clinical presentation, the American Uveitis Society adopted the following criteria in 1978 for the diagnosis of VKH[12]:

1. No history of ocular trauma or surgery
2. At least three of four of the following signs:
   a. Bilateral chronic iridocyclitis
   b. Posterior uveitis, including exudative retinal detachment, disc hyperemia or edema, and sunset glow fundus
   c. Neurologic signs of tinnitus, neck stiffness, headache, cranial nerve or central nervous system problems or CSF pleocytosis
   d. Dermatologic manifestations of alopecia, poliosis, or vitiligo

These criteria were offered as general guidelines for the diagnosis of VKH.

INVESTIGATION
Although the diagnosis of VKH is made by clinical examination, laboratory tests may be useful for supporting the diagnosis and assisting management.

Fluorescein Angiography
Fluorescein angiography (FA) in the acute stage of VKH is characteristic and typically demonstrates multiple punctate hyperfluorescent dots at the level of the RPE. These hyperfluorescent dots gradually enlarge and pool in the subretinal fluid underlying areas of exudative retinal detachment.[76–78] Seventy percent of the patients have disc leakage in the acute phase (Fig. 67–7).[76] In the chronic stage, the angiogram shows multiple hyperfluorescent RPE window defects or areas of blocked fluorescence corresponding to RPE atrophy or hyperpigmentation. Alternating hyper- and hypofluorescence from RPE alteration may give a moth-eaten appearance.[29] SRNVM, retinochoroidal anastomoses, and neovascularization of the disc were also documented.[76] Vascular leakage, sheathing, and staining are rare.[12, 18, 76, 79]

Indocyanine Green Angiography
Indocyanine green angiography shows a dark background in the early phase.[80] This finding may be detected as early as the prodromal stage of the disease.[81] During the midphase of the angiogram, multiple patchy hypofluorescent lesions in the posterior fundus, which may represent areas of choroidal inflammation and circulatory disturbance, have been described. These lesions are more numerous than areas either of serous retinal detachment or of punctate hyperfluorescence seen on FA. In severe cases, hyperfluorescent spots are also visible throughout the entire fundus. In the recovery stage of the disease, the dark background resolves and the patchy hypofluorescent lesions slowly disappear after the disease activity has subsided in most cases.[80]

Ultrasonography and Ultrasound Biomicroscopy
Ultrasonography is often helpful in making a diagnosis and planning management when the fundus view is ob-

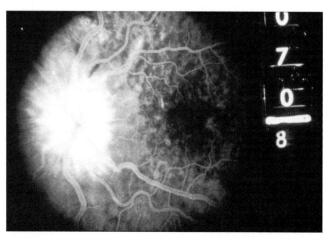

FIGURE 67–7. Fluorescein angiogram of a patient with VKH. Note the characteristic starry night appearance produced by the multitude of hot spots of active choroiditis.

scure, when presentation is atypical, or if extraocular signs are absent. Echographic manifestations of VKH were described by Forster and colleagues as follows[82]:

1. Diffuse thickening of the posterior choroid with low to medium reflectivity
2. Serous retinal detachment around posterior pole or inferiorly
3. Vitreous opacities without posterior vitreous detachment
4. Posterior thickening of the sclera or episclera

Scleritis, tuberculosis, sarcoidosis, leukemia, and lymphoma are other diseases with similar ultrasonographic findings.

Ultrasound biomicroscopy of the anterior chamber by several investigators has demonstrated ciliochoroidal detachment, which directly explains the shallow anterior chamber encountered in the early stage of VKH.[22–25]

Lumbar Puncture

Lumbar puncture has not been used routinely as a diagnostic procedure in most recent studies. In a report by Ohno and coworkers,[11] more than 80% of patients had CSF pleocytosis composed mainly of lymphocytes. CSF pleocytosis has been shown to occur within 1 week and to resolve within 8 weeks. Eighty-five percent of the lymphocytes in the CSF were OKT11+, and 65% were OKT4+.[83] Melanin-laden macrophages have been found in the CSF of patients with this disease.[84]

ELECTROENCEPHALOGRAPHY, ELECTRORETINOGRAPHY, AND ELECTROOCULOGRAPHY

Electrophysiologic tests are nondiagnostic in the setting of VKH. Abnormalities vary greatly, although worsening generally accompanies disease recurrence.[85]

Magnetic Resonance Imaging

Magnetic resonance imaging discriminates sclera from choroid and permits the differentiation of VKH from primary scleral disease. It also allows the detection of subclinical ocular and central nervous system (CNS) disease. Choroidal thickening can be demonstrated even when the fundus and FA appear normal.[86] Nonspecific punctate areas of high signal in the periventricular white matter and brain parenchyma have been reported.[86, 87]

Serologic Tests

No serologic tests have been proved useful in diagnosing VKH.

DIFFERENTIAL DIAGNOSIS

The differential diagnosis of VKH includes conditions that involve granulomatous inflammation, exudative retinal detachment, and white dot syndromes:

- Sympathetic ophthalmia
- Primary intraocular B-cell lymphoma
- Ocular Lyme disease
- Sarcoidosis
- Acute posterior multifocal placoid pigment epitheliopathy

- Multiple evanescent white dot syndrome
- Bilateral diffuse melanocytic hyperplasia
- Lupus choroidopathy
- Uveal effusion syndrome
- Posterior scleritis
- Other systemic disorders causing exudative retinal detachment, such as toxemia of pregnancy and renal disease

TREATMENT

Corticosteroids

The treatment of VKH usually begins with early and aggressive use of systemic steroids, to which this disease is quite responsive, particularly in the early stages. These may be tapered slowly, usually over 3 to 6 months. In severe cases, some investigators have employed high-dose pulsed steroid therapy intravenously (1 g of methylprednisolone) followed by oral prednisone 1 mg/kg/day is recommended.[88] The oral dosage may be as high as 2 mg/kg/day.[9] Hayasaka and colleagues[89] suggested that lower-dose steroids may be needed for the Harada form of the disease compared with the Vogt-Koyanagi type. Early and aggressive treatment appears to be associated with a shorter duration and less progression of the disease. A recent study by Sakaguchi and coworkers reported that hydrocortisone significantly suppressed the production of IL-6, IL-8, and granulocyte-macrophage colony-stimulating factor by T-cell clones from aqueous humor of VKH patients.[64]

Duration of treatment and rate of drug tapering is case specific depending on the clinical response. Rubsamen and Gass treated their patients with steroids for 6 months on average.[16] The average initial dosage was 80 to 100 mg/day. They found that recurrences occurred in 43% and 52% of their patients in the first 3 to 6 months, respectively, and these were associated with rapid tapering of the steroids. In the same study, 66% of their patients had a visual acuity of 20/30 or better at an average follow-up of 53 months. Nussenblatt and colleagues suggested that steroid treatment may continue for a year in some severe cases, with a slow and gradual taper.[9]

Associated anterior segment inflammation should also be treated with topical prednisolone 1% and cycloplegic drugs to lessen the inflammation and to reduce pain and synechiae. Topical steroids should be tapered according to the response.

Cytotoxic and Immunosuppressive Agents

Cytotoxic and immunosuppressive agents are reserved for patients who are refractory to corticosteroid therapy or for those who have developed unacceptable side effects thereof. Their use may also provide steroid-sparing effect, whereby the dose of steroid necessary to achieve quiescence is dramatically reduced or discontinued altogether.[90] Immunosuppressive or cytotoxic agents used in the management of VKH have been recommended by Moorthy and colleagues as follows[91]:

- Cyclophosphamide 1 to 2 mg/kg/day
- Chlorambucil 0.1 to 0.2 mg/kg/day; adjust every 3 weeks to maximum of 18 mg/day
- Azathioprine 1 to 2.5 mg/kg/day

- Cyclosporine 5 mg/kg/day, trough 0.1 to 0.4 μg/ml
- Tacrolimus (FK506) 0.1 to 0.15 mg/kg/day, trough <20 ng/ml

As previously discussed, the T-cell–mediated damage to melanocytes might be an immunopathologic basis of this disease. It is therefore appropriate to consider cyclosporine, which inhibits T-cell response and thus cell-mediated immunity, in treating VKH disease. Several studies support the use of cyclosporine in refractory cases, either alone or with low-dose steroids.[16, 90–95] Nussenblatt and colleagues reported such a steroid-sparing effect after using cyclosporine A.[90, 92] Similar results were described by Wakatsuki and coworkers[93] and Moorthy and coworkers.[91]

Cytotoxic agents have been used in the treatment of VKH and sympathetic ophthalmia with a positive therapeutic response, but the number of patients treated is small.[91, 96] Concerns regarding their myelosuppressive and toxic side effects may have limited their use.

A case report by Helveston and Gilmore described the use of azathioprine and intravenous immunoglobulin therapy with encouraging results.[97]

Nonmedical Treatment

In patients whose detachment did not resolve after adequate medical treatment, drainage of the nonrhegmatogenous detachment might prove beneficial. Rhegmatogenous retinal detachment can also occur and should be treated properly as quickly as the condition permits.

COMPLICATIONS

Three major complications of VKH for which therapy or surgical intervention may be required include cataracts, glaucoma, and SRNVM. Optic atrophy and pigmentary changes are also common.

Cataracts

Cataracts are reported to occur in 11% to 38% of the eyes involved as the result of both longstanding inflammation and steroid therapy.[11, 12, 16, 64, 98] Moorthy and coworkers found that cataracts developed in 26 of their 65 patients over the course of therapy.[98] In their study, steroid therapy for longer than 6 months and chronic recurrent anterior segment inflammation appeared to be significant determinants of cataract development.

Cataract extraction can be performed safely and can result in significant visual improvement in these patients, provided that pre- and postoperative management are judicious. Inflammation should be controlled for at least 3 months prior to surgery. In the same study by Moorthy and colleagues,[98] 19 eyes underwent cataract surgery after 3 months of minimal or no inflammation. These patients were also treated with pre- and postoperative steroids. After surgery, median visual acuity improved significantly from 20/400 to 20/40 after a median follow-up time of 13 months. Some investigators have suggested that intraocular lens placement can be performed safely in selected cases without exacerbation of the disease.[98–102] However, it should be kept in mind that extensive synechiae and lens capture by iris, as well as precipitates on the surface of the lens may develop after the surgery.

Glaucoma

Glaucoma is a common complication of VKH. Acute angle-closure glaucoma has been reported, presumably as a result of ciliary body edema with anterior displacement of the lens-iris diaphragm in the acute stage of the disease.[20, 21, 26] In chronic cases, glaucoma secondary to chronic angle closure from extensive peripheral anterior synechiae and posterior synechiae has been reported in 6% to 45% of patients (see Fig. 67–5).[11, 16, 34, 103] Open-angle glaucoma secondary to corticosteroid use can occur during the treatment. In a study by Forster and colleagues,[103] evidence of glaucoma was noted in 16 (38%) of 42 patients. Eleven patients (69%) required surgical intervention. In patients with angle closure secondary to pupillary block, laser iridotomy appears to have a lower success rate than surgical iridectomy. Adjunctive 5-fluorouracil or mitomycin C may increase the success rate of trabeculectomy when filtering surgery was required.[12, 26] Implantation of aqueous drainage devices may be preferred in patients with persistent inflammation.[103]

Subretinal Neovascularization

Along with cataracts and glaucoma, SRNVM formation is an important cause of late visual loss in patients with VKH. Snyder and Tessler[12] reported an incidence of 5% in their patients, and Ober and coworkers found 36% in their series. In a recent study by Moorthy and colleagues,[104] SRNVM developed in 10 (9%) of 116 eyes with VKH disease, which was consistent with an earlier report by Rubsamen and Gass.[16] The presence of extensive fundus pigmentary derangement or chronically recurrent inflammation, and recurrence of predominantly anterior segment inflammation appear to be risk factors for the development of SRNVM in VKH.[104] There is a propensity for the SRNVM to develop in the peripapillary, subfoveal, and extrafoveal macular regions, where inflammatory foci appear to be concentrated in these areas.[51, 104] The visual outcome of eyes with SRNVMs is generally poor. The use of indocyanine green angiography may be a useful adjunct in the laser treatment of these patients. With early recognition and appropriate intervention, visual acuity may be preserved in some cases.

PROGNOSIS

The use of corticosteroids and immunosuppressive agents has greatly improved the visual outcome in VKH patients. Overall prognosis of VKH is fair, with 48% to 93% of patients retaining visual acuity of 20/40 or better. Moorthy and colleagues showed that 53% of 130 eyes studied had final visual acuity of 20/30 or better after treatment for a mean of 5.6 months.[91] Rubsamen and Gass reported that 66% of the patients had a final visual acuity of 20/30 or better with corticosteroids and/or immunosuppressive treatment with a mean follow-up time of 53 months.[16] Seven percent of the eyes followed had a visual acuity of less than 20/400. These investigators cited three factors to be predictive of poor visual outcome: (1) increased age at the onset of the disease, (2) chronic inflammation requiring prolonged treatment with corticosteroids, and (3) SRNVM.[16]

CONCLUSIONS

VKH is a systemic disorder involving multiple organ systems, including the ocular, auditory, nervous, and integumentary systems. The etiology is unknown. Autoimmunity to melanocytes in the uveal tract and integumentary system is believed to be the pathogenesis. In the early stage of the disease, patients usually present with bilateral panuveitis, exudative retinal detachment, and optic disc hyperemia. Neurologic involvement such as headache, meningismus, and CSF pleocytosis is common. Fundus and skin depigmentation occurs months after the initial onset of the disease. The diagnosis of VKH is a clinical one, with FA, B-scan ultrasonography, and lumbar puncture being useful adjuvants diagnostically and in following the course of the disease. Systemic corticosteroids are the mainstay of treatment, with immunosuppressive agents being useful in refractory cases or as steroid-sparing agents in patients who have become intolerant of steroids or who have developed unacceptable steroid-induced side effects. The overall prognosis is fair, with a substantial number of patients achieving visual acuity of 20/50 or better with early and aggressive treatment. Ultimate visual potential may be limited by the development of cataract, glaucoma, and choroidal neovascular membrane.

References

1. Pattison EM: Uveo-meningoencephalitic syndrome (Vogt-Koyanagi-Harada). Arch Neurol 1965;12:197–205.
2. Schenkl A: Ein Fall von plotzlich aufgetretener poliosis circumscripta der wimpern. Arch Dermatol Syph 1873;5:137–139.
3. Hutchinson J: A case of blanched eyelashes. Arch Surg 1892;4:357.
4. Vogt A: Fruhzeitiges ergrauen der Zilien und bemerkungen uber den sogenannten plotzlichen eintritt dieser veranderung. Klin Monatsbl Augenheilkd 1906;4:228–242.
5. Harada E: Beitrag zur klinischen kenntnis von michteitriger choroiditis (choroiditis diffusa acta). Acta Soc Ophthalmol Jpn 1926;30:356–378.
6. Koyanagi Y: Dysakusis, alopecia und poliosis bei schwerer uveitis nicht traumatischen ursprungs. Klin Monatsbl Augenheilkd 1929;82:194–211.
7. Babel J: Syndrome de Vogt-Koyanagi (Uveite bilaterale, poliosis, alopecie, vitiligo et dysacousie). Schweiz Med Wochenschr Nr 1932;44:1136–1140.
8. Bruno MG, McPherson SD Jr: Harada's disease. Am J Ophthalmol 1949;32:513–522.
9. Nussenblatt RB, Whitcup SM, Palestine AG: Vogt-Koyanagi-Harada syndrome. In: Nussenblatt RB, Whitcup SM, Palestine AG, eds: Uveitis: Fundamental and Clinical Practice, 2nd ed. St. Louis, Mosby, 1996, pp 312–324.
10. Sugiura S: Vogt-Koyanagi-Harada disease. Jpn J Ophthalmol 1978;22:9–35.
11. Ohno S, Char DH, Kimura SJ, et al: Vogt-Koyanagi-Harada syndrome. Am J Ophthalmol 1977;87:735–740.
12. Snyder DA, Tessler HH: Vogt-Koyanagi-Harada syndrome. Am J Ophthalmol 1980;90:69–75.
13. Beniz J, Forster DJ, Lean JS, et al: Variations in clinical features of the Vogt-Koyanagi-Harada syndrome. Retina 1991;11:275–280.
14. Murakami S, Inaba Y, Mochizuki M, et al: A nationwide survey on the occurrence of Vogt-Koyanagi-Harada disease in Japan. Jpn J Ophthalmol 1994;38:208–213.
15. Nussenblatt RB: Clinical studies of Vogt-Koyanagi-Harada's disease at the National Eye Institute, NIH USA. Jpn J Ophthalmol 1988;32:330–333.
16. Rubsamen PE, Gass JDM: Vogt-Koyanagi-Harada syndrome: Clinical course, therapy, and long-term visual outcome. Arch Ophthalmol 1991;109:682–687.
17. Cunningham ET, Demetrius R, Frieden IJ, et al: Vogt-Koyanagi-Harada syndrome in a 4-year-old child. Am J Ophthalmol 1995;5:675–677.
18. Goto H, Rao NA: Sympathetic ophthalmia and Vogt-Koyanagi-Harada syndrome. Int Ophthalmol Clin 1990;30:279–285.
19. Ohno S, Minakawa R, Matsuda H: Clinical studies on Vogt-Koyanagi-Harada disease. Jpn J Ophthalmol 1988;32:334–343.
20. Kimura R, Sakai M, Okabe H: Transient shallow anterior chamber as initial symptom in Harada's syndrome. Arch Ophthalmol 1981;99:1604–1606.
21. Kimura R, Kasai M, Shoji K, et al: Swollen ciliary processes as an initial symptom in Vogt-Koyanagi-Harada syndrome. Am J Ophthalmol 1983;95:402–403.
22. Kishi A, Nao-i N, Sawada A: Ultrasound biomicroscopic findings of acute angle-closure glaucoma in Vogt-Koyanagi-Harada syndrome. Am J Ophthalmol 1996;122:735–737.
23. Gohdo T, Tsukahara S: Ultrasound biomicroscopy of shallow anterior chamber in the Vogt-Koyanagi-Harada syndrome. Am J Ophthalmol 1996;122:112–114.
24. Kawano YI, Tawara A, Niishioka Y, et al: Ultrasound biomicroscopic analysis of transient shallow anterior chamber in the Vogt-Koyanagi-Harada syndrome. Am J Ophthalmol 1996;121:720–722.
25. Maruyama Y, Kimura Y, Kishi S, et al: Serous detachment of the ciliary body in Harada disease. Am J Ophthalmol 1998;125:666–672.
26. Shirato S, Hayashi K, Masuda K: Acute angle closure glaucoma as an initial sign of Harada's disease—Report of 2 cases. Jpn J Ophthalmol 1980;24:260–266.
27. Brouzas D, Chatzoulis D, Galina E, et al: Corneal anesthesia in a case with Vogt-Koyanagi-Harada syndrome. Acta Ophthalmol Scand 1997;75:464–465.
28. Friedman AH, Deutsch-Sokol RH: Sugiura's sign: Perilimbal vitiligo in the Vogt-Koyanagi-Harada syndrome. Ophthalmology 1981;88:1159–1165.
29. Kanter PJ, Goldberg MF: Bilateral uveitis with exudative retinal detachment: Angiographic appearance. Arch Ophthalmol 1974;91:13–19.
30. Manager CC III, Ober RR: Retinal arteriovenous anastomoses in the Vogt-Koyanagi-Harada syndrome. Am J Ophthalmol 1980;89:186–191.
31. Rosen E: Uveitis with poliosis, vitiligo, alopecia and dysacusia (Vogt-Koyanagi syndrome). Arch Ophthalmol 1945;33:281–292.
32. Lubin JR, Lowenstein JI, Frederick AR Jr: Vogt-Koyanagi-Harada syndrome with focal neurologic signs. Am J Ophthalmol 1981;91:332–341.
33. Trebini F, Appiotti A, Bacci R, et al: Vogt-Koyanagi-Harada syndrome: Clinical and instrumental contribution. Ital J Neurol Sci 1991;12:479–484.
34. Minnakawa R, Ohno S, Hirose S, et al: Clinical manifestations of Vogt-Koyanagi-Harada disease. Jpn J Clin Ophthalmol 1985;39:1249–1253.
35. Hoshi H, Tamada Y, Murata Y, et al: Changes in audiogram in the course of Harada's disease. Jpn J Clin Ophthalmol 1977;31:23–30.
36. Matsuda H, Sugiura S: Ultrastructural changes of the melanocyte in Vogt-Koyanagi-Harada syndrome and sympathetic ophthalmia. Jpn J Ophthalmol 1971;15:69–80.
37. Norose K, Yano A, Aosai F, et al: Immunologic analysis of cerebrospinal fluid lymphocytes in Vogt-Koyanagi-Harada disease. Invest Ophthalmol Vis Sci 1990;31:1210–1216.
38. Sakamoto T, Murata T, Inomata H: Class II major histocompatibility complex on melanocytes of Vogt-Koyanagi-Harada disease. Arch Ophthalmol 1991;109:1270–1274.
39. Tagawa Y: Lymphocyte-mediated cytotoxicity against melanocyte antigens in Vogt-Koyanagi-Harada syndrome. Jpn J Ophthalmol 1978;22:36–41.
40. Ariga H, Ohno S, Higuchi M, et al: Immunological studies on lymphocytes in the cerebrospinal fluid of patients with Vogt-Koyanagi-Harada disease and sympathetic ophthalmia. Nippon Ganka Ogakkai Zasshi 1988;92:225–228.
41. McClellan KA, MacDonald M, Hersey P, et al: Vogt-Koyanagi-Harada syndrome—Isolation of cloned T cells with specificity for melanocytes and melanoma cells. Aust N Z J Ophthalmol 1989;17:347–352.
42. DeSmet MD, Yamamoto JH, Mochizuki M, et al: Cellular immune responses of patients with uveitis to retinal antigens and their fragments. Am J Ophthalmol 1990;110:135–142.
43. Naidu YM, Pararajasegaram G, Sun Y, et al: Predominant expression of T-cell antigen receptor (TCR) Vα10 in Vogt-Koyanagi-

Harada syndrome (abstract). Invest Ophthalmol Vis Sci 1991; 32(suppl):934.

44. Chan CC, Palestine AG, Nussenblatt RB, et al: Antiretinal auto-antibodies in Vogt-Koyanagi-Harada syndrome, Behçet's disease, and sympathetic ophthalmia. Ophthalmology 1985;92:1025–1028.

45. Chan CC, Palestine AG, Kuwabara T, et al: Immunopathologic study of Vogt-Koyanagi-Harada syndrome. Am J Ophthalmol 1988;105:607–611.

46. Inomata H, Sakamoto T: Immunohistochemical studies of Vogt-Koyanagi-Harada disease with sunset sky fundus. Curr Eye Res 1990;9(suppl):35–40.

47. Lubin JR, Ni C, Albert DM: A clinicopathological study of the Vogt-Koyanagi-Harada syndrome. Int Ophthalmol Clin 1982; 22:141–156.

48. Perry HD, Font RL: Clinical and histopathologic observations in severe Vogt-Koyanagi-Harada syndrome. Am J Ophthalmol 1977;83:242–254.

49. Rao NA, Marak GE: Sympathetic ophthalmia simulating Vogt-Koyanagi-Harada's disease: A clinico-pathologic study of four cases. Jpn J Ophthalmol 1983;27:506–511.

50. Spencer WH: Ophthalmic Pathology: An Atlas and Textbook, vol 3. Philadelphia, W.B. Saunders, 1985, pp 1956–1966.

51. Inomata H, Minei M, Taniguchi Y, et al: Choroidal neovascularization in long-standing case of Vogt-Koyanagi-Harada disease. Jpn J Ophthalmol 1983;27:9–26.

52. Rao NA: Mechanisms of inflammatory response in sympathetic ophthalmia and VKH syndrome. Eye 1997;11:213–216.

53. Kahn M, Pepose JS, Green R, et al: Immunocytologic findings in a case of Vogt-Koyanagi-Harada syndrome. Ophthalmology 1993;100:1191–1198.

54. Okada T, Sakamoto T, Ishibashi T, et al: Vitiligo in Vogt-Koyanagi-Harada disease: Immunohistological analysis of inflammatory site. Graefes Arch Clin Exp Ophthalmol 1996;234:359–363.

55. Sakamoto T, Inomata H, Sueishi K: Immunohistochemical analysis of Vogt-Koyanagi-Harada disease at the clinically convalescent stage. In: Usui M, Ohno S, Aoki K, eds: Ocular Immunology Today. Amsterdam, Elsevier, 1990, pp 371–374.

56. Ariga H, Ohno S, Higuchi M, et al: Immunohistochemical study on corneal limbus and vitiligo in Vogt-Koyanagi-Harada disease. Clin Immunol 1988;20:279–281.

57. Nonaka S, Takamura K, Goto H, et al: Lymphocyte subsets in the iris tissue with uveitis. Jpn J Ophthalmol 1986;40:447–451.

58. Norose K, Yano A, Wang X, et al: Dominance of activated T cells and interleukin-6 in aqueous humor in Vogt-Koyanagi-Harada disease. Invest Ophthalmol Vis Sci 1994;35:33–39.

59. Ohta K, Norose K, Wang XC, et al: Apoptosis-related fas antigen on memory T cells in aqueous humor of uveitis patients. Curr Eye Res 1996;15:299–306.

60. Ohta K, Yoshimura N: Expression of fas antigen on helper T lymphocytes in Vogt-Koyanagi-Harada disease. Graefes Arch Clin Exp Ophthalmol 1998;236:434–439.

61. Okubo K, Kurimoto S, Okubo K, et al: Surface markers of peripheral blood lymphocytes in Vogt-Koyanagi-Harada disease. J Clin Lab Immunol 1985;17:49–52.

62. Liu T, Sun SM: Peripheral lymphocyte subsets in patients with Vogt-Koyanagi-Harada syndrome (VKH). Chung Hua Yen Ko Tsa Chih 1993;29:138–140.

63. Rahi A, Rahi S, Rahi J: Phospholipid autoimmunity in the pathogenesis of vascular retinopathy. In: Usue M, Ohno S, Aoki K, eds: Ocular Immunology Today. Amsterdam, Elsevier, 1990, pp 317–320.

64. Sakaguchi M, Sugita S, Sagawa K, et al: Cytokine production by T cells infiltrating in the eye of uveitis patients. Jpn J Ophthalmol 1998;42:262–268.

65. Ohno S: Immunological aspects of Behçet's and Vogt-Koyanagi-Harada disease. Trans Ophthalmol Soc U K 1981;101:335–341.

66. Shindo Y, Inoko H, Yamamoto T, et al: HLA-DRBI typing of Vogt-Koyanagi-Harada disease by PCR-RFLP and the strong association with DRBI 0405 and DRBI 0410. Br J Ophthalmol 1994;78:223–226.

67. Weisz JM, Holland GN, Roer LN, et al: HLA associations in Hispanic patients with Vogt-Koyanagi-Harada syndrome. ARVO Abstracts. Invest Ophthalmol Vis Sci 1994;35(suppl):2097.

68. Zhang WY, Wang XM, Hu TS: Profiling human leukocyte antigens in Vogt-Koyanagi-Harada syndrome. Am J Ophthalmol 1992; 113:567–572.

69. Zhao M, Jiang Y, Abrahams IW: Association of HLA antigens with Vogt-Koyanagi-Harada syndrome in a Han Chinese population. Arch Ophthalmol 1991;109:368–370.

70. Goldberg AC, Yamamoto JH, Chiarella JM, et al: HLA-DRB1*0405 is the predominant allele in Brazilian patients with Vogt-Koyanagi-Harada disease. Hum Immunol 1998;59:183–188.

71. Pivetti-Pezzi P, Accorinti M, Colabelli-Gisoldi RA, et al: Vogt-Koyanagi-Harada disease and HLA type in Italians. Am J Ophthalmol 1996;122:889–891.

72. Martinez JA, Lopez PF, Sternberg P, et al: Vogt-Koyanagi-Harada syndrome in patients with Cherokee Indian ancestry. Am J Ophthalmol 1992;114:615.

73. Ishikawa A, Shino T, Uchida S: Vogt-Koyanagi-Harada disease in identical twins. Retina 1994;14:435–437.

74. Itho S, Kurimato S, Kouno T: Vogt-Koyanagi-Harada disease in monozygotic twins. Int Ophthalmol 1992;16:49–54.

75. Rutzen AR, Ortega-Larrocea G, Schwab IR, et al: Simultaneous onset of Vogt-Koyanagi-Harada syndrome in monozygotic twins. Am J Ophthalmol 1995;119:239–240.

76. Brinkley JR, Dugel PU, Rao NA: Fluorescein angiographic findings in Vogt-Koyanagi-Harada syndrome (abstract). Ophthalmology 1992;99(suppl):151.

77. Gass JDM: Harada's disease. In: Gass JDM, ed: Stereoscopic Atlas of Macular Disease. Diagnosis and Treatment. St. Louis, Mosby, 1987, pp 150–153.

78. Yoshioka H: Early fundus changes in Harada's syndrome. Jpn J Clin Ophthalmol 1967;21:135–141.

79. Okamura S: Harada's disease. Acta Soc Ophthalmol Jpn 1938;42:196.

80. Oshima Y, Harino S, Hara Y, et al: Indocyanine green angiographic findings in Vogt-Koyanagi-Harada disease. Am J Ophthalmol 1996;122:58–66.

81. Yuzawa M, Kawamura A, Matsui M: Indocyanine green video-angiographic findings in Harada's disease. Jpn J Ophthalmol 1993; 37:456–466.

82. Forster DJ, Cano MR, Green RL, et al: Echographic features of the Vogt-Koyanagi-Harada syndrome. Arch Ophthalmol 1990;108:1421–1426.

83. Okubo K, Kurimoto S, Okubo K, et al: Surface marker studies of cerebrospinal fluid lymphocytes in Vogt-Koyanagi-Harada disease. Nippon Ganka Gakkai Zasshi 1985;89:726–732.

84. Nakamura S, Nakazawa M, Yoshioka M, et al: Melanin-laden macrophages in cerebrospinal fluid in Vogt-Koyanagi-Harada syndrome. Arch Ophthalmol 1996;114:1184–1188.

85. Nagaya T: Use of the electro-oculogram for diagnosing and following the development of Harada's disease. Am J Ophthalmol 1972;74:99–109.

86. Ibanez HE, Grand MG, Meredith TA, et al: Magnetic resonance imaging findings in Vogt-Koyanagi-Harada syndrome. Retina 1994;14:164–168.

87. Ikeda M, Tsukagoshi H: Vogt-Koyanagi-Harada disease presenting meningoencephalitis. Report of a case with magnetic resonance imaging. Eur Neurol 1992;32:83–85.

88. Sasamoto Y, Ohno S, Matsuda H: Studies on corticosteroid therapy in Vogt-Koyanagi-Harada disease. Ophthalmologica 1990;201:162–167.

89. Hayasaka S, Okabe H, Takahashi J: Systemic corticosteroid treatment in Vogt-Koyanagi-Harada disease. Graefes Arch Clin Exp Ophthalmol 1982;218:9–13.

90. Nussenblatt RB, Palestine AG, Chan CC: Cyclosporin A therapy in the treatment of intraocular inflammatory disease resistant to systemic corticosteroids and cytotoxic agents. Am J Ophthalmol 1983;96:275–282.

91. Moorthy RS, Inomata H, Rao N: Vogt-Koyanagi-Harada syndrome. Surv Ophthalmol 1995;39:269–292.

92. Nussenblatt RB, Palestine AG, Rook AH, et al: Treatment of intraocular inflammatory disease with cyclosporin A. Lancet 1983; 2:235–238.

93. Wakatsuki Y, Kogure M, Takahashi Y, et al: Combination therapy with cyclosporin A and steroid in severe case of Vogt-Koyanagi-Harada disease. Jpn J Ophthalmol 1988;32:358–360.

94. Wakefield D, McCluskey P: Cyclosporin A therapy in inflammatory eye disease. J Ocul Pharmacol 1991;7:221–226.

95. Walton RC, Nussenblatt RB, Whitcup S: Cyclosporine therapy for severe sight-threatening uveitis in children and adolescents. Ophthalmology 1998;105:2028–2034.

96. Limon S, Girard P, Bloch-Michel E, et al: Les aspects actuels du syndrome du Vogt Koyanagi Harada. Apropos de 9 cas. J Fr Ophtalmol 1985;8:29–35.
97. Helveston WR, Gilmore R: Treatment of Vogt-Koyanagi-Harada syndrome with intravenous immunoglobulin. Neurology 1996;46:584–585.
98. Moorthy R, Rajeev B, Smith RE, et al: Incidence and management of cataracts in Vogt-Koyanagi-Harada syndrome. Am J Ophthalmol 1994;118:197–204.
99. Chung YM, Yeh TS: Intraocular lens implantation following extracapsular cataract extraction in uveitis. Ophthalmic Surg 1990;21:272–276.
100. Foster CS, Fong LP, Singh G: Cataract surgery and intraocular lens implantation in patients with uveitis. Ophthalmology 1989;96:281–288.
101. Foster RE, Lowder CY, Meisler DM, et al: Extracapsular cataract extraction and posterior chamber intraocular lens implantation in uveitis patients. Ophthalmology 1992;99:1234–1241.
102. Harada T, Takeuchi T, Kuno H, et al: Results of cataract surgery in patients with uveitis. J Fr Ophtalmol 1996;19:170–174.
103. Forster DJ, Rao NA, Hill RA, et al: Incidence and management of glaucoma in Vogt-Koyanagi-Harada syndrome. Ophthalmology 1993;100:613–618.
104. Moorthy RS, Chong LP, Smith RE, et al: Subretinal neovascular membranes in Vogt-Koyanagi-Harada syndrome. Am J Ophthalmol 1993;116:164–170.

68

MULTIFOCAL CHOROIDITIS AND PANUVEITIS

Albert T. Vitale and James G. Kalpaxis

DEFINITION

Multifocal choroiditis and panuveitis (MCP) is a posterior chorioretinal inflammatory disease of unknown etiology with prominent elements of vitritis and anterior segment uveitis. The acute chorioretinal lesions subsequently scar with proliferation of retinal pigment epithelium (RPE) and fibrosis, which may, in turn, lead to the frequent occurrence of choroidal neovascular membranes (CNVMs) and irreversible visual loss. Enlargement of the blind spot occurs frequently with MCP. This, together with multifocal chorioretinal pathology, with or without scarring, are features shared by a group of possibly related inflammatory syndromes of unknown etiology, namely, multiple evanescent white dot syndrome (MEWDS), punctate inner choroidopathy (PIC), and subretinal fibrosis and uveitis syndrome (SFU). Whether these syndromes represent distinct clinical entities or are a spectrum of a single disease remains controversial.

HISTORY

Nozik and Dorsch[1] first reported two distinctive cases of bilateral chorioretinopathy with anterior uveitis in late 1973, which resembled the presumed ocular histoplasmosis syndrome (POHS). By 1984, 28 additional patients with anterior uveitis, vitritis and multiple lesions at the level of the RPE were described by Dreyer and Gass,[2] who coined the descriptive term multifocal choroiditis and panuveitis, in contradistinction to POHS. Subsequently, Deutsch and Tessler[3] described 28 patients with inflammatory pseudohistoplasmosis, a condition that featured vitritis; however, systemically, the majority of these cases were presumed to have sarcoidosis, syphilis, or tuberculosis. Coincidentally, in 1984, Jampol and colleagues[4] used the term multiple evanescent white dot syndrome to describe a series of 11 young, predominantly female patients with acute, transient, monocular visual loss accompanied by numerous white dots in the fundus. In the same year, Watzke and colleagues[5] described punctate inner choroidopathy occurring in 10 healthy, young, myopic women who presented with visual symptoms in the absence of vitreous or anterior chamber inflammation, inner chorioretinal lesions that subsequently evolved into pigmented scars, and the frequent development of CNVMs. Subsequently, Morgan and Schatz[6] described a series of 11 patients with features of both MCP and PIC, which they termed recurrent multifocal choroiditis.

The syndrome of diffuse subretinal fibrosis was initially described in 1982 by Doran and Hamilton[7] in four patients with antecedent CNVMs. Palestine and associates[8] and later Cantrill and Folk[9] described two series of patients with progressive chorioretinal fibrosis, which appeared to be the terminal manifestation of a multifocal choroiditis of unknown etiology in young, healthy women, which could not be attributed to pre-existing CNVMs alone. We prefer the term subretinal fibrosis and uveitis for this entity, to underscore its inflammatory nature.

Recently, Reddy and colleagues[10] described the association of enlargement of the blind spot, together with other clinical, angiographic and electroretinographic features, in a group of 79 patients comprised of 41 with MCP, 16 with PIC, 6 with SFU, and 16 with MEWDS. Finally, the visual prognosis, incidence, treatment and natural history of CNVMs, and the medical management of this same group of patients were reviewed by Brown and colleagues.[11]

EPIDEMIOLOGY

MCP affects predominantly young, otherwise healthy adults in their mid-30s, with a range of 9 to 69 years.[2, 6, 10] In several series, patients were either exclusively women,[6] or women outnumbered men by more than 3:1.[2, 10] Moderate myopia was present in 10 of 11 women examined by Morgan and Schatz,[6] whereas a range of refractive errors from -9.00 to +2.50 diopters was reported by Reddy and colleagues.[10] There is no apparent racial or familial predilection. The geographic distribution and epidemiologic background of patients with MCP are distinctly different from those with POHS,[2] which is endemic to North American river valleys and other areas with a historically high prevalence of histoplasmin skin test positivity.[12]

CLINICAL CHARACTERISTICS

The majority of patients have bilateral disease, albeit asymmetric, with the involved fellow eye at times being totally quiescent and asymptomatic. Bilaterality ranged from 66% to 79% as reported by Reddy and coworkers[10] and Dreyer and Gass[2] respectively, whereas, this figure was only 45% in the series of Morgan and Schatz.[6]

Patients commonly present with blurred or decreased central vision and scotomata. Photopsias and floaters are less common complaints. Although the mean initial visual acuity in the 68 eyes of 41 patients with MCP reported by Brown and colleagues[11] was 20/50, the range may be considerable, varying from 20/20 to light perception.

Signs of mild to moderate anterior uveitis, including nongranulomatous keratic precipitates, posterior synechiae, and cells and flare, were observed in 52% of patients studied by Dreyer and Gass,[2] whereas 32% of those reported by Reddy and associates[10] exhibited anterior chamber cells. Similarly, mild to moderate vitreous cellular activity was more commonly observed in both series, and was present in 76%[10] and 100%[2] of patients, respectively. Biomicroscopic examination during the acute phase of MCP reveals multiple round to oval, yellow-gray lesions at the level of the RPE, ranging in size from 50 to 350 μm, and in number from several to more than 100, scattered

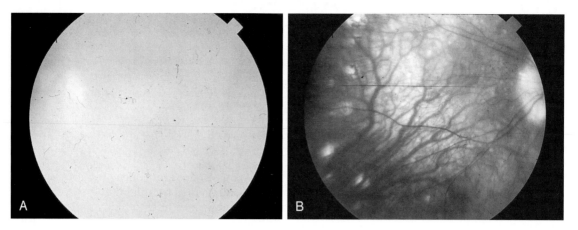

FIGURE 68–1. *A,* Typical picture of an eye affected by MCP, with vitreous cells (note the obscuration of a view of the retina) and multifocal lesions of inflammation in the choroid. *B,* Same eye as in 1*A* after successful control of the inflammation. Note the clearing of the vitreous, disclosing the multiple foci of prior inflammation in the choroid.

throughout the posterior pole and midperiphery (Fig. 68–1).[13] They may occur singly, in clusters, or in streak configuration, parallel to the ora serrata retinae as seen in POHS (Fig. 68–2).[14] A distinct propensity for a peripapillary and nasal midperipheral and peripheral distribution of these lesions has been observed.[10] The active lesions evolve into round, atrophic chorioretinal scars with a punched-out appearance and varying degrees of hyperpigmentation.

Optic disc swelling and hyperemia are not uncommon, occurring in 34% of 68 eyes examined by Reddy and associates.[10] Peripapillary atrophy, similar to that seen in POHS, is frequently seen on follow-up examination (Fig. 68–3). The development of cystoid macular edema (CME) is variable, occurring in 14% of eyes reported by Dreyer and Gass,[2] as opposed to 41% of patients with MCP studied at the National Eye Institute.[15] CNVMs, in either a macular or peripapillary location, have been observed in 32% to 46% of patients with MCP.[2, 6, 11]

Less commonly observed findings include retinal vasculitis[16] and retinal and optic disc neovascularization.[2]

Perimetry

Acute symptomatic enlargement of the blind spot in the absence of disc edema was initially described in three patients with MCP by Korram and coworkers,[17] who attributed the defect to peripapillary retinal dysfunction. Callanan and Gass[18] subsequently reported acute enlargement of the blind spot in seven patients who later developed findings consistent with MCP, four of whom had transient white dots typically seen in MEWDS, and suggested a common link in their etiology. Indeed, enlargement of the blind spot not solely attributable to disc swelling or peripapillary scarring was the most common visual field defect observed by Reddy and colleagues,[10] occurring in 47% of 51 eyes examined. In the same study, 22 eyes (43%) were found to have full visual fields, whereas 13 (25%), 4 (8%) and 2 (4%) eyes had central or paracentral, peripheral, and cecocentral field abnormalities, respectively, with a distinct predilection for involvement of the nasal retinal quadrant (Fig. 68–4).

Although the etiology of the blind spot enlargement in MCP is unknown, Brown and Folk have offered two possible explanations—the first involving the vascular arborization to the nasal retina, and the second relating to regional variation in the distribution of photoreceptors. In the first scenario, should MCP arise from hematogenous dissemination of an etiologic pathogen, the nasal retina may be more likely to be involved by preferential shedding of this agent to the medial posterior ciliary

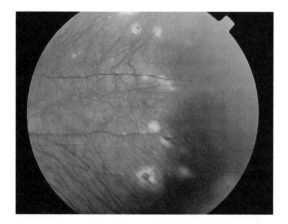

FIGURE 68–2. A photograph of a patient with MCP showing a linear peripheral arrangement of the spots of now inactive choroiditis.

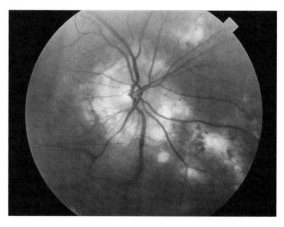

FIGURE 68–3. Extensive peripapillary atrophy in a patient with MCP.

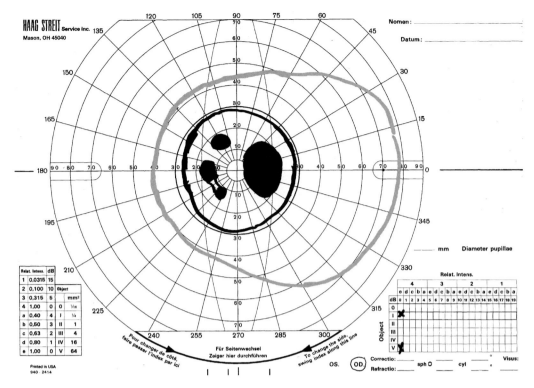

FIGURE 68–4. Goldmann field showing the cecocentral scotomata in a patient with MCP.

artery, which supplies the peripapillary choroid extending nasally to the equator.[19] More immediate access to this vessel could be achieved by virtue of its earlier and more acute bifurcation from the ophthalmic artery, as compared to the lateral posterior ciliary artery, which nourishes the temporal retina.[20, 21]

The second explanation for enlargement of the blind spot posits preferential involvement of rod photoreceptors in MCP, owing to their topographic distribution in the retina. Cuccio and colleagues[22] have found that the highest relative density of the rods to cones in the retina is in a peripapillary distribution extending nasally. Hence, if rods are more severely affected than cones in MCP, as electroretinography (ERG) suggests,[10] enlargement of the blind spot may be explained.

Electroretinography

ERG suggests that MCP is a diffuse disease process, with the degree of dysfunction relating to the severity and the extent of chorioretinal involvement. Normal to borderline ERGs were seen in 16 eyes (41%) of 16 patients (29 eyes) studied by Dreyer and Gass,[2] whereas moderately reduced and severely depressed ERG amplitudes were found in five and six eyes, respectively. Similarly, Reddy and coworkers[10] reported ERG data on 10 patients in relation to the number of chorioretinal lesions observed. Two patients with mild disease (20 or fewer lesions per eye) had essentially normal ERGs. Five patients with moderate disease (21 to 50 lesions per eye) exhibited abnormal ERG responses characterized by rod dysfunction, prolonged cone B-wave implicit times, and poor oscillatory potentials. Three patients with more than 50 lesions per eye were judged to have severe chorioretinal involve-

ment and were found to have markedly depressed rod and cone function with poor oscillatory potentials.

COURSE AND COMPLICATIONS

MCP is a chronic disease that may persist for many years, with the vast majority of patients experiencing multiple inflammatory recurrences in one or both eyes. Indeed, of 21 patients with MCP followed for 1 year or more, 18 (86%) demonstrated symptomatic, recurrent inflammation.[10] Inflammatory reactivation may manifest as vitreous or anterior chamber cellular infiltration and swelling of the choroidal scars with surrounding subretinal fluid, with the rare appearance of distinctly new lesions. Although recurrent lesions become larger and more pigmented with time, no new chorioretinal lesions were noted by Folk and Reddy,[10] who were able to trace these recurrent foci to previous lesions seen on color photographs or fluorescein angiograms.

As previously noted, although CME may complicate the course of MCP in a variable though significant number of patients, the most serious threat to central vision is the development of CNVMs, which are found in 32% to 46% of patients at some point in time during the course.[2, 6, 11] Typically, CNVMs arise either from atrophic scars or from yellow, nodular subretinal lesions, frequently in association with active inflammation. They may occur in a subfoveal, juxtafoveal, extrafoveal, or peripapillary location, ranging in number from one to as many as eight foci in a single eye, and varying in size from less than 100 μm in diameter to large lesions exceeding 200 μm.[11] In some of these eyes, the CNVMs appear to be anterior to the RPE. In others, Brown and colleagues[11] have noted that areas of neovascularization may be sur-

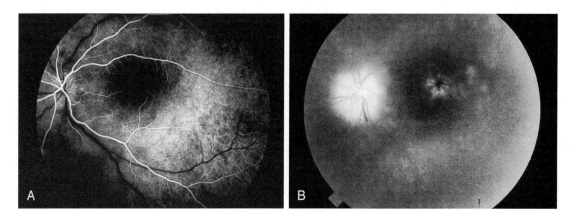

FIGURE 68–5. *A*, Fluorescein angiogram in a patient with MCP, early (arterial) phase. Note in particular the areas of choroidal fluorescence "blocking" temporal to the macula. *B*, Fluorescein angiogram in a patient with MCP, late phase. Note, in addition to the macular edema, the extensive areas of staining in the areas previously "blocking" the choroidal fluorescence pattern.

rounded by thick, hypofluorescent rings as seen on fundus fluorescein angiography and probably correlate to hyperplasia of the RPE. This pattern of proliferating RPE cells and small size (≦100 μm) of CNVMs was associated with spontaneous involution of the neovascular complex.[11, 19]

DIAGNOSIS

The diagnosis of MCP is in essence clinical, based on a thorough ophthalmic and medical history, review of systems, and ocular examination revealing the characteristic funduscopic findings in the presence of vitritis or anterior segment inflammation. As previously noted, choroidal neovascularization is common, may be apparent at presentation, or may evolve at any time during the disease course. There are no typical systemic disease associations, and features characterizing other ocular disorders (e.g., HLA-A29 suggestive of birdshot retinochoroidopathy) are absent. In fact, there are no specific laboratory or ancillary tests that establish the diagnosis of MCP; rather, they are most useful in excluding other differential diagnostic entities.

Fluorescein Angiography

The active yellow-gray lesions that are characteristic of the acute phase of MCP may be nonfluorescent in the early phase of the fluorescein angiogram (FA), with gradual staining and late leakage (Fig. 68–5). Atrophic, punched-out scars behave as window defects with early hyperfluorescence that fades in the late phase of the study. Disc swelling and hyperemia, together with CME, manifest angiographically by late dye leakage from retinal and optic disc capillaries.

Characteristic angiographic features of choroidal neovascularization include early hyperfluorescence with late leakage (Fig. 68–6). In addition, as previously noted, Brown and associates[11, 19] have observed that some of these foci may be surrounded by thick hypofluorescent rings corresponding to hyperplastic RPE, a pattern that may be indicative of spontaneous involution of the neovascular complex.[23, 24]

Indocyanine Green Angiography

Indocyanine green (ICG) angiography may provide additional information that is not detectable by clinical examination or FA. This feature may be useful not only in the differentiation of MCP from other inflammatory multifocal chorioretinal entities but may also serve to improve our understanding of the underlying nature of the disease, its progression, and its response to therapeutic intervention. In a study of 28 eyes with active inflammation associated with MCP, Slakter and colleagues[25] observed that 14 (50%) had large (200 to 500 μm) and 17 (61%) had small (50μm) hyperfluorescent lesions in the posterior pole on ICG angiography, which were more numerous and involved a more extensive area than those appreciated on FA or clinical examination (Fig. 68–7). These hyperfluorescent spots were thought to be indica-

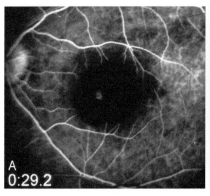
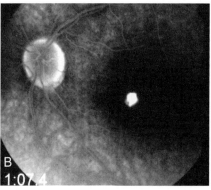

FIGURE 68–6. *A*, Fluorescein angiogram in a person with a choroidal neovascular membrane in the macula, exhibiting early fluorescence. *B*, Fluorescein angiogram in a person with a choroidal neovascular membrane in the macula, exhibiting late staining.

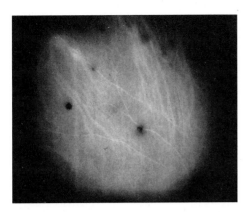

FIGURE 68–7. Indocyanine green angiogram, showing the areas of hypofluorescence in the choroid, indicative of foci of active inflammation in the choroid in a patient with MCP.

tive of acute or subacute disease, with an increase in their density and number corresponding to periods of increased vitritis and visual field loss. Conversely, hypofluorescent lesions were seen to resolve, either spontaneously as the acute disease process waned, or in response to systemic therapy with oral prednisone.

In five eyes, a dense confluence of hypofluorescent spots surrounding the optic nerve was associated with enlargement of the blind spot on visual field examination. Interestingly, in four of these cases, resolution of the hypofluorescence was associated with resolution of the visual field defect, representing for the first time a direct relationship between enlargement of the blind spot and a structural or functional defect in the peripapillary choroidal anatomy.[25]

Although the nature of these hypofluorescent spots could conceivably be attributed to underlying perfusion abnormalities of the choroid or choriocapillaris, no such defects were noted in areas of acute disease during the early phase of the ICG study in any of the eyes studied.[25] Rather, the authors implicate focal collections of inflammatory cells or postinflammatory debris, either at the level of the choriocapillaris as blocking fluorescence, or in the middle layers of the choroid producing a space-occupying effect, and so, preventing the egress of dye and diluting its concentration in the inflamed areas. The latter effect would produce an area of relative hypofluorescence in the mid- and late phase of the ICG study.[25] Finally, Slakter and coworkers[25] have identified certain patterns on ICG angiography that may serve to distinguish MCP from POHS and may provide insight into fundamental differences between these two entities. Although hypofluorescent spots are a characteristic feature of active disease in eyes with MCP, patients with POHS fail to manifest this finding, despite repeated examinations at various intervals during the course of their disease. In fact, some patients with POHS demonstrated focal areas of hyperfluorescence in the posterior pole during the midphase of the ICG study, presumably representing subclinical inflammatory activity. No hypofluorescent lesions, characteristic of MCP, were noted in eyes with POHS.

DIFFERENTIAL DIAGNOSIS

The differential diagnosis of MPC includes those infectious and noninfectious causes of white dot syndromes

(Table 68–1). Although it shares many similar morphologic features with POHS, MCP was originally described, in contradistinction to this entity, as exhibiting anterior chamber and vitreous cells, a female predilection, subnormal ERGs, and recurrent inflammatory disease. POHS has a significant association with HLA-DR2 (76%), whereas this genetic background is apparently absent in patients with MCP.[26] Furthermore, as previously mentioned, there are certain patterns on ICG angiography that may be useful in distinguishing these two diseases.[25]

MEWDS, like MCP, may present in young women with acute blind spot enlargement and vitreous inflammation. However, although important exceptions exist, MEWDS is predominantly a unilateral disease. As its name implies, it rarely produces permanent funduscopic pigmentary changes and resolves in most cases with resolution of the visual field abnormality and a favorable visual outcome.[18, 27] In MCP, resolution of the blind spot and peripapillary dysfunction are less certain.[17]

Although it has been suggested that SFU represents a terminal stage of MCP, because both share multifocality early in the disease course and recurrent inflammatory episodes, the pathology in SFU is limited to the posterior pole and eventuates in severe subretinal scarring not seen in MCP or PIC. Despite these changes, full-field ERGs were normal in the two patients with SFU studied by Reddy and colleagues.[10] This is in contrast to the markedly abnormal ERGs in patients with more advanced MCP, which are indicative of a more diffuse disease process.

Perhaps PIC is most closely related to MCP, with the frequent development of CNVMs and with its tendency toward bilaterality.[5, 11] Although by definition PIC has no vitreous or anterior cellular inflammation, it differs from MCP in that the chorioretinal lesions tend to be smaller than those seen in MCP, enlargement and recurrent inflammation around the chorioretinal scars are not observed, and electrophysiology is normal.

Other noninfectious entities to be considered in the

TABLE 68–1. MULTIFOCAL CHOROIDITIS AND PANUVEITIS: DIFFERENTIAL DIAGNOSIS OF WHITE DOT SYNDROMES

INFECTIOUS:
  Tuberculosis
  Syphilis
  Presumed ocular histoplasmosis syndrome (POHS)
  Diffuse unilateral subacute neuroretinitis (DUSN)
  Lyme disease
  Outer retinal toxoplasmosis
  Viral retinitis (cytomegalovirus, herpes simplex, herpes zoster)
  Septic choroiditis
NONINFECTIOUS:
  Multiple evanescent white dot syndrome (MEWDS)
  Punctate inner choroidopathy (PIC)
  Subretinal fibrosis and uveitis (SFU)
  Sarcoidosis
  Birdshot retinochoroidopathy
  Sympathetic ophthalmia
  Acute posterior multifocal placoid pigment epitheliopathy
    (APMPPE)
  Vogt-Koyanagi-Harada syndrome (VKH)
  Masquerade syndrome (CNS/intraocular large cell lymphoma)

differential diagnosis of MCP include sarcoidosis, birdshot retinochoroidopathy, APMPPE, and intraocular large-cell lymphoma. Although the diagnosis of sarcoidosis is suggested by elevation of the angiotensin-converting enzyme (ACE) level, together with characteristic findings on chest x-ray study and gallium scanning, these studies may be negative, with the definitive diagnosis depending on the demonstration of noncaseating granulomata on tissue biopsy. Birdshot retinochoroidopathy tends to occur in older patients, with characteristic hypopigmented fundus lesions, the frequent occurrence of optic neuropathy, CME, HLA-A29 positivity, and the rare development of CNVMs. APMPPE is a self-limited chorioretinal inflammation presenting in young adults, usually with a viral prodrome. In contrast to MCP, there is less vitreous and no anterior segment inflammation, the lesions of APMPPE tend to be larger, and the disease resolves within 2 to 3 months without recurrences and with a good visual outcome in most patients.[28] Furthermore, the visual field defects in APMPPE vary, and there is a higher prevalence of HLA-B27 and HLA-DR2.[28] Finally, the diagnosis of intraocular large cell lymphoma should be entertained, especially in elderly patients presenting with vitritis and multifocal choroidal infiltrates.

Patients presenting with an MCP-like picture and a rapidly progressive clinical course may, in fact, have an underlying infectious disease. Entities to be considered are listed in Table 68-1 and include, but are not limited to, diffuse unilateral subacute neuroretinitis (DUSN), septic choroiditis, and viral retinitis due to cytomegalovirus, herpes simplex, or herpes zoster. Timely diagnosis and institution of specific antimicrobial therapy are essential in these cases, which otherwise carry a very poor prognosis.

ETIOPATHOGENESIS

The etiology of MCP is unknown. Patients with MCP have no systemic disease associations, a negative history for living in areas where histoplasmosis is endemic, and in general, negative histoplasmin skin tests. In one study, although HLA-DR2 was found in 76% of patients with POHS[26] and may represent a risk factor for the development of this disease, particularly in association with choroidal neovascularization,[26, 29] no patients with MCP were found to express this antigen.

A viral etiology has been suggested by some investigators. Grutzmacher and colleagues cultured herpes simplex type I from separate chorioretinal and vitreous samples in a 20-year-old previously healthy patient, with funduscopic findings consistent with MCP.[30] Likewise, among seven patients with MCP, Frau and associates demonstrated the intraocular synthesis of specific antibodies against varicella zoster in two cases and against herpes simplex virus in one case.[31]

Tiedeman[32] described 10 patients with MCP, all of whom had serologic evidence suggestive of chronic or persistent Epstein-Barr virus (EBV) infection. All were generally healthy individuals, with no evidence of systemic disease consistent with infectious mononucleosis. In this study, patients with MCP, but none of the eight controls, had positive viral capsid antigen IgM or the Epstein-Barr early antigen antibody titers. All patients with MCP, and most of the controls, had viral capsid antigen IgG and Epstein-Barr nuclear antigen antibodies indicative of previous exposure to the virus. This serologic pattern is in contradistinction to that produced by infectious mononucleosis, in which the viral capsid antigen IgM followed by the viral capsid antigen IgG titers rise in a parallel fashion during viral incubation, 4 to 5 weeks following exposure to the virus. The early antigen rises with the onset of clinical disease, usually within 5 to 10 weeks of exposure, rises to a maximum, and then falls to undetectable levels 6 to 12 months after resolution of the infection. The Epstein-Barr nuclear antigen antibody appears slowly, within 2 months, and persists for life, whereas the viral capsid antigen IgM titer falls to undetectable levels after resolution of infection.

Because the diagnosis of chronic EBV infection is best supported by abnormally elevated antiviral capsid antigen IgM and anti-early antigen antibody levels,[33, 34] Tiedeman suggested that individuals with MCP might be immunologically unable to resolve the infection and may represent a subgroup of patients with chronic Epstein-Barr syndrome with manifestations limited to the eye. A reappraisal of the association between chronic EBV infection and MCP by Spaide and colleagues[35] failed to support this hypothesis. They found that neither the antiviral capsid antigen IgG nor the antinuclear antigen titers of 11 patients with MCP were significantly different from those of 11 sex- and age-matched controls. Furthermore, one would expect that a state of chronic EBV infection would eventually produce systemic signs and symptoms. This has not been the case in patients with MCP. Finally, the intraocular inflammatory manifestations of chronic EBV, as described by Wong and colleagues,[36] are distinct from those of MCP.

Pathologic examination of MCP lesions has revealed inflamed choroidal vessels in association with early neovascular membrane formation, retinal pigment epithelial hyperplasia, and immunocytochemical evidence of a mixed population of lymphocytes.[37–40] One study demonstrated a large number of B cells in the choroid,[39] whereas another pointed to a T-cell predominance in the choroid[37] and vitreous.[40] Ultrastructural studies and in situ hybridization failed to disclose herpes virus or other microbes.

Although a causal link between an external infectious pathogen has not been conclusively demonstrated, we believe, as do others,[15] that MCP probably develops in the genetically susceptible individual after contact with an inciting microbe, viral or otherwise, with the subsequent development of autoimmune choroiditis that is only amenable to anti-inflammatory and immunosuppressive chemotherapy. It is quite possible that MCP may have more than one cause producing a pattern morphologically indistinguishable on clinical examination.

Whether MCP, PIC, SFU, and MEWDS represent distinct clinical entities, or various manifestations of a single disease, remains controversial. Although MCP and PIC are ipso facto distinct by definition, the presence or absence of anterior chamber or vitreous cells in these two particular entities may indeed reflect essential differences in their nature, as the visual prognosis and response to treatment seem to indicate. Likewise, MEWDS and SFU are distinguishable on clinical grounds; they carry prognoses sufficiently distinct from each other, and from MCP and PIC, that it is sensible, from a clinical point of view, to treat these diseases as separate entities.

From an etiopathogenetic viewpoint, these distinctions may prove to be artificial. The retina and choroid have a sufficiently varied but definitively limited repertoire of morphologic responses to inflammatory disease, irrespective of primary etiology. Underlying host immunologic and genetic factors are likely to be equally important in determining the eye's response to a particular inciting pathogen, the clinical course of disease, and the morphologic manifestations thereof. For example, as previously noted, individuals who express HLA-DR2 antigen may be at greater risk for developing POHS and CNVMs.[26, 29] In a nonhuman primate model of histoplasmic choroiditis, Smith and colleagues[41–43] demonstrated that lymphocytic infiltrates may persist around choroidal lesions for as long as 10 years following the initial infection, and that these lesions may be reactivated with antigenic challenge. Similarly, the lesions of MCP, PIC, and SFU may evolve from a primary exposure to a single antigen or group of closely related antigens, with future reactivations depending on the host's underlying immunologic response to a particular antigen, the induction of autoimmunity, or subsequent exposure to other cross-reacting inflammatory stimuli.

TREATMENT

Steroids and Immunomodulatory Therapy

Systemic and periocular administration of corticosteroids may be of value, at least in the short term, in controlling intraocular inflammation and that associated with CNVMs and in preventing visual loss in some patients with MCP. However, our experience and that published in the literature suggest that MCP is more often resistant to protracted effective treatment with systemic and regional steroids.

Dreyer and Gass[2] treated 18 of 28 patients with either systemic or periocular steroids, noting an improvement in vision in six, no change in nine, and the prevention of rapid visual deterioration in two. Morgan and Schatz[6] reported visual improvement in all nine of their patients treated with steroids.

In contrast, Cantrill and Folk[9] noted that in their series of patients with multifocal choroiditis associated with progressive subretinal fibrosis, the acute lesions responded to systemic steroids initially in approximately 40% of cases, whereas some progressed to the fibrotic stage despite treatment. Brown and colleagues[11] treated 17 patients (28 eyes) with oral or subtenon corticosteroids, with 12 patients (16 eyes) showing definite improvement in visual acuity or decreased vitritis. Of the 16 eyes that showed visual improvement, four had CME. Nevertheless, on extended follow-up, 11 of 28 eyes had a final visual acuity of 20/200 or worse, with the majority of these eyes (8 of 11) having developed CNVMs. Nölle and colleagues[44] noted that the benefit of corticosteroids in their group of 20 patients with MCP was temporary and limited, with most patients eventually becoming refractory to treatment, with deterioration in visual acuity during corticosteroid therapy in the vast majority of patients. Finally, Nussenblatt and colleagues[15] described a moderately good initial response to steroid therapy in their patients with MCP, particularly those with CME, but advocated the addition of other immunosuppressive agents, because this disease is frequently recalcitrant to therapy.

Given the chronic and recurrent nature of MCP, its refractory response to long-term tolerable steroid treatment, and the well-known undesirable side effects of such therapy, we offer our patients the option of long-term immunomodulatory therapy as an alternative therapeutic approach. Our criteria for the selection of patients for immunomodulatory therapy and the guidelines for collaboration for proper monitoring are described in Chapter 12. The immunomodulatory agents that we have employed in the care of our patients with MCP have included methotrexate, azathioprine, cyclosporine, cyclophosphamide, chlorambucil, tacrolimus, leflunomide, mycophenolate mofetil, and etanercept. The dosage ranges, routes of administration, and major potential side effects of these agents are presented in Chapter 12.

Of the 19 patients with MCP followed on the Immunology and Uveitis Service of the Massachusetts Eye and Ear Infirmary for a mean of 72.7 months (range 5 to 278 months), 15 patients (30 eyes) were treated with immunomodulatory therapy.[45] This regimen was not associated with any significant medication-related complications and was effective in controlling inflammation and preserving good vision in patients with this potentially blinding disease. Ten of these 15 patients had previously been treated with systemic steroids. Four patients were treated with systemic nonsteroidal anti-inflammatory drugs (NSAIDs) or systemic steroids alone, and topical and regional steroids were used as adjunctive treatment. Systemic complications related to steroid treatment included duodenal perforation in one patient and cushingoid changes in three patients, whereas 12 patients developed cataract or glaucoma related to topical, regional, or systemic use of this drug. In contrast, an immunomodulatory-related complication was seen in only one patient, who experienced transient and reversible elevation of liver enzymes in association with methotrexate therapy.

Of the 15 patients (30 eyes) who received immunomodulatory therapy at some point during their disease course, seven patients (seven eyes) lost considerable vision in one eye while on steroid therapy alone. However, good vision in the fellow eye was preserved when immunomodulatory therapy was commenced. There was no visual loss among any of the eyes treated with immunomodulatory agents. Of the 30 eyes in this group, 20 have maintained a visual acuity of 20/80 or better, with one eye at 20/80, another at 20/60, and 18 eyes at 20/40 or better.

Laser Photocoagulation

No study has been performed that specifically addresses the safety and efficacy of laser photocoagulation for the treatment of CNVMs complicating MCP. Nevertheless, based on the experience with other macular diseases complicated by CNVMs for which abundant data exist, laser photocoagulation under fluorescein or ICG guidance is recommended for extrafoveal and juxtafoveal but not for subfoveal membranes, to prevent loss of central vision. Although the natural history of choroidal neovascularization in MCP is unknown, regression of CNVMs has occurred, either in association with corticosteroid therapy or spontaneously.[6, 11, 19] Brown and colleagues[11] observed that regression was more likely to occur with small (<100 μm in diameter) as opposed to large (>200 μm in diameter) areas of neovascularization, and that those which did regress were not infrequently associated with a hypofluorescent rim surrounding the CNVM, due to hyperplastic RPE, on fluorescein angiography. Accordingly, these investigators recommend laser photocoagulation for areas of neovascularization greater than 200 μm in diameter in an extrafoveal or juxtafoveal location, whereas lesions less than 100 μm in diameter may either be observed closely for signs of regression or treated with laser.[19] Subfoveal lesions should be observed and not treated. Extrafoveal and juxtafoveal CNVMs arising in four eyes of four patients with MCP treated with laser photocoagulation regressed nicely, with preservation of central vision in three and visual loss in one due to late expansions of scar.[11, 19]

Pars Plana Vitrectomy and Subfoveal Surgery

The efficacy of pars plana vitrectomy (PPV), with or without lensectomy, in the treatment of uveitis in general and specifically with respect to MCP, remains an open question, especially in light of the fact that, to date, no controlled randomized data in a homogenous population of uveitics are available to begin to answer this question. With this in mind, Nölle and Eckardt[40] found no impressive or sustained therapeutic benefit from PPV in nine patients (10 eyes) with MCP who were refractory to medical therapy. Although a modest visual improvement was achieved immediately postoperatively in most cases, the visual acuity decreased to preoperative values or less within 6 months. Neither the intensity nor the frequency of inflammatory relapses was altered by vitrectomy.

CNVMs associated with MCP, like those of POHS, are thought to arise from acquired damage to the choriocapillaris—Bruch's membrane—RPE complex due to focal choroiditis, with the growth of new blood vessels through these defects in Bruch's membrane extending laterally in the subretinal space, anterior to the RPE. Gass was the first to differentiate this path of advancing neovascularization (type II subretinal choroidal neovascularization) from that directed beneath the RPE as seen in age-related macular degeneration (type I sub-RPE neovascularization) and suggested that type II subretinal choroidal neovascularization may be amenable to surgical excision.[46] In the Rosenthal Lecture to the Macula Society in 1995, Thomas[47] presented his experience with subretinal surgery for the management of subfoveal CNVMs in 247 consecutive cases of eyes with various underlying disease entities, including 17 with MCP. With a median follow-up of 8 months (range: 2 to 31 months), 59% of eyes were 20/40 or better postoperatively, compared with none preoperatively. Sixty-five percent of eyes had an improvement of three or more Snellen lines postoperatively. Recurrent neovascularization occurred within 3 months in 18% of eyes during the follow-up period, 67%

of these being subfoveal. Although these initial results are encouraging, they are neither randomized nor controlled, and more extended follow-up is necessary to assess the impact of recurrent neovascularization on the ultimate visual prognosis. Therefore, at the present time, submacular surgery for subfoveal choroidal neovascularization in general, and that complicating MCP, is best performed in the context of a multicentered, randomized, prospective clinical trial, as is ongoing in the Submacular Surgery Trial (SST).

PROGNOSIS

Given the chronic, bilateral and recurrent nature of MCP, its visual prognosis is clearly guarded despite steroid treatment, with progression to permanent visual loss in 60% to 75% of reported cases.[2, 8, 9, 11, 44] Indeed, although Brown and colleagues[11] have reported an average final visual acuity of 20/54 in their 25 patients (47 eyes) with MCP followed for 6 months or more, with 26 eyes (60%) having 20/40 visual acuity or better, overall, 14 eyes (32%) had a final visual acuity of 20/200 or worse. Visual loss from CME, epiretinal membrane formation, RPE atrophy and macular scarring, optic neuropathy, neovascular glaucoma, subretinal fibrosis, and choroidal neovascularization occur as a consequence of chronic and recurrent inflammation or from complications of steroid use (secondary glaucoma and cataract). Our experience suggests that the early introduction of immunomodulatory therapy in MCP poses less risk for medication-related morbidity compared with the use of systemic steroids, and is effective in controlling inflammation, and so, preserving those ocular structures that are vital for good visual function.

Laser photocoagulation appears to be an effective treatment modality for larger juxtafoveal and extrafoveal CNVMs, with preservation of good visual function. The natural history of smaller foci of choroidal neovascularization is not known; however, as previously discussed, some have a tendency to regress spontaneously or with anti-inflammatory treatment. Vigilant monitoring of such lesions may be the prudent choice in an effort to obviate the inherent risks and putative proinflammatory stimulus of laser photocoagulation, particularly when these lesions are multiple, are not a direct threat to central vision, or are associated with inflammation. The ultimate role of submacular surgery with respect to the visual prognosis in MCP awaits further evaluation in the context of the SST.

CONCLUSIONS

MCP is a relatively newly recognized, chronic, recurrent, bilateral, potentially blinding uveitic syndrome of unknown etiology. The clinical features, visual prognosis, and response to treatment suggest that it is a distinct clinical entity, developing perhaps in genetically susceptible individuals following exposure to an inciting microbe, viral or otherwise, with subsequent development of an autoimmune choroiditis. The visual prognosis is guarded, with visual loss as a direct consequence of the sequelae of chronic and recurrent inflammation. Steroid therapy for MCP is only transiently effective, with most patients becoming refractory to conventional treatment or suffering intolerable side effects thereof. Our experience suggests that the early introduction of immunomodulatory therapy is a safe and effective alternative to the use of steroids that impacts positively on the ultimate visual prognosis in eyes with MCP.

References

1. Nozik RA, Dorsch W: A new chorioretinopathy associated with anterior uveitis. Am J Ophthalmol 1973;76:758.
2. Dreyer RF, Gass JDM: Multifocal choroiditis and panuveitis: A syndrome that mimics ocular histoplasmosis. Arch Ophthalmol 1984;102:1776.
3. Deutsch TA, Tessler HH: Inflammatory pseudohistoplasmosis. Ann Ophthalmol 1985;17:461.
4. Jampol LM, Sieving PA, Pugh D, et al: Multiple evanescent white dot syndrome. I. Clinical findings. Arch Ophthalmol 1984;102.
5. Watzke RC et al: Punctate inner choroidopathy. Am J Ophthalmol 1984;98:572.
6. Morgan CM, Schatz H: Recurrent multifocal choroiditis. Ophthalmology 1986;93:1138.
7. Doran R, Hamilton A: Disciform macular degeneration in young adults. Trans Ophthalmol Soc UK 1972;102:471.
8. Palestine AG, Nussenblatt RB, Garver LM, et al: Progressive subretinal fibrosis and uveitis. Br J Ophthalmol 1984;68:667.
9. Cantrill HL, Folk JC: Multifocal choroiditis associated with progressive subretinal fibrosis. Am J Ophthalmol 1986;101:70.
10. Reddy CV, Brown J, Folk JC, et al: Enlarged blind spots in chorioretinal inflammatory disorders. Ophthalmology 1996;103:606.
11. Brown J Jr, Folk JC, Reddy CV, et al: Visual prognosis of multifocal choroiditis, punctate inner choroidopathy, and the diffuse subretinal fibrosis syndrome. Ophthalmology 1996;103:1100.
12. Smith RE, Ganley JP: An epidemiological study of presumed ocular histoplasmosis. Trans Am Acad Ophthalmol Otolaryngol 1971;75:994.
13. Joondeph BC, Tessler HH. Multifocal choroiditis. Int Ophthalmol Clin 1990;30:286.
14. Spaide RF, Yannuzzi LA, Freund KB: Linear streaks in multifocal choroiditis and panuveitis. Retina 1991;11:229.
15. Nussenblatt RB, Whitcup SM, Palestine AG: White dot syndromes. In: Nussenblatt RB, Whitcup SM, Palestine AG: Fundamentals and Clinical Practice, 2nd ed. St. Louis, Mosby–Year Book, Inc., 1996, p 373.
16. Schener F, Böke N: Retinal vasculitis with multifocal retinochoroiditis. Int Ophthalmol 1990;14:401.
17. Korram KD, Jampol LM, Rosenberg MA: Blind spot enlargement as a manifestation of multifocal choroiditis. Arch Ophthalmol 1991;109:1403.
18. Callanan D, Gass JDM: Multifocal choroiditis and choroidal neovascularization associated with the multiple evanescent white dot and acute idiopathic blind spot enlargement syndrome. Ophthalmology 1992;99:1678–1685.
19. Brown J Jr, Folk JC: Multifocal choroiditis, punctate inner choroidopathy, and other related conditions. In: Guyer DR, Yannuzzi LA, Chang S, Shields JA, Green RW, eds. Retina, Vitreous, Macula. Vol. 1. Philadelphia, WB Saunders Co., 1999, p 614.
20. Hayreh SS: Segmental nature of the choroidal vasculature. Br J Ophthalmol 1975;59:631.
21. Hayreh SS: The ophthalmic artery. III. Branches. Br J Ophthalmol 1962;46:212.
22. Cuccio DA, Sloan KR, Kalina RE, et al: Human photoreceptor topography. J Comp Neurol 1990;292:497.
23. Millar N, Millar B, Ryan SJ: The role of retinal pigment epithelium in the involution of subretinal neovascularization. Invest Ophthalmol Vis Sci 1986;27:1644.
24. Glaser BM, Campochiaro PA, Davis JL: Retinal pigment epithelial cells release inhibitors of neovascularization. Ophthalmology 1987;94:780.
25. Slakter JS, Giovannini A, Yannuzzi LA, et al: Indocyanine green angiography of multifocal choroiditis. Ophthalmology 1997; 104:1813.
26. Spaide RF, Skerry JE, Yannuzzi LA, et al: Lack of the HLA-DR2 specificity in multifocal choroiditis and panuveitis. Br J Ophthalmol 1990;74:536.
27. Daniele S, Daniele C, Ferri CA: Association of peripapillary scars with lesions characteristic of multiple evanescent white-dot syndrome. Ophthalmologica 1995;209:217.
28. Wolf MD, Folk JC, Nelson JA, Peeples ME: Acute posterior multifocal placoid pigment epitheliopathy and Lyme disease [letter]. Arch Ophthalmol 1992;110:750.
29. Meredith TA, Smith RE, Duquesnoy RJ: Association of HLA-DRw2 antigen with presumed ocular histoplasmosis. Am J Ophthalmol 1980;89:70.
30. Grutzmacher RD, Henderson D, McDonald PJ, et al: Herpes simplex chorioretinitis in a healthy adult. Am J Ophthalmol 1983;96:788.
31. Frau E, Dussaix E, Offret H, et al: The possible role of herpes viruses in multifocal choroiditis and panuveitis. Int Ophthalmol 1990;14:365.
32. Tiedeman JS: Epstein-Barr virus antibodies in multifocal choroiditis and panuveitis. Am J Ophthalmol 1987;103:659.
33. Tosato G: The Epstein-Barr virus and the immune system. Adv Cancer Res 1987;49:75.
34. Thorley-Lawson DA: Immunological responses to Epstein-Barr virus infection and the pathogenesis of EBV-induced diseases. Biochem Biophys Acta 1988;948:263.
35. Spaide RF, Suqin S, Yannuzzi LA: Epstein-Barr virus antibodies in multifocal choroiditis and panuveitis. Am J Ophthalmol 1991; 112:410.
36. Wong KW, D'Amico DJ, Hedges TR, et al: Ocular involvement associated with chronic Epstein-Barr virus disease. Arch Ophthalmol 1987;105:788.
37. Charteris DG, Lee WR: Multifocal posterior uveitis: Clinical and pathological findings. Br J Ophthalmol 1990;74:688.
38. Dunlop AA, Cree IA, Hague S, et al: Multifocal choroiditis: Clinicopathologic correlation. Arch Ophthalmol 1998;116:801.
39. Martin DF, Chan CC, deSmet MD, et al: The role of chorioretinal biopsy in the management of posterior uveitis. Ophthalmology 1993;100:705.
40. Nölle B, Eckardt C: Vitrectomy in multifocal choroiditis. Ger J Ophthalmol 1993;2:14.
41. Anderson A, Clifford W, Palvolgy I, et al: Immunopathology of chronic experimental histoplasmic choroiditis in the primate. Invest Ophthalmol Vis Sci 1992;33:1637.
42. Smith RE, Dunn S, Jester JV: Natural history of experimental histoplasmic choroiditis in the primate. II. Histopathologic features. Invest Ophthalmol Vis Sci 1984;25:810.
43. Palvolgy I, Anderson A, Rife L, et al: Immunopathology of reactivation of experimental ocular histoplasmosis. Exp Eye Res 1993; 57:169.
44. Nölle B, Faul S, Jenisch S, et al: Peripheral multifocal chorioretinitis with panuveitis: Clinical and immunogenetic characterization in older patients. Graefes Arch Clin Exp Ophthalmol 1998;236:451.
45. Michel SS, Ekong A, Baltatzis S, et al: Multifocal choroiditis and panuveitis (MCP): Immunomodulatory therapy. Ophthalmology, in press.
46. Gass JDM: Biomicroscopic and histopathologic considerations regarding the feasibility of surgical excision of subfoveal neovascular membranes. Ann Ophthalmol 1994;118:285.
47. Thomas MA. Updated results in subfoveal surgery. Rosenthal Lecture. Macula Society, Palm Beach, Florida, 1995. Macula Society, Tucson, Arizona, 1996.

69 | MULTIPLE EVANESCENT WHITE DOT SYNDROME

Harvey Siy Uy and Pik Sha Chan

DEFINITION

Multiple evanescent white dot syndrome (MEWDS) is a rare disorder of unknown etiology characterized by the presence of white lesions deep in the outer retina or at the level of the retinal pigment epithelium (RPE). Other RPE inflammatory disorders, such as acute posterior multifocal placoid pigment epitheliopathy (APMPPE), birdshot retinochoroidopathy (BSRC), multifocal choroiditis and panuveitis, punctate inner choroidopathy (PIC), and presumed ocular histoplasmosis syndrome (POHS), may present with white dots in the fundus. However, the lesions of MEWDS are distinguished by their distinct morphology, associated macular granularity, transient nature, characteristic angiographic appearance, unilaterality, self-limiting course, lack of significant sequelae, absence of associated systemic involvement, rapid recovery, and excellent visual outcome.

HISTORY AND EPIDEMIOLOGY

The term multiple evanescent white dot syndrome was first used by Jampol and coworkers in 1984[1] to describe a series of 11 young adults with transient loss of vision accompanied by white dots in the fundus. MEWDS is an uncommon ocular disease. Over the following decade, 69 additional cases were reported worldwide, with the largest series published to date consisting of 11 patients. Just as with most of the other white dot syndrome entities, the majority of patients with MEWDS are within the younger age groups. The average age at presentation is 28, with a range of 17 to 47 years. A definite female predominance is observed (male to female ratio of approximately 1:3). The significance of this age and sex distribution is unknown. White, black, Hispanic, Chinese, and Japanese[1-3] patients have been reported, and it is likely that other races are susceptible to this condition as well.

CLINICAL CHARACTERISTICS

The lesions of MEWDS appear as multiple small (100 to 200 µm), round, slightly indistinct, white to yellow-white spots distributed over the posterior fundus, especially at the perifoveal and peripapillary regions (Fig. 69–1). Each "dot" is composed of aggregates of many smaller dots found deep in the retina or at the level of the RPE. These lesions are best appreciated by slit-lamp biomicroscopy using a contact or noncontact lens. Typically, these lesions tend to concentrate around the vascular arcades or the optic nerve head and extend to the midperiphery. Foveal involvement by these white dots is relatively rare; however, the fovea may exhibit fine mottling or hyperpigmentation. Macular granularity is a uniform and distinguishing feature of MEWDS and appears as multiple, minute, white or light orange specks (see Fig. 69–1). Other common clinical features include visual acuity reduction, anterior chamber cells, vitreous cells, an afferent pupillary defect,

irregularity of the internal limiting-membrane reflex, and mild optic disc swelling. Anterior chamber inflammation is occasionally observed and is mild; vitritis is also usually mild and may be present in about half of all affected eyes. Associated retinal findings are infrequent and may include retinal splinter hemorrhages and mild venous sheathing.[1, 4–10]

Although the majority of cases are unilateral and nonrecurrent, there have been at least 10 reported cases of bilateral involvement[11–12] and at least five cases of chronic recurrence.[4, 13] In bilateral involvement, the findings are usually asymmetric.

Patients may describe blurred or dim vision or the presence of floaters during an episode of MEWDS. The visual acuity may acutely deteriorate, even to 20/200. There is rapid recovery of visual function to normal or near normal levels, with some patients improving within 1 to 2 weeks of disease onset. The majority of patients achieve visual acuities of 20/30 to 20/20 within 4 to 8 weeks after onset of the disease.[1, 7] Regression of retinal lesions is coincident with visual recovery. The white dots and granularity of the macula tend to fade, leaving subtle RPE pigment alterations seen as window defects.[1]

Several authors have reported an association of MEWDS with the acute idiopathic blind-spot enlargement syndrome (AIBES).[5, 14, 15] This subset of patients may additionally manifest disc edema, afferent pupillary defect, loss of central vision, blind-spot enlargement, other visual field defects, color vision disturbance, and optic disc hyperfluorescence on fluorescein angiography. The optic nerve disturbances may be more prominent than the chorioretinal manifestations; however, in these instances, the diagnosis of MEWDS can be established by fluorescein angiography. AIBES can occur in patients with multifocal chorioretinitis and panuveitis and punctate inner choroidopathy (PIC) and may represent a common ocular response to chorioretinal inflammation.[16]

Late sequelae of MEWDS are rare and include subfoveal neovascular membrane formation, which may develop weeks or months after initial symptoms and may spontaneously resolve.[17, 18] Two cases of acute macular neuroretinopathy in association with MEWDS in the same eye have also been reported, suggesting common pathogenic mechanisms.[19]

PATHOGENESIS

The pathogenesis of MEWDS is currently unknown. An infectious etiology is suggested by the prodromal flulike symptoms experienced by some patients and by findings of elevated total serum IgM and IgG in at least one patient.[2] No specific etiologic agent has yet been identified despite extensive laboratory testing by different authors. An autoimmune or immunologic mechanism is suspected and is supported by reports of MEWDS developing after hepatitis B vaccination[20] and by detection

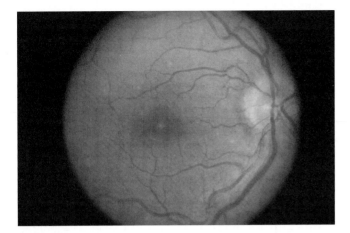

FIGURE 69–1. Fundus photograph of a patient with MEWDS. Note the deep, slightly indistinct, yellow-white lesions in the posterior pole. (See color insert.)

TABLE 69–1. DIAGNOSTIC FEATURES OF MULTIPLE EVANESCENT WHITE DOT SYNDROME

Patient characteristics
    Young
    Female predominance
    Unilateral involvement usually
    Viral prodrome possible
Ocular characteristics
    Anterior segment
        Mild anterior chamber inflammation
    Posterior segment
        Acute onset
        Visual dysfunction variable: 6/6 to 6/60
        Rapid recovery with return of good visual function
        Mild vitritis in 50%
        Multiple grainy white dots, mostly in posterior pole with foveal sparing
        Macular granularity
        Optic disc edema or hyperemia
Ancillary testing
    Fluorescein angiography: early hyperfluorescence with late staining; optic disc hyperfluorescence
    Indocyanine green angiography: hypofluorescent spots all over the fundus
    Perimetry: blind-spot enlargement and central, cecocentral, and arcuate scotomas
    Electrophysiology: abnormal ERG, ERP, and EOG
    Test results return to normal with visual recovery

ERG, electroretinogram; ERP, early receptor potential; EOG, electro-oculogram.

of HLA-B51 haplotype in 4 of 9 (44.4%) patients with MEWDS.[21]

It is well known that autoimmune diseases can be incited by normal immune responses to foreign antigens such as microbial agents. Infectious prodromes often precede the onset of autoimmune disease. Infectious agents can cause dysregulation of the immune system by several mechanisms. Inflammation caused by an infectious agent can lead to local tissue injury with resulting alteration of self-antigens to create cross-reactive new antigens. Tissue injury can also lead to exposure of self antigens that were previously concealed from the immune system. An infectious process can also heighten immune responses by means of polyclonal lymphocyte activation and proliferation and by release of inflammatory costimulators. Last, normal antibodies or T cells directed against the initiating viral or bacterial antigen can cross react with self proteins, resulting in autoimmune disease. These processes may be at work in the pathogenesis of MEWDS and other white dot syndromes, such as acute posterior multifocal placoid pigment epitheliopathy, in which viral prodromes have been reported. Molecular mimicry, wherein short homologous sequences exist between microbial antigens and self–major histocompatibility antigens, is another theoretical mechanism by which an infectious agent can cause autoimmunity.

The subset of patients with relapsing MEWDS is reminiscent of the recurrences experienced by patients with autoimmune uveitis or with herpetic disease and further strengthens the case for an autoimmune or infectious pathogenic mechanism. Likewise, the frequent presence of optic nerve involvement in patients with MEWDS occurs in other autoimmune or infectious uveitis entities, with posterior segment findings associated with optic nerve dysfunction, such as sarcoidosis, multiple sclerosis, syphilis, Lyme disease, cat scratch disease, toxoplasmosis, and herpetic eye disease. Further studies are needed to elucidate the pathogenesis of MEWDS.

DIAGNOSIS

The diagnosis of MEWDS is primarily based on its characteristic clinical findings, transient course, and excellent visual outcome (Table 69–1). As part of the uveitis evalua-

tion, a thorough review of systems should be conducted. A targeted medical work-up is advisable to rule out potentially treatable infectious or inflammatory disease such as syphilis, sarcoidosis, and toxoplasmosis. The most useful diagnostic examinations are fluorescein angiography and indocyanine green (ICG) angiography. These imaging studies are particularly useful when the clinical findings are equivocal, when the disease is relapsing or recurrent, and when atypical features are encountered such as optic nerve involvement or subretinal neovascularization.

During the acute phase of MEWDS, fluorescein angiography shows patchy or punctate, early hyperfluorescence of the white dots (Fig. 69–2) with late deep staining

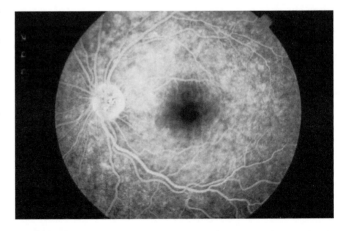

FIGURE 69–2. Fluorescein angiogram, midphase, of a patient with MEWDS. Note the extensive grouped granular lesions which, although they blocked choroidal fluorescence in the early phases of the transit, are beginning to stain at this midpoint of the transit.

of the RPE and peripapillary area (Fig. 69–3). These lesions are mostly located in the posterior pole. Occasional leakage from the optic disc and retinal capillaries may be observed. RPE window defects may also be noted in severe cases. The choroidal background fluorescence between lesions is usually normal. As the fundus returns to normal, the angiographic changes become less noticeable and the angiogram may return to normal.[1, 4–7]

ICG angiography has several advantages over fluorescein angiography in visualizing the choroidal circulation. Because ICG dye is a larger molecule than sodium fluorescein and binds more tightly to serum albumin, ICG does not significantly leak from the choriocapillaris and thus is able to provide improved images of the choroidal vasculature. In addition, ICG absorbs and emits infrared light with resulting improved light transmission through melanin, xanthophyll, blood, and infiltrates present in the layers of the retina. ICG angiography of MEWDS in the acute phase is characteristic and has not only been used to provide additional supportive evidence for the diagnosis of MEWDS but has also provided insight as to the pathophysiology of this disease.

The arteriovenous phase of the ICG study typically does not reveal any distinct abnormal findings (Fig. 69–4), with the first lesions appearing at the 10-minute phase of the angiogram and persisting to the late phases. A pattern of multiple deep, small, round, hypofluorescent spots are appreciated in the posterior pole extending to the periphery (Fig. 69–5). The lesions are denser and may be confluent in the posterior pole and become less concentrated as they radiate out into the midperiphery. Upon resolution of the disease, the hypofluorescent spots become smaller and eventually disappear.[22, 23] The nature and location of these spots are suggestive of deep choroidal lesions. Some of these spots may correspond to lesions seen on ophthalmoscopy or fluorescein angiography. Typically, many more spots are visible on ICG angiography than on fluorescein angiography.[22–24] The pattern of hypofluorescent spots in MEWDS suggests that there is choriocapillaris or choroidal precapillary arteriole injury in addition to RPE and photoreceptor involvement. The absence of early-phase lesions indicates that the larger

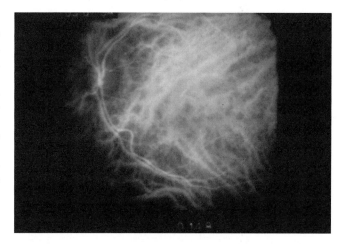

FIGURE 69–4. Indocyanine green angiogram, early phase, of a patient with MEWDS. Note the subtle block-early spots, which become much more apparent in the later transit. (Courtesy of John I. Loewenstein, M.D.)

choroidal vessels are spared. Several theories have been proposed by Obana and colleagues[23] to explain the apparent discrepancy between hyperfluorescence visible on fluorescein angiography and hypofluorescence during ICG angiography. A retinal lesion is unlikely to selectively block ICG transmission without blocking fluorescein transmission. A filling defect of the choriocapillaris would result in simultaneous fluorescein and ICG hypofluorescence. Inflammatory thickening of the choriocapillaris vessel walls with narrowing of the precapillary arterioles may result in decreased blood circulation with decreased entry or retention of the larger ICG molecule yet allow fluorescein transmission. A further possibility is that increased numbers of inflammatory cells in the choroidal interstitial tissue may result in tissue changes that may prevent entry or retention of the ICG molecule but not the smaller fluorescein molecule. A definitive explanation of this phenomenon awaits further studies.

Visual field testing will frequently reveal enlargement of the blind spot. Visual field defects associated with

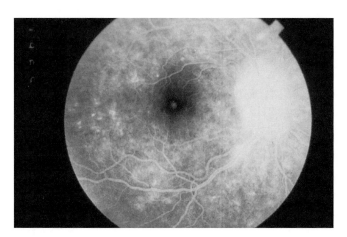

FIGURE 69–3. Fluorescein angiogram, late phase, of a patient with MEWDS. Note the staining pattern, with ring, wreath, and halo hyperfluorescence around the macula, and staining of the disc.

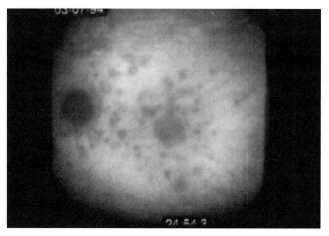

FIGURE 69–5. Indocyanine green angiogram, late phase, same case as seen in Figure 69–4. Note the multiple prominent foci of choroidal nonperfusion. (Courtesy of John I. Loewenstein, M.D.)

MEWDS include blind-spot enlargement, and central, cecocentral, and arcuate scotomas. These scotomas may be the presenting complaint. Many of these patients manifest mild disc swelling, vascular congestion, and optic disc hyperfluorescence on fluorescein angiography. The size of the visual field defect may be disproportionately large or may not be commensurate with ophthalmoscopic findings. The enlarged blind spot may persist longer than the other symptoms, but the size of the blind spot almost always returns to normal. Blind-spot enlargement is not unique to MEWDS but is found in other posterior segment inflammatory disorders, such as multifocal choroiditis and panuveitis, pseudo-presumed ocular histoplasmosis, acute macular retinopathy, and the acute idiopathic blind spot syndrome. This has prompted some authors to speculate on whether these conditions comprise a spectrum of disease or share a common pathogenesis.[5, 14, 15, 25]

Electrophysiologic abnormalities are observed in patients with acute MEWDS. Electroretinogram (ERG) and early receptor potential (ERP) amplitudes are often profoundly decreased, and ERP regeneration times are prolonged. These changes indicate pathology at the photoreceptor-RPE-Bruch membrane complex.[1] Foveal densitometry and color-matching testing during the active stage of MEWDS demonstrate gross abnormalities at the level of the cone photoreceptor outer segments.[26] Scanning laser densitometry studies reveal reduction of visual pigments during active MEWDS.[27] These two studies support the theory that there are metabolic disturbances at the level of the pigment epithelium-photoreceptor complex in patients with active MEWDS.

Prolonged latency and decreased amplitude of P100 complexes on electro-oculography, when optic disc swelling is present, indicate concomitant optic nerve dysfunction.[28] Focal electroretinography, however, reveals that macular ERG amplitude reduction is associated with central scotoma formation and that peripapillary ERG reduction is related to blind-spot enlargement.[29] This finding suggests that visual field disturbances in MEWDS primarily result from retinal rather than optic nerve dysfunction. Collectively, the results of these laboratory investigations indicate that the pathophysiologic mechanisms of MEWDS are complex and have yet to be fully elucidated.

DIFFERENTIAL DIAGNOSIS
The differential diagnosis of MEWDS includes acute posterior multifocal placoid pigment epitheliopathy (APMPPE), multifocal choroiditis and panuveitis (MCP), BSRC, acute retinal pigment epitheliitis (ARPE), PIC, sarcoidosis, and diffuse unilateral subacute neuroretinitis. A targeted medical work-up is advisable to rule out treatable infectious or inflammatory diseases such as syphilis, toxoplasmosis, tuberculosis, and sarcoidosis.

APMPPE is characterized by transient visual loss in young patients, rapid and full visual recovery, and resolution of the RPE placoid lesions. APMPPE may also be associated with viral prodromes, papillitis, and mild anterior chamber and vitreous inflammation. However, APMPPE is usually bilateral. APMPPE lesions are larger and exhibit blocked fluorescence early in the angiogram, as opposed to early hyperfluorescence in MEWDS. RPE pigmentary changes are more prominent in APMPPE than in MEWDS.

Multifocal choroiditis and uveitis is a disease of young, healthy, myopic women that may cause acute loss of vision. MCP is an RPE-choroidal inflammatory disorder characterized by multiple relapses and prominent vitreous cavity and anterior chamber inflammation. The lesions of MCP are usually more concentrated in the periphery and resolve, leaving atrophic punched-out scars with hyperpigmented borders. Treatment of MCP may require corticosteroid or immunosuppressive agents. Visual prognosis is guarded, with visual function frequently compromised by cystoid macular edema and choroidal neovascular membrane formation.

BSRC manifests as multiple cream-colored lesions at the level of RPE or deeper. BSRC is accompanied by prominent anterior chamber inflammation and vitritis. BSRC occurs mainly in older patients, and it is usually bilateral. The HLA A29 phenotype is highly (90%) associated with BSRC. Acute BSRC lesions may be angiographically silent, whereas older lesions may demonstrate early blocked fluorescence and late hyperfluorescence.

ARPE is similar to MEWDS in that it affects relatively young patients and causes acute visual loss followed by almost total recovery in 7 to 10 weeks. However, the macular lesions of ARPE are dark spots surrounded by a halo of depigmentation at the level of the RPE. The lesions, as seen on angiography, are hypofluorescent areas surrounded by hyperfluorescence. The ERG and cortical evoked responses are normal.

PIC predominantly affects young women and is usually bilateral. Small yellow-white lesions (100 to 300 μm) of the inner choroid and RPE are visible and may later form pigmented, atrophic, cylindrical lesions from which choroidal neovascular membranes often arise. Inflammation is characteristically absent in PIC. Recurrences are common but vision is not usually affected unless the fovea is directly involved.

Sarcoidosis may present with deep, small, white lesions of the retina, but it is easily distinguishable from MEWDS by the presence of Dalen-Fuchs nodules, choroidal granulomas, retinal vasculitis, pars planitis, and vitreous snowballs. Diffuse unilateral subacute neuroretinitis is caused by an intraocular nematode and occurs in young adults presenting with loss of vision and, occasionally, white dots in the retina. The clinical course is marked by progressive loss of vision, optic atrophy, retinal vessel narrowing, and diffuse and focal RPE degeneration.

TREATMENT
The lesions of MEWDS spontaneously resolve without treatment. Patients should be reassured of the self-limiting course of this disease and of the good visual prognosis.

SUMMARY
MEWDS is an uncommon disorder of the RPE and choroid. It should be considered in the differential diagnosis of young, healthy patients who present with unilateral or bilateral acute visual loss or optic neuritis. A correct diagnosis of MEWDS can be made after careful history taking and biomicroscopic examination of the fundus.

The presence of characteristic fundus findings and the transient clinical course are usually sufficient to establish the diagnosis. Fluorescein and ICG angiography, perimetry, and electrophysiologic studies may help distinguish MEWDS from other disease entities that present with white dots. This disorder is characterized by spontaneous, rapid, and full recovery of visual function; however, careful follow-up of these patients is necessary for detection of potential, albeit rare, complications. The pathogenesis of this disease is not well understood and awaits further investigation.

References

1. Jampol LM, Sieving PA, Pugh D, et al: Multiple evanescent white dot syndrome. I. Clinical findings. Arch Ophthalmol 1984;102:671.
2. Chung YM, Yeh TS, Liu JH: Increased serum IgM and IgG in the multiple evanescent white-dot syndrome. Am J Ophthalmol 1987;104:187.
3. Nakao K, Isashiki M: Multiple evanescent white dot syndrome. Jpn J Ophthalmol 1986;30:376.
4. Aaberg TM, Campo RV, Joffe L: Recurrences and bilaterality in the multiple evanescent white dot syndrome. Am J Ophthalmol 1986;101:489.
5. Dodwell DD, Jampol LM, Rosenberg M, et al: Optic nerve involvement associated with multiple evanescent white dot syndrome. Ophthalmology 1990;97:862.
6. Laatikainen L, Immonen I: Multiple evanescent white dot syndrome. Graefe's Arch Clin Exp Ophthalmol 1988;226:37.
7. Mamalis N, Daily MJ: Multiple evanescent white dot syndrome. A report of eight cases. Ophthalmology 1987;94:1209.
8. Palacios PT, Hurtado EP, Ramos MJM: Multiple evanescent white dot syndrome. Ann Ophthalmol 1993;25:216.
9. Slusher MM, Weaver RG: Multiple evanescent white dot syndrome. Retina 1988;8:132.
10. Jost BF, Olk RJ, McGaughy A: Bilateral symptomatic multiple evanescent white-dot syndrome. Am J Ophthalmol 1986;101:489–490.
11. Lefrancois A, Hamard H, Corbe C, et al: A case of MEWDS, the multiple evanescent white-dot syndrome. J Fr Ophthalmol 1989;12:103.
12. Meyer RJ, Jampol LM: Recurrences and bilaterality in the multiple evanescent white dot syndrome. Am J Ophthalmol 1985;100:29.
13. Tsai L, Jampol LM, Pollock SC, Olk J: Chronic recurrent multiple evanescent white dot syndrome. Retina 1994;14:160.
14. Kimmel AS, Folk JC, Thompson HS, Strand LS: The multiple evanescent white-dot syndrome with acute blind spot enlargement. Am J Ophthalmol 1989;107:425.
15. Singh K, de Frank MP, Shults WT, Watzke RC: Acute idiopathic blind spot enlargement. A spectrum of disease. Ophthalmology 1991;98:497.
16. Reddy CV, Brown J Jr, Folk JC, et al: Enlarged blind spots in chorioretinal inflammatory disorders. Ophthalmology 1996;103:606.
17. Barile GB, Reppucci VS, Schiff WM, Wong DT: Circumpapillary chorioretinopathy in multiple evanescent white-dot syndrome. Retina 1997;17:75.
18. Wyhinny GJ, Jackson JL, Jampol LM, Caro NC: Subretinal neovascularization following multiple evanescent white-dot syndrome [letter]. Arch Ophthalmol 1990;108:1384.
19. Gass JDM, Hamed LM: Acute macular neuroretinopathy and multiple evanescent white dot syndrome occurring in the same patients. Arch Ophthalmol 1989;107:189.
20. Baglivo E, Safran AB, Borruat FX: Multiple evanescent white dot syndrome after hepatitis B vaccine. Am J Ophthalmol 1996;122:431.
21. Desarnaulds AB, Borruat FX, Herbort CP, Spertini F: Le multiple evanescent white dot symdrome: Une predisposition genetique? Klin Monatsbl Augenheilkd 1996;208:301.
22. Ie D, Glaser BM, Murphy RP, et al: Indocyanine green angiography in multiple evanescent white-dot syndrome. Am J Ophthalmol 1994;117:7.
23. Obana A, Kusumi M, Tokuhiko M: Indocyanine green angiographic aspects of multiple evanescent white dot syndrome. Retina 1996;16:97.
24. Borruat FX, Auer C, Piguet B: Choroidopathy in multiple evanescent white dot syndrome. Arch Ophthalmol 1995;113:1569.
25. Callanan D, Gass JDM: Multifocal choroiditis and choroidal neovascularization associated with the multiple evanescent white dot and acute idiopathic blind spot enlargement syndrome. Ophthalmology 1992;99:1678.
26. Keunen JEE, van Norren D: Foveal densitometry in the multiple evanescent white-dot syndrome. Am J Ophthalmol 1988;105:561.
27. Van Meel GJ, Keunen JEE, van Norren D, van de Kraats J: Scanning laser densitometry in multiple evanescent white dot syndrome. Retina 1993;13:29.
28. Takeda N, Numata K, Yamamoto S: Electrophysiologic findings in optic nerve dysfunction associated with multiple evanescent white-dot syndrome. Doc Ophthalmol 1992;79:295.
29. Horigchi M, Miyake Y, Nakamura M, Fujii Y: Focal electroretinogram and visual field defect in multiple evanescent white dot syndrome. Br J Ophthalmol 1993;77:452.

ACUTE POSTERIOR MULTIFOCAL PLACOID PIGMENT EPITHELIOPATHY

Miguel Pedroza-Seres

DEFINITION

Acute posterior multifocal placoid pigment epitheliopathy (APMPPE) is an inflammatory retinal/choroidal disease characterized by sudden loss of vision caused by the sudden appearance of multiple yellow-white, flat inflammatory lesions lying deep within the sensory retina, most notably at the level of the retinal pigment epithelium (RPE) and choriocapillaris. Characteristically, patients with APMPPE experience a rapid recovery in vision, with resolution of the acute lesions, leaving a permanently altered RPE. APMPPE affects otherwise healthy, young individuals. In addition, the etiology is unknown, and there is considerable controversy about the pathogenesis.

HISTORY

APMPPE was originally described by Gass in 1968.[1] He reported the clinical and angiographic findings in three young women who presented with loss of central vision associated with multiple round and confluent yellow-white placoid lesions at the level of the RPE and choroid. These lesions resolved spontaneously over a few weeks, leaving scarring of the RPE with substantial return of visual acuity and continued improvement over several months.[1] Two of the patients reported by Gass showed a positive skin test for tuberculin, and one had a family history of pulmonary tuberculosis. All were taking some kind of medical drug before the onset of their eye symptoms.

Gass[1] named this disease pigment epitheliopathy because the pigment epithelium appears to be the tissue most significantly affected. He postulated that the clinical course of APMPPE suggests the presence of an acute pigment epithelial cellular response to some local injurious agent, rather than to transient pathology of choroidal vascular insufficiency or to a primary degeneration of the pigment epithelium.

Maumenee[2] reported in 1970 that he had six patients with lesions similar to those described by Gass, and he classified APMPPE as a distinct clinical uveitis entity.

Van Buskirk and colleagues,[3] in 1971, reported on a 15-year-old girl who developed blurred vision in both eyes, 1 day after she was diagnosed with pretibial erythema nodosum on both legs. They suggested, for the first time, that the delay in filling seen at the choriocapillaris represented a focal choroidal vasculopathy rather than a primary pigment epitheliopathy.

Deutman and coworkers[4] suggested, based on their own and previous reports, that APMPPE may be caused by a general hypersensitivity vasculitis. Retinal vasculitis associated with APMPPE in two patients reported by Kirkham and colleagues[5] in 1972 additionally support the idea that this disease is probably caused by a choroidal vasculitis.

Since then, more than 250 articles have appeared discussing patients with ocular findings consistent with APMPPE. In addition, numerous case reports have appeared reporting various ocular and systemic associations with this disease.

EPIDEMIOLOGY

APMPPE has been recognized as a distinct entity only for the past 30 years, and it represents an infrequent diagnosis in uveitis clinics. It was diagnosed in only five patients, representing 2% of the 240 with posterior uveitis, seen at the Immunology Service of the Massachusetts Eye and Ear Infirmary over one 10-year period.[6] This is an underrepresentation of cases, however, since at least as many cases of APMPPE were also treated by the Retina Service of the same hospital without referral to the Immunology Service.

APMPPE has a predilection for young adults, with peak occurrence between the ages of 20 and 30 years (mean age at onset, 26.5 years) and a range of 8 to 66 years.[7] Both sexes are equally affected. It has been observed primarily in whites, although dark-pigmented racial groups develop this disease as well.[8-11] Some authors believe that APMPPE cases appear to occur in clusters.[12] The true incidence and prevalence are unknown.

CLINICAL CHARACTERISTICS

APMPPE patients suddenly develop painless loss of vision in one or both eyes without external evidence of ocular inflammation. Retinal fundus examination discloses multiple round, circumscribed, flat, yellow-white, subretinal lesions involving the RPE. Depending on the localization of the lesions, patients may develop central or paracentral loss of vision. The overlying retina usually appears normal. The lesions are usually well circumscribed and discrete; they may be multiple and confluent, forming large patches (Fig. 70–1). After several days to weeks, the lesions begin to disappear, and these areas are replaced by scattered areas of depigmentation and fine to coarse clumping of the pigment epithelium (Fig. 70–2). After several weeks, some patients develop new lesions; these new lesions may appear in the peripheral fundus, tending to be round or linearly oriented radially (Fig. 70–3). Indeed, new lesions may develop in areas of unaffected retina, but they also may appear adjacent to healing lesions. These new lesions adjacent to healing lesions have a characteristic fluorescein angiographic appearance, the early phase of the angiogram showing a ring of choroidal hypofluorescence representing the acute APMPPE lesion and surrounding an area of choroidal hyperfluorescence representing the healed APMPPE lesion.

Ocular findings in patients with APMPPE include anterior or posterior chamber cells,[13, 14] keratic precipitates,[13, 15] episcleritis,[8, 14, 16] corneal melting,[17] retinal vasculitis,[5] pap-

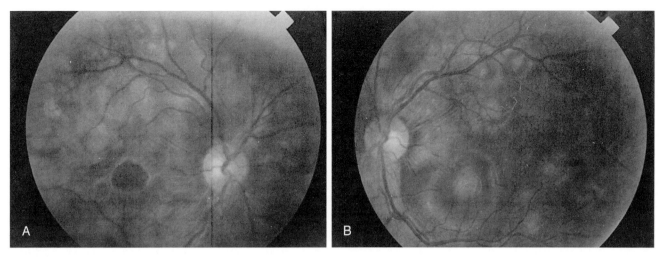

FIGURE 70–1. Acute posterior multifocal placoid pigment epitheliopathy (APMPPE). *A* and *B*, Fundus photograph of APMPPE. A 25-year-old Hispanic man presented to our clinic after 10 days of blurred vision in both eyes. Headache was the only symptom that preceded his eye disease. His visual acuity in the right eye was counting fingers (CF) to 12 ft and in the left eye was 20/30. Note the multiple round lesions. The right eye was the more affected (*A*) compared with the left eye (*B*). Note the well-circumscribed multifocal placoid lesion in the left eye (*B*).

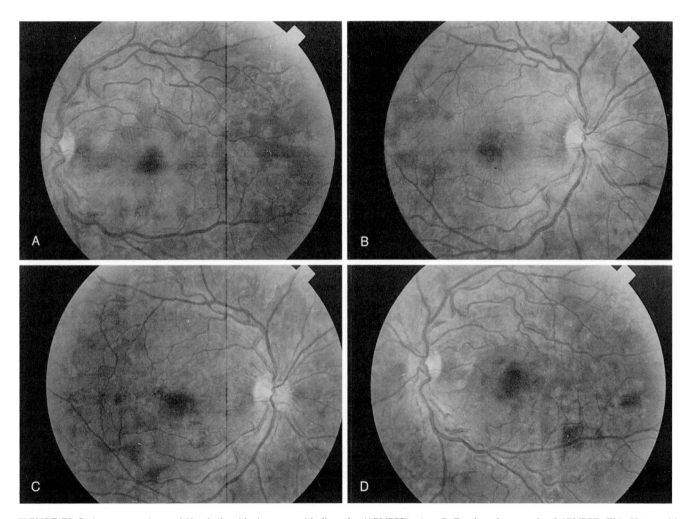

FIGURE 70–2. Acute posterior multifocal placoid pigment epitheliopathy (APMPPE). *A* to *D*, Fundus photograph of APMPPE. This 22-year-old Hispanic man presented with sudden loss of vision in his right eye (*A*) 2 weeks before his first visit to our clinic. The left eye (*B*) was affected one week after his right eye started with symptoms. Three weeks before his eye symptoms, he had severe headache accompanied by loss of appetite and nausea. He lost 11 pounds in that period. His initial visual acuity in the right eye (*A*) was CF 1 ft and his visual acuity in his left eye (*B*) was CF 3 ft. Nine months later, his visual acuity was 20/20 in both eyes (*C* and *D*). Note that the acute creamy lesions seen in the acute stage of the disease (*A* and *B*) were replaced by areas of depigmented RPE, and irregular clumping of pigment occurs (dark areas in *C* and *D*).

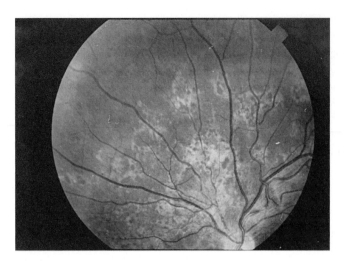

FIGURE 70–3. Acute posterior multifocal placoid pigment epitheliopathy (APMPPE). Fundus photograph. Some round irregular lesions are oriented radially following the direction of retinal vessels.

illitis,[5, 14] serious retinal detachment,[14, 15, 18] subretinal hemorrhages,[15] optic neuritis,[12] and vein occlusion.[19] Most of the patients with APMPPE have a history of a flulike syndrome before the onset of ocular symptoms. Fever, malaise, and headache may precede the ocular symptoms, suggesting a viral disease. APMPPE has been reported in patients with adenovirus type 5.[9] Systemic associations include cerebral vasculitis,[15, 20, 21] erythema nodosum,[3, 4] thyroiditis,[17] sarcoidosis,[22] microvascular nephropathy,[23] Lyme disease,[24] and elevated protein and pleocytosis in spinal fluid.[15, 21, 25]

APMPPE is most commonly bilateral, although unilateral cases have been described.[8, 7, 14] Patients complain of visual symptoms in one eye or both eyes simultaneously, although sometimes the fellow eye is involved within days or weeks after the first eye is affected. The loss of vision is sudden, and patients recover their vision after several weeks of the onset of visual loss, usually to 20/30 or even better (20/20). Recurrences are rare.[26, 27]

Fluorescein angiography in patients with APMPPE during the acute, active stage shows hypofluorescence during the early transit phase of the dye through the choroidal vasculature because the lesions block fluorescence resulting from RPE swelling, the presence of inflammatory cells, and tissue or choriocapillaris nonperfusion. In the late venous phase, they become hyperfluorescent, with fluorescence persisting up to 30 minutes (Fig. 70–4). This late hyperfluorescence is thought to represent diffusion of the fluorescein from the choroid into or between damaged pigment epithelial cells. The finding of leakage of dye from the periphery to the center of the lesions had been thought to support the theory that blockage is caused by inflammatory cells and inflamed tissue.

In the inactive stage of APMPPE, the fluorescein angiogram shows fluorescence in the background of areas of RPE atrophy and depigmentation. The late phases of the angiogram are remarkable for the lack of persistent fluorescence (Fig. 70–5). In those patients in whom acute lesions begin to resolve, the transition from the active to the inactive lesion can be useful in determining the presence and amount of residual activity.

Indocyanine green angiography (ICG) in APMPPE patients with acute lesions shows marked choroidal hypofluorescence in both the early and the late phases of the angiogram. In the early phases, large choroidal vessels can be seen in the hypofluorescent areas. In the late phases, the hypofluorescent lesions become well demarcated and irregularly shaped. Healed APMPPE lesions on ICG demonstrate choroidal hypofluorescence in the early and late phases. These lesions are smaller and less pronounced than the acute lesions of APMPPE.[28, 29]

Patients with APMPPE may have different responses in electrophysiologic studies. Although some patients have a normal electroretinogram (ERG) and electro-oculogram (EOG),[30] others have abnormal responses. Smith and colleagues[31] reported one patient with APMPPE who had abnormalities in color vision testing, subnormal EOG and subnormal β-wave in ERG, abnormally dark adaptation, and disorientation of the photoreceptors as demonstrated by an abnormal Stiles Crawford effect in the acute stage of APMPPE. Three weeks after the acute episode, they found normal visual acuity and normal EOG. One year later, the visual field, color testing, the Stiles Crawford effect, and dark adaptation were almost normal. Additional studies demonstrated abnormal densitometric results in parafoveal fixating APMPPE patients.[32] These findings, together with variation in the visual field abnormalities seen in patients with APMPPE, suggest that there may be a widespread, albeit transient, disruption to the RPE-photoreceptor complex in this disease.

In general, the visual prognosis in patients with APMPPE is good. Patients may experience a sudden drop in their vision ranging from a distorted 20/20 to counting fingers[1, 8, 23] at the onset of the disease, with recovery even to 20/20; the time between the onset of visual loss to improvement may take as long as 6 months.

PATHOPHYSIOLOGY/IMMUNOLOGY/PATHOLOGY

The etiology of APMPPE is unknown. An infectious etiology is suspected by the frequent occurrence of an antecedent viral illness. Some patients have developed APMPPE after swine flu vaccination,[33] hepatitis B vaccination,[34] mumps,[35] or bacterial infection.[36, 37] An increased incidence of a positive tuberculin skin test has also been reported in patients with APMPPE.[1, 5, 9] It is conceivable that a hypersensitivity reaction to antigens from different pathogens or antimicrobial agents[15] participates in the pathophysiology, leading to choroidal vasculitis and changes in the RPE.

The anatomic site of primary involvement in APMPPE is controversial. Some authors have favored the RPE. Gass[38] suggests that the primary area of pathology is in the RPE and perhaps retinal and receptor cells, but others have documented abnormal choroidal perfusion, indicating the choroid as the primary site of involvement. Deutman and Lion[28] propose that an acute inflammation resulting from a hypersensitivity reaction leads to occlusion of the precapillary choroidal arterioles feeding the lobules of the choriocapillaris, with subsequent secondary RPE changes. ICG angiography studies in patients with active and healed APMPPE support the hypothesis that the main cause of the placoid lesions is a partial choroidal

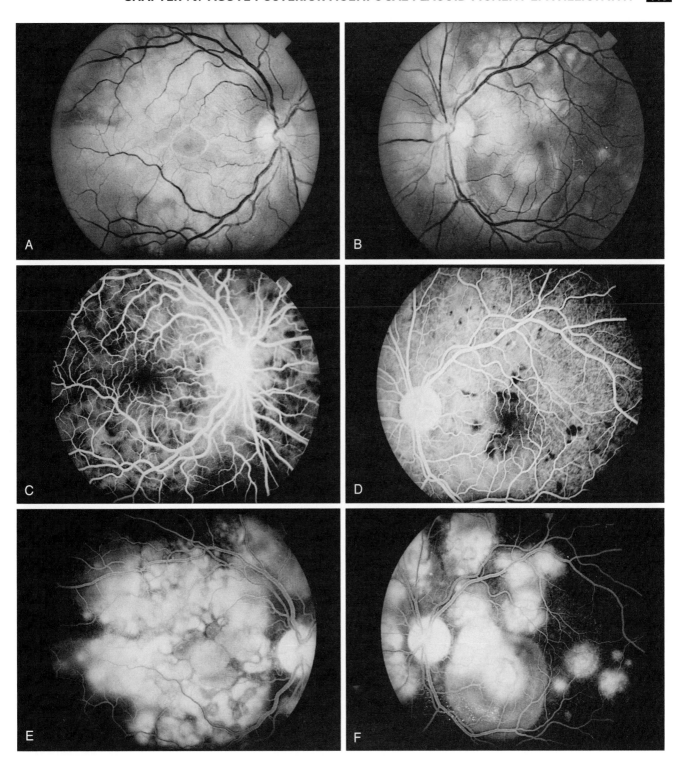

FIGURE 70–4. Acute posterior multifocal placoid pigment epitheliopathy (APMPPE). *A* to *F,* Fluorescein angiography in the acute stage of APMPPE. Same patient as in Figure 70–1. Red free photographs show clearly the multifocal placoid lesions in the right (*A*) and the left (*B*) eyes. Early transit of fluorescein revealed blockage of fluorescence in the region of the acute placoid lesions in the right (*C*) and the left (*D*) eyes. After several minutes of the injection of fluorescein, late staining of the acute lesions is evident in both eyes (*E* and *F*).

vascular occlusion, explaining the persistent pattern of choroidal hypofluorescence in the active or healed stages of APMPPE.[29, 39]

Wolf and coworkers[40] studied both human leukocyte antigen (HLA) classes I and II antigens in a series of 30 patients with APMPPE. They found HLA-B7 in 40% of patients compared with 16.6% of controls and HLA-DR2 in 56.7% of patients compared with 28.2% of controls. The immune system responds to a peptidic fragment of a foreign protein, which binds to specific major histocompatibility complex (MHC) molecules. Genes of MHC molecules are highly polymorphic: Diverse alleles exist within

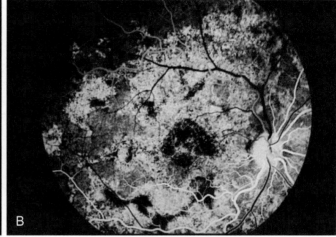

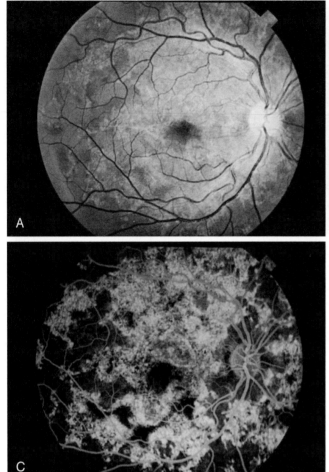

FIGURE 70–5. Acute posterior multifocal placoid pigment epitheliopathy (APMPPE). *A to C*, Fluorescein angiogram in the inactive stage of APMPPE. Same patient as in Figure 70–2. The red free photographs (*A*) show clearly the inactive stage of APMPPE. Comparing the early (*B*) and late (*C*) phases of the angiogram's lack of persistent fluorescence is evident. This angiogram was obtained nine months after the acute stage of APMPPE.

the population, and they are different in their ability to bind and present different antigenic determinants of proteins. If a peptidic determinant (e.g., one derived from an infectious agent) does not bind to any allelic MHC molecules expressed by an individual, that person's T cells cannot respond to that antigen. It is probable that certain HLAs predispose to develop certain diseases. HLA-B7 and HLA-DR2 were previously reported in high frequency in presumed ocular histoplasmosis[41] and HLA-B7 in serpiginous choroiditis.[42] It is possible that HLA-DR2 and HLA-B7 bind certain peptides from an infectious protein (viral or bacterial) predisposing to a specific pathophysiology event in APMPPE: choroidal nonperfusion secondary to vasculitis with subsequent RPE changes.

PATHOGENESIS

Delayed-type hypersensitivity (DTH) or type IV hypersensitivity has been implicated in the pathogenesis of APMPPE.[43] In a DTH response, antigen-specific CD4 + T_H1 cells secrete cytokines that recruit and activate effector cells such as macrophages and natural killer cells. One of the most important effector cytokines produced by T_H1 cells is interferon-γ, which stimulates microbicidal activities of phagocytes, promoting the intracellular destruction of phagocytosed microbes. T_H1 cells also secrete interleukin-2, which functions as an autocrine growth factor and stimulates the proliferation and differentiation

of CD8 + T cells. Additionally, T_H1 cells secrete lymphotoxin, which promotes the recruitment and activation of neutrophils. Cytokines function to (1) activate venular endothelial cells to recruit monocytes and other leukocytes at the level of the antigen challenge and (2) activate macrophages, enhancing their killing functions directed against intracellular microbes or viruses. Cytokines produced by CD8 + T cells can initiate the same reaction. In response to viral infections mediated by cytolytic T lymphocytes (CTLs), CD8 + T cells differentiate into functional CTLs. This process of differentiation requires cytokines secreted by antigen-active T cells. The function of CTLs is to destroy cells, other than macrophages, with intracellular viruses.[44]

Park and colleagues[43] cite several lines of indirect evidence, including the histopathology of some associated diseases seen in patients with APMPPE, that suggest that the pathogenesis was mediated by a DTH response:

1. The histopathologic findings in a patient with cerebral vasculitis showed cerebral arterial walls infiltrated with cells composed of monocytes, lymphocytes, histiocytes, epithelioid cells, and multinucleated giant cells.
2. Renal biopsy in a patient with sarcoidosis and APMPPE disclosed granulomatous cellular infiltration.
3. Tuberculin skin tests were positive in some patients with APMPPE.

4. Histopathologic results were positive in a patient with an ischemic infarct in the pons 6 months after he had APMPPE.

Additionally, fluorescein and ICG angiographic findings showing choroidal hypofluorescence could be explained because a DTH response with infiltrating T cells on the choroidal vessels leads to a partially obstructive vasculitis. This partial choroidal vascular occlusion explains the ICG choroidal hypofluorescence of acute and healed APMPPE lesions.[29, 39]

Other systemic vasculitic disorders reported in association with APMPPE can be on the basis of cell-mediated immunity. These include thyroiditis,[17] erythema nodosum,[3, 4] and microvascular nephropathy,[23] retinal vasculitis,[5] papillitis,[5, 14] and choroidal periphlebitis. Additionally, the frequent prodromal flulike syndrome suffered by most patients suggests a viral disease. It is well known that cell-mediated immunity is most important against microbes and viruses that live intracellularly.[44]

DIAGNOSIS

The diagnosis of APMPPE is clinical. A thorough diagnostic evaluation must include medical history, review of systems, and ocular examination. Careful questioning for a prodromal viral disease is important. Patients may complain that they have had headache, fever, malaise, myalgia, or upper respiratory symptoms weeks before the onset of eye symptoms. Approximately one third of patients with APMPPE have a history of recent viral illness.[15, 36]

Because some patients may have neurologic symptoms, admission to the hospital may be necessary. Usually patients with neurologic manifestations of the disease need rapid medical treatment and studies, including magnetic resonance imaging of the brain, computed tomography, and cerebrospinal fluid studies.

DIFFERENTIAL DIAGNOSIS

Many entities must be considered in the differential diagnosis of APMPPE. The presenting features of the disease will determine the focus of the differential diagnosis. The following diseases must frequently be excluded in diagnosing APMPPE: serpiginous choroidopathy, diffuse unilateral subacute neuroretinitis, multiple evanescent white dot syndrome, multifocal choroiditis with panuveitis, vitiliginous choroiditis, acute retinal pigment epitheliopathy (ARPE), punctate inner choroidopathy, sarcoidosis, syphilis, Harada's disease, sympathetic uveitis, primary or metastasic neoplastic infiltrates of the choroid or sub-RPE space, and choriocapillaris infarcts secondary to systemic hypertension (e.g., toxemia of pregnancy).

Because of clinical similarities at presentation, it is important to differentiate APMPPE from serpiginous choroiditis and Harada's disease. Serpiginous choroiditis usually begins in the third decade of life, it resolves slowly compared with APMPPE, and it produces profound choroid atrophy. Lesions in serpiginous choroiditis are localized around the optic nerve involving the macular area. In APMPPE, lesions are localized mainly at the postequatorial area. These lesions are isolated and multifocal, and fluorescein angiography shows similar patterns in both

serpiginous choroiditis and APMPPE. Visual recovery is poorer and recurrences are more frequent in serpiginous choroiditis.

Patients with Harada's disease develop an initial acute bilateral visual loss caused by serous retinal detachment, which may be preceded by headache, malaise, vomiting, and occasionally neurologic signs and symptoms. Commonly, patients have vitreous cells, iridocyclitis, and a hyperemic optic nerve. Some patients with Harada's disease eventually develop severe anterior uveitis, alopecia, poliosis, cutaneous and perilimbal vitiligo, and dysacousis (Vogt-Koyanagi-Harada syndrome). Some patients with Harada's disease may have multifocal, gray-white patches at the level of the RPE similar to, although less well defined than, those seen in patients with APMPPE. Fluorescein angiography findings in patients with Harada's disease can be identical to those in patients with APMPPE, but patients with Harada's disease show an accumulation of the fluorescein dye in the subretinal space in the late phases of the angiogram. Harada's disease and APMPPE are different mainly in the course of the disease. Although in a few patients with Harada's disease the retinal detachment may resolve spontaneously within several weeks, usually the course is prolonged and patients need systemic corticosteroid therapy to shorten the duration of the retinal detachment and to improve the visual prognosis. Additionally, other immunosuppressive drugs may be required. Recurrences are common in patients with Harada's disease and uncommon in patients with APMPPE.

ASSOCIATED DISEASES

APMPPE has been associated with systemic viral illness, different transient cerebral disturbances, cerebral vasculitis, eythema nodosum, subclinical nephropathy, thyroiditis, sarcoidosis, juvenile rheumatoid arthritis, tuberculosis, and streptococcal infection.

TREATMENT

APMPPE has a self-limiting clinical course. Prednisolone has been used effectively by many authors, but patients who did not receive steroids also showed improvement in their final visual acuity.[46] Therefore, it is often argued that APMPPE needs no treatment: it resolves without treatment, with 80% of patients enjoying 20/40 or better vision. However, 20% are left with impaired vision, and 20/40 is not good enough.

Patients with APMPPE and neurologic disease (e.g., cerebral vasculitis) improve with steroid therapy and cytotoxic drug therapy.[21] Bridges and colleagues[47] reported on a 16-year-old girl who had juvenile rheumatoid arthritis and developed APMPPE. She was treated initially with steroids but did not improve. Cyclosporin A therapy produced improvement in visual acuity within 14 days.

I suggest that systemic steroid therapy be considered in APMPPE patients with macular involvement because it is an inflammatory problem, 20% of eyes affected by APMPPE never recover vision above 20/40, even many patients with a final acuity of better than 20/40 are affected by the imperfect recovery of vision, and uncontrolled experience suggests that prompt systemic steroid therapy is effective in rapidly resolving the retinal inflammation.

CONCLUSIONS

APMPPE is a recently recognized posterior uveitis presenting mainly in young patients. Characteristically, patients with APMPPE experience a rapid loss of vision in one eye or both eyes simultaneously, and funduscopic examination shows multiple round, creamy subretinal lesions. After several days or weeks, these lesions disappear and are replaced by areas of pigment epithelium. The fluorescein angiographic and ICG findings are characteristic of this disorder and are frequently helpful in differentiating it from other entities. Although the pathogenesis and etiology are indeed unknown, recent ICG findings and systemic associations suggest that a hypersensitivity-mediated obstructive vasculitis resulting in partial choroidal vascular occlusion may be responsible for the lesions seen in APMPPE. The visual prognosis is generally good without treatment, but it may well be that early and aggressive treatment may result in altering the natural history of the disease and improvement of visual outcome. Future histopathologic and immunopathologic study may prove valuable in understanding the pathogenesis and in developing treatment strategies for patients with this disease.

References

1. Gass JDM: Acute posterior multifocal placoid pigment epitheliopathy. Arch Ophthalmol 1968;80:177–185.
2. Maumenee AE: Clinical entities in "uveitis": An approach to the study of intraocular inflammation. Am J Ophthalmol 1970;69:1–27.
3. Van Buskirk EM, Lessell S, Friedman E: Pigmentary epitheliopathy and erythema nodosum. Arch Ophthalmol 1971;85:369–372.
4. Deutman AF, Oosterhuis JA, Boen-Tan TN, Aan De Kerk AL: Acute posterior multifocal placoid pigment epitheliopathy. Br J Ophthalmol 1972;56:863–874.
5. Kirkham TH, Ffytche TJ, Sanders MD: Placoid pigment epitheliopathy with retinal vasculitis and papillitis. Br J Ophthalmol 1972;56:875–880.
6. Rodriguez A, Calonge M, Pedroza-Seres M, et al: Referral patterns of uveitis in a tertiary eye care center. Arch Ophthalmol 1996;114:593–599.
7. Ryan SJ, Maumenee AE: Acute posterior multifocal placoid pigment epitheliopathy. Am J Ophthalmol 1972;74:1066–1074.
8. Annesley WH, Tomer TL, Shields JA: Multifocal placoid pigment epitheliopathy. Am J Ophthalmol 1973;76:511–518.
9. Azar P, Gohd RS, Waltman D, Gitter KA: Acute posterior multifocal placoid pigment epitheliopathy associated with an adenovirus type 5 infection. Am J Ophthalmol 1975;80:1003–1005.
10. Isashiki M, Koide H, Yamashita T, et al: Acute posterior multifocal placoid pigment epitheliopathy associated with diffuse retinal vasculitis and late haemorrhagic macular detachment. Br J Ophthalmol 1986;70:255–259.
11. Kim RY, Holz FG, Gregor Z, et al: Recurrent acute multifocal placoid pigment epitheliopathy in two cousins. Am J Ophthalmol 1995;119:660–662.
12. Wolf MD, Folk JC, Goeken EN: Acute placoid multifocal epitheliopathy and optic neuritis in a family. Am J Ophthalmol 1990;110:89–90.
13. Fitzpatrick PJ, Robertson DM: Acute placoid multifocal pigment epitheliopathy. Arch Ophthalmol 1973;89:373–376.
14. Savino PJ, Weinberg RJ, Yassin JG, Pilkerton AR: Diverse manifestations of acute posterior multifocal placoid pigment epitheliopathy. Am J Ophthalmol 1974;77:659–662.
15. Holt WS, Regan CDJ, Trempe C: Acute placoid multifocal pigment epitheliopathy. Am J Ophthalmol 1976;81:403–412.
16. Gass JDM: Acute posterior multifocal pigment epitheliopathy: A long term follow-up study. In: Fine SL, Owens SL, eds: Management of Retinal Vascular and Macular Disorders. Baltimore, Williams & Wilkins, 1983, p 176.
17. Jacklin HN: Acute posterior multifocal placoid pigment epitheliopathy and thyroiditis. Arch Ophthalmol 1977;95:189–194.
18. Bird AC, Hamilton AM: Placoid pigment epitheliopathy presenting with bilateral serous retinal detachment. Br J Ophthalmol 1972;56:881–886.
19. Alle SD, Marks SJ: Acute posterior multifocal placoid pigment epitheliopathy with bilateral central retinal vein occlusion. Am J Ophthalmol 1998;126:309–312.
20. Sigelman J, Behrens M, Hilal S: Acute posterior multifocal placoid pigment epitheliopathy associated with cerebral vasculitis and homonymous hemianopsia. Am J Ophthalmol 1979;88:919–924.
21. Sinan C, Thierry V, Jeffrey SR, Neil AB: Neurological manifestations of acute posterior multifocal placoid pigment epitheliopathy. Stroke 1996;27:996–1001.
22. Dick DJ, Newman PK, Richardson J, et al: Acute posterior multifocal placoid pigment epitheliopathy and sarcoidosis. Br J Ophthalmol 1988;72:74–77.
23. Laatikainen LT, Immonen IJR: Acute posterior multifocal placoid pigment epitheliopathy in connection with acute nephritis. Retina 1988;8:122–124.
24. Bodine SR, Marino J, Camisa TJ, Salvate AJ: Multifocal choroiditis with evidence of Lyme disease. Ann Ophthalmol 1992;24:169–173.
25. Bullock JD, Fletcher RL: Cerebrospinal fluid abnormalities in acute posterior multifocal placoid pigment epitheliopathy. Am J Ophthalmol 1977;84:45–49.
26. Lewis R, Martonyi CL: Acute posterior multifocal placoid pigment epitheliopathy: A recurrence. Arch Ophthalmol 1975;93:235–238.
27. Lyness AL, Bird AC: Recurrences of acute posterior multifocal placoid pigment epitheliopathy. Am J Ophthalmol 1984;98:203–207.
28. Deutman AF, Lion F: Choriocapillaris nonperfusion in acute posterior multifocal placoid pigment epitheliopathy. Am J Ophthalmol 1977;84:652–658.
29. Howe LJ, Woon H, Graham EM, et al: Choroidal hypoperfusion in acute placoid multifocal pigment epitheliopathy: An indocyanine green angiography study. Ophthalmology 1995;102:790–798.
30. Fishman GA, Rabb MF, Kaplan J: Acute posterior multifocal placoid pigment epitheliopathy. Arch Ophthalmol 1974;92:173.
31. Smith VC, Dokorny J, Ernest JT, et al: Visual function in acute placoid multifocal pigment epitheliopathy. Am J Ophthalmol 1978;85:192.
32. Keunen JEE, van Meel GJ, van Norren D, et al: Retinal densitometry in acute posterior multifocal placoid pigment epitheliopathy. Invest Ophthalmol Vis Sci 1989;30:1515–1521.
33. Hector RE: Acute posterior multifocal placoid pigment epitheliopathy. Am J Ophthalmol 1978;86:424–425.
34. Brézin AP, Massin-Korobelnik P, Boudin M, et al: Acute posterior multifocal placoid pigment epitheliopathy after hepatitis B vaccine. Arch Ophthalmol 1995;113:297–300.
35. Borruat FX, Piguet B, Herbort CP: Acute posterior multifocal placoid pigment epitheliopathy following mumps. Ocul Immunol Inflamm 1998;6:189–193.
36. Brown M, Eberdt A, Lodos G: Pigment epitheliopathy in a patient with mycobacterial infection. J Pediatr Ophthalmol 1973;10:278.
37. Lowder CY, Foster RE, Gordon SM, et al: Acute posterior multifocal placoid pigment epitheliopathy after acute group A streptococcal infection. Am J Ophthalmol 1996;122:115–117.
38. Gass JDM: Inflammatory diseases of the retina and choroid. In: Stereoscopic Atlas of Macular Diseases. Diagnosis and Treatment, 4th ed. St. Louis, C.V. Mosby, 1997, pp 668–675.
39. Park D, Schatz H, McDunald R, Johnson RN: Indocyanine green angiography of acute placoid multifocal pigment epitheliopathy. Ophthalmology 1995;102:1877–1883.
40. Wolf MD, Folk JC, Panknene CA, Goeken EN: HLA-B7 and HLA-DR2 antigens and acute placoid multifocal pigment epitheliopathy. Arch Ophthalmol 1990;108:698–700.
41. Meredith TA, Smith RE, Duquesnoy RJ: Association of HLA-DRw2 antigen with presumed ocular histoplasmosis. Am J Ophthalmol 1980;89:70–76.
42. Chan CC, Hooks JJ, Nussenblatt RB, et al: Expression of Ia antigen

on retinal pigment epithelium in experimental autoimmune uveitis. Curr Eye Res 1988;5:325–330.

43. Park D, Schatz H, McDonald HR, et al: Acute multifocal posterior placoid pigment epitheliopathy: A theory of pathogenesis. Retina 1995;15:351–352.

44. Abbas AK, Lichtman AH, Pober JS: Cytokines. In: Abbas AK, Lichtman AH, Pober JS, eds: Cellular and Molecular Immunology. Philadelphia, W.B. Saunders, 1997, p 249.

45. Anderson K, Patel KR, Webb L, et al: Acute placoid multifocal pigment epitheliopathy associated with pulmonary tuberculosis. Br J Ophthalmol 1996;80:186.

46. Williams DF, Mieler WF: Long-term follow-up of acute placoid multifocal pigment epitheliopathy. Br J Ophthalmol 1989;73:985–990.

47. Bridges WJ, Saadeh C, Gerald R: Acute placoid multifocal pigment epitheliopathy in a patient with systemic-onset juvenile rheumatoid arthritis: Treatment with cyclosporin A and prednisone. Arthritis Rheum 1995;38:446–447.

Benalexander A. Pedro

DEFINITION

Acute retinal pigment epitheliitis (ARPE) is a distinct clinical entity characterized by acute inflammation of the retinal pigment epithelium (RPE) and manifested by transient and relatively subtle alterations at the level of the RPE. These are seen ophthalmoscopically as discrete clusters of small, dark-gray spots at the macular area, which clinically cause blurring of vision. Each of these spots appears to be surrounded by a yellow, halo-like zone. These lesions spontaneously resolve within weeks to months, accompanied by recovery of vision. Although there are many theories as to the nature of this transient RPE inflammation, its etiology currently remains unknown. A viral etiology seems plausible in light of the acute yet transient clinical course of this disorder.

HISTORY

Acute retinal pigment epitheliitis (ARPE), or Krill's disease, is a rare, yet relatively new, clinical entity, first described by Krill and Deutman[1] in six patients less than three decades ago (1972). Deutman[2] described two additional patients 2 years later in 1974. Since the publication of these two reports, other cases with similar clinical findings and courses have been described in the ophthalmic literature.[3-9] Some atypical cases believed to be ARPE were also reported.[5, 10-12]

EPIDEMIOLOGY

Patients with ARPE are typically young, healthy adults in the second to fourth decade of life. This condition has been reported to affect individuals from 16 to 75 years of age. The median age of onset is about 45 years. There appears to be neither a racial nor a genetic predilection. Of the more than 70 well-documented cases of ARPE, it appears that more than two thirds occur in male patients.[1, 2, 4, 5, 8, 13] The perturbation of the RPE in these patients may be bilateral or unilateral.

Acute retinal pigment epitheliitis (ARPE) is not a common disease. It is likely that this condition is underreported, given the transient nature of the disease and the often mild and negligible symptoms noted by patients, who may not seek ophthalmologic consultation. Furthermore, the inexperienced examiner may easily miss the subtle clinical findings in the macula and posterior pole. These factors increase the likelihood that the acute phase of the disorder will be missed. It is likely that, because of these factors, ARPE went unrecognized before Krill first described the condition in 1972.

CLINICAL FEATURES

Typically, ARPE is characterized by a patient history of acute visual disturbance characterized by unilateral blurred vision or metamorphopsia. A small proportion of patients end up complaining of a central scotoma.[1, 2] In one study, 15% of affected individuals were asymptomatic.[4] There is usually no preceding history of illness or flulike symptoms in the otherwise healthy patient. The systems review is generally unremarkable.

On clinical examination, the visual acuities of patients with ARPE are typically 20/20 to 20/100 at the time of presentation; visual acuity is 20/30 or better in about three fourths of patients. Bilateral ocular involvement is seen in about 40% of cases.[1, 2, 4, 5, 8, 13] The anterior segment examination is usually normal, without stigmata of acute inflammation. On the Amsler grid, patients may show a central scotoma or metamorphopsia. These findings may also be reflected in visual field examinations. Color vision abnormalities have been detected.[1, 2]

Funduscopy early in the disease shows the typical round macular lesions that are the hallmark of the disease. These are discrete clusters of small, hyperpigmented, dark-gray spots at the level of the retinal pigment epithelium surrounded by a yellowish white "halo" or area of depigmentation[1, 2] (Fig. 71-1). Each cluster typically contains one to four spots. As the condition resolves, the dark, grayish spots may further darken, displaying a pattern of pigment migration, or they may fade and become difficult to detect clinically. The halo noted around these spots also becomes less distinct as the disease resolves.[1-3, 5, 7] The lesions are generally confined to the macular region. However, extramacular lesions may also be observed, albeit rarely.[1] Other structures such as the optic nerve, retina, and retinal vasculature are normal, with absence of subretinal fluid, retinal edema, or perivasculitis. Infrequently, in some cases, a mild vitritis may be seen.[4, 7, 9]

A case of a 36-year-old male is shown in Figure 71-1. He initially complained of acute-onset blurring of vision in both eyes, which he described as a "haze." There was no history of illness or flulike symptoms. Review of systems was unremarkable except for a history of thyroiditis.

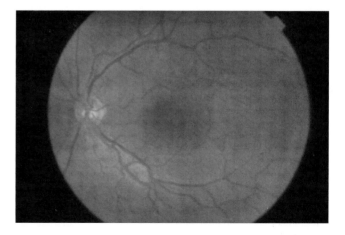

FIGURE 71-1. This photograph shows the left fundus of a 36-year-old male who complained of acute onset blurring of vision in both eyes. There are discrete clusters of small, hyperpigmented gray spots with a yellowish white halo at the level of the RPE at the macular area.

The patient's visual acuity was 20/20 in both eyes. A "doughnut"-shaped scotoma was elicited on Amsler grid. The anterior segment was quiet.

COMPLICATIONS

No significant ocular complications have been described in association with ARPE; the typical course of the disease is one of complete resolution of the symptoms. This natural history is so characteristic that an alternative diagnosis should be considered, should there be significant ocular complications or sequelae in a suspected case of ARPE.

ETIOLOGY, PATHOGENESIS, AND PATHOLOGY

The precise etiology and pathogenesis of ARPE are still unknown. It has been thought that this disorder represents an inflammatory condition at the level of the retinal pigment epithelium. Owing to the similarity of the retinal lesions of ARPE to those of rubella retinopathy, some have postulated a viral etiology. This notion is supported by cases of ARPE that were discovered to have an association with hepatitis C,[14, 15] and by the case of a woman with bilateral ARPE who had concurrent fever, chills, and myalgia of unknown etiology.[12]

The EAPU Animal Model

Experimental autoimmune pigment epithelial membrane protein–induced uveitis (EAPU) has been induced in Lewis rats by immunization with RPE membrane protein.[16] EAPU is mainly characterized by retinal pigment epithelial inflammation; this animal model provides new insight into the pathology of pigment epitheliitis. Clinical signs of EAPU begin to manifest at days 7 and 9 after immunization and peak by days 12 and 14. Histologic studies show typical plaque-shaped cell accumulations containing macrophages along the RPE.

Broekhuyse and colleagues studied the effect of macrophage depletion on EAPU.[16] They found that systemic treatment with a macrophage-depleting substance, C12MDP-containing liposomes (dichloromethylene diphosphate), immediately before the expected onset of the clinical signs of EAPU (days 7 and 9 after immunization) considerably delayed the inflammatory process. However, 2 weeks after treatment, a rebound EAPU was noted. Systemic treatment at the peak stage of EAPU (days 12 and 14 after immunization) resulted in rapid disappearance of the clinical signs of uveitis. Previously deposited cellular accumulations along the RPE neither regressed nor demonstrated further progression. Broekhuyse and associates concluded that hematogenous macrophages appear to play a crucial role in the development of EAPU, but that the effect of early macrophage depletion on EAPU appears temporary owing to blood repopulation of this cell line.

As further studies on animal models of pigment epitheliitis continue to be performed, new insights into the pathophysiology of this condition are sure to evolve.[16, 17]

DIAGNOSIS

The diagnosis of ARPE is clinical and is based on a history of acute visual decline or metamorphopsia in an otherwise healthy adult in the second or third decade of life, coupled with the characteristic retinal findings described previously. The review of systems typically is noncontributory.

Aside from the changes noted in Amsler grid and visual field examinations, other ancillary procedures such as fluorescein angiography (FA) and electrophysiologic studies aid in the diagnosis of this condition.

In the early phases of the fluorescein angiogram, multiple, small hyperfluorescent spots at the level of the RPE in the posterior pole and macula are noted. This hyperfluorescence corresponds to the depigmented halo around the hypofluorescent central dark spot. The dark spot central to the halo shows hypofluorescence, consistent with dye blockage from hyperpigmentation (Fig. 71–2). The hyperfluorescence increases mildly in mid-transit, consistent with window defect transmission, without late leakage or staining.[1–4, 5] Rarely, the FA fails to highlight this macular lesion.[2]

At times, the peripapillary area may be involved; rarely, in the late frames, the hyperfluorescent dots may appear to have slightly fuzzy margins, which may be indicative of mild leakage.

Electro-oculography (EOG) performed in patients with ARPE is abnormal in the acute stages.[1, 2] With clinical resolution of the disease, the EOG reverts to normal.[1, 2, 5] This abnormality in the acute stages appears to imply a more widespread dysfunction at the level of the RPE despite the paucity of findings on ophthalmoscopy or angiography. Electroretinography (ERG) and visual evoked response (VER) are normal.[1, 2, 5]

Figure 71–2 shows the FA of the patient in the previous figure (Fig. 71–1). Hyperfluorescence at the macular area and posterior pole mildly increases at the mid-phase of the angiogram and fades slightly in late frames with no late leakage or staining. EOG performed on this patient was abnormal, showing a low Arden's ratio. ERG was normal.

A summary of the diagnostic features of ARPE is shown in Table 71–1.

DIFFERENTIAL DIAGNOSIS

The differential diagnoses of ARPE appear in Table 71–2. These include acute macular neuroretinopathy (AMN), acute posterior multifocal placoid pigment epitheliopathy (APMPPE), central serous chorioretinopathy (CSCR), and viral retinitides (particularly rubella retinitis).

Acute Macular Neuroretinopathy

Bos and Deutman first described acute macular neuroretinopathy in 1975.[18] This is another rare condition that typically afflicts young adults, with acute onset of decreased central or paracentral vision and a history of a flulike prodrome. In AMN, there are subtle findings of superficial, dark, reddish-brown, petalloid or wedge-shaped retinal lesions in the macular area that resolve over several weeks to months. Acute macular neuroretinopathy is bilateral. Vision generally improves to baseline acuity over time, although paracentral scotomata may persist.

On fluorescein angiography, the clinician may detect no abnormalities.[18] More commonly, however, nonleaking

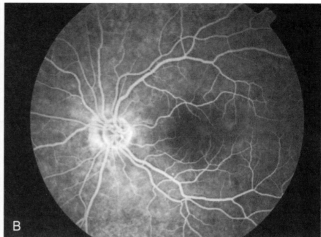

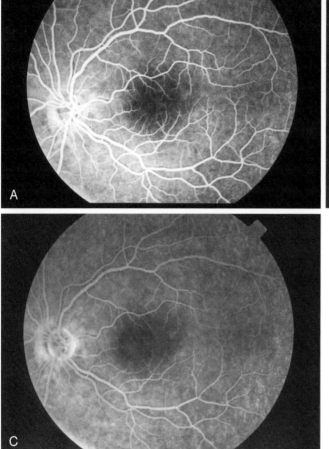

FIGURE 71–2. Fluorescein angiography of the patient seen in Figure 71–1 shows *(A)* the early phase of the angiogram in which hyperfluorescence that corresponds to the yellowish halo and hypofluorescence of the central dark spot is seen at the macular area in clusters. *B,* In mid-films, there is little change in the characteristics seen in the early films. *C,* Late films show no leakage from the pigment epithelial defects, which slightly fade.

dilated perifoveal capillaries[18] may be noted or early hyperfluorescence, followed by late staining of the macular lesions.[19–21]

Acute Posterior Multifocal Placoid Pigment Epitheliopathy

APMPPE is another condition typically included in the differential diagnosis of ARPE. Gass first described APMPPE in 1968.[22] This syndrome has been well characterized clinically by an acute decrease in central visual acuity in association with yellow-white placoid lesions at the level of the RPE and scattered throughout the posterior pole. As in ARPE, this is followed by spontaneous recovery.

APMPPE usually presents in the third decade of life, but has been reported in patients from 8 to 57 years of age.[23–26] It has neither racial nor sexual predilection. It is most commonly bilateral but may be unilateral at initial presentation. Vision may range from 20/20 to count fingers at the acute stage.

Unlike in ARPE, the anterior segment of patients with APMPPE may show episcleritis,[24, 25, 27, 28] marginal corneal thinning,[29] and iritis.[23–28, 30–33] Fundic findings are distinctly different from those of ARPE. Multiple, flat, cream-colored patches at the level of the pigment epithelium and choriocapillaris are the ophthalmoscopic hallmarks of APMPPE.[22, 23] The lesions are round and ovoid, with indistinct borders, and they are larger than ARPE

lesions. They vary in size from 1/8- to 1/4-disc diameters.[34] The lesions may become confluent and plaquelike. Initial lesions usually involve the posterior pole. As the disease evolves, fresh patches tend to arise in the periphery. Typically, there is a mild vitritis.[26–28, 30, 35] Less common fundic findings include retinal edema or hemorrhage,[24, 25, 36] retinal vasculitis,[25, 28, 36, 37] papillitis,[27, 29, 36, 38, 39] and serous retinal detachment.[25–27, 40–42]

Resolution of these subretinal lesions takes around 2 to 5 weeks. Pigment clumping and depigmentation occur with resolution. Recurrences are not common but have been noted.[40, 43–45]

APMPPE may occur as a solitary entity or, unlike ARPE, it may be associated with other systemic inflammatory disorders.[26, 46–52] Like ARPE, although an infectious etiology is postulated, no specific agents have been isolated. APMPPE may represent a nonspecific ocular manifestation of a systemic inflammatory disease, possibly affecting the central nervous system.[27, 46, 47]

Fluorescein angiography of the placoid lesions of APMPPE is distinctive and cannot be confused with ARPE. Hypofluorescence is observed early, followed by hyperfluorescence in the late venous phase. Each individual placoid lesion seen clinically may represent an area of focal swelling of the pigment epithelium overlying a nonperfused lobule of choriocapillaris.

No treatments specific for APMPPE have been discov-

TABLE 71–1. ACUTE RETINAL PIGMENT EPITHELIITIS: DIAGNOSTIC FEATURES

PATIENT CHARACTERISTICS
- Average age 45 years
- Sex incidence shows slight male-to-female preponderance
- No race or genetic predilection

OCULAR EXAMINATION
Anterior segment
- Typically quiet
Posterior segment
- Only fundus lesions noted
- Mild vitritis seen rarely
- Fundus lesions with round gray-black spots surrounded by yellow-white halo

ANCILLARY TESTS
- Amsler grid may show central metamorphopsia or central scotoma
- Visual field examinations may show a central scotoma
- Color vision abnormalities have been detected
- Angiographic findings show hypofluorescence of gray-black spots with surrounding early hyperfluorescent halo that fades later
- Electrophysiologic tests may show an abnormal electro-oculogram (EOG) with typically normal electroretinogram (ERG) and visual evoked response (VER)

DISEASE CHARACTERISTICS
- Visual acuity may range from 20/20 to 20/100 on presentation
- Occasionally bilateral
- Visual resolution noted within 6 to 12 weeks
- Recurrence has been noted but is atypical
- No systemic disease involvement
- Etiology is unknown, presumed viral
- Currently needs no therapy

ered, but high-dose systemic prednisone may hasten resolution of the problem. Overall, the visual prognosis of APMPPE is favorable, with about 80% of affected eyes having a final visual acuity of 20/40 or better.[53] However, persistent paracentral scotomata have been observed[23, 32, 36, 43, 44, 49, 54] and, unlike ARPE, cases with foveal involvement or recurrent inflammation tend to have poorer final visual acuities.[23, 24, 28, 45] The overall favorable natural history of APMPPE may breed complacency among ophthalmologists, who may treat this entity less aggressively than ARPE. Although the decision to treat with systemic steroids may be straightforward in patients presenting with severe or recurrent disease, it may well be that early and aggressive systemic treatment in patients with less severe disease may hasten visual recovery and improve overall visual outcome. Such is not the case with ARPE, in which adverse sequelae of inflammation are not described and excellent visual recovery is the rule.

Central Serous Chorioretinopathy
Among the differential diagnoses of ARPE, CSCR is probably the most difficult and important to exclude in the latter stages of disease.

TABLE 71–2. ACUTE RETINAL PIGMENT EPITHELIITIS: DIFFERENTIAL DIAGNOSES

Acute macular neuroretinopathy
Acute posterior multifocal placoid pigment epitheliopathy (APMPPE)
Central serous chorioretinopathy (CSCR)
Rubella retinitis (and other viral retinitides)

Von Graefe first described CSCR in 1866.[55] It is typically seen in young adults to middle-aged individuals, with ages ranging from 20 to 45 years.[55–66] There is a greater male-to-female preponderance of 8 to 10:1.[56, 66, 67–70] Patients with CSCR may occasionally complain of migraine-like headaches.[57] Additionally, they typically have type A personality traits.[71] Unilateral or bilateral involvement may be seen clinically.

Like with ARPE, patients may complain of decreased or blurred vision, metamorphopsia, paracentral scotomata, and chromatopsias. Vision in the acute stage of this disorder may range from 20/20 to 20/200.[66] The ophthalmoscopic hallmark of CSCR is a neurosensory retinal detachment. In addition, serous RPE detachment, subretinal precipitates, extramacular RPE atrophic tracts, multiple bullous serous retinal and RPE detachments, and RPE atrophic changes have been described.[57, 58, 66]

Fluorescein angiography in the acute stage typically shows a hyperfluorescent focal RPE defect that leaks dye. The dye accumulates beneath a neurosensory retinal detachment, which manifests as dye pooling in the late phases of the angiogram. This finding is the most important differentiating point between ARPE and CSCR in the acute stages. Unlike nonleaking focal RPE defects seen in ARPE, angiography in CSCR shows leakage of dye in the early stages, with pooling of dye within the serous detachment in the late frames. In the resolution phase of both diseases, it is difficult to differentiate CSCR from ARPE. Like ARPE, CSCR may, upon its resolution, leave pigmentary changes in the macula.

Krill and Deutman postulated that the RPE disturbance may lead to serous fluid leakage due to the breakdown of the pigment epithelial blood-ocular barrier.[1] Earlier studies have also shown a link between ARPE and CSCR in nine patients.[4] Piermarocchi and coworkers documented a case of ARPE that developed into CSCR with focal leakage in areas where ARPE lesions were initially noted.[13] It remains a possibility that in the pathogenesis of CSCR, retinal pigment epitheliitis may play a significant role. Other authors, however, prefer that CSCR-related ARPE be considered as a "secondary" form of CSCR, distinct from the idiopathic form of CSCR.[72]

Viral Retinitides
Viral retinitides, particularly rubella retinitis, show remarkably similar pigmentary changes in the retina compared with those of ARPE.[73] The most common ocular finding in ocular rubella syndrome is retinopathy, which occurs in 25% to 50% of eyes.[74] It is most commonly seen in children and may be unilateral or bilateral.[75] When there is no significant coexisting pathologic condition, visual acuity may range from 20/20 to 20/60, with a median range of 20/25.[76]

The pigmentary changes appear as fine, granular, symmetric mottling of the pigment epithelium, with a "salt-and-pepper" fundus appearance. However, one may differentiate rubella retinopathy from ARPE by the coarser pigmentation, the more widespread involvement of the retina, and the associated systemic findings associated with the former syndrome. Occasionally, pigment spicules and choroidal vascular changes are seen in rubella reti-

TABLE 71–3. DIFFERENTIATING FEATURES AMONG ARPE, AMN, APMPPE, AND CSCR

	ACUTE RETINAL PIGMENT EPITHELIITIS (ARPE)	ACUTE MACULAR NEURORETINOPATHY (AMN)	ACUTE POSTERIOR MULTIFOCAL PLACOID PIGMENT EPITHELIOPATHY (APMPPE)	CENTRAL SEROUS CHORIORETINOPATHY (CSCR)
Age	16–75 years (median, 45)	Young adults	8–57 years (3rd decade)	20–45 years
Sex	M>F	F>M	M = F	M>F
Systemic Association	None	Flulike (viral) prodrome	May have associated cerebral vasculitis, CSF pleocytosis, tinnitus, sarcoidosis, etc.	Migraine-type headaches, type A personality, hysteria, and hypochondriasis
Laterality	Unilateral/bilateral	Usually bilateral	Usually bilateral but may initially be unilateral	Unilateral/bilateral
Anterior Segment Findings	None	None	Occasionally, episcleritis, marginal corneal thinning, and iridocyclitis may be seen	None
Funduscopic Findings	Discrete clusters of small, dark-gray spots in the RPE surrounded by a yellowish halo	Superficial dark, reddish-brown, petalloid or wedge-shaped lesions	Multiple yellowish-white placoid lesions at the level of pigment epithelium or choriocapillaris	Serous retinal detachment, serous RPE detachment, subretinal precipitates, extramacular RE atrophic tracts, multiple bullous serous retinal and RPE detachment, and RPE atrophic changes
Associated Posterior Segment Findings	None. Vitritis has been reported	None	Mild vitritis, occasional retinal hemorrhage, retinal edema, vasculitis, serous RD, and papillitis may be seen	None
Fluorescein Angiogram Findings	Central hypofluorescence with a surrounding hyperfluorescence, corresponding to the central gray spot and surrounding yellowish halo, respectively	May present as: 1. Normal angiogram 2. Nonleaking dilated perifoveal capillaries 3. Hyperfluorescence followed by late staining of the macular lesions	Hypofluorescence of the placoid lesions seen early, followed by hyperfluorescence in the late venous phase	Hyperfluorescent focal RPE defect that leaks, with pooling and accumulation of dye within a serous detachment in late films
Resolution	6–12 weeks	Weeks to months	2–5 weeks; recurrence noted	3–12 months; recurrence noted
Visual Recovery	Good	Minimal	Good, if fovea not involved	Fair (25% with VA <20/200)

RD, retinal detachment; RPE, retinal pigment epithelium; VA, visual acuity.

nopathy. Patients usually have a normal electroretinogram and electro-oculogram.[77]

Other viral retinitides include those caused by herpes simplex, measles, and cytomegalovirus. Reports also implicate hepatitis C in cases of ARPE.[14, 15] However, despite a strong suspicion of a viral etiology, systemic evaluations have failed to reveal conclusive evidence pointing to a viral etiology in ARPE.

The differentiating characteristics among ARPE, acute macular neuroretinopathy, APMPPE, and CSCR appear in Table 71–3.

TREATMENT

Owing to the spontaneous resolution of the disease, its self-limited course, and associated favorable outcomes, no therapy is advocated. Furthermore, the brief clinical course of ARPE makes the assessment and evaluation of any therapeutic intervention very difficult to study scientifically.

Steroid treatment has been used in some cases, but the efficacy of steroid therapy is difficult to differentiate from the natural history of the disease.[1, 12, 13] Whether

steroid therapy has a salutary effect on the vitritis seen in some cases of ARPE is unknown; however, the risks of such an approach seem to be outweighed by any potential benefit.

Studies performed on Lewis rats with induced retinal pigment epitheliitis showed that systemic treatment with a macrophage-depleting agent at the peak stage of experimental pigment epitheliitis resulted in the rapid disappearance of the clinical signs of uveitis.[16] Such an approach may prove useful in the future for the prevention and treatment of other inflammatory conditions affecting the RPE that potentially have a greater number of destructive ocular sequelae, such as APMPPE.

NATURAL HISTORY AND PROGNOSIS

ARPE is typically benign. Its natural course demonstrates a total or near-total resolution of the symptoms, particularly with respect to vision. Return to baseline visual acuity and normalization of visual field defects are usually observed within 6 to 12 weeks without treatment.

In a study of eight patients with ARPE, who were followed by Chittum and Kalina[3] for an average of 4.2

years, all recovered 20/20 vision. In another study by Prost,[7] five patients were followed for 6 years and likewise showed complete recovery of previous visual acuity.

There have been a few reports of recurrent,[5] as well as bilateral cases, but these cases are very atypical.[1, 5, 7]

CONCLUSIONS

Acute retinal pigment epitheliitis is a rare, yet relatively new clinical entity, which was first described less than three decades ago. It is characterized clinically by an acute disturbance in central vision, metamorphopsia, or scotomata. There appears to be no underlying systemic involvement, and the patient's review of systems and medical history are typically noncontributory. The anterior segment examination is quiet. The funduscopic findings reveal the hallmark of this disease—discrete clusters of small, dark-gray spots at the level of the retinal pigment epithelium, surrounded by a round, yellowish halo in the central macula. Fluorescein angiography shows a central hypofluorescence with a surrounding hyperfluorescence, corresponding to the central gray spot and surrounding yellowish halo, respectively. Although its etiology is unknown, a viral etiology is highly suspected. The disease is typically benign with total or near-total resolution of the symptoms and complete visual recovery within 12 weeks, even without treatment. Studies of animal models with pigment epitheliitis are ongoing, and it is hoped that they will provide new insight into the pathogenesis of this disease entity and other related inflammatory conditions.

References

1. Krill AE, Deutman AF: Acute retinal pigment epitheliitis. Am J Ophthalmol 1972;74:193–205.
2. Deutman AF: Acute retinal pigment epitheliitis. Am J Ophthalmol 1974;78:571–578.
3. Chittum ME, Kalina RE: Acute retinal pigment epitheliitis. Ophthalmology 1987;94:1114–1119.
4. Eifrig DE, Knobloch WH, Moran JA: Retinal pigment epitheliitis. Ann Ophthalmol 1977;9:639–642.
5. Friedman MW: Bilateral recurrent acute retinal pigment epitheliitis. Am J Ophthalmol 1975;79:567–570.
6. Luttrul JK: Acute retinal pigment epitheliitis. Am J Ophthalmol 1997;123(1):127–129.
7. Prost M: Long term observations of patients with retinal pigment epitheliitis. Ophthalmologica 1989;199:84–89.
8. Deutman AF: Acute retinal pigment epitheliitis. Ophthalmologica 1975;171:361.
9. Luttrul JK, Chittum ME: Acute retinal pigment epitheliitis. Am J Ophthalmol 1995;120:389–391.
10. Jamison RR: Acute retinal pigment epitheliitis with macular edema. Ann Ophthalmol 1979;11:359.
11. Suzuki R, Suga Y, Teranishi H, et al: Diffuse midperipheral acute retinal pigment epitheliopathy. Ann Ophthalmol 1988;20:17.
12. Schwartz PL, Rosen DA, Lerner DS, et al: Acute retinal pigment epitheliopathies. Ann Ophthalmol 1981;13:1139–1141.
13. Piermarocchi S, Corradini R, Midena E, et al: Correlation between retinal pigment epitheliitis and central serous chorioretinopathy. Ann Ophthalmol 1983;15:425–428.
14. Quillen DA, Zurlo JJ, Cunningham D, et al: Acute retinal pigment epitheliitis and hepatitis C. Am J Ophthalmol 1994;118:120–121.
15. Tahri H, Chaoui Z, Berbicho, et al: The eye and hepatitis C. J Fr Ophtalmol 1997;20(6):453–455.
16. Broekhuyse RM, Huitinga I, Kuhlman ED, et al: Differential effect of macrophage depletion on two forms of experimental uveitis evoked by pigment epithelial membrane protein (EAPU), and by melanin-protein (EMIU). Exp Eye Res 1997;65(6):841–848.
17. Broekhuyse RM, Kuhlmann ED: Uveitogenic 28/20 kD and 43 kD polypeptides in pigment epithelial membranes of the retina. Ocul Immunol Inflamm 1997;5(1):19–26.
18. Bos PJM, Deutman AF: Acute macular neuroretinopathy. Am J Ophthalmol 1975;80:573.
19. Rush JA: Acute macular neuroretinopathy. Am J Ophthalmol 1977;83:490.
20. Priluck IA, Buettner H, Robertson DM: Acute macular neuroretinopathy. Am J Ophthalmol 1978;86:775.
21. Sieving PA, Fishman CA, Salzano T, Rabb MF: Acute macular neuroretinopathy: Early receptor potential changes suggest photoreceptor pathology. Br J Ophthalmol 1984;68:229.
22. Gass JD: Acute posterior multifocal placoid pigment epitheliopathy. Arch Ophthalmol 1968;80:177.
23. Ryan SJ, Maumenee AE: Acute posterior multifocal placoid pigment epitheliopathy. Am J Ophthalmol 1972;74:1066.
24. Annesley WH, Tomer TL, Shields JA: Multifocal placoid pigment epitheliopathy. Am J Ophthalmol 1973;76:511.
25. Gass JDM: Acute posterior multifocal placoid pigment epitheliopathy: A long term follow-up. In: Fine SL, Owens SL, eds: Management of Retinal Vascular and Macular Disorders. Baltimore, Williams & Wilkins, 1983, pp 176–181.
26. Holt WS, Regan CD, Trempe C: Acute posterior multifocal placoid pigment epitheliopathy. Am J Ophthalmol 1976;81:403.
27. Savino PJ, Weinberg RJ, Yassin JG, et al: Diverse manifestations of acute posterior multifocal placoid pigment epitheliopathy. Am J Ophthalmol 1974;77:659.
28. Damata BE, Nanjiani M, Foulds WS: Acute posterior multifocal placoid pigment epitheliopathy: A follow-up study. Trans Ophthalmol Soc UK 1983;103:517.
29. Jacklin HN: Acute posterior multifocal placoid pigment epitheliopathy and thyroiditis. Arch Ophthalmol 1977;95:995.
30. Fitzpatrick PJ, Robertson DM: Acute posterior multifocal placoid pigment epitheliopathy. Arch Ophthalmol 1973;89:373.
31. Van Buskirk EM, Lessel S, Friedman E: Pigment epitheliopathy and erythema nodosum. Arch Ophthalmol 1971;85:369.
32. Deutman AF, Oosterhuis JA, Boen-Tan TN: Acute posterior multifocal placoid pigment epitheliopathy: Pigment epitheliopathy or choriocapillaritis? Br J Ophthalmol 1972;56:863.
33. Lowes M: Placoid pigment epitheliopathy presenting as an anterior uveitis: A case report. Acta Ophthalmol Scand 1977;55:800.
34. Hedges TR III, Sinclair SH, Gragoudas ES: Evidence for vasculitis in acute posterior multifocal placoid pigment epitheliopathy. Ann Ophthalmol 1979;11:539.
35. Priluck IA, Robertson DM, Buettner H: Acute posterior multifocal placoid pigment epitheliopathy: Urinary findings. Arch Ophthalmol 1981;99:1560.
36. Kirkham TH, Ffytche TJ, Sanders MD: Placoid pigment epitheliopathy with retinal vasculitis and papillitis. Br J Ophthalmol 1972;56:875.
37. Isashiki M, Koide H, Yamashita T, Ohba N: Acute posterior multifocal placoid pigment epitheliopathy associated with diffuse retinal vasculitis and late haemorrhagic macular detachment. Br J Ophthalmol 1986;70:255.
38. Frohman LP, Klung R, Bielory L, et al: Acute posterior multifocal placoid pigment epitheliopathy with unilateral retinal lesions and bilateral disk edema. Am J Ophthalmol 1987;104:548.
39. Jenkins RB, Savino PJ, Pilkerton AR: Placoid pigment epitheliopathy with swelling of the optic disks. Arch Neurol 1973;29:204.
40. Kayazawa F, Takahashi H: Acute posterior multifocal placoid pigment epitheliopathy and Harada's disease. Ann Ophthalmol 1983;15:58.
41. Bird AC, Hamilton AM: Placoid pigment epitheliopathy presenting with bilateral serous retinal detachment. Br J Ophthalmol 1972;56:881.
42. Young NJ, Bird AC, Schmi K: Pigment epithelial diseases with abnormal choroidal perfusion. Am J Ophthalmol 1980;90:607.
43. Lyness AL, Bird AC: Recurrences of acute posterior multifocal placoid pigment epitheliopathy. Am J Ophthalmol 1984;98:203.
44. Lewis RA: Acute posterior multifocal placoid pigment epitheliopathy. A recurrence. Arch Ophthalmol 1975;93:235.
45. Saraux H, Pelosse B: Acute posterior multifocal placoid pigment epitheliopathy: A long term follow-up. Ophthalmologica 1987;194:161.
46. Smith CH, Savino PJ, Beck RW, et al: Acute posterior multifocal placoid pigment epitheliopathy and cerebral vasculitis. Arch Neurol 1987;40:48.
47. Kersten DH, Lessell S, Carlow TJ: Acute posterior multifocal placoid

pigment epitheliopathy and late-onset meningoencephalitis. Ophthalmology 1987;94:393.

48. Wilson CA, Choromokos EA, Sheppard R: Acute posterior multifocal placoid pigment epitheliopathy and cerebral vasculitis. Arch Ophthalmol 1987;106:796.

49. Sigelman J, Behrens M, Hilal S: Acute posterior multifocal placoid pigment epitheliopathy associated with cerebral vasculitis and homonymous hemianopia. Am J Ophthalmol 1979;88:919.

50. Bullock JD, Fletcher RL: Cerebrospinal fluid abnormalities in acute posterior multifocal placoid pigment epitheliopathy. Am J Ophthalmol 1977;84:45.

51. Fishman GA, Baskin M, Jednock N: Spinal fluid pleocytosis in acute posterior multifocal placoid pigment epitheliopathy. Ann Ophthalmol 1977;9:33.

52. Dick DJ, Newman PK, Richardson J, et al: Acute posterior multifocal placoid pigment epitheliopathy and sarcoidosis. Br J Ophthalmol 1988;72:74.

53. Brown M, Eberdt A, Ladas G: Pigment epitheliopathy in a patient with mycobacterial infection. J Pediatr Ophthalmol Strabismus 1973;10:278.

54. Hansen RM, Fulton AB: Cone pigments in acute posterior multifocal placoid pigment epitheliopathy. Am J Ophthalmol 1981;91:465.

55. Von Graefe A: Ueber centrale recidivierende retinitis. Graefes Arch Clin Exp Ophthalmol 1866;12:211–215.

56. Bennet G: Central serous retinopathy. Br J Ophthalmol 1995; 39:605–618.

57. Gass JDM: Pathogenesis of disciform detachment of the neuroepithelium. II. Idiopathic serous central choroidopathy. Am J Ophthalmol 1967;63:587–615.

58. Gass JDM: Stereoscopic Atlas of Macular Diseases. St. Louis, CV Mosby, 1987.

59. Burton TC: Central serous retinopathy. In: Blodi FC, ed: Current Concepts in Ophthalmology, vol 3. St. Louis, CV Mosby, 1972.

60. Edwards TS, Proestly BS: Central angiospastic retinopathy. Am J Ophthalmol 1964;57:9888–9996.

61. Gass JDM, Norton EWD, Justice J: Serous detachment of the retinal pigment epithelium. Trans Am Acad Ophthalmol Otolaryngol 1966;70:990–1015.

62. Gass JDM: Bullous retinal detachment: An unusual manifestation of idiopathic central serous choroidopathy. Am J Ophthalmol 1973;75:810–821.

63. Klein BA: Symposium: Macular diseases, clinical manifestations. I. Central serous retinopathy and chorioretinopathy. Trans Am Acad Ophthalmol Otolaryngol 1965;69:614–620.

64. Mitsui Y, Sakanishi R: Central angiospastic retinopathy. Am J Ophthalmol 1956;41:105–114.

65. Straatsma BR, Allen RA, Petit TH: Central serous retinopathy. Trans Pacific Coast Oto-Ophthalmol Soc 1966;47:107–127.

66. Klein ML, van Buskirk EM, Friedman E, et al: Experience with non-treatment of central serous choroidopathy. Arch Ophthalmol 1974;91:247–250.

67. Cohen D, Gaudric A, Coscas G, et al: Epitheliopathie retinienne diffuse et chorioretinopathie sereuse centrale. J Fr Ophtalmol 1983;6:339–349.

68. Gilbert M, Owen SL, Smith PD, et al: Long-term follow-up of central serous chorioretinopathy. Br J Ophthalmol 1984;68:815–820.

69. Spitznas M: Central serous chorioretinopathy. Ophthalmology 1980;87(8S):88.

70. Wessing A: Grundsatzliches zum diagnostochen Fortschritt durch die Fluoreszenzangiographie. Ber Zusammenkunft Dtsch Ophthalmol Ges 1973;73:566–568.

71. Yannuzi LA: Type A behavior and central serous chorioretinopathy. Trans Am Ophthalmol Soc 1986;84:799–845.

72. Piccolino FC: Central serous chorioretinopathy: some considerations on the pathogenesis. Ophthalmologica 1981;182(4):204–210.

73. Hayashi M, Yoshimura N, Kondo T: Acute rubella retinal pigment epitheliitis in an adult. Am J Ophthalmol 1982;93(3):285–288.

74. Fischer DH: Viral disease and the retina. In: Tabarra KF, Hyndiuk RA, eds: Infections of the Eye. Boston, Little, Brown, 1986, 487–497.

75. Alfano JE: Ocular aspects of the maternal rubella syndrome. Trans Am Acad Ophthalmol Otolaryngol 1966;70:235.

76. Wolff SM: The ocular manifestations of congenital rubella. Trans Am Ophthalmol Soc 1972;70:577.

77. Obenour LC: The electroretinogram in rubella retinopathy. Int Ophthalmol Clin 1972;12:105.

72 — SERPIGINOUS CHOROIDITIS

Alejandro Rodriguez-Garcia

DEFINITION

Serpiginous choroiditis is a rare, chronic, progressive, and recurrent bilateral inflammatory disease involving the retinal pigment epithelium (RPE), the choriocapillaries, and the choroid.[1, 2] The cause of serpiginous choroiditis is unknown.[2–4] The disease is characterized acutely by irregular, gray-white or cream-yellow subretinal infiltrates at the level of the choriocapillaries and the RPE.[3, 4] These lesions show a propensity for developing near the optic disc, extending centrifugally in a pseudopodial or serpentine fashion.[5] A pattern of inflammatory quiescence followed by recurrence is common,[6, 7] with the recurrences appearing at the edges of the atrophic chorioretinal scars from prior attacks, occurring weeks, months, or even years after a prior attack. With time, atrophy of the RPE, choriocapillaries, and overlying retina occurs, leaving scarred tissue in the wake of the lesions.[4–6] It is this final serpentine-shaped appearance of extended chorioretinal atrophy that gives this disease its name, serpiginous choroiditis. The disease has also been described in the literature as helicoid peripapillary chorioretinal degeneration,[8] geographic choroiditis[9] or choroidopathy,[4, 10] geographic helicoid peripapillary choroidopathy,[2] macular geographic helicoid choroidopathy,[3] choroiditis geographica,[11] and serpiginous choroidopathy.[12]

HISTORY

Serpiginous choroiditis was first described in 1932 by Junius,[13] who followed a 39-year-old patient for 14 years and described the clinical features that we now recognize as serpiginous choroiditis. He termed the condition peripapillary and central retinochoroiditis. Sorsby[14] described a series of patients who appeared to have serpiginous choroiditis in 1939 but classified them as a peripapillary type of choroidal sclerosis.

Franceschetti[15] pointed out that there were two groups of diseases that had similar appearances but different clinical courses. One group was probably degenerative in origin, whereas the other was characterized by progressive disease, probably representing serpiginous choroiditis. In his report, Franceschetti collected 16 cases of circumscribed atrophy of the RPE and choroid from his own practice and from previous reports in the literature, and he termed the condition helicoid peripapillary chorioretinal degeneration.[15] In this collection of cases, there was a considerable amount of parity in the clinical course and the probable cause of the disease. Although some patients were shown to have progressive disease, in others the disorder was static. Some patients were considered to have a primary hereditary degeneration, whereas others were thought to have an inflammatory disease.[4]

In 1974, Hamilton and Bird[4] described a series of patients with serpiginous choroiditis. They emphasized the recurrent and progressive course of the disease, with a final appearance of atrophy of the RPE and choriocapillaries in the posterior pole, similar to that described by Krill and Archer[16] in 1971.

Different reports of small series of patients with serpiginous choroiditis, describing the clinical presentation,[1, 3] fluorescein angiographic findings,[2, 4] clinical course,[5–7] treatment,[17–19] and complications[20–23] of the disease, have sporadically appeared in the literature thereafter.

EPIDEMIOLOGY

Serpiginous choroiditis is rare. Of 1237 patients with uveitis referred to the Ocular Immunology and Uveitis Service of the Massachusetts Eye and Ear Infirmary over a 10-year period, serpiginous choroiditis accounted for only 0.3% of all patients with intraocular inflammation seen and 1.6% of a total of 240 patients with posterior uveitis.[24] The largest series reported to date, by Chisholm, Gass, and Hutton,[5] consisted of 20 patients, all of whom were white. In this series, there were 11 men and 9 women, with a mean age at presentation of 47.5 years (range, 29 to 70 years). Other reports have also found a male predominance, with most patients being whites. Schatz and coworkers[2] reported serpiginous choroiditis in seven men and two women with a mean age at presentation of 51.6 years (range, 41 to 68 years). Identical sex distribution was reported by Weiss and coworkers.[7] In their series, the mean age at presentation was 46.0 years (range, 22 to 58 years). In another series of 15 Finnish patients, Laatikainen and Erkkilä[6] also found male predominance (eight men and six women) but with a younger mean age at presentation of 35.0 years (range, 20 to 65 years). According to these findings, the clinical presentation of serpiginous choroiditis occurs most commonly between the third and sixth decades of life.

Although the great majority of patients reported to have serpiginous choroiditis have been whites,[5, 7] the disease has also been noted in Asians,[25] blacks,[7] and Hispanics.[26]

CLINICAL CHARACTERISTICS

Patients with serpiginous choroiditis typically present with a painless unilateral decrease in central vision, metamorphopsia, and/or small central or paracentral scotomas (Table 72–1). The latter may by either absolute (particularly during the active stage of the disease) or relative, as the acute lesions resolve.[1, 2, 5, 7] Amsler grid testing reveals scotomas that correspond precisely to visible funduscopic lesions.[27]

On examination the anterior segment usually appears quiet, although a nongranulomatous anterior uveitis has been described in some cases.[4, 28] A mild vitritis and/or fine pigmented cells within the vitreous have been seen in up to 50% of eyes in some series.[5, 7, 29, 30]

On funduscopic examination, active disease manifests gray-green or cream-colored, deep-within-the-retina lesions with irregular borders involving the RPE and the choriocapillaris.[1, 2, 7] The overlying retina is usually edema-

TABLE 72–1. CLINICAL DIAGNOSTIC FINDINGS IN SERPIGINOUS CHOROIDITIS

Demographics
  Mostly whites
  Male to female ratio, 1:1
  Age at presentation, 30 to 60 years
Ocular findings
  Symptoms: Blurred vision, metamorphopsia, and central or
    paracentral scotomas
  Funduscopic appearance: Sharply demarcated gray-green or cream-
    colored deep-within-the-retina lesions with irregular borders,
    involving the RPE and choriocapillaris. Lesions extend in a
    pseudopodial pattern, leaving extensive chorioretinal atrophy.
  Disease progression: Centripetal (most common), macular (poor
    prognosis), centrifugal, and isolated peripheral lesions
Additional tests
  Visual fields: Absolute scotomas (active phase), relative scotomas
    (resolution) corresponding precisely to visible funduscopic lesions
  Fluorescein angiography
    Active phase: Early hypofluorescence and late hyperfluorescence
      (leakage) at borders of lesions.
    Inactive phase: Mottled hyperfluorescence and late staining of the
      scar
  ERG and EOG: Frequently normal, except for patients with
    extensive disease, particularly if macula is involved (abnormal
    recordings corresponding to extent of damage)

RPE, retinal pigment epithelium; ERG, electroretinogram; EOG, electro-oculogram.

tous and an associated neurosensory retinal detachment may occur[2, 4, 5] (Fig. 72–1).

The fundus lesions may vary in size from one to several disc diameters, having variable distribution and shape.[1–10] Multiple areas of inflammation may be seen, most frequently at the distal edges of inactive scars and extending in a pseudopodial fashion. Noncontiguous "skip" lesions have also been observed and may represent de novo foci of involvement.[2, 4, 5] Involved areas of each eye frequently show different stages of progression.[6, 7]

Classically, as described by Chisholm and colleagues,[5] lesions develop first in the peripapillary area and tend to spread centrifugally[2, 4] (Fig. 72–2). In such cases, the central vision is unaffected in the beginning of the

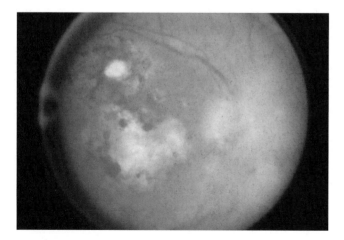

FIGURE 72–1. Serpiginous choroiditis, with both active and inactive lesions. Note the peripapillary involvement, with active foci nasal to the disc and the inactive areas of chorioretinal scarring in the macula. (Courtesy of C. Stephen Foster, MD.) (See color insert.)

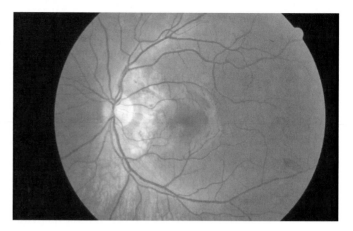

FIGURE 72–2. Residuum of the earliest lesions of serpiginous choroiditis around the disc. Note, however, that the disease is now inactive and that the vitreous is crystal clear. (Courtesy of C. Stephen Foster, MD.) (See color insert.)

process, and it is not until the fovea becomes involved that visual acuity diminishes, frequently to counting fingers.[1–5] Weiss and colleagues[7] found a substantial reduction in visual acuity in 15 of 17 eyes affected by serpiginous choroiditis, although in nine of these eyes, visual acuity recovered to variable degrees.

Improvement of vision following foveal involvement by an active lesion is variable, with a few patients demonstrating complete recovery and many others showing only partial improvement of one or two Snellen lines of visual acuity.[1, 6, 7] In their series, Laatikainen and Erkkilä[1] recorded visual recovery in only 6 of the 18 eyes affected. Hamilton and Bird[4] reported a visual improvement from 20/200 to 20/30 in one eye of the five patients they described, and Schatz and coworkers[2] did not find visual improvement in any of the nine patients in their series.

Hardy and Schatz,[3] and later Mansour and colleagues,[26] as well as others,[1, 13] have described a series of cases of serpiginous choroiditis in which the disease appeared initially in the macular area; they therefore termed this condition macular serpiginous choroiditis. In Hardy and Schatz's series of 31 patients, eight (11 eyes) had the macular form.[3] This form of the disease may be unilateral, or bilateral and simultaneous.[3] Although the clinical characteristics of eyes with the macular form differ little from those with the typical peripapillary form, patients with the macular form present early in the course of the disease with an acute onset of central visual loss.[1, 3, 26] Subretinal neovascularization, resulting in further visual loss, is relatively common in this type of serpiginous choroiditis.[20, 21]

Less frequently, midperipheral lesions, which tend to progress centripetally, may occur. Weiss and colleagues[7] described 3 of 17 eyes in which new lesions appeared in an extrapapillary location and progressed toward the optic disc. None of these patients had isolated macular disease. Finally, a few cases of isolated peripheral lesions have also been described.[7]

During active disease, the RPE appears edematous and inflamed.[4] Over a 2- to 3-month period, the edema resolves and atrophy of the RPE and choriocapillaris are observed.[2, 5] In time, coarse, irregular clumps of RPE hyperpigmentation develop within the lesions, and the large choroidal vessels become increasingly prominent.[5-7]

As the disease progresses, large geographic-type or serpentine-shaped areas of chorioretinal atrophy are produced, which extend into the far retinal periphery[6, 7] (Fig. 72–3). Subretinal fibrosis may eventually develop within the atrophic scars in up to 50% of eyes according to one series.[5]

Generally, the optic nerve is not affected,[5, 6] although Wu and colleagues[31] described a patient with temporal sectorial atrophy of the optic nerve. Fujisawa and colleagues[25] reported a patient with recurrent disease who developed optic neuritis, and Wojno and Meredith[22] reported two patients with optic disc neovascularization.

PATHOGENESIS/IMMUNOLOGY/ PATHOLOGY

The pathogenesis of serpiginous choroiditis is unknown. Although no definitive systemic involvement has been found, there have been reports of the disease in association with neurologic disorders. Richardson and colleagues[32] described a patient who had acquired extrapyramidal dystonia and two other cases suggesting a link between serpiginous choroiditis disorders, including a young man with a relative absence of arm swing while walking and another patient whose sister had multiple sclerosis.

King and colleagues[33] reported elevated von Willebrand factor VIII (VIII-VWF) antigen in eight patients with serpiginous choroiditis without evidence of rheumatic disease. Elevated levels of VWF have been associated with vascular occlusive disease, such as polymyalgia rheumatica, Raynaud's phenomenon, and progressive systemic sclerosis.[34] Other systemic associations reported in patients with serpiginous choroiditis include hypoglycemia, celiac disease, and autoimmune thrombocytopenic purpura.[35]

The slow progression and long duration of the disease might implicate some ubiquitous but relatively mild etiologic stimulus. Attempts to demonstrate a microbial etiology have been unsuccessful. Tuberculosis or other foci

of infection were initially assumed to be the cause of serpiginous choroiditis by Witmer[36] in 1952 and by Schlaegel[37] in 1969. Laatikainen and Erkkilä[1] found two patients with active pulmonary tuberculosis that preceded the appearance of clinical serpiginous choroiditis, and all nine patients in their series had a positive purified protein derivative (PPD) skin test. At that time, these authors suggested that a tubercular allergic etiology could be a possible mechanism in the pathogenesis of serpiginous choroiditis. In addition to the tuberculosis cases, a patient with viral meningitis, three patients with increased antistreptolysin antibody titers, and single cases of active serpiginous choroiditis with concurrent maxillary sinusitis and influenza have been described by the same investigators.[1]

No subsequent cases of serpiginous choroiditis have been associated with an infectious cause. Antibody determinations have been performed in patients with serpiginous choroiditis against the following infectious agents, all with negative results: vaccinia virus; herpes simplex and herpes zoster; cytomegalovirus; adenovirus; influenza viruses A and B; parainfluenza viruses 1, 2, and 3; respiratory syncytial virus, rubella and rubeola viruses; reovirus; polioviruses 1, 2, and 3; and coxsackieviruses A7, A9, B5, as well as other microorganisms, such as *Toxoplasma gondii* and *Mycoplasma pneumoniae*.[34]

Maumenee[38] has suggested that the disease is the result of a vascular abiotrophy and therefore could be considered a degenerative disorder. Indeed, the prominent choroidal vascular obliteration initially led to the inclusion of serpiginous choroiditis in the group of choroidal dystrophies. However, the late onset, the acuteness of visual loss, the marked asymmetry, and the absence of familial cases tend not to support this notion.[9]

On the other hand, the occasional presence of anterior uveitis, retinal vasculitis, and vitreous cellular reaction in patients with serpiginous choroiditis suggests an inflammatory cause.[7, 23, 28] Jampol and colleagues,[20] as well as others,[9, 37] suggest that an inflammatory process causes a disruption of Bruch's membrane, permitting the development of subretinal neovascularization, a not uncommon cause of visual loss in patients with serpiginous choroiditis. Wojno and Meredith[22] also support the inflammatory hypothesis, noting that optic disc neovascularization and vitritis are more readily explained by this type of mechanism.

Erkkilä and colleagues[39] have suggested that a localized immune vasculitis induces occlusion of the choroidal vessels. In addition, the demonstration of elevated VIII-VWF by King and colleagues suggests endothelial injury from a vaso-occlusive event, perhaps caused by a vasculitis.[33] In favor of this hypothesis are the fluorescein angiographic characteristics found in serpiginous choroiditis, in which interference with choroidal fluorescence is apparent, especially during the active phase of the disease.[2, 7, 10] In other areas, however, the remaining abnormal choroidal vasculature is visible on fluorescein angiography, indicating loss of integrity of the RPE barrier.[2] This finding, in addition to the lack of choriocapillaris flush, suggests that the choriocapillaris is obliterated within the margins of the lesion. The margins become hyperfluorescent from leakage of normal choriocapillaries at the borders. Large

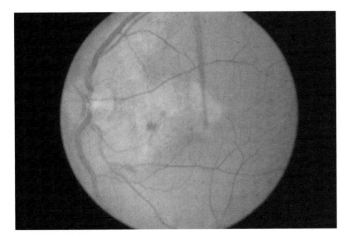

FIGURE 72–3. Progressive, active serpiginous choroiditis, which first began in the peripapillary region but now has spread in a serpiginous way superiorly and temporally in this left eye, now involving the macula. (Courtesy of C. Stephen Foster, MD.) (See color insert.)

remaining choroidal vessels within the lesion fill slowly and leak moderately, indicating that these vessels have also lost endothelial integrity.[2, 10]

Secchi and colleagues[18] have suggested that there is a vascular inflammatory lesion beginning at the choriocapillaris as a focal vasculitis. Type III (immune complex) and type IV (cell-mediated) hypersensitivity reactions may play a role. These authors also believe that in the course of the disease, type II (cytotoxic) reactions may also take place, possibly elicited by autoantibodies to retinal autoantigens (S and interphotoreceptor retinoid binding protein).

Broekhuyse and colleagues[40] found responsiveness to retinal S-antigen by lymphocytes from patients with serpiginous choroiditis, and they suggested that autoimmune reactivity probably depends on the damage of RPE cells, release of autoantigens, and leakage of S-antigen through the blood-retina barrier at the level of the RPE.

According to Nussenblatt and Palestine,[12] a possible mechanism for this disease entails abiotrophy with the release of potentially antigenic molecules, which, in genetically susceptible individuals, leads to an inflammatory response. Indeed, a statistically significant increase in the frequency of human leukocyte antigen (HLA)–B7 in 15 patients with serpiginous choroiditis compared with a control Finnish population (54.5% versus 24.3%; $p > .05$) was found by Erkkilä and colleagues.[39]

Very few eyes with serpiginous choroiditis have been studied histopathologically. Histologic examination shows extensive loss of the RPE and destruction of the overlying retina.[29, 31] The choriocapillaris as well as part of the choroid is filled with a mononuclear cell infiltrate, suggesting an inflammatory component to this disorder. A diffuse and focal accumulation of lymphocytes in the choroid has been observed.[31] This accumulation was greatest at the margins of the atrophic scars. Within the scars themselves, the RPE and photoreceptor layers are lost, with focal defects of the underlying Bruch membrane occurring at various sites within the lesions. Fibroglial tissue is seen at the inner surface of Bruch's membrane, with some migrating through breaks in Bruch's membrane into the choroid.[31]

DIAGNOSIS

The diagnosis of serpiginous choroiditis is made mainly on its clinical features in patients between their second and sixth decades of life, with a funduscopic appearance typical of active disease in one eye together with the characteristic bilateral distribution of pre-existing inactive disease.[2, 4]

Fluorescein Angiography

Active Phase

Fluorescein angiography of active lesions shows hypofluorescence during the early phases of the angiogram. The hypofluorescence of the interior lesion represents either blockage by swollen RPE cells or nonperfusion of the choriocapillaris, or both.[26] As the angiogram proceeds, hyperfluorescent borders, representing leakage of fluorescein from the surrounding choriocapillaris, may be seen.[2, 4, 10] Later in the angiogram, the inner portions of

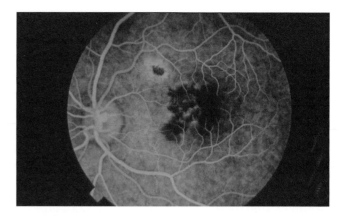

FIGURE 72–4. Fluorescein angiogram, midphase, in a patient with serpiginous choroiditis. Note the hyperfluorescence around the satellite lesion supratemporal to the macula, along the supratemporal arcade. (Courtesy of C. Stephen Foster, MD.)

a lesion may show spotty hyperfluorescence. The areas of active inflammation eventually stain late in the study.[5]

Inactive Phase

During the inactive stage of the disease, the fluorescein angiogram shows mottled hyperfluorescence, the result of pigment clumping with some late staining.[3, 10] In early phases of inactive disease, the scars are hypofluorescent because most of the choriocapillaris is absent (Fig. 72–4). As the angiogram proceeds, an increasing hyperfluorescence is seen at the margins of the scar as fluorescein diffuses into the scarred area from the bordering normal choriocapillaris (Fig. 72–5). Late staining of the sclera and fibrous tissue follows.[6, 7]

Indocyanine Green Angiography

Our experience with indocyanine green (ICG) angiography in serpiginous choroiditis is limited to one patient, in whom we found severe, diffuse atrophy of the choriocapillaris and increased visualization of the large choroidal vessels within the lesions. Middle and large choroidal vessels also appeared narrower and fewer in number (Fig. 72–6).

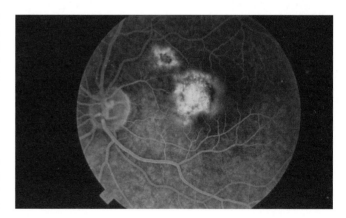

FIGURE 72–5. Fluorescein angiogram, same patient as shown in Figure 72–4, late phase, with late staining of the inactive macular lesion and perilesional halo staining of a mildly active satellite lesion superotemporal to the macula. (Courtesy of C. Stephen Foster, MD.)

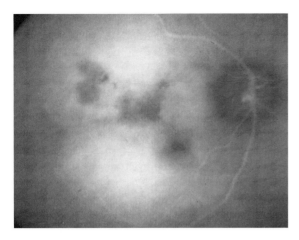

FIGURE 72–6. ICG angiogram in a patient with serpiginous choroiditis, showing diffuse leakage in the choroid during active inflammation. (Courtesy of C. Stephen Foster, MD.)

Giovannini and colleagues have recently described the ICG findings of patients with serpiginous choroiditis during the acute, subacute, and healed phases of the disease. Early hypofluorescence followed by late staining was observed with acute lesions, similar to that seen on fluorescein angiography. In addition, ICG revealed active choroidal involvement beyond that delimited by fluorescein angiography or visualized by biomicroscopy, suggesting more widespread ischemic or inflammatory pathology than what was apparent clinically. Healed lesions stain with both ICG and fluorescein angiography in areas of scarring and fibrovascular tissue. As in our patient, choroidal atrophy is sharply circumscribed, with absence of the choriocapillaris.[41]

Visual Fields

Visual field testing in active serpiginous choroiditis often demonstrates dense scotomas, corresponding in size, shape, and location to active lesions, and less dense scotomas as disease activity subsides.[5, 7] Frequently, scotomas are not uniformly absolute and may have a dense center with a light surrounding area.[7]

The regular use of Amsler grid testing is recommended to follow the central progression of the disease.[3, 26] Because of the slow and recurrent nature of serpiginous choroiditis, serial fundus photographs are also very helpful in documenting progression of the disease, particularly if this is subclinical.[34]

Electrophysiology

Electrophysiologic testing is frequently normal in serpiginous choroiditis. Weiss and colleagues[7] performed electroretinogram (ERG) and electro-oculogram (EOG) testing on eight of their nine patients with serpiginous choroiditis, and both tests were recorded within normal limits for all eyes. Abnormalities may be seen in patients with extensive disease, correlating with the degree of retinal damage.[1, 4, 5] When extensive disease is present, ERG values have been shown to fall to 70% to 80% of normal for total retinal illumination and to 20% to 30% of normal for focal macular illumination.[5, 9] Chisholm and colleagues[5] found that the ERG was abnormal in 3

of 26 eyes. Only the eye with the most extensive posterior pole involvement showed a marked reduction of the ERG. In their series, the EOG light rise ratio was normal in 17 eyes, moderately abnormal in one eye (1.45:1.65), and severely abnormal in eight eyes (<1.45). The reduced levels of the EOG appeared to correlate well with the extent of the funduscopic changes.[5]

This pattern differs from that seen in hereditary dystrophies, where electrophysiologic abnormalities are frequently found to reflect global pathology, and the degree of dysfunction is often greater than expected from the clinical appearance.[42]

DIFFERENTIAL DIAGNOSIS

When serpiginous choroiditis develops in the absence of previous lesions, the diagnosis can be a clinical challenge. A number of infectious, inflammatory, degenerative, and hereditary conditions may produce a clinical picture compatible with a diagnosis of serpiginous choroiditis (Table 72–2).

The differential diagnosis of macular serpiginous choroiditis involves many clinical entities, including age-related macular degeneration, idiopathic subretinal neovascularization, retinal pigment epitheliitis, presumed ocular histoplasmosis syndrome, multifocal choroiditis and panuveitis (MCP), and acute posterior multifocal placoid pigment epitheliopathy (APMPPE). Other causes of choroiditis, such as tuberculosis, sarcoidosis, Harada's disease, and sympathetic ophthalmia, may also resemble serpiginous choroiditis.[2]

The disease most likely to be confused with the initial acute presentation of serpiginous choroiditis is APMPPE, as the acute lesions in APMPPE involve the RPE and choriocapillaris and have a coloration and appearance similar to those of serpiginous choroiditis. Indeed, the fluorescein angiographic findings are similar in both diseases during the acute phase, with early blockage and late staining of the lesions. However, in APMPPE, the disease usually occurs bilaterally and simultaneously. The lesions are discrete, round to oval or placoid, usually confined to the posterior pole, and more randomly distributed; they tend not to coalesce, as do those of serpiginous choroiditis.[43] The lesions of APMPPE regress over a period of 1 to 2 weeks, usually with significant visual improvement, leaving scars which, while pigmented, are less atrophic and less destructive to the choroid and overlying neurosensory retina.[43–45] Recurrences, which are

TABLE 72–2. DIFFERENTIAL DIAGNOSIS OF SERPIGINOUS CHOROIDITIS

White dot syndromes
    Acute posterior multifocal placoid pigment epitheliopathy
    Multifocal choroiditis and panuveitis
    Presumed ocular histoplasmosis syndrome
    Acute retinal pigment epitheliitis
Infectious diseases
    Outer-layer retinal toxoplasmosis
    Tuberculous choroiditis
Miscellaneous
    Sarcoidosis choroiditis
    Harada's disease
    Sympathetic ophthalmia

distinctly unusual in APMPPE, are the rule in serpiginous choroiditis; with resolution of the lesions, there is profound derangement in the RPE, marked choroidal atrophy, and frequently impaired vision.

A diagnosis of APMPPE should be questioned in patients with unilateral, recurrent, or progressive macular lesions, especially if visual recovery does not occur. Visual acuity, even following foveal involvement, often recovers dramatically in APMPPE, but recovery is less common in serpiginous choroiditis.[27] Choroidal neovascularization has been reported in both entities but is more common in serpiginous choroiditis.[27, 29] Moreover, patients suffering from APMPPE are usually younger, and patients with serpiginous choroiditis are more frequently middle-aged.

Despite the clinical differences between APMPPE and serpiginous choroiditis, the recurrent form of APMPPE described by Lyness and Bird[46] resembles macular serpiginous choroiditis in its bilateral nature, fluorescein angiographic characteristics, and the resultant pigmentary disturbance. Whether APMPPE and serpiginous choroiditis represent extreme manifestations of a single disease or are in fact separate and distinct entities remains speculative.

Patients with MCP differ from those with serpiginous choroiditis in that they are young, mostly female, and frequently have moderate myopia.[47, 48] Choroidal lesions found in MCP are round, of variable size, more numerous, and more widely distributed than those seen in serpiginous choroiditis.[47] Vitreous inflammation is prominent in MCP, and late-stage subretinal fibrosis is quite common.[49]

Outer retinal toxoplasmosis may also mimic serpiginous choroiditis. Lesions in this disorder do not coalesce and are virtually always unilateral. Vitreous inflammation usually develops, and the overlying retina eventually becomes involved.[50, 51]

Disseminated tuberculous choroiditis may present with a yellowish gray, round lesion of the choroid with overlying necrotic retina, associated opacities of the vitreous, and, frequently, granulomatous uveitis.[52] Systemic findings include a positive PPD skin test and systemic manifestations of miliary tuberculosis.[1, 30] In serpiginous choroiditis, vitritis is not a prominent feature, nor is it granulomatous in nature.[28]

Biopsy-proven sarcoidosis in the clinical form of extensive, confluent choroiditis with RPE changes resembling serpiginous choroiditis has been reported by Edelsten and colleagues[53] in two patients. In their report, the patients presented with active lesions on the posterior pole associated with marked RPE changes, with fluorescein angiographic features of early masking and late staining of the edges of the lesions.

Several systemic diseases may cause choroidal ischemia in the posterior pole. These include hypertensive vascular disease, systemic lupus erythematosus, polyarteritis nodosa, toxemia of pregnancy, disseminated intravascular coagulation, and thrombotic thrombocytopenic purpura.[54–56] The fluorescein angiogram pattern in these conditions may resemble that of serpiginous choroiditis, but the clinical course is different and associated systemic findings are the rule in these cases.[54–56]

Choroidal neovascularization may be seen with many inflammatory, degenerative, and neoplastic conditions. Damage to Bruch's membrane with the occurrence of choroidal neovascularization may be seen in degenerative diseases, including angioid streaks, drusen, and myopia; dystrophic diseases such as Best's disease and fundus flavimaculatus may also produce choroidal neovascularization.[2, 3] Angioid streaks have a distinct funduscopic appearance, including "leopard-skin change" (peau d'orange), hemorrhage, and "salmon spot" changes quite typical for this condition, and together with the not infrequent association with pseudoxanthoma elasticum, they may be easily distinguished from serpiginous choroiditis.[2]

In older patients, metastatic tumors, non–Hodgkin's lymphoma, and choroidal osteoma may mimic the appearance of the acute unilateral lesion of serpiginous choroiditis. Stepwise progression with severe loss of the RPE and choriocapillaris are unusual in these disorders.[42]

TREATMENT

Medical Treatment

Serpiginous choroiditis is a chronic, recurrent, and progressive disease that is particularly resistant to treatment. Despite the use of a variety of anti-inflammatory and immunosuppressive drugs in the treatment of serpiginous choroiditis, most therapeutic regimens reported thus far do not seem to be totally efficacious in controlling the recurrent and progressive nature of the disease.

In their first report on serpiginous choroiditis, Laatikainen and Erkkilä[1] found a high incidence of active or presumed tuberculosis in their patients and decided to treat most of them with aggressive antituberculous therapy (streptomycin, isonicotinic acid hydrazide, and para-amino salicylic acid), with poor results.

The reports on the use of oral or periocular corticosteroids in the treatment of the acute phase or recurrences of serpiginous choroiditis have produced mixed results, with some authors reporting a beneficial effect while others were failing to demonstrate a good therapeutic response. Systemic prednisone at 60 to 80 mg/day has not been shown to affect the recurrence rate or the long-term outcome of the disease.[1, 7] Moreover, reports advocating corticosteroid therapy have recorded favorable responses over the same 1- to 2-month period as that in untreated lesions in other studies, making the treatment effect difficult to differentiate from the natural history of the lesion.[12]

Laatikainen and Erkkilä[1] did not find prednisone to be useful in preventing progression of the disease. Oral prednisone was given as a monotherapy to six patients with serpiginous choroiditis. In three patients, the lesions remained confined, whereas in the other three, considerable progression occurred in spite of therapy. Five of these six patients had one or more recurrences while on therapy.[6]

Chisholm and colleagues[5] treated 18 serpiginous choroiditis patients with periocular or systemic corticosteroids at some stage of the disease. Even though some patients felt clinical improvement, the authors could not find objective evidence of improvement as a result of the use of corticosteroids. They also noted that in patients with foveal involvement, there was no rapid resolution of disease activity with this same therapy.[5]

On the other hand, Hardy and Schatz[3] noted an apparently favorable response to early treatment with corticosteroids. Of eight episodes of acute disease treated with oral prednisone or sub-Tenon's injection of 40 mg of triamcinolone acetonide, all patients seemed to respond promptly, with resolution of disease activity and preservation or improvement of visual acuity.

Treatment of serpiginous choroiditis with cyclosporine-A (CsA) as monotherapy has also produced conflicting results. Failure of CsA therapy with respect to both progression of the disease[17, 57] and induction of disease regression and visual improvement has been observed.[18] Secchi and colleagues[18] treated seven patients (seven eyes) with active serpiginous choroiditis with CsA monotherapy at a starting dose of 4 to 7 mg/kg/day for a period of 6 to 21 months (mean duration of therapy, 10 months). Six of the seven eyes studied showed a significant improvement in visual acuity within the first few months of therapy and remained stable during the whole course of treatment. Moreover, four of the seven remaining inactive eyes showed some improvement in visual acuity. The results of this study, in which 80% of patients maintained vision equal to or better than baseline, indicate that CsA compares favorably with corticosteroids alone or in combination with immunosuppressive agents, for which the average rate of visual loss reported in the literature is 36%.[42] Accordingly, Secchi and colleagues[18] recommended CsA monotherapy as the first line of treatment for serpiginous choroiditis, particularly in the active phase of the disease and when the macula was threatened or involved.

On the other hand, separate therapeutic regimens using CsA or azathioprine in combination with prednisone have been tried in small numbers of patients with serpiginous choroiditis with disappointing results.[17]

Hooper and Kaplan[19] have shown that triple-agent immunosuppression, using azathioprine (1.5 mg/kg/day), CsA (5 mg/kg/day), and prednisone (1 mg/kg/day) combined, is effective in controlling disease progression. In their study, patients with serpiginous choroiditis were considered for treatment if visual acuity was reduced to 20/200 or less in one eye, or an active lesion was seen within 500 μm of the fovea centralis in the remaining eye. Five patients were treated with this regimen, and active lesions resolved within 2 weeks of therapy in all five patients. Vision remained stable in three eyes and improved in two as edema and subretinal fluid resolved. As the medications were weaned or discontinued, recurrences developed in two patients. Both recurrences responded rapidly to reinstitution of therapy and remained inactive over an 18-month period. These authors also observed less destruction of the RPE and choriocapillaris, with less pigment hyperplasia and intraretinal pigment migration in eyes treated during the active phase of the disease.[19]

Despite the apparent therapeutic efficacy shown by triple-agent immunosuppression in this study, there are several uncertainties with respect to this type of regimen: (1) the length of time patients remain relapse free while undergoing therapy; (2) the effect of therapy on the incidence of malignancy; and (3) the appropriate length of time that patients should be treated after stabilization of disease activity.[19] Because of this, the authors recommend this triple-agent therapeutic regimen only for serpiginous choroiditis patients with bilateral disease who have active lesions that threaten the central vision or do not respond to other forms of therapy.[19] Unfortunately, a definitive therapy for serpiginous choroiditis will require a long-term, well-controlled, prospective study including a large cohort of patients, a goal that seems very difficult if not impossible to accomplish, given the rarity of this disease.

Our group at the Massachusetts Eye and Ear Infirmary studied the clinical courses of six patients (12 eyes) with vision-threatening, steroid-dependent/resistant serpiginous choroiditis treated with the triple-agent immunosuppression regimen (prednisone, CsA, azathioprine) or with cyclophosphamide monotherapy.[58] All patients were treated for a minimum of 12 months (range, 12 to 87 months; mean, 43 months), with follow-up of 19 to 111 months (average, 62 months). All patients were able to successfully taper off from the oral steroids on which they had been dependent, and all were eventually able to taper off and discontinue the immunomodulatory agents as well. Ten eyes had improved visual acuity, none had progressive loss of vision during follow-up, and two with macular scars were stable. Cyclophosphamide was the most effective treatment, enabling long-term remission with much shorter treatment course (12 and 19 months in the two patients thus treated) than that required with combination triple therapy (average, 59 months).

Treatment of Choroidal Neovascularization

There are no reports on the therapeutic response of choroidal neovascularization to anti-inflammatory treatment in patients with serpiginous choroiditis.[42] On the other hand, subretinal neovascular membranes have been treated successfully with intense argon laser photocoagulation.[20, 21, 27, 59] Jampol and colleagues[20] were the first to report the successful treatment of subretinal neovascular membranes in serpiginous choroiditis using argon laser photocoagulation. In their report, two of three eyes with choroidal neovascularization in the macular area were photocoagulated with preservation of central vision. The third patient could not be treated because of the proximity of the neovascular membrane to the fovea centralis.

Laatikainen and Erkkilä[21] reported on two serpiginous choroiditis patients (three eyes) with subretinal neovascularization. One eye was treated with argon laser photocoagulation with recurrence of the neovascular net; the second eye could not be treated because of the subfoveal location of the lesion; and in the third eye, the neovascularization regressed spontaneously without therapy.

Recurrence of subretinal neovascularization following argon laser photocoagulation (which was further treated successfully with krypton laser) has also been reported by Mansour and colleagues.[26]

An early diagnosis of subretinal neovascularization is critical, because new vessels outside the fovea centralis may be suitable for treatment with laser.[20, 21] Subretinal neovascular membranes located in the foveal avascular zone of any etiology are now being treated with photodynamic therapy with verteporfin with promising results.

COMPLICATIONS

In earlier reports of serpiginous choroiditis in the literature, the occurrence of subretinal neovascular membranes (choroidal neovascularization) was not observed or was considered to be rare.[4, 5, 7, 29, 59] Although Gass[29] described one patient with an atypical case of serpiginous choroiditis characterized by subretinal neovascularization with exudation and hemorrhage, the first report that specifically addressed the occurrence of subretinal neovascularization in patients with serpiginous choroiditis was made by Jampol and colleagues.[20] Since then, choroidal neovascularization with secondary hemorrhage, exudation, or serous retinal detachment has been described to occur in approximately 13% to 20% of eyes with serpiginous choroiditis in long-term studies.[20, 21, 27, 59]

The neovascularization usually develops at the border of an old scar. The development of a subretinal membrane is not easily detectable on funduscopic examination or color fundus photographs. This is because the early formation of a neovascular membrane beside an old scar resembles a recurrent serpiginous choroiditis lesion.[20] In this case, the differentiation can best be made by fluorescein angiography findings.[21] Schatz and McDonald[27] emphasized that new lesions in patients with serpiginous choroiditis should be carefully assessed to determine whether they represent an inflammatory recurrence or a choroidal neovascular membrane.

Serous retinal detachment during the active phase of the disease has been observed in a few patients with serpiginous choroiditis.[2, 7] This shallow exudative detachment of the retina resolves as disease activity subsides.[7, 21] Another serpiginous choroiditis patient experienced an RPE detachment, as described and demonstrated angiographically by Wojno and Meredith.[22]

Cystoid macular edema has been demonstrated angiographically by Steinmetz and colleagues[60] in a patient with active macular serpiginous choroiditis. The patient was successfully treated with a significant improvement in visual acuity using 500 mg/day of acetazolamide for 2 weeks.

Retinal vasculitis and inflammation of the optic disc during active serpiginous choroiditis have also been described.[1, 5, 7, 28] Branch retinal vein or artery occlusions[23] and neovascularization of the optic disc[21, 22] have been seen uncommonly in association with active serpiginous choroiditis.

PROGNOSIS

Between 12% and 38% of eyes suffering from serpiginous choroiditis will end up with a central vision of less than 20/200 to counting fingers. Conversely, fewer than 5% of patients will have a final visual acuity of less than 20/200 in both eyes.[2–7]

If it occurs, visual recovery after foveal involvement in serpiginous choroiditis may be delayed by 1 year or more, and neither correlates with the degree of initial visual loss or with the appearance of the lesion. This notwithstanding, the great majority of affected eyes will end up with a poor central vision following foveal disease.[1, 2, 5–7]

The visual prognosis of macular serpiginous choroiditis is less favorable than that of peripapillary serpiginous choroiditis, probably because of early involvement of the macula in the former.[26] In addition, subretinal neovascularization may contribute to further loss of vision.[26] Patients with bilateral macular disease exhibit a tendency toward progression of the disease and recurrence, as well as to the development of subretinal neovascularization and neurosensory retinal detachment of the macula.[3] On the other hand, Hardy and Schatz[3] found that patients with unilateral macular serpiginous choroiditis have a better visual prognosis and, at least in their series, did not develop macular disease in the uninvolved eye during their entire follow-up (mean, 46.0 months).

Long-term follow-up studies of patients with serpiginous choroiditis are necessary to monitor disease activity and to assess the potential for macular involvement. In such cases, serial fundus photographs are very helpful to record progression of the disease. Patients with serpiginous choroiditis should also be instructed to perform self-testing with the Amsler grid to monitor the appearance of metamorphopsia or central scotomas between regular visits to the ophthalmologist.

CONCLUSIONS

Serpiginous choroiditis is a rare, chronic, and recurrent bilateral disease affecting the RPE, the choriocapillaris, and the choroid. The disease occurs more frequently in whites, with both sexes affected in equal proportion. The onset of the disease is between the third and sixth decades of life.

The etiology of serpiginous choroiditis is uncertain. Neither has a definitive systemic disease been associated with the disease, nor has an infectious agent been proven to be the cause. The contention that the disease could represent a dystrophy or a degenerative process can be dismissed by the lack of familial cases, the late onset of the disease, and the marked asymmetry observed in most cases.

On the other hand, the occasional presence of anterior uveitis, retinal vasculitis, and vitreous cellular reaction in these patients suggests an inflammatory cause. In addition, histopathologic examination of eyes suffering from serpiginous choroiditis has shown the choriocapillaris and part of the choroid filled with a round-cell infiltrate consisting of focal accumulations of lymphocytes. Finally, some patients have been shown to respond to anti-inflammatory therapy.

Patients with serpiginous choroiditis typically present with painless, unilateral decrease in central vision, metamorphopsia, and/or small central or paracentral scotomas. On examination, the anterior segment and vitreous usually appear quiet, although a nongranulomatous anterior uveitis and mild vitritis may be present.

Active disease manifests sharply demarcated, gray-green or cream-colored lesions deep within the retina with irregular borders involving the RPE and the choriocapillaris. The fundus lesions may vary in size from one to several disc diameters, having a variable distribution and shape. Multiple areas of disease activity may be seen, most frequently at the distal edges of inactive scars and extending in a pseudopodial fashion, usually from the optic disc.

The clinical course of the disease is one of long periods of quiescence, lasting months to years, followed by recurrent episodes of activity. Disease activity may last for 2 to 3 months before resolution. The end stage of the disease is characterized by the formation of a large serpentine-shaped area of chorioretinal atrophy, extending into the far retinal periphery.

The diagnosis of serpiginous choroiditis is based on clinical grounds. The typical funduscopic appearance of active lesions in one eye, in conjunction with a characteristic bilateral distribution of inactive chorioretinal scars, makes the suspicion of serpiginous choroiditis a very strong one. The fluorescein angiographic appearance of active lesions is typical, showing early hypofluorescence of the lesions and late hyperfluorescent borders, representing leakage of fluorescein from the surrounding choriocapillaris. During the inactive phase of the disease, the fluorescein angiogram shows mottled hyperfluorescence with some late staining of the sclera and fibrous tissue.

Serpiginous choroiditis is particularly resistant to treatment. Systemic steroids do not appear to be totally efficacious in controlling the recurrent and progressive nature of the disease. Even the use of oral or periocular corticosteroids in the treatment of the acute phase or recurrences of serpiginous choroiditis is controversial. There are reports showing a beneficial effect, but others fail to demonstrate a good therapeutic response.

Treatment of serpiginous choroiditis with CsA monotherapy has also produced conflicting results. Both failure of CsA therapy with progression of the disease, and inflammatory regression and visual improvement have been observed.

Triple-agent immunosuppression using azathioprine, CsA, and prednisone has been shown to be effective in controlling disease progression in a small number of patients. However, this therapeutic regimen has been recommended only for patients with bilateral disease who have active lesions that threaten central vision or those who do not respond to other forms of therapy.

Despite the promising results with triple-agent immunosuppression, a definitive therapeutic strategy for serpiginous choroiditis remains elusive and awaits a better understanding of the pathogenesis of the disease.

References

1. Laatikainen L, Erkkilä H: Serpiginous choroiditis. Br J Ophthalmol 1974;58:777.
2. Schatz H, Maumenee AE, Patz A: Geographic helicoid peripapillary choroidopathy: Clinical presentation and fluorescein angiographic findings. Trans Am Acad Ophthalmol Otolaryngol 1974;78:747.
3. Hardy RA, Schatz H: Macular geographic helicoid choroidopathy. Arch Ophthalmol 1987;105:1237.
4. Hamilton AM, Bird AC: Geographical choroidopathy. Br J Ophthalmol 1974;58:784.
5. Chisholm H, Gass JDM, Hutton WL: The late stage of serpiginous (geographic) choroiditis. Am J Ophthalmol 1876;82:343.
6. Laatikainen L, Erkkilä H: A follow-up study on serpiginous choroiditis. Acta Ophthalmol 1981;59:707.
7. Weiss H, Annesley WH, Shields JA, et al: The clinical course of serpiginous choroiditis. Am J Ophthalmol 1979;87:133.
8. Sveinsson K: Helicoidal peripapillary chorioretinal degeneration. Acta Ophthalmol 1979;57:69.
9. Baarsma GS, Deutman AF: Serpiginous (geographic) choroiditis. Doc Ophthalmol 1976;40:269.
10. Carr RE, Noble KG: Geographic (serpiginous) choroidopathy. Ophthalmology 1980;87:1065.
11. Pham-Duy T, Miszalok V: Choroiditis geographica. Klin Monatsbl Augenheilkd 1983;183:278.
12. Nussenblatt RB, Palestine AG: Serpiginous choroidopathy (choroiditis). In: Uveitis. Fundamentals and Clinical Practice. Chicago, Year Book Medical, 1989, p 309.
13. Junius P: Seltene augenspiegelbilder zum klinischen phanomen der retinitis exsudativa coats und der retino-choroiditis "parapapillaris." Arch Augenheilkd 1932;106:475.
14. Sorsby A: Choroidal angio-sclerosis with special reference to its hereditary character. Br J Ophthalmol 1939;23:433.
15. Franceschetti A: A curious affection of the fundus oculi. Helicoid peripapillary chorioretinal degeneration. Its relation to pigmentary paravenous chorioretinal degeneration. Doc Ophthalmol 1962;16:81.
16. Krill AE, Archer D: Classification of the choroidal atrophies. Am J Ophthalmol 1971;72:562.
17. Laatikainen L, Tarkkanen A: Failure of cyclosporine A in serpiginous choroiditis. J Ocular Ther Surg 1984;3:280.
18. Secchi AG, Tognon MS, Maselli C: Cyclosporine-A in the treatment of serpiginous choroiditis. Int Ophthalmol 1990;14:395.
19. Hooper PL, Kaplan HJ: Triple agent immunosuppression in serpiginous choroiditis. Ophthalmology 1991;98:944.
20. Jampol LM, Orth D, Daily MJ, et al: Subretinal neovascularization with geographic (serpiginous) choroiditis. Am J Ophthalmol 1979;88:683.
21. Laatikainen L, Erkkilä H: Subretinal and disc neovascularization in serpiginous choroiditis. Br J Ophthalmol 1982;66:326.
22. Wojno T, Meredith TA: Unusual findings in serpiginous choroiditis. Am J Ophthalmol 1982;94:650.
23. Friberg TR: Serpiginous choroiditis with branch vein occlusion and bilateral periphlebitis. Arch Ophthalmol 1988;81:481.
24. Rodriguez A, Calonge M, Pedroza-Seres M, et al: Referral patterns of uveitis in a tertiary eye care center. Arch Ophthalmol 1996;114:593.
25. Fujisawa C, Fujiwara H, Hasegawa E, et al: The cases of serpiginous choroiditis [Japanese, English abstract]. Nippon Ganka Gakkai Zasshi 1978;82:135.
26. Mansour AM, Jampol LM, Packo KH, et al: Macular serpiginous choroiditis. Retina 1988;8:125.
27. Schatz H, McDonald HR: Geographic helicoid peripapillary choroidopathy (serpiginous choroiditis). In: Ryan SJ, Schachat AP, Murphy RB, Patz A, eds: Retina. St. Louis, C.V. Mosby, 1989, p 705.
28. Masi RJ, O'Connor GR, Kimura SJ: Anterior uveitis in geographic or serpiginous choroiditis. Am J Ophthalmol 1978;86:228.
29. Gass JDM: Inflammatory diseases of the retina and choroid. In: Stereoscopic Atlas of Macular Diseases: Diagnosis and Treatment, 4th ed, vol II. St. Louis, Mosby, 1987, p 710.
30. Jampol LM: The retina: Inflammatory diseases. In: Miller S, ed: Clinical Ophthalmology. Bristol, Wright, 1987, p 186.
31. Wu IS, Lewis H, Fine SL, et al: Clinicopathologic findings in a patient with serpiginous choroiditis and treated choroidal neovascularization. Retina 1989;9:292.
32. Richardson RR, Cooper IS, Smith JL: Serpiginous choroiditis and unilateral extrapyramidal dystonia. Ann Ophthalmol 1981;13:15.
33. King DG, Grizzard WS, Sever RJ, Espinoza L: Serpiginous choroidopathy associated with elevated factor VIII–von Willebrand factor antigen. Retina 1990;10:97.
34. Bock CJ, Jampol LM: Serpiginous choroiditis. In: Albert DM, Jakobiec FA, eds: Principles and Practice of Ophthalmology. Philadelphia, W.B. Saunders, 1987, p 517.
35. Mulder CJJ, Pena AS, Jansen J, Oosterhuis JA: Celiac disease and geographic (serpiginous) choroidopathy with occurrence of thrombocytopenic purpura. Arch Intern Med 1983;143:842.
36. Witmer R: Fine spezielle Form rezidivierendir choroiditis. Ophthalmologica 1952;123:353.
37. Schlaegel TF: Metastatic nonsuppurative uveitis. In: Schlaegel TF, ed: Essentials of Uveitis. Boston, Little, Brown, 1969, p 77.
38. Maumenee AE: Clinical entities in "uveitis": An approach to the study of intraocular inflammation. XXVI Edward Jackson Memorial Lecture. Am J Ophthalmol 1970;69:1.
39. Erkkilä H, Laatikainen L, Jokinen E: Immunological studies on

serpiginous choroiditis. Graefes Arch Clin Exp Ophthalmol 1982;219:131.

40. Broekhuyse RM, Van Herck M, Pinckers AJLG, et al: Immune responsiveness to retinal S-antigen and opsin in serpiginous choroiditis and other retinal diseases. Doc Ophthalmol 1988;69:83.

41. Giovannini A, Mariotti C, Ripa E, et al: Indocyanine green angiographic findings in serpiginous choroidopathy. Br J Ophthalmol 1996;80:536–540.

42. Hooper PL, Secchi AG, Kaplan HJ: Serpiginous choroiditis. In: Pepose JS, Holland GN, Wilhelmus KR, eds: Ocular Infection and Immunity. St. Louis, Mosby 1996, p 579.

43. Gass JDM: Acute posterior placoid pigment epitheliopathy. Arch Ophthalmol 1968;80:177.

44. Deutman AF, Lion F: Choriocapillaris nonperfusion in acute multifocal placoid pigment epitheliopathy. Am J Ophthalmol 1977;84:652.

45. Ryan SJ, Maumenee AE: Acute posterior multifocal placoid pigment epitheliopathy. Am J Ophthalmol 1972;74:1066.

46. Lyness AL, Bird AC: Recurrences of acute posterior multifocal placoid pigment epitheliopathy. Am J Ophthalmol 1984;98:203.

47. Dreye RF, Gass JDM: Multifocal choroiditis and panuveitis. A syndrome that mimics ocular histoplasmosis. Arch Ophthalmol 1984;102:1776.

48. Nozik RA, Dorsch W: A new chorioretinopathy associated with anterior uveitis. Am J Ophthalmol 1973;76:758.

49. Cantrill HL, Folk JR: Multifocal choroiditis associated with progressive subretinal fibrosis. Am J Ophthalmol 1986;101:170.

50. Doft BH, Gass JDM: Outer retinal layer toxoplasmosis. Graefes Arch Clin Exp Ophthalmol 1986;224:78.

51. Friedman CT, Knox DL: Variations in recurrent active toxoplasmic retinochoroiditis. Arch Ophthalmol 1969;81:481.

52. Helm CJ, Holland GN: Ocular tuberculosis. Surv Ophthalmol 1993;38:229.

53. Edelsten C, Stanford MR, Graham EM: Serpiginous choroiditis: An unusual presentation of ocular sarcoidosis. Br J Ophthalmol 1994;78:70–71.

54. Gaudric A, Coscas G, Bird AC: Choroidal ischemia. Am J Ophthalmol 1982;94:489.

55. Spolaore R, Gaudric A, Coscas G, et al: Acute sectorial choroidal ischemia. Am J Ophthalmol 1984;98:707.

56. Kinyoun JL, Kalina RE: Visual loss from choroidal ischemia. Am J Ophthalmol 1986;101:650.

57. Nussenblatt RB, Palestine AG, Chan CC: Cyclosporine-A therapy in the treatment of intraocular inflammatory disease resistant to systemic corticosteroids and cytotoxic agents. Am J Ophthalmol 1983;96:275.

58. Yang J, Akpek E, Foster CS: Long-term immunosuppressive treatment of serpiginous choroiditis. Ophthalmology. In press.

59. Blumenkranz MS, Gass JDM, Clarkson JG: Atypical serpiginous choroiditis. Arch Ophthalmol 1982;100:1773.

60. Steinmetz RL, Fitzke FW, Bird AC: Treatment of cystoid macular edema with acetazolamide in a patient with serpiginous choroidopathy. Retina 1991;11:412.

SUBRETINAL FIBROSIS AND UVEITIS SYNDROME

Blanca Rojas

DEFINITION

Many inflammatory disorders of the posterior segment of the eye have been described. These include disorders with a known etiology and others in which the etiology has not been established. In general, a specific cause is rarely found in inflammatory disturbances involving retinal pigment epithelium (RPE) or choroid. As a result, classification of these disorders is established on the basis of the clinical course, the ophthalmoscopic appearance, or the angiographic findings.

During the inflammatory process, numerous cytokines, growth factors, and other proteins released by either inflammatory or ocular resident cells influence each other and produce various reactions in the eye. Subretinal fibrosis, a feature that can disrupt the normal intercellular relationship between the photoreceptors and the RPE,[1] is one such reaction.

The subretinal fibrosis and uveitis syndrome (SFU) is a rare clinical entity that presents with a distinctive posterior uveitis and progresses to subretinal fibrosis. It belongs to a group of inflammatory conditions characterized by the presence of multifocal lesions of the RPE and choroid and includes such entities as punctate inner choroidopathy and recurrent multifocal choroiditis and panuveitis. Although in some cases steroids have proved beneficial, the syndrome leads to progressive fibrotic subretinal lesions with severe and permanent visual loss.

HISTORY

Palestine and coworkers reported an entity characterized by chronic inflammation in the vitreous in association with whitish fibrotic-like subretinal lesions that progressively enlarged and coalesced.[2] They termed that entity progressive subretinal fibrosis and uveitis because the subretinal lesions had an appearance similar to the subretinal fibrosis seen in other retinal diseases such as complications of retinal detachment. The same group[3, 4] subsequently described the histopathology and immunohistopathology of this condition. This clinical picture could be the same as that of choroiditis proliferans, a rare disease reported by Fuchs (in 1949[5, 6]), in which large areas of connective tissue formed on the inner side of the choroid and led to a profound loss of vision despite slight changes in the retina. In 1982, Doran and Hamilton[7] reported ophthalmoscopic findings similar to those noted by Palestine and colleagues[2] and called the entity disciform macular degeneration in young adults. Later, Cantrill and Folk[8] reported a series of patients with multifocal choroiditis, uveitis, and progressive subretinal fibrosis; they called the clinical picture multifocal choroiditis with progressive subretinal fibrosis. Based on these reports, it seemed that an unusual form of multifocal choroiditis was preferentially affecting a group of young, healthy, myopic women. This condition differed from other multifocal choroidal diseases in that instead of forming chorioretinal scars, the acute lesion healed with the formation of discrete, sharply angulated subretinal scars that could coalesce, forming broad zones of subretinal fibrosis.[8] Recent reports in the literature refer to this entity as diffuse subretinal fibrosis syndrome (DSF).[9, 10]

It has been proposed that SFU may simply be a rarely observed late stage of any multifocal choroiditis, rather than being a unique entity.[9] Thus, the spectrum of this disease might include an early stage that is seen in reports describing recurrent multifocal choroiditis and panuveitis. This could be the case in the series of Morgan and Schatz,[9] who reported 11 cases of an inflammatory disorder involving the RPE and the choroid, characterized by multiple relapses.

Cases of progressive subretinal fibrosis have been included in reports of other clinical entities. Dreyer and Gass,[11] in a series of 28 patients with multifocal choroiditis and panuveitis, described three patients with "retinal pigment metaplasia" and "large subretinal bands" (cases 7, 9, and 10). Similarly, the report of Watzke and coworkers[12] on punctate inner choroiditis contained one example (case 7) in which hyperplastic scarring developed. Additionally, progressive subretinal fibrosis has been reported in the setting of multifocal inflammatory involvement of the RPE and inner choroid without concomitant vitreous or anterior chamber inflammation.[12–14] I have observed this same pattern of subretinal fibrosis in patients with sympathetic ophthalmia (Fig. 73–1).

EPIDEMIOLOGY

Patients affected by SFU as described by Palestine and colleagues[2] and Cantrill and Folk[8] are predominantly young, otherwise healthy myopic women. Taking into account those cases considered to be early stages of the disease, the patients are usually under 35 years old.[2–4, 8, 9, 11, 13, 15, 6] The youngest reported patient was 6 years old.[15] Some reports include patients older than 35.[9, 10, 14, 17] However, two series of patients have been reported that differ from all previous reports. Gass and coworkers[18] described three elderly patients, two men and one woman, with a mean age of 71 years (range, 69 to 76), with biopsy-proven SFU. Similarly, the report of Matsuo and Matsuo[14] includes a 71-year-old patient. Whether this is an indication that patients of all ages can develop the syndrome, and most patients were younger in previous series by chance, or there truly is a bimodal distribution of ages with both young and old susceptible to the syndrome remains to be seen.[19]

The vast majority of patients reported with SFU are women.[2–4, 8, 9, 11–13, 17, 20] In some series, most of the patients were myopic.[9, 10, 12, 13] Thus, the 10 patients reported by Watzke and associates[12] had a spherical equivalent rang-

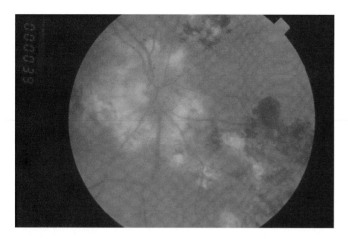

FIGURE 73–1. Soft yellow-white subretinal lesions, at the level of the choroid, of various ages and stages. (Courtesy of C. Stephen Foster, MD.) (See color insert.)

ing from −3.50 to −10 diopters. The refractive error of 10 of the 11 patients included in Morgan and Schatz's series ranged from −2.75 to −8.50.[9] There appears to be no racial predilection, and most systemic evaluations have been unremarkable.[2–4, 8, 13, 17, 18, 20] However, positive purified protein derivative test, for tuberculosis,[8, 12] histoplasmin skin test positivity,[2, 11] anomalies on chest radiograph,[11, 12] or the presence of *Histoplasma* on tissue section[2] have all been described in a few cases. In isolated cases, flulike symptoms preceded the onset of visual complaints.[11–13, 15]

CLINICAL FEATURES

Patients usually present complaining of acute or progressive unilateral visual loss[2, 3, 9–11, 13–15, 18, 20] or blurred vision.[2, 8, 13–15] However, visual acuity may be normal or slightly affected even though the fundus is involved.[2, 8, 9, 11–15, 17] Central or multiple scotomas,[8, 12, 13, 15] metamorphopsias,[9, 10, 14] and photopsias may also occur. The disease is usually bilateral, although the ocular involvement may be asymmetric.[2, 4, 8, 10–15, 17] The fellow eye may be simultaneously affected on clinical examination despite being asymptomatic.[2, 8, 9, 11, 12, 14, 16] Some cases of unilateral disease have been reported.[3, 8, 11–13, 16, 17]

The degree of visual loss depends on the stage of the disease at which the patient presents. Patients with mild disease can have 20/20 acuity, and severe disease may reduce visual acuity to light perception.

Whether a patient has the full clinical picture of SFU or only the early stages of the disease, mild to moderate anterior chamber[2, 8, 10, 11, 15, 18] and vitreous inflammation[2, 4, 8–11, 15, 17, 18, 20] is present. However, some cases of SFU without concomitant vitreous or anterior chamber inflammation have been reported, including one patient in the series of Cantrill and Folk[8] (case 1) and the patients reported by Salvador and coworkers[13] and Matsuo and Matsuo.[14] Occasionally, slit-lamp examination reveals other signs of inflammation, including episcleritis, scleritis, limbal phlyctenula, posterior synechiae, keratic precipitates, or iris atrophy.[2, 7–9, 11, 12, 15]

In the early stage of the syndrome, the funduscopic findings consist of multiple small, round, discrete, whitish yellow, hypopigmented lesions with soft, indistinct borders at the level of the RPE or inner choroid in the posterior pole and midperiphery (see Fig. 73–1). The lesions range in size from 50 to 500 μm in diameter,[2, 3, 8, 9, 11–13] and they occur singly, in clumps,[12] and in linear clusters.[12, 15] Lesions showing a swordlike pattern have also been reported.[15, 16] RPE disturbances at the posterior pole, adopting a crumpled and mottled pattern, may also be seen early in the course of the disease.[8, 14] The evolution of the acute whitish yellow hypopigmented lesions may adopt different patterns. Some lesions may fade over time without any alteration of the RPE, suggesting that they were located beneath the RPE.[8, 12] Others heal, leaving a punched-out atrophy suggesting involvement of the RPE,[3, 8, 11, 13, 15] or they become pigmented chorioretinal scars.[2, 3, 8, 9, 12, 15] But what gives distinctiveness to this syndrome is the fact that many of the acute lesions enlarge and coalesce, forming stellate irregular zones of subretinal fibrosis scattered throughout the posterior pole and mid periphery,[2, 8–10, 13, 14, 18, 20] occasionally having irregular, slightly pigmented borders (Fig. 73–2).[2, 8] The progression to fibrosis may take months to years to occur. The funduscopic appearance may evolve to form radial bands of fibrosis extending peripherally (Fig. 73–3).[3, 8]

Additional funduscopic findings can be seen in the setting of SFU. Serous detachment may develop with or without cloudy subretinal exudate.[2, 8, 9, 12, 14, 15, 18, 20, 21] Subretinal neovascular membranes,[8–12, 18] cystoid macular edema,[2, 8, 11, 15] and optic disc edema[8, 10, 13, 15] have all been reported. Perivascular infiltrate and vascular sheathing were noted in two reports.[2, 3]

HISTOPATHOLOGY

The histopathology and immunohistopathology for patients with SFU have been reported from chorioretinal biopsy in five cases[3, 18, 21] and from enucleation in five cases.[4, 18, 21] Palestine and associates[3] described for the first time the findings in a chorioretinal biopsy taken from a young woman with SFU syndrome who had progressive visual loss despite chronic steroid therapy. The vitreous aspirate contained a few lymphocytes that were identified as being T–helper-inducer lymphocytes and B cells.[3]

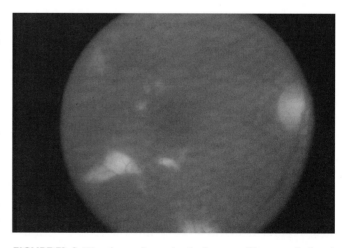

FIGURE 73–2. Fibrotic scar formation in the area of former soft choroidal lesions. (Courtesy of C. Stephen Foster, MD.) (See color insert.)

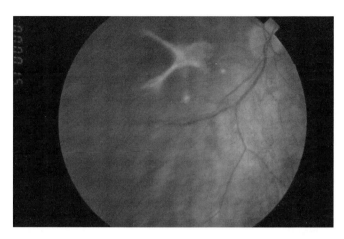

FIGURE 73–3. Expanding fibrotic bands, now beginning to contract in a patient with SFU. (Courtesy of C. Stephen Foster, MD.) (See color insert.)

The cases reported in the literature all exhibited choroidal inflammation on histopathology. The cellular infiltration of the choroid ranged from moderate to marked and consisted of lymphocytes and plasma cells.[3, 17] Retinal involvement varied from scattered infiltration of plasma cells and mostly a normal appearance on routine histologic examination[17] to one in which the RPE was essentially replaced by amorphous connective tissue, with lymphocytes extending to Bruch's membrane.[3, 17, 21]

The white, fibrous-like material was composed of fibrous amorphous tissue with islands of cells that had the histologic characteristics of pigment epithelial cells,[3] fibroblasts, and glial cells.[17]

The granulomatous inflammation reported by Kim and colleagues,[4] Gass and colleagues,[18] and Chan and colleagues[21] differs from the initial case reported by Palestine and associates[3] and those subsequently reported by others,[17, 21] in which the inflammatory infiltrate was not granulomatous. Kim and associates[4] studied the histopathologic and immunopathologic findings in one eye of a young woman who over a few months developed complete blindness caused by SFU, despite intensive anti-inflammatory and immunosuppressive therapy. The pathologic study of the subretinal tissue demonstrated a marked granulomatous reaction consisting of mononuclear cells, plasma cells, and some multinucleated giant cells.[4] In a report by Chan and associates,[21] the enucleated eye of a 24-year-old woman with multifocal choroiditis and subretinal whitish lesions that progressed to bilateral blindness in a short period of time despite immunosuppressive treatment, showed a marked gliotic retina and a thick subretinal fibrotic tissue. A diffuse granulomatous and T- and B-lymphocytic infiltration was present.

Additionally, in the report by Gass and coworkers,[18] three elderly patients with no evidence of systemic disease experienced ongoing loss of vision associated with multifocal choroiditis and SFU. The disease process resulted in blindness despite systemic corticosteroids and, in one patient, cyclophosphamide. Histopathologic examination of the four blind eyes disclosed findings involving the inner choroid and the outer retina. These included diffuse lymphocytic and plasma cell infiltration of the choroid, multifocal areas of degeneration, and focal de-

struction of Bruch's membrane associated with epithelioid and giant-cell proliferation, widespread destruction of RPE and retinal receptor cells, and multiple large, thick plaques of subretinal fibrosis. In cases 2 and 3,[18] there were concerns of the possibility of sympathetic uveitis because of the multiple operative procedures undergone by the patients. However, the histologic findings were not characteristic of sympathetic ophthalmia. Histopathologic findings of cases 1 and 2[18] were similar to those reported by Kim and colleagues.[4] The choroid was infiltrated by a mixture of T and B lymphocytes, with a relative predominance of B cells.[3, 4, 17, 21] The T–helper-inducer/suppressor-cytotoxic ratio was 1.8:1 in the study of Palestine and associates[3] and 4:1 in the case reported by Kim and coworkers.[4] Occasional monocytes and natural killer cells were also present.[3, 4] Immunofluorescence studies revealed complement and IgG deposition above Bruch's membrane[3, 17] as well as types I, III, and V collagen.[3]

The majority of large cells in the subretinal tissue demonstrated specific antigenic determinants of Müller cells.[3] The islands of cells within the white amorphous fibrous tissue stained with a monoclonal antibody specific for Müller cells. Some cells also stained with phosphatase and alphanapthylacetate esterase, which is a characteristic of RPE and macrophages.[3] In the case reported by Kim and coworkers,[4] Müller cells expressed the class II antigen of the major histocompatibility complex. Additionally, the interleukin-2 receptor marker (a marker of T-cell activation) was present in the locus of T-cell infiltration.[4]

Electron microscopic findings reported by Palestine and colleagues[3] disclosed that the subretinal amorphous connective tissue appeared to consist of collagen fibrils. The islands of cells within this amorphous connective tissue were surrounded by a basement membrane and by groups of numerous cells that were closely attached to each other with many desmosomes and tight junctions.[3] Altered pigmented cells were seen by electron microscopy in the fibrotic tissue of the eye studied by Kim and colleagues.[4] Special stains for microorganisms were negative.[4, 17, 18] Electron microscopy disclosed negative results for viral particles.[18]

PATHOGENESIS

In 1975, Mandelcorn and his group[22] showed that RPE cells had the ability to form membranes while proliferating. In their experiment, RPE cells from one eye were transplanted into the vitreous cavity of the fellow eye of owl monkeys, where they proliferated and underwent metaplastic changes. They observed long spindle cells forming membranes that resembled fibroblasts, although by electron microscopy these cells retained epithelial characteristics such as basement membranes and cell junctions (fibrous metaplasia). The metaplastic cells looked like pigmented macrophages, membrane-forming fibrocyte-like cells, and frank epithelial cells. The authors hypothesized that pigment epithelial cells could be the source of the intraocular proliferation seen in massive periretinal proliferation.

It is now widely believed that both RPE and Müller cells are the principal cell types responsible for the formation of abnormal cellular assemblage or "membranes" in the vitreous cavity and the subretinal space.[1] The subretinal membranes grow as sheets with or without pigmentation, depending on derivation from RPE or glial cells, respectively.[23] The proliferation of astrocytes is a common event in many injuries of the central nervous system. Müller cells are highly specialized astrocytes, and they react to injuries such as retinal detachment. Additionally, one or more localized factors may mediate the proliferative response. A number of growth factors are potential candidates for that role.[1] It has been reported that all non-neuronal cell types participate in retinal proliferation, including cells associated with the retinal vasculature, glia, and invading and "resident" macrophages (microglia).[1] The potential role of microglia in the regulation of the proliferation of other cell types has been suggested. The origin of subretinal fibrosis may lie in the early proliferation of cells in the retina, the migration of some fraction of these cells into the subretinal space, and their subsequent proliferation at those locations.[1]

The cause of SFU, like the causes of many other inflammatory conditions affecting the retina and choroid, is unknown. Histopathologic and immunohistopathologic findings in eyes with SFU seem to indicate that the disease is a result of inflammation leading to RPE destruction and transformation, with consequent fibrotic tissue formation and participation of Müller cells. An immune-mediated response could be involved in the pathogenesis of the disease. Palestine and colleagues[3] have postulated an autoimmune cause for SFU. They consider the disease to be an antibody-mediated inflammation in which local antibody production, possibly to the RPE structures, leads to the significant alterations seen. Their theory is supported by the presence of B cells and plasma cells in the inflammatory infiltrate, the deposition of immunoglobulin and complement in the outer subretinal tissue, the absence of circulating antibodies to the retina, and the marked decrease in the electro-oculogram (EOG).

The presence of granulomatous inflammation, consisting of a delayed-type hypersensitivity reaction (epithelioid cells, multinucleated giant cells, and fibrosis), supports the idea of an immune-mediated mechanism participating in the pathogenesis of the disease.

In the immune response, *Fas-FasL* interactions induce T-cell apoptosis, thus eliminating the potential autoreactive and activated T cells. Recent studies have indicated that apoptosis plays a role in immune-mediated inflammatory lesions in target organs.[24, 25] An enucleated eye and a chorioretinal biopsy from patients with SFU were included in the study of Chan and colleagues[21] investigating the expression of apoptotic markers in the eyes of patients with uveitis. The authors found an increased expression of *Fas* and *FasL* in the retina, the chorioretinal scars, and choroidal granulomas. Additionally, DNA fragmentation, which labels the particular cells undergoing apoptosis, was present in the gliotic retina, subretinal fibrotic tissue, and chorioretinal scars in eyes with SFU. Chan and colleagues stated that there might be pathologic consequences of *Fas-FasL* interactions in gliotic and fibrotic tissue, and they proposed that a dysregulation of the *Fas-FasL* pathway may lead to gliosis and fibrosis.

In summary, the fibrous portion of the amorphous connective tissue observed in the subretinal space of patients with SFU seems to be derived from RPE cells that have proliferated to form membranes. The RPE cell is pluripotent and can have fibroblastic activity when proliferating.[22, 26] Thus, it may be responding with fibroblastic activity to a yet unknown stimulus causing the subretinal fibrosis. Müller cells expressed class II antigens, which are not expressed by these cells in the normal retina.[4] RPE cells also expressed class II antigen, as it has been observed in other types of uveitis.[27, 28] The expression of such antigens may indicate that the cells are activated and proliferating, which could result in marked retinal gliosis and subretinal fibrosis formation.

DIAGNOSIS

Laboratory Investigations

Posterior involvement of the eye is considered to be one of the criteria to expand laboratory investigations from the minimal work-up required in a patient with uveitis to a more extensive evaluation. Laboratory and ancillary test selection is based on the diagnosis suggested by clinical examination and a careful review of systems.

It is mainly during the early phase of SFU, before subretinal fibrosis is present, that the clinician faces a diagnostic problem, as shown in the differential diagnosis section of this chapter. In that setting, it is essential to exclude treatable infectious (i.e., syphilis, tuberculosis, toxoplasmosis) and noninfectious (i.e., sarcoidosis) causes of choroidal and outer retinal involvement. But it should be kept in mind that, as in many other inflammatory processes involving the retina and choroid, the diagnosis of SFU is essentially based on clinical examination (Table 73–1).

Patients with SFU generally have no evidence of systemic disease.[2–4, 8–13, 15, 17, 18, 20] However, a flulike illness preceding ocular complaints has been reported in six patients.[11, 12] Extensive investigations reported in the literature, including complete blood cell count, erythrocyte sedimentation rate, antinuclear antibodies, complement

TABLE 73–1. SUBRETINAL FIBROSIS AND UVEITIS SYNDROME: DIAGNOSTIC FEATURES

Patient characteristics
  Female
  Young*
  Healthy
  Myopic
Early ocular manifestations
  Acute or rapidly progressive visual disturbances
  Unilateral symptoms despite bilateral involvement on clinical
    examination
Ocular examination
  Mild to moderate vitreous and anterior chamber inflammation
  Whitish yellow lesions (50–500 μm) in the posterior pole and
    midperiphery affecting RPE or inner choroid
  Lesions over time
    Fade without any RPE alteration
    Leave a punched-out atrophy
    Enlarge and coalesce, forming stellate zones of subretinal fibrosis
  Serous detachment, macular edema, disc edema

*Elderly patients have been described.
RPE, retinal pigment epithelium.

levels, serum protein electrophoresis, rheumatoid factor, angiotensin-converting enzyme, and lumbar puncture, were noncontributory. The chest radiograph was normal except for five patients with a positive skin test for histoplasmosis (three of these were from areas endemic for histoplasmosis).[11] A fourth patient showed hilar adenopathy, skin test positivity for histoplasmosis, and *Histoplasma* organisms on tissue section after mediastinal biopsy.[2] Serologic tests for syphilis, toxoplasmosis, toxocariasis, cryptococcosis, blastomycosis, coccidioidomycosis, herpes virus, cytomegalovirus, Epstein-Barr virus, Lyme disease, and *Histoplasma* titers were unrevealing. A histoplasmin skin test and purified protein derivative skin test were negative, except for isolated patients who displayed a positive result.[8, 11, 12] Examination of family members did not reveal any detectable abnormality.[13, 15]

Angiographic Findings

On fluorescein angiography (FA), acute lesions show hyperfluorescence during the early phase of the angiogram,[2, 9] with a mottled appearance in some instances.[8, 13, 14] Late in the course of the angiogram, staining of the lesions with[2, 8, 9, 14] or without[2, 13] leakage is observed. Late views show staining in the zones of subretinal fibrosis.[8] Resolving lesions show pigment epithelium window defects.[4, 8, 9, 15] The old resolved lesions (scars) demonstrate fluorescein staining. One of the patients reported by Palestine and associates[2] showed blockage of background choroidal fluorescence. Optic disc leakage and macular edema have also been reported.[8, 11]

Onoda and colleagues[16] reported the findings on FA and indocyanine-green angiography (ICG) of two young (14 and 18 years) myopic girls with multifocal choroiditis and subretinal fibrosis. On FA, the center of the lesions hypofluoresced and the edges hyperfluoresced. On ICG, the entire lesion hypofluoresced from an early stage and some major choroidal vessels were visible through them. The hypofluorescent areas persisted into the late phase and were larger than those seen in FA and in funduscopy.

Electrophysiology

Electrophysiologic features from 29 patients have been reported.[2, 3, 8–11, 13, 15] There were more anomalies in both the electroretinogram (ERG) and the EOG (23 patients)[2, 3, 8, 9, 11, 13] than normal responses (six patients).[9, 10, 13, 15] One patient in the series of Salvador and colleagues exhibited abnormal pattern ERG with normal EOG.[13]

Overall, patients with abnormal findings on electrophysiology had subretinal fibrosis on fundus examination,[2, 3, 8–11, 13] with a visual acuity of less than or equal to 20/100[2, 3, 8, 13] and chronic requirements or no response to systemic corticosteroids.[2, 3, 8, 11, 13] However, some patients had normal responses[8, 9, 11, 15] despite impaired visual acuity (less than or equal to 20/100)[8, 15] and diffuse fundus abnormalities, including three patients[8, 10] with subretinal fibrosis confined to the posterior pole.

Visual Field

Visual field testing sometimes shows marked scotomas that encompass an area somewhat larger than the area of subretinal lesions.[3] In the six patients studied by Reddy and coworkers[10] affected by what they called DSF, visual

field defects involved fixation at some time during the course of the disease in most patients. Enlarged blind spots were less frequent. With treatment, the size of the field defect improved, but it typically worsened with recurrence of inflammation. Other diseases affecting the choroid were included in their study. Overall, visual field defects improved in most patients with multiple evanescent white dot syndrome (MEWDS) and punctate inner choroidopathy (PIC), whereas most patients with multifocal choroiditis and panuveitis (MCP) and DSF did not improve.

Ancillary Tests

Unlike patients with other posterior uveitides, these patients did not exhibit in vitro lymphocyte proliferation in response to the retinal S-antigen.[2]

OTHER DISEASES WITH SUBRETINAL FIBROSIS

Subretinal fibrosis has been reported in other inflammatory conditions, such as the late stage of serpiginous choroiditis,[29] systemic lupus erythematosus associated central serous chorioretinopathy,[30] and onchocerciasis.[31] A 34-year-old man with acquired immunodeficiency syndrome (AIDS) presented with a choroidal mass, exudative retinal detachment, and vitritis. The patient underwent a choroidal biopsy to elucidate the infectious or malignant nature of the lesion. The specimen showed a subretinal eosinophilic infiltrate and subretinal fibrosis.[32]

Of interest are two cases recently reported by Matsuo and Matsuo,[14] who described two patients with subretinal fibrosis in the setting of rheumatoid arthritis. In both instances, subretinal fibrosis developed in parallel with exacerbation of rheumatoid arthritis and deteriorating renal function. The subretinal fibrosis in the right eye of the first patient developed abruptly in the course of active multifocal choroiditis with serous retinal detachment in both eyes, in parallel with rapid, progressive glomerulonephritis. In contrast, subretinal fibrosis in the second patient developed insidiously in the left eye and there was slowly progressive RPE atrophy in both eyes in the presence of stable, chronic renal failure.

Interestingly, a case of progressive subretinal fibrosis with fundus flavimaculatus has been reported.[33] A 20-year-old mildly myopic woman was under ophthalmologic care for fundus flavimaculatus. During 9 years of follow-up, an increasing number of chorioretinal punched-out spots in the posterior pole and midperiphery were noted, with progressive development of subretinal fibrosis. The anterior segment and vitreous were quiet, and systemic evaluation was unremarkable. FA demonstrated hypofluorescence and subsequent hyperfluorescence of the punched-out lesions, and staining of the fibrous tissue.

Lersutmikul and colleagues[34] have reported on the presence of subretinal fibrosis in Voght-Koyanagi-Harada (VKH) syndrome. In their retrospective study, 40% of patients (30 of 75) developed subretinal fibrosis defined as a yellow to white linear or polygonal fibrotic tissue at least one quarter of a disc diameter. For those patients having fibrotic lesions, these were located in the peripapillary and macular areas in 80% (22 of 30) of the cases. Subretinal fibrosis was not correlated with the presence of an exudative retinal detachment but with longer duration of the disease and more severe ocular inflammation. Additionally, presence of subretinal fibrosis was associated with a poor visual prognosis, as are choroidal neovascularization and the number of recurrences.

DIFFERENTIAL DIAGNOSIS

During the early stages of the disease, several entities may be confused with SFU. However, over time, the characteristic subretinal fibrosis helps to differentiate the disease from other conditions, including white dot syndromes, a collection of ocular disorders that share in common the presence of discrete, light-colored lesions in the fundus during at least one phase of the disease. Acute posterior multifocal placoid pigment epitheliopathy (APMPPE), MEWDS, birdshot retinochoroidopathy (BSRC), MCP, the presumed ocular histoplasmosis syndrome (POHS), and PIC[35] are the major members of this group of syndromes. Other entities, however, like acute retinal pigment epitheliitis (ARPE) and diffuse unilateral subacute neuroretinitis (DUSN), must also be included in this differential diagnosis (Table 73–2).

APMPPE[36] is a distinct entity often preceded by a viral illness. The disease is usually bilateral. Vitritis is rare, as are recurrences. Acute lesions consist of multiple yellow-white placoid or irregular lesions that are predominantly located in the posterior pole. FA features are characterized by early hypofluorescence of the plaques, followed by late hyperfluorescence. The lesions usually resolve, leaving a residual RPE stippling. Vision begins to improve spontaneously a few weeks after the onset of the symptoms; most patients recover 20/40 or better vision.

MEWDS[9] differs from SFU with respect to the lesions, with discrete white dots (100 to 200 μm) at the level of the outer retina or RPE. MEWDS lesions are mainly located in the macula, and they regress in a few weeks, leaving only very minor RPE defects. A macular granularity is often present. The patients' visual acuity returns to normal or near normal within a few weeks after the onset. Most patients suffering from BSRC[37] are human leukocyte antigen (HLA)–A29 positive. BSRC generally appears in middle-aged patients 40 to 60 years old. Multiple discrete, depigmented, or cream-colored spots in the midperiphery and posterior pole are seen. Most patients have chronic vitritis, papillitis, and retinal vascular leakage that results in macular edema. Problems with night vision and color discrimination are common complaints of patients with BSRC.

Patients with MCP[9, 11, 15] have numerous presumed ocular histoplasmosis syndrome (POHS)–like lesions, predominantly in the midperiphery of the retina, and vitreous cells are always present. MCP is characterized by bouts of recurrent inflammation, consisting of vitreous and anterior chamber cells and swelling around previously noted lesions. Subretinal neovascularization is common. Early hyperfluorescence on FA is a feature of the diagnosis.

POHS is a multifocal choroiditis characterized by atrophic peripheral "histo spots" (200 μm), peripapillary pigmented changes, and a disciform macular scar.[38] Patients with POHS may develop new choroidal lesions, but they do not have an appreciable associated vitritis; they may have pigment cells in the vitreous that can be confused for "vitritis."

PIC[12] is characterized by the absence of anterior chamber and vitreous cells. During its acute stage, 100 to 200 μm yellow, well-defined lesions at the level of the RPE or the inner choroid are observed in the posterior pole and midperiphery. Recurrent swelling around old lesions is rare. Patients with PIC do not develop new lesions on prolonged follow-up (Table 73–3).

ARPE[39] is a benign, self-limiting condition characterized by sudden, unilateral (75%), decreased visual acuity. The fundus picture consists of dark gray spots surrounded by a yellow-white halo without overlying vitritis in the acute stage. The lesions are usually located in the macula and they are smaller and subtler in appearance than those seen in SFU. There is typically complete resolution in 6 to 12 weeks, with a return to normal vision and no recurrences, although enlargement of the blind spot may be permanent.

Features of early DUSN[40] that distinguish it from SFU are diffuse RPE changes between the punched-out lesions, worms or worm tracks, the presence of outer retinal inflammation, vasculitis, vitritis, and papillitis. The biphasic nature of this immune or toxic reaction to worm byproducts leads to a progressive loss of the visual field, optic disc atrophy, and narrowing of the retinal vessels that can be seen late in the course of the disease.

The dark gray lesions and their normal or hypofluorescent appearance on FA help to differentiate acute macular retinopathy[41, 42] from SFU.

The exclusion of a potentially treatable infectious cause of uveitis is essential in any patient for whom systemic steroid therapy is contemplated. Both syphilis and tuberculosis can manifest inflammation involving the vitreous, outer retina, and choroid. Laboratory studies for syphilis and tuberculosis help to exclude these diagnoses, as do signs and symptoms of systemic disease that may coexist with the ophthalmic manifestations. Punctate

TABLE 73–2. SUBRETINAL FIBROSIS AND UVEITIS SYNDROME: DIFFERENTIAL DIAGNOSIS OF FUNDUSCOPIC APPEARANCE

Early phase
  Infectious
    Syphilis
    Tuberculosis
    Diffuse unilateral subacute neuroretinitis (DUSN)
    Punctate outer retinal toxoplasmosis
  Noninfectious
    Acute posterior multifocal placoid epitheliopathy (APMPPE)
    Multiple evanescent white dot syndrome (MEWDS)
    Birdshot retinochoroidopathy (BSRC)
    Multifocal choroiditis panuveitis (MCP)
    Presumed ocular histoplasmosis syndrome (POHS)
    Punctate inner choroidopathy (PIC)
    Acute retinal pigment epitheliitis (ARPE)
    Acute macular retinopathy
    Sarcoidosis
    Myopia
Late stage
    Serpiginous choroiditis
    Age-related macular degeneration (ARMD)

TABLE 73–3. PIC, MCP, AND SFU: DIFFERENCES AND SIMILARITIES

	PIC	MCP	SFU
Demographics	Young, female, myopic	Young to adult, female, myopic	Young, female, myopic
Location	RPE, choroid; posterior pole and midperiphery	RPE, choroid; posterior to equator > posterior pole	RPE, choroid; posterior pole and midperiphery
Laterality	Bilateral	Bilateral	Bilateral
Symptoms	Blurred vision, flashes, central scotomas	Blurred vision, flashes, central scotomas, floaters, metamorphopsias	Blurred vision, flashes, central scotomas, metamorphopsias
Anterior segment	No	Typically	Yes
Vitritis	Rare	Marked	Present >> absent
Acute lesions	100–300 μm, yellow, well-defined lesions	POHS-like lesions, 50–200 μm	50–500 μm white-yellow hypopigmented lesions
Evolving lesions	Atrophic cylindrical scars	Atrophic scars bigger and more pigmented than in PIC	Irregular zones of subretinal fibrosis
Other fundus findings	Serous RD	CME, serous RD, peripapillary pigmentary changes	CME, serous RD, papillitis
CNV	Rare	Common	Possible
Chronology	Unique episode	Chronic, recurrent	Chronic, recurrent
Fluorescein angiography	Early hyperfluorescence, late leakage	Early hyperfluorescence, fade late	Early hyperfluorescence, late leakage
Visual field	Usually normal	Enlarged blind spots, full fields, involving fixation	Enlarged blind spots, involving fixation
Electrophysiology	Normal	Abnormal-to-extinguished ERG responses	Abnormal ERG/EOG > WNL
Visual prognosis	Good unless CNV	Fair	Poor
Treatment	No	Yes: immunosuppressors, laser photocoagulation (CNV)	Yes: immunosuppressors, laser photocoagulation (CNV)
Response to therapy	Poor	Variable	Very poor if subretinal fibrosis is present

PIC, punctate inner choroidopathy; MCP, recurrent multifocal choroiditis and uveitis; SFU, subretinal fibrosis and uveitis syndrome; RPE, retinal pigment epithelium; RD, retinal detachment; POHS, presumed ocular histoplasmosis syndrome; CME, cystoid macular edema; ERG, electroretinogram; EOG, electro-oculogram; CNV, choroidal neovascular membrane; WNL, within normal limits.

outer retinal toxoplasmosis[43] is a subset of ocular toxoplasmosis in which patients present with acute, multifocal, gray-white lesions involving the outer retina and RPE, with little or no vitreous involvement. The lesions may recur next to each other in a satellite fashion and slowly resolve with scar formation. Serology for *Toxoplasma* is positive.

Sarcoidosis is a chronic multisystem disease, classically with candle-wax drippings around retinal vessels, retinal hemorrhages, "snowball" vitreous opacities, chorioretinal granulomas, and response to corticosteroid treatment. It must be included in the differential diagnosis of SFU.

Although many patients in the reports of SFU are myopic, the SFU differs from pathologic myopia, as there are no staphylomas, lacquer-cracks, straightening of the retinal vessels, or Fuchs' spots.

The late stage of SFU has an appearance similar to choroidopathies with subretinal neovascular membranes and disciform scarring, such as serpiginous choroiditis and age-related macular degeneration. Serpiginous choroiditis is a progressive disorder that affects the peripapillary RPE, choriocapillaris, and choroid. Lesions consist of large, well-circumscribed areas that extend from the disc in a progressive pseudopodial fashion. The FA pattern is quite characteristic, with hypofluorescence of the acute lesion early in the angiogram and late hyperfluorescence that begins along the margins of the lesion.[9]

TREATMENT

Although in some cases systemic corticosteroids may be of benefit during the acute phase of the disease, once the subretinal fibrosis occurs, there appears to be no effective treatment. In one series,[9] the nine patients who were treated with systemic and periocular injections of corticosteroids during the acute phase of the disease responded well to treatment. Even a subretinal neovascular membrane regressed with the steroid therapy. Unfortunately, most other studies describe variable responses, with a few patients showing improvement[8, 14, 20] and most exhibiting progression of the disease or, at best, questionable results.[2, 3, 8, 10, 11, 13, 17, 20, 21] Similarly, a combination of corticosteroid and therapy with immunomodulators (cyclophosphamide, azathioprine, or cyclosporine-A) has also shown variable benefit, with some cases showing no response[4, 17, 21] and some others in which the inflammation was controlled.[10, 17, 20]

Laser photocoagulation has been attempted to treat neovascular membranes without success.[7, 11, 12]

PROGNOSIS AND EVOLUTION

The visual prognosis of patients with SFU is poor.[20] Impaired visual acuity depends on the presence of subretinal fibrosis, atrophy, or subretinal neovascular membranes affecting the macula. The natural course of the disease consists of numerous bouts of inflammation, typically in and around previous lesions, with most of the affected eyes developing severe visual loss over a period of months[2, 3, 8, 9, 17, 18] to years.[4, 13, 21] In some cases, the disease may affect visual acuity in a short period. The case of a 24-year-old woman with a rapid and severe onset of the disease, which led to no light perception bilaterally in 6 months despite treatment with corticosteroids and cyclophosphamide,[4] is illustrative of this rapidly progressive form. Similarly, the case of a 31-year-old woman with visual acuity in her left eye decreasing to counting fingers in 3 weeks and further dropping to hand movements and unresponsive to systemic corticosteroids illustrates the same phenomenon.[13]

In most series reported, final visual acuity ranges from 20/200 to no light perception.[2, 3, 4, 8, 10, 11, 13, 17, 18, 20, 21] Reddy and colleagues[10] included in their series patients with MCP, PIC, MEWDS, and what they called DSF. Patients with DSF had the worst initial visual acuity (20/291) in comparison with MCP (20/45), PIC (20/41), and MEWDS (20/26). Additionally, the group with clinical features of DSF had the worst final visual acuity (20/163) in comparison with MCP (20/33), PIC (20/33), and MEWDS (20/20). Similarly, the patients with DSF had the worst visual prognosis of the three groups (the other two being MCP and PIC) in the study of Brown and coworkers.[20]

CONCLUSIONS

Inflammatory conditions causing multifocal lesions of the choroid and pigment epithelium are a confusing group of diseases. SFU differs from other multifocal choroidal or RPE diseases in that instead of forming atrophic or pigmented chorioretinal scars, the acute lesions heal with the formation of multiple zones of subretinal fibrosis that enlarge and coalesce, forming large placoid lesions with irregular margins. This rare condition usually affects young, myopic, otherwise healthy women, although middle-aged and older patients have been reported. Initially, only one eye may become symptomatic, but bilateral involvement is typical. Symptoms include unilateral visual loss, scotomas, metamorphopsias, and photopsias. Mild vitritis is normally present. In the acute stage, the funduscopic picture consists of multiple, small, white-yellow RPE or choroidal lesions. The visual prognosis is poor and recurrences are common, typically involving previously affected sites. Treatment is controversial, with some authors finding a beneficial effect of early steroids and chemotherapy treatment. The etiology is unknown, but SFU is believed to be a localized autoimmune reaction to the RPE. It may be a common response of the retina to different offending stimuli.

References

1. Fisher SK, Erickson PA, Lewis GP, Anderson DH: Intraretinal proliferation induced by retinal detachment. Invest Ophthalmol Vis Sci 1991;32:1739.
2. Palestine AG, Nussenblatt RB, Parver LM, et al: Progressive subretinal fibrosis and uveitis. Br J Ophthalmol 1984;68:667.
3. Palestine AG, Nussenblatt RB, Chan CC, et al: Histopathology of the subretinal fibrosis and uveitis syndrome. Ophthalmology 1985;92:838.
4. Kim MK, Chan CC, Belfort R, et al: Histopathologic and immunohistopathologic features of subretinal fibrosis and uveitis syndrome. Am J Ophthalmol 1987;104:15.
5. Fuchs A: Diseases of the Fundus Oculi with Atlas. Philadelphia, Blakiston, 1949, p 125.
6. Calixto N: Histopathologic and immunohistopathologic features of subretinal fibrosis and uveitis syndrome. Am J Ophthalmol 1988;105:220.
7. Doran R, Hamilton A: Disciform macular degeneration in young adults. Trans Ophthalmol Soc U K 1982;102:471.
8. Cantrill HL, Folk JC: Multifocal choroiditis associated with progressive subretinal fibrosis. Am J Ophthalmol 1986;101:170.
9. Morgan CM, Schatz H: Recurrent multifocal choroiditis. Ophthalmology 1986;93:1138.
10. Reddy CV, Brown J, Folk JC, et al: Enlarged blind spot in chorioretinal inflammatory disorders. Ophthalmology 1996;103:606.
11. Dreyer RF, Gass JDM: Multifocal uveitis and panuveitis. A syndrome that mimics ocular histoplasmosis. Arch Ophthalmol 1984;102:1776.
12. Watzke RC, Packer AJ, Folk JC, et al: Punctate inner choroidopathy. Am J Ophthalmol 1984;98:572.
13. Salvador F, García-Arumí J, Mateo C, et al: Multifocal choroiditis with subretinal fibrosis. Report of two cases. Ophthalmologica 1994;208:163.
14. Matsuo T, Matsuo N: Progressive subretinal fibrosis in patients with rheumatoid arthritis and renal dysfunction. Ophthalmologica 1998;212:289.
15. Nozik RA, Dorsch W: A new chorioretinopathy associated with anterior uveitis. Am J Ophthalmol 1973;76:758.
16. Onoda S, Shibuya K, Miyasaka H, et al: Multifocal choroiditis with subretinal fibrosis. Nippon Ganka Gakkai Zasshi 1997;101:711.
17. Martin DF, Chan CC, Smet MD, et al: The role of chorioretinal biopsy in the management of posterior uveitis. Ophthalmology 1993;100:705.
18. Gass JDM, Margo CE, Levy MH: Progressive subretinal fibrosis and blindness in patients with multifocal granulomatous chorioretinitis. Am J Ophthalmol 1996;122:76.
19. Kaiser PK, Gragoudas ES: The subretinal fibrosis and uveitis syndrome. Int Ophthalmol Clin 1996;36:145.
20. Brown J, Folk JC, Reddy CV, et al: Visual prognosis of multifocal choroiditis, punctate inner choroidopathy, and the diffuse subretinal fibrosis syndrome. Ophthalmology 1996;103:1100.
21. Chan CC, Matteson DM, Li Q, et al: Apoptosis in patients with posterior uveitis. Arch Ophthalmol 1997;115:1559.
22. Mandelcorn MS, Machemer R, Fineberg E, et al: Proliferation and metaplasia of intravitreal retinal pigment epithelium cell autotransplants. Am J Ophthalmol 1975;80:227.
23. Sternberg P, Machemer R: Subretinal proliferation. Am J Ophthalmol 1984;98:456.
24. D'Souza SD, Bonetti B, Balasingam V, et al: Multiple sclerosis: *Fas* signaling in oligodendrocyte cell death. J Exp Med 1996;184:2361.
25. Giordano C, Stassi G, Galluzo A: Potential involvement of *Fas* and its ligand in the pathogenesis of Hashimoto's thyroiditis. Science 1997;275:960.
26. Machemer R, Laqua H: Pigment epithelium proliferation in retinal detachment (massive periretinal proliferation). Am J Ophthalmol 1975;80:1.
27. Chan CC, Hooks JJ, Nussenblatt RB, et al: Expression of Ia antigen on retinal pigment epithelium in experimental autoimmune uveoretinitis. Curr Eye Res 1986;5:325.
28. Chan CC, Detrick B, Nussenblatt RB, et al: HLA-DR in retinal pigment epithelial cells from patients with uveitis. Arch Ophthalmol 1986;104:725.
29. Chisholm IH, Gass JDM, Hutton WL: The late stage of serpiginous (geographic) choroiditis. Am J Ophthalmol 1976;82:343.
30. Cunningham ET, Alfred PR, Irvine AR: Central serous chorioretinopathy in patients with systemic lupus erythematosus. Ophthalmology 1996;103:2081.
31. Newland HS, White AT, Greene BM, et al: Ocular manifestations of onchocerciasis in a rain forest area of West Africa. Br J Ophthalmol 1991;75:163.
32. Rutzen AR, Ortega-Larrocea G, Dugel PU, et al: Clinicopathological study of retinal and choroidal biopsies in intraocular inflammation. Am J Ophthalmol 1995;119:597.
33. Parodi MB: Progressive subretinal fibrosis in fundus flavimaculatus. Acta Ophthalmol 1994;72:260.
34. Lertsumitkul S, Whitcup SM, Nussenblatt RB, Chan CC: Subretinal

fibrosis and choroidal neovascularization in Voght-Koyanagi-Harada syndrome. Graefes Arch Clin Exp Ophthalmol 1999;12:1039–1045.

35. Brown J, Folk JC: Current controversies in the white dot syndromes. Multifocal choroiditis, punctate inner choroidopathy and diffuse subretinal fibrosis syndrome. Ocul Immunol Inflamm 1998;6:125.

36. Gass JDM: Acute posterior multifocal placoid pigment epitheliopathy. Arch Ophthalmol 1968;80:177.

37. Ryan SJ, Maumenee AE: Birdshot retinochoroidopathy. Am J Ophthalmol 1980;89:31.

38. Gass JMD: Presumed ocular histoplasmosis syndrome. In: Gass JMD, ed: Stereoscopic Atlas of Macular Diseases. Diagnosis and Treatment, 4th ed, vol I. St. Louis, Mosby–Year Book, 1997, p 130.

39. Krill AE, Deutman AF: Acute retinal pigment epitheliitis. Am J Ophthalmol 1972;74:193.

40. Gass JDM, Braunstein RA: Further observations concerning the diffuse unilateral subacute neuroretinitis syndrome. Arch Ophthalmol 1983;101:1689.

41. Priluck IA, Buettner H, Robertson DM: Acute macular neuroretinopathy. Am J Ophthalmol 1978;86:775.

42. Gass JMD: Acute macular neuroretinopathy. In: Gass JMD, ed: Stereoscopic Atlas of Macular Diseases. Diagnosis and Treatment, 4th ed, vol II. St. Louis, Mosby–Year Book, 1997, p 693.

43. Doft BH, Gass JDM: Punctate outer retinal toxoplasmosis. Arch Ophthalmol 1985;103:1332.

Carl H. Park and Michael B. Raizman

DEFINITION

Punctate inner choroidopathy (PIC) is an inflammatory multifocal chorioretinopathy of unknown cause. It is categorized with other inflammatory chorioretinopathies of unknown etiologies, including acute posterior multifocal placoid pigment epitheliopathy (APMPPE), multiple evanescent white dot syndrome (MEWDS), birdshot retinochoroidopathy (BSRC), serpiginous choroiditis, multifocal choroiditis and panuveitis (MCP), and subretinal fibrosis. PIC mainly affects myopic women who present with symptoms of blurry vision and/or scotoma. As suggested by the name, ophthalmoscopy reveals discrete, white-yellow lesions in the inner choroid, concentrated in the posterior pole. Examination of the eye is otherwise unremarkable, with no evidence of either anterior or posterior uveitis. PIC is thought to be a self-limited process, and the visual outcome is usually good, although it can result in the formation of choroidal neovascular membranes, which can lead to a poor visual outcome.

HISTORY

In 1984, Watzke and colleagues presented a series of 10 moderately myopic women (-3.25 to -10.00 diopters), ranging in age from 21 to 37, who presented with blurred vision, flashes, and paracentral scotomas.[1] Examination revealed small (100 to 300 μm) yellow-white lesions at the level of the inner choroid, often associated with small serous retinal detachments. Eight of the 10 patients presented with bilateral lesions, and six developed subretinal neovascular membranes. None of the 10 had vitreous or anterior chamber inflammation, and the laboratory evaluation failed to reveal evidence of a microbial cause (including histoplasmosis, blastomycosis, or coccidioidomycosis). The authors suggested that this was a new clinical entity, distinct from other chorioretinal inflammatory diseases, and they proposed the term punctate inner choroidopathy.

Watzke and colleagues felt that PIC was a distinct entity in the category of multifocal choroiditis of unknown etiologies, or the so-called white dot syndromes. Interestingly, several reports between 1984 and 1986 described other conditions predominantly affecting myopic women presenting with multifocal choroiditis with varying degrees of uveitis. In 1984, Dreyer and Gass presented 28 cases of multifocal choroiditis with vitreous inflammation and chorioretinal scars similar to those seen in presumed ocular histoplasmosis (POHS).[2] Average age at presentation was 33 years old, with a 3:1 female-to-male preponderance. Anterior chamber inflammation was seen in 52% of the eyes, and vitreous cells were seen in 94% of the eyes. Ophthalmoscopic examinations revealed deep choroidal lesions of varying size (50 to 300 μm) located both in the posterior pole and in the periphery. Choroidal neovascular membranes (CNVM) were observed in 30% of the eyes. Only 5 of 16 patients tested positive on the histoplasmosis skin test. Dreyer and Gass[2] suggested

that the presence of vitritis (and, in some, anterior uveitis), the size of the choroidal and retinal pigment epithelium (RPE) lesions (smaller than seen with POHS), and the lack of evidence for histoplasmosis exposure pointed toward a distinct clinical entity which they called MCP.

In 1986, Cantrill and Folk described a case series of five healthy women (ages 14 to 34) who presented with blurred vision or scotomas.[3] Four of the five patients showed no anterior chamber or vitreous inflammation. Funduscopic examination revealed clusters of hypopigmented lesions (100 to 200 μm) located in the posterior pole. Over time, these lesions faded, leaving either punched-out atrophic lesions or RPE pigment changes. The distinct characteristic of this series of patients was the development of progressive subretinal fibrosis, apparently formed by coalescence and evolution of the acute lesions. The authors reintroduced the term progressive subretinal fibrosis, initially coined by Palestine and coworkers,[4] to describe this unique outcome of what appeared to be a multifocal choroiditis of unknown etiology in young healthy women.

Cantrill and Folk suggested that the three entities just described may have a significant overlap in presentation, clinical finding, and clinical course.[3] There is clearly a preponderance of young women in these three series, and in most cases both eyes are affected. All three diseases can present (at least initially) as small, punctate, outer retinal lesions in the posterior pole and the periphery. Serologic and laboratory evaluations are typically negative. The clinical course of these three entities may also share certain features. Cantrill and Folk pointed out that one patient in the Dreyer and Gass series[2] demonstrated "large subretinal bands of metaplastic RPE," consistent with progressive subretinal fibrosis. A case series of Watzke and coworkers[1] included a patient with late formation of "a fibrotic hyperplastic central scar." And all three conditions are associated with formation of CNVM, which can lead to significant visual impairment.

These three diseases, PIC, MCP, and progressive (diffuse) subretinal fibrosis, are now thought to be a clinical spectrum of a single disease, a choroiditis that affects the choroid and the RPE of (mostly) young healthy women. MCP and subretinal fibrosis and uveitis syndrome (SFU) will be discussed in other chapters. This chapter will focus on the unique presentation and clinical course of PIC, as well as the clinical features shared with the other forms of multifocal choroiditis.

EPIDEMIOLOGY

It is difficult to estimate the incidence or the prevalence of PIC or other multifocal choroiditis entities, and good demographic data are also lacking. An estimate can be made from the studies of Brown and colleagues,[5] the largest published series on multifocal choroiditis. Their study reviewed all diagnoses for PIC, MCP, and SFU from 1980 and 1994 at the University of Iowa, a major regional tertiary eye care referral center in the midwestern United States. A total of 161 patients were identified with these three diagnoses in a period of 15 years, or approximately 11 cases per year. Assuming that the referral population of the University of Iowa is the population of Iowa (2.8 million), then a national incidence of multifocal choroiditis could be about 1000 to 2000 cases per year. Only 16 patients of the 161 case series patients had the diagnosis of PIC (10%). The national incidence of PIC could therefore be estimated as about 100 to 200 cases per year. It should be noted that many cases of PIC may be subclinical (i.e., minimal visual disturbances, lack of central foveal lesions, lack of foveal CNVM), so these numbers may be an underestimate.

PIC tends to affect young, apparently healthy women. However, case series of PIC are usually small and there may be a predisposition or bias against diagnosing PIC in men. Brown and colleagues[5] presented 16 cases of PIC with only one male patient. The average ages of the patients in the two studies were 27 and 30 years.[1, 5] No studies (or case series with sufficient numbers) exist that suggest a racial or cultural predisposition for PIC. However, most cases are in white women.[1, 5]

CLINICAL CHARACTERISTICS

The predominant symptoms at presentation for these young women are blurred central vision or scotomas. Also documented are complaints of flashes, floaters, and photopsias.[1, 5, 6] Visual disturbances are usually unilateral, although, as will be described later, funduscopic examinations usually reveal bilateral lesions.[1] There is usually no concurrent or recent systemic illness or viral prodrome, as often documented in cases of APMPPE or MEWDS.

The visual acuity at presentation is usually decreased. Reddy and colleagues[6] analyzed 16 patients with PIC (the same group as in the Brown and colleagues series[5]) and the initial average visual acuity was 20/41 with a range of 20/15 to 20/500. Over 75% of the patients were 20/40 or better. Their analyses of the refractive errors for the different chorioretinitis cases are of interest. PIC had the highest refractive error at −3.67 diopters, versus −2.19, −1.25, and −1.25 for MCP, SFU, and MEWDS, respectively.

The external examination of patients with PIC is unremarkable. The anterior segment examination is also normal, with a quiet anterior chamber and no stigmata of prior uveitis. The vitreous is clear without inflammatory cells. The lack of vitreous inflammation is a hallmark of PIC, and the presence of vitritis should suggest a different diagnosis. Fundus examination usually reveals multiple discrete, flat, yellow, round lesions (50 to 300 μm in size) at the level of the RPE and the inner choroid (Figs. 74–1 to 74–4). The number of lesions is variable (12 to 25 in the Watzke and coworkers series[1]). They are concentrated in the posterior pole, which is in distinct contrast to MCP and SFU, where mid-peripheral lesions are more apparent. Initially, some of these yellow spots may be associated with serous detachment of the neurosensory retina (see Fig. 74–1). Visual disturbances are usually associated with foveal choroidal lesions with or without an associated serous detachment. The acute lesions usually evolve over a few months to become either faded

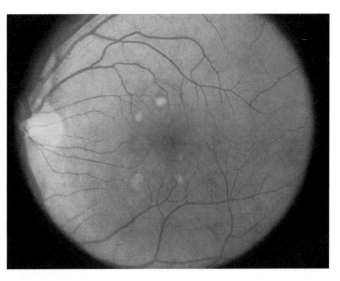

FIGURE 74–1. Case 1. Thirty-two-year-old white, myopic woman presented with a 2-week history of metamorphopsia OS. Fundus examination revealed several punctate chorioretinal lesions with overlying neurosensory retinal detachments. (See color insert.)

chorioretinal lesions or atrophic chorioretinal scars. Watzke and colleagues[1] found that some scars became pigmented over a period of years, often resembling old punched-out POHS scars (see Fig. 74–3). An important differentiating feature is the distinct absence of cystoid macular edema or disc edema in PIC as opposed to MCP or MEWDS.[1, 5, 6]

As previously stated, although visual symptoms are usually unilateral at presentation, fundus abnormalities are usually bilateral. Eight of 10 patients (80%) in the Watzke and coworkers' series[1] and 14 of 16 patients (88%) in the Brown and coworkers' series[5] had bilateral disease. In comparison, 27 of 41 (66%) patients with MCP, 5 of 5

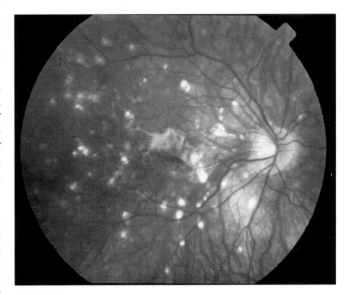

FIGURE 74–2. Case 2. Twenty-three-year-old white, myopic woman was referred with a 3-month history of central vision loss OD. Fundus examination showed numerous punctate, white chorioretinal atrophic lesions in the posterior pole. A fibrovascular CNVM was evident in the macular. (Courtesy of Jay S. Duker, M.D.) (See color insert.)

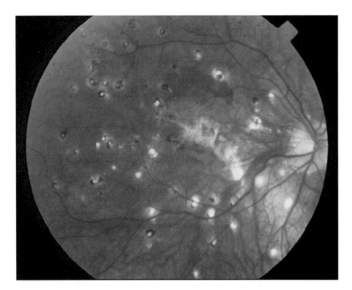

FIGURE 74–3. Case 2. One year later, the patient returned for a follow-up examination. Note that many of the chorioretinal lesions have become pigmented. A new CNVM with an associated subretinal hemorrhage is evident superior to the old macular scar. (See color insert.)

patients with SFU (100%), and only 4 of 16 (25%) patients with MEWDS had bilateral fundus lesions in the study by Reddy and colleagues.[6]

The most significant clinical sequela of PIC is the formation of CNVM. It is estimated that the 17% to 40% of eyes with PIC lesions will develop CNVM.[1, 5] CNVM may be present on the first examination or it may form up to 1 year later.[1, 5] It is the leading cause of poor visual outcome (less than 20/200) in patients with PIC.[5] It is thought that CNVM arises from focal chorioretinal scars in response to choroidal injury.[7] This may be in contrast to the formation of CNVM in age-related macular degeneration, where generalized deterioration of the RPE-

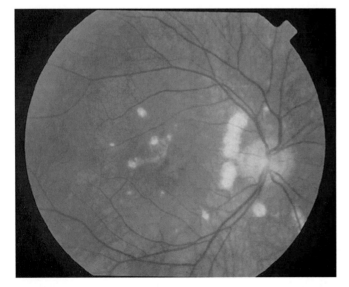

FIGURE 74–4. Case 3. Twenty-four-year-old white, myopic woman was referred with an 8-month history of a central scotoma. Fundus examination revealed multiple, punctate perifoveal lesions with a fibrovascular CNVM in the fovea. (Courtesy of Jay S. Duker, M.D.) (See color insert.)

Bruch membrane interface causes a nondistinct, nonfocal neovascularization to occur. The therapeutic implications of different types of CNVM and its relevance to PIC will be discussed later. The clinical characteristics of PIC are summarized in Table 74–1.

PATHOPHYSIOLOGY

No studies to date have examined the histopathology of the characteristic PIC lesions. Unfortunately, little is known about the etiology or pathogenesis of PIC. Watzke and colleagues[1] were not able to find an infectious cause for their patients with PIC. Their rather extensive evaluation included serologies for fungi (histoplasmosis, blastomycosis, and coccidioidomycosis), toxoplasmosis, herpes virus, and cytomegalovirus without revealing any candidate causative organism. Most patients with PIC have normal systemic studies, including complete blood cell count, erythrocyte sedimentation rate, angiotensin-converting enzyme, and antinuclear antibody titers.[1]

Watzke and colleagues[1] have speculated that PIC may be a special and limited spectrum of myopic degeneration. Clearly, most patients with PIC have a history of at least moderate myopia, and many of the PIC lesions appear in a linear configuration, which suggests a pathogenesis possibly similar to that of the lacquer cracks seen in myopic degeneration.

The histopathology of CNVM in PIC is important, as most visual loss from PIC results from the formation of a neovascular membrane. Olsen and colleagues[8] examined the clinical course and evolution of CNVM in five patients with PIC. They subsequently examined the surgical specimens following submacular extraction of these neovascular membranes. They described the typical PIC neovascular membranes as "multiple, small (<300 μm), yellow-white, or yellow-green foci deep to the retina with pigmented borders and an accompanying shallow overlying neurosensory retinal detachment." They observed that, with time, these smaller CNVMs coalesce to form a larger neovascular membrane with multiple "feeder vessels" from the choroid. These membranes, lying anterior to the RPE and below the neurosensory retina, have been termed type II membranes by Gass.[7] Type II membranes are more amenable to surgical removal than type I membranes, which are beneath the RPE as seen in age-related macular degeneration. The anatomic configuration of type II membranes in POHS and PIC may confer a better prognosis following surgical excision. Histopathologic examination showed a fibrovascular tissue bordered by RPE,

TABLE 74–1. CLINICAL CHARACTERISTICS OF PUNCTATE INNER CHOROIDOPATHY

FEATURES	COMMENTS
Female >> male	93% to 100% female
Young, healthy	20–30 years old, no prodrome
Myopic	Average, −4.00 diopters
Unilateral symptoms	Bilateral lesions
No anterior chamber reaction	A key element
No posterior inflammation	A key element
White punctate lesions	Mostly posterior pole
Choroidal neovascular membranes	17% to 40%

TABLE 74–2. DIFFERENTIAL DIAGNOSIS OF PUNCTATE INNER CHOROIDOPATHY

Presumed ocular histoplasmosis syndrome
Multiple evanescent white dot syndrome
Acute posterior multifocal placoid pigment epitheliopathy
Multifocal choroiditis and panuveitis
Subretinal fibrosis and uveitis
Birdshot retinochoroidopathy
Sarcoidosis
Myopic degeneration maculopathy
Ocular toxoplasmosis
Lyme disease
Vogt-Koyanagi-Harada syndrome

infiltrated with few lymphocytes. There was no evidence of Bruch's membrane or choriocapillaris. In this manner, the CNVM of PIC may be similar to the CNVM seen in POHS in that the membrane lies anterior to the RPE layer.[7] Surgical specimens from submacular CNVM extraction in POHS show a similar histology.

DIAGNOSIS

The differential diagnosis of PIC is extensive and is summarized in Table 74–2. However, the key element in the diagnosis of PIC, the absence of anterior and posterior segment inflammation, eliminates most of the diagnoses listed, including MFC, SFU, sarcoidosis, BSRC, toxoplasmosis, and Vogt-Koyanagi-Harada. PIC can be differenti-

ated from POHS by the lack of peripapillary atrophic changes and peripheral retinal lesions.

Other retinal white dot syndromes of unknown etiologies must be differentiated from PIC. MEWDS lesions are also concentrated in the posterior pole as in PIC, but the lesions have a less distinct border and do not have an associated serous detachment.[9] Also, patients with MEWDS have the characteristic granular appearance of the macula. APMPPE does not affect women predominantly, and patients with APMPPE may have associated systemic manifestations, including cerebral vasculitis and encephalitis.[10, 11] In contrast to PIC lesions, APMPPE lesions are typically placoid, large, and often confluent to each other.[12] Patients with BSRC have an associated vitritis, and the lesions are typically seen throughout the fundus to the periphery.[13, 14] Table 74–3 summarizes the clinical characteristics of the white dot syndromes, or multifocal choroiditis of unknown etiology.

Although the diagnosis of PIC usually can be made based on clinical examination, ancillary testing, including visual field testing and retinal angiography, can be helpful in confirming the diagnosis, following the clinical course of the disease, and making therapeutic decisions. Because patients present with a scotoma, visual field testing may be helpful in documenting and following this symptom. Reddy and colleagues[6] performed visual field testing on 22 eyes with PIC and they were able to document a defect in 12 of the 22 (55%). The predominant finding was an enlarged blind spot, seen in 41% of patients. Enlarge-

TABLE 74–3. SUMMARY OF WHITE DOT SYNDROMES OF UNKNOWN ETIOLOGIES

	APMPPE[12–12]	MEWDS[9]	BSRC[13, 14, 22]	SC[23, 24]	MCP/PU[2, 3, 5]	PIC[1, 5]
Age	20–30	20–40	30–60	20–60	20–60	20–40
Sex	M = F	F>>M	F>>M	M = F	F>>M	F>>M
Viral prodrome	Often severe[a]	50%	[d]	Rarely	Not typical	Rarely
Unilateral or bilateral	Bilateral	Asymmetric	Bilateral	Bilateral	Bilateral	Variable
Typical findings	Yellow, creamy, flat, placoid lesions	Multiple white lesions at level of RPE or choroid[b]	Vitritis; creamy, white lesions entire fundus[e]	Yellow/gray peripapillary lesion; progress in serpentine fashion[f]	Iritis, vitritis; peripapillary fibrosis; multiple yellow lesions	Multiple punctate, white chorioretinal lesions
Fluorescein angiography	Early hypo, then late hyper	Early hyper of lesions; disc hyper	Subtle late stain of lesions; disc stain	Late hyper of lesion; retinal vascular stain	Early block; late stain; cystoid macular edema	Early hyper of lesions
Indocyanine green angiography	Hypo lesions	Multiple hypo lesions[c]	Hypo lesions	Hypo lesions	Hypo lesions	Hypo lesions
Choroidal neovascularization	Rarely	Rarely	Rarely	Yes	Yes	Yes
Recurrent	Rarely	Rarely	Can be progressive	Chronic/ progressive	Can be progressive	Self limited
Visual outcome	Baseline	Baseline	Often decreased	Usually decreased	Variable	Usually decreased

RPE, retinal pigment epithelium; hypo, hypofluorescent or hypofluorescence; hyper, hyperfluorescent or hyperfluorescence; APMPPE, acute posterior multifocal placoid pigment epitheliopathy; MEWDS, multiple evanescent white dot syndrome; BSRC, birdshot chorioretinopathy; SC, serpiginous choroiditis; MCP/PU, multifocal choroiditis/panuveitis; PIC, punctate inner choroidopathy.
[a]Associated with cerebrovasculitis; CSF abnormalities
[b]Often disc edema, granular foveal changes
[c]ERG—decreased a-wave amplitude
[d]90% HLA-A29 positive; lymphocyte active against retinal S-Ag[15]
[e]Also disc edema and cystoid macula edema
[f]Often anterior/posterior inflammation; eventual atrophy of lesions

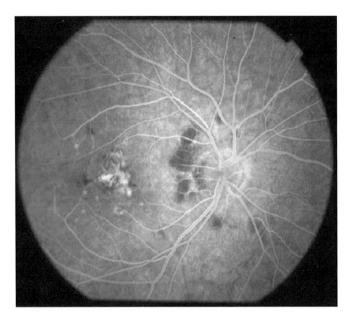

FIGURE 74–5. Case 3. Early transit fluorescein angiography revealed multiple punctate hyperfluorescent lesions with early staining of the fibrovascular CNVM.

ment of blind spots are well documented in other instances of multifocal choroiditis, such as MEWDS and MCP.[9, 15, 16]

Fluorescein angiography (FA) of acute PIC lesions usually shows an early hyperfluorescence in the arteriovenous phase with a variable amount of leakage in the late arteriovenous phase. Some lesions have been shown to block fluorescence in the early arteriovenous phase and stain thereafter. If a serous detachment is present, the spots leak dye into the subretinal space (Figs. 74–5 and

74–6).[1] Older PIC lesions can show transmission defect hyperfluorescence, reflecting the evolution of acute lesions to atrophic chorioretinal scars.

Indocyanine green (ICG) angiography of PIC lesions shows hypofluorescent spots in the posterior pole (Fig. 74–7). These spots may correspond to the areas of visible lesions. Slakter and colleagues have suggested that ICG angiography may be helpful in the diagnosis of MCP.[17] They have shown that in the active phase of MCP, ICG angiography shows hypofluorescent spots in the posterior pole, which gradually resolve with clinical improvement of the choroiditis. The same may perhaps also be true for PIC.

FA is invaluable in localizing and characterizing the CNVM seen in PIC. Most CNVM in PIC begins as multiple, smaller, yellow-green lesions in the deep retina with surrounding pigment changes.[8] FA of these lesions shows early hyperfluorescence with late leakage. Over time (weeks to months), these lesions coalesce to form a larger CNVM with bridging networks developing between the smaller membranes (see Fig. 74–6).[5, 8]

TREATMENT

No treatment is advised for the majority of patients without evidence of CNVM, as patients without CNVM have excellent visual outcomes.[1, 5] However, corticosteroids may be considered in some patients who present with poor initial visual acuity (less than 20/200) with an abundance of acute PIC lesions (with or without an associated serous detachment) concentrated in the fovea. There are two rationales for treating acute foveal PIC lesions. First, it may be possible that corticosteroids can limit the extent of RPE disturbance and choroidal scar formation following the insult of the acute PIC lesions. Significant RPE disturbances and scar formation in the fovea may lead to a relatively poor visual outcome when compared to eyes without extensive foveal changes. Second, it is thought

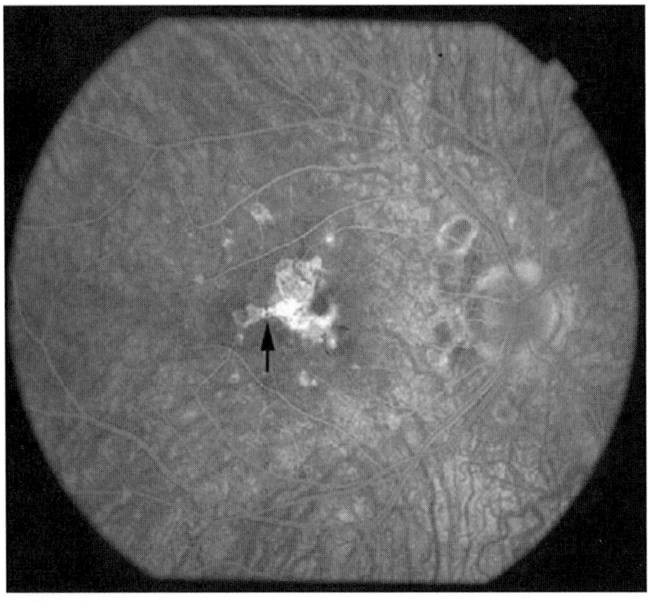

FIGURE 74–6. Case 3: Late-phase fluorescein angiography demonstrated further hyperfluorescence of the fibrovascular CNVM. The branched out configuration of this older, evolved CNVM with the small "bridging vessels" (*arrow*) is typical for PIC.

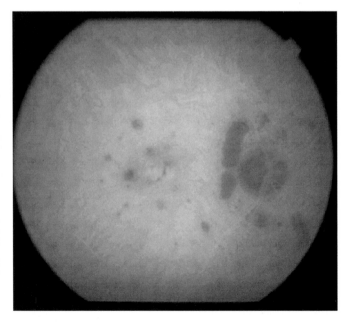

FIGURE 74–7. Case 3. Indocyanine green angiography demonstrated multiple perifoveal and peripapillary hypofluorescent lesions.

that most CNVMs arise from evolved PIC lesions and scars. Because the formation of a foveal CNVM portends a poor visual outcome, it may be possible to reduce the incidence of neovascularization by limiting foveal scar formation. These are theoretical arguments, and no studies have been performed to test the hypothesis that there is a benefit of corticosteroid use in treating acute PIC lesions without evidence of CNVM, and other immunosuppressive therapy has not been tried in the treatment of PIC. However, if the acute lesions are inflammatory (and we believe they are), and if CNVM generally results from inflammatory damage to an area (as in POHS), then anti-inflammatory therapy may prevent such damage and thereby reduce the likelihood of CNVM formation, provided such therapy is instituted at a time and at a dose that could reasonably be expected to rapidly reverse the inflammation. Testing this hypothesis in a rare disorder will be very difficult at best.

The treatment of CNVM probably represents the most significant challenge in the management of patients with PIC. The three available treatment modalities include laser photocoagulation, corticosteroids, and subfoveal surgery. Most clinicians would choose to treat the extrafoveal (greater than 200 μm from the foveal avascular zone [FAZ]) CNVM and the juxtafoveal (from 20 to 200 μm from the FAZ) CNVM with laser photocoagulation. Reports by Brown and colleagues and Watzke and colleagues demonstrate favorable regression response from laser photocoagulation of extrafoveal and juxtafoveal CNVM.[1, 5] No prospective studies have compared laser treatment with observation of these lesions or treatment with sub-Tenon's or systemic steroid for that matter. The outcome studies of the Macular Photocoagulation Study Group[18] showing a favorable response in the POHS subgroup may be extrapolated to the laser treatment of the CNVM associated with PIC, as much similarity exists (clinically, surgically, and histologically) between these two types of neovascular membranes.

Patients with subfoveal CNVM represent the greatest therapeutic challenge. Flaxel and colleagues have examined the use of oral corticosteroids in the treatment of subfoveal CNVM in patients with either PIC or MFC.[19] They treated 10 patients (12 eyes) with oral prednisolone at 1 mg/kg for 3 to 5 days with a gradual taper. In 10 eyes, the vision improved or stabilized, and in nine eyes, the authors were able to demonstrate resolution of the CNVM on FA. Brown and colleagues found that corticosteroids (oral and sub-tenon) may be helpful in slowing the growth of smaller CNVMs (less than 200 μm) associated with PIC and MCP.[5] Although these studies are of interest, they did not include control groups and may not be better than the natural history of the disease. Hence, well-designed comparative studies are needed. A trial of oral corticosteroids may be reasonable in PIC patients with a smaller (around 100 μm) subfoveal CNVM or an actively growing subfoveal CNVM.

In the near future, the best treatment for the larger subfoveal CNVMs in PIC may be submacular surgery. Although the technology and techniques of submacular surgery are currently state of the art and the early results are promising, especially in the subgroup of patients with POHS, and more recently in patients with PIC, more

long-term follow-up data are needed to assess this modality for these diseases.[8, 20] This is especially true in the light of recent data that were presented by Matt Thomas at the American Academy of Ophthalmology in October, 1998, in which he reported that the visual acuity outcome following macular surgery for POHS trend back toward baseline over 3 years of follow-up and a staggering 56% recurrence rate. The anatomy and the histopathology of the CNVM of POHS and PIC (see pathophysiology section) may be more favorable for surgical extraction than the CNVM of age-related macular degeneration.[8] Olsen and colleagues performed subfoveal CNVM extractions on six eyes in five patients with PIC, and they were able to show visual improvements in all six eyes.[8] However, the rate of recurrence was high (six events in four eyes), often requiring a repeat surgical or laser procedure.

COMPLICATIONS

Complications of the medical or surgical therapies for PIC are not unique to this disease. Vision loss and recurrence of the CNVM are complications of laser photocoagulation of CNVM in PIC. Complications of steroid therapy can be local (ocular hypertension and cataract) or systemic (e.g., hyperglycemia, immunosuppression, weight gain, peptic ulcer disease). The general health of the patient should be carefully reviewed prior to initiation of systemic corticosteroid therapy. As most patients with PIC are young and healthy, a course of corticosteroids is usually safe.

Although Olsen and colleagues did not report serious postsurgical complications, subfoveal surgery can result in macular hemorrhage, retinal tears, retinal detachment, scar formation, cataracts, epiretinal membrane, and endophthalmitis.[20, 21]

PROGNOSIS

Many patients with PIC will have a visual outcome of 20/40 or better. The case series of Brown and colleagues showed that 77% of the eyes with PIC had a visual acuity of 20/40 or better,[5] and Watzke and colleagues showed a similar outcome.[1] The main reason for poor vision was the formation of CNVM within the macula. Other causes for poor vision in PIC include extensive foveal RPE changes or scar formation, complications of the therapy, and late recurrences of the CNVM.

CONCLUSION

PIC is a relatively recently described condition characterized by discrete, posterior pole lesions in otherwise healthy, myopic women. The cause of PIC is unknown and the pathophysiology is poorly understood. Many clinicians believe that PIC is a subset of the broader spectrum of diseases including MCP and SFU. The visual outcome can be good unless complicated by the formation of CNVM. Treatment of subfoveal CNVM is controversial, although steroids and subfoveal surgeries may help to improve visual outcome. However, a prospective, randomized trial is needed, comparing the different treatment options (observation, corticosteroids, laser and subfoveal surgery) for subfoveal CNVM in PIC and other inflammatory chorioretinal diseases to allow for rational therapeutic decisions.

References

1. Watzke RC, Packer AJ, Folk JC, et al: Punctate inner choroidopathy. Am J Ophthalmol 1984;98:572–584.
2. Dreyer RF, Gass JDM: Multifocal choroiditis and panuveitis: A syndrome that mimics ocular histoplasmosis. Arch Ophthalmol 1984;102:1776–1784.
3. Cantrill HL, Folk JC: Multifocal choroiditis associated with progressive subretinal fibrosis. Am J Ophthalmol 1986;101:170–180.
4. Palestine A, Nussenblatt R, Parver L, Knox D: Progressive subretinal fibrosis and uveitis. Br J Ophthalmol 1984;68:667–673.
5. Brown J Jr, Folk JC, Reddy CV, Kimura AE: Visual prognosis of multifocal choroiditis, punctate inner choroidopathy, and the diffuse subretinal fibrosis syndrome. Ophthalmology 1996;103:1100–1105.
6. Reddy CV, Brown J Jr, Folk JC, et al: Enlarged blind spots in chorioretinal inflammatory disorders. Ophthalmology 1996;103:606–617.
7. Gass JDM: Biomicroscopic and histopathologic consideration regarding the feasibility of surgical excision of subfoveal membranes. Am J Ophthalmol 1994;118:285–298.
8. Olsen TW, Capone A Jr, Sternberg P Jr, et al: Subfoveal choroidal neovascularization in punctate inner choroidopathy. Ophthalmology 1996;103:2061–2069.
9. Jampol LM, Sieving PA, Pugh D, et al: Multiple evanescent white dot syndrome. I. Clinical findings. Arch Ophthalmol 1984;102:671–674.
10. Fishman GA, Baskin M, Jednock N: Spinal fluid pleocytosis in acute posterior multifocal placoid pigment epitheliopathy. Ann Ophthalmol 1977;9:36–46.
11. Weinstein JM, Bresnick GH, Bell CL, et al: Acute posterior multifocal placoid pigment epitheliopathy associated with cerebral vasculitis. J Clin Neuroophthalmol 1988;8:195–201.
12. Gass JDM: Acute posterior multifocal placoid pigment epitheliopathy. Arch Ophthalmol 1968;80:177–185.
13. Kaplan HJ, Aaberg TM: Birdshot retinochoroidopathy. Am J Ophthalmol 1980;90:773–782.
14. Ryan SJ, Maumenee AE: Birdshot retinochoroidopathy. Am J Ophthalmol 1980;89:31–45.
15. Hamed LM, Glaser JS, Gass JDM, et al: Protracted enlargement of the blind spot in multiple evanescent white dot syndrome. Arch Ophthalmol 1989;107:194–198.
16. Khorram KD, Jampol LM, Rosenberg MA: Blind spot enlargement as manifestation of multifocal choroiditis. Arch Ophthalmol 1991;109:1403–1407.
17. Slakter JS, Giovannini A, Yannuzzi LA, et al: Indocyanine green angiography of multifocal choroiditis. Ophthalmology 1997;104:1813–1819.
18. Macular Photocoagulation Study Group. Argon laser photocoagulation for ocular histoplasmosis. Results of a randomized clinical trial. Arch Ophthalmol 1983;101:1347–1357.
19. Flaxel CJ, Owens SL, Mulholland B, et al: The use of corticosteroids for choroidal neovascularization in young patients. Eye 1998;12:266–272.
20. Thomas MA, Dickinson JD, Melberg NS, et al: Visual results after surgical removal of subfoveal choroidal neovascular membranes. Ophthalmology 1994;101:1384–1396.
21. Thomas MA, Grand MG, Williams DF, et al: Surgical management of subfoveal choroidal neovascularization. Ophthalmology 1992;99:952–968.
22. Nussenblatt RB, Mittal KK, Ryan S, et al: Birdshot retinochoroidopathy associated with HLA-A29 antigen and immune responsiveness to retinal S-antigen. Am J Ophthalmol 1982;94:147–158.
23. Chisholm IH, Gass JD, Hutton WL: The late stage of serpiginous (geographic) choroiditis. Am J Ophthalmol 1976;82:343–351.
24. Jampol LM, Orth D, Daily MJ, et al: Subretinal neovascularization with geographic (serpiginous) choroiditis. Am J Ophthalmol 1979;88:683–689.

75 | ACUTE ZONAL OCCULT OUTER RETINOPATHY

Helen Wu

DEFINITION

Acute zonal occult outer retinopathy (AZOOR) is a syndrome characterized by rapid loss of retinal function in one or more regions, photopsias, mild vitritis, electroretinographic (ERG) abnormalities, an enlarged blind spot on visual field testing, and minimal initial ophthalmoscopic changes with late development of retinal degenerative changes. Similar findings have been seen in patients with multiple evanescent white dot syndrome (MEWDS), acute idiopathic blind spot enlargement syndrome (AIBSES), multifocal choroiditis and panuveitis (MCP, or pseudo-presumed ocular histoplasmosis syndrome), and acute macular neuroretinopathy (AMN). It has been suggested that these diseases are not separate entities, but rather constitute a spectrum of a single disorder. However, we believe this is probably not a correct notion because the natural histories and responses to treatment differ among these disorders. The etiology of AZOOR is unclear.

HISTORY

Although MEWDS, AIBSES, MCP, and AMN have been described as independent entities,[1-7] there have been reported cases in which certain features of these syndromes overlap,[8-12] prompting Gass to suggest that they are related diseases.[13] He reported on 13 young white adults, predominantly females, with acute loss of outer retinal function in one or more large retinal zones. Two of these patients had fundus lesions typical of both MEWDS and MCP. He proposed the term *acute zonal occult outer retinopathy* (AZOOR) to describe the findings in these 13 patients, and speculated that all of these seemingly heterogeneous disorders are closely related or perhaps manifestations of the same disorder.

In 1995, Gass reported on a patient he had previously diagnosed with acute progressive zonal inner retinitis and degeneration.[14] The patient had presented with an acute scotoma associated with a gray intraretinal ring corresponding to the scotoma. After years of follow-up, the patient was found to have depigmentation and migration of pigment epithelium into the overlying retina, similar to the earlier 13 patients with AZOOR. Gass termed this condition *acute annular outer retinopathy* and speculated that it was most likely a variant of AZOOR. He also presented another possible variant of AZOOR in 1997,[15] in which patients demonstrated acute disruption of the retinal pigment epithelium (RPE) and whitening of the outer retina and RPE.

Other published reports suggest that the full clinical spectrum of AZOOR may not yet be established. In 1994, Holz and colleagues presented a case of AZOOR associated with multifocal choroidopathy.[16] In 1996, Jacobson presented an atypical case of AZOOR with macular involvement, recurrences, and central nervous system inflammation.[17]

CLINICAL FEATURES

A significant percentage of patients with AZOOR may have flulike symptoms before the onset of ocular symptoms. Interestingly, two patients in Gass' original report were diagnosed with infectious mononucleosis 2 years prior to developing AZOOR. Photopsia and visual field loss in one or both eyes are the predominant presenting ocular symptoms of AZOOR. The photopsias have often been described as multicolored and are associated with shimmering or ameboid micromovements. The photopsias and scotomata may be exacerbated by bright light, exercise, stress, and fatigue.

Early in the course of the disease, the majority of eyes have 20/30 or better visual acuity. The visual field defects are most commonly noted in the superior and temporal quadrants, and they often include enlargement of the blind spot. The visual field loss is usually asymmetric. Typically, the scotomata increase in size within days to weeks, although progression of visual field defects has been documented up to 6 months after the onset of symptoms. The fundus appears normal in a majority of patients on presentation. Subtle pigment epithelial changes may be seen initially; depigmentation of the RPE layer corresponds to the areas of visual field loss in the later stages of the disease (Fig. 75–1). Retinal vessels may narrow in the areas of atrophy. Late pigment migration into the overlying retina can mimic the bone spicule appearance of retinitis pigmentosa. Focal perivenous infiltration or sheathing of the retinal vessels may occur. Several of Gass' original 13 patients had leakage at the optic nerve and macula on fluorescein angiography. In four of these patients, no funduscopic changes were found throughout the course of the disease, despite the presence of dense scotomata.

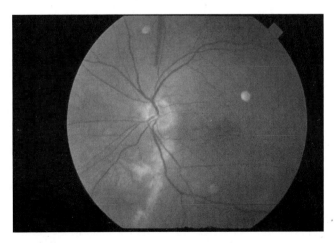

FIGURE 75–1. Patient with AZOOR. Status postresolution of the acute phase. Note the zone of RPE disturbance extending inferiorly from the disc.

Vitritis, which is present in approximately half of the cases, is generally mild. The degree of vitritis appears to be related to the degree of visual field loss. A relative afferent pupillary defect occurs in approximately half of reported cases. Optic disc swelling was seen in only one patient, although its appearance did not change over years. Optic atrophy has not been reported in any patient. Other ocular manifestations may include retinal lesions similar to those of MEWDS, AMN, or MCP.[13, 15, 16] Choroidal neovascularization has been observed in two patients, who subsequently developed impaired central vision.[16] Cystoid macular edema has also been reported.[13]

In the acute annular outer retinopathy variant of AZOOR, photopsias may not be a presenting symptom. In the first published case, the patient experienced sudden onset of a scotoma. A circular ring of gray-white retinal opacification was seen in the superotemporal fundus of the left eye, with narrowing of the retinal vessels within the ring.[14] The ring slowly enlarged over a period of several weeks and then disappeared. Pigmentary changes characteristic of AZOOR then occurred over months, demonstrating that the receptor cells and the RPE were the damaged layers. It is interesting to note that, in this index case, visual acuity remained 20/20 throughout, and the initial relative afferent pupillary defect vanished over the 6-year follow-up period. In other cases, RPE disruption occurred early in the course of the disease, with variable degrees of whitening of the outer retina and RPE.[14]

Although antecedent systemic disease is not uncommon in patients with AZOOR, concomitant systemic inflammation is rare. One patient was reported to have cerebrospinal fluid pleocytosis and multiple brain magnetic resonance imaging (MRI) signal abnormalities.[17] She subsequently developed an acute cervical myelopathy, which resolved after intravenous steroid therapy. Her ocular course was also unusual, with central macular involvement and recurrent bouts of an AZOOR picture over several years. It is unclear whether this case represents a true association between AZOOR and central nervous system (CNS) inflammation, a chance occurrence of AZOOR and possible multiple sclerosis, or an ocular problem that was not AZOOR to begin with.

ETIOLOGY

The etiology of AZOOR is unclear but it is presumed to be of inflammatory origin. Although patients with MEWDS, AIBSES, AMN, and MCP all share the common feature of occult visual field loss secondary to receptor cell and RPE damage, there is no known cause for these disorders. Because many of these patients are young women, who are more likely in general to have autoimmune disorders, it is tempting to propose an autoimmune etiology for AZOOR. Currently, there is no evidence for autoantibodies to any retinal cell type in any of these patients.[18] Gass speculates that in AZOOR, a viral infection latent in a region of the outer retina is activated, causing acute retinal dysfunction and death of the retinal receptors with no effect on retinal transparency or the outer and inner blood-retinal barrier in the early stages of disease. The ring seen in acute annular outer retinopathy may be caused either by the loss of transparency of the most recently affected area of the retina, or by an immune reaction at the junction between normal vascularized inner retina and the leading edge of the infected outer avascularized retina.[15] The presence of iritis in some, but not all, of the affected patients suggests that inflammation may be secondary to the underlying disease process. Patients with greater degrees of visual field loss appear to have associated iritis more often. One can speculate that vitritis occurs in response to factors released by damaged RPE and receptor cells.

DIAGNOSIS

The characteristic history of photopsias and the rapid onset of one or more large peripheral scotomata suggest the diagnosis of AZOOR. Funduscopic findings may be normal or subtle initially, and vitritis may or may not be present. Over time, characteristic pigmentary changes in the outer retina and RPE substantiate the diagnosis. In the acute phase, however, ERG abnormalities are essential to confirm the diagnosis and avoid additional unnecessary neurologic testing. In some patients, a focal ERG may be required to detect the abnormalities. Multifocal ERG[19] and scanning laser ophthalmoscopy[20] have also been used as adjunctive tools to confirm the diagnosis of AZOOR.

Laboratory Investigations

A laboratory work-up should be performed in all suspected AZOOR patients to rule out infectious etiologies, such as syphilis and Lyme disease. Noninfectious etiologies, including retinitis pigmentosa and cancer-associated retinopathy (CAR), should be considered. Medical and neurologic consultation should be obtained. Before the initiation of systemic therapy, the following tests should be obtained: complete blood count with differential, fluorescent treponemal antibody absorption and rapid plasma reagin tests, chest x-ray, blood urea nitrogen (BUN), and creatinine, and skin testing for anergy. Serologic titers for Epstein-Barr virus, herpes simplex virus, varicella zoster virus, and Lyme disease may be helpful. Testing for retinal antigens, including the CAR antigen, may be obtained. An MRI of the brain may be necessary to rule out CNS inflammation or a compressive mass lesion. If CAR is strongly suspected, further imaging of the chest, abdomen, and pelvis may be required to rule out a malignancy.

Fluorescein Angiography

Fluorescein angiography is typically normal in the acute phase of AZOOR, but it may show an increase in retinal circulation time in the affected area.[13–15, 20, 21] One patient demonstrated evidence of juxtapapillary choroidal neovascularization 4 weeks after the onset of symptoms.[16] After several months, fluorescein angiography demonstrates hyperfluorescence corresponding to the choriocapillaris underlying areas of depigmented RPE. Narrowing of the retinal vessels may occur in these areas as well, particularly when the affected region is large and peripheral in location.

In contrast, in patients with fundus lesions typical of MEWDS, fluorescein angiography shows early pinpoint hyperfluorescence and late staining of the lesions, with staining of the optic disc.[13]

Electrophysiology

Electroretinographic changes show dysfunction of the photoreceptors, which are patchy in distribution, with mildly to moderately decreased rod and cone amplitudes in most cases.[13, 15, 16, 18–21] In the initial report by Gass,[13] the ERG was extinguished in only one patient who later displayed some evidence of cone function by ERG testing. The cone responses were affected to a greater extent than the rod responses in the less-affected eyes, whereas the opposite was found in severely affected eyes. Overall, 81% of eyes had ERG abnormalities. Electro-oculography showed a reduced or absent response in all three eyes tested in this study. Two of 11 eyes had visual evoked-response abnormalities as well.

In one study that analyzed ERG changes in 24 patients with AZOOR, almost one third had normal ERG results in both eyes but showed abnormal interocular differences for some of the measured parameters.[18] Full-field ERG was typically adequate for detecting the abnormality in most patients with AZOOR. More than half of the patients tested had abnormalities 10 months to 20 years after the onset of symptoms, suggesting persistent retinal damage. The ERG is not only important in the diagnosis of AZOOR; it may also have a role in monitoring both the course of the disease and the outcomes of therapeutic intervention.

Multifocal ERG, which records primarily cone responses, was used in one published case to further define the exact topographic distribution of the retinal dysfunction in a patient with AZOOR.[19] The study confirms that the visual field defect in AZOOR results from outer retinal dysfunction, predominantly in the cones. The standard ERGs in that patient showed impairment of almost all cones and slight rod impairment, but they could not detect the precise location of the defect. The multifocal ERG demonstrated recordable responses only from the central macular area.

Ancillary Tests

Visual field testing should be performed in all suspected AZOOR patients; it generally shows temporal and superior field defects, with involvement of the blind spot. Visual field testing should be repeated regularly to monitor the course of the disease. Color vision testing using the Farnsworth D-15 color panel was abnormal in 25% of patients in Gass' initial report.[13]

Scanning laser ophthalmoscopy with a 514-nm wavelength laser performed in a single reported case[20] demonstrated retinal abnormalities undetectable by fundus examinations, fluorescein angiography, and computed tomography. The 630-nm wavelength laser was unable to demonstrate any abnormalities. This result localizes damage to the retinal layer because the 514-nm laser shows primarily the retinal layer, and the 630-nm laser visualizes the choroidal layer. Furthermore, the laser was able to demonstrate abnormal retinal lesions in the asymptomatic eye as well.

DIFFERENTIAL DIAGNOSIS

The differential diagnosis of patients with acute visual loss and visual field defects includes retrobulbar neuritis, pituitary tumors, and other intracranial lesions. Although the absence of local neurologic signs or symptoms may be reassuring, an MRI of the brain is frequently performed in this clinical setting to rule out these potentially devastating possibilities. The presence of cone or rod dysfunction on ERG testing, however, points to the diagnosis of AZOOR.

In patients who manifest abnormal cone function on ERG testing, the diagnoses of acquired cone dystrophy and paraneoplastic retinopathy, including CAR and melanoma-associated retinopathy (MAR), should be considered in addition to AZOOR.

Patients with paraneoplastic retinopathy may present with photopsias, visual field defects, color vision abnormalities, or nyctalopia. These patients may experience visual symptoms prior to the discovery of the carcinoma, which is most frequently a small-cell carcinoma of the lung. Paraneoplastic disorders have also been found in patients with other types of neoplasia, including melanoma and cervical, colon, prostate, and breast cancer. Most patients with CAR develop bilateral, progressive retinal degeneration with significant arteriolar narrowing.[22, 23] Vision loss is thought to be secondary to a cancer-evoked autoimmune retinopathy. Serum antibodies to a specific 23-kd retinal antigen (CAR antigen) have been identified, and the retina-specific immunologic reaction is located within the retinal receptors.[24–26] Patients with MAR may have acute nyctalopia, associated with anterior and posterior uveitis, depigmentation of the choroid, vitiligo, and dysacusis. Vision loss may be severe. Patients with MAR generally have central vision loss, as opposed to the ring scotomata seen with CAR and the peripheral vision field defects seen in AZOOR. The ERG early in the course of MAR does not show evidence of photoreceptor dysfunction, which is typically seen in CAR and AZOOR.

Bilateral diffuse uveal melanocytic proliferation associated with systemic occult carcinoma may also cause loss of retinal receptor function. Metastatic cutaneous melanoma and retinitis pigmentosa may also mimic the retinal changes seen in patients with the late stage of AZOOR, but the clinical course of the entities is much different from that of AZOOR.

A variety of diseases may produce white dots in the retina that may resemble those seen in some reported cases of AZOOR. Diffuse unilateral subacute neuroretinitis (DUSN) and the ocular histoplasmosis syndrome may produce white dots in the retina, resembling those seen in MEWDS or MCP. DUSN is caused by subretinal nematodes and may present with visual loss, vitritis, papillitis, retinal vasculitis, and gray-white outer retinal lesions early in the course of the disease. Later, patients may show diffuse RPE degeneration, with progressive visual loss, retinal vessel narrowing, and optic atrophy. This syndrome is always unilateral, however.

Syphilis and tuberculosis may also produce chorioretinitis and vitritis. In patients with luetic chorioretinitis, migration of pigment into the overlying retina may produce a bone-spicule pattern, similar to that seen in retinitis pigmentosa or AZOOR. Generally, the acute pattern of inflammation is quite different from that of patients with AZOOR, and geographic pale chorioretinal lesions are frequently confluent in the posterior pole and the mid-periphery of the fundus.

Sarcoidosis may produce retinal vasculitis, as well as vitritis and choroidal granulomata. Other white dot syndromes to be distinguished from MEWDS and MCP include punctate inner choroidopathy (PIC) and acute posterior multifocal placoid pigment epitheliopathy (APMPPE).

TREATMENT

Treatment is based on the patient's medical history, review of systems, and the presence or lack of inflammation. In general, patients with severe vitritis have been treated with systemic corticosteroids. Although inflammation has been resolved in all cases, it is unclear whether the treatment alters the course of the disease. The visual field defects have persisted in many patients despite therapy. Several patients have been treated with oral acyclovir, with mixed results. One patient was treated with ceftriaxone sodium and vancomycin hydrochloride because of suspected Lyme disease, with stabilization of the visual fields.

NATURAL HISTORY AND PROGNOSIS

For most patients with AZOOR, the visual prognosis appears good. All 13 patients in Gass' initial series maintained 20/25 or better visual acuity in at least one eye. One patient, however, is legally blind from a severe visual field defect. No progression of visual field defect was noted after 6 months in the original series, but the patient with combined ocular and CNS symptoms has had recurrences over several years. Other patients had more severe visual loss, with deterioration of ERG findings over time.[16] The photopsias may be chronic in some patients. In all reported cases, inflammation of the vitreous resolved over time. Cystoid macular edema may persist for months.[13] Permanent central visual loss may occur in cases with associated choroidal neovascularization.[16]

CONCLUSION

Acute zonal occult outer retinopathy (AZOOR) is a syndrome characterized by rapid loss of one or more broad zones of retinal function; it is associated with the acute onset of photopsias and scotomata. The ERG abnormalities are critical to an early diagnosis. Because these clinical and ERG findings may be seen in several other syndromes, such as MEWDS and MCP, Gass has coined the term AZOOR to describe this disease and postulates a possible common etiology of these clinical entities. The natural history of this disorder generally is one of stabilization of the visual field defects within days to weeks, with preservation of good central visual acuity. Treatment should be based on the patient's medical history and a review of systems. Systemic corticosteroids may be used to treat patients with severe vitritis; resolution of inflammation and stabilization of the visual field defects result in most cases. It is unclear, however, whether systemic treatment alters the course of the disease. Further work needs to be done to elucidate the etiology of this interesting and poorly understood syndrome.

References

1. Jampol LM, Sieving PA, Pugh D, et al: Multiple evanescent white dot syndrome. I. Clinical findings. Arch Ophthalmol 1984;102:671–674.
2. Sieving PA, Fishman LA, Jampol LM, et al: Multiple evanescent white dot syndrome: II. Electrophysiology of the photoreceptors during retinal pigment epithelial disease. Arch Ophthalmol 1984;102:675–679.
3. Fletcher WA, Imes RK, Goodman D, et al: Acute idiopathic blind spot enlargement: a big blind spot syndrome without optic disc edema. Arch Ophthalmol 1988;106:44–49.
4. Nozik RA, Dorsch W: A new chorioretinopathy associated with anterior uveitis. Am J Ophthalmol 1973;76:758–762.
5. Bos PJM, Deutman AF: Acute macular neuroretinopathy. Am J Ophthalmol 1975;80:573–584.
6. Dreyer RF, Gass JDM: Multifocal choroiditis and panuveitis; a syndrome that mimics ocular histoplasmosis. Arch Ophthalmol 1984;102:1776–1784.
7. Tessler HH, Deutsch TA: Multifocal choroiditis (inflammatory pseudo-histoplasmosis). In: Saari KM, ed: Uveitis Update: Proceedings of the First International Symposium on Uveitis, May 16–19, 1984, Hanasaan, Espoo, Finland. Amsterdam, Excerpta Medica, 1984, pp 221–226.
8. Gass JDM, Hamed L: Acute macular neuroretinopathy and MEWDS occurring in the same patient. Arch Ophthalmol 1989;107:189–193.
9. Hamed LM, Glaser JS, Gass JDM, et al: Protracted enlargement of the blind spot in multiple evanescent white dot syndrome. Arch Ophthalmol 1989;107:194–198.
10. Khorram KD, Jampol LM, Rosenberg MA: Blind spot enlargement as a manifestation of multifocal choroiditis. Arch Ophthalmol 1991;109:1403–1407.
11. Singh K, de Frank M, Shults WT, et al: Acute idiopathic blind spot enlargement: a spectrum of disease. Ophthalmology 1991;98:497–502.
12. Callanan D, Gass JDM: Multifocal choroiditis and choroidal neovascularization associated with the multiple evanescent white dot and acute idiopathic blind spot enlargement syndrome. Ophthalmology 1992;99:1678–1685.
13. Gass JDM: Acute zonal occult outer retinopathy. J Clin Neuroophthalmol 1993;13:79–97.
14. Gass JDM, Stern C: Acute annular outer retinopathy as a variant of acute zonal occult outer retinopathy. Am J Ophthalmol 1995;119:330–334.
15. Gass JDM: Stereoscopic Atlas of Macular Diseases: Diagnosis and Treatment, vol 2, 4th ed. St. Louis, CV Mosby, 1997, pp 682–687.
16. Holz FG, Kim RY, Schwartz SD, et al: Acute zonal occult outer retinopathy (AZOOR) associated with multifocal choroidopathy. Eye 1994;8:77–83.
17. Jacobson DM: Acute zonal occult outer retinopathy and central nervous system inflammation. J Neuroophthalmol 1996;16:172–177.
18. Jacobson SG, Morales DS, Sun XK, et al: Pattern of retinal dysfunction in acute zonal occult outer retinopathy. Ophthalmology 1995;102:1187–1198.
19. Arai M, Naoi N, Sawada A, et al: Multifocal electroretinogram indicates visual field loss in acute zonal occult outer retinopathy. Am J Ophthalmol 1998;126:466–469.
20. Nishio M, Suzuki T, Chikuda M, et al: Scanning laser ophthalmoscopic findings in a patient with acute zonal occult outer retinopathy. Am J Ophthalmol 1998;125:712–715.
21. Lee AG, Prager TC: Acute zonal occult outer retinopathy. Acta Ophthalmol Scand 1996;74:93–95.
22. Thirkill CE, Roth AM, Keltner JL: Cancer-associated retinopathy. Arch Ophthalmol 1987;105:372–375.
23. Thirkill CE: Cancer associated retinopathy: the CAR syndrome. J Neuroophthalmol 1994;14:297–323.
24. Thirkill CE, FitzGerald P, Sergott RC, et al: Cancer-associated retinopathy (CAR syndrome) with antibodies reacting with retinal, optic-nerve, and cancer cells. N Engl J Med 1989;321:1589–1594.
25. Thirkill CE, Keltner JL, Tyler NK, et al: Antibody reactions with retina and cancer-associated antigens in 10 patients with cancer-associated retinopathy. Arch Ophthalmol 1993;111:931–937.
26. Thirkill CE, Tait RC, Tyler NK, et al: Intraperitoneal cultivation of small-cell carcinoma induces expression of the retinal cancer-associated retinopathy antigen. Arch Ophthalmol 1993;111:974–978.

76

LENS-INDUCED UVEITIS

Shawkat Shafik Michel and C. Stephen Foster

DEFINITION

The terms phacogenic uveitis and lens-induced uveitis (LIU) will be used synonymously and interchangeably in this chapter for all cases of uveitis caused by lens material. Previously, these cases were called phacolytic, phacotoxic, or phacoantigenic uveitis, or endophthalmitis phacoanaphylactica. The old terms are not accurate and can be confusing. Now it is well established that anaphylaxis[1] is mediated by immunoglobulin E (IgE) antibodies attached to high-affinity receptors on the surface of basophils and mast cells. Cross-linking of these antibodies by a specific antigen leads to activation of mast cells and basophils. Activated mast cells secrete certain cytokines (interleukins 4 and 5 [IL-4 and IL-5]) and also release their stored and newly formed granules (degranulation). The result of this type of reaction (type I hypersensitivity reaction) is typically an acute eosinophil-rich inflammation. It is clear that phacogenic uveitis is completely different from the aforementioned mechanism, without participation of IgE, basophils, mast cells, or eosinophils.

Additional confusion rather than enlightenment developed in the medical literature regarding the terminology of phacogenic uveitis as a consequence of descriptive histopathology of LIU and other related or unrelated entities, including sympathetic ophthalmia, phacolytic glaucoma, and infectious postoperative endophthalmitis (e.g., secondary to *Propionibacterium acnes*). Thus, although earlier authors described the pathologic picture of zonal granulomatous inflammation around lens capsule ruptures and called it endophthalmitis phacoanaphylactica,[2, 3] more recently some ophthalmologists suggested the use of the term phacoanaphylactic endophthalmitis for cases showing a preponderance of polymorphonuclear leukocyte infiltration, and the term phacolytic uveitis for cases showing a predominance of macrophage infiltration.[4]

We suggest (and choose this approach here) the term phacogenic or lens-induced as a more simplified approach to the matter. We believe that the uveitis that develops as a consequence of mature cataract leakage, or residual cortex following cataract surgery, or lens material lost into the vitreous is caused by the presence of the lens material. Removal of this lens material is curative. The details, both clinical and histopathologic, may differ between cases, but the cause, mechanism, and cure are the same.

Although lens-induced or phacogenic uveitis is a curable type of uveitis, it is a frequently missed diagnosis.[5] Many of the cases mentioned in the literature have been histologically[6, 7] confirmed in eyes that had been enucleated for being blind and painful. If the diagnosis is missed and proper treatment not initiated, the condition usually progresses to secondary glaucoma, and ultimately the eye must be removed because of intractable pain. The resurgence of extracapsular cataract extraction and phacoemulsification should heighten the ophthalmologist's awareness of the possibility of this condition as a cause of protracted, sometimes stormy, postoperative uveitis.[8, 9]

HISTORY

Phacoanaphylactic endophthalmitis was initially recognized as a distinct entity by Straub in 1919. The nature of the process was further clarified by Verhoff and Lemoine 1922.[2] The clinical picture of phacolytic glaucoma was first described by Gifford as early as 1900, but the term phacolytic was coined by Flocks and coworkers[10] in 1955.

EPIDEMIOLOGY

There are no estimates for the incidence and prevalence of LIU in the medical literature. When compared with other causes of anterior uveitis (e.g., human leukocyte antigen B27–associated), phacogenic uveitis is not common, but it is an important and a frequently missed type of uveitis. Phacogenic uveitis is expected to be more prevalent in developing countries where cataract is the leading cause of blindness.[11, 12] The relationship between cataract (hypermature and mature) and phacogenic uveitis is well established. Uveitis as a cause of blindness is underestimated in developing countries.[11, 12] And in developed countries, where extracapsular cataract extraction is now the most common technique for cataract surgery, it may be expected that the incidence of phacogenic uveitis will increase. Regrettably, the diagnosis will probably often not be suspected.

In a retrospective study[13, 14] of 144 eyes that were characterized histopathologically, it was found that only 5% of cases had been clinically suspected. It was also found that the age range was between 60 and 70 years, with a peak corresponding to the most frequent time of cataract surgery. Men were slightly more prone to LIU than women, probably related to an increased history of trauma. But 20% of cases had neither history of trauma nor histopathologic evidence of a penetrating wound; 5% of the cases were shown to have gram-positive organisms in the histopathologic sections, raising the possibility, at least in this small number of cases, that a microbial adjuvant[14] effect with the lens material may enhance the possibility of escape from tolerance and development of an inflammatory immune response to lens protein.

ETIOLOGY AND PATHOGENESIS

Until the 1970s, it was taught that the lens proteins are sequestered[15] within the lens capsule with no opportunity to be recognized as self proteins by the cells of the immune system. Consequently, leakage of lens proteins was believed to result, essentially, in a foreign body reaction as a consequence of these proteins being recognized as foreign by cells of the immune system.

During the 1970s,[16–18] it was shown that lens proteins are neither organ- nor species-specific and that the lens proteins leak into the aqueous humor even under normal conditions (i.e., a clear lens with an intact capsule). Lens proteins, especially the soluble proteins, have been experimentally shown to be weak antigens (α- and β-crystallins) or to be frankly nonantigenic (γ-crystallin). Additional experiments showed that some animals were more tolerant than others to injected lens material. It is possible that differences in the immune response (Ir), or the immune-associated (Ia) β genes (various alleles of the major histocompatibility complex I and II molecules[1] account, at least in part, for this individual susceptibility to an inflammatory response to lens material in the anterior chamber.

Although the exact mechanism is not yet known, it is generally agreed that LIU is a localized form of autoimmune disease. It may be that tolerance to lens protein is lost or altered as a result of excessive leakage of lens material, and possibly as a result of some other factors, with IgG lens autoantibodies or autoreactive T cells initiating the inflammation. Anterior chamber–associated immune deviation (ACAID; see Chapter 5: Inflammation/Immunology) plays the important role of protecting the eye from the damaging effect of delayed-type hypersensitivity and complement-fixing antibodies. What role ACAID plays, or fails to play, in the pathogenesis of phacogenic uveitis is still to be answered.

Triggering Factors

Typically phacogenic uveitis is seen in the setting of trauma or mature cataract (also hypermature cataract); both of these conditions can be associated with rupture of the lens capsule. The trauma may be surgical (following cataract or glaucoma surgery), or nonsurgical, following blunt or penetrating trauma.

There have even been reports from pathologically examined eyes that phacogenic uveitis may occur in developmentally abnormal eyes (e.g., microcornea or persistent hyperplastic primary vitreous).[14] There are no associated systemic conditions.

PATHOLOGY

The characteristic histology[13, 14, 19] of phacogenic uveitis consists of zonal inflammation in and around the lens (Fig. 76–1), especially at the area of capsular rupture. The inflammatory cells are composed of lymphocytes, neutrophils, macrophages, epithelioid cells, and giant cells (Fig. 76–2). Eosinophils may be seen, but rarely.

In severe, neglected cases,[6, 7] as seen in badly damaged enucleated eyes, granulation tissue (newly formed blood vessels and fibroblasts) is seen in the center of the damaged lens. The iris and ciliary body are moderately to densely infiltrated by lymphocytes, plasma cells, and macrophages; nongranulomatous lymphocyte infiltration may be found in the limbus. Peripheral anterior synechiae, pupillary membranes, cyclitic membranes, glaucomatous optic atrophy, and other complications of the initial trauma, or of phacogenic uveitis, may be seen in such cases.

CLINICAL FEATURES

Clinically, a spectrum of different disease patterns can be seen after lens damage. The particular reaction appears to be determined by multiple factors, many of which are largely unknown.[19] Clinical observations and experimental evidence show that not only local factors (e.g., kind

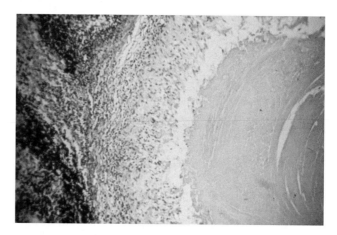

FIGURE 76–1. A case of phacogenic uveitis showing lens material in the anterior chamber. The uveitis in this patient did not respond to topical steroids but dramatically improved after complete surgical removal of lens material. (See color insert.)

of trauma, physical composition of the lens, degree of immunologic presensitization, amount and period of antigen liberation, vascularization), but also genetic and individual factors (e.g., age, degree of immunologic responsiveness) contribute to the individual response.

A history of a recent or old trauma to the eye, whether blunt or penetrating, is usually elicited from a patient with LIU. Similarly, a history of prior cataract or glaucoma surgery may be obtained. Phacogenic uveitis reportedly can develop between 24 hours and 59 years[13, 14] after the causative event.

The clinical picture is that of anterior uveitis, which may be granulomatous or nongranulomatous, depending on severity. It is usually associated with keratic precipitates (KPs), which may be small and white in the early stage but coalesce into large mutton-fat KPs in severe granulomatous inflammation. The anterior chamber usually shows thick flare and abundant cells. Hypopyon or pseudohypopyon (admixed with lens material) may be seen; here the horizontal fluid level is usually absent (Fig.

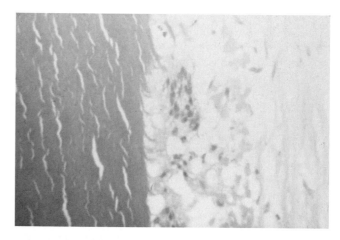

FIGURE 76–2. Pathology of phacogenic uveitis: zonal inflammation around the lens especially at the site of capsular rupture. Mononuclears are seen together with epithelioid cells and giant epithelial cells. (See color insert.)

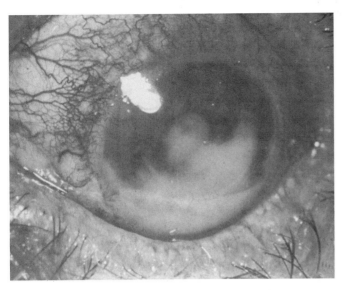

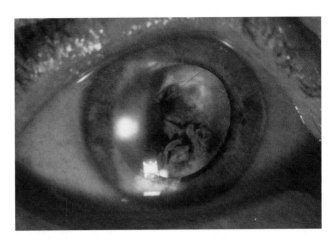

FIGURE 76–4. Significant amount of residual lens matter following extracapsular cataract extraction with lens implantation. This patient is at higher risk of developing phacogenic uveitis. (See color insert.)

FIGURE 76–3. Pathology of phacogenic uveitis: epithelioid and multinucleated giant cells engulfing lens material. (See color insert.)

76–3). The anterior lens surface may appear ragged (i.e., irregular anterior lens capsule), and the lens is always opaque. The intraocular pressure is usually elevated.

Vitreous inflammatory cells are the rule rather than the exception, especially in longstanding cases; this has been confirmed in enucleated eyes. For this reason, phacogenic uveitis is appropriately classified as an intermediate uveitis. Although the anterior segment inflammation and the opaque lens may obscure the view of the vitreous, ophthalmologists should be aware of accompanying vitritis. Phacogenic uveitis caused by lens material in the vitreous cavity following extracapsular cataract extraction may be associated with an especially intense vitritis.

DIAGNOSIS

The history and clinical features of phacogenic uveitis are characteristic (some published data clearly indicate that the diagnosis of LIU is often missed[5–7, 13, 14]). In case of doubt, anterior chamber tap may be diagnostic. Giant macrophages full of lens material will confirm the diagnosis. The aspirated aqueous can also be examined bacteriologically and with polymerase chain reaction to exclude the possibility of any microbial infection. The dramatic resolution of the inflammation following surgical removal of all lens material would also confirm the diagnosis.

A- and B-scan ultrasonography[9] are valuable tools for confirming the diagnosis when phacogenic uveitis is caused by lens material in the vitreous cavity, as may occur following extracapsular cataract extraction.

DIFFERENTIAL DIAGNOSIS

Phacogenic uveitis should not be difficult to diagnose in most cases. But apparently it continues to this day to escape the notice of many ophthalmologists. Thach and colleagues,[14] for example, found that only 5% of the cases in their study had been suspected as being LIU clinically. The main differential diagnosis in cases following trauma is sympathetic ophthalmia.[20–23] In cases following extracapsular cataract extraction, the main differential diagno-

sis is postoperative endophthalmitis, caused by *P. acnes.*[23–25] As a cause of anterior and intermediate uveitis, phacogenic uveitis should be differentiated from other causes of anterior and intermediate uveitis.

Sympathetic ophthalmia follows penetrating trauma or intraocular surgery in one eye. It is always a bilateral disease: Both eyes are usually affected at the same time, or within a short time interval. Phacogenic uveitis usually follows trauma to the eye, but it may also occur in nontraumatic mature cataract. Phacogenic uveitis is usually a unilateral disease; occasionally it is bilateral, as when it follows extracapsular cataract extraction or cases of trauma to both eyes. Extra attention to complete removal of all lens material should attend cataract surgery in a patient who has had phacogenic uveitis in the opposite eye (Fig. 76–4). Whereas sympathetic ophthalmia causes panuveitis, phacogenic uveitis typically causes anterior and intermediate uveitis. Lens material may be seen in the anterior chamber of patients with phacogenic uveitis but not in sympathetic ophthalmia. Phacogenic uveitis is

TABLE 76–1. DIFFERENTIAL DIAGNOSIS: PHACOGENIC UVEITIS AND SYMPATHETIC OPHTHALMIA

SYMPATHETIC OPHTHALMIA	PHACOGENIC UVEITIS
Always bilateral and simultaneous or within a short interval (days or a few weeks)	Usually unilateral. When it follows extracapsular extraction, care should be taken when removing the cataract in the other eye
Panuveitis	Anterior uveitis
Always follows a penetrating trauma or an intraocular surgical procedure	Usually but not always
No lens fragments in anterior chamber	Usually lens fragments in anterior chamber
Relapses are characteristic	No relapses once the lens is completely removed from the eye
Antigenic reaction to photoreceptor protein	Antigenic reaction to lens protein

TABLE 76–2. CHARACTERISTIC FEATURES OF EACH OF THE CAUSES OF ANTERIOR UVEITIS

	HISTORY	CORNEA	A.C.	IRIS	LENS	VITREOUS	ASS. DIS.	DIAG.
LIU	Trauma, surgery, or cataract	Fine or mutton fat KPs	Giant cells, pseudohypopyon		Cataract, ragged or ruptured capsule	Inflammatory infiltrates	None	Clinical features; A.C. tap
Idiopathic	Acute, recurrent	Fine KPs	Cells	± PS	Pigment on lens, PS		None	By exclusion
HLA-B27 ass.	Acute, recurrent	Fine KPs	Cells	± PS	Pigment		Spondylo-arthropathies	HLA-B27
JRA assoc.	Chronic, quiet eye	Band-shape keratop.	Flare and cells		Cataract	Inflammatory exudates	JRA	ANA on 2 substrates
Fuchs	Present late with cataract or glaucoma	Small-medium size KPs all over, specially inferior	Minimal inflammation	Heterochromia, prominent vessels, neovessels	Cataract (posterior subcapsular, progresses quickly)	Cells and debris	None	Clinical
Herpetic	± Preceding corneal involvement	± Corneal anesthesia	Cells	Transillumination defects, sector atrophy			None	Sector atrophy, transillumination
Syphilis	Sexual transmission	Fine or mutton fat KPs	Cells	Roseata		Exudates	Secondary or late latent	FTA-ABS test
Tuberculosis	± Exposure to disease	Mutton fat KPs	Cells	Nodules (granulomas)		Exudates	± Tuberculosis	+ PPD
Intraocular lens induced	Surgery	KPs	Cells, ± IOL, ± hyphema 1–2 + cells		IOL		Glaucoma	Clinical
Posner Schlossman	Acute, recurrent, self-limited	KPs, edema					High IOT	Clinical
Traumatic	History	Fine KPs	Cells, hyphema	± Lacerations	± Cataract	± Hemorrhage	None	Clinical

A.C., anterior chamber; Vit., vitreous; Ass. Dis., associated disease; FTA-ABS, fluorescent treponemal antibody-absorption test; HLA-B27 ass., HLA-B27 associated; IOL, intraocular lens; IOT, intraocular tension; JRA-assoc., juvenile rheumatoid arthritis associated; KPs, keratic precipitates; PPD, purified protein derivative; PS, posterior synechia; ±, may be associated with.

cured once the lens material is completely removed from the eye; sympathetic ophthalmia is characterized by frequent relapses and, if not properly diagnosed and treated, may ultimately lead to significant visual loss or complete blindness. In some cases, both phacogenic uveitis and sympathetic ophthalmia occur in the same eye[23] (Table 76–1).

P. acnes[23–25] is one cause of chronic infectious postoperative endophthalmitis. It usually occurs 3 months or more after extracapsular cataract extraction. It causes a granulomatous uveitis (mutton-fat KPs), small hypopyon, mild vitritis, and characteristic plaques on the posterior capsule. Residual lens material may be seen in the capsular bag. *P. acnes* in vitro culture may require up to 2 weeks of incubation under anaerobic conditions; samples of vitreous and posterior capsule should be obtained for such culture. Other causes of chronic infectious postoperative endophthalmitis include *Staphylococcus epidermidis* (between 2 and 6 weeks) and fungus (usually *Candida*, 1 to 3 months). Steroid-resistant or persistent postoperative inflammation is clearly an indication for aqueous and vitreous specimen harvesting for microbiologic stains and cultures.

Other causes of anterior uveitis that might, in very rare instances, be confused with phacogenic uveitis are shown in Table 76–2.

TREATMENT

Phacogenic uveitis typically responds completely to removal of all lens material. Removal of the inciting lens material is the prescribed treatment. Adjunctive therapy may include systemic and topical steroid and cycloplegics. If phacogenic uveitis follows extracapsular extraction, steroid treatment might be sufficient if the residual cortex is minimal; treatment should continue until all lens material is resorbed. Lens material that is unlikely to be quickly resorbed must be removed surgically. Surgical removal of lens material will be either through a limbal approach (when the residual material is in the anterior chamber) or a three-port pars plana vitrectomy (for lens material in the vitreous cavity). Pars plana vitrectomy is also the best way, of course, to obtain vitreous material for culture purposes.

Failure of the uveitis to respond completely to surgical removal of all lens material should alert the clinician to the possibility of sympathetic ophthalmia or another coexistent disorder (e.g., infectious endophthalmitis).

COMPLICATIONS

If the lens is not promptly removed from an eye suffering from phacogenic uveitis, the following complications may occur: glaucoma, pupillary membrane, cyclitic membrane, hypotony, corneal edema, macular edema or scarring, and even retinal detachment secondary to contraction of the cyclitic membrane. Ultimately, the eye may be blind and painful, eventually becoming phthisis bulbi.

CONCLUSION

Phacogenic uveitis is an important but frequently missed cause of uveitis. It should be suspected in all cases of traumatic or postoperative uveitis and in cases associated with mature or hypermature cataract. Once the lens material is completely removed from the eye, the inflammation resolves. Failure to remove the lens material from the eye may lead to serious complications and total loss of useful vision. The resurgence of extracapsular cataract extraction may be accompanied by a corresponding increase in cases of phacogenic uveitis.

References

1. Abbas AK, Lichtman AH, Pober JS: Cellular and Molecular Immunology, 3rd ed. Philadelphia, WB Saunders, 1997.
2. Verhoff FH, Lemoine AN: Endophthalmitis phacoanaphylactica. Proceedings of the International Congress of Ophthalmologists 1922;1:234–284.
3. Irvine SR, Irvine AR: Lens-induced uveitis and glaucoma. Part I: Endophthalmitis phacoanaphylactica. Am J Ophthalmol 1952;35:177–186.
4. Khalil MK, Lorenzetti DW: Lens-induced inflammation. Can J Ophthalmol 1986;21:96–102.
5. Chandler P: Problems in the diagnosis and treatment of lens-induced uveitis and glaucoma. Arch Ophthalmol 1958;60:828–841.
6. deVeer A: Bilateral endophthalmitis phacoanaphylactica. Arch Ophthalmol 1953;49:606–632.
7. Easom HA, Zimmerman LE: Sympathetic ophthalmia and bilateral phacoanaphylaxis. Arch Ophthalmol 1964;72:9–15.
8. Irvine WD, Flynn HW, Murray TG, et al: Retained lens fragments after phacoemulsification manifesting as marked intraocular inflammation with hypopyon. Am J Ophthalmol 1992;114:610–614.
9. Hodes BL, Stern G: Echographic diagnosis of phacoanaphylactic endophthalmitis. Ophthalmic Surg 1976;7:60–65.
10. Flocks M, Littwin CS, Zimmerman LE: Phacolytic glaucoma. Arch Ophthalmol 1955;54:37–45.
11. Ronday MJH, Stilman JS, Rothova A, et al: Blindness from uveitis in a hospital population in Sierra Leone. Br J Ophthalmol 1994;78:690–693.
12. Ronday M: Uveitis in Africa with emphasis on toxoplasmosis. Netherlands Ophthalmic Research Institute of the Royal Netherlands Academy of Arts and Sciences, Dept. of Ophthalmology, Amsterdam, 1996. ISBN 90-393-1467-5.
13. Marak G: Phacoanaphylactic endophthalmitis. Surv Ophthalmol 1992;36:325–339.
14. Thach AB, Marak GE, McLean IW, et al: Phacoanaphylactic endophthalmitis: A clinicopathologic review. Int Ophthalmol 1991;15:271–279.
15. Law F: Ocular reaction to lens protein. Br J Ophthalmol 1953;37:157–164.
16. Rahi AHD, Misra RN, Morgan G: Immunopathology of the lens. I. Humoral and cellular immune responses to heterologous lens antigens and their roles in ocular inflammation. Br J Ophthalmol 1977;61:164–176.
17. Rahi AHD, Misra RN, Morgan G: Immunopathology of the lens. II. Humoral and cellular immune responses to homologous lens antigens and their roles in ocular inflammation. Br J Ophthalmol 1977;61:285–296.
18. Rahi AHD, Misra RN, Morgan G: Immunopathology of the lens. III. Humoral and cellular immune responses to autologous lens antigens and their roles in ocular inflammation. Br J Ophthalmol 1977;61:371–379.
19. Muller-Hermelink HK: Recent topics in the pathology of uveitis. In: Kraus-Mackiwe E, O'Connor GR, eds: Uveitis: Pathophysiology and therapy. Stuttgart, Thieme, 1986, pp 155–203.
20. Blodi FC: Sympathetic uveitis as allergic phenomenon. Trans Am Acad Ophthalmol Otolaryngol 1959;63:642–656.
21. Easom HA, Zimmerman LE: Sympathetic ophthalmia and bilateral phacoanaphylaxis. Arch Ophthalmol 1964;72:9–15.
22. Allen JC: Sympathetic ophthalmia and phacoanaphylaxis. Am J Ophthalmol 1967;63:281.
23. Meisler AM, Mandelbaum S: *P. acnes* associated endophthalmitis after extracapsular cataract extraction. Ophthalmology 1989;96:56–61.
24. Winward KE: Postoperative *P. acnes* endophthalmitis. Treatment strategies and long-term results. Ophthalmology 1993;100:447–451.
25. Zambrano W: Management options for *P. acnes* endophthalmitis. Ophthalmology 1989;96:1100–1105.

77

RETINAL VASCULITIS

Will Ayliffe

DEFINITION

Retinal vasculitis is a sight-threatening inflammatory eye disease involving the retinal blood vessels.[1, 2] The terms retinal vasculitis and retinal perivasculitis are used interchangeably as clinical descriptions of the funduscopic sign of exudative gray-white sheathing of the retinal blood vessels (Fig. 77–1A).[3] Most frequently, the retinal veins are involved and the term retinal periphlebitis is used to describe this condition.

Retinal vasculitis may occur as a primary syndrome called idiopathic retinal vasculitis, which affects the eye vasculature without any evidence of any systemic or other eye disease. More commonly, retinal vasculitis is seen as a manifestation of systemic diseases including sarcoidosis, collagen-vascular autoimmune disorders, malignancy, neurologic conditions, and systemic infections.[4, 5] It also occurs in ocular inflammatory conditions such as pars planitis or birdshot retinochoroidopathy, as well as in infections of the eye (Table 77–1).

The clinically observable signs of retinal vasculitis are caused by inflammation in or around the walls of retinal blood vessels.[1, 4] Vasculitis in other organ systems is confirmed and classified on histopathologic findings. This is not routinely possible for eye disease, so retinal vasculitis is a diagnosis made by ophthalmoscopic observation of sheathing of the retinal vessels. Often this is a correct supposition and pathologic examination of the few enucleated eyes from patients with retinal vasculitis has confirmed leukocytic infiltration of the vessel walls and surrounding tissues.[1, 6–8]

However, there are noninflammatory causes of retinal vessel sheathing.[1, 9] These sclerotic changes do not cause leaking or staining of the vessel wall and are not associated with inflammatory changes in the vitreous. Perivascular sheathing that is not associated with angiographic evidence of leakage may merely represent long-term changes of blood vessels, which can develop following a variety of pathologic changes including vascular occlusion, atherosclerosis, and even previous vasculitis.

Inflammatory sheathing often occurs as focal fluffy cuffing with diffuse edges enveloping the vessel, contrasting with the well-defined long segments of sheathing seen as a consequence of noninflammatory vascular disease. The term perivascular cuffing, indicating inflammatory retinal vasculitis, may therefore be a more accurate term than sheathing to describe foci of active retinal vasculitis.

The clinical diagnosis of retinal vasculitis is supported by evidence of inflammation in the anterior chamber or vitreous and leakage or staining of the vessel wall seen by fluorescein angiography (Fig. 77–1B).[5, 10]

In addition to ophthalmoscopic observation of perivascular cuffing, many other fundal changes can also be seen. These include retinal hemorrhage, branch retinal vein occlusion, neovascularization, and vitreous hemorrhage.[4, 11]

HISTORY

The clinical picture of retinal periphlebitis was first described in 1887 by Wadsworth in a discussion of a case report on recurrent retinal hemorrhages by Theobald.[12] However, Perls had already performed histologic examination of periphlebitis in a case of tuberculosis (TB) affecting the eyes in 1873.[13] Even earlier, the dramatic

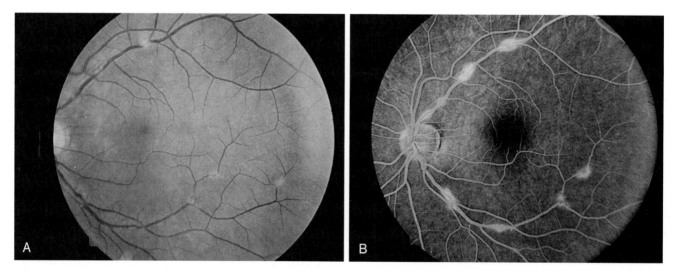

FIGURE 77–1. *A)* Red-free photograph of the left eye of a patient with retinal vasculitis. There are multiple foci of sheathing around the veins, periphlebitis. These are caused by inflammatory cells within and around the vessel giving the appearance of cuffing. *B)* Fluorescein angiogram of the same eye as in Figure 77–1A, showing leakage of dye from the inflamed vessel segments. Areas that are not apparently sheathed in Figure 77–1A are revealed by fluorescein angiography to be involved. For example, staining of the vessel wall and dye leakage is seen in a clinically normal portion of the inferior arcade.

TABLE 77–1. DISORDERS ASSOCIATED WITH RETINAL VASCULITIS

Ocular disorders
　Idiopathic retinal vasculitis
　Eales' disease
　Idiopathic retinal vasculitic aneurysms and neuroretinitis (IRVAN)
　Bilateral iridocyclitis with retinal capillaritis (BIRC)
　Acute multifocal hemorrhagic retinal vasculitis
　Frosted branch angiitis
　Idiopathic recurrent branch retinal arteriolar occlusion
　Pars planitis
　Primary ocular disease
　Birdshot retinochoroidopathy
　Sympathetic ophthalmia
　Vogt-Koyanagi-Harada syndrome
Neurologic disorders
　Multiple sclerosis
　Microangiopathic encephalopathy, hearing loss, and retinal
　　arteriolar occlusions
　Isolated central nervous system angiitis
Systemic autoimmune diseases
　Sarcoidosis
　Adamantiades-Behçet's disease
　Buerger's disease
　Crohn's disease
　Rheumatoid disease
　Human leukocyte antigen B27–associated uveitis
　Sjögren's syndrome A antigen
Retinal vasculopathy in systemic vasculitis
　Systemic erythematosus
　Wegener's granulomatosis
　Polyarteritis nodosa
Infections associated with retinal vasculitis
　Tuberculosis
　Syphilis
　Borreliosis (Lyme disease)
　Whipple's disease
　Brucellosis
　Cat scratch disease
　Rickettsia
　Toxoplasmosis
　Herpes virus
　Cytomegalovirus
　HIV
　Human T-cell lymphoma virus type 1
　Rift Valley fever virus
　Retinal periphlebitis and uveitis with viral-like upper respiratory
　　disease
　Epstein-Barr virus
　Candidiasis
　Endophthalmitis
Drug-induced retinal vasculitis
Retinal vasculitis secondary to malignancy
Miscellaneous causes of retinal vasculitis

complication of recurrent vitreous and retinal hemorrhages had previously brought the condition of retinal vasculitis to the attention of ophthalmologists using the first ophthalmoscopes. The observation by van Trigt in 1852 was followed by numerous subsequent descriptions in the literature[12, 14] and in several 19th century textbooks and atlases such as McKenzie's *Practical Treatise on Diseases of the Eye,* 4th edition, 1854.[1]

The first attempt to describe the syndrome was by Henry Eales in 1880.[15] He associated epistaxis and constipation with recurrent vitreous hemorrhage and, in a later paper, excluded known systemic diseases including diabetes, clotting abnormalities, blood dyscrasias, and syphilis.[16] In 1887, a 52-year-old nondiabetic woman with recur-

rent retinal hemorrhages was noted to have disc neovascularization.[12] Subsequently, the presence of periphlebitis in cases of recurrent vitreous hemorrhage was noted.[14]

A possible relationship with TB was suggested at the beginning of this century. In India, *Mycobacterium tuberculosis* is still believed to be the etiologic agent or involved by hypersensitivity in Eales' disease.[17]

Duke-Elder regarded Eales' disease as a clinical manifestation of inflammatory retinal vein occlusion or periphlebitis.[1] This accords with the modern view of many authorities not recognizing the eponymous condition as a distinct clinical entity. However, the disease is uncommon in the western hemisphere, and clinicians in areas where Eales' disease occurs frequently, such as in India, find it helpful to distinguish this condition from other types of retinal vasculitis.[17]

The association of retinal vasculitis with systemic disease became increasingly recognized in the middle of the 20th century. Retinal venous sheathing was observed in some patients with multiple sclerosis.[18] Subsequently, many more conditions, from eye infections to systemic inflammatory diseases, were found to be associated with retinal vasculitis.[1, 2, 4]

EPIDEMIOLOGY

In a prospective epidemiologic study in Savoy, France, the prevalence of uveitis was 38 per 100,000 with an annual incidence of 17 per 100,000 per year.[19] Only 13% of these cases were retinal vasculitis, giving an estimated incidence of 2 per 100,000 per year, which is similar to that in other areas.[5]

So, primary retinal vasculitis is rare and always has been. In the year 1980 to 1981, no cases of primary retinal hemorrhage were identified in the 12,000 eye patients who were treated at the Birmingham and Midland Eye Hospital in England.[16] More recently, the diagnosis was made in 25 patients seen at the National Eye Institute (NEI), Bethesda, between 1984 and 1994.[20]

Retinal vasculitis affects young adults and there may be female preponderance, although not all studies agree. In a series of 150 patients with retinal vasculitis seen over 10 years at St. Thomas' Hospital in London, the disease was confined to the eye in 40% of cases.[10] Most of these patients with primary retinal vasculitis were between 15 and 40 years of age and there was a female-to-male ratio of 4:2.7. A similar age distribution of 14 to 52 years but with an equal female-to-male ratio was found in the NEI group.[20]

However, retinal vasculitis is seen more commonly as a manifestation of ocular infections or systemic disorders such as Adamantiades-Behçet's Disease (ABD),[4, 5] and the incidence of these diseases varies throughout the world. Therefore, data from centers with a predominantly white population do not reflect the incidence of retinal vasculitis in other regions such as Brazil or Japan.

CLINICAL CHARACTERISTICS

Symptoms

Inflammation of the peripheral retinal vessels may be completely asymptomatic even in those patients with associated systemic disease.[4, 21] However, patients with retinal vasculitis often complain of painless blurring or loss of vision. Large scotomata corresponding to areas of ischemia may also be noticed. These symptoms may be accompanied by floaters. Some patients, particularly those with Eales' disease, may present with sudden loss of vision due to vitreous hemorrhage.

Symptoms and signs suggestive of systemic involvement should be identified. These include, but are not limited to, orogenital ulceration, arthritis, skin rashes, thrombosis, and neurologic and respiratory symptoms. It is often helpful to ask the patient to complete a standard uveitis questionnaire, and further inquiry with respect to positive answers enables the ophthalmologist to focus on specific systemic entities.

Visual acuity is variably affected. In the St. Thomas study, two thirds of patients had an acuity of 6/18 in at least one eye, and only 22% had bilateral acuities of less than 6/18.[10] Similarly, the NEI group reported a median visual acuity of 20/63 (range, 20/16—light perception) at the time of referral.[20] The disease affected both eyes in all cases.

Signs

Slit-lamp examination of the anterior segment is useful to detect anterior uveitis, which is found in about one third of cases.[10] Occasionally, evaluation of associated scleritis is required. Cellular infiltration of the vitreous is present in nearly all patients and it can be severe. Collections of inflammatory cells, or snowballs, are typically found in the inferior vitreous cavity, and a posterior vitreous detachment is usually present.

The striking vascular changes are the hallmark of retinal vasculitis. During the active phase, sheathing of the vessels occurs, which is seen by ophthalmoscopy as focal fluffy-white cuffing, in approximately two thirds of patients (Table 77–2).[10, 20] The sheathing may develop around long stretches of the vessel or it may occur as skip lesions. The sheathing is most often seen around retinal veins but can also affect arteries. Some authors have attempted to differentiate sheathing, seen in peripheral

retina and not necessarily associated with fluorescein leakage, from periphlebitis, identified as cuffing of retinal veins, with leakage of fluorescein at these sites.[10] This fine distinction may help to separate active disease from chronic changes, but it is not universally recognized, and we regard perivascular exudates or cuffing as active vascular disease.[3]

An extreme form of exaggerated sheathing of the vessels gives a clinical picture that resembles tree branches in winter. This sign is called frosted branch angiitis.[22] As well as vasculitis, other perivascular changes may occur in certain conditions. These need to be differentiated from true retinal vasculitis. For example, in some patients with sarcoidosis, discrete waxy nodules may be seen adjacent to the retinal vessels.[23] These yellow perivenous exudates, originally described by Walsh in 1939, were likened to candle wax drippings and called taches de bougie by Franceschetti and Babel in the French literature.[7, 23] This change represents perivascular granulomatous tissue with associated exudation.[7] It is seen in eyes with sarcoidosis but it is not necessarily pathognomonic for that condition.

Likewise, characteristic gray-white granular deposits are seen on the retinal vessels in human T-cell lymphoma virus type-1 (HTLV-1)–associated uveitis, and if recognized they may help establish the diagnosis.[24]

Retinal vascular occlusions are particularly associated with ABD,[10] but they are also seen in other types of retinal vasculitis.[20] Occlusive vasculopathy leads to retinal hemorrhage, cotton-wool spots, and pallor in areas of retinal ischemia. The vessels in these areas eventually become sclerotic and attenuated,[20] with large areas of capillary nonperfusion and retinal ischemia. Subsequent retinal neovascularization, occurring in 16% to 40% of all cases of retinal vasculitis, may develop, along with vitreous hemorrhage.

Alterations in the vascular architecture have also been described. These develop just temporal to the macula and include arteriolar-venous anastomoses and traversing of retinal vessels across the horizontal raphe.[4]

In addition to vascular changes, retinal pathology may also occur. Retinal edema is common and may precede vascular cuffing.[4] Deep retinal infiltrates are seen in some patients with ABD, and atrophic retinal pigment epithelial lesions may be seen in patients with isolated retinal vasculitis.[10]

TABLE 77–2. POSTERIOR FINDINGS AT PRESENTATION IN 25 PATIENTS

FINDINGS	NUMBER OF PATIENTS (%)
Vascular sheathing	16 (64)
Arteries and veins	4 (16)
Arteries	2 (8)
Veins	1 (4)
Not specified	9 (36)
Neovascularization	10 (40)
Intraretinal hemorrhage	9 (36)
Sclerotic/attenuated vessels	8 (32)
Vitreous hemorrhage	6 (24)
Vascular occlusion	5 (20)
Cystoid macular edema	4 (16)
Branch retinal vein occlusion	2 (8)
Optic atrophy	2 (8)
Retinal detachment	1 (4)

Modified from George T, Walton RC, Whitcup SM: Primary retinal vasculitis: Systemic associations and diagnostic evaluation. Ophthalmology 1996;103:384–389.

Fluorescein Angiographic Findings

Diffuse capillary leakage is a common finding in patients with idiopathic retinal vasculitis.[10] Macular ischemia is most readily identified on fluorescein angiography, and it is important to recognize, particularly in patients whose visual acuity fails to improve despite aggressive medical therapy and inflammatory control. Late staining of vessels occurs in two thirds of patients, and it affects arteries, veins, or both (Fig. 77–2).

Patients with ischemic disease have retinal capillary closure and nonperfusion.[20] When this affects the macula, it causes an enlarged or irregular foveal avascular zone.[25] Using fluorescein angiography to separate patients into ischemic and nonischemic groups has been shown to predict the visual outcome.[25]

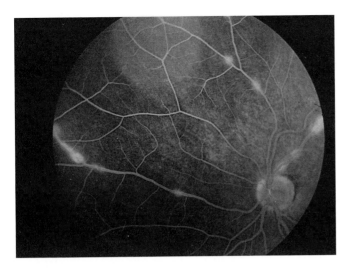

FIGURE 77–2. Late-phase fluorescein angiogram demonstrating staining of blood vessel walls.

Neovascularization is identified in 12% to 16% of patients with idiopathic retinal vasculitis.[20] The new vessels are flat and sometimes difficult to detect clinically. They leak fluorescein profusely and are readily detectable by fluorescein angiography, providing that peripheral areas of the fundus are imaged (Fig. 77–3). It is found more frequently in those patients with retinal vasculitis associated with sarcoid or uveomeningitis.[10] Neovascularization may often develop as a consequence of inflammatory mediators rather than of retinal ischemia, which is found in only one third of cases.[10]

DISORDERS ASSOCIATED WITH RETINAL VASCULITIS

The disorders associated with retinal vasculitis are multiple and diverse. A summary of the main diseases is found in Table 77–1. Many of the conditions are dealt with in detail in other chapters. The purpose of this survey is to highlight the retinal vascular changes and differential diagnosis of patients who have retinal vasculitis.

Retinal Vasculitis in Ocular Disease

Idiopathic Retinal Vasculitis

Primary retinal vasculitis is a rare disease but it affects young adults and can cause blindness.[20, 25] It is a clinical diagnosis based on the ophthalmoscopic findings of sheathing of the retinal vessels and vitritis. The diagnosis is supported by fluorescein angiography, which may also reveal areas of clinically invisible disease (Fig. 77–4). In the absence of systemic clinical findings by history and examination, an extensive laboratory investigation is not required.[20] In these cases, investigation can be limited to a full blood count and sedimentation rate, serology for syphilis, and a chest radiograph. However, in those patients with symptoms or signs indicating an underlying systemic condition, a work-up tailored to the suspected diagnosis is required. The visual outcome is variable and depends on the presence of retinal ischemia.[25] The ischemic group fared less well over a 5-year follow-up, with 34% having vision of 6/60 or worse compared to only 6% of the eyes deemed to be nonischemic at the start of the study.[25] Although retinal vasculitis may appear to be confined to the eye at presentation, it must be remembered that serious systemic illness may subsequently develop in some of these patients. In a retrospective study of 67 patients with at least 5 years follow-up, those with ischemic retinal vasculitis had a 59% chance of developing systemic disease. Over half of these had a major vascular event such as cerebrovascular accident or stroke.[26] This is of some consequence because these patients are young. So, although intensive investigations are not required to pursue a diagnosis in patients with isolated retinal vasculitis,[20] it is prudent to pay attention to cardiovascular risk factors including blood pressure, lipids, and particularly smoking.[26]

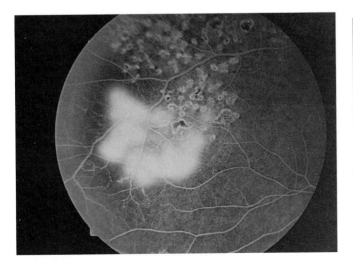

FIGURE 77–3. Fluorescein angiogram of retinal neovascularization in a patient with retinal vasculitis. Scars from laser that had been previously applied on the adjacent retina can be seen superiorly. The photograph is of the right eye of the same patient as in Figure 77–1 and was taken on the same day.

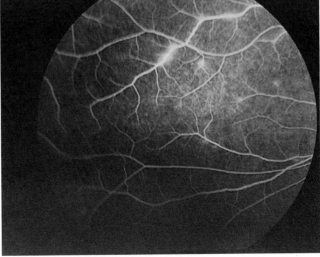

FIGURE 77–4. Fluorescein angiogram of the midperipheral fundus in another patient with retinal vasculitis revealing active disease in small vessels that was not detectable by ophthalmoscopy.

Eales' Disease

A syndrome of recurrent retinal and vitreous hemorrhage in young men, associated with constipation and epistaxis, was first described by Henry Eales in 1880[15] and was later shown to be associated with retinal periphlebitis. Classically, this entity manifests as an obliterative periphlebitis, anterior to the equator, involving multiple quadrants, with progression posteriorly. Neovascularization elsewhere (commonly occurring at the border between perfused and nonperfused retina), neovascularization of the disk, and rubeosis iridis may occur with or without vitritis.[5] While these changes may simulate those seen in idiopathic branch retinal vein occlusion, the retinal vascular changes associated with Eales' disease do not commonly occur at arteriovenous crossing sites and may or may not be associated with extensive cotton-wool spots. In addition to the retinal venous changes, choroidal inflammation develops under inflamed vein segments, and anterior, posterior, or intermediate uveitis may be present.[17] Eales' disease typically presents in young, healthy adult men between 30 and 40 years of age. It is most prevalent in India, Pakistan, and Afghanistan.[27] In India it is common, with an incidence of 1:200 ophthalmic patients.[17] In that subcontinent, the disease is associated with TB, and concomitant therapy with oral steroids and antitubercular chemotherapy is recommended if evidence of this infection is found. In other patients, the disease responds to oral steroids with sector laser panretinal ablation or cryotherapy to areas of nonperfused retina in the presence of neovascularization involving the retinal periphery or posterior pole. Some investigators have recommended full panretinal photocoagulation and early vitrectomy, in an effort to improve the visual prognosis in patients with Eales' disease.[28] Vitreoretinal surgery is necessary in cases with prolonged vitreous hemorrhage or complications arising from vitreoretinal traction (Fig. 77–5).

The diagnosis of Eales' disease is essentially one of exclusion. Fluorescein angiography is extremely valuable in revealing the degree of retinal capillary nonperfusion and the presence of neovascularization, and as a guide to laser photocoagulation for sector ablation.

The strong association of Eales' disease with purified

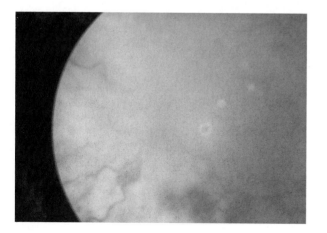

FIGURE 77–5. Recurrent vitreous hemorrhage in a patient with periphlebitis Eales' disease. (See color insert.)

protein derivative skin positivity,[29] and the demonstration of circulating immune complexes in these patients[30] suggests that Eales' disease is an immune-driven process. However, it is hard to reconcile this theory with the relative paucity of this disease in populations who are immunized with Bacille Calmette-Guérin vaccine. A long-term follow-up study of patients with Eales' disease found that a proportion developed vestibuloauditory dysfunction.[31] This complication occurs in other idiopathic retinal vasculitis subgroups,[32] which suggests that Eales' disease may in fact be a part of a spectrum of related conditions. Indeed, it is debatable whether Eales' disease represents a separate condition or is merely part of a spectrum of retinal vasculitis. The condition is probably identical to ischemic idiopathic retinal vasculitis,[25] and the eponym is less frequently used in the modern literature.

Idiopathic Retinal Vasculitis Aneurysms and Neuroretinitis

Two patients with bilateral retinal arteritis, multiple microaneurysms, neuroretinitis, and uveitis were described in 1983.[33] Ten more cases were subsequently described, in more detail, and the name idiopathic retinal vasculitis aneurysms and neuroretinitis (IRVAN) was proposed.[34] The distinctive retinal findings are numerous aneurysmal dilations (75 to 300 μm in diameter) of the retinal and optic nerve head arterioles. The sight-threatening complications are exudative retinopathy and peripheral capillary nonperfusion, leading to neovascularization and vitreous hemorrhage. Neuroretinitis (manifested by late diffuse staining of the optic nerve head) and retinal vasculitis (staining of the vessel walls seen in the late stages of the angiogram) were used as inclusion criteria for the study.

Despite the apparently inflammatory nature of this syndrome, steroids had little effect on the degree of uveitis or retinal ischemia.[34] Retinal photocoagulation is recommended if neovascularization or rubeosis iridis develops.

The condition is limited to the eye and inappropriate investigation can be avoided by tailoring the work-up to the review of systems.

Bilateral Iridocyclitis with Retinal Capillaritis

In addition to causing inflammation in arterioles and veins, retinal vasculitis can affect the capillary bed. A group of 18 juvenile patients with bilateral granulomatous uveitis and retinal capillaritis has been described.[35] The patients with this disease were between 9 and 17 years of age and presented with red eyes and photophobia. Examination revealed a variable extent of cloudy edematous retina. Fluorescein dye leakage and pooling from the retinal capillaries underlying the cloudy retina was the characteristic finding on angiography. Leakage from arterioles and veins was not observed, and this helped to distinguish the condition from other causes of retinal vasculitis associated with uveitis. Although leakage restricted to the retinal capillaries has been described in acute tubular interstitial nephritis, none of the patients with bilateral iridocyclitis with retinal capillaritis (BIRC) had any evidence of systemic disease. The condition was associated with human leukocyte antigen (HLA)-DR6 and

HLA-Cw7, but HLA-B27 was not found in any of the patients and there was no increased incidence of HLA-DR8, which is associated with juvenile rheumatoid arthritis.

Retinal vasculitis associated with seronegative spondyloarthritis also presents with diffuse capillary leakage and macular edema.[10] The capillaries and postcapillary venules are the preferential sites for inflammation in these patients.

Acute Multifocal Hemorrhagic Retinal Vasculitis

In 1988, a group of seven patients with acute bilateral loss of vision, retinal vasculitis (predominantly venular), variable retinal hemorrhage, posterior retinal infiltrates, vitritis, and papillitis was described.[36] The vasculitis was predominantly an occlusive phlebitis. These patients were otherwise fit and well. Treatment with oral prednisone was of some benefit but acyclovir was ineffective. Five of the patients developed neovascularization of the posterior pole and required laser photocoagulation. The major differential diagnostic considerations were acute retinal necrosis, sarcoidosis, toxoplasmosis, and ABD, all of which were excluded. This condition, like Eales' disease, appears to be yet another presentation of idiopathic retinal vasculitis, but whether it truly represents a distinct pathologic process is far from clear.

Frosted Branch Angiitis

In some patients with retinal vasculitis, the sheathing of the blood vessels is so extensive that the underlying vessels are obscured. This clinical picture, which looks like the branches of trees in winter, was first reported in a healthy 6-year-old Japanese boy and was called frosted branch angiitis.[22] Although initially described as affecting both arteries and veins, it predominantly involves the veins.[37]

Patients report with acute decrease in visual acuity. On examination, cells are detected in the anterior chamber and vitreous. Prominent sheathing of retinal veins is the hallmark of this condition, but in younger patients, the arteries may also be involved. In severe cases, macular edema develops. No clinical or laboratory evidence of systemic disease is detected.

Treatment is with systemic steroids. The condition resolves with treatment over 2 to 3 weeks, and most patients return to 20/20 acuity.

The initial cases were idiopathic, but subsequently cases have been described in patients with acquired immunodeficiency disease (AIDS) and early cytomegalovirus (CMV) retinitis.[38] After anti-CMV treatment is started, the sheathing resolves in 2 weeks, before the retinal opacification clears. The need to add steroid is debatable.

Frosted branch angiitis is a clinical sign representing an exaggerated sheathing of retinal vessels. It will probably be reported to occur in many other conditions that cause retinal vasculitis such as sarcoidosis, in infectious disorders,[39] and even in neoplastic disease.[40]

Idiopathic Recurrent Branch Retinal Arteriolar Occlusion

A small number of reports have described healthy middle-aged patients who developed recurrent branch retinal artery occlusions of unknown cause in one or both eyes.[41] These patients do not have underlying inflammatory disease or evidence of embolism. Ophthalmoscopy reveals focal periarterial sheathing, and fluorescein angiography shows multiple segments of arteriolar staining, suggesting that arteritis is the cause of the obstructions. Preretinal neovascularization occurs in areas of ischemia, but the prognosis for vision is generally good. Although no systemic cause was found, 50% of the patients had vestibuloauditory or transient sensorimotor symptoms or both.[32] It has been suggested[2] that these patients may have a partial manifestation of the microangiopathic syndrome of encephalopathy, hearing loss, and retinal arteriolar occlusions.[42] However, patients with the microangiopathic syndrome do not show evidence of true retinal vasculitis.

Pars Planitis

Pars planitis is a type of intermediate uveitis characterized by vitritis and snowballs, peripheral retinal vasculitis, and exudate at the pars plana. Although initially described as inflammation of the ora serrata, the term pars planitis was subsequently more commonly adopted.[43] The disease is usually bilateral at presentation and can vary from a mild inflammation, requiring no treatment, to a severe blinding condition.

The pars plana exudate is composed of collapsed vitreous, blood vessels, fibroglial tissue, and infiltrating lymphocytes. Pathologically, the exudates are collections of multinucleated giant cells and epithelioid cells. It remains uncertain whether the disease is primarily a retinal vasculitis, with the associated features being a consequence of the blood–retinal barrier breakdown, or whether it is a vitritis.

Primary Ocular Diseases

Retinal vasculitis, primarily affecting the retinal venules, is a prominent and consistent feature of birdshot retinochoroidopathy. Birdshot retinochoroidopathy may present as idiopathic retinal vasculitis with the development of the characteristic focal cream-colored lesions.[44, 45]

Sympathetic ophthalmia also has striking choroidal changes (Dalen-Fuchs nodules) with panuveitis. Some patients also have retinal vasculitis.[46] In Vogt-Koyanagi-Harada syndrome, retinal periphlebitis[47] and peripapillary venous sheathing are occasionally seen.[48] All these conditions are described in detail in other chapters.

Retinal Vasculitis as a Manifestation of Neurologic Disease

Multiple Sclerosis

A variety of ocular inflammatory signs have been described in patients with multiple sclerosis (MS), including iritis, intermediate uveitis, posterior uveitis, periphlebitis, and optic neuritis.[49] The association of retinal venous sheathing and MS was first reported by Rucker, who found the sign in 20% of patients.[18] The reported incidence of retinal periphlebitis in MS varies from 8.5% of eyes at autopsy,[50] to 33% of patients with MS undergoing ophthalmic examination.[51] In most cases, the periphlebitis is subtle, peripheral, and of no visual consequence. It is also transient, explaining the wide variability of its reported incidence. However, in other patients the periphlebitis can be severe, leading to occlusive vasculitis, ischemia, and retinal neovascularization.[49]

Patches of fluffy perivascular cuffing represent areas of active disease, whereas sclerotic whitening of the venular wall with no leakage is probably a chronic change. The periphlebitis consists of a lymphoplasmacytic infiltrate, occasionally with a granulomatous component.[50] The changes are similar to those seen in the brain of MS patients, which suggests that the finding of retinal vasculitis might have important implications.

In a study of 54 patients with pars planitis, 22% developed MS or optic neuritis after a 7.5-year follow-up.[52] The presence of retinal vasculitis at the time of diagnosis was associated with earlier onset of MS or optic neuritis.

The presence of retinal periphlebitis might also be an indicator of active neurologic disease. In a study of 282 patients with MS, retinal vasculitis was found in 43% of those with active disease compared to 25% of the group in remission.[53] In contrast, a more recent study did not find this correlation with disease activity.[54]

The relationship between MS and retinal vasculitis is therefore complex. About 25% of patients with retinal vasculitis or pars planitis will develop MS, particularly if they are female and carry the HLA-B7 or HLA-DR2 alleles. About 15% of patients with MS will have asymptomatic retinal vasculitis, and 25% will develop a symptomatic uveitis.

A Microangiopathic Syndrome of Encephalopathy, Hearing Loss, and Retinal Arteriolar Occlusions

This occlusive arterial disease affecting the brain, inner ear, and retina affects young women.[42] Patients present with encephalopathy manifesting as behavioral change and memory disturbance with hearing loss and tinnitus. Eye examination reveals bilateral retinal arterial occlusions and retinal infarctions. Although the arterioles are occluded with white matter, there is no clinical or angiographic evidence of vasculitis, and brain biopsies show multiple noninflammatory arteriolar occlusions. The disease may therefore not be a true retinal vasculitis, as is also the case for many patients with cerebral lupus and "retinal vasculitis."[55]

Isolated Central Nervous System Angiitis

This rare disorder can affect all age groups. It is characterized by granulomatous inflammation of intracerebral and leptomeningeal vessels.[56] The disease may be a nonspecific immunopathologic response to a variety of antigens. It has been reported to occur in some patients with malignant lymphoma and in patients with varicella zoster virus infections.[49] Some patients with isolated central nervous system (CNS) angiitis have occlusive retinal vasculitis.[49]

Retinal Vasculitis in Association with Systemic Autoimmune Disease

Sarcoidosis

Sarcoidosis is a granulomatous disease of unknown origin that affects many organs. Ophthalmic involvement occurs in 25% to 50% of patients.[57] Although anterior uveitis is the most common eye association, retinal vasculitis is a characteristic feature of sarcoidosis. It is nearly always a retinal periphlebitis, and retinal arteries are only rarely involved. It is the most common fundal finding and occurs in 10% to 45% of patients with active disease.[58]

The involvement of vessels is discontinuous, and this appears clinically as skip lesions. It may be mild and associated with peripheral retinal and focal vitreal infiltrates indistinguishable from idiopathic intermediate uveitis. Indeed, pars planitis may be the presenting sign in patients who develop sarcoidosis many years later.

In other patients, a more severe periphlebitis develops (Fig. 77–6). In the acute stage, this can be accompanied by retinal hemorrhage and edema. Retinal pigment epithelial atrophy may subsequently develop under the sites of periphlebitis.[10, 58] With systemic corticosteroid treatment, periphlebitis resolves, but some residual sheathing can persist.

Yellow perivenous exudates, described as taches de bougie (candle wax drippings), are also sometimes seen.[8] They are not, however, pathognomonic for sarcoidosis.

Neovascularization develops in 20% of cases[10] and may lead to vitreous hemorrhage or retinal detachment. It is often associated with ischemia and responds to panretinal laser photocoagulation.

Adamantiades-Behçet's Disease

ABD is a multisystem inflammatory illness presenting with recurrent orogenital ulceration, skin lesions, and intraocular inflammation. It is the leading cause of endogenous uveitis and acquired blindness in Turkey and Japan, and it is associated with HLA-B51.[4]

Retinal vasculitis is a major cause of visual loss in this multisystem disease, and it is difficult to treat. Relapses are frequent, leading eventually to a final stage of retinal and optic disc atrophy, variable chorioretinal and retinal pigment epithelial change, sheathed vessels, and chronic mild vitritis.

The acute stage of retinal vasculitis is associated with yellow-white retinal infiltrates.[10] Recurrent branch retinal vein occlusions are more common in ABD than in any

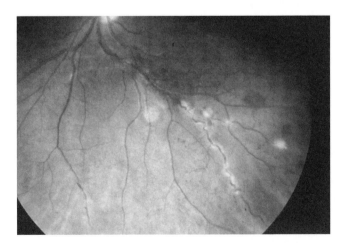

FIGURE 77–6. The fundus of a patient with sarcoidosis and retinal vasculitis showing creamy white sheathing of the retinal veins. (See color insert.)

other type of retinal vasculitis.[10] Capillary closure causes macular ischemia and, if extensive, can lead to neovascularization of the retina, disc, and iris. Arteriolar sheathing and occlusion may also develop. The vascular events are accompanied by vitritis, diffuse capillary leakage, macular edema, and optic disc swelling.

Buerger's Disease

Thromboangiitis obliterans (Buerger's disease) is an inflammatory obliterative vascular disease of unknown etiology that preferentially affects male smokers. The arterial lesions are segmental. The arterial wall is infiltrated with polymorphonuclear leukocytes and lymphocytes, and the inflammation extends into the surrounding tissues involving the veins. Fibrosis and proliferation of the intima follows and the lumen becomes obliterated with thrombus.[59] The disease follows a relapsing course with paroxysmal episodes of pain, cyanosis, and even gangrene. Ocular involvement may be preceded by a prodromal phase of visual obscurations that may result in complete blindness. The periarteritis of the retinal vessels results in obliterative endarteritis with thrombosis. The vessels eventually become densely sheathed, appearing as white strands. Occlusion of the central retinal artery is rare. Retinal vein occlusions and recurrent hemorrhages also occur.[60]

Crohn's Disease

Crohn's disease is a focal granulomatous disease affecting any part of the alimentary tract. Systemic vasculitis can occur in inflammatory bowel disease and several organs including the eyes may be affected. Uveitis occurs in 2% to 9% of patients with inflammatory bowel disease.[61] Retinal vasculitis associated with Crohn's disease is rare. In a study of 17 patients with uveitis and inflammatory bowel disease, a pars plana exudate occurred in one patient and retinal vasculitis was found in two (11%).[61] However, the retinal disease can be severe, affecting both retinal arteries and veins.[62, 63] Treatment may require both systemic corticosteroids and cyclophosphamide.[62]

Rheumatoid Disease

Rheumatoid arthritis is the most common rheumatic disorder and affects 1% to 2% of the adult population. Although it is recognized as a symmetric deforming polyarthritis, extra-articular manifestations are common and affect a variety of tissues.

Retinal vasculitis is rarely associated with rheumatoid arthritis, but several cases have been reported.[64] However, it may occur more frequently than is suspected by clinical examination alone. It has been found by fluorescein angiography to affect 17 patients with rheumatoid arthritis, even if no ophthalmoscopic signs were present.[65]

Retinal vasculitis has also been reported in juvenile rheumatoid arthritis and in severe seronegative arthritis, although it is a very rare complication.[10]

HLA-B27–Associated Uveitis

Although acute iritis is the most common manifestation of HLA-B27–associated uveitis, retinal vasculitis may occur.[66] It may be overlooked on clinical examination and detected only by fluorescein angiography. Some patients have more severe vasculitis, with multiple retinal infarcts, intraretinal hemorrhage, disc swelling, vitritis, and macular edema.[21]

Sjögren's Syndrome A Antigen

Sjögren's syndrome is a multisystem disease that is often overlooked. Some of these patients are at risk of severe systemic manifestations, which may require immunosuppression.

In a study of eight patients with primary Sjögren's disease and uveitis, four had pars planitis and one had a history of retinal periphlebitis and branch retinal vein occlusion.[67]

Patients with antibodies to Sjögren's syndrome A (SS-A) antigen, who may have mild or presumptive systemic lupus erythematosus (SLE), can also develop peripheral retinal vasculitis (arteriolitis) and neovascularization.[68] It seems that retinal vasculitis (arteriolitis) is more commonly seen in lupus-like illnesses if SS-A antigen is present.

It is important to recognize the existence of this syndrome to prevent confusing the neurologic manifestations of Sjögren's disease with MS. In addition, primary Sjögren's syndrome is associated with malignancy, and there are other aspects of this autoimmune disease that may require attention.

Retinal Vasculopathy in Systemic Vasculitis

Systemic Lupus Erythematosus

Retinopathy is the most frequent ocular complication of SLE, occurring in 7.5% of well-controlled patients.[69] The majority of these patients have mild small-vessel disease manifesting as multiple cotton-wool spots and intraretinal hemorrhages. The cotton-wool spot is the hallmark of the classic retinopathy of SLE. In contrast to hypertension and diabetes, arteriolar dilation, rather than constriction, may be observed. In some patients with SLE, especially those with elevated antiphospholipid antibodies, severe retinal vaso-occlusive disease may develop with occlusion of both arterioles and venules, causing retinal ischemia and proliferative retinopathy.[70]

The vessel occlusion may be caused by true vasculitis with perivascular inflammatory sheathing.[49] However, the retinopathy is more commonly not a true vasculitis but is caused by nonvasculitic occlusion, which is not associated with an inflammatory cell infiltrate, and is seen clinically as multiple cotton-wool spots.[55] The cause of these noninflammatory microvascular occlusions is contentious. A study in mice with lupus-like diseases suggests that occlusion of capillaries is by large immune complexes.[71] If these complexes are able to penetrate the vessel wall as in the choroid, then an intense inflammatory reaction will occur. It is suggested that the tight endothelial barriers in the retinal vasculature prevent either egress of the complexes or ingress of the leukocytes, and therefore inflammation is not initiated.[55]

The cause of occlusions in larger vessels is also uncertain but they may be initiated by lupus anticoagulant, anticardiolipin antibodies, or antiendothelial antibodies.

Occlusion of capillaries and small to medium-sized

arteries and veins may lead to proliferative retinopathy.[49] Proliferative lupus retinopathy may progress despite absent antinuclear antibody and normal serum complement levels. There does not have to be serologic evidence of active SLE for neovascularization to develop, particularly in the presence of retinal ischemia. Regression can be induced by panretinal scatter laser photocoagulation.[49, 70]

Wegener's Granulomatosis

Wegener's granulomatosis is a granulomatous, necrotizing, vasculitic condition that primarily affects the upper and lower respiratory tract and the kidneys. Ocular manifestations are common and may precede involvement of other organs.[72] Ophthalmic disease is the presenting feature in 8% to 16% of cases, and it may eventually develop in up to 87% of patients.[73] The eye disease mostly affects the orbits, causing proptosis, and the anterior segment, causing necrotizing sclerokeratitis.[74] Vitritis and optic nerve vasculitis occasionally develop.[74] Surprisingly, retinal vasculitis is an extremely uncommon manifestation of Wegener's granulomatosis.[73] The cytoplasmic pattern of the antineutrophil cytoplasmic antibody (cANCA) is highly specific for this disease.[75]

Polyarteritis Nodosa

Polyarteritis nodosa has protean manifestations depending on the site of vasculitis. There are disseminated inflammatory lesions involving medium and small-sized arteries, commonly affecting the heart, kidneys, liver, gastrointestinal tract, and CNS. Ocular involvement is infrequent, affecting 10% to 20% of patients and typically involving the choroidal arteries.[76] Retinal arteritis can occur and patients may present initially with uveitis.[76]

Relapsing Polychondritis

Relapsing polychondritis is a rare connective tissue disease characterized by inflammatory episodes involving the cartilage of the nose, ears, larynx, and trachea, together with an inflammatory arthritis. In a review of 112 patients, ocular disease was noted in 21 patients at the time of diagnosis, with episcleritis and scleritis being the most common manifestations. Retinal vasculitis, often associated with retinal vascular occlusion, was noted in 9% of the patients.[77]

Infections Associated with Retinal Vasculitis

Bacterial

TUBERCULOSIS

TB of the retina occurs via hematogenous spread from infections elsewhere, which may be occult. Choroiditis is the most frequent ocular feature of TB,[78] but periphlebitis is the most common retinal sign and, rarely, it can be the presenting sign of disseminated TB.[79, 80] There is usually associated vitritis and retinal hemorrhage.[79]

Branch or central retinal vein occlusion may occur, and this causes peripheral capillary closure. Neovascularization and vitreous hemorrhage may then develop.

This infection must be considered when evaluating patients with idiopathic retinitis. In India, the infection

or hypersensitivity to *Mycobacterium* antigens can cause a clinical picture identical to that of Eales' disease.[17]

The diagnosis is often difficult because it is hazardous to obtain biopsy material from these inflamed eyes. Smears and cultures from aqueous and vitreous have a low yield of positive results.[78] Polymerase chain reaction to amplify *Mycobacterium* DNA from intraocular fluids can be used. Most often, the diagnosis of intraocular TB is presumed in indirect evidence even in the presence of systemic disease. A 2-week trial of antitubercular drugs without steroids is recommended by some authors in cases of retinal vasculitis with a high sedimentation rate and a positive Mantoux reaction or suspicious chest radiographic findings.[17] However, single-agent treatment with isoniazid is not advised because of the risk for development of drug-resistant organisms.

Neovascularization of the disc and retina can be treated with panretinal scatter photocoagulation.

SYPHILIS

Because syphilis can mimic a variety of eye diseases, the infection should be excluded in any patient with retinal vasculitis. Syphilis causes vitritis, chorioretinitis, venous and arterial occlusions, retinal vasculitis, neuroretinitis, optic neuritis, subretinal neovascularization, and exudative retinal detachments.[81] Syphilitic retinal vasculitis is rare and is usually an arteritis, but isolated periphlebitis can also occur.[82]

Spirochetes cannot be routinely isolated, so the diagnosis is made by clinical history, examination, and laboratory tests, including the Venereal Disease Reference Laboratory (VDRL), fluorescent treponemal antibody absorption (FTA-ABS), and microhemagglutination *T. pallidum* tests. The uveitis may occur late in the course of the disease and the VDRL can be negative, so confirmatory FTA-ABS and microhemagglutination assay–*T. pallidum* should be performed.[2]

BORRELIOSIS (LYME DISEASE)

Lyme disease is caused by the tick-borne spirochete *Borrelia burgdorferi*. It is transmitted to humans via the bite of an infected tick, whose normal hosts include deer, birds, and field mice. The acute stage of Lyme disease is a localized annular skin rash with influenza-like symptoms. If left untreated, a variety of systemic symptoms may develop over the subsequent few weeks, affecting the integumentary, cardiovascular, musculoskeletal, and neurologic systems. Eventually, chronic arthritis and neurologic symptoms develop. The patients susceptible to arthritis have the HLA-DRb1*0401 allele, which is also found in rheumatoid arthritis. This allele binds a peptide derived from an outer surface protein of *Borrelia* called protein A. This peptide shows sequence homology with a human protein (LFA-1) and this may generate an autoimmune T-cell response to the self antigen.

Posterior uveitis occurs in the disseminated and chronic phases. Pars planitis, vitritis, choroiditis, exudative retinal detachment, branch retinal artery occlusion, and retinal vasculitis have all been described.[83] Retinal vessel sheathing and occlusion may lead to disc or retinal neovascularization and vitreous hemorrhage.

The diagnosis is made with the clinical history and

serologic evidence of *B. burgdorferi* infection. Cytologic examination of the vitreous may reveal the organism.[84] Serologic tests including immunofluorescence and enzyme-linked immunosorbent assay have limited sensitivity, but a rising titer of immunoglobulin G (IgG) supports the diagnosis of active disease. Western blot assay of vitreous specimens may also be helpful.

WHIPPLE'S DISEASE

Whipple's disease is a multisystem chronic inflammatory disorder that mainly affects men in their fifth decade. It causes fever, arthralgia, weight loss, anemia, diarrhea, and abdominal pain. An infectious cause is supported by histopathology demonstrating macrophages containing gram-negative bacilli that stain intensely with periodic acid–Schiff reagent.

Intraocular involvement is rare, but uveitis, retinal vasculitis, retinal hemorrhage, capillary nonperfusion, vitreous hemorrhage, and papilledema have all been described.[85] These intraocular complications may occur in the absence of CNS disease.

Treatment is with oral tetracycline or intravenous chloramphenicol to eradicate the bacterium.

BRUCELLOSIS

Brucellosis is a zoonotic systemic infection caused by members of the bacterial genus *Brucella*. It was first identified in British soldiers serving on the Mediterranean island of Malta. The infection is transmitted by direct contact with infected animals but mostly by consumption of unpasteurized dairy products.

Brucellosis presents acutely with fever, fatigue, weight loss, abdominal pain, and arthralgia. If not treated, it enters a chronic phase with arthritis, sacroiliitis, and neurologic complications. Many other symptoms and signs can also occur.

The eye may be involved in either the acute or the chronic phase, and uveitis is the most common manifestation. Inflammation may cause granulomatous or nongranulomatous anterior uveitis, vitritis, retinitis, and choroiditis.[86] Retinal vasculitis may also occur. The diagnosis is easily overlooked in patients with chronic uveitis, and this condition remains an important health hazard in many developing countries.[86]

CAT SCRATCH DISEASE

Cat scratch disease is a zoonotic infection with *Bartonella henselae* (formerly classified under the genus *Rochalimaea*), a small gram-negative rod of the Rickettsiaceae family of the Proteobacteria. It causes asymptomatic bacteremia in domestic kittens. Infection in humans is nearly always a mild self-limiting condition[87]; it is considered to be the most common cause of chronic regional lymphadenopathy in children and young adults. A local papule or vesicle occurs at the inoculation site, followed in a few weeks by a tender regional lymphadenopathy that resolves over several months. Extranodal dissemination causes severe and sometimes widespread complications.

Primary infection affecting the ocular surface causes Parinaud's syndrome. More severe eye sequelae include neuroretinitis, optic neuritis, uveitis, retinitis, and focal choroiditis.[87]

Retinal vasculitis is not typically associated with cat scratch disease, although a few cases are being recognized.[88] The role of antibiotic treatment for the systemic disease is controversial.[87] It is advisable to treat the posterior segment manifestations with antibiotics to minimize visual loss from retinal and optic nerve damage, and ciprofloxacin has been used to treat retinal vasculitis and pars planitis with good effect.[88]

ROCKY MOUNTAIN SPOTTED FEVER

Rickettsia rickettsii, the cause of Rocky Mountain spotted fever, is transmitted to humans by the bite of an infected tick. It is the most common rickettsial disease in the United States, with up to 12,000 reported cases annually, the majority of which are from North Carolina.[88] Retinal involvement is uncommon and includes vascular occlusions, retinal edema, multiple cotton-wool spots, hemorrhages, vitritis, and retinal vasculitis.[89] The condition responds to intravenous doxycycline.

Protozoal

TOXOPLASMOSIS

The major features of toxoplasmosis chorioretinitis are described in detail elsewhere (see Chapter 33). As well as retinal and choroidal inflammation, retinal vascular involvement occurs, observed ophthalmoscopically as perivascular sheathing. The retinal veins may show continuous sheathing over long segments, with narrowing near acute lesions or segmental cuffing. Vessels adjacent to areas of active retinitis may be involved, but vessels at remote locations may also be sheathed.[90] Periarteritis may also be seen and it occasionally occurs without associated periphlebitis.[91] The perivasculitis is believed to be caused by an Arthus-type reaction.[92] Locally produced antigens diffuse into the vessel walls where they react with circulating antibodies, activate complement, and thereby recruit inflammatory cells that form a cuff of mononuclear cells around and in the vessel wall.[92]

Focal periarterial exudates or plaques, called Kyrieleis arteriolitis, are not associated with vessel leakage or obstruction, and their pathogenesis is unknown.[3]

The vasculitis resolves quickly with resolution of the disease and disappearance of the antigen.

Viral

CYTOMEGALOVIRUS

CMV retinitis is a common ocular infections in AIDS patients. Since the introduction of highly active antiretroviral therapy (HAART) with a combination of reverse transcriptases and protease inhibitors, the incidence of CMV retinitis is falling. Most patients are asymptomatic in the early stages. CMV causes fluffy white necrotic lesions along the vascular arcades of the posterior pole. The lesions have discrete edges. Retinal hemorrhages and vessel sheathing are also seen.[93] The vasculitis is caused by perivascular neutrophil infiltration of both the arteries and veins. There is usually little vitritis associated with CMV retinitis, but in HAART-treated patients inflammation is a prominent feature.

Treatment is with antiviral drugs ganciclovir, cidofovir,

or foscarnet. Lifelong maintenance therapy is required to prevent recurrence of retinitis, but it may be possible to discontinue this in some patients on HAART who have had prolonged remission, CD4+ counts above 100 cells/mm³, and negative CMV plasma load.

A recent report described CMV causing peripheral necrotizing retinitis, occlusive retinal vasculitis, and pan-uveitis in an immunocompromised patient.[94] This clinical picture is called acute retinal necrosis and is usually caused by herpes virus infection in immunocompetent individuals.

HERPES VIRUS

Retinal infections with herpes simplex or zoster viruses result in necrotizing retinitis, vasculitis, and retinal hemorrhage.[93] Acute retinal necrosis occurs in healthy people but has also been described in immunocompromised patients. A peripheral full-thickness necrotizing retinitis with a marked vitreal inflammatory reaction is associated with a severe occlusive vasculitis affecting arteries in the retina and choroid. The causative organism can be detected from intraocular fluids. Retinal detachment is a common late complication.

A severe, rapidly progressive form of herpetic retinopathy, progressive outer retinal necrosis, occurs in AIDS patients.[93] The retinal necrosis develops in multiple patches in the posterior pole and, in contrast to acute retinal necrosis, there is not a prominent vitritis. Retinal arteritis is not a prominent feature, although vessel sheathing occurs in and adjacent to areas of retinal necrosis. Severe periphlebitis similar to frosted branch angiitis is seen in immunocompromised patients with CMV or herpes simplex virus infections. It may also occur as a finding in immunocompetent patients with herpes simplex infection. In this instance, polymerase chain reaction analysis of intraocular fluids is helpful in identifying the correct diagnosis.[39]

HUMAN IMMUNODEFICIENCY VIRUS

Retinal vasculopathy occurs in up to 50% of patients with AIDS. It is usually a microvasculopathy with cotton-wool spots and retinal hemorrhages, but, particularly in African patients, isolated retinal vasculitis can occur.[95]

HUMAN T-CELL LYMPHOMA VIRUS TYPE I

This retrovirus causes two systemic diseases. One is adult T-cell malignancy, and the other is a chronic progressive neurologic disease called HTLV-1–associated myelopathy or tropical spastic paraparesis.[24] The virus is widespread and endemic in the Caribbean, South America, Central Africa, and southwestern Japan. It is also found in immigrants from these areas.

In a report of 12 female patients with adult-onset, slowly progressive myelopathy and anti–HTLV-1 antibodies, three were found to have peripheral retinal phlebitis.[96]

More recently, HTLV-1 antibodies were found in 44% of patients with idiopathic endogenous uveitis.[97] This incidence of seropositivity was much higher than that in the general population. In these patients with anterior uveitis, vitreous opacities were common. A mild retinal vascular change consisting of punctate white or yellow deposits scattered on the vessel wall was seen in 13 of the 32 cases. In addition, some patients had more classic retinal vasculitis consisting of perivascular sheathing associated with dye leakage and staining on fluorescein angiography.

RIFT VALLEY FEVER VIRUS

Rift Valley fever is an arthropod-borne RNA-virus disease of livestock that is widespread in eastern and southern Africa. Humans are infected by handling diseased and dead animals or their products. Epidemics affecting humans occasionally occur. From 1977 to 1978, an outbreak in Egypt killed 600 people.[98] In humans, the disease is an acute febrile illness with biphasic temperature elevations mimicking dengue fever. There are muscle and joint pains, headache, and nausea. Conjunctivitis and photophobia are common in the early phase.

Visual loss develops some days or weeks after subsidence of the fever. Ophthalmoscopy reveals acute necrotizing retinitis with cotton-wool spots, retinal hemorrhages, retinal edema, and occlusive retinal vasculitis.[98]

ACUTE RETINAL PERIPHLEBITIS AND UVEITIS ASSOCIATED WITH VIRAL-LIKE UPPER RESPIRATORY DISEASE

Following an upper respiratory or flu-like illness, some patients develop panuveitis and retinal periphlebitis. Patients complain of blurred vision, which usually resolves over a fortnight. The fundal and angiographic changes revert to normal appearance. An adenovirus has been cultured from the throat of one 9-year-old boy who had this presentation in association with pleocytosis in the cerebrospinal fluid.[3]

Drug-Induced Retinal Vasculitis

Retinal vasculitis has been reported in association with inhalation of methamphetamine,[99] rifabutin treatment,[100] and with intravenous immunoglobulin therapy.[101, 102] The latter association is of concern because intravenous immunoglobulins have been suggested as a treatment for refractory uveitis.

Retinal Vasculitis Secondary to Malignancy

CANCER-ASSOCIATED RETINOPATHY

Cancer-associated retinopathy is an uncommon paraneoplastic condition that develops in patients with neoplasia remote from the eye, typically small cell lung cancer. Patients present with visual loss and progressive night blindness, and examination reveals attenuated retinal vessels.

Retinal phlebitis and vitritis have been reported in a Japanese man with small cell lung cancer.[103] However, despite sheathing of retinal veins and staining of the vessel walls on fluorescein angiography, no inflammatory cells were identified in the retinal vessels at autopsy 6 months later. This may have been because of resolution of the vasculitis with systemic prednisolone therapy.

Another case with dramatic fluorescein angiographic evidence of retinal vasculitis was reported in a woman with lung cancer.[104] She had an antibody to a 62-kD bovine retinal protein but no reactivity to 23-kD retinal protein (recoverin).

Cancer-associated retinopathy is probably an autoimmune condition, and circulating antibodies to retinal cells and retinal antigens including recoverin have been identified in most of these patients.[105]

OCULAR LYMPHOMA

In elderly patients, ocular lymphoma presents as chronic uveitis, which is poorly responsive to steroid therapy.[106] Manifestations are variable and include subretinal plaques, retinal infiltrates, and hemorrhage. It may present as retinal vasculitis,[107] and subretinal pigment epithelial infiltrates, retinochoroiditis, and vasculitis were found in 60% patients who underwent vitrectomy for intraocular lymphoma.[108] Retinal vasculitis leads to vitritis, vessel sheathing, and perivascular exudates that can mimic frosted branch angiitis.

The tumor cells are clustered in the perivascular regions of the retina, and there is destruction of pigment epithelium and Bruch's membrane.[109]

ACUTE LEUKEMIA

Some patients with acute leukemia have retinal sheathing that can be extensive, presenting as acute unilateral frosted branch angiitis.[40]

Miscellaneous Causes of Retinal Vasculitis

Retinal vasculitis has been described in association with a variety of conditions. These include IgA nephritis,[110] uveitis associated with particular HLA phenotypes (HLA-B5 and HLA-DR4),[111] hemifacial atrophy,[112] and adult Kawasaki disease.[113]

COMPLICATIONS

The complications of retinal vasculitis are diverse (Table 77–2).[10, 20] Neovascularization occurs in about 10% to 15% of patients with retinal vasculitis.[10] The new vessels are sometimes associated with capillary closure identified by fluorescein angiography (see Fig. 77–3).[25] It is believed that angiogenic factors are released from the ischemic retina. These factors induce blood vessel growth, which is the cause of ischemic diabetic eye disease.[114]

In contrast, some eyes with retinal vasculitis and neovascularization do not show vessel closure, and fluorescein angiography reveals diffuse capillary leakage.[11] Thus, new vessels may develop perhaps as a response to hypoxia, or possibly from stimuli derived from inflamed retina or inflammatory cells.[11] In such cases, neovascularization may be seen to involute with anti-inflammatory therapy alone.

In addition to new vessels, arteriolar-venular anastomoses and other vascular architectural changes can also occur, often just temporal to the macula.[4]

Macular ischemia due to closure of perifoveal capillaries is seen in some patients.[115] Fluorescein angiography, which reveals an enlarged and irregular foveal avascular zone, confirms the diagnosis. This complication should be considered if vision remains poor despite adequate immunosuppression.

Severe ischemic disease may also lead to rubeosis of the iris and subsequent glaucoma. Untreated new vessels in the disc and retina bleed easily, and vitreous hemorrhage is an important cause of visual loss in patients with retinal vasculitis (see Fig. 77–5).[11, 20, 25] The hemorrhage absorbs without the tendency to tractional retinal detachments seen in diabetic maculopathy. This may be because of the posterior vitreous detachment that occurs in eyes with vitritis. Retinal detachment is a rare complication. However, when it develops, it is accompanied by severe proliferative vitreoretinopathy, particularly in eyes with active inflammation. Perioperative systemic corticosteroids are therefore recommended.[116]

Those patients who have retinal vasculitis as part of a systemic condition may also have nonophthalmic complications of their systemic disease. However, it must be remembered that sometimes the retinal vasculitis may precede the onset of systemic disease by many months or years, as in MS and sarcoidosis. These patients will be initially diagnosed as having idiopathic retinal vasculitis. The amount of investigation required to exclude systemic disease in patients presenting with retinal vasculitis is controversial. Recent evidence suggests that those patients without any relevant systemic history or clinical signs suggestive of an underlying disease do not require an extensive laboratory work-up.[20] The patients who do have clinical evidence suggesting systemic illness should have investigations tailored to those symptoms and signs. This approach is unlikely to miss serious disease and will prevent the expensive, sometimes misleading and occasionally dangerous, overinvestigation of patients who will not necessarily benefit from it. Appropriate investigations can be performed at any time if suggestive features develop.

Even those patients with true idiopathic retinal vasculitis without any evidence of any systemic disease are at increased risk of developing serious systemic morbidity, including stroke and myocardial infarction at a relatively young age.[26]

PATHOPHYSIOLOGY

Retinal vasculitis is believed to be an immunologically mediated condition. Direct evidence to support this proposition in humans is scarce, as biopsy in eyes with potentially useful vision is not practicable and peripheral blood investigations are not helpful in patients without systemic disease. However, isolated pathologic reports of eyes with retinal vasculitis in sarcoidosis[117] and ABD[6, 7, 118] have provided some valuable insight. Most of these eyes were removed because of secondary complications such as phthisis, pain, or glaucoma. The results therefore reflect end stages of the disease.

Some studies have examined eyes obtained after the death of the patient.[6] Although the inflammation will have been modulated by immunosuppressive treatment, these reports may more accurately reflect the pathology than studies of enucleated eyes.

The evidence of an autoimmune pathogenesis for retinal vasculitis is derived from experimental work in animals and indirectly from clinical studies.[119] The retina contains a number of tissue-specific antigens, one of which is retinal S-antigen. Experimental autoimmune uveoretinitis can be produced by immunizing animals with S-antigen.[120] The ocular inflammation induced by S-antigen is a marked retinal vasculitis accompanied by focal mononuclear cell infiltrate and necrosis of the photoreceptor cell layer. Interestingly, patients with retinal vasculitis also develop autoimmunity to this molecule.[120, 121]

Patients who have a systemic inflammatory disease could develop retinal vasculitis because of the presence of circulating immune complexes, non–organ-specific autoimmunity, or abnormal white cell function.[119] On the other hand, isolated retinal vasculitis may be an organ-specific autoimmune disease of the retina. In either case, the disease responds to immunosuppressive therapy.

The major component of the immune response is cell-mediated immunity, with cell adhesion molecules playing a critical role in recruiting leukocytes to the site of inflammation. Humoral immunity may also be an important component, but its role may be that of immunomodulation.[121]

Cell-Mediated Immunity

The cause of idiopathic retinal vasculitis is probably a disorder of immunity, which generates self-reacting T cells. It has been known for some time that patients with the clinical features of retinal perivasculitis have lymphocytes infiltrating in and around the retinal veins.[122] These lymphocytes are predominantly T cells[6, 117] of the CD4+ subtype.[7, 118] In one study a proportion of these T cells were found to be activated, expressing interleukin (IL)-2 receptors, which is remarkable considering that

the patient had been heavily immunosuppressed at the time of death.[6] CD8+ T cells were not found in the uvea or vasculitic lesions.[6, 118] A few cells in the hyalinized vessel walls were positive for the macrophage primary antibody but neutrophils were not present.[6]

The presence of CD4+ T cells as the predominant cell in the vascular lesions of the eye supports the assumption that retinal vasculitis is a cell-mediated condition. The absence of B cells and neutrophils is evidence that humoral immunity does not play a major role in the tissue damage. However, one study of five eyes found infiltrating B cells but only infrequently.[7] A more recent report on an enucleated eye from a patient with ABD identified focal clusters of CD19+ B cells in the uvea and retina.[118]

Adhesion Molecules

Cell adhesion molecules of the selectin, integrin, and immunoglobulin supergene families play an essential role in the development of inflammation. To produce vasculitis, circulating leukocytes must be recruited to the site of inflammation, where their speed is curbed by tethering of selectin molecules to carbohydrate moieties. The leukocytes move toward the vessel walls and begin to roll along the endothelium. This enables adherence to the vascular endothelium, and activation of the leukocyte. The sequential interactions of leukocyte adhesion mole-

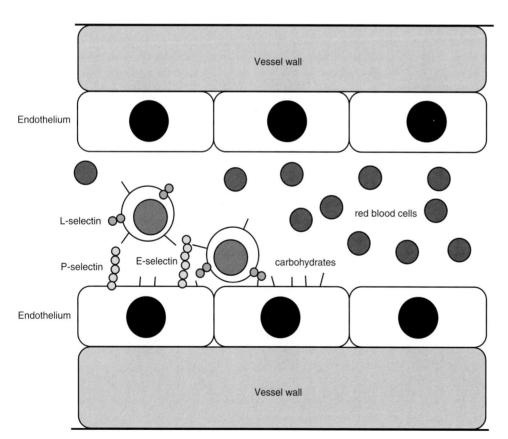

FIGURE 77–7. The cellular process involved in retinal vasculitis. *A,* Recruitment of inflammatory cells from the circulation.

Initial adhesion by selectins and carbohydrates slows the leukocytes. Once tethered the leukocytes begin to roll on the surface of the endothelium. The arrested leukocytes are to respond to cytokines and endothelial cell surface molecules.

A

cules with their receptors on the blood vessel wall are involved in each of these steps. Local action of chemokines also plays an important role (Fig. 77–7).[123]

Tethering and Rolling

The initial adhesion of leukocytes to the vascular endothelium is mediated by lectin-carbohydrate interactions (see Fig. 77–7A). The leukocyte L-selectin (CD62L) interacts with carbohydrates called addressins, which are present on the cell surface of vascular endothelial cells and are involved with cell trafficking in lymph nodes. These carbohydrate molecules are also induced at other sites during inflammation.

Activated vascular endothelium expresses P-selectin (CD62P) and later E-selectin (CD62E). Interaction of these selectins with carbohydrate moieties on the leukocyte, such as the sialyl Lewis-X carbohydrate associated with CD15 present on many leukocytes, slows their speed. Initial adhesion is followed by rolling of the white cells along the vascular endothelium.[124] Expression of P-selectin is up-regulated by inflammatory mediators including histamine. E-selectin is a cell surface glycoprotein that predominantly binds neutrophils. It is not normally expressed by vascular endothelium or ocular tissues. However, certain cytokines, including IL-1, interferon gamma,

and tumor necrosis factor alpha (TNF-α), induce expression of this molecule. In the rat endotoxin-uveitis model, E-selectin is up-regulated on corneal endothelium and vascular endothelium of the ciliary body within 12 hours and precedes the binding of neutrophils to inflamed tissues.[125] It is expressed only transiently and is mainly involved in the initial phases of leukocyte recruitment. E-selectin was not found in human eyes with chronic posterior uveitis except in the choroidal vasculature of one patient with sympathetic ophthalmia that exhibited choroidal neutrophil infiltration.[126]

Latching and Activation

Stronger attachment of the leukocytes then occurs via the β2 integrin family of adhesion molecules (see Fig. 77–7B). The integrins are composed of an α and a β subunit, which are each recognized by different antibodies. Thus, the CD11a antibody is directed against the α subunit and CD18 antibody against the β subunit of lymphocyte function–associated adhesion molecule-1, abbreviated LFA-1 (CD11a/CD18).

LFA-1 (CD11a/CD18) binds to an endothelial cell ligand called intercellular adhesion molecule-1 (ICAM-1 [CD54]). LFA-1 also binds to ICAM-2 (CD102) and ICAM-3 (CD50), so antibodies against all three ligands are

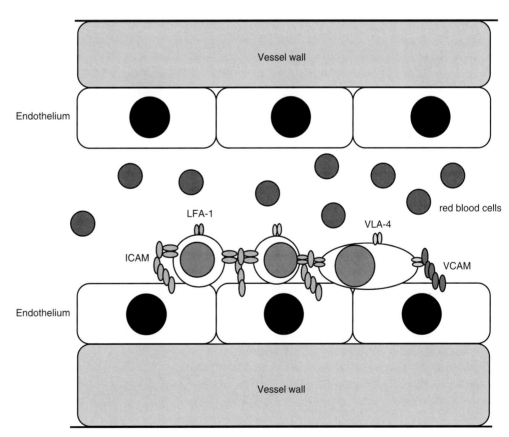

FIGURE 77–7 *Continued. B,* Adhesion and activation of lymphocytes.

Illustration continued on following page

Firm adhesion of the leukocyte, by interaction of its integrin receptors with members of the immunoglobulin supergene family on the endothelium, latches the cell to the vessel wall.

Activation of the leukocyte then occurs and it flattens onto the endothelium. The affinity of the leukocyte integrins is upregulated and expression of late binding proteins occurs. Binding to the cell adhesion molecules on the endothelium initiates migration.

B

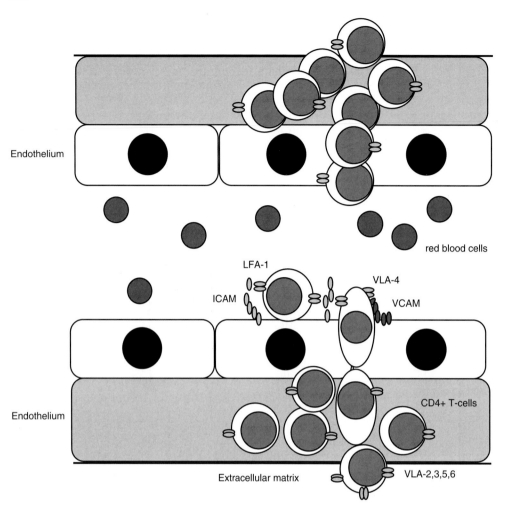

FIGURE 77–7 *Continued. C,* Transmigration of lymphocytes through the vascular endothelium and formation of perivascular inflammatory cell cuffing.

C
Cells migrate through the endothelium and basement membrane to form a perivascular cuff of inflammatory cells.
Lymphocytes interact with the extracellular matrix using β-integrins (VLA antigens).

required to completely block LFA-1–dependent, antigen-specific, T-cell responses. However, antibodies blocking LFA-1 or ICAM-1 alone are able to prevent lymphocyte proliferation in vivo and they also prevent lymphocyte homing and migration into the eye.[124] ICAM-1 is constitutively but weakly expressed by retinal vascular endothelium.[127] However, ICAM-1 is strongly expressed by retinal vascular endothelial cells in animals with experimental autoimmune uveitis.[124] Retinal and ciliary body vessels express ICAM-1 7 days after immunization with uveitogenic antigen, and this precedes retinal inflammatory cell infiltration. LFA-1 + leukocytes are subsequently recruited into the eye but are not observed for 9 days.[124] Furthermore, antibodies against β2 integrins prevent the development of endotoxin-induced uveitis.[128]

Similarly, ICAM-1 is strongly expressed on the vascular endothelium of retinal and choroidal blood vessels in patients with active posterior uveitis[126]; furthermore, the retinal cellular infiltrate is limited to those sites where ICAM-1 was expressed. ICAM-1 has also been demonstrated on the vascular endothelium of human eyes with retinal vasculitis.[118] Other adhesion molecules are also important, particularly in chronic disease. Those ex-

pressed in the later phases of lymphocyte activation are called very late antigens (VLA) and include VLA-4 (CD49d), which interacts with vascular cell adhesion molecule-1 (VCAM-1 [CD106]).

The expression of supergene family members by the vascular endothelium, ICAM-1 and VCAM-1, is up-regulated by inflammatory cytokines, TNF-α, interferon gamma, and IL-1.[128] TNF-α is found in human eyes with posterior uveitis localized to the areas of inflammation, and it may increase ICAM-1 expression by adjacent vascular endothelium.[126]

Migration

After passing through the vascular endothelium, the leukocytes lose L-selectin by enzymatic cleavage and begin to express the β1 family of integrins (the β-chain common to all of this family is recognized by anti-CD29). These receptors are the VLA, expressed only in the late stages of lymphocyte activation. They interact with collagen (VLA-2, VLA-3), laminin (VLA-3, VLA-6), and fibronectin (VLA-3, VLA-4, VLA-5) of the extracellular matrix. The migrated leukocytes form a cuff of cells around the vessel wall, which is visible ophthalmoscopically (see Fig 77–7C).

This evidence from animals and humans emphasizes the important role of CAMs for the recruitment of lymphocytes into the eye. It also suggests the therapeutic possibility of using antibodies against these molecules to treat retinal vasculitis.

Humoral Immunity and Immune Complexes

The role of antibodies and immune complexes in retinal vasculitis remains controversial, although type III hypersensitivity is a mechanism of tissue damage in systemic vasculitides. Antiretinal antibodies are found in 3.8% of normal individuals.[121] The prevalence of these autoantibodies is very much higher in patients with retinal vasculitis. In a large study of 150 patients with retinal vasculitis, antiretinal autoantibodies were found in 58% of patients.[121] It had previously been reported that patients with isolated retinal vasculitis who had more severe disease also had high levels of serum antiretinal antibodies.[119]

These same patients were also investigated for the presence of circulating immune complexes. Serum from patients with retinal vasculitis and systemic inflammatory disease (other than ABD) had elevated immune complexes and antiretinal antibodies.[121] Interestingly, these patients had lower disease severity scores, suggesting that immune complex formation may be a protective measure that mops up potentially dangerous antiretinal antibodies: Their presence may be the response to the inflammation, not the cause. Furthermore, those patients with ABD and sarcoidosis who had antiretinal antibodies but no immune complexes had the more severe disease.

The affinity of anti–S-antigen antibodies in patients with retinal vasculitis is lower than that of these antibodies when found in healthy control subjects.[129] It was suggested that high-affinity antibodies, which are also found in immune complexes, may be protective, and that patients who make low-affinity antibody are at increased risk of developing retinal vasculitis.

Thus, although overlooked in the presence of a dominating CD4+ T-cell response, retinal vasculitis may also have a humoral response, and this may have an immunoregulatory function perhaps influenced by immune complex formation.

TREATMENT

Historically, the treatment of retinal vasculitis has included deliberate infection with malaria, intravenous injection of milk or diphtheria proteins to induce shock, removal of teeth or appendectomy to clear possible infective foci, and paracentesis or deliberate injection of blood into the eye to introduce antibodies.[5] The introduction of steroids in the 1950s changed the management of uveitis. Oral corticosteroids remain the main therapeutic drugs, but other immunosuppressive agents have an increasing role.

Not all patients with retinal vasculitis require treatment. Treatment is indicated for cystoid macular edema, for severe vitritis affecting vision, for severe ischemia identified by fluorescein angiography as large areas of capillary drop-out, or if capillary destruction is identified around the foveal avascular zone.

It is important to have assessed the patient for infection with a careful history and eye and physical exams. Laboratory tests including serology, chest radiograph, and, if necessary, vitreous humor analysis are tailored, according to any findings on history and examination.[20]

If infection is identified, appropriate antimicrobial or antiviral therapy is mandatory before attempting immunosuppression. Likewise, identification of any underlying systemic disease is important, not only to help direct therapy for the ocular inflammation but also to control life-threatening complications of autoimmune diseases.

Thrombophilic abnormalities are present in about one third of patients with retinal vasculitis.[130]

Observation

If the patient has only mild vascular changes with little vitritis and no cystoid macular edema, then careful clinical observation is often all that is required. At all times the risks of systemic treatment must be borne in mind; because most patients will require treatment for years and be put at risk of developing iatrogenic complications, treatment may be unnecessary.

There is an increased risk of cardiovascular events in patients with retinal vasculitis. It is therefore important to minimize the impact of other risk factors for cardiovascular disease, even in patients who are not being treated, by checking for hypertension, hyperlipidemia, and diabetes. Patients should also be advised to stop smoking.

Medical Therapy

Several immunosuppressive drugs are available to the physician to modulate the inflammatory response in retinal vasculitis. No formal randomized controlled trials have been conducted on these treatments for retinal vasculitis because of the rarity of the conditions and the variety and complications of associated systemic diseases, which may also direct treatment choices. However, literature on series of cases exists and extrapolation of data from controlled trials for the treatment of panuveitis enables rational decisions to be made in treating patients with retinal vasculitis.

Corticosteroids

The choice of drug to use has traditionally centered on corticosteroids as the first line of therapy. They may be administered topically to control anterior uveitis, regionally (as sub-Tenon's or peribulbar injections) for mild unilateral disease, or systemically, usually by mouth but also by intravenous pulse therapy.

Oral corticosteroids have been shown to be an effective treatment for retinal vasculitis.[131] Treatment was initiated in a high dose: 80 mg of prednisolone for 4 days, then 60 mg for 4 days, followed by 40 mg for 1 month, tapering thereafter according to clinical response. Myles[132] felt that the failure to control retinal vasculitis was commonly caused by instituting therapy at too low a dose.

However, steroid treatment is potentially dangerous, and the incidence of serious side effects of high-dose or long-term treatment is frequently underestimated. For example, the main cause of death and morbidity in patients with giant cell arteritis is the corticosteroid treatment.[133] An excellent summary of complications of steroid therapy in the treatment of inflammatory eye disease has recently been published.[133] In the United Kingdom, the expert working group of the Medicines Control Agency and the Committee on Safety of Medicines has revised their guidelines for the use of systemic steroids. It now recommends that patients should be given treatment for the shortest time at the lowest dose that is clinically necessary.[134]

Immunosuppressive Drugs

Because of these concerns, many uveitis specialists are moving away from systemic steroids, or at least they use protocols that minimize dose and duration of treatment.[135] To reduce the total steroid dose, or in cases where retinal vasculitis is poorly controlled, steroid-sparing immunosuppressive drugs are required. Furthermore, steroids alone are insufficient treatment for certain specific conditions, and other immunosuppressive drugs are required to control both the ocular inflammation and the systemic manifestations of the disease.[136] However, the potentially serious side effects and bewildering array of immunosuppressive drugs have limited their use despite the undoubted benefits of immunosuppression in inflammatory eye disease, including retinal vasculitis. Much light has been shed on the issue with reviews from Boston[136] and more recently from Aberdeen[135] that have described clear guidelines for the use of immunosuppression in ocular inflammatory disease and posterior uveitis.

Following early trials that demonstrated its efficacy in high doses,[137] low-dose cyclosporine A has become the most common steroid-sparing agent for the treatment of retinal vasculitis.[135, 138] The starting dose is 2.5 to 5 mg/kg/day, usually given as a twice-daily regime. The major side effects include nephrotoxicity, hypertension, hirsutism, and gum hypertrophy.[133, 135, 136] However, a plethora of other problems may occur, including elevated serum levels of cyclosporin A caused by drugs or dietary grapefruit juice and the ominous possibility of increasing the risk of skin or lymphoid tumors in the distant future.

For patients who are unable to tolerate cyclosporine, tacrolimus (formerly known as FK506) is a good alternative with a similar mode of action.[139] Other immunosuppressive agents, including methotrexate, azathioprine, colchicine, chlorambucil, and cyclophosphamide, are used in treating retinal vasculitis. These agents also have a role in managing ABD.[136]

More recently, mycophenolate mofetil (CellCept) has become available. It is rapidly hydrolyzed in vivo by plasma esterases to mycophenolic acid, the active molecule, which inhibits inosine monophosphate dehydrogenase. This inhibition of the de novo pathway of purine synthesis is relatively selective to lymphocyte proliferation, sparing other cells such as neutrophils, which can use an alternative salvage pathway to obtain purines.[140] It is also useful in some patients with autoimmune disease, in whom it has been used to treat cases of refractory uveitis, intermediate uveitis, and ABD panuveitis.[141, 142] It has a particular use for patients who fail to respond, have toxicity, or are intolerant of cyclosporin.[141]

Systemic vasculitis is sometimes treated using intrave-

nous immunoglobulin.[143] If it is administered within 10 days of onset of Kawasaki disease, the incidence of coronary aneurysms is reduced. Intravenous immunoglobulins may also be helpful for treating the occasional patient with intractable retinal vasculitis. The mode of action is incompletely understood. It may act by directly bonding autoantibody, blocking crystallizable fragment (Fc) receptors, modulating cytokine interactions, and inhibiting complement.[143] Potential toxicity, the possibility for transmission of viruses, and reports of retinal vasculitis associated with this therapy limit its widespread use.[102]

Plasma exchange has been used to interrupt the acute inflammatory activity of retinal vasculitis in cases of ABD.[144] However, it does not prevent relapse, and the long-term prognosis in the four patients in that study was poor. Plasma exchange is also expensive and invasive, so it is not recommended for routine use.

Immunoregulation

More specific immunoregulation of autoimmune disease is becoming a reality with the advent of specific monoclonal antibodies (mAb) against lymphocytes and cytokine receptors.[145, 146] Another approach, based on successful experiments in animals, is to use retinal antigens to induce tolerance in the recipient.[147] These methods are being adapted to treat inflammatory eye disease including retinal vasculitis.

A panlymphocyte mAb, Campath 1H, controlled retinal vasculitis that had been refractory to all prior treatments.[148] Long-term benefit resulted from the short-term treatment, suggesting that modulating the immune system in this fashion could potentially induce tolerance.

TNF plays a crucial role in inflammation. Recently, the use of anticytokine therapy in Crohn's disease and rheumatoid arthritis has shown potential.[149] Two approaches are being used. One uses a human-mouse chimeric antibody, called infliximab, directed against TNF-α. The other uses a soluble TNF receptor called etanercept. Infliximab combined with methotrexate prevents antibodies against infliximab being formed and produces significant clinical benefit. Etanercept is a fusion protein made up of two recombinant p75 TNF receptors fused with the Fc portion of human IgG1. It binds both TNF-α and TNF-β (lymphotoxin). Again, impressive results in patients with rheumatoid arthritis have been reported.

It seems very likely that blocking adhesion molecules, antilymphocyte, or anticytokine therapy will also have a role for patients with refractory retinal vasculitis.

In the future, it may be possible to make the patient tolerant to retinal autoantigens given by mouth or intranasally. Inhibition of experimental autoimmune uveitis can be achieved by feeding animals S-antigen orally.[149] Tolerance to an autoantigen can spread to other antigens because of the local release of suppressor cytokines (such as transforming growth factor-β, IL-4, IL-10). Therefore, although many potential retinal autoantigens are involved in producing retinal vasculitis, immunization against one or a few may be enough to prevent disease. On this basis, a randomized, masked trial of oral tolerance has been conducted, with demonstration of an effect with an absence of side effects.[150] Although not statistically significant, the results are promising, but they must be interpreted cautiously because of the late stage of disease treated. Furthermore, the confounding effect of concurrent immunosuppressive therapy could easily influence the active mechanism by which tolerance is produced.

Laser Treatment

The use of laser photocoagulation in retinal vasculitis is controversial. It is rarely required for treating retinal vasculitis, and the main indication is for persistent neovascularization causing recurrent vitreous hemorrhage, and less frequently for treating rubeotic glaucoma.[5, 11] Retinal neovascularization associated with ocular inflammation is quite different from other proliferative retinopathies. First, the visual prognosis is better in patients with retinal vasculitis, possibly because of the associated posterior vitreous detachment, which removes the scaffold for elevated new vessels. In addition, new vessels regress with medical treatment in many cases.[11] There is a high incidence of macular edema developing after laser treatment in retinal vasculitis. Laser treatment is therefore reserved to treat those eyes with recurrent vitreous hemorrhage once adequate immunosuppressive treatment has been used.[11] In contrast to these recommendations, other authorities suggest that aggressive retinal laser should be used more frequently, even in those patients without neovascularization.[4] However, there is a risk of provoking further inflammatory episodes with retinal photocoagulation.

In India, laser treatment of retinal vasculitis is used more commonly, often as a primary therapy to manage the complications of Eales' disease.[151] Photocoagulation of proliferative retinopathy in Eales' disease has been used for over 30 years. Meyer-Schwickerath used xenon–arc light photocoagulation in a series of 176 eyes with Eales' disease and proliferative retinopathy.[152] Of the treated eyes, 124 remained symptom free over the follow-up period of 1 to 8 years. Eales' disease mainly affects the peripheral retina, and xenon-arc is not an ideal method of photocoagulation. Laser photocoagulation has therefore become the treatment of choice for the proliferative phase of Eales' disease,[151] but it is not useful for controlling the inflammatory phase. Laser burns are placed in areas of retinal neovascularization, capillary nonperfusion, microaneurysms, and arteriovenous shunt vessels (Fig. 77–8).[151] Direct treatment of flat retinal neovascularization is performed with argon laser spots of moderate intensity (2 to 500 μm diameter and 0.1 sec duration). Elevated new vessels are treated by coagulation of their feeder vessels. Panretinal photocoagulation is required if there are disc new vessels. Spot size is 500 μm for 0.1 sec duration and 1500 to 2000 burns are applied over two or three treatment sessions.

Vitrectomy

Recurrent vitreous hemorrhage is a major cause of visual loss in retinal vasculitis, and this is particularly the case for patients with Eales' disease. The first vitreous hemorrhage usually settles inferiorly with gravity and is absorbed over a few weeks or months, with restoration of central vision. Recurrent vitreous hemorrhages are a greater problem and lead to traction bands and membranes in the vitreous, which cause further complications.[151] The

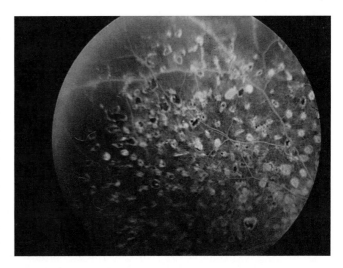

FIGURE 77–8. Sector retinal laser burns on an area of capillary nonperfusion and previous neovascularization in a patient with retinal vasculitis.

objective of surgery is to remove the vitreous opacity and the posterior vitreous face. Other surgical procedures are often required at the same sitting, including lensectomy to enable a clear view. Epiretinal membrane removal, endolaser, and cryotherapy with scleral buckling are frequently required.[151, 153] The prognosis following surgery is generally good, and most patients can expect to have a significant improvement of vision. Patients who have had fewer episodes of recurrent hemorrhage of shorter duration and who have had laser photocoagulation prior to vitrectomy fare better than patients with longstanding vitreous hemorrhage.[151]

PROGNOSIS

The diagnosis of retinal vasculitis has implications for general health as well as for sight. Appropriate counseling and management is therefore important to prevent complications or at least to minimize their impact.

To a large extent, the prognosis for the health of patients who have apparently isolated retinal vasculitis depends on whether an associated systemic disease subsequently develops. An extended 6-year follow-up study of 67 patients who had retinal vasculitis and intermediate uveitis found significant systemic morbidity.[26] These patients were divided on the basis of fluorescein angiography into two groups: ischemic, or nonischemic and leaky. Of the 45 patients in the nonischemic group, 28% subsequently developed MS. Most of these were women with HLA-B7. No patients in the ischemic group developed MS, but a third developed premature cardiovascular disease including stroke and myocardial infarction. Thus, even retinal vasculitis that is not associated with systemic autoimmune disease may still affect the prognosis for the patient's general health or longevity. This is important to recognize, as patients with retinal vasculitis are usually young.[10, 20]

More recently, studies of soluble ICAM-1 and IL-8 in the serum of patients with intermediate uveitis have been correlated with a predisposition to developing an associated systemic disease.[154] Using such tools will help to limit expensive and invasive diagnostic tests to those patients who are most likely to benefit from them.

Other patients develop retinal vasculitis as a component of a preexisting generalized disease. In such cases, the management of their systemic condition largely determines the prognosis for health.

The prognosis for sight varies among many different diseases, with most patients who have mild peripheral retinal phlebitis retaining good vision, often without treatment. In contrast, those patients with ABD often have a dire long-term prospect for sight despite aggressive immunosuppression.

Visual prognosis in retinal vasculitis also depends on whether there is ischemia noted on fluorescein angiography. A retrospective study of 54 patients found that 24% of patients with ischemic disease had a visual acuity of less than 6/60 at presentation. The percentage increased to 34% of patients over a mean follow-up period of 8.2 years.[25] In contrast, only 10% of the nonischemic group had a visual acuity of less than 6/60 and this percentage did not increase over the follow-up. Thus, patients with ischemic disease have a much poorer visual outcome because of cystoid macular edema, recurrent vitreous hemorrhage, and branch retinal vein occlusions. The worst visual outcome occurred despite aggressive immunosuppression, which suggests that other treatment, including anticoagulation, might also be needed in these patients. Interestingly, smoking was more prevalent in the ischemic group. It was postulated that von Willebrand's factor and fibrinogen, which are elevated in smokers, could put them at particular risk of capillary closure if they develop retinal vasculitis.[131] However, smoking also damages vascular endothelium directly and this mechanism could also be involved.

CONCLUSIONS
Retinal vasculitis is an important condition that is a component of many systemic inflammatory and infectious diseases. Idiopathic retinal vasculitis is uncommon in the western hemisphere, but Eales' disease (a type of retinal vasculitis associated with capillary shut-down and neovascular proliferation) occurs more frequently in India.

Whom to Investigate
Although retinal vasculitis can occur as part of a systemic disease, extensive investigation to uncover occult disease is not often required. A careful history, physical, and ocular exam will usually indicate which patients require a more extensive work-up.[20] Those with systemic disease need assessment for treatment, which often requires a multidisciplinary team approach for the best outcome. The role of the ophthalmologist is to preserve sight and to highlight the importance of the eye as a major target for organ damage.

Exclude Infection
Retinal vasculitis commonly occurs in toxoplasmosis and in posterior segment infections caused by viruses. If infection is identified, appropriate antimicrobial therapy is instituted, often with steroids to reduce the collateral damage from the inflammatory response.

Recommended Treatment Protocol
Patients with isolated retinal vasculitis do not necessarily require treatment. Those with sight-threatening complications are started on a regime designed to minimize the total dose of steroids.[135]

1. *The acute stage.* Systemic steroids are started at a dose of 0.5 to 1.0 mg/kg/day. Occasionally, intravenous pulse methylprednisolone 1 g/day for 3 days is required.
2. *Long-term control.* To allow steroid dosage to be reduced, low-dose cyclosporin therapy 5 mg/kg/day is also given. After 3 to 6 weeks, when control has been achieved, the dose of systemic steroid is tapered and if possible discontinued. Monotherapy with cyclosporin or combination therapy with low-dose steroid can be continued for months or years if necessary.
3. *Additional immunosuppression.* Other drugs are required if inflammation persists despite cyclosporin and low-dose steroid. A variety of agents can be used in combination or as alternatives to the maintenance regime. In certain special instances, patients with specific diagnoses such as Wegener's disease will require additional immunosuppression to control the life-threatening complications of their systemic disease.

Patients who are not responding to therapy also require the attention of specialists to exclude rare infections or malignancy. This may require unusual investigations that are not routinely available.

References
1. Duke-Elder S: Diseases of the retina. In: System of Ophthalmology. London, Henry Kimpton, 1967, pp 218–236.
2. AbuEl-Asrar A, Tabbara K: Retinal vasculitis. Curr Opin Ophthalmol 1997;8:68–79.
3. Gass JDM: The Macula. St. Louis, C.V. Mosby, 1997, pp 663–665.
4. Nussenblatt R, Whitcup S, Palestine A: Retinal vasculitis. In: Uveitis: Fundamentals and Clinical Practice. St. Louis, Mosby, 1996, pp 354–363.
5. Charteris D, Champ C, Rosenthal AR, et al: Behçet's disease–activated T lymphocytes in retinal perivasculitis. Br J Ophthalmol 1992;76:499–501.
6. Charteris D, Barton K, McCartney AC, et al: CD4+ lymphocyte involvement in ocular Behçet's disease. Autoimmunity 1992;12:201–206.
7. Gass JDM, Olson C: Sarcoidosis with optic nerve and retinal involvement. Arch Ophthalmol 1976;94:945–950.
8. Bisighini S, Pagliuso L: Retinal vasculitis: A diagnostic dilemma. Clin Eye Vis Care 1997;9:71–84.
9. Graham E, Stanford M, Whitcup S: Retinal vasculitis. In: Pepose J, Holland G, Wihelmus K, eds: Ocular Infection and Immunity. St. Louis, Mosby, 1996, pp 538–551.
10. Graham E, Stanford MR, Sanders MD, et al: A point prevalence study of 150 patients with retinal vasculitis: 1. Diagnostic value of ophthalmological features. Br J Ophthalmol 1989;73:714–721.
11. Graham E, Stanford MR, Shilling JS, et al: Neovascularization associated with posterior uveitis. Br J Ophthalmol 1987;71:826–833.
12. Theobald S: A case of recurrent retinal hemorrhages followed by the outgrowth of numerous blood vessels from the optic disc into the vitreous humor. Trans Am Ophthalmol Soc 1887;4:542.
13. Perls M: Zur Kenntniss der Tuberculose des Auges. Graefes Arch Ophthalmol 1873;19:221–246.
14. Wadsworth: Recurrent retinal hemorrhage followed by the development of blood vessels in the vitreous. Ophthalmol Rev 1887;6:289.
15. Eales H: Retinal hemorrhages associated with epistaxis and constipation. Birmingham Med Rev 1880;9:262–273.

16. Eales H: Primary retinal hemorrhage in young men. Ophthalmol Rev 1881;1:41–46.

17. Patnaik B, et al: Eales disease: Clinical features, pathophysiology, etiopathogenesis. Ophthalmol Clin North Am 1998;11:601–617.

18. Rucker C: Sheathing of retinal veins in multiple sclerosis. Mayo Clin Proc 1944;19:176–178.

19. Vadot E: Epidemiology of intermediate uveitis: a prospective study in Savoy. In: Boke W, Manthey K, Nussenblatt R, eds: Intermediate Uveitis. Basel, Karger, 1990, pp 33–34.

20. George T, Walton RC, Whitcup SM, et al: Primary retinal vasculitis: Systemic associations and diagnostic evaluation. Ophthalmology 1996;103:384–389.

21. Chee S: Retinal disease associated with systemic disease. Ophthalmol Clin North Am 1998;11:655–671.

22. Ito Y, et al: Frosted branch angiitis in a child. Jpn J Clin Ophthalmol 1976;30:797–803.

23. Duke-Elder S: Diseases of the uveal tract. In: System of Ophthalmology. London, Kimpton, 1966, pp 525–531.

24. Nakao K, Ohba N: HTLV-1 associated uveitis revisited: Characteristic gray white granular deposits on retinal vessels. Br J Ophthalmol 1996;80:719–722.

25. Palmer HE, Stanford MR, Sanders MD, et al: Visual outcome of patients with idiopathic ischemic and non-ischemic retinal vasculitis. Eye 1996;10:343–348.

26. Palmer HE, Zaman AG, Edelsten CE, et al: Systemic morbidity in patients with isolated idiopathic retinal vasculitis. Lancet 1995;346:505–506.

27. Helm CJ, Holland GN: Ocular tuberculosis. Surv Ophthalmol 1993;38:229.

28. Kharashi SA, Asrar AM: Full panretinal photocoagulation and early vitrectomy improve prognosis of Eales' disease. Saudi J Ophthalmol 1998;12:175.

29. Ashton N: Pathogenesis and aetiology of Eales' disease. In: Pandit YK, ed: Nineteenth International Congress of Ophthalmology. Bombay, 1962, p 20.

30. Muthukkaruppan V, Rengarajan K, Chakkalath HR, et al: Immunological status of patients of Eales' disease. Indian J Med Res 1989;90:351.

31. Renie WA, Murphy RP, Anderson KC, et al: The evaluation of patients with Eales' disease. Retina 1983;3:243–248.

32. Johnson MW, Thomley ML, Huang SS, et al: Idiopathic recurrent branch artery occlusion: Natural history and laboratory investigations. Ophthalmology 1994;101:480–489.

33. Kincaid J, Schatz H: Bilateral retinal arteritis with multiple aneurysmal dilatations. Retina 1983;3:171–178.

34. Chang TS, Aylward GW, David JL, et al: Idiopathic retinal vasculitis, aneurysms and neuroretinitis. Ophthalmology 1995;102:1089–1097.

35. Matsuo T, Matsuo N: Bilateral iridocyclitis and retinal capillaritis in juveniles. Ophthalmology 1997;104:939–944.

36. Blumenkrantz MS, Kaplan HJ, Clarkson JG, et al: Acute multifocal hemorrhagic retinal vasculitis. Ophthalmology 1988;95:1663–1672.

37. Kleiner RC, Kaplan HL, Shakin JL, et al: Acute frosted retinal periphlebitis. Am J Ophthalmol 1988;106:27–34.

38. Spaide RF, Vitale AT, Toth IR, et al: Frosted branch angiitis associated with cytomegalovirus retinitis. Am J Ophthalmol 1992;113:522–528.

39. Chatzoulis DM, Thesdosiadis PG, Apostolopoulos MN, et al: Retinal perivasculitis in an immunocompetent patient with systemic herpes simplex infection. Am J Ophthalmol 1997;123:699–702.

40. Kim T, Duker J, Hedges T: Retinal angiopathy resembling unilateral frosted branch angiitis in a patient with relapsing acute lymphoblastic leukemia. Am J Ophthalmol 1994;117:806–808.

41. Gass J, Tiedeman J, Thomas M: Idiopathic recurrent branch retinal arterial occlusion. Ophthalmology 1986;93:1148–1157.

42. Coppeto JR, Currie JN, Monteiro ML, et al: A syndrome of arterial-occlusive retinopathy and encephalopathy. Am J Ophthalmol 1984;98:189–202.

43. Welch R, Maumenee A, Wahlen H: Peripheral posterior segment inflammation, vitreous opacities and edema of the posterior pole. Arch Ophthalmol 1960;64:540–549.

44. Priem H, Oosterhuis J: Birdshot chorioretinopathy: Clinical characteristics and evolution. Br J Ophthalmol 1988;72:646–659.

45. Soubrane G, Bokobza R, Coscas G: Late developing lesions in birdshot retinochoroidopathy. Am J Ophthalmol 1990;109:204–210.

46. Lubin J, Albert D, Weinstein M: Sixty-five years of sympathetic ophthalmia: A clinicopathologic review of cases (1913–1978). Ophthalmology 1980;87:109–121.

47. Okamura S: Harada's disease. Acta Soc Ophthalmol Jpn 1938;42:196.

48. Snyder D, Tessler H: Vogt-Koyanagi-Harada syndrome. Am J Ophthalmol 1980;90:69–75.

49. Vine A: Retinal vasculitis. Semin Neurol 1994;14:354–360.

50. Arnold AC, Pepose JS, Hepler RS, et al: Retinal periphlebitis and retinitis in multiple sclerosis: 1. Pathological characteristics. Ophthalmology 1984;91:255–262.

51. Tola M, Granieri E, Casetta I: Retinal periphlebitis in multiple sclerosis: A marker of disease activity? Eur Neurol 1993;33:93–96.

52. Malinowski S, Pulido J, Folk J: Long-term visual outcome and complications associated with pars planitis. Ophthalmology 1993;100:818–825.

53. Engell T, Anderson P: The frequency of periphlebitis retinae in multiple sclerosis. Acta Neurol Scand 1982;65:601–608.

54. Birch MK, Barbosa S, Blumhardt LD, et al: Retinal venous sheathing and the blood retinal barrier in multiple sclerosis. Arch Ophthalmol 1996;114:34–39.

55. Graham EM, Spalton DJ, Barnard RO, et al: Cerebral and retinal vascular changes in systemic lupus erythematosus. Ophthalmology 1985;92:444–448.

56. Bettoni L, Juvarra G, Bortone E, et al: Isolated benign cerebral vasculitis. Case report and review. Acta Neurol Belg 1984;84:161–173.

57. Jabs D, Johns C: Ocular involvement in chronic sarcoidosis. Am J Ophthalmol 1986;102:297–301.

58. Spalton D, Sanders M: Fundus changes in histologically confirmed sarcoidosis. Br J Ophthalmol 1981;65:348–358.

59. Birnbaum W, Prinzmetal M, Connor C: Generalized thromboangiitis obliterans: Report of a case with involvement of retinal vessels and suprarenal infarction. Arch Intern Med 1934;53:410–422.

60. Gresser E: Partial occlusion of retinal vessels in a case of thromboangiitis obliterans. Am J Ophthalmol 1932;15:235–237.

61. Lyons J, Rosenbaum J: Uveitis associated with inflammatory bowel disease. Arch Ophthalmol 1997;115:61–64.

62. Duker J, Brown G, Brooks L: Retinal vasculitis in Crohn's disease. Am J Ophthalmol 1987;103:664–668.

63. Ruby A, Jampol L: Crohn's disease and retinal vascular disease. Am J Ophthalmol 1990;110:349–353.

64. Matsuo T, Koyama T, Morimoto N, et al: Retinal vasculitis as a complication of rheumatoid arthritis. Ophthalmologica 1990;201:196–200.

65. Giordano N, D'Ettore M, Biasi G, et al: Retinal vasculitis in rheumatoid arthritis: An angiographic study. Clin Exp Rheumatol 1990;8:121–125.

66. Stanford M, Graham E: Systemic associations of retinal vasculitis. Int Ophthalmol Clin 1991;31:23–33.

67. Rosenbaum J, Bennett R: Chronic anterior and posterior uveitis and primary Sjögren's syndrome. Am J Ophthalmol 1987;104:346–352.

68. Farmer S, Kinysua JL, Nelson JL, et al: Retinal vasculitis associated with autoantibodies to Sjögren's syndrome A antigen. Am J Ophthalmol 1985;100:814–821.

69. Stafford-Brady F, Urowitz MB, Gladman DD, et al: Lupus retinopathy. Patterns, associations and prognosis. Arthritis Rheum 1988;31:1105–1110.

70. Jabs D, Fine SL, Hochberg MC, et al: Severe retinal vaso-occlusive disease in systemic lupus erythematosus. Arch Ophthalmol 1986;104:558–563.

71. Accinni L, Dixon F: Degenerative vascular disease and myocardial infarction in mice with lupus-like syndrome. Am J Pathol 1979;96:477–492.

72. Bullen C, Liesegang TJ, McDonald TJ, et al: Ocular complications of Wegener's granulomatosis. Ophthalmology 1983;90:279–290.

73. Harman L, Margo C: Wegener's granulomatosis. Surv Ophthalmol 1998;42:458–480.

74. Haynes B, Fishman ML, Fauci AS, et al: The ocular manifestations of Wegener's granulomatosis: Fifteen years experience and a review of the literature. Am J Med 1977;63:131–141.

75. Soukiasian SH, Foster CS, Niles JL, et al: Diagnostic value of anti-neutrophil cytoplasmic antibodies in scleritis associated with Wegener's granulomatosis. Ophthalmology 1992;99:125.

76. Morgan C, Foster CS, D'Amico DJ, et al: Retinal vasculitis in polyarteritis nodosa. Retina 1986;6:205–209.

77. Isaak BL, Liesegang TJ, Michet CJ: Ocular and systemic findings in relapsing polychondritis. Ophthalmology 1986;93:681.

78. Helm C, Holland G: Ocular tuberculosis. Surv Ophthalmol 1993;38:229–256.

79. Rosen P, Spalton D, Graham E: Intraocular tuberculosis. Eye 1990;4:486–492.

80. Shah S, Howard RS, Sarkies NJ, et al: Tuberculosis presenting as retinal vasculitis. J R Soc Med 1988;81:232–233.

81. Margo C, Hamed A: Ocular syphilis. Surv Ophthalmol 1992;37:203–220.

82. Lobes L, Folk J: Syphilitic phlebitis simulating branch vein occlusion. Ann Ophthalmol 1981;13:127–135.

83. Karma A, Seppala I, Mikkila H, et al: Diagnosis and clinical characteristics of ocular Lyme borreliosis. Am J Ophthalmol 1995;119:127–135.

84. Schubert H, Greenbaum E, Neu HC: Cytologically proven seronegative Lyme choroiditis and vitritis. Retina 1994;14:39–42.

85. Avila M, Jalkh AE, Feldman E, et al: Manifestations of Whipple's disease in the posterior segment of the eye. Arch Ophthalmol 1984;102:384–390.

86. Tabbara K, Al-Kassimi H: Ocular borreliosis. Br J Ophthalmol 1990;74:249–250.

87. Ormerod L, Skolnick KA, Menosky MM, et al: Retinal and choroidal manifestations of cat-scratch disease. Ophthalmology 1998;105:1024–1031.

88. Soheilian M, Markomichelakis N, Foster CS: Intermediate uveitis and retinal vasculitis as manifestations of cat scratch disease. Am J Ophthalmol 1996;122:582–584.

89. Duffey R, Hammer M: The ocular manifestations of Rocky Mountain spotted fever. Ann Ophthalmol 1987;19:301–313.

90. Pavesion C, Lightman S: *Toxoplasma gondii* and ocular toxoplasmosis: Pathogenesis. Br J Ophthalmol 1996;80:1099–1107.

91. Schwartz P: Segmental retinal periarteritis as a complication of toxoplasmosis. Ann Ophthalmol 1977;9:157–162.

92. O'Connor G: The influence of hypersensitivity on the pathogenesis of ocular toxoplasmosis. Trans Am Ophthalmol Soc 1970;68:501–547.

93. Yoser S, Forster D, Rao N: Systemic viral infections and their retinal and choroidal manifestations. Surv Ophthalmol 1993;37:313–352.

94. Akpek E, Kent C, Jakobiec F, et al: Bilateral acute retinal necrosis caused by cytomegalovirus in an immunocompromised patient. Am J Ophthalmol 1999;127:93–95.

95. Kestelyn P, Lepage L, Perre PV: Perivasculitis of the retinal vessels as an important sign in children with the AIDS-related complex. Am J Ophthalmol 1985;100:614–615.

96. Sasaki K, Morooka I, Inomata H, et al: Retinal vasculitis in human T-lymphotrophic virus type-1 associated myelopathy. Br J Ophthalmol 1989;73:812–815.

97. Nakao K, Ohba N: Clinical features of HTLV-1 associated uveitis. Br J Ophthalmol 1993;77:274–279.

98. Siam A, Meegan H, Gharbawi K: Rift Valley fever ocular manifestations: Observations during the 1977 epidemic in Egypt. Br J Ophthalmol 1980;64:366–374.

99. Shaw H, Lawson J, Stulting R: Amaurosis fugax and retinal vasculitis associated with methamphetamine inhalation. J Clin Neuroophthalmol 1985;5:169–176.

100. Arevalo J, Russack V, Freeman W: New ophthalmic manifestations of presumed rifabutin-related uveitis. Ophthalmic Surg Lasers 1997;28:321–324.

101. Ayliffe W, Haeney M, Roberts SC, et al: Uveitis after antineutrophil cytoplasmic antibody contamination of immunoglobulin replacement therapy. Lancet 1992;339:558–559.

102. Vogele C, Andrassy K, Schmidbauer JM, et al: Retinal vasculitis and uveitis—An adverse reaction to intravenous immunoglobulins. Nephron 1994;67:363.

103. Ohnishi Y, Ohara S, Sakamoto T, et al: Cancer associated retinopathy with presumed periphlebitis. Br J Ophthalmol 1993;77:795–798.

104. Suzuki T, Obara Y, Sato Y, et al: Cancer-associated retinopathy with presumed vasculitis. Am J Ophthalmol 1996;122:125–126.

105. Keltner J, Thirkill CE, Tyler NK, et al: Management and monitoring of cancer-associated retinopathy. Arch Ophthalmol 1992;110:48–53.

106. Ridley M, McDonald HR, Sternberg P, et al: Retinal manifestations of ocular lymphoma (reticulum cell sarcoma). Ophthalmology 1992;99:1153–1161.

107. Brown S, Jampol L, Cantrill H: Intraocular lymphoma presenting as retinal vasculitis. Surv Ophthalmol 1994;39:133–140.

108. Akpek EK, Ahmed I, Hochberg FH, et al: Intraocular central nervous system lymphoma: Clinical features, diagnosis and outcomes. Ophthalmology 1999;106:1805–1810.

109. Barr C, Green WR, Payne JW, et al: Intraocular reticulum-cell sarcoma: Clinicopathological study of four cases and review of the literature. Surv Ophthalmol 1975;19:224–239.

110. O'Neill D, Brown C: Retinal vasculitis and uveitis in IgA nephritis. Eye 1994;8:711–713.

111. Wakefield D, Lane J, Penny R: Retinal vasculitis associated with HLA DR4. Brief definitive report. Hum Immunol 1985;14:11–17.

112. Ong K, Billson FA, Pathirana DS, et al: A case of progressive hemifacial atrophy with uveitis and retinal vasculitis. Aust N Z J Ophthalmol 1991;19:295–298.

113. Jackson J, Kunkel MR, Libow L, et al: Adult Kawasaki disease. Report of two cases treated with intravenous gamma globulin. Arch Intern Med 1994;154:1398–1405.

114. Jampol L, Ebroon D, Goldbaum M: Peripheral proliferative retinopathies: An update on angiogenesis, etiologies and management. Surv Ophthalmol 1994;38:519–540.

115. Bentley C, Stanford MR, Shilling JS, et al: Macular ischemia in posterior uveitis. Eye 1993;7:411–414.

116. Brockhurst R, Schepens C: Uveitis 4: Peripheral uveitis: The complication of retinal detachment. Arch Ophthalmol 1986;80:747–753.

117. Chan C, Wetzig RP, Palestine AG, et al: Immunopathology of ocular sarcoidosis. Arch Ophthalmol 1987;105:1398–1402.

118. George R, Chan CC, Whitcup SM, et al: Ocular immunopathology of Behçet's disease. Surv Ophthalmol 1997;42:157–162.

119. Dumonde D, Kasp-Grochowska E, Graham E, et al: Anti-retinal autoimmunity and circulating immune complexes in patients with retinal vasculitis. Lancet 1982;2:787–792.

120. Rao N, Wacker W, Marak G: Experimental allergic uveitis: Clinicopathological features associated with varying doses of S-antigen. Arch Ophthalmol 1979;97:1954–1958.

121. Kasp E, Graham EM, Stanford MR, et al: A point prevalence study of 150 patients with idiopathic retinal vasculitis: 2. Clinical relevance of antiretinal autoimmunity and circulating immune complexes. Br J Ophthalmol 1989;73:722–730.

122. Ballantyne A, Michaelson I: A case of perivasculitis retinae associated with symptoms of cerebral disease. Br J Ophthalmol 1937;21:22.

123. Whitcup S: Involvement of cell adhesion molecules in the pathogenesis of experimental autoimmune uveoretinitis. Ocul Immunol Inflamm 1995;3:53–56.

124. Whitcup S: Endothelial leukocyte adhesion molecule-1 in endotoxin-induced uveitis. Invest Ophthalmol Vis Sci 1992;33:2626–2630.

125. Whitcup S, Chan CC, Li Q, et al: Expression of cell adhesion molecules in posterior uveitis. Arch Ophthalmol 1992;110:662–666.

126. Hill T, Stanford MR, Graham EM, et al: A new method for studying the selective adherence of blood lymphocytes to the microvasculature of human retina. Invest Ophthalmol Vis Sci 1997;38:2608–2618.

127. Whitcup S, Hikita N, Shirao M, et al: Monoclonal antibodies against CD54 (ICAM-1) and CD11a (LFA-1) prevent and inhibit endotoxin-induced uveitis. Exp Eye Res 1995;60:597–601.

128. Springer T: Adhesion receptors of the immune system. Nature 1990;346:425–434.

129. Kasp E, Whiston R, Dumonde D, et al: Antibody affinity to retinal S-antigen in patients with retinal vasculitis. Am J Ophthalmol 1992;113:697–701.

130. Palmer H, Jurd KM, Hunt BJ, et al: Thrombophilic factors in ischemic and non-ischemic idiopathic retinal vasculitis. Eye 1995;9:507–512.

131. Howe L, Stanford MR, Edelsten C, et al: The efficacy of systemic corticosteroids in sight threatening retinal vasculitis. Eye 1994;8:443–447.

132. Myles A: Polymyalgia rheumatica and giant cell arteritis (letter). Br Med J 1995;311:1232.

133. Stanbury R, Graham E: Systemic corticosteroid therapy: Side effects and their management. Br J Ophthalmol 1998;82:704–708.

134. Anon and CSM/MCA: Withdrawal of systemic corticosteroid. Curr Probl Pharmacovig 1998;24:5–7.

135. Dick A, Azim M, Forrester J: Immunosuppressive therapy for chronic uveitis: Optimizing therapy with steroids and cyclosporin A. Br J Ophthalmol 1997;81:1107–1112.

136. Hemady R, Tauber J, Foster CS: Immunosuppressive drugs in immune and inflammatory ocular disease. Surv Ophthalmol 1991;35:369–385.

137. Nussenblatt R, Palestine A, Chan C: Cyclosporin A therapy in the treatment of intraocular inflammatory disease resistant to systemic corticosteroids and cytotoxic agents. Am J Ophthalmol 1983;96:275–282.

138. Towler H, Whiting P, Forrester J: Combination low dose cyclosporin A and steroid therapy in chronic intraocular inflammation. Eye 1990;4:514–520.

139. Mochizuki M, Masuda K, Sakane T, et al: A clinical trial of FK506 in refractory uveitis. Am J Ophthalmol 1993;115:763–769.

140. Allison A, Eugui E: Purine metabolism and immunosuppressive effects of mycophenolate mofetil (MMF). Clin Transplant 1996;10:77–84.

141. Kilmartin D, Dick A: Rescue therapy with mycophenolate mofetil in refractory uveitis. Lancet 1998;352:35–36.

142. Larkin G, Lightman S: Mycophenolate mofetil: A useful immunosuppressive in inflammatory eye disease. Ophthalmology 1999;106:370–374.

143. Mollnes T, Harboe M: Clinical immunology: Recent advances. Br Med J 1996;312:1456–1469.

144. Raizman M, Foster CS: Plasma exchange in the therapy of Behçet's disease. Graefes Arch Clin Exp Ophthalmol 1989;227:360–363.

145. Isaacs J, Dick A: Short-term immunosuppressive therapy and long-term immunoregulation: Promises and problems. Br J Ophthalmol 1996;80:1035–1036.

146. O'Dell J: Anticytokine therapy: A new era in the treatment of rheumatoid arthritis. N Engl J Med 1999;340:311–312.

147. Bach J: Tolerance and uveitis. Am J Ophthalmol 1997;123:684–687.

148. Isaacs J, Hale G, Waldmann H, et al: Monoclonal antibody therapy of chronic intraocular inflammation using Campath-1H. Br J Ophthalmol 1995;79:1054–1055.

149. Nussenblatt R, Caspi RR, Mahdi R, et al: Inhibition of S-antigen induced experimental autoimmune uveoretinitis by oral induction of tolerance with S-antigen. J Immunol 1990;144:1689–1695.

150. Nussenblatt R, Gery I, Weiner HL, et al: Treatment of uveitis by oral administration of retinal antigens: Results of phase I/II randomized masked trial. Am J Ophthalmol 1997;123:583–592.

151. Atmaca L, Nagpal P: Eales' disease: Medical, laser and surgical treatments. Ophthalmol Clin North Am 1998;11:619–626.

152. Meyer-Schwickerath G: Eales' disease: Treatment with light coagulation. Mod Probl Ophthalmol 1966;4:10.

153. Oyakawa R, Michels R, Blase W: Vitrectomy for nondiabetic vitreous hemorrhage. Am J Ophthalmol 1983;96:517–525.

154. Klok A, Luyendijk L, Zaal MJ, et al: Soluble ICAM-1 serum levels in patients with intermediate uveitis. Br J Ophthalmol 1999;83:847–851.

78 — INTERMEDIATE UVEITIS

Albert T. Vitale, Manfred Zierhut, and C. Stephen Foster

DEFINITION

The term intermediate uveitis (IU) was suggested by the International Uveitis Study Group (IUSG) to denote an idiopathic inflammatory syndrome, mainly involving the anterior vitreous, peripheral retina, and ciliary body, with minimal or no anterior segment or chorioretinal inflammatory signs.[1] Other names previously used in the literature to describe this entity include chronic cyclitis, peripheral uveitis, vitritis, cyclochorioretinitis, chronic posterior cyclitis and peripheral uveoretinitis. IU may or may not be associated with specific infections (Lyme disease, toxocariasis, Whipple's disease, cat-scratch disease) and noninfectious diseases (multiple sclerosis and sarcoidosis). The term pars planitis has been retained and used to describe the characteristic exudates that can be seen on the pars plana in some patients with IU, and may or may not represent a distinct clinical entity.

HISTORY

The first description of what probably was IU was reported by Fuchs in 1908.[2] At that time, he used the term chronic cyclitis. Schepens[3] described the disease entity of peripheral uveitis in 1950, which captured most of the classic clinical characteristics of IU. Subsequently, his group reported different aspects of this disease,[4–7] including peripheral vascular abnormalities and exudation along the pars plana. In 1960, Welch and associates[8] coined the term pars planitis. In 1987, the IUSG adopted the term IU as a part of its anatomic classification scheme for intraocular inflammation.[1]

EPIDEMIOLOGY

IU has been reported in 8% to 22% of uveitis patients.[8–18] There is only one report published regarding its incidence and prevalence. Vadot[17] found an incidence of 1.4/100,000 (0.64 to 2.64 confidence intervals) in a prospective epidemiologic study of 215 uveitis patients in Savoy, France. The prevalence was estimated to be 5.9/100,000. Of 1237 patients with uveitis referred to the Immunology and Uveitis Service of the Massachusetts Eye and Ear Infirmary over a 10-year period, 162 (13.0%) were classified as IU.[15] The disease seems to affect patients primarily from childhood through the fourth decade, but it has also been reported in older patients. There seems to be no clear gender or race predilection. Good epidemiologic studies that include a few hundred patients with IU are still lacking. Approximately 70% to 90% of cases are bilateral, albeit asymmetric, with symptoms frequently being confined to one eye.

IU is not a hereditary disorder. However, there have been some reports (thus far approximately a dozen cases) of IU occurring in families.[19–27] Human leukocyte antigen (HLA) studies in these families have not shown common HLA haplotypes, except for one report concerning two affected brothers with identical HLA-type.[26]

CLINICAL FEATURES

Patients with IU often present with minimal symptoms, which may include floaters or blurred vision, but no pain, photophobia or obvious external inflammation. In more severe cases, floaters aggregate and visual acuity may be significantly reduced. Sometimes, patients present with abrupt loss of vision owing to acute vitreous hemorrhage or retinal detachment.

Clinical signs of anterior segment inflammation may be present or absent. There may be mild anterior chamber cells, keratic precipitates, and even rarely posterior synechiae. The less-than-thorough clinician may simply treat these anterior findings, without performing a dilated, depressed peripheral retinal examination, thereby missing the diagnosis. Band keratopathy has been reported in children with IU, as may occur in uveitis of nearly any chronic kind in children.

Autoimmune endotheliopathy has been reported by Khodadoust and colleagues[28] in four of 10 patients with pars planitis. He described peripheral corneal edema with keratic precipitates that were arranged linearly on the border between edematous and normal cornea, suggesting that IU may also be an autoimmune disease–like transplant rejection. Similar findings have been described by other authors,[29, 30] and we, too, have observed this.

Vitreous cells are the most characteristic sign for IU (Fig. 78–1), ranging from 1+ to 4+ cells.[31] In severe cases, the cellular infiltration is so dense that it may obscure the view of the retina, and it is impossible for one to exclude the diagnosis of posterior uveitis. Vitreal yellowish white aggregates, the so-called snowballs, are typical and are mostly found in the inferior periphery (Fig. 78–2). Signs of vasculitis are seen in 10% to 32% of patients,[10, 32–34] depending on the method of diagnosis (Fig. 78–3). This includes vascular venous sheathing (periphlebitis), probably leading to occlusion[35] and sometimes peripheral retinal neovascularization (Fig. 78–4).

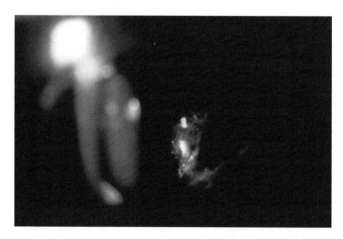

FIGURE 78–1. Vitreous inflammation, with dense vitreal cellular infiltrate seen on slit lamp biomicroscopy. (See color insert.)

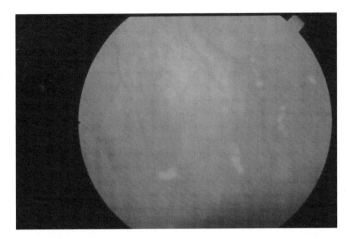

FIGURE 78–2. Vitreal cellular aggregates anterior to the retina ("snow-balls"). (See color insert.)

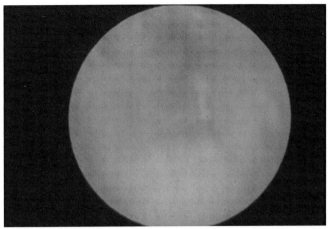

FIGURE 78–4. Neovascularization after occlusive vasculitis in intermediate uveitis. (See color insert.)

In addition, frank exudates on the pars plana can be found. The acute stage of the disease is characterized by white exudations, which may become extensive and confluent. In the later stages, the stimulation of collagen production results in the formation of the so-called snowbank. Snowbanks can be found mostly inferiorly, but may also extend to encompass 360 degrees of the retinal periphery. Their presence seems to be associated with worse visual outcome.[36, 37] Much confusion and loose usage have evolved regarding the terms snowballs and snowbank; because of this, we generally eschew the usage of these terms, preferring more precise language. We know of those who use the term snowbank to denote confluent pars plana exudates, which is present during active pars planitis, and also use the same term to describe the white collagen band (Fig. 78–5) at the pars plana seen chronically in some patients, even during periods of quiescence. Clearly, it is clinically useful to be more precise than this. We suggest that one simply say what one sees, in an effort to be precise. For example, if we observe a white, sharp-edged band at the pars plana in the absence of cells or exudates indicative of active inflammation, we speak of finding pars plana fibrosis,[38] rather than of a snowbank. Conversely, if we discover vitreal cells surrounding collections of exudates on the pars plana or on an area of pars plana fibrosis, we speak of active pars planitis, with pars plana exudates and vitreal cells.

A thorough peripheral retinal examination with scleral depression is an important exercise in the evaluation of all patients with IU.

COMPLICATIONS

Despite the fact that many studies have suggested that IU tends to be one of the most benign forms of uveitis, severe complications secondary to chronic, indolent inflammation may arise, which may eventuate in blindness. Even those authors who emphasize the generally good prognosis of this disease admit that 20% of patients have visual acuity of less than 20/40. Deane and Rosenthal[36] showed that *only* 63% of the 86 eyes followed for a mean of 48 months had a visual acuity of 20/20 or better.

Ocular hypertension, sometimes leading to glaucoma, has been reported in approximately 8% of patients with IU. In most cases, this ocular hypertension seems to be corticosteroid induced.[7, 16, 35] Interestingly, most studies have not reported on elevated intraocular pressure.[39]

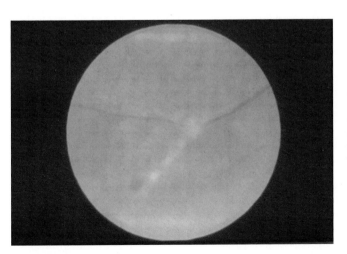

FIGURE 78–3. Vasculitis of peripheral retinal vein in a patient with intermediate uveitis. (See color insert.)

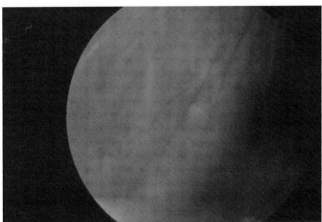

FIGURE 78–5. White collagen band at pars plana. (See color insert.)

In contrast, cataract formation is found in approximately 50% of patients with IU. Previous studies suggest that cataract formation tends to be less severe in patients who have been treated early with immunosuppressive drugs, rather than corticosteroids.*

Macular edema and maculopathy are the most common causes of severe visual loss in IU. The incidence may range from 12% to 50%† (Fig. 78–6) and seems to increase with severity and duration of inflammation.[40–42]

Retinal vasculitis is a frequent finding in many patients. Sometimes, this problem may induce neovascularization (5% to 15%)[41, 43] and cyclitic membrane formation. Although vitreous hemorrhages may occur in patients with peripheral neovascularization, it seems to be uncommon, occurring in 3% to 5% of patients.[7, 42] Shields and associates[44] described 113 vasoproliferative tumors of different origin. Of these, the underlying ocular disease was IU or pars planitis in 15 eyes.

Retinal detachment may occur in patients with IU. Characteristically, inflammation in IU may lead to exudative retinal detachment (Fig. 78–7) in 5% to 17% of patients,[10, 33, 41, 42] a finding uncommonly seen in other uveitic entities except for Vogt-Koyanagi-Harada syndrome. Vitreoretinal traction, reported in 3% to 22% of patients, may lead to retinal breaks, and combined rhegmatogenous-tractional retinal detachments.[5, 16] Brockhurst and Schepens[7] described four types of rhegmatogenous retinal detachment in patients with IU, the complexity of which varied directly with the duration and severity of the inflammatory disease. *Type I detachments* are low lying, chronic, associated with demarcation lines, and may resolve spontaneously. They occur in patients with a benign course and are secondary to small breaks near the ora serrata associated with exudate. *Type II detachments* resemble large dialyses at the posterior edge of the pars plana exudate. Similarly, these breaks are usually slowly progressive and may resolve spontaneously if vitreoretinal exudation occludes the break. Such detachments are seen in patients with a mild chronic inflammatory course. *Type III detachments* are rapidly progressive

---

*See references 3, 7, 10, 16, 24, 25, 36, 40, and 41.
†See references 7, 10, 25, 33, 36, 41, and 42.

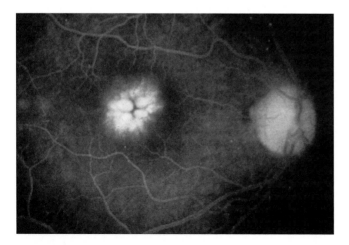

FIGURE 78–6. Macular edema in a patient with intermediate uveitis.

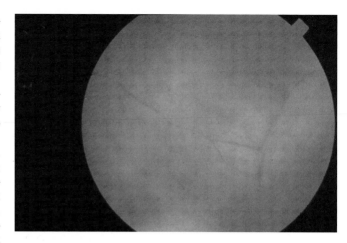

FIGURE 78–7. Exudative retinal detachment in intermediate uveitis, demonstrated by fluorescein angiography. (See color insert.)

due to large breaks associated with neovascularization of the vitreous base and circumferential pars plana exudation. These detachments are associated with severe, chronic uveitis. *Type IV detachments* are associated with anterior proliferative vitreoretinopathy associated with vascular cicatricial tissue, which produces circumferential traction, fixed folds extending from the periphery to the optic nerve, and total retinal detachment. The breaks in such eyes are difficult to visualize, because they are covered by the extensive pars plana exudate. These detachments occur in patients with the rapidly progressive form of IU, are extremely difficult to repair, and have an extremely poor functional and anatomic prognosis. Malinowski and coworkers[41] recently reported an 8.3% rate of retinal detachment in 54 patients with pars planitis followed for slightly more than 7.5 years.

Optic nerve involvement is not uncommon in IU. Disc edema is present in 3% to 20% of eyes.[10, 25, 33] It is less common in adult patients with IU,[10, 24, 25, 33, 45] and it is observed much more often in children.[46] In these cases, disc edema, rarely optic atrophy, and optic disc neovascularization arising from profound retinal ischemia have been reported. Optic neuritis, with or without associated multiple sclerosis (MS), has been reported to develop in 7.4% of 54 patients with pars planitis.[41]

ETIOLOGY

The etiology of IU remains unclear. As with many other forms of uveitis, IU may be initiated by an antigen (probably of infectious origin) leading to a uniform clinical picture with vasculitis and vitreous cells. Probably multiple stimuli can finally lead to the same clinical picture of IU.

The hypothesis now widely accepted is that some cases of IU may represent an autoimmune disorder of the eye. The initiating antigen may be of infectious origin. Only a few infectious agents have been described that lead to the clinical picture of IU, notably Lyme disease, syphilis, and cat-scratch disease. But for the most part, the nature of the antigen remains unclear. The hypothesis of autoimmune disease is supported by the fact that IU is sometimes associated with MS and with sarcoidosis. Furthermore, IU appears to be a T-cell–mediated disease, because it can be reproduced in experimental models and responds well to immunosuppressive treatment. And finally, Opremcak has shown that lymphocytes from patients with IU but not from patients with other uveitis respond in vitro to exposure to type II collagen, with proliferation and cytokine production, suggesting that type II collagen, richly present in the vitreous, may be an autoantigen in some patients with IU.[47]

Various studies have looked for a predominant association to an HLA antigen. Most of these studies have used serologic tests only. Recently, Martin and associates[48] reported that 28% of their patients with IU were HLA-A-28 positive, compared with 8.1% of their healthy control population and 8.6% of patients with posterior uveitis. These findings have not been confirmed by others. Tang and colleagues[49] found a positive, significant association of pars planitis to HLA-DR15, concluding that these patients have a higher risk for the development of systemic diseases. Two years later, researchers at The Johns Hopkins University School of Medicine confirmed these observations, suggesting that HLA-DR15 or some closely linked gene may play a role in both multiple sclerosis and pars planitis.[50] In an ongoing study with 150 patients, we were not able to find a predominant HLA class I– or class II–antigen association using molecular biology approaches.

Recently, Bora and coworkers[51, 52] described a protein from the serum of patients with active IU that may serve as a marker for, and play a potential role in the etiology of this disease.

It may become possible in the future to subdivide IU further concerning its etiology. Today, we do not have enough data for such a subdivision.

PATHOGENESIS AND PATHOLOGY

The pathogenesis of IU remains unclear. Because of improved treatment modalities, very few eyes have been enucleated, extending our knowledge regarding the pathogenesis and pathology of this disease.[25, 26, 38, 53–56] Additionally enucleated eyes are mostly blind eyes with longstanding, severe disease, hampering histologic and immunohistologic investigation such that predominant findings are limited to secondary changes, masking the primary pathologic mechanisms.

Various anatomic studies of the pars plana region show that this region is characterized by relatively low oxygen tension. In case of retinal hypoxia and ischemia, such findings may be relevant with respect to the initiation of inflammation at the pars plana.

In addition, there is evidence to suggest that the venules in the pars plana region may be modified in active disease in such a way as to promote lymphocyte trafficking. These venules are characterized by isolated, enlarged endothelial cells, a specialized modification known as high endothelial venule.[56] In one of the few histologic studies, Pederson and colleagues[38] demonstrated that pars plana exudates appear to consist of a loose fibrovascular layer containing occasional fibrocyte-like cells and scattered mononuclear inflammatory cells adjacent to the hyperplastic nonpigmented epithelium of the pars plana.

The fibroglial tissue consists of vitreous collagen and probably fibrous astrocytes, producing larger diameter collagen fibers.

Lymphocyte infiltration of retinal veins leads to the clinical signs of vasculitis, but histologically, arterioles are not involved. Choroidal involvement has been demonstrated only in severe cases.[53] These findings clearly demonstrate that IU is not a primary chorioretinal disease. Active vitreal inflammatory cell exudates, which are highly characteristic for IU, were found to be composed of epithelioid cells and multinucleated giant cells.[53] Wetzig and associates[26] found extensive MHC class II antigen expression on vascular epithelium. This could be part of the initiating process in the recruitment of activated T cells to stimulate a local vasculitis, leading to vitreal inflammation.

T cells have been shown to be the predominant cell type in the vitreous in IU, ranging from 11% to 95% of all vitreous cells.[26, 57] CD4-positive T cells account for 5% to 75% of all T cells. In the study by Davis and coworkers[58] involving three human vitreous biopsy specimens, the authors found similar results: 35% to 90% CD4-positive cells and 5% to 15% CD8-positive T cells. Macrophages were found to be the second most important cell type. The role of B cells remains unclear. Although Nölle and Eckardt[57] were able to demonstrate B cells only rarely, they were the dominant cells in the study of Kaplan and coworkers.[59]

Studies of the blood of patients with IU have not extended our knowledge of the pathogenesis of IU. Although the number of T lymphocytes and B lymphocytes in the peripheral blood was normal, an increased ratio of CD4 lymphocytes to CD8 lymphocytes was found in six patients with pars planitis.[60] α_2-Microglobulin, β_2-microglobulin, and complement components were also normal, but serum IgD levels and antiganglioside antibodies[61] were elevated. Klok and associates[62] have shown elevated interleukin (IL) 8 levels in the serum of patients with active IU, concluding that elevated IL-8 may predispose these patients to the development of associated systemic disease.

Increased levels of soluble IL-2 receptors[63] and intercellular adhesion molecule 1 (ICAM-1)[64] have been found in the serum of patients with IU. BenEzra and colleagues[65] recently demonstrated that serum IL-1–receptor antagonist levels in patients with active pars planitis do not differ from those of control patients.

In several studies, a search for an antibody response against ocular antigens was performed. Antibodies against Mueller cells were present in 10% of patients with IU but in only 2.3% of healthy controls and in 7.4% of patients with other autoimmune disorders.[66] Serum immunoglobulin has been found to bind frozen human retinal sections of patients with IU in 8 of 12 cases of IU,[67] whereas staining of retinal vessel walls was demonstrated in 5 of the 12 patients.[67] Antibody production against retinal S-antigen did not differ from normal controls.[68] Using the lymphocyte proliferation test, cellular immunity against retinal-S and interphotoreceptor-retinoid-binding protein (IRBP) was demonstrated in 22% to 43% of patients with IU, which is less frequent than that which has been shown for posterior uveitis patients.[68–70]

Previous studies from our group, investigating a cluster of autoantibodies nonspecific for the eye, disclosed typical patterns for acute anterior uveitis (antibodies against sarcolemma 59%, sinusoids 18%, laminin 41% and microsomes 59%) and posterior uveitis (antibodies against endothelial cells 33% and microsomes 33%) but only a very low production of any of the investigated autoantibodies in patients with IU.[71]

To study the pathology and immunohistology of uveitis, experimental models have clearly improved our knowledge. Using retinal S-antigen or IRBP, it is possible to induce a model that is very similar to clinical IU. Vasculitis of retinal vessels with vitreous inflammation is produced. The disadvantage of these models is that IU seems to be only a dose-dependent subgroup of panuveitis, implying that the detectable effects are nonspecific manifestations of inflammation. An IU-like model can also be induced in monkeys after intravitreal injection of hyaluronic acid.[72] Experimental models have shown the importance of T cells and the influence of drugs like cyclosporine A on the course of disease, findings that have been verified in clinical IU.

DIAGNOSIS

The diagnosis of IU is based on clinical findings. The absence of chorioretinal infiltration, together with vitreous cells that outnumber anterior chamber cell infiltration, vitreous snowballs, and the presence of pars plana exudation, suggest IU. Laboratory and ancillary tests are not necessary to establish the diagnosis; however, together with a careful review of systems, laboratory studies may be able to exclude an associated disorder, including Lyme disease, tuberculosis, syphilis, cat-scratch disease, multiple sclerosis, and sarcoid.

Review of Systems

The patient's history should concentrate on the duration of symptoms, the number of recurrences, and findings that might be associated with systemic disorders. Fever, fatigue, or night sweats are typical signs of sarcoidosis and tuberculosis, whereas loss of sensitivity or paresthesias of the hands, arms, or legs are suggestive of possible multiple sclerosis. Signs of dermatitis may point to Lyme disease, tuberculosis, or syphilis, whereas arthritis of the knee may suggest the possibility of Lyme disease, and contact with cats may raise the possibility of *Bartonella* infection.

Clinical Investigation

In addition to the measurement of visual acuity and slit-lamp biomicroscopy, measurement of the intraocular pressure and fundus examination with scleral depression is mandatory in patients with uveitis. The Amsler grid has been shown to mirror the presence of macular edema quite well, and we always suggest the grid to patients for self-monitoring.

Chest X-ray Studies

Chest x-ray studies may disclose findings indicative of sarcoidosis or tuberculosis.

Serology and Laboratory Testing

In cases of IU, only a few laboratory and serologic tests are necessary. These tests include determination of the angiotensin-converting enzyme (ACE) level.[73, 74] ACE is mainly produced by granuloma-forming epitheloid cells and is elevated in 60% to 90% of active sarcoid patients and rarely in other lung disorders. It should be remembered that ACE in children, as well as in smokers, is nearly always higher than in normal adults. Steroids can suppress elevated ACE activity. Elevated lysozyme levels are also found in the serum of patients with granulomatous disorders like sarcoid, tuberculosis, and leprosy. Serologic testing for cat-scratch disease, syphilis, and Lyme disease should be seriously considered in cases of IU.

Gallium-Scan and Chest Computed Tomography Scan

Subclinical pulmonary sarcoidosis, undetectable by chest x-ray study, may be detected via computed tomography (CT) of the chest or by gallium scan, or both. Abnormalities discovered through these modalities may be biopsied for definitive diagnosis. A positive gallium scan of the lacrimal gland is found in 60% to 75% of all sarcoid patients.[75] Studies from our group have shown that the combination of serum ACE level and whole-body gallium scan increases the diagnostic specificity without affecting sensitivity in patients with clinically suspicious ocular sarcoidosis who have normal or equivocal chest radiographs. Although the sensitivity of an elevated ACE in diagnosing sarcoidosis was found to be 73% and the specificity was 83%, the combination of a positive gallium scan and an elevated ACE raised the specificity for diagnosis to 100%, whereas the sensitivity remained unchanged at 73%.[76] Furthermore, elevated ACE levels were found in patients with uveitis due to diseases other than sarcoidosis, including Adamantiades-Behçet disease, HLA-B27–associated uveitis, syphilis, systemic lupus erythematosus, juvenile rheumatoid arthritis, tuberculosis, sympathetic ophthalmia, acute retinal necrosis, intraocular lymphoma, birdshot retinochoroidopathy, Lyme disease, Vogt-Koyanagi-Harada syndrome, and Wegener's granulomatosis.

Fluorescein Angiography

Fluorescein angiography can illustrate the extent of vasculitis and disclose areas of retinal nonperfusion and neovascularization.[16, 33, 34, 45] One can see staining of major veins, segmental hyperfluorescence, optic disc hyperfluorescence, and leakage of veins or venules in 40% to 50% of the eyes. In addition to the Amsler grid, fluorescein angiography is the definitive way to detect cystoid macular edema (CME); however, CME is usually apparent and is diagnosed on biomicroscopic examination of the macula.

Echography

In cases of typical pars planitis or IU, echography adds no information to the above-mentioned evaluation. However, severe vitreous infiltration, retinal detachment, posterior scleritis, *Toxocara canis* granuloma, and intraocular tumors can be excluded by this modality. Using ultrasound biomicroscopy (UBM), it is possible to demonstrate pars plana exudates and even inflammatory cell aggregates in the vitreous.[77]

Electrophysiology

Only a few electrophysiologic studies concerning IU have been published.[78–81] Cantrill and colleagues[78] found mild changes, especially supernormal B-wave implicit times on the electroretinogram (ERG), followed by absence or reduction of scotopic B-wave oscillations in most patients. In mild disease, the B-wave amplitude was found to be increased,[81] which may indicate active retinal inflammation or improvement of the inflammation under therapy. Electrophysiology is not a routinely recommended study in the diagnostic work-up of patients with IU.

Diagnostic Vitrectomy

Diagnostic vitrectomy is appropriate only in cases with severe vitreal infiltration when posterior uveitis, retinitis, endophthalmitis, or tumors cannot definitely be excluded and when the response to medical therapy is refractory.

DIFFERENTIAL DIAGNOSIS

The differential diagnosis of IU includes many causes of vitreous inflammation. It is imperative to exclude infectious causes, because specific treatment is indicated and may be curative. Infectious entities in the differential diagnosis include Lyme disease, toxocariasis, Whipple's disease, tuberculosis, syphilis, human T-cell leukemia virus type 1 (HTLV-1), Epstein-Barr virus, and cat-scratch disease. Equally important is the association of IU with underlying systemic diseases, particularly intraocular lymphoma, sarcoidosis, and MS, because timely diagnosis impacts not only ocular morbidity but also quality of life and potentially mortality. Finally, some other ocular diseases may be difficult to differentiate from typical IU, especially if the patient has already commenced treatment or is in the beginning stage of the disease, or if vitreous inflammation prevents examination of the fundus to exclude chorioretinal disease.

Multiple Sclerosis

Breger and Leopold[82] prospectively reported on 14 of 52 MS patients who developed pars planitis. Giles[83] described three patients with MS who later developed pars planitis. Porter[84] found only two cases of pars planitis in 60 patients with MS. Conversely, Chester and associates[85] studied the incidence of MS developing in patients with pars planitis and found that 4 of 51 patients with pars planitis developed MS. Zierhut and Foster[86] confirmed these findings in their study, which included 62 patients with pars planitis. Seven of these patients had MS, ranging from 17 years before the onset of pars planitis to 7 years after the development of pars planitis. Three additional patients (19%) were MS suspects. In their study, they additionally compared the incidence of CME, optic disc swelling, periphlebitis and retrobulbar neuritis in patients with pars planitis, with or without MS. Only retrobulbar neuritis was found to be significantly greater in the MS group compared with the control group without MS.

The association between MS and IU was studied by Engell, who positively correlated the level of clinical severity of MS with the presence of vascular sheathing.[87] All but one of these patients had active disease, with vascular sheathing being present in 43% of patients having a rapid progression of disease. Indeed, Malinowski and cowork-

ers[41] reported a 14.8% incidence of MS in 54 patients with pars planitis who were followed for a little over 7.5 years. Moreover, periphlebitis at the time of diagnosis of pars planitis appeared to be associated with an increased risk of developing MS or optic neuritis, or both.[41] Most recently, Raja and colleagues reported their findings of a long-term follow-up (mean 2 years) study of 53 patients with pars planitis.[50] Of 37 pars planitis patients who had had medical or neurologic follow-up evaluation, six (16.2%) developed MS. Moreover, the HLA-DR15 allele, coding for one of the two HLA-DR2 subtypes (a phenotype known to be linked to multiple sclerosis), was associated with pars planitis. These findings, together with the previous demonstration of the presence of HLA-DR2 in a homogeneous population of pars planitis patients by Malinowski and coauthors, further support an association between pars planitis and MS, implicating the HLA-DR locus in the pathogenesis of both entities.[88]

We recommend that, if symptoms or clinical signs are suggestive for MS on the patient's review of systems and examination, an magnetic resonance imaging (MRI) scan should be performed. This study may be followed by referral to a neurologist for evaluation, including examination of the cerebrospinal fluid.

Sarcoidosis

Landers[89] described three of 13 patients with sarcoidosis who developed IU. Similarly, Crick[90] reported the development of IU in all 13 of his patients with sarcoidosis. Conversely, Chester and colleagues[85] studied the incidence of sarcoidosis in a group of 51 pars planitis patients and found it to be only 2%. On the other hand, Jabs and Johns[91] studied 183 patients with known sarcoidosis, and they found 26% with ocular involvement. Eleven of those patients had IU. Other studies have shown that 2% to 10% of patients with IU have sarcoidosis.

In their study of 62 patients with pars planitis, Zierhut and Foster[86] found six cases of biopsy-proven sarcoid; an additional nine patients were suspected of having sarcoidosis because of elevated ACE levels. The onset of sarcoidosis had begun with pars planitis in two patients, with one patient developing pulmonary sarcoid 4 to 5 years after the onset of the pars planitis. On comparing the typical ocular findings seen in pars planitis patients, such as CME, optic disc swelling, periphlebitis, and retrobulbar optic neuritis, the IU patients with sarcoid did not show significant differences from IU patients without sarcoid.

In contradistinction to patients with IU, those with sarcoid uveitis have a different demographic: There is a slight female preponderance, an older age group, and a different racial predilection (blacks), at least in the United States. Furthermore, anterior uveitis is more common than posterior involvement, with more pronounced anterior segment pathology. Chorioretinitis is a distinctive feature of posterior segment disease in ocular sarcoidosis. As intraocular inflammation may precede by many years the onset of systemic disease in sarcoidosis, complete periodic examinations may be of value.

Infectious Disorders

Tuberculosis

Infection with *Mycobacterium tuberculosis* can induce a clinical picture similar to that of IU. It should be excluded by accurate history and review of systems, chest x-ray study, and skin testing. Nodules of the iris or granulomata of the choroid are distinctive findings that may lead to a higher suspicion for tuberculosis.

Syphilis

Infection with *Treponema pallidum* is known to mimic various ocular disorders and to affect nearly every ocular structure.[92] IU seems to be only rarely imitated by syphilis. History and systemic and ocular examinations, together with serologic testing (Venereal Disease and Research Laboratory [VDRL] and fluorescent treponemal antibody absorption [FTA-ABS]), should exclude the diagnosis of syphilis. The VDRL test is not used as the screening test, because 30% of patients with latent secondary syphilis associated with uveitis are VDRL negative but are FTA-ABS positive. Therefore, the FTA-ABS test is an essential part of the laboratory evaluation.

Lyme Disease

Lyme disease has been described as causing IU in a small number of studies.[93–96] The history of a tick bite (often unknown to the patient), erythema migrans, or migratory arthralgias (especially involving the knee) in an individual living in an endemic area, with or without neurologic symptoms (eighth cranial nerve palsy or chronic meningitis), strongly implicates infection with *Borrelia burgdorferi*. The diagnosis may be supported by serologic testing; however, such studies are not without problems, especially with respect to false-negative and false-positive findings. After the first several weeks of infection, IgG and IgM antibodies as detected by enzyme-linked immunosorbent assay (ELISA) should be positive. However, falsely negative cases of Lyme disease, in which the antigen has been isolated later, have been reported. False-positive results, especially with IgM, may occur in healthy subjects and in patients with a variety of other diseases, including syphilis.

Human T-Cell Leukemia Virus Type I

Infection with HTLV-1 has been shown to induce IU.[97, 98] Similar to sarcoidosis, HTLV-1 uveitis may lead to granulomatous uveitis with iris nodules, vitreous exudates, and periphlebitis. Differentiating between sarcoid and HTLV-1 virus uveitides may be difficult. HTLV-1 antibody production is found in serum and also in the aqueous humor and in cerebrospinal fluid. Although HTLV-1 is endemic in Japan and Haiti, the relevance of this microbe in other parts of the world is unclear.

Cat-Scratch Disease

Cat-scratch disease has been described by Soheilian and associates[99] as causing IU with focal vasculitis. The disease, caused by *Bartonella*, typically leads to conjunctivitis and neuroretinitis.[100] Laboratory tests may identify *Bartonella* directly from primary inoculation site, lymph nodes, or blood, or by detecting antibodies[101] against *Bartonella*. The skin test from which antigen is prepared from the purulent aspirate of a lymph node from a patient with proven cat-scratch disease, has a sensitivity of 79% to 100% with a specificity of 90% to 98% and negative predictive values of 78% to 100%.

Epstein-Barr Virus

Zierhut and Foster,[86] in their series of 62 patients with pars planitis, found one patient with acute Epstein-Barr virus (EBV) infection, one with serology suggestive for an old EBV infection and findings consistent with sarcoidosis, and one with serology suggestive for an old EBV infection and retinitis pigmentosa. The relevance of EBV in IU remains unclear at the present time.

Intraocular Lymphoma

IU can be the first sign of intraocular lymphoma.[102] If the vitreous inflammation becomes more dense, the chorioretinal lesions may not be visible. A poor or partial response to therapy (corticosteroids or immunosuppressive treatment) should alert the ophthalmologist to consider intraocular lymphoma, a disorder that mostly affects older patients but that has been described in younger patients as well. The diagnostic procedures of choice are vitreal biopsy, careful neurologic history, cerebrospinal fluid investigations, and brain MRI scanning if there is any evidence of a central nervous system (CNS) abnormality.

Anterior Uveitis

Anterior uveitis, by definition, has the predominance of inflammatory activity confined to the anterior chamber, with minimal vitreous reaction. If patients with severe anterior uveitis have been treated aggressively with topical corticosteroids, the anterior chamber cells may have cleared, leaving the anterior vitreous with residual spill-over inflammatory cells, presenting the illusion of IU for the moment. If the history is not typical for acute anterior uveitis (e.g., the presence of pain, photophobia, or red eye), one probably must observe the course of the disease, because a clear differentiation to IU may be impossible at that moment. Although posterior synechiae are not proof of anterior uveitis, cellular aggregates in the vitreous are found much more often in IU, only rarely in iridocyclitis, and never in iritis. Pars plana exudation is pathognomonic for pars planitis, completely excluding anterior uveitis.

Other Uveitic Syndromes

In certain instances, typical posterior uveitic entities must be differentiated from IU. In cases of severe vitreous infiltration, chorioretinitis may be overlooked, and so toxoplasmosis, toxocariasis, and also endogenous endophthalmitis must be excluded. On the other hand, mild vitritis seen in conjunction with subtle chorioretinal involvement in Vogt-Koyanagi-Harada syndrome, arteriolar vasculitis in Adamantiades-Behçet's disease, and occlusive vasculopathy in Eales' disease may rarely simulate IU. The history, review of systems, ocular examination, and clinical context serve to differentiate these entities.

Chester and associates,[85] in his report of 51 patients with pars planitis, described six as having retinitis pigmentosa. One additional patient was reported by Zierhut and Foster.[86] This young female patient, who also had serology suggestive of previous EBV infection, developed IU that evolved years later to retinitis pigmentosa, which had been previously diagnosed in her sister. The relevance of these findings remains unclear at the present time.

Recently, a patient with tubulointerstitial nephritis with uveitis (TINU) syndrome was reported to develop IU, not the anterior uveitis, which is more typically reported in patients with TINU.[103] Dann and coworkers[104] have reported a patient with Gaucher's disease, a sphingolipidose defect syndrome, who developed IU and showed good response to alglucerase substitution therapy. Ormerod and associates[105] reported a patient with pars planitis after cataract surgery. *Proprionibacterium acnes* was isolated from the vitreous.

TREATMENT

The rationale for treatment of IU is slightly different from that of most other uveitic entities. Before commencing therapy, one must have a clear idea of the best indication for treatment and, later, to decide if medication or surgery is the wiser approach in the patient with chronic disease.

Indication for Treatment

Whether acute IU should be treated depends on the presence of inflammation, the extent of vasculitis, coexisting macular edema, and finally, the degree of pars plana infiltration. Although the current consensus is that inflammation producing a decrease in visual acuity to 20/30 (some have suggested 20/40 as the point to begin therapy) is an indication for treatment,[46, 106] we do not subscribe to this view. It has been our experience that treating inflammation early and aggressively, rather than an arbitrary level of visual acuity, is more effective in both the short term and in the long run in preserving those ocular structures (the macula and optic nerve) that are critical for good visual function. We have pointed out that a significant number (20%) of patients with IU, who are allowed to lose vision to the 20/40 level before being offered treatment, are never able to recover normal vision even with treatment. Therefore, we believe that it is not reasonable to deny therapy to patients with IU with active inflammation who have lost some vision. The treatment itself carries some risk; however, given our philosophy of a limit to the total amount of steroid used for any individual, and given our belief that we personally would want treatment if we had IU and lost vision to the 20/30 level, we offer treatment to such patients. We also treat patients with a large extent of vasculitis, for example, involving more than 270 degrees of the retinal circumference, and patients with acute infiltration of the pars plana. If the macula is already involved, immediate and aggressive treatment seems to be the only way to prevent progressive visual loss.

Having excluded treatable infectious and noninfectious entities that may simulate or present a clinical picture of IU, we follow a modification of the four-step approach initially described by Kaplan.[107] In this regimen, a series of periocular steroid injections is recommended, followed by oral prednisone for those individuals who continue to experience recurrence of uveitis as the effect of each steroid injection declines, followed by vitrectomy or immunosuppressive drugs. We have modified this to a five-step program, because observing that some individu-

als, treated with oral nonsteroidal anti-inflammatory drugs (NSAIDs) during the administration of a series of periocular steroid injections and continued indefinitely thereafter, will remain relapse free. We also have suggested relatively strict limits to the total amount of steroid therapy: No more than six periocular steroid injections, and no more than 3 months of a tapering oral steroid regimen.

Our approach is to commence therapy with (1) topical corticosteroids in the presence of anterior segment inflammation, together with regional corticosteroid injections (triamcinolone, 40 mg); (2) oral NSAIDs, should inflammation recur following the third injection, and topical NSAIDs in the presence of CME; (3) a short course of systemic corticosteroids should inflammation persist or recur despite the previous interventions; (4) peripheral retinal cryopexy or indirect laser photocoagulation should pars planitis recur following the sixth regional steroid injection; and (5) offer therapeutic pars plana vitrectomy (PPV) versus immunosuppressive chemotherapy should inflammation be recalcitrant to the preceding modalities.

Cyclosporin A (CSA) and methotrexate are the immunosuppressives of choice at present, whereas mycophenolate mofetil appears to be a promising drug. Azathioprine generally is the second choice, whereas cyclophosphamide and chlorambucil are the drugs of last resort. Although some centers prefer to perform vitrectomy before immunosuppressive treatment, various reports show long-lasting improvement after therapy with immunosuppressants, reserving vitrectomy for cases of intolerable side effects or nonresponsiveness. We are flexible on this point and are conducting a randomized study comparing therapeutic PPV with low-dose once-weekly methotrexate for pars planitis.

There have been no controlled randomized studies assessing the efficacy of various immunosuppressive drugs or for vitrectomy in the treatment of IU. Most have been small retrospective reports, making comparison between treatment modalities nearly impossible owing to the heterogeneity of the uveitis populations, the nonuniformity of diagnostic criteria and treatment protocols, and because frequently immunosuppressive therapy was terminated too early in the course of the disease, before a remission could have developed.

Drug Therapy

Corticosteroids

Corticosteroids are still the mainstay of therapy for patients with IU and pars planitis. Although topical corticosteroids may be effective in some aphakic eyes, generally peribulbar or systemic corticosteroids are required. The optimal dosage is still unknown, but triamcinolone periocularly (40 mg every 3 to 5 weeks) seems to be effective,[35, 108] as is prednisolone orally for systemic administration (75 mg daily for 5 days followed by 50 mg for one week and reduced by 10 mg weekly thereafter).[108, 109] Our preference is to commence systemic steroid therapy at 1 mg/kg daily, with the initiation of tapering after 2 weeks of treatment, and guided thereafter by the clinical response. Treatment is rarely extended beyond 3 months.

When macular edema is present, we also add acetazolamide (250 bid for 3 to 6 weeks), and very slowly taper over a period of months and on a systemic NSAID, such as diflunisal, 500 mg PO bid.[110] Even using this regimen, recurrences are common. Godfrey and associates[35] found a greater effect on CME in patients with IU after periocular corticosteroid injections (71%) than after systemic treatment (41%).

Nonsteroidal Anti-inflammatory Drugs

Although the efficacy of NSAIDs in uveitic disease has not been firmly established, we have employed systemic NSAIDs successfully in our patients with pars planitis in an effort to spare the total amount of corticosteroids used and to maintain inflammatory remission. In addition, a variety of studies have shown reduced ocular inflammation following cataract extraction, a salutory effect on CME, and improvement in other forms of inflammation with the use of these agents.[111]

Cyclosporine A

Reports on the use of CSA for the treatment of IU, or comparison of its use for IU versus other forms of uveitis, are few. Schlote and colleagues[112] reported good results for uveitis in childhood. Similar positive results were obtained by Walton and coworkers,[113] who treated severe sight-threatening uveitis in children and adolescence, some of whom had IU. They concluded that CSA was a safe and effective therapy for this group of patients. CSA has also been the preferred immunosuppressive at the National Eye Institute for adults with IU who are intolerant of, or do not respond to, corticosteroid therapy. It should be pointed out that the dosage that is used in uveitis has been reduced from 5 to 10 mg/kg of body weight daily, down to 2 to 5 mg/kg of body weight daily, in an effort to curtail the nearly uniform occurrence of hypertension and renal side effects seen at the higher doses.[114] However, this dosage reduction has also resulted in diminished anti-inflammatory efficacy compared with that initially claimed for higher dosage regimens.

Methotrexate

Concerns regarding adverse side effects of methotrexate may have limited its use in the management of uveitis. In their initial reports, Wong and Hersh reported favorable responses in nine of 10 patients with steroid-resistant uveitis, including IU, who were treated with high-dose (25 mg/m² body surface area) intravenous methotrexate every 4 hours for 6 weeks. Although few serious adverse reactions occurred, inflammatory symptoms recurred in more than half of the patients when therapy was discontinued.[115–117] Lazar and associates[101] obtained similarly encouraging results in 14 of 17 patients with various steroid-resistant uveitides, including four with sympathetic ophthalmia who were treated with intravenous methotrexate. However, this success was associated with significant drug-induced toxicity, including gastrointestinal complications, secondary infections, and laboratory evidence of liver damage.[101] More recently, the reduced frequency and severity of adverse reactions reported with oral or intramuscular low-dose, pulsed (weekly) methotrexate therapy and folic acid supplementation have been exploited in the management of a variety of ocular inflammatory disorders, with favorable results.[118–120]

Azathioprine

Newell and Krill[121] employed azathioprine in the treatment of 20 patients with uveitis of various etiologies and found visual improvement in all treated eyes. Apparently, the drug was most effective in those patients with pars planitis. We use azathioprine as a second-line drug, mainly as a steroid-sparing agent.

Cyclophosphamide, Chlorambucil, and 6-Mercaptopurine

Cyclophosphamide and chlorambucil are both alkylating agents. Although they are highly effective in vasculitic diseases such as Adamantiades-Behçet's disease and Wegener's granulomatosis, these drugs carry the potential for serious toxicity and have been used in the therapy of IU only occasionally. Gills[122] described beneficial results after cyclophosphamide treatment in eight patients. Chlorambucil was used successfully by Godfrey and associates,[123] who achieved improvement in 10 of 31 patients with intractable uveitis. Likewise, 6-mercaptopurine was employed by Newell and Krill,[121] with improvement in four of five cases. Alopecia, bone marrow toxicity, sterility, and increased risk of malignancy late in life must taper one's enthusiasm for the use of alkylating agents in the care of patients with a disorder (e.g., IU) that carries a relatively good prognosis.

New Drugs

A new agent with significant therapeutic promise, a very low toxicity profile and virtually no mutagenic potential is mycophenolate mofetil (CellCept). This drug has been used in uncontrolled, open-label studies, at a dose of 1 g twice daily, in conjunction with corticosteroids as a steroid-sparing agent or as an adjunct to a pre-existing immunosuppressive regimen (CSA), with improvement in symptoms and reduction in inflammation in a variety of uveitic entities, including at least one patient with pars planitis.[124, 125] Masked, controlled, randomized clinical trials are required to evaluate the full potential of this drug, as compared with other immunosuppressive agents.

Surgical Therapy

Cryotherapy and scatter laser photocoagulation of the peripheral retina, as well as PPV with or without pars plana lensectomy (PPL), have been shown to be effective in the treatment of IU. Likewise, visual rehabilitation through cataract extraction with intraocular lens implantation is a safe and effective procedure, provided vigilant perioperative control of inflammation is achieved.

Cryotherapy

Patients in whom drug therapy has failed or who exhibit recurrent inflammation despite the administration of topical, regional, and systemic steroids, or NSAIDs, as previously outlined, may require cryotherapy or laser photocoagulation in order to control the disease. These patients have developed neovascularization of the vitreous base, which, although frequently obscured by pars plana exudation and vitritis, can sometimes be appreciated as thick, ropy vessels extending over the ora serrata on scleral depression. The rationale for both cryotherapy and for laser photocoagulation is to induce regression of this vitreous base neovascularization and consequently to stabilize inflammation. In two separate reports, Aaberg and colleagues[126, 127] demonstrated the efficacy of cryotherapy, with 35% of eyes showing complete inflammatory quiescence, with an additional 57% achieving marked reduction in inflammatory activity. Subsequently, Devenyi and associates[128] and Mieler and Aaberg[129] recommended cryotherapy for neovascularization of the vitreous base in patients with pars planitis following their experience in achieving inflammatory quiescence in 24 of 30 eyes (80%), with 67% enjoying visual improvement. However, six eyes (20%) required vitreous surgery following cryotherapy, with two developing a retinal detachment. Similarly favorable results were reported by Okinami,[130] with 61% regression of inflammation after one cryotherapy treatment, and from Berg and Kroll,[131] who, despite a 48% improvement of visual acuity, also reported a 39% relapse rate over a period of 1.2 years. In a small randomized study in which cryotherapy was compared with corticosteroids, cryotherapy was superior.[132] Favorable results notwithstanding, cryotherapy may produce significant adverse sequelae, including epiretinal membranes, cataract formation, exacerbation of macular edema, and retinal detachment.[106, 130] Although retinal detachment is observed as a part of the natural history of IU, and the incidence of retinal detachment seems no higher with cryotherapy than without it,[130] it is thought that cryotherapy causes more disruption of the blood-ocular barrier and adjacent inflammation, and may induce vitreous gel contraction, possibly accelerating the rate of retinal detachment in a predisposed eye.

Our technique is to apply a double row, single freeze, of cryopexy applications to the pars plana and posterior to it, extending one clock hour to either side of all areas affected by the inflammation.

Scatter Laser Photocoagulation

Recently, panretinal photocoagulation (PRP) has been shown to be effective in the treatment of peripheral neovascularization associated with IU.[133, 134] Park and colleagues demonstrated regression of neovascularization with stabilization of inflammation, reduction in CME, and improvement in visual acuity in eight of 10 eyes following PRP alone or in combination with PPV. Advantages of laser photocoagulation include ease of treatment delivery, fewer complications, and reduced ocular morbidity as compared with cryotherapy. This modality is obviously limited by the extent of vitreous opacification, but appears to be a safe and effective alternative to cryotherapy and is an especially useful adjunctive procedure when applied during therapeutic pars plana vitrectomy.

Vitrectomy

PPV, with or without PPL, is not only the modality of choice to treat certain complications of IU (vitreous opacification, tractional or rhegmatogenous retinal detachment, vitreous hemorrhage, and epiretinal membrane formation), but it may also have a salutory effect on active disease refractive to medical treatment and on

CME, and may ultimately alter the natural history of the disease. Diamond and Kaplan[135] were the first to demonstrate beneficial effect of PPV and PPL in patients with uveitis: Specifically, three of four IU patients achieved a visual acuity of 20/40 or better. Subsequently, Mieler and coworkers,[136] Heimann and associates,[137] and Eckardt and Bacskulin[138] reported the use of PPV with or without PPL for the treatment of vitreous and lenticular opacification, vitreous hemorrhage, tractional retinal detachment, and epiretinal membrane formation complicating pars planitis, and they demonstrated significant improvement in visual acuity. In addition, inflammatory recurrences were reduced with respect to both frequency and severity in 88% of patients,[138] preoperative hypotony was normalized in eight patients,[138] and CME regression was noted in 14 of 17 patients, while one patient experienced new postoperative CME.[136] The presence of active neovascularization of the vitreous base was associated with a poorer outcome, whereas preoperative cryotherapy appeared to improve the prognosis.[136] Likewise, a large retrospective review by Heiligenhaus and colleagues[60] included 16 patients with IU who underwent PPV with or without PPL. In this review, not only were the frequency and severity of inflammatory episodes reduced but CME was seen to resolve in three eyes. In addition, all six patients requiring prednisone preoperatively to achieve inflammatory quiescence were able to stop taking this medication during the postoperative period. Dugel and colleagues[139] reported visual acuity improvement and attenuation of CME in the majority of 11 eyes of nine patients who underwent PPV for CME and intraocular inflammation unresponsive to corticosteroids. Of the six eyes with pars planitis specifically, however, only three were among those noted to improve. Indeed, Schönfeld and coworkers[140] reported a visual acuity of 20/200 in 75% of their patients with IU undergoing pars plana vitrectomy, suggesting that pre-existing macular pathology limited the visual outcome.

The efficacy of PPV, with or without PPL, in the treatment of uveitis in general and specifically with respect to IU, remains an open question, especially considering that many of the aforementioned studies were uncontrolled, comparisons were frequently only made between preoperative and postoperative visual acuities, observation times were short, and sample sizes were small. The potential risks of PPV, including epiretinal gliosis, retinal detachment, and cataract, are also not to be trivialized, and hence the folly of being fixed in opinion on the matter of "vitrectomy versus immunomodulation" for any given patient. Definitive efficacy awaits randomized controlled study in a homogeneous population of uveitic patients.

Cataract Surgery

Cataract formation is one of the most significant complications of IU. Generally, it appears that cataract extraction is a safe procedure if any active inflammation is controlled with corticosteroids or immunosuppressives for a minimum of 3 months before surgery.[141] Cataract extraction can be achieved through PPL, in combination with PPV,[135] but also through extracapsular cataract technique[141] or phacoemulsification with consecutive intraocular lens implantation. Cataract extraction can also be followed by PPV in a single or two-step procedure.[142, 143] Fourteen of 17 eyes (88%) of patients with pars planitis reported by Kaufman and Foster[144] achieved a visual acuity of 20/40 or better following cataract extraction, for those in whom active inflammation had been suppressed before surgery for a minimum of 3 months. Most eyes underwent intraocular lens implantation, and those with significant vitreous opacification also had PPV performed. Problems may arise if ocular inflammation is not completely controlled preoperatively.[144] Indeed, in one series of 15 eyes of eight patients with pars planitis who underwent extracapsular cataract extraction with intraocular lens implantation, two eyes required lens explantation and five eyes required multiple laser or surgical procedures to clear posterior capsular membranes. Postoperatively, severe inflammation may lead to additional complications such as lens dislocation, symblepharon formation, or even phthisis. Despite these complications, 60% of eyes achieved a postoperative visual acuity of 20/40 or better.[143]

Alternative Therapies

In addition to drugs and surgical procedures, a few interesting alternatives have been suggested for the treatment of IU.

PLASMAPHERESIS

Brunner and associates[145] compared plasma exchange treatment with (25 patients) or without (24 patients) infusion of preserved serum in patients with IU. Additional corticosteroid pulse therapy was given to five patients in each group. The authors showed that in both groups, reduction of inflammatory signs was achieved. There was no control group.

TOLERANCE INDUCTION

We recently published our first results[146] using oral administration of retinal autoantigens in a phase I and II randomized masked trial. Sixteen of the 45 patients had IU. Patients who were dependent on immunosuppressive agents were assigned to one of four groups: Some patients received retinal-S antigen alone (10 patients); a second group received retinal-S antigen in a mixture of soluble retinal-S antigens (10 patients); a third group received a mixture of soluble retinal-S antigen alone (10 patients); and a fourth group received a placebo (15 patients). Although not statistically significant, the group receiving the purified S-antigen alone were able to be tapered off their immunosuppressive medications more successfully than were the other groups tested. Because of the small sample size, the authors did not show whether patients with IU responded differently from the other patients with uveitis.

NATURAL HISTORY AND PROGNOSIS

IU is often considered one of the most benign forms of uveitis. But Brockhurst and Schepens[7] described four different groups as defined by clinical course. A mild course was seen in 31% of patients, a mild chronic course in 49%, a severe chronic course in 15%, and a relentlessly progressive course in 10%. Smith and colleagues[16] found 19% to have mild, 42% moderate, and 39% severe in-

flammation in their group of patients with IU who were studied more than 10 years later. Obviously, such percentages depend greatly on the patient characteristics and referral patterns to a tertiary eye care center, where severe cases will be overrepresented.

At the moment, there are no well-defined parameters to predict the natural course of the disease. The presence of a pars plana exudate may have poor prognostic significance.[36, 37] Other studies have shown that the severity of inflammation is more important for the visual outcome than the duration of the disease. Smith and associates[16] found a 5% remission rate after a follow-up of 4 to 26 years. It seems that in most patients, the disease goes into remission after 10 to 15 years. The presence of periphlebitis at the time of diagnosis of pars planitis appears to be associated with an increased risk of developing multiple sclerosis or optic neuritis.[41] Moreover, there appears to be a clinically significant association between MS and pars planitis, a link strengthened by common tissue typing to HLA-DR2, and, by implication, a possible shared pathogenesis.[41, 50]

Regarding the prognosis of IU, no truly excellent studies are available. At presentation, approximately 50% of patients have a visual acuity of 20/30 or better.[37] More recent follow-up studies have shown that the majority of patients maintain their good initial visual acuity,[41] with up to 90% retaining a visual acuity of 20/40 or better over 2 years in one study.[50] Nevertheless, as previously mentioned, Smith and colleagues observed significant visual disability in over one third of their patients, and it is likely that, with more long-term follow-up, patients described in more recent studies will manifest visually limiting sequela. The clinician must ask the question, "Would I find such sequela acceptable for myself?" Aggressive treatment, before ocular complications arise, is a rational approach to this problem; however, the identification of patients who would benefit most from this approach remains to be determined with more certainty. This conundrum is underscored by the fact that, to date, no controlled data have been gathered to suggest which of the many therapeutic options, either medical or surgical, are most appropriate, impacting positively on the prognosis and natural history of the disease.

CONCLUSIONS

Patients with IU represent approximately 10% to 20% of all uveitis patients. Typical vitreous infiltration with cellular exudates and, in cases of pars planitis, pars plana exudates, are found. Potentially blinding complications include glaucoma, cataract, CME, and maculopathy. IU probably represents an autoimmune disease in most cases. Although the initiating antigen may be a microbial agent, its nature remains unknown. In the pathogenesis, CD4+ T-cells seem to play a major role. The diagnosis is based on clinical findings. Associated systemic disorders, such as sarcoid, multiple sclerosis, and infectious diseases including syphilis, Lyme disease, and tuberculosis, must be excluded. For the treatment of severe IU, a modified five-step approach has proven to be effective: (1) topical and periorbital steroids; (2) oral NSAIDs; (3) systemic corticosteroids; (4) cryotherapy or scatter laser photocoagulation; and (5) immunosuppressive chemotherapy or

PPV, with or without PPL. First-choice immunomodulators include CSA and methotrexate. Visual rehabilitation through cataract surgery with intraocular lens implantation, with or without PPV, appears to be safe, provided that proper patient selection and vigilant control of preoperative and postoperative inflammation are exercised. The visual prognosis is, in general, quite good; however, significant visual debility can result. Aggressive treatment of intraocular inflammation may be important in improving the prognosis. There appears to be a clinically significant association between IU and multiple sclerosis.

References

1. Bloch-Michel E, Nussenblatt RB: International uveitis study group recommendations for the evaluation of intraocular inflammatory disease. Am J Ophthalmol 1987;103:234–235.
2. Fuchs E: Textbook of Ophthalmology. Duane A (trans) Philadelphia, J.B. Lippincott, 1908, pp 381–390.
3. Schepens CL: L'inflammation de la région de l'"ora serrata" et ses séquelles. Bull Soc Ophtalmol Fr 1950;73:113–124.
4. Brockhurst RJ, Schepens CL, Okamura ID. Uveitis. I. Gonioscopy. Am J Ophthalmol 1956;42:545–554.
5. Brockhurst RJ, Schepens CL, Okamura ID: Uveitis. II. Peripheral uveitis: Clinical description, complications and differential diagnosis. Am J Ophthalmol 1960;49:1257–1266.
6. Brockhurst RJ, Schepens CL, Okamura ID: Uveitis. III. Peripheral uveitis: Pathogenesis, etiology and treatment. Am J Ophthalmol 1961;51:19–26.
7. Brockhurst RJ, Schepens CL: Uveitis. IV. Peripheral uveitis: The complication of retinal detachment. Arch Ophthalmol 1968;80:747–753.
8. Welch RB, Maumenee AE, Wahlen HR: Peripheral posterior segment inflammation, vitreous opacities and edema of the posterior pole: Pars planitis. Arch Ophthalmol 1960;64:540–549.
9. Abrahams IW, Jiang Y: Ophthalmology in China. Arch Ophthalmol 104:444–446, 1986.
10. Bec P, Arne JL, Philippot V, et al: L'uvéo-rétinite basale et les autres inflammations de la périphérie rétinienne. Arch Ophtalmol (Paris) 1977;37:169–196.
11. Chung H, Choi DG: Clinical analysis of uveitis. Korean J Ophthalmol 1989;3:33–37.
12. Henderly DE, Genstler AJ, Smith RE, Rao NA: Changing patterns of uveitis. Am J Ophthalmol 1987;103:131–136.
13. Martenet AC: Les cyclites chroniques. Arch Ophtalmol (Paris) 1973;33:533–540.
14. Martenet AC: Uveitis intermédiares. Bull Soc Belge Ophtalmol 1989;230:33–39.
15. Rodriguez A, Calonge M, Pedroza-Seres M, et al: Referral patterns of uveitis in a tertiary eye care center. Arch Ophthalmol 1996;114:593–599.
16. Smith RE, Godfrey WA, Kimura SJ: Chronic cyclitis. I. Course and visual prognosis. Trans Am Acad Ophthalmol Otolaryngol 1973;77:760–768.
17. Vadot E: Epidemiology of intermediate uveitis: A prospective study in Savoy. Dev Ophthalmol 1992;23:33–34.
18. Weiner A, BenEzra D: Clinical patterns and associated conditions in chronic uveitis. Am J Ophthalmol 1991;112:151–159.
19. Augsberger JJ, Annesley WH, Sergott RC, et al: Familial pars planitis. Ann Ophthalmol 1981;13:553–557.
20. Culbertson WW, Giles CL, West C, Stafford T: Familial pars planitis. Retina 1983;3:179–181.
21. Doft BH: Pars planitis in identical twins. Retina 1983;3:32–33.
22. Duinkerke-Eerola KU, Pinckers A, Cruysberg JRM: Pars planitis in father and son. Ophthalmic Pediatr Genet 1990;11:305–308.
23. Giles CL, Tranton JH: Peripheral uveitis in three children of one family. J Pediatr Ophthalmol Strabismus 1980;17:297–299.
24. Hogan MJ, Kimura SJ, O'Connor GR: Peripheral retinitis and chronic cyclitis in children. Trans Ophthalmol Soc UK 1965;85:39–51.
25. Kimura SJ, Hogan MJ: Chronic cyclitis. Trans Am Ophthalmol Soc 1963;61:397–413.
26. Wetzig RP, Chan CC, Nussenblatt RB, et al: Clinical and immuno-
27. Witmer VR, Körner G: Uveitis im Kindesalter. Ophthalmologica 1966;152:277–282.
28. Khodadoust AA, Attarzadeh A: Presumed autoimmune corneal endotheliopathy. Am J Ophthalmol 1982;93:718–722.
29. Pivetti-Pezzi P, Tamburi S: Pars planitis and autoimmune endotheliopathy. Am J Ophthalmol 1987;104:311–312.
30. Tessler HH: Pars planitis and autoimmune endotheliopathy. Am J Ophthalmol 1987;103:599.
31. Nussenblatt RB, Palestine AG, Chan CC, et al: Standardization of vitreal inflammatory activity in intermediate and posterior uveitis. Ophthalmology 1985;92:467–471.
32. Arellanes L, García LM, Morales V, et al: Report of characteristic angiographic findings in a series of pars planitis patients. Invest Ophthalmol Vis Sci 1992;33:743.
33. Pruett RC, Brockhurst RJ, Letts NF: Fluorescein angiography of peripheral uveitis. Am J Ophthalmol 1974;77:448–453.
34. Schmidt F: Fluorescein angiography in intermediate uveitis. Dev Ophthalmol 1992;23:139–144.
35. Godfrey WA, Smith RE, Kimura SJ: Chronic cyclitis: Corticosteroid therapy. Trans Am Ophthalmol Soc 1976;74:178–188.
36. Deane JS, Rosenthal AR: Course and complications of intermediate uveitis. Acta Ophthalmol Scand 1997;75:82–84.
37. Henderly DE, Haymond RS, Rao NS, et al: The significance of the pars plana exudate in pars planitis. Am J Ophthalmol 1987;103:669–671.
38. Pederson JE, Kenyon KR, Green WR, Maumenee AE: Pathology of pars planitis. Am J Ophthalmol 1978;86:762–774.
39. Schlote T, Zierhut M: Ocular hypertension and glaucoma associated with scleritis and uveitis: Aspects of epidemiology, pathogenesis, and therapy. Dev Ophthalmol, 1999;30:91–109.
40. Giles CL: Pediatric intermediate uveitis. J Pediatr Ophthalmol Strabismus 1989;26:136–139.
41. Malinowski SM, Pulido JS, Folk JC: Long term visual outcome and complications associated with pars planitis. Ophthalmology 1993;100:818–824.
42. Smith RE, Godfrey WA, Kimura SJ: Complications of chronic cyclitis. Am J Ophthalmol 1976;82:277–282.
43. Davis JL, Palestine AG, Nussenblatt RB: Neovascularization in uveitis. Ophthalmology 1988;95:171.
44. Shields CL, Shields JA, Barrett J, De Potter P: Vasoproliferative tumors of the ocular fundus—classification and clinical manifestation in 103 patients. Arch Ophthalmol 1995;113:615–623.
45. Schenck F, Böke W: Fluoreszenzangiographische Befunde bei intermediärer Uveitis. Klin Mbl Augenheilkd 1988;193:261–265.
46. Nussenblatt RB, Whitcup SM, Palestine AG: Intermediate uveitis. In: Uveitis. Fundamentals and Clinical Practice, 2nd ed. St. Louis, Mosby, 1996, pp 279–288.
47. Opremcak EM, Cowans AB, Orosz CG, et al: Enumeration of autoreactive helper T lymphocytes in uveitis. Invest Ophthalmol Vis Sci 1991;32:2561–2567.
48. Martin T, Weber M, Schmitt C, et al: Association of intermediate uveitis with HLA-A28: Definition of a new systemic syndrome? Graefe's Arch Clin Exp Ophthalmol 1995;233:269–274.
49. Tang WM, Pulido JS, Eckels DD, et al: The association of HLA-DR15 and intermediate uveitis. Am J Ophthalmol 1997;123:70–75.
50. Raja SC, Jabs DA, Dunn JP, et al: Pars planitis: Clinical features and class II HLA associations. Ophthalmology 1999;106:594–599.
51. Bora NS, Bora PS, Kaplan HJ: Identification, quantitation, and purification of a 36 kda circulating protein associated with active pars planitis. Invest Ophthalmol Vis Sci 1996;37:1870–1876.
52. Bora NS, Bora PS, Tandhasetti MT, et al: Molecular cloning, sequencing, and expression of the 36 kDa protein present in pars planitis. Invest Ophthalmol Vis Sci 1996;37:1877–1883.
53. Green WR, Kincaid MC, Michels RG, et al: Pars planitis. Trans Ophthalmol Soc UK 1981;101:361–367.
54. Kenyon KR, Pederson JE, Green WR, Maumenee AE: Fibroglial proliferation in pars planitis. Trans Ophthalmol Soc UK 1975;95:391–397.
55. Green RW: Retina: Inflammatory diseases and conditions. In: Spencer WH, ed: Ophthalmic Pathology, An Atlas and Textbook, vol 2, 3rd ed. Philadelphia: W.B. Saunders Co, 1985, pp 790–792.
56. Yoser SL, Forster DJ, Rao NA: Pathology of intermediate uveitis. Dev Ophthalmol 1992;23:60–70.

57. Nölle B, Eckardt C: Cellular phenotype of vitreous cells in intermediate uveitis. Dev Ophthalmol 1992;23:145–149.

58. Davis JL, Solomon D, Nussenblatt RB, et al: Immunocytochemical staining of vitreous cells: Indications, techniques, and results. Ophthalmology 1992;99:250–256.

59. Kaplan HJ, Waldrep JC, Nicholson JKA, Gordon D: Immunologic analysis of intraocular mononuclear cell infiltrates in uveitis. Arch Ophthalmol 1984;102:572–575.

60. Heiligenhaus A, Bornfeld N, Foerster MH, Wessing A: Long term results of pars plana vitrectomy in the management of complicated uveitis. Br J Ophthalmol 1994;78:549–554.

61. Yokoyama MM, Matsui Y, Yamashiroya HM, et al.: Humoral and cellular immunity studies in patients with Vogt-Koyanagi-Harada syndrome and pars planitis. Invest Ophthalmol Vis Sci 1981;20:364–370.

62. Klok AM, Luyendijk L, Zaal MJ, et al: Elevated serum IL-8 levels are associated with disease activity in idiopathic intermediate uveitis. Br J Ophthalmol 1998;82:871–874.

63. Murray PI, Young DW: Soluble interleukin-2 receptors in retinal vasculitis. Curr Eye Res 1992;11(Suppl):193–195.

64. Arocker-Mettinger E, Steurer-Georgiew L, Steurer M, et al: Circulating ICAM-1 levels in serum of uveitis patients. Curr Eye Res 1992;11(Suppl):161–166.

65. BenEzra D, Maftzir G, Barak V: Blood serum interleukin-1 receptor antagonist in pars planitis and ocular Behçet disease. Am J Ophthalmol 1997;123:593–598.

66. Nölle B: Antiretinal autoantibodies in intermediate uveitis. Dev Ophthalmol 1992;23:94–98.

67. Davis JL, Chan CC, Nussenblatt RB: HLA in intermediate uveitis. Dev Ophthalmol 1992;23:71–85.

68. Doekes G, vanderGaag R, Rothova A, et al: Humoral and cellular immune responsiveness to human S-antigen in uveitis. Curr Eye Res 1987;6:909–919.

69. DeSmet MD, Yamamoto JH, Mochizuki M, et al: Cellular immune responses of patients with uveitis to retinal antigens and their fragments. Am J Ophthalmol 1990;110:135–142.

70. Nussenblatt RB, Salinas-Carmona M, Leake W, Scher I: T lymphocyte subsets in uveitis. Am J Ophthalmol 1983;95:614–621.

71. Zierhut M, Klein R, Berg P, et al: Augenunspezifische Autoantikörper bei Uveitis. Fortschr Ophthalmol 1989;86:482–485.

72. Hultsch E: Peripheral uveitis in the owl monkey. Mod Probl Ophthalmol 1977;18:247–251.

73. Lieberman J: Enzymes in sarcoidosis: Angiotensin converting enzyme (ACE). Clin Lab Med 1989;9:745.

74. Zierhut M: Uveitis, Vol I. Differential Diagnosis. Buren, Netherlands, Aeolus Press, 1995.

75. Weinreb RN, Yavitz EQ, O'Connor GR, Barth RA: Lacrimal gland uptake of gallium citrate Ga 67. Am J Ophthalmol 1981;92:16–20.

76. Power WJ, Neves RA, Rodriguez A, et al: The value of combined serum angiotensin-converting enzyme and gallium scan in diagnosing ocular sarcoidosis. Ophthalmology 1995;102:2007–2011.

77. Haring G, Nolle B, Wiechens B: Ultrasound biomicroscopic imaging in intermediate uveitis. Br J Ophthalmol 1998;82:625–629.

78. Cantrill HL, Ramsay RC, Knobloch WH, Purple RL: Electrophysiologic changes in chronic pars planitis. Am J Ophthalmol 1981;91:505–512.

79. Ortega C, Jimenez JM, Arellanes L, Angel E: Electrophysiologic changes in chronic pars planitis. Invest Ophthalmol Vis Sci 1992;33:743.

80. Tetsuka S, Katsumi O, Mehta MC, et al: Electrophysiological findings in peripheral uveitis. Ophthalmologica 1991;203:89–98.

81. Zimmerman MD, Dawson WW, Fitzgerald CR: Part I: Electroretinographic changes in normal eyes during administration of prednisone. Ann Ophthalmol 1973;5:757–765.

82. Breger BC, Leopold IH: The incidence of uveitis in multiple sclerosis. Am J Ophthalmol 1966;62:540–545.

83. Giles CL: Peripheral uveitis in patients with multiple sclerosis. Am J Ophthalmol 1970;70:17–19.

84. Porter R: Uveitis in association with multiple sclerosis. Br J Ophthalmol 1972;56:478–481.

85. Chester GH, Blach RK, Cleary PE: Inflammation in the region of the vitreous base: Pars planitis. Trans Ophthalmol Soc UK 1976;96:151–197.

86. Zierhut M, Foster S: Multiple sclerosis, sarcoidosis and other diseases in patients with pars planitis. Dev Ophthalmol 1992;23:41–47.

87. Engell T: Neurological disease activity in multiple sclerosis patients with periphlebitis retinae. Acta Neurol Scand 1986;73:168–172.

88. Malinowski SM, Pulido JS, Goeken ME, et al: The association of HLA-B8, B51, DR2, and multiple sclerosis in pars planitis patients. Ophthalmology 1993;100:1199–1204.

89. Landers PH: Vitreous lesions in Boeck's sarcoid. Am J Ophthalmol 1949;32:1740–1741.

90. Crick RP: Ocular sarcoidosis. Trans Ophthalmol Soc UK 1955;75:189–206.

91. Jabs DA, Johns CJ: Ocular involvement in chronic sarcoidosis. Am J Ophthalmol 1990;102:297–301.

92. Tamesis RR, Foster CS: Ocular syphilis. Ophthalmology 1990;97:1281–1287.

93. Breeveld J, Rothova A, Kuiper H: Intermediate uveitis and Lyme borreliosis. Br J Ophthalmol 1992;76:181–182.

94. Guex-Crosier Y, Herbort CP: Maladie de Lyme en Suisse: Atteintes oculaires. Klin Monatsbl Augenheilkd 1992;200:545–546.

95. Nölle B: Serological evidence of an association between Lyme borreliosis and intermediate uveitis. Dev Ophthalmol 1992;23:115–117.

96. Winward KE, Hamed LM, Glaser JS: The spectrum of optic nerve disease in human immunodeficiency virus infection. Am J Ophthalmol 1989;107:373–380.

97. Mochizuki M, Watanabe T, Yamaguchi K, et al: Uveitis associated with human T-cell lymphotropic virus type I. Am J Ophthalmol 1992;114:123–129.

98. Mochizuki M, Watanabe T, Yamaguchi K, Tajima K: Human T-lymphotropic virus type I associated disease. In: Pepose JS, Holland GN, Wilhelmus KR, eds: Ocular Infection and Immunity. St. Louis, Mosby, 1996, pp 1366–1387.

99. Soheilian M, Markomichelakis N, Foster CS: Intermediate uveitis and retinal vasculitis as manifestations of cat scratch disease. Am J Ophthalmol 1996;122:582–584.

100. Jones DB: Cat scratch disease. In: Pepose JS, Holland GN, Wilhelmus KR, eds: Ocular Infection and Immunity. St. Louis, Mosby, 1996, pp 1389–1397.

101. Lazar M, Weiner MH, Leopold IH: Treatment of uveitis with methotrexate. Am J Ophthalmol 1969;67:383–387.

102. Michels RG, Knox DL, Erozan YS, Green WR: Intraocular reticulum cell sarcoma. Diagnosis by pars plana vitrectomy. Arch Ophthalmol 1975;93:1331–1335.

103. Sherman MD, Own KH: Interstitial nephritis and uveitis syndrome presenting with bilateral optic disk edema. Am J Ophthalmol 1999;127:609–610.

104. Dann K, Althaus C, Kersten A, et al: Uveitis-Masquerade-Syndrom bei M.Gaucher. Kausale Behandlung durch Alglucerase-Substitutionstherapie. Klin Monatsbl Augenheilkd 1998;213:358–361.

105. Ormerod LD, Puklin JE, Giles CL: Chronic *Propionibacterium acnes* endophthalmitis as a cause of intermediate uveitis. Ocul Immunol Inflamm 1997;5:67–68.

106. Davis JL, Bloch-Michel E: Intermediate uveitis. In: Pepose JS, Holland GN, Wilhelmus KR, eds: Ocular Infection and Immunity. St. Louis, Mosby, 1996, pp 676–693.

107. Kaplan HJ: Intermediate uveitis (pars planitis, chronic cyclitis)—a four step approach to treatment. In: Saari KM, ed: Uveitis Update. Amsterdam, Excerpta Medica, 1984, pp 169–172.

108. Helm CJ, Holland GN: The effects of posterior subtenon injection of triamcinolone acetonide in patients with intermediate uveitis. Am J Ophthalmol 1995;120:55–64.

109. Tanner V, Kanski JJ, Frith PA: Posterior sub-Tenon's triamcinolone injections in the treatment of uveitis. Eye 1998;12:679–685.

110. Schlote T, Zierhut M: Treatment of uveitic macular edema with acetazolamide. Doc Ophthalmol 1999;97:409–413.

111. Flach AJ: Cyclo-oxygenase inhibitors in ophthalmology. Surv Ophthalmol 1992;36:259–284.

112. Schlote T, Dannecker G, Thiel HJ, Zierhut M: Cyclosporin A in der Therapie der chronischen Uveitis im Kindesalter. Ophthalmologe 1996;93:745–748.

113. Walton RC, Nussenblatt RB, Whitcup SM: Cyclosporine therapy for severe sight-threatening uveitis in children and adolescents. Ophthalmology 1998;105:2028–2034.

114. Zierhut M: Uveitis, Vol 2. Therapy. Buren, The Netherlands, Aeolus Press, 1996.

115. Wong VG: Immunosuppressive therapy of ocular inflammatory diseases. Arch Ophthalmol 1969;81:628–637.

116. Wong VG, Hersh EM: Methotrexate in the treatment of cyclitis. Trans Am Acad Ophthalmol Otolaryngol 1965;69:279–293.

117. Wong VG: Methotrexate treatment of uveal disease. Am J Med Sci 1966;251:239–241.

118. Holz FG, Krastel H, Breitbart A, et al: Low-dose methotrexate treatment in noninfectious uveitis resistant to corticosteroids. German J Ophthalmol 1992;1:142–144.

119. Shah SS, Lowder CY, Schmitt MA, et al: Low-dose methotrexate therapy for ocular inflammatory disease. Ophthalmology 1992;99:1419–1423.

120. Dev S, McCallum RM, Jaffee GJ: Methotrexate treatment for sarcoid-associated panuveitis. Ophthalmology 1999;106:111–118.

121. Newell FW, Krill AE: Treatment of uveitis with azathioprine (Imuran). Trans Ophthalmol Soc UK 1967;87:499–511.

122. Gills JP, Durham NC: Combined medical and surgical therapy for complicated cases of peripheral uveitis. Arch Ophthalmol 1968;79:723–728.

123. Godfrey WA, Epstein WV, O'Connor GR, et al: The use of chlorambucil in intractable idiopathic uveitis. Am J Ophthalmol 1974;78:415–428.

124. Kilmartin DJ, Forrester JV, Dick AD: Rescue therapy with mycophenolate mofetil in refractory uveitis. Lancet 1998;352:35–36.

125. Larkin G, Lightman S: Mycophenolate mofetil—a useful immunosuppressive in inflammatory eye disease. Ophthalmology 1999;106:370–374.

126. Aaberg TM, Cesarz TJ, Flickinger RR: Treatment of peripheral uveoretinitis by cryotherapy. Am J Ophthalmol 1973;75:685–688.

127. Aaberg TM, Cesarz TJ, Flickinger RR: Treatment of pars planitis. Cryotherapy. Surv Ophthalmol 1977;22:120–130.

128. Devenyi RG, Mieler WF, Lambrou FH, et al: Cryopexy of the vitreous base in the management of peripheral uveitis. Am J Ophthalmol 1988;106:135–138.

129. Mieler WF, Aaberg TM: Further observations on cryotherapy on the vitreous base in the management of peripheral uveitis. Dev Ophthalmol 1992;23:190–195.

130. Okinami S, Sunakawa M, Arai I, et al: Treatment of pars planitis with cryotherapy. Ophthalmologica 1991;202:180–186.

131. Berg P, Kroll P: Cryotherapy in uveitis. Dev Ophthalmol, Basel, Karger, 1992;23:219–225.

132. Verma L, Kumar A, Garg S, et al: Cryopexy in pars planitis. Can J Ophthalmol 1991;26:313–315.

133. Franklin RM: Laser photocoagulation of retinal neovascularization in intermediate uveitis. Dev Ophthalmol 1992;23:251–260.

134. Park WE, Mieler WF, Pulido JS: Peripheral scatter photocoagulation for neovascularization associated with pars planitis. Arch Ophthalmol 1995;113:1277.

135. Diamond JG, Kaplan HJ: Lensectomy and vitrectomy for complicated cataract secondary to uveitis. Arch Ophthalmol 1978;96:1798–1804.

136. Mieler WF, Will BR, Lewis H, Aaberg TM: Vitrectomy in the management of peripheral uveitis. Ophthalmology 1988;95:859–864.

137. Heimann K, Schmanke L, Brunner R, et al: Pars plana vitrectomy in the treatment of chronic uveitis. Dev Ophthalmol 1992;23:196–203.

138. Eckardt C, Bacskulin A: Vitrectomy in intermediate uveitis. Dev Ophthalmol 1992;23:232–238.

139. Dugel PU, Rao NA, Ozler S, et al: Pars plana vitrectomy for intraocular inflammation related to cystoid macular edema unresponsive to corticosteroids: A preliminary study. Ophthalmology 1992;99:1535–1541.

140. Schönfeld CL, Weißschädel S, Heidenkummer HP, Kampik A: Vitreoretinal surgery in intermediate uveitis. German J Ophthalmol 1995;4:37–42.

141. Foster CS, Fong LP, Singh G: Cataract surgery and intraocular lens implantation in patients with uveitis. Ophthalmology 1989;96:281–287.

142. Fogla R, Biswas J, Ganesh SK, Ravishankar K: Evaluation of cataract surgery in intermediate uveitis. Ophthalmic Surg Lasers 1999;30:191–198.

143. Michelson JB, Friedlaender MH, Nozik RA: Lens implant surgery in pars planitis. Ophthalmology 1990;97:1023–1026.

144. Kaufman AH, Foster CS: Cataract extraction in patients with pars planitis. Ophthalmology 1993;100:1210–1217.

145. Brunner R, Borberg H, Kadar J, et al: Plasma exchange and immunoglobulins in the treatment of intermediate uveitis. Dev Ophthalmol 1992;23:275–284.

146. Nussenblatt RB, Gery I, Weiner HL, et al: Treatment of uveitis by oral administration of retinal antigens: Results of a phase I/II randomized masked trial. Am J Ophthalmol 1997;123:583–592.

Part VII

THE UVEITIS SYNDROMES: Medication Induced

79 MEDICATION-INDUCED UVEITIS

Margarita Calonge

DEFINITION

Medication-induced or drug-induced uveitis is a well-described and yet uncommon adverse reaction to medications. Under this designation, intraocular inflammation (cells and flare in the anterior chamber or vitreous cavity, or both) induced not just by medications but also by vaccines, toxins, or other substances is also included, regardless of the route of administration.[1, 2]

There are many medications that may cause uveitis (Table 79–1).[1–3] These medications have been reported to cause intraocular inflammation when injected into the anterior chamber or the vitreous cavity, or both. In addition, many of the substances and drugs mentioned in Table 79–1 are only possibly associated with uveitis, and because their causality in the production of uveitis is so weak, they will not be mentioned in this review. This chapter addresses uveitis caused by medications administered systemically or topically for which a cause-and-effect relationship with intraocular inflammation is proven or, at least, probable. These medications include systemic biphosphonates (pamidronic acid), intravitreous and systemic cidofovir, topical corticosteroids, topical latanoprost and metipranolol, systemic rifabutin, and systemic sulfonamides.[1, 2] A brief description of uveitis reported for many other agents that may possibly cause uveitis is listed in Table 79–1.

HISTORY

There are many reports in the ophthalmic literature over the past 35 years that have implicated medications, drugs, and vaccines as causes of intraocular inflammation.[1–3] Despite this fact, however, medication-induced uveitis is usually neglected in the differential diagnosis of uveitis. Of late, there is an increasing interest in the putative role of drugs as causes of intraocular inflammation because of reports of uveitis in patients with the acquired immunodeficiency syndrome (AIDS) receiving rifabutin and glaucoma patients treated with the recently marketed topical latanoprost.

Most reports of drug-induced uveitis are merely clinical observations with no histopathologic proof, and therefore, it is difficult to attribute causality of the inflammation to one particular drug or medication. In 1981, Naranjo and colleagues[4] proposed seven criteria to help establish causality of adverse events by drugs. Recently, Moorthy and associates[2, 5] applied these criteria to some drugs that the authors believed to be the cause of uveitis to evaluate causality; they found that it is rare that drugs

implicated in the induction of uveitis meet all of those criteria.

EPIDEMIOLOGY

Because medication-induced uveitis is an adverse drug reaction, it may be considered an iatrogenic eye disease.[6] Iatrogenic illness in general is a relevant problem, because it affects as many as one third of all hospitalized patients, and 3% to 7% of hospitalizations are attributable to adverse reactions to medications.[7] Drug-induced uveitis, however, seems to be a rare event: Fraunfelder and Rosenbaum[1] recently reported an incidence of less that 0.5% in their patient database. There is, however, an unavoidable bias because this figure refers to patients cared for in a tertiary referral Uveitis Clinic, while many patients with medication-induced uveitis are likely to go to general ophthalmology clinics or to AIDS and glaucoma specialists.

In general, there does not seem to be an age or sex predilection, and no HLA association has been described for any drug-related uveitis.

ETIOLOGY

Drugs implicated in the induction of uveitis include systemically administered drugs, topically applied medications and substances injected intraocularly. Intradermal vaccines, such as those used for influenza, hepatitis B, and bacille Calmette-Guérin (BCG) have been implicated in producing uveitis, as has skin testing with tuberculin protein (see Table 79–1).[1–3]

It is far from clear, however, that all of these agents are the real cause of the uveitis. Many of the reports are merely clinical observations without confirmation. In this sense, Naranjo and colleagues[4] proposed the following seven criteria, which should be fulfilled to attribute causality of adverse effects by drugs:

1. The adverse reaction should be a frequently described event and hence be well documented.
2. Recovery should occur on withdrawal of the drug.
3. Other possible causes for the event should be excluded.
4. The event should become more severe with increased dosage of the drug.
5. The adverse reaction should be documented by objective evidence.
6. The patients should experience a similar effect with similar drugs.

TABLE 79–1. DRUGS ASSOCIATED WITH INTRAOCULAR INFLAMMATION AND TYPE OF UVEITIS INDUCED

MEDICATION	UVEITIS CHARACTERISTICS/OTHER FINDINGS
SYSTEMIC DRUGS (ORAL, INTRAVENOUS, SUBCUTANEOUS)	
Antiproteases (ritonavir, indinavir, saquinavir)	Anterior
Biphosphonates* (pamidronate, risedronate, alendronate)	Anterior, mild-severe/episcleritis, scleritis, general symptoms
Chlorpromazine	Anterior, mild/lens pigment deposits
Cidofovir*	Anterior, mild-moderate/hypotony
Cobalt	Anterior, mild-moderate
Contraceptives (oral)	Anterior, retinal vasculitis, papilledema
Diethylcarbamazine	Anterior, chorioretinitis
Hydralazine	Lupus-like syndrome with episcleritis and retinal vasculitis
Ibuprofen	Anterior, mild/aseptic meningitis
Interleukin-3/interleukin-6	Anterior, moderate-intense
Nitrogen mustard	Necrotizing uveitis with retinal vasculitis
Procainamide	Lupus-like syndrome with episcleritis
Quinidine	Anterior, mild-moderate
Rifabutin*	Anterior, moderate-severe, hypopyon, vitritis/retinal vasculitis, general symptoms
Streptokinase	Anterior/serum sickness
Sulfonamides*	Anterior/systemic findings
Trimethoprim	Retinal hemorrhages
TOPICAL OCULAR DRUGS	
Amphotericin B	Anterior, mild
Anesthetics (topical) (benoxinate, butacaine, dibucaine, dyclonine, phenacaine)	Anterior, mild
β-blockers (other than metipranolol) (betaxolol, levobunolol, timolol)	Anterior, mild
Cholinesterase inhibitors (diisopropyl fluorophosphate, phospholine iodide, isoflurophate (demecarium bromide, echothiophate)	Anterior mild
Corticosteroids*	Anterior, mild-moderate, after withdrawal
Latanoprost*	Anterior, mild-moderate, predisposed eyes/cystoid macular edema
Metipranolol*	Anterior, moderate, granulomatous
Mitomycin C	Anterior, mild
Thiotepa	Anterior, mild
INTRAOCULAR DRUGS/SUBSTANCES FOR SURGERY	
Anesthesics (local) (bupivacaine, chloroprocaine, etidocaine, lidocaine, mepivacaine, prilocaine, propoxycaine)	Anterior, mild to severe
Antibiotics (amphotericin B, bacitracin, tetracycline, chlortetracycline, colistin, erythromycin, neomycin, penicillins, polymixin B, streptomycin, chloramphenicol)	Anterior, mild-moderate
Cidofovir*	Anterior, mild to moderate/hypotony
Urokinase	Sterile hypopyon, vitreous hemorrhage
Air	Anterior, mild
Perfluorocarbons	Anterior, severe
Silicone oil	Anterior, mild to moderate
Alpha-chymotrypsin	Vitritis, severe
VACCINES	
Bacille Calmette-Guérin (BCG)	Anterior, retinal pigment epithelium anomalies/iris atrophy
Influenza	Anterior, vitritis/optic neuritis, scleritis
Hepatitis B	Acute multifocal placoid epitheliopathy
Purified protein derivative (PPD) skin test	Anterior, vitritis, multifocal choroiditis, serous retinal detachment
OTHER	
Petty spurge sap (*Euphorbia peplus*)	Anterior/keratitis
Skin tattoos	Anterior, mild to moderate/skin granuloma

*Drugs associated with uveitis. These are the only drugs that probably cause uveitis. The remainder drugs are possibly related to uveitis, reported in single case reports and/or that causation has not been proven.

7. The event should recur on rechallenge with the suspected drug.

Using these criteria, Fraunfelder and Rosenbaum consider that medications reported to cause uveitis are the probable cause if many of the above-mentioned criteria are met, whereas the remainder of the medications that do not fulfill many of those criteria can possibly have a causative effect.[1] Moorthy and associates consider a probable cause of uveitis those drugs meeting at least five criteria.[2] For these authors, only systemic biphosphonates (pamidronic acid) and topical metipranolol fulfill all seven criteria, whereas systemic sulfonamides, rifabutin, and topical corticosteroids meet at least five criteria; the remaining drugs meet less than five. These authors did not include topical latanoprost in their initial evaluation,[2] although later they believed that this drug is also a probable cause of medication-induced uveitis.[5]

All authors agree that the most convincing criterion to be met is that the adverse event recurs on rechallenge.

The main drugs and substances reported to have caused intraocular inflammation are listed in Table 79–1. Some of them produced uveitis primarily, because confounding variables were eliminated and double-blind randomized rechallenge testing was performed. Some other drugs reported to have caused uveitis in single case reports lack accurate documentation or causation cannot be fully attributed.

PATHOGENESIS

Many of the adverse reactions to medications are idiosyncratic, unexpected, or unavoidable. But others result from medications used incorrectly or prescribed inappropriately.

Just as uveitis has multiple causes, so, too, multiple mechanisms could account for drug-induced uveitis. In most cases, the pathogenesis of the drug-induced intraocular inflammation is unknown or ill understood owing in part to the absence of histopathologic specimens.

Although the described mechanisms that produce drug-induced ocular toxicity may well be involved in drug-induced uveitis, there is no convincing evidence so far to demonstrate that drugs may induce uveitis by any of these reported multiple mechanisms.[8] Therefore, the pathogenic mechanisms mentioned later remain speculative and have not been fully proved to produce uveitis.

At least from a theoretical point of view, medications and other substances can cause intraocular inflammation by direct or indirect mechanisms, as recently pointed out by Moorthy and associates.[2] A direct mechanism, meaning that the drug must enter the eye, can usually be implicated for those drugs topically applied or intraocularly injected, and the inflammation usually develops soon after drug delivery. The drug can cause direct toxicity by itself or through its metabolites.[8] In general, topical drugs and those injected into the anterior chamber appear to induce uveitis by a direct disruption of the blood-aqueous barrier, whereas drugs applied intravitreally can cause a breakdown of both blood-aqueous and blood-retinal barriers.[2]

A drug can also cause uveitis by several indirect mechanisms, mainly by stimulation of the immune system via different routes.[2] First, the drug either by itself or combined with tissue or serum proteins may stimulate the production of antidrug antibodies. Thus, immune complexes may form and deposit in uveal blood vessels, producing uveitis weeks or even months after initial contact with the drug. Second, it is possible that the drug nonspecifically stimulates the immune system acting as an adjuvant. For example, secondary immunologic mechanisms can be enhanced by drugs, causing death of microbes located in the eye if antigens are released. The subsequent immune reaction can produce uveitis in the first 24 hours, but sometimes the process can take longer.[2] Third, melanin-related mechanisms, although more speculative, are also possible causes of inflammation weeks or months after drug exposure. There are certain drugs that, in addition to having an intrinsic high affinity for melanin, can also induce the release of toxic free radicals, which are partly detoxified by melanin. The consequence

of both is an impairment of melanin's capacity as a scavenger of free radicals, thus potentiating these drugs' toxicity and that from other sources of free radical production, with the induction of intraocular inflammation being the eventual consequence. Alternatively, if a drug combines with melanin, the intrinsic uveitogenicity of this pigment may be enhanced.[2, 8]

CLINICAL CHARACTERISTICS

Common Clinical Features

Drug-induced uveitis usually causes mild to moderate symptoms such as a mild decrease in visual acuity (in the range of 20/50 to 20/40, provided there was a previous good visual acuity). Some drugs, however, such as oral rifabutin, can cause severe uveitis if high doses are used (especially in combination with drugs that increase rifabutin's blood levels) and if the drug is not discontinued.[9–11]

Uveitis induced by drugs is characterized by cellular infiltration in the anterior chamber and, more infrequently, the vitreous. Inflammation in the anterior chamber may range from mild to intense, and it is usually nongranulomatous. Occasionally, posterior synechiae develop and hypopyon can also be seen.[10–12] In the vitreous, the cell reaction is usually mild, although some cases of severe vitritis, mainly attributed to oral rifabutin, have been reported.[9–11] There is usually an absence of retinal or choroidal lesions with a few exceptions.[13]

Drugs inducing uveitis by systemic routes can produce both unilateral or bilateral inflammation. Obviously, topical or intraocular drugs produce uveitis only in the targeted eye.

There is no recurrence of inflammation when the uveitis is purely due to a drug adverse effect, provided such drug is discontinued. Therefore, complications are not usually encountered and prognosis is favorable. Yet, uveitis can recur, either in the previously affected eye or in the contralateral one if the drug is not stopped. In these cases, involvement of all structures of the eye may occur, developing into a sterile endophthalmitis or panophthalmitis. This is a rare event, however, and has only been reported in oral rifabutin-induced cases.[9, 11, 12]

Usually, drug-induced uveitis has no systemic associations, although some drugs have been described to produce extraocular manifestations, such as the arthralgias or arthritis syndrome produced by high doses of rifabutin[14] or the mild general malaise associated with systemic biphosphonates.[15]

Distinct Clinical Pictures

The clinical picture of drug-induced uveitis can logically be different depending on the offending drug. A general overview is given in Table 79–1, and a more extensive review is given below only for those medications whose association with uveitis is proven or probable, but not for those with a possible association.

Biphosphonates (Pamidronate, Risedronate)

Biphosphonates (alendronate, clodronate, etidronate, pamidronate, risedronate) are inhibitors of bone resorption that are used in the management of Paget's disease of the bone, metastatic bone pain, tumor-induced hypercalcemia, and osteoporosis.[15] Two of these agents, oral risedronate and especially intravenous pamidronate, have been associated with anterior uveitis. The majority of those cases have been reported by Macarol and Fraunfelder,[15] who analyzed 23 reports of suspected ocular adverse reactions associated with the use of intravenous pamidronate disodium in a review from the Ciba-Geigy Central Epidemiology and Drug Safety Center.[16–21] Thirteen patients had nonspecific transitory conjunctivitis, three cases involved episcleritis or scleritis, and seven patients developed anterior uveitis. Most of the reported cases developed within the first 24 to 48 hours, and the severity ranged from mild (either clearing spontaneously or with topical corticosteroids) to severe, recurring when steroids were tapered.[15–21] More recently, three cases of alendronate-associated scleritis with possible contiguous myositis and orbital inflammation have been reported.[22]

The uveitis usually recurs when patients are rechallenged with the same or a similar biphosphonate.[15, 20] There are, however, two of these compounds that have not been associated with uveitis (disodium clodronate and disodium etidronate), which may be alternative therapies for patients developing uveitis after treatment with pamidronate or risedronate.[15, 20]

The acute ocular inflammatory response has also been associated in some patients with transient fever and a flulike episode, and it seems not to be related with the route of administration, the dosage or the activity of the baseline disease.[15]

The mechanism by which these biphosphonates cause anterior uveitis is not known. The precipitation of a type III hypersensitivity reaction by the drug has been hypothesized by some authors,[15] reasoning that these compounds are known to release interleukin 1 and 6, which can cause lymphocyte proliferation and enhancement of immune complex disease.

Cidofovir

Studies on cidofovir, a nucleotide analogue that inhibits viral DNA polymerase, have demonstrated its efficacy and safety when used intravenously for the treatment of both previously untreated[23] and treated but relapsing[24] cytomegalovirus (CMV) retinitis in patients with the AIDS. Uncontrolled case series have shown that intravitreous cidofovir seems to also be effective in preventing the relapse of CMV retinitis.[25–27] Anterior uveitis hypotony has been described in patients receiving intravenous and intravitreal cidofovir from the initial use of this drug and it seems to be independent of whether patients were or were not on immunodeficiency virus protease inhibitor therapy.[23–38]

Anterior nongranulomatous uveitis associated with intravitreal cidofovir injections ranges from mild to moderate, and its frequency seems to be dose dependent. The initial injections of 100-μg and 40-μg doses were always associated with uveitis and severe hypotony associated with loss of vision.[32] Consecutive series showed that a 20-μg dose of cidofovir (with concomitant oral probenecid) was highly effective but still produced uveitis in 14% of injections[26, 27] and in 23% to 32% of patients after the first injection.[29, 33, 34] Severe hypotony with irreversible

visual loss also occurred in 1% of injections and 3% of eyes, and transient hypotony with recoverable visual loss in 14% of eyes.[34] Iritis accompanied all cases of transient and chronic hypotony, but there were instances of iritis with no hypotony.[34] A first episode of uveitis seems to facilitate subsequent episodes with a second injection in the same or in the contralateral eye.[29] Kersten and coworkers[31] have found that 15 μg was effective but still found iritis and hypotony in 25% of eyes. Although 10-μg injections produced fewer side effects, with only a 2.2% frequency of iritis, this dose was less effective.[33]

Intravenous cidofovir produces a similar intraocular inflammatory response in 26%[30] to 59% of patients,[38] which occurs after 5 days, following four doses and may be bilateral. The reported rate of hypotony with visual consequences is similar to that reported for intravitreal injections.[28, 30]

Cidofovir seems to cause hypotony by damaging the nonpigmented epithelium of the ciliary body,[34, 39] with the subsequent possibility of ciliary body atrophy,[40] although the exact cause of iritis and its relation to hypotony is not well understood. Iritis accompanied all transient and chronic hypotony cases after both intraocular and intravenous cidofovir, but there were cases of iritis with no hypotony.[30, 34] However, intraocular pressure in eyes with iritis after a first injection of cidofovir was lower than in eyes with no anterior uveitis.[40]

Oral probenecid has been shown to reduce the incidence of uveitis effectively after the first injection from 71% to 18%. The explanation given is that this drug reduces the absorption of cidofovir into the ciliary body, thus decreasing the chance of developing uveitis.[29]

Most uveitis cases attributed to cidofovir have resolved within 2 weeks with frequent administration of topical corticosteroids and cycloplegics,[29] but some cases recurred, necessitating cidofovir discontinuation.[37] Topical steroids, however, have not been effective in preventing iritis after cidofovir injections of 20 μg.[29] Posterior synechiae, cataract, and hypotonous maculopathy cystoid macular edema (CME) vitritis have all been described as long-term sequelae of the uveitis.[29, 31, 34, 36, 37]

In summary, anterior uveitis and hypotony are common complications after cidofovir therapy. These complications may not preclude the use of this drug, because the response to topical treatment is usually rapid and satisfactory. However, if inflammation recurs or hypotony persists, cidofovir may have to be discontinued.

Corticosteroids

It is often difficult to ascertain whether uveitis reported to be induced by topical corticosteroids is, in fact, due to the use of these drugs because these agents are so widely used for the treatment of uveitis and for many other ocular inflammatory conditions. Nonetheless, there seems to be strong evidence that nongranulomatous anterior uveitis can be elicited on withdrawal of topical steroids.[41–45] This observation was first made by Krupin in 1970,[42] who published two cases of ipsilateral anterior uveitis found in a population of 2000 patients who were receiving topical dexamethasone sodium phosphate to test the response of their intraocular pressure (IOP) to topical steroids. In these two patients, topical steroid therapy was discontinued after 30 days because of a decrease in IOP and periocular pain. Two to five days later, anterior uveitis was diagnosed, which responded well to cycloplegics and intensive topical treatment with dexamethasone, the same agent that presumably had provoked the inflammation. Four years later, Martins and associates[43] reported 16 cases out a population of 621 patients who developed mild anterior uveitis after 2.5 to 6 weeks of treatment with dexamethasone sodium phosphate (except one patient, who received topical triamcinolone acetonide) and 1 to 16 days after topical corticosteroids had been stopped. Inflammation vanished within 3 to 10 days with cycloplegics and with no steroid treatment. One case was rechallenged with prednisolone acetate 1% for 15 days, and inflammation recurred 2 days after drops were discontinued because of steroid-induced pressure elevation, whereas no recurrences were observed upon rechallenge with the vehicles.

Similar experiences reported in three more publications[41, 44, 45] allow one to conclude that withdrawal of different corticosteroids drops may produce a subsequent episode of uveitis, fulfilling five of the seven criteria of Naranjo and associates to attribute causality.[4] There is not enough information in the cases reported as to whether corticosteroids were discontinued abruptly or slowly tapered, but abrupt stoppage is presumed in most cases because it is not specified otherwise.[41-45]

Most cases reported occurred in patients with glaucoma and ocular hypertension while they were being screened for steroid-induced IOP elevation,[41-45] but there seems not to be an association between IOP responsiveness and the development of uveitis.[43] The incidence of uveitis was similar in men and women,[43] and no special HLA locus for corticosteroid-induced uveitis was found.[45] Interestingly, four sisters out of seven black siblings developed uveitis when they were tested with dexamethasone to determine the response of their IOP to topical steroids.[41] No details were provided on age, duration of treatment, or whether uveitis occurred while these four patients were on treatment or after discontinuation. Whether this familial occurrence represents an inherited or a shared acquired tendency to develop corticosteroid-induce uveitis remains unknown.

It has been speculated that the development of corticosteroid-induced uveitis might correlate with a high prevalence of positive fluorescent treponemal antibody absorption test (FTA-ABS),[45] but there is not proof of such an assertion. In most cases of corticosteroid-induced uveitis that have been reported, other causes of intraocular inflammation were excluded and some authors believe that corticosteroids could have increased ocular susceptibility to an already pre-existing latent intraocular inflammation or infection.[1, 42] Additionally, melanin might have a role, because cases reported are far more frequent in black patients.[43]

In summary, uveitis elicited after corticosteroid withdrawal is anterior, nongranulomatous, and usually mild, responding to cycloplegics. Only if inflammation is more severe, corticosteroids must be resumed until inflammation subsides and then the steroid should be slowly tapered.

LATANOPROST

Latanoprost, a new prostaglandin F2α analogue, has been shown to be a safe and efficacious hypotensive agent in phase III clinical trials.[46-48] Adverse side effects reported with use of latanoprost include facial rash, conjunctival hyperemia, blurred vision, choroidal effusion, eye irritation, darkening of the iris color, iris cyst, hypertrichosis and hyperpigmentation of eyelashes.[46, 49-51] Corneal toxicity associated with latanoprost use ranges from not clinically significant superficial punctate keratopathy[46] or pseudodendrite formation,[52] to stimulation of recurrence of herpes simplex keratitis.[53, 54] It seems that uroprostone, another commercially available prostaglandin analogue, has the same adverse effect profile, but with more corneal toxicity.[55]

Two more probable side effects of latanoprost therapy have been reported lately: cystoid macular edema[51, 56-66] and anterior uveitis.[66, 67]

Although rare cases of anterior chamber flare and cells were documented after 12-month therapy with latanoprost in 1996,[47, 48] the first case reports of uveitis in patients treated with latanoprost were not published until 1998.[66, 67] Warwar and associates[66] first reported six cases of uveitis in a series of 94 patients (163 eyes) using latanoprost therapy. Uveitis was anterior and mild, and appeared within 1 day to 6 months after starting latanoprost. Inflammation resolved within 1 week after latanoprost discontinuation in three cases and with concurrent steroids drops in the remaining three patients. Three of the six patients with anterior uveitis were rechallenged, and two of them had a recurrence, which cleared solely with cessation of latanoprost. All six of these patients had had previous intraocular surgeries in the eye that developed uveitis. Two additional patients in this series receiving latanoprost bilaterally developed CME, one in both pseudophakic eyes and the other patient in the pseudophakic eye but not in the fellow phakic eye.

Fechtner and colleagues[67] have also reported four patients (five eyes) who developed iritis associated with latanoprost use. Four of five eyes had a history of prior inflammation or intraocular surgery and the fifth eye had had uncomplicated focal laser applied to the retina 5 years before. Uveitis developed within 1 day to 3 weeks, and its intensity ranged from mild to moderately severe (+3 cells in anterior chamber). In all cases, iritis improved after cessation of the drug and topical steroid therapy. All of these patients were rechallenged, and iritis recurred in all eyes within 3 days to 6 weeks. No adverse sequelae were produced by uveitis in any patient. An interesting recent report describes a frequency for latanoprost-induced uveitis of 1.0% in glaucoma patients with no previous history of uveitis, 23.1% for patients with prior uveitis but inactive at the time of the study, and 0% of worsening for glaucomatous eyes with active uveitis, the drug having no effect on intraocular pressure in this group. In all cases, intraocular anterior inflammation was mild (trace to + cells).[68]

The explanation given for these two side effects, uveitis and CME, is a breakdown of the blood-ocular barrier by latanoprost in predisposed eyes in which coexisting ocular conditions associated with an altered blood-ocular barrier had previously occurred.[50, 56-66] Whether latanoprost can also produce this disruption in normal eyes is yet unknown.

At least in the development of CME, it seems that the elapsed time between surgery and the onset of treatment with latanoprost could be determinant. One study has demonstrated that the initiation of latanoprost at least 3 months after incisional surgery seems not to cause angiographic CME,[61] whereas another study demonstrated CME 5 weeks after surgery when latanoprost was given before surgery and during the five subsequent weeks.[62] Therefore, it seems that latanoprost therapy should be avoided at least during the first 5 weeks after surgery. Most CME cases reported resolved or improved after cessation of drug and concurrent use of steroidal or nonsteroidal anti-inflammatory agents.[51, 55–66] Conversely, elapsed time between previous surgery and latanoprost-related uveitis does not seem to be relevant. All cases reported by Flechtner and colleagues had surgery at least 4 years before,[67] and no information in this regard is provided by Warwar and coworkers.[66]

Taken together, the published data[66, 67] indicate that latanoprost meets five of the seven criteria described by Naranjo and coworkers[4] to attribute causality of medication-induced uveitis to latanoprost but only in predisposed patients who have had previous episodes of intraocular inflammation or previous incisional ocular surgery.[5, 69] Although some authors disagree with the probable association of latanoprost and induction of uveitis and CME,[70–72] it may be wise not to choose this hypotensive agent in patients with a history of incisional surgery or intraocular inflammation.

METIPRANOLOL

Metipranolol, a nonselective β-blocker that lowers IOP by suppressing aqueous humor production, was introduced in the United Kingdom (UK) in 1986 to treat glaucoma and was marketed in three strengths: 0.1%, 0.3%, and 0.6%. The first cases of anterior granulomatous uveitis were reported in 1991, 15 patients (26 eyes) by Akingbehin and Villada[73] and eight by Kinshuck.[74] By the end of that year, more than 60 cases had been reported in the UK, with an incidence of 0.38% for metipranolol 0.6% solution and 0.11% for the 0.3% solution[73]; therefore, the multidose preparation of metipranolol was withdrawn from the market in the UK. The incidence of metipranolol-related uveitis seems to be less in the United States, and Melles and Wong[75] calculated an incidence of 0.49% for patients taking the 0.3% strength of metipranolol for more than 6 months at their institution.

The etiology of uveitis induced by metipranolol remains unknown. The fact that the incidence in the United States seems to be less has been explained by differences in the commercial preparation[76] or the strength, or both.[77] Metipranolol is marketed in the United States in a 0.3% concentration. It contains less benzalkonium chloride (0.044%), and bottles are prepared in a sterile fashion, whereas in the UK, the 0.6% strength was more commonly used, benzalkonium chloride concentration was 0.1% and bottles were sterilized by gamma radiation.[76]

The uveitis caused by metipranolol is anterior and granulomatous, with prominent mutton fat keratic precipitates,[73–75] although a case has been reported as mild nongranulomatous in a patient being treated with 0.3% metipranolol.[78] It has been more commonly reported in women, usually starting after 7 to 31 months of metipranolol treatment and causing elevation of IOP in about half of the patients,[73–75, 78] possibly explained by a decrease in outflow facility. Rechallenge with metipranolol in eyes that previously developed metipranol-induced uveitis caused a recurrence of the inflammation within 4 to 14 days in all cases.[75, 78, 79] All uveitis reactions reported have resolved after withdrawal of the drug plus additional topical steroids in some.[73–75, 78, 79]

Metipranolol fulfills the seven criteria proposed by Naranjo and coworkers,[4] and therefore its causality in the production of uveitis can be considered as certain. However, metipranolol-induced uveitis seems to be an uncommon reaction,[80] and in fact, single-dose units are still available in the UK and multidose preparations are also available in the United States, in some European countries, and in some other countries.[81]

Although there are rare descriptions of uveitis caused by other β-blockers such as timolol[82] or betaxolol,[83] causality has not been demonstrated; therefore, these agents remain as only a possible rare cause of uveitis.[1, 80]

RIFABUTIN

Rifabutin-induced intraocular inflammation is perhaps the best-documented form of uveitis among all drug-related types of uveitis. Rifabutin is a macrophage-penetrating lipophilic semisynthetic derivative of rifamycin and rifampin used as oral prophylactic treatment for disseminated *Mycobacterium avium* complex (MAC) infection in patients with AIDS. Other approved uses include treatment of refractory cases of pulmonary tuberculosis and inflammatory bowel disease.

As early as 1990, Siegal and colleagues[11] described a reversible syndrome of arthralgia and arthritis in 10 of 16 patients with AIDS treated with more than 1000 mg daily of oral rifabutin, two of whom developed uveitis. The uveitis was unilateral and mild in the first patient, although this increased to severe panophthalmitis on resuming rifabutin treatment at higher doses. The second case had a bilateral anterior uveitis. Both cases resolved with corticosteroid therapy after 6 to 10 weeks of permanent discontinuation of rifabutin and were thought to be caused by the high doses employed. When rifabutin was found to be efficacious in the prophylaxis against MAC infection in AIDS patients at lower maintenance dosages (300–600 mg/day) 3 years later,[84] more uveitis cases were reported.[9, 10, 12, 85–92]

The use of 600 mg of rifabutin daily in combination with other drugs has been reported to produce uveitis in 8% of patients.[93] In this same report, a diffuse polyarthralgia syndrome occurred in 19%, gastrointestinal symptoms in 42%, abnormal liver enzymes in 12%, and reduction in the total blood cell count in 100% of patients making rifabutin-related adverse effects quite frequent, occurring in 77% of patients. Uveitis induced by rifabutin develops sometimes in combination with arthralgia, arthritis, jaundice, pseudojaundice, and a transient rash.[14, 92]

In 1996, Shafran and coworkers[93] reported an incidence of uveitis of 5.6% for doses of 300 mg/day and a fourfold increase in the incidence when doses were 600 mg daily. A case-control study published by the same authors in 1998[94] found that baseline body weight predicted the development of uveitis, with an incidence of 14%, 45%, and 64% in patients weighing more than 45 kg, 55 to 65 kg, and less than 55 kg, respectively.

The most frequent rifabutin-induced uveitis type reported is mild-to-moderate unilateral anterior uveitis with concomitant mild vitritis, developing after 2 weeks to even 9 months of treatment.[85, 91, 92, 95, 96] Severe hypopyon uveitis and bilateral cases have also been reported.[10-12] Occasional reports have found vitreous opacities, developing sometimes into a pars planitis–like syndrome[10, 86] or even dense vitritis obscuring fundus visualization and mimicking infectious endophthalmitis or panophthalmitis if rifabutin had not been stopped.[9-11] In general, no chorioretinal involvement has been reported, although Arevalo and associates[13] described a patient with retinal vasculitis while being treated with rifabutin. Another rare event recently reported is bilateral corneal endothelial peripheral deposits in the absence of uveitis, found in 15% to 24% of children infected with the human immunodeficiency virus (HIV) and prophylactically treated with rifabutin[97, 98]; this event seems to be independent of the CD4 counts and the concomitant presence of cytomegalovirus retinitis, uveitis, and other medications.[98]

Rifabutin associated uveitis has also been reported in a nonimmunosuppressed patient who did not have AIDS with a pulmonary infection caused by MAC[99] and in immunosuppressed patients due to transplantation antirejection medication.[100, 101] However, uveitis did not develop in 25 patients followed for 2 years in whom 300 mg daily of rifabutin were administered because of inflammatory bowel disease.[102]

It seems clear now that uveitis is a dose-related toxicity of rifabutin therapy. The adverse reactions probably depend on the dose, metabolism, and excretion of the drug, and inhibition of cytochrome P450 seems to be an important mechanism.[14]

Using rifabutin at doses of 300 mg daily, the risk of uveitis is markedly reduced.[11, 94] Interactions with azoles and macrolides increase blood levels of rifabutin and can lead to the development of uveitis in patients with low doses of rifabutin in whom concomitant medications, especially fluconazole or clarithromycin, or both, are often used and so contribute to enhanced rifabutin ocular toxicity.[11, 103] For this reason, rifabutin is recommended not to be used at doses greater than 300 mg/day in multidrug regimens that include a macrolide, whereas it is less clear whether the same precaution needs to be taken when rifabutin is combined with fluconazole; in spite of being a drug known to raise rifabutin serum concentration, this combination has not been associated with increased incidence of uveitis in one study.[94]

It seems unlikely that the immune status or concomitant MAC infection plays a role in the pathogenesis of rifabutin-induced uveitis, because it has also been described in patients who did not have AIDS and who were treated with rifabutin for other indications and in the absence of MAC infection.[100-102] No etiologic infectious agent has ever been isolated from any patient, and only

acute infllammatory cells have been identified in a vitreous cytology specimen.[13, 95]

Although its pathogenic mechanism remains unknown and keeping in mind the present information about rifabutin-induced uveitis, a working hypothesis for the production of uveitis is that the drug kills the mycobacteria present in the eye, and that the dead bacteria might elicit an immune response similar to that produced by complete Freund's adjuvant (enhancer of the immune response consisting of dead mycobacteria in a water in oil emulsion). The greater incidence in patients with AIDS could be explained by increased rifabutin serum levels provoked by the azoles and macrolides that these patients usually receive concomitantly.

Rifabutin-induced uveitis responds rapidly to drug discontinuation, resolving within 1 to 2 months. Topical corticosteroids and cycloplegics are often used, leading to resolution, provided the drug is stopped.[95] In those cases that develop into panophthalmitis, systemic corticosteroids are required.[11] In general, if uveitis develops, rifabutin treatment must be discontinued promptly, because the inflammation is usually refractory to treatment if rifabutin is continued. In addition, recurrences are common in the first affected eye or in the contralateral eye if the drug is not stopped.

SULFONAMIDES

Systemic sulfonamides are antimicrobial drugs used for the treatment of many gram-positive and some gram-negative bacteria. In addition, the combination trimethoprim-sulfamethoxazole (TMP-SMX) is frequently used for ocular toxoplasmosis, cat-scratch disease, and is also the best prophylaxis for *Pneumocystis carinii* infection in HIV-infected patients. In general, adverse reactions to sulfonamides are frequently reported, but because these drugs are so commonly prescribed, adverse effects, including uveitis, may in fact be uncommon.[1, 2]

There are about 15 cases reported in the literature of sulfonamide-induced uveitis. Fourteen cases were collected by Tilden and associates and reported in 1991.[104] Twelve of those were treated with TMP-SMX, one with sulfacytine and one with an unspecified sulfonamide. Uveitis was always anterior, developed within 1 to 8 days, and it was bilateral in six cases. All patients developed acute bilateral iritis 24 hours after rechallenge with TMP-SMZ, which constitutes strong evidence that systemic sulfonamides are a cause of uveitis. Another case of bilateral anterior uveitis has been recently reported in association with the use of TMP-SMZ and TMP alone, in addition to retinal hemorrhages after the use of TMP alone.[105-107]

The mechanism by which sulfonamides cause uveitis remains speculative and could be the result of the development of a systemic vasculitis, similar to that produced in drug-induced Stevens-Johnson syndrome or as the result of direct immunogenicity of sulfonamides.[2] The majority of the reported cases had been associated with the frequently prescribed fixed combination TMP-SMZ, and because TMP alone can also be a possible cause of ocular toxicity,[105-107] the contribution of each component of the combination to the development of uveitis can be difficult to ascertain.

DIAGNOSIS

It is important to be aware that medications and other substances can be a cause of intraocular inflammation. This usually makes the physician confront the dilemma as to whether the inflammation is caused by inadequate or insufficient therapy, or is actually caused by the therapy itself.

It helps to be familiar with the main drugs that have historically been associated with uveitis[1-3] (see Table 79–1) and compare this list with the patient's medications and possible recent vaccinations. It is also advisable to record the patient's habits that might be associated, such as skin tattoos, for instance (see Table 79–1). When possible, the drug in question must be stopped and the patient rechallenged later when all inflammation has disappeared. Should inflammation recur, the suspected drug is most likely to be the cause.[4] It must be considered, however, that in many instances, the reported association may not necessarily mean that the patient developed uveitis because of the medication taken. Only well-controlled, large-scale epidemiologic studies can firmly establish a cause-and-effect relationship.[6]

In principle, even if the patient is highly suspected of having a drug-induced uveitis, he or she should undergo the same diagnostic approach followed for any other uveitis: a detailed clinical history, a uveitis questionnaire, a careful review of systems, and ancillary tests and consultations dictated by the differential diagnosis elaborated for that particular case. Exclusion of other possible causes of uveitis is, in fact, one of the seven criteria required by Naranjo and associates[4] to establish causality. This is most important, because the physician needs to be aware of all medications and putative toxins to which the patient has been or is currently being exposed. In addition, some drugs may produce pathology extraocularly, which may be unknown to the patient. Moreover, clinical history and examination may prove that the initially suspected medication-induced uveitis has in fact a different origin.

TREATMENT

Treatment of drug-induced uveitis begins with recognition of a drug-related event and usually, subsequent avoidance of the drug. Patients respond promptly to the classic topical treatment of uveitis (corticosteroids and cycloplegics) provided discontinuation of the causative medication is accomplished.[1, 2]

PROGNOSIS

In general, drug-induced intraocular inflammation is mild to moderate and causes no recurrence provided the drug is discontinued. Therefore, complications are not usually encountered and consequently the prognosis is favorable. In the few early cases of rifabutin-induced uveitis in which high doses were used, severe inflammation did occur, and recurrences were observed, sometimes developing into severe inflammation. Even in these less favorable cases, uveitis responded well to treatment and discontinuation of the drug.[9-11] The key point then, to ensure a good prognosis in medication-induced uveitis is to stop the offending drug.

CONCLUSIONS

Uveitis has been associated with a number of systemic and topical medications, and may also occur after vaccination and the use of other substances. However, drug-induced uveitis is a relatively rare event. Only a few drugs have been proven to cause uveitis, whereas many others may not represent a direct causal effect relationship. Anterior uveitis is the most common clinical presentation, and therefore, patients with a new onset anterior uveitis should be asked whether they have recently started any new medications. These patients need to undergo the same diagnostic protocol followed for any uveitis case.

Drug-induced uveitis is almost always reversible within weeks of cessation of the medication and the institution of topical treatment of the inflammation.

References

1. Fraunfelder FW, Rosenbaum JT: Drug-induced uveitis. Incidence, prevention and treatment. Drug Saf 1997;17:197.
2. Moorthy RS, Valluri S, Jampol LM: Drug-induced uveitis. Surv Ophthalmol 1998;42:557.
3. Fraunfelder FT, Grove JA, eds: Drug-Induced Ocular Side Effects and Drug Interactions. Philadelphia, Williams and Wilkins, 1996.
4. Naranjo CA, Busto U, Sellers EM, et al: A method for estimating the probablity of adverse drug reactions. Clin Pharmacol Ther 1981;39:239.
5. Moorthy RS, Valluri S, Jampol LM: Latanoprost-induced uveitis. Surv Ophthalmol 1999;43:466.
6. Rosenbaum JT: Drug-induced uveitis: Reporting inflammation while avoiding inflammatory reports. Am J Ophthalmol 1994;118:805.
7. Justiniani FR: Iatrogenic disease: An overview. Mount Sinai J Med 1984;51:210.
8. Koneru PB, Lien EJ, Koda RT: Oculotoxicities of systemically administered drugs. J Ocul Pharmacol 1986;2:385.
9. Akduman L, Del Priore LV, Kaplan HJ, et al: Rifabutin induced vitritis in AIDS patients. Ocul Immunol Inflamm 1996;4:219.
10. Schimkat M, Althaus C, Becker K, et al: Rifabutin-associated anterior uveitis in patients infected with human immunodeficiency virus. Ger J Ophthalmol 1996;5:195.
11. Siegal FP, Eilbott D, Burger H, et al: Dose-limiting toxicity of rifabutin in AIDS-related complex: Syndrome of arthralgia/arthritis. AIDS 1990;4:433.
12. Saran BR, Maguire AM, Nichols C, et al: Hypopyon uveitis in patients with acquired immunodeficiency syndrome treated for systemic *Mycobacterium avium* complex infection with rifabutin. Arch Ophthalmol 1994;112:1159.
13. Arevalo JF, Russack V, Freeman WR: New ophthalmic manifestations of presumed rifabutin-related uveitis. Ophthalmic Surg Lasers 1997;28:321.
14. Lowe SH, Kroon FP, Bollemeyer JG, et al: Uveitis during treatment of disseminated *Mycobacteria avium-intracellulare* complex infection with the combination of rifabutin, clarithromycin and ethambutol. Neth J Med 1996;48:211.
15. Macarol V, Fraunfelder FT: Pamidronate disodium and possible ocular adverse drug reaction. Am J Ophthalmol 1994;118:220.
16. Adami S, Zamberlan N: Adverse effects of biphosphonates. A comparative review. Drug Saf 1996;14:158.
17. De S, Meyer P, Crisp AJ: Pamidronate and uveitis. [Letter.] Br J Ophthalmol 1995;34:479.
18. Ghose K, Waterworth R, Trolove P, et al: Uveitis associated with pamidronate. [Letter.] Aust N Z J Med 1994;24:320.
19. O'Donnel NP, Rao GP, Aguis-Fernandez A: Paget's disease: Ocular complications of disodium pamidronate treatment. Br J Clin Pract 1995;49:272.
20. Siris ES: Biphosphonates and iritis. Lancet 1993;342:436.
21. Stewart GO, Stuckey BG, Ward LC, et al: Iritis following intravenous pamidronate. Aust N Z J Med 1996;26:414.
22. Mbekeani JN, Slamovits TL, Schwartz BH, Sauer HL: Ocular inflammation associated with alendronate therapy. Arch Ophthalmol 1999;117:837.
23. Studies of Ocular Complications of AIDS Research Group, AIDS

Clinical Trials Group: Parenteral cidofovir for cytomegalovirus retinitis in patients with AIDS: The HPMPC Peripheral cytomegalovirus retinitis trial. Ann Intern Med 1997;126:264.

24. Lalezari JP, Holland GN, Kramer F, et al: Randomized, controlled study of the safety and efficacy of intravenous cidofovir for the treatment of relapsing cytomegalovirus retinitis in patients with AIDS. J Acquir Immune Defic Syndr Hum Retrovirol 1998;17:339.

25. Kirsch LS, Arevalo JF, Chavez de la Paz E, et al: Intravitreal cidofovir (HPMPC) treatment of cytomegalovirus retinitis in patients with acquired immunodeficiency syndrome. Ophthalmology 1995;102:533.

26. Rahhal FM, Arevalo JF, Chavez de la Paz E, et al: Treatment of cytomegalovirus retinitis with intravitreous cidofovir in patients with AIDS. Ann Intern Med 1996;125:98.

27. Rahhal FM, Arevalo JF, Munguia D, et al: Intravitreal cidofovir for the maintenance treatment of cytomegalovirus retinitis. Ophthalmology 1996;103:1078.

28. Akler ME, Johnson DW, Burman WJ, et al: Anterior uveitis and hypotony after intravenous cidofovir for the treatment of cytomegalovirus retinitis. Ophthalmology 1998;105:651.

29. Chavez de la Paz E, Arevalo JF, Kirsch LS, et al: Anterior nongranulomatous uveitis after intravitreal HPMPC (cidofovir) for the treatment of cytomegalovirus retinitis. Ophthalmology 1997:104:539.

30. Davis JL, Taskintuna I, Freeman WR, et al: Iritis and hypotony after treatment with intravenous cidofovir for cytomegalovirus retinitis. Arch Ophthalmol 1997;115:733.

31. Kersten A, Althaus C, Hudde T, et al: Intravitreal injection of cidofovir in cytomegalovirus retinitis. Ophthalmologe 1998;95:602.

32. Kirsch LS, Arevalo JF, De Clercq E, et al: Phase I/II study of intravitreal cidofovir for the treatment of cytomegalovirus retinitis in patients with the acquired immunodeficiency syndrome. Am J Ophthalmol 1995;119:466.

33. Taskintuna I, Rahhal FM, Arevalo JF, et al: Low-dose intravitreal cidofovir (HPMPC) therapy of cytomegalovirus retinitis in patients with acquired immune deficiency syndrome. Ophthalmology 1997;104:1049.

34. Taskintuna I, Rahhal FM, Rao NA, et al: Adverse events and autopsy findings after intravitreous cidofovir (HPMPC) therapy in patients with acquired immune deficiency syndrome (AIDS). Ophthalmology 1997;104:1827.

35. Akler ME, Johnson DW, Burman WJ, Johnson SC: Anterior uveitis and hypotony after intravenous cidofovir for the treatment of cytomegalovirus retinitis. Ophthalmology 1998;105:651–657.

36. Bainbridge JW, Raina J, Shah SM, Ainsworth J, Pinching AJ: Ocular complications of intravenous cidofovir for cytomegalovirus retinitis in patients with AIDS. Eye 1999;13:353–356.

37. Cochereau I, Doan S, Diraison MC, et al: Uveitis in patients treated with intravenous cidofovir. OC Immunol Inflamm 1999;7:223.

38. Ambati J, Wynne KB, Angerame MC, Robinson MR: Anterior uveitis associated with intravenous cidofovir use in patients with cytomegalovirus retinitis. Br J Ophthalmol 1999;83:1153.

39. Taskintuna I, Banker AS, Rao NA, et al: An animal model for cidofovir (HPMPC) toxicity: Intraocular pressure and histopathologic findings. Exp Eye Res 1997;64:795.

40. Banker AS, Arevalo JF, Munguia D, et al: Intraocular pressure and aqueous humor dynamics in patients with AIDS treated with intravitreal cidofovir (HPMPC) for cytomegalovirus retinitis. Am J Ophthalmol 1997;124:168.

41. Kass MA, Gieser DK, Hodapp E, et al: Corticosteroid-induced iridocyclitis in a family. Am J Ophthalmol 1982;93:368.

42. Krupin T, LeBlanc RP, Becker B, et al: Uveitis in association with topically administered corticosteroid. Am J Ophthalmol 1970;70:883.

43. Martins JC, Wilensky JT, Asseff CF, et al: Corticosteroid-induced uveitis. Am J Ophthalmol 1974;77:433.

44. Mindel JS, Goldberg J, Tavitian HO: Similarity of the intraocular pressure response to different corticosteroid esters when compliance is controlled. Ophthalmology 1979;86:99.

45. Shin DH, Kass MA, Kolker AE, et al: Positive FTA-ABS tests in subjects with corticosteroid-induced uveitis. Am J Ophthalmol 1976;82:259.

46. Alm A, Camras CB, Watson PG. Phase III latanoprost studies in Scandinavia, the United Kingdom and the United States. Surv Ophthalmol 1997;41(Suppl 2):S105.

47. Camras CB, Alm A, Watson P: Latanoprost, a prostaglandin analog,

48. Mishima HK, Masuda K, Kitazawa Y, et al: A comparison of latanoprost and timolol in primary open-angle glaucoma and ocular hypertension. Arch Ophthalmol 1996;114:929.

49. Johnstone MA: Hypertrichosis and increased pigmentation of eyelashes and adjacent hair in the region of the ipsilateral eyelids of patients treated with unilateral topical latanoprost. Am J Ophthalmol 1997;124:544.

50. Krohn J, Hove VK: Iris cyst associated with topical administration of latanoprost. Am J Ophthalmol 1999;127:91.

51. Rowe JA, Hattenhauer MG, Herman DC: Adverse side effects associated with latanoprost. Am J Ophthalmol 1997;124:683.

52. Sudesh S, Cohen EJ, Rapuano CJ, et al: Corneal toxicity associated with latanoprost. Arch Ophthalmol 1999;117:539.

53. Kaufman HE, Varnell DE, Thompson HW: Latanoprost increases the severity and recurrence of herpetic keratitis in the rabbit. Am J Ophthalmol 1999;127:531.

54. Wand M, Gilbert CM, Liesegang TJ: Latanoprost and herpes simplex keratitis. Am J Ophthalmol 1999;127:602.

55. Eisenberg DL, Camras CB: A preliminary risk-benefit assessment of latanoprost and uroprostone in open-angle glaucoma and ocular hypertension. Drug Saf 1999;20:505.

56. Avakian A, Renier SA, Butler PJ: Adverse effects of latanoprost on patients with medically resistant glaucoma. Arch Ophthalmol 1998;116:679.

57. Ayyala RS, Cruz DA, Margo CE, et al: Cystoid macular edema associated with latanoprost in aphakic and pseudophakic eyes. Am J Ophthalmol 1998;126:602.

58. Callanan D, Fellman RL, Savage JA: Latanoprost-associated cystoid macular edema. Am J Ophthalmol 1998;126:134.

59. Gaddie IB, Bennett DW: Cystoid macular edema associated with the use of latanoprost. J Am Optom Assoc 1998;69:122.

60. Heier JS, Steinert RF, Frederick AR: Cystoid macular edema associated with latanoprost use. Arch Ophthalmol 1998;116:680.

61. Hoyng PF, Rulo AH, Greve EL, et al: Fluorescein angiographic evaluation of the effect of latanoprost treatment on blood-retinal barrier integrity: A review of studies conducted on pseudophakic glaucoma patients and on phakic and aphakic monkeys. Surv Ophthalmol 1997;41:S83.

62. Miyake K, Ota I, Maekubo K, et al: Latanoprost accelerates disruption of the blood-aqueous barrier and the incidence of angiographic cystoid macular edema in early postoperative pseudophakias. Arch Ophthalmol 1999;117:34.

63. Moroi SE, Gottfredsdottir MS, Schteingart MT, et al: Cystoid macular edema associated with latanoprost therapy in a case series of patients with glaucoma and ocular hypertension. Ophthalmology 1999;106:1024.

64. Reis A, Althaus C, Sundmacher R: Latanoprost (Xalatan)–induced macular edema. Klin Monatsbl Augenheilkd 1998;213:63.

65. Wardrop DR, Wishart PK: Latanoprost and cystoid macular oedema in a pseudophake. Br J Ophthalmol 1998;82:843.

66. Warwar RE, Bullock JD, Ballal D: Cystoid macular edema and anterior uveitis associated with latanoprost use. Ophthalmology 1998;105:263.

67. Fechtner RD, Khouri AS, Zimmerman TJ, el at: Anterior uveitis associated with latanoprost. Am J Ophthalmol 1998;126:37.

68. Smith SL, Pruit CA, Sine CS, et al: Latanoprost 0.005% and anterior segment uveitis. Acta Ophthalmol Scand 1999;77:668.

69. Warwar RE, Bullock JD: Latanoprost-induced uveitis. Surv Ophthalmol 1999;43:466.

70. Camras CB: CME and anterior uveitis with latanoprost use. Ophthalmology 1998;105:1978.

71. Eisenberg D: CME and anterior uveitis with latanoprost use. Ophthalmology 1998;105:1980.

72. Thorne JE, Maguire AM, Lanciano R: CME and anterior uveitis with latanoprost use. Ophthalmology 1998;105:1981.

73. Akingbehin T, Villada JR: Metipranolol-associated granulomatous anterior uveitis. Br J Ophthalmol 1991;75:519.

74. Kinshuck D: Glauline (metipranolol) induced uveitis and increase in intraocular pressure. Br J Ophthalmol 1991;75:575.

75. Melles RB, Wong IG: Metipranolol-associated granulomatous iritis. Am J Ophthalmol 1994;118:712.

76. O'Connor GR. Granulomatous uveitis and metipranolol. Br J Ophthalmol 1993;77:536.

77. Akingbehin AO: In discussion: O'Connor GR. Granulomatous uveitis and metipranolol. Br J Ophthalmol 1993;77:536.

78. Patel NP, Patel KH, Moster MR, et al: Metipranolol-associated nongranulomatous anterior uveitis. Am J Ophthalmol 1997;123:843.

79. Akingbehin T, Villada JR, Walley T: Metipranolol-induced adverse reactions: I. The rechallenge study. Eye 1992;6:277.

80. Beck RW, Moke P, Blair RC, et al: Uveitis associated with topical beta-blockers. Arch Ophthalmol 1996;114:1181.

81. KeBler C: Possible bilateral anterior uveitis secondary to metipranolol (OptiPranolol) therapy. Arch Ophthalmol 1994;112:1277.

82. Zimmerman TJ, Baumann JD, Hetherington J: Side effects of timolol. Surv Ophthalmol 1983;28:243.

83. Jain S: Betaxolol-associated anterior uveitis. Eye 1994;8:708.

84. Nightingale SD, Cameron DW, Gordin FM, et al: Two controlled trials of rifabutin prophylaxis against *Mycobacterium avium* complex infection in AIDS. N Engl J Med 1993;329:828.

85. Becker K, Schimkat M, Jablonowski H, et al: Anterior uveitis associated with rifabutin medication in AIDS patients. Infection 1996;24:34.

86. Chaknis MJ, Brooks SE, Mitchell KT, et al: Inflammatory opacities of the vitreous in rifabutin-associated uveitis. Am J Ophthalmol 1996;122:580.

87. Fuller JD, Stanfield LED, Craven DE: Rifabutin prophylaxis and uveitis. [Letter.] N Engl J Med 1994;330:1315.

88. Havlir D, Torriani F, Dube M: Uveitis associated with rifabutin prophylaxis. Ann Intern Med 1994;121:510.

89. Jacobs DS, Piliero PJ, Kuperwaser MG, et al: Acute uveitis associated with rifabutin use in patients with human immunodeficiency virus infection. Am J Ophthalmol 1994;118:716.

90. Karbassi M, Nikou S: Acute uveitis in patients with acquired immunodeficiency syndrome receiving prophylactic rifabutin. Arch Ophthalmol 1995;113:699.

91. Shafran SD, Deschenes J, Miller M, et al: Uveitis and pseudojaundice during a regimen of clarithromycin, rifabutin, and ethambutol. [Letter.] MAC Study Group of the Canadian HIV Trials Network. N Engl J Med 1994;330:438.

92. Shafran SD, Singer J, Zarowny DP, et al: A comparison of two regimens for the treatment of *Mycobacterium avium* complex bacteremia in AIDS: Rifabutin, ethambutol, and clarithromycin versus rifampin, ethambutol, clofazimine, and ciprofloxacin. Canadian HIV Trials Network Protocol 010 Study Group. N Engl J Med 1996;335:377.

93. Griffith DE, Brown BA, Girard WM, et al: Adverse events associated with high-dose rifabutin in macrolide-containing regimens for the treatment of *Mycobacterium avium* complex lung disease. Clin Infect Dis 1995;21:594.

94. Shafran SD, Singer J, Zarowny DP, et al: Determinants of rifabutin-associated uveitis in patients treated with rifabutin, clarithromycin, and ethambutol for *Mycobacterium avium* complex bacteremia: A multivariate analysis. Canadian HIV Trials Network Protocol 010 Study Group. J Infect Dis 1998;177:252.

95. Nichols CW: Mycobacterium avium complex infection, rifabutin, and uveitis: Is there a connection? Clin Infect Dis 1996;22(Suppl 1):S43.

96. Tseng AL, Walmsley SL: Rifabutin-associated uveitis. Ann Pharmacother 1995;29:1149.

97. Smith JA, Mueller BU, Nussenblatt RB, et al: Corneal endothelial deposits in children positive for human immunodeficiency virus receiving rifabutin prophylaxis for *Mycobacterium avium* complex bacteremia. Am J Ophthalmol 1999;127:164.

98. Holland JP, Chang CW, Vagh M, Cartright P: Corneal endothelial deposits in patients with HIV infection or AIDS: Epidemiologic evidence of the contribution of rifabutin. Can J Ophthalmol 1999;34:204.

99. Ramon PM, Tillie-Leblond I, Labalette P, et al: Uveitis, arthralgia and pseudo-jaundice in a HIV seronegative patient due to rifabutin. Rev Mal Respir 1998;15:204.

100. Jewelewicz DA, Schiff WM, Brown S, et al: Rifabutin-associated uveitis in an immunosuppressed pediatric patient without acquired immunodeficiency syndrome. Am J Ophthalmol 1998;125:872.

101. Ng P, McCluskey P, McCaughan G, et al: Ocular complications of heart, lung, and liver transplantation. Br J Ophthalmol 1998;82:423.

102. To KW, Tsiaras WS, Thayer WR: Rifabutin use in inflammatory bowel disease. Arch Ophthalmol 1995;113:1354.

103. Hafner R, Bethel J, Power M, et al: Tolerance and pharmacokinetic interactions of rifabutin and clarithromycin in human immunodeficiency virus–infected volunteers. Antimicrob Agents Chemother 1998;42:631.

104. Tilden ME, Rosenbaum JT, Fraunfelder FT: Systemic sulfonamides as a cause of bilateral, anterior uveitis. Arch Ophthalmol 1991;109:67.

105. Arola O, Peltoner R, Rossi T, et al: Arthritis, uveitis, and Stevens-Johnson syndrome induced by trimethoprim. Lancet 1998;351:1102.

106. Gilroy N, Gottlieb T, Spring P, et al: Trimethoprim-induced aseptic meningitis and uveitis. Lancet 1997;350:112.

107. Kristinsson JK, Hannesson OB, Sveinsson O, et al: Bilateral anterior uveitis and retinal haemorrhages after administration of trimethoprim. Acta Ophthalmol Scand 1997;75:314.

INDEX

Note: Page numbers followed by the letter f refer to figures; those followed by the letter t refer to tables.

A

ABD. *See* Adamantiades-Behçet's disease (ABD).
Abdominal pain in polyarteritis nodosa, 654
Absorptiometry for rheumatoid arthritis, 111
ACAID. *See* Anterior chamber–associated immune deviation (ACAID).
Acanthamoeba keratitis, 412
Accommodation, 10–11
ACE. *See* Angiotensin-converting enzyme (ACE).
Acetaminophen, 29t, 167t
Acetazolamide for intermediate uveitis, 852
Acetonide, 28t
α_1-Acid protein in uveitis testing, 95t, 96
Acid-fast staining and culture for tuberculosis, 267
Acneiform eruptions in Adamantiades-Behçet's disease, 632. *See also* Adamantiades-Behçet's disease.
Acquired immunodeficiency syndrome (AIDS). *See also* Human immunodeficiency virus (HIV).
  acute retinal necrosis in, 319
  bartonella in, 261
  cryptococcosis in, 377
  cytomegalovirus in, 323
  necrotizing herpetic retinopathy in, 318
  Pneumocystic carinii choroidopathy in, 425
  toxoplasmosis in, 390–391
  Whipple's disease in, 289
Acquired measles, 336–338
Acquired rubella, 345–346
Acquired toxoplasmosis, 389–390
  diagnosis of, 398–400
Acrodermatitis chronica atrophicans in Lyme borreliosis, 247
Activation proteins in multiple sclerosis, 704
Acute glomerulonephritis in Adamantiades-Behçet's disease, 636
Acute idiopathic blind-spot enlargement syndrome (AIBES), 767
  zonal occult outer retinopathy and, 813–816
Acute inflammation, 17
Acute leukemia in retinal vasculitis, 833
Acute lymphocytic leukemia (ALL), 506–509, 507f
Acute macular neuroretinopathy (AMN)
  retinal pigment epitheliitis versus, 781–782, 783t, 784t
  zonal occult outer retinopathy and, 813–816
Acute macular retinopathy, 802, 802t
Acute multifocal hemorrhagic retinal vasculitis, 827
Acute myelocytic leukemia (AML), 506–509, 507f

Acute nonsuppurative inflammation, 87–88, 88t
Acute papular onchodermatitis (APOD), 446, 447f
Acute periphlebitis in Adamantiades-Behçet's disease, 637
Acute posterior multifocal placoid pigment epitheliopathy (APMPPE), 20, 772–779
  angiography in, 121, 122f
  associated diseases of, 777
  birdshot retinochoroidopathy versus, 736t, 737
  clinical characteristics of, 772–774, 773f–776f
  definition of, 772
  diagnosis of, 79, 777
  differential diagnosis of, 777
  diffuse unilateral subacute neuroretinitis versus, 477
  epidemiology of, 772
  history of, 772
  multifocal choroiditis and panuveitis versus, 762
  pathogenesis of, 776–777
  pathophysiology/immunology/pathology of, 774–776
  retinal pigment epitheliitis versus, 782–783, 783t, 784t
  serpiginous choroiditis versus, 791–792
  subretinal fibrosis and uveitis syndrome versus, 802, 802t
  summary of, 809, 809t
  treatment of, 777–778
Acute postoperative endophthalmitis, 528, 528t. *See also* Endophthalmitis.
Acute retinal necrosis (ARN)
  glaucoma surgery and, 228, 228f
  in herpes simplex virus
    clinical characteristics of, 317–318, 318f
    diagnosis of, 320–321
    pathogenesis of, 319–320
    treatment of, 321–322
Acute retinal pigment epitheliitis (ARPE), 20, 780–786
  clinical features of, 780–781, 780f
  complications of, 781
  definition of, 780
  diagnosis of, 780f, 781f, 782, 783t
    differential, 781–784, 783t, 784t
  epidemiology of, 780
  etiology, pathogenesis, and pathology of, 781
  history of, 780
  natural history and prognosis for, 784–785
  subretinal fibrosis and uveitis syndrome versus, 802, 802t
  treatment of, 784

Acute tubulointerstitial nephritis (ATIN), 726. *See also* Tubulointerstitial nephritis and uveitis (TINU) syndrome.
Acute zonal occult outer retinopathy (AZOOR), 813–816
Acyclovir
  for acute retinal necrosis, 321
  for iridocyclitis and trabeculitis, 321
  mycophenolate mofetil and, 190
Adamantiades-Behçet's disease (ABD), 632–652
  acute retinal necrosis versus, 321
  angiography for, 127, 128f
  azathioprine for, 188
  chlorambucil for, 183–184
  clinical features of, 633–638
    diagnostic system in, 633–634, 633t
    nonocular, 634–636, 634f, 635f
    ocular, 636–638, 637f–639f
  colchicine for, 208
  complications of, 646–647
  cyclophosphamide for, 181
  cyclosporine A for, 194
  definition of, 632
  diagnosis of, 641–642, 641f, 642f
    imaging for, 112
  epidemiology of, 24, 632–633, 633t
  extraocular examination in, 94
  history of, 632
  in children, 638
  in pregnancy, 638–639
  multiple sclerosis and, 706
  pathogenesis and immunology of, 639–640
  pathology of, 640–641
  prognosis for, 647
  retinal vasculitis in, 828–829
  treatment of, 642–646, 643f, 644f
  Whipple's disease versus, 293
Adenopathy, hilar, 109
Adhesion molecules, 42t
  in retinal vasculitis, 834, 834f–836f
Adjuvants to immunosuppressive therapy, 204–209
α-Adrenergic agonists, 159
Adrenergic mydriatics, 159
Adrenocorticotropic hormone (ACTH)
  for multiple sclerosis, 706
  introduction and history of, 142
Adventitia proper, 6
Advil. *See* Ibuprofen (Advil, Motrin, Nuprin, Rufen).
Africa, onchocerciasis in, 443, 444f, 445t
African Americans, uveitis in, 88
African tick-bite fever, 298, 298t
  clinical characteristics of, 301t
  epidemiology of, 299
African trypanosomiasis, 420. *See also* Trypanosomiasis.

Brucellosis *(Continued)*
in retinal vasculitis, 831
molecular genetics, pathology, and immunology of, 278–279
prevention of, 283
prognosis for, 283
treatment for, 282–283
Bruch's membrane, in malignant melanoma, 510, 511f
Brugia malayi
in loiasis, 463
in onchocerciasis, 450–451
B-scan ultrasonography, 107
for intraocular foreign bodies, 548, 548f
for sympathetic ophthalmia, 743, 743f
BSHL (bilateral symmetrical hilar lymphadenopathy), in sarcoidosis, 717–718, 717f, 718t
BSRC. *See* Birdshot retinochoroidopathy (BSRC).
Buerger's disease
in Adamantiades-Behçet's disease, 637
retinal vasculitis in, 829
Busacca nodules, in Fuchs' heterochromic iridocyclitis, 694
Butazolidin. *See* Phenylbutazone (Azolid, Butazolidin).
Butterfly rash, in systemic lupus erythematosus, 601, 602f

C

Calabar swelling, in loiasis, 463–464
Calcaneal periostitis, in Reiter's syndrome, 584, 585f
Calcification, in congenital toxoplasmosis, 389, 390f
Calcitonin gene–related peptide (CGRP), 18–19, 19t
Calcitriol (1,25-dihydroxy-vitamin D₃), in sarcoidosis, 720
Calcium metabolism, corticosteroids and, 143
Calcofluor white stain, for ameba infection, 413
Calliphora, in ophthalmomyiasis, 485–487, 486f
Calreticulin, antibodies to, 453
CALT. *See* Conjunctival and lacrimal gland–associated lymphoid tissue (CALT).
Cancer-associated retinopathy (CAR), 520–522
acute zonal occult outer retinopathy versus, 815
in retinal vasculitis, 832–833
Candida, in endophthalmitis, 531–532
Candidiasis, 364–372
clinical characteristics of, 365–366, 365f
complications of, 366
definition of, 364
diagnosis of, 367–368
differential, 368, 368t
epidemiology of, 364–365
history of, 364
in human immunodeficiency virus, 499
pathogenesis/histopathology/immunology of, 366–367
Pneumocystic carinii choroidopathy versus, 426
prognosis for, 370
treatment of, 368–370
Canine ehrlichiosis, 299
Capillary dropout, in systemic lupus erythematosus, 605, 605f
Capillary permeability, corticosteroids and, 144
Capsulotomy, uveitis after, 575
CAR. *See* Cancer-associated retinopathy (CAR).

Carbohydrate metabolism, corticosteroids and, 143
Carboxyl terminus, 49
Card agglutination test, for trypanosomiasis (CATT), 422
Cardiac output, corticosteroids and, 144
Cardiac system
in Adamantiades-Behçet's disease, 634–635
in antiphospholipid syndrome, 684, 684t
in Lyme borreliosis, 247
in sarcoidosis, 711
in scleroderma, 612
in systemic lupus erythematosus, 602
in Wegener's granulomatosis, 663
Cardiolipin, in syphilis diagnosis, 240
Cardiomyopathy, in loiasis, 464
Cardiopulmonary schistosomiasis, 481
Cardiovascular disease
from ocular ischemic syndromes, 556
in relapsing polychondritis, 677
Cardiovascular syphilis, 238, 238t
Cardiovascular system
corticosteroids and, 144
in giant cell arteritis, 620
in Lyme borreliosis, 251, 251t
in polyarteritis nodosa, 653
Carotid endarterectomy, for ocular ischemic syndromes, 556
Carrión's disease, 260–263
Cartilage
in extraocular examination, 94
in relapsing polychondritis, 676, 677f, 678
CAT (computerized axial tomography), for cysticercosis, 470–471
Cataracts, 92
after radiotherapy, 517
ameba infection and, 413
endophthalmitis and, 534
from ocular toxoplasmosis, 397
from syphilis, 242
from Vogt-Koyanagi-Harada syndrome, 753
in Adamantiades-Behçet's disease, 646
in ciliary body melanoma, 510, 511f
in congenital rubella, 343, 343t
in Fuchs' heterochromic iridocyclitis, 693, 695, 698
in intermediate uveitis, 846
in juvenile rheumatoid arthritis, 594
in leprosy, 308
surgery for, 224–226, 225f, 226f
candidiasis and, 366
endophthalmitis after, 528–529, 530f
for intermediate uveitis, 853–854
for sarcoidosis, 723
nonsteroidal anti-inflammatory drugs for, 170, 171
varicella zoster infection and, 318
Caterpillar hairs, in ophthalmia nodosa, 488–491, 489f
Cats
in toxoplasmosis transmission, 387
uveitis and, 88
Cat-scratch disease (CSD), 260–263, 831
intermediate uveitis versus, 850
CATT. *See* Card agglutination test, for trypanosomiasis (CATT).
CD. *See* Clusters of differentiation (CD); Crohn's disease (CD).
CD46, 18, 19t
CD59, 18
CD4 cells, 36
CD4+ cells, 750–751
CD8 cells, 36
CD8+ cells, 750–751
CD4+ effector cells, 63
CD4+ lymphocytes
in human immunodeficiency virus, 493, 494f

CD4+ lymphocytes *(Continued)*
CMV retinitis and, 495
herpes zoster ophthalmicus and, 499
ocular toxoplasmosis and, 497
pneumocystosis and, 498
syphilis and, 499
VZV retinitis and, 497–498
in retinal vasculitis, 834
in sarcoidosis, 717
CD8+ T cells, in toxoplasmosis, 388
CD4+ Th cells
in ascariasis, 440
in toxoplasmosis, 387–388
CDRs. *See* Complementarity-determining regions (CDRs).
Ceftriaxone
for Lyme borreliosis, 253
for Whipple's disease, 294
Cefuroxime for Lyme borreliosis, 253
Celecoxib (Celebrex)
for cataract surgery, 224–225
systemic preparation of, 29t, 167t
Cell(s)
immune-mediated tissue injury by, 62–64, 63f
of pigmented epithelium, 9
Cell surface antigens in toxoplasmosis, 388, 388f
CellCept. *See* Mycophenolate mofetil (CellCept).
Cell-mediated immunity, 55
in Adamantiades-Behçet's disease, 641
in giant cell arteritis, 623
in Lyme borreliosis, 251
in retinal vasculitis, 834
in toxoplasmosis, 387–388
Cellular response to ameba infection, 412
Cellulitis, orbital, 534
Central lymphoid organs, 40, 41f, 42f, 42t
Central nervous system (CNS)
corticosteroids and, 143
cyclopentolate and, 164
in Lyme borreliosis, 247
in multiple sclerosis, 701. *See also* Multiple sclerosis (MS).
in sarcoidosis, 714–715, 714f
in schistosomiasis, 481
in Whipple's disease, 291, 291t
lymphoma of, 503–506, 504f
mydriatic-cycloplegic agents and, 163–164
Central retinal artery occlusion (CRAO), 621
Central retinal vein obstruction, 555–556
Central serous chorioretinopathy (CSCR), 783, 783t, 784t
Cephalexin, for bartonella, 262
Cerebral cysticercosis, 469
Cerebral involvement, in systemic lupus erythematosus, 606
Cerebrospinal fluid (CSF) analysis
for cryptococcosis, 378
for cysticercosis, 470–471
for intraocular-central nervous system lymphoma, 505
for leptospirosis, 275
for syphilis, 241
Cerebrovascular disease, in giant cell arteritis, 619
Cervical spine films, for rheumatoid arthritis, 111
Cervical spondylitis, 592
CF (complement fixation)
for cysticercosis, 471
for toxoplasmosis, 398
CGRP. *See* Calcitonin gene–related peptide (CGRP).
Chagas' disease, 420

ISBN 0-7216-6338-9

90038